NURSING CARE PLANS

Patient with depression, 63
Death and dying, 93
Patient with alcohol dependence, 117
Patient with hypokalemia, 199
Patient with epidural analgesia for pain management, 221
Patient with lung cancer, 261
Patient with a community-acquired infection, 295
Patient with a nosocomial infection, 320
Patient with acquired immunodeficiency syndrome, 340
Care of the stroke patient, 419
Patient with a heat-related emergency, 522
Patient following thoracotomy, 560
Patient with pneumonia, 580
Patient with congestive heart failure and oliguria, 650
Patient with aplastic anemia, 682
Patient with cirrhosis, 755
Patient with chronic renal failure, 801
Patient having surgery for implantation of penile prosthesis, 880
Patient with hyperthyroidism, 915
Patient who is confused, 959
Patient with detached retina, 1006
Patient with below-the-knee amputation, 1129

NURSING PROCESS BOXES

Manipulative patient, 50
Psychotic patient, 51
Depressed patient, 56
Spiritual distress, 88
Pain, 90
Alcohol-substance abuse or dependence, 116
Risk for infection, 137
Prevention of severe insect sting reaction, 144
Anaphylactic shock, 146
Fluid volume deficit: hypovolemia, 168
Fluid volume deficit: dehydration, 169
Fluid volume excess: hypervolemia, 170
Fluid volume excess: overhydration, 171
Sodium deficit: hyponatremia, 172
Sodium excess: hypernatremia, 173
Potassium deficit: hypokalemia, 177
Potassium excess: hyperkalemia, 178
Calcium deficit: hypocalcemia, 181
Calcium excess: hypercalcemia, 182
Magnesium deficit: hypomagnesemia, 183
Magnesium excess: hypermagnesemia, 184
Metabolic acidosis: base bicarbonate deficit or metabolic acid excess, 187
Metabolic alkalosis: base bicarbonate excess, 188
Respiratory alkalosis: carbonic acid deficit, 189
Respiratory acidosis: carbonic acid excess, 190
Emergency care of individuals in anaphylactic shock, 198, 504
Patient in pain, 220
External radiation therapy, 242
Sealed internal radiation therapy, 244
Unsealed internal radiation therapy, 246
Tuberculosis (community), 277
Acute food poisoning, 282
Sexually transmitted disease, 291
Urinary tract infection, 303
AIDS patient, 335
Alzheimer's disease, 362
Rehabilitation of the immobile patient, 392
Pressure sore, 402, 440
Rehabilitation of the incc
Rehabilitation of the dysphagic patient, 410
Preoperative preparation, 465
Postoperative care, 483
Emergency care of individuals in anaphylactic shock, 504
Influenza, 564
Chronic obstructive pulmonary disease, 570
Chronic bronchitis, 575
Bronchiectasis, 576
Asthma, 577
Active tuberculosis, 583
Pulmonary embolism, 587
Adult respiratory distress syndrome, 592
Patient undergoing permanent pacemaker placement, 612
Myocardial infarction, 630
Cardiac surgery, 634
Congestive heart failure, 637
Anemias, 675
Leukemia, 679
Total parenteral nutrition, 703
Inflammatory bowel disease, 718
Appendicitis/appendectomy, 722
Diverticulosis/diverticulitis, 724
Peptic ulcer disease, 732
Gastrectomy, 736
Hepatitis, 742
Cirrhosis, 744
Cholecystectomy, cholecystotomy, or choledochostomy—postoperative care, 753
Acute poststreptococcal glomerulonephritis, 781
Renal calculi, 785
Acute renal failure, 789
Urinary diversion—postoperative phase, 799
Lithotomy—postoperative phase (ureterolithotomy, pyelolithotomy, nephrolithotomy), 800
Colporrhaphy (repair of relaxed perineal muscles), 843
Hysterectomy, 848
Mastectomy, 856
Abortion or ectopic pregnancy, 861
Prostatectomy, 873
Hyperthyroidism, 893
Hypothyroidism, 895
Diabetes mellitus, 914
The unconscious patient, 928
Increased intracranial pressure, 931
Acute head injury, 933
Spinal cord injury, 936
Postoperative care—laminectomy patient, 941
Postoperative care—craniotomy patient, 943
Problems associated with cerebrovascular accident, 946
Cerebral aneurysm, 948
Seizures, 952
Parkinson's disease, 957
Intraocular surgery, 988
Glaucoma, 992
Extraocular surgery, 998
Otitis media, 1024
Pressure ulcers, 1050
Bacterial infection, 1059
Fungal infection, 1062
Viral infections, 1065
Disease of epidermal origin, 1069
Burn injuries, 1081
Neurovascular integrity, 1097
Patient with a cast, 1100
Patient in traction, 1107
Hip fracture/total hip replacement/total knee replacement, 1122

MEDICAL-SURGICAL NURSING

TOTAL PATIENT CARE

MEDICAL-SURGICAL NURSING

TOTAL PATIENT CARE

GAIL A. HARKNESS, RN, DrPH, FAAN
Chair, Health Promotion Unit;
Professor,
University of Connecticut, School of Nursing,
Storrs, Connecticut

JUDITH R. DINCHER, RN, BSN, MSEd
Director, Nursing and Related Programs;
Associate Professor, Department of Nursing,
William Rainey Harper College,
Palatine, Illinois

NINTH EDITION

with 385 illustrations

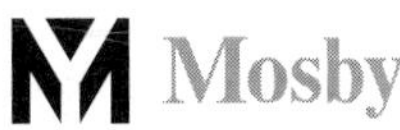

St. Louis Baltimore Boston Carlsbad Chicago Naples New York Philadelphia Portland
London Madrid Mexico City Singapore Sydney Tokyo Toronto Wiesbaden

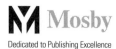

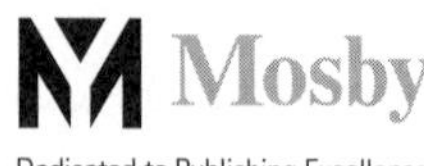

Dedicated to Publishing Excellence

Publisher: Nancy L. Coon
Senior Editor: Susan Epstein
Senior Developmental Editor: Beverly J. Copland
Project Manager: Deborah L. Vogel
Production Editor: Jodi Willard
Designer: Pati Pye
Manufacturing Managers: Theresa Fuchs, Tony McAllister
Some illustrations drawn by Karen Merrill

NINTH EDITION

A NOTE TO THE READER
The authors and publisher have made every attempt to check dosages and nursing content for accuracy. Because the science of pharmacology and healthcare is continually advancing, our knowledge base continues to expand. Therefore, we recommend that the reader always check product information for changes in dosage or administration before administering any medication. This is particularly important with new or rarely used drugs.

Printed in the United States of America.

Composition by Graphic World, Inc.
Color separating by Jefferson Keeler Printing Co.
Printing/binding by Rand McNally Book Services Group

Mosby-Year Book, Inc.
11830 Westline Industrial Drive
St. Louis, MO 63146

Library of Congress Cataloging-in-Publication Data
Harkness, Gail A.
Medical-surgical nursing : total patient care / Gail A. Harkness, Judith R. Dincher. — 9th ed.
p. cm.
Rev. ed. of: Total patient care. 8th ed. c1992.
Includes bibliographical references and index.
ISBN 0-8151-4084-3 (hardcover)
1. Nursing. I. Dincher, Judith R., 1937- . II. Harkness, Gail A. Total patient care. III. Title.
[DNLM: 1. Nursing Care. WY 100 H282 1995]
RT41.H65 1995
610.73—dc20
DNLM/DLC
for Library of Congress 95-20507
CIP

95 96 97 98 99 / 9 8 7 6 5 4 3 2 1

CONTRIBUTORS

Anne M. Acquila, RN, MSN, CCRN
Surgical Clinical Nurse Specialist
Hospital of St. Raphael,
New Haven, Connecticut

Sandra Blake, RN, MS, CIC
Infection Control Epidemiologist,
Loyola University Medical Center,
Maywood, Illinois

Catherine Borkowski Benoit, RNc, MSN, CNRN
Nurse Practitioner,
Beth Israel Hospital,
Boston, Massachusetts

Margaret F. Burbach, RN, BSN, MS, EdD, CS
Professor of Nursing,
William Rainey Harper College,
Palatine, Illinois

Karyl J. Burns, RN, PhD, CS
Assistant Professor of Nursing,
University of Connecticut,
Storrs, Connecticut

Helen Burton, RN, BS, CDE
Diabetes Clinical Case Manager,
Deaconess Hospital,
Boston, Massachusetts

Julie A. D'Agostino, RN, BSN, MSN, CEN, TNS
Trauma Nurse Specialist,
Glenbrook Hospital,
Glenview, Illinois
Adjunct Faculty, Nursing,
William Rainey Harper College,
Palatine, Illinois

Heyward Michael Dreher, RN, BSN, MN
Assistant Professor,
LaSalle University,
Philadelphia, Pennsylvania

Cheryl L. Durkee, RN, BSN, MS
Clinical Nurse Specialist,
Lutheran General Hospital,
Park Ridge, Illinois

Marian Frerichs, RN, EdD
Professor and Associate Chair, Emeritus,
Northern Illinois University,
DeKalb, Illinois

Elaine M. Geissler, RN, PhD, CTN
Associate Professor of Nursing,
University of Connecticut,
Storrs, Connecticut

Jean H. Genster, RN, BSN
Associate Professor,
William Rainey Harper College,
Palatine, Illinois

Marcia J. Hill, RN, BSN, MSN
Vice President,
Innovative Wound Care, Incorporated,
Houston, Texas

Joanne Leski, RN, BSN, MSN
Associate Professor,
William Rainey Harper College,
Palatine, Illinois

Jeanne LeVasseur, RN, C, MSN, FNP
Lecturer,
University of Connecticut School of Nursing,
Storrs, Connecticut

Mary Lou McNiff, RN, MS
Administrator,
Brockton Visiting Nurse Association,
Brockton, Massachusetts

Mary "Dee" Miller, RN, BSN, MS, CIC
Clinical Nurse Specialist, Infection Control/Epidemiology,
Mercy Health Care System;
Faculty, University of Phoenix,
Phoenix, Arizona

Mildred Owings, RN, MSN, CS
Associate Professor,
Patrick Henry Community College,
Martinsville, Virginia

Marion Phipps, RN, MS, CRRN, FAAN
Rehabilitation Nurse Specialist,
Beth Israel Hospital,
Boston, Massachusetts

Joanne Pier, RN, BSN, MA
Assistant Director of Nursing,
Medical College of Wisconsin,
Milwaukee, Wisconsin

Cleo J. Richard, RN, BS, BA, MSN
Consultant, Nephrology, Holistic Health and Biology,
Missoula, Montana

Andrea D'Amato Quinn, RN, MS, CCRN, CS
Clinical Specialist, Surgical Nursing,
Yale-New Haven Hospital,
New Haven, Connecticut

Pamela J. Schultz, RN, CRNO
Clinical Nurse Coordinator for Ophthalmology,
Rush-Presbyterian-St. Luke's Medical Center,
Chicago, Illinois

Helen Stupak Shah, RN, BSN, MSN, DNSc
Associate Professor of Nursing,
University of Connecticut,
Storrs, Connecticut

Donna Starsiak, RN, C, BS, MSN
Assistant Professor of Nursing,
Loyola University of Chicago,
Chicago, Illinois

Jean E. Steel, RN, PhD, FAAN
Associate Professor,
University of Connecticut,
Storrs, Connecticut

Patricia A. Tabloski, RN, PhD, CS
Assistant Professor of Nursing;
Director, Travelers Center on Aging,
University of Connecticut,
Storrs, Connecticut

Patricia Trotta, RN, BSc, MSN, ONC
Oncology Clinical Nurse Specialist,
Veteran's Memorial Medical Center,
Meriden, Connecticut

Mary Gretchen Vancura, RN, BSN, MN, CPN
Associate Professor of Nursing,
William Rainey Harper College,
Palatine, Illinois

Robin Whittemore, RN, MSN
Instructor of Nursing,
University of Connecticut,
Storrs, Connecticut

Clara Williams, RN, MA
Associate Professor Emeritus,
University of Connecticut, School of Nursing,
Storrs, Connecticut

REVIEWERS

Elizabeth A. Ayello, RN, BSN, MS, PhD, CS, CETN
Clinical Assistant Professor of Nursing,
New York, University,
New York, New York

Sharon Beasley, RN, MSN
Instructor,
Rend Lake College,
Ina, Illinois

Kathy Black, RN, MSN
Coordinator, PN Program,
Iowa Western Community College,
Harlan, Iowa

Catherine B. Burke, RN, MS
Nursing Faculty, Hospice Nurse,
Kankakee Community College,
Kankakee, Illinois

Kathlyn M. Carlson, RN, BSN, MA, CPAN
Postanesthesia Care Unit,
Abbott Northwestern Hospital,
Minneapolis, Minnesota

Patricia Castaldi, RN, BSN, MSN
Assistant Dean,
Elizabeth General Medical Center School of Nursing,
Elizabeth, New Jersey

Lynne Dearing, RN, MSN, MA
Nursing Instructor,
Grays Harbour College,
Aberdeen, Washington

Serita Dickey, RN, BSN, MS
Assistant Program Coordinator;
Instructor,
San Jacinto College North,
Houston, Texas

Cathy Franklin-Griffin, RN, BSN, MA
Dean, Nursing and Allied Health,
Rockingham Community College,
Wentworth, North Carolina

Mary Ann Fritz, RN, BSN, MS, EdD
Chair, Nursing Education,
South Florida Community College,
Avon Park, Florida

Faye H. Gaugler, RN, BSPA, ONC
Medical-Surgical Instructor,
Franklin County Area Vocational-Technical School,
Chambersburg, Pennsylvania

Hayward S. Gill, Jr., RN, BS, MS
BOE Office of Adult/Continuing Education Nursing Program; and
Faculty,
St. Joseph's College,
New York, New York

Patricia M. Jacobson, RN, BSN, MSN
Nursing Instructor,
Bullard Havens Regional Vocational-Technical School,
Bridgeport, Connecticut

Jacquelyn A. Lux, RN, BA, MA
Instructor, Nursing Department,
Northeast Iowa Community College,
Peosta, Iowa

Kaye L. Marfell, RN, BSN, MA
Instructor, VN Program,
Central Texas College,
Killeen, Texas

Michelle Naplin, RN, BAN, PHN
Instructor, Practical Nursing,
Northwest Technical College,
Thief River Falls, Minnesota

Nellie Nelson, RN, BSN, MSN, CARN
Nursing Faculty,
Scottsdale Community College; and
University of Phoenix,
Phoenix, Arizona

Linda North, RN, BSN, MSN, EdS
ADN Instructor,
Athens Area Technical Institute,
Athens, Georgia

Joann E. Potts Peuterbaugh, RN, MSN
LPN Coordinator,
FW Olin Vocational School of Practical Nursing,
Alton, Illinois

Kathleen Poindexter, RN, BA, MSN
Assistant Professor,
Northern Michigan University,
Marquette, Michigan

Cleo Richard, RN, BS, BA, MS
Nephrology and Holistic Nurse Consultant,
Missoula, Montana

A. Elaine Schmidt, RN, MSN
Faculty, PN Program,
Ivy Technical State College,
Evansville, Indiana

Cynthia A. Steury-Lattz, RN, BSN, MSN
Nursing Instructor,
Kankakee Community College,
Kankakee, Illinois

Dorothy Thomas, RN, BSN, MSN
Associate Professor of Nursing,
St. Louis Community College at Florissant Valley,
St. Louis, Missouri

Mona White, RN, BSN, MSN, CNS
Assistant Professor,
Delta College,
University Center, Michigan

Rose Wilcox, RN, BSN, MEd
Instructor,
Columbus Public Schools;
School of Practical Nursing,
Columbus, Ohio

Beverly Post Yeshion, RN, BSN, MA
Nursing Instructor,
Hillsborough Community College,
Tampa, Florida

PREFACE

Medical-Surgical Nursing: Total Patient Care has been a market favorite for more than 30 years and has served as a comprehensive text of adult health nursing for thousands of nursing students. The ninth edition builds on the strengths of this classic, addressing issues of contemporary practice and the needs of today's student.

This extensive revision features substantially expanded content that includes new chapters on AIDS, emergency and trauma care, substance abuse, nursing process and ethical decision making, nursing within the healthcare system, and cultural considerations. The text continues to focus on the nursing process, with increased emphasis on patient teaching and older adult considerations.

A contemporary new look and many new illustrations provide visual appeal and enhance learning. Boxes, tables, and numerous learning aids help students identify and retain important content. Each chapter contains new critical thinking exercises, nurse alerts, older adult considerations, and ethical dilemma boxes to help prepare students for the realities of practice.

FEATURES

- Completely revised and substantially expanded text throughout that provides current coverage of all content that is appropriate for today's practical/vocational nursing students
  - —New chapters are included on nursing within the healthcare system, nursing process and ethical decision making, cultural considerations, substance abuse, HIV Infection and AIDS, and emergency and trauma care.
  - —Expanded coverage is reflected by the separate chapters on reproductive health for women and men, as well as problems related to vision and hearing.
- An increased focus on the nursing process that better prepares students for applying the process in practice
  - —Nursing Process Boxes for key conditions include assessment, nursing diagnoses, nursing interventions, and evaluation of expected outcomes.
  - —Care Plans are based on case studies and include nursing diagnoses, nursing interventions, and evaluation of expected outcomes.
- Consistent organization of disorder chapters, including a review of anatomy and physiology, diagnostic tests, and commonly occurring conditions
- Inclusion of psychosocial factors that affect health and illness, which reminds students to address patients' emotional as well as physiologic needs
- Objectives, key words, and key concepts that help students identify and retain essential content
- A clear, readable writing style that promotes learning and understanding
- Numerous boxes and tables that spotlight valuable information in a concise, easily retrievable format

NEW FEATURES

- **New** medication tables throughout the text present information regarding routes of administration, normal dosage, and nursing considerations in a consistent format that is easily retrieved for reference.
- **New** patient/family teaching boxes and discussions emphasize this essential nursing responsibility.
- **New** older adult considerations boxes summarize and supplement narrative discussions to provide expanded focus on this growing and important patient population.
- **Unique** ethical dilemma boxes are based on realistic clinical scenarios and help students learn to examine their own values and to make good decisions in difficult situations. Guidelines for the decision-making process are provided in the instructor's manual.
- **New** nurse alerts offer practical, helpful tips and are designed to assist students in making the transition from the classroom to the clinical setting.
- **New** critical thinking exercises promote the development of clinical decision-making skills.
- An attractive, open two-color design and an expanded illustration program add visual appeal and instructional value.

TEACHING/LEARNING PACKAGE

The expanded, unsurpassed teaching-learning package includes the following:

- The workbook helps students reinforce and evaluate their understanding of important concepts in the text. The new edition offers a variety of learning activities and exercises, including chapter objectives and reviews, key word exercises, clinical

situations and questions, matching exercises, crossword puzzles, chapter review questions, anatomy labeling, and ethical dilemmas with guidelines for analysis.
- The instructor's manual with test bank provides invaluable support and assistance to instructors. Each chapter features a summary outline to aid faculty in class preparation. Critical thinking exercises for either group discussion or written exercises are included. The chapter ethical dilemmas with guidelines for analysis are a unique feature and highlight contemporary practice realities. The revised test bank contains nearly 500 questions with answers. Included also are the answers to the chapter activities from the student workbook.
- **New** 54 two-color transparency acetates feature key illustrations from the text to enhance lectures and to reinforce learning.
- **New** *Mosby's Instructor's Resource Kit* is a 3-ring binder that organizes all teaching materials in one handy location.
- **New** *Mosby's Medical-Surgical Nursing Computest* lets you generate your own tests on IBM or MacIntosh computers.

ACKNOWLEDGMENTS

Many people contributed to the ninth edition of *Medical-Surgical Nursing: Total Patient Care* in a variety of ways. A special tribute belongs to our contributing authors, who accepted the challenge of presenting complicated technical information in an understandable and interesting manner. Their work was enhanced by Robin Whittemore, who developed and revised nursing care plans and nursing process boxes; Joanne Pier, who created the series of ethical dilemmas; and Michael Dreher, who constructed the drug tables. Leona Mattson assisted with revision of the home healthcare chapter. We are grateful to all of our students, our fellow faculty members, our associates in clinical agencies, and the reviewers, whose efforts contributed significantly to the clarity of the text.

Our work could not have been completed without the love, patience, and understanding we have received from our families. Karen Merrill assisted with illustrations and editing. Mike and Melanie Merrill and little Michael Asa; Doris and Ron Kerbs; Tom Dincher; John, Donna, Megan, Ryan, and Bridget Rose Dincher; Liz, Todd, Zach, and Samantha Bjur; Julie, Bob, and Laura Breschock; and Pam and Tom Kavanaugh all provided encouragement and motivation.

CONTENTS

PART I NURSING AND HEALTHCARE

1 Nursing Within the Healthcare System, 2
Jean E. Steel, RN, PhD, FAAN

Total patient care, 3
Health, 3
Healthcare reform, 4
Healthcare delivery, 6
Healthcare team, 9
Nursing practice, 10
Patient rights, 16
Key concepts, 19
Critical thinking exercises, 19
References and additional readings, 19

2 Nursing Process and Ethical Decision Making, 21
Mary Gretchen Vancura, RN, BSN, MN, CPN
Joanne Pier, RN, BSN, MA

Critical thinking/decision making, 22
Nursing process, 22
Ethical analysis, 32
Patient respect, 35
Role of the ethics committee, 37
ANA code of ethics, 37
Key concepts, 38
Critical thinking exercises, 38
References and additional readings, 39

PART II PSYCHOSOCIAL ASPECTS OF PATIENT CARE

3 Psychosocial Effects, 42
Clara Williams, RN, MA

Needs of individuals, 43
Personality, 45
Mental health, 45
Anxiety, 45
Emotional disorders, 49
Psychoses, 51
Personality disorders, 53
Organic brain syndromes: dementia, 53
Somatic disorders, 54
Depression, 54
The therapeutic relationship in nursing, 56
Psychopharmacology, 59
Electroconvulsive therapy, 62
Key concepts, 64
Critical thinking exercises, 65
References and additional readings, 65

4 Cultural Considerations, 66
Elaine M. Geissler, RN, PhD, CTN

The phenomenon of culture, 67
Transcultural nursing, 69
Cultural variability, 71
Nursing diagnoses, 75

Patient and family teaching, 76
Key concepts, 77
Critical thinking exercises, 77
References and additional readings, 78

5 Death and Dying, 79
Mildred Owings, RN, MSN, CS

Death, 80
Grief and bereavement, 85
Nursing care of the dying patient, 86
Key concepts, 94
Critical thinking exercises, 94
References and additional readings, 94

6 Substance Abuse, 96
Jean H. Genster, RN, BSN

Terminology, 97
Etiology, 98
Substance abuse as a disease, 99
The dysfunctional family, 99
Central nervous system depressants, 100
Central nervous system stimulants, 109
Inhalants, 111
Hallucinogens, 111
PCP, 112
Treatment and rehabilitation, 112
Nursing management, 114
Chemically impaired nurses, 115
Key concepts, 119
Critical thinking exercises, 120
References and additional readings, 120

PART III PHYSIOLOGIC ASPECTS OF PATIENT CARE

7 Physiologic Responses, 124
Karyl J. Burns, RN, PhD, CS

Causes of disease, 125
Physiologic defense mechanisms, 132
Excessive immune responses, 141
Chemotherapeutic agents, 156
Key concepts, 159
Critical thinking exercises, 159
References and additional readings, 159

8 Fluids and Electrolytes, 161
Judith R. Dincher, RN, BSN, MSEd

Body fluids, 162
Fluid and electrolyte exchange, 164
Regulation of fluid and electrolytes, 167
Fluid and electrolyte imbalances, 167
Protein imbalances, 185
Acid-base imbalance, 185
Intravenous therapy, 190
Shock, 195
Psychosocial support, 198
Key concepts, 202
Critical thinking exercises, 203
References and additional readings, 203

9 The Patient With Pain, 204
Marian Frerichs, RN, EdD

The nature of pain, 205
Interventions for pain relief, 211

Key concepts, 224
Critical thinking exercises, 224
References and additional readings, 224

10 The Patient With Cancer, 226
Patricia Trotta, RN, BSc, MSN, ONC

Pathophysiology, 228
Causes of cancer, 230
Prevention and control, 231
Diagnostic tests and procedures, 233
Treatment of cancer, 238
Emotional care, 258
Rehabilitation, 259
Key concepts, 264
Critical thinking exercises, 264
References and additional readings, 264

11 Community-Acquired Infections, 266
Gail A. Harkness, RN, DrPH, FAAN

Characteristics of the infectious process, 267
Control of communicable disease, 269
The patient with a bacterial infection, 273
The patient with a viral infection, 283
The patient with a protozoal disease, 287
The patient with helminthic infestations, 288
Sexually transmitted diseases, 289
Emerging infections, 294
Key concepts, 297
Critical thinking exercises, 297
References and additional readings, 297

12 Nosocomial Infections, 299
Sandra Blake, RN, MS, CIC

Hospital infections, 300
Types of nosocomial infections, 302
Prevention and control, 308
Emotional support, 319
Key concepts, 323
Critical thinking exercises, 323
References and additional readings, 323

13 HIV Infection and AIDS, 325
Mary "Dee" Miller, RN, BSN, MS, CIC

Acquired immunodeficiency syndrome, 326
Clinical manifestations, 328
Nursing process, 333
Precautions to prevent transmission of HIV, 337
HIV/AIDS legal issues, 338
Burnout, 339
Key concepts, 343
Critical thinking exercises, 343
References and additional readings, 344

14 The Older Adult, 345
Patricia A. Tabloski, RN, PhD, CS

Demographics, 346
Progress and research, 347
Factors affecting aging, 348
Physiology of aging, 353
Nursing the elderly, 364
Care of the hospitalized elderly patient, 371
Nursing homes, 373
Alternatives to institutional care, 373
Key concepts, 374

Critical thinking exercises, 375
References and additional readings, 375

PART IV SPECIAL CARE SETTINGS

15 Rehabilitation, 380
Marion Phipps, RN, MS, CRRN, FAAN

Definition of disability, 381
Rehabilitation nursing, 382
Rehabilitation in each phase of healthcare, 382
The rehabilitation team, 385
Rehabilitation legislation, 387
Emotional response to disability, 388
Nursing approaches to rehabilitation care, 390
Patient teaching in rehabilitation, 415
Continuity of care, 418
Key concepts, 423
Critical thinking exercises, 423
References and additional readings, 423

16 Long-term Care, 425
Patricia A. Tabloski, RN, PhD, CS

Ethical dilemmas in long-term care, 427
General assessment guidelines, 428
Risk and specific care issues, 430
Key concepts, 442
Critical thinking exercises, 442
References and additional readings, 442

17 Home Healthcare, 444
Mary Lou McNiff, RN, MS

Home health services, 446
Supportive services in the community, 447
The home healthcare team, 447
Nursing in the home setting, 447
Healthcare reform, 451
Long-term care and home healthcare, 452
Key concepts, 453
Critical thinking exercises, 453
References and additional readings, 453

18 Care of the Surgical Patient, 454
Margaret F. Burbach, RN, BSN, MS, EdD, CS

The surgical experience, 455
Admission of the patient, 457
Informed consent, 457
Preoperative preparation, 458
Day of surgery, 463
Intraoperative care, 469
Postoperative assessment and interventions, 476
Postoperative complaints and complications, 482
Patient and family teaching and planning for discharge, 487
Key concepts, 487
Critical thinking exercises, 488
References and additional readings, 488

19 Emergency and Trauma Care, 489
Julie A. D'Agostino, RN, BSN, MSN, CEN, TNS

Emergency department, 490
Emergency nursing, 491
Patient arrival/consent, 492
Triage, 493
Physical assessment, 494

Violence, 509
Psychiatric emergencies, 514
Overdose emergency management, 515
Poisonings, 516
Environmental emergencies, 517
Disaster preparedness, 519
Sudden death, 520
Discharge and teaching, 521
Trends, 521
Key concepts, 524
Critical thinking exercises, 524
References and additional readings, 525

PART V MEDICAL-SURGICAL PROBLEMS

20 Respiration, 528
Anne M. Acquila, RN, MSN, CCRN

Structure and function of the respiratory system, 529
Assessment of signs and symptoms of respiratory disease, 531
Nursing assessment of the patient with a respiratory problem, 533
Laboratory diagnostic evaluation, 540
Nursing strategies for common respiratory problems, 544
The patient who requires airway management, 552
The patient undergoing thoracic surgery, 554
The patient with diseases and disorders of the respiratory system, 559
Respiratory infections, 577
Pleural conditions, 584
Tumors of the lung, 588
Chest wounds, 590
Adult respiratory distress syndrome, 591
Key concepts, 593
Critical thinking exercises, 594
References and additional readings, 594

21 Circulation, 596
Helen Stupak Shah, RN, BSN, MSN, DNSc

Cardiovascular structure and function, 597
Nursing assessment of the patient with a cardiovascular problem, 600
Electrocardiography, 604
Disorders of rate and rhythm of the heart, 606
Coronary care unit, 612
The patient with diseases and disorders of the cardiovascular system, 617
The patient with operative conditions of the cardiovascular system, 629
Cardiac rehabilitation, 635
Complications of myocardial infarction, 636
Heart disease complicated by pregnancy, 641
Diseases and disorders of the arteries, veins, and lymphatics, 641
Basic cardiac life support, 646
Advanced cardiac life support, 647
Airway obstruction, 648
Key concepts, 653
Critical thinking exercises, 653
References and additional readings, 654

22 Blood, 655
Joanne Leski, RN, BSN, MSN

Function of blood, 656
Structure of blood, 656
Therapeutic blood fractions, 658
Collection of blood, 662
Nursing responsibilities for diagnostic tests, 662
Nursing responsibilities for therapeutic procedures, 666
The patient with blood dyscrasias, 668

Key concepts, 686
Critical thinking exercises, 687
References and additional readings, 687

23 Gastrointestinal Function, 688
Andrea D'Amato Quinn, RN, MS, CCRN, CS

Structure and function of the gastrointestinal system, 689
Digestion and absorption, 690
Assessment of the gastrointestinal system, 691
Diagnostic procedures, 691
Laboratory studies, 697
Therapeutic techniques of the gastrointestinal tract, 699
Surgery of the GI tract and accessory organs, 704
Colostomy and ileostomy nursing care, 705
Continent pouch ileostomy and ileoanal reservoir, 710
Gastrointestinal manifestations of illness, 711
Eating disorders, 715
Specific diseases and disorders of the gastrointestinal system, 716
Diseases and disorders of the accessory organs of digestion, 740
Key concepts, 758
Critical thinking exercises, 759
References and additional readings, 759

24 Urinary Function, 760
Cleo J. Richard, RN, BS, BA, MSN

Structure and function of the urinary system, 761
Nursing assessment—history and physical examination, 764
Diagnostic tests and nursing responsibilities, 765
Therapeutic procedures and nursing implications, 770
Urinary incontinency, 778
Diseases and disorders of the urinary system, 779
Dialysis, 791
Renal transplantation, 794
Operative conditions of the urinary system, 795
Key concepts, 805
Critical thinking exercises, 805
References and additional readings, 806

25 Women's Reproductive Health, 807
Jeanne LeVasseur, RN, C, MSN, FNP

Structure and function of the reproductive system, 808
Phases of reproductive function throughout the life cycle, 816
Nursing assessment of the patient with problems of the reproductive system, 835
Nursing responsibilities for diagnostic procedures, 836
The patient with diseases and disorders of the reproductive system, 841
Conditions of pregnancy, 857
Key concepts, 862
Critical thinking exercises, 862
References and additional readings, 863

26 Men's Reproductive Health, 864
Mildred Owings, RN, MSN, CS

Structure and function of the reproductive system, 865
Nursing assessment of men with problems of the reproductive system, 866
Phases of reproductive function throughout the life cycle, 866
Examination of the male patient, 867
Conditions affecting the male genitalia, 868
Key concepts, 882
Critical thinking exercises, 883
References and additional readings, 883

27 Endocrine Function, 884
Helen Burton, RN, BS, CDE

Endocrine glands and their function, 885
Nursing assessment of the patient with endocrine problems, 887

Nursing responsibilities for diagnostic tests and procedures, 888
Nursing responsibilities for therapeutic procedures, 889
The patient with diseases and disorders of the endocrine system, 891
Key concepts, 918
Critical thinking exercises, 919
References and additional readings, 919

28 Neurologic Function, 921
Catherine Borkowski Benoit, RNc, MSN, CNRN

Structure and function of the nervous system, 922
Assessment of the patient with neurologic dysfunction, 923
General considerations in neurologic nursing, 927
Care of the patient with trauma to the nervous system, 930
Care of the patient with a tumor of the brain and spinal cord, 941
Care of the patient with cerebrovascular disease, 942
Cerebral artery aneurysm, 947
Care of the patient with a seizure disorder, 948
Care of the patient with central nervous system infection, 952
Nursing care of the patient with degenerative diseases involving the central nervous system, 954
Rehabilitation for neurologic disorders, 958
Key concepts, 964
Critical thinking exercises, 964
References and additional readings, 965

29 Vision, 966
Pamela J. Schultz, RN, CRNO

Structure and function of the eye, 967
Nursing assessment of the patient with eye problems, 969
The patient with vision problems, 975
Nursing interventions for eye disorders, 979
Eye emergencies and trauma, 1002
Eye safety, 1003
Normal aging and the eye, 1005
Key concepts, 1009
Critical thinking exercises, 1010
References and additional readings, 1010

30 Hearing, 1012
Cheryl L. Durkee, RN, BSN, MS

Structure and function, 1013
Nursing assessment of hearing loss, 1014
Diagnostic testing, 1015
Hearing loss, 1017
Disorders of the external ear, 1020
Disorders of the middle ear, 1023
Disorders of the inner ear, 1027
Key concepts, 1028
Critical thinking exercises, 1029
References and additional readings, 1029

31 Skin Integrity, 1031
Marcia J. Hill, RN, BSN, MSN
Donna Starsiak, RN, C, BS, MSN

Structure and function of the skin, 1032
Nursing assessment of the skin, 1034
Assessment and description of skin lesions, 1034
Nursing responsibilities for diagnostic tests and procedures, 1036
Nursing responsibilities for therapeutic procedures, 1037
Pressure ulcers, 1043
The patient with diseases and disorders of the skin, 1050
Burns, 1074
Key concepts, 1087
Critical thinking exercises, 1089
References and additional readings, 1089

32 Mobility, 1091
Mildred Owings, RN, MSN, CS

Structure and function of the musculoskeletal system, 1092
Position, exercise, and body mechanics, 1095
Neurovascular integrity, 1096
The patient with a cast, 1097
The patient with an orthopedic device, 1102
The patient with diseases and disorders of the musculoskeletal system, 1110
Neuromuscular conditions, 1128
Key concepts, 1131
Critical thinking exercises, 1131
References and additional readings, 1132

APPENDICES

A Abbreviations and Symbols for Units of Measurement, 1133

B 1994 NANDA-Approved Nursing Diagnoses, 1135

C Normal Reference Laboratory Values, 1137

GLOSSARY, 1145

INDEX, 1161

MEDICAL-SURGICAL NURSING

TOTAL PATIENT CARE

Part I

1 Nursing Within the Healthcare System

2 Nursing Process and Ethical Decision Making

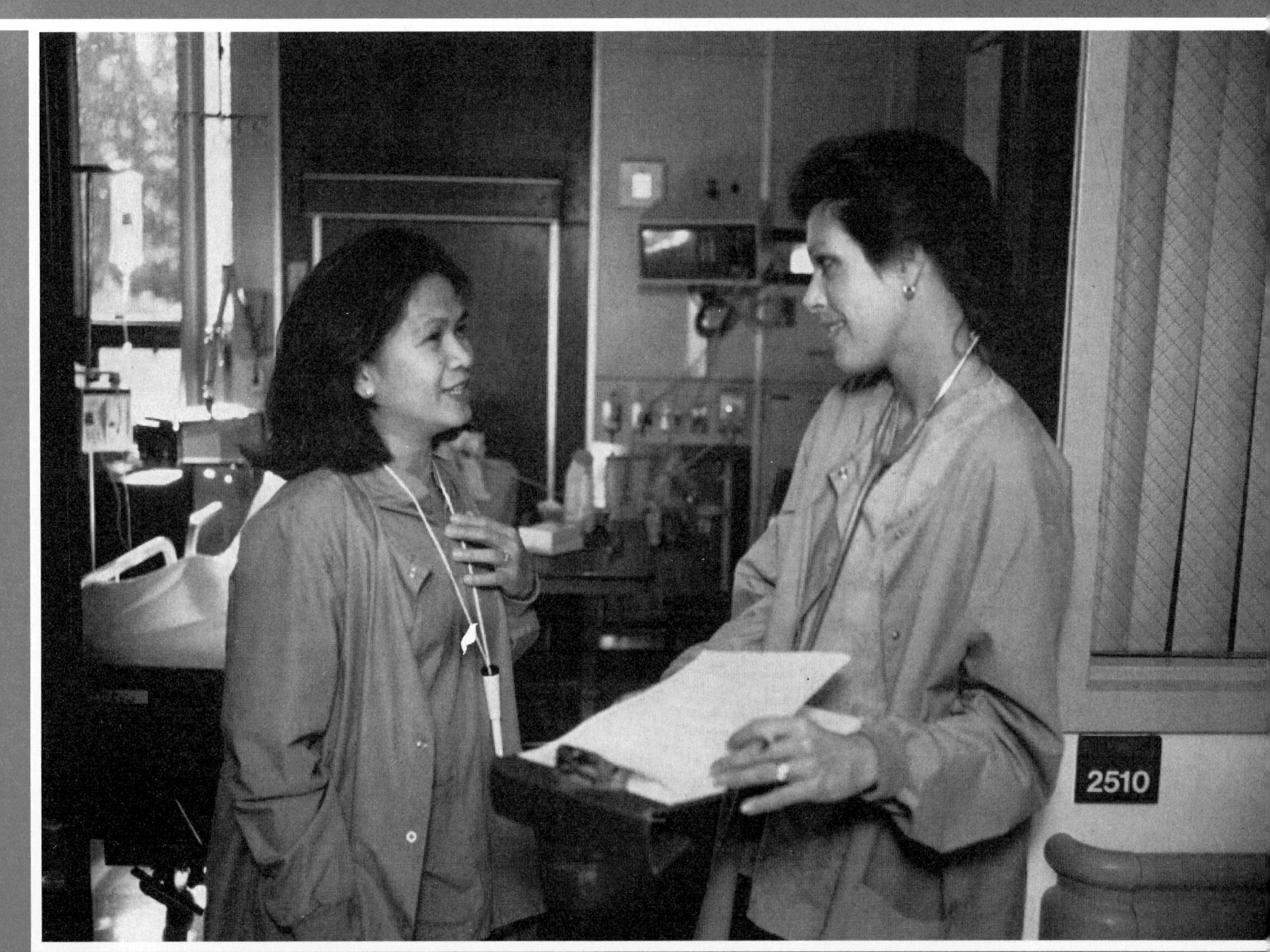

NURSING AND HEALTHCARE

CHAPTER 1

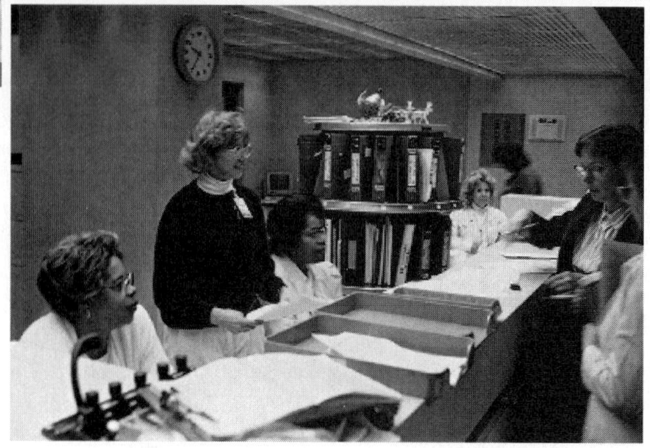

Nursing Within the Healthcare System

CHAPTER OBJECTIVES

1 Discuss the concept of "total patient care."
2 Define "health."
3 Discuss contemporary trends affecting healthcare in the United States.
4 Discuss the costs of healthcare and identify various reimbursement systems.
5 Identify the components of the healthcare delivery system in the United States.
6 Differentiate between a skilled nursing facility and an intermediate care facility.
7 Describe the services of a health maintenance organization (HMO).
8 Account for the increase in ambulatory care and home health agencies.
9 Discuss the concept of holistic care as provided by the healthcare team.
10 Differentiate between the levels of practice of licensed vocational/practical nurses and registered nurses with an associate degree, baccalaureate degree, or diploma.
11 Discuss the application of professional nursing standards.
12 Discuss the importance of quality assurance programs.
13 Contrast functional, team, and primary nursing patterns.
14 Discuss the value of theory in clinical application.
15 Identify the patient's rights.

KEY WORDS

ambulatory care
case management
diagnosis-related group (DRG)
extended-care facility
functional nursing
health maintenance organization (HMO)
Healthy People 2000
holistic care
intermediate care facility (ICF)
Medicaid
Medicare
multisystem
preferred provider organization (PPO)
primary care
primary nursing
primary prevention
proprietary
prospective payment
quality assurance/quality improvement
retrospective payment
secondary prevention
skilled nursing facility (SNF)
standards
team nursing
tertiary prevention
total quality management

TOTAL PATIENT CARE

Total patient care is a concept that provides a basis for nursing practice. The word *total* means **holistic,** or whole, and is used here to imply consideration of all human needs: physiologic, psychologic, and socio-cultural, develpmental, and spiritual. The nurse alone is not equipped to meet all needs but plays a major role in identifying them and coordinating services and personnel within and outside of the hospital. A patient is an individual who is seeking healthcare. The word *patient* formerly implied a passive acceptance of services, but now the patient is viewed as an active participant in care and a thinking consumer of health services. Continued use of the term *patient* does not imply acceptance of a less active role for the healthcare consumer. The meaning of a word may change with time, and *patient* is used here to describe an individual who initiates, plans, and actively participates in his or her care. The word *care* refers to those services that help the patient maintain or restore optimum health. This text focuses on the nursing care provided to the medical and/or surgical patient who is hospitalized in an acute- or extended-care facility to be cured, to improve after a specific illness or crisis, or to maintain optimum health.

HEALTH

The World Health Organization, an agency of the United Nations that was established in 1948, defines health as "a state of complete physical, mental, and social well-being and not merely the absence of disease" (Figure 1-1). Illness is considered to be an acute or chronic lack of adaptation to internal and environmental stressors. Implied in this concept is the belief that the body is constantly working to balance the internal environment (endocrine secretions, water, electrolytes, proteins, vitamins, minerals, oxygen) as it responds to the stressors of the external environment. When the body is able to maintain this balance, or equilibrium, it is in a state of homeostasis. Homeostasis is a dynamic process and requires constant body activity in response to change.

Because illness can result from deficiency or excess, the body must obtain needed materials and convert or eliminate excess materials. Stressors may be biologic (hemorrhage, bacterial toxins), psychologic (fear, worry), or sociologic (financial problems, marital difficulties), but all stressors produce a specific physiologic condition that requires adaptation. An individual's ability to adapt to stressors varies and depends on personal resources, the strength or amount of the stressor, the time at which it appears, and the gradual or sudden nature of its onset.

Society itself has begun to place greater emphasis on this complete state of well-being and on the values of preventive healthcare, health maintenance, physical fitness, and mental vigor. One national program that works to increase the healthy state of Americans is **Healthy People 2000.** This program identifies the objectives of national health promotion and disease prevention that are to be incorporated into any national health program. Healthy People 2000 addresses prevention of a wide range of disease conditions or the reduction of serious complications. It is intended to form the foundation of any health plan and emphasizes the prevention of disease and the promotion of a healthy lifestyle (U.S. Department of Health and Human Services, 1990a). Illness prevention can be classified as primary, secondary, and tertiary. **Primary prevention** involves activities that promote general well-being and specific protection for selected diseases, such as immunizations for diphtheria, measles, and tetanus. **Secondary prevention** focuses on early diagnosis and the implementation of measures that stop the progression of disease or handicapping disabilities. **Tertiary**

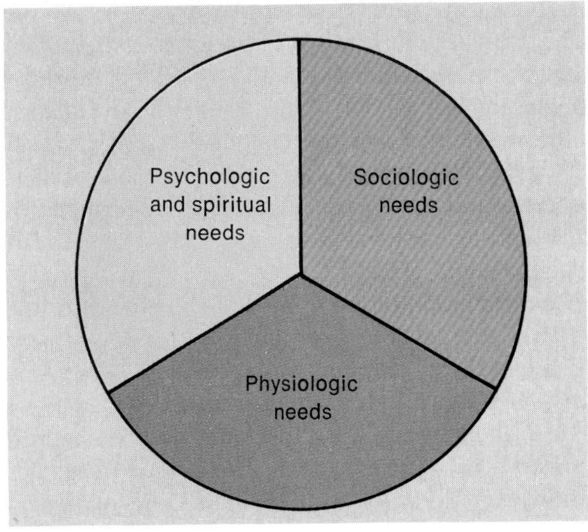

Figure 1-1 The total needs of the patient.

prevention deals with the rehabilitation of disabled patients to return them to a level of maximum usefulness (Stanhope, 1992).

HEALTHCARE REFORM

The United States currently does not have a national healthcare system but is developing new ways to provide universal care to all citizens. A variety of reform proposals exist, and each varies slightly in funding, implementation, and authority. President Clinton's Health Security Act of 1993 called for universal access to affordable and appropriate healthcare. President Clinton believes that any system must incorporate "security, simplicity, savings, choice, quality, and responsibility" (Health Security Act of 1993, 1993).

More than 60 national nursing organizations have developed and agreed to a Nursing Agenda for Health Care (American Nurses Association, 1991a). This agenda asks the public, legislators, and providers to reform their philosophy of care and to change their attitudes and systems to accommodate the public's demand for basic and equitable services. These services must be not only universally accessible, but also appropriate, affordable, and of high-quality.

Some type of healthcare reform will be initiated by the beginning of the 21st century. Nurse providers will be intimately involved with and affected by the new direction of healthcare. A large number of nurses currently employed in hospitals will be relocated into community settings. It is estimated that by 2015, 33% of all nurses will be in a hospital setting compared to the current report of 66%. Obviously this shift will affect the nursing profession, including where its members are educated and employed.

Trends Affecting Healthcare

The growing emphasis on illness prevention stems from the public's increasing awareness of healthcare. This awareness is only one of the trends affecting healthcare delivery in the United States. During the 1980s and 1990s considerable changes have occurred in society and healthcare. Demographic changes, scientific and technologic advances, and economic shifts have also taken place.

The population of the United States is maturing. In 1900 the average life expectancy was 47 years, and only 4% of the population was age 65 and older. However, a baby born today can expect to live past age 70. In 1994, the average life expectancy was 78 years for women and 76 years for men. The United States population was 255 million in 1992 and will exceed 274 million by the year 2000. In 1991, the majority of the population was female. The median age was 33.1 years, and slightly more than 13% of the population was over 65. A significant increase in persons over age 65 will be noted by the turn of the century. This increase can be attributed to the fact that the "baby boomers," the 76 million children born between 1946 and 1964, almost one third of the total population, are getting older. New technologies have also extended life expectancy. Scientific technology has seen a tremendous growth in the last 20 years, and these advances are reflected in modern healthcare. As death rates continue to decline, the number of frail elderly, generally considered to be 85 years and older, will increase dramatically. Such increases in the older population will require more long-term–care facilities and more personnel who are trained in geriatric care. The Census Bureau reports many statistics that are valuable in understanding the current demographics and permit some latitude in projecting future changes. (Box 1-1) (U.S. Department of Commerce, 1993).

BOX 1-1

UNITED STATES POPULATION STATISTICS
(available monthly from the National Center for Health Statistics)

VITAL STATISTICS: MARCH 1993-MARCH 1994	
Births	4,040,000
Deaths	2,294,000
Marriages	2,329,000
Divorces	1,182,000
LEADING CAUSES OF DEATH: FEBRUARY 1993-FEBRUARY 1994	
Heart disease	750,560
Cancer	535,420
Cerebrovascular disease	152,280
Chronic lung disease	105,660
Accidents	88,240

From US National Center for Health Statistics: *Monthly Vital Statistics Report,* 43:3, August 19, 1994, The Center.

Table 1-1 compares the leading causes of death in the United States in 1900 and 1990. A shift in causes of death from infectious diseases to noninfectious conditions is evident.

Emerging medical technologies are permitting an increasing number of outpatient diagnostic and therapeutic interventions. These technologies are drastically reducing inpatient stay requirements for some procedures. A significant increase in same-day surgery has been noted, which prevents high-cost hospitalizations. Many acute care requirements can be provided in the home. New pharmaceuticals are developed al-

TABLE 1-1

Comparison of the Leading Causes of Death in the United States Between 1900 and 1990*

1900	1990
1. Major cardiovascular-renal diseases	1. Diseases of the heart
2. Influenza and pneumonia	2. Malignant neoplasms
3. Tuberculosis	3. Cardiovascular accidents
4. Gastritis, duodenitis, enteritis, and colitis	4. Accidents
5. Accidents	5. Chronic obstructive pulmonary diseases
6. Malignant neoplasms	6. Pneumonia and influenza
7. Diphtheria	7. Diabetes mellitus
8. Typhoid and paratyphoid fever	8. Suicide
9. Measles	9. Chronic liver disease and cirrhosis
10. Cirrhosis of liver	10. HIV infection
11. Whooping cough	11. Homicide and legal intervention
12. Syphilis and its sequelae	12. Nephritis, nephrotic syndrome, and nephrosis

*Excludes fetal deaths.
From US Bureau of the Census: *Historical statistics of the United States, colonial times to 1970, bicentennial edition,* Part 2, Washington DC, 1975, US Government Printing Office; US Bureau of the Census: *Statistical abstracts of the United States: 1993,* ed 113, Washington DC, 1993, US Government Printing Office.

most weekly. Computerized information systems aid greatly in testing, interpretation, and diagnosis and are bringing preventive healthcare closer to reality. Computers are also used for scheduling, billing, payroll, budgeting, surveillance, ordering, documentation, and care plans. The list is endless.

Technologic advances have also affected the economy of healthcare. Although many of these advances have reduced the cost of some services, the research, development, and initial cost of such technologies is very expensive. The rising cost of healthcare and changes in reimbursement systems have greatly impacted healthcare delivery and are discussed in more detail in the next section.

The increased corporatization of healthcare has brought pervasive business orientation to the industry. Corporatization refers to the development of healthcare **multisystems** that manage a large network of facilities out of a single corporate office. Such multisystems can contain costs more efficiently than single institutions. Multisystem chains can include anything that concerns healthcare such as hospitals, **extended-care facilities, health maintenance organizations (HMOs),** clinics, outpatient facilities, pharmacies, medical supply distributors, and health insurance companies. Multisystem chains include both national and regional systems that operate on a for-profit or nonprofit basis.

The economy has also seen a steady increase in the standard of living and a concurrent rise in the demand for healthcare services. Inner cities and rural communities are particularly vulnerable to limited healthcare services and facilities, and both providers and residents are very concerned about access to affordable and appropriate care.

Healthcare Cost and Reimbursement

The gross national product (GNP) for healthcare was 10.7% in 1983 and rose to more than 12% by 1994. The United States currently spends more each year on healthcare than it does on national defense (Profile of Older Americans, 1990). It is estimated that expenses will exceed $700 billion per year in the 1990s and continue to grow. Although people over age 65 represent only 11% of the total population, they account for 29% of the total healthcare expenses (American Nurses Association, 1985).

Since the inception of **Medicare** and **Medicaid,** the GNP for healthcare has more than tripled (Profile of Older Americans, 1990). Medicare and Medicaid are government programs that were created in 1965 through an amendment to the Social Security Act. These programs are funded by taxes on the earnings of those currently employed. Medicare is a federally administered health insurance program and is available to those over age 65 (regardless of income), to the disabled who have received Social Security benefits for more than 2 years, and to individuals with severe kidney disease. Full Medicare coverage, like most private insurance plans, requires a monthly premium and involves a deductible charge for most services that must be paid by the individual or through supplemental private insurance. In 1994, this deductible was $6.96

for Part A (hospital care) and $41.40 for Part B (out-of-hospital care). The regulations for paid services constantly change and are difficult to interpret for both provider and consumer (U.S. Department of Health and Human Services, 1990b). Medicaid is a cooperative federal and state medical assistance program for the poor. It is designed to cover areas that Medicare does not and to defray expenses for those who have exhausted their Medicare benefits or cannot meet the cost of Medicare contributions. The program is operated on a state level, but the federal government provides guidelines and a portion of the funds on the basis of the per capita income of each state. A variety of benefits are available and differ in each state. Medicare and Medicaid currently cover only 40% of health costs for the elderly and the poor (Bower, 1992). Medicare provisions change often. For up-to-date information in an individual state, contact the local state welfare office for Medicaid or the local social security office for Medicare.

Federal and state agencies and private insurers have implemented various regulations to curtail the upward spiral of healthcare costs through new incentive programs and payment systems. Until 1984 the traditional method of reimbursement for healthcare services was **retrospective** (i.e., all the costs of care were added up after they were incurred and were eventually paid by the government, private insurance companies, and the individual). In 1984, **prospective** reimbursement systems were initiated in an attempt to curtail rising healthcare costs. This system was implemented by the Health Care Financing Agency (HCFA) and requires hospitals to assign **diagnosis-related groups (DRGs)** to all admitted patients as an incentive to reduce costs. The DRG system is currently in effect for acute-care hospitals and long-term–care institutions and will soon cover any inpatient and outpatient healthcare service. The HCFA has established several hundred DRG codes on the basis of the physician's diagnosis, the patient's age and sex, and the required treatments. The DRGs specify the number of hospital days that will be paid by Medicare. When a patient is discharged sooner than predicted for that DRG, the hospital profits. However, if a patient requires a longer admission, the hospital pays for the excess days. The DRG codes do not consider the intensity of nursing care that some patients require. Managing patients with high nursing care intensity has negatively affected institutional budgets.

Initially the implementation of DRGs affected only the hospitalized Medicare patient. The use of DRGs has now spread to the various prospective payment systems (PPSs) of many other government and private payers, including Medicaid, and is being extended to healthcare providers other than hospitals. Each type of PPS has a slightly different impact and its own advantages and disadvantages. DRGs have increased the emphasis on hospital discharge planning and hospital alternatives such as skilled extended care, outpatient services, and home care. Although evidence shows that DRGs have helped cut some healthcare costs, critics find many shortcomings in the system. Their greatest concern is that DRGs put an emphasis on cost efficiency, perhaps at the expense of quality of care.

The new payment systems have vast implications for nursing because nurses represent the major personnel expense in any hospital. The PPS provides an opportunity for nursing to demonstrate its value by clearly identifying nursing costs and by relating nursing care to positive patient outcomes. Nurses are in a position to maintain quality and cost-effective care, especially if they have managerial and financial capabilities.

New methods of prepayment cannot provide all the answers to the problems of the troubled healthcare system. Designing systems that provide needed services to the uninsured is a major subject in state and federal legislatures and in healthcare reform. An estimated 39% of the total U.S. population has no health insurance and therefore has limited access to available services. Of those over age 65, approximately 18% are not part of any healthcare insurance program. People significantly handicapped by the current healthcare payment system include single parents, the young, the homeless, acquired immunodeficiency syndrome (AIDS) victims, and the elderly.

HEALTHCARE DELIVERY

Healthcare is provided in a variety of settings. These settings include hospitals, extended-care facilities, HMOs, **ambulatory-care** facilities, government and community health clinics, physicians' offices, nurses' offices, and patients' homes. More than five million people, including more than two million nurses, are involved in healthcare.

The healthcare system is divided into three areas of care: primary (not to be confused with primary prevention), acute, and long-term care. **Primary care** is the first contact in a given episode of illness and leads to a decision of how to resolve the problem. It is provided by the individual responsible for the continuum of care, which includes maintenance of health, evaluations, management of symptoms, and appropriate referrals. Primary care is provided by physicians and advanced-practice nurses, including nurse practitioners and clincial nurse specialists. They assume responsibility for the management of acute and chronic disease and for a variety of health promotion activities and services. Acute care consists of services that treat the acute phase of illness or disability, and it emphasizes the restoration of normal life processes and functions. Long-term care consists of services that provide symptomatic treatment, maintenance, and rehabilitative services for patients of all ages in a variety of healthcare settings. These definitions of primary, acute, and long-term care describe three areas of nursing practice and the three levels of care in the healthcare system.

Hospitals

The hospital is the largest employer of nurses and other healthcare workers (Figure 1-2). The size of a hospital varies from under 25 to over 2000 beds. It may be governmental or nongovernmental, nonproprietary (nonprofit) or **proprietary** (for profit), and general or specialized, such as a children's hospital or cancer hospital. More than one third of all U.S. hospitals are either owned, leased, managed, or sponsored by a multisystem.

The hospital has numerous departments, and each is related to the total care of patients or the operation of support services. Most hospitals have departments for dietary and food service; laundry; business and finance; physical plant (maintenance, housekeeping); nursing service; and other professional services such as radiology, pharmacy, social service, speech therapy, respiratory therapy, laboratory, and medical records. Many hospitals have education departments that conduct the orientation and continuing education of employees. Education may be within a specific department such as nursing, or it may be central to the entire hospital. The volunteer department is also important and includes auxiliary members, teenage volunteers, and friendly visitors. Volunteer workers provide support services and contribute to care without increasing costs.

Most hospitals provide both inpatient and outpatient services. Surgery, diagnostics, dialysis, and physical therapy are a few of the services that may be offered on an outpatient basis. Many hospitals also offer various wellness programs to the community.

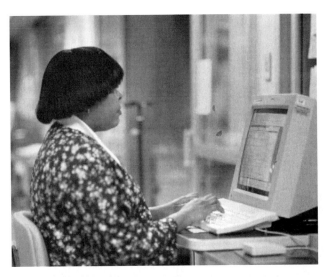

Figure 1-2 Nurses and other healthcare workers manage patient information on a daily basis.

Extended-care Facilities

Extended-care facilities, also called long-term care health centers or nursing homes, may be part of a hospital, but most are separate institutions. Some are nonproprietary, but most are proprietary. These facilities provide nursing, medical, and rehabilitation care and furnish residential and personal services to the elderly and the disabled. Residential care means providing a pleasant, healthy, and comfortable place to live; nutritious meals; clean laundry; barber and beautician services; and companionship. Personal care involves assistance with functional tasks such as dressing, bathing, toileting, eating, and walking. It also includes helping the resident to follow prescribed programs of medication, diet, and exercise and to attend scheduled activities. About 5% of those people age 65 to 85 and 20% of those over age 85 make their homes in long-term care centers. The increase in the older population and the magnitude of their health needs has led to a proliferation of extended-care facilities.

Long-term care centers can offer different levels of care. The Medicare and Medicaid programs have established two categories of extended-care facilities. A **skilled nursing facility (SNF)** is a long-term facility that has been certified in compliance with federal standards. These facilities provide 24-hour nursing services, regular medical supervision, and rehabilitation therapy. An SNF cares for the recuperating patient who no longer needs acute nursing and medical attention but who still requires skilled nursing care. An **intermediate care facility (ICF)** is also certified in compliance with federal standards but provides less extensive health-related services and nursing supervision. These facilities primarily serve people who cannot live alone yet who are not necessarily dependent on 24-hour nursing care (U.S. Department of Health, Education, and Welfare, 1976).

The terms *skilled nursing facility* and *intermediate care facility* describe the intensity of nursing care rather than the quality. Many extended-care facilities are certified and licensed to provide their residents with both skilled nursing and intermediate care. Medicare and other third-party payers (insurance plans) do not pay to keep a patient in a hospital beyond their need for hospital services. Therefore it is more cost-effective to move a patient to an extended-care facility that provides skilled nursing care. Medicare covers at least part of a "period of illness," or up to 100 days of care in an SNF, but only after a hospital stay of at least 3 days. Medicaid also assists with the cost of care in an SNF and an ICF. For example, if care is needed beyond 100 days, the cost may be supplemented by Medicaid and private insurance programs.

Medicare and Medicaid programs are instituting a type of PPS for extended-care facilities that is similar to the DRG categories currently used in hospitals. New York already uses such a system for some Medicaid reimbursement for long-term care (Mitty, 1987). These impending changes necessitate contacting local, federal, and state offices for up-to-date information.

Care is also provided by continuing care retirement communities (CCRCs), which provide private housing to residents and access to an adjacent SNF. Preventing temporary or permanent moves away from one's home is viewed as a significant benefit for senior citizens. This housing trend is expected to continue.

HMOs and PPOs

HMOs provide comprehensive health services to their members for a prepaid, fixed payment, regardless of the quantity of services provided. The distinguishing feature of HMOs is prepayment, or a type of annual prospective payment. Because the cost is fixed, the HMO profits more if the enrollee stays well or if unnecessary diagnostic tests and treatments are avoided. Health services may be provided directly or through arrangements with others and include the services of physicians, nurses, and other healthcare providers. HMOs also provide routine phsyical examinations, health maintenance programs (health education, fitness programs), and illness management. HMOs have grown rapidly in some parts of the country, primarily in the urban areas of the West and Midwest. More than 425 HMOs serve approximately 11% of the U.S. population. Most HMOs are part of a proprietary multisystem. Although the cost-effectiveness of HMOs is widely debated, HMO members do have 30% to 40% fewer inpatient days, which does not appear to be at the expense of quality of care.

Preferred provider organizations (PPOs) offer a delivery system that is similar to the HMO. A PPO is a group of physicians and nurses who have joined together to provide care as a group. Group members are not necessarily located in the same office but make referrals for each other. PPOs may or may not require a standard annual fee from each enrollee. Providers in the PPO furnish services on a discounted reimbursement basis in return for prompt payment and guaranteed volume. PPO enrollees are encouraged to use "preferred" providers through incentives such as lower insurance rates.

Ambulatory Care and Home Health Agencies

The shift in emphasis away from overnight stays in the hospital has generated a proliferation of ambulatory care and home health agencies, and many of them are part of health multisystems. Freestanding ambulatory care centers may be associated with a hospital or operated by a group of physicians on an extended-hour basis. These centers provide immediate and convenient access to episodic care at a relatively reasonable cost. There are more than 3000 ambulatory care centers in the United States, and some are open 24 hours.

Although most hospitals now have expanded outpatient surgery departments, freestanding outpatient surgery centers are also prevalent. These facilities may or may not be hospital owned. In 1975 the first "surgicenter" opened in Phoenix, Arizona, and now there are well over 600 of them. The relatively low complication rates associated with procedures performed at these surgicenters have been attributed both to the minor nature of the surgeries and to careful screening of the patients before surgery.

Community nursing centers have been established throughout the country in recent years. Their development is often stimulated by a university school of nursing, and they offer a variety of services needed by the community. These centers feature professional nursing as a benefit and may have other healthcare professionals available to patients. The centers are managed by professional nurses and work very closely with community residents. Because of this close association, the services of the center are directly related to the needs of the community. The staff in these centers have many collaborative relationships or contracts with other healthcare providers. More opportunities to fund the start-up for these systems are developing. It is anticipated that the community nursing center will be a major provider of primary care services, including management of acute and chronic disease and health promotion activities.

Home healthcare has long been provided by agencies such as the Visiting Nurse Association and county health departments. This field has greatly expanded to approximately 6000 such agencies. The number of private proprietary and nonproprietary home health agencies has increased, but the number of government-based agencies has remained the same or declined. Many home health agencies are hospital- or SNF-based. Hospitals are offering home healthcare more often than any other alternative service. Home health agencies provide services such as nursing, physical therapy, occupational therapy, social service, and home health aide/homemaker services in the patient's home. Because more complicated and invasive procedures are being performed in the home setting, the need for skilled nurses in these agencies has increased. The home health nurse may enjoy a greater sense of autonomy when functioning in this more independent role.

Hospice care is available to the dying patient who wishes to remain at home. Hospice care addresses the physical, spiritual, emotional, psychologic, financial, and legal needs of the dying patient and his or her family. This type of care is provided by an interdisciplinary team of professionals and volunteers.

Government Health Departments

Health departments are found on the federal, state, and local levels. The federal system is widespread and offers many services, most notably through the Department of Veterans Affairs. State health deparments have broad functions, usually in cooperation with federal agencies and local health departments. The average healthcare consumer deals most often with the local health department. Local boards of health vary in the services they provide. Their functions usually include communicable disease control, laboratory testing, environmental sanitation services, health screening, and health education. Public health nurses may provide clinic services or care in the home or school.

Other Healthcare Facilities

Healthcare is provided in many settings beyond the walls of the hospital or nursing home. Physicians, dentists, and nurses in private practice and incorporated group practice centers offer a variety of services and expertise and play a major role in the healthcare system. Schools provide examinations and health teaching. Industries offer emergency services and physical examinations and are becoming more involved in programs that promote prevention and health maintenance. Community health centers are playing a major role in bringing healthcare closer to the people. The goal of the community health center is to provide the needed services in an atmosphere of concern and understanding that is tailored to meet the needs of the community.

HEALTHCARE TEAM

Regardless of the setting, comprehensive healthcare requires the efforts of a team that includes health professionals and paraprofessionals. In the center of the team is the patient to whom the team is ultimately responsible. Often the patient lacks the ability or resources to lead and coordinate the health team. It is the nurse, who spends the greatest amount of time with the patient, who must assist the patient and act as the patient advocate. Often the nurse represents the patient and coordinates the efforts of the physician, physical therapist, social worker, clergy, dietician, respiratory therapist, psychologist, home care coordinator, occupational therapist, and others (Figure 1-3). The nurse assumes responsibility as a patient *advocate* and promotes patient needs, beliefs, and values for the development of a care plan. Each member of the health team is essential to the total, or holistic, care of the patient (Figure 1-4).

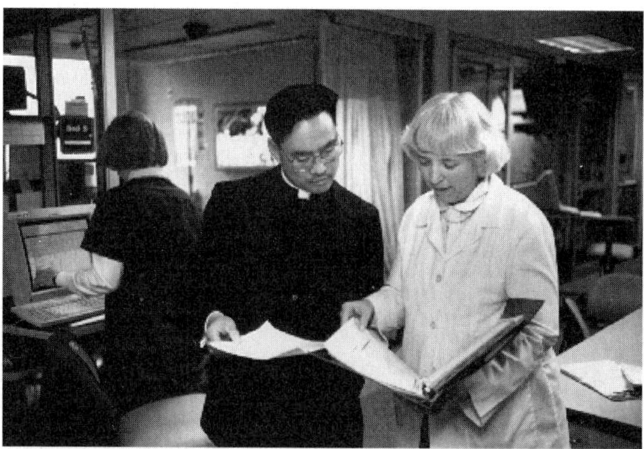

Figure 1-3 The nurse is a patient advocate and coordinates the work of others in meeting the varied needs of patients.

Collaboration Between Nurses and Physicians

The relationship between nurses and physicians has a significant impact on patient care outcomes (Steel, 1986). This relationship is receiving more and more attention as healthcare organizations look at systems and models for effective and efficient quality care. Healthcare organizations are realizing that the nurse-physician relationship significantly affects the provision of effective and efficient care. The most desirable relationship between nurses and physicians is a collaborative one. Collaboration is defined as a relationship of interdependence and an understanding that joint planning of care improves its quality and quantity. Collaboration requires trust between the nurse and the physician and respect for the care each provides. Such a relationship improves patient outcomes and, in many situations, reduces patient cost. Collaboration is essential to effectively evaluate patient care outcomes, analyze variances in outcomes, and modify necessary practice patterns.

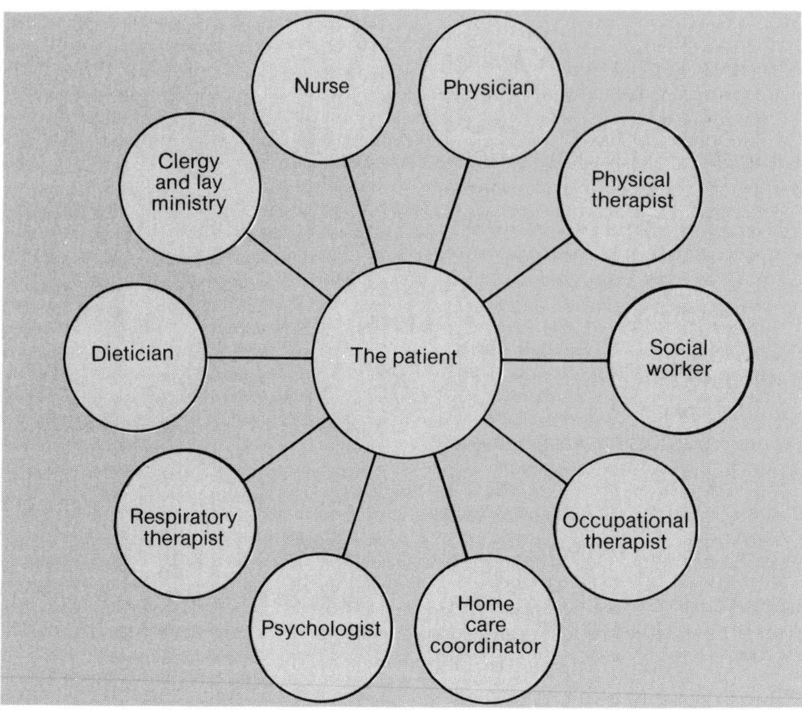

Figure 1-4 The healthcare team.

NURSING PRACTICE

The act of nursing was once a simple function performed by the untrained. The individual who nursed the sick was called a nurse. There was no formal preparation for nursing until Florence Nightingale opened her school with a prescribed curriculum of study and practical experience. As nursing evolved as a profession, nursing leaders attempted to define it. Florence Nightingale wrote that the goal of nursing is "to put the patient in the best condition for nature to act upon him." Virginia Henderson (1966) developed a classic definition of nursing. She wrote that the nurse's purpose is "to assist the individual, sick or well, in the performance of those activities contributing to health or its recovery (or to peaceful death) that he would perform unaided if he had the necessary strength, will, or knowledge. And to do this in such a way as to help him gain independence as rapidly as possible." The American Nurses Association (ANA) has defined nursing as "the diagnosis and treatment of human responses to actual or potential health problems" (American Nurses Association, 1980, p. 9). All of these definitions illustrate the nurses' consistent orientation to providing nursing care that promotes the well-being of the people served.

Nursing has long been described as an art and a science. Early definitions emphasized the care of the sick, whereas more recent descriptions stress the role of the nurse in disease prevention and health maintenance. These modern definitions stress the need to view the patient as a whole person, including physiologic, emotional, psychologic, intellectual, and social and spiritual factors and the interrelationship and interdependence of these factors as they affect health. Modern definitions also include references to the patient's family and significant others. The functions of the nurse are likely to be categorized according to the degree of dependence or independence of the patient. Dorothy Orem goes beyond a definition to a theory of nursing when she describes the "locus of decision making" and places it with the nurse, with the patient, or with the nurse and patient together, depending on the ability of the patient to make decisions or perform health-related activities.

Medical-Surgical Nursing

Medical-surgical nursing deals with any illness or disease that affects the physiology of adults. The illness may have begun in childhood, during or after pregnancy, or as a result of a psychiatric problem. Once the illness interferes with normal physiology, the patient is said to have a medical problem and is termed a *medical patient*. When the problem is treated by surgical intervention, the patient is termed *surgical*. Social and behavioral problems can affect or be affected by the physical illness and are therefore an important aspect of medical-surgical nursing. The content of medical-surgical nursing is complex and vast in scope.

The medical service in a hospital usually includes patients with serious conditions such as a myocardial infarction, terminal cancer, congestive heart failure, leukemia, and AIDS. The medical patient may have entered the hospital for a work-up, which includes diagnostic tests and examinations. After completion of the examinations and the establishment of a medical diagnosis, the patient may be treated and discharged or prepared for surgery. The patient may be transferred to a surgical service unless medical and surgical patients are admitted to the same units. Many patients have medical and surgical conditions at the same time, such as a diabetic patient who is admitted to the hospital to have his or her gallbladder removed.

The goal of medical-surgical nursing is to help patients help themselves. The degree of assistance required for each patient varies with the stage of illness. Nurses are often tempted to "do for" patients rather than encourage and assist with self-care. Sometimes it is faster to "do-for" patients, sometimes there is concern that the patient will not perform the activity well, and most often the need to help others prompts the nurse to do what the patient should be doing independently or with assistance. Most nurses express the desire to help others as a reason for entering nursing. Promoting independence while providing support and understanding to the patient is essential for the maintenance and restoration of optimum health (i.e., the patient's greatest possible level of health).

Regulation of Nursing Practice

Control or regulation of nursing practice is achieved through credentialing of the individual nurse. Credentialing includes licensure, certification, and accreditation.

Licensure

The state Boards of Nursing protect the public through approval of educational nursing programs and state licensure of individuals. In recent years the Boards of Nursing have achieved greater national standardization of requirements. This standardization provides nurses with gives nurses expanded choices in the job market by giving them easier access across state boundaries. The development and implementation of the state board licensing examination (NCLEX) assures the public that individuals are minimally safe to render nursing care. Each state has established broad definitions and standards for nursing care and monitors individuals through a renewal process that at this time does not require retesting. Some states require evidence of continuing education to secure the renewed license.

Certification

Certification is the validation of a body of knowledge in a specialized or occupational field. Initially the individual is tested and then maintains certification through a variety of mechanisms. This validation is based on professional standards of practice. Certification systems have been developed and implemented by national professional associations, including the ANA and specialty nursing organizations such as American Operating Room Nurses (AORN). Eligibility for certification varies among organizations. Although certification did not originate as a form of entry into practice, many state boards of nursing now require it to practice in advanced roles (e.g., nurse practitioners, clinical nurse specialists). Prescriptive authority and reimbursement may be permitted to individuals who have national certification.

Accreditation

Accreditation is another form of regulation of nursing practice. Accreditation is a system of review and approval of organized nursing education programs to ensure that basic minimum expectations are included in the curriculum. Educational programs that provide continuing education credits may also be accredited. Programs are approved for a period and are subject to reaccreditation. Individual nurses are not accredited.

Nursing Education and Scope of Practice

Education within the nursing profession has evolved and changed since Florence Nightingale established the first school of nursing. Today, to become a licensed vocational nurse (LVN) or a licensed practical nurse (LPN), one attends a 9- to 12-month program. To become a registered nurse (RN), one can attend a 2- to 3-year hospital diploma school, a 2-year community college associate degree program, a 4-year university baccalaureate program, or a "generic master's" program. Graduates of these programs complete their education with varying degrees of knowledge and differing skills and abilities.

The LVN/LPN is authorized to provide direct nursing care under the supervision and direction of an RN, physician, dentist, or podiatrist. Supervision need not be direct and is often quite distant, but the supervisor is responsible for authorizing the LVN/LPN to provide care. The LVN/LPN is prepared to provide nursing care to patients with predictable nursing care problems in well-defined situations. LVN/LPN programs are offered by hospitals, community colleges, vocational centers, and some high schools. The program must be state-approved for its graduates to be eligible to take the state board examination for practical nursing. All states except California use the National Council of State Boards of Nursing Licensing Examination for Vocational/Practical Nursing. California develops and administers its own examination.

Hospital-based diploma schools were the first educational programs offered in nursing. The functions and responsibilities of diploma school of nursing graduates include direct patient care in hospitals, extended-care facilities, and other healthcare agencies. The number of diploma schools has declined in recent years because of the high cost of maintaining such programs and the trend of moving nursing education into the academic setting.

The nursing graduate with an associate degree is prepared to give direct care to patients with well-defined acute or chronic health problems or to those who need information or support to maintain health. Such patients are usually found in hospitals, nursing homes, and other healthcare agencies. Practice is focused on the individual patient in consideration of that patient's relationships within a family, group, or community. The nurse with an associate degree can pursue study toward the baccalaureate degree. Some programs are designed to build directly on the associate degree program. Other baccalaureate programs admit associate degree graduates with advanced standing after evaluating transfer credit in the liberal arts and sciences. College credit can also be earned by passing standardized nursing examinations.

The nurse with a bachelor of science in nursing degree (BSN) is prepared to function in the acute- and extended-care facility and in the community. The academic background provided in the baccalaureate program prepares the graduate to assume a greater share of responsibility for healthcare and for directing other members of the health team. The curriculum emphasizes primary healthcare, preventive and rehabilitative services, acute and long-term services, health counseling, and education. Students are required to study such areas as nursing leadership, community health nursing, and nursing theory and research.

Several schools have established a generic master's program for students who have earned a bachelor's degree in a field other than nursing. The 3-year curriculum includes nursing knowledge and skill, with a focus in an area of specialty. The student earns a master's degree in nursing and is eligible for the RN examination. These programs attract people who may have pursued another field before choosing nursing.

Graduate education in nursing is available to those who have earned a bachelor's degree in nursing and who meet the entrance requirements of a university graduate school. The master's degree allows a nurse to focus in an area of specialty and become an advanced practice nurse. The term *advanced practice nurse* refers to the roles of nurse practitioner and clinical nurse specialist and may also include nurse midwife and nurse anesthetist. Other programs prepare nurse administrators to manage healthcare delivery systems.

Although there are a variety of educational entry points in nursing, each type of graduate provides a unique service to patients and their families. The profession continues to differentiate the various types of practice for the future according to education and experience (American Nurses Association, 1987).

Collaboration Between Nursing Practice and Nursing Education

The many changes in the healthcare delivery system and pressures on educational institutions are forcing the issue of increased collaboration between education and practice. There has been some movement toward such collaboration for the past 25 years, but today's pressures are causing practitioners and educators to examine the issues more seriously. Several good reasons exist for collaboration: (1) both groups of nurses have the patient as their focus, (2) nursing education requires a practice laboratory for students, and (3) healthcare agencies must rely on nursing schools to produce practitioners to work in their agencies. Practicing nurses may not have the preparation or the time to perform their own nursing research, but they can work closely with those already engaged in research to identify phenomena encountered in practice.

Standards of Nursing Practice

Standards are broad statements that encompass the full range of nursing's scope of practice. Standards reflect the values and priorities of the profession and provide a way to measure the effectiveness of care. Clinical standards provide the public with a way to determine the quality of care provided. The ANA is responsible for establishing and maintaining the generic, or general, standards of nursing practice. Many nursing specialty organizations work collaboratively with the ANA to issue joint standards. Specialty organizations also develop standards related to each area of expertise. Nurses are responsible for incorporating these standards into their ongoing care.

BOX 1-2

COMPONENTS OF CLINICAL NURSING PRACTICE STANDARDS

IMPLEMENT THE NURSING PROCESS
- Assessment of patient health information.
- Establish a nursing diagnosis.
- Determine expected outcomes.
- Create a plan of care.
- Implement the plan of care.
- Evaluate outcomes and quality of care.

MAINTAIN A PROFESSIONAL PRACTICE
- Self-evaluate clinical practice.
- Engage in continuous professional learning and apply findings to practice.
- Uphold a code of ethics in caring for patients.
- Collaborate with patients, significant others, and peers in providing care.
- Use healthcare resources effectively.

Modified from American Nurses Association: *ANA Standards of Clinical Nursing Practice,* Kansas City, MO, 1991, The Association.

BOX 1-3

COMPONENTS OF THE JOINT COMMISSION'S STANDARDS FOR QUALITY ASSESSMENT AND IMPROVEMENT

1 The organization has a planned, systematic, organizationwide approach to designing, measuring, assessing, and improving its performance.
2 New processes are designed well.
3 The organization has in place a systematic process to collect needed data.
4 Patient care services are appropriately integrated throughout the organization.
5 The organization's leaders set expectations, develop plans, and manage processes to assess, improve, and maintain the quality of the organization's governance, management, clinical, and support activities.

Modified from Joint Commission on Accreditation of Healthcare Organizations: *Accreditation manual for hospitals,* Volume 1 Chicago, 1995, The Commission.

The ANA (1991b) has published the generic standards and organized them into Standards of Clinical Nursing Practice, which contain the standards of patient care and the standards of professional performance. These standards are used as the basis for quality assurance systems, databases, healthcare reimbursement policies, certification programs, and many other measurement systems. These standards are periodically modernized in an effort to keep current with contemporary practice (Box 1-2).

Quality Assurance and Quality Improvement in Nursing

A significant component of nursing care delivery is the measurement or evaluation of the outcome of that care. Although the phrase *quality of care* is difficult to define, it has been one of the hallmarks of professional nursing practice. Most formal nursing systems have developed some form of measuring the care provided. Nationally **quality assurance (QA)** has been defined by the Joint Commission and Accreditation of Health Care Organizations (JCAHO) (1986) as a planned and systematic process for monitoring and evaluating the appropriateness of care, evaluating quality of service, and resolving existing problems. Delivery systems appoint a QA committee whose members are from a clinical practice unit. In this way direct providers of care are involved in QA measurement. Some systems incorporate a **quality improvement (QI)** system or a total quality management system (TQM). In all of these designs the major objective is to measure and evaluate the effectiveness and quality of care.

The characteristics of these systems include a focus on care, a variety of professionals who are involved in the system of measurement, a focus on a particular problem and continuing problems, and the integration of quality and cost of care. The JCAHO (1993) recommends a systematic approach to identify how care can be improved in the future (Box 1-3). The ultimate goals for quality assurance programs are to assure the public that the highest level of care is being provided and that there is a system to constantly monitor care. The professional provider and healthcare systems are involved in this monitoring. As a result of measurement and evaluation, systems redesign their policies or methods of providing service, and individual care is improved.

Nursing Delivery Systems

In the early days of nursing, each nurse cared for and provided all necessary services to one patient, or "case," or a group of patients. This was known as the "case method" of patient assignment. As medicine and technology advanced, the responsibilities and duties of the nurse became more complex. As a result of the nursing shortage during World War II, **functional**

nursing was developed. This system uses auxiliary health workers who are trained in a variety of skills. Each person is assigned specific duties or functions that are performed on all patients in a given unit. RNs give medications, LVNs/LPNs give treatments, and aides and orderlies make beds and distribute meals. Functional nursing is still used in some institutions throughout the United States.

In the early 1950s, **team nursing** was proposed to take advantage of the skills of a variety of nursing personnel while providing more comprehensive care to the patient. The RN acts as the leader of a nursing team that is responsible for a predetermined group of patients. LPNs/LVNs, nursing assistants, and other nurses assist the RN in the care of those patients. The team leader knows and understands the condition of each patient and provides care by assigning team members according to their individual capabilities and personalities. The team leader also assimilates and dispenses knowledge and is the contact between the head nurse and the physician. The team leader also has certain responsibilities for promoting team morale, suggesting changes for team members, and evaluating individual work. Essential to the team nursing concept is the team conference, in which team members discuss patient needs and jointly establish a plan of care under the direction of the team leader. The team conference includes the patient whenever possible. The use of a mixture of healthcare personnel coordinated by the RN is a modern version of team nursing (Figure 1-5).

Another type of nursing delivery system is **primary nursing.** Each nurse is assigned a group of patients, preferably no more than five, and is responsible for their total care from admission to discharge. The initial assessment is performed by the primary nurse, who plans the care to be given. When the primary nurse is off duty, other nurses follow the directives of this plan of care. The primary nurse involves the patient in the care, identification of goals, and discharge planning. This method provides continuity of care and enables the nurse to become better acquainted with and specifically provide for the needs of patients and their families. As a result, patient-centered care becomes a reality. The primary nurse accepts responsibility for the care of the patient and establishes accountability (Nenner, 1977). The primary nursing approach to patient care is not to be confused or equated with the concepts of primary care or primary prevention, which were discussed earlier in this chapter.

Primary nursing requires all care to be delivered by RNs. However, there is a trend to delegate less complex tasks to lesser prepared personnel, with the RN maintaining responsibility for the complete care of the patient. Pairing an RN with a nursing assistant or technician (partners in practice) is a modification of primary nursing.

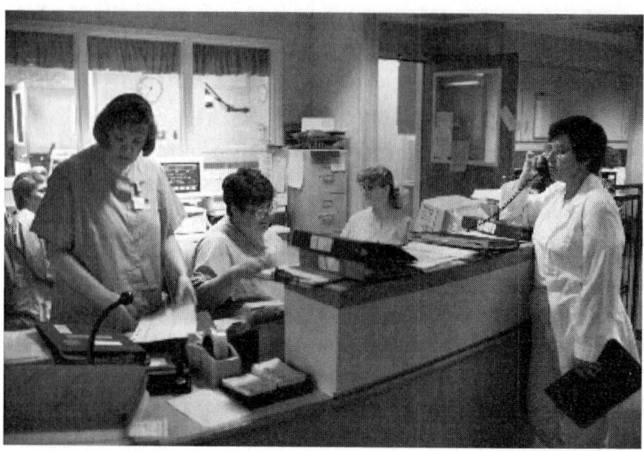

Figure 1-5 Patient care is delivered by a mixture of healthcare personnel.

Other nursing delivery systems have evolved from the primary nursing concept. Among these are the collaborative practice model and its variations and the new **case management** model. Collaborative practice models encourage effective communication between the physician and primary nurse and emphasize their interdependent roles and the independent role of the professional nurse. The case management concept incorporates primary and team nursing and holds the RN, as case manager, accountable for specific clinical outcomes. Each agency must examine its resources, develop and state its philosophy of nursing care, and organize its approach to nursing accordingly. Because of prospective reimbursement, the decision regarding which nursing delivery system to use may well rest on which approach is the most cost-effective.

Theory in Practice

Many theories or beliefs explain, predict, or describe the action of the nurse. Today, nursing practice is based on a wide range of theories developed by nurse scientists and others (Table 1-2) (Potter, 1993). These theorists have made significant contributions to the nursing profession and society.

Other theories developed by those outside of nursing have contributed to the understanding of behaviors and actions appropriate to the profession. For example, Maslow's work on understanding human need has contributed to the field of nursing. Maslow identified the needs basic to all humans, including physiologic, safety, love and belongingness, esteem and self-actualization. His work has helped give meaning to the concept of holism and the treatment of the patient's many needs as one mission. Others have also contributed theories that help nurses understand and

TABLE 1-2
Summary of Nursing Theories

Theorist	Goal of Nursing	Framework for Practice
Nightingale (1860)	To facilitate "the body's reparative processes" by manipulating client's environment (Torres, 1986)	Client's environment is manipulated to include appropriate noise, nutrition, hygiene, light, comfort, socialization, and hope.
Peplau (1952)	To develop interactions between nurse and client (Peplau, 1952)	Nursing is a significant, therapeutic, interpersonal process (Peplau, 1952). Nurses participate in structuring healthcare systems to facilitate natural ongoing tendency of humans to develop interpersonal relationships (Marriner-Tomey, 1989).
Henderson (1955)	To work interdependently with other healthcare workers (Marriner-Tomey, 1989); assisting client to gain independence as quickly as possible (Henderson, 1964); to help client gain lacking strength (Torres, 1986)	Nurses help client to perform Henderson's 14 basic needs (Henderson, 1966).
Abdellah (1960)	To provide service to individuals, families, and society; to be kind and caring but also intelligent, competent, and technically well prepared to provide this service (Marriner-Tomey, 1989)	This theory involves Abdellah's 21 nursing problems (Abdellah et al, 1960).
Orlando (1961)	To respond to client's behavior in terms of immediate needs; to interact with client to meet immediate needs by identifying client behavior, reaction of nurse, and nursing action to be taken (Torres, 1986; Chinn, Jacobs, 1987)	Three elements, including client behavior, nurse reaction, and nurse action, compose nursing situation (Orlando, 1961).
Hall (1962)	To provide care and comfort to client during disease process (Torres, 1986)	The client is composed of the following overlapping parts: person (core), pathologic state and treatment (cure), and body (care). Nurse is caregiver (Chinn, Jacobs, 1987; Marriner-Tomey, 1989).
Wiedenbach (1964)	To assist individuals in overcoming obstacles that interfere with the ability to meet demands or needs brought about by condition, environment, situation, or time (Torres, 1986)	Nursing as practice is related to individuals who need help because of behavioral stimulus. Clinical nursing has the following components: philosophy, purpose, practice, and art (Chinn, Jacobs, 1987).
Levine (1966)	To use conservation activities aimed at optimal use of client's resources	This adaptation model of human as integral whole is based on "four conservation principles of nursing" (Levine, 1973).
Johnson (1968)	To reduce stress so that client can move more easily through recovery process	This basic needs framework focuses on seven categories of behavior. Individual's goal is to achieve behavioral balance and steady state by adjustment and adaptation to certain forces (Johnson, 1980; Torres, 1986).
Rogers (1970)	To maintain and promote health, prevent illness, and care for and rehabilitate ill and disabled client through "humanistic science of nursing" (Rogers, 1970)	"Unitary man" evolves along life process. Client continuously changes and coexists with environment.

From Potter PA, Perry AG: *Fundamentals of nursing,* ed 3, St Louis, 1993, Mosby.

Continued.

TABLE 1-2—cont'd

Summary of Nursing Theories

Theorist	Goal of Nursing	Framework for Practice
Orem (1971)	To care for and help client attain total self-care	This is self-care deficit theory. Nursing care becomes necessary when client is unable to fulfill biological, psychological, developmental, or social needs (Orem, 1985).
King (1971)	To use communication to help client reestablish positive adaptation to environment	Nursing process is defined as dynamic interpersonal process between nurse, client, and healthcare system.
Travelbee (1971)	To assist individual or family to prevent or cope with illness, regain health, find meaning in illness, or maintain maximal degree of health (Marriner-Tomey, 1989)	Interpersonal process is viewed as human-to-human relationship formed during illness and "experience of suffering."
Neuman (1972)	To assist individuals, families, and groups to attain and maintain maximal level of total wellness by purposeful interventions	Stress reduction is goal of systems model nursing practice (Torres, 1986). Nursing actions are in primary, secondary, or tertiary level of prevention.
Roy (1979)	To identify types of demands placed on client, assess adaptation to demands, and help client adapt	This adaptation model is based on the physiological, psychological, sociological, and dependence-independence adaptive modes (Roy, 1980).
Patterson and Zderad (1976)	To respond to human needs and build humanistic nursing science (Patterson, Zderad, 1986; Chinn, Jacobs, 1987)	Humanistic nursing requires participants be aware of their "uniqueness" and "commonality" with others (Chinn, Jacobs, 1987).
Leininger (1978)	To provide care consistent with nursing's emerging science and knowledge with caring as central focus (Chinn, Jacobs, 1987)	With this transcultural care theory, caring is central and unifying domain for nursing knowledge and practice (Leininger, 1980).
Watson (1979)	To promote health, restore client to health, and prevent illness (Marriner-Tomey, 1989)	This theory involves philosophy and science of caring; caring is interpersonal process comprising interventions that result in meeting human needs (Torres, 1986).
Parse (1981)	To focus on man as living unity and man's qualitative participation with health experience (Parse, 1981) (Nursing as science and art [Marriner-Tomey, 1989])	Man continually interacts with environment and participates in maintenance of health (Marriner-Tomey, 1989). Health is continual, open process rather than state of well-being or absence of disease (Parsen, 1981; Marriner-Tomey, 1989; Chinn, Jacobs, 1987).

plan for change. Each description offers guidelines to nursing systems and individual nurses for making useful and timely changes.

PATIENT RIGHTS

Emphasis on the patient as an active participant in personal healthcare has prompted a variety of groups and individuals to make public statements about patient rights. The House of Delegates of the American Hospital Association adopted a "Patient's Bill of Rights" during its 1973 convention and revised this in 1992. It was believed that these rights would contribute to more effective patient care and greater satisfaction for the patient, physician, and hospital (Box 1-4) (American Hospital Association, 1992).

BOX 1-4

A PATIENT'S BILL OF RIGHTS

INTRODUCTION

Effective health care requires collaboration between patients and physicians and other health care professionals. Open and honest communication, respect for personal and professional values, and sensitivity to differences are integral to optimal patient care. As the setting for the provision of health services, hospitals must provide a foundation for understanding and respecting the rights and responsibilities of patients, their families, physicians, and other caregivers. Hospitals must ensure a health care ethic that respects the role of patients in decision making about treatment choices and other aspects of their care. Hospitals must be sensitive to cultural, racial, linguistic, religious, age, gender, and other differences, as well as the needs of persons with disabilities.

The American Hospital Association presents *A Patient's Bill of Rights* with the expectation that it will contribute to more effective patient care and be supported by the hospital on behalf of the institution, its medical staff, employees, and patients. The American Hospital Association encourages health care institutions to tailor this bill of rights to their patient community by translating and/or simplifying the language of this bill of rights as may be necessary to ensure that patients and their families understand their rights and responsibilities.

BILL OF RIGHTS*

1 The patient has the right to considerate and respectful care.

2 The patient has the right to and is encouraged to obtain from physicians and other direct caregivers relevant, current, and understandable information concerning diagnosis, treatment, and prognosis.

Except in emergencies when the patient lacks decision-making capacity and the need for treatment is urgent, the patient is entitled to the opportunity to discuss and request information related to the specific procedures and/or treatments, the risks involved, possible length of recuperation, and the medically reasonable alternatives and their accompanying risks and benefits.

Patients have the right to know the identity of physicians, nurses, and others involved in their care, as well as when those involved are students, residents, or other trainees. The patient also has the right to know the immediate and long-term financial implications of treatment choices, insofar as they are known.

3 The patient has the right to make decisions about the plan of care prior to and during the course of treatment and to refuse a recommended treatment or plan of care to the extent permitted by law and hospital policy and to be informed of the medical consequences of this action. In case of such refusal, the patient is entitled to other appropriate care and services that the hospital provides or transfer to another hospital. The hospital should notify patients of any policy that might affect patient choice within the institution.

4 The patient has the right to have an advance directive (such as a living will, health care proxy, or durable power of attorney for health care) concerning treatment or designating a surrogate decision maker with the expectation that the hospital will honor the intent of that directive to the extent permitted by law and hospital policy.

Health care institutions must advise patients of their rights under state law and hospital policy to make informed medical choices, ask if the patient has an advance directive, and include that information in patient records. The patient has the right to timely information about hospital policy that may limit the hospital's ability to implement fully a legally valid advance directive.

5 The patient has the right to every consideration of privacy. Case discussion, consultation, examination, and treatment should be conducted so as to protect each patient's privacy.

6 The patient has the right to expect that all communications and records pertaining to care will be treated as confidential by the hospital, except in cases such as suspected abuse and public health hazards when reporting is permitted or required by law. The patient has the right to expect that the hospital will emphasize the confidentiality of this information when it releases it to any other parties entitled to review information in these records.

7 The patient has the right to review the records pertaining to medical care and to have the information explained or interpreted as necessary, except when restricted by law.

8 The patient has the right to expect that, within its capacity and policies, a hospital will make reasonable response to the request of a patient for appropriate and medically indicated care and services. The hospital must provide evaluation, service, and/or referral as indicated by the ur-

**These rights can be exercised on the patient's behalf by a designated surrogate or proxy decision maker if the patient lacks decision-making capacity, is legally incompetent, or is a minor.*

Continued.

BOX 1-4

A PATIENT'S BILL OF RIGHTS—cont'd

gency of the case. When medically appropriate and legally permissible, or when a patient has so requested, a patient may be transferred to another facility. The institution to which the patient is to be transferred must first have accepted the patient for transfer. The patient must also have the benefit of complete information and explanation concerning the need for, risks, benefits, and alternatives to such a transfer.

9 The patient has the right to ask and be informed of the existence of business relationships among the hospital, educational institutions, other health care providers, or payors that may influence the patient's treatment and care.

10 The patient has the right to consent to or decline to participate in proposed research studies or human experimentation affecting care and treatment or requiring direct patient involvement, and to have those studies fully explained prior to consent. A patient who declines to participate in research or experimentation is entitled to the most effective care that the hospital can otherwise provide.

11 The patient has the right to expect reasonable continuity of care when appropriate and to be informed by physicians and other caregivers of available and realistic patient care options when hospital care is no longer appropriate.

12 The patient has the right to be informed of hospital policies and practices that relate to patient care, treatment, and responsibilities. The patient has the right to be informed of available resources for resolving disputes, grievances, and conflicts, such as ethics committees, patient representatives, or other mechanisms available in the institution. The patient has the right to be informed of the hospital's charges for services and available payment methods.

The collaborative nature of health care requires that patients, or their families/surrogates, participate in their care. The effectiveness of care and patient satisfaction with the course of treatment depend, in part, on the patient fulfilling certain responsibilities. Patients are responsible for providing information about past illnesses, hospitalizations, medications, and other matters related to health status. To participate effectively in decision making, patients must be encouraged to take responsibility for requesting additional information or clarification about their health status or treatment when they do not fully understand information and instructions. Patients are also responsible for ensuring that the health care institution has a copy of their written advance directive if they have one. Patients are responsible for informing their physicians and other caregivers if they anticipate problems in following prescribed treatment.

Patients should also be aware of the hospital's obligation to be reasonably efficient and equitable in providing care to other patients and the community. The hospital's rules and regulations are designed to help the hospital meet this obligation. Patients and their families are responsible for making reasonable accommodations to the needs of the hospital, other patients, medical staff, and hospital employees. Patients are responsible for providing necessary information for insurance claims and for working with the hospital to make payment arrangements, when necessary.

A person's health depends on much more than health care services. Patients are responsible for recognizing the impact of their life-style on their personal health.

CONCLUSION

Hospitals have many functions to perform, including the enhancement of health status, health promotion, and the prevention and treatment of injury and disease; the immediate and ongoing care and rehabilitation of patients; the education of health professionals, patients, and the community; and research. All these activities must be conducted with an overriding concern for the values and dignity of patients.

A *Patient's Bill of Rights* was first adopted by the American Hospital Association in 1973. This revision was approved by the AHA Board of Trustees on October 21, 1992.

KEY CONCEPTS

- ➢ Total patient care includes the application of physiologic, psychologic, socio-cultural, developmental, and spiritual.
- ➢ The World Health Organization's definition of health is "a state of complete physical, mental and social well-being and not merely the absence of disease".
- ➢ Nursing's Agenda for Health Care Reform calls for universal access to affordable and appropriate quality care.
- ➢ Public politics, demographics, and economics affect the future of nursing as a profession and nurses as providers of care.
- ➢ A wide variety of healthcare delivery systems are available.
- ➢ Total patient care depends on collaboration between and among healthcare professionals and assistants.
- ➢ Entry into the practice of nursing is regulated by licensure and certification, which is organized by State Boards of Nursing and Professional Associations.
- ➢ Standards of care reflect the profession's values and priorities and provide a way to measure the care and competence of the nurse.
- ➢ Theories that explain, predict, and describe nursing actions are generated by nurse scientists and other theorists outside of nursing.

CRITICAL THINKING EXERCISES

1 Select five key points from the chapter and write a paragraph that describes or explains each.
2 What examples can you give that demonstrate a violation of patient rights as identified by the American Hospital Association?
3 Discuss the factors that led to healthcare reform.

REFERENCES AND ADDITIONAL READINGS

American Academy of Nursing: *Differentiating nursing practice: into the 21st century,* Kansas City, 1991, The Association.

American Association of Retired Persons: Profile of older Americans, Washington, DC, 1990, The Association.

American Hospital Association: *Cost and compassion: recommendations for avoiding a crisis in care for the medically indigent,* Chicago, 1986, The Association.

American Hospital Association: *Patient's bill of rights,* Chicago, 1992, The Association.

American Nurses Association: *Nursing: a social policy statement,* Kansas City, 1980, The Association.

American Nurses Association: *Registered professional nurses and unlicensed assistive personnel,* Washington, DC, 1984, The Association.

American Nurses Association: *Environmental assessment: factors affecting long-range planning for nursing and health care,* Kansas City, 1985, The Association.

American Nurses Association: *Scope of nursing practice,* Kansas City, 1987, The Association.

American Nurses Association: *Classification systems for describing nursing practice: working papers,* Kansas City, 1989, The Association.

American Nurses Association: *Nursing's agenda for health care reform,* Kansas City, 1991a, The Association.

American Nurses Association: *Standards of clinical practice,* Kansas City, 1991b, The Association.

American Nurses Association: *Directory of RN to BSN programs,* Kansas City, 1992, The Association.

American Nurses Association: *Managed care and national health care reform,* Kansas City, 1992, The Association

Benner P: *From novice to expert,* Menlo Park, Calif, 1984, Addison-Wesley Publishing.

Benner P, Tanner C: Clinical judgment: how expert nurses use intuition, *Am J Nurs* 87(1):23-31, 1987.

Benner P, Wrubel J: *The primacy of caring,* Menlo Park, Calif, 1989, Addison-Wesley Publishing.

Bower K: *Case management by nurses,* Kansas City, 1992, The American Nurses Association.

Butts PA, Berger BS, Brooten DA: Tracking down the right degree, *Nurs Health Care* 7(2):90-95, 1986.

Dienemann J, editor: *Continuous quality improvement in nursing,* Kansas City, 1992, The American Nurses Association.

Easterbrook G: The revolution in medicine, *Newsweek,* pp 40-74, Jan 26, 1987.

Ebersole P, Hess PL: *Toward healthy aging: human needs and nursing response,* ed 4, St Louis, 1994, Mosby.

Enthoven A, Kronick R. The consumer-choice health plan for the 1990's, *N Engl J Med* 320(1):29-37, 1989.

Farley E: How we survived a redesign, *Am J Nurs* 94(3)43-45, 1994.

Health Security Act of 1993: The White House, Sept 20, 1993.

Henderson V: *The nature of nursing,* New York, 1966, Macmillan Publishing.

Ismeurt R and others: *Concepts fundamental to nursing,* Springhouse, Pa, 1990, Springhouse.

Joint Commission on Accreditation of Hospitals: *Accreditation manual for hospitals,* Chicago, 1986, The Commission.

Joint Commission on Accreditation of Health Care Organizations: Quality assessment and improvement. In *Accreditation manual for hospitals,* Chicago, 1993, The Commission.

Kelley L: *The nursing experience: trends, challenges, and transitions,* New York, 1987, Macmillian Publishing.

Lindeman C, McAthie M: *Nursing trends and issues,* Springhouse, Pa, 1990, Springhouse Corp.

Lynaugh J, Fagin C: Nursing comes of age, *Image J Nurs Sch* 20(4):184-189, 1988.

Lysought JP: *An abstract for action,* New York, 1970, McGraw-Hill.

Maglacas A: Health for all: nursing's role. *Nurs Outlook* 36(2):66-71, 1988.

Mitty E: Prospective payment and long-term care: linking payments to resource use, *Nurs Health Care* 8(1):15-21, 1987.

National Commission of Nursing: *Executive summary of final report,* Chicago, 1988, The Commission.

National Commission on Nursing Implemention Project: *Characteristics of professional and technical nurses of the future and their educational programs,* Chicago, 1987, The Commission.

Phipps WJ and others: *Medical surgical nursing: concepts and clinical practice,* ed 5, St Louis, 1995, Mosby.

Potter P, Perry A: *Fundamentals of nursing,* ed 3, St Louis, 1993, Mosby.

Primm P: Differentiated practice for ADN and BSN prepared nurses. *J Prof Nurs* 3(4):218-225, 1987.

Smith CE: DRGs: making them work for you, *Nursing* 15(1):34-41, 1985.

Stanhope M, Lancaster J: *Community health nursing,* ed 3, St Louis, 1992, Mosby.

Steel JE: *Issues in collaborative practice,* Philadelphia, 1986, WB Saunders.

Steel JE: Advanced nursing practice, *AACN Clin Issues* 5(1):71-76, 1994.

US Department of Commerce, Bureau of Census: *Statistical abstract of the US: 1993,* Washington DC, 1994, US Government Printing Office.

US Department of Health and Human Services, Division of Nursing: *Report to the President and the Congress on the status of health personnel in the United States,* vol 1, Part C: Nursing Personnel, Washington DC, 1984, US Government Printing Office.

US Department of Health and Human Services: *Healthy people 2000: national health promotion and disease prevention objectives,* Washington DC, 1990a, US Government Printing Office.

US Department of Health and Human Services: *The Medicare handbook,* Washington, DC, 1990b, US Government Printing Office.

Yorker B: Nurses accused of murder, *Am J Nurs* 88(10):1327-1332, 1988.

Zander K: Second generation primary nursing: a new agenda, *J Nurs Adm* 15(3):18-22, 1985.

CHAPTER 2

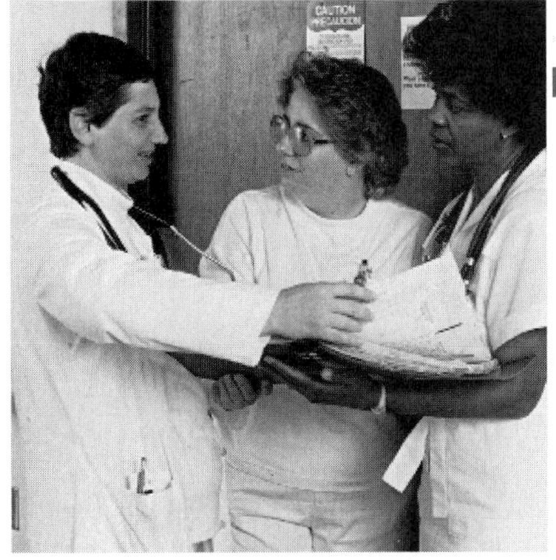

Nursing Process and Ethical Decision Making

CHAPTER OBJECTIVES

1 Define critical thinking.
2 Describe the steps in the nursing process: assessment, analysis, planning, implementation, and evaluation.
3 List techniques for effective interviewing.
4 Define nursing diagnosis and discuss the status of a universally accepted taxonomy of nursing diagnoses.
5 Discuss the role of the written care plan in providing individualized care to patients.
6 Differentiate between standardized care plans, care maps, and individualized care plans.
7 Discuss the importance of documentation.
8 Describe the "problem-oriented record" system.
9 Define ethics.
10 Define clinical ethics.
11 Discuss the principles that serve as a foundation for ethical decision making.
12 Discuss the concepts of respect and the nurse-patient relationship as a foundation for nursing ethics.
13 Use the nursing process as a framework for ethical analysis and decision making.
14 Discuss the purpose and importance of advance directives.
15 Apply the ANA Code of Ethics to the nursing experience.

KEY WORDS

advance directives
assessment
autonomy
beneficence
bioethics
care map
clinical ethics
critical thinking
dilemma
documentation
ethics
evaluation
fidelity
implementation
justice
living will
morals
nonmaleficence
nursing care plan
nursing diagnosis
nursing history
nursing process
outcomes
power of attorney for healthcare
planning
problem-oriented record
SOAP (IE)
standardized care plan
values
veracity

The practice of nursing requires the ability to think and act critically and ethically. As the nursing profession has evolved, the process of nursing has been studied and analyzed. This chapter discusses current ideas related to that process.

CRITICAL THINKING/DECISION MAKING

There is no universally accepted definition of **critical thinking.** Alfaro-LeFevre (1985) gives a one-word explanation: reasoning. She further describes critical thinking as "purposeful, goal-directed thinking that aims to make judgments based on evidence (fact), rather than conjecture (guesswork). It is based on principles of science and scientific method and requires strategies that maximize human potential and compensate for problems caused by human nature" (pp. 8-9).

Many elements of critical thinking are commonly used by nurses as they provide care. Critical thinking is a process that is used to make sound, accurate, and reasonable decisions on the basis of thorough data collection and analysis. It includes elements of the scientific method such as data collection, analysis, deductive and inductive reasoning, hypothesis testing, and evaluation. Continuous development and improvement of critical thinking skills is essential at all levels of nursing practice. Nurses use critical thinking skills when they use the **nursing process** to make decisions in all areas of patient care delivery.

NURSING PROCESS

Nursing is a dynamic and interpersonal problem-solving process that facilitates an individual's potential for health. The five-step nursing process includes (1) assessment, (2) analysis/nursing diagnosis, (3) planning/outcomes, (4) implementation, and (5) evaluation (Figure 2-1).

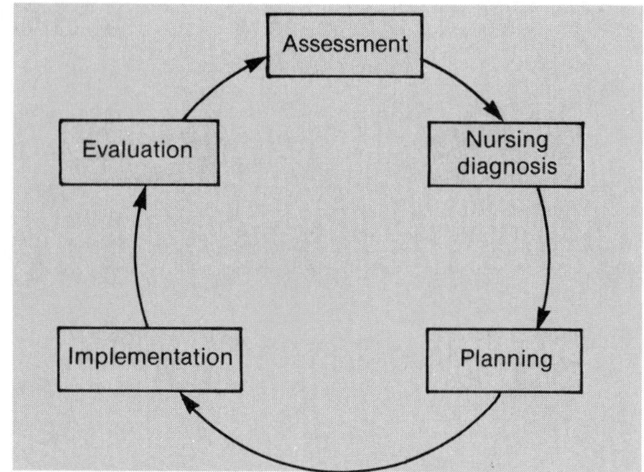

Figure 2-1 The nursing process.

Assessment

Assessment requires collecting and recording patient-related data and grouping it into meaningful categories. It includes the patient's physical and emotional signs and symptoms as well as information obtained from other sources such as the patient's chart, other nurses, laboratory reports, family, and visitors. A thorough nursing assessment requires systematic and careful observation of and interviews with the patient. Assessment is performed at the first encounter with the patient, and data are recorded as part of the **nursing history.** Assessment is also performed during every subsequent interaction with the patient to expand data and evaluate responses to illness or treatment. The quality of the nursing history and patient interviews can be enhanced by the use of effective interviewing techniques (Box 2-1).

Analysis/Nursing Diagnosis

Data analysis is required in the next step of the process, which is the development of the **nursing diagnosis.** The nurse uses elements of critical thinking and the scientific method to analyze assessment data so that valid conclusions about the patient are reached and accurate diagnoses are made.

A nursing diagnosis describes a combination of signs and symptoms that indicate an actual or potential health problem that nurses are licensed to treat and are capable of treating (Gordon, 1994). It is a concise statement that brings to mind the same behaviors to everyone. A common characteristic of a nursing diagnosis is the determination of human function or behavior. Behavior is used here in its broadest sense and refers to an observable response that may be physiologic, psychologic, intellectual, emotional, or spiritual. The nursing diagnosis uses a common language and enables nurses to communicate effectively and effi-

BOX 2-1

EFFECTIVE INTERVIEWING TECHNIQUES

- Approach the patient calmly and empathetically.
- Explain that the purpose of the questions is to provide better care by knowing more about the patient and family.
- Use terminology that is familiar to the patient.
- First ask about the patient's immediate concerns or complaints. Save delicate, personal questions until later.
- Call the patient by name.
- Speak clearly, slowly, and distinctly.
- *Listen.* Maintain the topic, but never interrupt.
- Ask open-ended questions that require more than a yes or no answer.
- Use signals such as a nod, uh-huh, or glance to encourage the patient to continue.
- Even if the institution uses a checklist, do not sound as if it is being used.
- Relying on memory is dangerous. Write brief notes during the interview, but do not be distracting.
- Be aware of own and patient's nonverbal communication.
- Remain open, accepting, and objective, even if the patient is hostile and uncooperative.
- Use good eye contact, but never stare.
- Be professional.

ciently the priority needs of the patient. It is the basis of the nursing care plan (Figure 2-2).

If a nursing diagnosis is to have universal meaning, it must be universally accepted. Nurses have been discussing the concept of the nursing diagnosis for over 30 years, and it continues to evolve as the common language of nursing. The National Conference Group on the Classification of Nursing Diagnosis began meeting in 1973. This group is now known as the North American Nursing Diagnosis Association (NANDA) and continues to meet annually to develop and validate nursing diagnoses. A list of accepted nursing diagnoses is published annually (see inside front cover). NANDA describes the diagnosis in a problem statement, which is followed by a statement that describes the etiology, signs, and symptoms. This format is referred to as the PES format: health problem (P), etiology (E), signs and symptoms (S).

Although different terms and philosophies exist, it is agreed that the nursing diagnosis must describe a behavior that is a problem for the patient and requires nursing interventions. The nurse's skill and knowledge in collecting and analyzing data are essential to establishing a nursing diagnosis. The problem must be stated in terms that give the nurse direction in selecting nursing interventions and identifying desired expected outcomes. For example, "ineffective airway clearance" is an accepted NANDA nursing diagnosis, but it is not complete without a statement of etiology, or a "related to" statement. Whether it is considered a part of or an addition to the nursing diagnosis, the "related to" statement is essential if the diagnosis is to be meaningful. To propose effective nursing interventions, one must know why the airway clearance is ineffective (the etiology). The nursing diagnosis statement can also be modified to fit each patient. For example, "impaired physical mobility" is an accepted nursing diagnosis that becomes more meaningful when the impairment is further described as an "impaired physical mobility of right hand." The complete diagnostic statement could read, "Impaired physical mobility, right hand, related to joint inflammation." According to the NANDA format, the nursing diagnosis is followed by a description of the signs and symptoms that led to the diagnosis. Whether this grouping of significant signs and symptoms appears on the actual care plan depends on the format adopted by a given agency.

Many healthcare institutions have developed Standard Nursing Care Plans. **Standardized care plans** are adapted and individualized to the particular client situation. The nurse selects from these plans only those elements that specifically apply to the patient (see Figure 2-2). In other healthcare settings, standardized care plans are used in conjunction with or are replaced by Standard Care Maps. **Care maps** cross all disciplines: nursing, medicine, laboratory, dietary, and physical and occupational therapy. Care maps give direction to appropriate nursing care and are also used by administrators and accreditors to evaluate quality and productivity and by insurers as the basis for reimbursement (Figure 2-3).

Although much progress has been made, the goal of a universally accepted system, or taxonomy, of nursing diagnoses has not yet been reached. This period of development is particularly confusing to nursing students who would like to be told precisely what is expected of them. While the nursing diagnosis continues to evolve, nurses will use diagnoses that have not been universally accepted, and they will not always agree on their appropriateness. Everyone in nursing must contribute ideas and be involved in testing the work of experts in the field. A universal taxonomy requires continual change to reflect current practice. The healthcare delivery system in the United States is rapidly expanding and changing. As nurses work

Text continued on p. 31.

DATE INITIALS	NURSING DIAGNOSIS	INTERVENTION/PLAN	OUTCOME	EVALUATION
	Actual/potential impaired mobility due to:	1. AROM/PROM $\bar{q}$ ______ 2. Reposition $\bar{q}$ ______ 3. Assist with ambulation as ordered 4. Assistive devices—define: 5. OOB ______ min. ______ times per day	1. Mobility as defined:	1. Date achieved: ______ 2. Not achieved–define discharge plan/follow-up: Initials
	Actual/potential alteration urinary elmination-incontinence/retention due to:	1. I & O 2. Record time and amount of voiding 3. Check for bladder distention 4. Assess urine for character, frequency, dysuria 5. Push fluids to ____ ml/day 6. Maintain skin integrity 7. Intermittent/indwelling cath. as ordered 8. Establish toilet regimen–define:	1. Bladder regimen established 2. No urinary retention 3. No skin breakdown 4. Urine output appropriate to fluid intake	1. Date achieved: ______ 2. Not achieved – define discharge plan/follow-up: Initials
	Actual/potential alteration bowel elimination–constipation due to:	1. Push fluids to ____ ml/day 2. Laxative/softeners as ordered 3. Enemas as ordered 4. Monitor frequency of stools 5. Ambulate ___ times/day 6. Instruct on fiber intake 7. Check bowel sounds $\bar{q}$ shift	1. Soft formed stools within patient's established pattern 2.	1. Date achieved: ______ 2. Not achieved–define discharge plan/follow-up: Initials
	Actual/potential alteration bowel elimination–diarrhea due to:	1. Assess frequency, appearance, volume of stools 2. Stool chart 3. Check for impaction 4. Monitor lytes–report abnormals 5. Maintain skin integrity 6. Obtain stool specimens as ordered	1. Soft formed stools within patient's established pattern 2. No skin breakdown	1. Date achieved: ______ 2. Not achieved–define discharge plan/follow-up: Initials
	Actual/potential ineffective coping due to:	1. Allow to verbalize 2. Offer support services A. Chaplain B. Reach for Recovery C. Stoma therapist D. Social service	1. Coping evidenced by:	1. Date achieved: ______ 2. Not achieved–define discharge plan/follow-up: Initials

Figure 2-2 Sample of a nursing care plan. (Permission authorized by Central Healthcare and Affiliates, October 1994.)

DATE INITIALS	NURSING DIAGNOSIS	INTERVENTION/PLAN	OUTCOME	EVALUATION
	Actual/potential impaired gas exchange due to:	1. Monitor ABG's–report abnormals 2. O_2 as ordered 3. H.O.B. up ______° 4. Describe rate, depth, lung sounds, rhythm, color & sensorium q̄ _____ 5. OOB ___ min. ___ times/day	1. Tolerates activity 2. Achieves optimum sensorium 3. Independent of O_2 therapy 4. Stable on O_2 at ____ l/min.	1. Date achieved: ________ 2. Not achieved–define discharge plan/follow-up: Initials
	Actual/potential alteration in cardiac output due to:	1. H.O.B. up ______° 2. Assess lung sounds 3. O_2 as ordered 4. Monitor lytes & ABGs–report abnormals 5. I & O assess fluid balance 6. Auscultate apical pulse 7. Plan activity with rest periods–define:	1. Tolerates activity 2. Independent of O_2 therapy 3. Stable on O_2 at ____ l/min.	1. Date achieved: ________ 2. Not achieved–define discharge plan/follow-up: Initials
	Actual/potential alteration in fluid volume–excess due to:	1. I & O 2. Weights q̄ _____ 3. VS q̄ _____ 4. Lung sounds q̄ _____ 5. Assess edema, L.O.C., orthopnea, neck vein distention 6. Monitor lytes & ABG's–report abnormals 7. Restrict fluids as ordered 8. Monitor reponse to diurectics	1. Resolution of fluid imbalance as evidenced by:	1. Date achieved: ________ 2. Not achieved–define discharge plan/follow-up: Initials
	Actual/potential alteration in fluid volume–deficit due to:	1. I & O 2. VS q̄ _____ 3. Monitor tissue turgor & skin condition 4. Push fluids to ____ ml/day 5. Oral hygiene q̄ ______	1. Resolution of fluid imbalance as evidenced by:	1. Date achieved: ________ 2. Not achieved–define discharge plan/follow-up: Initials
	Actual/potential self-care deficit due to:	1. Assist with feeding or feed 2. Assist/complete hygiene 3. Assist with self-care activities–define:	1. Performs self-care activities within limitations–define: 2.	1. Date achieved: ________ 2. Not achieved–define discharge plan/follow-up: Initials

NORTHWEST COMMUNITY HOSPITAL, Arlington Heights, Illinois

PATIENT CARE PLAN

Nurse–identify initials with signature	Initials	Signatures	Initials	Signatures

Figure 2-2, cont'd. For legend see opposite page.

Northwest Community Hospital Coordinated Caremap Summary

DRG: #174
Diagnosis: Upper GI Hemorrhage cCC
National LOS: 5.5
NWCH LOS: ______
Allergies: ______
Code status: ______

Physician: ______
Demographics: Adult with onset of GI Bleeding

AREA OF TREATMENT	TIMEFRAME	CLINICAL FOCUS	EXPECTED OUTCOMES
ER/T.C.	1-3 hr	Hydration status Hemodynamic stability • Identification and treatment of source of bleeding (ER or ICU)	TXC c̄ blood available Vital Signs within safety range for present condition—to ICU if unstable GI consult if needed V/S
ICU	1-2 days	Same as ER Circulatory/GI status • Anxiety • Pt./Family support offered	No evidence of bleeding Stable H & H Hemodynamics stable c̄ Normovolemia Taking diet Support given
Med/Surg. Unit	2-3 days	GI Status/function Blood volume Pt./family teaching • Meds • Lifestyle • Diet	Stable V/S and H & H Tolerating diet No bleeding Verbalizes understanding of teaching
Physician's Office	Within 7-10 days (1-2 hr)	Follow-up exam and evaluation Plan for follow-up endoscopy 4-6 weeks (Gastric Ulcer)	Stable Following dietary and lifestyle modifications Independence ADL

Figure 2-3 Coordinated care map summary. (Care Map is a registered trademark of The Center of Case Management, Inc., South Natick, MA. These care maps are copyrighted and are the property of Northwest Community Hospital, Arlington Heights, IL. They have been reprinted with permission of Northwest Community Hospital. Any reproduction or facsimile of these items without express permission of Northwest Community Hospital is prohibited.)

Northwest Community Hospital Coordinated Caremap Summary

TIMEFRAME (minutes, hours, days, weeks, visits)

Categories of Care	Date ER 1-3°	Date ICU – (1st 24°)
Consults	Primary physician Gastroenterologist	Care Coordinator PRN General Surgeon PRN
Tests	• CBC • PT/PTT • BUN/Creat • TXC3uPC	**Outcome:** Hb > 8 and coagulation WNL. • H & H q 4-6° × 24° as ord.
Specimens		
Treatments/therapy • Hemodynamics and hydration	**Outcome:** Stabilizing volemic and hemodynamic status. Date ____ Initials ____ • if unstable → to ICU • if stable → to Med/Surg. • IV (2 if unstable) •I&O • PC if unstable of Hb < 8 • O_2 • Cardiac monitor **Outcome:** Decompression of stomach Date ____ Initials ____ • NPO • NG → suction • Monitor bleeding • Lavage (as ord) • ICE, as ord. **Assess:** Vital signs (upright & supine) q 15-30 min, skin & mucous membranes/hydration, color and amt of NG, abdomen for firmness/distension, stools, urine output 30 cc/° or more **Consider:** Endoscopy within 6° → • If ulcer, continue with this path → • If varices, use varices pathway	**Outcome:** Within 24° hemodynamics stable with adequate hydration/no evidence of bleeding Date ____ Initials ____ • If unstable, continue: O_2, NG decompression (lavage as ord), volume resuscitation with adjustment as needed, V/S q 1-2°, NPO, 2 IV's, UO q 1° (30 cc/°) or as ord. Assess: UO, continue I&O • If stable: - V/S q 4° Range B/P $\frac{110\text{-}120}{70\text{-}80}$ - Clear liquids–p 60-100 - Saline lock–temp<99° **Outcome:** Soft abdomen • Auscultate/palpate abdomen q 8° and PRN • Assess stools
Meds	**Outcome:** Decreasing gastric acidity. Date ____ Initials ____ • H2 blocker • Other types of meds	**Outcome:** Decreasing gastric acidity with increased gastric pH. Date ____ Initials ____ - PO meds • H2 Blockers • Antiulcer meds (as ord) • Other ________
Activity	Bedrest	**Outcome:** tolerates getting OOB with help Date ____ Initials ____ • Up c̄ help
Miscellaneous	Blood consent Endoscopy consent PRN	Keep blood on hold
Teaching	**Outcome:** Verbalizes understanding of procedures Date ____ Initials ____ • Explain procedures • Pt/family support offered	**Outcome:** Understands plan of care Date ____ Initials ____
Discharge planning		

Continued.

Figure 2-3, cont'd. For legend see opposite page.

TIMEFRAME (minutes, hours, days, weeks, visits)

Categories of Care	Day 2 Date Unit		Day 3 Date Unit		Day 4-5 Date Unit	
Consults	Discharge planner PRN Social service PRN					
Tests	**Outcome:** Hb > 8.0. • H&H q 12° × 2 days as ord	Date _____ Initials _____	**Outcome:** Hb > 8.0. • H&H q 12° unitl day 4	Date _____ Initials _____	**Outcome:** Stable H&H • H&H daily	Date _____ Initials _____
Specimens						
Treatments/therapy	**Outcome:** Hemodynamics & hydration stable with no evidence of bleeding. • V/S q 4° as ord • IV saline lock • D/C **Outcome:** Soft abdomen. • Auscultate/palpate abdomen for distention, bowel sounds, flatus • Assess stools • Tolerates full liquids	Date _____ Initials _____ Date _____ Initials _____	**Outcome:** Hemodynamics & hydration stable with no evidence of bleeding-V/S WNL • Routine vital signs (as ord) **Outcome:** Soft abdomen. • Assess stools • Soft diet	Date _____ Initials _____ Date _____ Initials _____	**Outcome:** Hemodynamically stable Routine V/S × 1/shift or q 8° **Outcome:** Maintains soft abdomen. • Assess stools • General diet	Date _____ Initials _____
Meds	**Outcome:** Gastric pH neutralized (5.0 or higher) • PO H2 Blockers • PO Antiulcer meds • Other _____	Date _____ Initials _____	**Outcome:** Gastric pH maintained > 5.0 • PO H2 Blockers • PO Antiulcer meds • Other _____ (as ordered)	Date _____ Initials _____	**Outcome:** Decreased gastric acidity/healing • Anti ulcer (as ordered) • PO H2 blockers • Other	Date _____ Initials _____
Activity	**Outcome:** Tolerates ambulation without assistance	Date _____ Initials _____	Up and about		Up	
Miscellaneous	**Outcome:** Absence of bleeding for 24° prior to transfer • Transfer	Date _____ Initials _____	If rebleed → to Endoscopy with Hemostasis: → If rebleeding → to surgery			
Teaching	S/S of rebleeding with interventions: • If feel faint, weak, racing pulse—call for help		**Outcome:** Verbalizes S/S of rebleeding **To avoid:** • NSAIDS • ASA or similar • caffeine • ETOH • Tobacco	Date _____ Initials _____	**Outcome:** Verbalizes when to report changes and seek help • Review/verify understanding of teaching • Physician: Pt to have follow-up endoscopy 4-6 wks (gastric ulcer)	Date _____ Initials _____
Discharge planning	Evaluate home support (Decrease readmissions)				Prepare/finalize discharge	

Figure 2-3, cont'd. For legend see page 26.

DETOURS

Admission date: ______________________
Actual discharge date: ______________________
Case type: ______________________
Secondary diagnosis: ______________________
Surgical procedures: ______________________
DRG: ______________
Expected LOS: ________

Directions for use: Please code each entry with one of the listed codes below.

DATE	TIME	SOURCE NO.	DESCRIPTION	ACTION TAKEN	INT.

DETOUR SOURCE CODE

A. PATIENT/FAMILY
1. Patient condition
2. Pt/family decision
3. Pt/family availability
4. Pt/family other

B. CARE GIVER/CLINICIAN
5. Physician order
6. Caregiver(s) decision
7. Caregiver(s) response timelity
8. Caregiver other

C. HOSPITAL SYSTEM
9. Bed/appt time availability
10. Information/data availability
11. Supplies/equipment availability
12. Department overbooked/closed
13. Hospital other

D. COMMUNITY
14. Placement/home care availability
15. Ambulance delay
16. Community other

Addressograph

Figure 2-3, cont'd. For legend see page 26.

Continued.

Idividual Care Mapping Plan

DATE	PATIENT PROBLEM	PLAN	OUTCOME

Figure 2-3, cont'd. For legend see page 26.

within their own settings, they use the nursing care process and critical thinking, judgment, and decision-making skills, regardless of which format their agency/system uses.

Planning/Outcomes

In the **planning** stage of the nursing process, a concise written design of action is developed on the basis of the nursing diagnosis. Specific behavioral outcomes are identified, priorities are set, and appropriate specific nursing actions or interventions are proposed. **Outcomes** are statements that describe specific, desired patient behaviors or results. An outcome comprises what one hopes to achieve.

Individualized care of the total patient requires a written plan of care. **Nursing care plans** are required by hospitals and other healthcare agencies for all patients and are used to communicate, prevent complications, ensure continuity of care, identify and ensure patient teaching, and provide for discharge planning. The nursing care plan includes the nursing diagnosis or statements that identify the patient's problems. It also includes proposed nursing interventions. Each diagnosis should have a statement of expected outcome criteria that is stated in specific and measurable behavioral terms. Each intervention may also have a statement of expected outcome criteria. Outcome criteria are the expected results of the interventions. Although for a hospitalized patient most of the care plan focuses on inpatient nursing service, it should also include a discharge plan. Ambulatory and home care services also need a formal plan of care to ensure that quality, comprehensive, and cost-effective care is provided to patients.

Implementation

Implementation is the actual performance of the nursing interventions identified in the plan of care. The interventions may include direct patient care, observations or assessments, health teaching, or the performance or supervision of other activities that are beneficial to the patient. Documentation is important to the implementation step and the entire nursing process. It involves charting periodic patient assessment and all nursing interventions in the nursing record. Documentation is an important part of the patient's permanent record and is considered a legal document. Under the auditing methods of DRGs, Medicare, and Medicaid, inadequate nursing documentation can cause healthcare agencies to lose reimbursement through disallowance of services. Different agencies use different methods of documenting nursing interventions. Methods may vary from a narrative type to simplified flow sheets. With the advent of standard care plans and case maps, the use of flow sheets for the documentation of nursing interventions is increasing rapidly. No matter what form is used, it is important that nursing documentation be complete and accurate.

One system of record keeping, the *problem-oriented* record, provides organization for the patient's chart. It demands that all progress notes and orders be directly related to patient problems that have been identified and assigned a number. All healthcare workers use the same progress notes and order sheets. Some institutions separate notes according to professional discipline and use a separate page for nurses, physicians, and other healthcare workers. The problem-oriented record consists of four parts: *s*ubjective data, *o*bjective data, *a*ssessment, and *p*lan. This is often referred to as the **SOAP** system. Others have expanded this to SOAPIE by adding *i*ntervention and *e*valuation. The subjective data are the information the patient provides, whereas the objective data are the information the nurse obtains through observation and other methods. Assessment is based on analysis of subjective and objective data. The plan is the action to be taken according to the data and diagnosis. The SOAP(IE) system is based on the nursing process and provides a mechanism for recording data (Box 2-2).

Evaluation

Evaluation is the final stage of the nursing process and requires a statement of expected outcome criteria, or goals, for each nursing diagnosis. Goals may or may not be prescribed for nursing interventions. The expected outcomes must be stated in terms of patient behavior, patient activities, or identified changes that indicate successful interventions and resolution of the problem. Action verbs and specific numbers are critical elements of measurable outcome statements and allow for precise measurement of outcome achievement. Evaluation requires continued assessment of the patient and comparison of progress toward the expected outcome. If expected changes do not occur, alternative nursing interventions are proposed and carried out. Evaluation also implies updating the care plan and providing appropriate documentation.

Although the nursing process has been described in five stages, they do not occur in rigid progression. Assessment is continuous, and all findings must be analyzed and may modify planning. If expected outcomes are not identified in the beginning, it is impossible to evaluate the effectiveness of the nursing interventions. With each change in patient behavior, the cycle begins again. Critical thinking skills are used by all nurses as they engage in decision making and the nursing

BOX 2-2

EXAMPLE OF A SOAP NOTE

Problem: Pain in abdomen

S: "I have a dull, full pain in my stomach." Present for 2 days. Ate spicy meal 2 days ago. No bowel movements × 2 days. Remainder of systems review negative.

O: Temp. 98.8. BP 120/80. Bowel sounds present but slow and infrequent. Stool guaiac negative.

A: Probable constipation. R/O mass.

P: Refer to physician
Observe intake and output
Record food intake

process. In a structured setting where there is an opportunity to consult with an RN, the LPN/LVN can determine needs and provide care for patients who have common, well-defined health problems. In this setting, the LPN/LVN is able to contribute to the plan of care, perform identified nursing interventions, assess patient progress, and evaluate the effectiveness of patient care.

ETHICAL ANALYSIS

For thousands of years, people have asked what it means to be good or excellent human beings. **Ethics** is concerned with doing a good job of being a good person. The fundamental question is: how does ethics help one become a good nurse, as well as a good person? Such a question touches on themes that run through all aspects of everyday life and work.

Ethics is a branch of philosophy that studies two facets of human existence: (1) how people should act, and (2) what sort of character they should have. **Bioethics,** sometimes referred to as healthcare ethics, is the application of ethical principles and rules to biologic and medical issues. **Clinical ethics** refers to the application of bioethics to the identification, analysis, and resolution of **moral** problems that arise when caring for a particular patient (Box 2-3).

BOX 2-3

ETHICS

Bioethics The application of normative ethics to biologic and medical issues; sometimes referred to as healthcare ethics

Clinical ethics The application of bioethics to the identification, analysis, and resolution of moral problems that arise when caring for a particular patient

Dilemma A situation in which a choice must be made among two or more equal alternatives; the reasons for the alternatives are valid and important, and none are obviously right or wrong; a dilemma occurs in a context in which the facts, as known, do not make it clear which is the right choice

Ethics A branch of philosophy that studies two facets of human existence: (1) how people should act, and (2) what sort of character they should have; ethics is both foundational (called metaethics) and normative (principles and rules)

Fidelity Faithfulness to one's duty, commitments, and promises

Morals The set of beliefs, values, and principles to which a person is committed; often used interchangeably with ethics

Values Used subjectively to identify what a person considers worthwhile; used objectively to identify the intrinsic quality (good) of a thing

Veracity Habitual truthfulness

The Role of Ethical Theory

Recently interest in the ethical issues that surround medicine and healthcare has been growing. The development of new and sophisticated technology raises new possibilities for treating disease, increasing the life span, and caring for the disabled. However, the use of increasingly expensive technology also has a dark side. The conflict between the benefits and burdens of these developments leaves healthcare professionals and their patients with many difficult questions: Is it always appropriate to use this technology? If not, why not? Who makes that decision? What are the benefits? What are the costs, both in human suffering and in resources? The answers to these questions bring significant consequences.

One problem in searching for these answers is that all members of society do not come from the same cultural background and do not hold the same moral values. Not everyone is committed to the same set of **values** or principles. This is known as a morally pluralistic society. Without a shared value system, how can one begin to discuss, let alone answer, these and other important questions? A second problem is that in

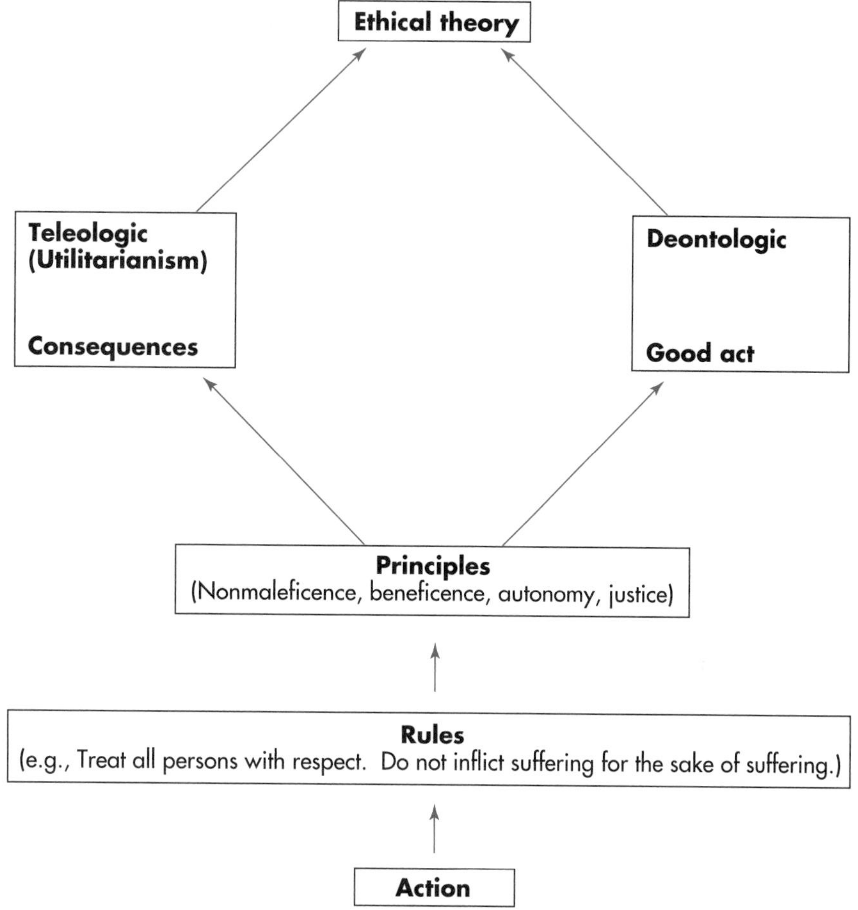

Figure 2-4 A framework for ethical decision making. The action in question is reviewed with rules in mind, which in turn are supported by the principles of nonmaleficence, beneficence, autonomy, and justice. Is the act good in itself (deontologic theory) or are the consequences good (teleologic theory/utilitarianism)? Answering all of these questions helps one determine if the action is ethical. (Modified from Beauchamp T, Childress J: *Principles of Biomedical Ethics,* ed 3, New York, 1989, Oxford University Press.)

many situations there can be a good reason to proceed in different and sometimes conflicting ways. When conflicting choices appear, how does a nurse decide which is the ethical way to proceed? A normative ethical theory can provide the nurse with principles and rules to guide actions.

Basic Ethical Principles, Theories, and Rules

Philosophers Tom Beauchamp (pronounced Beecham) and James Childress (1989) have developed a normative ethical framework that uses four basic principles: nonmaleficence, beneficence, autonomy, and justice (Figure 2-4). **Nonmaleficence** means "to do no harm." It also means the prevention and removal of harm. **Beneficence** directs one to do good on the patient's behalf. The principle of **autonomy** affirms the right of persons to govern their own lives, including how they are treated as patients. This obligates one to refrain from interfering with another person's autonomy without substantial reason. The principle of **justice** is concerned with the distribution of social benefits and burdens. It is a difficult principle to use in making decisions about individual patients because it requires consideration of society as a whole, such as who gets the benefits and who pays the burdens. Justice more often involves broad societal issues such as allocation of resources (e.g., who will pay for healthcare?). The question of spending healthcare dollars for organ transplants while some children lack simple im-

BOX 2-4

ETHICAL THEORIES

UTILITARIANISM:

- Is found in the works of Jeremy Bentham and John Stuart Mill.
- Is referred to as teleologic theory from the Greek word *telos,* which menas "end."
- Has the basic concept that an act is right if it helps bring about a good outcome or end.
- Involves weighing competing issues to determine which will bring the greatest good for the greatest number.

DEONTOLOGY:

- Involves the concept of moral duty or obligation.
- Stems from *deon,* the Greek word for "duty."
- Takes the position of philosopher Immanuel Kant.
- Believes that moral rightness or wrongness of a human action should be considered independently of its consequences.
- States that it is not consequences that make an action right or wrong but the principles or motivation on which the action is based.

munizations is a question of justice. When one must decide which patient gets the only open bed in intensive care, one is applying the principle of justice on a more individual level.

These four basic principles are supported by more general ethical theories. Utilitarianism and deontology are two common theories. Utilitarianism determines the morality of an act by viewing the consequences. It asks if the action provides more good than harm. Utilitarianism is also referred to as teleologic theory and stems from the Greek word *telos;* which means "end." Deontology determines the ethical appropriateness of an action by looking only at the action itself and not the consequences. It views acts as good or bad in themselves (Box 2-4). Principles of justice also serve as supporting mechanisms for more specific rules and guidelines such as **veracity** (habitual truthfulness) and **fidelity** (faithfulness to one's duty, commitment, and promises). Beauchamp and Childress' principles and the theories of utilitarianism and deontology together serve as a framework to guide decision making in ethical issues and to justify ethical decisions (see Figure 2-4).

Nursing Ethics

There is a recent movement among healthcare ethicists to center ethical principles within the practice itself. In other words, the ethics of the practice would flow from the practice itself rather than from justification. (Pellegrino, 1988). The current treatment of nursing ethics follows this recent initiative and is compatible with the belief that the nurse-patient relationship is the foundation of nursing practice. (Catalano, 1992; Fry, 1989; Watson, 1988). Using this approach, the outcomes of ethical decision making remain compatible with Beauchamp and Childress' four principles, although a different framework is used for justification. (Box 2-5).

Nursing as an inherently moral enterprise

The process of nursing includes the diagnosis and treatment of human responses to actual or potential health problems. The purpose of nursing is to enhance the well-being of others. Because this is an inherently good human goal, nursing is an inherently moral enterprise. Nursing is a science that is based on scientific knowledge and is directed by the need to help others. Applying this knowledge in a wise and humane manner is the art of nursing. The patient, as a unique person with individual needs, is the central focus of nursing. Such a focus is based on the virtually universal moral obligation to respect all human beings. The belief underlying this obligation is that human beings possess a dignity and an inherent worth on the basis of who they are as distinct human beings. The moral requirement to respect a person is not lessened for any reason, including socioeconomic status, personal attributes, and the nature of the health problem (American Nurses Association, 1985).

Personal and professional values

In addition to knowing the values of the nursing profession, nurses need to identify their personal values. Such knowledge helps them respect the values of others and understand how to influence the nurse-patient relationship. It is important to try to prevent values and prejudices from affecting patient care. For example, a nurse who is opposed to elective abortions may want to avoid working in a setting that requires contact with those receiving abortions or that requires assisting with the abortion procedure.

Ethics in daily practice

Understanding the nurse-patient relationship and its foundation of respect for human dignity is essential to the daily provision of compassionate nursing care. Too frequently "life and death" issues garner much at-

BOX 2-5

A METHOD FOR ETHICAL ANALYSIS AND DECISION MAKING

ASSESSMENT

- Collect information and know as much as possible about the situation.
- Identify the medical facts; treatment options; nursing diagnosis; and the patient's values, beliefs, and religious preference.
- Determine how the patient's family is involved in the decision.
- Identify the decision maker(s).
- Determine if there are any legal considerations.
- Use these and any other pertinent data to identify the problem.

ANALYSIS

- Identify the ethical components.
- Determine if there is any conflict.
- Identify the source of the conflict (e.g., conflicting values, conflict between professional duties, lying or withholding the truth).

PLANNING

- List options for resolving the conflict and their projected outcomes.
- Assess the benefit/burden ratio of the projected outcomes.
- Analyze each option in reference to the principle of respect for the patient.
- Determine which option can best fulfill that principle.

IMPLEMENTATION

- Choose the option that best fulfills the principle of respect and begin justifying that option.
- Use the ANA Code of Ethics and the Beauchamp/Childress principles (nonmaleficence, beneficence, autonomy, justice), which may be helpful in thinking through these difficult issues.
- Apply each principle to the chosen alternative.
- Justify or list the ethical reasons for the decision.
- Formulate and consider the ethical reasons that would oppose the decision.
- Weigh the reasons that support and oppose the decision.
- Test other options in the same way if necessary.
- Make a decision.

EVALUATION

- Determine if the patient's goals have been accomplished.
- Determine if the result is effective and realistic.
- Determine if the results are supported (justified) by ethical principles and theories.
- Determine what can be learned from this outcome for future situations.

tention, and ordinary but important issues receive little attention. Levine (1977) writes:

> There are overlooked ethical challenges in the mundane everyday routine activities of professional practice, and these have largely gone unexamined. Ethical behavior is not the display of one's moral rectitude in times of crisis. It is the day-by-day commitment to other persons and the ways in which human beings relate to one another in their daily interactions (p. 846).

This view of ethics encompasses a holistic framework that demands consideration of the patient's physical, psychologic, sociocultural, developmental, and spiritual dimensions.

PATIENT RESPECT

The Impact of Illness on Respect

Any illness or injury breaks up the daily pattern of life, which is often taken for granted. It affects jobs, daily activities, and family relationships. It can cause anxiety, frustration, suffering, and loss. Illness is marked by uncertainty. The patient asks, "What is wrong with me? Will I get better?" The forbidding and unfamiliar environment of the hospital or nursing home and the number of people involved in care adds to the patient's uncertainty. The patient must also trust and rely on all of these caregivers, who are almost always strangers. Hospital and nursing home care is intimate and personal, which places the patient in a very vulnerable position. Patients' needs are best served when they believe that the nurse and other caregivers respect them and address their legitimate needs, hopes, and fears.

Demonstrating Respect

Showing respect requires serious consideration of the values and goals of others. It also demands that care not be limited by personal attitudes, beliefs, or values. Respect is shown when one attempts to provide freedom from anxiety and pain and when one protects a person's right to privacy and confidentiality. Respect is not a reward for good behavior. It is an inherent right of patients, co-workers, and self.

Respect as the Application of Fidelity

The nurse's promise is a commitment to care that extends from respect for the patient. Nurses are morally committed to help care for patients in their living and dying. To do this effectively requires knowledge and skill that are appropriate to the particular level of nursing. This promise also requires honesty and integrity to accept responsibility for providing the best possible patient care. Respecting a patient is often referred to as "following the principle of fidelity."

Implication of DNR Orders

Some patients and/or their families are often concerned that if they choose not to be resuscitated (DNR orders), they will receive no further treatment and less intense nursing care. These patients often require significant medical and nursing care, and the principle of respect demands that they receive this care. It is important to provide essential nursing care and assure the patient and family that they will not be abandoned because of a DNR order.

Advance Directives

The principle of respect requires nurses to help the patient understand the concept of **advance directives,** which includes a **living will** and **power of attorney for healthcare** (Box 2-6). Except in extremely rare situations with substantial overriding reasons, respect for the patient demands than an advance directive be followed.

Need for Patient Involvement in Decision Making

The nurse is also required to act in the patient's best interest, a concept that is identified as beneficence. Ethical **dilemmas,** or problems, may arise when nurses determine what is best for the patient without getting patient input or agreement. The patient's best interest can be fully explored only by involving the patient. When patient involvement is not possible, the family and/or significant others must convey the patient's wishes.

Respect for Privacy/Confidentiality

Respect for the patient demands respect for privacy and confidentiality. All information regarding a patient belongs to that patient. A nurse may not give out any information without the permission of the patient or legal guardian. Giving information without permission discounts the patient's unique dignity, infringes on his or her autonomy, and may do significant harm. Breaches of confidentiality occur more frequently as a result of carelessness in elevators and cafeterias than as a result of purposeful and malicious violation of the patient's rights. As patient records become computerized, nurses need to be attentive to new possibilities for inadvertent violation of patient privacy.

BOX 2-6

ADVANCE DIRECTIVES

Definition: A written document that indicates your choices regarding the medical treatments you do or do not want and who you want to act on your behalf as your healthcare agent. This written directive becomes effective if and when you become incapacitated and cannot express your wishes.

TWO KINDS OF ADVANCE DIRECTIVES

A living will:

- Informs your doctor whether or not you want life-sustaining procedures if you are terminally ill or injured and your death is imminent or if you are in a persistent vegetative state.
- Goes into effect only when you are near death and are unable to understand your healthcare options or express your wishes to others.

A power of attorney for healthcare

- Informs your healthcare provider that you have appointed another person (a "healthcare agent") to make healthcare decisions for you if you are not capable of making them yourself. You give authority to your healthcare agent to make a wide range of healthcare decisions for you such as surgery, medications, or life support.
- Goes into effect only when two physicians or a physician and a psychologist agree in writing that you are no longer able to understand your treatment options or express your wishes to others.

FACTS ABOUT ADVANCE DIRECTIVES

- You must be 18 years old and of "sound mind" to have an advance directive.
- You can revoke or change your advance directive at any time.
- Your doctor(s) and family members should have copies of your advance directive. It should be kept where it can be easily found.
- You do not need a lawyer to complete the forms. However, two persons must witness your signature to these forms.
- Advance directives may vary from state to state; check your state for legal variations.

Pain Control

A major goal of nursing is to alleviate pain and promote comfort. However, the use of narcotics to alleviate pain can raise ethical issues. Patients in severe pain may require large doses of pain medication, which can cause respiratory depression. It is crucial for the nurse to understand the patient's situation, to be very well informed about the effects of pain medication, and to

ETHICAL DILEMMA

Mr. Stewart is a 71-year-old man who has been admitted to a general medical-surgical floor of a small community hospital. He is diagnosed with metastatic cancer that has spread from his prostate to his spinal column and hip.

Mr. Stewart has been admitted to the hospital because he is too weak to walk, cannot care for himself, and can barely feed himself. With his physician's concurrence he has decided not to have chemotherapy. Because he is in the terminal stages of cancer, he is to be kept comfortable with continuous IV infusion of narcotics.

Because of his emaciated condition, the skin over his coccyx has begun to break down. When staff attempts to turn Mr. Stewart every 2 hours, he cries out in pain to such an extent that the nurse wonders if this nursing intervention is really helping him. Finally the staff decides to hold a care conference to discuss what they should do about Mr. Stewart's care. The head nurse insists that Mr. Stewart be turned at least every 2 hours because it is routine and minimal nursing care for bedridden patients. If he is not turned every 2 hours, his coccyx will become necrotic and possibly cause an infection. Ms. Jones, his primary nurse, said she cannot stand to hear Mr. Stewart cry out in agony every time he is turned. Ms. Smith, another team member, suggests that Mr. Stewart have some say regarding his care. She claims that turning or not turning will hardly make a difference in the overall outcome of his terminal illness. How should they decide?

observe the patient for the effects. The nurse should discuss with the supervisor any questions regarding the use of the medication.

ROLE OF THE ETHICS COMMITTEE

Sometimes an ethical dilemma is so difficult that consulting an institutional ethics committee may be helpful. Most hospitals and many long-term care institutions have an ethics committee. Such committees usually comprise many individuals with a variety of backgrounds and expertise (including ethics). These groups are skilled and experienced in assisting patients, families, and healthcare professionals in ethical decision making.

ANA CODE OF ETHICS

Nursing is related to society. The state has given the profession the power to regulate and control its own practice. In turn the profession is obligated to see that acceptable standards are maintained. One important way to uphold this duty is provided by the American Nurses Association Code of Ethics (Box 2-7). This code is a public expression of the values and goals of the nursing profession and consists of 11 statements. Members of the nursing profession are required to follow this code, which is explicit about the importance of respect for patients (American Nurses Association, 1985).

BOX 2-7

CODE FOR NURSES

1 The nurse provides services with respect for human dignity and the uniqueness of the client, unrestricted by considerations of social or economic status, personal attributes, or the nature of health problems.
2 The nurse safeguards the client's right to privacy by judiciously protecting information of a confidential nature.
3 The nurse acts to safeguard the client and the public when health care and safety are affected by the incompetent, unethical, or illegal practice of any person.
4 The nurse assumes responsibility and accountability for individual nursing judgments and actions.
5 The nurse maintains competence in nursing.
6 The nurse exercises informed judgment and uses individual competence and qualifications as criteria in seeking consultation, accepting responsibilities, and delegating nursing activities to others.
7 The nurse participates in activities that contribute to the ongoing development of the profession's body of knowledge.
8 The nurse participates in the profession's efforts to implement and improve standards of nursing.
9 The nurse participates in the profession's efforts to establish and maintain conditions of employment conducive to high quality nursing care.
10 The nurse participates in the profession's effort to protect the public from misinformation and misrepresentation and to maintain the integrity of nursing.
11 The nurse collaborates with members of the health professions and other citizens in promoting community and national efforts to meet the health needs of the public.

Reprinted with permission from *Code for Nurses with Interpretive Statements*, 1985, American Nurses Association, Washington, D.C.

KEY CONCEPTS

- Critical thinking is a process used to make sound, accurate, and reasonable decisions on the basis of thorough data collection and analysis.
- Critical thinking includes five elements: (1) data collection, (2) analysis, (3) deductive and inductive reasoning, (4) hypothesis testing, and (5) evaluation.
- The nursing process is a dynamic problem-solving process that includes five steps: (1) assessment, (2) analysis/nursing diagnosis, (3) planning/outcomes, (4) implementation (performance and documentation), and (5) evaluation.
- A nursing diagnosis describes a combination of signs and symptoms that indicate actual or potential health problems that nurses are licensed to treat and are capable of treating.
- The use of nursing diagnoses provides a common language for nurses.
- In the planning phase of the nursing process, a concise, written design of action is developed on the basis of the nursing diagnosis. Outcomes are identified, priorities are set, and interventions are proposed.
- Outcomes are statements that describe specific, objective, and desired patient behaviors or results.
- Implementation involves the actual performance of the prescribed nursing interventions, which includes direct care, observations, and health teaching. Documentation of interventions is essential.
- Evaluation is the final stage of the nursing process. The outcomes established in the planning phase are compared to patient behavior and symptoms.
- Ethics is the branch of philosophy that studies how people should act and what sort of character they should have.
- The patient is the central focus of nursing. This focus is based on the universal moral obligation to respect all human beings because they possess dignity and inherent worth.
- Ethics requires consideration of the whole patient in daily relationships.
- One demonstrates respect when one seriously considers others' values and goals and how these goals impact the nurse-patient relationship. Illness can threaten a patient's sense of respect.
- The nurse's promise states that nurses are morally committed to help care for patients. This promise extends from respect for the patient.
- DNR orders do not justify abandonment. Respect demands that care be given.
- An advance directive is a written document that indicates a patient's choices regarding medical treatment. It must be followed out of respect for the patient.
- Patients must be involved in decision making.
- Respect for privacy and confidentiality grows out of respect for the patient.
- The American Nurses Association Code of Ethics describes a generally accepted set of behaviors. Behavior that is inconsistent with these established guidelines may be deemed unethical.

CRITICAL THINKING EXERCISES

1. Write a paragraph that explains what a nursing diagnosis is and how it differs from a medical diagnosis.
2. Mrs. Corona has been admitted from the emergency room with a diagnosis of congestive heart failure. In the emergency room, she was asked if she had an advance directive. She does not and asks you to tell her what it is. Explain advance directives to Mrs. Corona and how they differ from a living will.
3. After paying the rent and electric bill, Mary has no money to feed her two young children. She steals 50 dollars from her employer. Apply the principles of utilitarianism and deontology to determine if this is an ethical action.

REFERENCES AND ADDITIONAL READINGS

Alfaro-LeFevre R: *Critical thinking in nursing: a practical approach,* Philadelphia, 1985, WB Saunders.

American Nurses Association: *Code for nurses with interpretive statements,* Kansas City, Mo, 1985, The Association.

Aroskar MA: Ethical decision-making in patient care, *Am Nurse* 26(3):10, 1994.

Bandman B, Bandman E: *Critical thinking in nursing,* Norwalk, Conn, 1988, Appleton & Lange.

Bandman E, Bandman B: *Nursing ethics in the lifespan,* Norwalk, Conn, 1985, Appleton, Century, Crofts.

Beauchamp T, Childress J: *Principles of biomedical ethics,* ed 3, New York, 1989, Oxford University Press.

Benner P: *From novice to expert,* Menlo Park, Calif, 1984, Addison-Wesley Publishing.

Catalano JT: Systems of ethics: a perspective, *Crit Care Nurse,* 12(8):91-96, 1992.

Churchill LR: Trust, autonomy, and advance directives, *J Religion Health* 28(3), 1989.

North American Nursing Diagnosis Association: *Classification of nursing diagnosis: proceedings of the tenth conference,* 1994, JB Lippincott.

Fry ST: Toward a theory of nursing ethics, *Adv Nurs Sci,* 11(4):9-22, 1989.

Fry ST: The ethic of caring: can it survive in nursing? *Nurs Outlook* 38(1), 1990.

Gordon M: *Nursing diagnosis: process and application,* ed 3, St Louis, 1994, Mosby.

Grant AB: Exploring an ethical dilemma, *Nurs 92* 22(12):52-54, 1992.

Husted GL, Husted JH: *Ethical dilemmas and nursing practice,* ed 2, St Louis, 1994, Mosby.

Hydo B: Designing an effective clinical pathway for stroke, *Am J Nurs,* 95(3):44-51, 1995.

Leski J: Critical literacy: new ways to think and learn, *Nursing Spect* 6(6):9, 1993.

Levine M: Nursing ethics and the ethical nurse, *Am J Nurs* 77(5):845-849, 1977.

Mezey M and others: The patient self-determination act: sources of concern for nurses, *Nurs Outlook* 42(1):30-38, 1994.

Miller M: *Critical thinking applied to nursing,* St Louis, 1996, Mosby.

Moore FD: Ethics at both ends of life. In *A miracle and a privilege: recounting a half century of surgical advances,* Washington, DC, 1995, Joseph Henry Press.

O'Mara RJ: Ethical dilemmas with advance directives: living wills and do not resuscitate orders, *Crit Care Nurs Q* 10(2):17-28, 1987.

Pellegrino E, Thomasma D: *For the patient's good: the restoration of beneficence in health care,* New York, 1988, Oxford University Press.

President's commission for the study of ethical problems in medicine and biomedical and behavioral research: *Summing up: final report on studies of the ethical and legal problems in medicine and biomedical and behavioral research,* Washington DC, 1983, US Government Printing Office.

Reigle J: Should the patient decide when to die? *RN* 58(5): 57-61, 1995.

Salladay SA, McDonnell MM: Facing ethical conflicts, *Nurs 92* 22(2):44-47, 1992.

Scanlon C: Developing ethical competence, *Am Nurse* 26(3):1; 11, 1994.

Thompson DL: Ethical case analysis using a hospital bill, *Nurse Educ* 16(4):20-23, 1991.

Watson J: *Human science and human care,* New York, 1988, National League for Nursing.

Part II

3 Psychosocial Effects
4 Cultural Considerations
5 Death and Dying
6 Substance Abuse

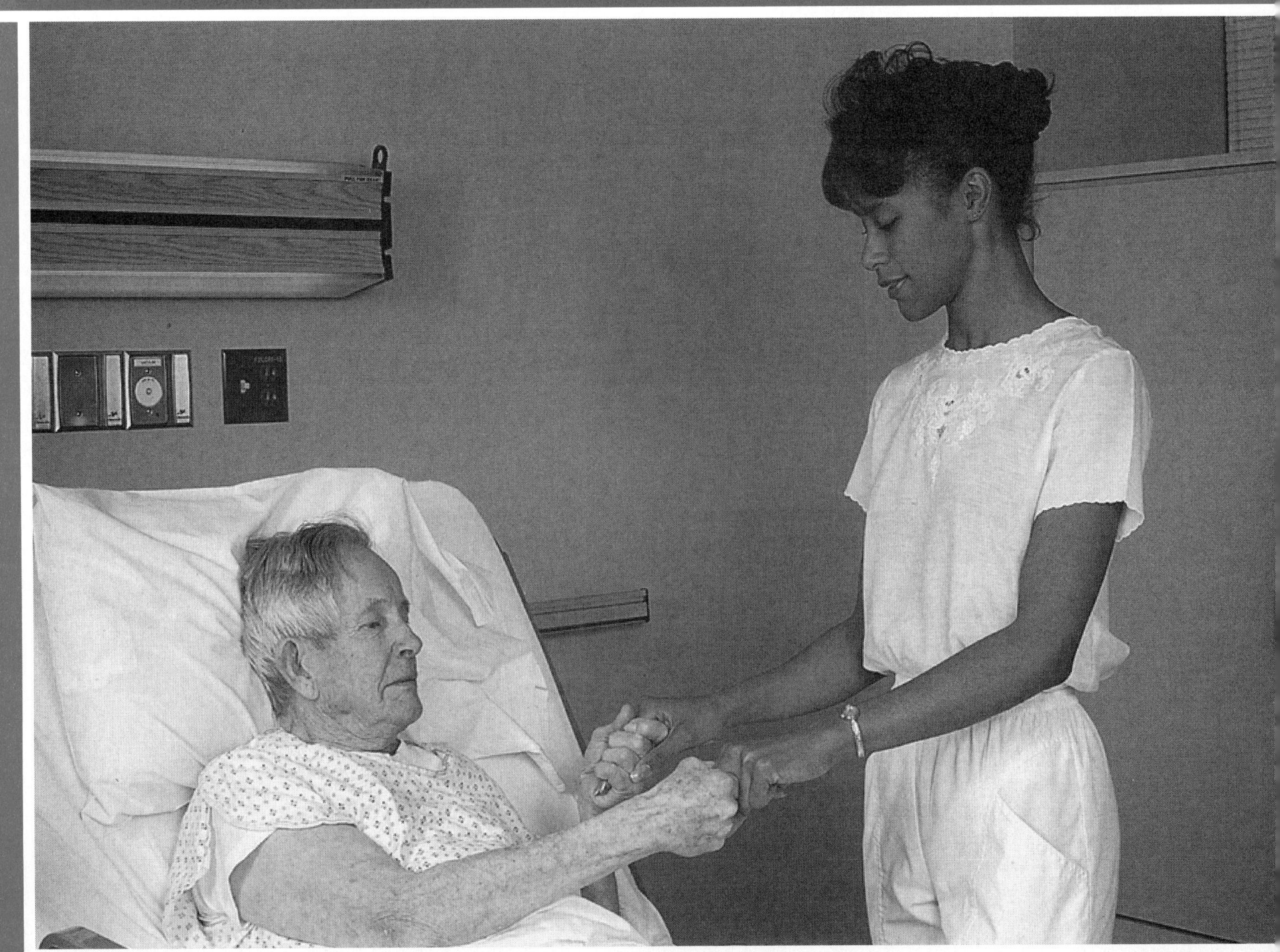

PSYCHOSOCIAL ASPECTS OF PATIENT CARE

CHAPTER 3

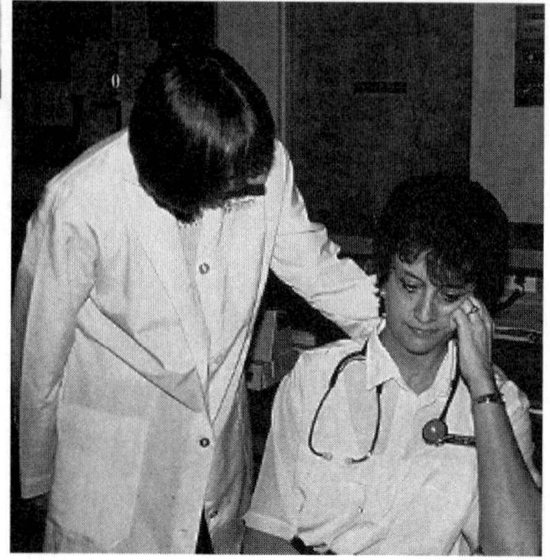

Psychosocial Effects

CHAPTER OBJECTIVES

1 Discuss stages of personality development.
2 Explain the normal use of defense mechanisms.
3 Define and differentiate between mood (affective) disorders, personality disorders, anxiety disorders, adjustment disorders, factitious disorders, dissociative disorders, and psychosomatic disorders.
4 Identify three types of each of the following: mood (affective) disorders, personality disorders, anxiety disorders, and psychosomatic disorders.
5 List five characteristics of schizophrenia.
6 Discuss the relationship between emotional and physical illness.
7 Describe regression and situational depression and the potential relationship of each to the ill or hospitalized nonpsychotic patient.
8 Identify four major sources of depression and list six symptoms of depression.
9 List signals often given by persons thinking about suicide.
10 List three behaviors that could signal emotional stress in a medically stressed patient.
11 List three common types of psychotropic drugs and one major side effect of each.
12 Describe, discuss, and demonstrate nursing techniques that are effective therapeutic tools for the care of both psychotic and nonpsychotic patients.

KEY WORDS

Alzheimer's disease
anxiety
anxiety disorders
conscious
defense mechanisms
delusion
depression
ego
endogenous depression
hallucination
Huntington's chorea
id
mental health
mental illness
mood (affective) disorders
organic brain syndrome
personality
personality disorder
posttraumatic stress disorder
psychoses
psychosomatic disorders
regression
schizophrenia
situational depression
subconscious
superego
unconscious

The nurse may choose to practice nursing in a variety of settings. Whatever the setting, it is important that the nurse have a knowledge and understanding of **mental health, mental illness,** and the ways in which illness can affect a patient's emotional well-being. Emotional reactions occur in all patients with a physical illness and increase a patient's need for emotional support. Mental health and mental illness are at opposite ends of an emotional spectrum. Without emotional support, the stress of a physical illness can move a patient toward mental illness.

There is no clear-cut division between physical illness and mental illness. Physical illness affects the emotional well-being of the patient, and mental illness affects the body. The mentally ill person may have physical problems, and the physically ill patient may develop emotional problems. It is never safe to assume that a patient has only one or the other type of problem. A great number of the patients currently seeking medical care have significant emotional problems that affect their physical states. Therefore almost all types of emotional problems can be seen in a general hospital, and many physical problems can be found in mentally ill patients. All persons have similar needs that must be met to maintain their ability to function.

NEEDS OF INDIVIDUALS

Each person is born with a definite set of basic needs, which are the same for everyone. These needs do not vary with age and are not changed by sex, color, race, religion, occupation, or marital status. They remain the same, regardless of the individual's emotional or physical health.

Maslow has identified physiologic, safety, love and a sense of belonging, esteem, and self-actualization needs as basic to all people (Figure 3-1). He refrains from identifying the physiologic needs more specifically. The concept of homeostasis and recent studies of appetite that have linked homeostasis in an imperfect way to an actual chemical insufficiency in the body have led Maslow to believe it impossible and useless to list fundamental physiologic needs. He believes the list could become endless. In his study of Maslow, physiologic needs are identified by Goble as food, liquid, shelter, sex, sleep, and oxygen. Physiologic needs are commonly identifed in nursing literature as nutrition, elimination, oxygenation, activity, rest, sleep, and sexuality. If physiologic needs are not met, the individual focuses on obtaining them. All other needs are ignored until the physiologic needs are adequately met.

The needs that emerge on the next level are the safety needs. Maslow describes safety needs as security; stability; dependency; protection; freedom from fear, anxiety, and chaos; and the need for structure, order, law, limits, and strength in the protector. The organism may be dominated by the safety needs. They may serve as the almost exclusive organizers of behavior and recruit all the capacities of the organism. This organism may be fairly described as a safety-seeking mechanism.

In children and adults, illness is a threat to safety and a disruption of order in their lives. This disruption is particularly threatening to children, who need an organized and structured world. The child who frantically clings to his or her parents, as is often seen in hospitals and other healthcare agencies, is testimony to the parent's role as protector. The average child and the average adult generally prefer a safe, orderly, predictable, lawful, and organized world on which they can depend and in which unexpected, unmanageable, chaotic, or other dangerous things do not happen. In such cases he or she has powerful parents or protectors who shield him or her from harm. The healthy and fortunate adult in our society is largely satisfied in his or her safety needs and no longer has any safety needs as active motivators. The tendency to have some religion or world philosophy that organizes the universe into a satisfactorily coherent, meaningful whole is also partly motivated by safety seeking. Science and philosophy are partially motivated by safety needs. The need for safety is seen as an active and dominant mobilizer of the organism's resources only in real emergencies such

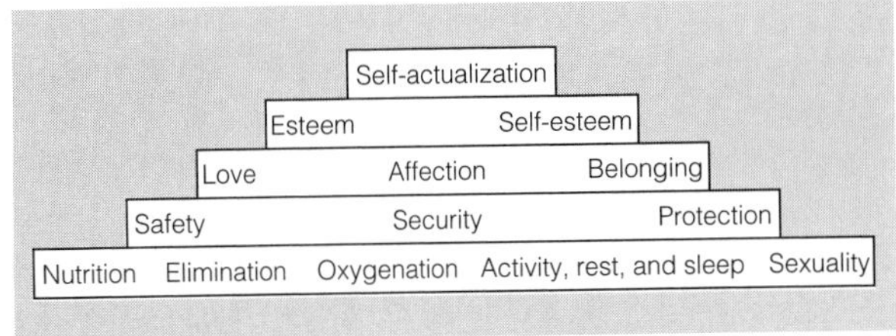

Figure 3-1 Maslow's hierarchy of human needs. (Modified from Goble FD: *The third force,* New York, 1970, Grossman Publishers.)

as war, disease, crime waves, neurosis, brain injury, and breakdown of authority.

If physiologic and safety needs are fairly well gratified, the need for love, affection, and belongingness emerges. The individual is now keenly aware of the absence of friends, a sweetheart, a spouse, or children and hungers for a place in a group or family. A sense of belonging has been underrated. Belonging to a group, neighborhood, or culture is now recognized as important. Society thwarts these needs, and these unmet needs are most commonly at the core of maladjustment and more severe illnesses.

Maslow believed that love and affection needs and their possible expression in sexuality are generally viewed with ambivalence and are customarily hindered by many restrictions and inhibitions. Most theorists of psychopathology have stressed the thwarting of love needs as a basic factor in maladjustment. Maslow stresses that love is not synonymous with sex. Sex may be studied as a purely physiologic need. Sexual behavior is usually multidetermined by sexual and other needs, namely love and affection. Love needs involve both giving and receiving love.

At the next level are the esteem needs. All people in society (with a few pathologic exceptions) need or desire a stable, firmly based, and high evaluation of themselves; self-respect and self-esteem; and the esteem of others. These needs may be classified into two subsidiary sets. First are the desires for strength, achievement, adequacy, mastery and competency, confidence in the face of the world, and independence and freedom. Second is the desire for reputation or prestige (respect or esteem from other people), status, fame, glory, dominance, recognition, attention, importance, dignity, and appreciation. Satisfaction of esteem needs leads to feelings of self-confidence, worth, strength, capability, adequacy, usefulness, and importance. Thwarting these needs produces feelings of inferiority, weakness, and helplessness. These feelings lead to basic discouragement or compensatory or neurotic trends. The most stable and healthy self-esteem is based on deserved respect from others rather than on external fame or celebrity and unwarranted adulation. Self-esteem must not be based on the opinions of others but on real capacity, competence, and adequacy for the task.

Even if all the previous needs are satisfied, discontent and restlessness soon develop unless the individual is acting according to personal capabilities. A musician must make music, and an artist must paint if he or she is to be ultimately at peace. What a person *can* be, he or she *must* be; one must be true to one's nature. Maslow calls this need self-actualization. It refers to a person's desire for self-fulfillment, namely, the tendency for one to become actualized in what one potentially is and to become all that one can. Individual differences are greatest at this level. The clear emergence of these needs usually rests on some prior satisfaction of the physiologic, safety, love, and esteem needs.

Maslow believes that there are different degrees of need satisfaction. Most members of society are both partially satisfied and partially unsatisfied with all their basic needs. A more realistic description of the hierarchy would be in terms of *decreasing* percentages of satisfaction at higher levels of the *hierarchy of prepotency* (superiority). The higher the level, the less often the need is satisfied by most members of society. Therefore emergence of a new need does not necessarily follow *total* satisfaction of the prepotent need. Instead, there is a gradual emergence by slow degrees from nothingness. As the degree of satisfaction increases, satisfaction of the next need will be increased. For example, if only 10% of prepotent need "A" is satisfied, then need "B" may not be visible at all. As 25% of "A" becomes satisfied, 5% of "B" may emerge. If 75% of need "A" becomes satisfied, 50% of need "B" may emerge.

Maslow does not claim that these needs are to be understood as exclusive determinants of certain types of behavior. Any behavior tends to be determined by several or all of the basic needs simultaneously rather than by only one of them. For example, eating may be partially for the sake of filling the stomach and partially for the sake of comfort and improvement of other needs.

Needs cease to play an active determining or organizing role as soon as they are gratified. Therefore, a perfectly healthy, normal, and fortunate person has *none* of these needs. One who is thwarted in any of these basic needs may be seen as sick or at least as less than fully human. A healthy individual is primarily motivated by needs to develop and actualize his or her fullest potentialities and capacities.

Although health evolves from the gratification of basic needs, it does not produce selfishness. It is not ego centered. On the contrary Maslow sees compassion and unselfishness in those who have had their basic needs gratified. Gratification assumes some positive growth tendency in the organism and drives it to fuller development.

If one subscribes to Maslow's theory, self-actualization and health or wellness can be equated. Self-actualization is a goal and the ultimate need of all human beings, and it occurs when all other needs are gratified. Persons involved with promoting wellness can therefore look to Maslow's theory of human motivation as a basis for their own theories. It treats the mind and body as a whole and has as its goal optimum wellness and self-actualization, which results in the most fully developed human individual.

PERSONALITY

Structure

Why do people appear to be so different? One person may be angry, aggressive, and ready to fight for the slightest reason, whereas another may be passive, submissive, and always ready to give in or compromise. An individual's response to a situation is based on **personality** structure, which is composed of a person's genetic makeup, life experiences, knowledge, and feelings.

Sigmund Freud is noted for deviating from the Viennese medical model by acknowledging the importance of emotions. He developed the concept of long-term psychotherapy called *psychoanalysis*. He referred to the awareness of the total environment as the **conscious** mind. He called the area just beneath consciousness where memories are stored the **subconscious** mind and named the reservoir of unremembered past experiences the **unconscious** mind. Because Freud was a scholar and a scientist, the goal he sought for his patients was not emotional happiness or mental health but self-knowledge and truth.

To describe and understand human behavior, Freud identified three parts of the personality: the id, the ego, and the superego. The **id** contains impulses and drives, and it operates at an unconscious level of thought. Id drives include hunger, sex, and warmth. Because the id operates on the pleasure principle, it demands almost immediate satisfaction. The **ego** deals with how one relates to the world. It is an awareness of the conscious self, or the "I." The ego has sometimes been called the executive of the personality because thoughts, feelings, compromises, and solutions are formed here. The ego attempts to satisfy the needs of the id, while at the same time considering the pressures from the superego. The **superego** controls, inhibits, and regulates the impulses. It contains the notions of right and wrong as taught by parents and society. The superego operates at both the conscious and unconscious levels and aids in critical self-evaluation, self-punishment, and self-love.

Development

All parts of the personality must achieve a balance before a person can function effectively and survive within a society. Like many theorists, Freud, Erikson, and Haviqhurst have attempted to explain how the personality develops.

Freud has described three principal stages that occur in the development of the individual: the *infantile stage*, which is divided into the *oral, anal,* and *phallic stage*, the *latent stage;* and the *genital stage*. Each of these stages contains its own centers of importance and has needs that must be met before the next stage can be entered successfully.

Personality development as conceived by Erik Erikson does not stress the psychosexual aspect of each stage of development. Instead he has proposed that each stage of development has a developmental task to be accomplished that not only contributes to some vital attribute of personality but also lays the groundwork for the next task. Erikson's first stages of emotional development are similar to those of Freud. Erikson has also described a sense of autonomy as the main emotional task of the early preschool years, a sense of initiative as the main task of the later preschool and early school years, and a sense of industry as the main task of the later childhood years. Similarly, Havighurst has developed a specific set of tasks that need to be accomplished in each developmental stage. Erikson's and Havighurst's theories together paint a mural of human development (Table 3-1).

MENTAL HEALTH

There is no easy formula for judging normality. What is considered normal can and does vary from culture to culture, country to country, and town to town. From any point of view, the concept of normality/abnormality is a relative one.

A variety of writers have attempted to define mental health. Glasser states that a normal human being is one who can function effectively, obtain some degree of happiness, and achieve something of benefit to himself or herself within the rules of the society. Morgan and Johnston define mental health as the ability to adjust to new situations, react to personal problems without marked distress, and productively contribute to society. An individual's degree of mental health may fluctuate from day to day and from situation to situation, but it maintains an overall consistency.

ANXIETY

Anxiety is a major motivating factor in a person's emotional life. A person usually takes the course of action that reduces the apprehension, tension, and uneasiness that threaten his or her sense of self or sense of control. These feelings stem from anticipated danger that may or may not be related to the reality of the situation. Some people are made anxious by love, some by hate, and some by the indifference of others.

Anxiety is first experienced in infancy when one's

TABLE 3-1

Comparison of Erikson's and Havighurst's Developmental Stages and Tasks

Developmental Stage	Erikson	Havighurst
	Trust versus mistrust 1. Oral needs of primary importance 2. Adequate mothering necessary to meet infant's needs 3. Acquisition of hope	1. Learning to walk 2. Learning to take solid foods 3. Learning to talk 4. Learning to control elimination of body wastes 5. Learning sex differences and sexual modesty 6. Achieving physiologic stability 7. Forming simple concepts of social and physical reality 8. Learning to relate oneself emotionally to parents, siblings, and other people 9. Learning to distinguish right and wrong and developing a conscience
Toddler years	*Autonomy vs. shame* 1. Anal needs of primary importance 2. Father emerges as important figure 3. Acquisition of will	
Early childhood	*Initiative vs. guilt* 1. Genital needs of primary importance 2. Family relationships contribute to early sense of responsibility and conscience 3. Acquisition of purpose	
Middle childhood	*Industry vs. inferiority* 1. Active period of socialization for child as he or she moves from family into society 2. Acquisition of competence	1. Learning physical skills necessary for ordinary games 2. Building wholesome attitudes toward oneself as a growing organism 3. Learning to get along with age mates 4. Learning an appropriate sex role 5. Developing fundamental skills in reading, writing, and calculating 6. Developing concepts necessary for everyday living 7. Developing conscience, morality, and scale of values 8. Developing attitudes toward social groups and institutions
Adolescence	*Identity vs. identity diffusion* 1. Search for self in which peers play important part 2. Psychosocial moratorium is provided by society 3. Acquisition of fidelity	1. Accepting one's physique and accepting a masculine or feminine role 2. New relations with age mates of both sexes 3. Emotional independence of parents and other adults 4. Achieving assurance of economic independence 5. Selecting and preparing for an occupation 6. Developing intellectual skills and concepts necessary for civic competence 7. Desiring and achieving socially responsible behavior 8. Preparing for marriage and family life 9. Building conscious values in harmony with adequate scientific world picture
Adulthood	*Intimacy vs. isolation* 1. Characterized by increasing importance of human closeness and sexual fulfillment 2. Acquisition of love	1. Selecting a mate 2. Learning to live with marriage partner 3. Starting family 4. Rearing children 5. Managing home 6. Getting started in occupation 7. Taking on civic responsibility 8. Finding congenial social group

From Sundeen SJ and others: *Nurse-client interaction: implementing the nursing process,* ed 5, St Louis, 1995, Mosby.

TABLE 3-1
Comparison of Erikson's and Havighurst's Developmental Stages and Tasks—cont'd

Developmental Stage	Erikson	Havighurst
Middle age	*Generativity vs. self-absorption* 1. Characterized by productivity, creativity, parental responsibility, and concern for new generation 2. Acquisition of care	1. Achieving adult civic and social responsibility 2. Establishing and maintaining economic standard of living 3. Assisting teenage children to become responsible and happy adults 4. Developing adult leisure activities 5. Relating oneself to one's spouse as a person 6. Accepting and adjusting to phsyiological changes of middle age 7. Adjusting to aging parents
Old age	*Integrity vs. despair* 1. Characterized by a unifying philosophy of life and a more profound love for mankind 2. Acquisition of wisdom	1. Adjusting to decreasing physical strength and health 2. Adjusting to retirement and reduced income 3. Adjusting to death of spouse 4. Establishing explicit affiliation with age group 5. Meeting social and civic obligations 6. Establishing satisfactory physical living arrangements

needs are not always met, and it continues to occur throughout the life cycle. Throughout life an individual faces many conflicts that lead to anxiety. This anxiety can be experienced in various degrees, from mild anxiety to a state of panic.

The sudden onset of an illness, a serious accident, or the death of a loved one may create anxiety and cause sleeplessness and other symptoms. An event that changes the family lifestyle or community status may cause a level of anxiety that makes a person feel helpless. The person who is in an acute state of panic and threatens to harm himself or herself or others may require the nurse to stay nearby until the panic is resolved.

Not all anxiety is harmful, nor is it to be avoided at all costs. Mild anxiety can actually increase one's alertness and improve performance. Moderate anxiety decreases one's ability to understand and makes learning difficult. Panic results in complete incapcitation. Anxiety also has many physiologic effects that prepare the body for the "fight or flight response."

Anxiety may be recognized through many physical symptoms and communicative manifestations. A person may experience restlessness, fatigue, palpitations, increased perspiration, increased respiration and pulse rates, a loss of appetite, an inability to sleep, tremors, frequent urination, a "lump in the throat," vomiting, diarrhea, and a change in abdominal sensations ("butterflies" in the stomach). Anxiety also affects communication. The anxious person may have a change in voice tone, speak at a higher pitch, or speak faster. The anxious person may be preoccupied with personal thoughts and either avoid certain topics or continually discuss a particular subject.

Defense Mechanisms

Because anxiety plays an essential role in influencing personality and behavior, it is helpful to explore the various mechanisms that people use to lower anxiety levels. **Defense mechanisms** are the attempts of the unconscious mind to protect the personality by controlling anxiety and reducing emotional pressures. Defense mechanisms are used by all people to reduce anxiety, and they consequently affect behavioral responses. The use of defense mechanisms is not intrinsically unhealthy. Because illness, hospitalization, and incapacitation are anxiety-producing experiences, an understanding of defense mechanisms is essential to those caring for the ill.

Daily frustrations and conflicts can usually be resolved by using conscious coping mechanisms. More complex frustrations and conflicts are dealt with through unconscious defense mechanisms. All people use defense mechanisms, and their use is not pathologic unless the individual's sense of reality is distorted. All defense mechanisms are automatic and are not consciously planned by the individual. Their purpose is to reduce emotional pressures and prevent anxiety. Table 3-2 lists some of the more common defense mechanisms.

TABLE 3-2
Defense Mechanisms

Mechanism	Definition	Example
Compensation	The individual attempts to make up for real or imagined feelings of inadequacy.	The girl who has been made to feel unattractive works very hard to excel in school or other areas.
Conversion	Emotional conflicts that cannot be dealt with mentally are expressed through physical means.	A soldier on the front lines of battle is very fearful, but the thought of being a coward is unacceptable. Unable to resolve this conflict through thought processes, he becomes paralyzed, thus escaping the combat situation. He truly is unable to walk.
Denial	A person avoids painful or anxiety-producing reality by unconsciously denying that it exists.	A person denies unpleasant traits such as dishonesty or stubborness or refuses to believe that a loved one has died or has a terminal illness.
Displacement	Pent-up emotions are redirected toward objects or people other than the primary source of the emotion.	A nursing student is chastised by the instructor. After returning home, the student may kick the cat, slam the door, and argue with family.
Identification	A person unconsciously enhances self-esteem by patterning himself or herself after another person.	A hospitalized teenager so admires one of the nurses that she decides to choose nursing as a career.
Projection	A person protects himself or herself from being aware of his or her own undesirable traits or feelings by attributing them to others.	The nurse believes that a particular patient does not like him or her, when in reality on an unconscious level he or she does not like the patient. The psychotic patient may state "He hates me" (I hate him) or "He thinks I am ugly" (I think I am ugly).
Rationalization	A person justifies inconsistent or undesirable behavior by giving acceptable explanations for them. (This has been called self-deception.)	A physician forgets to reorder medication for the patient and then criticizes the nurse for not giving a reminder.
Reaction formation	A person reverses unacceptable true feelings in exactly the opposite direction.	An overprotective and hovering mother actually resents and feels hostility toward her child.
Regression	A person returns to an earlier, less mature level of adaptation. Regression often results from lack of satisfaction or a threat to security. This behavior is seen to some extent in most hospitalized patients.	The 4-year-old boy suddenly starts to wet his pants and asks for a bottle after the arrival of a new baby at home. In some psychotic patients there can be a return to infantile behavior.
Repression	A person completely excludes from the conscious mind any impulses, experiences, and feelings that are psychologically disturbing because they arouse feelings of guilt or anxiety. Conflicts that remain repressed usually seek expression, as in one's dreams.	A daughter has very intense feelings of hatred for her father and wishes he would die. This thought is very unacceptable to the daughter and she excludes it from her conscious thought, yet she frequently has dreams of funerals and cemeteries.
Sublimation	Unconscious or unacceptable desires are channeled into socially acceptable activities. These desires are often sexual in nature.	A person may channel sexual drives into creating artwork or composing music.
Undoing	A person symbolically acts out in reverse something already done or thought that was unacceptable. The person attempts to erase the act or the guilt.	After slapping her child's hand, a mother keeps kissing her child's fingers.

Anxiety Disorders

Anxiety disorders are characterized by an anxious worrying that can result in a state of panic. Physical symptoms such as palpitations, shortness of breath, heavy perspiration, an inability to concentrate, and sleeplessness may be experienced and accompanied by unfocused feelings of dread. Anxiety disorders include panic disorders, phobic disorders, obsessive-compulsive disorders, conversion disorders, and **posttraumatic stress disorders** (Table 3-3).

EMOTIONAL DISORDERS

Emotional disorders are difficult to define. They range from mild to severe, and definitions may vary according to the experiences of the person who is doing the defining and the cultural attributes and context of the patient in question. A person who is uncomfortable with the powerful expression of feelings may see a very angry person as being emotionally disturbed. A very emotionally expressive person may see a reserved person as being depressed. A nursing home patient who says, "I have stars on my ceiling and a monkey who eats orchids in my greenhouse," may be thought of by the nurse as being senile or psychotic unless the nurse takes time to discover that the patient is recalling childhood memories when he or she did indeed have a ceiling with stars and an orchid-eating monkey in the greenhouse.

A person who is emotionally distressed is less able to act and behave in a useful and productive way. He or she may be well oriented to persons, places, and things but may not know the reasons underlying a particular behavior and so cannot modify behavior merely by willing change.

Whenever a person reaches a period of role change, new social and biologic pressures are brought to the surface. How well the transition occurs depends on the interpersonal resources, appropriate role models, and the acceptance by society of the new role. The harder it is to make a smooth adjustment, the greater the conflict, the more intense the stress, and the more vulnerable the individual is to emotional and physical illness. Examples of difficult role changes are a job loss, a death in a family, a career change, a divorce, an unwanted pregnancy, and school problems.

A patient with a physiologic illness may be termed by nursing staff as a "difficult patient." This is a patient whose emotional response to illness and hospitalization makes him or her behave in ways that challenge the nurse to get past the negative emotional response and identify the behavioral needs. The emotional responses that can be exhibited by a patient are hostility, manipulation, anxiety, and dependency.

TABLE 3-3

Anxiety Disorders

Disorder	Description	Example
Panic disorder	General symptoms of anxiety	A person driving a car suddenly feels terrified and may have to stop driving.
Phobic disorder	Enormous fear of an object or situation, even though the person recognizes that it cannot really do any harm	A person may have a fear of open spaces (agoraphobia), closed spaces (claustrophobia), or heights (acrophobia).
Obsessive-compulsive disorder	Obsession: repetitive thoughts Compulsion: repetitive acts that a person is unable to stop doing	A person constantly thinks about a love object, constantly drives by the love object's house, and makes him or her the total focus of all thoughts and activities.
Conversion disorder	Conversion type: blindness, deafness, paralysis Dissociative type: split from the memory of the trauma and development of amnesia or multiple personalities	A person sees a shooting and suddenly goes blind. A person is a victim of incest and remembers nothing of the incident.
Posttraumatic stress disorder	Numbness and decreased responses following trauma: flashbacks Acute: within 6 months of event Delayed: more than 6 months after the event Chronic: symptoms last more than 6 months	A person experiences a traumatic event such as rape, earthquakes, being held hostage, or war.

ETHICAL DILEMMA

A noncompliant patient and a hostile patient on your medical-surgical unit have been labeled as "difficult patients," and staff members are avoiding them. What would you do in this circumstance?

The hostile patient exhibits anger and rage that usually masks feelings of fear and loss of control. In an effort to regain power or to control the situation, the patient resorts to a barrage of abusive language, threats, and constant complaints about the quality of care. Sometimes this behavior escalates to physical activity to relieve the pent-up anger. The nurse can detect the early warning signs of hostile behavior: a loud and menacing tone of voice, clenched hands, facial taughtness, increased restlessness, pacing (if mobile), and listlessness (if in bed). The nurse should not personalize the patient's expressions of anger. The nurse should allow the patient to make choices and suggestions about his or her care. It is imperative to maintain open communication and avoid getting caught in a power struggle. The nurse should also ensure that the environment is safe. If the situation gets out of control, help should be obtained immediately. The nurse should never try to manage a violent situation alone. Rapid tranqulization with chlorpromazine (Thorazine), lorazepam (Ativan), or haloperidol (Haldol) may be effective. Mechanical restraints may be needed to prevent the individual from harming himself or herself or others. The nurse needs to know hospital protocols for initiating such an action. The nurse must remember to maintain the patient's dignity and show respect even in the most chaotic time.

The manipulative patient presents an interesting dynamic. This type of patient may use charm, threats, flattery, or demands, and he or she may evoke feelings of guilt or pity. The manipulative patient is adept at splitting the staff by playing one staff member against the other. The main purpose of this behavior is to gain control of the situation to have individual needs met. When dealing with a manipulative patient, the nurse should set realistic limits, be consistent, and be firm. This enables the patient to have set boundaries and decreases ideas of loss of control (Box 3-1). The nurse must not get trapped into taking the insults or threats personally. The nurse should explore the anger by accepting the patient but not the behavior. The nurse should also meet with other staff members to develop a consistent pattern of interaction. This strategy decreases the risk of splitting the staff and provides a common basis for interaction.

BOX 3-1 **Nursing Process**

MANIPULATIVE PATIENT

ASSESSMENT

Charming
Intelligent
Entertaining
Too insistent
Demanding/threatening

NURSING DIAGNOSIS

Ineffective individual coping related to manipulation of others

NURSING INTERVENTIONS

Identify the problem and who generated it.
Provide a consistent environment.
Point out manipulative behavior.
Set clear, reasonable, firm limits.
Reinforce positive regard.

EVALUATION OF EXPECTED OUTCOMES

Identifies self-behavior
Decreases anxiety
Trusting environment exists

The anxious patient has an unpleasant feeling of apprehension and dread and may be unaware of the causes of these feelings. The nurse should explore with the patient his or her perception of harm, and should use reality testing to test the perceived danger. The nurse should help the patient to verbalize perceptions of events and their causes. The nurse should also teach the patient the signs and symptoms of anxiety and should demonstrate ways to relieve anxiety such as relaxation, meditation, and diversional activities. The nurse should teach the patient about anxiolytics and minor tranquilizers.

The dependent patient exhibits an inability to do things for himself or herself, may be demanding, and constantly rings for the nurse. Dependency may be exhibited during hospitalization because the patient loses self-confidence in functioning successfully. The nurse's first goal is to foster independence. This is done by ensuring that dependency needs are met and by gradually transferring daily care tasks to the patient. Setting a schedule with the patient and adhering to it enables the patient and nurse to develop a trusting relationship and reassures the patient that his or her needs will be met. Praise and encouragement must be given after the patient completes even the most basic task.

PSYCHOSES

It has been said that the neurotic person builds castles, whereas the psychotic person lives in them. **Psychoses** are a group of major emotional disorders that are characterized by derangement of the personality and loss of ability to function realistically in the world.

Psychoses resulting from or associated with organic brain syndromes are mental disorders caused by brain damage. These psychoses include those associated with chronic brain syndromes, alcoholic psychoses, intracranial infections, and a variety of other physical conditions.

Psychoses can also result from the stress of being in an intensive care unit. To decrease the potential for an ICU psychosis the nurse should decrease the noise level, dim lights as necessary, and provide constant explanations of what is being done. The nurse should keep the patient oriented to time, place, and current events and should keep explanations simple. If hallucinations develop, the nurse should not repeat them but should continue to reorient the patient to reality. The nurse should assure the patient that this is a temporary state and that the hallucinations will go away as he or she gets better. Treatment varies according to the underlying physical situation (Box 3-2).

Psychoses that are not directly related to physical processes are termed functional psychoses. Functional psychoses can be divided into three categories: schizophrenia, mood disorders, and paranoid disorders.

Schizophrenia

Schizophrenia is the most widespread form of psychosis and includes a large group of disorders in which there are disturbances in thinking, mood, and behavior. Although there are five major subdivisions of schizophrenia, each with its own unique characteristics, several overall characteristics are possessed by all subgroups (Table 3-4).

The secondary symptoms of schizophrenia are those that characterize the five major subdivisions of the disorder. These symptoms are a person's last desperate attempt to reduce enormous anxiety. Three of the major subdivisions of schizophrenia are disorganized, catatonic, and paranoid schizophrenia.

Disorganized schizophrenia

Disorganized schizophrenia often begins in adolescence. A patient with this disorder begins to demonstrate inappropriate emotions. The patient often withdraws from social contact and smiles and giggles in a silly manner. There is severe **regression** until the patient's behavior becomes very childlike.

Catatonic schizophrenia

The catatonic type of schizophrenia has two forms. In one form the patient is completely inactive and mute and appears to be in a stupor. The

BOX 3-2 **Nursing Process**

PSYCHOTIC PATIENT

ASSESSMENT

Bizarre remarks
Internal preoccupation
Distractibility
Mumbling to self
Vacant look
Tension
Agitation

NURSING DIAGNOSES

Anxiety related to mistrust
Altered thought processes
Sensory/perceptual alterations: visual, auditory
Impaired verbal communication

NURSING INTERVENTIONS

Provide safe environment.
Decrease stimulation.
Understand what patient means.
Use physical contact sparingly.

EVALUATION OF EXPECTED OUTCOMES

Protected from self-injuries
Relaxed, restful environment decreases patient stressors
Enters into a trusting relationship
Interprets physical contact appropriately

TABLE 3-4

Characteristics of Schizophrenia

Characteristic	Description	Example
Thought and behavioral disturbances	The individual exhibits confused thought processes that are easily sidetracked or fragmented. The individual's speech lacks unity and clarity, and his or her behavior may be odd, sudden, and unreasonable.	Instead of thinking, "I'm cold. The window is open, and a breeze is blowing on me. I'll close the window," the schizophrenic person may think, "I'm hungry. Why is she staring at me? I see a red balloon."
Lack of affect	The individual does not display emotions, or displayed emotions are inappropriate. He or she fails to react to others in a meaningful way.	When informed of the death of a loved one, the individual may laugh.
Withdrawal	The individual becomes secluded from the rest of the world and exhibits decreased interest and initiative. He or she may have feelings of hopelessness, fear, and despair but remains acutely aware of the surroundings.	The individual may sit for hours staring into space without speaking to anyone.
Autism	The individual is detached from both reality and the world.	The individual is extremely withdrawn and involved with his or her own inner thoughts. He or she ignores all that is occurring in the immediate area and fails to relate to others.
Regression	The individual retreats to past levels of behavior.	The individual's behavior becomes more infantile.
Delusions	An individual with delusional thoughts has false beliefs based on misconceptions.	The individual may refuse all food, fearing that it may be poisoned.
Hallucinations	The individual has sensory perceptions that cannot be explained by external stimuli. Any sense may be involved.	The individual may hear voices or exhibit unusual behavior such as talking to himself, listening, or making unusual movements.

other form is characterized by an agitated state. Behavior is often impulsive and sometimes destructive.

Paranoid schizophrenia

In addition to displaying the other basic characteristics of schizophrenia, the paranoid schizophrenic is suspicious and aggressive and has **delusions** of persecution. The patient may hear voices that sometimes command action, or may believe that the police are following his or her movements. This type of patient can be very convincing and often demonstrates manipulative behavior.

Mood Disorders

This category includes a group of emotional illnesses that is characterized by a disorder of mood. There is either extreme depression or elation. **Mood (affective) disorders** include major depression, bipolar disorders, postpartum depression, and cyclothymic disorders.

Major depression

A major **depression** often occurs in middle age and occurs in people who have no previous history of depression. It is also called *involutional melancholia* and is often associated with menopause or with changes in a person's life situations. It is characterized by worrying, agitation, guilt, and hopelessness.

Bipolar disorder

Bipolar disorder, also called manic-depressive illness, is usually characterized by wide mood swings that alternate between elation and depression. In the manic phase the patient may make grandiose schemes and may not eat or sleep for days. The specific treatment of choice is lithium.

Postpartum depression

Postpartum depression can occur in the first 6 months of the postpartum period. It is characterized by weeping; lethargy; and feelings of being overwhelmed, incompetent, and helpless. Endocrine and hormonal changes, role changes, stress, or a combination of these have been proposed as causative factors.

Cyclothymic disorder

A cyclothymic disorder is characterized by mood swings between elation and depression. These mood swings are not as severe as those in a manic-depressive illness.

Paranoid Disorders

The paranoid patient has no **hallucinations** but has fixed delusions of grandeur or persecution that often center around religion. Other than the occurrence of these delusions, the personality is well balanced. There is some question as to whether paranoia is a separate disorder or is simply a branch of schizophrenia.

PERSONALITY DISORDERS

Personality disturbances fall somewhere in the middle of emotional disorders. The behavior of people with **personality disorders** indicates serious inner problems. However, those people are in contact with reality, and most of them are able to adapt socially. People with personality disorders do not demonstrate the anxiety that is characteristic of other types of emotional problems. The more common personality disorders include the paranoid personality, schizoid personality, obsessive-compulsive personality, antisocial personality, and passive-aggressive personality.

Paranoid Personality

People with a paranoid personality tend to be overly sensitive, suspicious, rigid, jealous, and envious. They sometimes demonstrate an exaggerated sense of their own importance, and they tend to blame others.

Schizoid Personality

People with a schizoid personality demonstrate emotional detachment, shyness, fearfulness, an inability to socialize well with others, and a tendency to daydream and withdraw.

Obsessive-Compulsive Personality

People classified as obsessive-compulsive are rigid, neat, inhibited, conforming, and overly conscientious. They may feel the need to perform some repetitive act to reduce anxiety.

Antisocial Personality

People with an antisocial personality (sociopathic personality) are unable to form meaningful attachments to other persons or groups or to society. They are selfish, irresponsible, impulsive, and unable to learn from punishment or past events. They feel no sense of guilt at causing harm or damage. Many prisoners are identified as having this personality type.

Passive-Aggressive Personality

People with a passive-aggressive personality have considerable difficulty fulfilling dependent needs and responding to authority. Their behavior includes pouting, stubborness, a failure to keep appointments, procrastination, intentional inefficiency, and tardiness. The person may evoke feelings of anger in family members, friends, and co-workers.

ORGANIC BRAIN SYNDROMES: DEMENTIA

Some forms of mental illness are caused by organic brain changes. These changes can result from a decreased blood supply to brain tissue, a traumatic destruction of brain cells by either trauma or disease, or the diminishing or destruction of brain tissue as a result of the aging process. It is sometimes possible to slow the symptoms of these **organic brain syndromes,** but such symptoms are irreversible, and patients with these disorders progressively deteriorate. Senility (senile dementia) is the pronounced loss of mental, physical, or emotional control in the elderly and was once thought to be a normal result of aging. It is now known to have a variety of organic causes, including neuron degeneration in the cerebral cortex.

Huntington's chorea is a genetically transmitted disease. Everyone who has the gene develops a psychosis around midlife and frequently requires institutionalization. Parkinson's disease is caused by a lack of dopamine in the basal ganglia. It is slowly progressive (see Chapter 28). **Alzheimer's disease,** a more recently discovered chronic brain disorder, can manifest itself as early as a person's mid-forties. This disease involves a progressive destruction of nervous system tissue and brain cells. The brain cells have a twisted shape. The symptoms of Alzheimer's disease include involuntary muscle movements, slurred speech, memory lapses and loss, and the gradual diminishing of thought processes and intellectual capabilities. Language disruption, emotional instability, an inability to carry out daily tasks, and difficulty in following a set of instructions may also occur.

To give effective care, the nurse should avoid overstimulating the patient and should provide consistency in care. The nurse should also use short, simple sentences when communicating with the patient and should give the patient time to respond. Patients with oganic brain syndromes are at high risk for injury when working around a stove or other potentially dangerous areas. Such patients may wander away and be unable to find their way back. Often these patients cannot state their name or address when asked.

SOMATIC DISORDERS

In the psychoses and personality disorders, an individual's anxiety is expressed through his or her behavior. In somatic reactions an individual's emotional conflict appears to be a major factor in the development of pathologic changes in a previously healthy organ of the body. The interaction between chronic anxiety and physical disease can be seen in a patient who develops essential hypertension as an adult. This person may have been raised in an environment that suppressed the expression of anger, and he or she may have lived for years with repressed hostility and underlying anxiety. Such a state can produce a slight but continual stimulation of the sympathetic nervous system and lead to a degree of arteriolar constriction in the kidneys, skin, and most visceral organs. A decreased blood supply to the kidney can lead to the development of hypertension. Other psychosomatic conditions include asthma, peptic ulcers, ulcerative colitis, hives, and migraine headaches. The specific causes of these disorders are unknown.

Not enough knowledge is presently available to provide conclusively that these diseases originate in the mind. The National Foundation of Ileitis and Colitis believes that ileitis and colitis have been incorrectly labeled as being psychosomatic. The foundation is involved in research to determine the cause of these diseases.

Whatever the cause of illness, it is the nurse's role to be supportive and caring. Those caring for patients with **psychosomatic disorders** may become impatient with or intolerant of a patient who they think is "doing it to himself or herself." Consequently an unsupportive and unsympathetic attitude may be conveyed to a patient who is truly suffering.

DEPRESSION

Because of the high incidence of depression in the general population (estimated to occur in 1 of every 12 people) one can assume that there is a high incidence of depression among patients requiring nursing care. The types of depression include grief, **situational/reactive depression, endogenous depression** (occurs without an identified precipitating event), chronic depression, and manic-depressive illness.

There are many signs and symptoms of depression, some of which can actually mask depression. All of these symptoms should be considered when evaluating a patient for depression and should include the following:

1 *Mood:* sad, unhappy, blue, crying, within the "normal" range
2 *Thoughts:* helplessness, hopelessness, pessimism, guilt, low self-esteem, loss of interest and motivation, decrease in efficiency and concentration, inability to make decisions and choices
3 *Behavior and appearance:* neglectful of personal appearance, angry/hostile, demanding, always smiling, seemingly the "good patient" (always compliant), perfectionistic, obsessive, anxious, hyperenergetic, withdrawn, dependent, indecisive, slowed in psychomotor capacities (speech and actions), agitated, apathetic
4 *Somatic or physical symptoms:* loss or increase of appetite, loss or increase in weight, constipation, insomnia, fatigue or sleeping too much, chronic pain (especially backache, headache, and adominal pains), menstrual changes, loss of interest in sex, sexual complaints or dysfunction, palpitations, hyperventilation, difficulty swallowing, rashes, asthma, colitis, hypertension

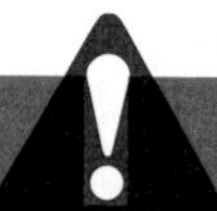

NURSE ALERT

A sudden elevation in a depressed patient's mood may indicate that he or she has developed a suicide plan and will act on it. A severely depressed person does not have the energy level or the ability to concentrate to effectively carry out a plan.

Many feelings underlie or contribute to depression, especially helplessness, hopelessness, and worthlessness. Other feelings that may cause depression include anger, despair, guilt, resentment, hostility, dependency, negativity, inferiority, low self-esteem, feelings of inadequacy, a poor self-image, a recent diagnosis of chronic or terminal disease, and loss. Loss can be defined in many ways and can include the loss of a significant other, a body part, a bodily function or its mobility, a dependent state *(success depression),* a symbolic object, self-esteem, or self-image.

Although feelings are significant factors in depression, depression can also be part of a symptom complex of certain diseases, including tapeworms, diabetes mellitus, thyroid disease, Addison's disease, Cushing's syndrome, systemic lupus, uremia, hypoglycemia, gallbladder disease, stroke, cardiac disease, and Alzheimer's disease. Certain medications can also induce depression, including reserpine, propranolol and other beta-blockers, methyldopa, diazepam, clonidine, corticosteroids, and oral contraceptives.

Nursing Assessment of Depression

A nursing assessment and interview is useful not only in developing a nursing care plan but also in helping the patient feel understood and cared for. A tool useful for evaluating whether a patient is depressed is the phrase "IN SAD CAGES" (Box 3-3). In assessing a patient for depression, it is important to differentiate among the types and severity of depression and to recognize the components of each:

1 *Grief:* involves a real loss; is weeks to years in duration; patient feels that everything has ended but knows better; reaction is proportionate to loss; no loss of self-esteem
2 *Reactive depression:* related to loss in current life situation (either real or imagined); comes and goes; can become chronic; patient manifests impaired functioning, has distorted perceptions, and may be suicidal; patient's reactions are disproportionate to loss; patient suffers loss of self-esteem; patient reacts to imagined losses as if they are real
3 *Endogenous depression:* stems from internal dynamics; same symptoms as reactive depression
4 *Psychotic depression:* not necessarily a loss involved; patient has distorted thought processes and severely impaired functioning and suffers gross distortion of perceptions (hallucinations, delusions, or both); patient reacts disproportionately, is suicidal, and suffers a loss of self-esteem

BOX 3-3

ASSESSING DEPRESSION

INterest—Have interests changed recently regarding work, family, hobbies, or friends? If so, how have they changed?
Sleep
Appetite
Depressed mood
Concentration
Activity
Guilt
Energy
Suicide

Nursing Assessment of Suicide

Suicide is one of the top five leading causes of death in the general population, is the second most frequent cause of death for 15- to 24-year-olds, and has a very high incidence among the elderly and the ill elderly. Therefore when a nurse assesses or suspects depression in a patient, it is extremely important to determine whether the patient is suicidal. It is always appropriate to ask the patient very directly if he or she is suicidal or has ever thought about hurting or killing himself or herself. Directly asking patients if they are suicidal does not increase the risk of suicide. Often patients feel relieved about having the opportunity to talk about how terrible they feel. The nurse should always believe a patient if he or she expresses suicidal thoughts. Not believing a patient may lead to his or her death. The nurse might ask the following questions when assessing a patient's risk for suicide:

- Do you feel that life is worth living?
- Have you thought about hurting yourself or committing suicide?
- What do you think you might do?
- Do you have a plan to kill yourself?
- Have you ever tried to harm yourself before? How far did you go?
- On a scale of 1 to 10, how suicidal are you?
- How do you see yourself in the future?
- Has any member of your family committed suicide?

Suicide is the ultimate expression of anger, hostility, hopelessness, and helplessness. Often the patient states the belief that "You have failed me." Many factors contribute to or increase the sense of hopelessness and helplessness and the risk of suicide in a patient:

- Previous suicide attempt
- Direct or disguised suicide threat (giving away belongings or stating, "My family won't have to worry about me much longer.")
- Chronic illness
- Isolation
- Bereavement/loss
- Financial stress
- Severe depression or psychosis
- Alcoholism/drug abuse
- Chronic use of hypnotics/sedatives
- Family history of suicide
- Suicide of a close friend

Whatever the setting, it is important for the nurse to avoid trying to cheer up a depressed patient or to make statements such as, "Things aren't that bad." The nurse should also avoid actions and attitudes that convey rejection, which can cause the patient to feel irritable and impatient and can lower self-esteem even further. Helpful actions include encouraging the patient to express anger and hostility; acknowledging the patient's statements about feeling depressed, sad, or worthless; and being nurturing, accepting, and respectful (Box 3-4). How would the nurse want to be treated if the roles were reversed?

NURSE ALERT

When dealing with a suicidal patient, ask specific questions about intent. Create a safe environment. Make a verbal contract that the patient will seek help of staff member and not harm self.

THE THERAPEUTIC RELATIONSHIP IN NURSING

Psychologist Carl Rogers is often credited with refining the use of a therapeutic relationship in the treatment of the emotionally ill. In a psychotherapeutic relationship, therapists use interpersonal relationships with the patients as a therapeutic tool. The therapists direct their own behavior in such a way as to effectively treat the patient. The patient's behavior is analyzed as an expression of individual needs.

Nurses also need to establish therapeutic relationships with their nonpsychiatric patients. Whatever the setting, the nurse needs to use the self as a therapeutic tool for patients and to develop a relationship that promotes healing. Nurses can develop meaningful and helpful relationships with their patients. Nurses have frequent opportunities to interact with them, observe their behavior, and react in a beneficial manner. Rogers has presented a variety of behaviors that are necessary for a helping relationship, including being genuine, offering warm acceptance of the person, and seeing the world as the patient sees it.

To work effectively with the psychologic needs of a patient, it is helpful to remember that the patient is attempting to communicate to the nurse verbally and behaviorally. The nurse is communicating with the patient in the same way. The cornerstone in any relationship is communication. Communication implies a meaningful verbal and nonverbal exchange between people.

Verbal communication involves an exchange of words on a variety of levels. Each day one may greet a neighbor by saying, "Hi, how are you?" The neighbor may reply, "Fine, thank you, how are you?" This exchange is not meaningful communication. Neither person is really interested in how the other is feeling. Often a nurse cheerfully enters a patient's room with a bright "Good morning. Isn't it a beautiful day?" without observing that the patient is lying in bed quietly crying. The nurse is not in tune with the patient's nonverbal communication (crying). There are four steps in successful communication:

BOX 3-4 **Nursing Process**

DEPRESSED PATIENT

ASSESSMENT

Anger
Helplessness
Hopelessness
Apathy
Crying
Approval seeking
Unkempt appearance
Vague pain
Fatigue
Agitation/retardation
Decreased social interest
Focus on negative
Appetite disturbance

NURSING DIAGNOSES

Ineffective individual coping
Altered thought processes
Altered nutrition
Potential for injury

NURSING INTERVENTIONS

Accept patient.
Be nonjudgmental.
Encourage verbalization.
Encourage patient to make own choices.
Help patient solve problems.
Encourage participation in groups.
Assess patient's ability to perform self-care tasks.

EVALUATION OF EXPECTED OUTCOMES

Increased feelings of self-worth
Trust is developed
Gains self-control/mastery
Receives positive feedback

1 *Listen.* Often one is so involved with one's own thoughts or beliefs that the other person is not really heard. When a patient attempts to talk with the nurse, the nurse should really try to listen to what the patient is saying.

2 *Support* what a patient is saying by not challenging or disagreeing with it. For example, a patient states, "I am really afraid to have surgery tomorrow. I wonder if my doctor knows what to do?" It would be easy to reply, "There is no reason to be afraid. The doctor knows what to do." This type of reply indicates that the nurse is not listening to the patient and supporting his or her feelings. Instead the nurse may say, "I can understand that the thought of surgery is scary. Let's talk about what worries you most." With this reply the nurse is supporting what the patient is saying and is offering the patient the opportunity to discuss and perhaps resolve some of his or her fears.

3 Demonstrate *empathy.* Empathy involves a sincere attempt by the nurse to understand situations as the patient perceives them. For example, it is easy for the nurse to becomeannoyed with the patient who refuses to learn to care for a colostomy. However, while talking with the patient the nurse may learn that the patient's mother died shortly after having a colostomy. It is not always possible to determine why patients perceive things as they do. Situations have a variety of meanings for people, and nurses should be tuned in to what each patient is expressing.

4 Use *therapeutic responses.* Therapeutic responses are ways of communicating that encourage further discussion and indicate that the nurse is listening to what the patient is saying (Table 3-5). It

TABLE 3-5

Therapeutic Communication Techniques

Technique: Listening
Definition: An active process of receiving information and examining reaction to the messages received
Example: Maintaining eye contact and receptive nonverbal communication
Therapeutic value: Nonverbally communicates to the patient the nurse's interest and acceptance
Nontherapeutic theat: Failure to listen

Technique: Broad Openings
Definition: Encouraging the patient to select topics for discussion
Example: "What are you thinking about?"
Therapeutic value: Indicates acceptance by the nurse and the value of the patient's initiative
Nontherapeutic threat: Domination of the interaction by the nurse; rejecting responses

Technique: Restating
Definition: Repeating the main thought the patient expressed
Example: "You say that your mother left you when you were 5 years old."
Therapeutic value: Indicates that the nurse is listening and validates, reinforces, or calls attention to something important that has been said
Nontherapeutic threat: Lack of validation of the nurse's interpretation of the message; being judgmental; reassuring, defending

Technique: Clarification
Definition: Attempting to put into words vague ideas or unclear thoughts of the patient to enhance the nurse's understanding or asking the patient to explain what he or she means
Example: "I'm not sure what you mean. Could you tell me about that again?"
Therapeutic value: Helps to clarify feelings, ideas, and perceptions of the patient and to provide an explicit correlation between them and the patient's actions
Nontherapeutic threat: Failure to probe; assumed understanding

Technique: Reflection
Definition: Directing back the patient's ideas, feelings, questions, and content
Example: "You're feeling tense and anxious and it's related to a conversation you had with your husband last night?"
Therapeutic value: Validates the nurse's understanding of what the patient is saying and signifies empathy, interest, and respect for the patient.
Nontherapeutic threat: Stereotyping the patient's responses; inappropriate timing of reflections; inappropriate depth of feeling of the reflections; inappropriate for the cultural experience and educational level of the patient

Technique: Humor
Definition: The discharge of energy through the comic enjoyment of the imperfect
Example: "That gives a whole new meaning to the word *nervous,*" said with shared kidding between the nurse and patient
Therapeutic value: Can promote insight by making conscious repressed material, resolving paradoxes, tempering aggression, and revealing new options, and is a socially acceptable form of sublimation
Nontherapeutic threat: Indiscriminate use; belittling patient; screen to avoid therapeutic intimacy

From Stuart GW, Sundeen SJ: *Principles and practice of psychiatric nursing,* ed 5, St Louis, 1995, Mosby.

continued

TABLE 3-5

Therapeutic Communication Techniques—cont'd

Technique: Informing
Definition: The skill of information giving
Example: "I think you need to know more about how your medication works."
Therapeutic value: Helpful in health teaching or patient education about relevant aspects of patient's well-being and self-care
Nontherapeutic threat: Giving advice

Technique: Focusing
Definition: Questions or statements that help the patient expand on a topic of importance
Example: "I think that we should talk more about your relationship with your father."
Therapeutic value: Allows the patient to discuss central issues and keeps the communication process goal-directed
Nontherapeutic threat: Allowing abstractions and generalizations; changing topics

Technique: Sharing Perceptions
Definition: Asking the patient to verify the nurse's understanding of what the patient is thinking or feeling
Example: "You're smiling but I sense that you are really very angry with me."
Therapeutic value: Conveys the nurse's understanding to the patient and has the potential for clearing up confusing communication
Nontherapeutic threat: Challenging the patient; accepting literal responses; reassuring; testing; defending

Technique: Theme Identification
Definition: Underlying issues or problems experienced by the patient that emerge repeatedly during the course of the nurse-patient relationship
Example: "I've noticed that in all of the relationships that you have described, you've been hurt or rejected by the man. Do you think this is an underlying issue?"
Therapeutic value: Allows the nurse to best promote the patient's exploration and understanding of important problems
Nontherapeutic threat: Giving advice; reassuring; disapproving

Technique: Silence
Definition: Lack of verbal communication for a therapeutic reason
Example: Sitting with a patient and nonverbally communicating interest and involvement
Therapeutic value: Allows the patient time to think and gain insights, slows the pace of the interaction and encourages the patient to initiate conversation, while conveying the nurse's support, understanding, and acceptance
Therapeutic threat: Questioning the patient; asking for "why" responses; failure to break a nontherapeutic silence

Technique: Suggesting
Definition: Presentation of alternative ideas for the patient's consideration relative to problem solving
Example: "Have you thought about responding to your boss in a different way when he raises that issue with you? For example, you could ask him if a specific problem has occurred."
Therapeutic value: Increases the patient's perceived options or choices
Nontherapeutic threat: Giving advice; inappropriate timing; being judgmental

is very important that the nurse respond to the patient's feelings, not just to his or her words. It is also very important that the nurse ask questions and not make assumptions about meaning. Fear and anxiety interfere with understanding. Therefore it is important for the nurse to realize that a patient who does not follow instructions is not attempting to "get the nurse" but may have difficulty understanding what the nurse wants. Because most patients want to please, the nurse's communications must be clear and easy to understand.

Nonverbal communication is also extremely important and is a form of communication that does not use words (Figure 3-2). It is "body language." Every move of the body and every gesture may convey one's true feelings.

The incontinent patient in a nursing home who needs to have the bed changed for the third time in one evening may become only too aware of how loudly nonverbal communication speaks. The patient says to the nurse who is changing the bed, "I'm so sorry, my dear, I hope you don't mind." The nurse replies, "Oh, that's all right," while pulling and tugging at the sheets with an uncharacteristic roughness. The patient has "heard" the anger, although not a word of anger was actually spoken.

It is helpful for nurses to observe nonverbal communication carefully. Is the husband really listening to his wife when he is seated 2 feet from the television with his eyes glued to the screen? His body language is saying he is not. What is the mother conveying to her child when the child wraps his arms around her and she stiffens and draws away, but says, "I love you"?

The use of verbal and nonverbal communication in nursing is as important as performing the proper tech-

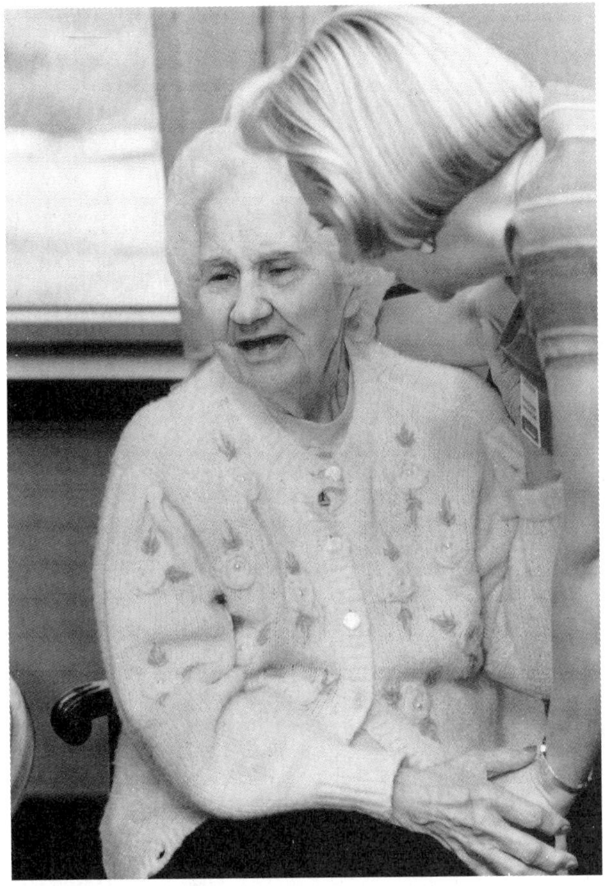

Figure 3-2 Touching a patient's shoulder and hand is an appropriate nonverbal gesture that expresses interest and support. (From Stuart GW, Sundeen SJ: *Principles and practice of psychiatric nursing,* ed 5, St Louis, 1995, Mosby.

niques. Those first entering the nursing field are often unsure of themselves when conversing with patients and fearful of saying the wrong thing. However, patients can sense when nurses are sincere in their attempts to communicate. That attempt alone will be appreciated. Successful communication is worthwhile. It takes practice and effort, but its end results may be more important than any medication.

Several general principles should be kept in mind when attempting to develop therapeutic relationships with patients. It is most important to accept the individual as he or she is. Patients should not be judged. Relationships are effective only if an individual perceives that the other party is interested in him or her as a human being worthy of dignity and respect.

The nurse should explain routines, procedures, and events according to the patient's level of understanding (Figure 3-3). Patients should be told that their feelings can be expressed and that they will be heard. Having patients participate in group sessions is often therapeutic. Mentally ill patients are usually anxious

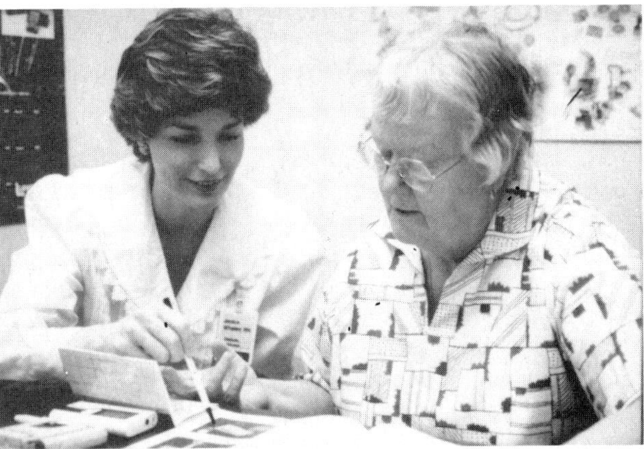

Figure 3-3 Explaining routines, procedures, and events help maintain therapeutic communication with patients. (From Potter PA, Perry AG: *Fundamentals of nursing,* ed 3, St Louis, 1993, Mosby.)

and should be treated with understanding and consistency. They should be offered reassurance for improvements in behavior, but false beliefs should not be supported. Any restrictions on behavior should be consistently enforced. Adhering to these principles can create a stable and supportive atmosphere that is conducive to mental health.

PSYCHOPHARMACOLOGY

The use of medications to treat mental illness has revolutionized the field of psychiatry. Before the major tranquilizers were discovered in the 1950s, patients often spent their entire lives in various institutions. Medications themselves do not necessarily cure the patient but often lessen symptoms sufficiently to allow the patient to participate more easily in other forms of treatment and to function more effectively in the community. As a result, the patient may be counseled in various community-based mental health centers rather than in an institutionalized setting.

Drugs that affect behavior are called *psychotropic* drugs. The two major drug groups in this category are the *tranquilizers* and the *antidepressants.* Tranquilizers affect the behavioral and the emotional tone of feeling (affect) of the individual. Antidepressants have a stimulating and energy-producing action that is particularly helpful in the treatment of depressive states (Table 3-6).

It is important to note that neuroleptic malignant syndrome may develop suddenly in people who are receiving antipsychotic drugs. Patients with fluid and electrolyte imbalances, nutritional deficiencies, and organic brain disorders may be at risk. Because this is a life-threatening situation, early recognition of this syndrome is vital. A fever greater than 103° F, hyper-

TABLE 3-6

Pharmacology of Drugs Used for Psychosocial Effects

Drug (Generic and Trade Name); Route and Dosage	Action/Indication	Common Side Effects and Nursing Considerations
ALPRAZOLAM (Xanax) **ROUTE:** PO **DOSAGE:** 0.25-0.5 mg 2-3 times daily as needed (not greater than 4 mg/day); decrease dosage in debilitated/elderly patients	Benzodiazepine used in the treatment of anxiety, depression, and "panic attacks"	Dizziness, drowsiness, and lethargy
AMITRIPTYLINE (Elavil) **ROUTE:** PO, IM **DOSAGE:** PO 30-100 mg/day single bedtime or divided dose, dose may be gradually increased up to 150-300 mg/day; IM 20-30 mg 4 times daily	Antianxiety drug used in treatment of depression	Drowsiness, sedation, lethargy, fatigue, dry mouth, dry eyes, blurred vision, hypotension, and constipation; potentially fatal reaction with MAO inhibitors; may adversely interfere with antihypertensive drugs
CHLORDIAZEPOXIDE (Librium) **ROUTE:** PO, IM, IV **DOSAGE:** For alcohol withdrawal PO 50-100 mg, repeated agitation up to 400 mg/day; for anxiety PO 5-25 mg 3-4 times daily, IM, IV 50-100 mg initially then 25-50 mg 3-4 times daily as required	Benzodiazepine used in treatment of anxiety, alcohol withdrawal, and preoperative sedative	Dizziness and drowsiness; use with caution in liver or kidney disease
CHLORPROMAZINE (Thorazine) **ROUTE:** PO, IM, IV, Rectal **DOSAGE:** For psychosis PO 10-25 mg 2-4 times daily, increase by 20-50 mg/day every 3-4 days (usual dose is 200 mg/day); for nausea and vomiting PO 10-25 mg q 4-6 hr, IM 25-50 mg q 3-4 hr; rectal 50-100 mg q 6-8 hr; for intractable hiccups PO, IM 25-50 mg 3-4 times daily	Antipsychotic and antiemetic used for acute and chronic psychosis, nausea and vomiting, preoperative sedation, and intractable hiccups	Sedation, extrapyramidal reactions, dry eyes, blurred vision, hypotension, constipation, dry mouth, and photosensitivity; use with caution in liver and cardiac disease; may cause bone marrow suppression; may have adverse reactions with other CNS depressants
CLORAZEPATE (Tranxene) **ROUTE:** PO **DOSAGE:** 15-60 mg/day in divided doses	Benzodiazepine used in treatment of anxiety, alcohol withdrawal, and management of seizures	Dizziness, drowsiness, and lethargy; use with caution in previously suicidal or addicted patients
DIAZEPAM (Valium) **ROUTE:** PO, IM, IV **DOSAGE:** For anxiety 2-10 mg 2-4 times daily or 14-30 mg extended release form once daily; for seizures IV 5-10 mg and may repeat q 10-15 minutes for total of 30 mg; for alcohol withdrawal 10 mg 3-4 times daily in first 24 hr, decrease to 5 mg 3-4 times daily	Benzodiazepine used in treatment of anxiety, seizures, and alcohol withdrawal; used as a muscle relaxant, light anesthetic, and for preoperative sedation	Dizziness, drowsiness, and lethargy; use with caution in debilitated, renal or hepatic dysfunction, and previously addicted or suicidal; drug has very few compatabilities

TABLE 3-6

Pharmacology of Drugs Used for Psychosocial Effects—cont'd

Drug (Generic and Trade Name); Route and Dosage	Action/Indication	Common Side Effects and Nursing Considerations
FLUOXETINE (Prozac) **ROUTE:** PO **DOSAGE:** 20 mg/day in the morning, after several weeks, may increase by 20 mg/day at weekly intervals (not to exceed 80 mg/day)	Antianxiety drug used in treatment of depression	Anxiety, insomnia, headache, drowsiness, tremor, diarrhea, excessive sweating, and pruritis; may cause anorexia and weight loss; use with caution in renal or hepatic dysfunction and in the elderly
HALOPERIDOL (Haldol) **ROUTE:** PO, IM, IV **DOSAGE:** PO 0.5-5 mg 2-3 times daily; patients with severe symptoms may require up to 100 mg/day; IM 2-5 mg q 1-8 hr, not to exceed 100 mg/day; IV 0.5-50 mg, may be repeated in 30 minutes	Antipsychotic drug used in treatment of acute and chronic psychoses	Extrapyramidal reactions, dry eyes, blurred vision, hypotension, constipation, dry mouth, and photosensitivity
LITHIUM (Lithium) **ROUTE:** PO **DOSAGE:** 900-1200 mg/day in 3-4 divided doses; blood level monitoring necessary to monitor therapeutic dose	Antimania drug used in the treatment of a variety of psychiatric disorders, especially bipolar affective disorders	Tremors, headache, impaired memory, lethargy, fatigue, ECG changes, nausea, anorexia, epigastric bloating, diarrhea, abdominal pain, polyuria dermatitis, hypothyroidism, leukocytosis, and muscle weakness; avoid in severe cardiac or renal dysfunction; known alcohol intolerance; must monitor drug levels closely
LORAZEPAM (Ativan) **ROUTE:** PO, IM, IV **DOSAGE:** PO 1-3 mg 2-3 times daily (up to 10 mg/day); decrease dosage in elderly	Benzodiazepine used in treatment of anxiety, insomnia; used preoperatively for sedation and anesthesia	Dizziness, drowsiness, and lethargy; use with caution in debilitated, renal or hepatic dysfunction, and previously addicted or suicidal patients
OXAZEPAM (Serax) **ROUTE:** PO **DOSAGE:** 10-30 mg 3-4 times daily; in older patients, initial dose should be 5 mg 1-2 times daily or 10 mg 3 times daily	Benzodiazepine used in treatment of anxiety and alcohol withdrawal	Dizziness, drowsiness, and lethargy; use cautiously with the elderly, hepatic dysfunction, and previously suicidal or addicted patients
PAROXETINE (Paxil) **ROUTE:** PO **DOSAGE:** 20 mg as a single morning dose; may increase dose by 10 mg/day at weekly intervals for maximum 50 mg/day dose	Antianxiety drug used in treatment of depression	Somnolence, dizziness, insomnia, tremor, nervousness, anxiety, headache, weakness, nausea, dry mouth, constipation, diarrhea, ejaculatory disturbance, male genital disorders, and sweating; potentially fatal reaction with MAO inhibitors; use with caution in the elderly and in renal or hepatic dysfunction

continued

TABLE 3-6

Pharmacology of Drugs Used for Psychosocial Effects—cont'd

Drug (Generic and Trade Name); Route and Dosage	Action/Indication	Common Side Effects and Nursing Considerations
SERTRALINE (Zoloft) **ROUTE:** PO **DOSAGE:** 50 mg/day as a single morning dose; may increase at weekly intervals for a maximum 200 mg/day	Antianxiety drug used in treatment of depression	Headache, dizziness, tremor, insomnia, drowsiness, fatigue, dry mouth, nausea, diarrhea, male sexual dysfunction, and increased sweating; potentially fatal reaction with MAO inhibitors; use with caution in elderly and renal or hepatic dysfunction
TRANYLCYPROMINE (Parnate) **ROUTE:** PO **DOSAGE:** 30 mg/day initially in single or divided doses; after 2 weeks can increase by 10 mg/day, up to maximum dose of 60 mg/day	Monamine oxidase inhibitor (MAO) used in treatment of neurotic or atypical depression	Restlessness, insomnia, dizziness, headache, blurred vision, orthostatic hypotension, arrhythmias, constipation, anorexia, nausea, vomiting, diarrhea, abdominal pain, and dry mouth; must watch for multiple drug reactions that could cause hypertensive crisis; foods containing tyramine (cheese, sour cream, beer, yogurt) can cause fatal hypertensive crisis; chocolate and caffeine can elevate BP

tension, tachycardia, diaphoresis, muscle rigidity, tremors, decreased consciousness, and incontinence may occur. Extrapyramidial symptoms and mental status changes may also be present. Neuroleptic malignant syndrome is a medical emergency, and the care delivered depends on the patient's symptoms. The neuroleptic drug should be discontinued immediately, and recovery may take 5 to 7 days.

NURSE ALERT

A sudden elevation in temperature, increased vital signs, diaphoresis, muscle rigidity, tremors, and an altered state of consciousness may herald neuroleptic malignant syndrome. This is a severe medical emergency that can occur in people who are taking antipsychotic drugs.

ELECTROCONVULSIVE THERAPY

Electroconvulsive therapy (ECT) is an effective treatment for patients with severe depression. Muscle relaxants, general anesthesia, and proper education before the administration of ECT have decreased fear of this treatment. The public's image of ECT as a mind-destroying, brutal, and indiscriminate therapy is gradually being replaced by the image of an effective therapy. Patients usually receive ECT three times per week for 2 to 4 weeks. They may experience temporary memory loss, learning loss, and confusion. Posttreatment nursing interventions help the patient perform routine and structured tasks and maintain adequate nutrition.

The goal of all treatments is to help people relieve their symptoms and learn new behaviors and different ways of relating to others. Some forms of psychotherapy can also help people to understand themselves better.

Nursing Care Plan

PATIENT WITH DEPRESSION

Marcus Overton is a 20-year-old college student who has been admitted to an acute inpatient psychiatric facility after an attempted suicide. He initiated hanging himself in his dorm room but halted it due to severe neck pain and a change of intent. A college professor noticed the markings on his neck and referred him to the Student Health Services, who recommended hospitalization.

Past History	Family History	Assessment Data
Marcus witnessed the violent deaths of both parents at a very young age and has recurring bouts of depression and feelings of hopelessness and helplessness. He recently has been struggling with college academics, has difficulty maintaining social relationships, and has feelings of profound apathy.	Marcus currently lives in a dorm on the campus of a large university. He is compatible with his roommate, but the two are not close friends. After his parents' death he lived with his grandparents, and he still lives there during summers and intersessions. He has one older sister who also was severely traumatized by the loss of her parents. Marcus has a close relationship with family members but has few close friends.	Thin, quiet, and withdrawn male Alert and oriented; responds appropriately to questions but has short answers Has flat affect and avoids eye contact Reports feeling inadequate in college and feels helpless regarding what to do Verbalizes difficulty concentrating due to hopelessness and constant reminders of loss of parents Acknowledges need for hospitalization and is interested in "getting better" Denies suicidal tendencies at present *Physical examination:* Within normal limits

NURSING DIAGNOSIS

Self-directed violence related to previous psychological trauma, low self-esteem, depression, and hopelessness

NURSING INTERVENTIONS	EVALUATION OF EXPECTED OUTCOMES
Explore suicidal thoughts and ideation. Provide safe environment and close supervision at all times. Develop contract that he will not act on impulse and harm himself. Encourage ventilation of feelings regarding previous loss and current difficulties. Encourage participation in individual and group therapy. Administer antidepressant medications as prescribed. Spend extra time when available and convey care and concern.	Participates in program to full extent No evidence of behavior that could harm self

continued

NURSING DIAGNOSIS

Hopelessness related to past trauma and current difficulties in college as evidenced by verbal comments such as "giving up" and "nothing to live for"

NURSING INTERVENTIONS	EVALUATION OF EXPECTED OUTCOMES
Assess for feelings such as hopelessness, lack of self-worth, and giving up. Assess for sources of hope, expectations of future, and social supports. Encourage and assist with physical care that communicates care, concern, and respect. Encourage expression of previous trauma and feelings of pessimism. Express hope for him appropriately and realistically. Help him to identify personal strengths, hopes, and future goals and to recognize accomplishments. Help him identify resources on campus that can help him with academics. Encourage and help him set realistic goals.	Recognizes personal strengths and accomplishments Expresses some optimism regarding the future

NURSING DIAGNOSIS

Social isolation related to withdrawn behavior, low self-esteem, and fear of failure as evidenced by lack of close friends, current hospitalization, and separation from environment

NURSING INTERVENTIONS	EVALUATION OF EXPECTED OUTCOMES
Assess involvement with staff, other patients, and family. Encourage relationships as appropriate and participation in activities. Provide positive reinforcement when interacting with others and participating in groups. Educate regarding social skills if indicated. Help him develop a plan to engage in social activities and pursue friendships of specific individuals after returning to school. This will enhance self-esteem. For example, encourage study groups, which will help academically and allow friendships to develop.	Recognizes need to be involved with others Identifies plan to get involved with activities

KEY CONCEPTS

- The successful completion of developmental stages and tasks helps the patient respond to physiologic illness.
- Broken-down defense mechanisms create aberrant behavior.
- Patients who are extremely angry and out of control are at risk for becoming violent.
- The most serious risk of depression is suicide.
- Psychotic patients exhibit irrational behavior because their thinking pattern is irrational.

CRITICAL THINKING EXERCISES

1. Why should a nurse who is planning to work in a medical-surgical area study psychology?
2. What are motivating factors in a person's life?
3. When does the use of defense mechanisms become pathologic?
4. How do somatic disorders differ from emotional, psychotic, personality, and anxiety disorders?
5. How does one use interpersonal relationships with patients as therapeutic tools?

REFERENCES AND ADDITIONAL READINGS

American Psychiatric Association: *Diagnostic and statistical manual of mental disorders,* ed 4, Washington, DC, 1994, The Association.

Buckwalter KC, Abraham IL: Alleviating the discharge crisis: the effects of a cognitive-behavioral nursing intervention for depressed patients and their families, *Arch Psychiatr Nurs* 1(5):350-358, 1987.

Castner E: Dealing with the "difficult patient," *J Pract Nurs* 32:30, 1992.

Collier S: Mrs. Hixon was more than "the C.V.A. in 251," *Nursing* 22(5):62-64, 1992.

Daley DC, Bowler K, Cahalane H: Approaches to patient and family education with affective disorders, *Patient Educ Couns* 19(2):163-174, 1992.

English J, Morse JM: The "difficult" elderly patient: adjustment or maladjustment? *Int J Nurs Stud* 25(1):23-39, 1988.

Field WE, Jr: Hearing voices, *J Psychosoc Nurs Ment Health Serv* 23(1):8-14, 1988.

Glasser W: *Mental health or illness: psychiatry for practical action,* New York, 1970, Harper & Row.

Gulesserian B, Warren CJ: Coping resources of depressed patients, *Arch Psychiatr Nurs* 1(6):392-398, 1987.

Hebert CP, Seifert MH, Jr: When the patient is a problem . . . managing the difficult patient, *Patient Care* 24(1):59-62; 64-66; 69-71, 1990.

Hirst SP: Understanding the difficult patient, *Nurs Manage* 14(2):68-70, 1983.

Jezierski M: Profile for depression, *JEN* 20(1):80-81, 1994.

Jones CP: Mr. Webb had a few reasonable requests, *Nursing* 22(1):60-62, 1992.

Kerr NJ: Signs and symptoms of depression and principles of nursing intervention, *Perspect Psychiatr Care* 24(2):48-63, 1988.

Linquist D: Frankie was never satisfied . . . until she made a new connection with life, *Nursing* 22(7):60-62, 1992.

McDonald S: An ethical dilemma: risk versus responsibility, *J Psychosoc Nurs Ment Health Serv* 32(1):19-25; 40-41, 1994.

McEnany GW: Psychobiological indices of bipolar mood disorder: future trends in nursing care, *Arch Psychiatr Nurs* 4(1):29-38, 1990.

Morgan AJ, Johnston MK: *Mental health and mental illness,* ed 2, 1976, JB Lippincott.

Nehls N: Brief hospital treatment plans: innovations in practice and research, *Issues Ment Health Nurs* 15(1):1-11, 1994.

Paiva Z: Sundown syndrome: calming the agitated patient, *RN* 53(7):50-51, 1990.

Petersen S: Dealing with the difficult patient-family and remaining sane, *Caring* 9(11):23-25, 1990.

Piccinino S: The nursing care challenge: borderline patients, *J Psychosoc Nurs Ment Health Serv* 28(4):22-27, 40-41, 1990.

Platt-Koch LM: Borderline personality disorder: a therapeutic approach, *Am J Nurs* 83(12):1666-1671, 1983.

Reed SA: Specific strategies: interventions for identified problem behaviors, *Nurse Managers' Bookshelf* 2(4):65-76, 1990.

Stafford LL: Dissociation multiple personality disorder: a challenge for psychosocial nurses, *J Psychosoc Nurs Ment Health Serv* 31(1):15-20; 30-31, 1993.

Stolley MM: When your patient has Alzheimer's disease, *Am J Nurs* 94(8): 34-41, 1994.

Stuart GW, Sundeen SJ: *Principles and practices of psychiatric nursing,* ed 5, St Louis, 1995, Mosby.

Wandal JC, Prince MR: Case studies . . . the care of patients with behavioral problems (including commentary by Mian P, Danis D), *J Prof Nurs* 7(2):126-135, 1991.

Whall AL: What is nursing treatment for depression? *J Gerontol Nurs* 20(1):42, 45, 1994.

CHAPTER 4

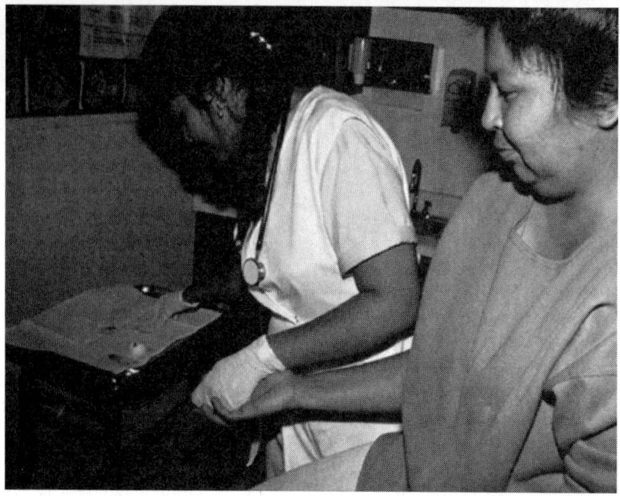

Cultural Considerations

CHAPTER OBJECTIVES

1 Gain beginning insight and skills into the delivery of culturally congruent nursing care.
2 Explain what culture is and is not.
3 Identify the differences between cultural customs, beliefs, and values.
4 Analyze own personal attitudes and values about common cultural concepts.
5 Identify the purpose of the field of transcultural nursing.
6 List two errors a nurse can make concerning patients who may be using alternative, nonconventional therapies.
7 Identify the three components of the transcultural triad.
8 Demonstrate the ability to use Leininger's three modes of nursing care decisions and actions.

KEY WORDS

beliefs
cultural blindness
cultural conflict
cultural imposition
cultural relativity
culture
customs
ethnocentrism
monochronic time
polychronic time
stereotyping
subculture
sync time
transcultural nursing
values

It is hard to believe that, for more than 100 years after the birth of modern nursing with Florence Nightingale around 1860, the culture of patients was ignored. Dr. Madeleine Leininger, the first nurse to earn a doctorate in anthropology, began a lifelong crusade to change the status quo. Leininger's first book *Nursing and Anthropology: Two Worlds to Blend* (1970) awakened the profession of nursing about the relevance of **culture** to beliefs regarding the causes and cures of illness and the cultural caring practices people expect when they are sick. It is now widely recognized that culture is a significant component of nursing care, but not all nurses know what *culturally congruent* nursing care is or how to provide it (Leininger, 1994). This chapter provides beginning insight into the delivery of culturally congruent nursing care.

THE PHENOMENON OF CULTURE

What Culture Is

When one thinks about culture, one often only visualizes people who live in distant exotic places and who behave in ways thought of as different and perhaps even strange or backward. However, culture is also the fabric of life. Every human being belongs to a culture.

Culture has been defined as values, beliefs, attitudes, and customs that are shared by a group and passed from one generation to the next (Potter, 1993). Culture can be compared to an old pair of shoes; one does not think about them but just wears them comfortably day after day. Only when one puts on a brand new pair of shoes (or is confronted with different cultural patterns) does one become uncomfortable.

Boyle and Andrews (1989) describe four essential characteristics of culture. First, as the definition of culture clearly implies, it is *learned* and transmitted. People begin learning their own culture from birth. Some who practice the Islamic faith whisper into the newborn's ear so that the first words he or she hears are from the Koran, the holy scriptures. Role relationships are part of culture. One may believe that the term *brother* means a biologic sibling born of the same set of parents. However, black/African Americans may have a different meaning and define brother or "bro" as any black/African American man. Other people may define a brother as any male first cousin on the maternal side of the family or even anyone who was breast-fed by the same woman. It soon becomes apparent that there are more cultural differences than there are similarities among the people of the world (Leininger, 1991). A patient may completely misinterpret a nurse's very simple question about the patient's brothers. Therefore to avoid misinterpretation, the nurse should be aware of these differences and clarify the meaning of the term with the client.

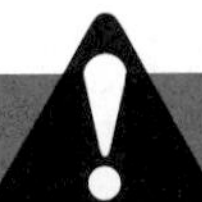

NURSE ALERT

Patients may misinterpret questions because of cultural definitions of words or phrases. Be sure the meaning of questions is clear to the patient.

Second, culture is *shared*. Members of the same group share culture both consciously and subconsciously. One may remember hearing as a child consciously shared rules such as, "Share your toys with your sister!" or "You can't have dessert until you eat your vegetables!" However, one probably does not remember learning that "baby boys don't wear the color pink." Such an idea was probably subconsciously transmitted. For most Americans it is culturally unacceptable for men to wear dresses. However, for people of Scottish heritage the skirt (kilt) is a symbol of pride and clan identity. In the Catholic religion priests wear cassocks that look like floor-length dresses. This sharing of common practices provides each group with part of its cultural identity. These exceptions to a so-called norm are culturally acceptable to most people, even if they do not belong to the group, often because these practices are widely recognized as a way of proclaiming who or what a person is.

Third, culture is an *adaptation* to one's environment that reflects the specific conditions and natural resources available to groups of people. For example, building homes with wide open spaces in the outer walls instead of covered doors and windows would not be appropriate for the environmental conditions of cold northern climates. "Kangaroo care," a relatively new strategy that began in Bogota, Colombia, is a means of survival for some low-birth-weight infants who are born into cultures where high-tech equipment, such as an incubator, is unavailable. In kangaroo care the mother and father serve as human incubators, like the kangaroo, which keeps its offspring warm in its pouch (Whitelaw, 1988). The mother holds the infant vertically between her breasts in skin-to-skin contact for as much time as possible. This cultural adaptation has been so successful that developed countries, including the United States, are adopting it along with high technology.

Fourth, culture is a *dynamic* and ever-changing process. Cultures do change, but they change slowly in response to the conditions and needs of the group. Not too long ago the United States was known as a "throw-away" society. Disposable needles and syringes replaced metal and glass ones, styrofoam dishes and containers and plastic eating utensils replaced reusable ones, and disposable diapers replaced cloth ones. However, that throw-away attitude is slowly changing as Americans become more aware of and responsive to the limited resources of the environment and the damage created by the reckless use of these finite resources. In many cultures the roles of both men and women are changing. The idea of the man as the sole wage earner and the woman as the homemaker and childrearer is no longer the norm, and people are exploring alternative patterns of behavior that fit better with their needs and beliefs. The nursing profession in America is equally slow in changing and is still perceived as a female profession. Although every nurse belongs to a larger culture, nurses share many norms, values, and practices that make them a distinct group known as **subculture** (Leininger, 1970). No culture can ultimately survive without being dynamic and adaptable to a changing world.

What Culture Is Not

The characteristics one acquires through genetics is not culture. Racial and biologic characteristics and variations are also part of the genetic legacy. When one member of a cultural group displays unique behaviors that are not common to the group, it is not a cultural characteristic. Just as there are more differences than similarities among cultures, so there are differences among individuals within one cultural group.

Common Concepts

When a nurse cares for a patient from a given culture and assumes that the patient will behave in exactly the same way as everyone else in that culture, he or she is **stereotyping.** Stereotyping prevents the nurse from performing an individualized assessment of the patient's potential differences. During her research with Mexican-American clinic patients, Shellenberger (1987) found that patients also stereotyped nurses. After interviewing her subjects about their healthcare practices, she noticed that no one had mentioned folk practices. She returned to interview them again and was told that they had not talked about their cultural health practices because they thought an Anglo nurse would not be interested in hearing about them. However, unlike stereotyping, generalizing about the commonalities clients from a certain cultue often hold increases a nurse's knowledge about that culture. Generalizing serves as a starting point for an individualized assessment of which cultural commonalities each individual client believes and practices and which he or she does not (Galanti, 1991; Geissler, 1994).

Almost everyone has been guilty at some time of harboring the **ethnocentric** attitude that one's own culture is the best one. Comparative judgments are made with other cultures that result in the conclusion that one's own culture is the only one that is normal and natural (Stewart, 1991). The opposite of ethnocentrism is **cultural relativity.** The nurse who approaches clients from the perspective of cultural relativity is open to the characteristics of culture and the wide variety of beliefs and practices that may result from being reared in different environments with different societal needs. According to Tripp-Reimer (1984), "the caregiver would attempt to understand the behavior of transcultural clients within the context of the clients' own culture" (p. 229).

Cultural Customs, Beliefs, and Values

Cultural customs, beliefs, and values are the building blocks of all cultures. Although it is impossible for any nurse to know about all of the thousands of cultures in the world, it is essential to learn about a few of the cultures that are encountered frequently in nursing. **Customs** are the easiest to learn and recognize because they are often easily seen. Customs are habitual practices, or the usual way of acting under certain circumstances. When a patient wears a string of special blue beads around his or her wrist, when a patient does not look anyone directly in the eye when spoken to, when a woman cannot sign a consent form because she is a woman, when a man resists having his body hair shaved before a surgical procedure, or when a woman refuses to bathe after giving birth, deeply rooted cultural customs are being demonstrated. **Beliefs,** or norms, are the rules that guide human behavior (Leininger, 1978). The rules tell a person what is appropriate or inappropriate behavior in a given situation or circumstance. Beliefs are more difficult to assess because they cannot be directly observed, but they can be learned by asking the right kind of questions, such as, "What do *you* think caused this problem you're having now?" Some of the more common answers may include familiar western biomedical explanations; or the problem may be explained as a punishment from God for a self-perceived transgression, as a loss of harmony or balance within the body, or as a hex cast on the patient either purposely or inadvertently by another person. Patients often believe that the cause of an illness dictates the type of treatment. Western biomedical caregivers cannot cure a magico-religious type of problem. Special help is sought from a folk practitioner who is knowledgeable about the cause of and cure for these special problems.

Values are "goals to which behavior is directed (Boyle, 1989, p.14)." Values are within the realm of the unconscious mind, and an individual may not even realize that he or she holds them. Therefore they are the most difficult to assess. Kluckholn (1953) conceptualized several options that different cultures commonly hold about the basic values of life. For example, one may be asked, "What is your basic value about the environment? Do you believe that the environment controls *you* or that you should live and coexist in harmony with the environment? Do you believe that man controls the environment?" One may wonder, "Do I just think that's the way it should be, or do my behaviors demonstrate my belief?" One may also be asked, "What do you believe about your relationship to others? Do you believe that it is an ordered succession with a continuity that is based primarily on heredity and kinship, that the family as a group is more important than any individual within it, or that independence and autonomy of the individual are paramount?" People differ in their views about health and illness. One person may believe that health is the result of choices and actions, another may believe that it is an inevitable balance of sickness and health throughout life, and another may believe that illness is sent by God or some supernatural force as punishment for wrongdoing. Such values have a subtle yet tremendous impact on patients' motivations and reactions to healthcare.

When a nurse and a patient and family believe and behave according to different values, beliefs, and customs, a **cultural conflict** can result. Figure 4-1 shows two icebergs. One iceberg represents the nurse, and the second iceberg represents the patient. Customs reside near the tip of the icebergs and above the waterline where they can be observed, acknowledged, and dealt with. Beliefs are close to the waterline and may or may not be observable. The greatest difficulty lies in the conflicting values, which are hidden well below the waterline. When these two icebergs collide, the collision is felt at this deepest level, where the impact actually occurs.

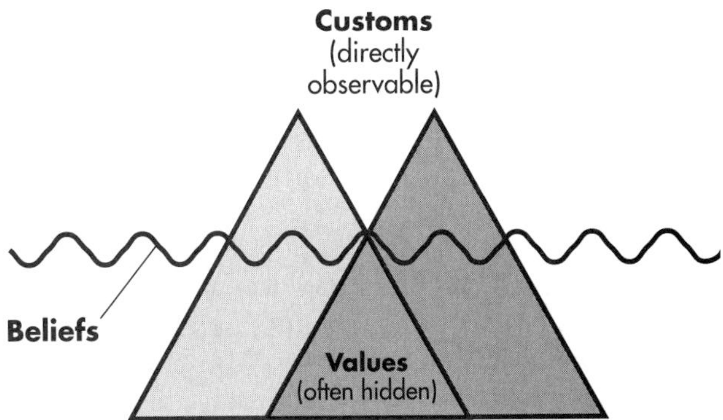

Figure 4-1 One iceberg symbolizes the nurse's cultural customs, beliefs, and values and the second iceberg symbolizes those of the patient and family. Cultural conflict may occur at any level but is most serious when deeply held and hidden values clash below the observable waterline and are not recognized by the participants.

TRANSCULTURAL NURSING

The field of **transcultural nursing** is a formal area of study and practice that was conceived by Leininger in the mid-1950s. Leininger (1978) defined transcultural nursing as "the area of nursing which focuses upon the comparative study and analysis of different cultures and subcultures with respect to nursing and health-illness caring practices, beliefs, and values with the goal of generating scientific and humanistic knowledge, and of using this knowledge to provide culture-specific and culture-universal nursing care practices" (p. 33). Since the 1960s, courses and programs have been established by nurse leaders who are trained in anthropology and transcultural nursing. The Transcultural Nursing Society was founded in 1974 as a worldwide organization for nurses interested in and prepared to advance transcultural nursing. The Society serves as a forum to bring nurses with common and diverse interests together to improve care to culturally diverse people. The *Journal of Transcultural Nursing,* founded in 1989, is focused on transcultural nursing theory, research, and practice. Since 1989, nurses have been certified as transcultural nurses (TCNs) (Transcultural Nursing Society).

Alternative Therapies

The *New England Journal of Medicine* reports that in 1990 one out of every three Americans, an estimated 61 million people, used alternative nontraditional therapies for problems such as cancer, arthritis, chronic back pain, AIDS, gastrointestinal problems, chronic renal failure, and eating disorders (Eisenberg, 1993). Of the various therapies studied, relaxation techniques, chiropractic care, and massage were most frequently used. The estimated number of visits to providers of these modalities was greater than the total number of visits to traditional Western physicians during the same year. These data become even more significant because the study did not include visits to herbalists, curanderas, medicine men and women, or other important folk practitioners. The message is clear. Large numbers of Americans are consulting nontraditional healthcare practitioners. Some people may use and combine nontraditional therapies with the biomedical regimens prescribed by their physicians. Other people may elope from the healthcare system because they are dissatisfied with the results obtained from Western medicine and want to seek help from folk practitioners. The nurse can make two serious errors regarding patients who may be using alternative therapies. The first error is failing to ask about alternative therapies that the patient may be using concurrently so that the effects of interaction between the two systems can be evaluated. The second error is assuming that the patient who has not kept Western appointments or sought Western treatments, has received no healthcare during this time. A nurse with an education in transcultural nursing can be a valuable resource when assessing, planning, and evaluating nursing care in situations involving culturally diverse patients.

The Transcultural Triad

The American Nurses Association position statement on cultural diversity in nursing practice identifies three interacting systems in nurse-patient encounters. They are "the culture of the nurse, the culture of the patient and the culture of the setting" (American Nurses Association, 1991, p. 1). The patient is not the only person in the nurse-patient relationship. Nurses bring their own customs, beliefs, and values into this *transcultural triadic relationship.* The nurse who understands the particular culture of a patient may still be missing part of the equation. Understanding self is the starting point for understanding the culturally diverse patient. When the two icebergs meet below the waterline, the nurse will be unable to fully understand why cultural conflict is occurring unless the nurse's own subconscious cultural behaviors are also recognized. Without cultural self-understanding, the nurse's negative reactions to cultural conflict may include ethnocentrism and stereotyping or **cultural blindness** and **cultural imposition.**

Cultural blindness occurs when the nurse ignores the differences of the patient and proceeds to give care as if the differences do not exist. Cultural blindness is a sign of ignorance to differences of cultural expression. Cultural imposition is closely tied to ethnocentrism. It occurs when the nurse expects the patient to conform to the cultural norms of the nurse and the hospital or healthcare agency. The nurse may be thinking, "You're here in my hospital, and you'll just have to do things our way." Such a negative reaction can create breakdowns in nurse-patient communication, the nurse-patient relationship, and even in patient compliance because of the patient's feelings of loss of trust and security. Some hospitals ask patients who are about to be discharged to fill out a questionnaire rating their satisfaction with the care they received during their hospitalization. Although patients may have received very high quality nursing care, some may respond that they are dissatisfied. One reason may be that their cultural needs have not been recognized and met.

The third part of the triad is the often bureaucratic healthcare setting with which the patient/family must interact and from which conformity with its norms may be expected. Some people believe that vigilance over their sick relative is a prescribed extended family role. Hospital rules that restrict visitors in an intensive care unit to two people for 15 minutes every hour are difficult to deal with. When a small waiting room becomes so full that other patients' families are complaining about not having a place to sit because of the presence of so many extended family members for one patient, the nurse becomes involved.

Nursing Care Decisions and Actions

Leininger's theory of cultural care diversity and universality offers three nursing strategies, called modes of action or decision, that guide nurses in providing culturally congruent care (Reynolds, 1993). These modes of action originate from the premise that "cultures have folk and professional care values, beliefs, and practices in Western and non-Western cultures" (Leininger, 1988, p. 155). Elements of two different health systems may be in operation at one time. The nurse is operating under a professional system that is influencing the nurse's decisions and actions. At the same time, a culturally diverse patient may be operating, at least in part, under a folk system that is guiding his or her decisions and actions. The potential for conflict between the two systems exists. To avoid conflict and to make decisions that result in more culturally congruent care, the nurse gathers information from the patient and family regarding the customs, beliefs, and values that are relevant to health promotion, health maintenance, or health restoration within the circumstances the patient is experiencing. The nurse then identifies one of the following modes of action that minimize cultural conflict and benefit the patient's needs:

1 "Cultural care preservation or maintenance refers to those assistive, supportive, or enabling professional actions and decisions that help clients of a particular culture to preserve or maintain a state of health or to recover from illness and to face death" (Leininger, 1988, p. 156).

For example, an East Asian female patient who has no dietary restrictions wants her family to bring her an herbal tea that she always uses to calm her "nervous stomach." The nurse asks what is in the tea and learns that it contains nothing that would be contraindicated with her medications. Her family is encouraged to bring the tea. The decision and mode of action are not harmful to the patient, and in her opinion may be beneficial. The worst that could happen is that the tea is medically neutral (i.e., neither harmful nor helpful). From the patient's point of view it is important that her cultural belief has been preserved.

2 "Cultural care accommodation or negotiation refers to those assistive, supporting, or enabling professional actions and decisions that help clients of a particular culture to adapt to or negotiate for a beneficial or satisfying health status or to face death" (Leininger, 1988, p. 156).

Either the patient, the hospital, or both may need to accommodate in this mode. A classic example of unknown origin concerns a hospitalized and dying gypsy king. The king's culture believed that he should die on the ground, but it was very cold outside and there was snow on the ground. Two solutions could resolve this dilemma: (1) close to death, the king would be placed on the floor beside his hospital bed; or (2) a long rope would be brought in, one end placed in the king's hand, and the other end of the rope lowered through an open window until it touched the ground outside. Either of these creative solutions would meet the patient's needs in a culturally satisfying way.

3 "Cultural care repatterning or restructuring refers to those assistive, supportive, or enabling professional actions or decisions that help patients change their lifeways for new or different patterns that are culturally meaningful and satisfying or that support beneficial and healthy life patterns" (Leininger, 1988, p. 156).

Nurses may be faced with situations in which they understand the patient's cultural belief but also believe that they cannot professionally or ethically support or negotiate the practice because it will be harmful to the patient. For example, some mothers believe that they should stop giving a baby fluids when the baby gets diarrhea. The nurse cannot preserve this belief, nor can the nurse negotiate that the mother only give the child half the fluids it so desperately needs. Both are potentially life-threatening alternatives. In a respectful and nonthreatening way, the nurse tries to work with the mother to restructure this aspect of her belief system. Perhaps there are one or two appropriate and culturally preferred fluids that the mother may be willing to give the child, or the mother may be willing to be taught to make an oral rehydration mixture from home ingredients as a special "medicine" for her child (Figure 4-2) (Werner, 1992).

CULTURAL VARIABILITY

In addition to cultural variations that involve healthcare beliefs and practices, there are variations in everyday behaviors to which little or no conscious thought is given (Figure 4-3). Being aware of such differences in nurse-patient interactions is essential for effective interpersonal interactions, the development of respect and trust between individuals, and the patient's satisfaction with the self-perceived quality of nursing care.

Perceptions of Time

Perception of time is one of the core values of culture. People are controlled by time and usually believe that everyone else perceives time in exactly the same way. However, there are many different perceptions of time. Anthropologist Edward T. Hall (1983) has extensively researched people's perceptions of time, and three forms are particularly relevant to nursing care.

Monochronic time is a form of time perception that is very familiar to many Americans (Hall, 1983). Time is linear and is clearly divided into yesterday, today, and tomorrow. People develop lists of priorities and concentrate on getting one thing done before moving on to the next. People often keep personal schedule books to organize their daily or weekly activities. Time is treated as a physical commodity that can be bought and sold. People who perceive time as monochronic speak about time that is spent, saved, killed, lost, wasted, or made up, and they use many other descriptive words that are usually used to refer to tangible objects. The primary goal for people with this perception of time is to get tasks done. As with all components of culture, this perception of time is arbitrary, learned, and transmitted from our early caregivers. It is neither

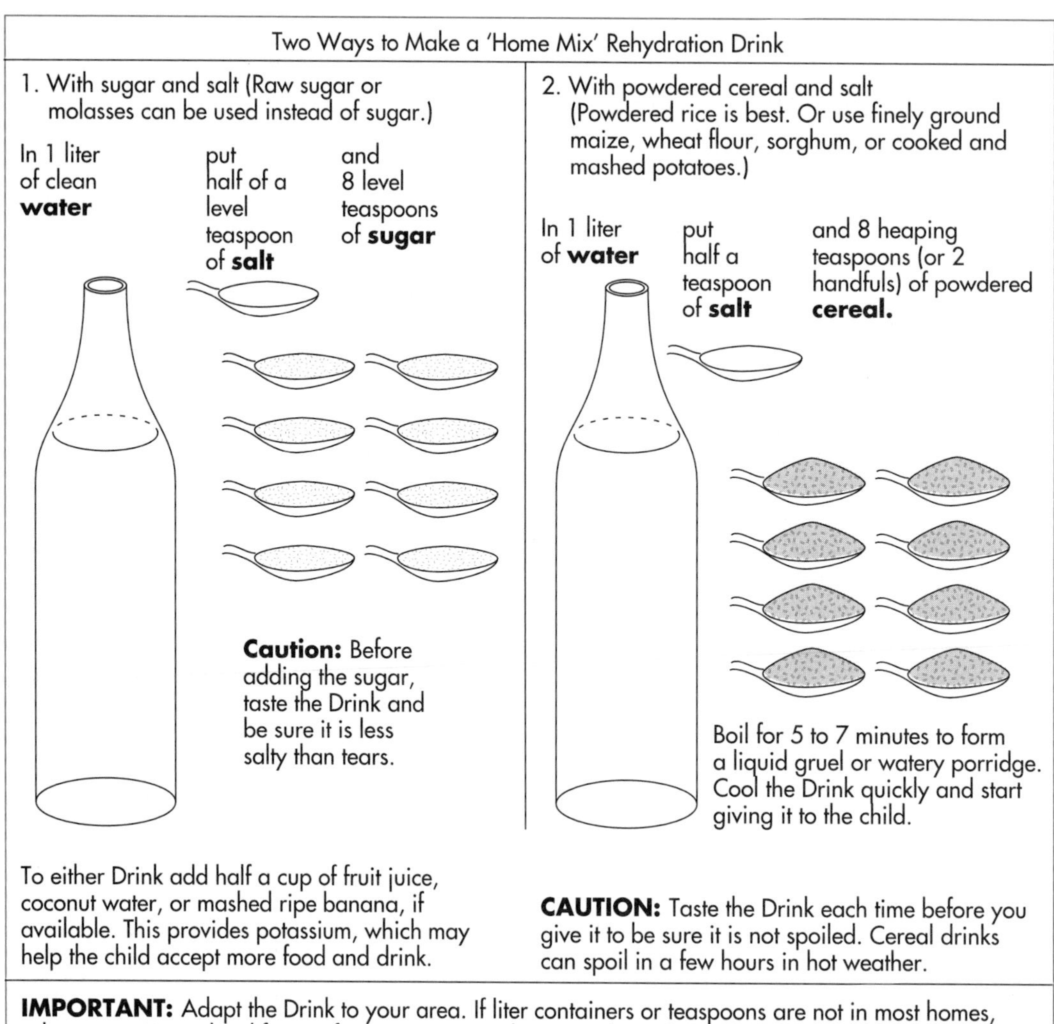

Two Ways to Make a 'Home Mix' Rehydration Drink
1. With sugar and salt (Raw sugar or molasses can be used instead of sugar.)
In 1 liter of clean **water**
put half of a level teaspoon of **salt**
and 8 level teaspoons of **sugar**
Caution: Before adding the sugar, taste the Drink and be sure it is less salty than tears.
2. With powdered cereal and salt (Powdered rice is best. Or use finely ground maize, wheat flour, sorghum, or cooked and mashed potatoes.)
In 1 liter of **water**
put half a teaspoon of **salt**
and 8 heaping teaspoons (or 2 handfuls) of powdered **cereal.**
Boil for 5 to 7 minutes to form a liquid gruel or watery porridge. Cool the Drink quickly and start giving it to the child.
To either Drink add half a cup of fruit juice, coconut water, or mashed ripe banana, if available. This provides potassium, which may help the child accept more food and drink.
CAUTION: Taste the Drink each time before you give it to be sure it is not spoiled. Cereal drinks can spoil in a few hours in hot weather.
IMPORTANT: Adapt the Drink to your area. If liter containers or teaspoons are not in most homes, adjust quantities to local forms of measurement. Where people traditionally give cereal gruels to young children, add enough water to make it liquid, and use that. Look for an easy and simple way.

Give the dehydrated person sips of this Drink every 5 minutes, day and night, until he or she begins to urinate normally. A large person needs 3 or more liters a day. A small child usually needs at least 1 liter a day, or 1 glass for each watery stool. Keep giving the Drink *often* in small sips, *even if the person vomits.* Not all of the Drink will be vomited.

Figure 4-2 A homemade or commercial oral rehydration mixture is an internationally recognized and potentially life-saving method for treating dehydration. (From Werner D: *Where there is no doctor,* Palo Alto, Calif, 1992, Hesperian Foundation.)

correct nor incorrect but is just how some people view time. When the nurse says to a patient, "I'll be back in 15 minutes," the patient with a monochronic time view expects the nurse to reappear within approximately 15 minutes, not an hour later. The patient gets more annoyed as more and more time passes and the nurse does not return. Nurses react the same way when the situation is reversed.

People sharing **polychronic** perceptions of time do not behave in a linear way. They prefer to be involved in and interacting with several people or things simultaneously. Schedules, if written at all, are not firm, and plans may be changed at the last second. Rather than focusing on tasks and what should come next, those with polychronic perceptions focus on people and relationships. Caring about interruptions in human relationships has a much higher priority. For such people it is much more important to stop and chat than it is to break off a conversation just to be on time for an appointment. These people do not constantly look at the clock. Some Latin American, Middle Eastern, and Mediterranean Sea area cultures value this less rigid, nonlinear perception of time (Hall, 1983). Patients may miss or be late for clinic appointments for many rea-

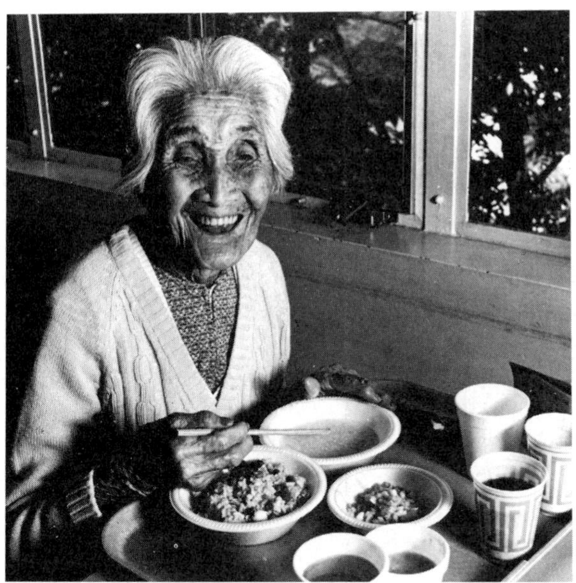

Figure 4-3 Oriental food and chopsticks make an enjoyable meal for this older Japanese woman. (Courtesy Ken Yamaguchi. From Castillo HM: *The nurse assistant in long-term care: a rehabilitative approach, St Louis, 1992, Mosby.)*

sons, including difficulties traveling to the clinic or in finding a responsible adult for child care, but another possibility is that the patient may be following a polychronic perception of time. The nurse may evaluate the late patient negatively, when in fact the patient is simply placing a higher value on people than on a bureaucractic and often rigid time schedule.

Sync (for synchrony) **time** is a form of time perception that has not been as widely researched but can be very significant in patient interactions. According to Hall (1983), greater awareness of sync time began when silent movies started to have soundtracks and it became necessary to synchronize the soundtrack with the moving pictures. Hall (1983) states that, "though it took the white man thousands of years to discover "sync time," the Mescalero Apaches have known its significance for centuries" (p. 25). Rhythm is the basic ingredient of synchrony and is an indispensable factor in nurse-patient relationships. Imagine a hospitalized patient who has been lying very quietly in bed for several hours. Suddenly a nurse who has been very busy running around the unit enters this patient's room and says, "I need to get you out of bed for a little walk once more before I go off duty in a few minutes. Are these your slippers? Where's your bathrobe? Do you want to use the bathroom while you're up?" At the same time the nurse is lowering the head of the bed and pulling down the patient's bedcovers. Nurse and patient are completely out of sync! To the patient, the nurse is trying to make him or her move at the speed of light, and to the nurse, the patient is not moving fast enough to accomplish this task in the time available. The entire mismatch can be avoided if the nurse lets the patient know in advance what is going to happen and gives the patient a chance to prepare mentally and physically and if the nurse recognizes the importance of being in sync with the patient on middle ground. The probable result is that the ambulation time will be more successful and satisfying for both. Hall (1983) credits the Japanese with a much higher recognition of the impact of synchrony and gives the example of a sumo wrestling match in which the referee will not allow a match to start until the two wrestlers synchronize their breathing. Nurses need to learn to become referees during the many nursing care interactions and interventions that are impacted by sync time.

For 15 years Levine (1990) researched people's attitudes toward time and the tempo of cultures, as well as the health consequences of each. The research was conducted in nine cities in each of the four regions of the United States. Results indicated that the pace of life is faster in the Northeast, followed by the Midwest, the South, and the West. There was a significant relationship between the pace of life, the rate of cigarette smoking, and death from ischemic heart disease. The same study was also conducted in six countries with Eastern and Western cultures and varying degrees of economic development. The fastest pace was measured in Japan, followed by the United States, England, Taiwan, Italy, and Indonesia. Therefore self-selection of a fast-track versus a slow-track pace of life can be one indicator of the environmental dimension of culture.

Use of Space

Hall (1966) coined the word *proxemics* to describe the study of people's use of social and personal space as a cultural phenomenon and nonverbal communication pattern. Within different cultures rather precise distances are considered appropriate or inappropriate and often depend on the role between individuals and the closeness of their social relationship. Breaking the unwritten and unspoken rules of culturally learned spatial distances can be very stressful. A number of body organs and receptors are involved in the use of space. Seeing, hearing, smelling, heat gain and loss, and touch are important barometers that determine the range of space that one finds comfortable in a variety of different situations. For example, being close enough to breathe on one another is a common behavior among many Arab cultures, whereas being close enough to detect body odor is avoided in other cultures (Hall, 1966). In some cultures being close enough to touch frequently is a vital component of communication, whereas in other cultures people stand in a crowded elevator with arms pressed in close to the body to avoid touching and feel relieved when some people exit the elevator and make more space available for their body.

Hall (1966) classifies the space envelopes, or protective personal invisible bubbles of space, into four general ranges. *Intimate space* is 6 to 18 inches and involves smell, heat, the feel of the other's breath, and distorted sight. In *personal space,* 18 inches to 4 feet, the visual distortion lessens, but one must still shift the gaze by looking into one eye at a time. Body heat is not detectable, but even at its farthest distance people can still touch each other at arm's length. Personal discussions occur within this range, and individual cultures determine the amount of closeness needed for satisfying communication to occur. *Social space,* from 4 to 12 feet, is often used for less personal business or social interactions. At its farther distances, the entire face can be taken in at a glance, and shifting from one eye to the other is not needed. Finally, *public space* is more than 12 feet and causes significant changes in one's behaviors. At this distance people are more careful of their choice of words; and phrasing, grammar, and syntax are calculated to serve a more "speech-making" type of interaction.

A family member or professional colleague may approach a nurse at the nurse's station, and the nurse may take small backward steps because the person seems to be moving too closely into the protective space bubble. As the nurse moves backward, the person moves in to close the gap because he or she is becoming uncomfortable with the distance. Americans use the phrase, "Get out of my face," to express the discomfort experienced with this degree of closeness. The nurse may perceive this family member or colleague as pushy, aggressive, demanding, or intrusive. In contrast, the other person may be perceiving the nurse as uncaring, cold, aloof, or disinterested. Communication is breaking down on a subconscious nonverbal level, regardless of how effectively the verbal words are being exchanged. Both parties come away dissatisfied and may not know why they feel as they do. However, the dissatisfaction may simply have been a result of the differences in cultural perceptions of space.

Each space category has both close and distant ranges that alter behavior and may overlap. For example, does the change of shift report occur in personal or social space? The size of the group, the size of the room, the presence of physical barriers such as a rectangular table around which everyone is seated, and how well the participants get along all mandate, or at least influence, the use of space. The rules may also be changed to accommodate the role of the individual. For example, a nurse must frequently enter into a patient's intimate or personal space during nursing care activities. For some patients this may be acceptable, but for others the nurse should be aware that permission may be needed for such necessary closeness. For example, during a female urinary catheterization a nurse might say to a patient, "I'm going to have to get really close to be able to see clearly the small hole where I need to insert this catheter. The better I can see, the more comfortable I can make this for you." As with all cultural variations, the use of space varies both among and within different cultural groups (Dolphin, 1994).

Use of Touch

As with space, there is considerable variation in the unspoken rules of and rather precise limits on the use of touch. The appropriateness of touch is determined by several variables, including duration, location, intensity, frequency, action, and the sensation conveyed. Touch must also be situationally appropriate. In the United States touch is believed to be an important part of nursing care. Lack of knowledge about the reaction of a specific culture to touch may inhibit the nurse-patient interaction and even cause fear. In the Vietnamese culture the head is considered to be the seat of the soul. Touching and performing invasive procedures on the head or in the various openings of the head may be highly stressful because of the fear that the soul may be lost (Geissler, 1994). Even placing on a pillow a piece of clothing that is worn on the lower body may be objectionable to some Southeast Asian patients. People of English, German, or Japanese heritage may prefer minimal touching during interactions, whereas Hispanics and Arabs may prefer more touching.

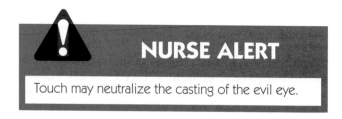

Touch may neutralize the casting of the evil eye.

According to Spector (1991) the evil eye is one of the oldest and most common superstitions that exist in many cultures of the world. It is a common Hispanic belief. The evil eye may be cast to project harm on an object or a person when something, especially a child, is admired or criticized. There are many differing beliefs among people and among cultures regarding who can cast the evil eye, the purpose for which it is cast, how it is cast, the effect it has on the person receiving it, and the cultural practices used to protect against it. Nurses may inadvertently cast the evil eye. Touch is one practice that may neutralize or undo the casting of the evil eye (Giger, 1991). For example, when telling a mother that her child is pretty or handsome, the nurse should simultaneously touch the child.

Nurses may or may not touch people frequently as a result of cultural values that guide their behaviors. Sensitivity to both the nurse's and the patient's desire for and reaction to touch should be assessed to deliver culturally congruent care. Touch should never be forced on or withheld from patients who have different perceptions of its meaning and importance.

Eye Contact

People from other cultures such as Arab cultures, have such prolonged eye contact that they may seem confrontational to the uninitiated. Others, particularly the Navajo people and Asians, use less eye contact or the lighthouse sweep during interactions (Geissler, 1994). Downcast eyes may partly reflect respect for authority figures. Some people are sensitive to the physiologic changes that occur in the pupil of the eye during interactions. Pupils tend to dilate slightly when one is interested and constrict slightly with disagreement or disinterest (Geissler, 1994). Cultures that prefer a narrower space between individuals may also be cultures that use more prolonged direct eye contact and have the ability to evaluate changes in pupil size.

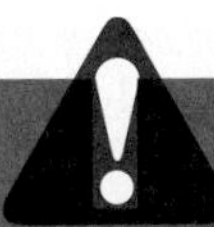

NURSE ALERT

The nurse may be perceived as an authority figure. Patients may believe that looking the nurse directly in the eye for a sustained period of time might challenge the nurse's authority and be considered unacceptable behavior.

Anglo-Americans use a moderate amount of direct eye contact during interactions. They are comfortable with some direct eye contact and may interpret a lack of eye contact as uncertainty, embarrassment, or even lying. These attitudes are reflected in the common phrase, "Now look me straight in the eye and tell me the truth." Yet Anglo-Americans are also comfortable with looking past the side of the face or away from the face. The former may be interpreted as "I'm thinking or considering what you are saying," and the latter, as long as it does not last very long, may be interpreted as a fleeting but acceptable momentary distraction. It is the total pattern that cultures find significant during an interaction rather than each discrete eye movement.

Time, space, touch, and eye contact are but a few examples of cultural variability. There are many other factors, including birth and death rites, reactions to pain, family dominance patterns, gender-specific roles, child-rearing beliefs and practices, communication patterns with authority figures such as healthcare professionals, and the family's role in hospital care. For example, some people from East Indian and Middle Eastern cultures insist on a professional caregiver of the same gender. Such restrictions should be honored whenever feasible by involving the family in care or by altering patient assignments. All of these factors play simultaneous roles within some cultures and help determine when and when not to use a particular variable. The patient or family is the best data source for the assessment of cultural differences and similarities. The nurse must be aware of potential differences that could be critical to the patient's responses to nursing care, health restoration, and health maintenance.

OLDER ADULT CONSIDERATIONS

Heritage Consistency

Some older adults may have immigrated to the United States many years or even decades ago. However, the nurse should not plan care under the potentially false assumption that these adults have integrated themselves into the American culture. In some American communities it is possible for older adults to shop at food stores, attend places of worship, communicate in their own language, attend social activities, and seek healthcare from traditional healers while remaining predominantly within the culture of their ethnic birthplace. Spector's *Heritage Assessment Tool* (1991) is a useful guide for assessing the extent to which an individual is engaged in a traditional lifestyle and planning appropriate nursing care.

NURSING DIAGNOSES

The use or misuse of nursing diagnoses with the culturally diverse patient has raised several questions in recent years (Leininger, 1990). Transcultural nursing recognizes that, regardless of a patient's medical diagnosis, it is important to plan nursing care that reflects the patient's own unique healthcare beliefs and practices. The official list of nursing diagnoses of the North American Nursing Diagnosis Association (NANDA) does not adequately address the cultural needs of patients (Geissler, 1992). Nursing diagnoses that have been used with patients include actual, high risk, or potential for spiritual distress, impaired verbal communication, social isolation, and noncompliance.

A few examples illustrate the problem. When a patient does not speak English, who has the actual problem with verbal communication? Is the patient or the nurse to blame when both are adequately fluent in their own languages? The problem is one of mutual understanding or lack of it, not the inability to communicate verbally. Patients with limited English skills can experience extreme stress when trying to communicate in English. It can be frustrating and exhausting to express oneself in such a circumstance, and the patient may never be sure that the message was understood accurately. The NANDA diagnosis is directed at verbal communication and does not address the critical role that nonverbal communication plays in human expression. Understanding nonverbal messages is very important to mutual understanding. The diagnosis of noncompliance implies that a patient has made an informed decision to comply or not comply, but for many the term *nonadherence* may be more acceptable. The term *compliance* implies that the patient must or should follow the medical and nursing regimens prescribed by the dominant healthcare system's practitioners. However, there are many valid ways of viewing health and illness. When a patient does not hold the same egocentric healthcare beliefs and values of the Western biomedical system, he or she may be falsely labeled as noncompliant. Therefore the nursing diagnosis of noncompliance can become a manifestation of the nurse's own culture, and a value conflict between the nurse and the patient may result.

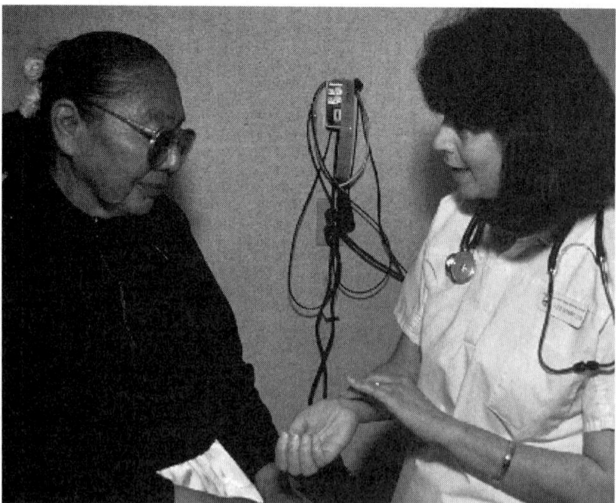

Figure 4-4 Nurse showing a non–English-speaking patient how to take a pulse. (Courtesy Michael Clement, MD, Mesa, Az.)

Until transcultural nursing is adequately incorporated into an official classification system of nursing diagnoses, the nurses may have to rely on their own creativity in writing culturally appropriate nursing diagnoses. Possible new nursing diagnoses have been suggested, including cultural distress, compromised health beliefs, broken beliefs, conflict in belief system, fear of witchcraft, biologic variations, alterations in caring patterns, and translocation syndrome.

PATIENT AND FAMILY TEACHING

Patient and family teaching may present some unique challenges for the nurse because the patient may not speak or be sufficiently fluent in English to ensure understanding of the material being taught (Figure 4-4). A translator or interpreter may be used. However, there may be significant differences in the information communicated by translators and interpreters. Also, needed translators or interpreters may not be available, and too frequently the nurse resorts to using visitors or even other patients as interpreters. Languages cannot be translated word for word, and the risk of failing to accurately communicate a message is high. Sometimes a patient's young children who attend English language schools are used very inappropriately as interpreters, such as using a young boy to interpret a discussion about birth control to his mother. Despite how well the boy seems to speak English, he may not have the sex education background to interpret the words, or cultural taboos may be violated regarding what a child, especially a male child, can speak about with his mother.

ETHICAL DILEMMA

1 How should a nurse respond to a patient who confides that he or she is also currently under the care of a folk healer because he or she does not fully trust the physician's ability to heal?
2 How should a nurse respond when the same patient opens a bag in the bedside stand and displays the folk medicines that he or she is taking while in the hospital?
3 What should the nurse do if the same patient refuses to let the nurse tell anyone about the folk treatments?

The nurse may also need to include the male spouse or eldest member of the family in any discussions. Family dominance patterns may require these individuals to be involved in any decision-making or teaching-learning activities. The American culture tends to value the autonomy and independence of the individual patient in deciding what is best for him or her. However, this is not true in many other cultures in which family members, particularly the elders or males, play an integral role in deciding what is best for the patient. Therefore both the patient and significant family members must be well informed. In this situation teaching sessions become a dialogue among all participants rather than just a lecture given to the patient. The patient needs to be asked beforehand who should be included in the discussion, and a time for the teaching must be scheduled when the important individuals can be present. If relevant teaching materials are available in the patient's own language, they can be obtained in advance.

KEY CONCEPTS

- Culture is defined as the homogeneous and learned patterns of behavior, values, and attitudes that are shared by a group of people and passed from one generation to the next.
- Culture is learned, shared, and dynamic behavior that represents an adaptation to the environment.
- Cultural definitions of words and phrases vary. Therefore it is essential that the meaning of questions is clear to patients.
- Generalizing about the commonalities that patients from a specific culture often hold is a starting point for individualized assessment.
- Cultural relativity implies that a person is open to the wide variety of beliefs and practices that are characteristic of a specific culture.
- Cultural customs, beliefs, and values are the building blocks of all cultures.
- Transcultural nursing focuses on the comparative study and analysis of different cultures and subcultures as a way of providing universal and culture-specific nursing care practices.
- Common alternative therapies practiced by various cultures include relaxation techniques, chiropractic care, and massage.
- Nurse-patient relationships include three interacting systems that together are termed the transcultural triad: the culture of the nurse, the culture of the patient, and the culture of the setting.
- Modes of action for nursing care decisions and actions include cultural care preservation or maintenance, cultural care accommodation or negotiation, and cultural care repatterning or restructuring.
- The nurse's understanding of cultural variability in the perception of time, the use of space, the use of touch, eye contact, and other factors is critical to the patient's response to nursing care, health restoration, and health maintenance.
- It is important to note that there may be significant differences in the communications that result from translators and interpreters.

CRITICAL THINKING EXERCISES

1 An Asian-American patient's family wants to prepare and bring all of her meals to the hospital. What must you consider and do to make this happen?

2 You are assigned to an alert patient who speaks no English. There is no family present when you give care, and no one on the unit speaks the patient's language. Although there is an interpreter in the hospital, she cannot be there when you are there. What creative ways might you devise to accomplish some very basic communication with your patient?

3 Your African-American patient closely follows his Islamic faith. Friday is his day of worship, certain foods are forbidden, and he prays to Mecca five times a day. Describe how you would facilitate his culturally congruent religious care.

4 Choose a culturally diverse patient on your unit, and examine the Kardex, nurses' notes, nursing diagnosis, and problem list. Are there any cultural considerations in these records? If yes, how are they actually carried over into the patient's nursing care? If no, should there be? What are your suggestions, and how would you put them into practice?

REFERENCES AND ADDITIONAL READINGS

American Nurses Association: *Position statement on cultural diversity in nursing practice,* Kansas City, Mo, 1991, The Association.

Boyle JS, Andrews MM: *Transcultural concepts in nursing care,* Glenview, Ill, 1989, Scott, Foresman.

Dolphin CZ: Variables in the use of personal space in intercultural transactions. In Samovar LA, Porter RE, editors: *Intercultural communication,* ed 4, Belmont, Calif, 1994, Wadsworth.

Eisenberg DM and others: Unconventional medicine in the United States, *N Engl J Med* 328(4):246-283, 1993.

Galanti GA: *Caring for patients from different cultures: case studies for American hospitals,* Philadelphia, 1991, University of Pennsylvania Press.

Geissler EM: Transcultural nursing and nursing diagnoses, *Nurs Health Care* 12(4):190-192; 203, 1991.

Geissler EM: Nursing diagnoses: a study of cultural relevance, *J Prof Nurs* 8(5):301-307, 1992.

Geissler EM: *Pocket guide to cultural assessment,* St Louis, 1994, Mosby.

Giger JN, Davidhizar RE: *Transcultural nursing: assessment and intervention,* St Louis, 1991, Mosby.

Hall ET: *The hidden dimension,* Garden City, New York, 1966, Doubleday.

Hall ET: *The dance of life: the other dimension of time,* New York, 1983, Anchor Books.

Kluckholn FR: Dominant and variant value orientations. In Kluckholn C, Murray HA, editors: *Personality in nature: society and culture,* New York, 1953, Alfred A Knopf.

Leininger MM: *Nursing and anthropology: two worlds to blend,* New York, 1970, John Wiley & Sons.

Leininger MM: *Transcultural nursing: concepts, theories, and practices,* New York, 1978, John Wiley & Sons.

Leininger MM: Leininger's theory of nursing: cultural care diversity and universality, *Nurs Sci Q* 1(4):155, 1988.

Leininger, MM: Issues, questions, and concerns related to the nursing diagnosis cultural movement from a transcultural nursing perspective, *J Transcult Nurs* 2(1):23-31, 1990.

Leininger *MM: Leininger's theory of cultural care diversity and universality,* Livonia, Mich, 1991, Madonna University (videotape).

Leininger MM: Are nurses prepared to function worldwide? *J Transcult Nurs* 5(2):2-4, 1994.

Levine, RV: The pace of life, *Am Scient* 78(5):450-459, 1990.

Potter PA, Perry AG: *Fundamentals of nursing: concepts, process, and practice,* ed 3, St Louis, 1993, Mosby.

Reynolds CL, Leininger MM: *Cultural care diversity and universality theory,* Newbury Park, Calif, 1993, Sage Publications.

Shellenberger JM: A practice model for culturally appropriate nursing care in a primary healthcare setting for Mexican-American persons, Doctoral Dissertation, 1987, University of Texas at Austin.

Sobralske M: *Suggested new transcultural nursing diagnoses,* Livonia, Mich, 1986, Transcultural Nursing Society.

Spector RE: *Cultural diversity in health and illness,* ed 3, Norwalk, Conn, 1991, Appleton & Lange.

Stewart EC, Bennett MJ: *American cultural patterns: a cross-cultural perspective,* Yarmouth, Me, 1991, Intercultural Press.

Transcultural Nursing Society: *Historical facts about the society,* Livonia, Mich, The Society (pamphlet).

Tripp-Reimer T: Cultural assessment. In Bellack JP, Bamford PA: *Nursing assessment: a multidimensional approach,* Monterey, Calif, 1984, Wadsworth.

Werner D: *Where there is no doctor,* Palo Alto, Calif, 1992, Hesperian Foundation.

Whitelaw A and others: Skin to skin contact for very low birth weight infants and their mothers, *Arch Dis Child* 63:1377-1381, 1988.

CHAPTER 5

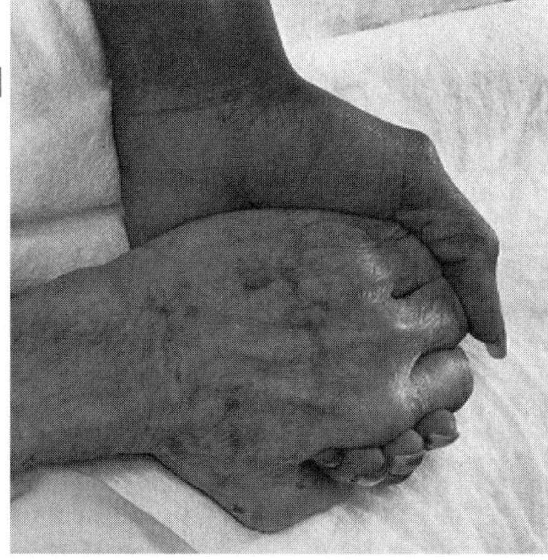

Death and Dying

CHAPTER OBJECTIVES

1 Discuss the changing attitude of society toward death.
2 Define the term *thanatology*.
3 Discuss the living will and explain how this document contributes to death with dignity.
4 Identify the behaviors characteristic of each stage of dying: denial, anger, bargaining, depression, and acceptance.
5 Discuss the phases of grief and bereavement.
6 Identify the physical, emotional, social, and spiritual needs that are common to the dying patient.
7 Identify nursing interventions that support the dying patient's needs.
8 Identify the needs of the family and friends of the dying patient and suggest interventions that support these needs.

KEY WORDS

acceptance
anger
anticipatory grief
bargaining
bereavement
denial
depression
grief
hospice
living will
respite
thanatology

DEATH

Until recently Americans have had the reputation of being a death-denying society. Ministers, nurses, and physicians have experienced long-standing frustrations in attempting to support dying patients and their families, who often deny the reality of the approaching death of their loved one.

In the 1960s and 1970s death, dying, grief, and bereavement became the focus of research in various disciplines. Through her writings concerning her work with dying patients, Elisabeth Kübler-Ross peaked the interest of the general public. **Thanatology,** the scientific study of death, found its way into the course offerings of many universities across the United States. Death has become a popular topic of books, articles, films, and videos. The **hospice** movement began in England and has rapidly developed in the United States as a support system for dying patients and their families.

Death and dying can be an everyday reality of nursing practice and must be addressed. Kübler-Ross states that death is the final stage of growth and development. If death is accepted as the final stage, it should be faced and experienced fully. The nurse has a unique opportunity and a major responsibility to help the patient and his or her family through the experience of dying and death (Kübler-Ross, 1975). It is necessary to understand how the physiologic and psychologic factors that surround death affect the individual. Many of the physiologic processes are well known, and the nurse or physician can predict death with reasonable accuracy. The psychologic and spiritual impact of the impending death is less understood.

The needs of the dying patient are complex, but it is important to acknowledge and deal with them. The biologic needs are the simplest to identify and include the need for adequate physical care, caring providers, prudent medical management, and comfort. Most nurses find the physical needs the easiest to acknowledge. The emotional and social aspects of death are much more difficult to identify. They are closely tied with the spiritual needs of the dying patient and his or her family. Meeting the spiritual needs of the patient and family is as important as meeting the biologic needs (Gravely, 1993). Spiritual distress is a nursing diagnosis characterized by expression of concern with the meaning of life and death and by the questioning of belief systems that provide strength, hope, and meaning to life (NANDA) (Box 5-1). The nurse must remember that all people have a spiritual dimension whether or not they participate in formal religious practices (Carpenito, 1993). As each patient moves toward his or her own death, each views the experience and accepts death in a unique way. There is no specific pattern that is applicable to all persons. By studying death and dying, nurses and other members of the healthcare team can improve their ability to understand the terminally ill person and to support the family and significant others. The nurse must be aware of his or her personal beliefs and values and acknowledge that these values may not be effective for others. To meet the needs of the patients, the nurse must be aware of the common religious and cultural practices regarding medical treatment and death in his or her area (Carson, 1989) (Box 5-2).

BOX 5-1

SIGNS OF SPIRITUAL DISTRESS

1 Questions credibility of belief system
2 Demonstrates discouragement or despair
3 Is unable to practice usual religious rituals
4 Has ambivalent feelings (doubts) about beliefs
5 Expresses that he or she has no reason for living
6 Feels a sense of spiritual emptiness
7 Shows emotional detachment from self and others
8 Expresses concern, anger, resentment, or fear regarding the meaning of life, suffering, and death
9 Requests spiritual assistance for a disturbance in the belief system

Modified from Carpenito LJ: *Nursing diagnosis application to clinical practice,* ed 5, Philadelphia, 1993, JB Lippincott.

When Does Death Occur?

The question of when death occurs is highly controversial. A diagnosis of death is usually made when there is an absence of heartbeat and a cessation of respiration. The use of these signs as the only criteria for determining death was questioned when the first human heart transplant was accomplished in 1967. Physicians who were interested in organ transplants

BOX 5-2

SELECTED RELIGIOUS PRACTICES AT TIME OF DEATH

Christian Science	An autopsy is usually declined unless required by law. Donating organs is unlikely but is an individual decision.
Church of the Nazarene	Cremation is permitted, and stillborn infants are buried.
Islam	It is preferred that the family wash, prepare, and place the body in a position that faces Mecca. If necessary, healthcare providers may perform these procedures as long as they wear gloves. Burial is performed as soon as possible. Cremation is forbidden. An autopsy is also prohibited except for legal reasons, and no body part is to be removed. Donating body parts or organs is not allowed because beliefs indicate that the person does not own his or her body.
Mennonite	Prayer is important at times of crisis. Therefore contacting a minister is important.
Muslim	The family is contacted before any care of the deceased is performed. There are special procedures for washing and shrouding the body.
Reform Jews	The use of life support without heroic measures is advocated. Cremation is allowed, but it is suggested that ashes be buried in a Jewish cemetery.
Roman Catholics	Each Roman Catholic should participate in the anointing of the sick and in the Eucharist and penance before death. The body should not be shrouded until these sacraments have been performed. All body parts that retain human quality must be appropriately buried or cremated.

Modified from Carson VB: *Spiritual dimensions of nursing practice,* Philadelphia, 1989, WB Saunders.

believed that a new definition was necessary, mainly because the donor organ must be removed as quickly as possible after death. Whether a person is actually dead, even though the heart may still be beating, is a question that has not yet been resolved.

In an effort to answer the question, "When is death?" physicians now use the electroencephalograph (EEG) to measure brain activity. They believe that the absence of brain activity on the EEG at three separate times, indicates that death has occurred, even though the heart may still be beating. Most physicians accept a definition of death that is based on the absence of brain waves. The Uniform Determination of Death Act (1982) indicates that death has occurred when there is no spontaneous brain activity and no spontaneous respirations.

The use of the EEG in determining death is now commonly used when a patient is being kept alive by extraordinary means and a decision to continue or discontinue life support must be made. In most situations in which life support has not been started, physicians determine death by the more traditional method: the absence of heartbeat and the cessation of respiration. Until recently this determination has been a medical responsibility and remains a medical responsibility within institutional settings.

Prolonging Life

New technologies and drugs have made it possible to prolong the lives of some terminally ill patients. However, after transferring from home to the hospital, dying patients find themselves surrounded by technologically advanced equipment. Such an environment is often lonely and sterile for the patient without the support of friends or family.

The use of life support is a common subject of television programs, magazine articles, and healthcare ethics committees. The following question is posed: if death is inevitable, should not care be directed toward making the patient as comfortable as possible rather than toward prolonging life? This problem is dealt with daily in hospitals and nursing homes. Using extraordinary means to prolong the life of a terminally ill patient becomes a tangled web of ethical, religious, legal, and moral questions to which there are no decisive answers. The use of the physician's "No Code" or "Do Not Resuscitate" orders is becoming more common now. For the nurse this means that cardiopulmonary resuscitation or other "heroic" measures will not be started if the patient's heartbeat or respirations stop. Terminally ill patients and their families discuss these treatment options with their physician before the order is written.

Living Wills and Advanced Medical Directives

The Patient Self-Determination Act became effective in December 1991. It requires hospitals, nursing homes, hospices, and home healthcare and provider agencies to advise patients at admission of their right to accept or refuse medical treatment and of their right to execute an advance directive. This step has become a routine part of many healthcare admission procedures. The advance directive can be in the form of a **living will** or a durable power of attorney.

Concern for Dying, a nonprofit educational council in New York, provides national leadership in addressing issues that involve the rights of the dying patient. The council has prepared a living will/advanced directive document that enables individuals to state in advance their wishes regarding the use of life-sustaining procedures in the event of terminal illness (Figures 5-1 and 5-2). Questions regarding the legality of a living will focus on when the will is drawn up and on the patient's mental status. Therefore nationwide support for living will legislation is one of the main goals of the council. Living will legislation, although still controversial, is one of the first steps in an attempt to regulate and standardize the criteria on which life-and-death decisions are made for the terminally ill (Davies, Martens, Reimer, 1991). All 50 states and the District of Columbia have enacted a living will legislation that offers guidelines for healthcare professionals who are involved in making decisions about life and death.

A durable power of attorney allows the patient to designate an individual who will make treatment decisions should the patient be unable to make them. It is a stronger legal document and is more specific than the living will. Unlike the living will the durable power of attorney covers all healthcare choices and is not limited to questions related to a terminal illness. It is not easy for most people to deal with this question, and hopefully public education will prepare individuals for this event. It is necessary that patients discuss with the individual who has been given durable power of attorney their wishes regarding treatment.

In situations in which the patient has not made and cannot make his or her wishes known, the physician is responsible for determining what measures to take. Patient and family input is sought whenever possible. The nurse's assessment of the patient and communication with the family contribute to the decision-making process. The nurse is not responsible for these decisions but should encourage communication between all parties so that they all agree to the plan of treatment. The decision to use any measure should be guided by what will contribute to the patient's comfort, safety, and well-being. If the use of oxygen relieves labored respiration, it should not be considered a heroic measure. However, administering a new antibiotic drug that can in no way alter the outcome would be considered questionable.

Fear of Dying and Death

A fear of dying is usually present when an individual's health is so compromised that there is a distinct possibility that he or she may die. This fear may lead the person to seek or accept extraordinary measures to prolong his or her life and prevent death. When all life-preserving measures have failed and death is imminent, an individual may fear death. This fear focuses on the physical cessation of vital functions and what will happen when mortal life ceases. The fear of death may also be related to frequently overlooked psychologic and spiritual factors, which are often of primary importance to the dying patient (Box 5-3).

Although research into the fear of dying is limited, there is some evidence that not all persons fear dying. Kastenbaum and Aisenberg (1992) report that fear and anxiety may be experienced by the dying patient but that depression is far more common. The patient with severe, painful physical symptoms may experience anxiety, whereas the patient who is aware of the terminal condition may experience a greater degree of depression.

Many variables are related to the fear of dying, including age, culture, social status, educational and occupational background, serious chronic diseases, and mental health status. The aged person who has undergone biologic changes that are characteristic of his or her age group appears to show less fear of dying than a younger person. Death means the end of everything that an individual has held dear and enjoyed throughout life. Although one mourns his or her loss, the fears are primarily related to the unknown. What happens after death? Is there an afterlife? Is death a painful experience? What will happen to the body after death? An individual who has well-developed spiritual or religious beliefs may have fewer fears about death. An individual may also have concerns regarding the losses and grief that family members will experience at the time of his or her death. Family discussions regarding the future help alleviate these concerns. Kübler-Ross (1969) found that death can more easily be accepted when there is the opportunity for communication, counseling, and resolution of problems. As death approaches and the sensorium changes, the fears tend to subside, and the individual often appears composed.

To My Family, My Physician, My Lawyer And All Others Whom It May Concern

Death is as much a reality as birth, growth, and aging—it is the one certainty of life. In anticipation of decisions that may have to be made about my own dying and as an expression of my right to refuse treatment, I, ______________________________, being of sound mind, make this statement of my wishes and instructions concerning treatment. (print name)

By means of this document, which I intend to be legally binding, I direct my physician and other care providers, my family, and any surrogate designated by me or appointed by a court, to carry out my wishes. If I become unable, by reason of physical or mental incapacity, to make decisions about my medical care, let this document provide the guidance and authority needed to make any and all such decisions.

If I am permanently unconscious or there is no reasonable expectation of my recovery from a seriously incapacitating or lethal illness or condition, I do not wish to be kept alive by artificial means. I request that I be given all care necessary to keep me comfortable and free of pain, even if pain-relieving medications may hasten my death, and I direct that no life-sustaining treatment be provided except as I or my surrogate specifically authorize.

This request may appear to place a heavy responsibility upon you, but by making this decision according to my strong convictions, I intend to ease that burden. I am acting after careful consideration and with understanding of the consequences of your carrying out my wishes. *List optional specific provisions in the space below. (See other side.)*

Durable Power of Attorney for Health Care Decisions (Cross out if you do not wish to use this section)

To effect my wishes, I designate ______________________________, residing at ______________________________

______________________________, (phone #) ______________________________, (or if he or she shall

for any reason fail to act, ______________________________, residing at ______________________________

______________________________, (phone #) ______________________________) as my health care surrogate—that is, my attorney-in-fact regarding any and all health care decisions to be made for me, including the decision to refuse life-sustaining treatment—if I am unable to make such decisions myself. This power shall remain effective during and not be affected by my subsequent illness, disability or incapacity. My surrogate shall have authority to interpret my Living Will, and shall make decisions about my health care as specified in my instructions or, when my wishes are not clear, as the surrogate believes to be in my best interests. I release and agree to hold harmless my health care surrogate from any and all claims whatsoever arising from decisions made in good faith in the exercise of this power.

I sign this document knowingly, voluntarily, and after careful deliberation, this ______ day of ______________________, 19_____.

____
(signature)

Address ______________________________

____

I do hereby certify that the within document was executed and acknowledged before me by the principal this ______ day of ______________________, 19_____.

____
Notary Public

Witness ______________________________

Printed Name ______________________________

Address ______________________________

____

Witness ______________________________

Printed Name ______________________________

Address ______________________________

____

Copies of this document have been given to:

This Living Will expresses my personal treatment preferences. The fact that I may have also executed a declaration in the form recommended by state law should not be construed to limit or contradict this Living Will, which is an expression of my common-law and constitutional rights.

(Optional) my Living Will is registered with Concern for Dying (Registry No. ______)

Distributed by Concern for Dying, 250 West 57th Street, New York, NY 10107 (212) 246-6962

Figure 5-1 A living will and durable power of attorney for healthcare decisions. (Reprinted with permission from Concern For Dying, 250 West 57th Street, New York, NY 10107.)

How to Use Your Living Will

The Living Will should clearly state your preferences about life-sustaining treatment. You may wish to add specific statements to the Living Will in the space provided for that purpose. Such statements might concern:

- Cardiopulmonary resuscitation
- Artificial or invasive measures for providing nutrition and hydration
- Kidney dialysis
- Mechanical or artificial respiration
- Blood transfusion
- Surgery (such as amputation)
- Antibiotics

You may also wish to indicate any preferences you may have about such matters as dying at home.

The Durable Power of Attorney for Health Care

This optional feature permits you to name a surrogate decision maker (also known as a proxy, health agent or attorney-in-fact), someone to make health care decisions on your behalf if you lose that ability. As this person should act according to your preferences and in your best interests, you should select this person with care and make certain that he or she knows what your wishes are and about your Living Will.

You should not name someone who is a witness to your Living Will. You may want to name an alternate agent in case the first person you select is unable or unwilling to serve. If you do name a surrogate decision maker, the form must be notarized. (It is a good idea to notarize the document in any case.)

Important Points to Remember

- Sign and date your Living Will.
- Your two witnesses should not be blood relatives, your spouse, potential beneficiaries of your estate or your health care proxy.
- Discuss your Living Will with your doctors; and give them copies of your Living Will for inclusion in your medical file, so they will know whom to contact in the event something happens to you.
- Make photo copies of your Living Will and give them to anyone who may be making decisions for you if you are unable to make them yourself.
- Place the original in a safe, accessible place, so that it can be located if needed—not in a safe deposit box.
- Look over your Living Will periodically (at least every five years), initial and redate it so that it will be clear that your wishes have not changed.

The Living Will Registry

In 1983, Concern for Dying instituted the Living Will Registry, a computerized file system where you may keep an up-to-date copy of your Living Will in our New York office.

What are the benefits of joining the Living Will Registry?

- Concern's staff will ensure that your form is filled out correctly, assign you a Registry number and maintain a copy of your Living Will.
- Concern's staff will be able to refer to *your* personal document, explain procedures and options, and provide you with the latest case law or state legislation should you, your proxy or anyone else acting on your behalf need counselling or legal guidance in implementing your Living Will.
- You will receive a permanent, credit card size plastic mini-will with your Registry number imprinted on it. The mini-will, which contains your address, Concern's address and a short version of the Living Will, indicates that you have already filled out a full-sized witnessed Living Will document.

How do you join the Living Will Registry?

- Review your Living Will, making sure it is up to date and contains any specific provisions that you want added.
- Mail a photo copy of your original, signed and witnessed document along with a check for $25.00 to: Living Will Registry, Concern for Dying, 250 West 57th Street, Room 831, New York, New York 10107.
- The one-time Registry enrollment fee will cover the costs of processing and maintaining your Living Will and of issuing your new plastic mini-will.
- If you live in a state with Living Will legislation, send copies of any required state documents as well.
- If you have any address changes or wish to add or delete special provisions that you have included in your Living Will, please write to the Registry so that we can keep your file up to date.

Revised March 1989

A LIVING WILL

And Appointment of a Surrogate Decision Maker

Prepared by

CONCERN FOR DYING

An Educational Council

Figure 5-2 Instructions for completing a living will and the durable power of attorney for healthcare decisions. (Reprinted with permission from Concern For Dying, 250 West 57th Street, New York, NY 10107.)

BOX 5-3

COMMON FEARS OF DYING PATIENTS

1 Unrelenting pain
2 Changes in body image
3 Loss of control of bodily functions
4 Lack of truth telling regarding physical condition
5 Loss of decision-making control in planning care and quality-of-life issues
6 Loss of privacy
7 Unresolved or unfinished business
8 Abandonment by family or significant others
9 Dying alone

Emotional Stages Experienced in the Dying Process

Observations of terminally ill patients indicate that patients experience stages of well-defined emotional feelings as they move through the dying process. These stages are identified as denial, anger, bargaining, depression, and acceptance (Kübler-Ross, 1969).

Denial

When patients are unable to face the diagnosis of terminal illness, they often deny its existence. They are essentially saying, "No, not me." **Denial** is a defense mechanism that protects individuals from thoughts that they are unable to accept at that time.

Anger

Patients who are not ready to accept that their illness is terminal become angry and displace that **anger** on those around them. Patients in this stage may be rude to their family, demanding of the nurse, and hostile to the physician. The patient who is experiencing anger asks, "Why me?"

Bargaining

Anger may subside and patients may begin **bargaining,** or deciding how they can buy additional time. Such patients are saying, "Yes me, but . . . ." Their first approach may be to God, negotiating for an extension of time in exchange for leading a better life so that they can achieve a long-sought goal or attend a special event such as a wedding or graduation.

Depression

Depression is marked by feelings of loss and despair. Depressed patients ask, "What is the use?" The ravages of disease and illness begin to take their toll. As the patient becomes weaker, the illness cannot be denied any longer. The patient becomes sad, may show less interest in visits from family and friends, may withdraw, and becomes uncommunicative.

Acceptance

The final emotional stage is **acceptance.** The patient says, "I am ready." This stage may either be one of active acceptance or of passive acceptance when the patient is too weak and tired to fight for life any longer. The struggle is over, and the patient longs for quiet and rest before the final journey (Kübler-Ross, 1969). However, the patient still needs contact from family and friends. Touch is a very important way to maintain contact and to support the patient during this time.

The sequence in which these emotions are experienced is varied. Some patients do not experience all of these emotional stages, and some do not exhibit the behavior characteristics of each stage. Not every patient will pass sequentially from denial to acceptance in the exact order. A patient often moves back and forth, entering the next stage and regressing to a previous stage. The patient's family and friends may experience the same stages but not necessarily in the same order or at the same time as the patient. Different family members may experience these stages at different times and in different orders. The patient may still be in the stage of anger when the family has progressed to bargaining. This difference may cause problems in communication and make it more difficult for everyone to be supportive of one another. Both the patient and the family need the nurse's assistance to help them work through their individual stages. The longer the period of dying, the more likely it is that the patient and family will move back and forth from one stage to another. Even if and when the patient reaches the stage of acceptance, hope still continues. Throughout the terminal illness the patient never loses hope that some new drug, treatment, or medical discovery will alter the outcome. Hope enables the patient to live as fully as possible despite weakness and vulnerability.

GRIEF AND BEREAVEMENT

Grief is a normal emotional reaction to the loss of material possessions, self-identity, or a body function or part. A separation from loved ones such as in war or incarceration may also cause one to grieve. The death

OLDER ADULT CONSIDERATIONS

It has been found that older adults, having accomplished many of their life's tasks, move through the grieving process more quickly than does a younger person. The older person has usually seen his or her family grow up, has completed a career, and has felt the biologic changes of aging occur. Such factors seem to make it easier to adjust to the idea of impending death.

of a close relative or friend may cause an intense emotional response. The dying patient may grieve over the loss of life, independence, and meaningful experiences of the past; life work left unfinished; and the separation from loved ones.

After the patient dies, attention is focused on the significance of the death to the patient's family and friends. A period of **bereavement** is experienced by the family and friends of the deceased. More distant members of the family group and nurses who have had a long association with the patient may also grieve the death. Studies of bereavement indicate that a wide range of behavioral patterns may accompany grief. Whereas some individuals are able to accept the situation and appear to have the emotional stability to adjust to the loss, others may develop psychosomatic complaints. In some instances a physical illness may develop after the loss of a close friend or relative. If grieving is not experienced at the time of an individual's death, it may be experienced later, at the time of another loss.

The loss of a loved one rates high on the stress scale. Support from friends and the community is important when working through the grieving process. Recently developed sources of help are available in many communities and include bereavement support groups, often affiliated with a hospital, funeral home, church, or hospice program.

According to the United States census, the number of widows far exceeds the number of widowers. Spouses who lose their partners are especially vulnerable to bereavement because of its consequences. An elderly person who loses a spouse may not experience the same problems as a younger person. Age, stage of development, and life experience affect how one adjusts to loss. When the loss of a loved one occurs, there is deprivation (Groenwald, 1991). Spiritually the individual is most acutely aware of the loss itself and may not think about deprivation until some time later. However, deprivation invariably follows loss. For example, the death of a mate can mean deprivation through loss of income, which lowers the standard of living to which the surviving spouse is accustomed. The younger person may also be left with the responsibility of raising a family alone. If the survivor is not already working, it may become necessary to seek employment to support the family.

Grieving is a psychologic process with three distinct phases. After the death of an individual, the survivor may be numb with grief and may protest the reality of the event. The survivor may experience physical changes such as a loss of appetite, nausea, an inability to sleep, weakness, and restlessness. A feeling of nonreality may exist, and the individual may be preoccupied with thoughts of the deceased. During this time the survivor is usually surrounded by friends and sympathizers. However, after the funeral the support systems often diminish. The individual is alone, and the second phase of grieving begins. This phase is characterized by despair. It is common to experience depression, decreased energy, a difficulty in making even simple decisions, and a sense of being slowed down in thought processes and actions. The final stage before recovery is characterized by detachment. Feelings of apathy, a loss of interest, and an absence of spontaneity may be present. The length of each of these stages varies and eventually culminates in some subtle "breakthrough" behaviors, such as reaching out to a new activity, interest, or person. These behaviors are accompanied by a fleeting sense of being able to enjoy some aspects of life once again (Box 5-4).

Many variables affect the grieving process, and no clear-cut pattern can be applied to every individual. The stages of grief are similar to the stages of dying. Grief is a response to a loss. Therefore it is logical that the bereaved, like the dying person, moves along a similar path. For a few people the period of grief lasts only a few weeks, but for most others it may last more than a year. The progression through the grief process is not steady and is characterized by up and down periods rather than a gradual progression of feeling better. The process may vary if the death is sudden and unexpected or if it occurs after a prolonged terminal illness. If the family or loved ones have cared for and supported the patient, part of the grief work will have occurred before the death. This phenomenon is referred to as **anticipatory grief** and helps the individual move more quickly through the grieving process.

NURSING CARE OF THE DYING PATIENT

The nurse is responsible for caring for not only a dying patient but also the patient's family and friends.

BOX 5-4

CHARACTERISTIC EXPERIENCES OF THE GRIEVING PROCESS

1 Feelings of nonreality
2 Despair
3 Detachment
4 Breakthrough behaviors
5 Recovery

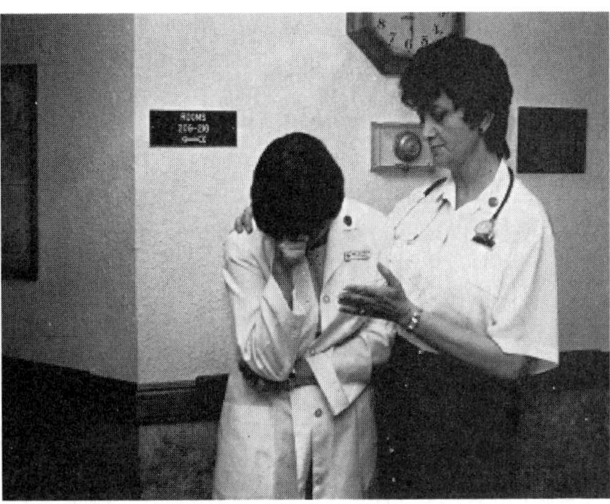

Figure 5-3 Colleagues can provide comfort for nurses.

Several studies indicate that nurses sometimes avoid dying patients. It has been proposed that caring for a dying patient stimulates nurses to think about their own deaths or unresolved grief. For some nurses the avoidance may be from the frustration of being unable to "make everything right."

When working with the terminally ill, the nurse moves through the same stages of grieving as the family and patient. To fulfill this emotionally demanding role, the nurse must receive support from some other source (Figure 5-3). Individual sessions with more experienced nursing personnel and group sessions with pastoral care staff, social workers, and psychologists can provide support to the nurse. Expanding this type of support system is desirable to prevent burnout and to help nurses grow from their experiences.

Caring for the terminally ill patient involves dealing with the physical, psychosocial, and spiritual health of the patient (Box 5-5). A terminal illness does not mean that the patient is facing immediate death. Many illnesses from which the patient is not expected to recover, such as acquired immunodeficiency syndrome (AIDS) and some types of cancer, are marked by long remissions that are punctuated by exacerbations.

During a patient's admission to the hospital, the nurse should get to know the patient and learn about his or her social and cultural background, religious or spiritual orientation, and personal problems that may be particularly concerning him or her. The nurse should assess how the patient is dealing with the illness and identify which emotional stages the patient and family are experiencing. In addition, the nurse can help the patient identify any unfinished business that the patient wishes to address before death.

Although many patients are aware of their prognosis, others may not be. Some patients who suspect that they have a terminal illness seek confirmation from the nurse. The nurse should be aware of this possibility and be prepared to handle it in a sensitive manner. It is especially important that the nurse know what the physician has told the patient and the family. Many experts in the field of death and dying believe that the patient always knows the truth, whether or not the family or physician has shared the prognosis. The nurse can be of greatest help to the patient by facilitating and encouraging open expressions of feelings and concerns. By conveying this information to the physician and the family, the nurse can help all parties involved to face the subject of death openly.

If staffing patterns permit, the same nurse should be assigned to care for the patient on each admission. When this is possible, the patient and family develop a feeling of trust, security, and confidence. When the patient is admitted for the last time, the personal relationship that has been established may help to bridge the gap between living and dying.

Patient and Family Teaching

The patient and family should be allowed to ask any questions they may have regarding treatments and the prognosis. The patient and family may repeat the same questions to different caregivers. They should be given as complete an explanation as they can deal with and understand.

Death Following Traumatic Injury

The nurse faces a special challenge when providing support to patients and families in the intensive care unit following a sudden and unanticipated traumatic injury in which death is imminent. In today's technologically advanced environment it is possible to lose sight of the patient as a person and to disregard what the patient considers to be in his or her best interests. Comfort and communication should be a high priority. The nurse is instrumental in ensuring that the family

BOX 5-5 **Nursing Process**

SPIRITUAL DISTRESS

ASSESSMENT

Presence of anxiety, doubt, anger, and depression
Rejection or neglect of previous religious practices
Increased interest in spiritual matters

NURSING DIAGNOSIS

Spiritual distress related to diagnosis of terminal disease

NURSING INTERVENTIONS

Make time to listen actively to patient and family.
Help the patient focus on successes and the value of the positive experiences in life.
Offer to contact a religious leader if the patient wants counseling, or refer the patient to hospital chaplin services.
Allow the patient to express feelings such as anger, guilt, despair.
Offer unconditional support to the patient and family.

EVALUATION OF EXPECTED OUTCOMES

Verbalizes feelings concerning the diagnosis
Talks with family and significant others about feelings
Able to put this life event in perspective with the rest of life
Works through the grief stages toward resolution
Expresses feelings of acceptance of impending death

has the opportunity to stay with the patient as much as possible. These elements are crucial to ensuring a dignified death for the patient. Often the nurse's role is to ask questions to help the patient, family, and physician steer the situation toward responsible and appropriate treatment (Pelliter, 1992)

Organ Donation

When death is inevitable, the patient and family have few choices. If the patient has the potential to be an organ or tissue donor, the option should be offered.

ETHICAL DILEMMA

1 Should a dying patient be told of his or her condition? Justify your answer and give reasons.
2 Should limited healthcare resources such as intensive care beds and dialysis machines be restricted to patients who have a chance of recovery?
3 Is a patient's refusal of life-sustaining treatment the same as suicide?
4 Who makes the decisions regarding life-sustaining treatment if the patient cannot?
5 How might a nurse's personal view of death affect the care of dying patients? Should personal views affect the care provided?

Offering this option to a grieving family can be a final way to help them through their grief (Chabalewski, Gaedeke-Norris, 1994). It may be difficult for the family to understand and accept death when their loved one is being maintained on a ventilator and still has a heartbeat. The nurse should be supportive and answer any questions. The most common information that the nurse provides regarding organ donation includes the surgical recovery of donated tissue and organs, the fact that open caskets are still possible after donation, and the fact that the family does not assume the cost of the surgical recovery (Chabalewski, Gaedeke-Norris, 1994). To provide this information to the family the nurse must be well informed about the policies and procedures of the hospital. The nurse may also help determine which family member to approach when a potential donor is identified. This individual should be the one who has demonstrated emotional strength and clear thinking throughout the ordeal. The consent of the next of kin is also required. Organs presently used for transplant include the kidney, heart, liver, pancreas, and lung. Tissues that can be donated include the cornea, skin, bone, and heart valves (Chabalewski, Gaedeke-Norris, 1994).

The Hospice Movement

The special needs of the dying patient and his or her family are addressed by the concept of **hospice.** The term *hospice* originally referred to a resting place for travelers on a difficult journey. The concept of care for the dying began in England and has rapidly spread throughout the United States in the last decade. There are three basic types of hospices: (1) home-based,

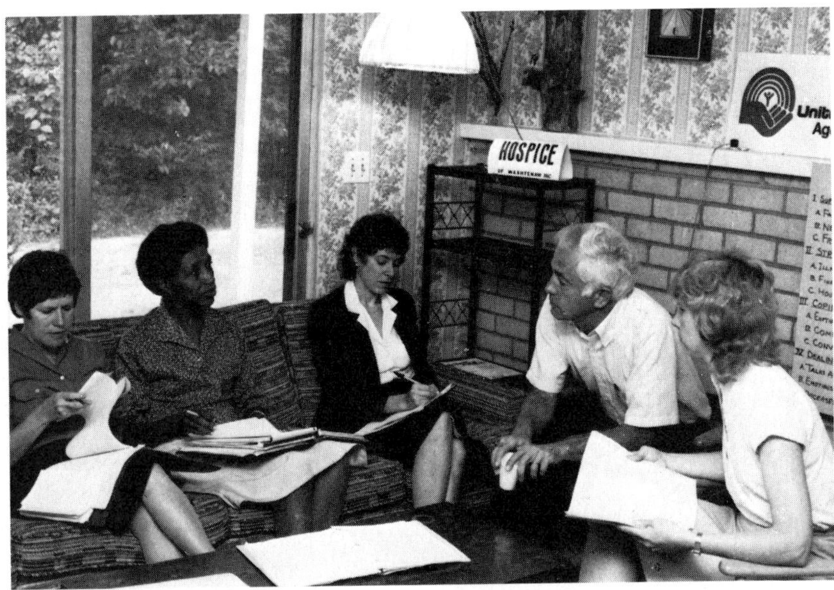

Figure 5-4 Hospice teams meet to plan care for their terminally ill patients and families. (Courtesy of Hospice of Washtenaw, Ann Arbor, Mich.)

which provides a support system that enables a patient to die at home; (2) freestanding, which is available as a haven for the terminally ill to come to die; and (3) defined areas or teams, which exist in the general hospital setting. The hospice concept requires the cooperation of various disciplines, including nurses, physicians, pharmacists, social workers, dieticians, clergy, and volunteers. All work together to address the patient's physical, emotional, and spiritual needs around the clock (Figure 5-4). The basic goals of hospice care are:

1 Maintaining the patient in as symptom-free a state as possible. In many cases this means addressing the problem of pain control. The nurse, physician, and pharmacist work together to keep the patient as nearly free of pain as possible and at a level of alertness that enables him or her to interact with family and friends.
2 Encouraging the patient to continue to define quality of life, maintain control, and make decisions about care.
3 Encouraging the patient to live fully and supporting his or her efforts to communicate with family and friends to complete the unfinished business of life. The nurse, social worker, and clergy often work together to attain this goal.
4 Being available to the family and providing them with individualized and appropriate support. Volunteers are important members of the hospice team and provide **respite** care for family members, help with household chores, and run errands.

If nurses are in tune with the patient's needs, many of these goals can be accomplished at home or in the hospital.

Each patient faces death in a unique way. In most cases he or she does not want to feel abandoned and desires the company of a close friend or relative. The family should be encouraged to spend as much time with the patient as possible. A nurse's frequent visits to the patient's room, a gently placed hand on the patient's shoulder, and a kind word convey to the patient that he or she is not alone (Figure 5-5). The nurse should serve as a role model for the family by demonstrating appropriate methods of comfort and support. Small objects belonging to the patient, such as family pictures, should be placed within easy viewing distance. The creative use of light, flowers, and music can provide a comforting atmosphere. The patient should be placed in an area where he or she can hear people and not feel alone.

Nursing Interventions

Physical care

The physical care of the patient must continue to the end. Such care is supportive and maintains the patient's comfort. As with all patients, it is appropriate to

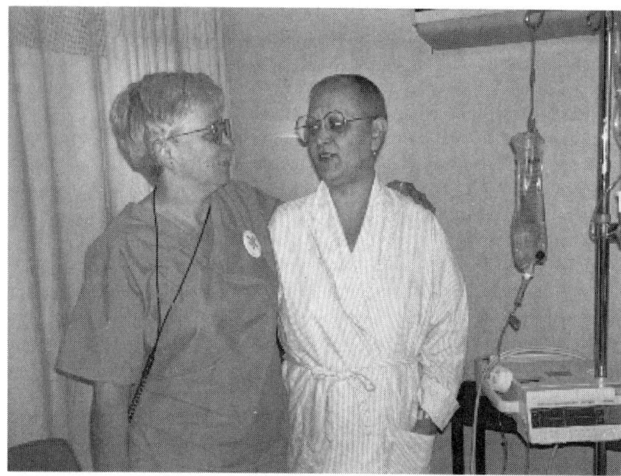

Figure 5-5 The nurse serves as a role model for the family by demonstrating appropriate methods of comfort and support.

use universal and body substance isolation precautions when providing care. The patient may be unable to care for his or her personal hygiene needs. Bathing, including perineal and skin care, is essential. It is also important to establish a regular schedule for turning the patient. The dying patient may experience edema, muscle atrophy, and/or decreased mobility, which makes good skin care essential for the patient's comfort. Oral care must not be neglected. Many terminally ill patients breathe through their mouths, which causes mucous membranes to become dry and sore. A poor oral condition interferes with speech and swallowing. When dentures cannot be worn, drooling occurs. Pathogenic organisms and oral secretions may cause stomatitis and maceration of tissues around the mouth, which may cause the patient actual pain (Buckley, and others, 1993). Oral care should be given regularly and be sufficient to keep the tissues clean and free of odor.

Because a terminal illness is often accompanied by pain, ongoing assessment of pain is important (Box 5-6). The patient's need for frequent pain medication, which is administered intravenously for greater effectiveness, is often the only reason the patient remains in the hospital rather than going home to die. Often the dose of pain medication given to a terminally ill patient far exceeds the normal ranges for the drug because the patient needs greater amounts to control the increasing pain. It is important for the nurse to recognize this need and be willing to adjust the dosage according to the patient's need for pain control.

BOX 5-6 **Nursing Process**

PAIN

ASSESSMENT

Physical pain
Levels of pain
Previous successful and unsuccessful pain relief measures

NURSING DIAGNOSIS

Pain related to physiologic processes

NURSING INTERVENTIONS

Administer pain relief medications as per orders; assess effectiveness frequently.
Reposition patient to a more comfortable position.
Attend to patient's personal hygiene needs.
Provide back rubs and massages prn for relief of muscular discomfort due to immobility.

EVALUATION OF EXPECTED OUTCOMES

Patient verbalizes that pain is decreased or absent.
Family participates in providing effective pain relief measures to patient.

PATIENT/FAMILY TEACHING

Pain

Teach patient how to rate pain on a scale of 1-10.
Teach family methods of comfort and relief such as massage.

Pain and the effects of pain medications affect the patient's appetite, which leads to poor nutritional status and further debilitation. A stool softener is an important adjunct to pain control medication and prevents the additional discomfort of constipation. The sensory effects of the pain medication can make it im-

PATIENT/FAMILY TEACHING

Dying

Teach patient and family the stages of the grief process.
Discuss with patient and family the resources available for support

possible for the patient to think clearly and to deal effectively with loved ones.

Recent developments in pain control include new methods of morphine use. The use of oral morphine has increased. Higher concentrated solutions of morphine and sustained-release morphine tablets are available for oral use. Transdermal patches with analgesics are also being used for pain control. However, transdermal patches have slow onset of effectiveness, and the patient may need some supplemental short-acting analgesics while waiting for the patch medication to reach effective levels.

Effective pain control is possible if medications are given around the clock. The dosage should be adjusted according to the patient's unique and changing needs. This method of medication administration replaces the demand, or prn, method and is more successful in controlling pain breakthrough and erasing pain memory. The nurse should check frequently with the patient and/or family to make sure the pain is being controlled effectively.

Emotional support

The patient or family may be demanding and angry, tearful, or withdrawn. It is important that the patient express his or her feelings. The nurse can best facilitate the expression of feelings by being an attentive listener. The nurse's continued presence and support conveys feelings of care and concern and lessens the fear of abandonment. Attentive listening enables the nurse to identify the family's and patient's specific concerns or unfinished business. If the nurse cannot assist in problem solving, the patient and family may be referred to a social worker, minister, or psychiatrist as appropriate.

Reminiscence therapy and relaxation techniques may also help provide emotional support to the patient and family. Humor also plays an important role in interacting with the terminally ill and is thought to provide a sense of power and self-worth when emotional pain is overwhelming. Herth (1990) states that humor is closely related to self-concept and provides a sense of perspective, hope, and joy, which empowers the individual and results in a sense of control. Shared humor also serves as a connecting mechanism and diminishes the feelings of isolation that are associated with dying.

Spiritual support

Before providing spiritual support to patients and their families, nurses must assess their feelings regarding their own deaths and dying experiences. The process of identifying personal spiritual beliefs continues throughout a nurse's lifetime and enables continued improvement in the nurse's supporting skills.

If the nurse can suspend judgment, interpretation, and analysis, an atmosphere of openness can be created, and the patient and family may feel more comfortable sharing their spiritual philosophy or religious beliefs. It is essential to listen, affirm beliefs, and help the patient and family participate in familiar religious rituals. When requested to do so, the nurse may pray with or read to the patient and family from the patient's personal religious text.

NURSE ALERT

Regardless of the nurse's beliefs, support should be provided within the patient's own spiritual or religious framework. With the patient's and family's permission, referrals can be made to the patient's minister or to the hospital pastoral care staff.

Support of the family

Attending to the family's needs is an extension of caring for the dying patient. Emotional support includes providing the family with as much uninterrupted time with the patient as possible. Providing a quiet and private place for the family to be together is also important. Family members should be given the opportunity to express their feelings as death approaches (Box 5-7).

BOX 5-7

GUIDELINES FOR THE CARE OF THE DYING PATIENT AND HIS OR HER FAMILY

1 Decisions concerning the use of extraordinary means to prolong life are the responsibility of the patient, the family, and the physician. Input from other members of the healthcare team may often be helpful.
2 Encouraging the patient to be a decision maker regarding his or her care and treatment for as long as the condition permits is basic to maintaining dignity and feelings of self-worth.
3 It is the nurse's responsibility to see that physical care and emotional and spiritual support are available to the dying patient. The nurse plays an important part in this care and should involve others of the healthcare team as appropriate.
4 The patient may identify one or two members of the family or the hospital staff with whom he or she feels most comfortable discussing feelings. The choices of individuals should be respected.
5 The nurse should assess how the patient's family members and friends are dealing with the impending loss of their loved one, encourage them to express their feelings, and direct them toward additional support from the healthcare team as necessary.
6 Various cultures and religions have ritualistic practices that help a bereaved individual move through the grief process. These practices should be encouraged and respected.
7 It is common for the bereaved to express feelings of guilt in regard to past life experiences with the deceased.
8 Family and friends should be made aware of local bereavement support groups.

Following Death

In addition to the legal requirements for autopsy, death certificates, and interstate transport of bodies, each hospital, county, and state has its own policies and procedures regarding death. The nurse should become familiar with these policies and procedures. When the patient dies, the family should have the opportunity to view and spend time with the deceased family member. If possible, the nurse should straighten the bedclothes and surroundings and place the deceased in a composed position before the viewing.

After the family has finished viewing the deceased, the body is prepared for removal. Unless there is to be an autopsy, all invasive tubes are removed. The eyes and mouth should be closed. To secure the jaw closed it may be necessary to place a roll of gauze under the chin and tie another piece of gauze under the chin and over the top of the head. Tags with identifying information are usually placed on the wrist, ankle, and shroud. After the body has been removed, the nurse should help the family gather the patient's belongings. Handling the patient's body and belongings with dignity conveys to the family respect for the deceased and concern for their feelings. Emotional support for the family should continue.

Nursing Care Plan

DEATH AND DYING

Mr. Duffy is a 66-year-old man who was diagnosed with oat cell carcinoma of the lungs 2 months ago. He has been hospitalized for 7 days because of recurring high fever; cachexia; and a persistent, debilitating cough. For several days Mr. Duffy has refused inhalation therapy and other treatments. He has requested to have the blinds drawn in his room during the day shift and has spent the last 2 days lying with his eyes closed and facing the wall when awake. Today he refused both his breakfast and lunch trays. When the nurse expressed concern he stated, "I feel sad and empty. How can God let this happen to me?" He asks the nurses to tell his family that he prefers not to see them during visiting hours.

Past Medical History

No previous surgeries
History of smoking × 40 years
Has had recurrent respiratory infections in the past but none serious enough to warrant hospitalization
No current meds except pain medications and cough suppressants
Has poor vision corrected somewhat by glasses

Psychosocial Data

Married for 29 years
Has four living children; closest is living 5 hours away; other children live out of state
Owns 3-story house with large yard
Is a retired attorney
Recreational activities include fishing, reading, crossword puzzles, gardening

Assessment Data

Alert and oriented × 3
Vital signs stable and within normal limits
Coughing productively at times; producing thick, white sputum tinged with blood
Respirations somewhat labored; nasal O_2 at 2 L/min administered via nasal cannula

NURSING DIAGNOSIS

Spiritual distress related to terminal disease diagnosis

NURSING INTERVENTIONS

Take time to sit with the patient and listen in a nonjudgmental manner.
Encourage the patient to reminisce about past experiences and their significance to his life. Help the patient focus on successes and the value of positive experiences.
Help the patient place the illness experience into the context of the total life experience. Pray with the patient as the patient desires.
Discuss the patient's significant family relationships and ways to maintain and strengthen them. Provide for privacy needs during visiting hours. Be available to the family with ideas regarding how to best support the patient, such as hospice or pastoral referral.
Help the patient with relaxation techniques. Suggest music therapy, meditation, and prayer.

EVALUATION OF EXPECTED OUTCOMES

Expresses anger and other feelings
Increases his level of acceptance of self, God, and others
Experiences an increased sense of meaning in living with an illness
Maintains communication with and accepts support from his family
Develops an increased sense of hope and inner peace
Describes what loss and death means to him
Shares his feelings and grief with his family and significant others

KEY CONCEPTS

- The nursing care of the terminally ill deals with the physical, psychosocial, and spiritual health of the patient.
- The nurse can facilitate communication between the patient and family members during these emotional times and provide for the physical needs of the patient.
- In working with the terminally ill and their families, the nurse often moves along the same stages of grief as the family and the patient.
- Supporting patients and families following a sudden and unanticipated traumatic injury in which death is imminent provides a special challenge.
- The nurse should serve as a role model for the family by demonstrating appropriate ways to comfort and support the patient.
- The physical care of the dying patient focuses on maintaining the comfort of the patient. This includes not only personal hygiene needs but also adequate pain control.
- The nurse can best provide emotional support by being an attentive listener.
- The nurse needs to provide the patient and family with an atmosphere of acceptance and openness in which to discuss spiritual concerns.
- Grief is the emotional response to loss.
- When moving through the dying process, terminally ill patients experience stages of denial, anger, bargaining, depression, and acceptance. Friends and families also experience these emotional stages.
- Terminally ill patients now discuss options with their physicians regarding prolonging life with extraordinary means. Advanced directives/living wills are documents that allow other individuals to state a patient's healthcare wishes if he or she is unable to do so.
- The nurse should discuss organ donation with the families of potential donors.
- The hospice movement developed as a support system for the dying and their families.
- The use of technology to prolong life has made the definition of death more difficult. Death is defined as the absence of spontaneous brain activity and spontaneous respirations.
- Using extraordinary means to prolong the life of terminally ill patients becomes a tangled web of ethical, religious, legal, and moral questions that have no clear answers.

CRITICAL THINKING EXERCISES

1 What factors have influenced the change in American society's attitudes regarding death?

2 How does anticipatory grief affect the period of bereavement?

3 What factors must be considered in selecting treatment measures for the patient who has completed an advance directive and designated a durable power of attorney for healthcare?

REFERENCES AND ADDITIONAL READINGS

Bersford J: *Hospice handbook,* Boston, 1993, Little, Brown.

Boutell K, Bozett F: Nurses' assessment of patients' spirituality: continuing education implications, *J Contin Educ Nurs* 21(4):172-176, 1990.

Buckley FP and others: Symptom management in the terminally ill, *Patient Care* 27(1):33-37, 41-44, 1993.

Carpenito LJ: *Nursing diagnosis application to clinical practice,* ed 5, Philadelphia, 1993, JB Lippincott.

Carson VB: *Spiritual dimensions of nursing practice,* Philadelphia, 1989, WB Saunders.

Chabalewski F, Gaedeke-Norris MK: The gift of life . . . talking to families about organ and tissue donation, *Am J Nurs* 94(6):28-33, 1994.

Clark C and others: Spirituality: integral to quality care, *Holistic Nurs Pract* 5(3):67-76, 1991.

Clarke J: The day after a death, *Nurs Time* 89(12):46-47, 1993.

Claxton JW: Paving the way to acceptance: psychological adaptation to death and dying in cancer, *Prof Nurse* 8(4):206-211, 1993.

Dart S, Taylor E: Talking it through, *Nurs Time* 89(16):50-52, 1993.

Davies G, Martens N, Reimer JC: Palliative care: the nurse's role in helping families through the transition of "fading away," *Cancer Nurs* 14(6):321-327, 1991.

Enck RE: The last few days, *Am J Hospice Palliat Care* 9(4):11-13, 1992.

Gravely JN, Jr: *Spirituality as a nursing diagnosis in the plan of care for terminally ill clients,* unpublished Master's Thesis, Radford, 1993, Radford University School of Nursing.

Groenwald SL: *Psychosocial dimensions of cancer,* Boston, 1991, Jones & Bartlett.

Groenwald SL and others: *Cancer nursing: principles and practice,* ed 3, Boston, 1993, Jones & Bartlett.

Hallal JC, Walsh MB: Loss, bereavement, and care of the dying person. In *Gerontologic nursing care of the frail elderly,* Burke MM and others, editors: St Louis, 1993, Mosby.

Herth K: Contributions of humor as perceived by the terminally ill, *Am J Hospice Care* 7(1):36-40, 1990.

Irvine B: Teaching palliative care to nursing students, *Nurs Stand* 7(50):37-39, 1993.

Johnson CJ, McGee MG: *How different religions view death and afterlife,* Philadelphia, 1991, The Charles Press.

Johnson SH: Saying "goodbye" . . . when a family member is near death, *Dimens Crit Care Nurs* 12(6):319, 1993.

Kastenbaum R, Aisenberg RB: *The psychology of death,* ed 2, New York, 1992, Springer Publishing.

Kaye P: *Notes on symptom control in hospice and palliative care,* Essex, Conn, 1991, Hospice Education Institute.

Kübler-Ross E: *On death and dying,* New York, 1969, Macmillan Publishing.

Kübler-Ross E: *Death: the final stage of growth,* Englewood Cliffs, NJ, 1975, Prentice Hall.

Leftridge DW and others: Helping Ben live and die his way . . . nursing grand rounds, *Nursing* 22(9):59-64, 1992.

MacInnis K: Making good-byes . . . dear dying person, *Am J Nurs* 92(3):120, 1992.

Madden E: *Carpe diem . . . enjoying every day with a terminal illness,* Boston, 1993, Jones & Bartlett.

Maher MF, Smith DC: Achieving a healthy death: the dying person's attitudinal contributions, *Hospice J* 9(1):21-32, 1993.

Mallison MB: Decoding the messages of the dying, *Am J Nurs* 93(1):7, 1993.

Marks M: Palliative care, *Nurs Stand* 6(33):9-16, 1992.

McCaffery M, Wolff M: Pain relief using cutaneous modalities, positioning, and movement, *Hospice J* 8(1, 2):121-153, 1992.

McFarland G, McFarland E: *Nursing diagnosis and intervention,* ed 2, St Louis, 1993, Mosby.

McMilliam CL, Burdock J, Wamsley J: The challenging experience of palliative care support-team nursing, *Oncol Nurs Forum* 20(5):779-785, 1993.

Mendyka BE: The dying patient in the intensive care unit: assisting the family in crisis, *AACN Clin Issues Crit Care Nurs* 4(3):550-557, 1993.

Moore FD: Ethics at both ends of life. In *A miracle and a privilege: recounting a half century of surgical advances,* Washington, DC, 1995, Joseph Henry Press.

Murphy PA, Price DM: "ACT": Taking a positive approach to end-of-life care, *Am J Nurs* 95(3):42-43, 1995.

North American Nursing Diagnosis Association: *NANDA nursing diagnoses: definitions and classification 1995-1996,* Philadelphia, 1994, The Association.

Nyatanga B: Emotional pain in terminal illness: a dilemma for nurses, *Senior Nurse* 13(3):46-48, 1993.

Pelliter M: The organ donor family members' perception of stressful situations during the organ donation experience, *J Adv Nurs* 17(1):90-97, 1992.

Rothkopf MM, Askanazi J: *Intensive home care,* Baltimore, 1992, Williams & Wilkins.

United States Department of Health and Human Services: *Clinical practice guidelines: management of cancer pain,* March 1994, Agency for Health Care Policy and Research.

CHAPTER 6

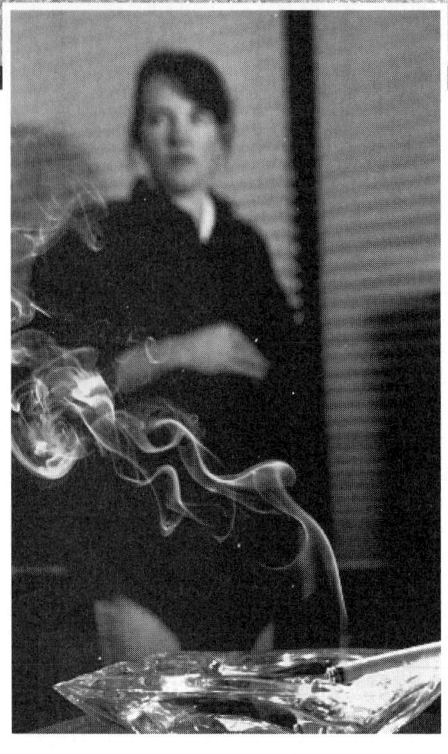

Substance Abuse

CHAPTER OBJECTIVES

1 Define the terms associated with substance abuse.
2 Discuss the causative factors associated with substance abuse and dependence.
3 Identify the substances most subject to abuse and the behaviors likely to be observed in an individual who is experiencing substance abuse or dependence.
4 Identify the major symptoms and interventions in the management of patients who are experiencing withdrawal.
5 Describe methods of ongoing treatment that are available to patients with substance dependence.
6 State examples of nursing diagnoses that are likely to apply to a patient with substance abuse or dependence.
7 Discuss how substance abuse and dependence impacts the family unit, the community, and society in general.
8 Identify own feelings about individuals who are substance abusers or substance dependent.

KEY WORDS

addiction
blackout
codependency
cross-tolerance
delerium tremens
denial
dry drunk
flashbacks
habituation
intervention
minimizing
progression
relapse
substance abuse
substance dependence
tolerance
withdrawal

Substance abuse is the pathologic use of a mind-altering chemical that is accompanied by a loss of control over how much and how often the chemical is used. Substance abuse results in impaired thinking and functioning. The user may abuse the chemical occasionally or continuously over a period, or months may elapse between episodes of abuse. Substance abuse differs from **substance dependence (addiction),** which describes the total psychophysical state of one who must receive an increasing amount of the chemical to prevent the onset of withdrawal symptoms. There is an overwhelming involvement with getting and using the drug.

The abuse of legal and illegal substances is a major health and socioeconomic problem worldwide. In the United States the abuse of mind-altering substances affects millions of users, their families, their co-workers, and the population in general. Alcohol abuse, smoking, and illegal drug use cause illness and death and are related to domestic violence, child abuse, lost productivity, and crime. Substance abuse places a tremendous burden on the economy because it strains the healthcare system, social services, and the criminal justice system. The total cost of substance abuse is staggering. It is estimated that the healthcare costs of alcoholics are twice as high as for nonalcoholics. Many dollars are spent on healthcare and social services for close family members of addicted persons, who often are at risk of developing physical and emotional illnesses. Money is also spent for services for the victims of substance-abuse–related crime.

Experts on substance abuse estimate that one out of every five people who seek medical treatment from a physician or clinic are substance abusers. Between 20% and 35% of all admissions to hospital medical-surgical units are substance abusers and possible candidates for withdrawal symptoms (Mendelson, Mello, 1992). The numbers are higher in critical care areas because of the link between alcohol and drug use and trauma (Sommers, 1994). Therefore it is wise to view every patient seen in a healthcare facility as a potential abuser. Mortality related to substance abuse remains high (Figure 6-1).

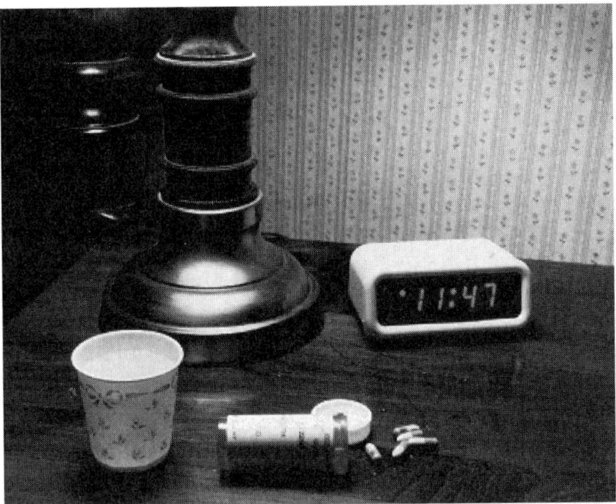

Figure 6-1 Abuse of prescription drugs is a major health problem. (Courtesy Michael Clement, MD, Mesa, Ariz.)

Fortunately the general public is becoming more intolerant of substance abuse, possibly because of an increased awareness of its health risks and the cost of social programs that deal with its associated problems. Tobacco use and alcohol-related motor vehicle accidents are decreasing. As more people become aware of the incidence and impact of substance abuse, perhaps the nationwide educational and treatment activities will have a positive effect on the problem.

TERMINOLOGY

To understand the problem of substance abuse, or chemical dependency, it is essential to become familiar with several terms. **Habituation** is an acquired tolerance that results from repeated exposure to a particular substance. Psychologic or emotional dependence may result from habituation, but there is little tendency to increase the dose, and withdrawal symptoms do not occur if the substance is discontinued. **Withdrawal** is a syndrome of potentially serious physical or psychologic symptoms that occurs when the use of a drug is severely decreased or discontinued. Symptoms vary with the substance and occur until the substance is eliminated from the body. It is important to note that with heavy users, withdrawal symptoms may begin before all of the drug has been eliminated from the body. **Tolerance** describes the physiologic adaptation to the effects of a chemical substance, which makes it necessary to increase the dose or frequency of use to obtain the original or desired effect. The ability of the human body to adjust to increasing doses of some chemicals is remarkable. Some heavy users ingest large amounts of drugs with seemingly few apparent effects, whereas the same dose may be life threatening to an individual who has not developed a tolerance. It is unclear how long tolerance lasts in an individual. With some mind-altering substances such as alcohol, tolerance may last for many years. **Cross-tolerance** occurs when a body that has developed a tolerance for one substance develops tolerance for substances in the same or similar categories. For example, a patient who is alcohol dependent can develop a tolerance for other central nervous system (CNS) depressants and may require larger doses of surgical anesthetics and pain medications to achieve the desired effects.

It is not possible to determine when a substance abuser becomes substance dependent. Estimates of the number of substance abusers who eventually become substance dependent varies, but some experts put the figure at approximately 50%. Substance abusers use mind-altering drugs for one reason: to change the way they feel. Initially substances are used to produce a feeling of well-being or pleasure. However, as dependence progresses the substance is used, in spite of the consequences, to function and to avoid withdrawal. Box 6-1 lists some alternate names for commonly abused substances.

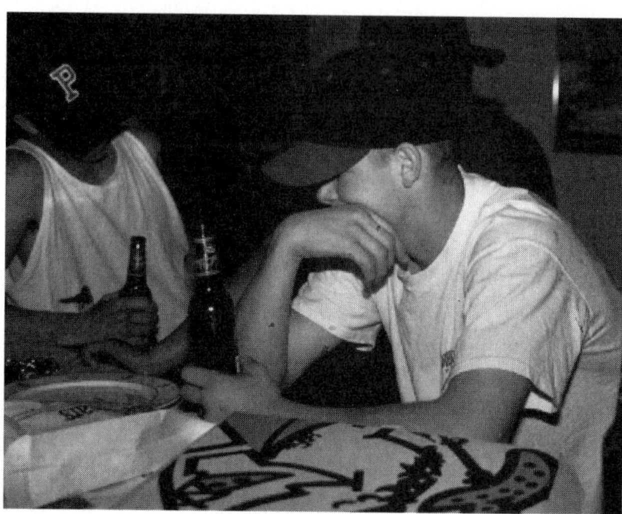

Figure 6-2 Peer pressure leads many teens to experiment with drugs and run the risk of becoming chemically dependent. (Courtesy Michael Clement, MD, Mesa, Ariz.)

ETIOLOGY

Much research has been and continues to be done in the attempt to explain why some people are prone to substance abuse and others are not. Various theories focus on the biologic, psychologic, sociocultural, and behavioral-cognitive aspects of the problem.

The biologic theory states that there is a physiologic cause for substance abuse. A genetic predisposition to alcoholism is evidenced by studies that reveal a high incidence of alcoholism in families of alcoholics. Sons of alcoholic men appear to be particularly at risk, because the chance of them developing alcoholism ranges between 30% and 50%. Children of alcoholic birth parents who were adopted as infants and raised apart from their birth parents have also been found to have higher rates of alcoholism. Studies of adopted twins have shown that identical twins of an alcoholic have a 60% chance of becoming alcoholics. For fraternal adopted twins of an alcoholic parent, the risk of becoming alcoholics is only 30%. There is also evidence of brain chemistry alterations among some substance abusers. Cocaine abusers show a deficiency in dopamine and norepinephrine. The enkephalins and endorphins are noted to be deficient in alcoholics and narcotic abusers. Studies continue regarding evidence of metabolic defects and the possibility of abnormal enzyme levels in some chemically dependent individuals.

The psychologic theory proposes that substance abusers are responding to depression, low self-esteem, and other stressors and are self-medicating to deal with tension, anxiety, and various kinds of psychic pain. For example, chemical use may initially relieve the loneliness that results from a lack of meaningful relationships.

The sociocultural theory recognizes the importance of group values and attitudes. The group can be relatively permanent, such as a biologic family or ethnic group, or temporary, such as junior high school classmates. Social expectations and encouragement may promote irresponsible use of even legal substances. Many teenagers become chemically dependent because peer pressure is particularly strong (Figure 6-2). Cultural beliefs can encourage or discourage the responsible use of substances (Mendelson, Mello, 1992). For example, people with an Irish, Scandinavian, or Native American heritage show a proclivity for substance abuse, whereas there is a low rate of abuse among Jewish and Asian people. Low socioeconomic status and racial inequality are also precursors of chemical dependency, such as with Native Americans and poor, black males. It has recently become evident that the geriatric population, which has been long ignored in substance abuse studies, is at high risk for becoming chemically dependent.

The behavioral-cognitive theory assumes that using and abusing patterns are learned and continue because of positive reinforcement. When the use of mind-altering substances within the family or peer group is accepted as normal behavior and encouraged, it is viewed as a way to manage stress, deal with problems, or have fun or celebrate. Therefore consumption provides the individual with short-term rewards, which reinforces the consumption pattern. As an individual becomes substance dependent, certain cues are associated with consumption, including the end of the work

BOX 6-1
"STREET" NAMES FOR COMMONLY ABUSED DRUGS

Marijuana
Acapulco gold
Grass
Joint
Mary Jane
Pot
Reefer
Roach
Tea
Weed

PCP
Angel dust
Cosmos
Jet
Mist
Peace pill
Rocket fuel
Superjoint
Tranq
Whack

Hashish
Ganja
Hash
Rope
Sweet Lucy

Hallucinogens
Acid (LSD)
Blue dots (LSD)
Cactus (mescaline)
Cube (LSD)
Magic mushroom (psilocybin)
Love drug (MDA)
Purple haze (LSD)

Cocaine
Blow
Coke
Flake
Gold dust
Nose candy
Rock
Snow
Speedball (heroin; cocaine)
White girl

Heroin
Brown
Hoise
Junk
Shag
Smack

Stimulants
Bennies
Dexies
Crystal
Meth
Pep pills
Speed
Ups

Barbiturates
Barbs
Blues
Downer
Goof balls
Rainbows
Yellow jacket (pentobarbital)
Red devil (secobarbital)
Blue devil (amobarbital)

Tranquilizers
Blues (10 mg Valium)
Yellows (5 mg Valium)
Tranks

day, a particular group of friends, or certain locations.

It is evident that substance abuse and dependence are the result of complex and incompletely understood processes. In some substance abusers no genetic link has been found. Many people believe that the interaction of genetic and environmental factors produce vulnerability to substance abuse. Therefore, even though a genetic propensity may exist, substance abuse or dependency is not inevitable.

SUBSTANCE ABUSE AS A DISEASE

In the United States Dr. Benjamin Rush recognized alcoholism as a disease as long ago as 1748. He described acute and chronic symptoms and observed hereditary and nongenetic influences. Beginning in the 1930s scientific studies of alcoholism were based on the understanding of alcoholism as a disease. In 1956 the American Medical Association officially accepted alcoholism as a disease (Report to Congress, 1990). The *Diagnostic and Statistical Manual of Mental Disorders IV* of the American Psychiatric Association identifies various forms of alcoholism and substance abuse, including not only illegal drugs but also nicotine and caffeine, as diseases.

The explanation of alcoholism and other substance abuses as diseases contrasts with historical moral explanations, in which any substance dependence is believed to come from a character defect that an individual can conquer by will power. Today even physicians and healthcare professionals only partially accept the idea that substance abuse is a disease. The reasons for this ambivalence are complex and may involve individual beliefs about moral judgment and free will and about the paradox of personal responsibility in the disease process. With some individuals this ambivalence may stem from having a substance abuser in the family (Miller, Toft, 1990).

THE DYSFUNCTIONAL FAMILY

Healthcare professionals who treat substance abusers view substance abusers and dependence as a disease process that is a problem not only for the individual but also for the family or significant others. Much has been written about the dysfunctional family, which results when a substance abuse problem is present. In a dysfunctional family, family members assume clearly defined roles and interact and communicate in predictable patterns to maintain the relationship or family structure.

Roles

As substance abuse progresses one or more family members begin to act in ways that protect the abuser from the consequences of substance abuse. This behavior is known as enabling. The enabler begins to assume the roles or duties that the addicted person can no longer perform. A spouse may take a second job to ease the financial burden that occurs when the abusing spouse gets fired from a job. A significant other may lie to an employer or to school authorities about absenteeism or poor performance. Family members may make excuses when social events or family gatherings are missed. Such enabling behaviors spare the abusers from embarrassment, financial consequences, and other negative effects of alcohol or drug abuse.

Other roles assumed by family members include the scapegoat, mascot, hero, and lost child. The scapegoat is the child who may act out to divert attention away from the using family member and toward himself or herself. The scapegoat is blamed for the problems within the family. The mascot is the funny, playful, or especially loving child who diverts attention to himself or herself in an attempt to shift the focus from the family pain. The hero is the good child who gets excellent grades, always acts responsibly, and possibly helps the nonusing parent meet family responsibilities. The lost or forgotten child withdraws and tries to avoid attention. The lost child does not expect his or her needs to be met. All of these roles help family members cope with the dynamics of substance abuse in the family. These roles are considered adaptive, yet they become a dysfunctional way of coping to maintain homeostasis or equilibrium within the alcoholic family system.

Codependency

Substance abuse affects all family members to some degree. As the substance abuser becomes more preoccupied with getting and using the chemical, family members become more focused on the abuser and his or her behavior and chemical use. They begin to change their own behaviors in response to the abuser's lifestyle. For example, family members may try to control the drinking, activities, or friends of the alcoholic. They may attempt to keep peace within the family system and may begin to withdraw from activities outside the family. Their lives begin to focus entirely on the substance abuser and his or her problem, and the disease of **codependency** develops. Codependency itself has predictable traits that may parallel those of the chemically dependent person (Box 6-2). The concept of codependency began in relation to the treatment of alcoholism as a family disease and the awareness that the alcoholic was not the only person affected by the disease. During the past 10 years the concept of codependency has grown to include a broad range of definitions.

BOX 6-2

SHARED TRAITS OF ALCOHOLISM AND CODEPENDENCY

Denial (dishonesty)
Alcoholic: I can stop drinking any time I want to.
Codependent: She doesn't get drunk every time she drinks.

Rationalization (confused thinking)
Alcoholic: I only drink because the boss doesn't like me and has it in for me.
Codependent: If I could keep the house cleaner and the children quiet when he gets home, he wouldn't drink so much.

Minimizing (denying the amount of alcohol consumed)
Alcoholic: I buy a lot of rounds at the bar, but I don't drink that much myself.
Codependent: She buys a lot of beer, but her friends drink most of that.

Fear
Alcoholic: I'm afraid to stop drinking. I've been doing it so long, what will I do instead?
Codependent: I can't make it on my own if he leaves me.

Self-centeredness
Alcoholic: I don't care what he wants to do. I work hard all week and deserve to go out and have a few drinks if I want to.
Codependent: After all I've done for her, how could she do this to me?

Loss of personal values
Alcoholic: I would never have taken that money from petty cash if I hadn't been buzzed from the drinks I had at lunch.
Codependent: I hate lying to his boss about him being sick, but if I don't he'll be fired because he's missed so many days.

Low self-esteem
Alcoholic: I'm really not as good as these other salesmen. I have to have a few drinks to loosen up before I can make my presentation.
Codependent: He's right. I can't do anything right.

Depression
Alcoholic: I'm sick and tired of feeling this way. My family would be better off if I just killed myself.
Codependent: I feel hopeless. Nothing is ever going to get better. No matter what I do, she still drinks.

CENTRAL NERVOUS SYSTEM DEPRESSANTS

Alcohol and Alcoholism

About two thirds of all adult Americans and a significant number of those under age 21 drink alcohol. Alcohol is rapidly absorbed from the gastrointestinal tract, beginning in the stomach and continuing in the small and large intestines. The rate of absorption is affected by the amount of food in the stomach and the concentration of alcohol in the drinks. Before reaching the bloodstream, some of the ethanol is metabolized in the stomach by gastric alcohol dehydrogenase. Men generally produce more of this protective stomach enzyme than women, which partially explains why women typically become intoxicated more quickly than men even considering women's smaller size. All of the ethanol absorbed from the stomach is carried to the liver, which is the primary site of alcohol metabolism. Here the alcohol is converted to acetaldehyde and then acetate with the help of enzymes known as alcohol dehydrogenases. The rate of metabolism depends on the weight and tolerance of the drinker. The amount of ethanol excreted through the liver varies and depends on the amount ingested. Usually 5% to 10% of ethanol is excreted unchanged through the lungs and kidneys without passing through the liver. If the blood alcohol level (BAL) is high, a relatively large amount of alcohol is excreted rather than metabolized (Mendelson, Mello, 1992).

The most serious effect of chronic excessive alcohol intake is alcoholism. There have been many terms used to describe alcoholism. Alcoholism is currently defined as a chronic, progressive, and potentially fatal biogenic and psychosocial disease that is characterized by tolerance and physical dependence and manifested by a loss of control, diverse personality changes, and social consequences.

Alcoholism is found in all socioeconomic levels, all occupations, and all age groups from preteen through the end of the life span. The average alcoholic takes his or her first drink between 12 and 14 years of age, first becomes intoxicated between age 14 and age 18, and experiences the first alcohol-related problem between 18 and 25 years of age. The first major problems with alcohol occur between 23 and 33 years of age. A variety of drinking patterns may occur. Alcoholics may drink on a daily basis, 2 or 3 times a week, only on weekends, or in sporadic binges that occur every few weeks or months. According to Schuchit and Marc (1989), "the average alcoholic has spontaneous periods of abstinence and marked decreases in drinking, which appear to alternate with times of heavy drinking" (p. 66). It is easier for the alcoholic not to drink at all than to try to control the amount of alcohol that he or she ingests. Any alcoholic substance may be used by the alcoholic: beer, wine, or distilled spirits. It is a myth that a person must drink "hard liquor" to become an alcoholic.

The effects of alcohol are related to the level of alcohol in the blood and brain. Symptoms of alcohol intoxication include impaired cognition (from drowsiness to stupor); ataxia; labile affect; slurred speech; diplopia; euphoria or violent, belligerent behavior; flushing; anorexia; and a depressed mood. An intoxicated individual may also experience **blackouts.** A blackout does not involve losing consciousness or passing out. It is a period of amnesia that occurs while a person seems to be functioning normally, and it is seen in someone who is or has been drinking heavily. The period of amnesia may range from a few minutes to several days. The blackout explains why a heavy drinker does not remember driving home, how a party ended, or what decisions were made at a business meeting.

If left untreated, alcoholism progresses through stages that Jellinek (1960) identified in his classic writings and studies (Box 6-3). Alcohol directly or indirectly affects every organ system in the body. Some people may be more predisposed than others to develop severe physical consequences from alcohol use (Box 6-4).

Because alcoholism involves a physical dependence, a significant decrease in the BAL or the sudden cessation of alcohol intake is likely to result in some withdrawal symptoms. Alcohol withdrawal is potentially life threatening, although a large number of alcoholics do not experience severe signs of withdrawal. Withdrawal symptoms begin as the BAL decreases (usually

BOX 6-3

JELLINEK'S STAGES OF ALCOHOLISM

Phase I: Prealcoholic
Uses alcohol to relax and deal with tension
Gradually increases tolerance
Phase II: Early Alcoholic
May begin experiencing blackouts
Sneaks drinks
Rationalizes drinking
Becomes defensive when someone mentions drinking
Has an increased preoccupation with drinking
Experiences guilt and denial
Phase III: Crucial Phase
Is fully addicted
Has lost control over drinking
Develops a physiologic dependence
Has severe problems with job, marriage, and interpersonal relationships
Phase IV: Chronic Phase
Experiences many physical and psychologic illnesses
Severe withdrawal results from abrupt cessation of drinking

Modified from Beare P, Myers J: *Principles and practice of adult health nursing,* ed 2, St Louis, 1994, Mosby.

from 4 to 12 hours after the last drink). Each alcoholic responds differently to withdrawal, and subsequent withdrawals in the same individual may progress differently. Mild physical symptoms are common, including an increase in pulse, blood pressure, respiratory rate, and temperature. Mild-to-moderate diaphoresis, anorexia, nausea and vomiting, diarrhea, irritability, anxiety, and insomnia are also common. Tremors are seen in more than half of the people who experience mild-to-moderate withdrawal symptoms. The inexperienced observer may confuse the tremors commonly seen in withdrawal with **delirium tremens (DTs).** Alcohol withdrawal syndrome, or delirium tremens, is the most serious stage of alcohol withdrawal and is characterized by severe autonomic nervous system dysfunction, confusion, hallucinations, and grand mal seizures. Table 6-1 summarizes the stages of alcohol withdrawal.

Because alcoholics are more prone to developing medical problems than the general population, a physical examination and assessment is essential as the first step in the treatment of alcohol withdrawal. However, many people with alcoholism go through withdrawal at home and without any medical supervision (Mendelson, Mellon, 1992). The goal of treatment during withdrawal is to provide a medically safe and reasonably comfortable period of detoxification (detox). Medications may be used to control the symptoms, make the patient more comfortable, and lessen the risk for seizures or DTs. Such treatment is especially important when the alcoholic has been diagnosed with hypertension or Type I diabetes or has a history of seizure activity. Although there are indications that almost any central nervous system (CNS) depressant can be used to detoxify a patient from alcohol, one or more of the benzodiazepines is generally used. Longer-acting benzodiazepines, such as diazepam (Valium) or chlordiazepoxide (Librium), are generally given in decreasing doses and provide a safe detox or withdrawal. Shorter-acting drugs from that class, such as oxazepam (Serax) or lorazepam (Ativan) are less likely to accumulate in someone with severe liver disease. However, if they are not given at least every 4 hours, they may add to the problem of alcohol withdrawal or precipitate seizures (Schuchit, Marc, 1989).

After alcohol withdrawal has been completed, most alcohol-dependent individuals require some form of ongoing treatment. During the first few weeks or months of recovery, disulfiram (Antabuse) may be prescribed to help prevent a **relapse** into drinking. Antabuse prevents the normal breakdown of alcohol in the liver. There are few side effects to disulfiram

BOX 6-4

PHYSIOLOGIC EFFECTS OF ALCOHOL ABUSE

Cardiovascular
Cardiomyopathy
Hypertension (systolic)
Beriberi
Heart disease

Gastrointestinal
Cancer of mouth, stomach, pancreas
Gastritis
Peptic ulcer
Esophagitis
Esophageal varices
Hypoglycemia
Cirrhosis of liver
Alcoholic hepatitis
Pancreatitis
Colitis
Malabsorption
Vitamin deficiencies
Malnutrition

Genitourinary
Impotence in males
Testicular atrophy
Gynecomastia in males
Menstrual irregularities in females

Hematologic
Anemia
Hyperlipidemia
Lactic acidosis
Impaired immune response

Musculoskeletal
Reduced bone density
Increased fracture risk
Skeletal myopathies

Neurologic
Cerebral atrophy
Impaired cognition and memory
Peripheral neuropathies
Wernicke-Korsakoff syndrome

Respiratory
Decreased resistance to chronic infections (e.g., tuberculosis, pneumonia)
Chronic obstructive pulmonary disease

Integumentary
Spider angiomas
Palmar erythema
Bruising

TABLE 6-1

Alcohol Withdrawal Symptoms and Interventions

Stage	Medications*	Interventions
Mild Tremors (begin 3-36 hr after last drink) Pulse < 92 BP < 140/90 Slight diaphoresis Slight flushing Anxiety **Moderate** Tremors Pulse between 90 and 130 BP between 140/90 and 160/110 Moderate to profuse diaphoresis Irritability; anxiety Agitation; anxiety Anorexia Nausea and vomiting **Hallucinosis** Moderate symptoms plus auditory or visual hallucinations	Librium Valium Librium Valium	1. Monitor vital signs (VS) q 1-3 hr. 2. Administer sedating medications as ordered, prn if needed. 3. Offer small, high CHO feedings q 2-3 hr. 4. Offer clear or nourishing liquids as tolerated. 5. Record intake and output (I&O). 6. Administer vitamins as ordered. 7. Assist with activities of daily living (ADLs) as needed. 8. Allow and encourage ambulation if VS and gait are stable. 9. Orient to time, place, and person if necessary. 10. Follow seizure precautions if any history of seizures. 11. Spend time with patient and family. Be nonjudgmental and reassuring.
Alcohol withdrawal syndrome (DTs) Begins 24-72 hr after last drink (mortality up to 35%) Pulse > 130 Confusion Delirium Severe agitation Hallucinations Seizures Cardiovascular collapse	Anticonvulsants intravenously (IV) per physician order	1. Check patient q 15 min. 2. Monitor VS q 1 hr. 3. Assess neuro status q 1 hr. 4. Restrain if necessary to prevent injury. 5. Monitor IV fluids and catheter. 6. Administer medication as ordered. 7. Assess for signs of trauma or skin breakdown. 8. Provide calm, quiet atmosphere.

*Each physician may have his or her own detox protocol. It is not uncommon to exceed usual medication parameters with a patient who is experiencing withdrawal from alcohol.

Maximum dosages:

Librium: 600 mg/24 hr
Valium: 120 mg/24 hr } administered by mouth (PO)

itself. Drowsiness may occur for a few days, but taking the daily dose at bedtime may help to alleviate the insomnia that many alcoholics experience for weeks after becoming sober. However, when Antabuse is in the body (up to 14 days after the last dose), as little as one-half ounce of alcohol in the bloodstream causes a physical reaction that begins with flushing, increased respirations, and an increased heart rate. This reaction begins within a few minutes and can progress to nausea and vomiting, aches, and weakness. Immediate medical help is needed if such symptoms occur.

Because of the potentially harmful effects of drinking or using alcohol-based products while taking Antabuse, a witnessed and signed consent form should be required of the patient. Teaching protocols are helpful for the nurse to use with a patient who is taking Antabuse, because he or she needs to know the important contraindications while on the medication. Some teaching issues include not giving blood while on Antabuse therapy and avoiding products such as vinegar and alcohol-based shaving lotions and cough medications. It is very important to instruct the patient that after quitting the medication, the effects of the drug remain in the system up to 14 days and therefore any use of alcohol or alcohol-based products will cause an adverse reaction.

OLDER ADULT CONSIDERATIONS

Alcohol problems are much more common among older adults than professionals in healthcare and aging services generally recognize. Manifestations of alcohol abuse in older adults are more subtle, atypical, and nonspecific than in younger populations. Many older patients consume smaller quantities of alcohol than younger patients and therefore may develop overt withdrawal states less often. Those who consume lesser quantities may not drink to the point of intoxication and therefore may appear to be more in control of their drinking. Because of the increased susceptibility to the toxic effects of alcohol with advancing age, a person can develop alcohol problems just by becoming older and without necessarily changing the amount of alcohol consumed. In such cases craving and compulsive use may not be apparent, but continued use in spite of negative consequences still defines problem drinking.

An alcohol intake that is considered moderate for a younger person may cause adverse consequences in an older adult, who has less physiologic reserve in meeting self-care needs such as grooming and housekeeping. A small, frail, older person who is barely functioning in terms of self-care capabilities and who consumes two or three drinks a day can tip the balance toward an inability to maintain himself or herself independently.

Approximately 80% of Americans over age 65 have at least one chronic disease. Many will have several chronic diseases, any or all of which may be complicated by even small amounts of alcohol. Unlike in younger adults, alcohol abuse in the older adult most likely manifests itself in the form of some combination of nonspecific, functional deficits, which makes it all the more difficult to diagnose.

Tranquilizers

The most common type of tranquilizers are the benzodiazepines, which are psychoactive drugs that are used to lessen anxiety and may also be used as anticonvulsants and muscle relaxants. They include diazepam (Valium), alprazolam (Xanax), lorazepam (Ativan), chlordiazepoxide (Librium), oxazepam (Serax), clorazepate (Tranxene) and triazolam (Halcion) (Table 6-2). Benzodiazepines are available in tablet, capsule, and liquid form and are widely prescribed. Therefore they are often abused. The antianxiety effects of the minor tranquilizers are short-lived, and when the effects wear off, an individual may experience an increased level of anxiety. Tolerance and physical and psychologic depen-

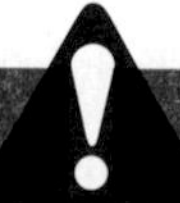

NURSE ALERT

Combining alcohol with different substances can produce serious effects.

Sedatives—anxiolytic

Produces additive or synergistic increases in the sedative actions.

Psychomatic impairment also occurs.

Tricyclic antidepressants

Both smoking and alcohol may accelerate the clearance of these antidepressants. Therefore depressed alcoholics may not achieve the appropriate blood levels of antidepressants.

Monoamine oxidase inhibitors (MAOIs)

Some MAOIs produce disulfiram-like (Antabuse-like) effects.

Dark beer and red wines contain tyramine and may produce hypertensive episodes.

Opioids

Respiratory depressant effects of both ethanol and opioids may be potentiated.

Cocaine

Cardiovascular effects may be potentiated.

Oral hypoglycemic agents

Significant decreases in blood sugar levels may be produced if agents are ingested with alcohol.

Acetaminophen

Accumulation of toxic metabolites may occur and increase susceptibility to acetaminophen-induced hepatotoxicity.

Salicylates and aspirin

Alcohol increases the tendency of salicylates to cause gastrointestinal (GI) bleeding. Aspirin increases alcohol absorption, which results in elevated BALs.

Anticoagulants

Chronic drinkers metabolize warfarin more rapidly, which makes very careful monitoring of anticoagulant effects necessary, especially when the drinking pattern varies substantially.

H2 antagonists

Cimetidine, ranitidine, and rizatidine (but not famotidine) may increase BALs by reducing ethanol metabolism in the stomach.

Antimicrobials/Antibiotics

Many antimicrobials (chloramphenicol, furazolidone, griseofulvin, metronidazole, some cephalosporins) may interact with acute alcohol consumption to produce a disulfiram-like (Antabuselike) reaction.

TABLE 6-2
Pharmacology of Drugs Used in Substance Abuse

Drug (Generic and Trade Name); Route and Dosage	Action/Indication	Common Side Effects and Nursing Considerations
ALPRAZOLAM (Xanax) **ROUTE:** PO **DOSAGE:** 0.25 mg-0.5 mg 2-3 times daily as needed (not greater than 4 mg/day); decrease dose in debilitated/elderly patients	Benzodiazepine used in the treatment of anxiety, depression, and "panic attacks"	Dizziness, drowsiness, and lethargy
AMITRIPTYLINE (Elavil) **ROUTE:** PO, IM **DOSAGE:** PO 30-100 mg/day single bedtime or divided dose, and dose may be gradually increased up to 150-300 mg/day; IM 20-30 mg 4 times daily	Antianxiety drug used in treatment of depression	Drowsiness, sedation, lethargy, fatigue, dry mouth, dry eyes, blurred vision, hypotension, and constipation; potentially fatal reaction with MAO inhibitors; may adversely interfere with antihypertensive drugs
CHLORDIAZEPOXIDE (Librium) **ROUTE:** PO, IM, IV **DOSAGE:** For alcohol withdrawal PO 50-100 mg, repeated agitation up to 400 mg/day; for anxiety PO 5-25 mg 3-4 times daily or IM, IV 50-100 mg initially, then 25-50 mg 3-4 times daily as required	Benzodiazepine used in treatment of anxiety, alcohol withdrawal, and preoperative sedative	Dizziness and drowsiness; use with caution in liver or kidney disease
CHLORPROMAZINE (Thorazine) **ROUTE:** PO, IM, IV, Rectal **DOSAGE:** For psychosis PO 10-25 mg 2-4 times daily, increase by 20-50 mg/day every 3-4 days (usual dose is 200 mg/day); for nausea and vomiting PO 10-25 mg q 4-6 hr, IM 25-50 mg q 3-4 h, rectal 50-100 mg q 6-8 hr; for intractable hiccups PO, IM 25-50 mg 3-4 times daily	Antipsychotic and antiemetic used for acute and chronic psychosis, nausea and vomiting, preoperative sedation, and intractable hiccups	Sedation, extrapyramidal reactions, dry eyes, blurred vision, hypotension, constipation, dry mouth, and photosensitivity; use with caution in liver and cardiac disease; may cause bone marrow suppression; may have adverse reactions with other CNS depressants
CHLORAZEPATE (Tranxene) **ROUTE:** PO **DOSAGE:** 15-60 mg/day in divided doses	Benzodiazepene used in treatment of anxiety, alcohol withdrawal, and management of seizures	Dizziness, drowsiness, and lethargy; use with caution in previously suicidal or addicted
DIAZEPAM (Valium) **ROUTE:** PO, IM, IV **DOSAGE:** For anxiety 2-10 mg 2-4 times daily or 14-30 mg extended-release form once daily; for seizures IV 5-10 mg and may repeat q 10-15 minutes for total of 30 mg; for alcohol withdrawal 10 mg 3-4 times daily in first 24 hr, decrease to 5 mg 3-4 times daily	Benzodiazepene used in treatment of anxiety, preoperative sedation, light anesthesia, seizures, muscle relaxant, and alcohol withdrawal	Dizziness, drowsiness, and lethargy; use with caution in debilitated, renal or hepatic dysfunction, and previously addicted or suicidal; drug has very few compatibilities

continued

TABLE 6-2

Pharmacology of Drugs Used in Substance Abuse—cont'd

Drug (Generic and Trade Name); Route and Dosage	Action/Indication	Common Side Effects and Nursing Considerations
FLUOXETINE (Prozac) **ROUTE:** PO **DOSAGE:** 20 mg/day in the morning; after several weeks, may increase by 20 mg/day at weekly intervals (not to exceed 80 mg/day)	Antianxiety drug used in treatment of depression	Anxiety, insomnia, headache, drowsiness, tremor, diarrhea, excessive sweating and pruritis; may cause anorexia and weight loss; use with caution in renal or hepatic dysfunction and in the elderly
HALOPERIDOL (Haldol) **ROUTE:** PO, IM, IV **DOSAGE:** PO 0.5-5 mg 2-3 times daily (patients with severe symptoms may require up to 100 mg/day); IM 2-5 mg q 1-8 hr, not to exceed 100 mg/day; IV 0.5-50 mg, may be repeated in 30 minutes	Antipsychotic drug used in treatment of acute and chronic psychoses	Extrapyramidal reactions, dry eyes, blurred vision, hypotension, constipation, dry mouth, and photosensitivity
LITHIUM (Lithium) **ROUTE:** PO **DOSAGE:** 900-1200 mg/day in 3-4 divided doses; blood level monitoring necessary to monitor therapeutic dose	Antimania drug used in the treatment of a variety of psychiatric disorders, especially bipolar affective disorders	Tremors, headache, impaired memory, lethargy, fatigue, ECG changes, nausea, anorexia, epigastric bloating, diarrhea, abdominal pain, polyuria, dermatitis, hypothyroidism, leukocytosis, and muscle weakness; avoid in severe cardiac or renal dysfunction, known alcohol intolerance; must monitor drug levels closely
LORAZEPAM (Ativan) **ROUTE:** PO, IM, IV **DOSAGE:** PO 1-3 mg 2-3 times daily (up to 10 mg/day); decrease dose in elderly	Benzodiazepene used in treatment of anxiety and insomnia, used preoperatively for sedation and anesthesia	Dizziness, drowsiness, and lethargy; use with caution in debilitated, renal or hepatic dysfunction, and previously addicted or suicidal
METHADONE (Dolophine) **ROUTE:** PO **DOSAGE:** 15-20 mg orally (up to 40 mg orally) to suppress symptoms; maintenance dose of 20-120 mg daily to control abstinence	Narcotic analgesic that replaces heroin or other opioid analgesics in detoxification/maintenance programs	Sedation, confusion, hypotension, and constipation; euphoria is much less prominent, and the addict may eventually overcome compulsive need for "narcotic high"
OXAZEPAM (Serax) **ROUTE:** PO **DOSAGE:** 10-30 mg 3-4 times daily; in older patients, initial dose should be 5 mg 1-2 times daily or 10 mg 3 times daily	Benzodiazepene used in treatment of anxiety and alcohol withdrawal	Dizziness, drowsiness, and lethargy; use cautiously with the elderly, hepatic dysfunction, and previously suicidal or addicted

TABLE 6-2

Pharmacology of Drugs Used in Substance Abuse—cont'd

Drug (Generic and Trade Name); Route and Dosage	Action/Indication	Common Side Effects and Nursing Considerations
PAROXETINE (Paxil) **ROUTE:** PO **DOSAGE:** 20 mg as a single morning dose; may increase dose by 10 mg/day at weekly intervals for maximum 50 mg/day dose	Antianxiety drug used in treatment of depression	Somnolence, dizziness, insomnia, tremor, nervousness, anxiety, headache, weakness, nausea, dry mouth, constipation, diarrhea, ejaculatory disturbance, male genital disorders, and sweating; potentially fatal reaction with MAO inhibitors; use with caution in the elderly and in renal or hepatic dysfunction
SERTRALINE (Zoloft) **ROUTE:** PO **DOSAGE:** 50 mg/day as a single morning dose; may increase at weekly intervals for a maximum 200 mg/day	Antianxiety drug used in treatment of depression	Headache, dizziness, tremor, insomnia, drowsiness, fatigue, dry mouth, nausea, diarrhea, male sexual dysfunction, and increased sweating; potentially fatal reaction with MAO inhibitors; use with caution in the elderly and in renal or hepatic dysfunction
TRANYLCYPROMINE (Pamate) **ROUTE:** PO **DOSAGE:** 30 mg/day initially in single or divided doses; after 2 weeks can increase by 10 mg/day, up to maximum dose of 60 mg/day	Monamine oxidase inhibitor (MAOI) used in treatment of neurotic or atypical depression	Restlessness, insomnia, dizziness, headache, blurred vision, orthostatic hypotension, arrhythmias, constipation, anorexia, nausea, vomiting, diarrhea, abdominal pain, and dry mouth; must watch for multiple drug reactions that could cause hypertensive crisis; foods containing tyramine can cause fatal hypertensive crisis (cheese, sour cream, beer, yogurt); chocolate and caffeine can elevate blood pressure

dence can develop. Withdrawal symptoms can develop within 12 to 24 hours. Many symptoms, including anxiety, insomnia, irritability, vomiting, diaphoresis, tremors, and seizures may occur during withdrawal, especially if the use has been prolonged. Therefore the dose is gradually reduced over time. Benzodiazepines have a synergistic effect with alcohol, and the combination may lead to an overdose (Box 6-5).

Barbiturates

Barbiturates are synthetic drugs that are used medically to treat insomnia and epilepsy and to sedate the surgical patient. Tolerance and physical and psychologic dependence can result from barbiturate use, regardless of whether it is a prescribed medication or a street drug. Barbiturates are available in oral forms (capsules or elixirs), in suppository form, or in a liquid form for injection. Taking another CNS depressant with a barbiturate may lead to an accidental overdose, which includes symptoms of slurred speech, disorientation, confusion, respiratory depression, cyanosis, hypotension, ataxia, a weak pulse, and death (Box 6-6). Withdrawal symptoms range from mild to life threatening and can include irritability, insomnia, weakness, anxiety, nausea and vomiting, headache, mental confusion, hallucinations, convulsions, and delirium. The patient is best hospitalized for this withdrawal, which may involve substituting a long-acting barbiturate for the original abused substance. The dosage is slowly tapered over a period of several weeks until the drug is discontinued.

Narcotics

Narcotics include opium and its derivatives, heroin, codeine, morphine, hydromorphone, and synthetic opiates, including meperidine, methadone, propoxyphene (Darvon) and pentazocine (Talwin). Tolerance and physical and psychologic dependency can occur rapidly. Heroin is the most commonly abused of the opiate drugs, but dependency can occur with any of the narcotics. Heroin users report an initial euphoria followed by the "nod," which is a feeling of almost complete physical and mental relaxation that can last for several hours (Box 6-7). Once a drug used primarily by minorities in the lower socioeconomic class, heroin has recently been increasingly used by middle class whites. It may be inhaled through the nose (snorted) or injected. The use of contaminated needles creates a risk for human immunodeficiency virus (HIV), hepatitis, and septicemia.

Withdrawal symptoms may begin within 8 to 12 hours of the last dose. Heroin withdrawal is rarely life threatening and may create mild flu-like symptoms such as diaphoresis, nausea, vomiting, a runny nose, increased lacrimation, yawning, and generalized musculoskeletal aches. More severe symptoms include anxiety, agitation, chills, fever, tremors, muscle spasms, and an elevated blood pressure and pulse. Clonidine may be used to treat some of the withdrawal symptoms. Naltrexone (Trexan), a long-acting narcotic antagonist, may be used after the patient has been free of opiates for at least 5 days. Administering Trexan to a patient who is using opiates can precipitate a relatively severe withdrawal syndrome, because Trexan negates the effects of the opiates. Therefore the patient must be properly screened to determine current opiate levels.

Methadone, a synthetic opiate, is sometimes used to decrease or eliminate the symptoms of heroin withdrawal. The patient may be enrolled in a methadone maintenance program in which he or she receives the drug over a prolonged period of weeks to years. Because methadone itself is addicting, its dosage must be tapered slowly. Not all professionals endorse the use of methadone and instead recommend symptomatic treatment of withdrawal to reach complete abstinence.

BOX 6-5

CLINICAL MANIFESTATIONS OF TRANQUILIZER USE

Side effects include the following:
1 Skin rash
2 Headache
3 Nausea
4 Impairment of sexual function
5 Dizziness
6 Lightheadedness

Signs of overdose include the following:
1 Sleepiness
2 Confusion
3 Loss of consciousness
4 Diminished reflexes

From Phipps WJ and others: *Medical-surgical nursing: concepts and clinical practice,* ed 5, St Louis, 1995, Mosby.

BOX 6-6

CLINICAL MANIFESTATIONS OF BARBITURATE USE

1 Feeling of well-being
2 Euphoria
3 Relief from anxiety
4 Side effects, including breathing difficulties, lethargy, allergic reactions, nausea, and dizziness

From Phipps WJ and others: *Medical-surgical nursing: concepts and clinical practice,* ed 5, St Louis, 1995, Mosby.

BOX 6-7

CLINICAL MANIFESTATIONS OF NARCOTIC USE

1 Relief of pain and feeling of well-being
2 Shallow breathing
3 Reduced hunger and thirst
4 Reduced sexual drive
5 Drowsiness
6 Euphoria
7 Lethargy
8 Heaviness of limbs
9 Apathy
10 Loss of ability to concentrate
11 Loss of judgment and self-control
12 Overdoses can cause coma, convulsions, respiratory arrest, and death

From Phipps WJ and others: *Medical-surgical nursing: concepts and clinical practice,* ed 5, St Louis, 1995, Mosby.

Marijuana

Marijuana, or cannabis, has been used as a mind-altering drug for thousands of years. It grows wild in many countries and is easily cultivated for street use. Marijuana comes from the dried leaves and flowers of the hemp plant, and it is smoked in a pipe or cigarette. "Bongs," or water-filled pipes, may also be used for smoking marijuana or hashish, which is a concentrated extract of the hemp plant. Marijuana is one of the most commonly abused illegal drugs in the United States and is particularly popular among young people. Cannabis is used in medicine to help control the side effects of chemotherapy and is occasionally used to reduce the eye pressure in glaucoma. Cannabis is a CNS depressant, and psychologic dependence may occur in users. The use of cannabis before or during activities that require concentration and motor coordination is dangerous. Driving a vehicle or operating machinery while under the influence increases the risk of injury or death to self or others (Boxes 6-8 and 6-9).

BOX 6-8

PHYSICAL MANIFESTATIONS OF MARIJUANA USE

1 Drying of the eyes and mouth
2 Increase in appetite and food consumption
3 Can produce glucose intolerance, leading to hyperglycemia, which can be a problem in those with diabetes
4 Reddening of eyes
5 Impairment of short-term memory
6 Increased heart rate and blood pressure
7 Decreased body temperature
8 Impairment of coordination

From Phipps WJ and others: *Medical-surgical nursing: concepts and clinical practice,* ed 5, St Louis, 1995, Mosby.

BOX 6-9

PSYCHOLOGIC MANIFESTATIONS OF MARIJUANA USE

1 Altering of perception (e.g., sight, sound, touch, sense of time, and taste)
2 Feeling of well-being and intoxication, although depression and panic may occur
3 Confusion and distortion of reality may occur

From Phipps WJ and others: *Medical-surgical nursing: concepts and clinical practice,* ed 5, St Louis, 1995, Mosby.

CENTRAL NERVOUS SYSTEM STIMULANTS

Amphetamines

Amphetamines are synthetic psychoactive drugs that are used to increase a sense of alertness and wakefulness and alter mood. They are legally available by prescription in tablet and capsule form. Methamphetamine is an illegal street drug that is produced in powdered form and mixed with a diluent for injection.

Amphetamines stimulate the brain and heart, which results in an increased blood pressure and pulse rate, dilated pupils, reduced fatigue, a reduced appetite, and increased concentration. Large doses or prolonged use results in an unnatural wakefulness and euphoria that is often followed by a "crash," or a period of physical and mental exhaustion and depression (Box 6-10). Amphetamines may produce tolerance and a psychologic dependence. It is unclear whether a physical dependence occurs.

Amphetamine withdrawal symptoms may include fatigue, lethargy, depression, muscle pain, and a toxic psychosis. Severe symptoms may require respiratory and cardiovascular support. Intravenous Valium (for sedation) and antihypertensives may also be ordered.

Cocaine

Cocaine is a highly addictive and potent CNS stimulant, and its use has increased greatly in the United States during the last decade. Cocaine can be used in a variety of ways. A powdered form of cocaine may be

BOX 6-10

CLINICAL MANIFESTATIONS OF AMPHETAMINE USE

1 Restlessness
2 Dizziness
3 Insomnia
4 Lack of appetite, dramatic weight loss
5 Diarrhea or constipation
6 Agitation and anxiety
7 Paranoia; paranoid psychosis
8 Cerebral hemorrhage
9 Myocardial infarction
10 Collapse from exhaustion

Withdrawal often leads to profound depression and may lead to suicide.

From Phipps WJ and others: *Medical-surgical nursing: concepts and clinical practice,* ed 5, St Louis, 1995, Mosby.

snorted or dissolved and injected intravenously. Crack cocaine is produced by heating cocaine with baking soda and water, which results in a purified substance that may contain as much as 90% pure cocaine. Crack is smoked in a pipe or mixed with tobacco and rolled and smoked as a cigarette. Freebasing involves heating the cocaine to separate it from the adulterants used to cut (or dilute) the drug. Freebase cocaine may be smoked or injected intravenously. Cocaine is a rapid but relatively short-acting drug. When it is snorted, the effects are felt within approximately 3 minutes and last from 15 to 30 minutes. A more intense euphoria occurs when crack cocaine is smoked. The euphoria begins within 4 to 6 seconds but lasts only 6 to 7 minutes.

Tolerance and psychologic dependence can occur rapidly with cocaine. The high is usually followed by a crash when the drug wears off. The feelings of well-being and confidence are replaced with fatigue and depression. The rapid and intense effects of cocaine motivate an individual to use more of the drug, which leads to repeated abuse. To relieve the sometimes uncomfortable effects of CNS stimulation, users often also abuse a CNS depressant such as alcohol or heroin. Physical dependence may occur in some cocaine users. Cocaine acts on the neurotransmitters of the brain and prolongs the effects of norepinephrine and dopamine. Repeated or habitual use may break down the neurotransmitters and eventually deplete the supply of norepinephrine and dopamine to the brain and peripheral nerves.

Severe physical problems occur with cocaine use. Soon after taking cocaine, the user's blood pressure and pulse increase rapidly, and the user may report chest pain and a pounding heart. Death may be caused by a ventricular arrhythmia, seizures, a cocaine-induced stroke, or respiratory paralysis. Some users describe a cocaine psychosis, which includes hallucinations, insomnia, and an increased potential for violent behavior in some persons (Box 6-11). Withdrawal treatment depends on the patient's symptoms and may include the use of sedatives, tranquilizers, anticonvulsants, and antiarrhythmic drugs.

BOX 6-11

CLINICAL MANIFESTATIONS OF COCAINE USE

1 Stimulation of respiration and heart rate
2 Raising of blood pressure and blood sugar levels
3 Suppression of appetite
4 Dilation of pupils
5 Constriction of certain blood vessels
6 Increase in levels of physical activity
7 Insomnia
8 Trembling
9 Sensations of extreme euphoria
10 Feelings of energy, power, confidence, and talkativeness

There is a letdown effect (cocaine crash) that occurs when the effect of the drug wears off.

From Phipps WJ and others: *Medical-surgical nursing: concepts and clinical practice,* ed 5, St Louis, 1995, Mosby.

Nicotine

Nicotine, which is found in tobacco, is used by 25% to 30% of all Americans. Tobacco may be smoked or chewed. Finely chopped tobacco in the form of snuff is placed between the gums and the cheek, and the nicotine is absorbed through the mucous membranes in the mouth. Nicotine is very addictive, perhaps more so than any other drug. It is both psychologically and physically addicting. The physically damaging effects of cigarette smoking are widely recognized (Figure 6-3). When tobacco smoke is inhaled, the effects are felt within seconds, and the nicotine is rapidly metabolized in the body. Because the effects of nicotine are brief, the user smokes from several times a day to several times an hour, depending on the tolerance that has developed and the opportunities for use. Laws and policies are increasingly limiting the opportunities for smoking in public places.

Although nicotine is a mild CNS stimulant, users report that smoking a cigarette may have an energizing or a calming effect, depending on the user's mood and the circumstances. Nicotine acts as a mild-to-moderate appetite suppressant and causes a temporary rise in blood pressure. In excessive doses it produces mild tremors and an increased respiratory rate. Withdrawal symptoms occur rapidly. Within 1 to 3 hours after smoking a cigarette, the craving for another may begin. Cravings may last for weeks or months after cessation but diminish in frequency and intensity over time. Other withdrawal symptoms include irritability, anxiety, poor concentration, headaches, fatigue, insomnia, and constipation or diarrhea.

A number of behavior modification programs that promote smoking cessation are available. Acupuncture and hypnosis have proven successful for some smokers. Transdermal nicotine patches lessen physical withdrawal symptoms by providing small amounts of nicotine continuously through the skin. The patches are most effective when used in conjunction with a behavior modification program.

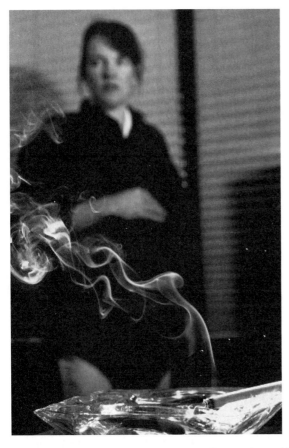

Figure 6-3 The physically damaging effects of smoking are widely recognized. Women are advised not to smoke during pregnancy to prevent effects that are potentially harmful to the infant. (Courtesy Michael Clement, MD, Mesa, Ariz.)

INHALANTS

Inhalants include a wide range of chemicals that emit vapors or fumes. Many household products such as glue, paint thinner, nail polish remover, spot remover, gasoline, kerosene, and cleaning products belong to this category. Aerosol products such as hair spray, stain protector, deodorants, and insecticides become drugs of abuse when the fumes are inhaled. Nitrous oxide and ether are anesthetics that are sometimes used recreationally. The user may sniff the vapors directly from an aerosol can or other container or may capture the fumes in a bag or balloon. Because these products are inexpensive and, except for the anesthetics, easily obtainable, most inhalant abusers are adolescents, and incidence is rapidly increasing in that age group (InTouch). Some inhalants cause tolerance and may cause physical dependency.

Most inhalants are CNS depressants. Box 6-12 lists the clinical manifestations of inhalant use. Serious consequences may occur from the excessive or repeated use of inhalants, including damage to the liver, kidneys, bone marrow, and brain. Death may result from cardiac arrest or from suffocation as a result of the displacement of oxygen in the lungs.

BOX 6-12

CLINICAL MANIFESTATIONS OF INHALANT USE

1 Slurred speech
2 Blurred vision, bloodshot eyes
3 Inflamed mucous membranes, nosebleeds
4 Bad breath/chemical odor
5 Lightheadedness
6 Ringing in the ears
7 Watering eyes
8 Loss of coordination/poor memory
9 Excessive nasal secretions
10 Loss of consciousness or seizures lasting 20 to 45 minutes with large doses

Modified from Phipps WJ and others: *Medical-surgical nursing: concepts and clinical practice*, ed 5, St Louis, 1995, Mosby.

HALLUCINOGENS

Hallucinogens are drugs that produce an acute change in thinking and in reality perception. Included in this group are lysergic acid diethylamide (LSD); mescaline; 2,5-dimethoxy-4-methamphetamine (STP); psilocybin; dimethyltryptamine (DMT); and methylenedioxyamphetamine (MDA). These street drugs became popular during the 1960s and 1970s. Hallucinogens are ingested orally and may be found in many forms, including tablets, capsules, powder, mushrooms, and peyote buttons. Sometimes they are mixed with food or put on sugar cubes. LSD is also found on blotter paper and on sheets of paper containing tattoos or pictures of cartoon characters.

Hallucinogens distort the user's perception of the environment and alter thought and emotional patterns (Box 6-13). Visual hallucinations and mood changes vary dramatically from person to person and also within the same person, depending on the circumstances in which the drug is ingested. Hallucinogenic effects may last from 6 to 12 hours. A "bad trip" occurs when frightening images, panic, terror, or depression is experienced. Paranoid or violent behavior or psychotic episodes may occur.

Tolerance develops quickly and often after only a few days' use. Psychologic dependence may occur with frequent use, but no physical dependence occurs.

BOX 6-13

CLINICAL MANIFESTATIONS OF HALLUCINOGEN USE

1 Initial stimulation followed by depression
2 Anxiety
3 Depressed appetite
4 Increased body temperature
5 Increased heart rate
6 Increased respiration
7 Dilated pupils; dizziness, numbness of face, and shivering may also occur with psilocybin
8 Altered sensory awareness
9 Senses become more acute
10 Thoughts that colors can be heard and sounds seen
11 Fantasies and illusions
12 Hallucination-like happenings
13 Unawareness that hallucinations are not real
14 Melding of past and present experiences, which leads to a feeling of oneness, compassion, and love for all things

From Phipps WJ and others: *Medical-surgical nursing: concepts and clinical practice,* ed 5, St Louis, 1995, Mosby.

Treatment aims at getting the patient into a quiet, nonstimulating environment and remaining with him or her until the effects of the drug wear off. Talking to the patient in a calm and reassuring way (i.e., talking him or her "down") may be helpful. **Flashbacks** occur when the user briefly experiences the original sensations experienced during use even when no drug has been ingested. Although the frequency of flashbacks varies, they may occur for many years after an individual's last use of hallucinogens.

PCP

Phencyclidine (PCP) is a psychoactive drug and is classified as an anesthetic-hallucinogen. It is available legally only as an animal anesthetic for use by veterinarians. It is available on the street in powder, capsule, or tablet form. It may be snorted, injected, or smoked with tobacco or marijuana.

PCP use results in symptoms that vary from person to person (Boxes 6-14 and 6-15). It may act as a CNS stimulant, a CNS depressant, or a hallucinogen. PCP ingestion may be viewed as a psychiatric emergency because of its unpredictable and volatile effects. There is the potential for harm to self or others. This drug is psychologically habit forming, but there is disagreement as to whether it is physically addicting.

BOX 6-14

DOSE-RELATED PHYSICAL MANIFESTATIONS OF PCP USE

Dose	Effects
5 mg	Physical sedation
	Numbness of extremities
	Loss of muscle coordination
	Dizziness
	Constricted pupils, blurred or double vision, and involuntary eye movements
	Flushing and profuse sweating
	Nausea and vomiting
	Increase in blood pressure, heart rate, and respiratory rate (breathing is shallow)
5 to 10 mg	Marked drop in blood pressure, breathing, and heart rate
	Shivering, increased salivation, and watering of the eyes
	Loss of balance, dizziness, and ridigity of muscles
	In some cases, repetitive movements such as rocking
	Analgesic and anesthetic properties apparent
> 10 mg	Extreme agitation, followed by seizures or coma
	Symptoms similar to mental confusion and delusion of schizophrenia

From Phipps WJ and others: *Medical-surgical nursing: concepts and clinical practice,* ed 5, St Louis, 1995, Mosby.

TREATMENT AND REHABILITATION

There is a difference between being sober and being a recovering alcoholic or substance abuser. To maintain sobriety and be in recovery, one must make major changes in attitudes, behavior, beliefs, and thinking. A **dry drunk** is one who abstains from alcohol completely but still exhibits the attitudes, impaired thinking, and behaviors of an active alcoholic.

It is frequently difficult to convince an abuser (who is often still in **denial**) that treatment is needed. In *I'll Quit Tomorrow,* Vernon Johnson (1980) states:

> It is a myth that alcoholics (drug abusers) have some spontaneous insight and then seek treatment. . . . Typically, in our experience they come to their recognition scenes

BOX 6-15

DOSE-RELATED PSYCHOLOGIC MANIFESTATIONS OF PCP USE

Dose	Effects
Low	Euphoria and a sense of alcohol-like intoxication Changes in body image Mood swings from ecstasy to panic Hallucinations and confusion regarding time and space In final stage in some cases, a sense of despair and emotional isolation, possibly leading to a feeling of paranoia and a sense of impending death
Moderate	Increase in effects felt at low dose Loss of sense of contact with environment
High	Symptoms of mental and emotional confusion similar to schizophrenia

From Scott L: *PCP* (pamphlet), Charlotte, NC, 1981, Charlotte Drug Educational Center.

through a buildup of crises that crash through their almost impenetrable defense systems. . . . They are forced to seek help . . . it was not only pointless but dangerous to wait until the (alcoholic/drug abuser) hit bottom. . . . We came to understand that crises could be used creatively to bring about intervention . . . in all the lives we studied, it was only through crisis that intervention had occurred (pp. 3-4).

An **intervention** occurs when the patient's significant others, family, friends, and a professional who works with addicts unite with the goal of breaking through the patient's denial and getting him or her into appropriate treatment. The intensity level and type of treatment that the patient is referred to depends on a number of factors, including how long the dependence problem has existed, medical problems, family support relationships, available facilities, and financial resources. Since 1990 many inpatient detoxification and treatment facilities have closed as a result of reduced reimbursement from insurers and changes in treatment modalities. In view of this, detoxification may be done as an inpatient on a hospital medical-surgical unit or on an outpatient basis in which the patient makes a daily visit to a clinic to be monitored. Initial treatment after detox may also occur as an inpatient or outpatient. Most alcohol and substance abuse rehabilitation (rehab) programs last from 3 to 8 weeks and include education about the disease process, an orientation to Alcoholics Anonymous, individual and group therapy, and the involvement of significant others.

BOX 6-16

TWELVE STEPS OF ALCOHOLICS ANONYMOUS

1 We admitted we were powerless over alcohol—that our lives had become unmanageable.
2 Came to believe that a power greater than ourselves could restore us to sanity.
3 Made a decision to turn our will and our lives over to the care of God as we understood Him.
4 Made a searching and fearless moral inventory of ourselves.
5 Admitted to God, to ourselves, and to another human being the exact nature of our wrongs.
6 Were entirely ready to have God remove all these defects of character.
7 Humbly asked Him to remove our shortcomings.
8 Made a list of all persons we had harmed, and became willing to make amends to them all.
9 Made direct amends to such people whenever possible, except when to do so would injure them or others.
10 Continued to take personal inventory and when we were wrong promptly admitted it.
11 Sought through prayer and meditation to improve our conscious contact with God as we understood Him, praying only for knowledge of His will for us and the power to carry that out.
12 Having had a spiritual awakening as a result of these steps, we tried to carry this message to alcoholics, and to practice these principles in all our affairs.

From *Alcoholics Anonymous,* New York, 1976, Alcoholics Anonymous World Sources.

Relapse, or the return of drinking or use of any mind-altering drugs, is common in recovering alcoholics. Follow-up treatment after the initial rehabilitation program significantly decreases the number of patients who relapse during their first year of recovery and for some time thereafter.

Alcoholics Anonymous (AA) plays an important part in the recovery of many alcoholics. Founded in 1935, it is the original self-help group and presently has more than 1 million members in the United States. Members follow 12 steps and 12 traditions in an attempt to stay sober one day at a time (Box 6-16). AA is a spiritual (not a religious) program that promotes reliance on a higher power and the responsibility to help each other maintain recovery after admitting to powerlessness over alcohol. Subgroups of AA, such as Al-Anon, Alateen, Alatot, and Adult Children of Alcoholics, recognize the family disease of alcoholism and provide assistance to family members in their own recovery from codependency.

Some recovering addicts benefit from spending a few weeks or months in a halfway house, which provides a support system during early recovery. The emphasis is on assuming responsibility for one's own well-being and adjusting to living in a drug-free community. Residents are expected to find employment, help maintain the residence, and work toward continued recovery by attending the appropriate self-help meetings and counseling.

NURSING MANAGEMENT

In the following sections, alcoholism is used as the model for all substance abuse and dependence disorders. The following information applies to the abuse of all mind-altering drugs.

Given the prevalence of alcoholism in the United States, all nurses may expect to encounter both diagnosed and undiagnosed alcoholics in any healthcare setting. It is important that the nurse recognize the signs and symptoms of alcoholism, its medical problems, and the physical symptoms of withdrawal and to identify the psychologic and social problems related to alcoholism.

The nurse may find it necessary to carefully examine his or her own views when dealing with alcoholics. As with any other disease, not all alcoholics will remain in recovery. Some will relapse once or repeatedly, and many will die as a result of the disease, which may cause feelings of anger or helplessness in the nurse. Without realizing it, nurses sometimes respond to the dysfunctional behavior of alcoholics and their family members in a rejecting, judgmental, or condescending way. Occasionally the nurse may become an enabler to the alcoholic or the family.

Assessment

Direct observation of the alcoholic patient and information gathered from a number of sources results in the most complete and accurate assessment possible. Because denial and impaired thinking are almost universally displayed in the untreated alcoholic, the information given by the patient may be inaccurate or incomplete. If possible, this information should be confirmed with a friend or family member.

The objective data helpful in assessing the alcoholic patient might include:

- General appearance: neat and clean or disheveled and dirty
- General behavior: loud, aggressive, euphoric, combative, uncooperative, depressed
- Speech: normal, slurred, incoherent
- Memory: evidence of memory loss
- Sensorium: clear, disoriented, hallucinations
- Tremors: tremors, motor incoordination
- Vital signs: depressed, elevated
- Eyes: dilated or pinpoint pupils, normal or blurred vision
- Skin color and integrity: well-oxygenated, jaundiced, cuts, bruises, petechiae, needle marks
- Gastrointestinal: nausea/vomiting, presence of ascites, blood in stools
- Breath: describe odor
- Laboratory reports: note any abnormal results

The following subjective data should be gathered:

- Date and time of last drink or use
- Substances used, quantity used
- History of blackouts, tremors, seizures, hallucinations, delirium tremens
- Usual drinking and/or using pattern

Box 6-17 lists additional signs of substance abuse.

Planning

The first priority in planning for the alcoholic patient is to ensure his or her medical safety if withdrawal

BOX 6-17

PSYCHOSOCIAL SIGNS AND SYMPTOMS OF ALCOHOL/SUBSTANCE ABUSE

1. Family history of substance abuse
2. History of physical or sexual abuse
3. History of ADD
4. Depression: current or past
5. History of suicide attempts
6. Risk-taking behavior (potentially destructive)
7. Work or school problems
8. Loss of friends
9. Withdrawal from family members
10. Legal problems: DUIs, possession of illegal substances, assault
11. Financial problems

From Phipps WJ and others: *Medical-surgical nursing: concepts and clinical practice,* ed 5, St Louis, 1995, Mosby.

symptoms are present or impending. Careful assessment may identify numerous problems that need attention. After withdrawal is complete, the nurse may help the patient accept his or her substance abuse problem and refer him or her to a substance abuse professional who can help clarify treatment options.

Teaching

Health teaching is an essential part of the nursing care of alcoholic (and other chemically dependent) patients. Patients need to learn about the physiologic effects of mind-altering drugs, the disease concept of substance abuse, and the environmental factors that may contribute to the development of a full-blown dependence problem. Information about cross-tolerance to drugs in the same general category is important in preventing the patient from developing a poly-abuse problem. Health teaching about HIV prevention is especially important in alcoholics. Alcoholics, especially women, are more likely to become sexually promiscuous while under the influence. They may deny that they are at high risk for exposure to the human immunodeficiency virus (HIV).

Pain Management

Another area of concern for the nurse and the patient is pain management. Even for a specific medical problem, patients committed to recovery are often hesitant to admit to the need for pain medication. However, some patients are drug seeking and demand more pain medication than they actually need so that they can get a mind-altering effect. The responsible nurse conducts a pain assessment and tries to determine the cause of pain. Even when the nurse has doubts about the credibility of the patient's record, it is wise to remember that the patient's report of pain must be considered the most reliable indicator of pain. Establishing a schedule for administering pain medication with input from the patient and physician may help resolve conflicts. Withholding pain medication as a result of distrust regarding the patient's report of pain usually serves no purpose.

The alcoholic and the chemically dependent patient have a higher tolerance for pain medication than do other patients. Therefore during periods of acute pain such as the first 2 to 3 days after major surgery, the physician often orders larger-than-usual doses of pain medication to be given at more frequent intervals. The patient is then rapidly weaned from the pain medication and probably should not be discharged with a prescription for pain medication. Any questions regarding safe dosages should be discussed with the physician to clarify the parameters for administration of the medication.

PATIENT/FAMILY TEACHING

Alcohol/Substance Abuse

The nurse should discuss the following concepts with the patient and family members:

- Disease concept of addiction
- Medical aspects of alcoholism/substance abuse
- Need for abstinence
- Defense mechanisms
- Coping mechanisms
- Importance of avoiding all mind-altering substances
- Products to avoid that contain alcohol
- Importance of expressing feelings
- Importance of honesty with healthcare personnel
- Importance of family support
- Importance of treatment program, including aftercare and AA
- Signs of impending relapse
- Prevention of transmission of HIV/Hepatitis B

Evaluation

It is important to evaluate the patient's responses to medical and nursing interventions on an ongoing basis during hospitalization and at the time of discharge (Box 6-18).

If withdrawal symptoms are or were present, consider the following:

- Stability of vital signs
- Status of respiratory function
- Fluid volume status
- Nutritional intake
- Cognition
- Potential for harm to self or others

To evaluate the patient's understanding and acceptance of the substance abuse problem, consider the following:

- Absence of current substance abuse
- Verbalization of a willingness to obtain treatment
- Understanding of potential mental and physical problems caused by substance abuse
- Verbalization of a desire to cope with problems caused by substance abuse

CHEMICALLY IMPAIRED NURSES

The rate of chemical dependency in nurses and other healthcare professionals is greater than in the

BOX 6-18

Nursing Process

ALCOHOL SUBSTANCE ABUSE OR DEPENDENCE

ASSESSMENT

Vital signs
Fluid volume status
Level of consciousness, mental status, and behavior
Respiratory rate, depth, and breath sounds as indicated
Nutritional status and presence of nausea, vomiting, or anorexia
Laboratory studies (electrolytes, liver function tests, ammonia, blood urea nitrogen [BUN], glucose, coagulation, arterial blood gases [ABGs]).
Effective coping mechanisms
Family relationships
Assess often during acute phase of withdrawal

NURSING DIAGNOSES

Risk for ineffective breathing pattern related to alcohol or drug toxicity and/or the sedative effect of drugs given to treat withdrawal
Risk for injury related to seizures, cessation of alcohol or drug intake, and impaired cognitive and motor ability
Risk for self- or other-directed violence related to altered thinking patterns, chemical alteration, and hostility
Sleep pattern disturbance related to withdrawal, anxiety, and insomnia
Altered nutrition: less than body requirements related to anorexia and inadequate intake
Fluid volume deficit related to anorexia, nausea, vomiting, diarrhea, and impaired cognition
Sensory/perceptual alterations related to withdrawal, memory impairment, and impaired judgment
Ineffective individual coping related to alcohol or drug dependence and loss of support system or employment
Powerlessness related to inability to control alcohol or drug use
Noncompliance related to alcoholic or drug-using lifestyle, denial, lack of resources, and physical or mental disability
Altered family processes related to situational crisis of alcohol/substance abuse
Knowledge deficit related to denial of the disease process, medical consequences of addiction, and treatment programs

NURSING INTERVENTIONS

Maintain patent airway.
Elevate head of bed.
Encourage patient to turn, cough, and deep breathe every 2 hours.
Have suction equipment and airways available.
Maintain nothing by mouth (NPO) until alert.
Avoid medications that cause respiratory depression.
Administer supplement oxygen as ordered.
Institute seizure precautions.
Assist with ambulation and self-care.
Administer medications for withdrawal as ordered.
Note onset of any hallucinations.
Provide quiet environment with lights low.
Restrict visitors.
Reorient as needed.
Restrain as necessary to prevent harm to self or others.
Remove dangerous objects from environment.
Approach patient nonthreateningly, take time to introduce self and describe procedures.
Maintain IV fluids until tolerating oral (po) intake.
Encourage diet high in protein and carbohydrates.
Provide small, frequent meals.
Develop a trusting relationship.
Project an accepting attitude toward patient.
Help patient identify feelings and express thoughts.
Confront patient with unacceptable behaviors.
Reward positive behaviors.
Involve patient/family in alcohol support groups.

EVALUATION OF EXPECTED OUTCOMES

Respiratory status stable with clear lungs and no evidence of hypoxia
Vital signs stable
No physical injury to self or others
Regains previous level of consciousness
Reports absence of hallucinations
Consumes adequate dietary intake
Verbalizes understanding of the effects of alcohol on nutrition
Begins to recognize effect of self-destructive behaviors
Refrains from alcohol/substance use
Participates in a support group
Identifies available resources

general public. The reasons may be complex, but the reality is that nurses generally have much greater access to mind-altering substances. Drug or alcohol abuse is a serious problem in any individual, but diminished judgment and performance in a caregiver threatens patient safety. Therefore if there is ever reason to suspect that another nurse is chemically dependent, there is only one option for action: document incidents and contact the state board of nursing or the State Nurses Association.

With the support of the American Nurses Association many states have developed peer assistance programs within the last decade that assist impaired nurses with treatment and recovery. Other goals of peer assistance programs include protecting the public from the untreated nurse, helping the recovering nurse safely reenter nursing, and helping monitor the recovering nurse for a period of time. Many states have laws that allow the impaired nurse to receive treatment without losing the professional license. Although practice may not be allowed for a period of time, the nurse is diverted from full disciplinary action.

ETHICAL DILEMMA

A registered nurse who is a co-worker on your unit confides to you that she was recently arrested and convicted of driving while under the influence and of possessing cannabis and drug paraphernalia. She was given probation, but no professional treatment program was mandated by the court. You have suspected her of being under the influence at work on two separate occasions. What are your ethical responsibilities in this situation?

Nursing Care Plan

PATIENT WITH ALCOHOL DEPENDENCE

Mr. DePaul is a 66-year-old male who has been admitted with carcinoma of the bladder for cystectomy and urinary diversion via urostomy. He has a past medical history of emphysema, has been a two-pack-per-day smoker for 45 years, and reports to consuming 6 beers every day since his retirement at age 58. His operation is uneventful and without complications. However, after surgery he is difficult to wean from the ventilator and requires 2 days in the critical care unit for respiratory management. It is now 2 days after his surgery, and he has been transferred to the medical-surgical unit.

Psychosocial Data	Postoperative Treatment	Assessment
Mother and father had a history of smoking and emphysema; both parents deceased No siblings Wife in very good health Married for 44 years with 2 grown children, who live out of state Limited contact with children and grandchildren Has few friends and describes himself as a "loner" Verbalizes difficulty adjusting to retirement *Hobbies:* Television and vegetable gardening	D5 ½ NS at 100 ml/hr CL diet Respiratory therapy with Alupent q 4 hr O_2 at 2L via nasal cannula Pulse oximetry q shift Urostomy to gravity drainage I & O	Barrel-chested pale male; alert and oriented; irritable and angry at times Height 5′10″, weight 204 lb *Skin:* Good condition; abdominal dressing dry and intact; staples intact; wound edges well approximated with no erythema or drainage at incision *Chest:* Increased AP diameter; scattered crackles/rhonchi throughout; respiratory rate 24-32; shallow, symmetrical respirations Apical pulse 112 regular; strong peripheral pulses; no peripheral edema; brisk capillary refill *Abdomen:* Obese; softly distended, positive bowel sounds

continued

Nursing Care Plan

PATIENT WITH ALCOHOL DEPENDENCE—CONT'D

Psychosocial Data	Postoperative Treatment	Assessment
		Urostomy patent and draining cloudy yellow urine, >30 ml/hr Full range of motion all extremities; out-of-bed with assist of one; dyspneic with exertion; tremors of upper extremities Further assessment of alcohol intake with wife reveals history of 24 beers/day, which has gradually increased since retirement Physician informed and Ativan 1 mg q 8 hr initiated

NURSING DIAGNOSIS

Risk for ineffective breathing pattern related to postoperative sedation, sedation from medication to prevent alcohol withdrawal, smoking history, and immobility

NURSING INTERVENTIONS	EVALUATION OF EXPECTED OUTCOMES
Monitor respiratory status q 2 hr. Auscultate breath sounds q 8 hr and prn. Keep head of bed elevated 30 degrees at all times. Encourage coughing and deep breathing. Encourage change of position q 2 hr. Encourage mobility. Have suction equipment and airway available. Administer/monitor O_2 at 2L via nasal cannula. Monitor pulse oximetry q 8 hr. Educate patient and wife regarding importance of aggressive respiratory management and prevention of complications	No evidence of respiratory distress Lungs clear O_2 saturation >90% on room air Effectively coughs and deep breathes with encouragement

NURSING DIAGNOSIS

Risk for injury related to cessation of alcohol intake and effect of medications

NURSING INTERVENTIONS	EVALUATION OF EXPECTED OUTCOMES
Monitor for evidence of alcohol withdrawal (e.g., tremors, tachycardia, diaphoresis, hypertension) q 8 hr. Monitor loss of consciousness and orientation and orient prn.	No evidence of withdrawal symptoms No evidence of injury

NURSING INTERVENTIONS	EVALUATION OF EXPECTED OUTCOMES
Maintain bed in low position, siderails up, padded rails, call light within reach and observe often. Provide quiet environment. Restrain prn. Maintain seizure precautions. Include wife in treatment plan. Administer medications as prescribed.	

NURSING DIAGNOSIS

Risk for impaired individual coping related to cessation of alcohol, denial of problem, withdrawal symptoms, and change in body image with urostomy

NURSING INTERVENTIONS	EVALUATION OF EXPECTED OUTCOMES
Assess coping mechanisms, and confer with wife if necessary. Have same staff care for patient to develop a trusting relationship. Spend time with patient every day. Encourage patient to openly discuss alcohol usage, feelings, fears, and concerns. Encourage support and involvement of wife. Provide positive support and encouragement. Provide with necessary instructions to care for ostomy. Refer to support groups in the community regarding alcohol and ostomy.	Begins to recognize maladaptive behaviors Verbalizes feelings and concerns Patient/wife demonstrate effective coping mechanisms Patient/wife verbalize potential benefit of support groups

KEY CONCEPTS

- Substance abuse is a complex disease and is most likely precipitated by a combination of etiologic factors.
- Alcoholism is a progressive, chronic, and debilitating disease that significantly shortens life expectancy.
- Substance abuse is found in every age group from childhood through the life span and in all health-care settings. It is often undiagnosed.
- Substance abuse is a family disease. Family members and significant others usually react in predictable ways that become increasingly dysfunctional.
- Withdrawal from alcohol and other mind-altering substances is a complex nursing problem and may require medical supervision or hospitalization.
- Substance abuse is not curable, but continuous recovery is possible, especially with the assistance of professional help and self-help groups such as Alcoholics Anonymous, Cocaine Anonymous, Narcotics Anonymous, and Pills Anonymous.
- Recovery requires abstinence from all mind-altering chemicals.
- A variety of treatment options are available to help the patient and family with recovery.
- Drugs of abuse are categorized as depressants, stimulants, hallucinogens, and inhalants.
- Nurses are at a greater risk of becoming chemically dependent than is the general public.

CRITICAL THINKING EXERCISES

1 During the second day of his hospitalization for detoxification, a patient complains to you that the nurse on the previous shift delayed each dose of his Valium, stating that, "The more uncomfortable you are, the less likely you will be to go out and drink again." One of your previous detox patients made a similar complaint about the same nurse. Is any action necessary on your part? Why?

2 You are a nurse working in a clinic. One of your patients states that her family is in turmoil because her 10-year-old son will not behave in school. You see in her record that she has a history of alcohol abuse. Identify a possible reason for the son's behavior.

3 Give examples of the behaviors you would expect of a child who has an alcoholic parent and who is assuming the role of "hero."

REFERENCES AND ADDITIONAL READINGS

Adams WL and others: Alcohol-related hospitalizations of elderly people, *JAMA* 270(10):1222, 1993.

Alcoholics Anonymous big book, ed 3, New York, 1976, AA World Services.

Antai-Otong D: Helping the alcoholic patient recover, *Am J Nurs* 95(8):22-30, 1995.

Boyle MH and others: Predicting substance abuse in late adolescence: results from the Ontario child health study follow-up, *Am J Psychiatr* 149(6): 761-767, 1992.

Diagnostic and statistical manual of mental disorders DSM-IV, ed 4, Washington, DC, 1994, American Psychiatric Association.

Huntington DD: Home care of the elderly alcoholic, *Home Healthcare Nurse,* 8(5):26-32, 1990.

InTouch Newsletter, Kenneth Young Centers, Elk Grove, Ill, Summer 1995.

Jellinek EM: *The disease concept of alcoholism,* New Brunswick, NJ, 1960, Hillhouse Press.

Johnson V: *I'll Quit Tomorrow: a practical guide to alcohol treatment, San Francisco,* 1990, Harper & Row.

Lawson GW, Lawson AW, editors: *Adolescent substance abuse: etiology, treatment and prevention,* Gaithersburg, Md, 1992, Aspen.

Lerner WD, Barr M, editors: *Hospital based substance abuse treatment,* New York, 1990, Pergamon Press.

Mendelson JH, Mello N, editors: *Medical diagnosis and treatment of alcoholism,* New York, 1992, McGraw-Hill.

Miller N, Toft D: *The disease concept of alcoholism and other drug addiction,* Minneapolis, 1990, Hazelden Foundation.

Moss HB, Tarter RE: Substance abuse, aggression and violence: what are the connections? *Am J Addiction* 2(2): 149-160, 1993.

Phipps WJ and others: *Medical surgical nursing: concepts and clinical practice,* ed 5, St Louis, 1994, Mosby.

Robin HS, Michelson JB: *Illustrated handbook of drug abuse, recognition, and diagnosis,* Chicago, Ill, 1988, Yearbook Medical.

Shaef AW: *Co-Dependence: misunderstood-mistreated,* New York, 1966, Harper Collins.

Schuchit MD, Marc A: *Drug and alcohol abuse: a clinical guide to diagnosis and treatment,* ed 3, New York, 1989, Plenum Medical Book.

Seventh Special Report to the US Congress on Alcohol and Health: Rockville, Md, Jan 1990, US Department of Health and Human Services.

Sommers M: Alcohol and trauma: the critical link, *Crit Care Nurse,* 14(4): 82-93, 1994.

Stimmel B: *The facts about drug use,* Binghamton, NY, 1993, The Hawarth Press.

Stuart G, Sundeen S: *Principles and practice of psychiatric nursing,* ed 4, St Louis, 1991, Mosby.

Taylor CM: *Mereness' essentials of psychiatric nursing,* ed 13, St Louis, 1990, Mosby.

Trimpey J: *The small book,* New York, 1992, Delacorte Press.

Twerski AJ: Avoiding relapse on medication, *Prof Couns,* p 10, Oct 1991.

Volkow ND and others: Decreased brain metabolism in neurologically intact healthy alcoholics, *Am J Psychiatr* 149(8):1016-1022, 1992.

Wang MQ and others: Tobacco use among American adolescents: geographic and demographic variations, *South Med J* 87(6): 607-610, 1994.

Wilson S: Can you spot an alcoholic parent? *RN* 57(1): 46-50, 1994.

Yates WR, Meller WH: Comparative validity of five alcoholism topologies, *Am J Addiction,* 2(2): 99-108, Spring 1993

Part III

7 Physiologic responses

8 Fluids and electrolytes

9 The patient with pain

10 The patient with cancer

11 Community-acquired infections

12 Nosocomial infections

13 HIV infection and AIDS

14 The older adult

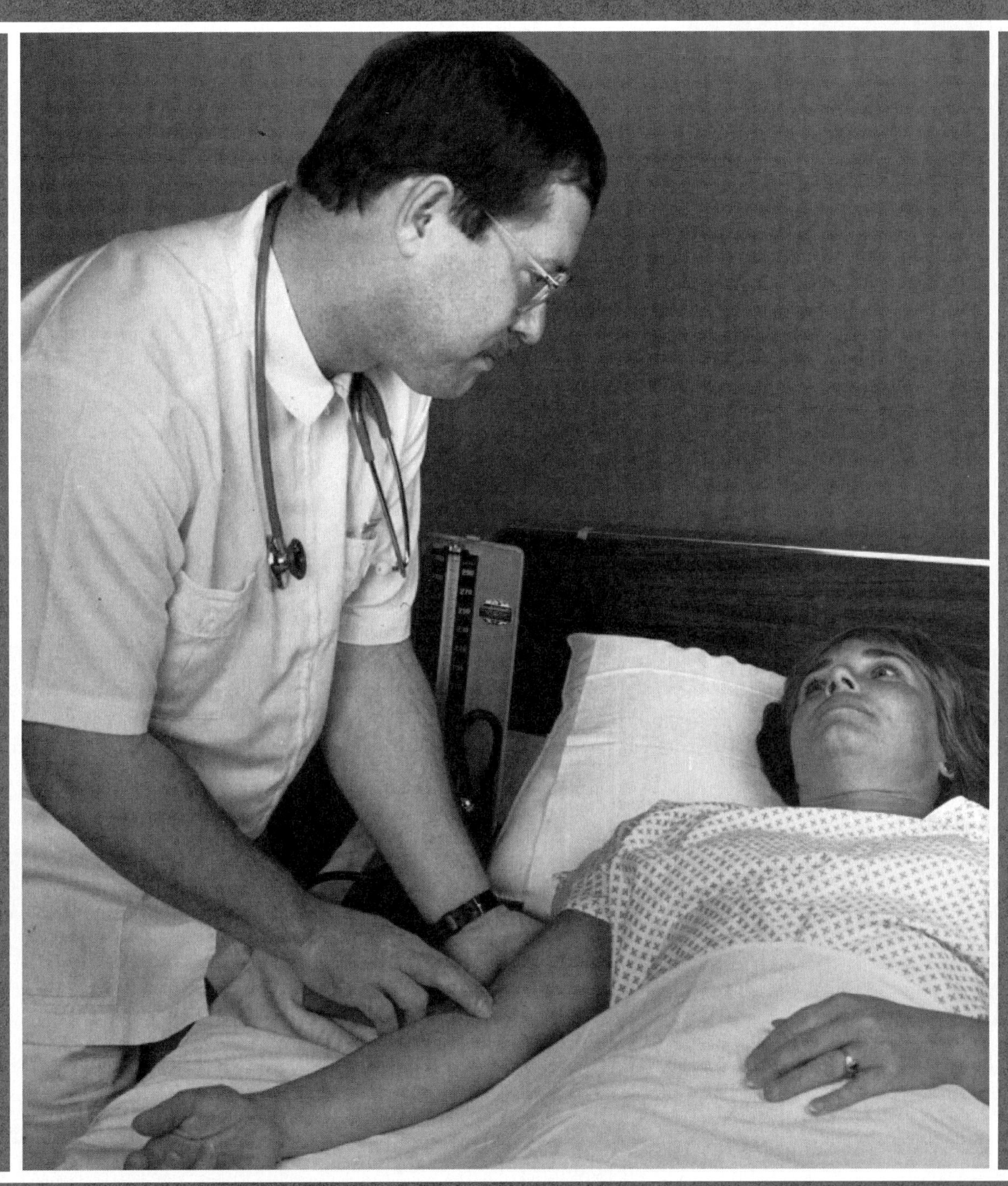

PHYSIOLOGIC ASPECTS OF PATIENT CARE

CHAPTER 7

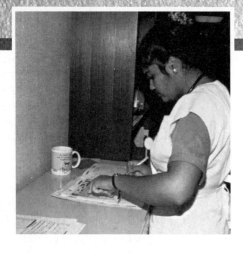

Physiologic Responses

CHAPTER OBJECTIVES

1 Identify the major causes of illness and disease.
2 Give an example of each of the major causes of disease.
3 Describe the major physiologic defense mechanisms of the body.
4 Identify the characteristics of the inflammatory process.
5 Describe nursing interventions for a patient with an inflammatory condition.
6 Explain the function of the immune system in combating and preventing disease.
7 Define hypersensitivity.
8 List the major assessment techniques used for allergic conditions.
9 Identify nursing interventions for people with allergies.
10 Discuss the nurse's responsibility in the intervention for a patient in anaphylactic shock.
11 Identify diseases attributed to autoimmunity.

KEY WORDS

allergen
antibody
antihistamine
autoimmune
bacteriostatic
cell-mediated immunity
corticosteroids
desensitization
endotoxin
epinephrine
exotoxin
gram negative
gram positive
humoral immunity
hypersensitivity
immunity
immunoglobulins
inflammation
leukocytes
normal flora
nosocomial infection
systemic infections
virulence

CAUSES OF DISEASE

Disease is any condition in which either the physiologic or psychologic functions of the body deviate significantly from what is regarded as normal. Health and disease are often viewed as a spectrum, with excellent health on one end of the scale and disease with permanent disability or death on the other end (Figure 7-1). In health a person successfully adapts to environmental stresses, but in illness the capacity to adapt has been limited in some way. Homeostasis is the maintenance of a balance of physiologic processes within the body, and adaptation is the maintenance of a balance while interacting with the environment (Anthony, Thibodeau, 1986).

Most diseases are characterized by specific signs and symptoms. These signals result from pathologic processes that interfere with normal body functioning. Because in a state of health the body functions as a whole with each part interdependent, the malfunctioning or abnormal condition of any part of the body may affect the entire body. Often more than one specific disease, each resulting from different causes, may be present in the same person at the same time. The most common causes of disease are (1) microorganisms, (2) nutritional imbalances, (3) physical agents, (4) chemical agents, and (5) cellular abnormalities.

Microorganisms

Microbiology is the study of microorganisms, or microbes. Microbes are living, minute organisms that usually have a one-cell structure. Many microbes live normally within the body without causing disease or illness. They are referred to as **normal flora** and are found in places such as the gastrointestinal tract, the upper respiratory system, the genitourinary tract, and the skin. However, some microbes can become pathogenic, or disease producing, and invade the body, multiply, and cause disease. When this occurs a person has an infection. Infections interfere with normal physiologic functioning and cause inflammation and possibly purulent discharge. The specific symptoms depend on the site of the infection. For example, an abscess in the brain tissue results in neurologic symptoms, whereas pneumonia results in respiratory distress. Microbes are classified as *bacteria, viruses, fungi,* and *protozoa.*

Bacteria

The study of bacteria has shown that they have many different characteristics. There are three basic shapes—round, oblong, and spiral—but there are also many variations of these shapes. Some may be elongated or have pointed ends, and some may be flattened on one side. Some are shaped like a comma, and others appear square. Spirilla may be tightly coiled like a corkscrew. During cell division some remain together to form pairs, whereas others may form long chains. All of these modifications are important in identifying specific types of bacteria.

Bacteria may also have different chemical compositions, require different nutrients, and form different waste products. *Aerobic* bacteria grow only in the presence of oxygen, whereas *anaerobic* bacteria grow only

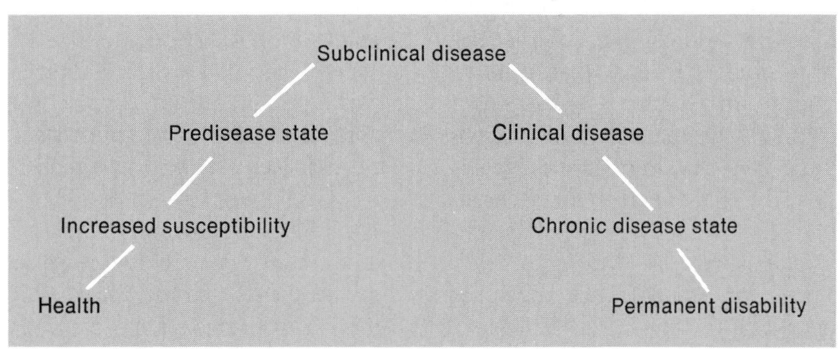

Figure 7-1 Health-illness spectrum.

in the absence of oxygen. Some bacteria are capable of movement. Their motility is possible because of fine, hairlike projections called *flagella* that arise from the bacterial cell (Figure 7-2). These projections cause a wavelike motion that moves the cell. A bacterium may have only one flagellum attached to one end of the cell, or there may be many flagella surrounding the cell. Locomotion of the spirochete is achieved by a wiggling motion that involves the entire cell body.

Some bacteria form a specialized structure called a *spore* (see Figure 7-2). Spore formation appears to occur when conditions are unfavorable for growth of the bacterium. A spore is a round body that is formed by the bacterium in the presence or absence of oxygen. The spore enlarges until it is as large as the bacterial cell and is surrounded by a capsule. Eventually the portion of the cell that surrounds the spore disintegrates. The spore remains dormant until environmental conditions become favorable for growth. At that time the spore germinates and begins to reproduce in a normal manner. Spores have a high degree of resistance to heat and disinfectants. They cannot be stained by the usual laboratory methods but require special staining techniques.

Some bacteria have the ability to form *capsules* around the cell wall (see Figure 7-2). These mucilaginous envelopes seem to form when the bacterial environment is unfavorable. The formation may also protect the bacteria. The composition of the capsule varies with the species of bacteria, but it may be composed of protein or fat substances or may contain nitrogen and phosphorus. As with spores, staining in the laboratory may require special procedures. When capsules are present, antibiotic therapy can be difficult because the capsule may prevent the drug from reaching the bacteria within the capsule.

Many diseases cannot be diagnosed and properly treated until the specific microorganism that is causing the illness has been identified by specially trained laboratory personnel. Most bacteria cannot be seen until a special staining process has been done. Staining is accomplished by applying dye to a specially prepared glass slide that contains a small amount of the material to be examined. Most bacteria can be identified by this simple process, but some bacteria require additional staining. Depending on whether a color can or cannot be removed by a solvent, the organism is identified as being **gram positive** or **gram negative.** This is a simple laboratory test that helps select effective antibiotics and is important in the treatment of the patient. Different bacteria may require different antibiotics for their destruction. Some bacteria are known as acid-fast bacteria, depending on the staining process. Special staining is required for bacteria having flagella, spores, or capsules.

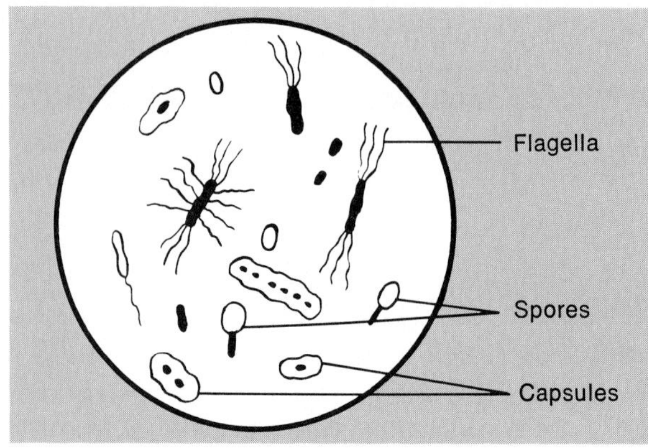

Figure 7-2 Specialized structures of bacteria: flagella, spores, and capsules.

Body fluids and secretions suspected of containing pathogenic organisms can be collected in sterile containers and sent to the laboratory for culture and sensitivity tests. In the laboratory the collected specimens are transferred to a special culture medium that promotes growth. The culture is studied, and the pathogens are identified. Sensitivity tests are performed to determine which antibiotics effectively inhibit the growth of the pathogens. Appropriate antibiotics are ordered on the basis of these tests.

Bacterial infections are transmitted from person to person by direct contact, by inhaling droplet nuclei, and by indirect contact with articles contaminated with the pathogen. Some infections are also transmitted through the ingestion of contaminated food and drink (see Chapter 11).

Bacteria are divided into three major groups: (1) cocci, (2) bacilli, and (3) spirilla (Figure 7-3). In addition, the rickettsiae are now classified as bacteria.

Streptococci, staphylococci, and diplococci. The streptococcus bacterium is responsible for more diseases than any other organism. Some strains produce serious or even fatal diseases, other strains produce disease only under special conditions, and other strains are nonpathogenic. Disease-producing strains include beta-hemolytic streptococci and the viridans group, which is also called alpha-hemolytic streptococci.

The beta-hemolytic group of streptococci is responsible for about 90% of streptococcal infections. Some of the diseases caused by this group are extremely serious and may be fatal. The diseases include osteomyelitis, septicemia, scarlet fever, rheumatic fever, and pneumonia. This group also causes relatively common diseases such as tonsillitis and impetigo. The organisms may also invade surgical wounds or malignant lesions. Wound infection may occur as a result of improper handwashing before changing dressings.

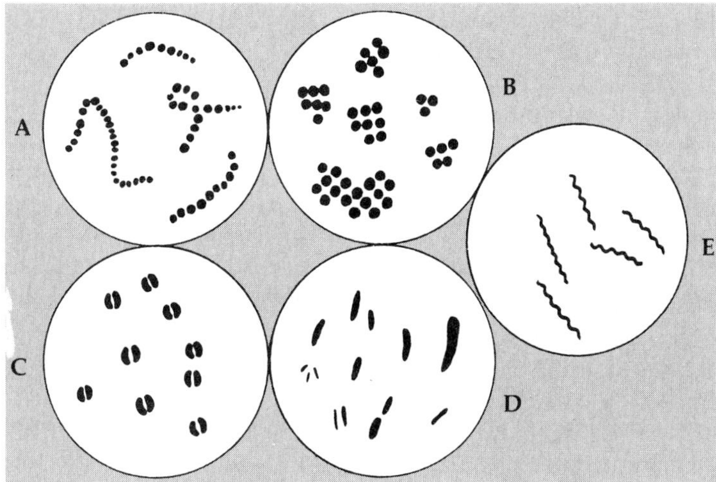

Figure 7-3 Common disease-producing bacteria. **A,** Streptococci. **B,** Staphylococci. **C,** Diplococci. **D,** Bacilli. **E,** Spirilla.

The organisms live in the upper respiratory tract and may be spread from one person to another by direct or indirect contact. Viridans streptococci may cause subacute bacterial endocarditis, which may affect the valves of the heart. Viridans streptococci may also be found in the nose and throat of healthy people.

There are two primary species of staphylococcus bacteria: *Staphylococcus aureus* and *Staphylococcus epidermidis. S. aureus* belongs to the pyogenic (pus-producing) group. Staphylococci may be found on the skin at all times and cause boils (furuncles), abscesses, and carbuncles. Sometimes they get into the bloodstream and cause serious complications (see Chapter 12). *S. epidermidis* is a nonpathogenic species of the staphylococcus organism and inhabits the human skin. Although this species may cause minor infections, the incidence of such infections is low.

There are several types of diplococcus bacteria. One type causes pneumonia and was previously called *pneumococcus.* It is now called *Streptococcus pneumoniae.* One characteristic of this organism is that it is encased in a capsule, or gelatinous envelope. Two other forms of diplococci cause gonorrhea *(gonococcus)* and meningitis *(meningococcus).*

Bacilli. The term *bacilli* means "little rod" (see Figure 7-3). Its rodlike shape is extremely variable. Certain forms of the bacillus produce spores, which are present in the intestinal tract of humans and animals and discharged onto the soil. These spore-forming bacilli produce tetanus, gas gangrene, and anthrax (see Chapter 11). Numerous other diseases are caused by these organisms, including tuberculosis, diphtheria, pertussis, typhoid fever, and bacillary dysentery.

Spirilla. Spirilla organsims are spiral and shaped like a corkscrew. Some forms of spirilla are rigid, whereas others are flexible (spirochetes). One form resembles a comma and is the cause of Asiatic cholera. Most diseases caused by the spirilla bacteria are uncommon. The spirochetes that cause syphilis are spiral shaped but have been separated and classified in a different order of bacteria. Lyme disease is also caused by a spirochete.

Rickettsiae. Rickettsiae are microorganisms that combine the characteristics of bacteria and viruses. They are parasites that flourish only within living susceptible cells, which provide a suitable environment and the nutrients needed for growth. The most serious diseases caused by rickettsiae are typhus fever and Rocky Mountain spotted fever. Typhus fever is spread from person to person through bites from infected body lice or from fleas that have been infected from rats. Epidemic typhus is an acute, severe disease that is associated with overcrowding, famine, and filth. It has caused devastating epidemics, resulting in the deaths of millions of people over the past centuries. Although it is rare, cases can be found in the southern United States along the Mexican border.

Rocky Mountain spotted fever has been found in almost every area of the United States, and its prevalence seems to be increasing. It is transmitted to humans through the bite of an infected tick. Several varieties of ticks carry the disease. The ticks live on many different types of animals in rural and wooded areas. They may also live on common house pets such as cats and dogs. Persons working in areas where ticks are known to be abundant are more likely to become infected. The tick attaches itself to the skin, and the longer it remains attached to the skin, the more likely the person is to become infected. When removing a tick from the skin, great care should be taken not to crush or squeeze it.

Symptoms of Rocky Mountain spotted fever and typhus fever are similar; in both diseases patients are usually extremely ill (see Chapter 11).

Viruses

Before 1900, scientists discovered that certain agents, unlike bacteria, would pass through a laboratory filter. Scientists were unable to observe these tiny bodies with the ordinary microscope. In 1898 Martinus W. Beijerinck called these small bodies viruses, and they became known as filterable viruses. Viruses are the smallest known agents that cause disease. They are not complete cells but consist of a protein coat around a nucleic acid core and depend on the metabolic processes of the cell they enter.

For years scientists knew little about viruses even though they were able to observe their effect on humans and animals. In 1941 the electron microscope became available, which opened a whole new era in the study of human disease. With this advancement the science of *virology* was born. In addition to the electron microscope, the use of certain dyes that become luminous when exposed to ultraviolet light (fluorescent microscopy), tissue culture methods, ultracentrifuges, cytochemistry, and the development of other technical laboratory aids have led to rapid advances in the study of viruses.

The virus may gain entrance to the body through the respiratory tract, the gastrointestinal tract, or the broken skin as a result of an animal bite. It may also be injected by a mosquito or hypodermic needle. Viruses are selective in the type of body cells they attack, but once they find cells that show affinity, they enter the cells and reproduce rapidly. As they multiply they interrupt cell activities and use cell material to produce new virus material.

Viral infections are usually self-limiting. They run a given course and the person recovers. One exception is rabies, which is almost always fatal. Other viral diseases may be fatal if complications occur or if they attack extremely weak, elderly, or debilitated persons. The common cold is caused by a virus, and the aches, fever, and chills may be relieved with rest and certain medicines. However, no medicine can cure the common cold. In nearly all viral diseases, antibiotics and sulfonamide agents do not alter the course of the disease.

Viruses are classified in various ways. They can be classified according to the human diseases they cause or by the characteristics of a specific group. In the latter classification system, each subgroup may have many types of strains (Box 7-1).

BOX 7-1

MAJOR GROUPS OF VIRUSES AND RELATED DISEASES

Papovavirus—papilloma (wart)
Adenovirus—bronchitis, pneumonitis, pharyngitis
Herpesvirus—herpes simplex (cold sore), herpes zoster (shingles)
Poxvirus—rubella, rabies, smallpox
Picornavirus—poliomyelitis, common cold
Reovirus—believed to cause acute respiratory tract diseases

Fungi

The fungal (mycotic) infections are among the most common diseases found in humans. Fungi belong to the plant kingdom, and although many of them are harmless, some are responsible for infections. Types of fungi that are familiar to everyone include the fuzzy, black, green, or white growth on stale bread, rotten fruit, or damp clothing. Fungi are among the most plentiful forms of life. Mycotic infections are diseases caused by yeasts and molds. They may be superficial and involve the skin and mucous membranes. The areas most frequently affected include the external layers of the skin, hair, and nails. These infections are called *dermatomycosis* (ringworm). The most frequent site of ringworm in children is the scalp. The condition is considered infectious, and the child may not be permitted to attend school until the infection has been cured. Other sites include men's beards (barber's itch) and the feet (athlete's foot). The infection may also occur on other parts of the body and often around the nails. Domestic pets may also have ringworm infection and are frequently the source of infection for humans.

Fungi also invade the deeper tissues of the body. Most of these infections produce no symptoms, but some become serious and may be fatal. Those most common in the United States are coccidioidomycosis (valley fever) and histoplasmosis. *Coccidioidomycosis* was discovered in southern California, although it is found in other areas of the Southwest where the climate is hot and dry. The disease affects the lungs and is believed to be contracted by inhaling the spores present in the soil, which are blown about by the wind. *Histoplasmosis* also affects the lungs. This disease is widespread throughout the world. In some areas 80% of the population may be infected. The disease occurs as the result of inhaling spores present in the soil, and there is also a possibility that ingestion of the spores may cause the disease. Histoplasmosis has often been associated with various kinds of birds. However, it is now believed that the only relationship between birds and this disease is that bird droppings enrich the soil and provide fertile media in which the fungi may proliferate.

Candida albicans may cause superficial or **systemic infections.** This fungus is a normal inhabitant of the gastrointestinal tract, the mouth, and the vagina. An infection develops when something, such as a change in pH, interferes with the balance of the normal flora and allows the organism to grow. This change in balance can occur as a result of antibiotic therapy.

Protozoa

Protozoa are single-celled animals that exist in some form everywhere in nature. Some of the parasitic forms of protozoa are found in the intestinal tract, genitourinary tract, and circulatory system of humans and animals. The disease-producing protozoa are responsible for malaria, amebic dysentery, and African sleeping sickness. Another form of protozoa causes vaginal trichomoniasis in women, often as a complication of pregnancy. It may also live in the male urethra and may be acquired or transmitted through coitus. Of the diseases caused by protozoa, the two of importance in the United States are malaria and amebic dysentery. The latter is more prevalent where sanitation is poor and personal hygiene is neglected. The source of infection can be the excreta of convalescent patients or carriers, and the disease is transmitted by food handlers or by contaminated food or water supplies. The common housefly may be an intermediary vector by transmitting the organism to food.

The malaria protozoan is transmitted to humans through the bite of the female *Anopheles* mosquito. Malaria is a worldwide health problem and is one of the most serious handicaps in the development of many countries (see Chapter 11).

Nutritional Imbalance

Nutritional imbalance may be caused by (1) an insufficient or excessive diet, (2) an unbalanced diet, (3) an increased use of a specific nutrient, and (4) a failure of the body to use nutrients. Both nutritional excesses and deficiencies lead to an inadequate supply of nutrients to the cell. The general classes of nutrients needed by the body to perform vital functions are water, carbohydrates, proteins, lipids, vitamins, and minerals. An individual's diet needs to include these essential nutrients for the body to be maintained, to grow, to repair, and to reproduce. The necessary amount of each nutrient varies from person to person and is influenced by such factors as age and amount of activity.

Nutritional imbalance lowers the body's resistance to infection. The very young, adolescents, pregnant women, the disabled, and the poor are especially vulnerable to malnutrition. There has never been greater emphasis on diet than now.

TABLE 7-1

Macrominerals

Mineral	Physiologic functions
Calcium	Structural and maintenance role in bones and teeth
Chloride	Regulates stomach pH; major anion of extracellular fluid
Magnesium	Important intracellular cation; acts as activator for many enzymes
Phosphorus	Helps in bone formation and maintenance; important in energy metabolism of adenosine triphosphate (ATP)
Potassium	Major intracellular cation; necessary for transmission of nerve impulses, an acid-base balance, and the formation of protein and glycogen
Sodium	Major cation of extracellular fluid; regulates body fluid osmolarity and volume

For years it has been known that a deficiency of certain vitamins can cause scurvy, beriberi, and pellagra. Lack of adequate iron in the diet can lead to anemia. Minerals serve many functions in the body. Those present in large amounts in the body are called *macrominerals* (Table 7-1). Twenty-two minerals are known to be essential. Those present in small amounts are called trace minerals. These are arsenic, chromium, cobalt, copper, fluoride, iodine, iron, manganese, molybdenum, nickel, selenium, silicon, tin, vanadium, and zinc (Thibodeau, 1993).

Obesity is a major health concern in affluent countries. Obesity is defined as an excessive amount of body fat and is caused when the calories consumed exceed the calories used in the production of energy. Two types of obesity have been described: upper-body (android or male) and lower-body (gynoid or female). Upper-body obesity is characterized by larger fat cells and is more prevalent among men. The lower-body type is more common among women. It is characterized by increased numbers of fat cells, especially in the gluteal-femoral region of the body. Obesity and diets high in saturated fats have been identified as risk factors in coronary artery disease. A high intake of dietary fats may also be associated with endometrial, breast, prostatic, ovarian, and rectal cancer (Carroll, 1991; Kelsey, Gammon, 1991). Obesity is also responsible for social isolation, glucose intolerance, hypertension, cholelithiasis, and menstrual irregularity.

Certain eating disorders are also becoming significant health concerns. Anorexia nervosa is a psychologic and physiologic syndrome that involves the fear of becoming overweight. This fear results in fat and muscle depletion and produces severe symptoms and sometimes death. Bulimia is another eating disorder and involves the consumption of food followed by vomiting or purging. Physical and psychologic problems can result.

Present research is concerned not only with the types of food necessary for health but also with how the body metabolizes and uses nutrients. A diet may be entirely adequate from a nutritional standpoint, but because of an organ or body part malfunction, the nutritional content of the food is not properly used and the person becomes ill. For example, in persons with diabetes, the body cannot use carbohydrates despite an adequate intake.

In some countries the lack of food is so serious that people are predisposed to developing various diseases or dying from starvation. Protein-calorie malnutrition (marasmus, kwashiorkor) is of particular concern for the children in developing countries. To help combat malnutrition, the United States has made millions of dollars worth of surplus food and grains available to many of these countries. The problem of hunger and malnutrition is still of concern in some areas of the United States. Programs such as food stamps for low-income families have been created to increase the purchasing power of those who qualify.

Physical Agents

Physical agents that result in injury to the body include trauma, changes in external temperature, electric current, exposure to radiation, changes in atmospheric pressure, mechanical factors, and noise. Injuries from trauma can result in closed or open wounds, fractured bones, injured organs, and disruption of blood flow. Exposure to high environmental temperatures can lead to heat exhaustion or heatstroke. Severe environmental heat can cause life-threatening problems if not quickly recognized and treated appropriately. Overexposure to the sun's rays may result in severe burns and skin cancer. Fever is an example of internal heat production. A fever is a body temperature above 100° F (38° C) when the body is at rest. Heat can also be used therapeutically in medicine. For example, cautery is used to treat wounds, stop bleeding, and even cut tissue during surgery.

Exposure to extreme cold may cause frostbite or actual freezing of body parts and possible death. Normally the body temperature never varies more than 1 degree from normal. The lethal limits for total body temperature range from approximately 71.6° F to 107.6° F (22° C to 42° C). Cold *(hypothermia)* is generally tolerated better than heat *(hyperthermia)*. Controlled hypothermia is used in medicine as an anesthetic for minor pain, freezing techniques can be used for surgical purposes *(cryosurgery)*, and profound hypothermia can be used for an extracorporeal bypass during cardiac surgery. General hypothermia may be used during surgery to decrease the activity of the body tissues. This decreased activity results in a reduced need for oxygen and nourishment that is circulated by the blood.

Electric current may cause slight tingling, such as may be experienced in the home as a result of faulty wiring, or it may result in severe shock, burns, or death when a person is exposed to high voltage. Severe and harmful radiation injury may occur from exposure to atomic radiation, and unless proper precautions are taken, injury may result from x-ray or radium therapy.

Deviation from normal atmospheric pressure to increased or decreased pressure may cause illness or death. Persons traveling by air may experience extreme pain in the ears because of the rapid changes in atmospheric pressure. A condition known as the *bends* can occur in divers if there is a rapid reduction in water pressure. The rapid reduction causes the gases in the blood to come out of solution. The gases can form emboli and result in obstruction of the blood vessels.

Mechanical injuries can be caused by physical impact or by irritation and are often related to occupational hazards. Occupational biomechanics deals with the prevention of overexertion disorders, which are caused by mechanical factors that affect the body (McCance, Huether, 1994). Noise is sound that can cause body injury. Noise-induced hearing loss can result from prolonged exposure to intense sound. Precautions in the workplace must be taken to prevent hearing loss. Acoustic trauma can result from a single loud sound such as a gunshot (McCance, Huether, 1994).

Chemical Agents

Studies indicate that poisoning constitutes a major health problem. Substances known to be toxic in large doses, such as medicines, may be taken accidentally or intentionally. There are many new drugs on the market for which no satisfactory antidote may be available. Overdoses of some drugs cause respiratory and cardiovascular depression.

Of great interest and concern in contemporary society is the prevalence of chemical dependency. The abuse of addictive and recreational substances, including drugs and alcohol, has long-term consequences that range from cardiac and liver disease to low-birth-weight and addicted newborns. Programs are available to help people with chemical dependence gain access to treatment plans. These programs are often located in hospitals and community agencies. Peer assistance programs are also available for health professionals to obtain treatment for their own chemical dependence.

Some chemical agents such as lye may be ingested, and others such as carbon monoxide are inhaled as gases. Carbon monoxide poisoning as a result of faulty heating systems is becoming a major concern. It is an odorless, colorless gas and can cause hypoxic injury and death. Carbon monoxide detectors are being recommended for home use to alert residents of dangerous levels of this gas.

Various industrial processes use chemicals that are injurious if inhaled or allowed to touch the skin. Other commonly available chemical agents that have been shown to cause harm include caffeine and tobacco. Cigarette smoking has been closely linked with coronary artery disease and an increased incidence of lung cancer. Of concern now is the risk to nonsmokers who breathe the secondhand smoke. Secondhand smoke has been linked to diminished pulmonary function, increased respiratory infections, and exacerbations of asthma in children (Chilmonczyk and others, 1993).

There is increasing concern that the environment is becoming contaminated by insecticides and herbicides, lead from gasoline combustion, and industrial wastes. In certain high-risk occupations such as mining, exposure to gases or dust may cause acute or chronic illness.

In some older homes the potential for lead poisoning in children from lead-based paint is of particular concern. The sweet taste of the paint attracts youngsters to ingest it. In children, lead is readily absorbed from the intestine (McCance, Huether, 1994).

Hospitals, clinics, and other institutions have established poison control centers, where information concerning a drug is available, usually on a 24-hour basis. Special educational displays, posters, and printed material have been placed in public buildings to inform the public about the harmful effects of poisons. The U.S. government has curtailed the use of once common food additives and some drugs because of the possible harmful effects that result from their use. State and local governments are becoming increasingly aware of the necessity for more public information and legislation for the control of hazardous drugs, chemicals, insecticides, and sprays.

Cellular Abnormalities

Cells are the smallest living structures capable of maintaining life functions and reproducing. Cells of varying structure and function form tissues, and tissues form organs, each of which contribute to the integrated holistic function of the body. In all pathologic conditions the cells that form tissues, organs, and other structures are affected.

Although there is a significant variation in types of cells, there are structures that are common to all. A typical animal cell structure is found in Figure 7-4. The *cell membrane* forms the outer boundary, maintains cell structure, and determines which substances may move into or out of the cell. *Protoplasm* is the internal substance of the cell and is composed primarily of the elements hydrogen, oxygen, carbon, and nitrogen. These elements are combined to form the major compounds—water, carbohydrates, proteins, lipids, and nucleic acids. Protoplasm minus nuclear material is called *cytoplasm*.

The specific internal structures of the cell are called *organelles* (Box 7-2). The number and types of organelles vary according to the type and specific function of each cell. For example, muscle cells have numerous mitochondria to provide energy for muscle contraction. Gland cells have extensive amounts of endoplasmic reticulum and Golgi complex to provide for secretion, and white blood cells have large numbers of lysosomes to destroy bacteria that have invaded the body.

Cells can be damaged in many ways. A lack of nutrients or oxygen may injure the cell membrane or other cell structures or cause cell death. An imbalance in the composition of the fluids surrounding the cells can also create cellular damage, and drugs or toxins can alter cell membrane function (see Chapter 8). Tumors are caused by cells that have been altered in some way (see Chapter 10).

Defects in genes that carry inherited traits can result in abnormal metabolism that may or may not be compatible with life. Hereditary disorders such as phenylketonuria, hemophilia, and some neuromuscular disorders are examples. Traits for these conditions are carried in the genes and passed from parents to offspring. Congenital defects may also be caused by environmental agents such as maternal disease and drugs. Many congenital defects are believed to occur during the first few weeks of embryonic life, even before the mother realizes she is pregnant. For example, if a mother has German measles during the first trimester of pregnancy, there is a possibility that the baby will have a congenital defect. There is increasing evidence that other infectious diseases, including mumps, infectious hepatitis, and influenza, may play some part in spontaneous abortion, premature birth, stillbirth, and birth defects.

Congenital birth defects may affect any organ or system of the body, and several defects that involve different organs or systems may often occur in the same child. In recent years certain drugs have been shown to cause alterations in fetal development. Excessive caffeine intake during pregnancy has been associated with increased fetal loss. Alcohol intake and

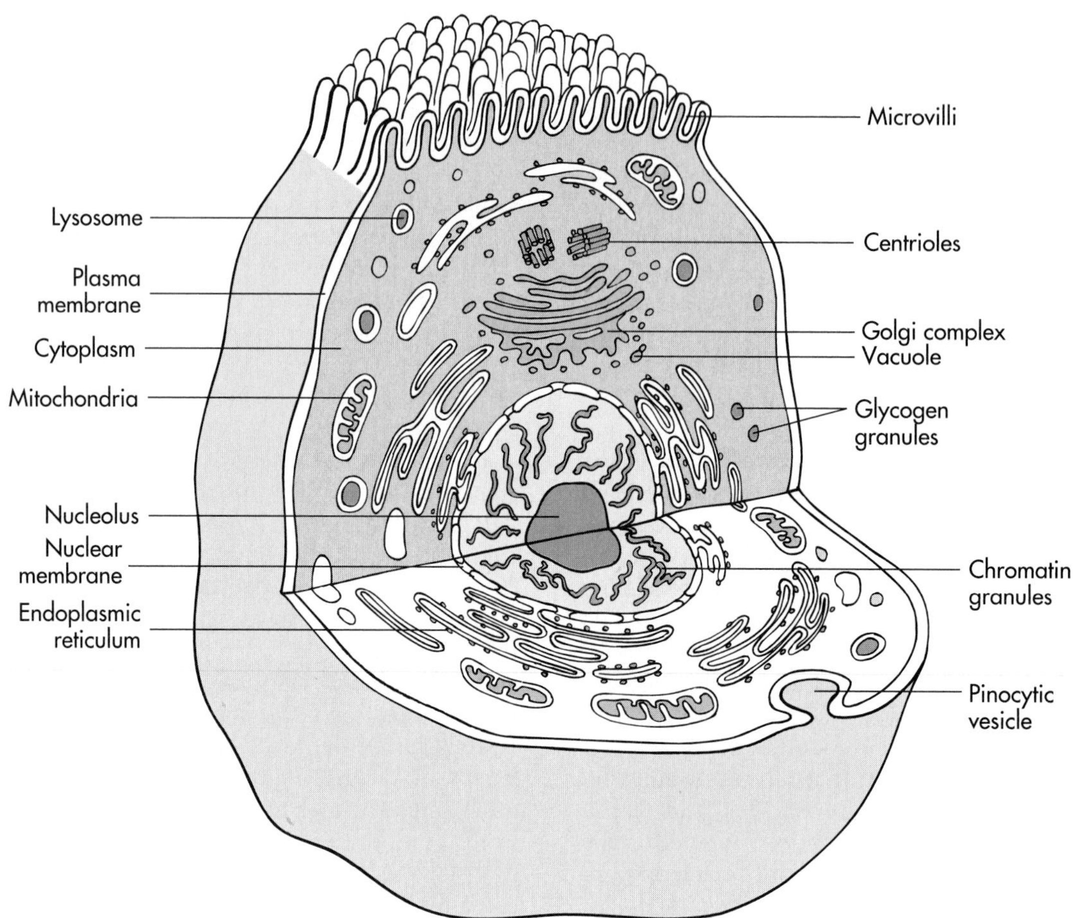

Figure 7-4 Structures of a typical body cell.

smoking also adversely affect fetal development (Clark, Queener, Karlo, 1993).

PHYSIOLOGIC DEFENSE MECHANISMS

Nature has provided the body with various physiologic defense mechanisms that limit the ability of microorganisms and other substances to invade the body and cause disease. The first line of defense is the unbroken skin and the mucous membranes, which serve as mechanical barriers against invaders. Perspiration, the excretion of the sudoriferous (sweat) glands, has an average acid content of 5.65% on the skin, which is lethal to many bacteria. Lysozyme, an antibacterial enzyme that is present on the skin, dissolves some bacteria and is also present in saliva and tears.

The mucous membranes lining the respiratory tract, gastrointestinal tract, and urinary tract secrete substances that are **bacteriostatic,** or able to inhibit bacteria growth. The lacrimal fluid (tears) has the ability to destroy some microorganisms, and the secretions continuously bathe and wash foreign materials, including pathogens, from the eye. The high acid content of the stomach acts as a formidable barrier for pathogens that are swallowed. Any pathogens that enter the intestines may be destroyed by certain enzymes that are secreted by cells along the intestinal route. Vaginal secretions are normally acidic, and pathogens entering the vagina are usually destroyed. Frequent vaginal irrigations reduce the pH (acid) concentration of the vagina and thereby reduce the effectiveness of the natural barrier.

The nasal cavities, trachea, and bronchi contain fine hairlike projections called *cilia,* which are in constant wavelike motion. The cilia sweep pathogens toward the pharynx, where they may be swallowed or expectorated. If swallowed, they are destroyed by the stomach acids. The fine hairs around the external nares help prevent pathogens from entering, and if they do enter, they are trapped by cavities. The mouth has a high concentration of microorganisms. Many are swallowed and destroyed. Pathogens in the mouth usually do no harm as long as the mucous membrane remains intact. Involuntary acts also help the body rid itself of pathogens. Through acts or reflexes such as sneezing and coughing, pathogens may be eliminated from the respiratory tract. Vomiting and diarrhea eliminate bacteria and their toxins from the gastrointestinal system.

Some cells constantly combat infectious agents and other substances that enter the body. Cells that line many of the vascular and lymph channels are capable of phagocytizing bacteria, viruses, and other foreign material. Lymph nodes are located intermittently along the course of the lymphatic vessels, which drain the excess interstitial fluid that surrounds the cells of the body. These lymph nodes contain many cells that phagocytize foreign materials and prevent their general dissemination throughout the body. The spleen filters blood and removes not only old red blood cells from the circulation but also abnormal platelets, blood parasites, bacteria, and other substances. Kupffer's cells in the liver remove large numbers of bacteria that succeed in entering the body through the gastrointestinal tract. The bone marrow has the ability to remove fine particles, such as protein toxins, from the bloodstream. Phagocytic cells in the tissues throughout the body also protect various organs against invading organsims or foreign material (Guyton, 1991).

The white blood cells **(leukocytes)** also combat invasion. The majority of these cells are *polymorphonuclear leukocytes*, or granulocytes. There are three types of polymorphonuclear leukocytes: the *neutrophils*, the *basophils*, and the *eosinophils*. The primary function of the neutrophils is phagocytosis, or the ingestion and digestion of debris and foreign material throughout the body. Neutrophils are the first cells to arrive at the scene when an inflammatory reaction is stimulated. The basophils do not phagocytize, but they contain powerful chemicals such as histamine that can be released locally and assist in the inflammatory process. The eosinophils appear to play a role in allergy and foreign protein reactions. The *mononuclear leukocytes*, or monocytes, become large phagocytic cells when stimulated and also play an important role in inflammation. The *lymphocytes* are the cells primarily concerned with the development of immunity (Guyton, 1991).

Inflammation

One of the most important defense mechanisms is the inflammatory response. **Inflammation** occurs when any agent, such as a chemical substance, foreign body, severe blow, or bacteria, injures the tissue. The inflammatory process is characterized by five classic signs: redness (rubor), heat (calor), swelling (tumor), pain (dolor), and limitation of movement (Box 7-3). When tissue is traumatized, a defensive process begins in which the body tries to localize or eliminate the injurious agent, neutralize or destroy its poisons, and, finally, repair the injured tissue (Figure 7-5). The inflammatory process begins with an increased flow of blood to the area. The tiny capillary blood vessels become dilated, which allows a larger amount of blood to pass through them. This dilation is primarily caused by the release of histamine from injured cells. The leukocytes have the power to move about and begin to migrate

BOX 7-2

CELL ORGANELLES

endoplasmic reticulum Network of interconnected canals that wind through the cytoplasm, form proteins, and serve as a means of transportation of substances throughout the cell

Golgi complex Tiny sacs that are believed to synthesize carbohydrate molecules that are combined with proteins, coated with membrane, and released from the cell as a secretion

mitochondria Delicate, double-layered structure with many partitions that contain enzymes for oxidizing glucose to form energy, which is subsequently stored as adenosine triphosphate (ATP); known as the powerhouses of the cell

lysosomes Small sacs containing enzymes that are capable of digesting any cell structure

ribosomes Small, round organelles that use genetic material to give directions for protein synthesis

centrioles Tubular cylinders that function during cell division

nucleus Largest cell structure, which stores, transmits, and transcribes genetic information (Adlercreutz, 1990)

BOX 7-3

CARDINAL SYMPTOMS OF INFLAMMATION

Redness	Hyperemia from vasodilation
Heat	Vasodilation—blood vessels closer to skin surface
Swelling	Fluid exudation into tissue
Pain	Chemical (bradykinin) irritation of nerve endings; pressure of fluid in tissues
Limitation of movement	Tissue swelling and pain

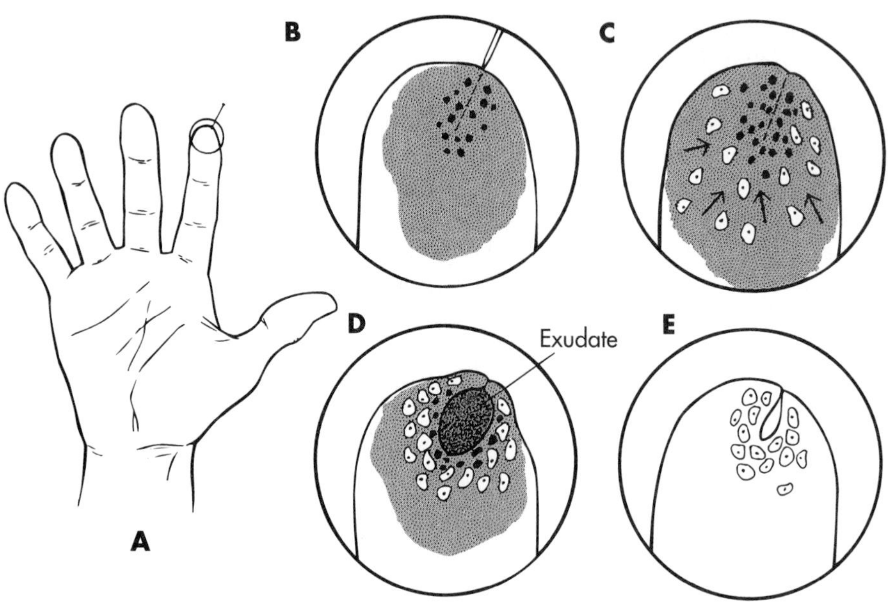

Figure 7-5 Inflammatory process. **A,** Pathogenic bacteria are introduced into tissue through portals of entry such as a pinprick. **B,** Blood supply to area begins to increase. **C,** Leukocytes begin to move out of blood capillaries. **D,** Phagocytes begin to engulf and digest bacteria; dead phagocytes, cells, and tissue fluid escape as exudate. **E,** When phagocytosis is complete, wound begins to heal.

out of the capillaries and into the area where the pathogen has invaded the tissue. The first cells to arrive at the scene are the neutrophils, which begin to engulf and ingest any bacteria or foreign material. After several hours the monocytes follow and are transformed into large phagocytic cells called *macrophages.* It is believed that monocytes are stimulated by substances draining from the site. If the injurious agent is not removed from the site within 24 to 48 hours, lymphocytes begin to predominate at the site and the immune process is stimulated.

During the inflammatory process some phagocytes are killed, and some tissue is destroyed. The phagocytes and destroyed cells and some tissue fluid accumulate at the site. This is called the exudate. If the area has been invaded by microbes, or pathogens, an infection can occur and purulent drainage may be present. The characteristic heat and redness at the site is caused by the increased flow of blood to the area. Swelling results from the accumulation of exudate, and stimulation of the nerves in the area causes the pain. Depending on the location, any effort to move the part may be painful and cause the individual to limit movement. When phagocytosis is complete, the inflammatory condition subsides and healing begins (see Figure 7-5).

Healing is the replacement of dead or damaged cells. Two overlapping stages occur in the process of healing: (1) the regeneration of lost cells with identical or similar tissue, and (2) the formation of scar tissue. The ability of the body to regenerate new tissue depends on the ability of the cells to multiply and form units that can function physiologically like the original cell. Damaged brain, myocardium, and nerve tissue cannot regenerate. Scar tissue is formed by the proliferation of fibroblasts, which secrete collagen precursors. This preliminary stage is called *granulation* tissue. Collagen is a fibrous protein and is present in the connective tissues of the body. Layers of collagen are deposited at the site of injury and form a dense area of scar tissue.

Wounds are repaired with a similar process. The three types of healing in wounds are labeled as primary, secondary, and tertiary intention. Healing by primary intention means that a wound heals with its edges close together or in close approximation and with a minimum of granulation tissue (Figure 7-6, *A*). Surgical wounds heal this way. A secondary intention healing occurs when a greater amount of tissue is damaged and necrotic debris or inflammatory exudate is formed (Figure 7-6, *B*). These wounds take longer to heal and produce more scar tissue. Tertiary intention is sometimes called delayed primary closure. A wound that is surgically closed several days after the injury heals by tertiary intention. For example, a heavily contaminated wound may be left open intentionally to drain and then closed.

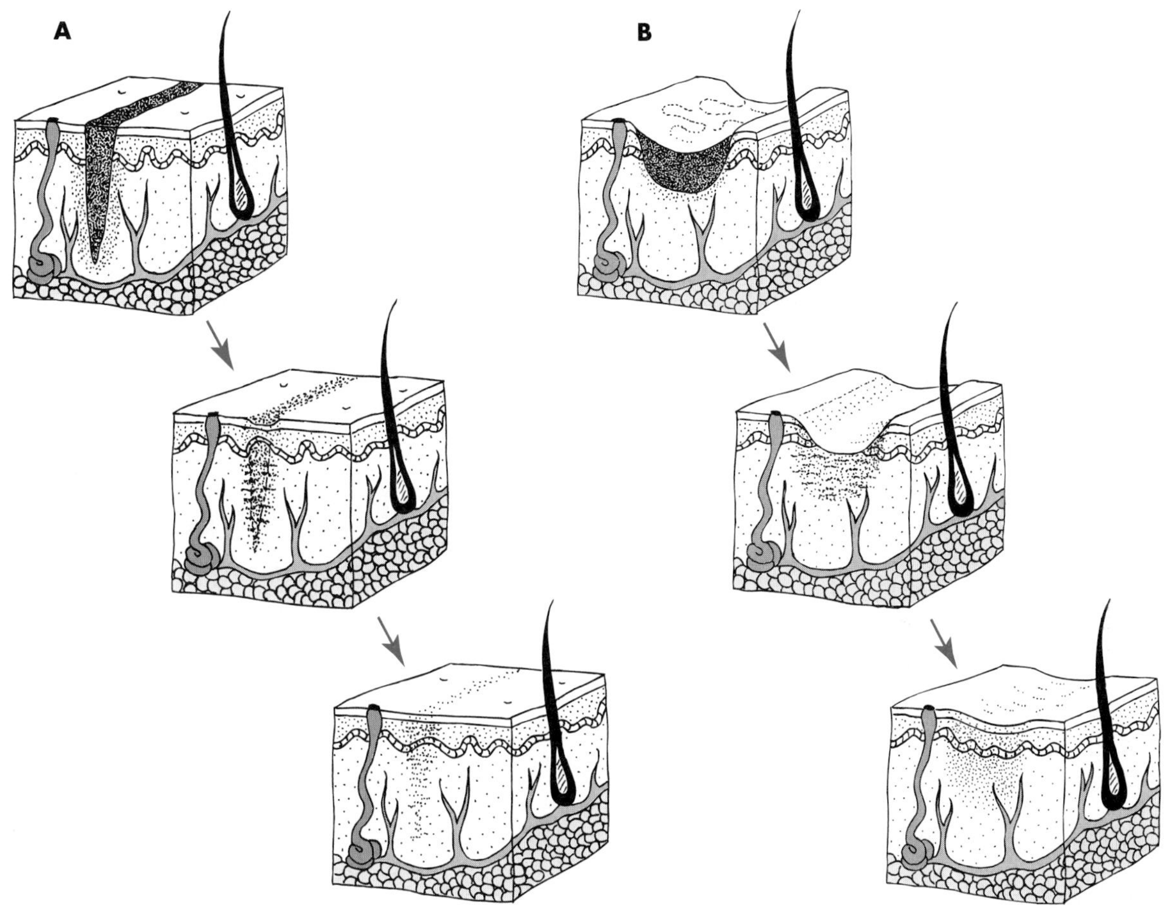

Figure 7-6 Types of wound healing. **A,** Primary. **B,** Secondary.

Infection

Pathogenic organsims may enter the body through the respiratory system, digestive system, reproductive system, urinary system, and skin. They may leave the body through vomitus, feces, urine, draining wounds, drainage tubes, or discharges from the nose and throat. Pathogens may also enter via the urethral meatus in men or the vaginal canal in women. Certain pathogenic organisms such as in malaria and hepatitis B may be transferred through a blood transfusion. Acquired immunodeficiency syndrome (AIDS) is transmitted by blood and some body fluids. Placental transfer of microorganisms to the fetus from the mother may occur in some cases such as syphilis. Individuals may enter a healthcare facility free of infection but may develop an infection during their stay. This is referred to as a **nosocomial infection.** An example of a nosocomial infection is oxacillin-resistant staphylococcal infection (see Chapter 12).

An *endogenous infection* may occur when microorganisms already present in the body produce disease as a result of compromised defense mechanisms. For example, patients with diabetes may develop monilial infections.

An *exogenous infection* occurs when pathogenic microorganisms gain entrance to the body from the outside such as in hepatitis B.

Another way in which bacteria may harm the body is by the production of powerful poisons, or toxins. These toxins are classified as **endotoxins** or **exotoxins.** Endotoxins are present in the cell walls of gram-negative rods and cocci. Most endotoxins are contained in organisms that cause enteric diseases such as typhoid fever and bacillary dysentery. Exotoxins are produced by bacteria and released outside the cell. They are the most poisonous substances that can injure humans. Diseases in which exotoxins are produced include diphtheria, tetanus, and botulism.

Some bacteria are powerful enough to resist the leukocytes and destroy many of them. Bacteria may also produce powerful toxins that kill the leukocytes. If this occurs, the bacteria causes disease, and either the bacteria or their toxins may be carried by the bloodstream and the lymphatic vessels to various parts of the body. The time factor is extremely important in an infection because the longer the bacteria have to multiply, the more severe the infection. The physician may prescribe bacteriostatic drugs for the patient to prevent rapid multiplication of bacteria.

Infection is classified in a number of different ways according to its location, extent, and severity (Box 7-4). When pathogenic microorganisms invade the body and cause inflammation or infection, they may cause certain symptoms or conditions with which the nurse should be familiar (Box 7-5).

The following five factors influence the ability of invading pathogens to survive and cause disease (pathogenicity):

1 Whether the pathogens gain entrance by their characteristic route
2 Whether the pathogens have an affinity for only certain types of tissue
3 The ability of the toxins to enter the body and produce toxins (virulence)
4 The number of pathogens that enter the body at a given time
5 The degree and character of resistance that the host offers the invading pathogens

Most bacteria enter the body by a specific route. Unless they are successful in gaining entrance by their characteristic route, they may not cause disease. For example, bacteria whose characteristic route is the respiratory system may be harmless if swallowed. Some pathogens have a particular affinity for certain types of tissue. Once they gain entrance to the body they go directly to that tissue and leave other tissues unaffected. The virus causing poliomyelitis attacks only nerve tissue, and other pathogens attack only the respiratory system.

Pathogens vary in their power to invade the body and produce toxins. This factor is called **virulence.** Pathogens may be highly virulent and possess a great

BOX 7-4

INFECTION CLASSIFICATION

primary infection An acute infection that appears, runs its course, and resolves in a short period of time
chronic infection Initial stages of the infection are the same as primary infections, but symptoms persist and run a prolonged course
secondary infection Usually a complication of the primary infection; bacteria causing a secondary infection may not always be the same as those causing the primary infection
local infection An infection confined to a single area
generalized infection An infection that spreads and involves the entire body
focal infection An infection in which bacteria has spread from the original site of the infection to other parts of the body
latent infection A condition in which bacteria are still present in the body but are not active and do not cause any symptoms
specific infection An infection caused by one type of microorganism
mixed infection An infection caused by more than one type of microorganism

BOX 7-5

MANIFESTATIONS OF INFECTION

abscess A walled-off area surrounded by inflamed tissue with a collection of pus in a cavity
bacteremia The presence of bacteria in the bloodstream
carbuncle An area of inflammation in the skin and deeper tissues that terminates with pus formation; sometimes constitutional symptoms accompany its presence
cellulitis An inflammatory process that is poorly defined and diffuse and usually involves the skin and subcutaneous tissue
exudate An accumulation of fluid within a cavity or area of inflammation that may contain cells, protein, and solid material
furuncle A boil or an inflamed, pus-filled swelling on the skin
gangrene Death of tissue because of poor arterial or venous circulation
granulation Budding projections formed on the surface of a wound that bring a rich blood supply to tissue
necrosis The death of tissue or small groups of cells
purulent discharge A discharge that contains pus
pyemia Pus in the bloodstream, which causes multiple abscesses in various parts of the body
sanguineous discharge A discharge that contains blood
septicemia The presence of pathogens or their toxins in the bloodstream
serous discharge A clear, watery, thin discharge

power to invade and the ability to produce deadly exotoxins. Other pathogens may be of low virulence and able to invade the body but too weak to produce disease.

The occurrence of disease may depend on the number of pathogens that enter the body at a given time. If a large number of pathogens enter the body, disease is more likely to occur than if only a few invade the host. However, the presence of a few highly virulent pathogens may result in disease, and a large number of pathogens of low virulence may be destroyed without causing disease (Box 7-6).

Intervention

An inflammation may occur without infection (e.g., sunburn), but an infection is usually accompanied by inflammation. Intervention depends on the type of injury, the extent of involvement, and the effectiveness of the defense mechanism An infection may be local (e.g., a boil), an entire body system (e.g., the respirat if there is a bloodstream infection, it may affect the entire body.

Local inflammatory conditions may be painful and may cause the patient considerable discomfort. The goals of patient care are directed toward relieving discomfort and terminating the inflammatory condition before it can affect other parts of the body. To achieve these goals it is necessary to monitor the injured or inflamed site, perform interventions that aid in the healing process and ensure adequate blood flow, and provide for adequate rest and nutrients. Treatment includes rest, elevation of the affected part, application of heat or cold, the use of analgesics, and occasionally incision and drainage (I & D). Antibiotic therapy is required when an infection is present. Elevating the affected part above the level of the heart

BOX 7-6 **Nursing Process**

RISK FOR INFECTION

ASSESSMENT

Vital signs q 4 h
Presence of risk factors such as inadequate defenses, invasive devices or procedures, chronic disease
Labs: White blood cell count, culture, and sensitivities
Signs and symptoms of infection:
- Respiratory status: adventitious sounds, sputum
- Urinary symptoms: urine color, consistency, burning with urination
- IV sites
- Wounds, skin condition, if applicable

Nutritional status
Immunization status
Recent exposure to individuals with acute infections
Immunosuppression

NURSING DIAGNOSIS

Risk for infection

NURSING INTERVENTIONS

Wash hands carefully before and after contact.
Maintain strict asepsis with required nursing care (e.g., IV therapy, Foley catheter care, suctioning).
Change equipment, tubings, and solutions used for nursing care according to hospital policy.
Maintain asepsis with invasive procedures.
Screen visitors and staff for colds, nausea, vomiting, and fever.
Keep patient in a private room or protective isolation if required.
Eliminate fresh flowers, fresh vegetables, or water-filled vases, if required.
Keep skin clean, dry, and well lubricated with daily bathing.
Encourage a high protein, high calorie diet (if not contraindicated).
Encourage liberal fluid intake (if not contraindicated).
Teach and/or provide perineal care.
Teach and/or provide oral hygiene.
Help patient to turn, cough, and deep breathe q 2 h.
Ambulate, if tolerated.
Perform range-of-motion exercises if mobility is limited.
Administer antimicrobials as ordered.

EVALUATION OF EXPECTED OUTCOMES

Absence of signs and symptoms of infection
Patient/family demonstrate preventive measures

OLDER ADULT CONSIDERATIONS

Infections

- Morbidity and mortality as a result of infections are greater in the elderly than in younger adults
- Factors that increase susceptibility to infection include the following:
  - Decreased function of the immune system
  - Slow response to antibiotic therapy
  - Physical changes that disrupt normal defense mechanisms, such as decreased cough reflex, atrophic skin, or decreased gastric acid production
  - Decreased serum albumin
  - Chronic diseases or drug therapy that produces immunosuppression
  - Lifestyle choices such as smoking or lack of exercise

ETHICAL DILEMMA

Do nurses have the right to refuse care to a patient who has an infectious disease that may put the healthcare worker at risk (e.g., tuberculosis, AIDS)?

relieves pain and throbbing, thus increasing patient comfort.

Heat and cold are applied to the body to aid in the healing process. Heat and cold cause different physiologic responses. The initial response to local heat application is vasodilation of skin blood vessels, which increases blood flow to the area. Increased blood flow helps reduce pain and swelling and increases the movement of nutrients, white blood cells, and antibiotics to the site. The application of cold reduces blood flow to the site of injury, which prevents additional swelling and decreases inflammation and pain.

Whether dry or moist heat or cold are used depends on the type of wound or injury, the location of the body part, and the presence of drainage or inflammation. Compresses and packs can be hot or cold. A compress is a moist gauze dressing that is applied to a specific area. If the skin is broken, a sterile technique is used. For a hot, moist compress the gauze is soaked in a solution that is 43° C to 46° C (110° F to 115° F) (Potter, Perry, 1993). For a cold, moist compress the temperature is 15° C (59° F). Moist heat may also be applied with soaks or baths. For example, a sitz bath is taken to immerse the pelvic area in warm water. Soaks aid in the debridement, or cleaning, of wounds and are useful for the application of medicated solutions.

PATIENT/FAMILY TEACHING 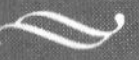

Risk for Infection

The patient and his or her family should be taught the following:

- Signs and symptoms of infection
- How to perform personal hygiene
- Antibiotic dosage, action, and side effects
- Importance of handwashing

Dry heat can be applied with an aquathermia pack, a hot water bottle, a heating pad, or a heat lamp. Aquathermia packs contain distilled water that circulates through tubes. The desired temperature is preset and is regulated by a temperature control unit. Hot water bottles are rarely used with hospitalized patients because they can injure the skin. Patients who use one at home should be instructed to fill it with warm tap water that is between 43° C and 46° C (110° F to 115° F), cover it with a towel or pillow case, and apply it for 20 to 30 minutes. Before applying any type of heat, the nurse should consult the appropriate procedure manual and assess the patient's physical and mental status regarding his or her ability to tolerate heat. Because of the danger of burning the patient, the nurse should frequently assess the area receiving the heat treatment (Potter, Perry, 1993).

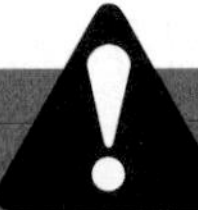

NURSE ALERT

When applying heat to the patient, assess the area often.

Moist cold is applied in the form of cold compresses, usually for short intervals and at specified periods. Dry cold is provided by an ice bag or ice collar. Because of the danger of injury to the tissues, an uncovered ice bag should never be applied directly to the skin and should not be used to cover wet dressings.

When local inflammation does not respond to treatment, a surgical incision may be required to allow the accumulated exudate to escape. This may be referred to as an I & D.

Patients with generalized infections may be very ill and have an extremely high temperature and a corresponding increase in the pulse and respiratory rates. The white-blood cell count is increased *(leukocytosis)*, and chills, loss of appetite, sweating, and delirium may occur. The patient is usually confined to bed.

Acetaminophen (Tylenol) or acetylsalicylic acid (aspirin) may be given to lower the temperature. Sometimes a cooling blanket may be applied. A tepid or cool sponge bath may also be used to remove waste products from the skin and provide comfort. Special mouth care should be given several times a day or as indicated. An emollient jelly may be used to lubricate the lips and nose to prevent dryness and crust formation. Accurate measurement of fluid intake and fluid loss from all sources is an important nursing intervention. Because the patient is losing greater amounts of fluid through the skin and respiratory system, adequate fluid intake should be encouraged. It is important that the patient continue to produce large amounts of urine to help eliminate toxins. Oral fluids should be high in nutrients, calories, and electrolytes. If sufficient fluids are not ingested, the physician may prescribe intravenous fluids. Periodic weighing of the patient provides information regarding loss of weight and body fluids. During the febrile period the diet should be liquid, followed by soft, easily digested foods and a gradual return to a general diet.

NURSE ALERT

Recording fluid intake and output accurately is essential for patients with generalized infections.

Back rubs, a quiet and well-ventilated room, and freedom from annoying disturbances adds to the patient's comfort. The nurse should ensure that young children, the elderly, and delirious patients are protected from injury. Because most patients generally feel ill, the number of visitors should be kept to a minimum. The nurse should be careful to maintain medical asepsis, with special attention to handwashing (see Chapter 12).

PATIENT/FAMILY TEACHING

Once the nurse has confirmed the order for heat or cold application, the nurse should explain the rationale for the treatment, review the procedure and the precautions, and give instructions to alert the nurse if any discomfort is experienced. After the patient has been taught, the nurse must ensure that he or she understands the instructions.

Immunity

Immunology includes the mechanisms by which the body's cellular and chemical systems recognize and react to foreign substances. This dynamic process occurs throughout life to counteract the effects of foreign materials, bacteria, viruses, foods, and chemicals that constantly enter the body. A person with an immune system that is functioning normally is immunocompetent.

Immunity can be natural or acquired. *Natural immunity* is present at birth and depends on species, race, and heritage. For example, humans do not suffer from foot and mouth disease, which is found in cattle.

Acquired immunity is gained actively or passively by the individual. To develop *active immunity,* a person must contract the disease or be infected with an attenuated form of the disease-producing organism. This process does not provide immediate protection against the organism because the body requires time to develop a sufficient response. *Passive immunity* is gained from another source. A newborn acquires passive immunity from the mother through the placenta and breast milk. Others gain passive immunity by receiving disease-specific antiserum or pooled gamma globulin that contains antibodies to a number of diseases. This is a temporary type of immunity and is used to protect an individual from disease immediately after exposure.

Any invading agent that can elicit an immune response is called an *antigen.* Antigens are usually large proteins or large polysaccharides, and many bacteria contain these substances. Some substances have a low molecular weight and cannot elicit a response by themselves. However, they do have antigenic sites and can combine with carrier substances. If these substances react with another material, they can stimulate an immune response. These substances are called *haptens* and include some drugs, chemicals in dust, and breakdown products from animal dander.

The immune system is composed of specialized cells, central lymphoid tissue (bone marrow and thymus), and peripheral lymphoid tissue (lymph nodes, tonsils, spleen, and intestinal lymphoid tissue such as Peyer's patches and the appendix). The cells responsible for the development of immunity include lymphocytes and macrophages. The lymphocytes are divided into two categories: (1) the B lymphocytes, which are responsible for antibody formation, or humoral immunity, and (2) the T lymphocytes, which are responsible for cellular, or cell-mediated immunity. Lymphocytes originate in hematopoietic tissue as stem cells and migrate to lymphoid tissue for maturation and expression of their immune functions (Figure 7-7). Another major component of the immune system is complement, which consists of approximately 20 proteins that are found in normal human serum. The term *complement* refers to the ability of these proteins to enhance the other components of the immune system (Levinson, Jawetz, 1994).

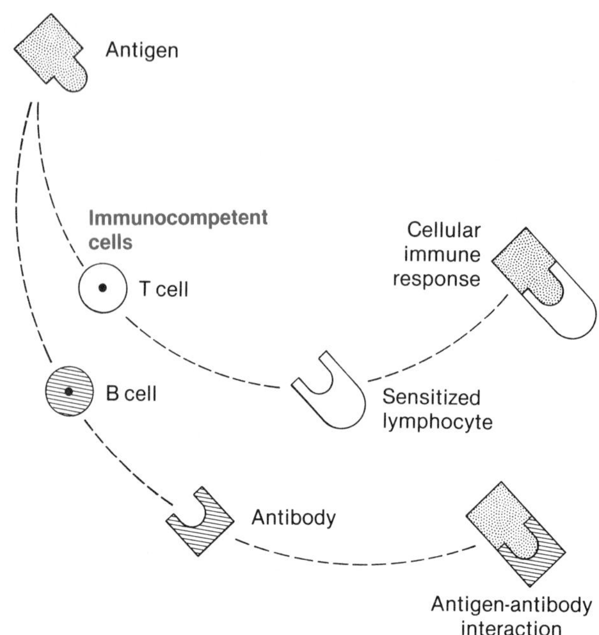

Figure 7-7 Humoral (B-cell) immunity results in antibody formation. Cellular (T-cell) immunity results in production of a sensitized lymphocyte.

Humoral immunity

Humoral immunity results when an invading agent stimulates dormant B lymphocytes in the lymph nodes to produce **antibodies.** Antibodies are proteins that are developed to react with a specific *antigen*. The invading agent also stimulates the B lymphocytes to produce new lymphocytes that will continue to manufacture antibodies in the future. Therefore, immunity to the agent may continue over long periods. The antibodies are called **immunoglobulins (Ig)** and can react only with the antigen that first stimulated the B cell. There are five classes of immunoglobulins—IgA, IgG, IgD, IgM, and IgE—and each has its own specific characteristics and functions. The IgE antibody is called the reaginic antibody and is primarily responsible for allergic reactions (Guyton, 1991) (Table 7-2).

The antigen-antibody reaction destroys or inactivates the invading agent through several processes. It can neutralize an antigen and decrease its toxic qualities, cause the agent to become insoluble in a solution or precipitate, cause agglutination or clumping of antigens, lyse cell membranes, or render the antigen susceptible to phagocytosis. Some antigen-antibody reactions have the ability to stimulate the activity of nine different enzymes that are normally inactive in plasma and body fluids. This is the complement system, which helps destroy and inactivate invading organisms.

Cellular immunity

The immune response referred to as **cell-mediated** or cellular is based on the function of T-lymphocytes. There are three major groups of T cells: *helper, suppressor,* and *killer* cells. The helper T cells enhance the function of the B cells. The suppressor cells inhibit the activities of other lymphocytes and provide feedback to the system. The killer cells destroy targeted enemy cells by directly binding to their surface.

Cellular immunity results when T cells are activated by an antigen. Whole cells become sensitized in a process similar to that which stimulates the B cells to form antibodies. Once sensitized, these T cells are released into the blood and body tissues, where they remain indefinitely. The cellular type of immunity is stimulated by fungi, viruses, parasites, and some bacteria that live inside other cells. Tuberculosis is a disease that stimulates cellular immunity. It is believed that there is an interaction between humoral immune processes and cellular immune processes that uses the helper T cells as a switch between the two processes.

There is no absolute immunity to any specific disease to which humans are susceptible. The degree of resistance to a certain disease or agent may vary from person to person and within the same person at different times.

TABLE 7-2

Classes of Immunoglobulins

Name	Characteristics
IgG	Present in serum and amniotic fluid; activates complement; protects newborns
IgA	Present in serum, tears, saliva, gastrointestinal (GI) tract, secretions, colostrum; protects mucous membranes
IgM	Present in serum; activates complement; forms antibodies for ABO blood antigens
IgD	Present in serum and umbilical cord; action unknown
IgE	Present in serum and tissues; functions in allergic and hypersensitivity reactions

EXCESSIVE IMMUNE RESPONSES

Allergy

The condition now known as **hypersensitivity,** or an *allergy,* was first observed in 1832 but not seriously studied until 1890. Koch was the first to observe and describe the allergic reaction after he administered the tuberculosis test for a diagnosis of tuberculosis. The term *allergy* was not used until 1906 when von Pirquet used it to describe the changes associated with repeated contact with various antigenic substances. Since that time the term *allergy* has been accepted to designate hypersensitivity in certain individuals. The terms *allergy* and *hypersensitivity* are used interchangeably.

An allergy is an inappropriate and excessive response of the immune system to certain substances that are not harmful to most persons. When an individual contacts the offending substance *(antigen),* the body is immediately stimulated to produce either antibodies or sensitized white blood cells, (T lymphocytes) to defend itself against the offending antigen. When the same antigen is contacted again, the antibodies or sensitized cells react with the antigen and destroy or neutralize the antigen, which results in a group of symptoms that are referred to as manifestations of an allergy.

Genetic transmission of predisposition to an allergy occurs in some families. If a parent has an allergic disorder, the offspring may develop an allergic condition at some period during their lifetime, but it will not necessarily be the same as the parent's allergy. The homeostasis of the body plays an important role when the individual has an inherited predisposition to allergy. Any episode that disturbs the homeostatic balance, such as a severe infection, a pregnancy, or an endocrine dysfunction, may cause or exacerbate an allergy.

An **allergen** may be transmitted directly from the mother to the fetus in utero by the placental blood supply. When the infant has been sensitized in utero to a specific allergen, contact with the allergen after birth may cause an allergic reaction.

Allergens can be classified as inhalants, ingestants, injectants, contactants, or infectants. The most common inhalants are pollens from grasses, weeds, trees, and grains, as well as dust. An allergy caused by inhaling pollens is usually seasonal and occurs when flowering and pollination occur. The most common type of allergy caused by pollens is hay fever. Ingestants are usually foods to which the individual may be hypersensitive. The most common offenders include the proteins of cow's milk, egg whites, chocolate, strawberries, shellfish, and nuts. Among the injectants are drugs such as antibiotics. Horse serum, which may be used in making antitoxins, may cause severe reactions. The venom from a snake bite or stings from some insects may cause a reaction in a hypersensitive person. Some individuals may be sensitive to contactants such as laundry powders, cosmetic preparations, nickel compounds used in costume jewelry, rubber compounds used in elastic, and the sap from plants such as poison ivy or poison oak (Figure 7-8). Factors related to infectants have been demonstrated in tuberculosis, typhoid fever, and anthrax.

Assessment includes an exposure history, signs, symptoms, and other relevant assessments should be recorded. A thorough physical examination is done and involves a complete blood count and differential count. *Eosinophils* are white blood cells that normally comprise 1% to 3% of all leukocytes. Frequently during an allergic reaction the number of circulating eosinophils frequently increases. They collect at sites of antigen-antibody reactions, such as in the nasal secretions. Another diagnostic blood study is the radioallergosorbent technique (RAST) test, which uses a sample of the patient's blood to test for the presence of reaginic (IgE) antibodies.

Pathophysiology

Most allergies are caused by an antigen-antibody reaction that damages some of the body's tissues. This type of response is called an *immediate* reaction. The body tissues commonly involved are called target organs and are those tissues that come in frequent contact with the external environment, such as the skin, mucous membranes, respiratory tract, and gastroin-

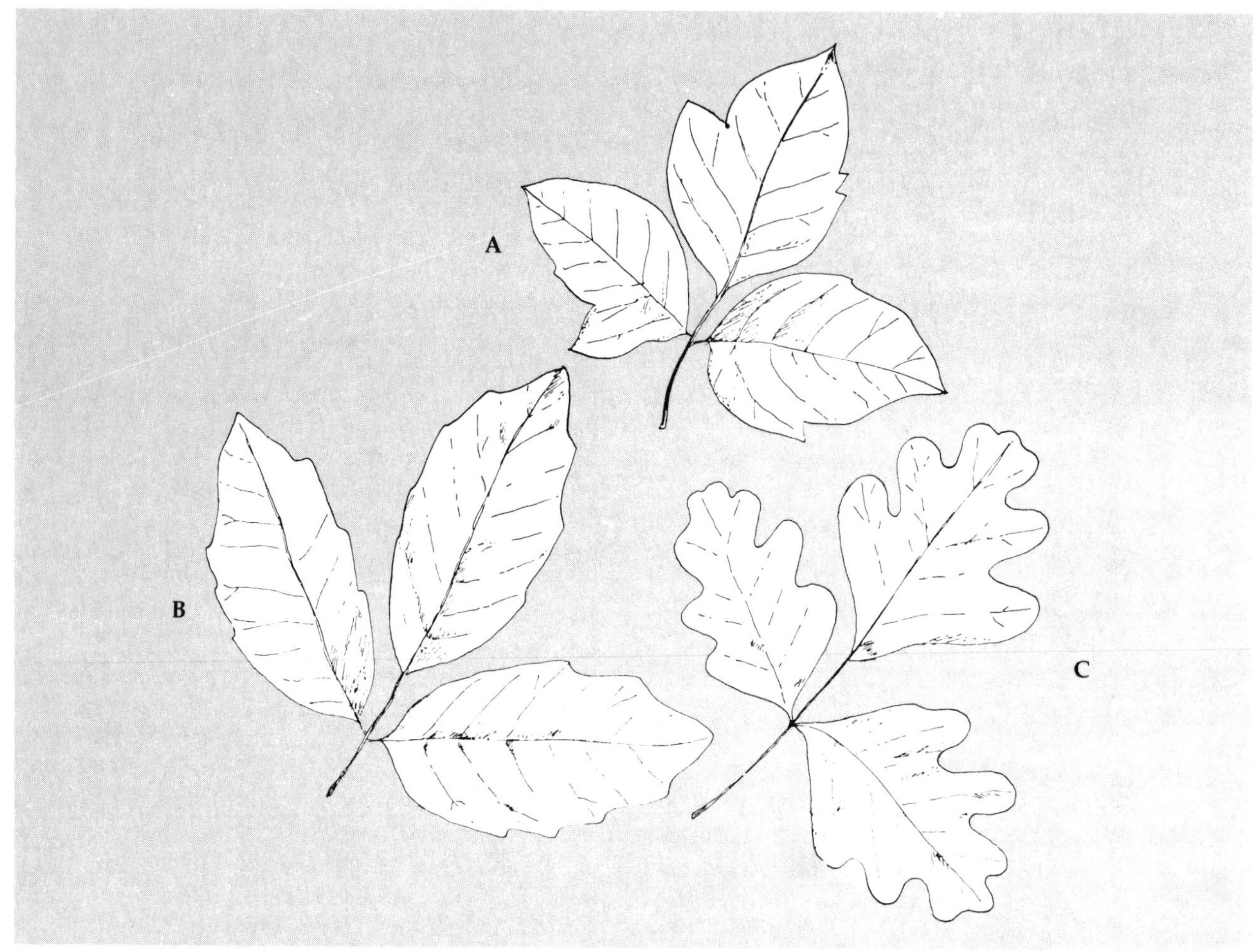

Figure 7-8 Plants and shrubs that commonly cause severe skin reaction. **A,** Poison ivy. **B,** and **C,** Types of poison oak. Note asymmetry in leaf formations.

testinal tract. A summary of hypersensitivity reactions in found in Table 7-3. Types I, II, and III reactions are related to humoral immunity and are the immediate result of interactions that involve circulating antibodies. Type IV reactions are delayed, related to cell-mediated immunity, and the direct result of interactions involving *sensitized* lymphocytes.

Immediate hypersensitivity. Individuals with a Type I immediate hypersensitivity reaction must first come into contact with an allergen. The body may respond by forming specific antibodies that react with the allergen. Although this is essentially a normal mechanism, the hypersensitive individual produces an altered form of an antibody called a *reaginic IgE antibody.* A nonallergic person would produce the IgG antibody. Subsequent contact with the allergen initiates an antigen-antibody reaction that damages tissues. Enzymes such as histamine and histamine-like substances are released from mast cells in the target organ to which the reaginic antibody and antigen have

TABLE 7-3

Hypersensitivity Reactions

Type	Reaction
Type I	Immediate reactions: IgE-mediated local or systemic anaphylaxis; atopic disorders
Type II	Cytotoxic reactions: IgG- and/or IgM-mediated destruction of cells; drug and transfusion reactions
Type III	Immune complex reactions: IgM- or IgG-mediated formation of antigen-antibody complexes; serum sickness; Arthus reactions
Type IV	Cell-mediated reactions: mediated by sensitized T cells; allergic contact dermatitis; delayed hypersensitivity reactions

From Beare P, Myers J: *Adult Health Nursing,* ed 2, 1994, Mosby.

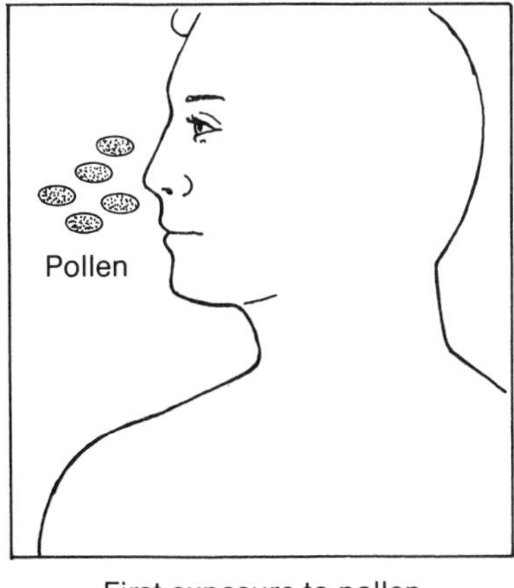

First exposure to pollen

B cells

IgE

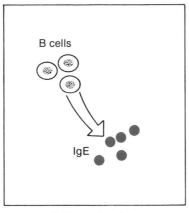

Antigen stimulates B-lymphocyte to produce IgE antibodies.

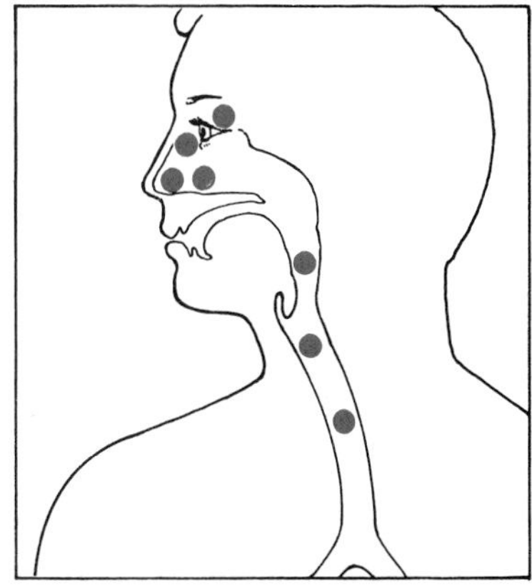

IgE lives on most cells located in upper respiratory tract, conjunctiva, and skin.

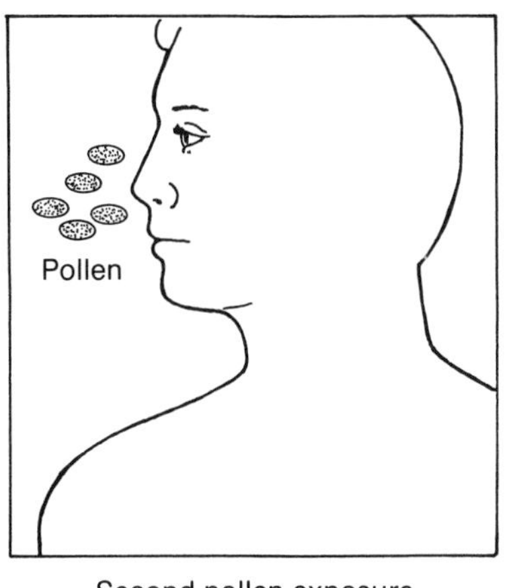

Second pollen exposure

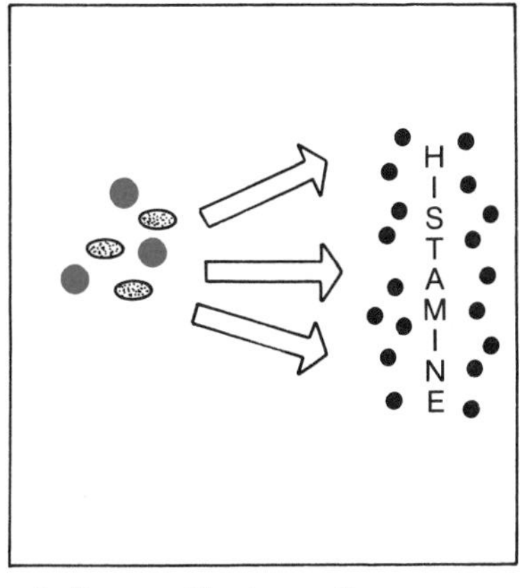

Antigen-antibody reaction occurs. Histamine and other chemical mediators are released.

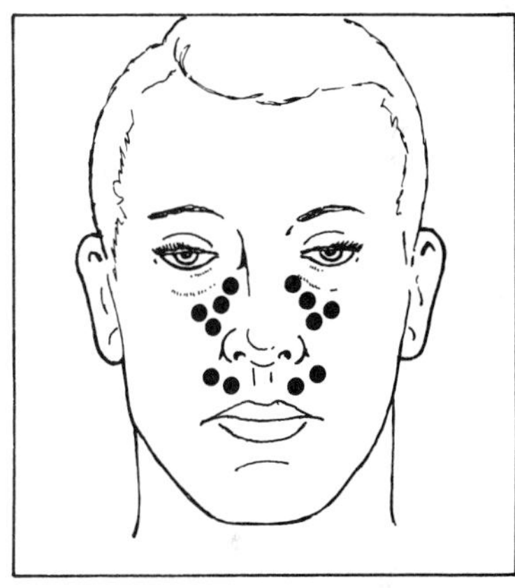

Symptoms of congestion, sneezing, coughing, and difficulty in breathing are exhibited.

Figure 7-9 Allergic response to ragweed pollen.

become attached. This process causes increased vascular permeability, constriction of smooth muscle, and an increased mucus secretion. A local inflammatory response is initiated.

The symptoms of this type of allergy depend on the chemicals and the lactation of the tissue in which the antigen-antibody reaction is occurring. If a sensitized person inhales ragweed pollen, the antigen-antibody reaction occurs in the respiratory tract. Histamine causes vasodilation. Vessels become more permeable, which allows fluids to escape into the body tissues and cause edema. Constriction of the smooth muscle lining the airway and increased mucus secretion may all lead to congestion, sneezing, coughing, and difficulty breathing (Figure 7-9).

Inhalants usually cause congestion of the nasal mucosa; sneezing; a thin, watery nasal discharge; red, itching conjunctivae; and increased lacrimation. Allergens entering through the digestive tract may produce nausea, vomiting, and diarrhea. Various contact substances cause urticaria and dermatitis. Typical skin reactions such as hives or wheals are localized areas of swelling that are red, hot, and itchy. Hives can also develop in the gastrointestinal tract, on the lining of the respiratory passageways, and along blood vessels. When histamine causes spasm and constriction of the bronchioles, bronchial asthma may occur. Many local Type I reactions are atopic or inherited. Usually the symptoms of atopic allergy are localized to the site of the antigen-antibody reaction. However, if large amounts of chemicals are released, they may enter the circulation and cause systemic effects. For example, drug allergies may cause a variety of reactions from fever and skin rash to urticaria, anaphylactic shock, and death.

Allergic reactions from insects. The bites or stings of various insects may cause local or systemic reactions. The local reaction that occurs at the site of the bite or sting is not considered to be an allergic reaction. However, the symptoms of systemic reactions are con-

143

rgy. Stings by bees, wasps, hornets, may produce systemic reactions urticaria and itching to respiratory of consciousness, and death. The action may occur with all insects with only one specific insect. The same process of antibody formation occurs as with other antigens. The first sting may cause no trouble, but a reaction may occur if the individual is stung again. The speed with which the reaction develops is in direct proportion to its severity. If a large number of stings occur at the same time, the reaction may be immediate and can be fatal as a result of the large amount of toxin injected. If the stinger is left in the skin, it should be scraped off. Squeezing should be avoided. The best treatment is prevention (Box 7-7). Patients with a known allergy to insect stings should carry an emergency medical information card or dog tag that explains the problem.

Anaphylactic shock. Anaphylactic shock is a systemic response to a Type I hypersensitivity reaction and follows exposure to a substance to which the individual is extremely sensitive. It is potentially fatal and can appear within minutes in people who have been previously sensitized to the allergen. It is a sudden, severe, systemic reaction and is a true medical emergency. Although it is relatively rare, anaphylactic shock occurs after the injection of vaccines, drugs, foreign sera, or allergenic extracts that are used in desensitization. Penicillin; bee or wasp venom; and substances containing iodine, which are frequently used as a contrast medium for x-ray examinations, are common causes of anaphylaxis. Foods containing iodine are often implicated.

Assessment. Initial symptoms of anaphylaxis are sneezing, apprehension, and edema and itching in the eyes and ears and/or at the site of injection. Edema of the face, hands, and other parts of the body can occur in seconds or minutes. Respiratory distress from bronchospasm, sneezing and coughing, wheezing, dysp-

PATIENT/FAMILY TEACHING

Prevention of Severe Insect Sting Reaction

- Instruct patient to carry emergency medical card or tag that identifies problem.
- Instruct patient to carry emergency kit that contains injectable epinephrine (note expiration dates), oral antihistamines, and tourniquets.
- Advise patient to avoid perfumes, brightly colored clothing, flowers, and fields and to wear shoes at all times.
- Advise patient always to seek follow-up emergency treatment.

BOX 7-7 **Nursing Process**

PREVENTION OF SEVERE INSECT STING REACTION

ASSESSMENT

Local reaction at site of sting
Evidence of systemic reaction
History of severe allergic reaction
Compliance with carrying emergency kit

NURSING DIAGNOSES

Knowledge deficit related to preventive measures
Risk for injury related to severe allergic insect sting reaction

NURSING INTERVENTIONS

Instruct the patient to carry an emergency medical card or tag that identifies condition.
Instruct the patient to carry an emergency kit that contains injectable epinephrine (note expiration dates), oral antihistamines, and tourniquets.
Advise the patient to avoid perfumes, brightly colored clothing, flowers, and fields and to wear shoes at all times.
Advise the patient to always seek follow-up emergency treatment.

EVALUATION OF EXPECTED OUTCOMES

Able to verbalize understanding of the need to avoid antigen in the future
Demonstrates ability to initiate emergency treatment for anaphylactic shock

nea, and cyanosis follow. Edema of the larynx and laryngospasm may lead to death. Gastrointestinal symptoms such as nausea and vomiting, abdominal pain, and diarrhea may be present. Cardiovascular signs such as dysrhythmia, tachycardia, or bradycardia may be followed by circulatory collapse, which is indicated by a falling blood pressure, pallor, and loss of consciousness. In extreme cases death may occur in 5 to 10 minutes after onset of the reaction (Table 7-4; Box 7-8).

PATIENT/FAMILY TEACHING

Anaphylactic Shock

The nurse should discuss the following topics with the patient and his or her family:

- Factors that may cause recurrence
- Interventions to prevent recurrence
- Insect sting kits, if indicated
- Importance of Medic-Alert tags
- Importance of communicating allergy to health-care providers

Cytotoxic hypersensitivity. Cytotoxic, or Type II, hypersensitivity occurs when antibodies directed against antigens of the cell membrane stimulate complement (Levinson, Jawetz, 1994). A cytotoxic hypersensitivity reaction occurs when an incompatible blood product is given to a patient. The antigen responsible for the antigen-antibody reaction is the donor red blood cell. This cell reacts with the recipient's antibody and complement to cause cell lysis (see Chapter 22). Some drug reactions are also cytotoxic reactions.

Immune complex hypersensitivity. Normally the products of the antigen-antibody reaction (immune complexes) are promptly removed, but sometimes they persist and become deposited in the tissues. This results in a Type III hypersensitivity reaction (Levinson, Jawetz, 1994). Inflammation results and damages the affected organ system. For example, a response to the beta hemolytic streptococcus can result in acute poststreptococcal glomerulonephritis, which damages the nephrons of the kidney (see Chapter 24).

Cell-mediated hypersensitivity. Delayed reactions, or Type IV hypersensitivity, may be local or systemic and may be delayed from hours to days. This type of hypersensitivity results from an alteration in the cell-mediated immune response, where entire lymphocytes (T cells) become sensitized to the antigen (see Table 7-3). Antibodies are not produced, but instead the

TABLE 7-4

Emergency Care of Individuals in Anaphylactic Shock

Signs and Symptoms	Nursing Interventions	Expected Patient Outcomes
Rapid, shallow breathing; bronchospasms; dyspnea; cyanosis; restlessness; "sense of doom"; irritability; laryngeal edema	Prepare for oropharyngeal intubation or surgical insertion of tracheotomy; oxygen therapy per order. Prepare for administration of antihistamines such as benadryl 25-50 mg IM, aminophylline IV drip; administer corticosteroids to decrease inflammation as ordered.	Maintains patent airway; demonstrates effective breathing pattern
Hypotension; rapid, thready pulse	Administer 0.1 ml to 0.5 ml 1:1000 epinephrine solution subcutaneously (SC) or intramuscularly (IM) into upper arm and massage site to hasten absorption; prepare to administer vasopressor drugs such as norepinephrine bitartrate (Levophed) and high-dose dopamine (Intropin); monitor pulse and blood pressure q 3-5 min until stable.	Maintains hemodynamic stability as evidenced by blood pressure and pulse in normal range
Edema and itching at site of injection or insect bite	Place a tourniquet above the site of the antigen. Remove tourniquet q 10-15 min or until reaction is under control; apply ice.	Reduces systemic absorption of the antigen

whole cell attacks the antigen and destroys it. The most common example of a delayed reaction is the tuberculin skin test. Individuals who have been previously sensitized to the antigen respond to an intradermal injection of old tuberculin with erythema and induration after 24 to 48 hours. Allergic contact dermatitis is the most common immunologic disorder that is treated by dermatologists. The most common sensitizing antigens are poison ivy, rubber compounds used in elastic, and nickel used in costume jewelry and buttons. These substances combine with skin proteins and create a non-self–antigen. A localized irritation of the skin (eczema) occurs and is characterized by redness, edema, and scaling. Organ transplant rejection is also believed to be a type of delayed sensitivity. An individual's history as it relates to tension-producing situations, infection, endocrine disturbance, and work-related activities may be significant. Geographic movement may be important because of change of climate or exposure to new types of allergens.

BOX 7-8

Nursing Process

ANAPHYLACTIC SHOCK

ASSESSMENT

Vital signs q 3-5 min until stable
Respiratory status (dyspnea, tachypnea, wheezing, stridor, hoarseness)
Breath sounds
Arterial blood gases (ABGs)
Level of consciousness, orientation
Urine output
Skin (temperature, flushing, urticaria, rash)
Presence of facial edema
Peripheral pulses
Level of anxiety
Coping mechanisms
Knowledge of condition/allergies

NURSING DIAGNOSES

Decreased cardiac output related to severe allergic reaction
Ineffective breathing pattern related to airway and facial edema, bronchospasm
Impaired skin integrity related to urticaria, dermatitis
Anxiety related to sudden, severe change in health status
Knowledge deficit related to new medical condition, need for future prevention
Ineffective individual coping related to variable nature of allergic reactions and necessity of altering lifestyle

NURSING INTERVENTIONS

If ingested food or drugs are the cause, help with forced emesis.
If injected agents or insect bites are the cause, place a tourniquet around the site and apply ice directly to site. Remove tourniquet q 10-15 min and reapply.
Administer medications as prescribed:
- Epinephrine 0.1 ml to 0.5 ml 1:1000 solution SC or IM into upper arm. Massage site to hasten absorption
- Benadryl 50-100 mg IM
- Aminophylline IV infusion
- Corticosteroids
- Vasopressor drugs (norepinephrine bitartrate, dopamine)

Place patient in position for shock with head and trunk horizontal and lower extremities elevated 20-30 degrees, if indicated.
Administer oxygen as prescribed.
Stay with patient during acute distress; constantly assess and provide reassurance.
Prepare for emergency intubation or tracheostomy if indicated.
Administer IV fluids as ordered.
Observe for rash development.
Explain all procedures and treatments.

EVALUATION OF EXPECTED OUTCOMES

Vital signs stable and within normal limits for patient
Urine output > 30 ml per hour
Alert and oriented
No evidence of respiratory distress
Strong peripheral pulses
Decrease in urticaria, rash
Verbalizes anxiety and fear
Verbalizes understanding of allergy cause, prevention, and treatment

Assessment of people with atopic allergies

Approximately 40 million Americans have some type of allergy (Jacobs, Meltzer, Selner, 1989). Because these hypersensitivity reactions occur so frequently, nurses in all fields must learn to appropriately assess the allergy patient. A careful and thorough allergy history is essential in identifying possible allergens (Figure 7-10). Genetic and congenital factors are extremely important in establishing a diagnosis. Patients should be asked about any family history of allergies and any previous allergic experiences. Past allergic reactions must be recorded and described in the assessment.

ALLERGY SURVEY SHEET

Name: John Richards Age: 36 Sex: m Date: Sept. 3, 1989

I. Chief complaint: stuffy nose & watery eyes
II. Present Illness: wheezing, clear nasal discharge, itchy eyes for 5 wks.
III. Collateral allergic symptoms: same symptoms last fall.

Eyes: Pruritus ✓ Burning — Lacrimation ✓
Swelling ✓ Infection — Discharge —
Ears: Pruritus — Fullness — Popping —
Frequent infections —
Nose: Sneezing ✓ Rhinorrhea ✓ Obstruction —
Pruritus ✓ Mouth breathing —
Purulent discharge —
Throat: Soreness — Post-nasal discharge ✓
Palatal pruritus ✓ Mucus in the morning —
Chest: Cough — Pain — Wheezing ✓
Sputum — Dyspnea —
Color — Rest —
Amount — Exertion —
Skin: Dermatitis — Eczema — Urticaria —

IV. Family allergies: Father had eczemas. Mother none.
V. Previous allergic treatment or testing: no
Prior skin testing: none

Drugs:		
Antihistamines	Improved yes	Unimproved
Bronchodilators	Improved yes	Unimproved
Nose drops	Improved yes	Unimproved
Hyposensitization	Improved not done	Unimproved —
Duration —		
Antigens —		
Reactions —		
Antibiotics (not used)	Improved —	Unimproved
Steroids (not used)	Improved —	Unimproved

VI. Physical agents and habits:

	Bothered by:	
Tobbaco for — years	Alcohol —	Air cond. —
Cigarettes — packs/day	Heat —	Muggy weath. —
Cigars — per day	Cold —	Weath. chngs. —
Pipe — per day	Perfumes —	Chemicals —
Never smoked ✓	Paints —	Hair spray —
Bothered by smoke yes	Insecticides —	Newspapers —
	Cosmetics —	

Figure 7-10 Allergy survey sheet. (From Patterson R: *Allergic diseases,* ed 4, Philadelphia, 1993, JB Lippincott.)

Continued.

VII. When symptoms occur:

Time and circumstances of 1st episode:
Prior health:
Course of illness over decades: progressing ✓ regressing
Time of year:
Perennial ✓ Exact dates Aug./Sept. 1988
Seasonal ✓
Seasonally exacerbated ✓ Aug. 1–present 1989
Monthly variations (menses, occupation): none
Time of week (weekend vs weekdays): no
Time of day or night: no
After insect stings: no

VIII. Where symptoms occur:

Living where at onset: Kansas City, Kansas
Living where since onset: Kansas City, Kansas
Effect of vacation or major geographic change: until June 1988 lived in N.W. Pennsylvania
Symptoms better indoors or outdoors: indoors
Effect of school or work: better at work inside
Effect of staying elsewhere nearby: none
Effect of hospitalization: –
Effect of specific environments: went to park with increased severity of symptoms
Do symptoms occur around:
old leaves ✓ hay ✓ lakeside – barns –
summer homes – damp basement – dry attic –
lawnmowing ✓ animals – other –
Do symptoms occur after eating: no
cheese – mushrooms – beer – melons –
bananas – fish – nuts – citrus fruits –
other foods (list) none
Home: city – rural ✓
house ✓ age 10 yrs
apartment – basement ✓ damp dry ✓
heating system ✓ Forced
pets (how long) none dog – cat – other –

Bedroom:	Type	Age	Living room:	Type	Age
Pillow	foam	3 yrs.	Rug	nylon	1 yr.
Mattress	foam	5 yrs.	Matting	nylon	1 yr.
Blankets	thermal	5 yrs.	Furniture	wood + nylon fabric	1 yr.
Quilts	none	–			
Furniture	wood	5 yrs.			

Anywhere in home symptoms are worse: no

IX. What does patient think makes him worse: outside Aug./Sept.

X. Under what circumstances is he free of symptoms: in air conditioning

XI. Summary and additional comments:

Figure 7-10, cont'd For legend see previous page.

Skin tests. Skin tests include the scratch test, intradermal test, and patch test. Testing often begins with the scratch test, in which a small scratch is made through the skin with a blunt instrument. The scratch is not deep enough to cause bleeding. The allergen may be a powder, liquid, or paste. When the test is done on the forearm, an inert substance (the control) is placed on the other arm. If the individual is sensitive to the antigen, an area of redness and a wheal appears in 15 to 30 minutes, and the control does not show any reaction.

The intradermal test may be used without prior use of the scratch test, or it may be used only for antigens

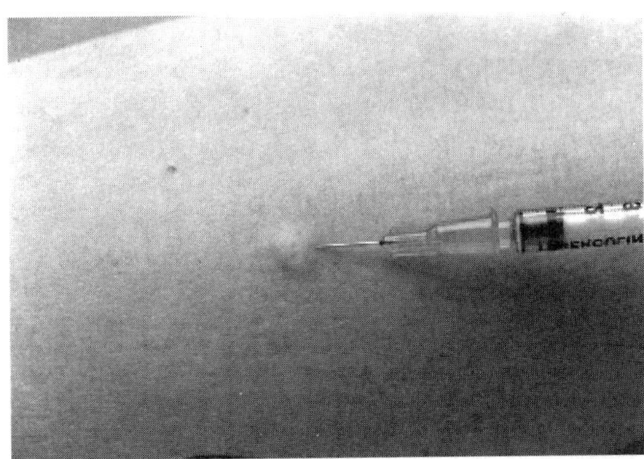

Figure 7-11 Intradermal skin testing for allergic response. (From Potter PA, Perry AG: *Fundamentals of nursing,* ed 3, St Louis, 1993, Mosby.)

that failed to react to the scratch test. A minute amount (0.01 to 0.02 ml) of an antigen is injected into but not through the skin with a tuberculin syringe and a No. 26-gauge needle (Figure 7-11). The sensitivity reaction is similar to that of the scratch test and occurs in approximately 10 minutes. With the prick test a drop of allergen and a control substance are placed approximately 2 cm apart. A No. 26-gauge needle carefully pricks the skin through the drop and gently lifts it upward (Gooi, Chapel, 1990). Both the intradermal and the prick test have grading systems to standardize their interpretation (Middleton and others, 1993).

Patch tests may be used for suspected allergies to specific substances for which commerical allergens are not available. The allergen is applied to the skin, covered, and secured with adhesive tape. The patch is removed in 2 to 3 days, and the skin is examined. The appearance of erythema or a wheal indicates sensitivity to the allergen.

The nurse must be alert for any reaction that might indicate that the patient is developing a generalized allergic reaction. Sudden difficulty in breathing, a change in vital signs, pallor, or dizziness should be reported to the physician immediately. A syringe of 1:1000 epineprhine (Adrenalin) should be available for immediate use. All patients undergoing testing should be kept under surveillance for at least 20 minutes after testing. If the patient has a reaction, follow the procedure previously outlined in Table 7-4.

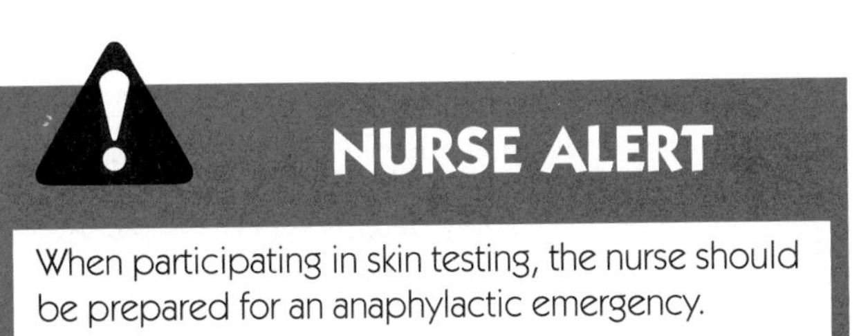

NURSE ALERT
When participating in skin testing, the nurse should be prepared for an anaphylactic emergency.

Mucous membrane sensitivity tests. Tests may also be performed by placing the allergen into the conjunctival sac of the eye. Nothing is placed in the opposite eye, which serves as a control. If the test is positive, itching of the conjunctiva and increased tearing *(lacrimation)* occur. The eyes are then flushed with physiologic saline solution to remove the allergen, and 1 or 2 drops of a 1:1000 aqueous solution of epinephrine is placed in the conjunctival sac. The nasal cavity may also be used for testing. The allergen is sprayed or sniffed into one nostril, and the opposite nostril serves as a control. A positive reaction causes sneezing; nasal congestion; and a thin, watery discharge. Because of the discomfort experienced by the patient, mucous membrane testing is not widely used.

Elimination tests. When food is believed to be the cause of an allergy, a patient may be given an elimination diet to determine the specific food causing the trouble. One of two methods may be used. The patient may be asked to keep a record of all food eaten for a given period. After this period one food such as milk, chocolate, or wheat products is eliminated from the diet. By gradually eliminating specific foods from the diet, the food causing the allergy may be identified. The other method is to give the patient a diet that consists of foods that usually do not cause allergy. The diet is followed for a week. If allergic symptoms continue, changes are made in the diet. If the symptoms continue, it is generally considered that food is not the cause of the allergic reaction. However, if the symptoms disappear, other foods are added to the diet until the patient develops allergic symptoms. That food is then considered to be the probable cause and is eliminated from the diet. This type of testing may be used to identify the cause of urticaria, or hives. Elimination testing is also used for patients with contact dermatitis. Offending agents such as cosmetics, hair spray, and certain types of clothing are eliminated until the dermatitis disappears. These agents are gradually reintroduced to identify the causative agent.

Nursing Interventions for People With Allergies

Nursing interventions for people with allergies include education on avoidance therapy, drug therapy, and help with immunotherapy **(desensitization).** Patients should be educated on the importance of maintaining optimal health, getting enough rest, and controlling stress. The emotional status of the patient influences the severity of the allergy symptoms and the effectiveness of the allergy treatment.

Allergen avoidance. The best treatment for an allergy is to prevent the person from coming in contact with the allergen. The specific allergen must be identified and necessary adaptations made. Adaptation may completely change a person's way of life and may also affect family members. It may mean moving to another environment, changing employment, or changing the type of clothing worn. When animal dander is a factor, it may be necessary to remove household pets or to avoid contact with farm animals. Picnicking or hiking into the woods may need to be eliminated. Air-conditioning, damp mopping, dusting, and closed windows may help prevent allergic attacks caused by household dust or other allergens in the air. Rainy, damp, humid weather is often associated with asthma. Using a dehumidifier to remove moisture from the air may be beneficial in preventing attacks of asthma. Individuals with allergies are advised to avoid exposure to infections. A common cold may precipitate an allergic reaction. It may be necessary for an individual to make many changes in environment and lifestyle.

Drug therapy. Antihistamines, epinephrine, topical decongestants, and corticosteroids are commonly used to treat allergies. Because of the antigen-antibody reaction, histamine is released from the cells and is primarily responsible for allergic symptoms. Drug therapy is designed to counteract the effects of histamine.

Antihistamines are most useful in allergic conditions that affect the nasal mucosa (e.g., hay fever), *rhinitis,* itching, and acute urticaria. They are also used for motion sickness, nausea and vomiting, vertigo, and sleeplessness. Antihistamines block the action of histamine on the bronchioles and blood vessels. The major side effect from these drugs is drowsiness. Therefore persons who are taking any of this group of drugs are advised not to drive motor vehicles. Other side effects include dizziness, dryness of mucous membranes, and weakness. There are many antihistaminic preparations on the market (Table 7-5). Antihistamines may be administered orally, and some are available for parenteral injection or rectal administration.

Epinephrine (Adrenalin) has several uses. It is used for serious hypersensitivity, such as anaphylactic shock. A 1:1000 aqueous solution is used for parenteral injection. Epinephrine counteracts the actions of histamine and helps reverse the pathology that has occurred. It increases the strength and force of the heartbeat, increases blood pressure, and relaxes the smooth muscles of the respiratory tract.

Topical decongestants exhibit an antiallergy effect and shrink congested nasal mucous membranes. Phenylephrine (NeoSynephrine) is one of the most widely prescribed topical nasal decongestants. It should be used at intervals of at least 4 hours to prevent rebound congestion. Rebound congestion can occur after prolonged and repeated vasoconstrictor stimulation initiates a compensatory vasodilation and subsequent increased secretions. When this occurs, the drug treatment should be discontinued (Williams, Baer, 1990).

Text continued on p. 155.

TABLE 7-5

Pharmacology of Drugs Used for Physiologic Responses

Drug (Generic & Trade Name); Route and Dosage	Action/Indication	Common Side Effects and Nursing Considerations
Antibiotics		
AMOXICILLIN (Augmentin) **ROUTE:** PO **DOSAGE:** 250-500 mg q 8 hr; gonorrhea, 3 g plus 1 g probenecid single dose	Antiinfective (extended-spectrum penicillin) used for the treatment of skin and skin structure infections, otitis media, sinusitis, respiratory and genitourinary infections, meningitis, septicemia, endocarditis prophylaxis, and Lyme disease	Rashes and diarrhea; contraindicated in hypersensitivity to penicillins; use with caution in severe renal insufficiency and infectious mononucleosis
AMPICILLIN (Principen, Totacillin, Omnipen, Polycillin) **ROUTE:** IM, IV, PO **DOSAGE:** All routes, 1-2 g/day in divided doses q 4-6 hr	Antiinfective (penicillin) used for all above except Lyme disease	Rashes and diarrhea; contraindicated in hypersensitivity to penicillin; use with caution in severe renal insufficiency

TABLE 7-5

Pharmacology of Drugs Used for Physiologic Responses—cont'd

Drug (Generic & Trade Name); Route and Dosage	Action/Indication	Common Side Effects and Nursing Considerations
CEFAZOLIN SODIUM (Ancef, Kefzol) **ROUTE:** IM, IV **DOSAGE:** Life-threatening infections, IM, IV, 1-1.5 g q 6 hr; mild/moderate infections, IM, IV, 250-500 mg q 8 hr	Antibiotic cephalosporin used to treat skin, skin structure urinary tract, and bone and joint infections; septicemia, intraabdominal and biliary tract infections, and as a perioperative prophylactic antiinfective	Nausea, vomiting, diarrhea, rashes, phlebitis and pain at IV site; contraindicated in hypersensitivity to cephalosporins and serious hypersensitivity to penicillins; use with caution in renal impairment
CEFOXITIN (Mefoxin) **ROUTE:** IM, IV **DOSAGE:** IM, IV. 1-2 g q 6-8 hr (up to 12 g/day); uncomplicated gonorrhea, 2 g IM single dose with 1 g probenecid PO	Antiinfective (second generation cephalosporin) used to treat respiratory tract, skin, skin structure, bone and joint, urinary tract, and gynecologic infections; also used in septicemia and for perioperative prophylaxis	Rashes, nausea, vomiting, diarrhea, phlebitis and pain at IV site, and anaphylaxis; contraindicated in hypersensitivity to cephalosporins and serious hypersensitivity to penicillins; use with caution in renal impairment
CEPHALEXIN (Keflex) **ROUTE:** PO **DOSAGE:** 250-500 mg q 6 hr (500 mg q 12 for cystitis)	Antiinfective (first generation cephalosporin) used in the treatment of serious skin, skin structure, urinary tract, bone and joint, and respiratory tract infections; septicemia; and otitis media	Nausea, vomiting, diarrhea, rashes, phlebitis and pain at IV site, and anaphylaxis; contraindicated in hypersensitivity to cephalosporins and serious hypersensitivity to penicillins; use with caution in renal impairment
DOXYCYCLINE (Vibramycin) **ROUTE:** PO, IV **DOSAGE:** PO, IV, 100-200 mg/day given once daily or in divided doses q 12 hr	Antiinfective (tetracycline) used most commonly to treat infections due to unusual organisms including *Mycoplasma, Chlamydia,* and *Rickettsia;* also useful in treatment of gonorrhea and syphilis in patients who are allergic to penicillin; has been used for "traveler's diarrhea," exacerbations of chronic bronchitis, and Lyme disease	Nausea, vomiting, and diarrhea; can cause permanent staining of teeth in children; use with caution in cachectic, debilitated, hepatic, or renal disease
ERYTHROMYCIN (Erythromycin, Ilotycin) **ROUTE:** PO, IV, topical, ophthalmic **DOSAGE:** PO, 250-500 mg q 6-12 hr, IV, 1-4 g/day in divided doses q 6 hr, or as continuous infusion; topical, 2% ointment, gel, or solution bid; ophthalmic, 0.5% ointment to conjunctiva 1 or more times daily	Antiinfective (macrolide) used in the treatment of upper and lower respiratory tract infections, otitis media, skin and skin structure infections, pertussis, diphtheria, intestinal amebiasis, pelvic inflammatory disease, nongonococcal urethritis, syphilis, rheumatic fever, and legionnaires' disease; used topically against acne and opthalmically against superficial ocular infections	Nausea, vomiting, and phlebitis at IV site; contraindicated in hepatic dysfunction; administer around the clock on an empty stomach, at least 1 hr before or 2 hr after meals; may be taken with food if GI irritation occurs; should not be taken with fruit juices

continued

TABLE 7-5

Pharmacology of Drugs Used for Physiologic Responses—cont'd

Drug (Generic & Trade Name); Route and Dosage	Action/Indication	Common Side Effects and Nursing Considerations
GENTAMICIN SULFATE (Garamycin) **ROUTE:** IM, IV, topical, ophthalmic **DOSAGE:** IM, IV, 3-5 mg/kg/day in divided doses q 8 hr; doses as low as 3 mg/kg/day given once daily or in divided doses q 12 hr have been used for uncomplicated urinary tract infection; topical, apply cream or ointment to cleansed area 3-4 times daily; ophthalmic, 1-2 drops of solution q 2-4 hr or ointment 2-3 times daily	Antiinfective (aminoglucoside) used in treatment of gram-negative bacillary infections and infections due to staphylococci when penicillins or other less toxic drugs are contraindicated; also used as part of a regimen for endocarditis prophylaxis	Ototoxicity and nephrotoxicity; use with caution in renal impairment; monitor serum electrolytes
NAFCILLIN SODIUM (Unipen) **ROUTE:** IM, IV, PO **DOSAGE:** PO, 250-1000 mg q 4-6 hr; IM, 500 mg q 4-6 hr; IV, 500-1500 mg q 4 hr	Antiinfective (penicillinase-resistant penicillin) used in the treatment of the infections due to susceptible strains of penicillinase-producing staphylococci	Nausea, vomiting, diarrhea, rashes, and allergic reactions; contraindicated in hypersensitivity to penicillins; use with caution in renal impairment
NEOMYCIN SULFATE (Myciguent, Mycifradin) **ROUTE:** PO, topical **DOSAGE:** Preparation for GI surgery, PO, 1 g q hr for 4 hr, then 1 g q 4 hr for 24 hr prior to surgery or 1 g given 19 hr, 18 hr, and 9 hr prior to surgery; minor skin infections, topical, 0.5% cream or ointment 1-3 times daily	Antiinfective (aminoglycoside) used to prepare the GI tract for surgery or to decrease the population of ammonia-producing bacteria in the management of hepatic encephalopathy; also used in treatment of minor skin infections	Ototoxicity and nephrotoxicity; contraindicated in renal impairment; use with caution in neuromuscular diseases
PENICILLIN G BENZATHINE (Bicillin) **ROUTE:** IM **DOSAGE:** Streptococcal infections, 1.2 million units single dose; syphilis, 2.4 million units single dose (primary, secondary, or latent syphilis of <1 yr duration) repeated q wk for 3 wk; patients with neurosyphilis should be initially treated with aqueous penicillin G plus probenecid, then 2.4 million units penicillin G benzathine weekly for 3 wk; prevention of rheumatic fever, 1.2 million units q 4 wk	Antiinfective (penicillin) used in the treatment of a wide variety of infections including pneumococcal pneumonia, streptococcal pharyngitis, syphilis, and prevention of rheumatic fever	Nausea, vomiting, diarrhea, epigastric distress, rashes, and pain at IV site; contraindicated in previous hypersensitivity to penicillins and benzathine; cross-sensitivity may exist with cephalosporins; use with caution in renal impairment

TABLE 7-5

Pharmacology of Drugs Used for Physiologic Responses—cont'd

Drug (Generic & Trade Name); Route and Dosage	Action/Indication	Common Side Effects and Nursing Considerations
PENICILLIN G POTASSIUM (Pentids) **ROUTE:** PO **DOSAGE:** Pneumococcal/streptococcal infections, 400,000-5,000,000 U q 6-8 hr × 10 days (streptococcal) or afebrile × 2 days (pneumococcal infections); prevention of recurrence of rheumatic fever, 200,000-250,000 U bid continuously; gingivitis/pharyngitis, 400,000-500,000 U q 6-8 hr	Broad-spectrum antibiotic-natural penicillin used for emphysema, gangrene, anthrax, gonorrhea, mastoiditis, pneumonia, tetanus, osteomyelitis, meningitis, and urinary tract infections; used prophylactically in rheumatic fever, and effective for non-penicillinase–producing gram-positive cocci	Coma, convulsions, increased bleeding time, bone marrow depression, granulocytopenia, hyper- and hypokalemia, alkalosis, and hypernatremia; contraindicated in hypersensitivity to penicillin; use with caution with hypersensitivity to cephalosporins
PENCILLIN G PROCAINE (Crysticillin, Wycillin) **ROUTE:** IM **DOSAGE:** Moderate to severe infections, 600,000-1.2 million U/day, single dose or 2 divided doses; uncomplicated gonorrhea, 4.8 million U divided into 2 injection sites, preceded by 1 g probenecid PO	Antiinfective (penicillin) used to treat pneumococcal pneumonia, streptococcal pneumonia, streptococcal pharyngitis, syphilis, gonorrhea; used in enterococcal infections (requires the addition of an aminoglycoside)	Nausea, vomiting, diarrhea, epigastric distress, rashes, and pain at injection site; contraindicated in hypersensitivity to penicillin and procaine; use with caution with hypersensitivity to cephalosporins and in renal insufficiency
PENICILLIN V (Pen-Vee-K) **ROUTE:** PO **DOSAGE:** 125-500 mg q 6 hr	Antiinfective (penicillin) used to treat such infections as pneumococcal pneumonia, skin and soft tissue infections, and streptococcal pharyngitis; used to prevent rheumatic fever	Nausea, vomiting, diarrhea, epigastric distress, rashes, and anaphylaxis; contraindicated in hypersensitivity to penicillin; use with caution with hypersensitivity to cephalosporins and in renal insufficiency; may be administered without regard to meals
Antihistamines		
CHLORPHENIRAMINE (Chlor-Trimeton, Tildrin) **ROUTE:** PO, SC, IM, IV **DOSAGE:** PO, 4 mg q 4-6 hr or 8-12 mg of extended-release formulation q 8-12 hr (not to exceed 24 mg/day); SC, IM, IV, 5-20 mg single dose (not to exceed 40 mg/day)	Antihistamine used for symptomatic relief of allergic symptoms caused by histamine release; most useful for nasal allergies and allergic dermatoses; also used for management of severe allergic or hypersensitivity reactions, including anaphylaxis and transfusion reactions	Drowsiness, sedation, hypertension, blurred vision, and dry mouth; contraindicated in acute attacks of asthma and alcohol intolerance; use with caution in glaucoma, liver disease, and the elderly
DIPHENHYDRAMINE (Benadryl) **ROUTE:** PO, IM, IV, topical **DOSAGE:** PO, 25-50 mg q 4-6 hr; IM, IV,10-50 mg single dose (may need up to 100 mg dose, not to exceed 400 mg/day); topical, 1%-2% cream, lotion, or spray 3-4 times daily	Antihistamine and antitussive used for relief of allergic symptoms caused by histamine release, including anaphylaxis, nasal allergies, allergic dermatoses, Parkinson's disease; and dystonic reactions from medication; used to prevent motion sickness	Drowsiness, dry mouth, and anorexia; contraindicated in acute attacks of asthma and intolerance to alcohol; use with caution in elderly, severe liver disease, glaucoma, seizure disorders, and prostatic hypertrophy

continued

TABLE 7-5

Pharmacology of Drugs Used for Physiologic Responses—cont'd

Drug (Generic & Trade Name); Route and Dosage	Action/Indication	Common Side Effects and Nursing Considerations
TERFENADINE (Seldane) **ROUTE:** PO **DOSAGE:** 60 mg twice daily	Antihistamine used for symptomatic relief of allergic symptoms, including nasal allergies and allergic dermatoses	Drowsiness, sedation, headache, nausea, vomiting, abdominal pain, and dry mouth; use with caution in prostatic hypertrophy, glaucoma, and cardiac disease
Corticosteroids		
HYDROCORTISONE (Cortef, Hydrocortone, Solu-Cortef) **ROUTE:** PO, IM, IV **DOSAGE:** PO, 10-320 mg/day in 1-4 divided doses; IM, IV, 100-500 mg q 2-6 hr (succinate, range 100-8000 mg/day); 15-240 mg (phosphate) q 12 hr	Short-acting glucocorticoid used in the management of adrenocortical insufficiency and short-term management of such inflammatory and allergic reactions as asthma and ulcerative colitis; chronic use is limited to mineralocorticoid activity; not suitable for alternate-day therapy	Depression, nausea, petechiae, decreased wound healing, adrenal suppression, decreased growth in children, hypokalemia, and sodium retention; contraindicated in serious infections; use with caution, chronic treatment with doses greater than 20 mg/day may result in adrenal suppression; do not discontinue abruptly; during periods of stress, dose may need to be increased; use lowest possible dose for shortest period of time; may mask infection
PREDNISOLONE (Delta-Cortef) **ROUTE:** PO, IM, IV, otic, ophthalmic **DOSAGE:** PO, 5-60 mg/day single dose or divided doses (maintenance doses may be given as a single dose or every other day); multiple sclerosis, 200 mg/day for 7 days, then 80 mg every other day for 1 mo; IM, IV, 4-60 mg/day; ophthalmic, 1 drop q hr initially, then decrease to 2-4 times daily; otic, 3-4 drops 2-3 times daily	Glucocorticoid (intermediate-acting) used systemically and locally for such chronic illnesses as inflammatory, allergic, hematologic, neoplastic, and autoimmune diseases; also used for replacement therapy in adrenal insufficiency	Depression, euphoria, hypertension, nausea, anorexia, decreased wound healing, petechiae, ecchymoses, fragility, hirsutism, acne, adrenal suppression, muscle wasting, osteoporosis, increased susceptibility to infections, and cushingoid appearance (moonface, buffalo hump); contraindicated in active, untreated infections and known alcohol intolerance; use with caution in children; chronic treatment with doses greater than 20 mg/day may result in adrenal suppression; do not discontinue abruptly; during periods of stress dose may need to be increased; use lowest possible dose for shortest period of time; may mask infection
PREDNISONE (Deltasone) **ROUTE:** PO **DOSAGE:** 5-60 mg/day single dose or divided doses; for multiple sclerosis, 200 mg/day for 1 wk, then 80 mg every other day for 1 mo	Glucocorticoid (intermediate-acting) used systemically and locally in a wide variety of chronic diseases, including inflammatory, allergic, hematologic, neoplastic, and autoimmune diseases; suitable for alternate-day	Same as above

TABLE 7-5

Pharmacology of Drugs Used for Physiologic Responses—cont'd

Drug (Generic & Trade Name); Route and Dosage	Action/Indication	Common Side Effects and Nursing Considerations
	dosing in the management of chronic illness; also used for replacement therapy in adrenal insufficiency	
TRIAMCINOLONE, ACETONIDE (Kenacort, Aristocort, Kenalog) **ROUTE:** PO, IM, inhalation **DOSAGE:** PO, 4-48 mg/day in divided doses qd-qid; IM, 40 mg q wk (acetonide), 5-48 mg into neoplasms, 2-40 mg into joint or soft tissue; inhalation, 2 sprays 3-4 times daily (up to 12-16 sprays per day); nasal inhalation, 2 sprays each nostril once daily (up to 2 sprays in each nostril twice daily or 1 spray in each nostril 4 times daily)	Glucocorticoid (intermediate-acting), antiinflammatory agent used systemically and locally to treat chronic inflammatory, allergic, hematologic, neoplastic, and autoimmune diseases; not suitable for alternate-day therapy	Same as above
Sulfonamides		
SULFAMETHOXAZOLE (Gantanol, Azo Gantanol) **ROUTE:** PO **DOSAGE:** 2 g initially, then 1 g q 8-12 hr	Antiinfective (sulfonamide) used in the treatment of urinary tract infections, nocardiosis, toxoplasmosis, and malaria	Nausea, vomiting, rashes, and fever; use with caution in severe renal or hepatic impairment
SULFISOXAZOLE (Gantrisin, Azo Gantrisin) **ROUTE:** PO, ophthalmic **DOSAGE:** PO, 2-4 g initially, then 4-8 g/day in divided doses q 4-6 hr (not to exceed 12 g/day); ophthalmic, 1 drop 3 or more times daily, may increase interval as infection resolves	Antiinfective (sulfonamide) used in the treatment of urinary tract infections, nocardiosis, and in combination with other antiinfectives for malaria and pelvic inflammatory disease in prepubescent adolescents; ophthalmic uses for treatment of eye infections such as chlamydia	Nausea, vomiting, rashes, aplastic anemia, agranulocytosis, and fever; contraindicated in hypersensitivity to sulfonamides; cross-sensitivity to Lasix, thiazides, sulfonylurea oral hypoglycemic agents, and carbonic anhydrase inhibitors may appear; use with caution in severe renal or hepatic impairment

Corticosteroids are not generally used for allergic disorders because of their serious side effects. However, steroid preparations are marketed as ointments, creams, and lotions for topical application. They are used in allergic dermatosis and applied two or three times a day. Corticosteroids may be given to a patient with life-threatening asthma but usually only after other forms of medication have failed. Corticosteroids are also administered in some immediate allergic reactions, including anaphylactic shock, an allergic reaction to penicillin, and other severe drug reactions. Corticosteroids help reduce the inflammatory reaction and help with recovery. Hydrocortisone succinate (Solu-Cortef) is often used.

Immunotherapy. Immunotherapy, or desensitization as it is sometimes called, is a form of immunization and is commonly referred to as "allergy shots." Immunotherapy involves the injection of increasing amounts of allergen to which the patient displays a Type I hypersensitivity. The goal is to improve tolerance with fewer symptoms after exposure to the allergen. The precise mechanism of the improvement has

PATIENT/FAMILY TEACHING

Once allergies have been identified, the nurse must educate the patient regarding all sources of the allergen to be avoided. The nurse may help the patient identify avoidance strategies and acceptable substitutions for the offending material. The nurse may educate the patient about drug therapy, including the name, dose, schedule, administration, storage, and side effects of the medication. For those with the potential for a severe allergic reaction, the nurse may teach the patient and family appropriate emergency measures, including the use of epinephrine. For those undergoing immunotherapy, the nurse must ensure that the patient understands the procedure and the schedule of treatments. As with all patient and family education, the nurse is responsible for reviewing the instructions and planning care.

not been definitively established (Patterson and others, 1993).

The extract is usually given weekly, and the amount is gradually increased with each injection until the largest dose that causes no reaction has been given. This last dose is considered to be the maintenance dose. Desensitization has been most effective with hay fever. Persons who have a seasonal allergy are advised to begin injections early, before allergic symptoms appear. Immunotherapy is not a lifetime regimen. Most allergists consider a routine course to last for 3 to 4 years (Jacobs, Meltzer, Selner, 1989).

Autoimmune Disease

Normally the adult host shows tolerance to tissue antigens recognized as "self." Sometimes this tolerance is lost, and immune reactions may develop against self-antigens and result in **autoimmune** diseases. These diseases tend to occur in genetically predisposed people who are exposed to an environmental agent that stimulates an immune response against normal tissue. Bacteria, viruses, and drugs may trigger the activation of T cells and B cells. Most reactions are mediated by antibodies (Levinson, Jawetz, 1994). Diseases and disorders that result from this reaction may affect the eyes, skin, joints, thyroid gland, kidneys, brain, and vascular system (Levinson, Jawetz, 1994) (Box 7-9). Intensive study and research are continuing to produce a better understanding of autoimmunity.

Autoimmune diseases are usually treated with drug therapy that is aimed at interfering with the immune response. Immunosuppressants such as azathioprine (Imuran) and corticosteroids such as prednisone (Deltasone) may be administered.

BOX 7-9

DISEASES CONSIDERED TO BE AUTOIMMUNE IN NATURE

Rheumatoid arthritis
Systemic lupus erythematosus
Idiopathic thrombocytopenic purpura
Myasthenia gravis
Pernicious anemia
Hashimoto's thyroiditis
Glomerulonephritis
Multiple sclerosis
Ulcerative colitis
Type I diabetes mellitus

CHEMOTHERAPEUTIC AGENTS

Chemotherapy refers to the treatment of disease with chemical drugs. Some chemotherapeutic drugs are *bacteriostatic* and arrest the multiplication of pathogenic bacteria, whereas others are *bactericidal* in action and kill bacteria. Other drugs suppress the inflammatory response when pathogens are not involved (Table 7-5).

Sulfonamides

The sulfonamide drugs were the first chemotherapeutic agents to be discovered and were first used in the 1930s. They were originally used in the treatment of both gram-negative and gram-positive infections. Thousands of sulfonamides have been developed, but only a few are in use today as a result of the development of bacterial resistance to sulfonamides and the discovery of newer, less toxic drugs (Lehne, 1994). Many other antimicrobial agents have now replaced or been used in combination with sulfonamides. The sulfonamides are primarily bacteriostatic and act by interfering with the metabolism of the invading microorganism to prevent further growth.

Some sulfonamide drugs are especially effective in treating uncomplicated infections of the urinary tract and preventing infection when long-term therapy is required. Sulfonamides are also common in the treatment of ulcerative colitis, chancroid, and burns (Clark, 1993). Patients receiving sulfonamide (sulfa) drugs should be encouraged to drink large amounts of fluids to provide from 1200 to 2000 ml of urinary output over a 24-hour period.

Persons receiving sulfonamides should be observed for side effects, the most common being anorexia and nausea and vomiting. These drugs can also cause a decrease in circulating red blood cells, white blood cells, and platelets, which can lead to the development of *purpura*, or bleeding into the skin. Any rash should be carefully observed. Signs of sensitivity such as sneezing or itching should be noted. Hematuria and the formation of crystals in the urine may be significant problems (Lehne, 1994). A severe hypersensitivity reaction (Stevens-Johnson Syndrome) is a rare reaction but has a mortality rate near 25% (Lehne, 1994).

Antibiotics

The development of antibiotic drugs began in 1928 when Alexander Fleming, a British bacteriologist, discovered a substance that he called *penicillin*. His findings were not immediately accepted, and it was not until about 1941 that the United States began intensive work in the development of penicillin. In the early days only penicillin and streptomycin were available, but today there are a large number of antibiotic agents. Some antibiotic drugs are effective against only gram-positive or gram-negative bacteria, and others are called broad-spectrum antibiotics because they are effective against both gram-positive and gram-negative bacteria.

The penicillins are the most effective and widely used antibiotics. The penicillins and their semisynthetic derivatives prevent the development of the cell wall in bacteria and therefore are bactericidal. Penicillins are used to treat a variety of illnesses, including pneumococcal pneumonia, streptococcal infections, meningococcal meningitis, gonorrhea, syphilis, and *Salmonella* infections. However, some organisms such as *S. aureus* and *Escherichia coli* are capable of producing penicillinases, which are enzymes that destroy certain penicillins. Many new penicillins have been developed that are effective against these penicillinase-producing bacteria and against other virulent organisms. The penicillins are inexpensive and have a low incidence of toxicity. The development of "super" antibiotics has shortened infection times. They are expensive but have fewer side effects, and the patient feels better sooner.

Penicillin is available in different forms and under a variety of trade names. It is administered through intramuscular injection, intravenously, or orally. Under usual conditions penicillin is nontoxic, but allergic reactions may occur in some patients. These reactions vary from mild skin rashes to fatal anaphylactic shock. The nurse administering penicillin should first make sure that the patient has had no previous reaction to it and should also observe the patient carefully for several hours after administering the drug. Reactions do not always develop immediately, and fatal reactions have occurred several hours after the drug has been given.

No penicillin should be administered to anyone with a previous history of an allergic reaction to any member of the penicillin family. Oral preparations should not be taken for at least an hour before or after eating because they are poorly absorbed if acid is present in the stomach. Acidic fruit juices should not be used to administer the drugs.

The cephalosporin antimicrobial agents were first developed and used in the early 1960s. Cephalosporins are structurally similar to penicillin and share many physical characteristics. They are expensive, semisynthetic, and broad-spectrum antibiotics. Because they inhibit cell wall synthesis in microbes, they are bactericidal in action. Cephalosporins are classified into groups, called generations, that reflect their introduction and use. The difference between each generation stems from its effectiveness against gram-positive and gram-negative organisms. Cephalosporins should be avoided in patients who have severe or immediate reactions to penicillins. About 5% to 10% of the individuals who are allergic to penicillin show a cross-sensitivity to cephalosporins (Lehne, 1994). Caution is recommended when using cephalosporins with patients who have preexisting renal conditions.

Tetracyclines were introduced in 1948 and were the first broad-spectrum antibiotics. They block the formation of proteins in microorganisms and are *bacteriostatic*. Their use has increased as resistant organisms have declined. Gastrointestinal disturbances can occur with tetracyclines, but generally the drugs are nontoxic, and allergic reactions are rare. The tetracyclines should not be administered with milk products, antacids, or iron preparations because the combination disturbs absorption of the drug. Tetracyclines are used in the treatment of adolescent acne, chlamydia, and other uncommon infections. They are the treatment of choice in rickettsial infections. Tetracyclines are not used in children and pregnant women because they bind to newly formed bones and teeth.

The group of antibiotics known as the *aminoglycosides* were in use as early as 1944 along with streptomycin but were further developed after 1952. Aminoglycosides also interfere with protein synthesis in invading microbes. They are bactericidal and have a widespread clinical use. However, toxic effects increase with increased dosage. The eighth cranial nerve can be affected and result in serious injury to the inner ear. Symptoms may include hearing loss, dizziness, ringing in the ears and imbalance. In addition, these drugs can be toxic to the kidney nephrons (Lehne, 1994). The nurse is responsible for carefully monitoring intake and output.

The *macrolides* (erythromycins) are bacteriostatic and inhibit protein synthesis. They are effective against gram-positive cocci and can be used as a penicillin substitute in persons allergic to penicillin. Gastrointestinal disturbances may occur. Allergic reactions may also occur but are not common.

Because a specific antibiotic may be ineffective against a particular organism, sensitivity tests should be done before any antibiotic is administered. By identifying the microorganisms causing the illness, the physician can prescribe the most suitable antibiotic to cure the disease.

Corticosteroids

The corticosteroids are used when inflammation is caused by some agent other than pathogens. They are hormones that are produced by the adrenal cortex and include cortisone and hydrocortisone, commonly referred to as adrenal steroids. One adrenal gland is located above each kidney and is composed of two parts. The inner part is the medulla, and its primary secretion is epinephrine. The outer part is the cortex, which produces several substances, some of which are necessary for life. The cortex also produces cortisone and hydrocortisone. When the adrenal glands fail to function or are surgically removed because of disease, hydrocortisone is administered to replace the normal secretion.

The first corticosteroids were prepared as glandular extracts around 1928. Today commercially available corticosteroids are of the same chemical composition but are made synthetically and have a higher potency. Chemical modification of the natural steroids has produced other, more selective synthetic steroids. They are used for replacement therapy and to suppress the inflammatory and immune response.

The beneficial effects of corticosteroid therapy are the relief of inflammation, reduction of fever, and production of a feeling of well-being. The latter effect is probably a result of symptom relief. For example, when cortisone is administered for an inflammatory condition, the classic signs of inflammation may be absent. Patients receiving cortisone feel encouraged because of the absence of symptoms. However, cortisone used therapeutically does not cure disease or alter its course and does not reverse any preexisting damage such as crippling in arthritis. When used systemically the corticosteroids are powerful and dangerous drugs and can cause serious side effects that can affect every system of the body. Most physicians prescribe these drugs extremely cautiously because of the toxic effects. Abrupt withdrawal and potentially life-threatening adrenal insufficiency is avoided by gradually decreasing the dosage. Corticosteroids may be administered orally, intravenously, intramuscularly; applied topically such as an ophthalmic preparation, or injected directly into an inflamed joint or lesion.

Patients receiving any of the corticosteroid preparations must be carefully observed for undesirable or toxic effects. Clear instructions regarding the drug must be given when patients are transferred to other home healthcare facilities or discharged home.

Other drugs used to relieve inflammatory conditions are the nonsteroidal antiinflammatory agents and aspirin. Aspirin is used to decrease the joint inflammation associated with arthritis. Nonsteroidal antiinflammatory drugs and aspirin have a basic effect on the biochemistry or inflammation. Both drugs can lead to serious bleeding complications and must be used cautiously. They should be avoided in combination.

NURSE ALERT

Check for patient allergies before giving any medication.

KEY CONCEPTS

- Causes of disease include microorganisms, nutritional imbalances, physical agents, chemical agents, and cellular abnormalities.
- Bacteria and viruses are examples of microorganisms. Nutritional imbalances include insufficient or excessive diet intake, an unbalanced diet, an excess use of a specific nutrient, and failure of the body to use nutrients. Physical agents include trauma, changes in external temperature, electric current, radiation, atmospheric pressure, mechanical factors, and noise. Chemical agents include harmful substances and gases. Cellular abnormalities include cell damage from a lack of nutrients or oxygen, an altered environment, tumors, and defective genes.
- The major defense mechanisms of the body are the skin, mucous membranes, cilia, stomach acids, reflexes, and the various cells and organs that participate in the inflammatory and immune responses.
- Characteristics of the inflammatory process include redness, heat, pain, swelling, and limitation of movement.
- Intervention for inflammation depends on the type of injury, the extent of involvement, and the effectiveness of the defense mechanisms of the body. Heat and cold can be applied to the body to aid in the healing process.
- The immune system works to counteract the effects of foreign materials, bacteria, viruses, foods, and chemicals that constantly enter the body.
- Hypersensitivity is an inappropriate and excessive response of the immune system to certain substances that are not harmful to most persons.
- Assessment techniques used for allergic conditions include a detailed history, skin testing, mucous membrane tests, and elimination testing.
- Nursing interventions for people with allergies include administering drug therapy, assisting with immunotherapy, and educating patients about avoidance therapy.
- In an anaphylactic emergency the nurse is responsible for administering ordered medications, preparing for procedures such as oropharyngeal intubation, applying oxygen per order, and taking measures as prescribed to prevent the absorption of the antigen.
- Autoimmune diseases include rheumatoid arthritis, systemic lupus erythematosus, idiopathic thrombocytopenia purpura, myasthenia gravis, pernicious anemia, Hashimoto's thyroiditis, glomerulonephritis, multiple sclerosis, ulcerative colitis, and Type I diabetes mellitus.

CRITICAL THINKING EXERCISES

1. Relate the classic signs of infection to the pathophysiologic changes that have occurred.
2. What factors influence the pathogenicity of invading organisms?
3. Perform an allergy assessment on a friend or relative.
4. Design a plan for prevention of insect stings for a small rural community.

REFERENCES AND ADDITIONAL READINGS

Adlercreutz H: Western diet and Western diseases: some hormonal and biochemical mechanisms and associations, *Scand J Clin Lab Invest* 50(suppl 201):3-23, 1990.

Beare P, Myers J: *Principles and practice of adult health nursing,* ed 2, St Louis, 1994, Mosby.

Carroll KK: Dietary fats and cancer, *Am J Clin Nutr* 53:1064s-1067s, 1991.

Chilmonczyk BA and others: Association between exposure to environmental tobacco smoke and exacerbations of asthma in children, *N Engl J Med* 328(23):1665-1669, 1993.

Clark SF, Queener SF, Karlo VB: *Pharmacologic basis of nursing practice,* ed 4, St Louis, 1993, Mosby.

Gooi HC, Chapel H: *Clinical immunology: a practical approach,* New York, 1990, Oxford University Press.

Guyton AC: *Textbook of medical physiology,* ed 8, Philadelphia, 1991, WB Saunders.

Hamilton GC: *Presenting signs and symptoms in the emergency department,* Baltimore, 1993, Williams & Wilkins.

Jacobs RL, Meltzer ED, Selner JC: Rhinitis: not just hay fever, *Patient Care* 23(6):168, 1989.

Kelsey JL, Gammon MD: The epidemiology of breast cancer, *CA: Cancer J Clin* 41(3):146-159, 1991.

Lederer J and others: *Care planning pocket guide: a nursing diagnosis approach,* ed 3, Redwood City, Calif, 1990, Addison-Wesley Publishing.

Lehne RA: *Pharmacology for nursing care,* ed 2, Philadelphia, 1994, WB Saunders.

Levinson WE, Jawetz E: *Medical microbiology and immunology examination and board review,* ed 3, Norwalk, Conn, 1994, Appleton & Lange.

Long BC and others: *Medical-surgical nursing,* ed 3, St Louis, 1993, Mosby.

McCance KL, Huether SE: *Pathophysiology: the biologic basis for disease in adults and children,* ed 2, St Louis, 1994, Mosby.

Middleton E and others: *Allergy principles and practice,* ed 4, St Louis, 1993, Mosby.

Muir BL: *Pathophysiology: an introduction to the mechanisms of disease,* ed 2, New York, 1988, John Wiley & Sons.

Patterson R and others: *Allergic diseases: diagnosis and treatment,* ed 4, Philadelphia, 1993, JB Lippincott.

Potter PA, Perry AG: *Fundamentals of nursing: concepts, process, and practice,* ed 3, St Louis, 1993, Mosby.

Roitt IM, Brostoff J, Male DK: *Immunology,* ed 3, St Louis, 1993, Mosby.

Thibodeau GA, Patton K: Anatomy and Physiology, ed 2, St. Louis, 1993, Mosby.

Williams B, Baer C: *Essentials of clinical pharmacology in nursing,* Springhouse, PA, 1990, Springhouse.

CHAPTER 8

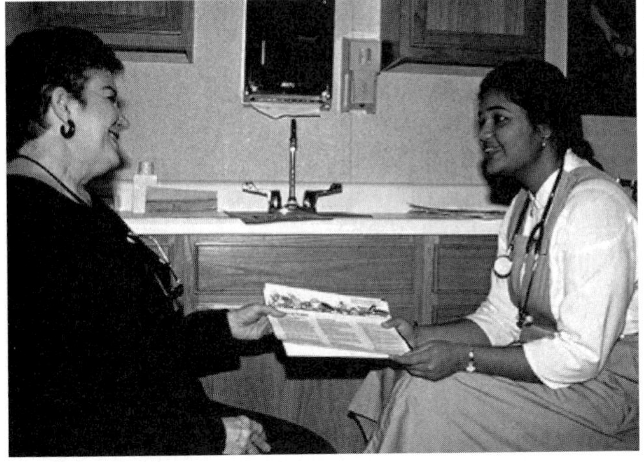

Fluids and Electrolytes

CHAPTER OBJECTIVES

1 Identify the compartments of body fluid.
2 Differentiate between intracellular and extracellular fluid.
3 Identify the major ways fluids are gained and lost from the body.
4 Explain the processes involved in fluid and electrolyte exchange throughout the body.
5 Identify the signs and symptoms of primary fluid and electrolyte imbalances.
6 Explain the role of body systems in controlling acid-base balance.
7 Discuss the causes of acid-base imbalance.
8 Describe the symptoms of acidosis and alkalosis.
9 Interpret blood gas values to determine the types of acid base imbalance.
10 State the primary nursing responsibilities in maintaining intravenous therapy.
11 Compare and contrast the types of solutions used for fluid and electrolyte therapy.
12 Differentiate among the major types of shock according to cause.
13 Identify the goals of drug therapy in the major types of shock.
14 Outline the nursing management of the patient in shock.

KEY WORDS

acidosis
alkalosis
anion
cardiogenic shock
cation
diffusion
disseminated intravascular coagulation
electrolyte
extracellular fluid
filtration
hypercalcemia
hyperchloremia
hyperkalemia
hypernatremia
hypophosphatemia
hypertonic (hyperosmolar)
hypervolemia
hypocalcemia
hypochloremia
hypokalemia
hyponatremia
hyperphosphatemia
hypotonic (hypoosmolar)
hypovolemia
hypovolemic shock
ion
interstitial fluid
intravascular fluid
intracellular fluid
isotonic (isoosmolar)
neurogenic shock
normovolemic shock
osmolarity
osmolality
osmosis
third spacing
vasogenic shock

BODY FLUIDS

Body fluids are essential to each of the billions of cells that make up the body. Body cells have been compared to the first cells that developed millions of years ago in ancient seas. Ancient cells used the ocean as a source for all their nutrients and as a means for carrying away discharged wastes. Body cells also receive nutrients and discharge wastes into the environment, but the fluid is trapped beneath the skin, and volume and chemical composition are regulated precisely by intricate and complicated homeostatic mechanisms. It is believed that body fluids resemble ancient seas; oceans today have become more concentrated from dissolved substances from land.

Water Content of the Body

Water is the *solvent* of the body, the liquid in which other substances such as electrolytes are dissolved. Although the human body appears solid, approximately two thirds of it is liquid. Approximately 75% of an infant's body weight is water, whereas average adult men have approximately 60% and women have approximately 50% water in their bodies. The percentage of body weight that is water decreases with age. Obese individuals have a smaller percentage of body weight in water because fat contains little water. Therefore the obese and the aged are at greater risk in situations that involve fluid loss because they have reduced fluid reserves. Infants and very young children are also at great risk because they have a higher ratio of body surface to body weight, immature kidneys that are less able to reabsorb water when necessary, and a higher percentage of fluid in the interstitial space, where water is more readily lost from the body.

OLDER ADULT CONSIDERATIONS

The percentage of total body water decreases with age if there is increased fat and decreased muscle. The kidney is less efficient in concentrating urine and slower in conserving sodium. Stress, fever, and loss of body fluids can be life threatening.

Body Fluid Compartments

Three fourths of the total amount of body fluid is located within the body cells as **intracellular fluid (ICF).** The remainder of the fluid is located outside the body cells as **extracellular fluid (ECF).** Approximately one fourth of the ECF is plasma of **intravascular fluid,** and three fourths is **interstitial fluid.** Interstitial fluid is found between the cells and in the lymph system. Intraocular fluid, cerebrospinal fluid, gastrointestinal tract fluids and fluids within body organs are considered transcellular and are part of the interstitial portion of the ECF. The ECF maintains the proper environment for cellular life. It supplies food, oxygen, water, vitamins, and electrolytes, and it carries away wastes. The ECF must be constantly monitored and controlled by sensitive homeostatic mechanisms to maintain appropriate volume and chemical composition and to keep the body healthy.

Fluid Spacing

The distribution of body water is also classified by the space it occupies. First spacing means that there is a normal distribution of fluid in both the extracellular and intracellular compartments. Second spacing refers to an excess accumulation of interstitial fluid (edema). *Third spacing* is fluid accumulation in areas that normally have no fluid or a minimal amount of fluid. Examples of third spacing include ascites, edema associated with burns, and the accumulation of fluid in bowel tissue that occurs with peritonitis. Third spacing can take fluid away from the normal fluid compartments and produce hypovolemia.

Electrolytes

Substances that are dissolved in body fluids are called *solutes.* Solutes are nonelectrolytes and electrolytes. Nonelectrolytes are compounds that do not separate into charged particles when dissolved in water. Glucose is a nonelectrolyte. **Electrolytes** separate into particles, called **ions,** that develop an electric charge when placed in water. For example, salt (NaCl) breaks up, or ionizes, into sodium (Na^+) and chloride (Cl^-). **Cations** are positively charged ions, and **anions** are negatively charged ions. The principal ions in the body are listed in Table 8-1. Oppositely charged ions attract each other, and like charges repel each other. All electrolytes are found inside and outside the cell. However, ECF contains large amounts of sodium, chloride, and bicarbonate ions. Sodium is the major cation, and chloride is the major anion. ICF contains large amounts of potassium, sulfate, and phosphate. Potassium is the major cation, and phosphate is the major anion. Protein is more concentrated in the plasma. Normally the total number of positive and negative charges is equal on both sides of the cell membrane.

To anticipate and prevent their depletion, it is helpful to know what electrolytes are found in which body fluids. For example, gastric secretions have a high concentration of hydrogen ions, and pancreatic secretions contain high bicarbonate concentrations. Sodium is abundant in bile and in gastric and pancreatic secretions.

Gains and Losses

Fluid and solutes, including electrolytes, are gained primarily through the intake of food and water. A small amount of water is also gained as a by-product of the metabolism of carbohydrates, fats, and proteins to produce energy for body functions. Normally, fluid gains approximately equal fluid losses. For example, the daily urinary output is approximately equal to the daily fluid intake, and the amount of water derived from solid foods and metabolic processes approximates the water lost via the lungs, stool, and skin (insensible loss). Patients can gain water and solutes from the use of nasogastric tubes, rectal tubes, and intravenous therapy. In renal failure, fluid loss does not compensate for fluid gain.

Fluid and electrolyte deficits are common because of the many abnormal states that contribute to fluid loss. Water and electrolyte loss occurs normally through respiration, urination, perspiration, lacrimation (crying), and defecation. Abnormal conditions that result in a loss of fluid and electrolytes include burns, wound drainage, hemorrhage, vomiting, and diarrhea. Therefore during an illness, gains and losses are not always equal. Abnormal losses accumulate during the illness and may cause serious problems.

Calculation of fluid gain or loss

A sudden weight change is the best indicator of a fluid gain or loss. One liter of water weighs 1 kg, or 2.2 lb. Drinking 1 cup of water (240 ml) results in a weight gain of about ½ lb. A patient who is on diuretic theraby and loses 2 kg (approximately 5 lb) in 24 hours has lost approximately 2 L of fluid (Beare, Myers, 1994).

Measurement of electrolytes

Electrolytes are measured both by weight and by combining power (the ability of the electyrolyte to combine with other electrolytes). Electrolyte weight is expressed in milligrams per deciliter (mg/dl). Com-

TABLE 8-1

Normal Electrolyte Content of Body Fluids

Electrolytes (anions and cations)	Extracellular* Intravascular (mEq/L)	Extracellular* Interstitial (mEq/L)	Intracellular (mEq/L)
Sodium (Na^+)	138-145	146	15-20
Potassium (K^+)	3.5-5.0	5	150-155
Calcium (Ca^{++})	4.5-5.5	3	1-2
Magnesium (Mg^{++})	1.5-2.5	1	27-29
Chloride (Cl^-)	96-106	114	1-4
Bicarbonate (HCO_3^-)	22-26	30	10-12
Protein ($Prot^-$)	16	1	63
Phosphate (HPO_4^{--})	1.7-4.6	2	100-104
Sulfate (SO_4^{--})	1	1	20
Organic acids	5	8	0

Modified from Phipps WJ and others: *Medical-surgical nursing,* ed 5, St Louis, 1995, Mosby.

*Note that the electrolyte level of the intravascular and interstitial (extracellular) fluids is approximately the same and that sodium and chloride contents are markedly higher in these fluids, whereas potassium, phosphate, and protein contents are markedly higher in intracellular fluid.

bining power is expressed in milliequivalents per liter (mEq/L).

FLUID AND ELECTROLYTE EXCHANGE

Passive Transport

Fluids and electrolytes move through the body by passive and active transport systems. Passive transport of fluid and electrolytes occurs through the **diffusion** (concentration differences), **filtration** (pressure differences), and **osmosis** (diffusion of water molecules).

Diffusion

Diffusion is based on the principle that molecules and ions flow through a semipermeable membrane from an area of higher concentration to an area of lower concentration (from where there is more of the substance to where there is less). Diffusion moves molecules (solutes, particles) into and out of cells.

Facilitated diffusion

Some molecules require a carrier to move more rapidly across the cell membrane. This process is called facilitated diffusion. Molecules move from higher to lower concentration as in simple diffusion. For example, in the transportation of glucose into the cell, insulin acts as the carrier molecule.

Filtration

Filtration is the movement of fluid and electrolytes by the pressure or force that is exerted as a result of the weight of the solution. Movement occurs from an area of higher pressure to an area of lower pressure.

Osmosis

Osmosis is the diffusion of water through a semipermeable membrane, which is a membrane that allows only particles of a certain size to pass through. A cell membrane is a semipermeable membrane. When solutions of different concentrations exist, one on each side of the semipermeable membrane, water passes through the semipermeable membrane from the weaker solution to the more concentrated solution in an attempt to equalize the strength of the solutions on each side of the membrane (Figure 8-1).

Diffusion, filtration, and osmosis are passive transport systems. Water and electrolytes continually move between the intravascular fluid, interstitial fluid, and intracellular fluid by all of these processes. Any change in the composition of one fluid is quickly reflected in changes in the others.

Active Transport

Some substances can also be moved through semipermeable membranes by an active transport system. In this process energy is needed to move ions from an area of low concentration to an area of high concentration. The sodium-potassium pump is an example of active transport. During neuromuscular function, sodium diffuses into the cell and potassium diffuses out of the cell. Each is returned to its original place with the aid of the energy source, adenosine triphosphate (ATP). This process maintains the majority of sodium outside the cell and potassium inside the cell (Figure 8-2).

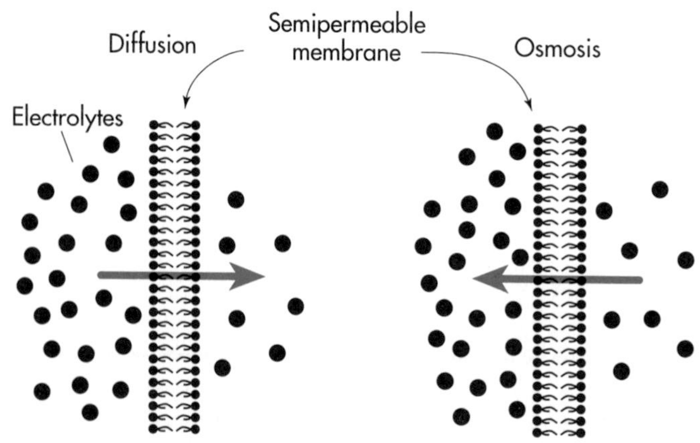

Figure 8-1 Osmosis and diffusion through semipermeable membrane.

Osmotic Pressure

Osmotic pressure or force is a term used to describe the "pulling" of water in the process of osmosis. Osmotic force is measured in units of milliosmoles (mOsm). Osmolarity and osmolality are both measurements of osmotic pressure. **Osmolality** measures the total milliosmoles of solute per *unit weight of solvent* (mOsm/kg). **Osmolarity** measures the total milliosmoles of solute per unit of *total volume of solution* (mOsm/L). Osmolality is the more acceptable term for body fluids because it allows for a comparison of body fluids that do not have the same weight for equal volume, such as plasma and urine. Osmolarity is used to compare solutions of equal weight and volume, such as plasma and intravenous (IV) solutions. Normal body fluid osmolality is between 275 and 295 mOsm/kg. A patient's body osmolality tells if he or she is adequately hydrated, overhydrated, or dehydrated.

Osmotic Movement of Fluids

Fluids added to the body that have the same osmolality as the fluid inside the cell are called **isotonic,** or **isomolar.** Solutions that contain more water (are more diluted) than the ICF are **hypotonic,** or **hypoosmolar.** Solutions with less water (more concentrated) than the cell are **hypertonic,** or **hyperosmolar.** Normally the ECF and ICF are isotonic to one another, and no movement of water occurs. Although there is a constant exchange of substances (including electrolytes) between the compartments, there is no net loss or gain of water. If a hypotonic fluid is introduced and surrounds the cell, water moves into the cell and causes it to swell and possibly burst. Hypertonic fluid that surrounds a cell draws water from the cell to dilute the ECF, which causes the cell to shrink and eventually die. IV fluids and their osmolarity are discussed later in this chapter.

Hydrostatic Pressure

Hydrostatic pressure is the force exerted by a fluid against the walls of its container. Pressure in the vascular system is generated primarily by the force of the pumping heart. The hydrostatic pressure in the vascular system is higher on the arterial side than it is on the vascular side. At the arterial end of the capilllary the pressure measures approximately 32 mm Hg. The size of the capillary bed and the movement of fluid out of the capillary and into the interstitial fluid decreases the pressure to approximately 15 mm Hg at the venous end of the capillary. Hydrostatic pressure is the major force in the movement of water out of the capillaries and into the interstitial fluid (Figure 8-3).

Oncotic Pressure

Oncotic pressure is also called colloidal osmotic pressure and is the pressure caused by colloids in solution. Colloids are particles that are too large to pass through a semipermeable membrane. Proteins are an example of a colloid. More protein is found in the plasma than in the interstitial space, so they create an osmotic force that pulls fluid from the interstitial space.

Capillary Fluid Movement

Fluid must leave the capillary to enter the interstitium (interstitial fluid) and bathe the cells. It must also return. The amount and the direction of fluid movement are determined by the interaction between (1) the hydrostatic pressure in the capillary and in the inter-

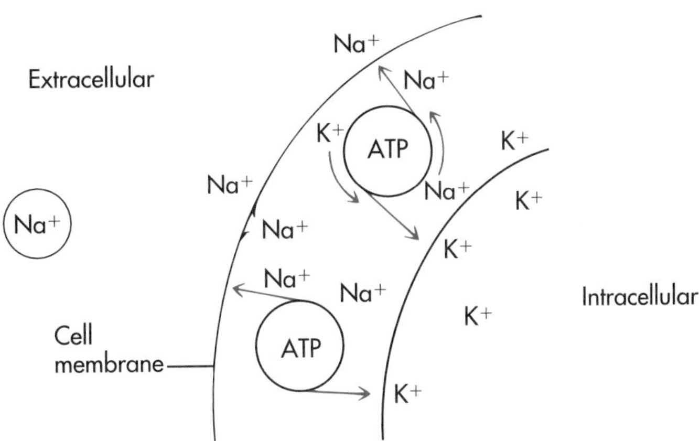

Figure 8-2 Sodium-potassium pump. As sodium diffuses into the cell and potassium out of the cell, an active transport system supplied with energy delivers sodium back to the extracellular compartment and potassium to the intracellular compartment.

stitial space, and (2) the oncotic pressure in the plasma and in the interstitial space. Hydrostatic pressure is higher than the oncotic pressure at the arterial end of the capillary and therefore forces fluid into the interstitium. At the venous end hydrostatic pressure is lower than the oncotic pressure, so fluid is drawn back into the capillary by plasma proteins (Figure 8-3).

Fluid Shifts

An alteration in capillary and/or interstitial pressure causes an abnormal shift of fluid from one compartment to another. Edema is caused by a shift of fluid from the plasma to the interstitial space. Dehydration occurs when fluid shifts from the interstitial space to the plasma.

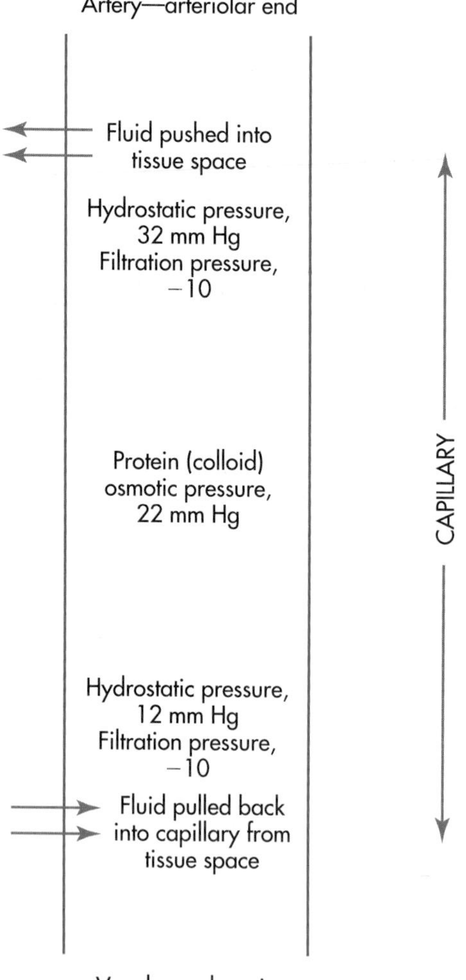

Figure 8-3 Control of fluid movement from intravascular to interstitial space and return to intravascular space. Hydrostatic pressure (HP): pressure of blood against blood vessel walls. Colloid osmotic pressure (COP): osmotic pressure exerted by plasma proteins, mainly albumin. Filtration pressure (FP): HP minus COP; FP may be positive or negative.

Shifts of plasma to interstitial fluid (edema)

Plasma shifts to the interstitial fluid if the hydrostatic pressure rises in the vascular system. It also shifts if colloidal osmotic pressure is decreased in the plasma, because an adequate "pull" is not exerted to keep fluid in the capillary or to draw it back from the interstitial space. If oncotic pressure rises in the interstitial space, fluid is pulled and remains there. All of these shifts result in edema.

Increase in venous hydrostatic pressure

If the pressure is higher than normal at the venous end of the capillary, the movement of fluid back into the capillary is inhibited. The high pressure can be caused by anything that obstructs venous return of blood to the heart, such as congestive heart failure, torniquets, thrombi in the venous system, fluid overload, or poor venous return resulting from varicose veins.

Decrease in plasma oncotic pressure

If the plasma oncotic pressure is too low, fluid is not drawn back to the capillary from the interstitium. Oncotic pressure decreases in several cases: (1) when protein is lost from the plasma, as seen in some kidney diseases; (2) when protein is not synthesized, as seen in liver disease; and (3) when insufficient protein is ingested, such as in malnutrition. Edema occurs in all of these cases.

Increase in interstitial oncotic pressure

Damage to capillary walls from trauma, burns, or inflammation allows plasma proteins to escape into the interstitial space. This shift results in an increase in interstitial oncotic pressure, which draws fluid into the interstitial space and retains it. This phenomenon explains the edema that occurs with tissue damage or inflammation.

Shifts of Interstitial Fluid to Plasma

An increase in the oncotic (osmotic) pressure of the plasma draws fluid from the interstitium. The administration of colloids, dextran, mannitol or hypertonic solutions may be ordered to achieve this result and relieve some patients of edema.

Hyperglycemia, as seen in uncontrolled diabetes mellitus, also pulls fluid from the interstitium. An increase in the hydrostatic pressure of the tissues shifts fluid into the plasma, as is seen when elastic bandages or hose are worn to decrease peripheral edema.

REGULATION OF FLUID AND ELECTROLYTES

Hypothalamus

The thirst mechanism is located in the hypothalamus and regulates the ingestion of water in the consicious person. The thirst mechanism is stimulated by hypotension and increased serum osmolality. A dry mouth causes the patient to drink.

Hormonal Regulation

Fluid and electrolyte balance is also maintained by three hormones: the *antidiuretic hormone (ADH), aldosterone,* and *parathormone.* ADH is produced in the hypothalamus and is stored and released from the posterior pituitary gland. It acts on the renal tubules to retain water and decrease urinary output. Aldosterone is produced by and secreted from the adrenal cortex. It increases sodium and water reabsorption while increasing postassium excretion in the renal tubules. The reabsorption of water and sodium results in increased circulatory volume (McCance, Huether, 1994).

Both ADH and aldosterone act in the kidney, which normally reabsorbs 99% of the fluid that is filtered in the glomerulus. Parathormone is produced by the parathyroidal glands. It promotes the absorption of calcium from the intestine, the release of calcium from the bones (bone resorption), and the excretion of phosphate ions by the kidneys.

FLUID AND ELECTROLYTE IMBALANCES

Fluid and electrolyte inbalances occur when the homeostatic mechanisms that normally control volume and concentraion are ineffective. Disturbances are primary when they are directly related to the amount of fluid or electrolyte. For example, a large amount of salt intake over a short time can result in sodium excess. Disturbances can also be of a secondary nature when other pathologic processes in the body contribute to fluid and electrolyte inbalances. Body fluid disturbances accompany many illnesses. Therefore every patient is a potential victim. The very young and the very old are at high risk.

To provide a basis for the understanding of these processes, the most important and most common imbalances are presented separately. However, because of the intricate and interacting nature of the mechanisms that control the body fluid composition, several types of imbalances usually occur at one time. Because ICF is inaccessible for analysis, fluid and electrolyte imbalances are determined by examining the ECF. The effects of a change in one fluid compartment are rapidly transmitted to the others. Therefore the ECF accurately reflects the state of all fluids throughout the body.

Extracellular Fluid Volume Imbalances

Volume distrubances of the ECF (the plasma and interstitial fluid) can be classified as a volume deficit or a volume excess.

Isotonic extracellular fluid deficit

Isotonic extracellular fluid deficit, or **hypovolemia,** occurs when both water and electrolytes have either been lost from the body or trapped in an area of the body in such a way that they are unavailable to the circulation, which occurs in second and third spacing. Examples of third spacing include fluid accumulation at the site of burns or massive soft tissue injury, the collection of fluid in the peritoneal cavity (ascites), and shifts of fluid from the intravascular space to the interstitial and intracellular spaces after abdominal and chest surgery.

Third spacing with tissue injury results from increased capillary membrane permeability, which allows fluid and albumin to leave the capillary and enter the interstitial space. This shift reduces colloid osmotic pressure in the plasma and increases colloid osmotic pressure in the interstitial space, which pulls greater amounts of fluid into the interstitial space and depletes the circulating volume. The patient requires fluid replacement and may need albumin to restore the plasma colloid osmotic pressure. In the patient with burns a normal reabsorption occurs in 48 to 72 hours. The capillaries begin to heal, and plasma proteins are replaced or reabsorbed through the lymphatic system. Therefore fluid is drawn back into the plasma, and hypervolemia can result if the return is too rapid or too much IV fluid is administered. Diuretics are administered if fluid volume becomes excessive (see Chapter 31).

Hypovolemia occurs with any abrupt decrease in fluid intake, an acute loss of secretions or excretions, or a sudden shift of fluid to the interstitial space. It often results from a combination of these forces. The most common cause of isotonic extracellular fluid deficit is loss of fluids through the gastrointestinal tract by vomiting and diarrhea. Other conditions that lead to hypovolemia include intestinal obstruction, peritonitis, and acute pancreatitis. All of these involve inflammation, which diverts fluid from the intravascular space to the inflamed tissues. Fistulas (abnormal channels between organs or parts) can cause fluid loss.

No specific laboratory tests can indicate when a fluid deficit is occurring. However, the patient's signs and symptoms plus results from other more nonspecific laboratory tests can indicate that the condition is developing. The isotonic extracellular fluid deficit can result in an acute weight loss, often in excess of 5% of body weight; decreased body temperature; low blood pressure; increased respiratory rate; delayed vein filling; anorexia; nausea; vomiting; and shock. *Oliguria,* a urinary output below 20 ml in 1 hour or 480 ml in 24 hours, can occur in severe cases. Treatment involves correcting the cause of the deficit and replacing the fluid with oral or parenteral solutions that have a normal balance of water and electrolytes, such as lactated Ringer's solution (Box 8-1).

Hypertonic extracellular fluid deficit

When body water loss exceeds electrolyte loss or when excess electrolytes are ingested or administered, the remaining fluid is hypertonic. Water moves out of the cell to dilute the ECF. Cell dehydration results, and this condition is referred to as *dehydration* (Box 8-2). The thirst response is triggered by the hypertonic ECF. The skin is flushed, the skin and mucous membranes are dry, and body temperature increases. Skin turgor is poor, and the skin produces a "tenting" effect when grasped between two fingers. Normal skin turgor prompts the skin to quickly return to its former position when released and can be described as "elastic." The best place to check skin turgor is over the sternum or on the inner thigh (Beare, Myers, 1994) (Figure 8-4).

A common cause of dehydration is the administration of concentrated tube feedings to an unconscious patient, who is unable to respond to the thirst mechanism. Hyperglycemia that occurs with uncontrolled diabetes mellitus also produces dehydration. A deficiency of ADH or a diseased kidney that does not respond to ADH results in profound diuresis, which leads to dehydration. Dehydration also results from excessive pulmonary water loss with high fever and diarrhea in infants, as well as excessive sweating without water replacement.

BOX 8-1 **Nursing Process**

FLUID VOLUME DEFICIT: HYPOVOLEMIA (ISOTONIC FLUID DEFICIT)

ASSESSMENT

Decreased temperature
Low blood pressure
Tachycardia
Weak pulse
Increased respiration
Delayed vein filling
Cold extremities
Weakness
Restlessness
Weight loss
Nausea and vomiting
Anorexia
Decreased urinary output
Shock
Increased hematocrit and hemoglobin values and red blood cell count

NURSING DIAGNOSIS

Risk for injury related to hypovolemia

NURSING INTERVENTIONS

Monitor administration of oral and IV fluids.
Monitor vital signs.
Observe for signs of shock.
Record body weight daily.
Observe skin turgor.
Maintain accurate intake and output (I&O) records.
Observe for oliguria.
Monitor and communicate laboratory results.
Observe fluid accumulation in "third spaces."

EVALUATION OF EXPECTED OUTCOMES

Correction of fluid deficit
Increased hydration
Shock prevented
Progressive weight loss prevented
Skin elastic
Renal function maintained; output 30 ml/hr
Therapy modified accordingly
Fluid remobilized

In either type of extracellular fluid deficit, the components of the blood are more concentrated as a result of the fluid loss. The increased concentration elevates the hematocrit and hemoglobin values and red blood cell count.

Extracellular fluid excess

When there is an excess of water and electrolytes in the ECF, a state of **hypervolemia** exists. Hypervolemia commonly occurs when the kidneys are not functioning properly or when isotonic intravenous solutions are being administered too rapidly. Congestive heart failure and malnutrition can also result in retention of water and electrolytes.

There are no specific tests to indicate excess ECF. However, the hematocrit and hemoglobin values and red blood cell count may decrease as a result of the dilution effect of the excess fluid. Patients most commonly display symptoms of pitting edema, dyspnea, hoarseness, a bounding pulse, acute weight gain, puffy eyelids, and engorgement of peripheral veins. All symptoms are caused by the accumulation of excess fluid throughout the body. The treatment for isotonic extracellular fluid excess involves correcting the underlying cause, withholding fluids, restricting sodium intake, and administering diuretics (Box 8-3).

Primary water excess

An excess of body water that occurs without excess electrolyte accumulation is called primary water excess (formerly termed "water intoxication"). The ECF is hypotonic, and water moves into the cells, causing them to swell. Cerebral edema occurs, which causes

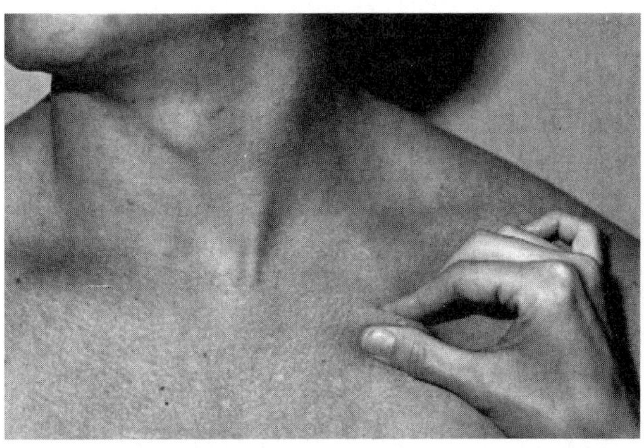

Figure 8-4 Assessment of skin turgor. When normal skin is pinched, it resumes shape within seconds. If the skin remains in a "tent" shape for 20 to 30 seconds, the client has poor skin turgor (tenting). (From Seidel HM and others: *Mosby's guide to physical examination,* ed 3, St Louis, 1995, Mosby.)

BOX 8-2 **Nursing Process**

FLUID VOLUME DEFICIT: DEHYDRATION (HYPERTONIC FLUID DEFICIT)

ASSESSMENT

Thirst
Flushed skin
Dry skin and mucous membranes
Decreased skin turgor; nonelastic (tenting)
Increased body temperature
Increased hematocrit and hemoglobin values and red blood cell count
Weight loss
Decreased urinary output

NURSING DIAGNOSIS

Risk for injury related to dehydration

NURSING INTERVENTIONS

Ask if thirsty.
Observe skin and mucous membranes.
Apply moisturizing creams.
Monitor vital signs (frequency determined by condition).

EVALUATION OF EXPECTED OUTCOMES

Correction of fluid deficit
Increased hydration
Shock prevented
Progressive weight loss prevented
Skin elastic
Renal function maintained; output 30 ml/hr
IV therapy modified accordingly
Fluid remobilized

BOX 8-3 **Nursing Process**

FLUID VOLUME EXCESS: HYPERVOLEMIA (ISOTONIC FLUID EXCESS)

ASSESSMENT

Acute weight gain
Decreased hemoglobin and hematocrit values and red blood cell count
Skin warm, moist
Pitting edema
Puffy eyelids
Bounding pulse
Engorged peripheral veins
Dyspnea, increased respiratory rate
Hoarseness
Moist rales in lungs
Cyanosis
Cardiac enlargement

NURSING DIAGNOSIS

Risk for injury related to hypervolemia

NURSING INTERVENTIONS

Record body weight daily.
Maintain accurate I&O records.
Monitor and communicate laboratory results.
Observe and document skin integrity.
Monitor vital signs.
Assess neck veins.
Observe for pulmonary edema.
Restrict fluids and sodium as ordered.
Administer medications as ordered.
Check lung sounds.
Elevate head of bed 45 degrees.

EVALUATION OF EXPECTED OUTCOMES

Fluid accumulation prevented; normal weight maintained
Laboratory values normal
Vital signs within normal limits
Neck veins flat
Adequate oxygenation

confusion, weakness, and lethargy. Seizures may also result. Increased volume results in increased central venous pressure (CVP) and jugular vein distention. The patient experiences a sudden weight gain. Skin will be warm and moist.

Water excess with hypotonicity is seen in patients with renal failure who have taken too much fluid by mouth or have been given excessive IV fluids. Administration of 5% dextrose in water after surgery or trauma can result in overhydration because the water is hypotonic after the glucose is metabolized. The water "dilutes" the plasma, and the hypotonic plasma enters the cells and overhydrates them. Balanced solutions are usually given and include dextrose to provide calories and isotonic fluids to maintain fluid volume after surgery (Box 8-4).

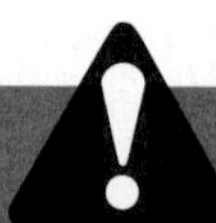

NURSE ALERT

Expect to administer balanced IV solutions to patients after surgery or trauma. Avoid dextrose in water if cerebral edema is present or probable because dextrose will metabolize and water will enter the brain cells and increase cerebral edema.

Electrolytes in Body Fluids

Electrolytes are measured in milliequivalents per liter (mEq/L), which indicates their chemical combining activity. For example, 1 mEq of a sodium cation can combine with 1 mEq of an anion such as chloride or bicarbonate. Cations and anions are found in equal milliequivalents in the plasma. The normal levels are usually given on laboratory reports, and normal ranges may vary slightly from one laboratory to the next, depending on the equipment. The normal ranges cited in this text are commonly accepted but may vary slightly when compared to a specific laboratory.

Electrolytes function as a group to promote neuromuscular irritability, maintain body fluid volume and osmolality, distribute body water between fluid compartments, and regulate acid-base balance (Long, Phipps, 1995). Each electrolyte has specific functions, which are affected when there is a deficit or a surplus. There are two basic ways by which changes in electrolyte concentration can be produced: (1) by altering the total quantity of the electrolyte in the body, and (2) by altering the total quantity of water in the ECF in which the electrolyte is dissolved. For example, an excess of sodium can be caused by an increased intake of sodium, decreased output of sodium, decreased intake of water, or increased output of water. Generally a combination of these factors produces the imbalance. This principle applies to all of the extracellular electrolytes.

BOX 8-4 **Nursing Process**

FLUID VOLUME EXCESS: OVERHYDRATION (HYPOTONIC FLUID EXCESS) (WATER INTOXICATION-PRIMARY WATER IMBALANCE)

ASSESSMENT

Acute weight gain
Decreased sodium
Decreased hemoglobin, hematocrit
Skin warm, moist
Edema
Full bounding pulse
Increased blood pressure, jugular distention
Increased CVP
Confusion
Lethargy
Seizures
Moist rales
Low urine specific gravity

NURSING DIAGNOSIS

Risk for injury related to overhydration

NURSING INTERVENTIONS

Weigh daily.
Obtain accurate I&O.
Restrict fluid intake as ordered.
Monitor laboratory results.
Observe and document skin integrity; protect from heat, cold, pressure.
Monitor vital signs.
Note central venous pressure.
Assess orientation.
Establish seizure precautions.
Monitor lung sounds.
Check specific gravity.

EVALUATION OF EXPECTED OUTCOMES

Weight loss; return to previous weight
Laboratory values normal
Skin warm, dry, elastic
Neck veins flat
Vital signs and CVP within normal limits
Oriented to time, place, person
Injury avoided
Lungs clear
Specific gravity within normal limits

Sodium

Sodium is the chief cation of the ECF and accounts for 90% of all the extracellular positive ions. It is largely responsible for maintaining the proper relationships of body fluids by regulating fluid balance and osmotic pressure. Sodium has several functions:

1. Plays a vital role in numerous chemical reactions
2. Participates in the generation and transmission of nerve impulses
3. Assists in maintaining acid-base balance
4. Is necessary for the regulation of water reabsorption and excretion in the kidney tubule

A normal serum sodium level of 138 to 145 mEq/L and intracellular sodium concentrations of 10 mEq/L are necessary to balance body fluids. If there is too much sodium outside the cell **(hypernatremia)** or too little inside, water leaves the cell and causes it to shrink. If intracellular sodium increases or extracellular sodium decreases **(hyponatremia),** water moves into the cell and causes it to swell. Both shrinking and swelling disturb normal cellular activity in the central nervous system. The major role of sodium in neuromuscular transmission is demonstrated by the changes in muscle tone that are seen as early signs of abnormalities. Shrinking or swelling in cerebral cells results in dysfunction.

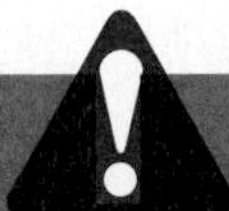

NURSE ALERT

Use normal saline to irrigate nasogastric tubes. Water draws sodium from the stomach tissues (diffusion).

Sodium levels are controlled by the hormone aldosterone, which is secreted by the adrenal cortex when sodium levels are low. Aldosterone stimulates the renal tubules to reabsorb more of the sodium, which could otherwise pass out of the body in the urine. Once normal levels of sodium are reached, aldosterone secretion decreases. In this way, the concentration of sodium is maintained in normal limits. A daily intake of 2 to 4 g sodium is needed to replenish stores. Because the body stores sodium well, a decreased intake does not immediately result in a deficit.

Sodium deficit. A sodium deficit, or hyponatremia, can be caused by loss of sodium or by an excess of water. It is usually caused by excessive perspiration associated with the drinking of plain water; losses from the gastrointestinal tract because of (or related to) vomiting, diarrhea, or nasogastric suction; or administration of a potent diuretic. Too much salt is lost, or the intake of water is excessive.

A sodium deficit can also be caused by adrenal insufficiency. The adrenals secrete aldosterone, and without sufficient aldosterone, the patient fails to retain sodium. Dilutional hyponatremia can occur with a fluid overload that is caused by congestive heart failure, cirrhosis of the liver, or by the administration of excessive hypotonic IV solutions.

In a sodium deficit there are too few particles in relation to the amount of water present. The ECF is therefore hypoosmolar, or hypotonic. In an attempt to create equilibrium, the water moves into the interstitial spaces and the cells by osmosis. The cells become swollen and cause symptoms of anorexia, headache, nausea, vomiting, mental disturbances, and confusion followed by disorientation, convulsions, and coma. The deficit affects transmission of nerve impulses, which causes abdominal cramps and muscle weakness. Treatment usually includes the administration of normal saline or, with a severe deficit, 3% or 5% hypertonic saline solution if the kidneys are healthy. Hypertonic solutions must be administered slowly to prevent pulmonary edema. If too much water is the cause of the sodium deficit, fluids are restricted while sodium is gradually added (Box 8-5).

If sodium is lost in equal proportions with water, the ECF remains isotonic but its volume is decreased. Serum sodium levels are normal, and the patient's symptoms are related to circulatory collapse caused by decreased ECF volume. Isotonic fluids are administered to replace fluid and electrolytes.

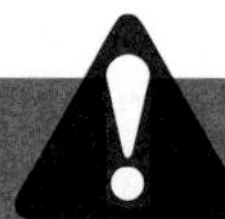

NURSE ALERT

Because sodium regulates fluid balance, expect a patient with a sodium imbalance to also have a fluid imbalance.

BOX 8-5

Nursing Process

SODIUM DEFICIT: HYPONATREMIA

ASSESSMENT

Plasma sodium less than 133 mEq/L
Low urine specific gravity
Anorexia, nausea, vomiting
Weakness
Headache
Muscle cramps
Abdominal cramps
Confusion
Disorientation
Convulsions
Coma with severe deficit

NURSING DIAGNOSIS

Risk for injury related to hyponatremia

NURSING INTERVENTIONS

Encourage diet high in sodium if ordered.
Weigh daily.
Check specific gravity q 8 hr.
Monitor neurologic status.
Monitor vital signs.
Monitor administration of IV fluids.
Monitor serum electrolyte levels as ordered q 2 to 4 hr.
Maintain accurate intake and output records.
Observe for a change in status.
Pad side rails of bed.
Place head in lateral position if seizure occurs.
Restrict fluids if deficit is caused by excess water.

EVALUATION OF EXPECTED OUTCOMES

Serum sodium level increased and within normal limits
Specific gravity within normal limits
Early symptoms observed
More severe symptoms prevented
Renal compensation for low serum sodium level determined
Volume overload prevented
Patient safety maintained
Airway maintained

Sodium excess. A sodium excess, or hypernatremia, can occur in any condition in which fluids that contain little sodium are lost in excess, such as the losses that accompany profuse watery diarrhea. When the water in the plasma is decreased, the electrolyte readings increase even though the total amount of the electrolyte in the body has not changed. Because sodium is the most abundant electrolyte, it is the first to show changes.

When a large amount of salt is ingested over a short time, acute sodium excess can occur. Following the laws of osmosis, water from the cells flows into the more concentrated ECF. This helps dilute the ECF but leaves the cells in need of water.

The high levels of sodium in the ECF draw fluid from the cells and result in cellular dehydration. Therefore the symptoms of hypernatremia are those of dehydration: dry, sticky mucous membranes; dry tongue; fever; thirst; flushed appearance; weakness; and irritability. Shallow, rapid breathing; fluttering eyelids; and muscle spasms that lead to stupor, seizures, and coma can occur. Laboratory data indicate increased levels of plasma sodium and chloride, and the specific gravity of the urine is elevated.

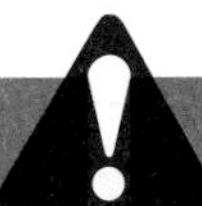

NURSE ALERT

Sodium and potassium imbalances often occur inversely. If sodium is high, potassium may be low and vice versa.

Hypernatremia occurs in victims of salt-water drowning; renal disease; and hyperaldosteronism, which results in reabsorption of too much sodium by the kidney. Normal sodium levels are restored by infusion of hypotonic saline solutions, administration of furosemide (Lasix) or hydrochlorothiazide (HydroDiuril) to promote sodium excretion, and dietary restriction of sodium (Box 8-6).

When sodium is gained over a longer period of time, water is also retained. Sodium and water increase together in similar proportions, so serum sodium levels are within normal limits. Because the ECF remains isotonic, the cells of the body do not swell or shrink and there are no symptoms of cerebral irritability or depression. The result of this isotonic imbalance is in-

BOX 8-6 **Nursing Process**

SODIUM EXCESS: HYPERNATREMIA

ASSESSMENT

Plasma sodium more than 150 mEq/L
Dry and sticky mucous membranes
Dry tongue
Flushed appearance
Thirst
Oliguria
Increased BP
Elevated temperature
Weakness
Irritability, excitability
Disorientation
Shallow, rapid breathing
Fluttering eyelids
Muscular spasm
Seizures
Stupor
Coma

NURSING DIAGNOSIS

Risk for injury related to hypernatremia

NURSING INTERVENTIONS

Encourage low-sodium diet if ordered.
Observe skin and mucous membranes.
Maintain accurate I&O records.
Monitor administration of IV fluids.
Monitor vital signs.
Administer muscle relaxants and/or diuretics as ordered.
Observe seizure precautions.
Maintain life support systems during therapy.

EVALUATION OF EXPECTED OUTCOMES

Serum sodium levels decreased
Deficit of water corrected
Rapid correction avoided
Efficacy of treatment determined
Temperature and BP within normal limits
Muscular spasms controlled

creased volume of ECF, which causes edema and circulatory overload. Patients who are retaining sodium and fluid are placed on a low-sodium diet (2 g/day or less). Processed foods, dairy products, and salty foods are high in sodium.

Potassium

Potassium (K^+) is the major intracellular cation. It is responsible for ICF balance, a regular heart rhythm, conduction of neuromuscular impulses, conversion of glucose to energy in the cell, protein synthesis, and regulation of acid-base balance. The normal potassium range is 3.5 to 5 mEq/L. This is the amount in the ECF that can be measured by diagnostic testing. It is an indirect measurement of the level of potassium found in the cell, where it is much more abundant.

NURSE ALERT

The body does not store potassium well, so a deficit can occur quickly if potassium intake is poor or the loss excessive.

Potassium affects acid-base balance because it acts as part of the body's buffer system. If the body becomes acidotic **(acidosis),** hydrogen ions move into the cell to reduce their number in the ECF. As hydrogen enters the cell, potassium exits in exchange for hydrogen ions, which raises the serum level of potassium. This elevated serum potassium level is called a false positive because actual levels of potassium in the body have not changed. In **alkalosis** the plasma is low in hydrogen ions, so hydrogen leaves the cell and enters the plasma to compensate. Potassium then leaves the plasma and enters the cell, and **hypokalemia** results. In these cases, the potassium imbalance is treated by correcting the acid or base imbalance.

Plasma potassium falls about 0.6 mEq/L for each 0.1 unit rise in blood pH. A level below 3 mEq/L is toxic. Plasma potassium increases about 0.6 mEq/L for each 0.1 unit fall in blood pH. Regardless of the cause, a serum potassium level below 3 mEq/L or above 5.5 mEq/L can produce toxic effects.

The role of potassium in neuromuscular function is to excite or irritate nerve cells, resulting in muscular contraction. Smooth, skeletal, and cardiac muscle depend on potassium for proper contraction and function. Heart muscle is particularly sensitive to an imbalance.

Large amounts of potassium are found in secretions and excretions of the body such as sweat, saliva, gastric juice, and stool. Unlike with sodium, the body has no effective mechanism for conserving potassium and continues to excrete potassium in the urine even when the levels are already low. Because 90% of the potassium is excreted in the urine, levels increase if kidney function is impaired. To replenish potassium stores, 40 to 60 mEq of potassium are needed daily.

Potassium deficit. Probably the most common cause of potassium deficit, or hypokalemia, in the United States is the use of diuretics without potassium supplementation. Loop and thiazide diuretics increase potassium excretion. Loop diuretics are drugs that act by inhibiting the active reabsorption of chloride ions in the ascending limb of Henle's loop. Because chloride draws sodium with it, sodium reabsorption is also prevented. Therefore sodium chloride is retained in the tubule and excreted in urine, carrying water with it. Thiazide diuretics block sodium and chloride reabsorption in the distal convoluted tubule, which results in increased excretion of sodium, chloride, and water. With both loop and thiazide diuretics, the high concentration of sodium in the distal convoluted tubule causes an increased exchange of sodium and potassium, which in turn causes additional potassium to be pulled in and excreted.

Some diuretics spare potassium because they act in ways that do not cause potassium excretion. An example is spironolactone (Aldactone), which inhibits the action of aldosterone in the distal tubule. Aldosterone normally causes more sodium to be reabsorbed in the distal tubule, and potassium is excreted. When its action is inhibited by Aldactone, less sodium is reabsorbed. It is excreted and at the same time potassium is "spared."

Other factors that contribute to potassium loss are insufficient potassium intake; inefficient gastrointestinal absorption; and abnormal gastrointestinal losses as a result of diarrhea, vomiting, and ileostomy drainage. Metabolic alkalosis causes potassium to move into the cell in exchange for hydrogen ions, which reduces extracellular potassium levels. This condition is corrected by treating the alkalosis rather than by administering potassium.

OLDER ADULT CONSIDERATIONS

A high percentage of older adults take diuretics to treat hypertension. This places them at high risk for a potassium deficit. Many older adults also take digitalis to strengthen heart function, which can produce toxic effects if potassium is low. Watch for signs of potassium deficit and digitalis toxicity. Anorexia may be the first sign for both.

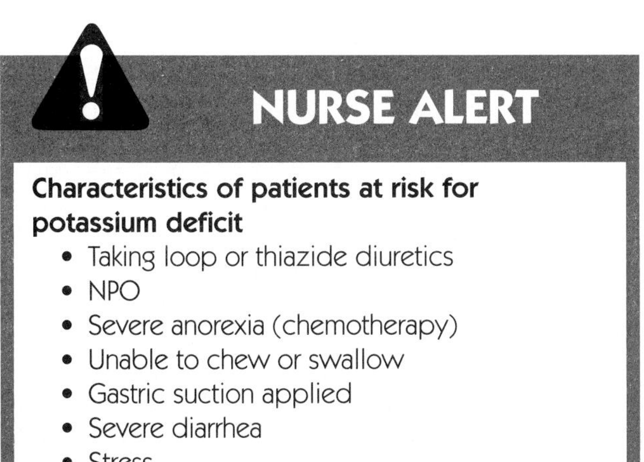

Characteristics of patients at risk for potassium deficit

- Taking loop or thiazide diuretics
- NPO
- Severe anorexia (chemotherapy)
- Unable to chew or swallow
- Gastric suction applied
- Severe diarrhea
- Stress

Effects of stress on serum potassium levels. Stress stimulates the pituitary gland, which causes the release of ADH from the posterior pituitary. ADH causes the body to retain water and sodium and to reduce urine output. This action maintains blood volume, which may be needed if one is threatened physiologically or psychologically. Stress also causes the adrenal cortex to secrete aldosterone, which results in the retention of sodium, chloride, and water and in the loss of potassium. Therefore stress can be a factor in hypokalemia.

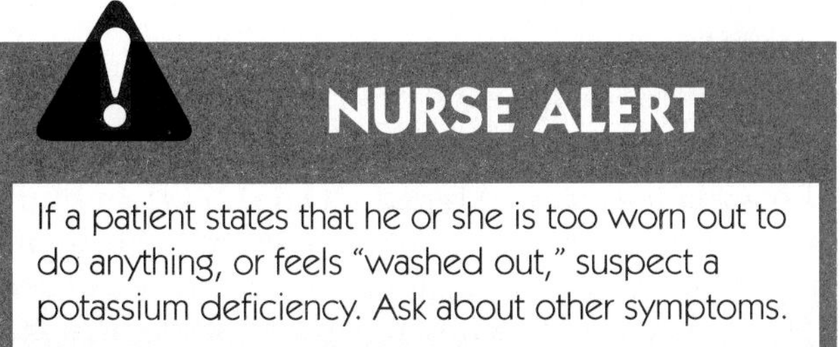

If a patient states that he or she is too worn out to do anything, or feels "washed out," suspect a potassium deficiency. Ask about other symptoms.

Assessment. Many of the signs and symptoms of potassium deficit result from its effect on the nervous and muscular systems. As a result of the deficit, the nerve cells are not as "excited" as they need to be to produce good muscle function. Skeletal muscle weakness and fatigue are common early complaints. The decreasing tone of the smooth muscle of the gastrointestinal tract can produce symptoms of anorexia, vomiting, distention, and possible paralytic ileus. Decreasing blood pressure, a weak pulse, faint heart sounds, and paralysis of the respiratory muscles are later signs. Cardiac arrhythmias are common, and the electrocardiogram may show a flattened T wave and the presence of a U wave (Figure 8-5). Ventricular tachycardia and cardiac arrest may occur when the levels are very low. Hypokalemia reduces the ability of the renal tubules to concentrate waste, which results in an increased fluid loss in urinary output. Laboratory data show low potassium levels in plasma.

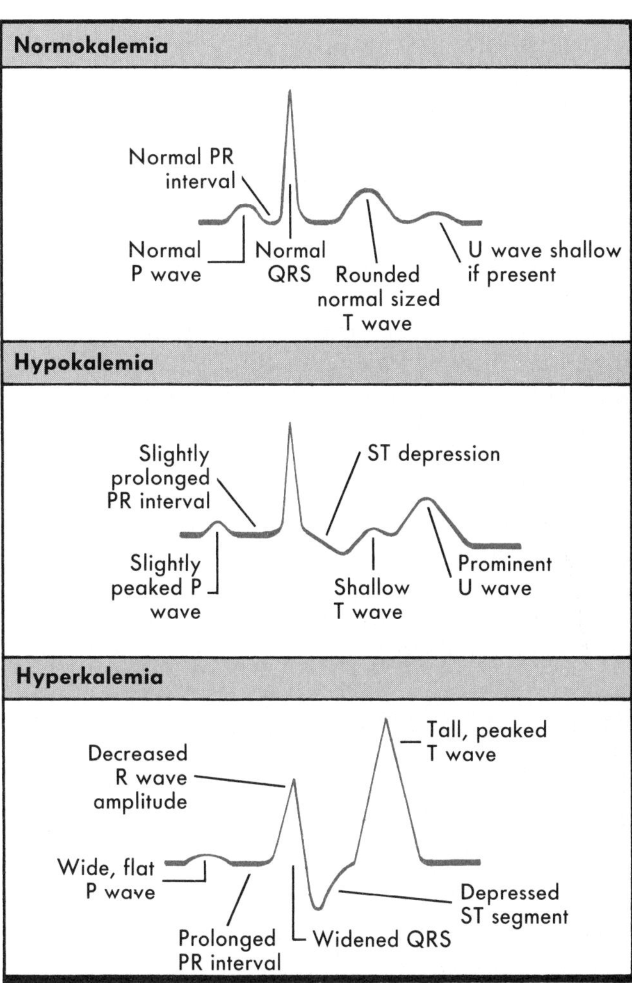

Figure 8-5 ECG changes with potassium imbalance. (From McCance KL, Huether SE: *Pathophysiology: the biologic basis for disease in adults and children,* ed 2, St Louis, 1994, Mosby.)

Intervention. Hypokalemia is treated with oral or IV supplements of potassium chloride (KCl). KCl should not be given if urine output is less than 30 ml/hr because excretion of potassium will be inadequate, which quickly results in an excess. Because of the effect of potassium on the cardiac muscle, a deficit should not be corrected rapidly. Correcting the deficit too rapidly can also cause tetany. KCl supplements added to IV solutions should never exceed 60 mEq/L, and 40 mEq/L is preferred. The rate of IV administration of KCl should not exceed 20 to 40 mEq/hr to prevent hyperkalemia and cardiac arrest. KCl is always diluted when administered intravenously. It is never given as a bolus IV push because the concentrated solution can cause cardiac arrest. Even in solution, KCl can be very irritating to the vein at the site of entry. Central venous lines inserted in the subclavian or a peripheral vein are preferred. Any underlying disease that is causing the potassium deficit must be identified and treated.

NURSE ALERT

When KCl is administered IV, it is always mixed in solution. Give slowly and never exceed 20 to 40 mEq/hr.

Mild deficits can be treated with a dietary intake of potassium. Preventing and treating deficits requires a knowledge of dietary sources of potassium (Box 8-7). Individuals who are taking diuretics that cause potassium loss, especially thiazide and loop diuretics, need to increase their dietary intake of potassium and need to know the signs and symptoms of a deficit. At the earliest sign they should increase intake and report their symptoms to their healthcare provider (Box 8-8).

Hypokalemia and the client taking digitalis. Digitalis is a cardiotonic drug that is used to slow and strengthen the heartbeat. It is given to a patient with a failing heart to increase the heart's capability as a pump. Frequently the same patient is taking diuretics, which act to reduce ECF volume and reduce the workload of the pumping heart. Loop and thiazide diuretics cause a loss of potassium, so the patient taking drugs of this type is at a greater risk of potassium deficiency. When the potassium level falls below normal, a patient who is taking digitalis is more likely to develop a toxic reaction to the drug.

Digitalis toxicity can be mild and cause anorexia, nausea, and visual disturbances in which the visual field appears to have a yellow cast. Symptoms can also be severe and lead to fatal arrhythmias (irregular heart rhythms). Most clients on digitalis and diuretics have diseased hearts that may be more likely to have irregular rhythms.

BOX 8-7

SOURCES OF POTASSIUM (in mg)

Butternut squash, 1 cup baked, 1200
Lima beans, dry, 1 cup cooked, 1200
Spinach, 1 cup cooked, 1160
Black beans, 1 cup cooked, 1000
Soybeans, 1 cup cooked, 970
Pinto beans, 1 cup cooked, 940
Navy beans, 1 cup cooked, 790
Acorn squash, ¼ baked, 750
Green lima beans, 1 cup cooked, 720
Papaya, medium, 710
Cantaloupe, ½ medium, 680
Avocado, ½ medium, 650
Raisins, ½ cup, 650
Kidney beans, 1 cup cooked, 630
Chard, 1 cup cooked, 600
Prune juice, 1 cup, 600
Parsnips, 1 cup cooked, 590
Split peas, 1 cup cooked, 590
Blackstrap molasses, 1 tablespoon, 580
Dates, 10 medium, 520
Potato, 1 medium, cooked, 500
Orange juice, 1 cup, 500
Skim milk powder, ¼ cup, 490
Beet greens, 1 cup, 480
Banana, medium, 440
Low-fat milk, 1 cup, 430
Kohlrabi, 1 cup cooked, 430
Peas, fresh, 1 cup, 420
Brussels sprouts, 1 cup cooked, 420
Nectarine, medium, 410

NURSE ALERT

A client who develops hypokalemia while taking digitalis is likely to develop a toxic reaction, which could be fatal. The nurse must observe the client for symptoms of potassium deficit and teach the client to do the same.

Potassium excess. **Hyperkalemia** occurs most often when the kidneys are unable to excrete potassium adequately (renal failure). It can also occur soon after massive injury, such as burns and crushing injuries. Cellular destruction releases large amounts of intracellular potassium into the ECF. Severe infections and chemotherapy with cytotoxic drugs can also cause cellular destruction (catabolism). The destroyed cells release their intracellular potassium into the interstitial fluid. Administering blood that is near its expiration date may also cause an excess of potassium as a result of the breakdown of old red blood cells. Metabolic acidosis causes potassium to leave the cell and enter the ECF in exchange for hydrogen ions, which results in an elevated serum potassium. Adrenal insufficiency leads to retention of potassium in the serum because aldosterone is deficient and sodium is not reabsorbed. Therefore the potassium that is normally excreted in exchange for sodium remains in the body. Administering IV potassium solutions too rapidly may also lead to a potassium excess.

Many of the early symptoms of potassium excess are nonspecific. Electrocardiogram (ECG) changes

BOX 8-8 **Nursing Process**

POTASSIUM DEFICIT: HYPOKALEMIA

ASSESSMENT

Plasma potassium < 3.5 mEq/L
Muscular weakness
Fatigue
Vertigo
Electrocardiographic changes
T wave flattened
U wave present/prominent
Anorexia
Vomiting
Distention
Paralytic ileus
Decreasing blood pressure
Weak pulse
Faint heart sounds
Respiratory muscle paralysis

NURSING DIAGNOSIS

Risk for injury related to hypokalemia

NURSING INTERVENTIONS

Note serum potassium results.
Encourage diet high in potassium if indicated.
Monitor administration of replacement solutions.
Assist if ambulating to prevent injury.
Monitor ECG results.
Monitor bowel sounds and palpate and measure abdomen for distention.
Maintain accurate I&O records.
Observe for metabolic alkalosis (secondary to hypokalemia causing shift of hydrogen to the cell so needed K^+ can move from cell to plasma; metabolic alkalosis can also cause hypokalemia).
Monitor vital signs.

EVALUATION OF EXPECTED OUTCOMES

Potassium level slowly returns to normal
No falls
Safety maintained
Changes in heart rhythm secondary to decreased potassium detected at onset; cardiac arrest prevented
Absence of tingling and twitching; pH normal
Bowel sounds present, all quadrants
Shock and respiratory arrest prevented

usually occur early, but often the patient is not monitored for these changes. Because potassium plays a major role in neuromuscular activity, muscle twitching is an early sign. Facial and respiratory muscles may become involved, and parethesias (numbness, tingling) of the face and tongue may develop. Gastrointestinal symptoms of nausea, diarrhea, and intestinal colic are also related to neuromuscular overexcitability. Flaccid paralysis may develop. The most serious effect of a high potassium level is on the cardiac muscles. Cell excitability is increased, but cardiac contractions are weaker, which can result in a dilated, flaccid heart. Tachycardia is seen and is followed by bradycardia and dysrhythmia, which may lead to cardiac arrest. The conduction system of the heart is disturbed, and ectopic beats appear on the ECG. Changes include tall, peaked T waves; a shortened Q-T interval; a prolonged PR interval followed by a disappearance of the P wave; and a widening of the QRS complex (see Figure 8-5). Laboratory data indicate levels of potassium in the plasma in excess of 5.5 mEq/L. ECG changes become more severe at higher levels.

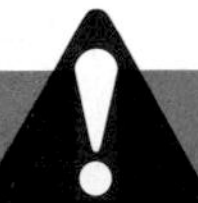

NURSE ALERT

Monitor cardiac function closely in hyperkalemia. Cardiac cell overstimulation leads to life-threatening changes in heart rate and rhythm. Tachycardia is followed by bradycardia. ECG monitoring is necessary.

The treatment of potassium excess varies according to the type and severity of the underlying problem. In mild cases potassium intake is avoided, and any IV solutions should omit potassium. An ion-exchange resin, sodium polystyrene sulfonate (Kayexalate), can be used orally, rectally, or by nasogastric tube to treat hyperkalemia. It binds with potassium in the gastrointestinal tract and is eliminated. When given rectally, it is administered as a retention enema and retained for 30 to 60 minutes. A potassium-wasting diuretic such as

BOX 8-9 **Nursing Process**

POTASSIUM EXCESS: HYPERKALEMIA

ASSESSMENT

Plasma potassium greater than 5.0 mEq/L
Electrocardiographic changes: tall, peaked T waves, shortened Q-T interval, prolonged PR interval followed by disappearance of the P wave, widened QRS complex; bradycardia, arrhythmias leading to cardiac arrest
Tachycardia followed by bradycardia
Muscle twitching and weakness
Hyperactive deep-tendon reflexes
Nausea, diarrhea, intestinal colic (abdominal cramps)
Paresthesias of the face, tongue, and extremities
Ascending paralysis in severe cases; could result in respiratory arrest

NURSING DIAGNOSIS

Risk for injury related to hyperkalemia

NURSING INTERVENTIONS

Note serum potassium results; encourage diet low in potassium if taking food.
Monitor ECG results; monitor vital signs.
Administer calcium solutions to neutralize potassium; use with caution if patient is receiving digitalis preparations.
Monitor muscle tone.
Monitor deep tendon reflexes.
Check bowel sounds; observe level of hydration.
Observe and report parathesia.
Check respirations q 15 min to q 1 hr.

EVALUATION OF EXPECTED OUTCOMES

Potassium level slowly returns to normal
Abnormal electrical conductions detected and treated at onset; normal sinus rhythm resumed
Muscle activity normotonic
Bowel sounds present, all quadrants; no report of nausea or diarrhea; well hydrated
No report of numbness
Respirations 14/min or above

furosemide (Lasix) also brings down potassium levels by causing potassium to be excreted.

If the condition is acute, 10 or 20 U of regular insulin is administered along with intravenous hypertonic dextrose solution (25% to 50%). As the dextrose accompanied by insulin enters the cell, potassium is carried along and lowers levels in the ECF. The effects are temporary but provide time for the other measures to restore balance.

Sodium bicarbonate may also be added to alkalinize the plasma. Sodium bicarbonate causes hydrogen to enter the plasma from the cells in an attempt to restore acidity. Potassium leaves the plasma and enters the cell in exchange for hydrogen, thus lowering serum potassium. Sodium bicarbonate also provides sodium, which antagonizes the effects of potassium on the myocardium. This effect also is only temporary. Peritoneal dialysis and hemodialysis can also be used in emergencies.

IV administration of calcium may be ordered to stimulate heart contraction by antagonizing the effects of excess potassium on heart muscle. However, calcium solutions should be used cautiously with patients who are receiving digitalis preparations. Calcium sensitizes the heart to digitalis, and digitalis toxicity can result and cause severe visual, gastrointestinal, neuropsychologic, and cardiac disturbances (Box 8-9).

Calcium

Calcium (Ca) is absorbed through the small intestine. Vitamin D is essential for the absorption of calcium. The majority of calcium in the body is stored in the teeth and bones. It is absorbed by the bones from the ECF (bone formation) and also flows from the bone back to the ECF (bone resorption) to be excreted. Although normal levels of serum calcium are low, it is an important ion for the transmission of nerve impulses. Intracellular calcium is essential for the contraction of muscle tissue. Extracellular calcium is necessary for blood clotting and for tooth and bone formation. It is needed for the absorption and use of vitamin B_{12} and is essential for maintaining a normal heart rhythm. Extracellular calcium stabilizes the cell membrane and blocks sodium transport into the cell, thus decreasing the excitability of the cell. A decreased serum calcium level causes increased nerve and muscle cell excitability. Many enzyme systems are activated by calcium.

BOX 8-10

FORMULA TO CORRECT CALCIUM READINGS DISTORTED BY ABNORMAL ALBUMIN LEVELS

Hypoalbuminemia

1 Subtract patient's serum albumin from the normal level (4.0 mg/dl)
2 Multiply that remainder by a correction factor of 0.8
3 Add that product to the total calcium level found in the laboratory results

Example:

1	4.0	mg/dl (normal serum albumin)
	− 1.7	mg/dl (patient's albumin level)
	2.3	mg/dl (remainder)
2	2.3	mg/dl (remainder)
	× 0.8	(correction factor)
	1.84	mg/dl (product)
3	1.84	
	+ 10.1	mg/dl (patient's total calcium level)
	11.94	mg/dl adjusted total calcium level, which indicates hypercalcemia

Hyperalbuminemia

1 Subtract normal albumin (4.0 mg/dl) from the patient's albumin level
2 Multiply the remainder by a correction factor of 0.8
3 Subtract that product from the total calcium level found in the laboratory results

Example:

1	6.4	mg/dl (patient's albumin)
	− 4.0	mg/dl (normal albumin)
	2.4	mg/dl (remainder)
2	2.4	mg/dl (remainder)
	× 0.8	(correction factor)
	1.92	mg/dl (product)
3	8.6	mg/dl (patient's total calcium level)
	− 1.92	
	6.68	mg/dl adusted total calcium level, which indicates hypocalcemia

Calcium levels are regulated by the parathyroid hormone and by calcitonin. When serum calcium levels drop, the parathyroid gland increases secretion of the parathyroid hormone, which draws calcium from the bones to the circulating serum (bone resorption). Parathyroid hormone also increases gastrointestinal absorption of calcium and increases renal tubule reabsorption of calcium.

Calcitonin is the other hormone that regulates calcium balance. It is produced by the thyroid and is stimulated by high serum calcium levels. It *opposes* the action of parathyroid hormone and thus lowers the serum calcium level by decreasing gastrointestinal absorption, by increasing bone mineralization (preventing bone resorption), and by promoting renal excretion.

Laboratory tests can measure ionized serum calcium or total serum calcium. It is more difficult to measure ionized calcium, so the routine test measures total calcium. Total calcium is measured in milligrams, and the normal level is 8.6 to 10.6 mg/dl. Ionized calcium is measured in milliequivalents, and the normal range is 4.5 to 5.5 mEq/L. Total calcium includes the calcium bound to albumin and other proteins, which is about 44% of the circulating calcium in the body. The remainder is ionized and is the portion that is biologically active and can cause problems by being too high or too low. The amount of *bound* calcium decreases when serum albumin drops, which causes a decrease in total serum calcium. Therefore a normal serum calcium level accompanied by low serum albumin is actually indicative of **hypercalcemia** because the ionized calcium now represents a higher percentage of the serum calcium. Conversely, a high albumin level causes bound calcium to increase. Therefore a normal total calcium level accompanied by hyperalbuminemia actually indicates an ionized calcium deficit, or **hypocalcemia.** Serum pH affects calcium binding to albumin. Acidosis decreases calcium binding, which leads to more ionized calcium. Alkalosis increases calcium binding (Lewis, Collier, 1992). Box 8-10 shows how to "correct" total calcium readings in the presence of hypoalbuminemia or hyperalbuminemia (Walpert, 1990).

Calcium deficit. A calcium deficit, or hypocalcemia, is often associated with excessive gastrointestinal losses. Because calcium levels in the serum are regulated by the parathyroid glands, hypoactive or absent glands can also lead to a calcium deficit. When a thyroidectomy is performed, the parathyroid glands can be removed inadvertently, or postoperative edema can temporarily restrict the flow of the parathyroid hormone and cause a calcium deficit. Pancreatic diseases (e.g., acute pancreatitis), massive subcutaneous infections, and peritonitis may lead to extraction of calcium from the ECF and cause a calcium deficit. Multiple blood transfusions can cause hypocalcemia because the citrate used to anticoagulate the blood binds with calcium.

Assessment. The signs and symptoms of calcium deficit result from neuromuscular irritability because there is not enough calcium to decrease the excitability of the nerve and muscle cells. Tetany occurs, which is characterized by tingling of the extremities, muscle cramps and twitching, carpopedal spasms (sharp flexion of the wrist and ankle joints), and convulsions. Tetany is a state of increased neuroexcitability and sustained muscle contraction. Because the peripheral nerves are affected first, carpopedal spasm is one of the first signs of tetany (Figure 8-6, *A*). Early signs of tetany are evident if *carpal* spasm occurs when the brachial artery is occluded by constriction, such as when a blood pressure cuff is applied to the upper arm and inflated. Carpal spasm is evident within 3 minutes if hypocalcemia is present. This phenomenon is called *Trousseau's sign.* Patients can also be checked for *Chvostek's sign,* which involves tapping the face over the facial nerve in front of the ear (Figure 8-6, *B, C*). If the face twitches, the results are positive and indicate a calcium deficit. Laryngeal stridor, dysphagia, dysarthria, cardiac dysrhythmia, and convulsions are also seen with tetany. ECG changes and x-ray films of bones are helpful in establishing a diagnosis. Changes in the blood clotting process can also be observed. Laboratory data indicate low calcium levels in the urine and plasma.

Intervention. Symptoms of calcium deficit must be treated immediately. Any patient who has had thyroid surgery must be watched closely for signs and symptoms of calcium deficit. Calcium levels must be returned to normal while the cause is being identified and treated. Calcium carbonate can be given orally if symptoms are less severe. IV calcium gluconate is administered if symptoms are life threatening. The IV infusion site must be checked frequently because calcium infiltration can cause sloughing of the tissue. Calcium is not given intramuscularly because it precipitates (separates out of solution) in the muscle. Calcium-rich foods are prescribed along with vitamin D supplements to help absorb calcium from the gastrointestinal tract. Synthetic parathyroid hormone (parathormone) can also be given (Box 8-11).

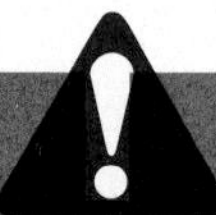

NURSE ALERT

Observe patient after a thyroidectomy for calcium deficit. Ask patient about tingling of the fingertips, and look for Trousseau's sign when taking blood pressure.

Calcium excess. Hypercalcemia is a state of excess calcium in the serum. It most often occurs as a result of a tumor of the parathyroid glands. However, it is also associated with excessive administration of vitamin D, multiple fractures, multiple myeloma, and prolonged immobilization. Renal diseases may prevent calcium excretion and result in abnormally high levels in the body fluids.

Calcium excess produces depression of neuromuscular activity. Signs and symptoms include lethargy and decreased muscle tone. The patient demonstrates decreased memory span, confusion, disorientation, and fatigue. Nausea, vomiting, and constipation may occur, and cardiac dysrhythmias are evident. Deep bone pain may be present if the excess serum calcium is caused by bone resorption. High levels of serum cal-

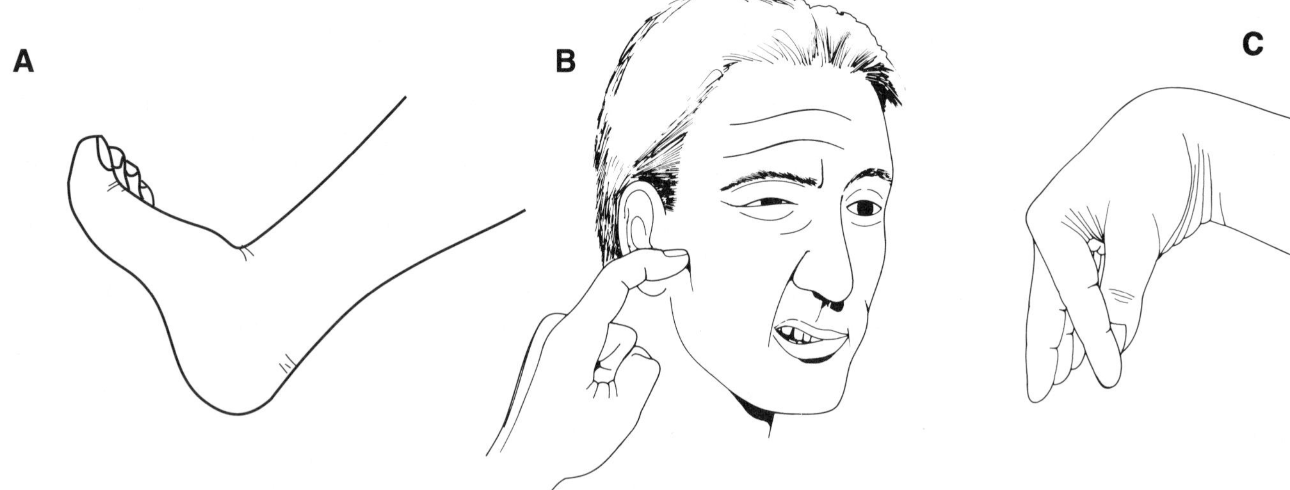

Figure 8-6 **A,** Carpopedal spasm—hyperflexion of wrist and ankle. **B,** Chvostek's sign—a contraction of the facial muscle elicited in response to a light tap over the facial nerve in front of the ear. **C,** Trousseau's sign—a carpal spasm (hyperflexion at the wrist) induced by inflating a blood pressure cuff above the systolic pressure.

BOX 8-11

Nursing Process

CALCIUM DEFICIT: HYPOCALCEMIA

ASSESSMENT

Serum calcium level less than 8 mg/dl
Tingling of extremities; abdominal cramps; carpopedal spasm
Positive Chvostek's sign
Positive Trousseau's sign
Convulsions
ECG changes
Delayed blood clotting

NURSING DIAGNOSIS

Risk for injury related to hypocalcemia

NURSING INTERVENTIONS

Encourage increased dietary intake of calcium.
Monitor administration of IV solutions containing calcium, monitor serum calcium.
Instruct patient regarding expected symptoms.
Establish and maintain communication with patient, encouraging symptom report.
Check for Chvostek's sign.
Compress brachial artery to check for Trousseau's sign.
Monitor neurologic status.
Maintain quiet environment, subdued lighting.
Establish seizure precautions.
Monitor vital signs.
Monitor clotting times.
Observe for hemorrhagic areas.

EVALUATION OF EXPECTED OUTCOMES

Mild calcium deficit corrected through dietary measures
Bradycardia, which is caused by giving too much IV calcium, is prevented
Patient will report altered neuromuscular sensations
Absence of facial twitch
Absence of carpal spasm
Absense of seizure activity
Prevention of injury
Control of arrhythmias
Bleeding avoided

cium can result in kidney stones, which cause flank pain. As calcium levels continue to rise, psychoses and coma may develop. Laboratory data indicate high levels of calcium in the urine and plasma.

Treatment of hypercalcemia involves promoting calcium excretion in the urine by administering a loop diuretic (furosemide or ethacrynic acid) and IV infusions of normal saline (Beare, Myers, 1994). If the patient can take fluids by mouth, he or she must drink 3000 to 4000 ml of fluid daily to promote renal excretion of calcium and decrease the possibility of renal calculi formation. Synthetic calcitonin may be given to reduce gastrointestinal absorption, increase return of calcium to the bone, and promote renal excretion. Mithramycin, a cytotoxic antibiotic, inhibits bone resorption and thus lowers serum calcium. Corticosteroids may be used to decrease bone turnover and reabsorption in the kidney tubules. Weight-bearing exercise is encouraged to enhance bone mineralization. The underlying cause must be identified and treated (Box 8-12).

Magnesium

Magnesium (Mg) is the second most abundant intracellular cation. Approximately half of the magnesium in the body is contained in the bone, and 40% to 50% is found in the cells of the heart, liver, and skeletal muscle. Approximately 1% is found in the ECF. Normal serum magnesium is 1.8 to 2.4 mEq/L, and approximately one third of that is bound to plasma proteins (McCance, Huether, 1994). Magnesium depletion may be present even if levels are normal because such a small percentage is in the ECF sample that is analyzed. Magnesium activates many enzymes that are needed for carbohydrate and protein metabolism. Without magnesium, potassium is excreted to excess. Magnesium also influences the use of calcium and protein. It is involved in the sodium-potassium pump, which moves sodium out and potassium into the cells. Therefore it plays a crucial role in maintaining normal muscle and nerve activity. Neuromuscular excitability is profoundly affected by alterations in serum magnesium. Recent studies indicate that magnesium protects the heart from damage by influencing cardiac enzyme activity and calcium and potassium levels in myocardial and vascular muscle tissue. Magnesium is now used to treat patients with myocardial infarction to prevent further damage and fatal arrhythmias (Owens, 1993).

BOX 8-12 **Nursing Process**

CALCIUM EXCESS: HYPERCALCEMIA

ASSESSMENT

Serum calcium greater than 11 mg/dl
Lethargy
Decreased muscle tone
Deep bone pain
Flank pain
Kidney stones (renal calculi)
Hypertension
Nausea and vomiting
Thirst
Anorexia
Constipation
Psychoses
Coma, cardiac arrest

NURSING DIAGNOSIS

Risk for injury related to hypercalcemia

NURSING INTERVENTIONS

Eliminate calcium from diet.
Use caution if patient taking digitalis.
Monitor neurologic status.
Encourage patient to communicate these symptoms.
Medicate for pain as ordered.
Observe for passage of calculi.
Strain urine.
Monitor vital signs.
Provide IV isotonic saline as ordered or PO fluids if tolerated (3000-4000 ml daily).
Provide small, frequent meals.
Encourage mobility as patient condition permit.
Reorient patient to reality.
Maintain life support systems.
Support family members.

EVALUATION OF EXPECTED OUTCOMES

Calcium level within normal limits
Myocardial response to digitalis monitored; arrythmias prevented
Able to perform activities of daily living
Stones sent to laboratory if passed
Blood pressure within normal limits
Ouput equals intake
Hydrated and able to take diet
Optimum nutritional status maintained
Constipation decreased
Patient feels more secure, less fearful
System integrity maintained throughout hypercalcemic period
Family members able to voice their concerns

Magnesium deficit. A magnesium deficit (hypomagnesemia) is rarely the result of diet but does occur in cases of severe malnutrition, chronic alcoholism, prolonged diarrhea, intestinal malabsorption, prolonged nasogastric suction, and prolonged IV therapy that lacks magnesium. It is believed that chronic alcoholism accompanied by liver disease leads to a lack of digestive enzymes, which reduces magnesium absorption and causes a deficit. Hypoparathyroidism, prolonged diuretic therapy as with congestive heart failure, and the diuresing phase of renal failure can also produce a magnesium deficit. Patients with gastrointestinal cancer who are receiving chemotherapy are also at increased risk. The cancer interferes with absorption, and the patient is often anorexic, which further reduces magnesium intake.

Increased neuromuscular and central nervous system irritiability result from a magnesium deficit and produce symptoms similar to those of a calcium deficit, such as agitation, paresthesia, hyperreflexia, tremors, leg cramps, muscle twitching, jerking, tetany, and convulsions. Cardiac arrhythmias occur in severe cases. Serum calcium and magnesium levels can provide an accurate diagnosis (Box 8-13).

The patient with a magnesium deficit has discomfort as a result of neuromuscular excitability. The nurse should move the patient and handle his or her extremities gently. The nurse should also keep the room quiet and the lighting subdued to reduce stimulation. A linen cradle should also be used to reduce the weight of bed linens, which could provoke spasms. If a diet is allowed, give soft foods to prevent choking and aspiration from laryngeal or esophageal spasms.

Treatment of a mild deficit requires oral supplements and an increased intake of magnesium-rich foods such as nuts, bananas, peanut butter, whole grains, and green vegetables. Diet can be supplemented with magnesium-based antacids such as Mylanta, Gelusil, Maalox, or Milk of Magnesia. A more se-

BOX 8-13 **Nursing Process**

MAGNESIUM DEFICIT: HYPOMAGNESEMIA

ASSESSMENT

Serum Mg 1.0 mEq/L or less
Leg cramps, agitation
Esophageal and laryngeal spasm
Muscle twitching, hyperreflexia, jerking (tetany)
Convulsions

NURSING DIAGNOSIS

Risk for injury related to hypomagnesemia

NURSING INTERVENTIONS

Monitor serum Mg levels daily or after each 16 mEq supplement of Mg is administered.
Provide a bed cradle for linens, a quiet room, and subdued lighting.
Provide a soft diet if PO food allowed.
Check deep-tendon reflexes.
Administer Mg as ordered.
Monitor urine output and vital signs.

EVALUATION OF EXPECTED OUTCOMES

Serum Mg between 1.0 and 3.0 mEq/L
Agitation reduced; cramps not evident
Swallows without choking or aspirating food
Normotonic muscle activity
Urine output greater than 30 ml/hr or physician notified
Respiratory rate greater than 12 or physician notified
BP within normal limits

vere deficit requires IV or intramuscular administration of magnesium sulfate. Oral replacement can be used to prevent a deficit in individuals who are predisposed to a deficit.

Magnesium given intravenously must be given slowly to prevent cardiac or respiratory arrest. The patient receiving magnesium sulfate intravenously or intramuscularly must be observed closely to avoid excess. Renal function must be observed and the physician notified if output falls below 30 ml/h. Without adequate renal function, an excess can develop easily because magnesium is excreted by the kidneys. Vital signs and deep-tendon reflexes must be checked hourly. A decrease in blood pressure, weak or absent deep tendon reflexes, or a decrease in respirations below 12 per minute indicate toxicity. In addition, symptoms of flushing, generalized warmth, thirst, sweating, anxiety followed by lethargy, and decreased motor function should be reported immediately, and the drug should be discontinued. Toxicity can produce coma. In the event that toxicity develops, calcium gluconate should be administered because it antagonizes the action of magnesium and reverses the symptoms of toxicity. If calcium gluconate is administered via the same IV line used for the magnesium, the line must be flushed thoroughly before the calcium gluconate is added because the calcium will precipitate with the sulfates of the magnesium preparation and stop the infusion.

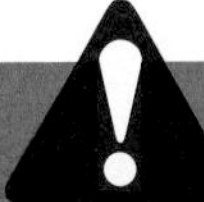

NURSE ALERT

Magnesium given intravenously must be administered slowly to prevent cardiac or respiratory arrest.

Magnesium excess. A magnesium excess (hypermagnesemia) is less common. It is found in patients with renal insufficiency who are unable to excrete magnesium adequately. It is also found in severely dehydrated patients who develop oliguria and magnesium retention. Patients with renal failure must avoid antacids that contain magnesium, such as Gelusil. A magnesium excess depresses neuromuscular and central nervous system functions. Symptoms include a generalized sense of warmth; decreased deep tendon reflexes, which lead to flaccid paralysis; low blood pressure; depressed respirations; and drowsiness and lethargy, which lead to coma and respiratory arrest (Box 8-14). The ECG reveals arrythmias, and cardiac arrest may result. Treatment must be aimed at correcting the underlying cause. Dialysis may be necessary to eliminate the excess and prevent life-threatening symptoms.

BOX 8-14 **Nursing Process**

MAGNESIUM EXCESS: HYPERMAGNESEMIA

ASSESSMENT

Serum Mg 3.0 mEq/L or more
Nausea and vomiting
Generalized sense of warmth
Decreased deep-tendon reflexes
Flaccid paralysis can develop
Low blood pressure
Depressed respirations
Respiratory arrest
Drowsiness and lethargy
Coma
Arrhythmias and cardiac arrest

NURSING DIAGNOSIS

Risk for injury related to hypermagnesemia

NURSING INTERVENTIONS

Monitor serum Mg levels.
Prepare patient for dialysis if ordered.
Observe and report sense of warmth.
Observe deep-tendon reflexes q 1 hr or as ordered.
Check movement of extremities.
Check BP q 1 hr or as ordered.
Monitor respirations; report drop to less than 14/min.
Monitor level of consciousness q 1 hr or as ordered.
Monitor cardiac rhythm.
Maintain life support systems.

EVALUATION OF EXPECTED OUTCOMES

Serum Mg between 1.0 and 3.0 mEq/L
Tolerating normal diet
No report of sense of warmth
Normotensive
Movement of extremities is retained
BP within normal limits
Respirations 14/min or above
Alert, oriented
Normal sinus rythym

Chloride

Chloride deficit. Chloride is the major extracellular anion. It is a component of hydrochloric acid in the stomach and plays a role in the transport of carbon dioxide by red blood cells. Chloride is excreted by the kidney and is affected by aldosterone secretion. When aldosterone is released to cause sodium reabsorption, chloride is also reabsorbed. Chloride is secreted into the gastrointestinal tract, and **hypochloremia** can occur if there is a loss of gastrointestinal secretions as seen in vomiting, diarrhea, and nasogastric suctioning. Plasma chloride levels change with and resemble sodium levels. Chloride is lost along with sodium in patients who are receiving diuretic therapy, but urinary loss of chloride may be greater than the loss of sodium. Gastric fluids contain a higher proportion of chloride, so a loss of gastrointestinal fluids causes more chloride than sodium to be lost. When chloride is depleted and unavailable for reabsorption with sodium, the bicarbonate ion is reabsorbed to maintain the cation-anion balance. The increase in bicarbonate may cause metabolic alkalosis. The normal chloride level is 96 to 106 mEq/L. Hypochloremia occurs at levels below 95 mEq/L. The symptoms of hypochloremia are the same as those of hyponatremia and metabolic alkalosis.

Chloride excess. **Hyperchloremia** occurs with hypernatremia because chloride ions move with sodium ions. Such movement occurs in a severely burned patient when fluid is remobilized from the edematous burned areas to the vascular compartments, usually a few days after the burn is sustained.

Hyperchloremia can also result from hyperaldosteronism or renal failure. Excessive aspirin ingestion and sodium polystyrene (Kayexalate), the drug used to treat hyperkalemia, can cause chloride excess. Excess chloride interferes with bicarbonate reabsorption and results in metabolic acidosis. Symptoms of hyperchloremia are those of acidosis: lethargy, confusion, weakness, and stupor. The patient's breathing becomes deep and labored as the lungs attempt to correct the problem by blowing off carbon dioxide to reduce carbonic acid. IV sodium bicarbonate is administered to return the pH to normal. The kidneys retain the bicarbonate and eliminate chloride. A change to slow, shallow breathing indicates that the patient has too much bicarbonate and is trying to conserve carbon dioxide to restore normal acidity. Frequent assessment is necessary.

Phosphates

Phosphate levels vary inversely with calcium levels. A high calcium level usually means a low phosphate level and vice versa. The parathyroid hormone that promotes calcium uptake also inhibits absorption of phosphate. Both electrolytes are deficient when the imbalance is caused by malnutrition or malabsorption.

Hypophosphatemia results from inadequate intake, poor absorption (e.g., shortening of the gastrointestinal tract), loss caused by thiazide diuretics, hyperparathyroidism, and lead poisoning. Alkalosis reduces serum phosphate levels. Hypophosphatemia is treated with supplements of oral sodium and potassium phosphates. (Neutra Phos K). Severe cases require the IV administration of sodium phosphate or potassium phosphate.

Hyperphosphatemia occurs most often in patients with renal failure. They also have hypocalcemia, and those symptoms are the most obvious. Patients with renal failure often take aluminum hydroxide or aluminum carbonate to bind phosphate in the gastrointestinal tract and prevent its absorption into the bloodstream.

PROTEIN IMBALANCES

Plasma proteins attract water and act as colloids, which creates colloidal osmotic pressure within the vascular system.

Hyperproteinemia (protein excess) is very rare but can occur with dehydration, which causes the blood to be more concentrated. Hypoproteinemia (protein deficit) can occur over a long period of time when intake is reduced, such as in anorexia, malnutrition, starvation, fad dieting, and true vegetarian diets. Gastrointestinal diseases involving poor absorption can result in a protein deficit. Surgery and severe burns require cell growth and repair, which increases the use of protein by the body. Inflammation can cause cell membrane changes, which allow protein to shift out of the ECF to a "third space," as is seen with ascites. The breakdown of protein increases with increased metabolic and catabolic states such as fever, infection, and certain malignancies. Hemorrhages can cause a protein deficit, and large amounts of protein, especially albumin, are lost through the kidneys in nephrotic syndrome.

Major abdominal or chest surgery (e.g., coronary bypass surgery) involves massive tissue trauma, inflammation, increased catabolism, and damage to red blood cells. This combination of factors may result in protein loss, and fluids may shift to tissues because of the reduction in colloidal osmotic pressure. Generalized edema develops (second spacing), and the blood pressure drops because of reduced intravascular volume. Urine output is low.

Symptoms of protein deficit include edema (from decreased colloidal osmotic pressure), slow healing, anorexia, fatigue, and anemia. The body eventually breaks down tissue to obtain needed protein, which results in muscle loss. Infusion of IV fluids most likely increases the edema rather than raises intravascular volume. Administration of albumin restores colloidal osmotic pressure, draws the fluids back from the tissues, raises blood volume and blood pressure, and increases urinary output. The nurse should be alert to the development of and increase in edema in a postsurgical patient. A high carbohydrate, high protein diet with protein supplements is required to treat a protein deficit. Hyperalimentation may be necessary if the patient is unable to eat a normal diet or if the gastrointestinal system is not functioning.

ACID-BASE IMBALANCE

Hydrogen Ion Concentration

The normal composition of body fluids depends not only on the volume of fluid and concentration of various electrolytes but also on the concentration of the acids and bases, or alkalies, in the body. *Acids* are substances that can release hydrogen ions (H^+), and *bases* are substances that can accept hydrogen ions. It is the concentration of hydrogen ions that determines whether a solution is acidic, basic, or neutral. The pH scale measures the amount of acidity or alkalinity of fluids. On a scale of 1 to 14, a pH of 7 is neutral. Anything below 7 is considered acidic, and anything above 7 is considered alkaline. The normal pH of ECF ranges from 7.35 to 7.45 and therefore is slightly alkaline. The normal range that can support life is from 6.8 to 7.8.

Acid-Base Regulation

The body controls pH with buffer systems, the lungs, and the kidneys. The buffers react immediately. The respiratory system responds within minutes and begins to lose effectiveness in a few hours. The kidneys take 2 to 3 days to reach maximum response but can maintain the balance for a long period of time. If a problem exists with respiratory or kidney function, the body may not be able to successfully regulate acid-base balance.

Buffer systems

The buffer system is the primary regulator of acid-base balance. Buffers react with an acid or base to prevent a large change in pH. They act chemically to change strong acids into weaker acids or to bind with acids to neutralize their effect.

The primary buffer is the carbonic acid/bicarbonate system. Bicarbonate neutralizes hydrochloric acid (HCl) by combining with it and changing it to a weaker acid (carbonic acid) and a salt (NaCl). A ratio of 20 parts of bicarbonate to 1 part carbonic acid maintains an adequate supply of bicarbonate to combine with and neutralize acids. The carbonic acid that is formed is broken down to water and carbon dioxide (CO_2). CO_2 is excreted by the lungs, and water is excreted by the lungs and kidneys. This action maintains the 20:1 ratio and the normal pH. A second buffer, the phosphate buffer system, works in a similar way.

The intracellular and extracellular proteins are also buffers. Their amino acids include free acid radicals, which can contribute hydrogen ions, and free basic radicals, which can dissociate and combine with hydrogen to form water. Hemoglobin is also a buffer. It regulates pH by shifting chloride in and out of red blood cells in exchange for bicarbonate. The level of oxygen in the blood triggers this chloride shift, which is capable of raising or lowering bicarbonate levels as needed. The cell acts as a buffer by shifting hydrogen into and out of the cell. If hydrogen is increased in the ECF, the cell accepts hydrogen in exchange for another cation, which is usually potassium because it is abundant in the cell.

Pulmonary system

The lungs help maintain acid-base balance by controlling the amount of carbon dioxide that is released into the air during respiration. Carbonic acid in the ECF of the pulmonary capillaries dissociates into CO_2 and water. When respiration is suppressed, carbonic acid accumulates in the body fluids because less CO_2 is excreted. When respirations are stimulated, the levels of carbonic acid within the body fall. The rate and depth of respiration and thus excretion is regulated by the respiratory center in the medulla in the brain, which is triggered by the level of CO_2 and hydrogen ions.

Renal system

The kidneys selectively excrete or resorb bicarbonate and excrete hydrogen ions as needed by the body.

Alterations in Acid-Base Balance

Two general types of disturbances in the body result in an upset of the balance between the base bicarbonate and the carbonic acid. Body metabolic processes add base bicarbonate to or subtract it from the ECF. The respiratory process adds carbonic acid to or subtracts it from the ECF. Metabolic processes can also produce acid. Therefore a state of acidosis can be caused by lowering the amount of base bicarbonate or by increasing the amount of carbonic acid or metabolic acids. A state of alkalosis can be caused by increasing the amount of base bicarbonate or decreasing the amount of carbonic acid. Each of these conditions alters the ratio of base bicarbonate to carbonic acid. Acid-base imbalances can take one or a combination of these forms, each of which alters the ratio of base bicarbonate to carbonic acid.

Metabolic acidosis

A base bicarbonate deficit, or metabolic acidosis, can result either from the accumulation of too many acid by-products of metabolism or from the loss of bicarbonate. Abnormal metabolic processes such as diabetes, renal insufficiency or failure, and shock produce metabolic acidosis by the accumulation of acids within the body. Anaerobic metabolism produces lactic acidosis, and fasting or starvation can produce ketosis. Excessive bicarbonate is lost in renal insufficiency and severe diarrhea; via ileostomies, ureterosigmoidostomy, intestinal or biliary fistulas, and intestinal suction; and as a result of increased chloride levels.

The laboratory test used to differentiate between the two types of metabolic acidosis is the *anion gap* (or *R factor*). The anion gap is the difference between the concentration of the cations (sodium and potassium) and the sum of the chloride and bicarbonate anions. This difference reflects the concentration of anions in the ECF. When metabolic acidosis is caused by a loss of bicarbonate, the anion gap is normal at 13 mEq/L or below. When the cause is an excess of metabolic acids, the gap is increased above 13 mEq/L. Acidosis resulting from bicarbonate loss is called *normal anion gap acidosis;* acidosis resulting from excess metabolic acid is called *high anion gap acidosis.*

Signs of metabolic acidosis include deep, rapid respirations; weakness; disorientation; diarrhea; and drowsiness leading to stupor and coma. Any state of acidosis depresses the central nervous system. The lungs attempt to compensate for the state of acidosis by increasing the rate and depth of respirations, which reduces the amount of carbonic acid in the system. This type of breathing is known as *Kussmaul's respiration.* The serum pH level is below 7.35, the pH of the urine is lower than normal, and the serum bicarbonate level is decreased or normal, depending on the cause. Serum potassium levels are elevated when acidosis occurs.

BOX 8-15 **Nursing Process**

METABOLIC ACIDOSIS: BASE BICARBONATE DEFICIT OR METABOLIC ACID EXCESS

ASSESSMENT

Serum pH less than 7.35
Low urine pH
Decreased serum bicarbonate
Increased serum potassium
Blood CO_2 decreased
Diarrhea
Increased rate and depth of respirations
Weakness, drowsiness
Disorientation
Shock
Stupor
Coma

NURSING DIAGNOSIS

Risk for injury related to metabolic acidosis

NURSING INTERVENTIONS

Monitor pH and potassium values.
Keep bicarbonate readily available.
Monitor laboratory results.
Monitor heart rhythm.
Maintain accurate I&O records.
Monitor vital signs.
Monitor neurologic status and level of consciousness.
Observe orientation.
Observe for decreased BP/increased pulse.
Administer medications as ordered to correct metabolic acidosis.
Maintain life support systems.

EVALUATION OF EXPECTED OUTCOMES

Patient's response monitored
pH within normal limits
Serum potassium within normal limits
IV fluids administered at prescribed rate
ECF volume deficit avoided
Respiratory compensation for metabolic imbalances observed
Alert and oriented
Safety maintained
Shock prevented
Patient more alert
Integrity of body systems maintained

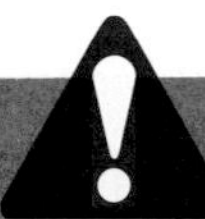

NURSE ALERT

A patient using an increased rate and depth of respirations (Kussmaul's respiration) is trying to correct metabolic acidosis by eliminating additional CO_2

Appropriate therapy for metabolic acidosis is treatment of the underlying cause. Bicarbonate can be given intravenously to counteract the excessive acids in the blood. Often sodium lactate is given because the liver metabolizes sodium lactate into bicarbonate. In renal failure, dialysis may be the treatment of choice (Box 8-15).

Metabolic alkalosis

A base bicarbonate excess, or metabolic alkalosis, can result either from the loss of acid in the body or from the accumulation of bases in the blood. Loss of acid can occur with excessive vomiting or from gastric suction, which removes the upper gastrointestinal secretions that are high in hydrochloric acid. Administration of potent diuretics can cause a loss of hydrogen and chloride ions and result in a relative increase of bicarbonate in the blood. Ingestion of an excessive amount of sodium bicarbonate or antacids causes accumulation of base in the ECF.

The major signs and symptoms of metabolic alkalosis include nausea, vomiting, and diarrhea. Muscles cramp and have increased tone, and symptoms similar to tetany may appear. Often patients are confused and irritable, and convulsions can occur. The lungs attempt to compensate by decreasing the rate and depth of respiration to conserve carbonic acid. Plasma bicarbonate levels, serum pH, and urine pH are increased. Plasma potassium levels are lowered in alkalosis.

The underlying cause of metabolic alkalosis must be determined and treated. Excessive losses should be replaced, and acidifying solutions can be given orally or intravenously. The specific treatment depends on the cause (Box 8-16).

BOX 8-16 **Nursing Process**

METABOLIC ALKALOSIS: BASE BICARBONATE EXCESS

ASSESSMENT

Serum pH greater than 7.45
Increased urine pH
Increased serum bicarbonate
Decreased serum potassium (<4 mE q/L)
Blood CO_2 tension increased
Nausea and vomiting
Diarrhea
Decreased rate and depth of respirations
Confusion
Irritability
Increased muscular tone and cramps
Twitching
Tingling, numbness (tetany)
Convulsions

NURSING DIAGNOSIS

Risk for injury related to metabolic alkalosis

NURSING INTERVENTIONS

Monitor laboratory values.
Observe for signs of hypokalemia.
Monitor administration of IV fluids.
Maintain accurate I&O records.
Monitor vital signs.
Monitor neurologic status.
Orient patient to reality.
Observe change in level of consciousness.
Maintain quiet environment.
Administer muscle relaxants as ordered.
Observe for signs of increased muscle tone and cramps, indicating tetany.
Establish seizure precautions.

EVALUATION OF EXPECTED OUTCOMES

Patient's response monitored
Abnormal laboratory results communicated
Serum potassium within normal limits
Fluid balance maintained
Respiratory compensation for metabolic imbalance observed
Patient more assured, less fearful
Decreased need for psychotropic agents
Decreased oxygen need; conservation of patient's energy
Injury prevented

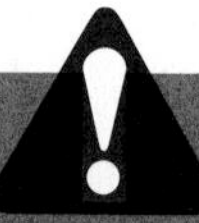

NURSE ALERT

Hyperventilation results in respiratory alkalosis. Have patient use a brown bag to rebreathe CO_2 and restore carbonic acid.

Respiratory alkalosis

A carbonic acid deficit, or respiratory alakalosis, is caused primarily by hyperventilation, which can result from anxiety, fever, or lack of oxygen. Some drugs can stimulate the respiratory center and cause hyperventilation. Too much CO_2 is excreted during hyperventilation, so carbonic acid levels decrease. Common symptoms of respiratory alkalosis are related to increased neuromuscular irritability and include headache, dizziness, paresthesias, tingling of the fingertips and around the mouth, and tetany. The blood pH is above normal, the blood gas CO_2 level is low, and the urine pH increased. The bicarbonate level of the plasma may be normal or slightly lowered. Serum potassium levels are usually lowered in alkalosis. Treatment consists of sedation, emotional support, and the use of a bag to rebreathe exhaled CO_2 (Box 8-17).

Respiratory acidosis

A carbonic acid excess, or respiratory acidosis, is caused by any condition that interferes with the normal release of CO_2 from the lungs. Emphysema, bronchitis, pneumonia, and asthma are conditions that interfere with the normal transport of gases across the pulmonary membrane. In addition, sedatives, narcotics (morphine), and brain trauma may affect the respiratory center in the medulla and depress respirations. Carbonic acid levels increase. Patients become weak, restless, drowsy, disoriented, and may lose consciousness. Headache and muscle twitching may lead to convulsions. The pulse rate increases, and arrhythmias may occur. Cyanosis is usually a late sign. The plasma pH is low, and the

BOX 8-17 **Nursing Process**

RESPIRATORY ALKALOSIS: CARBONIC ACID DEFICIT

ASSESSMENT

Elevated blood pH
Decreased serum CO_2
Increased urine pH
Plasma bicarbonate normal or slightly decreased
Serum potassium lowered
Headache
Dizziness
Paresthesias
Tingling, numbness (tetany)

NURSING DIAGNOSIS

Risk for injury related to respiratory alkalosis

NURSING INTERVENTIONS

Monitor laboratory values.
Observe patient for signs and symptoms of primary disease process that could contribute to respiratory alkalosis.
Administer pain medication as ordered.
Reassure patient.
Educate patient concerning breathing techniques.
Monitor sensorium.
Observe for signs of tetany.

EVALUATION OF EXPECTED OUTCOMES

Patient's response monitored
Treatment of primary disease with correction of carbonic acid deficit
Headache controlled
Hyperventilation decreased
Oxygenation improved
Alert/oriented
Injury prevented

blood gas CO_2 level is elevated. The bicarbonate level is normal or elevated in an attempt to compensate. Serum potassium is usually elevated during acidotic states.

Severe respiratory acidosis can be an emergency. Treatment measures should first involve improvement of ventilation, and mechanical ventilation may be necessary (Box 8-18).

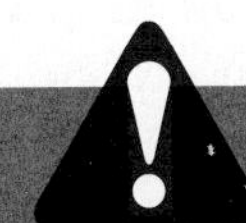

NURSE ALERT

Hypoventilation results in respiratory acidosis. If patient demonstrates slow, weak respirations or signs of hypoxia, look for respiratory acidosis.

Interpretation of Blood Gas Values

When evaluating laboratory reports of blood gas values, the nurse should first determine if the pH level is normal or indicates acidosis (below 7.35) or alkalosis (above 7.45). The nurse should next evaluate the bicarbonate and carbonic acid levels. Normal bicarbonate is 22 to 26 mEq/L. Carbonic acid is measured by the $PaCO_2$, and its normal range is 35 to 45. If the pH indicates acidosis and the bicarbonate level is low and the carbonic acid or $PaCO_2$ level is normal, the patient has a base bicarbonate deficit, or metabolic acidosis. If the pH indicates acidosis and both bicarbonate and carbonic acid are normal, the cause is excess metabolic acid, or metabolic acidosis. If the pH level indicates acidosis and the carbonic acid level is high while the bicarbonate is normal, the patient has a carbonic acid excess, or respiratory acidosis. With an alkaline pH level, a high bicarbonate level indicates metabolic alkalosis, and a low carbonic acid level indicates respiratory alkalosis (Box 8-19).

Compensation

The "normal" value in each of these situations gradually becomes abnormal in an attempt to compensate by balancing carbonic acid and base bicarbonate levels. This compensation causes the pH to move toward normal. Because balance is being attempted but has not yet been achieved (pH is still abnormal), this state is termed *partially compensated*. Once the pH has returned to normal, the state is called *compensated* because even though the bicarbonate and carbonic acid levels may be abnormal, they have achieved a proper balance. With continued treatment, these levels are returned to normal while a normal pH is maintained.

BOX 8-18 **Nursing Process**

RESPIRATORY ACIDOSIS: CARBONIC ACID EXCESS

ASSESSMENT

Decreased blood pH
Increased serum CO_2
Plasma bicarbonate normal or increased
Serum potassium increased
Weakness
Restlessness
Disorientation, drowsy
Headache
Muscle twitching
Convulsions
Increased pulse
Arrhythmias
Cyanosis

NURSING DIAGNOSIS

Risk for injury related to respiratory acidosis

NURSING INTERVENTIONS

Monitor laboratory values.
Maintain patent airway.
Provide suction as necessary.
Monitor administration of IV fluids.
Assist with transfer.
Provide oxygen as ordered.
Provide emotional support.
Monitor neurologic status.
Provide reorientation.
Establish seizure precautions.
Monitor vital signs.
Administer medications as ordered.
Perform chest percussion and postural drainage as ordered.
Place patient in semi-Fowler's position if indicated.

EVALUATION OF EXPECTED OUTCOMES

Arterial blood gases within normal limits
Serum potassium decreased via the dilutional effect of IV fluids
Prevention of injury
Oxygen level increased
Patient verbalizes increased awareness of environment
Prevention of injury
Arrhythmias avoided
Transport of gases across the pulmonary membrane facilitated

INTRAVENOUS THERAPY

IV therapy is a primary therapeutic technique that is used to treat patients with fluid and electrolyte imbalances or to prevent their occurence. Three types of solutions are commonly used and are categorized according to the strength of their composition, or their osmolarity (Box 8-20).

Types of Solutions

Isotonic, or isoosmolar, solutions have the same tonicity as plasma. No osmosis occurs between two isotonic solutions when they are separated by a membrane, such as a cell membrane. These solutions are similar to normal blood plasma. They provide water, electrolytes, and carbohydrates and do not change body osmolarity.

Hypertonic, or hyperosmolar, solutions are stronger than isotonic solutions because they have more solutes dissolved in them per unit of volume. When introduced into the plasma they send electrolytes into the cell via diffusion and draw water from the interstitial space and from the cells via osmosis, thus expanding plasma volume even more.

Hypotonic, or hypoosmolar, solutions are weaker than isotonic and hypertonic solutions. Osmosis causes the fluid to enter the cell in an attempt to equalize the concentration of solutes on either side of the cell membrane. Therefore these fluids cause cellular hydration and stimulate kidney function. These solutions usually contain carbohydrates in water or hypotonic saline. The carbohydrate is metabolized, and the water is free to be absorbed by the cells or is eliminated.

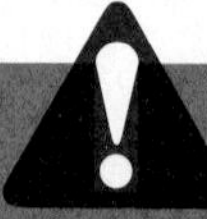

NURSE ALERT

Do not administer 5% dextrose/water or other hypotonic intravenous solutions to patients with stroke or head injury. Such solutions enter the cell and increase cerebral edema and intracranial pressure.

BOX 8-19

BLOOD GAS INTERPRETATION*

1 Is pH acid or alkaline? (normal range 7.35-7.45)
Give it a name: acidosis or alkalosis
2 Look for the cause: acidosis results from ⇑ acid or ⇓base; alkalosis results from ⇓acid or ⇑ base.
Therefore check the levels of bicarbonate and carbonic acid.
3 Is bicarbonate (HCO_3^-) normal? (22-26 mEg/L)
If yes, go on.
If no, is it high or low? Does it explain the condition named in step 1? (Example: If acidosis, a low bicarb could explain the cause; a high bicarb would not *cause* acidosis)
4 Is carbonic acid ($Paco_2$) normal? (35-45 mm Hg)
If yes, go back to bicarb level.
If no, is it high or low? Does it explain the condition? (Example: If acidosis, a high carbonic acid level could explain the cause; a low carbonic acid level would not cause acidosis)
5 Give it another name related to the possible cause. If it is caused by a change in bicarb, it is a metabolic imbalance. If it is caused by a change in carbonic acid, it is a respiratory imbalance.
Acidosis with bicarb ⇓ = metabolic acidosis
Acidosis with carbonic acid ⇑ = respiratory acidosis
Alkalosis with bicarb ⇑ = metabolic alkalosis
Alakalosis with carbonic acid ⇓ = respiratory alkalosis
The second name comes from the possible cause.
6 Look for compensation.
Metabolic acidosis, carbonic acid ⇓ (to compensate)
Metabolic alkalosis, carbonic acid ⇑
Respiratory acidosis, bicarb ⇑
Respiratory alkalosis, bicarb ⇓
If pH is abnormal, it is uncompensated.
If pH is normal and carbonic acid or bicarb abnormal, it is compensated.
7 There are now three names:

Compensated or Uncompensated	choose this name last
Respiratory or Metabolic	choose one of these names second
Acidosis or Alkalosis	choose one of these names first

Exercises: Assign three names to the following:

	pH	HCO_3^-	CO_2
	7.23	14	32
	7.10	28	63
	7.51	25	26
	7.55	34	43
	7.36	34	56

*Answers are in Instructor's Resource Manual.

When administering IV fluids, it is important to provide adequate fluids for hydration while preventing fluid overload. Too much fluid (fluid overload) decreases the normal body osmolality. A high body osmolality indicates dehydration. A patient's osmolality can be determined by a formula that is based on sodium, blood urea nitrogen (BUN), and blood glucose levels (Box 8-21). A shortcut calculation is based on the sodium level only (sodium level × 2 = approximate body osmolality). Normal body osmolality is between 275 and 295 mOsm/L.

Techniques and Equipment

Fluids are introduced into veins through metal needles or through plastic cannulas that are inserted by sliding them over a metal needle. If a vein cannot be accessed, a cutdown may be necessary, which requires making a small incision into the vein to insert the catheter. An IV infusion tubing set and a bottle or plastic bag filled with the appropriate solution are prepared before the procedure is started (Figure 8-7). The clamp on the tubing is closed, the tubing is connected to the bag, and the clamp is opened to fill the tubing with fluid. A vein is selected and the site is cleansed. Any long hairs in the area are cut. Figure 8-8 illustrates the sites commonly used for intravenous infusion. The needle is inserted, and the over-the-needle cannula, if present, is advanced into the vein. The needle adapter of the infusion set is connected to the hub of the catheter. The fluid is started, and a proper flow rate is established. The catheter is secured with narrow

BOX 8-20

PARENTERAL SOLUTIONS

Hypotonic solutions (0.45% saline, D5%/0.45% saline, 2.5% dextrose, 0.33% saline), D5%/W*)
- Decrease intravascular osmolarity
- Result in intracellular hydration
- Used for cellular dehydration
- Complications: shock and increased intracranial pressure
- Contraindications: anasarca (total body edema), cerebral edema, hypotension

Hypertonic solutions (D10%/NS, D5%/NS, D5%/RL, 8% amino acids)
- Increase intravascular osmolarity
- Result in intracellular and interstitial dehydration
- Used for intravascular expansion by shifting intracellular and interstitial fluids
- Complications: circulatory overload
- Contraindications: intracellular dehydration, hyperosmolar states

Istonic solutions (Normal saline, Ringer's solution, lactated Ringer's solution, 10% Dextran 40 in 0.9% sodium chloride)
- Do not change osmolarity
- Results in total body water (TBW) expansion
- Complications: circulatory overload
- Contraindications: circulatory overload; do not give Ringer's lactate in alkalosis

BOX 8-21

NORMAL BODY OSMOLALITY

To calculate serum osmolality, use this formula:

$$2\ \text{Na} + \frac{\text{BUN}}{5} + \frac{\text{Glucose}}{20} = 275 \text{ to } 295 \text{ mOsm/L}.$$

Or use this shortcut:

$2 \times \text{Na} = \text{osmolality}$

Example: if Na = 139, osmolality = 278

Serum osmolality < 275 mOsm/L, fluid overload

Serum osmolality > 295 mOsm/L, dehydration

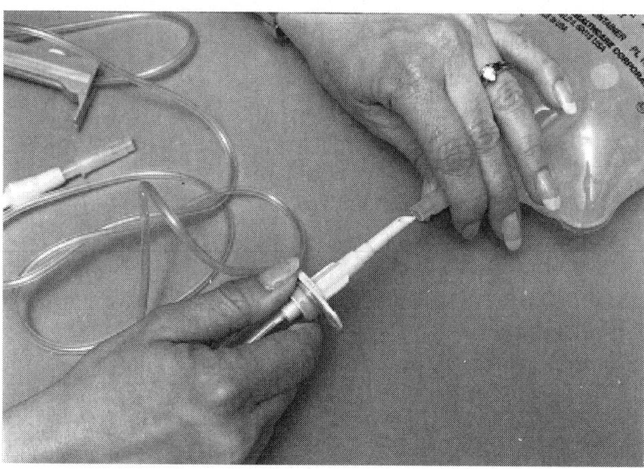

Figure 8-7 Tubing insertion site is inserted into bag. Tubing clamp is opened slowly. Tubing is filled with IV fluid in preparation for attachment of the needle adapter of the infusion set to the hub of the cannula that is inserted in the vein. (From Potter PA, Perry AG: *Basic nursing: theory and practice,* ed 3, St Louis, 1995, Mosby.)

tape and covered with a transparent or gauze dressing (Figure 8-9).

Complications

Local

The nurse observes and monitors the patient's IV fluids. The prescribed flow rate must be regulated. The IV site is watched for infiltration, which is caused by displacement of the IV needle from the vein into the surrounding tissue. Infiltration is characterized by swelling of the affected tissue. The patient may experience a burning sensation at the needle site. The infiltrated site is pale, cool, edematous, and is firm or hard to the touch. To confirm infiltration, a tourniquet can be applied above the infusion site. The solution continues to flow if the solution is infiltrating the surrounding tissues but will stop flowing if the needle is still in the vein. If infiltration is confirmed, the IV line must be discontinued and restarted at another site. Warm compresses can be applied to the infiltrated site to promote reabsorption of the IV fluid.

Thrombophlebitis is a more common complication in which the vein becomes inflamed and a clot forms. Redness, warmth, and edema occur at the injection site, and the patient complains of pain along the vein. When thrombophlebitis occurs, the IV infusion should be discontinued, and warm, moist compresses should be applied to reduce pain and stimulate healing.

Systemic

Systemic complications may occur from IV infusions and include fluid overload (circulatory overhead), embolism, and infection. Nurses should be continuously alert for symptoms of circulatory overload, which include respiratory distress and increased venous pressure. Shortness of breath, increased respirations, coughing, increased blood pressure, bounding pulse, and distended veins can also signal circulatory overload. If infusion continues, pulmonary edema can result.

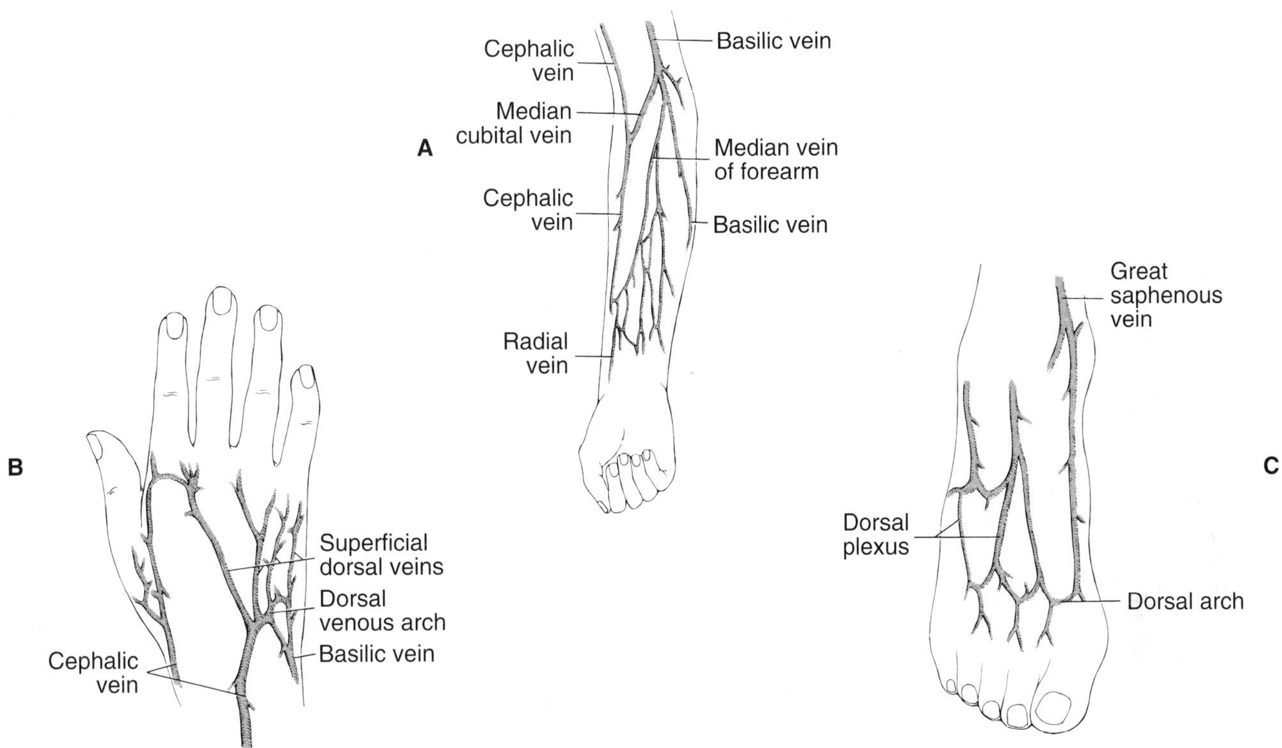

Figure 8-8 Common intravenous sites. **A,** Inner arm. **B,** Dorsal surface of hand. **C,** Dorsal surface of foot (used primarily for pediatric clients). (From Potter PA, Perry AG: *Basic nursing: theory and practice,* ed 3, St Louis, 1995, Mosby.)

Air embolism occasionally occurs when substantial amounts of air enter the blood through an improperly running infusion. The apparatus should be checked often, and the infusion should be stopped or the solution changed before the bottle and tubing are empty. Such actions prevent air from entering the vein. Sudden vascular collapse can occur from air embolism, with the patient showing signs of shock and loss of consciousness.

A pulmonary embolism results if the clot that forms in the process of thrombophlebitis breaks loose and travels to the lungs. Sudden and severe respiratory distress is an indication of pulmonary embolism and requires emergency treatment. If nausea, vomiting, an increased pulse rate, and chills occur, the patient may be experiencing a systemic infection. The infusion is stopped immediately, and the physician is called.

Central Venous Lines

Fluids can also be infused through central venous lines. In the operating room the doctor inserts a catheter into the right atrium of the heart, usually through the subclavian vein. These catheters can remain in place for long periods, which reduces the need for frequent venipuncture. These catheters can have more than one lumen to allow infusion of multiple solutions and/or medications. Using strict aseptic technique, the site must be cleansed and dressed regularly and observed for signs of infection (Figures 8-10, *A* and 8-11).

Peripherally Inserted Central Catheter

Central lines can also be introduced in a peripheral brachial vein and inserted into the right atrium. These can be inserted by the registered nurse, but correct placement must be verified by x-ray before the line is used (Figure 8-10, *B*).

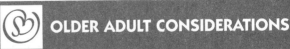

OLDER ADULT CONSIDERATIONS

Cardiac function may be compromised in an older adult, resulting in a reduced ability to pump normal fluid volume. IV fluids must be given more slowly to avoid fluid overload. Monitor respirations and neck vein distention closely during IV administration to avoid fluid overload and pulmonary edema.

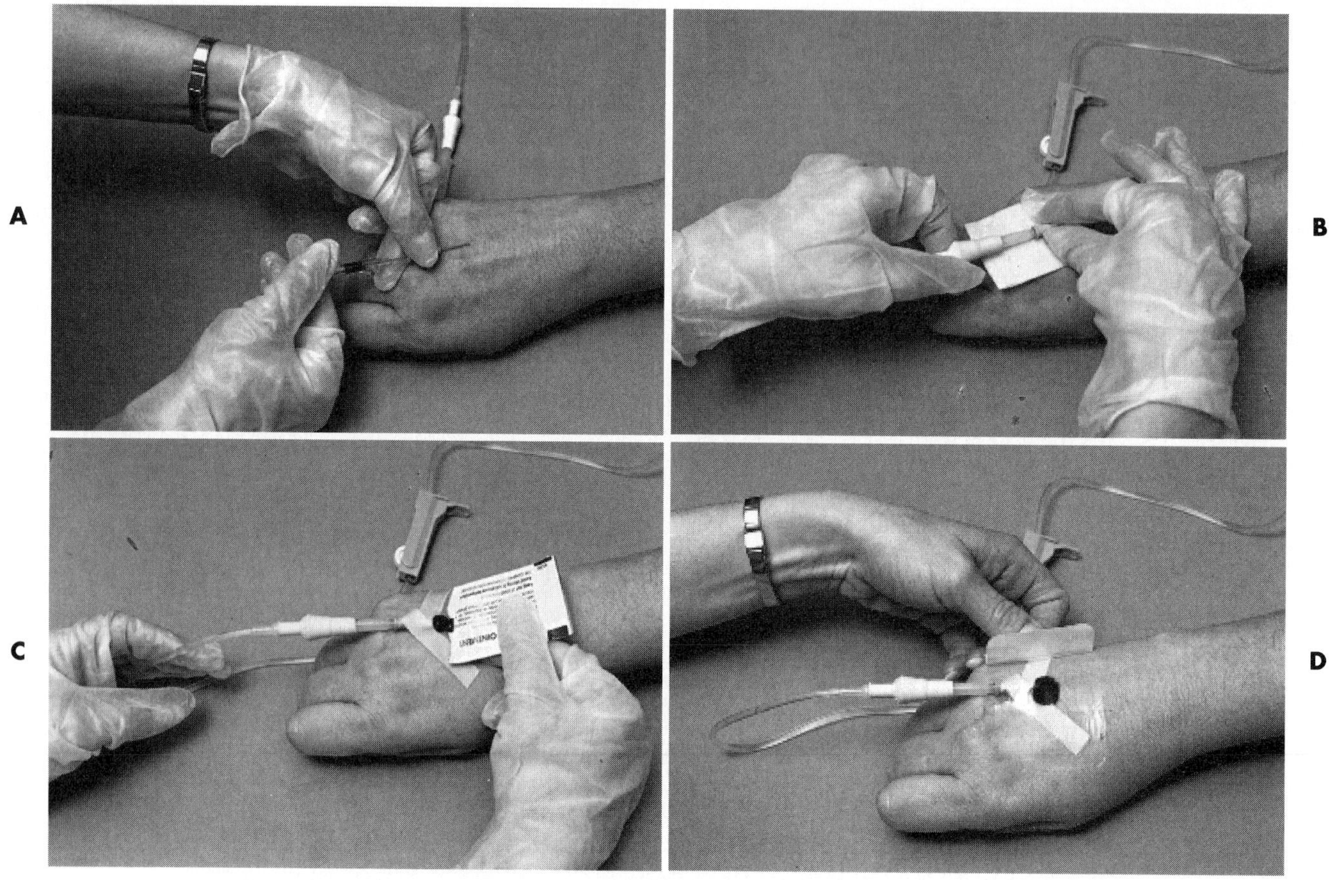

Figure 8-9 **A,** Venipuncture, using needle. An over-the-needle catheter (ONC) will be advanced into the vein. **B,** Needle adapter of infusion set is connected to hub of ONC. **C,** Needle hub is secured with a narrow (½ inch) piece of tape. Tape is placed adhesive-side-up under hub, then crossed over catheter hub. Povidine-iodine ointment may be placed on insertion site. A second piece of narrow tape may be placed over hub. **D,** Transparent dressing is placed over IV site in direction of hair growth (e.g., from inner to outer aspect of hand). The connection between the IV tubing and catheter hub should not be covered with the clear dressing. (From Potter PA, Perry AG: *Basic nursing: theory and practice,* ed 3, St Louis, 1995, Mosby.)

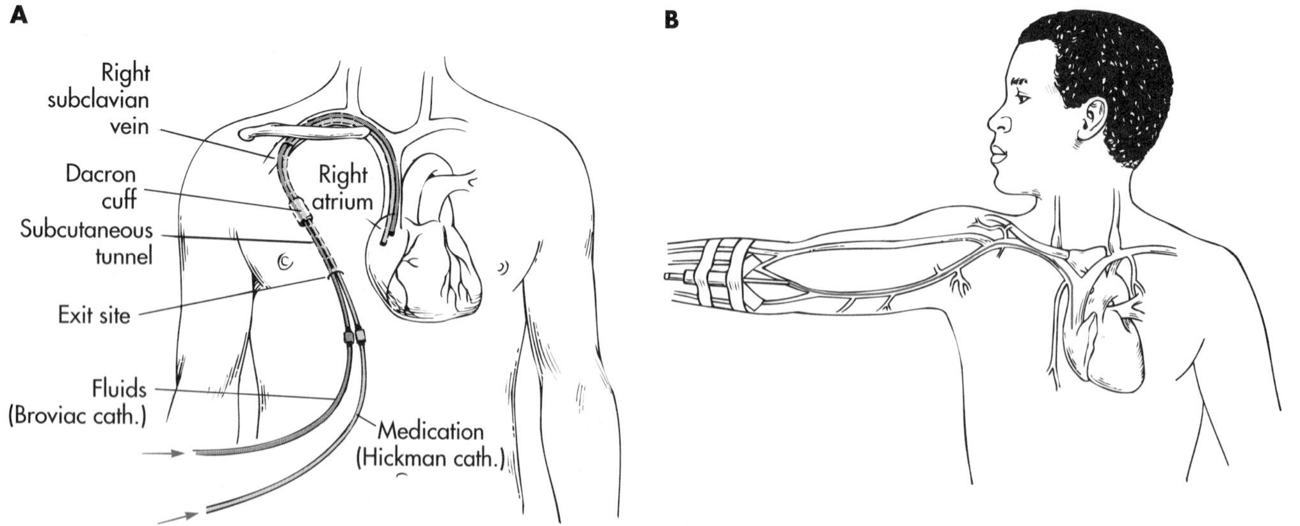

Figure 8-10 **A,** Central venous catheter. Double lumen. **B,** Peripherally inserted central catheter.

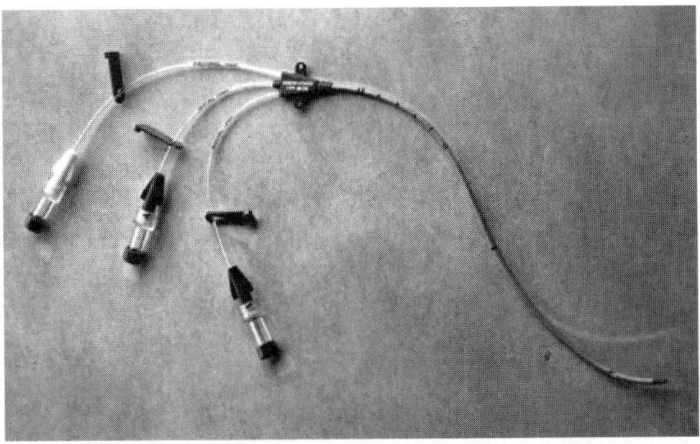

Figure 8-11 ARROWg+arg Blue™ Antiseptic Surface Triple Lumen Catheter. (Printed with permission by Arrow International, Inc.)

SHOCK

The basic abnormality that occurs when a state of shock develops is an imbalance between the tissue needs and its supply of adequately oxygenated blood. Contributing to this is a disproportion between the volume of blood and the vascular space in which it is circulating. Lack of oxygen results and leads to altered chemical activity within all the cells of the body. Normal metabolic processes that produce the energy needed for work within the cell are interrupted. Lactic acid is produced, which diffuses out of the cells into the ECF, causing a state of acidosis.

Body Response to Shock

Although the causes of various forms of shock differ, many of the compensatory mechanisms that counteract the effects of shock are the same. Loss of fluid volume or a disproportion between fluid volume and the size of the vascular space causes the blood pressure regulatory mechanisms to react.

Decreasing blood pressure excites the vasoconstrictor center of the brain (medulla oblongata), and epinephrine and norepinephrine are released from the adrenal medulla. The effect is vasoconstriction of the peripheral blood vessels and an increased heart rate and strength of the contraction. These mechanisms may be successful in elevating the blood pressure and increasing the cardiac output in mild shock. The kidneys secrete the hormone renin when the blood pressure falls. Renin produces angiotensin, which is a powerful vasoconstrictor for peripheral arterioles (Immunosuppression: septic shock in the E.D., 1993). To return the blood volume to normal, the body releases aldosterone from the adrenal cortex, which causes sodium reabsorption and water retention by the kidney tubules. This increases ECF and blood volume and decreases urinary output.

Assessment of Shock

The signs and symptoms of shock are similar, regardless of the cause. The basic property of shock is decreased blood flow and therefore decreased delivery of oxygen, nutrients, hormones, and electrolytes to the cells. There is also a decreased removal of metabolic wastes. Signs of shock are a direct result of the body's attempt to counteract the effects of decreasing cardiac output.

Subtle, early signs of shock include an increased pulse rate, increased respirations, a mild drop in blood pressure, oliguria, and restlessness. Weakness; lethargy; pallor; cool, moist skin; rapid, shallow respirations; decreasing body temperature; a rapid, thready pulse; and progressively decreasing blood pressure with a narrowing pulse pressure occur later. Pulse pressure is the difference between the systolic and diastolic blood pressures. A normal pulse pressure is 40 mm Hg. For example, a blood pressure of 128/88 would produce a pulse pressure of 40. Pulse pressure narrows in early shock because of a decreased systolic blood pressure.

Types of Shock

Hypovolemic shock

Shock can be classified in several ways. **Hypovolemic shock** results from a loss of fluid available to the circulation. It is caused most often by hemorrhage but can also result from the loss of body fluids such as in dehydration caused by diabetic ketoacidosis; severe, extended vomiting; or diarrhea. Burns and other trauma can trap fluid at the site of the injury and decrease the volume of the bloodstream. Tissue injury that occurs during trauma or surgery can increase the permeability of capillary membranes and allow albumin to leave the circulating blood. This disturbs plasma colloid osmotic pressure and allows fluid to shift from the circulation to the tissues (see Figure 8-3). Hypovolemia results, and shock is a potential danger.

Hypovolemic shock is an extension of fluid volume deficit. Loss of plasma results in hemoconcentration. Loss of fluid volume results in less venous blood returning to the right side of the heart. Therefore less blood is pumped out of the heart into the vascular system. Insufficient oxygen is provided to the body cells and abnormal metabolic processes result, which leads to metabolic acidosis.

Assessment. An objective assessment includes location, quality, and rate of pulse. The location of a pulse that can be palpated can give an estimate of the patient's blood pressure (Box 8-22).

Signs and symptoms of hypovolemic shock are decreased level of consciousness; uncontrolled bleeding; tachycardia; hypotension; prolonged capillary refill; and cool, pale skin. A person in hypovolemic shock

BOX 8-22

ESTIMATING BLOOD PRESSURE

Pulse Site	Estimated Systolic Blood Pressure
Carotid	60 mm Hg
Femoral	70 mm Hg
Radial	80 mm Hg

If a radial pulse is present, the systolic pressure is at least 80 mm Hg. If a radial pulse is absent but a femoral pulse is present, the estimated systolic pressure is 70 mm Hg. If radial and femoral pulses are absent but a carotid pulse is present, the estimated systolic pressure is 60 mm Hg.

has flat neck veins. A condition that mimics shock, such as a cardiac tamponade, results in distended neck veins and distant (muffled or quieter) heart sounds.

Intervention. Prevention of shock is the best possible treatment. Shock must be anticipated as a possible complication afer surgery or in any condition that involves a significant blood loss. Early signs of shock should be observed and treatment instituted before the condition becomes life threatening.

The primary objective in treatment is to restore adequate tissue perfusion of oxygenated blood. The blood volume must be restored and the hemorrhage controlled. If uncontrolled bleeding is the cause of hypovolemic shock, bleeding must be controlled or stopped. Applying pressure to the artery that supplies the area of uncontrolled bleeding reduces blood flow (see Chapter 19). The hand or an additional firm object is held on the artery to compress it against the bone that lays behind it. A tourniquet is a last resort because it is likely to result in loss of the extremity. The patient is given oxygen at a rate of at least 6 L/min. A large bore needle is used to initiate an IV line, usually in the antecubital space, because it is likely that blood products will be given. Ringer's lactate or normal saline are the usual fluids ordered.

Patients should be kept flat, and those who do not have head injuries may have their lower extremities slightly elevated. Trendelenburg's position is avoided because gravity pushes the abdominal organs up against the chest, which interferes with diaphragmatic excursions and cardiac contractions. Position changes should be made slowly and gently. Observations should be made systematically and recorded in written form. Pertinent observations include blood pressure, pulse, respirations, skin color, temperature, IV and oral fluid intake, urinary and other forms of fluid loss, a running balance of I & O, and level of consciousness.

Care should be taken to avoid factors that increase the severity of shock. External heat should not be applied to a patient who is in shock unless the patient is shivering. Shivering increases the metabolic need for oxygen and causes vasodilation, so the patient should be covered just enough to stop the shivering. External heat would also cause peripheral vasodilation, thus supplying the peripheral tissues with blood at the expense of the vital organs and contributing to the progression of shock. Pain medications should be administered carefully to avoid extreme vasoconstriction, which can result from increased stimulation of the sympathetic nervous system.

A central venous catheter is inserted. Frequent monitoring of central venous pressure is done to prevent the danger of overhydrating the patient. Overloading the patient's circulatory system can lead to pulmonary edema, which further impedes the amount of oxygenation and CO_2 removal that can occur in the lungs. Patients receiving high-humidity oxygen can absorb some of the humidity through their lungs. Daily chest x-ray films are beneficial in monitoring the development of pulmonary edema. Diuretics, such as furosemide, may help prevent fluid accumulation in the pulmonary bed. Arterial blood-gas determinations indicate the patient's oxygen and CO_2 levels, as well as acid-base balance.

Military antishock trousers (MASTs) or pneumatic antishock garments (PASGs) may be applied. These garments apply pressure to the lower extremities and abdomen to help increase the blood return to the vital organs and decrease the blood volume in the lower extremities. They are used to keep the systolic blood pressure above 80 mm Hg. MASTs and PASGs are contraindicated in patients with severe head injury, congestive heart failure, or an intrathoracic bleed. When the garment is inflated, the pulse must be checked in the lower extremities. The garment should never obscure the pulse. Once the blood volume has been restored with fluids and blood products, the garment can be removed by first deflating the area over the abdomen and then over one leg at a time. If the blood pressure drops more than 5 mm Hg, the deflation is stopped until the blood pressure returns to the previous reading. If the patient requires surgery to control bleeding, these garments may be left in place and removed in the operating room after the surgery is complete.

Normovolemic shock

Shock that results from causes other than fluid loss is termed **normovolemic shock. Cardiogenic shock** results from a failure of the heart to pump adequate amounts of blood into the systemic circulation to fully perfuse and therefore oxygenate the body tissues. Cardiogenic shock is easiest to treat in its early stages but is *not* easily identified. It is not easily reversed if it is not identified early. The seriousness of the precipitating factors tends to shadow the impending shock. Precipitating factors include arrhythmias, myocardial infarction, or congestive heart failure. Decreased blood pressure, a decreased level of alertness, and decreased renal function are all present in cardiogenic shock and reflect the failure of the heart as a pump.

Neurogenic shock or **vasogenic shock** both result from vasodilation, or an increase in the size of the vascular bed with a normal blood volume. Blood pressure decreases and therefore venous blood returned to the heart is decreased, which contributes to decreased cardiac output. In both types of shock, venous pooling results, and tissue hypoxia and cell death occur.

Although vasodilation occurs in both neurogenic and vasogenic shock, the causative factors of each differ. The cause of *neurogenic* shock is nerve stimulation or nerve blocks, such as those arising from deep general anesthesia, spinal anesthesia, postural hypotension, drug reactions, brain damage, or insulin shock. *Vasogenic* shock occurs as a result of factors that directly affect the blood vessels. Vasodilation in vasogenic shock is followed by a decrease in venous return, cardiac output, blood pressure, and volume of blood to the tissues. Cellular anoxia and destruction occur. Anaphylactic shock and septic shock are examples of vasogenic shock.

Anaphylactic shock results from an abnormal antigen-antibody response. The IgE antibody produced causes the release of histamine from mast cells and basophils (see Chapter 7). The release of histamine results in arterial and venous dilation and increased capillary permeability. Vasodilation and decreased cardiac output cause a decrease in systolic and diastolic blood pressure. Plasma leaks through the vascular bed into the interstitial space, which leads to circulatory collapse. Histamine contracts the smooth muscle of the bronchi and causes bronchospasms, asthma, and panting. The bronchioles constrict and contribute to hypoxemia. The patient initially complains of dizziness, drowsiness, and itching of the eyes and ears. Confusion; diaphoresis; edema of the hands, lips, and eyelids and tongue; and laryngospasm quickly appear. The reaction rapidly progresses to complete respiratory obstruction and distress and circulatory collapse.

Treatment requires immediate elimination of the antigen, such as removing a bee stinger or stopping an infusion that caused the reaction. The patient should be placed in a supine position to increase blood flow to the brain. An open airway must be maintained, and oxygen is given at 5 to 10 L/min. IV fluids should be started, and the patient is placed on a cardiac monitor. Epinephrine is given to block the release of histamine, counteract bronchospasms, and prevent circulatory collapse. Antihistamines, corticosteroids, and aminophylline are given to supplement the effects of epinephrine. After recovering from the acute episode, the patient must be fully informed of the allergy to avoid future exposure (Box 8-23).

Septic shock is caused by the metabolic end-products of bacteria. During the early phase of septic shock, the vessels are dilated and the patient may have a fever. There is still adequate blood flow to the brain, as indicated by the patient's alertness. Urinary output, which reflects renal perfusion, is adequate. The pulse may be moderately elevated, but the increase in heart rate does not support an adequate cardiac output, and systolic blood pressure slowly falls. Hyperventilation results in metabolic alkalosis.

The late phase of septic shock is marked by decreased mentation, which may lead to confusion and stupor. The sluggish blood is prone to clot, especially within the smaller vessels. This condition is known as **disseminated intravascular coagulation.** The clotted vessels are unable to deliver oxygen and nutrients to the affected tissues. The widespread clotting depletes blood clotting factors, and the patient begins to hemorrhage. Metabolic acidosis results from cellular hypoxia and the inability of the clotted vessels to carry cellular waste products from the affected areas. Arterial and venous constriction contribute to cold, pale, and clammy skin with a below-normal body temperature. Constriction of the renal arteries leads to decreased perfusion of the kidneys, and little urine is produced. Acute or chronic renal failure is the second most common cause of death in septic shock.

Drug Therapy for Shock

Various types of drug therapy are ordered according to the cause of shock. Vasoactive drugs, which affect vascular tone, can be categorized into various groups according to the following actions: constriction/dilation of arterioles, constriction/dilation of veins, or increasing myocardial contractability. Vasoactive drugs include norepinephrine, nitroprusside, and dopamine. For example, a patient in cardiogenic shock might be given norepinephrine, which would cause the cardiac muscles to contract with greater force, a condition that is also called a *positive inotropic effect*. The result would be an increase in cardiac output. Management is actually more complex than this. For example, an increase in cardiac contractility also increases myocardial oxygen demand. The patient's condition must be closely monitored.

Noninotropic drugs, such as nitroprusside, that equally dilate arterioles and veins also decrease cardiac

BOX 8-23 **Nursing Process**

EMERGENCY CARE OF INDIVIDUALS IN ANAPHYLACTIC SHOCK

ASSESSMENT

Rapid, shallow breathing; bronchospasms; dyspnea; cyanosis; restlessness; "sense of doom"; irritability; laryngeal edema
Hypotension
Rapid, thready pulse
Edema and itching at site of injection or insect bite

NURSING DIAGNOSIS

Risk for injury related to anaphylatic shock

NURSING INTERVENTIONS

Prepare for oropharyngeal intubation or surgical insertion of tracheotomy; provide oxygen therapy per order.
Prepare for administration of antihistamines such as Benadryl 50-100 mg IM, aminophylline IV drip; administer corticosteroids to decrease inflammation as ordered.
Administer 0.1 ml to 0.5 ml 1:1000 epinephrine solution SC or IM into upper arm and massage site to hasten absorption; prepare to administer vasopressor drugs such as levarterenol bitartrate (Levophed) and high-dose dopamine (Intropin); monitor pulse and blood pressure q 3-5 min until stable.
Place a tourniquet above the site of the injected antigen; remove tourniquet q 10-15 min or until reaction is under control; apply ice.

EVALUATION OF EXPECTED OUTCOMES

Maintains patent airway
Demonstrates effective breathing pattern
Maintains hemodynamic stability, as evidenced by blood pressure and pulse in normal range
Reduces systemic absorption of the antigen

oxygen demand and increase perfusion of peripheral vessels. However, perfusion of the vital organs is decreased. Other drugs used in shock include antiarrhythmics (lidocaine, procainamide), antibiotics (tobramycin, gentamicin), and diuretics (ethacrynic acid).

PSYCHOSOCIAL SUPPORT

This chapter has considered the biologic alterations in a patient who has fluid and electrolyte imbalances or one who is in a state of shock. However, the patient leads a biopsychosocial existence. Therefore biologic alterations are likely to affect both psychologic and social spheres.

Many of the conditions previously discussed affect mentation to various degrees. Progressive lethargy and weakness or intermittent confusion may frighten one patient, cause another to withdraw, and inspire anger and hostility in yet another. Various family members also have diverse responses. Responding to patients and their families in a calm, reassuring manner is often all that is needed to decrease fears, encourage communication, and lessen anger.

Patients and family members will have many questions, both verbalized and nonverbalized: Why does he twitch so uncontrollably? He was normally so active, why is he so sleepy all the time? Why doesn't my wife recognize me? Why are all those needles in her

ETHICAL DILEMMA

Mrs. Smith is an 88-year-old women who has been admitted for dehydration, anemia, and a deteriorated cognitive state. She has a long history of depression and has expressed over many years her apparent wish to die. She is also nearly deaf. According to her daughter, Mrs. Smith has lost approximately 25 pounds over the past year. The patient had a mastectomy for breast cancer 25 years ago. Before admission, Mrs. Smith was living in her own apartment. Family members visited often and provided cooked meals and other necessities.

One problem in treating Mrs. Smith is that she refuses to eat with any regularity. During rehydration she had to be restrained because of combativeness. She has also refused IV and nasogastric (NG) tube feedings. Her family is concerned about her lack of nutrition and hydration, but they do not want to see her physically restrained and fed against her wishes. There is also the problem of placement. Mrs. Smith's apartment has been relinquished by her family, and family members state that they are not in a position to provide the necessary care to their mother within their homes.

What are the ethical questions related to the care of Mrs. Smith? Should she be fed via an IV and/or an NG tube?

arm? What is that machine for? Often the only answer required is factual information that is communicated in words that are understood by the patient or family member. However, sometimes it is not information that is sought, but rather someone to listen attentively. Emotional support is not necessarily exclusively verbal. It can be a gentle touch on the shoulder or maintained eye contact when someone trusts the nurse enough to ask a question or share his or her anxieties.

As a member of the healthcare team, the nurse knows each team member's talents well enough to consult with them at appropriate times. When a family member wants to know a patient's prognosis, the physician is often the most appropriate team member to consult and refer to the family member. When a patient has financial concerns, the nurse draws from the expertise of the social worker.

The nurse, aware that the patient's psychosocial health can influence biologic health and affect responses to medical and nursing therapy, incorporates this aspect of the patient's health into the plan of care.

Nursing Care Plan

PATIENT WITH HYPOKALEMIA

Mr. Baxter is a 73-year-old male who has been admitted from the emergency room with a diagnosis of dehydration, abdominal pain, and hypokalemia. He had been well at home until the past week, when he began experiencing nausea, vomiting, and abdominal discomfort. He attributed this to a flu until 6 days had passed and the abdominal pain increased in severity. He has not moved his bowels in 3 days. Abdominal x-ray examinations reveal a small bowel obstruction.

Past Medical History	Psychosocial Data	Assessment Data
Myocardial infarction × 2, most recent 2 years ago; has participated in cardiac rehabilitation and is able to continue moderate activities around the house Congestive heart failure, which is under control with medications; very compliant with taking his cardiac medications and has continued to take them despite nausea this past week Hypertension for 20 years Colectomy 3 years ago for adenocarcinoma No known allergies Wife has severe osteoarthritis but has remained active; no cardiopulmonary disease Children are healthy Father died of heart disease Mother had diabetes	Lives independently in own single-level home with wife of 52 years Active lifestyle; is avid gardener Very involved with extended family; has 4 children, 10 grandchildren, and 6 great-grandchildren Religious affiliation is Baptist; he and his wife attend church every week and are involved in activities of the church Nonsmoker; minimal alcohol usage	Height 5'10", weight 155 lb Vital signs: T 99.2, P 100, R 18, BP 102/64 Alert and oriented × 3 In moderate distress; pleasant and personable *Skin:* intact, pink, warm, and dry; poor skin turgor Eye-ear-nose-throat (EENT): mucous membranes dry; lips dry and cracked *Respiratory:* lungs clear to auscultation; diminished breath sounds bilateral bases; respirations nonlabored, shallow, and symmetrical *Cardiovascular:* apical pulse 100, slightly irregular; no jugular vein distention or edema; weak peripheral pulses bilaterally *Abdomen:* firm, distended abdomen; bowel sounds absent; NG tube inserted in the ER is draining a moderate amount of bile-colored fluid *Musculoskeletal:* full, active range-of-motion (ROM) all extremities. Soft, slightly flabby muscles; gait even, slow, and steady. *Urinary:* decreased urine output; indwelling urinary catheter inserted in the ER is draining 30 ml/hr; urine is clear, dark amber color ***Laboratory data*** Hemoglobin 12.2, Hematocrit (HCT) 38.3, BUN 31, Chromium (Cr) 1.3, WBC 12,000 Na, 134 K 2.3, Cl 92 Chest x-ray: Clear, no evidence of infiltration, atelectasis, or vascular congestion

continued

Nursing Care Plan

PATIENT WITH HYPOKALEMIA–CONT'D

Past Medical History	Psychosocial Data	Assessment Data
		ECG: Normal sinus rhythm; occasional unifocal premature ventricular contraction (PVC); flattened T wave; U wave present ***Medications*** *Home:* Lasix 40 mg qd NitroDur 0.4 mg patch qd digoxin 0.25 mg qd Cardizem 30 mg qid *Hospital:* Demerol 50-75 mg IM q 3 hr prn Compazine 10 mg IM q 6 hr prn D5 ½ normal saline with 40 mEq KCl at 125 ml/hr Nasogastric tube to low intermittent suction

NURSING DIAGNOSIS

Fluid volume deficit related to nausea, vomiting, diuretic therapy, NG tube as evidenced by poor skin turgor, dry mucous membranes, decreased urine output, concentrated urine, decreased blood pressure

NURSING INTERVENTIONS	EVALUATION OF EXPECTED OUTCOMES
Assess skin turgor, mucous membranes, vital signs, and level of consciousness. Maintain accurate I&O. Monitor urine output q 2 h during acute illness. Maintain IV fluids at prescribed rate. Observe for signs of orthostatic hypotension. Monitor serum electrolytes, primarily K, and report abnormal values. Explain all treatments and procedures to patient and family.	Vital signs stable and within normal limits for patient Urine output > 30 ml/hr and urine yellow in color Supple (elastic) skin turgor Moist mucous membranes Tolerating diet and fluids without nausea and vomiting

NURSING DIAGNOSIS

Risk for decreased cardiac output related to hypokalemia and potential effect on cardiac conduction system

NURSING INTERVENTIONS	EVALUATION OF EXPECTED OUTCOMES
Monitor vital signs, level of consciousness, and peripheral pulses. Monitor heart rhythm for arrythmia, and report irregularities immediately. Administer potassium as prescribed. Provide rest to reduce oxygen demands. Monitor for signs and symptoms of digitalis toxicity because hypokalemia enhances action of digitalis.	BP and pulse within normal limits for patient Regular cardiac rhythm Strong and equal peripheral pulses Serum potassium within normal limits

NURSING DIAGNOSIS

Pain related to gastric distention, decreased GI motility, vomiting as evidenced by verbal complaints and nonverbal pain behavior

NURSING INTERVENTIONS	EVALUATION OF EXPECTED OUTCOMES
Assess pain for severity, location, duration and quality q 2-4 hr. Assess abdominal distention and bowel sounds q 8 hr. Medicate as needed with analgesic. Respond immediately to complaint of pain, and monitor effectiveness of analgesic. Help patient assume a comfortable position. Maintain elevation of head of bed. Medicate as needed with antiemetic. Maintain patency of NG tube, and irrigate prn with 30 ml normal saline. Provide comfort measures (massage, relaxation).	Abdominal distention and pain decreased Reports tolerable level of pain NG tube patent and functioning while in place Nausea and vomiting resolved

NURSING DIAGNOSIS

Knowledge deficit related to complication of diuretic therapy and acute illness

NURSING INTERVENTIONS	EVALUATION OF EXPECTED OUTCOMES
Assess patient and family level of understanding of illness. Review the correlation between diuretic use, vomiting, and hypokalemia. Review other conditions that may lead to hypokalemia. Instruct on medication action, dosage, and side effects. Teach the importance of ingesting potassium-rich foods (oranges, bananas, tomatoes, dark green leafy vegetables, milk). Review signs and symptoms to report to primary physician.	Verbalizes causes of hypokalemia Identifies potassium-rich foods Verbalizes understanding of medication administration

KEY CONCEPTS

- Infants, the aged, and the obese are at higher risk in situations that involve fluid loss.
- A 5-lb weight gain represents 2L of fluid retained.
- A solution that is equal in concentration to fluid in the cell is hypotonic. A solution that is higher in concentration is hypertonic, and a solution that is lower in concentration is hypotonic.
- Shifts of plasma to interstitial fluid (edema) result from elevation of venous hydrostatic pressure, a decrease in plasma oncotic pressure, or an elevation of interstitial oncotic pressure.
- Shifts of interstitial fluid to plasma result from an increase in oncotic pressure of plasma or an increase in hydrostatic pressure of the tissues.
- An isotonic ECF deficit (hypovolemia) occurs when fluids and electrolytes are lost equally. Symptoms are low blood pressure, a weak pulse, weight loss, and shock.
- A hypertonic ECF deficit (dehydration) occurs when more water is lost than electrolytes, which causes water to leave the cell to dilute the ECF. Symptoms are tenting and dry mucous membranes.
- An isotonic ECF excess occurs when water and electrolytes are retained. Symptoms are edema, a bounding pulse, and dyspnea.
- A hypotonic ECF excess (primary water excess) occurs when water intake exceeds electrolyte intake. Symptoms of confusion, lethargy, and seizures result from cerebral edema.
- The following is a list of symptoms of electrolyte imbalances:
  - Hyponatremia: anorexia, nausea, vomiting diarrhea, muscle cramps, abdominal cramps
  - Hypernatremia: same as dehydration
  - Hypokalemia: weakness, anorexia, nausea, vomiting, abdominal distention, prominent U wave on ECG
  - Hyperkalemia: muscle twitching, paresthesia of the face and tongue, tachycardia followed by bradycardia, peaked T waves on ECG
  - Hypocalcemia: tingling, twitching, tetany, carpopedal spasm, positive Chvostek's sign and positive Trousseau's sign as a result of increased nerve and muscle cell excitability
  - Hypercalcemia: lethargy and decreased muscle tone as a result of depressed neuromuscular activity
  - Hypomagnesemia: similar to hypocalcemia
  - Hypermagnesemia: lethargy, decreased tendon reflexes, depressed respiratory rate, low blood pressure
  - Hypochloremia: same as hyponatremia and metabolic alkalosis
  - Hyperchloremia: same as acidosis (lethargy, confusion, weakness, stupor)
- Phosphate levels vary inversely with calcium levels. If calcium is high, phosphate is low and vice versa.
- Hypoproteinemia results in reduced colloidal osmotic pressure in the plasma, which causes edema.
- Acid-base balance is regulated by the buffer systems, the lungs, and the kidneys. The primary buffer system is carbonic acid/bicarbonate. The cells are buffers. The lungs control CO_2. The kidneys excrete or reabsorb bicarbonate and excrete hydrogen ions as needed.
- Metabolic acidosis is caused by a deficit of base bicarbonate or an excess of acid byproducts from metabolism. Symptoms of metabolic acidosis are Kussmaul's respiration, weakness, disorientation, drowsiness, stupor, and coma.
- Metabolic alkalosis is caused by an excess in base bicarbonate. Symptoms of metabolic alkalosis are nausea, vomiting, diarrhea, muscle cramps, twitching, and tetany.
- Respiratory alkalosis is caused by a carbonic acid deficit. Symptoms of respiratory alkalosis are paresthesia, numbness, headache, tingling, and tetany.
- Respiratory acidosis is caused by an excess in carbonic acid. Symptoms of respiratory acidosis are weakness, restlessness, drowsiness, disorientation, headache, muscle twitching, and convulsions.
- Interpreting blood gas values requires three steps:
  - Step 1. Name the pH level (acidosis or alkalosis)
  - Step 2. Look at bicarbonate and carbonic acid levels. Identify the abnormality that can cause what was found in Step 1. Add either "respiratory" or "metabolic" to the name.
  - Step 3. Look for compensation. Add "compensated" or "uncompensated" to the name.
- A quick formula to determine body serum osmolarity is 2 × sodium level.
- The following is a list of types of shock:
  - Hypovolemic shock: caused by a loss of fluid available to circulation
  - Cardiogenic shock: caused by pump failure (heart is the pump)
  - Neurogenic shock: caused by vasodilation following nerve stimulation or nerve block
  - Vasogenic shock: involves vasodilation resulting from factors affecting blood vessels
  - Anaphylactic shock: results from an abnormal antigen-antibody response
  - Septic shock: results when the metabolic end products of bacteria cause vasodilation; can result in disseminated intravascular coagulation
- To treat shock, remove or treat the cause, replace blood volume, provide oxygen, and position patient flat or with feet elevated if cerebral edema is not present or likely

CRITICAL THINKING EXERCISES

1 Mr. Graham has been admitted to the Veterans Administration Hospital after suffering a myocardial infarction 2 days ago. While giving him medications, the nurse observes that he is slightly less alert than earlier in the day, yet he is restless. When taking his blood pressure, which is 30 mm Hg lower systolic than normal, the nurse also notices that his skin appears to be clammy.

a What complication may be occurring? In what position should Mr. Graham be placed immediately, and why?

b The medical service orders include bedrest, high-humidity oxygen, and a sodium nitroprusside (Nipride) IV drip. Explain the rationale behind each of these disorders.

c The nursing care plan for Mr. Graham includes patient assessments and observations. What should be observed and documented regarding the circulatory system? The respiratory system? The urinary system?

2 Mrs. Jordan is admitted to the university hospital with a diagnosis of acute renal failure. Because potassium is excreted via the kidneys, Mrs. Jordan must be observed for signs and symptoms of hyperkalemia. Mrs. Jordan's complete blood count (CBC) indicates decreased hemoglobin, hematocrit, and red blood cell counts. A nursing observation reveals warm, moist skin; pitting edema of dependent extremities; and full, engorged peripheral veins. What are the signs and symptoms of hyperkalemia? What is Mrs. Jordan's state of fluid balance? What nursing goals should be incorporated into Mrs. Jordan's nursing care plan?

3 Mrs. Wilson is a 46-year-old female who had a small bowel resection for a malignant tumor 2 days ago. She has an NG tube in place, an abdominal dressing, and a Jackson-Pratt drain inserted next to the abdominal wound. When you approach her to discuss plans for nursing care, she tells you that she is just too tired to do anything today and that she definitely is too weak to get out of bed. She is also feeling a little nauseated.

a List the additional assessments you would make before reporting your observations to the physician.

b What electrolyte imbalance(s) might you suspect in Mrs. Wilson?

REFERENCES AND ADDITIONAL READINGS

Angelucci, D, Todaro A: Reversing acute dehydration: how to restore fluids and electrolytes to prevent further dehydration, *Nursing* 23(1):33, 1993.

Beare PG, Myers JL: *Principles and practice of adult health Nursing*, St Louis, 1994, Mosby.

Bove LA: How fluids and electrolytes shift after surgery, *Nursing* 24(6):34, 1994.

Carroll P: Speed: the essential response to anaphylaxis, *RN* 57(6):26-31, 1994.

Cerrato PL: Magnesium: don't overlook this mineral deficiency, *RN* 55(7):61-62, 1992.

Dennison RD, Blevins BN: About acid-base imbalance: myths and facts, Part 3, *Nursing* 22(3):69, 1992.

Dennison RD, Blevins BN: About electrolyte imbalance, Part 2, *Nursing* 22(2):26, 1992.

Dennison RD, Blevins BN: About fluid imbalance, *Nursing* 22(1):22, 1992.

Flavel CM: Combating hemorrhagic shock, *RN* 57(12):26-30, 1994.

Hastings-Tolsma M, Yucha C: IV infiltration: no clear signs, no clear treatment? *RN* 57(12):34-38, 1994.

Howard PM, Eisenberg PG, Gianino MS: Dressing a central venous catheter a better way, *Nursing* 22(2):60, 1992.

Immunosuppression: septic shock in the ED, *Nurs 93* 23:63, September 1993.

Lewis SM, Collier IC: *Medical-surgical nursing: assessment and management of clinical problems*, St Louis, 1992, Mosby.

Mays DA: Turn ABGs into child's play, *RN* 58(1):36-40, 1995.

McCance KL, Huether SE: *Pathophysiology: the biologic basis for disease in adults and children*, St Louis, 1994, Mosby.

Nelson WP: Any flashing 'lytes? *Patient Care* 26(1):172, 1992.

Norris MKG: Evaluating sodium levels, *Nursing* 22(7):20, 1992.

O'Neal PV: How to spot early signs of cardiogenic shock, *Am J Nurs* 94(5):36-41, 1994.

Owens MW: Keeping an eye on magnesium, *Am J Nurs*, 93(2):66, 1993.

Phipps WJ and others: Medical-surgical nursing: concepts and clinical practice, ed 5, St Louis, 1995, Mosby.

Raimen F: How to identify electrolyte imbalances on your patient's ECG, *Nursing* 24(6):54-58, 1994.

Russell S: Hypovolemic shock: is your patient at risk? *Nursing* 24(6):34, 1994.

Russell S: Septic shock: can you recognize the clues? *Nursing* 24(4):24:40-46, 1994.

Sheldon JE: What you should know about IV dressings: learn the pros and cons of three major types, *Nursing* 24(1):32, 1994.

Stringfield YN: Back to basics: acidosis, alkalosis, and ABGs, *Am J Nurs* 93(11):43-44, 1993.

Tasuta FJ, Wesmiller SW: Assessing ABGs: maintaining the delicate balance, *Nursing* 24(5):34, 1994.

Taylor DL: Respiratory acidosis: pathophysiology, signs, and symptoms, *Nursing* 20(9):52-53, 1990.

Venfrolio LG: Would you hang these IV solutions? *Am J Nurs* 95(6): 37-39, 1995.

Wolpert N: An orderly look at calcium metabolism disorders, *Nursing* 20(7):60-64, 1990.

Yarnell RP and others: Detecting hypomagnesemia: the most overlooked electrolyte imbalance, *Nursing* 21(7):55-57, 1991.

CHAPTER 9

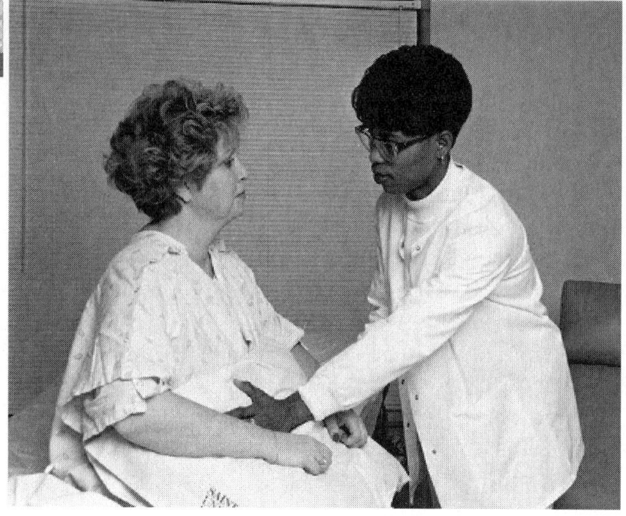

The Patient With Pain

CHAPTER OBJECTIVES

1 Discuss the nature of pain.
2 Identify applications of the gate control theory to pain management.
3 Discuss the role of the nurse in pain management.
4 Identify the components of a pain assessment.
5 Describe medications appropriate for mild, moderate, and severe pain.
6 Discuss the nurse's role in administering pain medications.
7 Describe nonpharmacologic measures appropriate for the nurse to use in pain relief.
8 Identify neurosurgical interventions for pain relief.

KEY WORDS

acute pain
addiction
chordotomy
chronic acute pain
chronic benign pain
distraction
endorphins
epidural analgesia
faces rating scale
gate control theory
intrathecal analgesia
neurectomy
neurotransmitters
pain
pain threshold
pain tolerance
patient-controlled analgesia
phantom pain
physical dependence
placebo
relaxation techniques
referred pain
rhizotomy
specificity theory
tolerance
transcutaneous electrical neural stimulation (TENS)
visual analog scale

The alleviation of **pain** is one of the most common problems faced by nurses when giving care to patients. Nurses have a well-established central role in the successful management of pain. Whether in a hospital, long-term care facility, physicians' office, or patient's home, the nurse has numerous opportunities to work with patients who are anticipating or experiencing pain. The nurse's role includes assessing an individual who has pain, administering therapeutic modalities, teaching the patient/family about pain and its control, and monitoring the effectiveness of the interventions. The nurse can be the key link in facilitating communication between a patient who has pain and the healthcare team.

Pain is often the symptom that brings the patient to the physician. The physician assumes primary responsibility for diagnosing the cause of the pain and for treating the disease that is causing the symptom. However, the nurse has the most direct contact with the patient during the long hours that he or she is experiencing pain. Therefore the nurse is in a position to make a major contribution to any program of pain relief. Nurses are held accountable for managing the pain program for patients under their care.

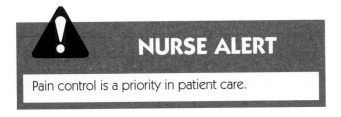

Pain control is a priority in patient care.

THE NATURE OF PAIN

The nature of pain has been of considerable interest throughout history. Pain is a nebulous sensation. Scientists cannot directly measure its intensity, nor can they see it in action. Patients often have trouble describing their pain and sometimes even have trouble pinpointing its location. Religion and culture may have a strong influence on an individual's experience of pain. Some people believe that they have pain because they have sinned and must suffer to make up for their wrongdoing. Others believe that they are suffering to improve or discipline themselves. The word *pain* is derived from the Latin word *poena,* which means punishment. Members of primitive cultures sometimes deliberately inflicted pain on themselves in an attempt to appease the gods and redeem their souls.

The beliefs, values, and customs that are passed from one generation to another (cultural factors) greatly influence how an individual reacts to pain. In some cultures/families, it is important to be stoic and suffer in silence. In other cultures, outward displays of emotion are acceptable. It is important for the nurse not to stereotype individuals because they belong to a certain ethnic group and not to assume that the characteristics common to a particular sociocultural group occur in all members of that group.

In more recent years scientists have come to realize that pain is both a physical and a psychologic phenomenon. Pain can be viewed as having two components: (1) the sensation, or *perception,* of pain; and (2) the response, or *reaction,* to pain. The perception of pain depends on the intactness of the nerve pathways and brain and on the degree of physical damage. The pain reaction is a complex response and involves the highest cognitive (thinking) mechanisms. Many factors influence an individual's reaction to pain, such as anxiety, previous pain experiences, age, culture, and the meaning of the pain-producing situation. Research has shown that the **pain threshold** (the point at which a sensation is perceived as pain) is essentially the same in all people under normal circumstances. However, **pain tolerance** (the point at which a pain sensation is no longer voluntarily endured) and the reaction to pain varies widely from one person to another and even in the same individual under different circumstances.

Defining Pain

Pain is an intensely personal and complex biochemical event. The International Association for the Study of Pain (1986) defines pain as an unpleasant sensory experience and emotional experience that arises from actual or potential tissue damage. Pain can also be considered as present if a person describes the experience in terms of such damage. Much of the difficulty in precisely defining pain occurs because it is a very personal, subjective phenomenon that can only be interpreted in terms of its meaning to the person who is experiencing it. To the patient, pain is simply "what hurts." Nurses can experience their own pain but can only make judgments about the pain of others. It is critical that the healthcare staff believe the patient's report of pain and not depend on their own perceptions of how a person in pain should act. McCaffrey and Beebe's (1989) definition of pain best meets the needs of nurses who are caring for patients in pain: "Pain is whatever the experiencing person says it is, existing wherever he says it exists." Using this definition, the nurse accepts that the patient is having pain. The patient does not have to prove that pain exists.

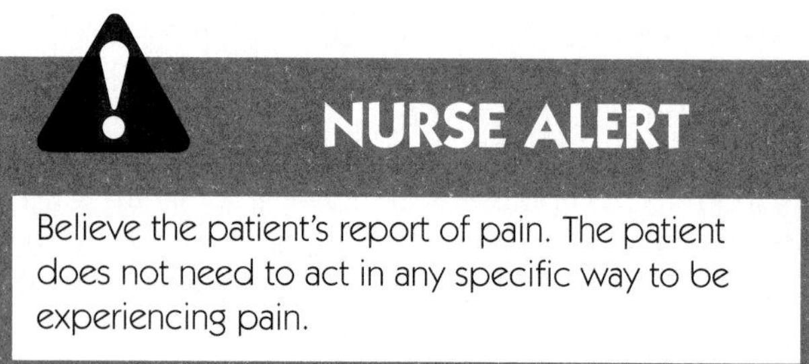

Believe the patient's report of pain. The patient does not need to act in any specific way to be experiencing pain.

Function of Pain

Pain can serve as a protective mechanism for the body by signaling that tissues are damaged or threatened with damage. Pain is often the first symptom that tells an individual that something is wrong with the body or urges that person to seek medical assistance. Pain can also protect the body from further injury. For example, the pain caused by contact with a hot object causes a person to withdraw from the object. However, the protective function of pain sometimes becomes lost or obscured, such as in long-term arthritis or chronic back pain. No longer is the pain a useful mechanism that warns of danger. In such individuals reactions to pain and methods of adapting to and living with pain become of great significance to the healthcare team.

Individuals who cannot feel and respond to pain because of a loss of sensation (e.g., spinal cord injury) or because of an absence of pain receptors (genetic deficiency) are very susceptible to injury. The nurse must be extremely vigilant when providing care to these patients. Whether a result of anesthesia, sedation, or neurologic damage, an unconscious patient is at great risk for skin integrity problems. The nurse is unaware of the pain that the unconscious patient is experiencing because he or she cannot communicate verbally or nonverbally.

Pain Theories

Science does not yet have a satisfactory explanation for pain transmission and pain relief. Therefore it must resort to theory, or the best guess available on the basis of current evidence. More than 200 years ago the **specificity theory** was proposed. This theory stated that pain was a sensation much like sight and hearing. It implied that there is a fixed, straight-through transmission system from pain receptors to the pain center in the brain. The specificity theory did not attempt to explain differences in individuals but concentrated on neurosurgical techniques to cut the pain pathway. Recent psychologic and neurologic data have demonstrated the incompleteness of the theory. Melzack and Wall (1965) proposed the **gate control theory,** which has generated much research and has provided a partial explanation of how pain is transmitted and perceived (Figure 9-1). According to this theory, pain sensations travel along small-diameter C-δ (C delta) fibers and go to the brain through a "gate" located in the spinal cord. Pain sensations can be blocked at this gate by stimulating the large-diameter A-δ (A delta) fibers, which carry generalized sensations. The gate can also be closed by brain activity. Psychologic factors, memories of previous pain experiences, and many physical or mental activities can also influence the perception of pain. Applications of this theory include the use of transcutaneous electrical neural stimulation (TENS), massage or backrubs, counterirritants such as Ben Gay and Deep Heat ointments, and heat or cold. In each case the fast-moving impulses coming from the peripheral nerve receptors reach the "gate" first and block the impulses traveling along the slower pain fibers. The brain receives and interprets the general sensation message and does not receive the pain message.

Current research on pain focuses on the neurochemical nature of pain. It is now known that the body is capable of secreting narcotic-like substances called **endorphins** (West, 1981). Endorphins lock into narcotic receptors on nerve endings in the brain and spinal cord and block the transmission of pain sensations. Different individuals have different amounts of endorphins, which may help explain differences in pain perception. Research has shown that such things as prolonged pain or constant stress can decrease the amount of endorphins. Brief pain or brief stress increases the amount. It is interesting to note that intense physical exercise, such as jogging, can temporarily increase an individual's endorphin level.

The body also produces a number of endogenous chemicals such as histamine, substance P, serotonin, and prostaglandins that act as **neurotransmitters** for the transmission of pain impulses (Paice, 1991). Much research is being done to discover medications that can block the actions of specific neurotransmitters. One such drug is ketorolac tromethamine (Toradol), which can inhibit the synthesis of prostaglandins. Further research on the roles of neurotransmitters will lead to better methods of inhibiting pain. Although

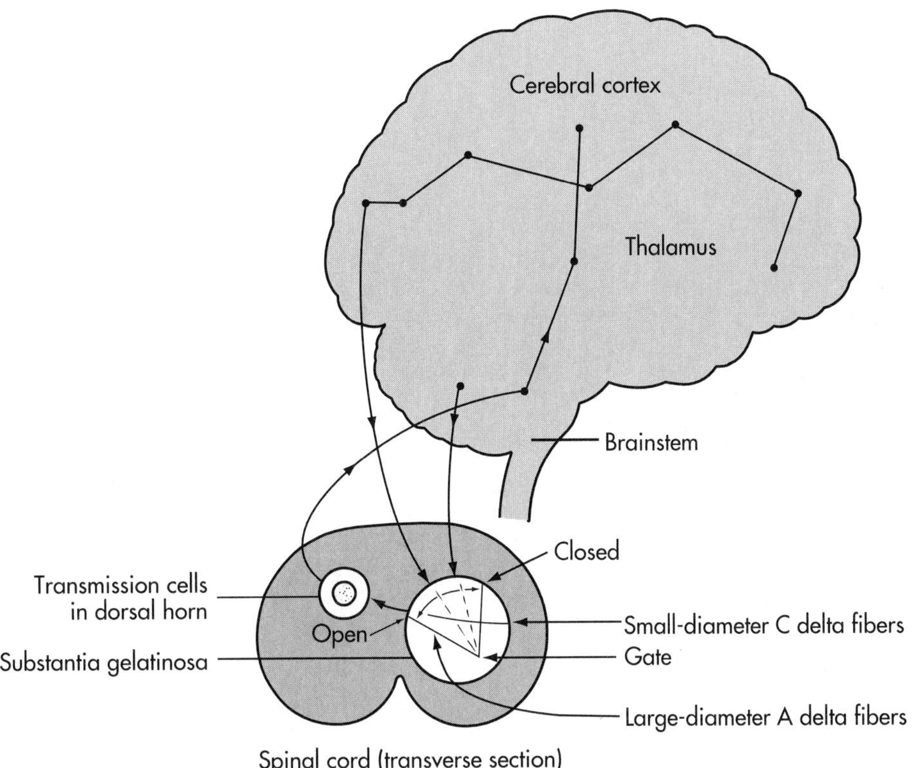

Figure 9-1 Gate control theory. Pain sensations, traveling along small-diameter C delta fibers, go through a "gate" (located in the substantia gelatinosa), through transmission cells, and to the brain. These sensations can be blocked at the gate by the stimulation of large-diameter A delta fibers, which carry general sensations. The gate can also be closed by brain activity.

much is known about the pain experience, more is yet to be discovered. For a person in pain, the answers cannot come quickly enough.

Types of Pain

Pain is often classified into three major categories on the basis of its cause (McCaffery, Beebe, 1989). **Acute pain** occurs after injury or surgery and usually subsides within a predictable time span (Figure 9-2). **Chronic acute pain** occurs almost daily over a long period. Examples of chronic acute pain include cancer, spinal injury, and burn pain. This type of pain may last for many months before being cured or controlled, and it may end only with the death of the patient. **Chronic benign pain** is persistent or recurs over a period of months or years. Examples of this type of pain include backaches, headaches, and arthritis. Living with pain on a daily basis can be destructive to an individual and lead to anger, chronic fatigue, and depression. Such patients need to be referred to pain management specialists. Something can be done to help them live more normal lives.

Pain can also be classified by its location or source. Superficial pain occurs when the skin or its surface structures are affected by a painful stimulus. The pain localizes to the site of the stimulation and is usually described as having a prickling or burning quality. Deep pain arises from deeper structures such as the muscles and visceral tissue. Deep pain may be localized to the site of the stimulus but more likely is poorly localized with a dull and aching quality. Deep pain is often felt at a site that is distant from the area of stimulation, which is an occurrence known as **referred pain** (Figure 9-3). Referred pain is projected from various internal organs of the body to the body surface, such as cardiac pain that arises in the heart but is projected to the jaw, left arm, or epigastric region. It is likely that referred pain occurs because the branches of the nerve fibers from the actual pain site and the fibers from the site of the perceived pain enter the spinal cord at the same place, which causes the brain to make

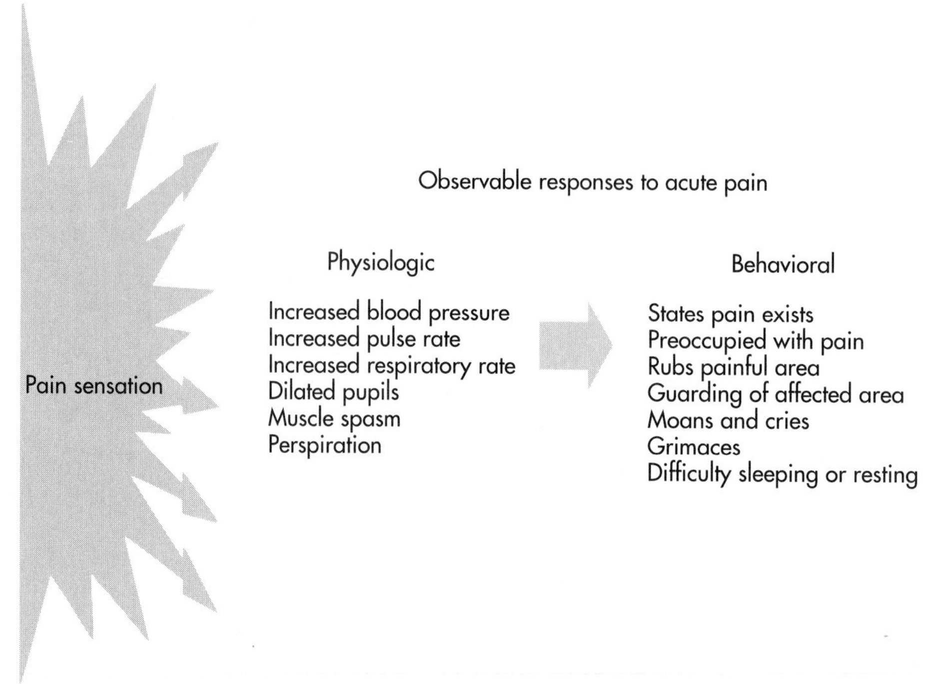

Figure 9-2 Observable responses of acute pain. (Modified from McCaffery M, Beebe A: *Pain: clinical manual of nursing care,* St Louis, 1989, Mosby.)

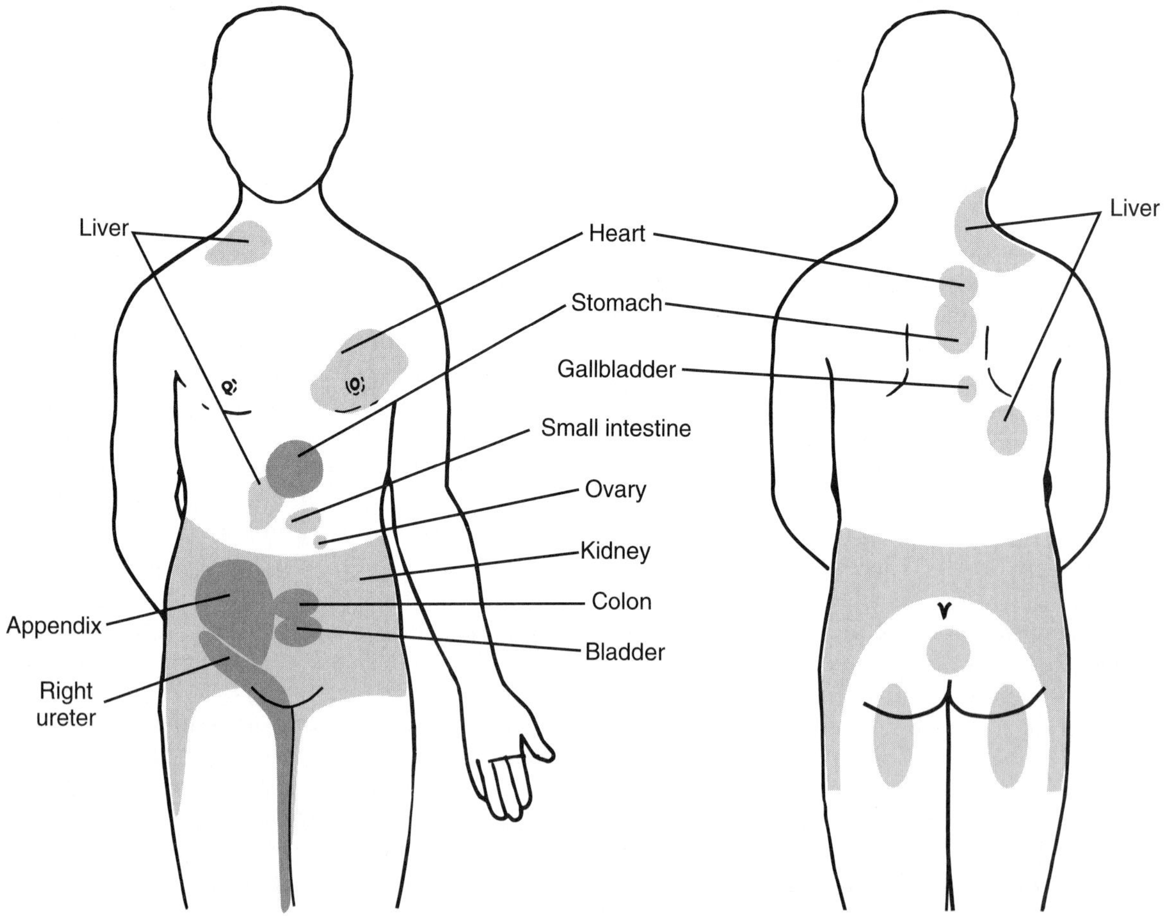

Figure 9-3 Areas of referred pain.

BOX 9-1

ASSESSMENT OF PAIN

1 **History of pain**—prior occurrences, factors that precipitated the pain, activities that increased or decreased the pain, methods used to relieve the pain, usual time of occurrence of pain episodes
2 **Physiologic characteristics**—increase in pulse and respiratory rates, increase in diastolic and systolic blood pressure, pallor, dilated pupils, diaphoresis, nausea; because of the ability of the body to adapt to abnormal situations, these physiologic signs may be absent or decreased in prolonged acute pain or chronic pain
3 **Verbal statements**—description of the quality or character of pain (aching, burning, prickling), severity of pain using a scale (mild, moderate, severe), location of pain (precisely located or diffuse), frequency and duration of pain, meaning of pain to the individual
4 **Facial expressions**—clenched teeth, tightly shut lips, tightening of jaw muscles, strained look
5 **Body movements**—lying quietly or rigidly, restless or purposeless movements, protective or guarding movements toward a specific area, rubbing movements

a faulty interpretation. **Phantom pain** is commonly felt by an individual after the amputation of a body part such as a limb or breast (Sherman, 1987). The person feels as if the part is still there and may feel tingling, burning, itching or other unpleasant sensations. Phantom pain is very disturbing to the patient and may be difficult to treat.

Assessment of Pain

A detailed and accurate description of the patient's pain is essential for a precise diagnosis and treatment of the underlying cause. Because pain is subjective, the patient should be encouraged to describe in detail the nature, intensity, and location of pain (Box 9-1; Figure 9-4). The nurse will find it helpful to follow a specific pattern for assessing each painful episode (McCaffery and others, 1989).

Quantifying the degree of pain before and after administering medications or performing other interventions is a useful way to monitor the effectiveness of the therapy. Two methods that are widely used to monitor treatment effectiveness are questionnaires and rating scales. The McGill-Melzack Pain Questionnaire measures both sensory and affective dimensions of pain (Melzack, Wall, 1988). Rating scales can be used in any patient care setting (McCaffrey, Beebe, 1989). The patient is asked to rate his or her pain on a scale of 1 to 5 or of 10 or 100, either verbally or on a **visual analog scale** (Figure 9-5). The visual analog scale is a 10 cm line that represents a continuum from no pain to the worst imaginable pain. The patient makes a pencil mark at the point on the line that describes the intensity of his or her pain at that time. A **faces rating scale** can be used for children or other persons who cannot speak (Figure 9-6). The patient points to the face that best illustrates his or her pain.

It is important that patients receive information regarding the use of rating scales and how their pain will be managed as part of their preoperative teaching. It is essential that all healthcare personnel use the same scale and the same pain management program with each patient.

It is standard practice in many hospitals to keep a rating scale on the patient's bed or door to make it convenient for the nurse to check the patient. It is important to remember that all pain measurements are subjective. A single measure is not significant in itself. What is important is the change over time.

A problem that nurses often face in pain assessment is the wide variation of how pain is experienced and reported by patients. The nurse may use the term *pain* to mean one thing, but the patient may interpret it to mean something quite different. A patient may respond "No" to a question about pain and yet be in need of assistance. To determine just what the patient is experiencing, it is helpful to use a variety of terms such as ache, pressure, hurt, and discomfort. It is also important to use the phrase "patient reports" pain rather than "patient complains of" pain. The negative connotation of the word *complain* may influence the responses of the patient or significant others.

The young child and the elderly patient present special problems when the nurse is assessing pain (Ferrell, 1991; Herr, Mobily, 1991; McCaffrey, Beebe, 1989; McGuire and others, 1982). The nurse needs to be especially alert to nonverbal cues. A child often cannot describe the pain or denies having pain for fear of receiving a "shot." An elderly patient often is reluctant to "complain" or fears being overmedicated or becoming addicted to narcotics. In either case, the nurse needs to play an active role to prevent undue suffering resulting from undertreatment of pain.

INITIAL PAIN ASSESSMENT TOOL Date___________

Patient's Name___________________________ Age________ Room________

Diagnosis___________________________ Physician___________________________

Nurse___________________________

I. LOCATION: Patient or nurse mark drawing.

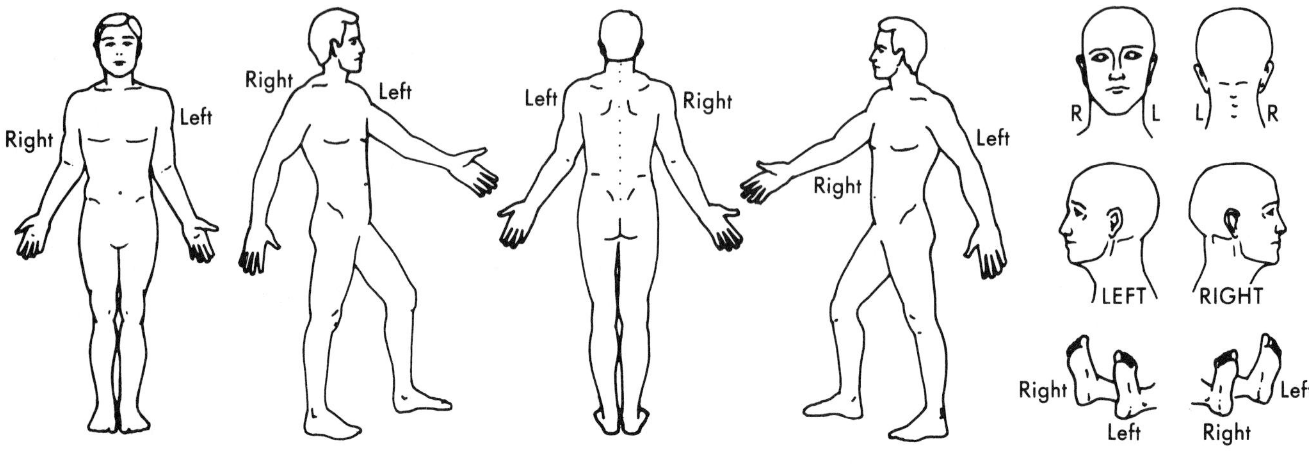

II. INTENSITY: Patient rates the pain. Scale used ___________________________

Present:___________________________

Worst pain gets:___________________________

Best pain gets:___________________________

Acceptable level of pain:___________________________

III. QUALITY: Use patient's own words (e.g., prick, ache, burn, throb, pull, sharp) ___________________________

IV. ONSET, DURATION, VARIATIONS, RHYTHMS:___________________________

V. MANNER OF EXPRESSING PAIN:___________________________

VI. WHAT RELIEVES THE PAIN?___________________________

VII. WHAT CAUSES OR INCREASES THE PAIN?___________________________

VIII. EFFECTS OF PAIN: Note decreased function, decreased quality of life.

Accompanying symptoms (e.g., nausea)___________________________

Sleep___________________________

Appetite___________________________

Physical activity___________________________

Relationship with others (e.g., irritability)___________________________

Emotions (e.g. anger, suicidal, crying)___________________________

Concentration___________________________

Other___________________________

IX. OTHER COMMENTS:___________________________

X. PLAN:___________________________

Figure 9-4 Initial pain assessment tool. (From McCaffery M, Beebe A: *Pain: clinical manual of nursing care,* St Louis, 1989, Mosby.)

INTERVENTIONS FOR PAIN RELIEF

When a specific underlying cause of the pain can be identified, medical management is directed toward eliminating it. For example, the pain of appendicitis or cholecystitis can be eliminated by surgically removing the involved organ, and the pain associated with infection can be relieved with antibiotics. When an underlying cause cannot be identified or eliminated, a patient may be referred to a pain clinic, where a multidisciplinary approach is used to diagnose and treat the pain. In such a clinic the major focus is to help patients learn a variety of methods, such as distraction, guided imagery, biofeedback and relaxation techniques, that help them to better manage their pain on a daily basis (Baque, 1989).

Nursing Interventions and Pain Medication

The administration of a drug should not be the only or even the first action considered by the nurse when responding to a patient's report of pain. Offering reassurance or using general comfort measures often reduces the need for pain medication or augments the pharmacologic intervention.

Various medications are used to alleviate pain by interacting with some aspect of the pain experience (Table 9-1) (Acute Pain Management Guideline Panel, 1992, 1994; McCaffery, Beebe, 1989; McCaffery and others, 1989; Willens, 1994). Aspirin and other nonsteroidal antiinflammatory drugs are commonly used for mild to moderate pain (Acute Pain Management

Worst
possible
pain

No
pain

Figure 9-5 Visual analog scale (VAS). Patients draw a line to indicate the amount of pain they are experiencing. The 10 cm line is measured against a patient's line, which provides an objective indication of perceived pain.

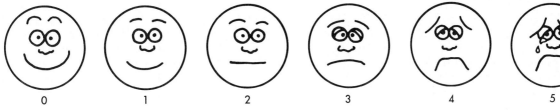

1) Explain to the child that each face is for a person who feels happy because he or she has no pain (hurt, or whatever word the child uses) or feels sad because he or she has some or a lot of pain.
2) Point to the appropriate face and state, "This face is . . .":
   0—"very happy because he doesn't hurt at all."
   1—"hurts just a little bit."
   2—"hurts a little more."
   3—"hurts even more."
   4—"hurts a whole lot."
   5—"hurts as much as you can imagine, although you don't have to be crying to feel this bad."
3) Ask the child to choose the face that best describes how he or she feels. Be specific about which pain (e.g., "shot" or incision) and what time (e.g., now? earlier before lunch?).

Figure 9-6 Wong-Baker faces rating scale. (From McCaffery M, Beebe A: *Pain: clinical manual of nursing care,* St Louis, 1989, Mosby.)

TABLE 9-1

Pharmacology of Drugs Used for the Patient With Pain

Drug (Generic and Trade Name); Route and Dosage	Action/Indication	Common Side Effects and Nursing Considerations
ACETAMINOPHEN (Liquiprin, Tempra, St. Joseph's tablets, Tylenol) **ROUTE:** PO, Rectal **DOSAGE:** PO, 325-650 mg q 3-4 hr prn (maximum of 4000 mg daily); may also be given rectally as a suppository	Mild analgesic and antipyretic (reduces fever)	Can mask fever/infection; overdose or chronic use can cause liver damage; monitor liver function tests
ACETAMINOPHEN AND CODEINE (Tylenol #3) **ROUTE:** PO **DOSAGE:** 1-2 q 3-4 hr prn	Contains acetaminophen 300 mg with codeine phosphate 30 mg; used for mild pain unrelieved by plain Tylenol	Not for use in addicted or in those with codeine allergies
ACETYLSALICYCLIC ACID (aspirin) **ROUTE:** PO, rectal **DOSAGE:** PO and rectal as analgesic and antipyretic, 325-1000 mg q 4-6 hr as needed (not to exceed 4 g/day); antiinflammatory, 2.6-6.2 g/day in divided doses	Mild analgesic, antipyretic, antiinflammatory	Increases prothrombin time and can cause gastric bleeding; give with full glass of water or milk to minimize gastrointestinal reactions
CODEINE (Codeine) **ROUTE:** PO, IM, SC **DOSAGE:** PO, IM, SC, 15-60 mg q 3-6 hr as needed	Mild-to-moderate analgesic narcotic	Most often used in combination with aspirin or acetaminophen; high doses (e.g., 60 mg) may cause restlessness and excitement; watch for constipation and urinary retention
FENTANYL (Sublimaze, Duragesic) **ROUTE:** IV, epidural, transdermal patch **DOSAGE:** IV, 15-50 μg per hour; epidural, 50-100 μg per hour; transdermal patch, 25, 50, 70, or 100 μg per patch q 72 hr	Potent analgesic; also used as anesthetic in operating room; bypasses gastrointestinal absorption	Nausea, mental clouding, and skin irritation; very potent; epidural or IV dose acts rapidly (4-10 min and action disappears in 3 hr or less); transdermal patch contains a 72-hr dose with peak effect in 12-18 hr; patient may need other opioid for breakthrough pain
HYDROMORPHONE (Dilaudid) **ROUTE:** IV, epidural, PO, IM, SC, rectal **DOSAGE:** Epidural, 0.15-0.3 mg each hour; SC, IM, IV, 1-2 mg q 2-3 hr; PO, 2-12 mg q 4-6 hr; rectal suppository, 3 mg q 6-8 hr	Very potent synthetic narcotic analgesic; is 8 to 10 times stronger than morphine; used for severe pain, especially cardiac pain	Sedation, confusion, hypotension, and constipation; use smallest dose possible; as tolerance develops, larger dose may be required; use with caution in head trauma, increased intracranial pressure, severe renal or hepatic disease, severe pulmonary disease, hypothyroidism, adrenal insufficiency, alcoholism, elderly or debilitated patients, undiagnosed abdominal pain, and prostatic hypertrophy.

TABLE 9-1

Pharmacology of Drugs Used for the Patient With Pain—cont'd

Drug (Generic and Trade Name); Route and Dosage	Action/Indication	Common Side Effects and Nursing Considerations
IBUPROFEN (Motrin, Nuprin) **ROUTE:** PO **DOSAGE:** Analgesia, 200-400 mg q 4-6 hr (not to exceed 3200 mg/day); antiinflammatory, 300-800 mg 3-4 times a day (not to exceed 3200 mg/day)	Nonsteroidal antiinflammatory, nonopioid analgesic, antipyretic agent used in the management of mild-to-moderate pain and such inflammatory disorders as rheumatoid and osteoarthritis; also used to lower fever	Headache, drowsiness, nausea, dyspepsia, vomiting, constipation, and gastrointestinal bleeding; additive adverse gastrointestinal effects with aspirin, other nonsteroidal antiinflammatory agents, potassium supplements, glucocorticoids, or alcohol
LEVORPHANOL (Levo-Dromoran) **ROUTE:** SC, PO **DOSAGE:** PO, SC, 2-3 mg q 4-6 hr	Very potent synthetic narcotic analgesic (4 to 6 times stronger than morphine); used for severe pain	Sedation, confusion, hypotension, and constipation; very strong sedative and respiratory depressant; slow onset of peak effect (60-90 min), but prolonged duration (6-8 hr)
MEPERDINE (Demerol) **ROUTE:** IM, IV, PO **DOSAGE:** Preoperatively, IM, 50-100 mg q 30-90 min before surgery, IM dose should be reduced; sometimes may be given PO	Narcotic analgesic used preoperatively and for moderate-to-severe pain	Increased ICP and respiratory depression; contraindicated if hypersensitive or previously addicted; use with caution in addictive personality, heart disease, respiratory depression, hepatic or renal disease; less spasmodic and constipating than most narcotics; significantly less effective orally
METHADONE (Dolophine) **ROUTE:** IM, SC, PO **DOSAGE:** IM, SC, PO, 2.5-10 mg q 3-4 hr	Synthetic narcotic used for severe pain	Sedation, confusion, hypotension, and constipation; administration may be painful; longer-acting and less sedating than morphine
MORPHINE (Morphine) **ROUTE:** PO, IM, IV **DOSAGE:** IM, 10 mg (range 5-20 mg) q 3-4 hr prn; PO, 10-30 mg q 4 hr prn; prolonged-release tablets, 15, 30, 60, and 100 mg q 12 hr; IV, 4-10 mg diluted in 4-5 ml H_2O for injection over 5 min	Narcotic analgesic used preoperatively and for severe pain; considered best first choice for relief of severe pain	Respiratory depression; contraindicated in the addicted, hemorrhage, bronchial asthma, and increased intracranial pressure; use with caution in addictive personality, severe heart disease, and hepatic and renal disease; standard narcotic to which all other narcotics are compared
NAPROXEN (Naprosyn) **NAPROXEN SODIUM** (Anaprox) **ROUTE:** PO **DOSAGE:** Naprosyn, 500 mg initially followed by 250 mg q 6-8 hr; Anaprox, 550 mg initially followed by 275 mg q 6-8 hr	Nonopioid analgesic; nonsteroid antiinflammatory drug used in the management of mild-to-moderate pain, the treatment of dysmenorrhea, and the management of inflammatory disorders, including rheumatoid arthritis and osteoarthritis	Headache, drowsiness, dizziness, nausea, dyspepsia, and constipation; contraindicated in active gastrointestinal bleeding or ulcer disease; possibility of cross-sensitivity to other nonsteroidal antiinflammatory drugs

continued

TABLE 9-1

Pharmacology of Drugs Used for the Patient With Pain—cont'd

Drug (Generic and Trade Name); Route and Dosage	Action/Indication	Common Side Effects and Nursing Considerations
OXYCODONE (Percodan) **ROUTE:** PO **DOSAGE:** 5 mg q 3-6 hr as needed or 10 mg 3-4 times daily as needed	Opioid analgesic used alone and in combination with nonopioid analgesics in the management of moderate-to-severe pain	Sedation, confusion, and constipation; use with caution in head trauma or increased intracranial pressure, severe hepatic or renal disease, severe pulmonary disease, hypothyroidism, adrenal insufficiency, alcoholism, addicted patients, elderly or debilitated patients, undiagnosed abdominal pain, and prostatic hypertrophy
PENTAZOCINE (Talwin) **ROUTE:** IV, IM, PO **DOSAGE:** IM, IV, 30 mg q 2-4 hr; PO, 50 mg q 3-4 hr (maximum dose of 600 mg/day)	Analgesic used for moderate pain (one-third as potent as morphine); often used as a preoperative medication or to supplement anesthesia	Sedation, headache, euphoria, hallucinations, dizziness, and nausea; can antagonize effect of morphine and other narcotics and may elicit withdrawal symptoms in patients who have been taking other narcotics regularly
PROPOXYPHENE (Darvon, Darvon-N) **PROPOXYPHENE/ACETAMINOPHEN** (Darvocet-N) **PROPOXYPHENE-N/ACETAMINOPHEN** (Darvocet-N-100) **ROUTE:** PO **DOSAGE:** 100 mg propoxyphene napsylate = 65 mg; propoxyphene hydrochloride: 65 mg q 4 hr (hydrochloride-Darvon) or 100 mg q 4 hr (napsylate-Darvocet-N with acetaminophen, Darvon-N) as needed (not to exceed 390 mg/day as hydrochloride or 600 mg/day as napsylate).	Nonopioid analgesic often used in combination with acetaminophen, aspirin, and caffeine for management of mild-to-moderate pain	Dizziness, weakness, drowsiness, nausea, and vomiting; use with extreme caution in patients receiving MAO inhibitors; same precautions as percodan (above)

Guideline Panel, 1992, 1994). These drugs block the production of neurotransmitters near the injury that activate nerve endings and send pain signals to the brain. Tricyclic antidepressant drugs (e.g., amitriptyline, doxepin) may be used to elevate mood and raise the levels of neurotransmitters that stimulate the production of endorphins.

Opiate drugs are often used for moderate-to-severe pain. Morphine molecules fit into receptor sites on certain cells in the brain and central nervous system and prevent pain messages from being received. Combinations of drugs are often used (e.g., aspirin and codeine) to attack the pain problem from several approaches. Long-acting versions of morphine, such as MS Contin, Oramorph SR, and "patches" of transdermal fentanyl (Duragesic), are often used in the home setting. Most analgesic drugs used to be administered on an "as needed" (prn) basis. The patient had to ask for pain relief. Current thinking is to suppress the pain "around the clock" (ATC). By giving medications according to a time schedule, the patient's body maintains a sufficient level of drug to keep the pain under control, prevents anxiety from building, and prevents the memory of suffering from becoming established.

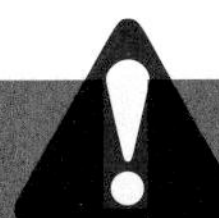

NURSE ALERT

Teach the patient to request pain medication as soon as pain occurs or before it increases.

It is critical that the nurse be aware of the significant variations in drugs, peak effects, duration of effects, and side effects. The nurse must also be alert to the differences that result from oral versus parenteral administration of a medication. The peak effect for most parenteral narcotics is 1 hour, whereas the peak effect of most oral forms of the same drug occurs 2 or more hours later. Oral analgesics usually have a longer duration of effect than parenteral drugs. A careful assessment of these factors must be made and incorporated into the plan of care for any patient who is receiving medications. If one analgesic is not providing satisfactory pain relief, another drug is likely to be substituted. Tables 9-2 and 9-3 provide examples of approximate equivalent doses and durations of pain relief for some commonly prescribed analgesic agents.

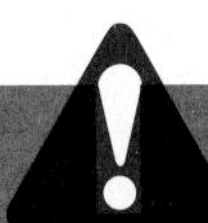

NURSE ALERT

The onset, peak effects, and duration of analgesia for each drug differs and may also vary with individuals.

TABLE 9-2

Equianalgesics for Mild-to-Moderate Pain. Approximate Oral Dose as Compared With Aspirin 650 mg.

Analgesic	Oral Dose (mg)	Duration of Analgesia (hours)
aspirin	650	4
acetaminophen (Tylenol)	650	4
codeine (Codeine)	32	4-6
meperidine (Demerol)	50	4
oxycodone (Percodan)	5	3-6

Patients should be monitored for side effects of all medications. This is especially true of opiate (narcotic) drugs. All narcotics have the potential to cause respiratory depression as a result of the decreased sensitivity of the respiratory center to carbon dioxide. The nurse must carefully assess the patient for respiratory changes. Treatments for respiratory depression include arousing the patient, establishing a patent airway, administering a narcotic antagonist such as naloxone, and providing artificial ventilation should it become necessary. The patient will develop a tolerance to respiratory depression if the opiate continues to be used.

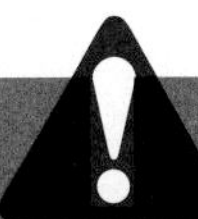

NURSE ALERT

The first sign of tolerance to a narcotic is decreased duration of pain relief, followed by decreased pain relief.

Constipation is a common side effect of opioid administration. Opiates cause decreased peristaltic contractions in the gastrointestinal tract, which allows increased absorption of water from bowel contents. Tolerance to this side effect does not occur, nor does it diminish over time. Because constipation can cause pain and discomfort, it is necessary to begin a program of constipation prevention when opioids are started.

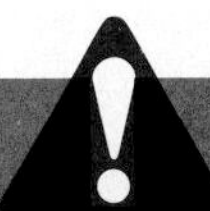

NURSE ALERT

Constipation, drowsiness, and nausea are all possible effects of narcotics. Something can be done about each of these.

Older adults often suffer multiple, chronic, and painful illnesses and often taken multiple medications. Therefore they are at greater risk for drug-drug and drug-disease interactions. Aging may also alter the function of organs that are vital to the use and elimination of drugs, such as the liver and kidneys. Older patients may need to be given lower doses of certain drugs, and the intervals between doses may need to be adjusted to compensate for the older patient's changed physiology (Acute Pain Management Guideline Panel, 1992; Ferrell, 1991; Ramsey, 1988).

TABLE 9-3

Equianalagesics for Moderate-to-Severe Pain. Approximate Equivalent IM and Oral Doses of Commonly Used Analgesics as Compared with Morphine 10 mg.

Analgesic	IM Route (mg)	Oral Route (mg)	Duration of Analgesia (hours)
morphine (Morphine)	10	30-60*	4-6
codeine (Codeine)	130	200	4-6
hydromorphone (Dilaudid)	1.5	7.5	2-3
levorphanol (Levo-Dromoran)	2	4	4-6
meperidine (Demerol)	75	300	2-3
oxycodone (Percodan)	15	30	4-5

*When used over a long period, the dose is usually 30 mg.

OLDER ADULT CONSIDERATIONS

Pain is not a normal part of aging. Older patients sometimes believe that pain cannot be relieved and are stoic in reporting their pain. The frail and those over age 85 are particularly at risk for undertreatment of pain. Aging need not alter pain thresholds or tolerance. The pain experiences between older and younger patients have far more similarities than differences.

Pain assessment can be difficult in the older adult. Cognitive impairment, delirium, dementia, and visual and hearing changes may interfere with the use of some pain assessment scales. When a verbal report is not possible, observe for behavioral clues to pain, such as restlessness or agitation. The absence of pain behaviors does not indicate the absence of pain. Older adults often suffer multiple, chronic, and painful illnesses and often take multiple medications. Therefore they are at risk for drug-drug and drug-disease interactions. Nonsteroidal antiinflammatory drugs (NSAIDs) can be used safely in older adults, but their use requires vigilance for side effects, especially gastric and renal toxicity. Opiates are safe and effective when used appropriately in older adults. However, they are more sensitive to the analgesic effects of opiate drugs and often experience higher peak effects and longer durations of pain relief.

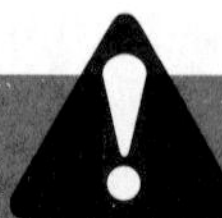

NURSE ALERT

A patient can be both sedated and in pain. Do not confuse sedation with analgesia.

Patients should be given analgesics before their pain becomes severe. If a patient must wait too long for relief, discomfort and anxiety increase, and significantly more medication is needed to adequately control the pain. Ideally the patient should not need to ask for analgesics for pain relief. The observant nurse assesses the patient's need and proceeds according to the principle of prevention rather than the treatment of already existing pain.

Addiction

Pain medications should not be withheld from patients because of fear of tolerance or dependence. **Addiction** (psychologic dependence) must be distinguished from physical dependence or drug tolerance (Ferrell and others, 1992; McCaffery, Beebe, 1989; Porter, Hick, 1980). With drug **tolerance,** increasingly larger doses are needed to provide the same effect as the original dose produced. The first sign of tolerance is that the duration of the drug's effect is shortened. The amount of pain relief obtained is then lessened. Tolerance can be handled by increasing the dose of the drug or occasionally by switching to another medication with an equivalent analgesic effect.

If a patient receives narcotics continuously for several weeks, it is assumed that physical dependence will occur (McCaffery, Beebe, 1989). **Physical dependence** is an altered state that is produced by the repeated administration of a drug. Withdrawal symptoms occur when the drug is stopped. In the clinical setting, pain seldom stops abruptly. Patients who become physically dependent can be weaned off the drug by gradually diminishing the doses as the pain subsides. Addiction is a behavioral pattern that is rooted in a psychologic desire for the euphoric effects of narcotics. It is characterized by an overwhelming need to get and use the drug. Most patients do not request analgesics unless they have pain. In fact it is far more common for patients with pain to refuse analgesics unnecessarily because of a fear of addiction. Most experts agree that psychologic dependence (addiction) is rare when narcotics are administered to patients who experience pain during short hospital stays.

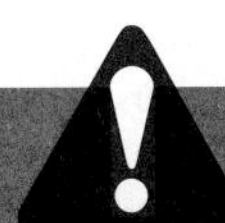

NURSE ALERT

Focus on the patient's response to a medication rather than on the size of the dose.

Placebos

Placebos have no role in clinical pain management. A **placebo** is an inactive substance or procedure that is prescribed by a physician for a patient as a supposedly effective treatment (McCaffery, Beebe, 1989; Perry, Heidrich, 1981). They are commonly used as control measures in research. A placebo is documented on the patient's chart just as any other drug or therapy. Approximately one third of the population reacts to placebos and experiences effects of pain relief. However, on successive uses, patients report less or no pain relief. Research has shown that the effects of placebos are physical, as well as psychologic. The exact mechanisms by which placebos work is not known, but research suggests that placebos stimulate the brain to produce endorphins and other chemicals, thus calling on "the doctor within." To a large extent the ability of a placebo to produce effects is a measure of the faith or confidence that the patient has in his or her physician or nurse. Administering placebos sometimes creates an ethical dilemma for the nurse. If a placebo is being given for an inappropriate purpose (e.g., to "prove" that the pain is not "real"), the nurse has the right to refuse to give it. In such a situation, the nurse should discuss the problem with the nursing supervisor so that the action has administrative support and the patient receives attention for his or her pain (McCaffery, Beebe, 1989). The obligation to manage pain and relieve the patient's suffering is at the core of a healthcare professional's commitment (Acute Pain Management Guideline Panel, 1992).

NURSE ALERT

The use of placebos can destroy a patient's trust in healthcare professionals.

ETHICAL DILEMMA

Mr. Jones, age 57, has come to the hospital with lung cancer that has spread to his bones and liver. Mr. Jones knows that he is dying and has signed an advance directive to prevent any "heroic measures." He has also made it clear that he does not want to die in pain. His medications include morphine every 3 hours.

One morning Miss Adams, his nurse, heard from the night nurse during report that Mr. Jones' respirations were only 8 per minute. Therefore the night nurse had withheld the last dose. Miss Adams discussed this situation with her fellow nurses, and they feared that another dose of morphine might kill him. Miss Adams talked to Mr. Jones and discovered that he was alert but fearful because his pain was getting worse.

1 Was it appropriate for the night nurse to withhold the medication?
2 How should Miss Adams follow up on this situation?

Patient-controlled analgesia

Patient-controlled analgesia (PCA) is a method of delivering painkilling drugs into an intravenous line (Figure 9-7) (Fitzgerald, Shamy, 1987; Jones, Brooks, 1990). A variety of intravenous infusion pumps are now used to allow patients to control pain by administering analgesic medications to themselves. The pumps are programmed to provide specific amounts of drugs at time intervals that are determined by the physician. The pumps are equipped with safety features that prevent overdoses. The patient should be told how often he or she can administer a dose and whether medications will be received after each attempt. It is important that the patient notify the nurse if pain relief is not satisfactory, because a different order may need to be obtained from the physician. Research has shown that PCA can often provide better pain relief than periodic injections because patients can receive relief at the first sign of pain. Studies also show that patients like the idea of controlling their own pain. Anxiety and tension are decreased, and often less narcotic is used. When using a PCA pump, it is important to assess the patient's pain at least every 4 hours and to maintain accurate records of the infusion on the flow sheet. The amount of medication used needs to be tailored to each patient's needs, regardless of how it is delivered.

Intraspinal analgesia

Opiates are sometimes administered via catheters into the epidural or subarachnoid space in the spinal

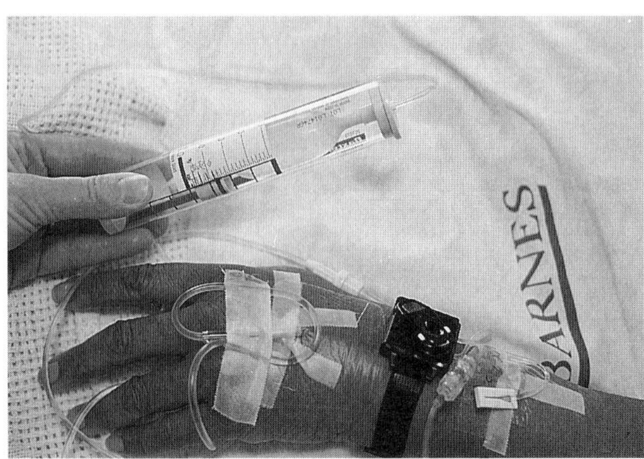

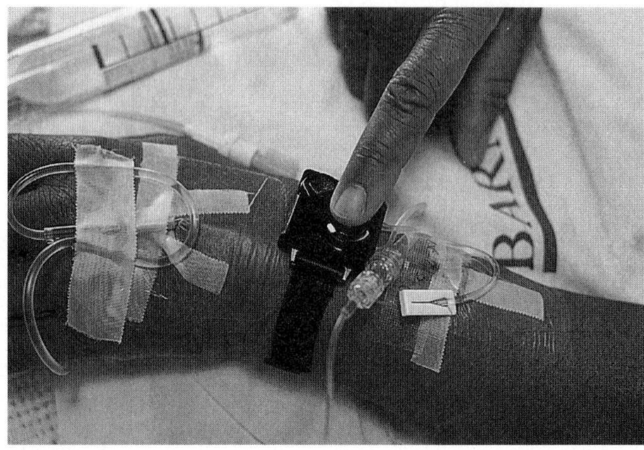

Figure 9-7 Patient-controlled analgesic (PCA) devices. (From Perry AC, Potter PA: *Clinical nursing skills and techniques*, ed 3, St Louis, 1994, Mosby.)

cord (Haight, 1987; Keeney, 1993; Wild, Coyne, 1992). Analgesia results from the drug's direct effect on receptors within the spinal cord instead of within the brain. Fewer side effects (e.g., sedation, disorientation) are seen by this route than with the systemic administration of narcotics. The spinal route can be used for both acute and chronic pain. Intraspinal analgesia is most commonly used for postoperative pain (e.g., cesarean section, orthopedic surgery) and for cancer pain that is poorly controlled by systemic medications. Nurses must have specific, additional inservice education on this method before being assigned to care for patients who have orders for **epidural** or **intrathecal analgesia.** Patients must be carefully monitored to be certain that the catheter remains in place and that no inflammation is present. The nurse must also monitor for side effects such as pruritus, urinary retention, nausea and vomiting, respiratory depression, and postural hypotension. Patients should be instructed to quickly report any side effects or lack of pain relief.

Transcutaneous electrical neural stimulation

Transcutaneous electrical neural stimulation (TENS) is most commonly used for pain that is fairly well localized (McCaffery, Beebe, 1989). TENS modulates pain by stimulating peripheral nerves with electrical current via electrodes that are applied to the skin and connected to a small battery-operated pulse generator (Figure 9-8). This stimulation enhances the production of endorphins and therefore mobilizes the pain defenses of the body. This method may be used alone or in conjunction with other modalities. TENS is most often used to control chronic pain but may also be used for acute pain, especially postoperative pain and pain from injuries such as sprains and lacerations. Using TENS with a postoperative patient often decreases (although not completely) the patient's need for narcotic analgesics and therefore decreases unwanted side effects such as respiratory depression, nausea and vomiting, and slow bowel functioning. In most clinical settings, the physician or physical therapist introduces the patient to TENS. The treatment is typically administered by nurses who have had special education in the use of TENS. The patient is encouraged to handle the equipment and experiment with the settings to determine the best location for the electrodes and the most comfortable frequency and duration of current. Before the electrodes are attached to the skin, the nurse should wash the area with soap and water to reduce resistance, rinse the area, and dry it. The nurse applies enough electrode gel to ensure adequate conduction but not so much that the gel oozes from under the electrode. The nurse tapes the electrodes in place, turns on the stimulator, and slowly advances the output control until the patient feels stimulation. Most patients describe the stimulation as a buzzing or tingling sensation. The nurse helps the patient adjust the controls to provide the most comfortable sensation that gives the most pain relief. Most patients obtain considerable relief from TENS. However, TENS does not work the same for everyone. Some patients experience great relief immediately. Others experience relief only after repeated applications. Some patients find that the analgesia may last for hours or even days after the current is turned off, whereas others experience relief only for a limited time. Nurses can provide support and encouragement to their patients while they experiment with this device.

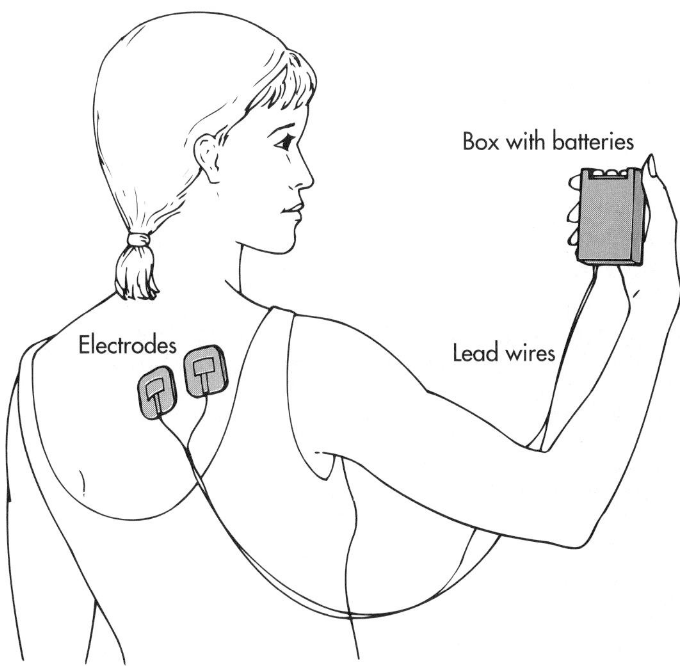

Figure 9-8 Three major components of a TENS unit, with two electrodes placed on the upper back of the patient to relieve shoulder pain. (From McCaffery M, Beebe A: *Pain: clinical manual of nursing care,* St Louis, 1989, Mosby.)

Noninvasive interventions

A number of physical or mental activities can be used to help the patient focus his or her attention on sensations other than pain (Acute Pain Management Guideline Panel, 1992; Barbour, McGuire, Kirchhoff, 1986; Mast and others, 1987; McCaffery, Beebe, 1989; Watt-Watson, Donovan, 1992). **Distraction** is a very useful technique if a patient is experiencing mild-to-moderate pain. With severe pain, distraction tends to increase anxiety and tension and thus increase pain. Examples of distraction include talking on the telephone, watching television, working on hobbies or crafts, and performing rhythmic breathing techniques. It is critical to remember that distraction does not make the pain go away but only makes it more bearable. Any procedure that helps the patient relax can help relieve emotional and muscular tension and lessen pain. A wide variety of **relaxation techniques** are available, such as progressive relaxation exercises, meditation, biofeedback, and self-hypnosis. The Lamaze method of childbirth is an example of a procedure that uses both distraction and relaxation procedures. Most relaxation techniques require time and effort to master but are very useful, especially for a patient who has chronic pain. Nurses who have a knowledge of relaxation techniques can help their patients tolerate short-term painful procedures. They can also provide encouragement and support as their patients practice new methods.

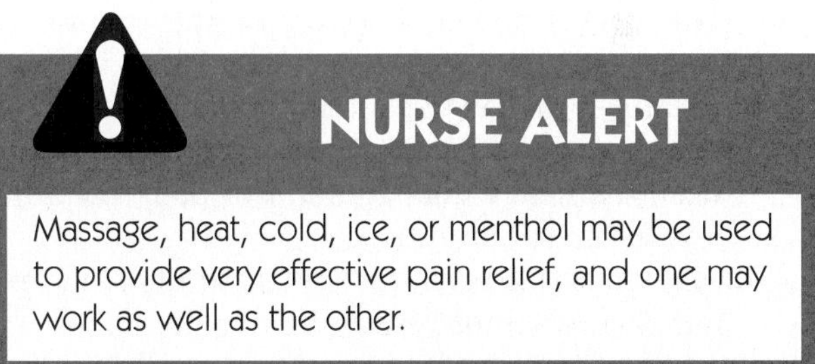

NURSE ALERT

Massage, heat, cold, ice, or menthol may be used to provide very effective pain relief, and one may work as well as the other.

Many patients have developed their own methods for coping with pain. The nurse should ask the patient to describe procedures that have helped in the past and should support and encourage the patient as he or she attempts to use them in the present pain situation. As with the use of analgesics, it is important to begin pain control methods before the pain becomes severe.

Neurosurgical interventions

A number of neurosurgical techniques for blocking pain transmission have been tried (Acute Pain Management Guideline Panel, 1992; McCaffery, Beebe, 1989; Miaskowski, 1993). Peripheral nerve blocks using local anesthetics such as lidocaine can temporarily relieve pain in some acute painful situations such as neuralgia, thrombophlebitis, or musculoskeletal conditions. Absolute alcohol or phenol may be used for longer effects (up to 6 months). However, these substances are not used often because of their toxic effects—they may produce necrosis and sloughing of superficial tissue. Surgical interruption of the pain pathways may be necessary if the pain becomes severe and cannot be controlled by any other means. A peripheral **neurectomy** (severing of a nerve) may be performed if the pain is localized to a specific area such as an arm or leg. When the pain is more diffuse (e.g., cancer pain), the pain pathways in the spinal cord may be interrupted. This procedure is known as a **chordotomy** and can be done at various levels depending on the location of the pain. Other procedures that may be performed include **rhizotomy** (resecting a portion of a spinal nerve root) or the destruction of small, specific sites in the brain by using radiation or by using a probe to apply a heating current. The nurse must be aware that the body is no longer protected from injury as a result of the loss of sensation in the area that was affected by the surgery. Therefore such patients are particularly susceptible to pressure sores. Box 9-2 de-

BOX 9-2 **Nursing Process**

PATIENT IN PAIN

ASSESSMENT

History of pain: prior pain experiences, factors that precipitated the pain, activities that increase or decrease the pain, methods used to relieve the pain, usual time of occurrence of pain episodes

Physiologic characteristics: increase in pulse and respiratory rates, increase in diastolic and systolic blood pressure, pallor, dilated pupils, diaphoresis, nausea; because of the body's ability to adapt to abnormal situations, these physiologic signs may be absent or decreased in prolonged acute pain or chronic pain

Verbal statements: description of the quality or character of the pain (aching, burning, prickling), severity of pain using a scale (mild, moderate, severe), location of pain (precisely located or diffuse), frequency and duration of pain, meaning of pain to the individual

Facial expressions: clenched teeth, tightly shut lips, tightened jaw muscles, strained look

Body movements: lying quietly or rigidly, restless or purposeless movements, protective or guarding movements toward a specific area, rubbing movements

NURSING DIAGNOSIS

Pain, chronic pain (additional diagnoses may occur as a result of pain, such as anxiety, constipation, fatigue, or fear) related to pathophysiologic condition

NURSING INTERVENTIONS

Assure the patient that it is known that the pain is real and that he or she will have help in dealing with it.

Provide general comfort measures such as turning, repositioning, providing back rubs, and changing damp dressings.

Provide support for painful areas when moving the patient, such as placing a pillow to the abdominal incision area.

Individualize pain control measures by considering a variety of approaches.

Use pain control measures before pain becomes severe; get ahead of the pain. Include measures that the patient believes will help.

Provide distraction and meaningful and interesting sensory stimulation such as radio, television, hobbies, and conversation.

Provide cutaneous stimulation to block pain transmission, such as gentle massage, pressure, application of menthol rubbing agents to skin or around painful area, application of heat or cold as indicated, and TENS.

Promote relaxation. Instruct the patient to breathe deeply and "let go" on expiration. Help patient to relax his or her body while contracting one muscle group (e.g., arm, leg).

Help patient use guided imagery and imagine a pleasant event as a substitute for the pain experience.

EVALUATION OF EXPECTED OUTCOMES

Pain reduced or eliminated

Understanding of the rationale for therapy

Use of effective measures for relief of discomfort

Anxiety and fear reduced or eliminated

Side effects of medications controlled or minimized

Demonstration of increased tolerance for pain by returning to work, using analgesics less often, or increasing daily activities

scribes nursing care guidelines for patients who are in pain.

Patient and Family Teaching

It is important to work routinely with both the patient and the family. Patients who understand their pain and the possible ways to reduce it feel more in control of their life and are better able to actively participate in the available interventions. Nurses provide a vital service by teaching patients ways to manage the pain or discomfort they may face.

Every patient education plan must start with an assessment of what the patient needs to know and how much he or she already does know. Assess the patient's readiness and ability to learn. The severity and duration of the patient's pain often dictates what he or she is ready to learn. Determine whether the patient has any barriers to learning, such as hearing or visual impairments, language difficulties, or a lack of reading skills. It is always wise to keep any instruction simple. Medical terminology may not be understood by patients or their families.

Prevention is a key concept that needs to be taught. Patients should ask for pain relief when the pain first begins. Make certain that patients (and their families) know how to use a pain rating scale and how to help with the pain relief by assessing and reporting their own pain. They should be assured that other measures of pain control are available and can be used if the current measures of pain control are not satisfactory.

Provide specific instructions for each pain relief measure and follow the procedures set forth by the physician or institution. Learn and practice as many noninvasive measures as possible to be prepared to help a patient when the need and opportunity arises.

PATIENT/FAMILY TEACHING 

Explain what pain to expect and what will be done about it.
Explain the concept of prevention; teach patient to take (or ask) for pain relief drugs when pain first begins.
Explain how to use the pain rating scale and how it helps the staff to determine the best way to control pain.
Provide instructions for who to notify if pain relief is not satisfactory.
Provide specific instructions for each pain relief measure (e.g., PCA, TENS, epidural, relaxation, distraction, medications).

Nursing Care Plan

PATIENT WITH EPIDURAL ANALGESIA FOR PAIN MANAGEMENT

The patient is a 52-year-old female who had an elective abdominal hysterectomy this morning. She is in good general health and has no known food or drug allergies. An epidural catheter is in place for pain management. Patient is a good candidate for epidural analgesia. Monitoring for actual or potential patient responses to epidural analgesia is an essential nursing responsibility.

Past Medical History	Psychosocial Data	Assessment Data
Good general health Discomfort from large uterine fibroids for 6 years Normal vaginal deliveries × 3 Menopause at age 50	Both parents and husband in good health Three grown children, living in vicinity Married, lives with husband in own home Employed as teacher in local high school Has good family support	Oriented to time, place, person *Respiratory:* Lungs clear to percussion and auscultation; chest movements symmetrical *Cardiovascular:* Apical pulse strong and regular at 78; vital signs stable (T 99.6, P 76-84, R 18, BP 114/74) *Abdomen:* Soft with slight distention; lower transverse incision, area clean and intact; dressings dry and clean

continued

Nursing Care Plan—cont'd

PATIENT WITH EPIDURAL ANALGESIA FOR PAIN MANAGEMENT

Past Medical History	Psychosocial Data	Assessment Data
		Epidural catheter: Taped in place at L3; transparent dressing-surgical tape dry and intact; catheter connected to a continuous infusion with label on it stating "for epidural use"; catheter looped over left shoulder and secured on the back with tape; connected to infusion pump. *Pain:* States feeling no pain. **Medications** droperidol (Inapsine) 0.625-1.23 mg IV q 4 hr prn for nausea IV fluids D5 with lactated Ringer's solution 1000 ml q 12 hr; may d/c when PO intake is adequate *Epidural infusion:* See Epidural Analgesia Order form

NURSING DIAGNOSIS

Potential for knowledge deficit related to process of epidural analgesia.

NURSING INTERVENTIONS	EVALUATION OF EXPECTED OUTCOMES
Ask patient if clarification of terms or procedures is needed; review the physician's explanation with the patient. Remind patient to take a slow and gradual approach to changing position or ambulating. Observe for signs that patient may be more active than is safe.	Verbalizes an understanding of procedures and reports any side effects and/or lack of pain relief After surgery, does not attempt activities beyond ability

NURSING DIAGNOSIS

Pain related to inadequate analgesia catheter problems, pruritus, or nausea and vomiting

NURSING INTERVENTIONS	EVALUATION OF EXPECTED OUTCOMES
Monitor and evaluate analgesic effect; ask patient about level of comfort; observe level of ease at which patient moves about. Notify anesthesiologist if pain relief not adequate with highest level of dose range ordered. Check catheter for breaks, knots, or leakage at dressing site or at catheter hub. Observe for patient scratching or rubbing, especially around the face or neck.	Verbalizes pain relief Verbalizes no pruritus or minimal pruritus that does not interfere with comfort Verbalizes no nausea and experiences no vomiting

NURSING INTERVENTIONS	EVALUATION OF EXPECTED OUTCOMES
Promptly notify primary care nurse and physician of edema, urticaria, or respiratory difficulties. Provide support measures such as lotions, cool/warm packs, or diversional activities as directed. Observe for signs of nausea or vomiting. Notify primary care nurse and physician; administer droperidol (Inapsine) per physician's order. Provide hygienic and emotional support; increase activities slowly.	

NURSING DIAGNOSIS

Risk for ineffective breathing pattern related to pathophysiologic condition

NURSING INTERVENTIONS	EVALUATION OF EXPECTED OUTCOMES
Administer narcotics, sedatives, and analgesics only as directed by physician. Assess respiratory function q 1 hr for first 24 hours, then q 2-8 hr and as necessary; assess level of consciousness/sedation and color of mucous membranes. Attach patient to apnea monitor if necessary. Obtain and evaluate blood gases as ordered. Notify physician if respiratory depression occurs; administer naloxone per physician's order.	Respiratory function maintained: Respiratory rate > 12 Respiratory depth adequate Baseline level of consciousness maintained Skin, nail beds, and mucous membranes pink Arterial blood gases within normal limits

NURSING DIAGNOSIS

Risk for altered urinary elimination/urinary retention related to pathophysiologic condition

NURSING INTERVENTIONS	EVALUATION OF EXPECTED OUTCOMES
Monitor output; observe for symptoms of discomfort, urgency, or decreased output; gently palpate bladder for distention if no urinary catheter is in place. Rule out other causes, such as fluid balance or positioning; assist patient with voiding. Catheterize per physician's order.	Verbalizes no complaints of distention; bladder is not palpable; patient voids within 8 hr of surgery

NURSING DIAGNOSIS

Risk for injury related to postural hypotension

NURSING INTERVENTIONS	EVALUATION OF EXPECTED OUTCOMES
Assess postural blood pressure and heart rate before ambulation. Assess fluid balance. Help patient sit up or ambulate the first time, then as needed.	Postural hypotension prevented or detected before ambulation Tolerates position changes without feeling dizzy or lightheaded

KEY CONCEPTS

- Pain is both a physical and a psychologic phenomenon.
- Pain is whatever a person says it is and exists wherever a person says it does.
- Nurses are held accountable for managing the pain program for patients under their care.
- The gate control theory at least partially explains how massage, heat and cold, counterirritants (e.g., Ben Gay), distraction, relaxation, and TENS affect the sensation of pain.
- A detailed and accurate description of the patient's pain is essential for accurately diagnosing and treating pain.
- Quantifying the amount of pain before and after administering medications or providing other interventions is a useful way to monitor the effectiveness of the therapy.
- Pain medications should be given on a set time schedule (ATC) to maintain a sufficient level of drug and control the pain, prevent anxiety, and prevent the memory of suffering.
- Pain medications should be given before the pain becomes severe. Prevention of pain is the goal of satisfactory pain management.
- The peak effect of most parenteral drugs is 1 hour. For oral drugs the peak effect is 2 or more hours later.
- Addiction (psychologic dependence) is rare in persons who are receiving narcotics for pain. Although physical dependence is to be expected if narcotics are used over a period of several weeks, the patient can be "weaned" off the drug.
- The ability of a placebo to cause effects is often a measure of the faith or confidence that the patient has in his or her physician or nurse.
- Patient-controlled analgesia can often provide better pain relief than injections because patients can receive relief at the first sign of pain.
- Nurses must have special education to care for patients who are receiving intraspinal analgesia.
- Distractions such as watching television and visiting with friends are helpful if the pain is mild or moderate.
- Any activity that helps a patient relax can help relieve emotional and muscular tension and lessen pain.

CRITICAL THINKING EXERCISES

1 How would you assess a non-English–speaking patient for pain following abdominal surgery?

2 Discuss at least one systemic effect that the acute pain of abdominal surgery could have on the cardiovascular, respiratory, and gastrointestinal systems.

3 List four medications that a patient could buy over-the-counter to help relieve the chronic pain of arthritis.

4 Discuss the use of meperidine (Demerol) for long-term use for a trauma patient.

REFERENCES AND ADDITIONAL READINGS

Acute Pain Management Guideline Panel: *Acute pain management: operative or medical procedures and trauma. Clinical practice guideline,* Rockville, Md, February 1992. Agency for Health Care Policy and Research, Public Health Service, US Department of Health and Human Services, AHCPR Publication No 92-0032.

Acute Pain Management Guideline Panel: Acute pain management in adults: operative procedures quick reference guide for clinicians, *MedSurg Nurs* 3(2):99-107, 1994.

Baque ML: What matters most in chronic pain management, *RN* 53(3):46-50, 1989.

Barbour LA, McGuire DB, Kirchoff KT: Nonanalgesic methods of pain control used by cancer patients, *Oncol Nurs Forum* 13(6):56-60, 1986.

DeWolf MS: The ethics of pain management, *MedSurg Nurs* 2(3):218-220, 1993.

Ferrell BA: Pain management in elderly people, *J Am Geriatr Soc* 39(1):64-73, 1991.

Ferrell AB and others: Pain and addiction: an urgent need for change in nursing education, *J Pain Symptom Manage* 7(2):117-124, 1992.

Fitzgerald J, Shamy P: Let your patient control his analgesia, *Nurs 87* 17(7): 48-51, 1987.

Haight K: What you should know about epidural analgesia, *Nurs 87* 17(9):58-59, 1987.

Herr KA, Mobily PR: Complexities of pain assessment in the elderly: clinical considerations, *J Gerontol Nurs* 17(4):12-19, 1991.

International Association for the Study of Pain: Pain terms: a current list with definitions and notes on usage, *Pain* 3(27):S215-S221, 1986.

Jones J, Brooks J: The ABC's of PCA, *RN* 54(5):54-60, 1990.

Keeney SA: Nursing care of the postoperative patient receiving epidural analgesia, *MedSurg Nurs* 2(3):191-196, 1993.

Mast D and others: Relaxation techniques: a self-learning module for nurses, *Cancer Nurs* 10(6):141-147, 1987.

McCaffery M, Beebe A: *Pain: clinical manual for nursing practice,* St Louis, 1989, Mosby.

McCaffery M, Ferrell BR: How to use the new ACHPR cancer pain guidelines, *Am J Nurs* 94(7):42-47, 1994.

McCaffery M and others: Giving narcotics for pain: the secrets to giving equianalgesic doses, *Nurs 89* 19(10):161-168, 1989.

McGuire L: The nurse's role in pain relief, *MedSurg Nurs* 3(2):91-98, 1994.

McGuire L and others: Managing pain in the young patient...in the elderly patient, *Nurs 82* 12(8):52-57, 1982.

Melzack R, Wall P: Pain mechanisms: a new theory, *Science* 150(3699):971-978, 1965.

Melzack R, Wall P: *The challenge of pain,* ed 2, London, 1988, Penguin Books.

Miaskowski C: Current concepts in the assessment and management of cancer-related pain, *MedSurg Nurs* 2(2):113-118, 1993.

Paice JA: Unraveling the mystery of pain, *Oncon Nurs Forum,* 18(5):843-849, 1991.

Perry S, Heidrich G: Placebo response: myth and matter, *Am J Nurs* 81(5):720-725, 1981.

Porter J, Hick H: Addiction rare in patients treated with narcotics, *N Engl J Med* 302(2):123, 1980.

Ramsey R: Adjusting drug dosages for critically ill elderly patients, *Nurs 88* 18(7):47-49, July 1988.

Sherman R: A survey of current phantom limb pain treatment in the United States, *Pain* 8(28):285-295, 1987.

Watt-Watson JH, Donovan MI: *Pain management: nursing perspective,* St Louis, 1992, Mosby.

West BA: Understanding endorphins: our natural pain relief system, *Nurs 81* 11(2):50-53, 1981.

Wild L, Coyne C: The basics and beyond: epidural analgesia, *Am J Nurs* 92(4):26-34, 1992.

Willens JS: Giving fentanyl for pain outside the OR, *Am J Nurs* 94(2):24-28, 1994.

CHAPTER 10

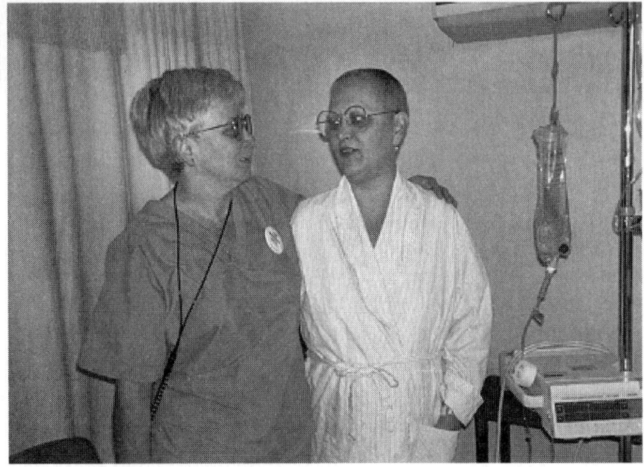

The Patient With Cancer

CHAPTER OBJECTIVES

1. Discuss cancer as a healthcare problem.
2. Describe the predominant characteristics of cancer.
3. Identify the major causes of cancer.
4. List recommended methods of prevention and early detection.
5. Describe the common methods of diagnosis and treatment of cancer.
6. Discuss nursing care of the patient receiving radiation therapy.
7. Discuss nursing care of the patient receiving chemotherapy.
8. Discuss the emotional impact of cancer on the patient and family.

KEY WORDS

benign
biologic response modifier
bone marrow transplantation
carcinogens
carcinoma
chemotherapy
desquamation
ionizing radiation
leukopenia
magnetic resonance imaging
malignant
metastasis
myelosuppression
neoplasm
oncogenes
oncology
palliative
radiation therapy
radioisotope
sarcoma
thrombocytopenia

Cancer is characterized by abnormal and unrestricted cell division and by the spread of these cells into healthy tissues of the body. Without appropriate medical intervention, this dissemination of cancer cells can become widespread and lead to tissue destruction, which may ultimately cause the death of the individual. Cancer is one of the oldest diseases known to humans. Its cause has been a puzzle for centuries and remains so.

In the United States, the annual number of deaths resulting from cancer each year is exceeded only by those resulting from heart disease. In 1994 it was estimated that approximately 1,208,000 new cancer cases would be diagnosed and that approximately 538,000 Americans would die of cancer that year (American Cancer Society, 1994). According to current trends, one out of every four persons and three out of every four families will be affected by cancer at some time. Cancer attacks rich and poor and young and old with equally devastating effects. The largest number of malignant tumors occurs in four areas of the body: the lungs, colon-rectum, breast, and prostate.

Lung cancer is the leading cause of cancer deaths in both men and women. Recently the incidence of lung cancer has been decreasing in men but continues to increase in women. Since 1987, more women have died each year from lung cancer than from breast cancer. In 1994 it was estimated that 153,000 people in the United States would die from lung cancer—94,000 men and 59,000 women. The survival rate for lung cancer is extremely low. Only approximately 13% of the victims live as long as 5 years after the disease has been diagnosed. These statistics are unfortunate because the disease is largely preventable. Cigarette smoking is directly related to at least 87% of the cases of lung cancer and accounts for approximately 30% of all cancer deaths (American Cancer Society, Inc., 1993).

According to 1994 estimates, colon-rectum cancer kills approximately 56,000 persons each year and ranks second as a cause of cancer deaths (American Cancer Society, 1993). There has been a small increase in survival rates during the past 2 decades. Approximately two out of every three patients may be saved by early diagnosis and prompt treatment, which are the keys to survival. Digital rectal examination, stool blood tests, and sigmoidoscopy are the methods recommended for early detection. Breast cancer is the most common cancer among women over the age of 40. In 1994 it was expected that 182,000 new cases of breast cancer would diagnosed and that 46,000 women would die from the disease. When cancer of the breast is diagnosed early and at a localized stage, 93% of those affected survive 5 years or longer. When diagnosis and treatment are delayed and regional spread occurs, the 5-year–survival rate drops to 72%. When women have distant metastases, the survival rate is 18% (American Cancer Society, 1993). Despite new methods of detection and treatment, the death rate from breast cancer has not been substantially reduced. Several prominent women have had breast surgery in recent years, which has resulted in better public awareness, and more women now perform breast self-examinations (BSEs), have screening mammograms, and seek healthcare early. Prostate cancer, the second leading cause of cancer death in men, was estimated to be responsible for 38,000 deaths in 1994. Between 1980 and 1990, prostate cancer incidence rates increased 50%, largely as a result of improved detection. Black men have a 30% higher incidence rate than white men. Digital rectal examinations and serum screening tests are recommended for early detection. Prostatic ultrasound is also being used to improve early detection. The most common sites and mortality rates of malignant neoplasms are found in Figure 10-1.

The U.S. Congress appropriates millions of dollars to the National Cancer Institute for research and training. Congress also provides grants and contracts to other organizations whose research activities may be applied to the prevention, detection, diagnosis, and treatment of malignant disease.

The National Cancer Act of 1971 provided funds for the establishment of cancer research centers throughout the nation. These centers are carefully reviewed by the National Cancer Advisory Board and receive funding from the National Cancer Institute, the American Cancer Society (ACS), and many other sources. The ACS is one of the oldest and largest voluntary health agencies in the United States. It is dedicated to eliminating cancer through research, education, patient service, and rehabilitation. In 1993 the ACS spent an estimated 100 million dollars in funding for research grants and fellowships (American Cancer Society, 1993).

The ultimate objective of all cancer research is the control of cancer in humans. Progress toward this goal is measured by (1) increased knowledge about malignant disease, (2) identification and control of factors

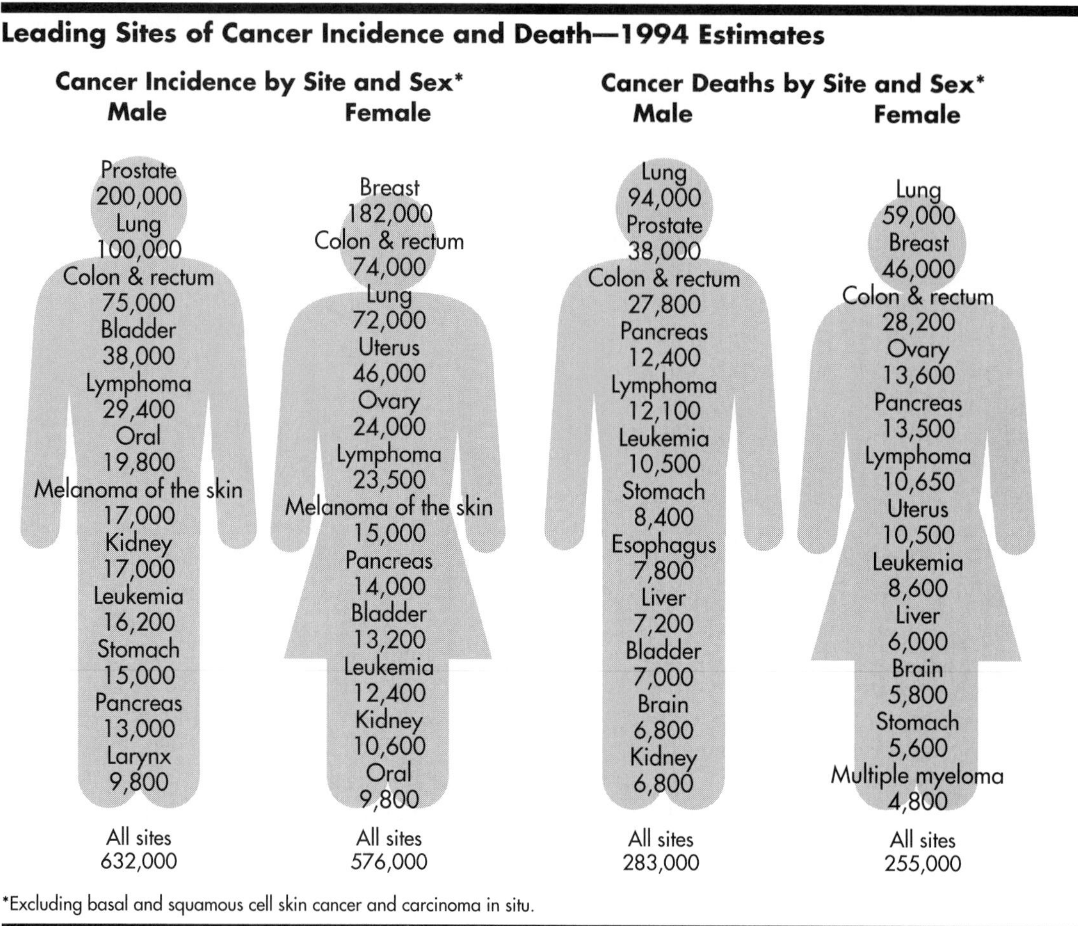

Figure 10-1 Leading sites of cancer incidence and death, 1994 estimates. (From American Cancer Society: *Cancer facts and figures,* 1994, Atlanta, 1994, The Society.)

related to cause and prevention, and (3) improvement in detection, diagnosis, and treatment.

The financial costs of cancer are exceedingly high and account for 10% of the total cost of disease in the United States. The National Cancer Institute estimates overall annual costs for cancer at $104 billion, which has a significant financial impact on both the individual and society as a whole. The current debate on healthcare reform has concentrated on ways to control the high cost of healthcare and ensure equal access for all Americans, including the 8 million Americans who have cancer (American Cancer Society, 1993).

PATHOPHYSIOLOGY

The basic structural unit of all forms of animal and plant life is the cell. Each organ of the body is composed of many different types of cells that are joined together to perform specific functions. It is the coordination of all cellular activities that allows the body to function as a whole organism. All cells have the genetic capability of dividing and multiplying, and they normally do so in response to a specific need of the body. However, a normal cell can undergo changes that transform it into a cancer cell. Cancer cells are able to divide and multiply, but not in a normal manner. Instead of limiting their growths to meet the specific needs of the body, cancer cells continue to reproduce in a disorderly and unrestricted manner. Whether benign or malignant, new growths of abnormal tissue are referred to as **neoplasms,** or tumors. **Benign** tumors normally do not progress or spread and are easily removed. **Malignant** tumors tend to become progressively worse, which often results in the death of the individual. Although benign tumors are usually harmless, they occasionally involve vital organs, such as the brain, with fatal results. The word ending *-oma* means "tumor," and the site of the tumor is indicated by the stem. Tumors are usually named according to the type of tissue from which they arise.

TABLE 10-1

General Characteristics of Neoplasms

Benign Tumor	Malignant Tumor
Slow, steady growth	Rate of growth varies, usually rapid
Remains localized	Metastasizes
Usually contained within a capsule	Rarely contained within a capsule
Smooth, well defined, movable when palpated	Irregular, more immobile when palpated
Resembles parent tissue	Little resemblance to parent tissue
Crowds normal tissue	Invades normal tissue
Rarely recurs after removal	May recur after removal
Rarely fatal	Fatal without treatment

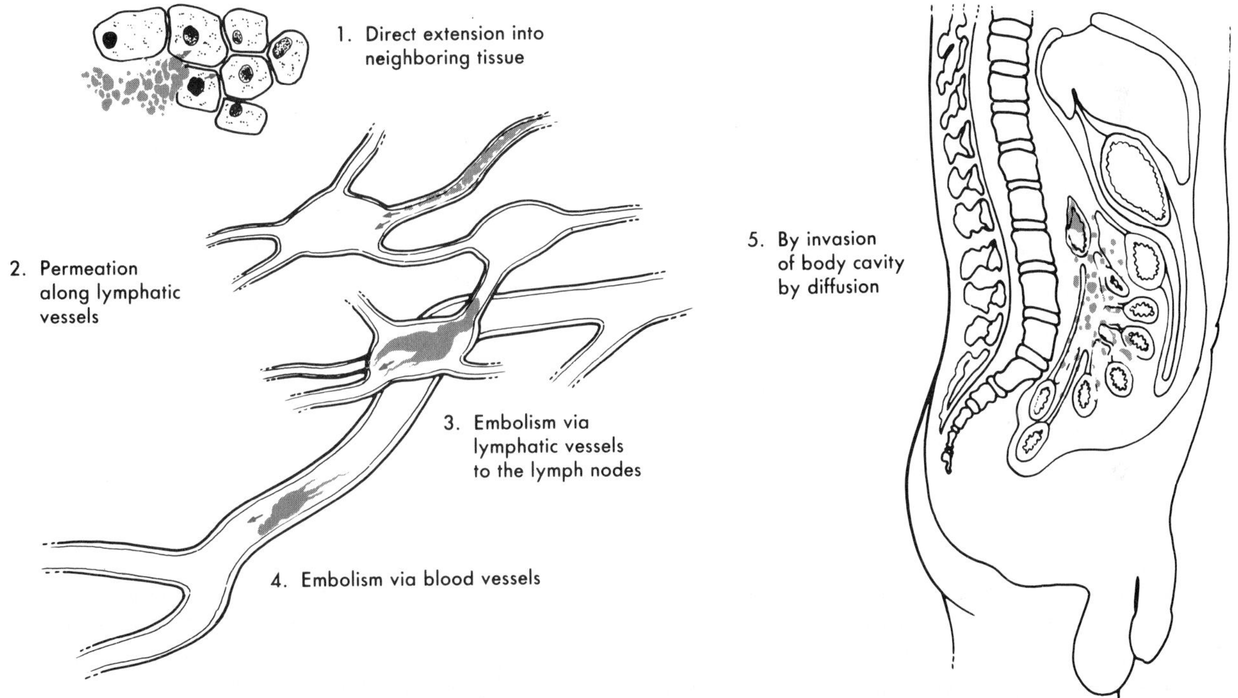

Figure 10–2 Modes of dissemination of cancer. (From Phipps WJ and others: *Medical-surgical nursing: concepts and clinical practice,* ed 5, St Louis, 1995, Mosby.)

Malignant tumors differ from benign tumors in several important aspects (Table 10-1). They are capable of continued growth that compresses, invades, and destroys normal tissue. Malignant cells break away from their original sites and are transported by the blood or lymph to new sites, where they begin to grow. This process is called **metastasis.** During metastasis, malignant cells are temporarily stopped by the lymph nodes, but they may grow and multiply there. The body's immune system constantly tries to rid the body of these metastasizing cells and is generally successful, with only a fraction of 1% surviving. However, this small percentage is sufficient to establish tumors in other portions of the body. Cancer spreads by the following processes (Figure 10-2):

1. Direct extension into adjacent tissue
2. Permeation along lymphatic vessels
3. Embolism through lymphatic or blood vessels
4. Diffusion or seeding within a body cavity

It is not known why a single body cell suddenly fails to divide and multiply in a normal manner, but tumors are found in all types of tissue and in all parts of the body. **Carcinoma,** a malignant tumor, is the most common form of cancer. Carcinomas arise from epithelial cells, which form coverings such as the skin and line cavities such as the mouth, stomach, and lungs. Other types of epithelial cells are found in glandular organs such as the breast. Another form of cancer is **sarcoma,** which occurs less often than carcinomas. Sarcomas arise from connective tissue such as bone, muscle, and cartilage. Carcinomas and sarcomas are called solid tumors. Cancer can also develop in the blood-forming and lymphoid organs. *Leukemia* is an abnormal, uncontrolled multiplication of white blood cells. *Lymphoma* arises in the lymph system, especially the lymph nodes and spleen, and is characterized by overproduction of lymphocytes. There are two main forms of lymphoma: Hodgkin's disease and non-Hodgkin's lymphoma. *Multiple myeloma* is caused by an overproduction of plasma cells in the blood and bone marrow.

CAUSES OF CANCER

Although the specific cause of cancer is unknown, many theories have been developed. Agents that can cause malignant changes in healthy cells after prolonged exposure are referred to as carcinogenic agents, or **carcinogens.** These include viruses, chemical agents, physical agents, hormones, and dietary factors. Hereditary factors are also important.

Although viruses are thought to cause some forms of human cancers, it has been difficult to isolate specific human–cancer-causing viruses. Cancer-causing viruses are able to enter the cell and alter the genetic material that controls cell growth. One virus has been shown to cause a rare adult leukemia, and other viruses have been linked with an increased risk of certain cancers.

Chemical agents include a wide variety of substances that are often found in increased amounts in certain occupations and in polluted environments. The most common chemical carcinogens include hydrocarbons found in cigarette smoke, air pollutants, tar, soot, aniline dyes, and benzene. Asbestos, vinyl chloride, cobalt, chromium, nickel, and arsenic compounds are other common chemical carcinogens. The relationship between cigarette smoke and lung cancer has been well established, and there is increased evidence that secondary smoke is a hazard. Snuff, a form of smokeless tobacco, has been implicated as a cause of mouth cancer and is a concern because of the increased use of "dipping snuff" by young males (American Cancer Society, 1994).

Physical agents include ultraviolet radiation from sunlight and **ionizing radiation** from natural gamma rays, x-rays, and radioactive isotopes. Skin cancer is found more often in persons who have had prolonged exposure to sunlight, and it is more common in fair-skinned persons. The greater pigmentation in dark skin appears to protect against the effects of ultraviolet rays. Persons acutely or often exposed to ionizing radiation have an increased incidence of cancers, especially leukemia. This phenomenon is seen in the survivors of the atom bomb, in persons cured of an earlier cancer by the use of radiation therapy, and in radiation workers before strict exposure precautions were enforced. Physical trauma from chronic irritation of parts of the body can also contribute to cancer. Bladder stones, chronic infections, and parasitic infestations can produce a chronic inflammatory condition that predisposes a person to cancer.

Hormones have been implicated in the development of some forms of cancer. Prolonged estrogen therapy has been linked to an increased incidence of endometrial cancer. Use of diethylstilbestrol (DES) during pregnancy has been related to the development of vaginal carcinoma in female children. In prostate cancer and in some breast cancers, tumor growth can be slowed by treatments that stop the natural production of sex hormones.

Dietary factors have been linked to the development of certain cancers. It is thought that some diets may increase the risk of cancer, whereas other diets may offer some protection from cancer. High-fat diets have been associated with an increased risk of colon, breast, prostate, and endometrial cancer, whereas fiber is thought to have a protective role against colon cancer. Various vitamins, particularly vitamins A and C, may decrease the risk of cancer (American Cancer Society, 1993; 1994). Some food additives have been suspected to be carcinogenic, and excessive alcohol use has been linked to an increased risk of cancer of the mouth, larynx, and esophagus.

Human cancer is thought to be caused by a combination of many environmental and genetic factors. Recent research suggests that each cell has certain genes that control cell growth. Some of these genes, called **oncogenes,** can somehow be activated to produce a protein that causes the cell to grow in an abnormal or malignant fashion (Gross, Johnson, 1994). What "switches on" the oncogenes is not yet known, but many of the carginogens previously discussed are being studied. Some scientists believe that cancer cells form in the body throughout life and that the immune system is constantly detecting and eliminating the abnormal cells. This concept has stimulated research involving the immune system of the body. Some immunologists suggest that cancer may be caused by a failure of this system and that strengthening the natural immune defenses of the body may help destroy malignant tissue.

PREVENTION AND CONTROL

Cancer usually begins as an alteration in one microscopic cell of the body, and the individual is asymptomatic and considered to be an active, healthy person. As the cancer cell begins to divide without restraint, symptoms eventually appear. The first symptoms are insidious and not readily apparent to the victim. A small, painless lump; a vague change in bowel habits; or a chronic cough may be the only warning sign of a devastating illness. Often these poorly defined symptoms are not considered valid reasons to seek healthcare. If left untreated, cancer cells continue to invade adjacent healthy tissue and eventually spread to other parts of the body, where new cancer growths are established. Because of this characteristic pattern of development, cancer is difficult to detect in its earliest stages. If the disease is not readily diagnosed, the chances for cure are greatly reduced because the disease has already spread. The current survival rate is four in ten patients. However, early diagnosis and prompt treatment could save more than 50% of all cancer patients. It is clear that cancer must be prevented or controlled at an early stage. Future efforts must concentrate on promoting research, controlling environmental carcinogens, and educating health professionals and the public about prevention and early detection.

Nurses can play a particularly important role in these efforts by promoting primary and secondary prevention. Primary prevention refers to the steps that can be taken to avoid those factors that might cause cancer (Box 10-1). Many of the risk factors are avoidable, and the risk decreases as positive behavioral changes occur. The ACS recommends 10 steps to a healthier life and a reduced cancer risk (Box 10-2) (Baird, McCorkle, Grant, 1991). Secondary prevention

BOX 10-1

RISK FACTORS FOR MAJOR CANCERS

Lung
Cigarette smoking
Exposure to some industrial chemicals such as arsenic or asbestos
Radiation exposure, including radon
Secondhand smoke

Colon-rectum
Personal or family history of cancer or polyps of colon or rectum
Inflammatory bowel disease
High-fat and/or low-fiber diet

Breast
Age over 40
Personal or family history of breast cancer
Early age at menarche
Late age at menopause
Never had children or late age at first birth
High-fat diet

Prostate
Increasing age
Living in northwestern Europe or North America
Being a black American
Family history of prostate cancer
High-fat diet

Uterus (cervix)
Early age at first intercourse
Multiple sex partners
Cigarette smoking
Infection with human papilloma virus (HPV)

Uterus (endometrium)
Early menarche
Late menopause
History of infertility
Failure to ovulate
Unopposed estrogen therapy (without progesterone)
Obesity

Ovary
Increasing age
Never had children
Family history of ovarian cancer

Mouth
Cigarette, cigar, pipe smoking
Smokeless tobacco
Excessive alcohol use

Skin
Excessive exposure to ultraviolet radiation
Fair complexion
Occupational exposure to coal tar, pitch, arsenic, radium

Bladder
Cigarette smoking
Urban living
Exposure to dye, rubber, or leather

Stomach
Diet heavy in smoked, salted, or pickled foods
Family history of stomach cancer

TABLE 10-2

American Cancer Society Guidelines for Cancer-Related Checkups in People Without Symptoms, According to Age

Site	Increasing Age →		
Basic	All persons 20 to 40 years of age should have a "cancer-related health checkup" every 3 years.	All persons age 40 and over should have a "cancer-related health checkup" every year.	
Breast	Women age 20 and over should perform BSE monthly. Women 20 to 40 years of age should have a physical breast examination every 3 years.	All women should have a baseline mammogram by age 40. Women 40 to 49 should have a mammogram and breast examination every 1 to 2 years.	Women age 50 and over should have a mammogram and breast examination every year.
Colon-rectum		Men and women over age 40 should have a digital rectal examination every year.	Men and women over age 50 should have a stool-blood test every year and a sigmoidoscopy every 3 to 5 years.
Cervix/uterus	Women age 18 and over and younger women who are sexually active should have an annual Pap smear and pelvic examination. After three or more consecutive normal annual examinations, a Pap smear may be done less frequently at the physician's discretion.		High-risk women should have an endometrial tissue sample at menopause.
Lung	Primary prevention should focus on helping smokers stop smoking and keeping nonsmokers from starting.		
Prostate		Men age 40 should have a digital rectal examination every year.	Men age 50 and over should have an annual prostate-specific antigen blood test every year. If either result is suspicious, a transrectal ultrasound is recommended.
Skin	Primary prevention involves avoiding exposure to sunlight, using sunscreens, and protecting children from traumatic sunburns. Skin self-examination should be practiced every month.		

Modified from American Cancer Society: *1994 cancer facts and figures,* Atlanta, 1994, The Society.

BOX 10-2

TEN STEPS TO REDUCE CANCER RISK

1 Do not smoke
2 Watch weight
3 Eat a varied diet
4 Eat a lot of fruits and vegetables
5 Add more high-fiber foods
6 Trim fat from diet
7 Cut down on salt-cured, smoked, and nitrite-cured foods
8 Restrict use of alcohol
9 Protect self from the sun
10 Protect self from harmful chemicals

(Modified from American Cancer Society: *Taking control: ten steps to a healthier life and reduced cancer risk,* Atlanta, 1994, The Society, publication no 201915.)

BOX 10-3

SEVEN WARNING SIGNALS OF CANCER

Change in bowel or bladder habits
A sore that does not heal
Unusual bleeding or discharge
Thickening or lump in breast or elsewhere
Indigestion or difficulty swallowing
Obvious change in wart or mole
Nagging cough or hoarseness
If a warning signal occurs, see a healthcare professional.

refers to the steps taken to diagnose cancer as soon as possible after it has developed and while it is still potentially curable. Early detection of cancer in people without symptoms is a major goal of all cancer organizations. The ACS and other agencies recommend certain guidelines for cancer-related checkups (Table 10-2). Simple steps to early diagnosis include a monthly BSE, testicular self-examination (TSE), and skin self-examination; as well as a regular mammogram, Papanicolaou's (Pap) smear, digital rectal examination, stool-blood test, and sigmoidoscopy. All nurses should urge their patients to practice these preventive health behaviors and should teach them the seven warning signs of cancer (Box 10-3).

Public awareness and concern is increasing regarding the prevention and early detection of cancer. Cigarette advertisments on radio and television have been banned; airlines no longer allow smoking on flights; and many businesses, government agencies, and restaurants have banned smoking. Educational programs in schools and spot filmstrips on television are designed to acquaint the public with the hazards of smoking and to encourage persons who smoke to discontinue the habit. Smoking-cessation classes and support groups are now widely available and often are provided by companies for their employees. Public education programs have also alerted more women to the benefits of BSE, mammograms, and Pap smears. Colorectal, skin, and prostate screening programs are often run by community agencies.

The National Cancer Institute and the ACS spend a large amount of money on public and professional education. The National Cancer Institute sponsors a toll-free information line, which is accessible in all parts of the country by dialing 1-800-4-CANCER. Trained counselors provide the most up-to-date answers regarding cancer prevention, detection, and treatment. The ACS has units in all states and provides free information to the public about cancer, as well as services to people with cancer. The ACS unit phone numbers can be found in local phone directories or by calling 1-800-ACS-2345.

DIAGNOSTIC TESTS AND PROCEDURES

Before a physician or pathologist can make a diagnosis of cancer, the patient must be carefully examined, a tissue sample must be obtained, and the primary location and anatomic spread (stage) of the cancer must be established. The degree of malignancy, or grade, is based on microscopic examination of the lesion. The higher the grade, the worse the prognosis. Staging is a classification that describes the extent of the spread of the tumor. Staging does not consider the microscopic characteristics of the lesion (Box 10-4).

Tissue Sampling

A definite diagnosis of cancer can only be made when a pathologist sees malignant cells in a tissue specimen that is viewed under a microscope. A number of techniques can be used to make a tissue diagnosis.

Exfoliative cytology

Exfoliative cytology, or the Pap smear test, is used to study cells that the body has shed during the normal sequence of body tissue growth and replacement. If cancer is present, cancer cells are also shed. By study-

BOX 10-4

CLASSIFICATION OF MALIGNANT LESIONS BY GRADE AND STAGE

Grade	Stage
Grade 0 Normal tissue	**Stage 0** Cancer in situ
Grade 1 Well-differentiated, with minimal deviation from tissue of origin	**Stage I** Tumor limited to tissue of origin
Grade 2 Moderately well-differentiated, with evidence of structural changes from normal tissue of origin	**Stage II** Limited local spread
Grade 3 Poorly differentiated, with extensive structural changes from normal tissue of origin	**Stage III** Extensive local and regional spread
Grade 4 Very anaplastic, with no resemblance to tissue of origin	**Stage IV** Widespread metastasis

From Phipps WJ and others: *Medical-surgical nursing: concepts and clinical practice,* ed 5, St Louis, 1995, Mosby.

ing these cells under the microscope, malignant conditions can be diagnosed before symptoms are noticed by the patient. The test was originally developed to diagnose early cancer of the cervix but can now be used effectively to study cells shed from the stomach, esophagus, lung, colon, and bladder, as well as discharge from the breasts. If cancer cells are found, a biopsy is always done.

Cervical secretions are obtained during a pelvic examination. The examination is a simple, painless procedure that should be performed annually in women age 18 and over. The nurse can help the patient by explaining how to prepare for the examination. The Pap smear is not done during the menstrual period. The patient should not douche for several hours before the test, and both coitus and tub bathing should be avoided for 24 hours before the test. A Pap smear is primarily a screening test, and further examination may be necessary to confirm a diagnosis. This simple test has resulted in a decreased death rate from cervical cancer.

Biopsy

A biopsy is the surgical removal of a piece of tissue for microscopic examination. There are several biopsy techniques. An *incisional* biopsy involves taking a small sample out of a tissue mass, whereas an *excisional* biopsy involves removing all of the known tumor. An incisional needle biopsy can be performed with tumors that are close to the skin, visible on x-ray films or scans, or seen during endoscopic procedures. Fine needle biopsies are easy to do but yield only a few cells. Larger bore needles give bigger tissue samples but are more difficult to perform.

Simple biopsies may be performed in a physician's office, but excisional biopsies that require sedation are performed in the hospital or in an outpatient surgery center. Needle biopsies of internal organs are often done in the radiology department with the guidance of x-ray films or ultrasound. If the biopsy is taken from an external lesion, preparation includes the use of an antiseptic and an injection of a local anesthetic such as 2% procaine solution. Using a special biopsy instrument, the physician removes a small amount of tissue for examination, after which a sterile dressing is applied. Although the biopsy is a simple procedure, it may not seem simple to a frightened, nervous patient.

The frozen-section biopsy enables a tissue specimen to be quickly examined during an operation to immediately determine whether the tissue is benign or malignant. The specimen is immediately frozen, cut, and stained. Although this technique is not satisfactory for a detailed study of the cells, possible malignancies can be promptly identified. Permanent sections of the tissue are prepared so that the pathologist can use special stains to make a definite diagnosis. Patients should be told that these biopsies usually take several days to process and that a diagnosis may be delayed until then.

Imaging Techniques—Direct Visualization

The primary location and anatomic spread of cancer can be determined by a number of imaging techniques that use direct or indirect visualization. Direct visualization techniques involve introducing fiber-optic endoscopy tubes into hollow organs to view internal surfaces. Fiber-optic tubes contain lighting, magnifying devices, and attachments that allow brushings or biopsies to be performed.

Bronchoscopy

Bronchoscopy involves the examination of the trachea and bronchi while the patient is under local or general anesthesia. The bronchoscope is inserted through the nose and advanced into the upper airway. Biopsies or brushings of suspicious areas can be done through the tube. The patient's throat is numbed during this procedure to prevent discomfort and gagging. After the procedure, the patient is warned not to eat or drink until the gag reflex returns, which should happen within 2 hours. The nurse monitors the patient for signs of breathing difficulties or bleeding after the procedure.

Esophagoscopy and gastroscopy

Esophagoscopy and gastroscopy involves the visualization of the esophagus and stomach by using a flexible tube that is inserted through the patient's mouth. Biopsies or washings can be taken during the procedure. Before the procedure, the patient is instructed not to eat or drink after midnight. The patient is given medication before the gastroscopy to permit relaxation and sleepiness. The patient is requested to arrange for someone else to take him or her home after the procedure.

Sigmoidoscopy

Sigmoidoscopy is the examination of the anus, rectum, and sigmoid colon by the use of a rigid tube that can be up to 10 inches long. Tumors, polyps, or ulcerations may be studied by examination and biopsy. It is extremely important that all fecal matter be removed before the examination, which is usually accomplished by cleansing enemas. Laxatives and cathartics are seldom given before the procedure, but the nurse should be familiar with the exact preparation desired by the physician. The patient is placed in the knee-chest position and is draped to expose only the anal area. In some situations it may be desirable to place the patient in a side-lying position. The patient should be given information about the examination and what to expect. He or she should know that there may be some discomfort but that the procedure is usually not painful. Because the examination is often fatiguing, especially for an elderly person, the nurse should arrange for the patient to rest after the procedure. Providing light nourishment may be appropriate.

Colonoscopy

Colonoscopy involves the examination of the entire colon by means of a long flexible tube. Preparation of the bowel for a colonoscopy is more extensive than for a sigmoidoscopy. The patient must be on a liquid diet and use laxatives and enemas before the examination.

Imaging Techniques—Indirect Visualization

Indirect visualization techniques include radiograpic tests such as chest x-ray examinations, mammograms, gastrointestinal series, barium enemas, computerized axial tomography (CAT) scans, and **radioisotope** studies; as well as nonradiographic tests such as ultrasounds and **magnetic resonance imaging (MRI).**

Radiographic studies can be done with or without contrast. Noncontrast x-ray examinations include chest x-ray examinations, mammograms, and abdomen and bone films. Contrast x-ray examinations use materials such as air, iodine-containing dyes, or barium to outline an organ. Contrast x-ray examinations include lymphangiograms, myelograms, and barium studies of the gastrointestinal tract.

X-rays are electromagnetic waves that are similar to light and heat waves and are produced in a vacuum tube. X-rays have the ability to penetrate most substances and alter a photographic plate, which produces an image of the substances through which the rays pass. The image reflects the varying densities of substances such as bone, soft tissue, fat, and air. Body cavities, organs, and bones can be visualized, which assists the physician in diagnosis and treatment. Fluoroscopy is an x-ray technique in which the radiologist views internal structures while they are functioning. For example, fluoroscopy of the chest enables the radiologist to view the expansion and contraction of the lungs. Nurses may be requested to assist while diagnostic x-ray films are being made. Precautions must be taken to avoid exposure to radiation. A nurse who remains in the room with the patient should wear a lead apron and possibly gloves.

Mammography

Mammography is a safe and simple technique for detecting the presence of breast tumors. Using a low-energy beam, films of the soft breast tissue are taken without the use of a radiopaque medium. It is often possible to differentiate between a benign and malignant tumor. To generate a good quality film, the breast must be compressed firmly. Therefore women who have sensitive breasts may find this an uncomfortable procedure. A mammography is recommended for women who have signs and symptoms of breast disease; a familial history of breast cancer; a previous breast biopsy or breast surgery; or large, pendulous breasts that make palpation difficult. At age 40, all women should have a baseline mammography and have one every 1 to 2 years until age 49. A yearly mammography is now recommended as a screening test for all women age 50 and over. Mammography is combined with BSE and physical examination of the breast by a healthcare provider to detect early breast cancer. The technique of BSE is shown in Figure 10-3.

Barium enema

A patient must be prepared carefully when the physician wishes to visualize the colon above the sigmoid. It is important that all fecal matter be removed from the colon, because any residue left in the colon may interfere with a correct diagnosis. Usually the patient takes nothing by mouth after midnight and is given laxatives, rectal suppositories, and enemas. Enemas are often given until the solution returns free of fecal material. A poorly prepared patient may delay the examination, which is an inconvenience to the x-ray department and results in additional expense to the patient. The patient reports to the x-ray department at the scheduled hour and is given an enema of barium, a radiopaque substance, which the patient is asked to retain. Using the fluoroscope, the radiologist observes the filling of the colon, after which x-ray films are taken. The patient is then allowed to evacuate the barium. Sometimes the radiologist has the patient return after evacuating the barium. The colon is distended with air, and additional x-ray films are taken. The patient may feel exhausted after the examination, and

How to do BSE

1. Lie down and put a pillow under your right shoulder. Place your right arm behind your head.
2. Use the finger pads of the three middle fingers on your left hand to feel for lumps or thickening. Your finger pads are the top third of each finger.

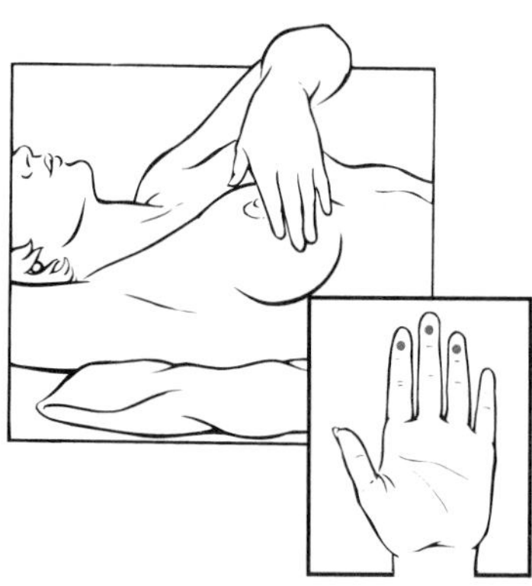

3. Press hard enough to know how your breast feels. If you're not sure how hard to press, ask your health care provider. Or try to copy the way your health care provider uses the finger pads during a breast exam. Learn what your breast feels like most of the time. A firm ridge in the lower curve of each breast is normal.

4. Move around the breast in a set way. You can choose either the circle (A), the up and down line (B), or the wedge (C). Do it the same way every time. It will help you to make sure that you've gone over the entire breast area, and to remember how your breast feels each month.

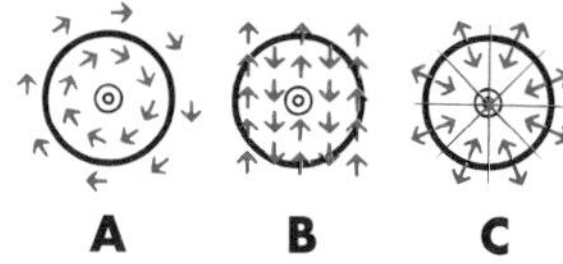

5. Now examine your left breast using right hand finger pads.

You might want to check your breasts while standing in front of a mirror right after you do your BSE each month. You might also want to do an extra BSE while you're in the shower. Your soapy hands will glide over the wet skin making it easy to check how your breasts feel.

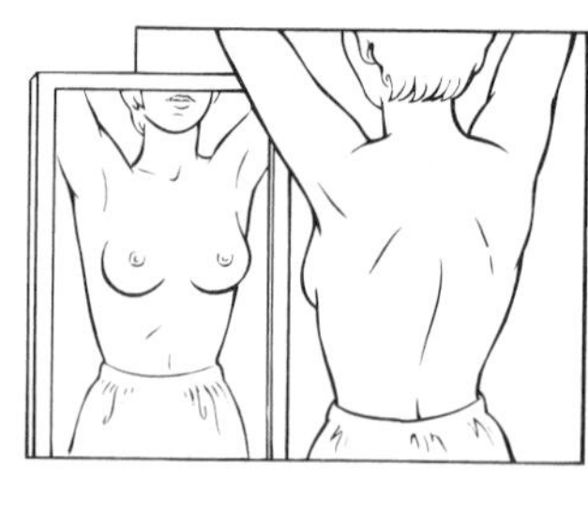

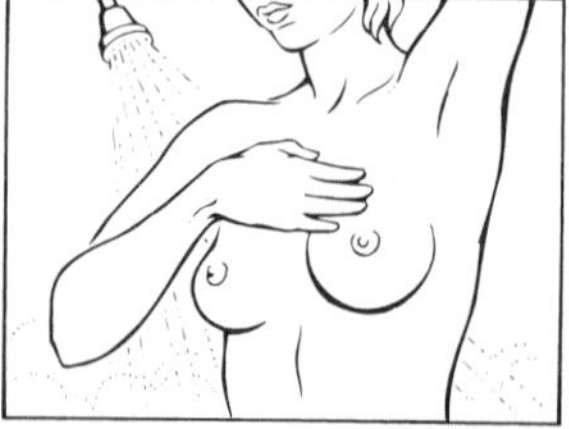

Figure 10–3 Breast self-examination. Courtesy of American Cancer Society, Atlanta.

therefore a period of rest is desirable. Because barium that has been retained in the bowel becomes difficult to expel, a warm oil retention enema or a laxative such as magnesium citrate may be ordered following the examination.

Gastrointestinal series

The gastrointestinal (GI) series is an x-ray examination of the upper GI tract using a radiopaque contrast medium. It is used to identify pathologic conditions in tissues of the stomach and duodenum. Because food in the stomach causes misleading x-ray films, the patient is told not to eat or drink for at least 6 to 8 hours before the examination. The patient reports to the x-ray department at the scheduled hour and is given a mixture of barium to drink. The fluoroscope is used to observe the barium as it passes through the esophagus and into the stomach. X-ray films are taken at specific intervals over several hours to study the movement of the barium from the stomach to the small intestine. The patient is not given any food until the x-ray department indicates that it is finished with the tests. Many patients, especially older adults, find the examination fatiguing. The patient is usually hungry and should be served a warm, appetizing meal; made comfortable; and allowed to rest undisturbed. In ambulatory settings, the patient may remain in the area for observation and stabilization. A cathartic may be included in the barium mixture or ordered following the examination to hasten the elimination of the barium from the intestines.

Computerized tomography

Computerized tomography (CT), also known as a CAT scan, is a computer-aided x-ray examination that has proven to be a major breakthrough in diagnostic technique. Conventional x-ray films can only differentiate between bone, soft tissue, fat, and air with any precision. The CT is 100 times more sensitive to differences in tissue densities, and individual organs and structures within organs can be seen. A narrow x-ray beam is rotated around the patient, and multiple exposures are made. Sensitive detectors record the results, which are processed by a computer. An image of the body section exposed to the x-ray beam, or a tomogram, is constructed. Each image represents a horizontal cross-section, or "slice," of the body. This diagnostic device can be used to detect tumors and other pathologic conditions without performing special procedures that are often painful, complicated, invasive, or risky.

Because the x-rays are focused on a few thin layers of the patient's body, patients receive no more radiation than with a conventional x-ray examination. The patient lies on an adjustable hydraulic couch, and the scanner rotates around the chosen site. As the scanner rotates, it makes a clicking noise, which may frighten the unsuspecting patient. Patients must remain completely still because motion will disturb the image. Snug-fitting restraints are often used as appropriate. The procedure is safe, painless, and usually requires no specific preparation or follow-up. Sometimes a contrast medium is given to highlight certain parts of the body. If the contrast medium is given intravenously, the patient is warned that it may produce a warm sensation. The x-ray personnel should be alerted if the patient is allergic to iodine or contrast mediums. If an oral or intravenous contrast medium is to be used, the patient is usually told not to eat or drink for several hours before the test. Check with the radiology department for specific instructions for each test.

Radioisotope studies

Radioisotopes are elements that emit rays of energy. They occur naturally as radium or uranium or can be artificially produced from other elements. The most widely used radioisotopes in medicine are altered forms of iodine, phosphorus, cobalt, iron, and gold. The patient needs no specific preparation other than an explanation of the procedure. At a specified time the patient is given an intravenous injection of an isotope that has a tendency to accumulate in the organ to be studied. In the radioisotope laboratory, a sensing device charts or maps the areas of the organ that have picked up the radioactive material. Variations from normal are seen as lighter or darker areas and indicate abnormality of the organ, which is often a malignancy. For example, radioactive iodine is readily assimiliated by the thyroid gland, and pathogenesis can be detected during a thyroid scan. It is now possible to scan most major organs such as the brain, kidneys, liver, pericardium, and bone. Because such minute amounts of radioactive material are used and because the material is eliminated so quickly, the patient is not considered radioactive.

Magnetic resonance imaging

MRIs are relatively new. An MRI uses a magnetic field and radiofrequency sound waves to produce excellent images of the soft tissues, veins, arteries, brain, and spinal cord. The procedure is not invasive and poses no risk for radiation exposure. However, an MRI is costly ($700 and up) and may last up to 1½ hours. The patient must remove all metal objects and lie still for periods of up to 20 minutes on a narrow stretcher that is rolled into a shallow tunnel. Despite efforts to prevent claustrophobia by providing mirrors, a call button, and a voice-activated intercom, the procedure is frightening to many people. Teaching by the nurse is essential for decreased anxiety. Guided imagery and rhythmic breathing may be useful for distraction and for giving the patient control (Kyba, Ogburn-Russel, Rutledge, 1987).

Ultrasound

Ultrasound uses high frequency sound waves instead of x-rays to show the structure and function of internal organs. A sound wave transducer (transmitter and receiver) is moved over the skin. The sound waves pass through the skin and send echoes back to the transducer as they strike various organs. Each tissue produces a distinctive echo that can be identified by the transducer. The sound waves are changed into electrical energy that forms an image on a screen. With the advent of CAT scans and MRIs, ultrasound has been used less but is still a good diagnostic test for some cancers and is often used to complement x-ray examinations. The advantages of ultrasound are that there is no radiation exposure, no discomfort, and no injections. Usually no special preparation is needed. The patient is asked to fast for several hours before a GI ultrasound and to drink fluids and keep the bladder full for pelvic ultrasounds.

Laboratory Studies

Analyzing chemicals in the blood may help diagnose the type and extent of cancer. Some cancers produce substances called tumor markers. For example, carcinoembryonic antigen (CEA) is commonly found in metastatic colon cancer, and CA-125 is usually elevated in ovarian cancer. Elevated acid phosphatase and prostate-specific antigen (PSA) levels may be found in persons with prostate cancer. Most of these tests are not very useful in screening for cancer because these chemicals are also elevated in many benign conditions. PSA is now recommended as a screen for prostate cancer, but many experts do not consider it a cost-effective screening test. Tumor markers are most useful in evaluating responses to treatment.

TREATMENT OF CANCER

Cancer may be treated in four ways: surgery, radiotherapy, chemotherapy, and biotherapy. Some leukemia patients may benefit from bone marrow transplantation. Early diagnosis and treatment may result in a cure, whereas delayed diagnosis and treatment may result in treatment that is **palliative** only, with death the inevitable outcome. For many, cancer becomes a chronic illness, and nursing care focuses on rehabilitation and efforts to optimize the patient's quality of life.

Surgery

Surgery is often the primary treatment for cancer and may be performed for various purposes. It may be preventive, diagnostic, curative, or palliative and may range from the removal of a small tumor to extensive surgical excision. Surgery is considered preventive if a premalignant lesion, such as a suspicious mole or a colon polyp, is removed. Diagnosis of cancer in internal organs often necessitates a surgical procedure. In recent years, laparoscopy has reduced the need for open surgical biopsies. Surgery is curative if a malignant tumor is completely removed before it spreads beyond the local area. If the cancer has metastasized, surgery is usually only palliative, such as for the relief of intestinal obstruction or the control of pain. Palliative surgery contributes to the patient's comfort and may prolong life. Surgery that is performed early, before metastasis occurs, offers the patient the best chance for cure.

Research is being conducted to find ways to increase the chances of cure by surgery. The effects of chemotherapy and/or radiation therapy administered before, during, or after surgery are being investigated. This is called "adjuvant therapy." Some inoperable tumors have been reduced in size by drugs or radiation so that surgery can be performed. A course of chemotherapy and/or radiation therapy that is given after all visible tumor has been removed may reduce the risk of recurrence in some cancers, such as some stages of breast and colon-rectum cancer. Adjuvant chemotherapy or hormonal therapy is commonly used for the treatment of early stage breast cancer after surgery and/or radiation therapy.

Newer surgical techniques and tools have been developed. Cryosurgery is used to treat some cancers of the skin and mouth, as well as other superficial lesions. Cryosurgery destroys tumors by freezing them with liquid nitrogen. Laser surgery uses intense light beams to vaporize some cancerous lesions such as those that are on the larynx or blocking the bronchi of the lung.

Reconstructive or plastic surgery may beused to correct defects caused by the original surgical intervention. Many women are now choosing to have breast reconstruction after a modified radical mastectomy for breast cancer.

The preoperative and postoperative nursing care of patients undergoing surgical procedures for cancer is essentially the same as for any other type of surgery and is reviewed in the appropriate sections. However, in this case psychosocial needs are often more intense because the potential or actual diagnosis of cancer exists.

Radiotherapy

Radiotherapy, or **radiation therapy,** refers to the use of ionizing radiation to treat tumors. Radiation is ionizing when it can break atoms of a substance into smaller parts that carry a positive or negative charge (ions). The most common types of radiation, such as heat and light, are not ionizing. X-rays, gamma rays, and radioactive particles (alpha and beta particles, neutrons, and protons) are types of ionizing radiation. When ionizing radiation passes through living tissue, it damages DNA molecules and disrupts cell function and division. The goal in using various forms of radiation to treat cancer is to give doses that are large enough to destroy cancer cells without causing irreparable damage to normal tissue that surrounds the tumor. Although both normal and malignant cells can be destroyed, most malignant cells are more susceptible to ionizing rays than are normal cells. Radiation therapy may be used to obtain a cure either alone or in combination with surgery and/or chemotherapy, or it may be used for palliation of symptoms when a cure is impossible.

Ionizing radiation is considered hazardous material because acute and chronic exposure causes cellular changes that can lead to gene mutation, birth defects, and carcinogenesis. Whether the radiation is for diagnostic or treatment purposes, precautions must be taken to minimize patient and personnel exposure. Persons who work in radiation areas are carefully monitored to ensure that they do not receive more than the maximum permissible dose each year (5 rem). Nurses are most at risk for radiation exposure when caring for patients receiving internal radiation therapy. Safety precautions are discussed later in this chapter. The symbol for a radiation area is shown in Figure 10-4. Two general types of radiation therapy are currently used: external beam radiaton (teletherapy) and internal radiation therapy (brachytherapy). External beam therapy is given from outside the body with various radiation-generating machines. Internal radiation therapy places a radiation source close to the tumor. Sealed radiation sources can be placed into the tumor-containing tissue or into a cavity close to the tumor. Unsealed internal radiation uses solutions of radioisotopes that emit ionizing radiation.

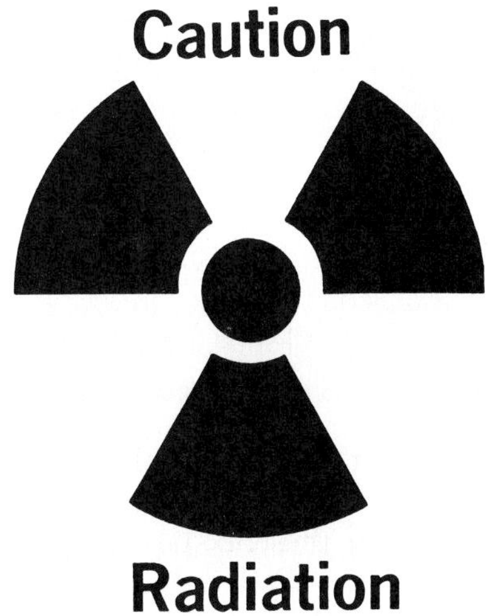

Figure 10–4 Radiation symbol.

External radiation therapy

External radiation is most often delivered to the patient by machines that generate x-rays or that contain radioisotopes, such as cobalt-60, that emit gamma rays. Most machines used today generate super-voltage radiation that can be accurately directed to deep tumors and spare the skin from damage. Before the first treatment is administered, the exact area to be radiated is carefully mapped during a process called *simulation.* Indelible ink or tattoo marks are placed on the skin and are used to position the machine before each treatment. Shielding is provided for the sites not being treated. Radiation is generally given in small doses over time, usually 5 days per week for 4 to 8 weeks. Palliative radiation takes less time. This method of delivering radiation is called *fractionation* and may increase cancer cell destruction while minimizing damage to normal tissues.

Assessment. Before starting a course of external radiation therapy, the patient is assessed for knowledge level, including misconceptions or anxiety about the therapy. Any self-care deficits are noted, especially restrictions in mobility that would affect the patient's ability to get to the daily treatments, or to get on and off the treatment table. The presence of significant symptoms, such as pain, is noted and addressed. A baseline assessment is made of nutritional status, as well as skin integrity in the radiation field. The nurse should be aware of the location of the radiation field and the side effects that might result from damage to the underlying tissues (Hassey-Dow, Hilderley, 1992; Strohl, 1988).

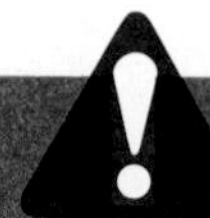

NURSE ALERT

A patient who is receiving external beam radiation therapy is never a source of radiation and will not experience "radiation sickness." The nurse can help reduce patient anxiety by dispelling any misconceptions about radiation therapy.

Nursing interventions. External radiation therapy is most often given on an outpatient basis. The course of therapy that has been prescribed for the patient is usually explained by the radiation oncologist. Nurses can often clarify uncertainties, answer questions, and explain the radiation procedure more fully. Teaching self-care measures to patients who are receiving external radiation therapy is essential, especially if the patient is receiving therapy as an outpatient. New patients are usually extremely apprehensive and need much reassurance and support. The term *radiation therapy* often incites fear in both the patient and family and often is viewed as the last resort when all else has failed.

It is helpful if the patient can be oriented to the radiation therapy department before the first treatment. It is important to explain to the patient that he or she will not become radioactive and that the treatments do not hurt. The nurse should explain that the patient lies very still on a table during the treatment and that the machine often rotates around the table making a clicking sound. Although the patient must be left alone during the 1-to-3 minute treatment, technicians observe and are in constant communication with the patient from outside the shielded room.

The patient is informed that during the course of treatment, there may be some reddening of the treated skin, which may turn dark in color, become dry, itch and slough (*dry* ***desquamation***). The nurse should avoid referring to the reddening as a burn. In cases where the radiation is directed close to the skin surface or includes skin folds or prominences, the area may blister, crack, or weep *(moist desquamation)* (Sitton, 1992; Strohl, 1988).

Whether the patient may shower or bathe depends on the policies of the radiation therapy department. If permitted, the patient is instructed to use a mild moisturizing soap such as unscented Dove, Ivory, Basis, or Neutrogena. The patient is also instructed to pat, not rub, the area dry. If ink markings are used, the patient must be careful not to remove them during bathing. Tattoo marks are permanent. Ointments, medications, perfumes, cosmetics, powders, shaving lotions, and deodorants are not used in the treatment field unless approved by the radiation therapy department. These products may contain alcohol or metals that can react with the radiation and cause skin problems. These restrictions do not apply to the rest of the patient's skin. Cornstarch or unscented lotions are usually allowed to alleviate itching on unbroken skin. If moist desquamation occurs, great care must be taken to avoid infection. All routine skin products are withheld, and the radiation oncologist or nurse is consulted for further treatment. If ointments or dressings are ordered, they often need to be removed and the skin cleansed before treatment is administered.

Extremes of heat or cold, such as ice packs, heat lamps, steam baths, whirlpools or saunas, should be avoided in the radiated area. The treatment skin should not be exposed to the sun for the rest of the patient's lifetime. The patient is strongly recommended to use protective clothing and sunscreen lotion. Tight-fitting or rough clothes over the treatment area may cause irritation. Soft, loose-fitting cotton undergarments or shirts may be more comfortable next to the skin. Radiation therapy is more effective when the patient's nutritional status is good. Therefore a high-calorie, high-protein diet is generally recommended. Patients receiving external radiation may experience nausea, vomiting, and diarrhea (Hassey-Dow, Hilderley, 1992; Strohl, 1988). These reactions are most common when radiation is given to or near the GI tract. Several small feedings per day may be tolerated better than regular meals. If vomiting is severe, food intake may be reduced to liquids only and increased to 3000 ml per day to compensate for fluid loss. Several drugs, including prochlorperazine (Compazine) and trimethobenzamide (Tigan) may help control nausea and vomiting. Diarrhea can usually be controlled with loperamide (Imodium) or diphenoxylate (Lomotil). Many radiation therapy departments have registered dieticians, who are available to counsel patients and families about optimizing nutrition during therapy. Fatigue is common and peaks during the fourth and fifth weeks of therapy. Extra rest periods are encouraged throughout therapy, but some planned exercise may help restore energy levels.

The cumulative effects of radiation may involve damage to the bone marrow, where blood cells are formed. White blood cells are highly sensitive to radiation and may be destroyed. The resulting **leukopenia** produces an increased susceptibility to infection. Low platelet levels produce **thrombocytopenia,** and an increased tendency to hemorrhage may result, which necessitates that the patient be protected from injury. Anemia may also occur from the depression of red blood cell formation. Complete blood counts are generally done every week.

Additional symptoms may occur and depend on the site being treated. Radiation to the scalp may cause alopecia, or loss of hair. Cystitis may occur with radiation to the pelvis, and pneumonitis may occur with radiation to the chest wall. Radiation to the mouth, throat, and neck often results in mouth soreness and ulceration (stomatitis) (Box 10-5).

Patients should be encouraged to report any symptoms that may occur so that appropriate comfort measures can be started (Box 10-6). Symptoms gradually get worse during the treatment course and usually resolve within a few weeks after treatment ends. Although great care is taken during treatment planning to minimize radiation effects on normal tissues, damage can occur. Radiation effects can be divided into acute (during treatment to 6 months after) and chronic (variable onset after 6 months) (Table 10-3) (Strohl, 1988). Many of the acute changes have been discussed previously and mostly involve tissues that contain many dividing cells, such as the skin, mucous membranes, hair follicles, and bone marrow. Acute reactions are often reversible. Chronic changes involve tissues with cells that divide more slowly, such as muscles and the vascular system. These changes are rarely reversible. Chronic effects include tissue fibrosis, tissue necrosis, fistula formation, and cataracts.

Sealed internal radiation therapy

Internal radiation therapy involves temporarily implanting sealed applicators that contain a radioactive substance into various organs of the body. Applicators may be inserted into the patient's tongue, neck, vagina, and cervix or other body cavity. Radium is a radioactive element that has been used for some time to treat cancerous lesions in this way. The supply of radium is limited and costly. However, radium remains almost unchanged over many years and therefore can be used repeatedly. As radium slowly disintegrates, it gives off a radioactive gas called radon. Although ra-

BOX 10-5 Guidelines for Care of Patient With Mouth and Throat Problems

The linings of the mouth and throat are among the most sensitive areas of the body. Cancer patients, especially those receiving chemotherapy or radiation treatments, often complain of soreness in these areas. These problems seem directly related to the treatment. Recent surgery in the head and neck area also may result in chewing and swallowing difficulties. Physicians may prescribe medicine that will control mouth and throat pain or infection. Dentists can also give tips for mouth care. Remember that part of the healing process in this area of the body depends on eating well and drinking fluids. Eating food and drinking fluids are imperative for patients who are undergoing treatment for mouth and throat lesions.

If the patient has a sore mouth or throat, suggest the following:

1. Try soft foods that are easy to chew and swallow such as milkshakes, soft fruits, cottage cheese, mashed potatoes, custards, puddings, gelatin, scrambled eggs, oatmeal, pureed foods, and liquids.
2. Cut food into small pieces.
3. Mix food with butter, thin gravies, and sauces to make it easier to swallow.
4. Use a blender or food processor to puree foods.
5. Use a straw to drink fluids.
6. Try foods cold or at room temperature. Hot and warm foods can irritate a tender mouth.
7. Avoid irritating foods such as citrus fruits or juices; spicy or salty foods; and rough, course, or dry foods.
8. Rinse mouth often with water to remove food and bacteria.
9. Do not wear dentures if sores are present.
10. Consult the physician about numbing medications that permit anesthesia while eating.

If the patient has a changed sense of taste, suggest the following:

1. Choose and prepare foods that look and smell good.
2. Avoid foods that have an unpleasant taste.
3. Try tart foods, which may have more taste.

If the patient has a dry mouth, suggest the following:

1. Try very sweet or tart foods and beverages, such as lemonade. These foods help the mouth produce more saliva. Do not use these if the mouth is sore.
2. Suck on sugar-free hard candy or popsicles or chew sugar-free gum.
3. Eat foods with sauces and gravies.
4. Sip water often.
5. Keep lips moist with lip salves.
6. Ask the physician or dentist about artificial saliva.

Modified from National Cancer Institute: *Eating hints,* Washington, DC, July 1992, The Institute. NIH Publication No 92-2079.

BOX 10-6 **Nursing Process**

EXTERNAL RADIATION THERAPY

ASSESSMENT

Level of knowledge and understanding
Anxiety level
Restrictions in mobility and activities of daily living (ADLs)
Skin condition in radiation field
Presence and level of pain
Nutritional status
Area of body to be irradiated

NURSING DIAGNOSES

Knowledge deficit related to treatment with external radiation
Anxiety related to the procedures and effects of radiation
Risk for impaired skin integrity related to radiation therapy
Risk for altered nutrition related to effects of radiation therapy

NURSING INTERVENTIONS

Observe for and manage radiation reactions:
- Nausea
- Vomiting
- Diarrhea
- Skin reddening
- Skin breakdown
- Fatigue
- Weakness
- Anorexia
- Leukopenia
- Thrombocytopenia
- Anemia
- Specific symptoms according to radiation site

Give reassurance and support
Patient teaching will include:
- Purposes and procedures
- Skin markings not to be removed
- Skin care instructions
- Diet high in calories, protein, fluids
- Rest/exercise planning
- Reporting infection and bleeding
- Site specific symptom management (e.g., nausea, diarrhea, mucositis)

EVALUATION OF EXPECTED OUTCOMES

Verbalizes understanding of the purposes of the therapy and procedures used
Verbalizes less anxiety related to fear of the unknown or to misconceptions
Verbalizes understanding of the importance and rationale of maintaining a high-calorie, high-protein diet and high-fluid intake during therapy
Skin markings present
Cares for skin; takes measures to prevent skin breakdown and infection
Reports signs and symptoms of radiation reactions
Adjusts activities to compensate for fatigue

dium is kept in a sealed container, a tiny pinhole can result in leakage of the gas and the consequent exposure of other patients and personnel. Therefore cesium-137, a radioactive isotope, is now being used instead of radium in hospitals. Other radioisotopes commonly used are iodine-125 and gold-198.

The radioactive isotope is prepared in a number of ways, including in needles, tubes, capsules, and wires. External molds created specifically for each patient can be applied to the skin and mucous membranes. The specific form used is determined by the area to which radiation is to be applied. For example, needles may be used to treat cancer of the mouth, whereas tubes or capsules are generally used for internal irradiation of the uterus. Whatever isotope is used, the radiologist determines the exact length of time that it should remain in place, and it must be removed at exactly the specified time. The isotope is removed by the physician using long-handled forceps, washed, and placed in a lead-lined container.

Nursing interventions. The patient who is to have an implanted radiation source is assessed and prepared in the same way as most surgical patients. For a cervical or uterine implantation, a cleansing enema is given the night before treatment. A douche may also be given. A bedtime sedative is administered to ensure sleep and rest, and the patient is not allowed anything by mouth after midnight.

During surgery, the physician positions the applicator and either inserts the radioactive substance at that time (preloading) or waits until the patient has returned to the hospital bed (afterloading). Afterloading is often preferred because fewer hospital personnel are exposed to the radiation.

The psychologic preparation of a patient who is receiving an implantation is important. Patient care dur-

TABLE 10-3

Side Effects of External Radiation Therapy

Time of Occurrence	Side Effects
Acute (during treatment and up to 6 months following treatment; usually reversible)	Skin reactions Erythema Dry desquamation Moist desquamation Nausea and vomiting Diarrhea Fatigue Bone marrow suppression Stomatitis Cystitis Pneumonitis
Chronic (after 6 months of radiation therapy; often permanent)	Fibrosis (lung, bladder, heart) Fistulas Necrosis (bone, nerve) Paresthesia Cataracts Cancer

ing the treatment is minimal, and the patient is usually in isolation. The nurse can provide the patient with quiet diversional activities while he or she is receiving treatment, can offer reassurance, and can help relieve the patient's anxiety by stopping often at his or her door. After returning to the unit, the patient is placed in a private room, and a sign is placed on the bed and door that indicates that the patient is receiving radiotherapy. The patient should be instructed to lie quietly to avoid displacing the radioactive source. The vital signs are checked often until they are stable. The temperature, pulse, and respiration are checked every 4 hours unless the nurse is directed otherwise. The patient should maintain a high-fluid intake. Talking should be discouraged when implants are placed in the mouth.

When applicators are placed in the cervix, the patient is positioned with the head and chest fairly low. The patient should be turned often and encouraged to breathe deeply. The legs should be held close together and straight, and the patient should be carefully rolled to the side when turning. No perineal care is given while the applicator is in place in the cervix. Usually the treatment lasts for only 1 or 2 days.

The patient may have a Foley catheter inserted into the bladder to prevent distention, and it should be checked at intervals to ensure that it is draining properly. Patients should be watched for any bleeding and leaking of urine around a Foley catheter, and the radiologist should be notified if such complications occur. Patients are usually given a low-residue diet and diphenoxylate to prevent bowel movements that might dislodge the implant. However, the patient should use the bedpan for bowel evacuation if necessary and should be instructed not to strain. The contents of the bedpan should be inspected carefully before disposing of them. All vomitus, clothing, and bed linens are inspected before they are removed from the unit.

Dark threads are attached to the applicator and brought to the outside, where they are fastened to the skin. The patient should be cautioned to avoid pulling on the threads, and they should be counted every 4 hours and recorded on the patient's chart. Long forceps and a lead carrier are kept in the patient's room in case the applicator is accidentally displaced. Dislodged applicators should never be picked up with the hands. The forceps and carrier can also be used to remove the implant, although this is often done in the radiology department. If any radioactive source becomes dislodged, the radiologist should be notified immediately.

The patient should be observed for symptoms of a radiation reaction. Nausea, vomiting, malaise, and anorexia may indicate that the treatment needs to be altered. An elevated temperature may indicate an infection. The physician must be notified of any unusual symptoms.

The radiologist calculates the dose of radioactive source necessary to destroy cancer cells. The exact hour that the radioactive source is to be removed is noted on the patient's chart, and it may also be noted on a tag that is placed on the patient's wrist. The radiologist should be notified at least 30 minutes before the time of removal, and a tray with the necessary equipment should be at the patient's bedside. After removal of the radioactive source, the patient should be given a warm cleansing bath and made comfortable on a freshly made bed. The equipment and utensils in the room are not radioactive and require only routine cleaning.

Postprocedure self-care instructions are given to the patient before discharge. Normal tissues in the area of the applicator often become irritated from the effects of the radiation. The patient is warned of the potential side effects and how to alleviate symptoms. Because mucositis may occur after implants in the mouth area, mouth care instructions are given to such patients. Women who have had vaginal or uterine applicators may experience dysuria and vaginal dryness. Sexual intercourse can be resumed in a few weeks with the physician's approval. Because vaginal stenosis can occur, routine vaginal dilation is usually recommended. The patient may need the nurse's help in dealing with

BOX 10-7

Nursing Process

SEALED INTERNAL RADIATION THERAPY

ASSESSMENT

Level of knowledge and understanding
Anxiety level
Area of body to receive sealed radiation

NURSING DIAGNOSES

Knowledge deficit related to treatment with sealed internal radiation
Anxiety related to the procedures and effects of radiation
Risk for altered nutrition related to effects of radiation therapy

NURSING INTERVENTIONS

Follow precautions as ordered.
Attach radiation symbol to door of room.
Check vital signs often.
Check position of applicator q 4 hr.
Observe for symptoms of radiation reaction.
Observe for specific symptoms according to radiation site.
Maintain measures for self-protection.
Limit the amount of time spent in the room. Organize well.
Approach patient only when necessary. Communicate from doorway.
Use shielding if available.
Never touch a radiation source with bare hands. If the applicator becomes dislodged, pick it up with long forceps, place it in a carrier, and notify the radiologist immediately.
Provide support and opportunities to communicate using the principles of time, shielding, and distance.
Patient education should include the following:
- Purpose and procedures
- Instructing patient to lie quietly
- Quiet diversional activities
- Encouraging high fluid intake
- Providing postprocedure self-care instructions

EVALUATION OF EXPECTED OUTCOMES

Verbalizes understanding of the purposes of the therapy and procedures
Verbalizes less anxiety related to fear of unknown or to misconceptions
Radioactive applicator remains in place
Describes appropriate postprocedure self-care

the physical and emotional impact of this procedure (Box 10-7).

It is important to realize that the patient does not become radioactive. When the sealed applicator is removed from the body, no radiation remains. Body excretions are not radioactive unless part of the source has become dislodged and is present in the excretion. Nurses cannot become radioactive by caring for a patient with sealed internal radiation therapy, and they cannot expose others to radiation. However, the sealed applicator *is* a source of radiation, and nurses and other hospital personnel are exposed to some radiation when caring for these patients. Radiation safety precautions must be taken by all those who come in contact with the patient. Visitors should be instructed to limit the length of their visits and stay at least 6 feet from the patient. Pregnant women and children should not be allowed to visit the patient.

Self-protection. There are three main factors that determine the amount of radiation the nurse receives while caring for the patient. The amount of *time* spent with the patient should be the absolute minimum required for whatever care is necessary. However, nursing care should be planned so that good care is provided without the nurse presenting a hurried appearance. As the *distance* from the source of radiation (the patient) is increased, the amount of radiation exposure significantly decreases (Hassey-Dow, Hilderley, 1992). When caring for a patient with a cesium source in the pelvis, the nurse should plan care so that no more than 30 minutes a day is spent at a distance of no less than 3 feet from the source. At a distance of 6 feet, 2 hours a day is safe. This general guideline also applies to visitors.

Speaking often to the patient from the doorway provides him or her with reassurance and gives him or her the opportunity to communicate without exposing personnel to undue radiation. A bedside telephone helps the patient keep in touch with family. When a radioisotope has been placed in the pelvic area, a drawsheet that is placed under the patient on the operating room table may be used to lift him or her from the table onto the stretcher and from the stretcher onto the bed, thus avoiding close contact. Walking at the head rather than at the side of the stretcher while transferring the patient also reduces exposure.

Shielding must also be considered for self-protection. Various materials, such as a lead sheet or shield, can be placed between the nurse and the patient to absorb the radiation. All personnel who spend considerable time in radiation areas should wear badges with small dental film inside. This film is developed at intervals and observed for fogging that might indicate overexposure. It is important to understand that these badges are to measure an *individual's* exposure to radiation. Therefore nurses should not use others' badges or lend their badge to others. Radiation safety officers are employed by most hospitals that provide radiation therapy. The officers monitor patient safety and calculate safe working times and distances for each isotope and dose.

Unsealed internal radiation therapy

Unsealed internal radiation therapy involves the administration of radioisotopes orally or by injection. Depending on the radioisotope used and its pattern of distribution in the body, the radioactivity may be localized or spread throughout the body.

Nursing intervention. Radioactive iodine (^{131}I) is commonly used for the treatment of thyroid diseases. Like many other isotopes, radioactive iodine circulates in the blood stream and is eliminated from the body by the kidneys. When large doses are given for treatment, special care must be taken in the handling and disposal of the patient's body fluids (e.g., blood, urine, feces, and vomitus). Sheets and dressings should be handled with gloves and stored until they may be disposed of safely. In the first day, 50% of the radioactive iodine is excreted from the patient's body, and the radioactivity of the retained iodine decreases by one-half every 8 days. Therefore precautions are rarely necessary after one week. Isotopes of phosphorus, cobalt, and gold are also used for therapeutic purposes. Each has specific characteristics and necessitate various protective measures.

It is important to note that the patient receiving therapeutic doses of a radioisotope *does* become a source of radioactivity as long as the radioisotope remains within the body and continues to emit radiation. Nursing personnel must know which radioisotope was used, how and when it was administered, how long it will continue to emit radiation, and how it is distributed and excreted by the body. The radiation safety principles of time, distance, and shielding must be used. Patients should be placed in isolation, and all body fluids are handled as contaminated fluids. The nursing actions for this radioisotope are similar to those used with other radioisotopes (Box 10-8).

Strontium-89 (Megastron), another radioactive isotope, is a promising new treatment in the palliation of bone pain that results from metastases. After injection into the patient, Strontium-89 is handled by the body like calcium and is carried into the bones, where it delivers radiation to the bony metastases precisely where it is needed. Pain relief may take 1 or 2 weeks and lasts several months. Side effects are minimal and mostly involve a drop in blood count. The effects of Strontium-89 are confined within the patient's body, and other people are not harmed through bodily contact. However, during the first week after injection, the radioisotope is present in blood and urine. The patient is instructed on precautions to take, such as flushing the toilet twice, washing hands after urination, and laundering urine- or blood-stained clothes separately. In the hospital setting, patients do not need to be isolated, but body fluid precautions are strictly enforced.

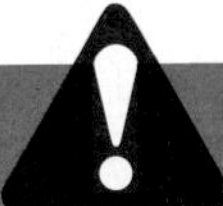

NURSE ALERT

A patient receiving any form of internal radiation therapy may be a source of radiation. Nurses caring for these patients must adhere to the safety principles of time, distance, and shielding.

Chemotherapy

Cancer is a disease that involves cellular metabolism. Much of the present cancer research is directed toward finding chemicals that control the growth and multiplication of malignant cells. **Chemotherapy** plays a major role in the early curative treatment of cancer patients and also provides palliative measures for the patient who has widespread metastasis. New drugs are continually being developed, and several may be combined to provide the most satisfactory results. Drugs may also be used in combination with surgery and/or radiotherapy.

Chemotherapeutic drugs disrupt the internal metabolism of cells so that they are either prevented from multiplying or are directly killed (Table 10-4). The drugs are usually classified according to their mechanism of action. *Alkylating agents* react with the nuclear material of cells to impair cell division and growth, and *plant alkaloids* disrupt the mechanics of cell division. *Antimetabolites* block the formation of normal nu-

BOX 10-8 **Nursing Process**

UNSEALED INTERNAL RADIATION THERAPY

ASSESSMENT

Level of knowledge and understanding
Anxiety level
Type of radioisotope, half-life, route of administration, distribution and excretion pattern

NURSING DIAGNOSES

Knowledge deficit related to treatment with unsealed internal radiation
Anxiety related to the procedure and effects of radiation
Risk for altered nutrition related to effects of radiation therapy

NURSING INTERVENTIONS

Follow precautions as ordered.
Attach radiation symbol to door of room when patient is receiving therapeutic doses of radioisotopes.
Check patient's room for the following items:
- Solid waste container
- Soiled linen container
- Other containers as directed by hospital radiation safety officer

Check that all meals are served on disposable items.
Maintain visitor restrictions (no one under age 18, no pregnant women).
Maintain measures for self-protection; use the principles of time, distance, and shielding.
Wear gloves when handling any body fluids.
Patient education includes the following:
- Purpose and procedure
- Reason to remain in the room
- Quiet diversional activities
- Use of the bathroom and waste containers
- Postprocedure instructions

EVALUATION OF EXPECTED OUTCOMES

Verbalizes understanding of the purposes of the therapy and procedures used
Verbalizes less anxiety related to fear of the unknown or to misconceptions
Remains in isolation and uses containers for urine, feces, and vomitus
Participates in maintaining nutrition and fluid intake

clear material. *Antibiotics* used in cancer therapy are highly toxic drugs and are not used to treat infections. Some antibiotics appear to destroy nuclear material, although their mechanisms of action vary. The action of *hormones* is largely unknown, but some block the action of the natural hormones that stimulate tumor growth. Steroid therapy is sometimes used as cancer therapy, generally to alter certain hormones.

Although chemotherapeutic drugs are effective in destroying or preventing the multiplication of cancer cells, normal tissue is also affected. Tissues that rapidly multiply are affected the most, such as cells in the gastrointestinal tract, hair follicles, and bone marrow. As a result, side effects can be expected from the administration of these drugs. The severity of the side effects is usually related to the strength of the dose. Reducing the dose or discontinuing the drug minimizes the symptoms (Walters, 1990).

Assessment

Chemotherapy may be given with curative or palliative intent. It is important to determine the patient's expectations regarding the outcome of the therapy. Although the physician is responsible for informing the patient of the risks and benefits of chemotherapy, the nurse needs to assess the patient's level of understanding and to reinforce teaching. Patients generally dread receiving chemotherapy, and it is not uncommon for them to refuse treatment because they fear side effects such as vomiting and hair loss. Nurses play an important role in helping patients find ways to cope with the physical and emotional reactions to chemotherapy.

Nursing interventions

Before treatment begins, the drug regimen is thoroughly reviewed, and the patient and family are given written information about the drugs and their side effects. The nurse can explain that significant side effects may not be experienced but that those that occur can usually be well controlled if treated promptly. Therefore early reporting of any symptoms is urged. The physician's 24-hour phone number should be given to the patient before discharge.

Continued on p. 254

TABLE 10-4

Pharmacology of Drugs Used for the Patient With Cancer

Drug (Generic and Trade Name); Route and Dosage	Action/Indication	Common Side Effects and Nursing Considerations
ASPARAGINASE (Elspar) **ROUTE:** IM, IV **DOSAGE:** In combination, IV 1000 IU/kg/day × 10 days given over 30 min; IM 6000 IU/m²/day; sole induction, IV 200 IU/kg/day × 28 days	Antineoplastic *Escherichia coli* enzyme agent used for acute lymphocytic leukemia	Hypersensitivity reactions, malaise, anorexia, nausea, and vomiting; nausea and vomiting usually mild; not toxic to bone marrow, oral mucosa, GI mucosa, or hair follicles; anaphylaxis may occur, especially with IV administration; epinpehrine, diphenhydramine, hydrocortisone, physician support, and resuscitation support must be available; hyperglycemia and coagulation disorders may occur
BLEOMYCIN SULFATE (Blenoxane) **ROUTE:** SC, IM, IV **DOSAGE:** SC, IV, IM 0.25-0.5 U/kg × 1-2 wk or 10-20 U/m², then 1 U/day or 5 U/wk; may also be given intraarterially; do not exceed total dose 400 U in lifetime	Antitumor, antibiotic antineoplastic agent used for testicular cancer	Stomatitis, anorexia, fever, chills, pulmonary fibrosis, and alopecia; fever can be controlled by premedication and around-the-clock administration of acetaminophen; skin changes include hyperpigmentation, erythema, nail changes and loss, inflammation of the palms and hands; oral changes include burning, erythema, and ulceration; pulmonary fibrosis occurs more often with a cumulative dose > 300 U; watch for dyspnea, dry cough, and rales; anaphylaxis can occur; increased pain at the tumor site may occur because of local cellular destruction
BUSULFAN (Myleran) **ROUTE:** PO **DOSAGE:** 4-12 mg/day initially until WBC levels fall to 10,000/mm³; then drug is stopped until WBC levels raise over 50,000/mm³; then 1-3 mg/day	Alkylating antineoplastic agent used for chronic myelocytic leukemia	Bone marrow suppression, nausea, vomiting, gonadal changes, pulmonary fibrosis; reproductive/sexual changes include impotence, azoospermia, amenorrhea, or gynecomastia; pulmonary fibrosis may occur much later (1 to 3 years); watch for dyspnea, dry cough, and rales
CARBOPLATIN (Paraplatin) **ROUTE:** IV **DOSAGE:** IV infusion 360 mg/m² given over >15 min on day 1 q 4 wk; do not repeat single intermittent courses until neutrophil count is > 2,000/mm³ and platelet count is > 100,000/mm³	Antineoplastic agent used for ovarian malignancies	Bone marrow suppression, nausea, vomiting, and mild renal toxicity; myelosuppression can be a dose-limiting toxicity; both thrombocytopenia and leukopenia may be delayed (14 to 18 days and 18 to 25 days, respectively); nausea and vomiting may have delayed onset and is usually of short duration

continued

TABLE 10-4

Pharmacology of Drugs Used for the Patient With Cancer—cont'd

Drug (Generic and Trade Name); Route and Dosage	Action/Indication	Common Side Effects and Nursing Considerations
CARMUSTINE (BiCNU) **ROUTE:** IV **DOSAGE:** IV 75-100 mg/m² over 1-2 hr × 2 days or 200 mg/m² × 1 dose q 6-8 wk; if leukocytes fall below 2000 or platelets below 75,000, only 50% of dose should be given	Nitrosourea antineoplastic agent used for brain malignancies	Nausea, vomiting, bone marrow suppression, facial flushing, and abnormal liver function tests; bone marrow suppression is usually delayed; nadir typically 3 to 5 weeks; burning and pain may occur along injection site during infusion; application of ice may provide relief; pulmonary fibrosis may occur with cumulative doses over 900 mg/m²
CHLORAMBUCIL (Leukeran) **ROUTE:** PO **DOSAGE:** 0.1-0.2 mg/kg/day for 3-6 wk initially, then 2-6 mg/day; maintenance 0.2 mg/kg for 2-4 wk; course may be repeated at 2-4 wk intervals	Alkylating antineoplastic agent used for chronic lymphocytic leukemia	Bone marrow suppression, gonadal changes, nausea and vomiting; myelosuppression usually moderate, gradual, and rapidly reversible; GI effects usually minimal or absent unless large doses given; increased toxicities occur with prior barbiturate use
CISPLATIN (Platinol) **ROUTE:** IV **DOSAGE:** Testicular cancer, IV 20 mg/m² q d × 5 days, then repeat q 3 wk for 3 cycles or more, depending on response; bladder cancer, IV 50-70 mg/m² q 3-4 wk; ovarian cancer, IV 100 mg/m² q 4 wk or 50 mg/m² q 3 wk with doxorubicin therapy; mix with 2 L of NaCL and 37.5 g mannitol over 6 hr	Inorganic heavy metal antineoplastic agent used for testicular, bladder, ovarian, and lung malignancies	Nausea, vomiting, renal toxicity, neurotoxicity, and anemia; at high doses, rigorous prehydration and mannitol (for osmotic diuresis) may be given to decrease risk of renal damage; monitor renal function, electrolytes, BUN, and creatinine; 24-hr urine collection for creatinine clearance may be evaluated before therapy; myelosuppression mild except at higher doses; ototoxicity is cumulative and may be permanent; anaphylaxis can occur
CYCLOPHOSPHAMIDE (Cytoxan) **ROUTE:** IV, PO **DOSAGE:** PO initially 1-5 mg/kg over 2-5 days, maintenance is 1-5 mg/kg; IV initially 40-50 mg/kg in divided doses over 2-5 days, maintenance 10-15 mg/kg q 7-10 days, or 3-5 mg/kg q 3 days	Alkylating neoplastic agent used for lymphoma and breast and ovarian malignancies	Bone marrow suppression, bladder toxicity, nausea, gonadal changes, and alopecia; push fluids (2-3 qt/day) to maintain urine output; manifestations of bladder toxicity include bladder fibrosis, hemorrhagic cystitis, and bladder carcinoma; check urine for blood at each void; administer drug early in day to prevent accumulation in bladder; encourage frequent voiding; myelosuppression usually recovers rapidly with sparing of platelets; cardiac damage and necrosis with very large single doses; may inhibit immune function

TABLE 10-4

Pharmacology of Drugs Used for the Patient With Cancer—cont'd

Drug (Generic and Trade Name); Route and Dosage	Action/Indication	Common Side Effects and Nursing Considerations
CYTARABINE (Ara-C) (Cytosar) **ROUTE:** IV **DOSAGE:** IV infusion 200 mg/m²/day × 5 days; intrathecal 5-50 mg/m²/ day × 3 days a week or 30 mg/m²/ day q 4 days	Antimetabolite antineoplastic agent used for leukemia	Bone marrow suppression, nausea, stomatitis, and headaches; nausea, vomiting, and diarrhea increase in severity with increasing doses; stomatitis and anorexia very common; watch for tumor lysis syndrome caused by rapid lysis of cells; rash, palmar erythema and desquamation, conjunctivitis, and cerebellar toxicities occur with larger doses
DACARBAZINE (DTIC-Dome) **ROUTE:** IV **DOSAGE:** Malignant melanoma, 2-4.5 mg/kg/day for 10 days q 4 wk or 250 mg/m²/day for 5 days q 3 wk; Hodgkin's disease, 150 mg/m²/day for 5 days (in combination with other agents) q 4 wk or 375 mg/m² (with other agents) q 15 days	Alkylating antineoplastic agent used for melanoma and Hodgkin's disease	Nausea, vomiting, bone marrow suppression, alopecia, hepatoxicity, and flu syndrome; flu-like syndrome (headache, malaise, fever, chills, and myalgias) may occur 7-10 days after treatment and persist 1-3 weeks; patient may experience burning sensation at IV site and metallic taste during infusion; vesicant agent—avoid extravasation; burning may or not indicate extravasation; nausea and vomiting (often severe) begins within 1-3 hours and lasts 1-12 hours
DACTINOMYCIN (Actinomycin-D) **ROUTE:** IV **DOSAGE:** 10-15 μg/kg/day for up to 5 days q 4-6 wk or 500 mcg/m² (up to 2 mo) weekly for 3 wk	Antitumor, antibiotic, antineoplastic agent used for Wilms' tumor	Bone marrow suppression, stomatitis, nausea and vomiting, skin rash, and alopecia; myelosuppression may be severe; vesicant agent—avoid extravasation; GI symptoms also may be severe; skin changes include patches of depigmentation with vitiligo, acne, and erythema; skin reactions may develop in previously irradiated areas ("radiation recall"); erythema and desquamation can occur; reversible skin discoloration may occur along veins used for drug administration
DAUNORUBICIN (Cerubidine) **ROUTE:** IV **DOSAGE:** Adult < 60 yr, 45 mg/m²/day for 1-3 days, as part of a combination regimen; adult > 60 yr 30 mg/m²/day for 1-3 days, as part of a combination regimen	Antitumor, antibiotic, antineoplastic agent used for acute leukemia	Bone marrow suppression, nausea, stomatitis, cardiac toxicity, and alopecia; vesicant agents—avoid extravasation; cumulative doses >550 mg/m² may cause cardiomyopathy; patient may experience reversible ECG changes, arrhythmias, and congestive heart failure; myelosuppression may be severe; alert patient that urine will turn red until drug is fully excreted and does not indicate bleeding; radiation recall may occur

continued

TABLE 10-4

Pharmacology of Drugs Used for the Patient With Cancer—cont'd

Drug (Generic and Trade Name); Route and Dosage	Action/Indication	Common Side Effects and Nursing Considerations
DIETHYLSTILBESTROL (DES, Honvol, Stilbestrol, Stilphostrol) **ROUTE:** PO, IV **DOSAGE:** Postmenopausal breast carcinoma, PO, 15 mg/day; prostate carcinoma, PO, 1-3 mg/day; IV, 500 mg-1 g/day initially until response is obtained (5 or more days), then 250-500 mg 1-2 times weekly	Estrogen hormone antineoplastic agent used for breast and prostate cancer	Headache, edema, hypertension, intolerance to contact lenses, nausea, weight changes, breakthrough bleeding, dysmenorrhea, amenorrhea, testicular atrophy, impotence, acne, oily skin, gynecomastia, and breast tenderness; contraindicated in thromboembolic disease and if possibly pregnant; use with caution in underlying cardiac disease and severe renal or hepatic disease; may increase risk of endometrial carcinoma
DOXORUBICIN (Adriamycin) **ROUTE:** IV **DOSAGE:** 60-75 mg/m^2 daily, repeat q 21 days or 25-30 mg/m^2 daily for 2-3 days, repeat q 3-4 wk or 20 mg/m^2/wk; total cumulative dose should not exceed 550 mg/m^2 without monitoring of cardiac function	Antitumor, antibiotic, antineoplastic agent used for acute leukemia, sarcoma, and breast cancer	Bone marrow suppression, nausea, vomiting, stomatitis, cardiac toxicity, and alopecia; vesicant agent—avoid extravasation; myelosuppression and nausea and vomiting may be severe; cardiotoxicity is dose-limiting; flare reaction (facial flushing and local flushing at IV site) may occur, especially during rapid infusion; alert patient that urine will turn red; radiation recall can occur.
ETOPOSIDE (VePesid) **ROUTE:** PO, IV **DOSAGE:** Testicular neoplasms, IV 50-100 mg/m^2 daily for 5 days, repeat every 3-4 wk, or 100 mg/m^2 on days 1, 3, and 5 every 3-4 wk; small cell carcinoma of the lung, PO, 70 mg/m^2 (rounded to the nearest 50 mg) every day for 4 days, repeated every 3-4 wk up to 100 mg/m^2 (rounded to the nearest 50 mg) every day for 5 days every 3-4 wk; IV, 35 mg/m^2 every day for 4 days up to 50 mg/m^2 every day for 5 days every 3-4 wk	Vinca alkaloid, antineoplastic agent used for lung and testicular cancer	Bone marrow suppression, neurotoxicity, and alopecia; orthostatic hypotension and bradycardia occur if infused too rapidly; most doses can safely be administered over 4 hours; radiation recall can occur
5-FLUOROURACIL (5-FU) **ROUTE:** IV **DOSAGE:** IV 12 mg/kg/day × 4 days, not to exceed 800 mg/day; may repeat with 6 mg/kg on day 6, 8, 10, 12; maintenance is 10-15 mg/kg/wk as a single dose, not to exceed 1 g/wk	Antimetabolite antineoplastic agent used for colon and breast cancer	Diarrhea, bone marrow suppression, stomatitis, nausea, and alopecia; stomatitis and diarrhea are dose-limiting and can be severe; skin changes include nail changes and loss, rash, darkening of the veins used for drug administration, and photosensitivity

TABLE 10-4

Pharmacology of Drugs Used for the Patient With Cancer—cont'd

Drug (Generic and Trade Name); Route and Dosage	Action/Indication	Common Side Effects and Nursing Considerations
FLUTAMIDE (Eulexin) **ROUTE:** PO **DOSAGE:** 250 mg q 8 hr tid, for a daily dosage of 750 mg	Antiandrogen, antineoplastic hormone used for prostate cancer	Hot flashes, decreased libido, impotence, gynecomastia, diarrhea, nausea, vomiting, and hepatitis; monitor liver function studies
IFOSFAMIDE (IFEX) **ROUTE:** IV **DOSAGE:** 1.2 g/m^2/day × 5 days, repeat course q 3 wk	Alkylating, antineoplastic agent used for lymphoma	Hemorrhagic cystitis, nausea, vomiting, alopecia, somnolence, confusion, and neurotoxicity; cystitis can be prevented by concomitant administration of mesna, a uroprotective agent; maintain rigorous hydration (at least 2 L/day) for 72 hr after treatment; myelosuppression may be dose-limiting
LOMUSTINE (CCNU) **ROUTE:** PO **DOSAGE:** 130 mg/m^2 as a single dose q 6 wk; titrate dose to WBC level; do not give repeat dose unless WBC are > 4000/mm^3, platelet count > 100,000/mm^3	Alkylating, antineoplastic agent used for brain and lymphoma malignancies	Bone marrow suppression, nausea, and vomiting; myelosuppression is cumulative and may be delayed; leukopenia may appear about 4-6 wk after a dose and lasts 1-2 wk
MECHLORETHAMINE, NITROGEN MUSTARD (Mustargen) **ROUTE:** IV **DOSAGE:** 0.4 mg/kg or 10 mg/m^2 as 1 dose or 2-4 divided doses over 2-4 days; second course after 3 wk depending on blood cell count	Alkylating, antineoplastic agent used for Hodgkin's disease	Bone marrow suppression, nausea, vomiting, gonadal changes, and stomatitis; drug has very short stability; use immediately after reconstitution; potent vesicant—avoid extravasation and any skin or mucous membrane contact; nausea and vomiting are usually severe; chills, fever, and diarrhea may occur immediately after administration; watch for hyperuricemia; maintain adequate hydration of at least 2 L/day for 48 hours after treatment; thrombophlebitis, local irritation, and burning may occur along veins used for administration; patient may experience metallic taste
MEGESTROL ACETATE (Megace) **ROUTE:** PO **DOSAGE:** 40-320 mg/day in divided doses	Progestin hormone, antineoplastic agent used for breast cancer	Nausea, vomiting, hypercalcemia, and thrombophlebitis at drug administration site; do not use if pregnant

continued

TABLE 10-4

Pharmacology of Drugs Used for the Patient With Cancer—cont'd

Drug (Generic and Trade Name); Route and Dosage	Action/Indication	Common Side Effects and Nursing Considerations
MELPHALAN (Alkeran) **ROUTE:** PO, IV **DOSAGE:** Multiple myeloma, PO, 150 μg/kg/day for 7 days, followed by 3 wk rest, then 50 μg/kg/day maintenance dose or 100-150 μg/kg/day for 2-3 wk followed by 2-4 wk rest, then 2-4 mg/day maintenance dose; other regimens are used; ovarian carcinoma, IV, 16 mg/m^2 q 2 wk for 4 doses, then q 4 wk; PO, 0.2 mg/kg/day for 5 days given every 4-5 wk	Alkylating, antineoplastic agent used for multiple myeloma and ovarian carcinoma	Bone marrow suppression, nausea, gonadal changes, secondary malignancies; myelosuppression may be delayed up to 30 days after treatment; thrombocytopenia can be persistent; thinning of hair with repeated doses; vomiting is uncommon
6-MERCAPTOPURINE (6-MP) **ROUTE:** PO **DOSAGE:** 1.5-2.5 mg/kg/day (up to 5 mg/kg/day) single dose or divided doses	Antimetabolite, antineoplastic agent used for leukemia	Bone marrow suppression, nausea, hepatic toxicity, and stomatitis; myelosuppression usually of gradual onset and persistent after drug discontinued; allopurinol may be given concomitantly to prevent uric nephropathy secondary to hyperuricemia; allopurinol inhibits 6-MP degradation, thus 6-MP dose must be reduced by ⅓ in presence of allopurinol administration; cholestatic jaundice may occur after 2-5 months of treatment and usually reversible after drug discontinued
METHOTREXATE (MTX) **ROUTE:** PO, IV **DOSAGE:** Leukemia, PO 3.3 mg/m^2/day, maintenance 30 mg/m^2/day twice a week; IV 2.5 mg/kg q 2 wk; choriocarcinoma, PO, 15-30 mg/m^2/q d $\times$ 5 days, then off 1 wk; may repeat	Antimetabolite, antineoplastic agent used for leukemia, breast cancer, and lymphoma	Stomatitis, bone marrow suppression, nausea, and renal toxicity; stomatitis and diarrhea may be severe and warrant interruption of treatment; renal tubular necrosis at high doses; during large dose administration, 100 mg leucovorin rescue is given to counteract the immediate hematopoietic toxicity by supplying normal cells with the form of folic acid needed for DNA synthesis; urine will turn bright yellow and will resolve after drug excreted; photosensitivity may occur even without sunlight exposure; patient may develop erythematous rash and must be cautioned to use sunscreen when outdoors

TABLE 10-4

Pharmacology of Drugs Used for the Patient With Cancer—cont'd

Drug (Generic and Trade Name); Route and Dosage	Action/Indication	Common Side Effects and Nursing Considerations
MITOMYCIN C (Mutamycin) **ROUTE:** IV **DOSAGE:** 2 mg/m²/day × 5 days, stop drug for 2 days, then repeat cycle; or 10-20 mg/m² as a single dose, repeat cycle in 6-8 wk; stop drug if platelets are < 75,000/mm³ or WBC < 3000/mm³	Antitumor, antibiotic, antineoplastic agent used for stomach and pancreatic malignancies	Bone marrow suppression, nausea, vomiting, stomatitis, renal toxicity, and alopecia; vesicant agent—avoid extravasation; myelosuppression often severe, cumulative, and delayed (up to 8 weeks after); thrombocytopenia can be prolonged; skin reactions include dermatitis, pruritis, dark half-circles in nailbeds, and severe phlebitis; nailbed discolorations disappear after drug is discontinued
MITOXANTRONE (Novantrone) **ROUTE:** IV **DOSAGE:** IV infusion 12 mg/m²/day on days 1-3, and 100 mg/m² cytosine arabinoside × 7 days as a continuous 24-hr infusion	Antitumor, antibiotic, antineoplastic agent used for leukemia and lymphoma	Nausea, vomiting, myelosuppression, alopecia, and stomatitis; drug is blue and may cause green discoloration of urine and blue streaking of vein; mild congestive heart failure may occur in patients previously treated with anthracycline antibiotics; transient elevation of hepatic enzymes is seen
TAMOXIFEN CITRATE (Nolvadex) **ROUTE:** PO **DOSAGE:** 10-20 mg bid	Antiestrogen hormone, antineoplastic agent used for advanced breast malignancies	Thrombocytopenia, leukopenia, nausea, vomiting, hot flashes, headache, and lightheadedness
TESTOSTERONE (Andro 100, Histerone 100, Tesamone) **ROUTE:** IM **DOSAGE:** Titrated dose; use lowest effective dose and give IM deep into gluteal muscle	Androgenic anabolic steroid given for breast cancer in postmenopausal women	Cholestatic jaundice; contraindicated in pregnancy and severe renal, cardiac, and hepatic disease; use with caution in diabetes and myocardial infarction; causes increased effect of anticoagulants and decreased effect of insulin
VINBLASTINE (Velban) **ROUTE:** IV **DOSAGE:** 0.1 mg/kg or 3.7 mg/m² q wk or q 2 wk, not to exceed 0.5 mg/kg or 18.5 mg/m² q wk	Vinca alkaloid, antineoplastic agent used for lymphoma	Bone marrow suppression, neurotoxicity, stomatitis, alopecia, mental depression, and nausea; potent vesicant—avoid extravasation; neurotoxicity can be manifested by abdominal pain, diarrhea, constipation, paralytic ileus and obstruction, urinary retention, numbness, parasthesias, loss of deep tendon reflexes, foot drop, headache, convulsions, depression, and Raynaud's disease
VINCRISTINE (Oncovin) **ROUTE:** IV **DOSAGE:** 1-2 mg/m²/wk, not to exceed 2 mg	Vinca alkaloid, antineoplastic agent used for acute leukemia and Kaposi's sarcoma	Renal and hepatic toxicity, skin rash, stomatitis, and alopecia; potent vesicant—avoid extravasation; no bone marrow toxicity; constipation, paralytic ileus, and abdominal pain can occur, as well as cranial nerve palsies

Common gastrointestinal reactions include nausea and vomiting, anorexia, diarrhea or constipation, and possibly distortion of taste. Nausea and vomiting most often occur within a few hours after administration of the drug, although it may not occur at all in some patients. When the physician orders an antiemetic medication, the nurse can encourage the patient to take it regularly before and after treatment to prevent nausea and vomiting. In the past few years, antiemetics that block serotonin uptake (ondansetron [Zofran], granisetron [Kytril]) have been developed (Distasio, 1993). These drugs have fewer side effects than previously used antiemetics and have significantly reduced the incidence and severity of chemotherapy-induced nausea and vomiting. Small, frequent feedings are suggested if nausea does occur, and patients are encouraged to increase their fluid intake. Most hospitals have registered dieticians, who are very knowledgeable about the effect of chemotherapy on the nutritional status of the cancer patient. Whenever possible, a nutritional consult should be obtained for patients who are receiving chemotherapy.

Soreness and ulceration of the mouth may also occur. Good oral hygiene, including frequent rinsing of the mouth, is encouraged. Antibacterial mouthwashes may be ordered. Dry, cracked lips may be soothed with petroleum jelly.

Alopecia, or loss of hair, may be a significant psychologic event. Wigs, scarves, and cosmetics can effectively conceal the hair loss. The patient should be encouraged to purchase a wig before the hair is lost, which is usually a few weeks after chemotherapy is first given. Some ACS units provide free wigs. The nurse should reassure the patient that the hair will grow back once the treatment is discontinued. Because not all chemotherapy drugs cause hair loss, first check which drugs the patient will be receiving. Nursing research has shown that "icing" the scalp before chemotherapy reduces hair loss. Several commercial caps are available to "ice" the scalp. However, this procedure may be uncomfortable to the patient. The treatment also cannot be used for patients with tumors that can metastasize to the skin, because the ice cap will prevent the chemotherapy from reaching this area and will create a sanctuary for the cancer cells.

Suppression of bone marrow **(myelosuppression)** produces the most serious side effects. The bone marrow continually produces the three major types of blood cells: white blood cells, platelets, and red blood cells. Chemotherapy temporarily stops the division of blood cells in the marrow, which leads to a drop in the number of circulating blood cells (nadir counts) 1 to 2 weeks after chemotherapy is given. Complete blood counts should be checked weekly, or more often if indicated. Leukopenia, the reduction in the number of white blood cells, can increase the risk of infection. To reduce this risk, patients undergoing chemotherapy should be instructed to do the following:

1. Inform the physician or nurse about any signs of infection such as fever, chills, cough, sore throat, urinary frequency, or skin rashes.
2. Maintain good hygiene techniques (e.g., having clean nails and hair, washing hands before meals).
3. Maintain good perineal care, including washing genitalia after urination or bowel movements.
4. Avoid individuals with colds and flu, and avoid crowds during the flu season.

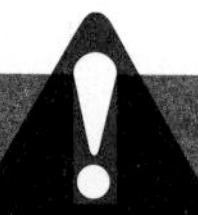

NURSE ALERT

Fever is the most reliable indicator of infection in a patient with leukopenia. Ensure that the patient has a thermometer at home and knows how to use it.

Antibiotics are given at the first sign of infection. Patients with very low white blood cell counts may be hospitalized and placed on "reverse isolation," with good handwashing precautions and masks for visitors with colds. Uncooked fruits and vegetables are eliminated from the diet while the white count is low. Strict reverse isolation using laminar air flow rooms, or plastic bubbles, is used in bone marrow transplant units only for patients with extreme and prolonged bone marrow suppression.

Thrombocytopenia, a low platelet count, increases the chance of hemorrhage. If the platelet count is low or the patient exhibits signs or symptoms of bleeding, platelet transfusions are needed. Anemia may require the transfusion of packed red blood cells.

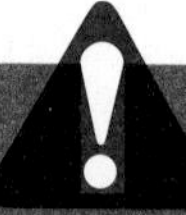

NURSE ALERT

A patient with a platelet count of less than 50,000 cells/mm^3 should be on bleeding precautions, which include instructing the patient to avoid trauma and to report unusual bleeding promptly. Nurses can teach patients safe behaviors such as using an electric razor instead of a straight-edged razor, avoiding rectal suppositories, and doing nonabrasive mouth care.

Hematopoietic growth factors are now often used to stimulate normal bone marrow recovery after chemotherapy. Growth factors are a form of biologic response modifier. Granulocyte colony stimulating factor (G-CSF, filgrastim [Neupogen]) stimulates the bone marrow to produce more of the bacterial-fighting white blood cells, called neutrophils. The patient experiences less leukopenia, and the risk of infection is reduced. Erythropoietin (Procrit) is another growth factor that is available for use in chemotherapy patients who become anemic. It specifically stimulates red blood cell production in the bone marrow. Both G-CSF and erythropoietin are given by subcutaneous injection, and nurses are responsible for teaching patients how to give themselves the injection.

Other side effects of chemotherapy can occur that are specific to the type of drug being given. For instance, cardiac toxicity and altered functioning of the reproductive system can occur with some types of antibiotic or hormone therapy. Other organs that can be damaged by some chemotherapeutic drugs include the kidneys, lungs, liver, and peripheral nerves. It is important to determine the expected side effects of the drugs the patient is receiving (Box 10-9) (Wujcik, 1993).

BOX 10-9 **Guidelines for Care of the Patient on Chemotherapy**

Side Effect	Intervention
Gastrointestinal	
Nausea	Provide small, frequent meals; have patient eat when least nauseated; suggest that patient avoid fatty, fried, sweet, or odorous foods.
Vomiting	Instruct patient not to eat or drink until vomiting is under control and then try clear liquids before progressing to full liquids.
Anorexia	Teach patient the need for increased protein, carbohydrates, and vitamins. Teach patient to have nutritious snacks.
Diarrhea	Inform physician if diarrhea is continual. Instruct patient about the importance of maintaining high fluid intake during episodes of diarrhea.
Skin—stomatitis (breakdown of the mucous membranes of the mouth)	Teach patient to avoid smoking, alcohol, and irritating food. Teach patient to brush teeth with soft toothbrush and rinse after brushing with baking soda and water at least twice a day. Encourage patient to report changes in skin of mouth (e.g., bleeding, ulcerations, severe stomatitis). Recommend high-protein liquids/blenderized food until mouth sores heal. Recommend cold food such as frozen fruit sticks or frozen ice cream sticks to ease pain of stomatitis.
Alopecia (loss of hair)	Encourage patient to use wigs, scarves, and hats. Provide opportunities to talk about change in patient's body image.
Bone marrow suppression	Obtain complete blood counts as ordered.
Leukopenia (reduced white blood cells)	Teach patient to report early symptoms of infection such as fever, cough, sore throat, and urinary frequency. Instruct patient in good hygiene practices, including perineal care. Teach patient to avoid crowds during flu season.
Thrombocytopenia (reduced platelets)	Teach patient to report early signs of bleeding such as easy bruising and blood in urine or stool. Teach patient to avoid physical trauma.
Anemia (reduced red blood cells and hematocrit)	Teach patient to report symptoms of anemia such as fatigue, shortness of breath, and dizziness. Encourage patient to set priorities for activities and to pace daily routine.

Chemotherapy is usually given intermittently to minimize side effects. A combination of several drugs is often used to maximize the killing of tumor cells without causing unacceptable side effects. A variety of routes of administration are used: oral, intramuscular, intravenous, intraarterial, intrathecal, and intraperitoneal. The intravenous route is a relatively short and painless procedure and is the most common route of administration. When chemotherapeutic drugs are administered intravenously, the drug flows through the entire circulatory system.

Some drugs are vesicants and cause tissue damage if they leak outside the vein. Intravenous sites must be observed carefully, and the integrity of the patient's veins must be preserved. Venous punctures should be done only when absolutely necessary. Blood for some tests can be obtained by fingerstick.

Most chemotherapy is administered in outpatient clinics or oncologists' offices. Regimens that involve high drug doses or multiple-day infusions may be given in the hospital, most often on **oncology** units, where the nurses are well prepared in chemotherapy administration. A new technique for delivering chemotherapy is by the use of ambulatory infusion pumps. These portable, battery-operated pumps are designed to deliver continuous drug therapy. The pump is small and light enough to attach to the patient's belt and enables the patient to receive continuous chemotherapy while engaged in daily activities in the community. Because chemotherapy drugs alter the genes of the cell, it is important for the nurse to prevent self-exposure when caring for a patient who is receiving chemotherapy. The nurse should wear latex gloves when handling any chemotherapy bags or tubing, waste, and patient excreta for 48 hours after drug administration, because some of the drugs are excreted in the urine and stool (Occupational Safety and Health Administration, 1986).

Bone Marrow Transplantation

In the 1980s, **bone marrow transplantation** became an important means of treating leukemia. Transplantation is currently being used in over 15 different diseases, including leukemias, lymphomas, multiple myeloma, and various solid tumors (Leukemia Society of America, 1992). A bone marrow transplant begins by using very large doses of drugs to kill all the cancer cells. The patient's bone marrow is then restored to prevent life-threatening bleeding or infection. High doses of chemotherapy and radiation are given to eradicate all tumor cells from the patient's body, as well as to suppress the patient's immunity to donor marrow. The patient's bone marrow is replaced by bone marrow from a compatible donor or from the patient. There are three basic types of bone marrow transplantation: *autologous* (patient is his or her own donor); *allogeneic* (person with compatible tissue is donor, usually a sibling); *syngeneic* (identical twin is donor).

The donor marrow is obtained from the hip bone with a special syringe and needle. Because the procedure can be painful, it is usually performed under general anesthesia. The donor may be stiff for a few weeks. The donated bone marrow is infused into the patient's blood stream and travels to the bone, where it begins to produce a new population of blood cells. If the marrow successfully grows, (engraftment) and no malignant cells recur, the patient may be potentially cured of the cancer.

For several weeks after the transplant, while the new marrow is developing, the patient is kept in the hospital in a bone marrow transplant unit. During this time he or she is very susceptible to infections and may bleed easily. Blood products, antibiotics, and antifungal medications can be used to support the patient. Germ-free precautions are strictly enforced. The patient is in the hospital for 1 to 2 months and is followed very closely as an outpatient. The immune system takes as long as 9 months to recover.

A complication of allogeneic, but not autologous or syngeneic, transplants is a graft-versus-host disease. This disease results when the donor T-lymphocytes recognize the patient's cells as foreign and attack them. Symptoms, which can range from minor to severe, include skin rash and peeling, nausea, vomiting, diarrhea, liver dysfunction, photophobia, and dryness and burning of the eyes. *Peripheral stem cell* transplants have become more common in the past few years. They are used instead of or in addition to autologous bone marrow transplants. Circulating blood contains some of the same stem cells that are harvested from the marrow. Peripheral stem cells are collected by apheresis, a process of separating blood into its different components. This collection procedure is better tolerated than bone marrow aspiration. Recovery from peripheral stem cell transplants is often quicker, hospital stays are shorter, and complications are fewer.

As bone marrow transplantation becomes increasingly available in different parts of the country, nurses will be caring for more pretransplant and posttransplant patients. The nurse needs to be prepared to help the patient and family cope with both the physical and emotional reactions that result from such an intensive treatment.

Biologic Response Modifiers

Although advances in the use of combinations of surgery, radiation therapy, and chemotherapy have resulted in increased survival for cancer patients, effective treatments remain unavailable for many types of cancer. In recent years, cancer treatment research has focused on the use of **biologic response modifiers (BRMs),** which include immunotherapy and biotherapy (Wujcik, 1993). BRMs are agents that make the cancer patient's biologic response to the tumor cells more effective. In addition to strengthening the patient's immunologic response, some BRMs have direct antitumor activity, and some have other biologic effects that help fight cancer. BRM research is a rapidly expanding field as a result of technologic advances in gene cloning and hybridoma technology. Gene cloning allows the production of large quantities of purified human BRMs, and hybridomas can produce monoclonal antibodies against specific tumors.

Earlier attempts at immunotherapy used nonspecific stimulation of the immune system with bacteria (bacille Calmette-Guérin [BCG]) or viruses. It also used active specific immunization with tumor cells. There were some tumor responses reported with these methods, but interest has now shifted to the newer BRMs (Box 10-10).

Nursing interventions

BRM therapy results in many of the same side effects as chemotherapy, but there are some unique nursing care problems associated with the use of biologic agents. Because many BRMs stimulate the immune system to function more efficiently, patients receiving this therapy have symptoms similar to those suffered during a bacterial or viral infection. These flulike symptoms include chills, fever, headache, malaise, and fatigue. Comfort measures include body temperature stabilization with the use of acetaminophen (Tylenol), appropriate clothing, cooling blankets, and tepid baths. Attention should be paid to proper fluid and nutritional intake, and the patient should be allowed plenty of rest. Gastrointestinal effects of nausea, vomiting, anorexia, and altered taste should be treated in ways similar to those recommended for chemotherapy patients. BRMs may also cause skin rashes and itchiness, subtle mental status changes, and cardiac and blood circulation dysfunction. Nurses must be alert for any of these physiologic changes in patients who are receiving BRMs (Wujcik, 1993).

Biotherapy has not achieved the success in treating cancer that was once expected. However, research on BRMs is progressing rapidly. Most biologic agents are still experimental but some, such as interferon, are being released for more general use. Nurses will become increasingly involved with caring for patients receiving BRMs and will need to be prepared to help manage the side effects.

BOX 10-10

BIOLOGIC RESPONSE MODIFIERS

interferons Naturally produced in response to viral infections; have many biologic actions, including antitumor effects; alpha, beta, and gamma are the three types of interferons

interleukins Large group of cytokines produced by activated lymphocytes; play an important part in regulating blood cell growth and the immune response; twelve interleukins have been identified (IL-1 to 12)

tumor necrosis factor (TNF) Substance produced by certain white blood cells that can directly kill the tumor cells causing necrosis but does not harm normal cells

monoclonal antibodies Antibodies that are produced by a single clone of B-lymphocytes and directed against an antigen on a tumor cell; have been called "magic bullets"

colony stimulating factors (CSFs) (hematopoietic growth factors) Proteins that stimulate growth of young blood cells in the bone marrow; granulocyte colony stimulating factor (G-CSF) stimulates granulocyte production; erythropoietin stimulates red blood cell production; growth factors might allow use of higher doses of chemotherapy drugs by preventing life-threatening bone marrow suppression

differentiating agents Agents that cause cancerous or precancerous cells to mature into normal cells; include growth factors and some hormones

Unproven Methods

Beyond the above treatment options, cancer patients may seek out alternate therapies. Most of these methods do not withstand scientific trials and have been referred to as quackery. In the last 20 years, *l*-mandelonitrile-β-glucuronic acid (Laetrile) has received extensive publicity as a treatment that might cure cancer. Laetrile was studied by the National Cancer Institute for several years and was found to be a toxic drug that was *not* effective as a cancer treatment. Many other "fad" treatments have come and gone. Shark cartilage and macrobiotic diets have received much coverage in the popular press. There is some very promising scientific research on gene therapy, but it is a long way from routine use. To date, the best hope of a cure for cancer lies with the standard treatments of surgery, radiation, chemotherapy, and biotherapy.

EMOTIONAL CARE

One of the most important aspects of care of the patient with cancer is psychologic support. Often this aspect is more important than the physical care of the patient. Anxiety and depression are common emotional reactions to cancer. Many patients suffer from feelings of guilt and see their illness as a punishment for their own past. Overt anger is also a common behavior pattern in cancer patients and usually is accompanied by acute anxiety. Although they may not be verbalized, these feelings are close to the surface, and hope is the one indispensable aspect of treatment that must permeate from all persons involved in the patient's care (National Cancer Institute, 1993).

OLDER ADULT CONSIDERATIONS

Modifications of cancer therapy may be necessary for older adults.

Skin and mucous membranes and bone marrow function may be more vulnerable as a result of the normal functional decreases associated with aging.

Fatigue may be compounded by a disruption of lifestyle patterns.

Anxiety and depression can be expected psychologic reactions to cancer therapy.

Referrals to community agencies can provide invaluable support for assistance in home care.

Public education has gone far in making people more conscious of the seriousness of cancer, and although many patients may know consciously or unconsciously that the diagnosis is cancer, they still hope that a cure may be found in time for them. In the past, many physicians believed that patients should not be told that they had cancer. Education has resulted in a greatly enlightened public. The modern communication media have been used to present fictional dramas concerning cancer. These factors have helped bring changes in the knowledge and understanding of cancer.

It is believed that a majority of patients suspect or know that they have cancer without being told. The nurse should be aware of statements made by the patient that indicate a need for some confirmation of the belief. The patient may say, "I'm sure that I have cancer," or may ask "Did the doctor tell you that I have cancer?" Answers to such statements and questions may not be easy to give. The patient must be allowed to fully express his or her concerns and be given the opportunity to ask questions. It is essential that nursing personnel be aware of the patient's understanding. However, the individual's knowledge or understanding does not eradicate the emotional impact when the cancer diagnosis is given. Cancer is a threat to survival, and most persons want to look forward to life, not death. The patient and family will need information during every phase of the illness (Table 10-5).

TABLE 10-5

Information Needed by Cancer Patients and Spouses Over the Course of Illness

Diagnostic Phase	Hospital Phase	Treatment Phase	Adaptation Phase	Recurrent Phase
Type and purpose of diagnostic procedures to be performed When test results can be expected The person who is coordinating the care The typical emotions that develop while awaiting diagnosis (e.g., anxiety, uncertainty)	Type of surgery planned When pathology report will be available Expected length of hospitalization Role limitations to anticipate when patient is discharged The effects of illness on other family members	Type and length of treatment planned Anticipated side effects and when they may occur Ways to minimize side effects Likelihood of temporary role changes Availability of cancer education and support groups	When follow-up exams or tests are necessary The typical concerns during this phase (e.g., fear of recurrence) Importance of balancing needs of patient and family members Availability of cancer education and support groups	Type of treatment planned Anticipated side effects and when they may occur The typical feelings during this phase (e.g., uncertainty, sadness, fear) Ways to maintain hope regardless of recurrence Availability of support groups and community resources

From Northouse LL, Peters-Golden H: Cancer and the family: strategies to assist spouses, *Semin Oncol Nurs* 9(2): 77, 1993. Used with permission.

When caring for the cancer patient, the nurse must objectively examine personal attitudes and beliefs. The nurse's own feelings about cancer can be projected both verbally and nonverbally to the patient and family. It is important that the nurse support the therapy being offered to the patient and reassure the patient and family. It is best to stress the progress and events of the day rather than refer to the future optimistically. The nurse must realize that cancer can be cured and that patients can live with cancer under control for many years.

The ability to communicate with the cancer patient does not always involve the spoken word. A soothing back rub, a change of position, or a refreshing drink may be more meaningful to the patient than any verbal conversation. Members of the patient's family also often need emotional support. Giving emotional support to the family may mean providing a blanket or a pillow at night or giving them a report of the patient's condition during surgery. Collaborative practice between the nurse and physician can be effective in gaining a joint understanding of the patient's fears and special problems. The patient with cancer, perhaps more than a patient with another condition, appreciates visits from the hospital chaplain or a minister (Figure 10-5). The nurse can help arrange for such visits. When everything has been done for the patient that is humanly possible and the physician has terminated therapeutic measures, the nurse should continue to provide physical comfort and emotional support to the patient and family.

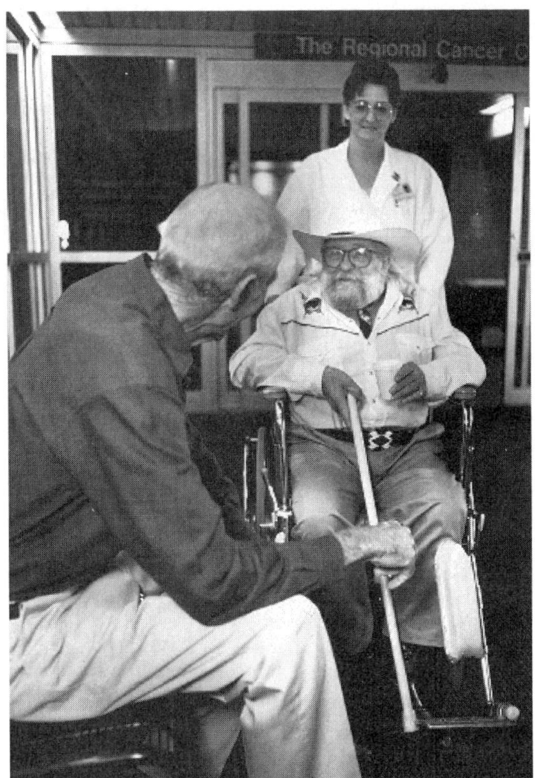

Figure 10–5 Visits are important to patient's comfort.

REHABILITATION

Rehabilitation of a patient who has cancer is an obligation of those responsible for care. The patient is confronted with unique problems that are seldom experienced by patients with other diseases. Adjustments in body image and self-concept must often be made. The patient may have a permanent colostomy, a permanent tracheostomy, a loss of voice, or a ureterostomy. The thought of facing life with the loss of these normal functions may be overwhelming to the patient. If mutilating surgery is to be performed, the patient should know before the surgery what to expect and should be assured that care and information regarding self-care will be provided. Patients who are to have laryngectomies should be visited by the speech therapist, who can explain how they will be taught to speak again. In preparation for eventual hospital discharge, patients should be permitted to assist with procedures. These procedures may include management of the tracheostomy, suctioning, colostomy irrigations, oral irrigations, or gastrostomy feedings. Patients who have had mastectomies should be taught arm exercises. All patients should be encouraged to return to their normal activities as soon as possible.

If patients are in a terminal phase of illness, they should remain ambulatory and perform the daily activities of self-care as long as possible. Many patients will be able to do this until the last stages of their terminal illness. Although the prognosis may be poor and only a few months may remain, many patients return to their normal work for weeks or months. Most can-

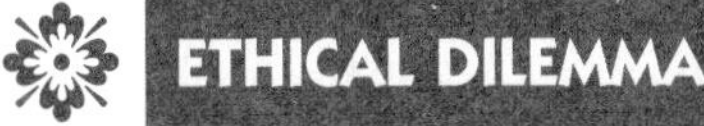

ETHICAL DILEMMA

You have been caring for Mr. Edwards, a 90-year-old gentleman with a history of gastrointestinal cancer. He has been a resident for 2 years in the nursing home in which you work. He has become increasingly confused and is also refusing to eat. He is sleeping a great deal during the day and arouses only with stimulation. His wife, Emma, asks you to talk to the doctor about writing an order for tube feedings. Discuss how you would respond to this request.

cer patients remain at home and often are employed. Hospitalizations are intermittent and only when necessary. Nursing care can be given in the home by a community health nurse, and hospice programs are available in many communities, often as part of the nursing agency (see Chapter 17). While the patient is still hospitalized, the home care nurse may visit the patient to jointly plan for the care that will be needed after discharge.

Patients are often helped and encouraged when given an opportunity to meet and talk with a person who has had a similar cancer or cancer treatment. These self-help groups may be very effective for the patient and family (Box 10-11).

BOX 10-11

SELF-HELF CANCER GROUPS*

Reach to Recovery

The ACS sponsors this organization. On receiving a physician's referral, a trained ACS volunteer who has had breast cancer surgery visits a woman who has just had this surgery. The volunteer teaches the woman exercises to help her recover and offers practical advice about adjusting to a mastectomy.

International Association of Laryngectomees

Also sponsored by the ACS, this organization helps persons with recent laryngectomies make early adjustments to loss of voice and to overcome psychosocial problems. Local clubs may be called "Lost Chord" or "New Voice."

I Can Cope

This ACS-sponsored educational program is designed to inform cancer patients and their families about the disease. Programs include classes on cancer and its treatments, how to live with the diagnosis of cancer, and the resources available to patients and families.

United Ostomy Association

Local chapters are composed primarily of persons with ostomies, with the purpose of providing mutual aid, moral support, and education to those who have had a colostomy, ileostomy, or urostomy. (National office: 36 Executive Park, Suite 120, Irvine, CA 92714 1-800-826-0826)

Candelighters Childhood Cancer Foundation

This national organization has local patient and family support networks. To find a nearby chapter, check local phone books or contact the national office. (Suite 1011, 1901 Pennsylvania Avenue, NW Washington, DC 20006 (202) 659-5136)

National Coalition for Cancer Survivorship (NCCS)

This network of independent groups and individuals is concerned with survivorship and the support of cancer survivors and their loved ones. (NCCS, 323 Eighth Street SW, Albuquerque, NM 87102 (505) 764-9956)

*More information on ACS-sponsored groups can be obtained from local ACS units or by calling 1-800-ACS-2345.

Nursing Care Plan

PATIENT WITH LUNG CANCER

Mr. Halton is a 76-year-old male who has been admitted from home with the diagnosis of squamous cell cancer of the right lung. He is currently undergoing outpatient radiation therapy and had a treatment today. He has a known right pleural effusion secondary to the cancer. He has been dyspneic for several days, but tonight the dyspnea increased in severity, and Mr. Halton has come to the emergency room with markedly reduced breath sounds in the right and middle-to-lower lobes, a low-grade fever, and dyspnea. His admitting diagnosis is pleural effusion and pneumonia/hypoxia secondary to cancer.

Past Medical History

No known allergies
Two-three pack a day smoker × 55 years
Hypertension
Peripheral vascular disease
Non–insulin-dependent diabetes mellitus
Chronic obstructive pulmonary disease
Osteoarthritis of the spine
Younger sister with hypercholesteremia and arteriosclerotic heart disease
Family history of heart disease

Psychosocial Data

Has 4 brothers and 2 sisters who are deceased
Widowed × 10 years; no children
Lives alone in mobile home
Retired factory worker
Has several male friends who live in neighboring mobile homes; they gather together for "smoking and playing cards"
Verbalizes doubts about seeing them anymore since he is not able to smoke

Assessment Data

Height: 5′6″; weight 128 lb
Recent weight loss of 20 lb
T 99.8; P 112; R 36; BP 156/86
Mental status: Alert and oriented; appears chronically ill
Skin: Warm, dry, intact; radiation markings on right anterior side of the chest
Eye, ear, nose, throat: Mucous membranes dry; full upper and lower dentures; lips slightly cyanotic
Respiratory: Thoracentesis performed in emergency room with drainage of 500 ml of clear, serosanguinous fluid; rate 36-40, shallow, almost absent breath sounds in right middle-to-lower lobe before thoracentesis; rate remains diminished after thoracentesis; left lung field has scattered crackles
Cardiovascular: Loud 3/6 holosystolic murmur; no gallop; peripheral pulses 1+ to lower extremities, 2+ to upper extremities; arterial pressure 112, irregular
Abdomen: Soft, nontender, nondistended; + bowel sounds

Laboratory Data

WBC 11.8, Hgb 7.3, Hct 28.2
Na 139, K 5.1, Cl 106, CO_2 22
BUN 48, Cr 1.3
ABGs: pH 7.45, Po_2 21, Po_2 106, HCO_3 24, O_2sat 95% on nonbreather O_2
cXr: preexisting right upper lobe effusion, wispy infiltrate right upper lobe
ECG: occasional PVC; left ventricle hypertrophy

Medications

Accucheck AC and HS
Regular insulin coverage
150-200 2 U
201-250 4 U
251-300 8 U
> 300 12 U
ceftazidine (Fortaz) 1 g IV q 8 hr
methylprednisolone (Solu-Medrol) 60 mg IV q 6 hr × 2 days
glyburide (DiaBeta) 5 mg before breakfast
enalapril maleate (Vasotec) 10 mg qd
alprazolam (Xanax) .5 mg tid
Transfuse 1 unit platelets and red blood cells

continued

NURSING DIAGNOSIS

Impaired gas exchange related to restricted lung expansion from pleural effusion; inflammation and tumor as evidenced by hypoxemia and dyspnea

NURSING INTERVENTIONS	EVALUATION OF EXPECTED OUTCOMES
Assess respiratory status q 4 hr and prn. Monitor pulse oximetry q 4 hr and prn. Maintain high Fowler's position. Maintain O_2 delivery to maintain O_2 saturation $> 90\%$. (Recently changed from non-rebreather to ventimask at 35%) Encourage coughing and deep breathing q 2 hr. Plan care in blocks of time and provide rest periods often. Increase activity as tolerated. Administer medications as ordered: Corticosteroids to decrease inflammation Antibiotics to decrease infection Administer blood transfusion according to hospital policy to increase oxygen-carrying components. Inform healthcare provider if respiratory status deteriorates.	No evidence of respiratory distress Maintains an O_2 saturation of $> 90\%$ Experiences no dyspnea at rest; mild dyspnea on exertion Able to assist with self-care activities without dyspnea Hgb is 10 or greater

NURSING DIAGNOSIS

Risk for impaired skin integrity related to effects of radiation

NURSING INTERVENTIONS	EVALUATION OF EXPECTED OUTCOMES
Assess skin condition in area of radiation. Bathe with mild soap. Avoid rubbing or using soap or lotion on chest area. Be careful not to wash the radiation marks placed on the skin to identify the area of radiation. Provide soft, loose clothing next to the chest area. Use mild water-based lubricant lotions.	Radiation marks on chest wall remain intact. Skin of chest wall is maintained intact without redness, drying, or excoriation

NURSING DIAGNOSIS

Altered nutrition: less than body requirements related to anorexia, dyspnea as evidenced by weight loss and inadequate consumption of meals

NURSING INTERVENTIONS	EVALUATION OF EXPECTED OUTCOMES
Place in high Fowler's position for meals and provide O_2 at 5 L during meals. Provide soft foods that are high in calories and high in protein. Monitor percentage of meals and snacks consumed.	No further weight loss Able to consume 75% of the meals Verbalizes importance of adequate nutrition

NURSING INTERVENTIONS	EVALUATION OF EXPECTED OUTCOMES
Provide rest periods before meals to minimize fatigue. Provide largest percentage of calories/protein for breakfast meal. Encourage sister to bring in favorite foods. Report this to dietician to plan subsequent American Dietetic Association (ADA) meals. Weigh every third day.	

NURSING DIAGNOSIS

Anticipatory grieving related to diagnosis of cancer and changes in lifestyle with friends as evidenced by patient statements

NURSING INTERVENTIONS	EVALUATION OF EXPECTED OUTCOMES
Provide an atmosphere of care and concern. Establish rapport and develop relationship. Encourage verbalization of anger, fear, sadness, and difficulties related to diagnosis and loss. Provide realistic hope regarding prognosis and diagnosis. Explain the process of grieving to the patient and sister; encourage her support. Encourage and facilitate communication between patient and significant friends. Encourage honesty in discussing issues of smoking. Arrange a visit from clergy if desired by patient.	Verbalizes feelings about diagnosis and changes in lifestyle Expresses grief with staff and/or family Uses available support systems

KEY CONCEPTS

- Cancer is characterized by abnormal, unrestricted cell division and the spread of these cells into healthy tissues of the body.
- One out of every four persons and three out of every four families in the United States will be affected by cancer at some time.
- The most common sites of cancer are the lungs, colon-rectum, breast, and prostate.
- Metastasis occurs when malignant cells break away from their original sites and are transported by the blood or lymph to new sites, where they begin to grow.
- The specific cause of cancer is unknown.
- Carcinogens are agents that can cause malignant changes in healthy cells after prolonged exposure. Carcinogens include viruses, chemical agents, physical agents, hormones, and dietary factors. Hereditary factors are also important.
- Risk factors for the major cancers have been identified. Many of these factors are potentially avoidable, and risk decreases as primary prevention is instituted and positive behaviors occur.
- Early detection and prompt treatment are secondary prevention goals.
- Multiple diagnostic tests are used and depend on the site of the tumor.
- Cancer is treated by four methods: surgery, radiotherapy, chemotherapy, and biotherapy.
- In addition to meeting the physical needs of patients, nurses are responsible for clarifying uncertainties, answering questions, and explaining procedures fully.
- Patients receiving external beam radiation therapy are never sources of radiation.
- Time, distance, and shielding are important determinants of the amount of radiation healthcare workers will receive when caring for patients who are undergoing internal radiation therapy. Self-protective measures should be used.
- A reduction in the number of white blood cells as a result of chemotherapy can increase the risk of infection. Fever is the most reliable indicator of this complication.
- Chemotherapy patients with a platelet count of less than 50,000 cells/mm^3 should be placed on bleeding precautions.
- Patients undergoing immunotherapy and biotherapy may experience flu-like symptoms.
- One of the most important aspects of care for the patient with cancer is psychologic support.
- Rehabilitation includes adjustments in body image and self-concept. Self-help groups may be very effective in the adjustment process.

CRITICAL THINKING EXERCISES

1 How do ACS recommendations for the early detection of cancer for a 20-year-old female compare with those for a 60-year-old female?

2 How does exfoliative cytology differ from a biopsy?

3 Why does chemotherapy result in gastrointestinal and mucosal side effects?

4 Why do some scientists think immunotherapy will help the body fight cancer?

5 Which community resources could be used to help the cancer patient and his or her family cope with the disease?

REFERENCES AND ADDITIONAL READINGS

American Cancer Society: *1994 cancer facts and figures,* Atlanta, 1993, The Society.

American Cancer Society: *Taking control: ten steps to a healthier life and reduced cancer risk,* Atlanta, 1994, The Society, Publication no 201915.

Baird SB, McCorkle R, Grant M, editors: *Cancer nursing: a comprehensive textbook,* 1991, Philadelphia, WB Saunders.

Distasio SA: Zofran makes chemo bearable, *RN* 56(5):56-59, 1993.

Greifzu S: Helping cancer patients fight infection, *RN* 54(7):24-29, 1991.

Groenwald SL and others, editors: *Cancer nursing: principles and practice,* ed 2, Boston, 1990, Jones & Bartlett.

Gross J, Johnson BL, editors: *Handbook of oncology nursing,* ed 2, Boston, 1994, Jones & Bartlett.

Hassey-Dow K, Hilderley LJ: *Nursing care in radiation oncology,* Philadelphia, 1992, WB Saunders.

Leukemia Society of America: *Bone marrow transplantation (BMT),* New York, 1992, The Society.

Morra M, Potts E: *Choices: Realistic alternatives in cancer treatment,* New York, 1987, Avon Books.

National Cancer Institute: *Eating hints,* Washington, DC, July 1992, The Institute NIH Publication no 92-2079.

National Cancer Institute: *Taking time: support for people with cancer and the people who care about them,* Washington, DC, 1993, The Institute NIH Publication no 93-2059.

Occupational Safety and Health Administration: *Work practice guidelines for personnel dealing with cytotoxic (antineoplastic) drugs,* Washington, DC, 1986, OSHA—US Department of Labor.

Sitton E: Early and late radiation-induced skin alterations, Part II: nursing care of irradiated skin, *Oncol Nurs Forum,* 19(6):907, 1992.

Strohl RA: The nursing role in radiation oncology: symptom management of acute and chronic reactions, *Oncol Nurs Forum* 15(4):429-434, 1988.

Walters P: Chemo: a nurse's guide to action, administration, and side effects, *RN* 53(2):52-66, 1990.

Wujcik D: An odyssey into biologic therapy, *Oncol Nurs Forum,* 20(6):879-887, 1993.

CHAPTER 11

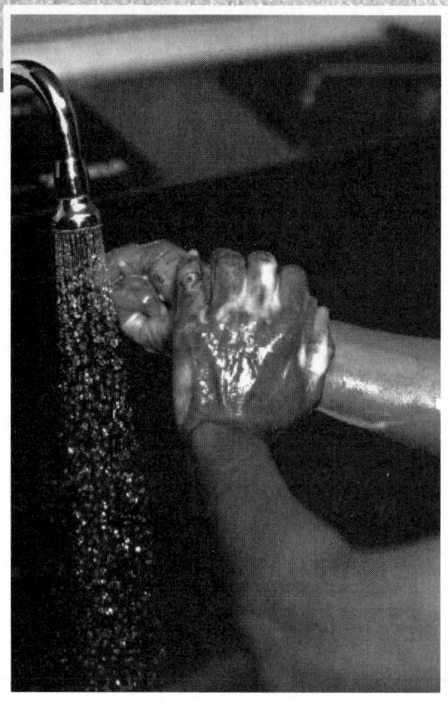

Community-Acquired Infections

CHAPTER OBJECTIVES

1 Discuss the interrelationships between the agent, host, and environment in the development of infectious disease.
2 Describe the major means of transmission of communicable diseases.
3 Explain the role of immunization in the prevention of communicable diseases.
4 Differentiate among the common infectious diseases in the community setting according to agent, host, and environmental characteristics.
5 Define the nurse's role in treatment, prevention, and control of communicable disease.

KEY WORDS

active immunity
agent
antitoxin
carrier
communicable disease
environment
  biologic
  physical
  socioeconomic
epidemiology
fomite
host
immunogenicity
immunoglobulins (Ig)
incubation period
infectious disease
infectivity
infestation
natural immunity
passive immunity
pathogen
pathogenicity
primary prevention
secondary prevention
tertiary prevention
toxoid
vaccine
vector
virulence

One of the greatest accomplishments of the twentieth century has been the control of communicable diseases in humans. There are remarkable contrasts when one examines health trends during the past 100 years. Those born at the beginning of the century had an average life expectancy of 47.5 years. In 1900, tuberculosis accounted for 25% of all deaths. Seventy-five percent of all major illnesses resulted from acute infectious diseases. These diseases took a particularly devastating toll on infants.

Public health measures, such as clean drinking water, effective waste control, availability of a variety of foods, better methods of food handling, and public enlightenment have been largely responsible for the remarkable decrease in these illness burdens. Medical advances have produced immunizing agents, such as serums and vaccines, that aid human immune processes in preventing disease or in modifying its severity. Antibiotics have reduced the impact of many diseases and have enhanced recovery with minimal complications. The result, over what is a relatively short period, has been a decline in disease-related deaths, particularly infant deaths, and an increase in life span.

Life expectancy is currently more than 75 years, and the population is not only increasing but is also growing older. Illnesses have changed. With the exception of acquired immunodeficiency syndrome (AIDS), chronic noninfectious diseases have replaced most infectious diseases as the leading causes of morbidity and mortality in the United States. Atherosclerosis, the underlying disease process in heart attacks and strokes, and conditions such as cancer, diabetes, emphysema, and arthritis now comprise the majority of the health burdens in the United States. These illnesses are long lasting, demand more monitoring and care, and have contributed, in part, to the increase in medical costs during the latter part of the century.

Despite the remarkable success in reducing the impact of infectious diseases on society, an ongoing program of infectious disease prevention and control must be maintained. Infectious processes continue to account for a major proportion of acute illnesses. Pneumonia has consistently remained among the ten highest causes of death, and lost schooldays and workdays per year from infectious diseases are significant. In 1990, AIDS resulting from infection with the human immunodeficiency virus (HIV) became the tenth leading cause of death in the United States. This is a testimony to the need for ongoing surveillance, prevention, and control.

CHARACTERISTICS OF THE INFECTIOUS PROCESS

A communicable disease is an **infectious disease** in which the causative organism is transmitted from where it lives and multiplies to another person or place. It can be transmitted directly from one person to another or indirectly through contaminated objects or infected insects or animals. The development of the infection depends on the interaction of the causative **agent,** or **host,** and the **environment** (Figure 11-1). The interaction among the agent, the host, and the environment must be correct for an infectious disease to develop. For instance, organisms such as tetanus spores cannot grow and multiply in oxygen-rich environments. Other organisms, such as the tubercle bacillus, thrive in persons who are malnourished, fatigued, and exposed to poor sanitary conditions (e.g., homeless persons).

Agent

The infectious agent is usually a microorganism called a **pathogen.** Parasites such as helminths (small wormlike animals) and insects such as lice are communicable **infestations.** Infectious agents are classified as bacteria, viruses, rickettsiae, protozoa, and helminths (see Chapter 7). All infectious agents have intrinsic properties that are unique to the microorganism or parasite. These characteristics include size, chemical character, growth requirements, antigenic properties, ability to produce toxin, ability to become resistant to chemicals, ability to live outside of the host, and other factors. Some organisms require moist, warm, dark breeding grounds. Others can survive in dry, warm, or cold settings until the proper conditions exist for them to grow and multiply. The virulence of the organism can vary, particularly in those organisms that are subject to change, such as the influenza viruses. Some organisms can exist in a dormant state. Knowledge of these intrinsic properties is essential to the prevention and control of infectious agents.

Some properties of infectious agents are not necessarily intrinsic to the agent but result from an interaction among the agent, the host, and the environment. These properties include the **infectivity, pathogenicity, virulence,** and **immunogenicity** of a specific infectious agent (Box 11-1). There are normal ranges of these properties for all infectious agents. However, host factors such as age, nutritional status, and under-

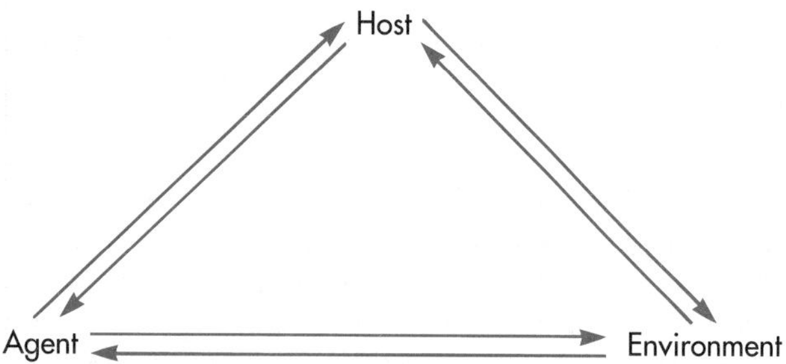

Figure 11-1 The interactions among the agent, host, and environment must be correct for an infectious disease to develop.

lying illness can result in an increased or decreased resistance to the agent. Similarly, environmental conditions can affect such factors as the amount of the dose and the ability of the agent to be transmitted to the host.

Host

The presence of an infectious agent does not always produce disease. A susceptible host must also be present. Many underlying host factors determine whether the person develops the infection. Factors that contribute to susceptibility include the person's general health, immune status, and age; the amount or dose of the infectious agent; and the duration of exposure.

Infectious processes can produce a variety of clinical effects in the host, ranging from inapparent (subclinical) infection to mild, moderate, or severe clinical illness or death. Inapparent infection can occur when the infectious agent invades the host and begins to grow and multiply but does not produce symptoms of illness. The host's immune system is able to combat the infection without visible effects. Such a person may become a **carrier** who is capable of infecting others without having evidence of the disease. This characteristic of early HIV infection, the causative agent in AIDS, has produced great problems for the prevention and control of its spread. Depending on the agent characteristics, people with active infections are communicable for varying periods, but an average for common infectious diseases is from 3 to 7 days.

Environment

The interaction between the agent and the host occurs in the environment. The environment includes all external influences that affect living organisms. The **physical** environment includes the characteristics of the place (geography), the climate, and the seasons. The **biologic** environment is composed of the living plants and animals that surround the host. The **socioeconomic** environment refers to the social and economic conditions that have an impact on the quality of life. These conditions determine the availability of safe drinking water, sanitary facilities, a variety of food, and medical care. Poor socioeconomic conditions commonly contribute to the spread of infectious diseases.

Modification of the environment is one way that the agent-host-environment interaction may be changed to prevent or control an infectious disease. Changing environmental conditions can alter the infectivity, pathogenicity, virulence, and immunogenic properties of the agent and decrease its ability to cause illness in human beings. For example, placing contaminated objects in boiling water has long been used to destroy organisms and prevent their spread.

BOX 11-1

PROPERTIES OF INFECTIOUS AGENTS INFLUENCED BY THE HOST AND THE ENVIRONMENT

Infectivity	Ability of the agent to invade the host and replicate
Pathogenicity	Ability of the agent to produce an infectious disease in a susceptible host
Virulence	Severity of the infectious disease that results from exposure to the agent
Immunogenicity	Ability of the agent to produce specific immunity within the host

Transmission

The transmission of infectious agents to a susceptible host occurs in the environment. The transmission of microorganisms involves many factors (Figure 11-2). There are four main modes of transmission: contact, airborne, vehicle, and vectorborne. A single microorganism may be transmitted by more than one route. For example, the varicella-zoster virus (chickenpox) can be spread either by the airborne route or by direct contact.

Contact transmission is the most common method by which microorganisms are transmitted from one person to another. Contact transmission can be divided into three subgroups: direct contact, indirect contact, and droplet contact. *Direct contact* involves person-to-person spread and occurs when there is physical contact between the source and the susceptible person. Contact occurs constantly during daily patient care, with hands having the most contact with the patient. Therefore thorough handwashing is the best way to

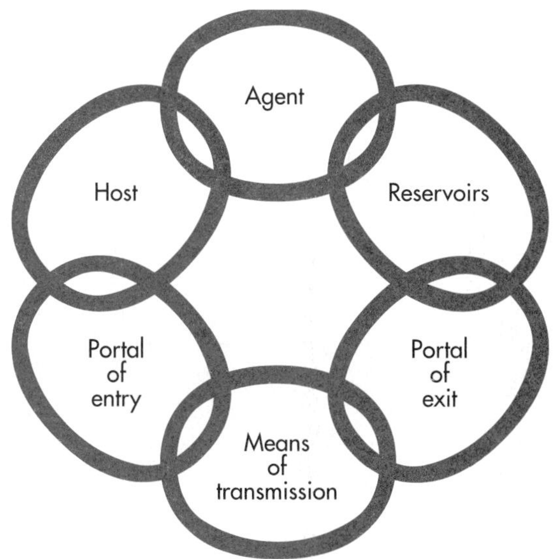

Figure 11-2 Chain of infection.

prevent transmission by direct contact. *Indirect contact* involves personal contact of the susceptible host with a contaminated intermediate object, or a **fomite.** For example, an inadequately disinfected endoscope can indirectly transfer organisms. *Droplet contact* occurs when an infectious agent briefly passes through the air. The infected sources and the susceptible host are usually within a few feet of each other. This is considered "contact" transmission rather than airborne, because droplets usually travel no more than 3 feet. Organisms are usually dispersed when an infected person coughs, sneezes, or talks.

Airborne transmission occurs when infectious agents remain suspended in the air for long periods. The organisms can be widely dispersed by air currents before being inhaled by or deposited on the susceptible host. Tuberculosis is a disease transmitted by this route. Good ventilation systems help prevent the transmission of infectious agents by the airborne route.

Vehicle transmission occurs when contaminated items such as blood, blood products, food, water, or drugs serve as the vector of transmission to multiple persons. An example of this type of transmission is the spread of salmonellosis from contaminated dairy products.

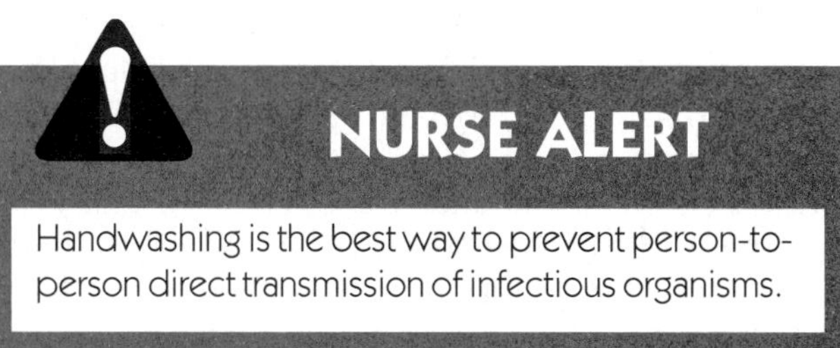

Handwashing is the best way to prevent person-to-person direct transmission of infectious organisms.

Vectorborne *transmission* occurs when insects or other animals serve as intermediate hosts for an infectious agent. For example, malaria is transmitted by mosquitos, and Rocky Mountain spotted fever is transmitted by ticks.

CONTROL OF COMMUNICABLE DISEASE

Prevention and control of communicable disease involves interfering with the normal pattern of transmission of the organism. This may be done by altering characteristics of the agent, the host, or the environment. One of the most common methods of breaking the chain of infectious events is to enhance the immunity of the host. Other methods involve altering or destroying the agent or interrupting the life cycle of the organism through environmental changes.

Immunity

Natural immunity is not produced by the immune response. It results from the passage of a mother's antibodies across the placental barrier into the circulation of the fetus. The mother's antibodies protect the newborn infant from specific infectious organisms. Natural immunity is transitory and protects the newborn infant for the first 3 to 6 months, when mortality is the greatest.

Acquired active immunity

Active immunity results from the stimulation of the body's immune system to produce either *antibodies* or specialized cells that have the ability to destroy or neutralize foreign microorganisms (see Chapter 7). Active immunity occurs after an infectious agent is introduced into the body, producing either an illness or an inapparent illness, or through *immunization.* Immunity is most durable if the person actually acquires the infectious disease. However, severe or fatal complications can result from some infections. It is also possible for a recovered person to become a carrier and harbor microorganisms and transmit them to others unknowingly.

Following exposure, part of the microoganism acts as an *antigen,* a substance that is usually composed of large protein or polysaccharide molecules and is capable of inducing a specific immune response (see Chapter 7). The body responds with the production of antibodies **(immunoglobulins),** which are protein molecules that are specific to the antigen and can interact with the antigen to interfere with the infectious process.

TABLE 11-1

Recommended Childhood Immunization Schedule*—United States, January 1995

Vaccine	Birth	2 Mo	4 Mo	6 Mo	12 Mo	15 Mo	18 Mo	4-6 Yr	11-12 Yr	14-16 Yr
Hepatitis B	HB-1									
		HB-2		HB-3						
Diphtheria, Tetanus, Pertussis		DTP	DTP	DTP		DTP or DTaP at ≥15 months		DTP or DTaP	Td	
H. influenzae type b		Hib	Hib	Hib		Hib				
				OPV						
Poliovirus		OPV	OPV					OPV		
						MMR				
Measles, Mumps, Rubella								MMR or	MMR	

From Centers for Disease Control and Prevention: Recommended childhood immunization schedule—United States, *MMWR* 43(51,52):960, 1995.
*Recommended vaccines are listed under the routinely recommended ages. Shaded bars indicate range of acceptable ages for vaccination.

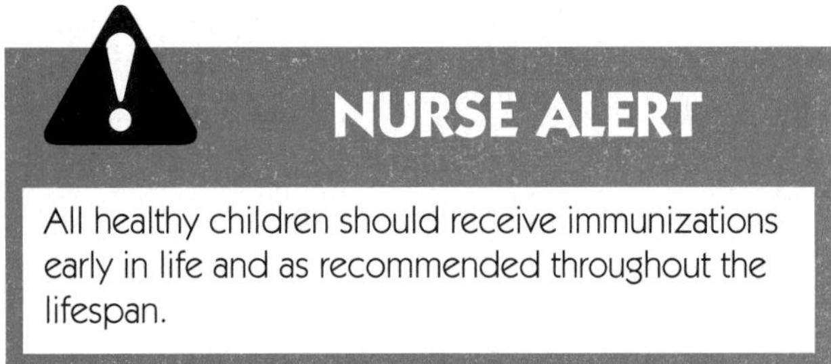

NURSE ALERT
All healthy children should receive immunizations early in life and as recommended throughout the lifespan.

Immunizations produce artificially acquired active immunity. The immunizing agents are **vaccines** or **toxoids.** Vaccines are suspensions of killed microorganisms or live, attenuated (altered) microorganisms. Toxoids are toxins produced by microorganisms that have been treated with chemicals or heat to decrease their toxic effect while retaining their ability to stimulate the immune system. Immunizations are given before the person has been exposed to the illness, if possible. Because the immune response that results from a vaccine or toxoid is not as strong as that which results from acquiring the acute illness, boosters are given periodically to maintain immunity.

Most children receive immunizations early in life, because young children can suffer severe complications from many infectious diseases (Table 11-1). These immunizations prevent diphtheria, pertussis, tetanus, polio, measles, mumps, rubella, *Haemophilus influenza* type B (Hib), and hepatitis B (Hb). Vaccines are available either singly or in combinations other than those indicated, such as measles-rubella (MR).

Measles is a serious contagious disease. It is common in the United States as a result of low immunization levels of the population. Every child and young adult should receive protection from this disease, because complications can lead to encephalitis, mental retardation, pneumonia, blindness, and death. Side effects of the vaccine do not occur often, but a mild temperature elevation may occur, or a skin rash may appear.

The measles vaccine is a live virus vaccine that has been attenuated, or reduced in virulence. It is believed that one dose is sufficient to produce long-lasting immunity, although some states require a second dose before entering school. The measles vaccine should not be administered to children who are sensitive to egg protein, because it is used in the manufacturing process. Contraindications for the administration of the measles virus vaccine include leukemia or other malignant disorders. Children whose resistance is low as a result of receiving steroid therapy, radiation, alkylating drugs, and antimetabolites should not be given the measles vaccine. Administration of the vaccine during pregnancy should be avoided.

Mumps can be a serious disease and lead to deafness and encephalitis in children and orchitis and oophoritis in adults. Sterility can occur. Administration of live mumps virus vaccine provides an active immunity against mumps. The vaccine is prepared in a chick embryo cell culture and therefore should not be given to persons sensitive to the proteins of eggs. Contraindications for its use are the same as for measles vaccine.

A live rubella virus vaccine provides active immunity against rubella (German measles). The vaccine should not be given to pregnant women because of the possibility of producing the disease in the unborn child. Rubella has caused defects of the heart, brain, eye, and ears in children whose mothers have had rubella during the first trimester of pregnancy. Rubella vaccine is given to all children to prevent the spread of the disease to pregnant women and their unborn children. The Centers for Disease Control and Prevention (CDC) in Atlanta recommends that educational and training institutions seek proof of rubella immunity from all female students and employees. The vaccine may be given to women of childbearing age only if pregnancy will be avoided for at least 2 months. It should not be given during febrile illnesses but should be postponed until recovery occurs. Other contraindications are the same as for measles and mumps. To prevent hypersensitivity reactions, the label on the bottle should be read before administering the vaccine to determine the type of cells from which the vaccine has been prepared. Box 11-2 presents a summary of the contraindications for immunization.

Poliomyelitis is an acute viral infection with a severity that ranges from a nonapparent, subclinical infection to paralytic disease and death. It occurs worldwide and is transmitted by close direct contact through a fecal-oral route. It is currently targeted for elimination, similar to the eradication of smallpox from the world as announced by the World Health Organization in 1980. Both a live attenuated oral poliovirus vaccine (OPV) and an inactivated poliovirus vaccine (IPV) are available and are administered by subcutaneous injection. Contraindications are pregnancy and immunocompromised states.

In recent years, Hib and HB have been added to the recommended schedule for routine vaccinations. Hib occurs worldwide and in the United States has been the most common type of bacterial meningitis in children under 5 years of age. Since 1988, when the vaccine was licensed, the incidence of Hib has decreased markedly. HB is also found worldwide, and the severity of this disease ranges from mild to severe liver disease. The vaccine is contraindicated for persons who have an allergy to yeast.

BOX 11-2

CONTRAINDICATIONS FOR IMMUNIZATIONS

- Hypersensitivity to egg protein, animal tissues, or antibiotics used in vaccine preparation
- Altered immune states
  - Lymphoma
  - Leukemia
  - Generalized malignancy
  - Dysgammaglobulinemia
- Immunosuppressive therapy
  - Steroids
  - Antimetabolites
  - Alkylating agents
  - Radiation
- Pregnancy in some instances, especially measles
- Febrile illness (immunization should be delayed until recovery)

Acquired passive immunity

Passive immunity is acquired by injecting a serum that contains antibodies to the infectious organism into the susceptible host. Because the person receives antibodies that have been formed elsewhere, there is no direct stimulation of the person's own immune system. The immunity that is acquired is temporary and rarely lasts longer than 3 weeks. It is useful in emergency situations and in the treatment of specific diseases. Administration of immunoglobulin (gamma globulin) to prevent hepatitis A in exposed people is an example.

Antitoxins contain antibodies that react against the toxin that is produced by the particular microorganism infecting the body. An antitoxin is administered to neutralize the poisons produced by pathogens and does not have any effect on the organism itself. Chemotherapeutic drugs may be given to the individual to destroy the organism. Examples of antitoxins include diphtheria antitoxin, tetanus antitoxin, and antisnake (antivenom) serum.

Immunoglobulin (immune gamma globulin) is the fraction of the plasma of human blood that contains antibodies against certain diseases. It is occasionally used to treat or modify measles in a nonimmune person. It may also be used to prevent infectious hepatitis in exposed persons. Other diseases for which it has been used include rubella, mumps, and poliomyelitis. Immunoglobulin is prepared in a sterile solution for subcutaneous or intramuscular injection. It is never given intravenously. Emphasis should be placed on active immunization to prevent those diseases for which vaccines are available.

Public Education

People today have less concern about communicable childhood diseases than in previous decades. The incidence of these diseases has decreased to such an extent that fear of them or their consequences has been lessened. Although this decrease in incidence has contributed to an increased quality of life, problems still exist. Immunization rates throughout the United States have gradually declined, especially among some religious groups. As a result there has been a rise in the incidence of some diseases, such as measles.

Many states have attempted to remedy this situation by passing laws that require immunizations for children before attending school. However, these laws do not reach all segments of the population. Preschool children and elderly people are not included. Some local health departments operate well-child clinics for the purpose of monitoring immunization status and general wellness. The United States has launched a nationwide campaign to increase the levels of immunity throughout the country. In some communities, immunization levels have fallen to 50% or less. There is a continual need for study and development of programs that will reach all members of the population.

There also is a need for public education programs regarding positive health practices that are important in the prevention of disease. Sociologic factors may have a profound effect on the incidence of certain infectious diseases. Reservoirs of infection may exist in areas that have a low socioeconomic status, inadequate housing, poor sanitary facilities, inadequate refuse collection, and possibly even contaminated water supplies.

Poor nutritional standards also decrease resistance to disease and provide the opportunity for pathogens to invade the human body. The social picture is often one of apathy and lack of motivation coupled with lack of transportation and inaccessible medical and clinical services. Such conditions contribute to a failure to secure immunization of young children and produce conditions for a potential epidemic of infectious disease.

The high mobility of some segments of the population means that a person who has been exposed to an infectious disease or who is a possible source of disease may be hundreds of miles away from the point of contact within a few hours. Therefore the worldwide spread of infectious diseases is more of a problem now than ever before.

Healthy People 2000 is a visionary agenda for the health of the nation that grew out of a health strategy that the Federal government initiated in 1979 (Healthy People 2000, 1991). It reflects a consensus of a consortium of almost 300 national organizations, the U.S. Public Health Service, state health departments, and the Institute of Medicine of the National Academy of Sciences. On the basis of measurable objectives, the report presents goals that will increase the span of healthy life and reduce health disparities for the American people. Some of the goals to be achieved include reducing the risk for infectious diseases (Box 11-3). To achieve these goals, several types of activities are recommended, including expanding immunization laws; increasing the proportion of primary care providers who provide information, counseling, and immunizations; and removing financial barriers to receiving immunizations. The CDC and state health departments monitor the accomplishment of these objectives through a series of surveillance activities.

Nursing's Role in Prevention

The development of an infection is multifactorial and results from complex interactions among many factors that are related to the agent, the host, and the environment. The development of appropriate interventions requires a complete analysis of these factors. The goal is to prevent the spread of the infectious agent from its reservoir, or source, to susceptible hosts and thereby break the chain of infection (see Figure 11-2). Interven-

BOX 11-3

HEALTHY PEOPLE 2000 OBJECTIVES FOR IMMUNIZATION AGAINST INFECTIOUS DISEASES

- Eliminate diphtheria, tetanus, polio, measles, and rubella among people age 25 and younger
- Reduce cases of mumps to 500 per year
- Reduce cases of pertussis to 1000 per year
- Increase the levels of basic immunization series among children under age 2 to at least 90%
- Increase the levels of basic immunization series among children in licensed child care facilities and kindergarten through postsecondary education institutions to at least 95%
- Increase immunization levels for pneumococcal pneumonia and influenza among institutionalized, chronically ill, or older people to at least 80%
- Increase immunization levels for pneumococcal pneumonia and influenza among noninstitutionalized, high-risk populations to at least 60%
- Increase hepatitis B immunization among high-risk populations to at least 90%
- Reduce postexposure rabies treatments to no more than 9000 per year

tions should be based on the natural history of the disease and be directed toward the link in the chain of infection that is the most susceptible to interruption.

Nurses are constantly involved with assessing patients for factors that indicate whether a patient requires preventive intervention, is at high risk for infection, or is experiencing an infection. **Primary prevention** strategies that prevent diseases from occurring include immunizations, healthy lifestyle behaviors (e.g., proper nutrition and exercise), and patient education. Nurses have a primary role in encouraging all people to keep immunizations current and to maintain proper records of their immunization history. Every nurse should engage in public information or education programs and provide information to individuals in their health practices whenever possible. For example, prevention of HIV infection should be a consideration of all nurses. Nurses often observe human behavior as it relates to health and illness and can offer solutions to problems that are related to disease prevention.

Secondary prevention measures are designed to detect disease and initiate early treatment to limit the spread and severity of infectious disease and to prevent complications. These activities include the assessment of individuals for signs and symptoms that indicate infectious disease, periodic examinations, and screening procedures. Nurses should encourage patients to seek medical attention whenever they observe unusual physical symptoms. Diagnosing a disease when early physiologic changes are occurring limits the complications. Too often the infections are well advanced before treatment is sought.

Tertiary prevention involves treatment to arrest the infectious process and minimize disability. Nurses are often responsible for the administration of medications and are expected to maintain proper handwashing techniques, as well as precautions with excretions, secretions, trash, and waste. These measures are specific to the characteristics of the infectious process and the limitations that face the patient (see Chapter 12). Residual disabilities do occur with some infections. For example, repeated ear infections can result in hearing loss, and chronic Lyme disease can produce cardiovascular problems.

THE PATIENT WITH A BACTERIAL INFECTION

Because of improved public health standards and the widespread use of immunizations, many infectious diseases have a less significant impact on the population now than at the beginning of the century. Four bacterial infectious diseases caused significant morbidity in the past: diphtheria, pertussis, tetanus, and typhoid fever. Other infectious diseases are prevalent among certain groups in specific geographic locations or on a seasonal or cyclic basis. New illnesses, such as Lyme disease, occasionally appear and can become widespread in a relatively short period.

Staphylococcal Infections

In many people, staphylococcal organisms are normal inhabitants of the upper respiratory tract, skin, and gastrointestinal (GI) tract. It is estimated that between 20% and 40% of all persons are asymptomatic carriers of *Staphylococcus aureus*, which provides a source of infection for themselves and for others when host resistance is lowered. Transmission usually occurs through direct contact with purulent discharge from an infected person. Transmission through fomites or airborne particles is rare. The **incubation period** is 4 to 10 days. The organism is communicable as long as purulent lesions continue to drain or the carrier state persists. Staphylococcal infections occur worldwide but are more prevalent in overcrowded areas where personal hygiene is poor. There are no specific preventive measures other than cleanliness and adherence to strict aseptic technique where appropriate.

In the community, *S. aureus* infections usually manifest as skin lesions such as impetigo, boils, carbuncles, abscesses, wound infections, and conjunctivitis. Some toxin-producing strains can cause a distinctive scaulded skin syndrome. Infection around the nose and mouth can spread backward into the cranial vault, where there are no mechanical barriers to halt the spread. For this reason, infected pimples or acne must not be squeezed or traumatized. Systemic disease is rare and usually occurs in those who are immunosuppressed or suffering from a debilitating illness. However, septicemia, pneumonitis, lung and brain abscesses, pneumonia, endocarditis, osteomyelitis, and other complications can occur. Staphylococcal pneumonia commonly complicates influenza.

Prevention is best accomplished through education in personal hygiene, especially in handwashing. Prompt treatment with topical antibiotics (or systemic antibiotics if the infection has disseminated) reduces transmission. Contaminated articles should be disinfected appropriately. Outbreaks in schools, camps, and other population groups should be reported to public health authorities.

Toxic shock syndrome

During 1980 and 1981 an epidemic of toxic shock syndrome (TSS) occurred that was associated with toxin-producing strains of *S. aureus*. TSS is a severe illness that is characterized by sudden onset of high fever, vomiting, profuse diarrhea, and myalgia. It can lead to hypotension, shock, and death. A deep red "sunburn" rash develops within a few hours and is followed by desquamation of the skin approximately 10 days after onset, especially on the palms of the hands and soles of the feet. Approximately 95% of the reported cases in women occurred during the menstrual period, and most cases were associated with use of vaginal tampons. In cases of TSS that are not associated with menstruation, including cases in men, *S. aureus* has been isolated from focal lesions of skin, bone, lung, and stool. Aggressive fluid, electrolyte, and antistaphylococcal antibiotic therapy is required.

Nurses in community and school settings should communicate information regarding the risk of TSS. Menstrual TSS can be prevented by avoiding vaginal tampons. However, using tampons intermittently, changing them often, and avoiding products that have the potential to irritate mucous membranes reduce the risk of TSS.

Streptococcal Infections

Streptococci, like staphylococci, are found almost everywhere in the environment. These infections probably cause more illnesses than any other group of organisms. They can attack any part of the body and cause both primary and secondary disease. Many distinct strains exist, but not all are pathogenic. Streptococci are normal inhabitants of the human respiratory tract. Group A beta-hemolytic *Streptococcus pyogenes* produces the most significant variety of diseases in man. Streptococcal sore throat and skin infections are the most common. Cellulitis, mastoiditis, otitis media, pneumonia, wound infections, septicemia, scarlet fever, and other diseases can also occur. These conditions can be particularly severe in the elderly.

Streptococcal sore throat is prevalent in temperate and semitropical regions. In the United States, epidemics in New England and in the Great Lakes region are common. Transmission results from direct contact with another infected person or object. Organisms usually enter the body through the respiratory tract or through a wound. Nasal carriers are often transmitters of the organism. Outbreaks of streptococcal sore throat may follow ingestion of contaminated foods, particularly milk and milk products. Following a short incubation period of 1 to 3 days, the organism becomes established in the lymphoid tissues, which causes a local cellulitis. The infectious process can easily spread, because toxins released by the organism prevent the normal inflammatory process from walling off the lesion.

Infected persons exhibit fever, sore throat, exudative tonsillitis or pharyngitis, and tender anterior cervical lymph nodes. Petechiae may be present in a diffusely red throat. However, symptoms can be minimal. Repeated attacks of streptococcal sore throat or other illnesses as a result of different types of streptococci are also relatively common. With antibiotic therapy, transmission is generally limited to 24 to 48 hours, but untreated cases can transmit the organisms for an indefinite period. Complications such as scarlet fever, rheumatic fever, or acute glomerulonephritis may appear in 1 to 5 weeks following infection, but this is rare when adequate treatment is begun at an early stage.

Scarlet fever includes all of the symptoms that occur with a streptococcal sore throat, although it may be associated with infections at other sites. It has an abrupt onset with chills, vomiting, headache, and high temperature. In approximately 24 hours a fine, erythematous rash occurs that blanches on pressure and feels like sandpaper. The rash occurs most often on the neck, chest, axillary folds, elbows, groin, and the surface of the inner thighs. Usually it does not affect the face. The tongue has a furred appearance that gradually disappears and becomes characteristically red (strawberry tongue). The incidence and severity of scarlet fever has decreased in recent years, although the mortality rate in some parts of the world has been as high as 3% (Beneson, 1990).

One of the most important factors in control of these infections is the identification and treatment of streptococcal infections before serious complications result. The treatment of choice is penicillin therapy for at least 10 days. Treatment that is initiated within the first 24 to 48 hours decreases severity, reduces complications, and prevents the development of most cases of acute rheumatic fever. Infected people should be observed carefully for complications that may appear throughout the course of the illness. Preventive measures that nurses should convey include education of the public regarding the transmission of the organism and the relationship of streptococcal infections to scarlet fever, acute rheumatic fever, and other complications.

Pulmonary Tuberculosis

Tuberculosis is one of the oldest known diseases and is one of the most devastating worldwide diseases of all time. It attacks any organ or tissue and results in years of chronic invalidism or death. In 1882, Robert Koch discovered *Mycobacterium tuberculosis* as the causative organism, and modern treatment became possible. Significant advances have been made in the treatment, prevention, and control of the disease, which has resulted in downward trends in morbidity and mortality in many countries. In 1993 the incidence rate in the United States was 9.8 new cases per 100,000 (Centers for Disease Control and Prevention, 1994). The incidence has risen in recent years, primarily as a complication of the immunosuppression that accompanies persons infected with the HIV virus. Resistant strains of the organism have also emerged. Morbidity and mortality increase with age, are higher in men than women, and are higher in nonwhites than whites (Centers for Disease Control and Prevention, 1994). Tuberculosis is also more common among people of a lower socioeconomic status, where factors such as overcrowding increase the risk of infection.

Transmission

Transmission of the *M. tuberculosis* organism occurs when a susceptible person inhales an airborne droplet nuclei that was derived from the sputum of an infected person. When a person with active tuberculosis coughs, sneezes, or expectorates, the infectious organisms are carried into the air as droplets, or droplet nuclei. Droplet nuclei are particles that contain the microorganisms that become suspended in the air. However, prolonged contact is usually necessary for infection to occur, and transmission through indirect contact is rare.

The incubation period for a primary tuberculosis lesion is approximately 4 to 12 weeks. Persons who have the microorganisms in their system react positively to a tuberculin skin test (10 mm or greater), although the disease may not be present. People can transmit the organism to others as long as the organism is being discharged from their bodies. Progressive development of the disease is greatest within 1 to 2 years of infection, although it may remain as a latent infection throughout a lifetime. Pulmonary tuberculosis is most common, although dissemination of the organism through lymphatic drainage and the circulation can lead to involvement of many parts of the body.

Assessment

Primary pulmonary infections usually go unnoticed by the individual. As a result of the stimulation of the immune system of the body, lesions containing the tubercule bacillus often become walled off and calcified, which isolates the organism and prevents spread of the disease. However, the organisms may remain viable, and if the person's resistance falls at a later time, an active case of tuberculosis may develop.

Clinical manifestations of active tuberculosis include infection, cavitation of lung tissue, and tissue destruction (Figure 11-3). Symptoms are often the result of toxic manifestations produced by the infection. Mild fever, fatigue, and gradual weight loss can occur

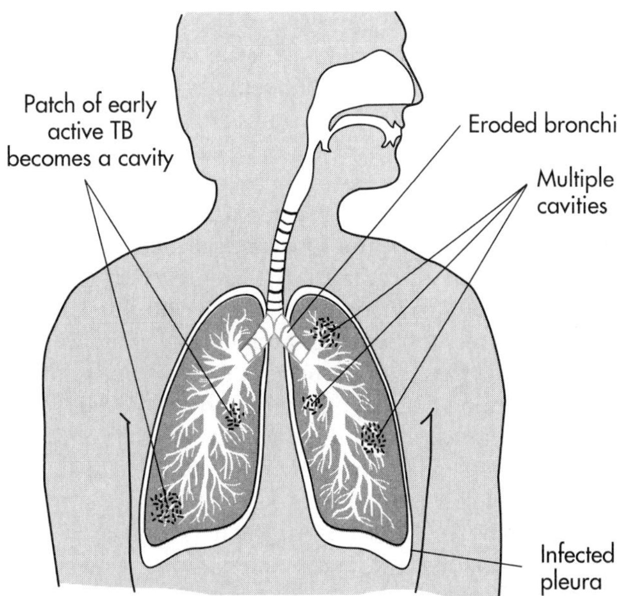

Figure 11-3 Infection, cavitation, and tissue destruction are characteristic of active tuberculosis infection. (From Beare P, Myers J: *Adult health nursing,* ed 2, St Louis,1994, Mosby.)

early, whereas cough, chest pain, dyspnea, and hemoptysis become prominent only when the disease has progressed. Profuse sweating may occur late in the day and at night. The spitting of blood (hemoptysis) may occur when cavitation extends into a blood vessel. A wide variety of symptoms can accompany tuberculosis, and there is no specific pattern in which they occur.

Case finding

When tuberculosis is suspected, the patient must have a complete history and physical examination, including routine laboratory examinations. A history of exposure is of special significance. A definitive diagnosis of active tuberculosis is made by finding the tubercle bacillus in smears of sputum. Regular sputum examinations are required to isolate the tubercle bacillus, and failure to find it does not always rule out the diagnosis of tuberculosis. Under some conditions it may not be possible to secure sputum for examination. In this case a gastric lavage is performed, and the gastric contents are examined. A bronchoscopic examination is often done to secure secretions from the bronchial tree or directly from portions of the lung. X-ray films visualize calcified nodules in the lung and can be used to follow the progression of the disease following diagnosis.

The tuberculin test is a diagnostic aid that indicates the presence of infection but does not necessarily indicate the presence of the disease. The tuberculin test is presently used as a screening method to detect persons with infection and to rule out persons who do not have tuberculosis.

The Mantoux test is the skin test of choice for identifying infected persons. It involves inoculation of tubercle bacillus extract (tuberculin) intradermally on the inner surface of the forearm. Purified protein derivative (PPD) is usually used. The reaction is an example of a delayed (cellular) hypersensitivity reaction. The test is read between 48 and 72 hours after administration. If the site of induration is 0 to 4 mm, the test is considered to be negative; if the induration is 5 to 9 mm, it is doubtful; and if it is 10 mm or more, it is positive. The amount of induration, or hardness, is important, not the amount of redness present. A positive reaction indicates that a patient has had contact with the tubercle bacillus, but active tuberculosis may not be present. Generally, the more intense the reaction to the test, the greater the likelihood that an active case of tuberculosis is present. Positive reactions may be suppressed in patients who are acutely ill with tuberculosis, receiving corticosteroid drugs, or infected with certain other infectious diseases such as measles.

Other skin tests are available for screening, but not diagnosing, large groups of people. These include the tine test and the Mono-vacc. These tests pierce the skin at several points at the same time. The reaction is considered negative if the areas of induration are less than 2 mm. If there is a meeting of the reactions of two or more puncture sites, the reaction is considered positive. Positive reactions should be tested further for presence of the disease.

Ideally, everyone should have an annual examination for tuberculosis. Periodic testing should be routine for all medical and nursing personnel. X-ray examinations should be restricted to those persons with positive reactions. The greatest emphasis in screening should be on high-risk groups, such as contacts of active tuberculosis cases, patients in general hospitals and mental institutions, immigrants from areas in which tuberculosis is common, and populations of lower socioeconomic status. All active cases must be reported to local health departments so that contacts may be examined and monitored.

OLDER ADULT CONSIDERATIONS

Tuberculosis

- An aging immune system and chronic health problems increase an older adult's susceptibility to tuberculosis.
- A cohort of older people exists who were either exposed to tuberculosis as children or who had active tuberculosis when they were young but did not receive treatment. Dormant infection can be activated at any time and expose others.
- Any older person with a history of untreated tuberculosis and a chest x-ray film that shows cavitation should be evaluated for drug therapy.
- Reactions to skin tests may not be typical in the older adult.
- The classic symptoms of tuberculosis may not be evident in older adults. Weight loss or anorexia may sometimes be the only observable symptoms.
- Older adults must be monitored carefully for side effects of drug therapy.
- People with a history of previous treatment for tuberculosis are at an increased risk for drug-resistant tuberculosis.

Drug therapy

Following diagnosis, the stage of the patient's disease is evaluated, and an individual schedule of treatment is planned. Effective chemotherapy reverses the infectiousness of tuberculosis within 2 weeks of initiation and prevents progression of the illness. A combination of agents is used to affect the organism in different stages of growth. Primary drugs include isoniazid (INH), rifampin (RIF), streptomycin (SM), pyrazinamide (PZA), and ethambutol (EMB) in varying combinations. The standard treatment is isoniazid plus rifampin and pyrazinamide for 6 months (Boskovich, 1994; Elpern and others, 1993; Moy, 1990). Secondary drugs are available for cases that are resistant to the primary drugs. Any treatment considers the stage of the disease, its activity, and the patient's resistance to the drug.

Patients must be monitored for the onset of toxic symptoms that would necessitate a change or discontinuance of the drug. Numbness, tingling, and weakness of the extremities are toxic signs that may be observed when isoniazid is being given. Streptomycin may cause deafness, dizziness, unsteadiness of gait, ringing in the ears, or severe headache. Toxic symptoms are more likely to occur in older persons or in those who have been taking the drug for several years. Because patients with tuberculosis often receive chemotherapeutic drugs over a prolonged time, regular laboratory examinations are important. In addition, visual acuity and hearing tests should be done at intervals if indicated. Patients receiving isoniazid should avoid alcohol while taking the drug.

Nursing interventions

Tuberculosis is not a highly infectious disease, and prompt specific chemotherapy limits the release of tubercle bacilli into the air within a few days after therapy is initiated. The patient needs instruction regarding the proper handling of sputum to prevent organisms from becoming airborne. When the patient coughs or sneezes, moist droplets are carried into the air. Some droplets fall into the immediate environment, whereas others remain suspended in the air as droplet nuclei. Good ventilation carries droplet nuclei on air currents, where they may be killed by sunlight or ultraviolet light. When the patient is taught to cover his or her nose and mouth when coughing or sneezing, the dissemination of moist droplets into the environment is reduced or eliminated. Cooperation can usually be expected when the patient understands the importance of this procedure. Tissues used to cover coughs or to collect sputum may be placed in public sewer systems or into a paper bag and burned.

Nurses should emphasize the importance of continuing to take the prescribed medications (Box 11-4). One of the main factors in the continued transmission of tuberculosis is lack of adequate patient education and follow-up to ensure that therapy is completed. Patients should understand the nature and extent of the illness and recognize that medications must be continued as prescribed. Failure to take medications regularly impedes the healing process and contributes to the development of resistant strains of the organism.

Prevention and control

In addition to drug therapy, a variety of other prevention and control measures are recommended that interfere with transmission patterns in other ways. A vaccine known as BCG (bacille Calmette-Guérin) is available. However, the amount of protection that it produces against tuberculosis is variable. In the United States, where the risk of infection is low, immunization is not generally indicated. It may be used for medical personnel who risk exposure to undiagnosed cases, for contacts of active tuberculosis cases, and for newborns whose mothers have active tuberculosis. If BCG is used, it is given only to persons who have a negative tuberculin test. Improving social conditions and educating the public about prevention of the spread of tuberculosis organisms can help control the transmission of the organisms. Tuberculin testing in high-risk groups, increased availability and accessibility of medical diagnosis and treatment, and nursing case management are important methods for casefinding and controlling the spread of tuberculosis. The use of chemotherapeutic drugs is now recommended for

BOX 11-4 **Nursing Process**

TUBERCULOSIS (COMMUNITY)

ASSESSMENT

Understanding of disease process and transmission
Compliance with medical therapy
Respiratory status (breath sounds, dyspnea, cough)
Hemoptysis
Temperature
Laboratory studies (sputum AFB, urinalysis, BUN, LFTs, SGOT)

NURSING DIAGNOSES

Risk for infection related to *M. tuberculosis* in respiratory secretions
Impaired home maintenance management, noncompliance, and inadequate handling of secretions related to long-term therapy
Noncompliance related to lack of understanding, lack financial resources, lack of emotional support
Knowledge deficit related to new medical condition and treatment
Ineffective breathing pattern related to respiratory secretions

NURSING INTERVENTIONS

Maintain/teach AFB isolation until antimicrobial therapy is initiated.
Maintain adequate nutrition and fluid intake.
Encourage rest and progressively increase activity as tolerated.
Administer/supervise medication use.
Monitor for symptoms of toxic side effects of medications.
Reinforce the importance of compliance with therapy.
Refer to Visiting Nurse Association for follow-up.
Examine close contacts at time of treatment and in 3 months.

EVALUATION OF EXPECTED OUTCOMES

No evidence of active infection or complications of tuberculosis
Self-administers medications as prescribed
No transmission of infection to close contacts
No evidence of dyspnea or hypoxia

known contacts who have been exposed to tuberculosis and tested positive but do not have the disease.

Tuberculosis has occurred among persons infected with the HIV virus. HIV infection causes immunosuppression, which allows latent tuberculosis infection to progress to a clinically apparent disease. *M. tuberculosis* infection in the presence of laboratory evidence for HIV infection and involving at least one site outside the lung is now diagnostic of AIDS. Prevention and control efforts need to focus on those with or at risk for HIV infection.

The U.S. Department of Health and Human Services released a strategic plan for the elimination of tuberculosis in the United States by the year 2010. The report also established an interim target case rate of 3.5 per 100,000 by the year 2000. The three-step plan includes: (1) more effective use of existing prevention and control measures, especially for high-risk populations; (2) development and evaluation of new technologies for diagnosis, treatment, and prevention; and (3) rapid assessment and transfer of newly developed technologies into healthcare practices (Centers for Disease Control and Prevention, 1989). An effective tuberculosis elimination effort such as this requires good **epidemiologic** surveillance data that target the affected populations and geographic areas. The emergence of resistant organisms and the increased incidence linked to HIV infection are barriers to achieving this goal.

Lyme Disease

Lyme disease was first identified by a Yale rheumatologist in 1975 when he analyzed an unusual cluster of arthritis cases that occurred in Lyme, Connecticut. Cases have spread rapidly in the Northeast, the Midwest, and the California coast and have reached epidemic proportions. Cases have been diagnosed in almost every state and in many other countries throughout the world. Cases have been recorded in Europe for several decades, which has led epidemiologists to suspect that the organism was introduced in this country through migratory birds. The true incidence is unknown because healthcare workers are not required to report the disease to public health authorities.

The organism *Borrelia burgdorferi* is the causative agent. The bacterial spirocete is transmitted to humans through the bite of a small tick vector the size of a poppy seed. Studies of the life cycle of the tick indicate that it commonly feeds on an infected white-footed mouse in its larval stage, medium-size mammals including people in its nymph stage, and white-tailed deer as adults (Hudacek, 1990) (Figure 11-4). The tick

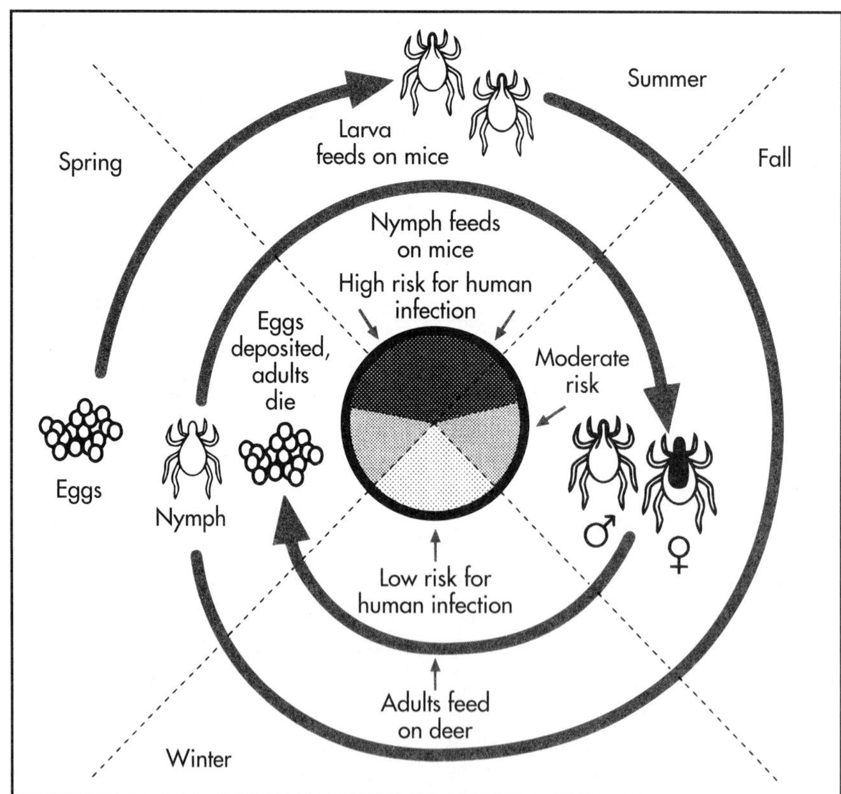

Figure 11-4 Life cycle of the *Ixodes dammini* tick. The tick is a vector and reservoir for *Borrelia burgdorferi,* the agent that produces Lyme disease in humans. (From Harkness GA: *Epidemiology in nursing practice,* St Louis, 1995, Mosby.)

deposits the organism in the capillary system as it feeds on the host's blood, often from 12 to 24 hours. The incubation period is from 3 to 21 days after tick exposure. The human immune system responds weakly to the infection, and antibodies do not appear in any quantity for 4 to 6 weeks. Because of this, laboratory tests are not helpful in early stages and may produce false negative results.

Like other spirocete infections such as syphilis, symptoms of Lyme disease resemble many other diseases. The majority of people may first realize they were bitten when a characteristic rash at the site of the bite appears. It is an expanding red circle that often has a small, white welt in the center. Flu-like symptoms such as fever, headache, fatigue, a stiff neck, and swelling of the knee joints are common. If Lyme disease is not treated promptly, generalized arthritis, severe fatigue, arrhythmias, and symptoms of central nervous system involvement such as numbness, facial paralysis, visual disturbance, and seizures may occur. Permanent structural damage to joints may develop. Early treatment with antibiotics usually prevents complications. Advanced cases may require prolonged intravenous or intramuscular antibiotics. Ceftriaxone (Rocephin) penetrates the blood-brain barrier and is used in people with central nervous system involvement.

Various measures have been used to interfere with the transmission of Lyme disease. However, the most effective measures so far involve preventing the bite of the tick. People are advised to (1) check their bodies for "moving freckles" when in an area known to be tick-infested; (2) tuck pants into long socks and wear a long-sleeved shirt in tick-infected areas; (3) wear light colors and tightly woven fabrics; (4) spray insect repellant containing the ingredient DEET on the clothes; (5) avoid tall grass and low brush; (6) keep pets free of ticks; (7) remove ticks with tweezers. Large-scale spraying has been ineffective in reducing the tick population, and efforts to treat infestations in mice with cotton-soaked insecticides are expensive and practical only in small areas (Hudacek, 1990).

Meningococcal Meningitis

Meningococcal meningitis is an acute bacterial infection of the membranes that cover the brain and spinal cord. The causative organism is *Neisseria meningitidis.* It occurs worldwide, most commonly in the winter and in the spring. Children and young adults are usually the victims, although outbreaks have occurred in adults who live in crowded conditions. Meningococcal infections may be asymptomatic or exhibit respiratory tract symptoms. The disease is not a significant health problem in the United States, although a vaccine is available that can be used under special circumstances. It is generally recommended for military personnel in the United States and for civilians who travel to areas of the world where the organism is prevalent. The treatment of choice is penicillin (see Chapter 28).

Legionellosis

Legionellosis (legionnaires' disease) is primarily a respiratory infection that is caused by bacterium recently named *Legionella pneumophilia.* Although occasional outbreaks occur, it is not considered a significant health problem in the United States. Recently nosocomial outbreaks of legionellosis have been documented (see Chapter 12). It is believed to be transmitted by airborne droplets from contaminated water sources. The sources of several outbreaks have involved various types of air-conditioning systems, although the organism has been isolated from a creek near a contaminated water-cooling system. It is believed that the organism is free-living in soil. Symptoms of infection include fever, malaise, a nonproductive cough, and respiratory difficulty. Some patients have complained of chest pain, abdominal pain, and other GI symptoms. Complications have included renal damage and encephalitis. The organism is sensitive to erythromycin.

Clostridium Infections

The *Clostridium* organisms include all anaerobic, gram-positive, spore-forming bacterial bacilli. They are widely distributed in nature and are found in soil, decaying vegetation, marine sediment, and in the intestinal tract of humans and animals. Several species produce toxins that are responsible for illness in humans.

Strains of *Clostridium perfringens* are common sources of food poisoning (Table 11-2), which is an intestinal disorder that is characterized by abdominal cramps, diarrhea, and nausea. Fever and vomiting are usually absent. Almost all outbreaks are associated with inadequately heated or reheated beef, chicken, or turkey. The spores can survive normal cooking temperatures and germinate and multiply with inadequate storage or rewarming. The illness is produced by the toxins released from the bacteria. *Clostridium botulinum* intoxication occurs sporadically and produces severe neurologic symptoms, including flaccid paralysis. It occurs predominantly from inadequate heating during home canning of fruits and vegetables. *C. perfringens* and other clostridial species can also cause myonecrosis or gas gangrene. Organisms may find their way into a wound that is contaminated with dirt or through soiled clothing. Penetrating wounds such as gunshot wounds, compound fractures, or lacerated wounds present the greatest risk, because these bacilli live and multiply in the absence of air.

The onset of symptoms is usually sudden and may occur 1 to 4 days after injury. Severe pain and edema develop, and although there may be little fever, the pulse rate may be rapid, weak, and thready. The respiratory rate is increased, and the blood pressure may fall. The wound may have a peculiar odor, which often is the first indication of the infection. The slightest unusual odor should be reported immediately to the physician. As the infection extends into the surrounding muscles, skin color change and gas bubbles may be seen at the site of the wound or may be expressed from the muscles. Unless it is treated promptly, the disease is fatal.

The most important aspect of treatment is the excision of all infected tissue. Gas gangrene antitoxin is given, and antibiotic therapy is started. Supportive treatment may include blood transfusion and intravenous fluids. When an extremity is involved, amputation may be necessary to save a patient's life. The patient must be isolated, and rigid medical asepsis must be carried out. The nurse must remember that spore-forming bacteria are not destroyed by ordinary disinfecting methods and that contaminated equipment and linens must be autoclaved. Gas gangrene is dangerous and may spread to other patients unless precautions are taken.

Clostridium difficile is a common organism in the GI tracts of children and is carried in the GI tract of approximately 5% of all adults. It does not normally result in illness. However, disease can occur when the organism is present and the normal flora of the bowel is disturbed. Disease can occur during antibiotic therapy, and colitis can result. *C. difficile* has become an increasing problem in institutions, where organisms can be transmitted from person-to-person by the hands of healthcare workers. Infections can be treated with metronidazole for 10 days.

Tetanus (lockjaw) is an acute neurointoxication induced by *Clostridium tetani.* Tetanus spores can enter the body through a trivial cut or an extensive wound. The anaerobic organism multiplies in the wound and produces a lethal toxin. Early symptoms of headache, restlessness, and irritability progress to opisthotonos (arching of the spine), generalized muscle spasms, and convulsions. Because most people have been immunized for this infectious disease, the incidence is low in the United States. However, adults who have not received a tetanus toxoid vaccine every 10 years to maintain immunization levels are at risk for the infection.

Food Poisoning

Food poisoning refers to illnesses that are acquired through consumption of food or liquids contaminated with chemicals, bacteria, bacterial toxins, or organic poisons that are naturally present in some edible substances. The bacteria often multiply in food that has been stored at improper temperatures. Food poisonings resulting from bacterial contamination occur shortly after ingestion of food. These illnesses are infectious but not communicable diseases and are not usually transmitted from one person to another (Table 11-2; Box 11-5).

Staphylococcal enteric intoxication

The *S. aureus* enterotoxin is one of the more common causes of food poisoning in the United States. The foods commonly involved are those touched by the food handler without subsequent cooking or those that are improperly heated. Foods such as pastries, custards, salad dressings, and sliced meats can be contaminated by purulent discharges. If the food stands at room temperature for several hours before eating, an environment favorable to reproduction of the organism and subsequent enterotoxin production is created. Acute gastroenteritis occurs approximately 1 to 6 hours after ingestion of the food. Severe nausea, cramps, vomiting, and diarrhea can occur and last for several hours. The duration of the illness is 1 or 2 days, and hospitalization may be required. Deaths are rare.

The food is often consumed by large groups of people, which causes an outbreak that is reportable to public health authorities. Individual cases are rarely identified. An epidemiologic investigation can determine the population at risk, the place and time of exposure, and ultimately the food item responsible for the attack. The implicated food will have the highest attack rates. Most of the ill will have eaten the food, and most of the well will have not eaten the food.

Prevention includes the reduction of food-handling time, with no more than 4 to 5 hours at room temperature, refrigeration of perishable foods at 40° F (4.4° C) or lower, and maintenance of hot foods above 140° F (60° C). Nurses should promote these practices as an everyday concern in all households. Persons with boils, abscesses, and other purulent lesions of the hands and face should be prohibited from handling food. All food handlers should be educated in proper hygiene techniques. These techniques include handwashing, cleaning fingernails, keeping the food preparation area clean, and using proper temperature control, therefore reducing the danger of infections.

Salmonella infections

Salmonellosis is an acute gastroenteritis caused by certain species of the genus *Salmonella.* It is usually classified with food poisoning because food is the

TABLE 11-2

Overview of Food Poisoning: Intoxications and Enteric Infections

	Intoxications		Enteric Infections		
	Staphylococcal Food Poisoning	**Botulism**	***Clostridium perfringens***	***Vibro parahaemolyticus***	***Bacillus cereus***
Occurrence	Widespread and frequent; one of the principal acute food poisonings in the United States	Sporadic; family-grouped cases occur	Widespread and frequent in countries with cooking practices that favor growth of organism	Sporadic cases and outbreaks occur in warm months of the year	Outbreaks in Europe and United States
Etiologic agent	Several enterotoxins of staphylococci; stable at boiling temperature	Toxins produced by *Clostridium botulinum* in anaerobic conditions; destroyed by boiling	Type A strains of *C. perfringens (C. welchii)*	*V. parahaemolyticus* (many types)	*B. cereus,* an aerobic spore former that produces two enterotoxins—one heat stable, causing vomiting, and one heat labile, causing diarrhea
Reservoir	Humans; cows with infected udders; dogs and fowl	Soil, water, and intestinal tract of animals and fish	Soil and gastrointestinal tract of humans and animals	Marine silt, coastal waters, fish, and shellfish	Soil; commonly found in raw, dried, and processed foods
Transmission	Ingestion of food containing staphylococcal toxin, which formed while food was held at room temperature	Ingestion of food in which toxin has formed; generally home-canned vegetables, fruits, and meats; also onions and potatoes cooked and held at room temperature	Ingestion of food, especially meat, contaminated by soil or feces; spores survive normal cooking temperatures, germinate, and multiply during cooking and reheating	Ingestion of raw or undercooked seafood; food contaminated with seawater	Ingestion of food that has been kept at ambient temperatures after cooking, permitting multiplication of the organism
Incubation period	30 min-7 hr, usually 2-4 hr	12-36 hr	6-24 hr; usually 10-12 hr	4-96 hr; usually 12-24 hr	1-6 hr for disease causing vomiting; 6-20 hr for disease causing diarrhea
Period of communicability	Noncommunicable	Noncommunicable	Noncommunicable	Noncommunicable	Noncommunicable
Susceptibility and resistance	General; no immune response	General; no immune response	General; no resistance develops from exposure	General	Unknown
Report to local health authority	Prompt report of outbreaks	Report of cases and outbreaks	Prompt report of outbreaks	Report outbreaks	Report cases and outbreaks

From Grimes D: *Infectious diseases,* St Louis, 1991, Mosby.

BOX 11-5 **Nursing Process**

ACUTE FOOD POISONING

ASSESSMENT

History of eating high-risk foods or under high-risk conditions
Nausea, vomiting, diarrhea, vertigo, abdominal pain, paralysis
Vital signs
Fluid volume status

NURSING DIAGNOSES

Fluid volume deficit related to prolonged vomiting and diarrhea
Diarrhea related to pathogens in intestinal tract
Ineffective breathing pattern related to neurologic effect
Impaired physical mobility related to neurologic effect

NURSING INTERVENTIONS

Encourage sips of clear fluids as tolerated.
Progress diet as tolerated.
Instruct patient to wash hands and lubricate anal opening after diarrhea.
Instruct patient to report and seek medical treatment immediately if having difficulty breathing or swallowing or if experiencing paralysis.
Report to local health authority, if indicated.

EVALUATION OF EXPECTED OUTCOMES

No evidence of dehydration
Returns to previous pattern of elimination
Verbalizes understanding of preventive measures
No respiratory compromise or neurologic deficits

most common vehicle of infection. The proportion of cases that are recognized and reported are probably very small. Outbreaks that are reported usually involve hospitals, schools, restaurants, and nursing homes. Infections usually occur as a result of food that has been contaminated at its source, cross-contaminated during processing, or contaminated at some point by an undetected carrier. Most chicken should be considered contaminated and should be handled and cooked accordingly. The organism is also found in cracked eggs, meat and meat products, and other types of poultry. Infection is prevented by thoroughly cooking all foodstuffs derived from animal sources and by educating all food handlers.

The incubation period is from 6 to 72 hours, usually from 12 to 36 hours. It is followed by a sudden onset of frequent, bulky stools and then watery diarrhea. Abdominal pain, nausea and vomiting, headache, and fever may occur. Anorexia and loose stools may persist for several days. The organism may localize in any part of the body and cause a variety of complications. Generally deaths are uncommon and occur only in the very young and the elderly.

Treatment is supportive. The infection is usually self-limiting, and antibiotic treatment may prolong the carrier state. However, antibiotics are indicated when complications occur. The primary objective in care is to maintain hydration. Lost fluids and electrolytes may need to be replaced intravenously.

Shigellosis

Shigellosis (bacillary dysentery) is an acute inflammatory diarrheal disease of the colon caused by the *Shigella* bacillus bacterium. The inflammatory condition, which may also involve portions of the ileum, results in severe ulceration and, if sufficiently intense, may destroy the mucous membrane of the colon, although perforation may not occur. The disease is spread by the fecal-oral route, often through contaminated water, food, or feces. The organism has been isolated from milk products and shrimp. It usually occurs in crowded areas where sanitary conditions are poor.

The incubation period is usually between 1 and 7 days, with an abrupt onset. The primary symptom is severe diarrhea with abdominal cramping. The diarrhea results in loss of fluids and electrolytes, and the patient becomes severely dehydrated. The stools contain blood, pus, and mucus. The temperature may range from low-grade elevation to between 102° F and 104° F (39° C or 40° C) in the afternoon. Urination may be painful, and the patient has a constant desire to defecate.

A problem in the treatment of bacillary dysentery has been the resistance of the organisms to various antimicrobial drugs. Tetracycline, ampicillin, and trimethoprim-sulfamethoxazole are considered to be effective. Intravenous fluids and electrolytes are given to combat dehydration. The patient should be isolated, and enteric precautions should be taken. A low-residue diet is offered, and the use of milk and cream should be avoided. The disease is considered to be self-limiting, and mortality is low when treatment is secured.

Rickettsial Infections

The rickettsia are small, round, or rod-shaped specialized bacteria that live as intracellular parasites in fleas, lice, ticks, and mites. They are transmitted to humans by bites from these insects. Illnesses resulting from rickettsial infections are infectious but not communicable diseases. Rickettsial diseases have been responsible for many severe epidemics, such as epidemic typhus. However, in parts of the world where insect and rodent populations are well controlled, rickettsial diseases are uncommon.

Rocky Mountain spotted fever

Rocky Mountain spotted fever is caused by *Rickettsia rickettsii* and is the most common rickettsial disease in the United States. The incidence of Rocky Mountain spotted fever is low and is greater along the eastern seaboard and in the southeastern states than in the Rocky Mountain area. Three types of ticks may be responsible for the disease: the American dog tick, the Rocky Mountain wood tick, and the Lone Star tick. The disease is seasonal and is more common from April to August. In some areas the disease presents an occupational hazard. When occupations take persons into areas that are heavily infested with ticks, the risk is greater. The disease is commonly contracted by persons vacationing or picnicking in areas in which ticks exist. The fatality rate is high if the disease is untreated. The incubation period is 3 to 14 days.

Assessment. The disease may be mild, with the person remaining ambulatory, or may be severe, with death occurring within a few days after its onset. Early symptoms may be loss of appetite, malaise, irritability, and vague aches and pains. The disease may have an abrupt onset, beginning with chills, a severe headache, an elevation of temperature to 104° F (40° C) or higher, and severe muscle aching. There may be an unproductive cough, nosebleeds, and abdominal pain with nausea and vomiting. The face is flushed, there is profuse sweating, the mouth is dry, and the tongue is coated. In severe cases there may be rigidity of the neck, mental confusion, delirium, incontinence, constipation, and severe prostration, and convulsions and coma may occur. On the third or fourth day a rash appears that begins on the wrists and ankles but gradually spreads over the body and may include the scalp and mucous membranes of the mouth and throat. The rash is petechial in type and tends to fade on pressure. It is rose colored in the beginning but darkens as the disease continues. The acute illness may last for 2 or 3 weeks, with the temperature remaining high for as long as 10 days. The pulse rate is usually slow in relation to the amount of fever present, but in persons with severe cases it may become weak and rapid.

Intervention. The treatment of Rocky Mountain spotted fever is with chloramphenicol (Chloromycetin) or tetracycline, and treatment should be administered early in the disease, preferably with the beginning of the skin rash. The use of antibiotic therapy may remarkably improve the symptoms and reduces the febrile period. Other treatment consists of administering intravenous fluids if sufficient fluid is not taken orally. Blood transfusions may sometimes be indicated.

Care is the same as that for any patient with a febrile disease. The patient is on a regimen of bed rest, and measures to control the temperature, such as sponge baths and antipyretic drugs, are instituted. Special mouth care and eye irrigations may be necessary. The diet should be high in protein with extra between-meal feedings that are also high in protein.

Prophylaxis. No vaccine is currently licensed in the United States. Preventive measures are similar to Lyme disease. Persons who work in tick-infested areas and persons who go camping or picnicking in areas in which they may be exposed to ticks should use tick repellents, avoid sleeping on the ground, wear long pants tucked into socks, and inspect clothing and skin carefully. Areas such as the hairline and under the arms should be given special attention. When removing ticks it is important to avoid crushing them or leaving their heads embedded in the skin. The greatest danger of infection occurs after the tick has fed for 6 to 8 hours.

THE PATIENT WITH A VIRAL INFECTION

Measles

Measles (rubeola) is a highly infectious and often severe viral disease that occurs in young children. Although measles is preventable through active immunization, the disease has occurred in a significant number of people in recent years. Before a measles vaccine was available, more than 400,000 cases were reported annually in the United States. Since the introduction of the vaccine in 1963, the incidence of cases per year has decreased by more than 90%. However, the incidence of measles has increased somewhat in all age groups, with the highest incidence in preschoolers who were never immunized. In 1990, 11.2 cases of measles occurred per 100,000 people (Centers for Disease Control and Prevention, 1994). This rate contrasts with 1.4 cases per 100,000 people in 1988. This remarkable increase stimulated federal- and state-funded primary prevention programs to immunize children throughout the United States. In 1993, the rate dropped to 0.12 cases per 100,000 people. Measles control in the future depends on the success of continuing programs to immunize all susceptible persons who can tolerate the vaccine.

The onset of measles is usually sudden after an incubation period of 7 to 14 days. It occurs most often in the late winter or early spring. In the beginning the disease is often mistaken for a severe cold. Coryza; lacrimation of the eyes, which are red and sensitive to light; sneezing; and a bronchial cough appear. The patient may have a fever, with temperatures ranging from 103° F to 105° F (39.5° C to 40.5° C), and often appears severely ill. During this period, examination of the throat will reveal small white spots with a reddened base (Koplik's spots). In approximately 4 days a macular type of rash begins to appear around the face and gradually extends over the entire body. The rash gradually coalesces to form a slightly elevated eruption that reaches its height in approximately 48 hours, after which it begins to fade. After the rash disappears, a fine desquamation of the skin occurs.

With the development of the rash, the acute symptoms begin to subside. If complications do not develop, recovery may be expected in 10 to 14 days. Measles is often complicated by bronchopneumonia, otitis media, and encephalitis. Encephalitis accompanies rubeola in approximately 1 in every 1000 children affected and may cause brain damage and mental retardation.

Intervention

There is no specific treatment for measles. The child with measles should be isolated from other children, and care should be taken in the disposal of nose and throat secretions. The patient is usually more comfortable in a darkened room because of the sensitivity to light. Sponge baths may be given to reduce fever, and fluids should be encouraged. Bed rest is indicated, and exposure to drafts or respiratory infections should be avoided. The nurse should be alert to complaints of earache or enlargement of the cervical lymph nodes, and the physician should be notified if these symptoms occur. During the febrile period, the diet should be liquid or soft. Cough medications have little effect on the cough, and antibiotic therapy does not alter the course of the disease.

Prophylaxis

For children who have not had measles, active immunization should be given at 15 months of age. Maternal measles antibodies in the serum of a child under age 1 limit the effectiveness of the measles vaccine in producing an active immunity. If an unvaccinated child has been exposed to measles, an immunization given within 72 hours may provide protection.

The measles vaccine produces a mild or subclinical, noncommunicable infection in 95% of susceptible children. It is recommended that persons who were immunized with a live measles vaccine before 12 months of age and those who received an inactivated vaccine that was available between 1963 and 1967 be reimmunized.

Rubella

Rubella (German measles) is sometimes called *3-day measles* because of the short duration of the disease. The symptoms may be similar to those of rubeola but are usually much milder, and Koplik's spots are absent. Some cases may be so mild that the rash is the first and only significant indication of the disease. The lymph nodes behind the ears are almost always enlarged.

The incubation period of the disease is from 12 to 23 days. Isolation and careful handling and disposal of respiratory secretions are important during the course of the disease.

Pregnancy

The occurrence of rubella during pregnancy has been found to present a major hazard to early fetal development. The rubella virus infects the placenta and spread to the fetal circulation. The time of gestation and the length of time that the virus survives and continues to grow in fetal tissue determines the effects on the fetus. The greatest incidence of defects takes place between the second and the sixth week of gestation. After 8 weeks, heart defects, cataracts, and glaucoma decrease, but brain and ear defects may continue to occur into the second trimester of pregnancy. Fetal defects do not develop during late pregnancy. Because 75% of rubella cases occur in school-age children, they represent the reservoir of infection for pregnant women and women of childbearing age.

Prophylaxis

In 1969 the U.S. government licensed a live rubella virus vaccine for general distribution. Children in kindergarten and early grades may be the source of community epidemics and should be high on the priority list for immunization. A single dose of rubella vaccine produces protective antibodies in approximately 95% of susceptible persons. It is often combined with measles or measles-mumps vaccines and given at 15 months of age.

The vaccine should not be given to pregnant women or to women who may become pregnant within 3 months of receiving the vaccine. Persons with febrile illness should not be immunized until they have recovered from their illness. The vaccine has not been reported to be associated with allergic reactions. However, some vaccines do contain trace amounts of antibiotics. Therefore label information on the vaccine bottle should be reviewed carefully before administering the vaccine to patients who are allergic to antibiotics.

The immunization of male adolescents and adults is useful in preventing and controlling epidemics. Because the rubella vaccine is in general use, several factors are important: (1) surveillance of epidemics, (2) accurate diagnosis and reporting of cases, and (3) reporting of all birth defects related to rubella.

Chickenpox

Chickenpox (varicella) is the second most commonly reported communicable disease (following gonorrhea) in the United States. The herpes varicella-zoster (V-Z) virus is the causative agent and is transmitted by direct contact with skin lesions or by airborne transmission of respiratory tract secretions. The incubation period is 2 to 3 weeks, and the period of communicability is usually 1 to 2 days before onset of the characteristic rash.

There is a sudden onset of slight fever with a maculopapular rash. The rash is superficial and first appears on the chest, abdomen, and back. It gradually extends to other parts of the body. The lesions appear in crops, and small reddened spots are often observed in the throat before the rash appears on the skin. The rash goes through a series of stages, beginning with a macule and progressing to a papule, vesicle, and crust. Headache, loss of appetite, and malaise are also common symptoms. Scratching the lesions may lead to secondary infections, and scar formations may result. The disease is self-limiting, and there is no specific treatment. Isolation is generally considered unnecessary, but items contaminated with nose and throat discharges should be carefully discarded.

Although chickenpox is usually a relatively benign disease, infection in a child who has leukemia may result in a widely disseminated infection. More children are surviving with leukemia because of the use of chemotherapeutic drugs. However, infection with chickenpox may be fatal. Live attenuated varicella vaccines can be administered safely to children with leukemia.

Herpes Zoster

Herpes zoster (shingles) is a local manifestation of a recurrent infection that occurs with the chickenpox virus, usually in an older adult. Vesicles erupt on the skin in crops or in irregular patterns along a sensory nerve. Eruptions commonly appear along the chest wall, and occasionally the ophthalmic branch of the trigeminal nerve may be involved. Severe pain and paresthesias can occur over the infected nerve. The pain is controlled with analgesics, and topical steroid applications may promote healing.

Mumps

Mumps (parotitis) is an infectious disease caused by a specific virus that primarily affects children. However, susceptible adults may contract the disease. It has continued to decrease in incidence since the vaccine was licensed in December 1967. In 1993, 0.66 cases per 100,000 people occurred (Centers for Disease Control and Prevention, 1994). Mumps is characterized by inflammation and swelling of the parotid glands on one or both sides, and the salivary glands may be affected. However, 40% of the cases are believed to be subclinical. The incubation period is 14 to 21 days but may extend beyond 21 days. The disease is transmitted through droplet infection from the upper respiratory tract.

Symptoms depend on the severity of the attack, may may include a slight-to-moderate temperature elevation, general malaise, and pain on moving the jaw or opening the mouth. A characteristic condition associated with mumps is an acute sensitivity to acidic substances.

Other glands in the body occasionally become involved, the most common being the testes in men past puberty. Encephalitis, aseptic meningitis, and unilateral nerve deafness are the most serious complications. The question of mumps occurring during early pregnancy as a possible cause of fetal malformations has come under investigation.

Intervention

The patient should be isolated until all symptoms of the infection have subsided. Warm or cold packs may be applied to swollen, tender salivary glands. The diet should be liquid or soft, and any food or drink with a tart or acidic taste should be avoided. If orchitis develops, bed rest, narcotic analgesics, support of the inflamed testis with a bridge, and ice packs may make the patient feel more comfortable. If the illness remains uncomplicated, it may run a course of approximately 7 to 10 days.

Prophylaxis

Although it is available independently, the mumps vaccine is usually combined with a measles-rubella vaccine and administered at age 15 months. Administration of the vaccine within 1 to 2 days after exposure offers some protection to the susceptible person.

Infectious Mononucleosis

Infectious mononucleosis is an acute infection caused by the Epstein-Barr (EB) virus, which is closely related to the herpes viruses. The name *mononucleosis* was derived from the atypical lymphocytes among the white blood cells. Infection with the virus is worldwide, but infectious mononucleosis occurs primarily in developed countries where contact with the virus is delayed from early childhood until the age of 15 to 25. Infection with the virus at an early age results in a subclinical infection that usually goes unnoticed. A syndrome resembling infectious mononucleosis may be caused by herpesvirus type 6 or the cytomegalovirus (another member of the herpesvirus group of organisms).

The disease appears to have a low degree of communicability and, often occurs among groups of young people living together, as in college dormitories. The disease has been referred to as the "kissing disease," because transmission appears to be by the oral route and the exchange of saliva.

The disease is characterized by sore throat, fever, enlarged lymph nodes, headache, and vomiting. In persons with severe cases the spleen may be enlarged or jaundice may occur. The incubation period is believed to be 4 to 14 days but may be as long as 6 weeks.

There is no specific treatment for the disease, which is self-limiting. During the acute phase, the patient should be confined to bed. Mild analgesics may be given to relieve the discomfort from the sore throat and enlarged glands. Antibiotics have no effect on the course or the outcome of the disease. In severe cases, steroid therapy may be recommended. Although serious complications, including neurologic problems, are possible, they are rare. Chronic fatigue syndrome may be an outcome of the infection.

Influenza

Influenza is an acute viral disease of the respiratory tract. Epidemics and pandemics of influenza have been known since the sixteenth century. The worst pandemic of modern times occurred in 1918 and 1919, when it was estimated that 20 million people died. More than half of these deaths occurred in the United States. Several serious epidemics have occurred since then. The disease occurs in cycles, but sporadic illness occurs during nonepidemic years. Each year, most states report cases of influenza to the CDC, although only epidemics are required to be reported. Attack rates during epidemics have been estimated from less than 15% of the population to 25% in large communities. True incidence data is difficult to obtain.

Three types of influenza viruses have been identified: A, B, and C. Type A and B have long been associated with epidemics. Type C has appeared only sporadically and in localized outbreaks. Strains of influenza A are described by geographic origin, strain number, year of isolation, and by an index that identifies the antigenic characteristics of the strain. Hemagglutinin (H) and neuraminidase (N) are surface antigens of the virus that stimulate antibody production. Each strain has specific configurations. For instance, the viral strain that caused the Hong Kong influenza epidemic in 1968 is described as A/Hong Kong/1/68 (H3N2).

The mode of transmission is by direct contact through droplet infection, which is often airborne in crowded, enclosed areas. The incubation period is short, usually from 24 to 72 hours, and the period of communicability is limited to 3 days from the onset of clinical symptoms. The typical onset is sudden with chills; a temperature of 102° F or above; aching of the head, back, and extremities; sore throat; coughing; sneezing; and weakness. In uncomplicated cases the acute period usually lasts from 3 to 5 days. Some cases begin with GI symptoms, bronchopneumonia, or sinusitis. Influenza is especially hazardous for the elderly, and mortality from influenza-related pneumonia is high. Generally the treatment is symptomatic. Antibiotics may be given if a secondary infection such as a bacterial pneumonia occurs.

Susceptibility to the influenza viruses is universal. Infection produces immunity to the specific infecting virus, and infections with related viruses broadens immunity. However, type A influenza viruses undergo "antigenic shifts" in which distinctive new hemagglutinin or neuraminidase surface antigens are formed. These shifts result from changes in the genetic material of the virus. These new variants of influenza create new epidemics when enough of the population is susceptible.

Vaccines have been created to immunize people at high risk, including healthcare workers. Because the antigenic characteristics of the current strains provide the basis for selecting the virus strains included in each year's vaccine, the vaccines may not be effective if new strains appear. Because the proportion of elderly people in the United States is increasing and chronic diseases are more prevalent, an increased emphasis on control measures is necessary for the future. It is recommended that the following groups be targeted for vaccination programs (in order of priority):

1. Children and adults with chronic disorders of the cardiovascular or pulmonary systems
2. Residents of chronic-care facilities
3. Healthy individuals 65 years or older
4. Children and adults with chronic metabolic diseases, renal dysfunction, anemia, or immunosuppression
5. Children and teenagers who are receiving long-term aspirin therapy, because they are at risk of Reye's syndrome following influenza infection
6. Physicians, nurses, and other personnel that have extensive contact with high-risk patients, because they may transmit the virus and cause nosocomial infections in patients
7. Providers of care to high-risk people in the home

Local health planning and education in schools and institutions and surveillance of the extent and progress of outbreaks are other means of prevention and control.

Hepatitis

Viral hepatitis is an infectious disease that attacks the liver and causes a diffuse inflammatory reaction. Several distinct infections actually occur and differ in etiologic and pathologic characteristics. Their prevention and control measures also vary (see Chapter 23).

Hepatitis A incidence was 9.4 cases per 100,000 people in 1993 (Centers for Disease Control and Prevention, 1994). The virus is transmitted from person to person by the fecal-oral route, and contaminated food is a common vehicle. The incubation period is from 15 to 50 days, and averages 28 to 30 days. The virus is excreted in the feces long before clinical symptoms appear, although the carrier is thought to be most infectious just before the onset of symptoms. Because the disease has a low incidence in infants and preschool children, mild, inapparent, and asymptomatic infections are probably common.

The onset of viral hepatitis is abrupt, with fever, malaise, nausea, and abdominal discomfort followed by jaundice within a few days. The illness varies from mild symptoms to a severely disabling disease that lasts several months. Severity increases with age, although complete recovery is normal. Presently, no vaccine for active immunization is available. Immunoglobulin (Ig) may be given as a prophylactic measure to exposed persons or to those who anticipate travel to highly endemic areas. All feces, blood, and body fluids from the infected individual should be treated as potentially infectious. Prevention and control measures focus on education of the public regarding good sanitation, personal hygiene, and handwashing.

Hepatitis B (HB) has a similar incidence to Hepatitis A: 5.18 cases per 100,000 people in 1993 (Centers for Disease Control and Prevention, 1994). The infection occurs worldwide with little seasonal variation. The virus is composed of a core surrounded by an outer coat that contains the surface antigen. Transmission occurs when blood, serum, or plasma from an infected person is introduced parenterally, often through venipuncture equipment or needle sticks. The infection can also be transmitted through contamination of open wounds or through exposure of mucous membranes to infected body fluids. Fecal-oral transmission has not been demonstrated. The average incubation period is 60 to 90 days. Blood is infectious weeks before the onset of symptoms, through the clinical course of the illness, and during the chronic carrier state, which may last for years. Surface antigens can be detected in the serum several weeks before onset of symptoms and into the carrier state.

The onset is usually insidious, with vague abdominal discomfort, anorexia, malaise, nausea and vomiting, and joint pain. Fever may be mild or absent. Jaundice is common and is accompanied by dark urine, clay-colored stools, and pruritus. The illness ranges from inapparent infection to acute hepatic necrosis, which may be fatal. Treatment is symptomatic only and is planned to strengthen the patient's resistance to infection. The patient's contacts and those who are accidentally exposed can be immunized with an inactive viral antigen (HB). Preventive measures include strict discipline in blood banks, use of blood and blood products only when essential, and sterilization of all reusable equipment.

Hepatitis C resembles HB clinically and epidemiologically. It is usually less severe in the acute stage, but asymptomatic or symptomatic chronicity is common. The incubation period is from 2 weeks to 6 months. Treatment, control, and prevention measures are similar to HB.

THE PATIENT WITH A PROTOZOAL DISEASE

There are approximately 30 known protozoal diseases. Most of them have a low incidence in the United States but are prevalent in other parts of the world. Most cases occur in travelers who have been to countries where the infections are endemic. Examples include amebiasis and giardiasis, which affect the intestine; toxoplasmosis and malarias, which are systemic diseases; and trichomoniasis, which affects the genitourinary tract and is considered a sexually transmitted disease. Trichomoniasis is widespread throughout the world. Malaria is a serious, worldwide disease and is reportable to the CDC.

Malaria is transmitted from person to person by a mosquito known as the *Anopheles quadrimaculatus*. Control of the disease in the United States has been brought about primarily through destruction of mosquito breeding places and adequate treatment of persons with malaria. Most cases in the United States have been in persons returning from areas of the world where the disease still exists.

There are four species of the parasite that cause malaria in humans. The most serious is known as *Plasmodium falciparum*. The parasite is injected into the body by a female mosquito who is seeking a blood meal before ovulation. The parasites invade the liver, where they grow and multiply. After 12 to 14 days (the incubation period), they enter the bloodstream and invade red blood cells. The symptoms that result are caused by the continual lysis of red blood cells.

Symptoms of malaria begin with a headache and a gradually increasing fever. The typical malaria pattern soon develops: severe chills followed by a high fever, with temperatures ranging from 103° F to 105° F (39.5° C to 40.5° C), followed by a rapid fall in temperature and profuse sweating. This sequence may repeat itself every 48 hours, and between the episodes the patient may be reasonably well. However, without adequate treatment, anemia and enlargement of the spleen gradually develop.

Oral administration of chloroquine (Aralen) is the treatment of choice for most cases of malaria. However, in areas where *P. falciparum* has become resistant to chloroquine, quinine sulfate is given along with tetracycline (Beneson, 1990). Travelers to Asia, Africa, or South America, where the chloroquine-resistant organisms are present, are advised to take mefloquine for prophylaxis. This drug is contraindicated for pregnant women, and other drug therapy is recommended. Administration of the drug should begin 2 weeks before departure and continue for 6 weeks after leaving the malarious area.

THE PATIENT WITH HELMINTHIC INFESTATIONS

Metazoa are parasites that belong to the animal kingdom. When they invade the human body, this is referred to as a *helminth infestation*. The Metazoa are divided into two groups: (1) Platyhelminthes, which includes tapeworms; and (2) Nematoda, or roundworms. Nematoda include *Ascaris* parasites, hookworms, pinworms, and *Trichinella* parasites.

Parasites often ingest nutrients in the GI tract of the infected person, which causes a state of malnutrition even though the person is eating a balanced diet. Some parasites feed on the host's blood, which causes severe anemia. Irritation and tissue damage can occur. If the parasites grow or increase in number, blood vessels, ducts, and even the GI tract can be blocked. Pinworms are sometimes found in the appendix when acute appendicitis has necessitated its removal. Some parasites produce toxins that injure tissue or cause severe allergic tissue reactions.

Platyhelminthes (Flatworms)

Tapeworms (Cestoda) are flatworms, and nearly all flatworms are segmented. At one end there is a head and a neck called the *scolex*. The head is tiny in relation to the size of the worm. The scolex contains a mechanism that enables the worm to attach itself to the mucous membrane of the intestinal tract. Three forms of the worm are known to infect humans in the United States: (1) dwarf tapeworm, (2) beef tapeworm, and (3) fish tapeworm.

The dwarf tapeworm is the smallest of the tapeworms. It is most prevalent in areas in which the sanitation is extremely poor. Infection occurs after ingesting the eggs of the worm, which hatch in the human intestinal tract. The cycle begins when the worms produce eggs that are discharged in the feces. Improper handwashing after using the toilet is the medium by which the eggs are conveyed to the mouth and thus to the intestinal tract.

The beef tapeworm, the most commonly found tapeworm in the United States, reaches the human intestinal tract through the ingestion of raw or insufficiently cooked beef that contains the larvae of the worm. The cycle begins when the larvae produce worms. The eggs produced by the worms are present in human feces and are deposited onto soil where cattle graze. A cow ingests the eggs, which hatch in the small intestine. The larvae (an intermediate stage in the development of the worm) lodge in the animal's tissues. A person who eats raw or undercooked beef that contains the larvae may become infected. The beef tapeworm is known to grow to a length of 25 feet, and as long as the head remains attached to the mucous membrane of the intestinal wall, it continues to grow and produce eggs.

The fish tapeworm, like the beef tapeworm, requires an intermediary host, and human infection occurs in a similar way. Human feces containing the eggs are deposited into fresh water, where the eggs mature into tiny embryos. The embryos are usually eaten by small shellfish, which are ultimately eaten by larger fish. The embryo then matures in the tissues of the fish. Infection may occur in areas where fish is eaten raw or is insufficiently cooked. The fish tapeworm may grow to

30 feet in length and may live for many years in the human intestine. Fish tapeworm infection is believed to be more prevalent than previously thought. Infection is known to result in severe anemia, and it is reported that the worm absorbs large amounts of vitamin B_{12} from the intestinal tract. Praziquantel (Biltricide) or niclosamide (Niclocide) is the drug of choice for both beef and fish tapeworm infestations.

Nematoda (Roundworms)

Ascaris is a genus of large roundworms that resemble the common earthworm (fishworm). Roundworms vary in length from 4 to 12 inches, and the female worm may produce as many as 27 million eggs. When human feces are deposited on the ground, they become mixed with the soil, where the eggs may live for indefinite periods. Infection results from ingestion of the eggs containing the larvae. The larvae reach the small intestine, where they mature. Infection with *Ascaris* may be serious and cause complications such as intestinal obstruction, perforation of ulcers, appendicitis, and similar conditions. Administration of mebendazole (Vermox), pyrantel pamoate (Antiminth) or piperazine salts provide effective treatment.

Hookworms

There are two species of hookworm, and both may cause human infection. One species is most common in the southern United States, and the other species is most prevalent in Europe and Asia. As with many other types of worms, the source of infection is soil that has been contaminated with human feces that contain the eggs. The larva of the hookworm penetrates the unbroken skin of the feet and legs and enters the body by way of the hair follicles and sweat glands. It penetrates lymph and blood vessels and may reach the lungs, where it is often coughed up and expectorated.

If larvae is swallowed, the larva reaches the small intestine, where the worms mature. The worm attaches itself to the intestinal mucosa by a pinching kind of hook. A mature worm produces from 5000 to 10,000 eggs daily. The hookworm is reported to ingest as much as 50 ml of the host's blood daily, which results in a severe iron-deficiency anemia. It also damages and ingests bits of tissue from the intestinal mucosa and commonly causes allergic reactions. Mebendazole (Vermox) and thiabendazole (Mintezol) are effective in testing the infestation. Examination of stool specimens should be repeated after 2 weeks.

Pinworms (Threadworms, Seatworms)

Pinworms are found worldwide and represent the most common helminth infection in the United States. Prevalence is highest in school-age children and lowest in adults. Often entire families are infected at the same time. The pinworm is a tiny worm, and infection is self-induced by the anal-oral route. The ingested eggs pass into the stomach, and the worm matures in the large intestine. When the mature worm is ready to lay its eggs, it crawls to the outside and deposits its eggs in folds around the rectum and anus, after which it dies. The life cycle is approximately 4 to 6 weeks. Severe itching occurs around the area. Through scratching, the hands become infected with the eggs, which are then carried to the mouth, and the entire cycle begins again. Reinfection may cause the number of worms present in the GI tract to increase over several months.

Several drugs are effective in eliminating the infestation, among them pyrantel pamoate, mebendazole, albendazole, and pyrvinium pamoate (Povan). Treatment is repeated after 2 weeks. Taking daily showers, changing underclothes and bedsheets often, washing hands often, discouraging nailbiting, and providing education in personal hygiene help prevent outbreaks.

Trichinellosis (Trichinosis)

Trichina is a parasitic organism of the genus *Trichinella* and is responsible for trichinosis. The primary source of trichinosis is insufficiently cooked pork and pork products that are infected with the worm. The larva that is present in the meat passes into the intestinal tract, and the worm matures in the intestine, where it becomes embedded in the mucosa. The larva is then released and eventually reaches the bloodstream. After entering the general circulation, the larva is carried to skeletal muscle tissue and becomes encased in a cyst. There are several stages of infection during the development of the worm and its passage through the body. During the various stages of the infection, symptoms may be acute, with fever, increased leukocyte count, allergic manifestations, and psychologic symptoms. After encasement, the primary symptom is rheumatic-like pain. The disease is serious, and 5% to 10% of the persons infected die.

Thiabendazole has been effective in treatment of the infestation when given during the very early, intestinal stage of the disease. Mebendazole is used in the muscular stage of the disease. Corticosteroids are indicated only in severe cases.

SEXUALLY TRANSMITTED DISEASES

Six diseases are classified as sexually transmitted diseases (STDs) and are reportable to public health authorities: AIDS, syphilis, gonorrhea, chancroid, lymphogranuloma venereum, and granuloma inguinale. AIDS is the epidemic of the twentieth century (see Chapter 13). Syphilis and gonorrhea remain significant health problems in the United States. The incidence rates of chancroid, lymphogranuloma venereum, and granuloma inguinale are less than one case per 100,000 people (Centers for Disease Control and Prevention, 1994).

Trichomoniasis, venereal warts, herpes simplex type 2, and some chlamydial infections can also be sexually transmitted, but reporting these conditions is not required. The most common conditions are discussed in the following sections. Table 11-3 outlines the characteristics of the less prevalent or less serious venereal diseases, and Box 11-6 outlines the care for patients with sexually transmitted diseases.

TABLE 11-3

Characteristics of Sexually Transmitted Diseases

Disease (Pathogen)	Transmission/ Incubation	Symptoms	Prevention and Control
Chancroid *(Haemophilus ducreyi)*	Direct contact; 3-5 days, up to 14 days	Painful ulcers at site; painful regional lymph nodes	Ceftriaxone or erythromycin; report to health authorities; prophylactic treatment of contacts
Condyloma acuminatum, genital warts (human papilloma virus)	Direct contact; 2-3 months average	Fleshy, cauliflower-like growths around genitalia	10%-25% podophyllin in tincture of benzoin; intralesional recombinant interferon alfa-2b (Intron A); sexual contacts should be examined and treated, if indicated
Granuloma inguinale *(Calymmatobacterium granulomatis)*	Direct contact through sexual activity; 8-80 days	Small, beefy-red nodule, slowly spreads; often painless; can spread to other parts of the skin, mucous membranes	Tetracycline, co-trimoxazole, or chloramphenicol for 3 weeks; report to health authorities; examine sexual contacts
Lymphogranuloma venereum *(Chlamydia trachomatis)*	Direct contact, usually sexual intercourse; 4-21 days, usually 7-12 days	Small, painless papule or nodule often unnoticed; suppuration of regional lymph nodes and invasion of adjacent tissues; fever, chills, headache, joint pain	Tetracycline; doxycycline; treatment of recent contacts; report to health authorities
Molluscum contagiosum (Molluscipoxvirus)	Direct sexual contact and indirect contact; 2-7 weeks	Smooth-surfaced, firm, spherical papules, white translucent or yellow; 2-5 mm in diameter	No drug therapy available; curettage with local anesthesia
Other chlamydial infections	Direct contact through sexual intercourse; 7-14 days or longer	Males: urethritis; females: mucopurulent cervicitis; itching, burning on urination	Tetracycline or doxycycline; prophylactic treatment of sexual partners; reportable in some states
Trichomoniasis *(Trichomonas vaginalis)*	Direct contact with vaginal and urethral discharges or contaminated articles; transmitted to infants during birth; 4-20 days, average 7 days	Petechial lesions; profuse, thin, foamy, yellow discharge with foul odor; sometimes asymptomatic vaginitis, and/or urethritis	Metronidazole (Flagyl); sexual partners should be treated concurrently

BOX 11-6 **Nursing Process**

SEXUALLY TRANSMITTED DISEASE

ASSESSMENT

Sexual history
Dysuria, discharge, rectal irritation, malaise
Posterior pharynx for inflammation, exudate
Temperature
External genitalia
Inguinal lymphadenopathy

NURSING DIAGNOSES

Risk for infection (patient contacts) related to pathogens in lesions and mode of transmission
Risk for infection (patient) related to untreated or inadequately treated disease
Anxiety/fear related to social stigma of venereal disease
Knowledge deficit related to new condition, transmission, prevention, and treatment

NURSING INTERVENTIONS

Administer medications (antivirals, antibiotics) as prescribed.
Monitor for symptoms of pelvic inflammatory disease with gonorrhea and chlamydia.
Keep lesions clean and dry.
Report to local health authority, if indicated.
Reexamine and treat pregnant women before delivery.
Examine and treat patient contacts.
Provide emotional support.

EVALUATION OF EXPECTED OUTCOMES

Describes medication regimen
Describes correct use of condom
Verbalizes avoidance of sexual contacts until lesions are healed
Infection resolved

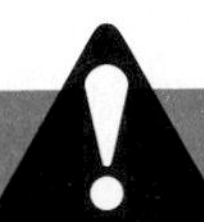

NURSE ALERT

AIDS, syphilis, gonorrhea, chancroid, lymphogranuloma venereum, and granuloma inguinale are reportable STDs.

Syphilis

Syphilis (lues) is a widespread communicable disease. Nearly 75,000 cases were reported in 1993, resulting in a case rate of 39.7 per 100,000 people (Centers for Disease Control and Prevention, 1994). Syphilis primarily involves people between 15 and 30 years of age. Social factors are significantly related to the disease. It is more common in urban settings and among male homosexuals in some areas. It also is more common in males than females.

Syphilis is contracted almost exclusively through direct sexual contact with exudates from a person infected with the bacterial spirocete *Treponema pallidum*. Susceptibility is universal. Saliva, semen, blood, and vaginal discharges may carry the organism. Fetal infection may occur through transfer of the organism through the placenta. The incubation period is from 10 days to 10 weeks, but usually 3 weeks. Four stages of development have been identified: the primary, secondary, latent, and late stages. The period of communicability of untreated patients is variable and indefinite.

Primary syphilis

The primary lesion appears as a painless papule that occurs on the male prepuce or female vulva, vagina, or cervix. It may become an indurated chancre. The serologic blood test is usually negative at this time. During the primary stage the disease is highly infectious. The primary lesion disappears in 3 to 4 weeks with or without treatment, and no topical application will hasten its healing. Positive identification of the specific spirochete may be made at this time by a dark-field examination (a special attachment on the microscope). When adequate treatment is given early during the primary stage, the serologic test may remain negative. Without treatment, the disease progresses to the secondary stage. The secondary stage usually begins 2 to 8 weeks after the appearance of the chancre.

Secondary syphilis

As a result of the invading organisms, several symptoms develop, including a rash. The rash may be a slight erythema or may be extensive, with macular, papular, or pustular lesions. The rash may involve the entire body and especially the palms and soles, which are locations that strongly suggest the diagnosis. Lesions called *mucus patches* appear around the mouth and lips, and the throat may be sore. A papular type of lesion (condyloma latum) appears around the genitals. All moist lesions are infectious, and positive dark-field examination may often be secured from these secondary lesions. Other symptoms include alopecia, pain in the bones, gastric disturbances, inflammation of the eyes, loss of appetite, and malaise. Without treatment, the symptoms of secondary syphilis may disappear slowly and recur at intervals for as long as 2 years, and the disease is considered highly infectious during this stage.

Latent syphilis

The latent stage is generally considered to cover 4 years or more from time of onset of the disease. During this period, there is no clinical evidence of the disease after the disappearance of secondary lesions, except for the reactive serologic test. However, it is during this time that the organism attacks the vital structures and causes an inflammatory condition. The body's defenses may be sufficient to overcome the destructiveness of the organism. However, there is no way to determine which individuals may ultimately suffer severe disability. The serologic test remains reactive, and the disease is potentially infectious through sexual contact. Latency sometimes continues throughout life, and spontaneous recovery may occur.

Late syphilis

The late stage occurs 5 to 20 years after initial infection. Disabling lesions occur in the cardiovascular system and central nervous system. This stage is often referred to as neurosyphilis, cardiovascular syphilis, or gummatous syphilis. These late manifestations impair health, limit occupational efficiency, and shorten life.

Congenital syphilis

Mothers with untreated syphilis often have a history of repeated abortions. If the pregnancy is completed, the fetus may be stillborn. If the infant survives, it may have syphilis. An infant with congenital syphilis may have a rash on the face, palms of the hands, soles of the feet, and buttocks, with the latter often mistaken for diaper rash. There may be mucus patches in the mouth and nasal stuffiness and rhinitis (snuffles). The bones and abdominal organs are often involved. The syphilitic lesions of the infant are infectious, just as are those of the adult. The child who survives may develop complications at any time before 16 years of age. These complications include changes in the bones, deformed permanent teeth, interstitial keratitis, and eighth nerve deafness. The central nervous system may be involved, and mental retardation may occur in a small number of children.

Intervention

The present treatment of syphilis is administration of long-acting penicillin G. There is no evidence that the syphilitic organism is becoming resistant to penicillin. However, caution must be exercised because more individuals are becoming sensitive to penicillin. The same care should be exercised as when administering penicillin to a patient for any condition. Treatment may extend over a period of several days or may be given in one initial dose. Patients who are sensitive to penicillin may be treated with tetracycline or erythromycin.

The fundamental approach to controlling syphilis is to interview patients to identify contacts. All identified contacts of confirmed syphilis cases should receive preventive penicillin therapy and be educated about the disease. The privacy of the individual must be protected. Preventive measures assumed by nurses include health and sex education, discouragement of sexual promiscuity, and encouragement of syphilis serology during prenatal examination. Control of prostitution and ensuring availability and accessibility of care are broader goals for healthcare personnel.

Gonorrhea

Gonorrhea remains an epidemic in the United States. It is an infection of the genitourinary tract with the organism *Neisseria gonorrhoeae* (gonococcus bacterium). Gonorrhea is the most commonly reported infectious disease and has a case rate of 323 per 100,000 people. It is very common in the United States among sexually promiscuous male homosexuals. With the introduction of resistant strains of the organism, the incidence has increased worldwide (Centers for Disease Control and Prevention, 1994).

Transmission of the organism occurs through direct contact with exudates from the mucous membranes of infected people. The incubation period is 2 to 7 days. Without treatment, the infection may be self-limiting or result in a chronic carrier state. In females, urethritis or cervicitis initially occurs. It is often mild and may go unnoticed. Chronic endocervical infection is common, and the uterus may be invaded as the infection progresses. Because of the sometimes mild nature of the disease in women, many cases go untreated and spread the infection to others. The period of communicability may extend for months if untreated. A diseminated gonococcal infection develops in approximately 5% of those infected and causes arthritis, fever, and skin lesions (Beneson, 1990).

The characteristic symptoms begin with burning, urgent, and painful urination. There may be redness and edema of the urinary meatus. After the initial symptoms, a purulent urethral discharge occurs in men, and a discharge may be expressed from the vaginal glands, ducts, and the urethra in women. In the absence of treatment or with inadequate treatment, the disease may become chronic and lead to complications. Epididymitis and prostatitis may occur in men, and salpingitis and pelvic inflammatory disease (PID) may occur in women. An acute inflammatory condition in the fallopian tubes leads to occlusion and sterility.

The treatment for gonorrhea consists of administering 4.8 million units of penicillin G during one visit. Ampicillin or tetracycline can also be used. However, certain strains of the gonococcus have become resistant to penicillin. For persons who are sensitive to penicillin, other antibiotics may be administered. Minocycline (Minocin), a semisynthetic derivative of tetracycline, has been used as an alternative treatment. Interviewing patients and tracing contacts are fundamental elements of a control program. Preventive measures are the same as for syphilis.

Herpes Simplex

There are four major types of herpes viruses. The herpes simplex virus (HSV) types 1 and 2 cause both genital and oral infections. Other viruses included in this family are the Epstein-Barr virus, which causes mononucleosis; the varicella-zoster virus, which causes chickenpox and shingles; and the cytomegalovirus (CMV), which can result in severe congenital abnormalities. The majority of oral HSV infections are caused by type 1, and most genital lesions are caused by type 2. However, either strain can be found in the oral and genital areas, as well as on other parts of the body as skin lesions. Recurring cold sores around the external surface of the mouth are considered oral herpes. HSV-1 and HSV-2 infections can be distinguished only by tissue culture.

Most people have been exposed to HSV-1 and/or HSV-2 infections. Random sampling of various populations for the presence of antibodies to the virus has estimated that 40% to 100% of the general population has been exposed at some time to the viruses.

Pathophysiology

HSV infections are believed to be transmitted by skin-to-skin contact with an infected lesion. The virus enters the body through a break in the skin or mucous membrane, and transmission is not necessarily sexual in nature. Incubation is from 2 to 12 days. The virus enters the nervous system at the site of infection, resides in that area permanently, and can remain dormant indefinitely. An outbreak of active infection can be triggered by such things as local trauma, sunlight, emotional stress, and the presence of other debilitating diseases. Asymptomatic transmission can also occur, which causes extensive problems for prevention and control of the infection.

The initial or primary infection is usually the most severe and lasts from 7 to 21 days. An initial infection in the mouth causes severe stomatitis, but the lesions do not recur. A fluid-filled vesicle forms first, followed by shallow ulcerations. When this occurs in the genital area, itching, burning, tingling, and sometimes severe pain may be present. Edema, swollen lymph glands, and a thin, white discharge may occur. The number of lesions may vary considerably. Moist lesions heal more slowly than dry lesions. Outbreaks may recur, although they become progressively more mild and less common, and lesions last from 4 to 10 days.

Prevention and control

There is no cure for oral or genital herpes. Topical 5-iodo-2′-deoxyozidine (idoxuridine) may modify acute symptoms. Acyclovir (Zovirax), used orally, intravenously, or topically may reveal shedding of the virus, diminish pain, and accelerate healing time. Keeping lesions dry and clean is essential. A vaccine for HSV is under study but will have little effect for those who have already been infected. Prevention of herpes focuses on the avoidance of contact with open lesions. Healthcare personnel should wear gloves when in contact with mucous membranes that may be infected with HSV. Using a condom during sexual activity may decrease the risk of infection.

HSV infections during pregnancy have devastating effects on the fetus, particularly if it is an initial infection. The infection in the infant can be systemic and result in death. A cesarean section may be performed to prevent infection in the newborn when the mother has an active infection. HSV-2 infections have also been related to cervical cancer.

The emotional problems associated with a herpes infection can be severe. Guilt and despair can result when a mother unknowingly infects her infant or when a person passes the infection to a sexual partner. The social stigma of venereal disease may be very destructive. Empathy and acceptance are imperative.

• • •

STDs have commonly been termed "social diseases" because of the factors in society that contribute to their existence, including poverty, poor housing, low income, ignorance, and in more recent times the high mobility of people, increased alcohol consumption, ease of treatment, and a change in value systems. All these factors contribute to the incidence of STDs.

Prevention and control continues to be a major health focus. Healthy People 2000 has created a list of

BOX 11-7

SUMMARY OF *HEALTHY PEOPLE 2000* OBJECTIVES FOR STDS

- Confine annual incidence of diagnosed AIDS cases to no more than 98,000 cases
- Confine the prevalence of HIV infections to no more than 800 per 100,000 people
- Reduce gonorrhea to an incidence of no more than 225 cases per 100,000 people; reduce repeat gonorrhea infections to no more than 15% within the previous year
- Reduce *Chlamydia trachomatis* infections to no more than 170 cases per 100,000 people
- Reduce primary and secondary syphilis to an incidence of no more than 10 cases per 100,000 people
- Reduce the annual number of first-time consultations with a physician for genital herpes and genital warts to 142,000 and 385,000
- Reduce sexually transmitted hepatitis B infections to no more than 30,500 cases

objectives (Box 11-7). Preventive measures include educational programs, especially in schools, on general health, sex education, and preparation for marriage (Box 11-8).

Most states require premarital and prenatal examinations, including blood serology. Discouraging sexual promiscuity and teaching methods of personal prophylaxis will help protect members of the community. Facilities for early diagnosis and treatment should be available in all communities. Control measures include mandatory reporting of all cases to local health departments so that all contacts can be investigated. Interviewing patients and tracing contacts are fundamental in controlling transmission.

BOX 11-8

PATIENT/FAMILY EDUCATION GUIDE FOR PREVENTION OF STDS

- Reduce the number of sexual partners, preferably to one person.
- Avoid sexual contact with people who have multiple partners or other high-risk behaviors, such as drug abuse.
- Know partner's present and past sexual activities.
- Avoid sexual contact with individuals known to be infected.
- Examine genital areas for sores, rashes, or pus before having sex, and avoid sexual contact if these signs are present.
- Use a water-based lubricant.
- Use latex condoms whenever having sex.
- Wash hands and genital area before and after sex.
- Use mouthwash or gargle with hydrogen peroxide or an antiseptic to reduce the risk of oropharyngeal infection.
- Urinate after intercourse.
- Avoid excessive douching.
- Seek medical help whenever there is any suspicion of an STD, and have periodic examinations.

EMERGING INFECTIONS

The CDC maintains an ongoing surveillance system for the detection of emerging infectious diseases. The term *emerging infectious diseases* refers to those infectious diseases that have an incidence in humans that has increased within the past two decades or threatens to increase in the near future. These diseases may be new, previously unrecognized, reemerging, or those that have developed a resistance to previously effective antimicrobial drugs. Several of these diseases are posing an increasing threat to public health. Strains of *Escherichia coli*, streptococcus, and hantavirus are examples (Centers for Disease Control and Prevention, 1994).

Escherichia Coli

An outbreak of a specific strain of *E. coli* found in contaminated meat affected more than 500 people in four western states and resulted in 56 cases of hemolytic uremic syndrome and four deaths. It is believed that the prevalence of this infection is much higher. It is recommended that this infection be made reportable by all states and territories.

Streptococcal Diseases

The prevalence of *Streptococcus pneumoniae* (pneumococcus) strains that are highly resistant to penicillin has increased significantly in recent years. This organism is the agent for much of the community-acquired pneumonia, particularly in the elderly. The CDC and other organizations are developing recommendations for the surveillance of these infections along with optimal treatment regimens. Surveillance for group A streptococcal disease is also being expanded. This organism is responsible for invasive diseases such as toxic shock syndrome and necrotizing fascitis. The incidence of these diseases appears to be increasing, particularly in the very young and the elderly.

Hantavirus Pulmonary Syndrome

Hantavirus pulmonary syndrome (HPS) is a newly recognized illness that is characterized by influenza-like symptoms followed by an acute onset of respiratory failure. It was first identified in the southwestern United States in 1993 following a cluster of unexplained deaths. A new Hantavirus was found to reside primarily in the deer mouse, and contact with mouse excreta has produced illness in humans. It has now been found in 20 states and has a case fatality rate of 53%.

ETHICAL DILEMMA

1. What are the ethical issues that arise in a situation in which a parent refuses to have his or her child immunized?
2. What are the ethical issues that arise in a situation in which a person with a diagnosis of drug-resistant tuberculosis refuses to take his or her medications and has admitted that he or she "is out and about" in the community?

Nursing Care Plan

PATIENT WITH A COMMUNITY-ACQUIRED INFECTION

Mrs. Johnson is an 84-year-old woman who lives independently in a senior citizen housing project. She tends to avoid physician visits and does not believe in immunizations. She refuses the influenza vaccine each year on the basis that she is allergic to eggs since she suffers diarrhea when she drinks eggnog. Until one week ago, Mrs. Johnson was alert, oriented, continent, and able to enjoy social activities with her friends and family.

One week ago, her son noticed that she was increasingly lethargic, spent more time in bed, and had occasional urinary incontinence. Her appetite was markedly decreased. Mrs. Johnson stated that she felt very weak but had no complaints of pain or shortness of breath. Her son took her to see her physician who after physical examination diagnosed pneumonia, probably caused by *Streptococcus pneumoniae*.

Past Medical History	Psychosocial Data	Assessment Data
Cerebrovascular accident 9 years ago with resultant left hemiparesis Osteoporosis with loss of height Decreased vital capacity related to vertebral shortening Hypertension	Parents deceased of unknown causes Two sons both healthy Lives in small apartment and manages well with the assistance of her son, who lives nearby and visits her 3-4 times a week Eats one meal a day in a communal dining room and attends many social activities sponsored by the housing project; approximately 300 other residents live in the building, and 50-75 residents typically congregate for social events	Height 5'1", weight 110 lb Alert and oriented × 3 Quiet, withdrawn, drowsy *Skin:* Intact, overall coloring very pale *Respiratory:* Diminished breath sounds bilaterally; crackles in the right lower lobe; respirations 22-26, slightly shallow, symmetrical; infrequent, dry, nonproductive cough *Cardiovascular:* Apical pulse 90 and regular; strong peripheral pulses *Abdomen:* Soft, nontender, nondistended abdomen; normoactive bowel sounds *Musculoskeletal:* Full range of motion right side; weakened active ROM left side; full passive ROM left side; ambulates with quad cane; gait slightly unsteady ***Laboratory data*** WBC 18,000 *Sputum:* Unable to obtain *Urinalysis:* Within normal limits *Chest x-ray:* Consistent with right lower lobe pneumonia ***Medications*** furosemide (Lasix) 40 mg qd amoxicillin 500 mg tid

continued

NURSING DIAGNOSIS

Ineffective airway clearance related to secretions, advanced age, decreased vital capacity as evidenced by increased respiratory rate, crackles in the right lower lobe, nonproductive cough

NURSING INTERVENTIONS	EVALUATION OF EXPECTED OUTCOMES
Teach proper self-administration of antibiotic. Encourage liberal fluid intake, adequate nutrition, and frequent rest periods and explain rationale. Encourage usage of humidifier in home. Instruct in proper disposal of contaminated tissues. Encourage visits from family to ensure ability to take medication, take adequate fluid and diet, and to monitor for improvement in status. Instruct patient and family to contact physician in 2 days if condition does not improve.	No evidence of respiratory distress Respirations $< 24/\text{min}$ No dyspnea Able to consume previous dietary intake and adequate fluid intake Energy and activity restored to level before illness

NURSING DIAGNOSIS

Risk for injury related to weakness, acute illness, advanced age, and hemiparesis

NURSING INTERVENTIONS	EVALUATION OF EXPECTED OUTCOMES
Identify effects of illness on ability to perform self-care activities. Assess ability to care for self independently. Explore possibility of family staying with patient until acute aspect of illness is resolved. Encourage provision of safe environment (e.g., use of quad cane, removal of throw rugs).	Patient/family able to identify potential for injury Safe environment Patient/family comfortable with assistance required during acute illness Recuperates from illness without further injury

NURSING DIAGNOSIS

Knowledge deficit related to acute illness and possible preventive measures

NURSING INTERVENTIONS	EVALUATION OF EXPECTED OUTCOMES
Explain the rationale for rest, increased fluids, and adequate nutrition during recuperation. Teach the action, dosage, and side effects of antibiotic. Discuss preventive strategies to avoid recurrence; discuss the importance of seeking early medical attention for subtle changes that may signify onset of pneumonia or worsening of condition. Reeducate patient regarding the influenza vaccine and the benefits versus the risks. Teach patient to avoid persons with coughs and colds during flu season.	Verbalizes understanding of disease prevention and treatment Verbalizes reportable symptoms Verbalizes understanding of influenza vaccine

KEY CONCEPTS

- Infectious diseases result from a complex interaction among the agent, the host, and the environment.
- Properties of infectious agents that are influenced by characteristics of the host and the environment include infectivity, pathogenicity, virulence, and immunogenicity.
- Transmission of infectious agents occurs through contact, airborne, vehicle, and vectorborne routes.
- Immunizations with vaccines or toxoids produce artificially acquired active immunity.
- Routine vaccination of infants and children include immunizations for diphtheria, tetanus, pertussis, polio, measles, mumps, rubella, *Haemophilus influenzae* type b, and hepatitis B.
- *Healthy People 2000* is a visionary agenda to increase the span of healthy life and to reduce health disparities for the American people.
- The nurse's role in prevention is multifaceted and includes primary, secondary, and tertiary prevention strategies.
- Common bacterial infections include staphylococcal and streptococcal infections, tuberculosis, and Lyme disease.
- Meningococcal infections, legionellosis, and clostridium infections are less prevalent but serious conditions.
- Food intoxications and infections are prevalent but are often not diagnosed.
- Measles, mumps, rubella, and chickenpox are viral infections that have a relatively low incidence in the United States.
- Infectious mononucleosis, influenza, and Hepatitis B are viral infections and are found worldwide.
- With the exception of pinworms, helminthic infestations are not common in the United States.
- Six STDs are reportable to public health authorities: AIDS, syphilis, gonorrhea, chancroid, lymphogranuloma venereum, and granuloma inguinale.
- Emerging community-acquired infections include strains of *E. coli,* resistant strains of *S. pneumoniae,* invasive Group A streptococcal infections, and the Hantavirus.

CRITICAL THINKING EXERCISES

1 What sociologic factors contribute to the spread of infectious disease?
2 Why is it a mistake to wait until a child begins school before having him or her immunized?
3 What is the danger of making pets of wild animals?
4 Why are STDs the most difficult to prevent and control?
5 What social factors are contributing to the emergence of new and resistant strains of microorganisms?

REFERENCES AND ADDITIONAL READINGS

Alder MB and others: Health promotion and disease prevention for the international traveler, *Nurse Pract* 16(5):10; 12-14; 16-18; 1991.

American Thoracic Society: Control of tuberculosis in the United States, *Am Rev Resp Dis* 146(6):1623-1633, 1992.

Beneson AS: *Control of communicable diseases in man,* ed 15, Washington, DC, 1990, American Public Health Association.

Bentley DW: Tuberculosis in long-term facilities, *Infect Control Hosp Epidemiol* 11(1):42-46, 1990.

Biester DJ: Childhood immunization: nursing's role and responsibility, *J Pediatr Nurs* 7(1):65-66, 1992.

Blaylock B: The aging immune system and common infections in elderly patients, *J Enter Nurs* 20(2):63-67, 1993.

Boley T and others: Herpes zoster: etiology, clinical course, and suggested management, *J Am Acad Nurse Pract* 2(2):64-68, 1990.

Boskovich SJ: New concepts in nursing management of the TB patient: a community training program, *J Community Health Nurs* 11(1):45-49, 1994.

Burgess W: The great white plague and other epidemics: lessons from early visiting nursing, *J Home Health Care Pract* 6(1):12-17, 1993.

Centers for Disease Control and Prevention: A strategic plan for the elimination of tuberculosis in the United States,

MMWR 38(Suppl S-3):1-25, 1989.

Centers for Disease Control and Prevention: Summary of notifiable diseases: United States, 1993, *MMWR*, 42(53), 1994.

Cuzzell JZ: Clues: pain, burning, and itching, *Am J Nurs* 90(7):15-16, 1990.

Czurylo KT and others: Dealing with a hidden hazard: methicillin-resistant staphylococcus aureus, *Nursing* 21(12):68-69, 1991.

Dawkins BJ: Genital herpes simplex infections, *Prim Care* 1(17):95-113, 1990.

Elpern EH and others: Tuberculosis update: new challenges of an old disease, *Medsurg Nurs* 2(3):176-183, 1993.

Embry FC: A guide through the maze of viral hepatitis, *J Home Health Care Pract* 6(1):18-26, 1993.

Falco V and others: Legionella pneumophilia: a cause of severe community-acquired pneumonia, *Chest* 100(4):1007-1011, 1991.

Gaffney KF and others: "Think TB": new focus for family assessment, *Pediatr Nurs* 20(1):36-38, 1994.

Glittenberg JE: Problems of global control of tuberculosis, *J Prof Nurs* 6(2):73, 129, 1990.

Graham JM and others: Chlamydial infections, *Prim Care* 17(1):85-93, 1990.

Gurevich I: Counseling the patient with herpes, *RN* 53(2):22-28, 1990.

Gurevich I: Varicella zoster and herpes simplex virus infections, *Heart Lung* 21(1):85-93, 1992.

Harkness GA and others: Streptococcus pyogenes outbreak in a long-term care facility, *Am J Infect Control* 209(3):142-148, 1992.

Harning AT: Stirring up trouble: food-related emergencies, *JEMS* 17(8):24-30, 79-83, 1992.

Healthy People 2000: National Health Promotion and Disease Prevention Objectives. Washington, DC, US Government Printing Office, 1991, DHHS Publication No (PHS) 91-50213.

Hudacek SS: Lyme disease: facts & essential assessments, *Adv Clin Care* 5(4):6-9, 1990.

Igoe JB and others: Meeting the challenge of immunizing the nation's children, *Pediatr Nurs* 17(6):583-585, 1991.

Ismeurt RL and others: Tuberculosis: a new threat from an old nemesis, *Home Healthc Nurse* 11(4):16-23, 1993.

Kamper C: Treatment of Rocky Mountain spotted fever, *J Pediatr Health Care* 5(4):216-222, 1991.

Lippman H: Taking the fight to the streets, *RN* 56(9):34-39, 1993.

Lisanti P and others: An overview of viral hepatitis: A through E, *AORN J* 59(5):997-998, 1000-1005, 1994.

Long CO and others: The tuberculin skin test, *Home Healthc Nurse* 11(3):13-18, 1993.

Mason JO: Food irradiation—promising technology for public health, *Public Health Rep* 107(5):489-490, 1992.

Melvin SY: Syphilis: resurgence of an old disease, *Prim Care* 17(1):47-57, 1990.

Moy JG: The patient with gonococcal infection, *Prim Care* 17(1):59-63, 1990.

Nettina SL: Syphilis: a new look at an old killer, *Am J Nurs* 90(4):68-70, 1990.

Nettina SL and others: Diagnosis and management of sexually transmitted genital lesions, *Nurse Pract* 15(1):20, 1990.

Noble RC: Sequelae of sexually transmitted diseases, *Prim Care* 17(1):173-181, 1990.

Powell MA: Question and answer: infectious mononucleosis, *J Am Acad Nurse Pract* 5(2):89-91, 1993.

Rapini RP: Venereal warts, *Prim Care* 17(1):127-144, 1990.

Richards MS and others: Investigation of a staphylococcal food poisoning outbreak in a centralized school lunch program, *Public Health Rep* 108(6):24-30, 79-83; 1993.

Richardson JP: Tetanus and tetanus immunization in long-term care facilities, *Infect Control Hosp Epidemiol* 14(10):591-594, 1993.

Robinson KR: The role of nursing in the influenza epidemic of 1918-1919, *Nurs Forum* 25(2):19-26, 1990.

Semonin-Holleran R: Taking the sting out of summer, *RN* 56(7):40-46, 1993.

Sharts-Engel NC: An overview of maternal-child infectious diseases, *MCN* 16(1):58, 1991.

Swanson JM and others: Psychosocial aspects of genital herpes: a review of the literature, *Public Health Nurs* 7(2):96-104, 1990.

Walsh ML and others: Update on antimicrobial agents, *Nurs Clin North Am* 26(2):341-360, 1991.

Weingarten CT and others: Measles: again an epidemic, *Pediatr Nurs* 18(4):369-371, 1992.

White MC: Infections and infection risks in home care settings, *Infect Control Hosp Epidemiol* 13(9):535-539, 1992.

Willis D: Lyme disease, *J Neurosci Nurs* 23(4):211-219, 1991.

Yu VL: Legionnaire's disease: new understanding of community-acquired pneumonia, *Hosp Pract* 28(10A):63-67, 1993.

CHAPTER 12

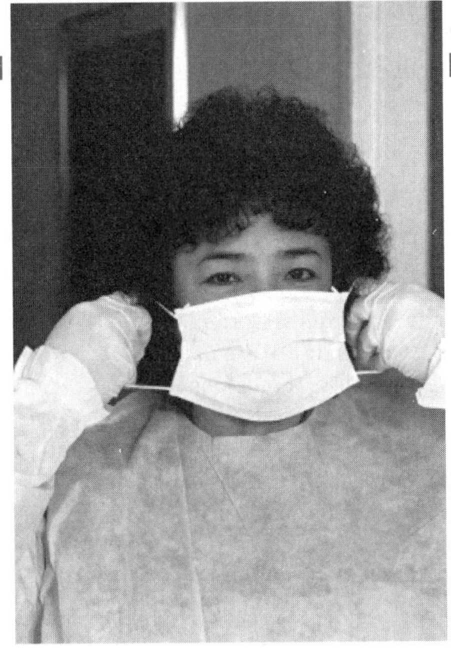

Nosocomial Infections

CHAPTER OBJECTIVES

1. Differentiate between nosocomial and community-acquired infections.
2. Name the most common sites, hospital services, and types of organisms associated with hospital-acquired infections.
3. List the risk factors that increase a patient's susceptibility to infection.
4. Identify measures to prevent and control urinary tract infections, surgical wound infections, pneumonia, and bacteremia.
5. Define antiseptic and disinfectant.
6. Identify effective surveillance methods for hospital-associated infections.
7. Contrast the differences among category-specific isolation, disease-specific isolation, universal precautions, and body substance isolation.
8. Discuss the emotional responses that may be experienced by persons with nosocomial infections.

KEY WORDS

abscess
antiseptic
bacteremia
colonize
control
disinfection
endemic
endogenous
Escherichia coli
etiologic
exogenous
fomite
high risk
infection
isolation
Klebsiella organisms
nosocomial
pathogen
pseudomonades
reservoir
source
spores
Staphylococcus
sterilization
Streptococcus
surveillance
universal precautions

HOSPITAL INFECTIONS

Infections have always been associated with hospitalization. A **nosocomial** infection is defined as a clinically active infection that occurs in a hospitalized patient and was not present or incubating at the time of admission. Residual infections that were acquired in the hospital but appear after discharge are also classified as nosocomial. The term *nosocomial* is derived from the Greek word *nosos* (illness or disease) and *komeo* (to take care of). One of the first private hospitals in ancient Greece was called a nosocomium.

In contrast to nosocomial infections, a *community-acquired* infection is found in patients who enter the hospital with a known or incubating infection. In this case, the symptoms of infection may be present or may appear during hospitalization. Any infection, whether hospital-acquired or community-acquired, may be serious if it spreads to other susceptible persons.

In all people, microorganisms are present in the nose, throat, and intestinal tract and on the skin. Although some microorganisms are harmless and some are beneficial, others have the potential to precipitate a hospital infection if the circumstances are favorable. Any patient or hospital employee may either be a source or a recipient of a nosocomial infection.

The hospital is an environment that is contaminated by patients, visitors, and hospital personnel. People admitted to hospitals are exposed to an increased variety and increased concentration of microbial agents. A **reservoir** is the location where an infection-causing microorganism is usually found. Patients, healthcare personnel, healthcare equipment, and the environment are reservoirs that have been associated with nosocomial infections. A **source** is the location from which the organism is transmitted to a host. The reservoir and the source may be the same location, such as an infected wound, or the source may be a piece of equipment which is contaminated and subsequently has contact with a susceptible host. Portals of exit for infectious agents from the human host include the respiratory, gastrointestinal, and genitourinary tracts. Skin, wounds, and blood can also serve as portals of exit.

All people, as well as the environment, are **colonized** with a multitude of microorganisms. Human beings live in harmony with a family of microorganisms that are referred to as normal flora. However, when these normal flora invade a body part in which they are not "normal," an infection may occur. For example, a serious bloodstream infection may occur when ***Staphylococcus* epidermidis,** which is part of the normal skin flora, invades the vascular system by way of a intravenous (IV) catheter. Patients are often exposed to new organisms that are peculiar to the hospital environment and that have developed increased virulence and drug resistance. Methicillin-resistant *Staphylococcus aureus* (MRSA), aminoglycoside-resistant gram-negative organisms, penicillin-resistant pneumococci, and, most recently, vancomycin-resistant enterococci (VRE) and multiple–drug-resistant tuberculosis (MDRTB) are examples of such organisms. Illness decreases the resistance of the body and therefore increases the patient's susceptibility to infection.

Diagnostic and treatment methods may also weaken or bypass normal defensive barriers and place some patients at **high risk** for nosocomial infections. Medical-surgical supplies and equipment may become contaminated while they are being used. Ventilators, respiratory therapy equipment, pressure monitoring devices, IV catheters, and urinary catheters are all examples of equipment that bypass normal body defenses and become a source of infection. Even prepackaged sterile supplies that are designed to protect the patient can become contaminated and serve as a source of nosocomial infection.

Incidence of Nosocomial Infections

In 1969 the Centers for Disease Control (CDC) initiated the National Nosocomial Infections Study (NNIS) to gather ongoing data from a variety of hospitals in the United States. Their statistics indicated that when all infections from all types of hospitals are considered, there are approximately 3.4 nosocomial infections per 100 discharged patients, or an infection rate of 3.4%. Infection rates appear to be associated with the type of facility and service that is offered. Large teaching hospitals have the highest reported incidence of nosocomial infections, and small nonteaching hospitals have the lowest. It has been suggested that this latter finding is partly a result of the severity of the illnesses and the increased length of hospitalization that is often found in larger hospitals (Centers for Disease Control, 1986).

The Study of the Efficacy of Nosocomial Infection Control (SENIC) represents a large-scale study conducted by the CDC during 1975 and 1976. In this study, a statistical sample of all U.S. hospitals was used. The national nosocomial infection rate was determined to be 5.7 nosocomial infections per 100 admissions (Haley and others, 1985b).

Other reported nosocomial rates range from 3% to 15% of all patients admitted to hospitals. However, the 6% rate established by the SENIC study is the generally quoted rate. It is estimated that more than 8 million extra hospital days are required every year to care for patients with nosocomial infections. The estimated annual cost of this care is approximately $4 billion nationwide. It is also estimated that 20,000 deaths per year are directly attributable, and another 60,000 are partly attributable to nosocomial infections. These figures indicate that nosocomial infections are a leading cause of death in the United States (Haley, 1986). Infection control programs can be a cost benefit to the hospital if the program results in decreased morbidity and mortality related to nosocomial infections.

The 1984 NNIS data show that the urinary tract is the most common site of infection in hospitalized patients, followed by lower respiratory tract and surgical wound infections. Infections of these three sites account for almost 75% of all nosocomial infections. The hospital services with the highest rates include surgical, medical, and gynecologic units, followed by obstetric and newborn nursery units. ***Escherichia coli***, *Pseudomonas aeruginosa*, *Enterococcus faecalis*, and *S. aureus* are the most frequently reported **pathogens.**

High-Risk Patients

Nosocomial infections can be classified as either exogenous or endogenous. **Exogenous** infections are acquired from sources outside the patient, or from the environment. **Endogenous** infections result when circumstances permit the potentially virulent normal flora that reside within the host to multiply, which causes a pathologic condition within the patient. When endogenous infections occur, the host's normal defense mechanisms are deficient or compromised. A person with deficient defense mechanisms is called a *compromised host*.

Many underlying host factors determine whether a person develops an infection. Age and underlying disease are two of the most important determinants. Newborn infants, especially those of low birth weight, have immature immune systems and therefore have fewer physical resources to combat infectious microorganisms. The elderly have less efficient immune systems and thus have a decreased resistance to infection. Chronic diseases such as renal failure, diabetes, or cancer, and conditions such as burns, malnutrition, or shock can all predispose a patient to infection. Treatment measures that invade body cavities bypass natural defense mechanisms and create a direct route for microorganisms to gain entrance to body organs and cause infection (Box 12-1). Urinary catheterization, IV infusions, peritoneal dialysis, and surgical incisions of

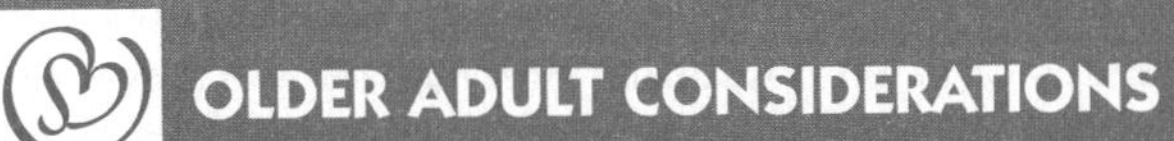

OLDER ADULT CONSIDERATIONS

Nosocomial Infections

- Older adults have less efficient immune systems and therefore a decreased resistance to infection.
- An older adult's response to antibiotic therapy may be slow.
- Chronic diseases predipose older adults to infection.
- Treatment measures that invade body cavities bypass natural defense mechanisms that may already be compromised in the older adult.

BOX 12-1

FACTORS THAT INCREASE THE RISK OF INFECTION

DISEASES OR DISORDERS

Burns
Chronic disease
Circulatory impairment
Cirrhosis
Diabetes mellitus
Extensive dermatitis
Hepatitis
Immune deficiencies
Malignancies
Malnutrition
Open wounds
Persons receiving immunosuppressant drugs
Renal failure
Shock
Transplant recipients
Trauma

THERAPEUTIC TECHNIQUES

Bladder catheterization
Central nervous system shunts
Decubitus care
Hyperalimentation
Immunosuppressive therapy
IV cannulation
Radiation therapy
Respiratory therapy
Surgery
Tracheostomy

the skin are examples of treatment interventions that can allow microbial access. Ionizing radiation and immunosuppressive drug therapy can depress the immune response and place the patient at a high risk for infection. The extensive use of antibiotics may also be responsible for the decrease in host resistance and the development of more virulent and resistant strains of organisms.

Methods of Transmission

Microorganisms are transmitted by various routes, and a single microorganism may be transmitted by more than one route. For example, the varicella-zoster virus (chickenpox) can spread by the airborne route and by direct contact. There are four main routes by which organisms are transmitted to a susceptible host: contact, airborne, vehicle, and vectorborne transmission.

Contact transmission is the most common method by which microorganisms are transmitted from one person to another. Contact transmission can be divided into three subgroups: direct contact, indirect contact, and droplet contact. *Direct contact* involves person-to-person contact between the source and the susceptible person. Contact occurs constantly during daily patient care, with hands having the most contact with the patient. Therefore, thorough handwashing, even when gloves have been worn, is the best means of preventing transmission by direct contact. *Indirect contact* involves personal contact of the susceptible host with a contaminated intermediate object, or a **fomite.** For example, an inadequately disinfected endoscope can indirectly transfer organisms. *Droplet contact* occurs when an infectious agent briefly passes through the air. The infected sources and susceptible host are usually within a few feet of each other. This is considered "contact" transmission rather than airborne, because droplets usually travel no more than 3 feet. Organisms are usually dispersed when an infected person coughs, sneezes, or talks and during the performance of certain procedures such as suctioning.

Airborne transmission occurs when infectious agents remain suspended in the air for long periods of time. Organisms carried in this manner can be widely dispersed by air currents before being inhaled by or deposited on the susceptible host. Tuberculosis (TB) is transmitted by this route. Good ventilation systems help prevent the airborne transmission of infectious agents.

Vehicle transmission occurs when contaminated items such as blood, blood products, food, water, or drugs serve as the vector of transmission to multiple persons. Examples of this type of transmission are the spread of salmonellosis from contaminated dairy products or hepatitis A from contaminated food.

Vectorborne transmission occurs when insects or other animals serve as intermediate hosts for an infectious agent. For example, malaria is transmitted by mosquitoes, and Rocky Mountain spotted fever is transmitted by ticks. Vectors have not played a significant role in the transmission of nosocomial infections in the United States.

TYPES OF NOSOCOMIAL INFECTIONS

Urinary Tract Infections

Urinary tract infections (UTIs) are the most common nosocomial infections that occur in hospitalized patients. Approximately 80% of the nosocomial UTIs are associated with urinary tract manipulations (Mandell, Douglas, Bennett, 1990). Catheter-associated UTIs are caused by a variety of pathogens, including *E. coli,* and ***Klebsiella*** **organisms,** *protei, enterococci,* **pseudomonades,** *Enterobacter, Serratia,* and *Candida organisms.* Many of these microorganisms are part of the patient's endogenous bowel flora but can also be acquired by cross-contamination from other patients, the hands of hospital personnel, contaminated solutions, or contaminated equipment.

Host factors that appear to increase a person's susceptibility to catheter-associated UTIs include debilitation, chronic disease, and the presence of pathogenic bacteria in the periurethral area. Women and the elderly have higher rates of such infections. Although most UTIs are of low morbidity and mortality, infections can occasionally lead to such complications as prostatitis, epididymitis, cystitis, pyelonephritis, and **bacteremia.**

Infecting microorganisms gain access by several routes. Microorganisms that colonize in the meatus or distal urethra can be introduced directly into the bladder when the catheter is inserted. Infecting microorganisms can also migrate to the bladder along the outside of the catheter and the periurethral mucous sheath or along the internal lumen of the catheter after the collection bag or catheter drainage tube junction has been contaminated.

Nursing measures that can prevent or control urinary catheter-associated infections relate to optimal catheter care for patients who require drainage systems. The most direct way to prevent catheter-associated bacteriuria is to avoid catheterization. Urinary catheters should be inserted only when necessary and should be left in place only as long as necessary. Indications for the use of an indwelling catheter include relief of urinary obstruction, a neurogenic bladder, and as a means of accurate measurement of output. Catheters must be inserted using aseptic technique and

BOX 12-2 **Nursing Process**

URINARY TRACT INFECTION (UTI)

ASSESSMENT

Frequency, urgency, burning on urination
Fever and chills
History of previous infections
Urine culture
Presence of occult blood

NURSING DIAGNOSES

Altered urinary elimination related to urinary tract infection
Pain related to inflammation
Knowledge deficit related to causes of urinary tract infection and prevention measures

NURSING INTERVENTIONS

Give antibiotic therapy regularly and on time even if symptoms cease.
Maintain 3 to 4 L/day of fluids if possible.
Discuss specific procedures such as x-ray examinations or catheterization if necessary.
Stress the need for follow-up care and additional urine cultures.
Teach female patients about good perineal hygeine and voiding after intercourse.

EVALUATION OF EXPECTED OUTCOMES

Urine bacteria count refects infection is not present; bacteria count less than 1×10^5 organisms/ml of urine
States that urinary symptoms are relieved
Correctly describes the signs and symptoms of UTI, the risk factors, the rationale for increasing fluids, the routine for taking medications, and the need for follow-up care

sterile equipment. The routine use of indwelling catheters for incontinence is not appropriate unless there is concern about massive skin breakdown (Box 12-2).

Once a urethral catheter is in place, UTIs are best avoided by maintaining a closed system and by minimizing the duration of catheterization. Urine specimens should be obtained without opening the catheter collection tube junction. Special ports in the system allow for aseptic collection of urinary specimens. These ports should be cleansed with a disinfectant before a sterile needle and syringe are used for aspiration of the urine.

Urinary flow should be unobstructed. The catheter and collecting tubing should be prevented from kinking, and the collecting bag should be emptied regularly, using a separate collecting container for each patient. Nosocomial transmission has occurred between patients when contaminated urine-collecting devices have been used for more than one patient (Rutala and others, 1981). Routine changing of indwelling catheters does not reduce the risk of UTIs.

NURSE ALERT

UTIs can best be avoided by maintaining an undisturbed closed drainage system and by minimizing the duration of catheterization.

Handwashing is extremely important and should be done immediately before and after any manipulation of the catheter, even if gloves have been worn. It is imperative that hands be washed between handling the catheters of different patients (Box 12-3).

Nosocomial Pneumonia

Nosocomial pneumonia is the second most common nosocomial infection. It accounts for 15% of all nosocomial infections in U.S. hospitals. Nosocomial pneumonia is associated with mortalities that range from 20% to 50% and is the most common fatal nosocomial infection (Mandell, Douglas, Bennett, 1990).

A majority of these pneumonias occur in intensive care unit settings or in postanesthesia care units. The NNIS consistently reports that more than 60% of all nosocomial pneumonias are caused by aerobic gram-negative bacilla. *P. aeruginosa* alone accounts for 16.9% of nosocomial pneumonias. *Klebsiella* and *Enterobacter* organisms, *E. coli*, *Serratia marcescens*, and protei are other gram-negative bacteria that may cause nosocomial pneumonia. *S. aureus*, a gram-positive organism, is the second most common **etiologic** agent that causes hospital-acquired pneumonia, and it accounts for 12.9% of the cases (Centers for Disease Control, 1986). Less common etiologic agents that cause hospital-acquired pneumonia include anaerobic mouth flora, ***Streptococcus*** *pneumonia*, *Branhamella catarrhalis*, Influenza A virus, *Haemophilus influenzae*, *legionellae*, and *Aspergillus* (Centers for Disease Control, 1982b).

BOX 12-3

CONTROL AND PREVENTION OF UTIs

- Wash hands before and after urinary manipulation.
- Catheterize only when necessary.
- Insert catheter using aseptic technique and sterile equipment.
- Secure catheter.
- Maintain a closed drainage system.
- Obtain urine samples aseptically.
- Maintain an unobstructed flow.

It is also now evident that *Legionella pneumophila* accounts for a small number of cases of nosocomial pneumonia. Because of the special testing techniques required to diagnose *L. pneumophila,* the true abundance of this pathogen is unknown. Some hospitals have experienced clusters of nosocomial *Legionella* pneumonia, which are usually related to environmental factors such as contamination of portable water- or air-conditioning systems.

Nosocomial lower respiratory viral infections can occur and often reflect the occurrence of a virus in the community. During community outbreaks, viruses are introduced into the hospital by patients, employees, and visitors. These viral infections may be particularly severe in high-risk, debilitated patients. Respiratory syncytial virus (RSV), parainfluenza virus, and influenza are responsible for a large portion of viral nosocomial pneumonia cases.

A number of factors predispose patients to hospital-acquired pneumonia. Intubation of the respiratory tract is associated with a high incidence of nosocomial pneumonia because endotracheal tubes bypass the protective defense mechanisms of the upper respiratory tract. Hospitalized patients also often have impaired host defenses as a result of clinical conditions such as chronic obstructive pulmonary disease, cystic fibrosis, leukemia, central nervous system depression (coma), and electrolyte imbalances. These patients can become colonized with potential pathogens from their own endogenous flora or from exogenous sources, such as contaminated respiratory therapy equipment and the hands of hospital personnel. A colonized patient may become infected through the aspiration of upper respiratory tract secretions.

Diagnosing nosocomial pneumonia may be difficult. A positive culture of respiratory tract secretions does not distinguish between **colonization** of the upper and lower respiratory tract. Therefore to make a diagnosis, the clinician must rely on a change in clinical symptoms, such as altered mental status, fever, chest x-ray films, cough, sputum production, and an elevated leukocyte count. However, these clinical conditions may be present without the occurrence of pneumonia.

The prevention of nosocomial respiratory tract infections is based on reducing the acquisition of potential bacterial pathogens in the upper airways and thereby decreasing the risk for aspiration of these organisms. Gloves should be worn during all contact with respiratory secretions. Hands should be washed after contact with respiratory secretions, even if gloves have been worn. Hands must be washed before and after contact with a patient who is intubated or who has had a recent tracheostomy.

General nursing techniques such as maintaining an open airway; having the patient turn, cough, and deep breathe; and early ambulation after surgery are important interventions in preventing postoperative pneumonia. Before surgery, patients should receive instructions regarding measures that will reduce the risk of nosocomial pneumonia. Patients should demonstrate and practice adequate coughing and deep breathing. It is improtant to control pain in a postoperative patient so that it does not interfere with coughing and deep breathing.

Closely adhering to the guidelines for the use of respiratory therapy equipment also decreases the incidence of nosocomial pneumonia. Only sterile fluids should be nebulized or used in a humidifier. Nebulizers (including medication nebulizers) and their reservoirs and cascade humidifiers should be changed or replaced with sterilized or disinfected equipment every 24 hours. Warm humidifiers that create droplets to humidify should not be used. Ventilator tubing was once routinely changed every 24 hours, but data now suggest that circuit changes every 48 hours or at even longer intervals do not increase the risk of nosocomial pneumonia (Wenzel, 1993).

Patients who have a tracheostomy should have it suctioned using sterile techniques. The risk of cross-contamination and excessive trauma increases with frequent suctioning. Therefore suctioning should be done using a "no-touch" technique and sterile gloves on both hands. A new sterile catheter should be used for each series of suctioning. If flushing the catheter is necessary because of tenacious mucus, sterile fluid should be used to remove the secretions. Fluid used for one series of suctioning should be discarded. A closed system multiuse catheter is now used in many hospitals. After the catheter is used, a sheath slides over it to protect it from environmental contamination. These catheters are usually changed every 24 hours (Wenzel, 1993).

Enteral feeding may increase the risk of aspiration and pneumonia. Using continuous rather than bolus feeding, maintaining and removing residual, and maintaining the patient in an upright position may decrease the risk of aspiration and subsequent pneumonia.

Patients in intensive care units are given one of several prophylactic regimens to prevent stress bleeding. Data suggest that patients who are receiving sucralfate have less risk of pneumonia than those receiving H_2O blockers or antacids but have the same protection against stress bleeding (Wenzel, 1993).

Patients with potentially transmissible respiratory infections should be isolated from other patients according to the hospital isolation guidelines. To prevent the acquisition of nosocomial viral infections from employees, healthcare workers with acute respiratory infections should not be assigned to the direct care of high-risk patients. In addition, all healthcare workers who are assigned to care for high-risk patients should receive an influenza vaccine annually to decrease the risk of transmission to patients (Box 12-4).

BOX 12-4

CONTROL AND PREVENTION OF NOSOCOMIAL PNEUMONIA

- Wear gloves for all contact with respiratory secretions.
- Wash hands after contact with respiratory secretions, even if gloves have been worn.
- Maintain open airways.
- Teach patients how to cough and deep breathe before surgery.
- Control pain.
- Follow guidelines for the use of respiratory therapy equipment.
- Use sterile technique when suctioning a tracheostomy.
- Wear sterile gloves on both hands and use a "no-touch" technique when suctioning.
- Elevate the head of a patient who is receiving enteral feedings.
- Isolate patients with potentially transmissible respiratory infections.

Surgical Wound Infections

In most hospitals, surgical wound infections are the third most common type of nosocomial infections. They are divided into categories of incision or deep infections. Incisional infections account for 60% to 80% of surgical wound infections, and the remainder are classified as deep infections.

A wound is considered to be infected if purulent material drains from it, even without a positive wound culture. Wounds are classified according to the likelihood and degree of wound contamination at the time of the operation. A widely accepted classification scheme outlined by the American College of Surgeons (1984) predicts the relative probability that a wound will become infected. Clean wounds are those in which neither the gastrointestinal, respiratory, or genitourinary tract nor the pharyngeal cavity is entered and in which no inflammation is found during surgery. Clean wounds are also cases in which no breaks in aseptic technique have occurred. These wounds have a 1% to 5% risk of infection. Clean-contaminated operations are those in which the gastrointestinal, respiratory, or genitourinary tract is entered but in which significant spillage did not occur during the procedure. These wounds have a 3% to 11% risk of infection. Contaminated wounds result from surgical procedures in which there has been a major break in aseptic technique, gross spillage from a contaminated system, or in which acute inflammation without pus has been encountered. Fresh traumatic wounds also fit in this category. Contaminated wounds have a 10% to 17% risk of infection. Dirty wounds include old traumatic wounds and wounds with pus or a perforated viscus. These wounds have more than a 27% risk of infection (Centers for Disease Control, 1985).

Another index to predict the likelihood of surgical wound infection is a multivariate index that was developed and tested during the SENIC study. This index includes four risk factors: (1) having an abdominal operation; (2) having an operation that lasts longer than 2 hours; (3) having a contaminated, dirty, or infected operation by the traditional classification system; and (4) having three or more discharge diagnoses (Haley and others, 1985a).

NNIS has developed a different surgical wound infection risk index, which includes the following elements: (1) if the patient's wound class was contaminated or dirty; (2) if the patient was assigned an American Society of Anesthesiology (ASA) score of 3, 4, or 5 by the anesthesiologist before surgery; and (3) if the procedure lasted longer than T hours, in which T is the approximate 75th percentile of the duration of surgery for an operative procedure as reported to the NNIS database. A patient's risk category is determined by adding the number of risk factors present. Therefore a patient's risk score may range from 0 to 3 (Centers for Disease Control, 1991). Investigators believe that the NNIS surgical wound infection index is a better indicator of patients who are at risk for surgical wound infections than wound class alone.

Age is one host factor that may influence the risk of infection. Persons over age 65 have twice the chance of contracting nosocomial surgical wound infections as younger persons. Obesity, severe malnutrition, infection at other sites, and extended preoperative stays in the hospital are other host factors that are associated with an increased risk of infection.

Gram-negative aerobic bacteria account for approximately 40% of the pathogens isolated from surgical wounds. However, *S. aureus* remains the most commonly isolated species from surgical wounds. Microorganisms that infect surgical wounds can be acquired from the patient, the hospital environment, or hospital personnel. However, the patient's own flora are responsible for most infections. Sources of infection include the gastrointestinal, respiratory, genital, and urinary tracts, as well as the skin and anterior nares. Whether acquired from the environment or the patient's own flora, most infections appear to be acquired in the operating room. Few infections are acquired after the operation if there is primary closure of the wound. Open wounds and the presence of drains increase the risk of infection in the postoperative period.

Measures to prevent surgical wound infection actually begin before the operation. An important preoperative measure is the treatment of any active infection before surgery. Shortening the patient's preoperative hospital stay also reduces the risk of infection. Historically, hair adjacent to or in the area of the proposed surgery has been removed to prevent it from contaminating the wound during the operation. However, several recent studies suggest that shaving with a razor can injure the skin and increase the risk of infection. Therefore clipping hair, using a depilatory, or not shaving at all have been suggested in place of shaving (Cruse, Foord, 1980).

Before surgery, skin at the operative site should be thoroughly cleansed with an **antiseptic** solution to remove all superficial skin flora, soil, and debris. The surgical team must also scrub their hands to minimize the normal flora on their skin. The surgical scub is designed to kill and remove as many bacteria as possible, including resident bacteria. After they have scrubbed their hands, the members of the surgical team wear sterile gloves, which act as an additional barrier against the transfer of microorganisms to the surgical wound.

To reduce airborne contamination, modern operating rooms have ventilation systems that produce 20 changes of highly filtered air per hour. Some operating rooms, especially those used for orthopedic surgeries that involve joint replacements, have installed laminar flow ventilation units.

Operative technique is the most important measure to prevent wound infection. For example, perforation of the bowel during surgery prolongs the operation and increases the risk of postoperative infection.

Another approach to preventing surgical wound infection is the use of prophylactic antimicrobial therapy. Prophylactic antibiotics are recommended for operations that are associated with a high risk of infection or for operations that are considered severe or life-threatening. Antibiotics used for prophylaxis should be started shortly before the operation and promptly discontinued after the operation. The area may also be irrigated with antibiotic solutions during the operative procedure. One highly recommended preventive measure, which has resulted from the findings on the SENIC study, is to report the surgical wound infection rates to individual surgeons. This reporting may decrease surgical wound infection rates by 20% (Haley, 1985a).

The postoperative period usually does not contribute greatly to the risk of surgical wound infections. However, wounds can become contaminated and infected if they are not handled with aseptic technique. Aseptic technique is especially important if the wound is not completely closed. Wounds should be kept covered with a sterile dressing until they are sealed, which is usually approximately 24 hours after the operation. Nursing personnel can reduce the risk of surgical wound infections by washing their hands and by using a "no-touch" technique when changing surgical wound dressings. If the wound becomes infected, patients should be placed on either drainage-secretion precautions or contact isolation (Box 12-5).

Nosocomial Bacteremia

Nosocomial **bacteremia** is defined as the isolation of an organism from a properly obtained blood culture specimen in a patient who has clinical signs of sepsis and who was admitted with neither signs and symptoms of infection nor a positive blood culture. Nosocomial bacteremia can be divided into two categories. Primary bacteremia occurs without any recognizable focus of infection with the same organism at another

BOX 12-5

CONTROL AND PREVENTION OF SURGICAL WOUND INFECTIONS

- Assess for infections that may need treatment before surgery is performed.
- Instead of using a razor, use a depilatory or clip hair before the surgery.
- Wash hands before and after changing a surgical wound dressing.
- Maintain aseptic technique and a "no-touch" technique when changing surgical wound dressings.
- Patients with infected wounds should be placed on drainage or secretion precautions or placed in isolation.

site. These infections are considered to be related to IV fluid therapy when an IV line is present. Secondary bacteremia results from an infection at another site. This section focuses on primary nosocomial bacteremia that is associated with intravascular devices. Secondary bacteremia is reduced by giving attention to the prevention and control of infections at other body sites.

Intravascular-related infections consist of those related to microbial contamination of the cannula, the cannula wound, or the infusate. Most of these infections are cannula-related. Factors that influence a patient's risk of acquiring cannula-related infection include the patient's susceptibility, type of cannula used, method of insertion, duration of cannulation, and purpose of the cannula. Plastic cannulas have been associated with a higher risk of infection than steel cannulas. Peripheral catheters that remain in place more than 72 hours are associated with a marked increase in infection rates. Central cannulas, which are used for monitoring central venous pressure, are also associated with high rates of infection.

Staphylococci are the most commonly encountered pathogens in catheter-related infections. *S. aureus* is a common cause of device-associated infection. However, coagulase-negative staphylococci (e.g., *S. epidermidis*) have become a more common cause of these infections in recent years. Staphylococci account for one half to two thirds of the bacteremia associated with these devices. Gram-negative bacteria and *Candida* organisms are also important pathogens in the cause of bacteremia (Centers for Disease Control, 1982a). Infections related to microbial contamination of infusate are far less common than cannula-related infections. Contamination can occur during the manufacturing process or during hospital preparation. Infections caused by contaminated infusate usually result from gram-negative bacilli.

Nursing interventions are important in preventing vascular-related infections. As with other nosocomial infections, handwashing is of major importance. Hands should always be washed before inserting an IV cannula and before performing any manipulation of the cannula or line. Gloves should be worn for cannula insertion.

Inserting the cannula into the upper extremity of an adult is preferred over the lower extremity. The IV site should be scrubbed with antiseptic before venipuncture. After insertion, the cannula should be secured to stabilize it at the insertion site, and sterile dressing should be applied over the insertion site. The date of the insertion should be recorded in a place in which it can be easily found. Many institutions record the date of insertion in both the medical record and on the dressing or tape at the IV site.

Patients with IV devices should be evaluated at least every 8 hours for evidence of cannula-related complications. An evaluation can be performed by palpating the insertion site through the dressing or by visually examining the site through a transparent polyurethane dressing. Pain or tenderness warrants the removal of the dressing and inspection of the site. Hospital policies usually require peripheral cannulas to be replaced every 48 to 72 hours. However, several studies have demonstrated that peripheral catheters can be left in place more than 72 hours without an increased risk of infection (Wenzel, 1993). If a peripheral IV remains in place more than 72 hours, the site should be inspected and cared for often. A silver-impregnated cuffed catheter and an antiseptic-impregnated catheter are now available and may be beneficial in preventing catheter-associated blood stream infections (Wenzel, 1993). Any cannula that has been inserted without proper asepsis, such as in an emergency setting, should be replaced at the earliest opportunity. If purulent thrombophlebitis, cellulitis, or IV-related bacteremia is diagnosed or strongly suspected, the entire IV system should be changed. No general guidelines are available to recommend a specific time interval for changing central lines, but many hospitals require changes every 5 to 7 days. The insertion and removal of all intravascular lines should be documented in the patient's medical record.

IV administration tubing is routinely changed every 72 hours. Tubing used for hyperalimentation sets should be changed every 24 to 48 hours. Tubing should be changed immediately after the administration of blood, blood products, or lipid emulsions. Once started, all parenteral fluids should be completely used or discarded in 24 hours. Blood should not hang for more than 4 hours.

Nurses who are caring for patients with intravascular devices must always remember to follow strict aseptic technique. Although nosocomial bacteremia does not occur often, it can be life threatening (Box 12-6).

Other Sites of Nosocomial Infections

Although the previously discussed sites of infection account for the majority of nosocomial infections, approximately 10% to 15% fall into the category of "other nosocomial infections." These infections include skin and subcutaneous infections, central nervous system infections, gastroenteritis, and endometritis. In preventing these infections, the nurse must always remember the routes of transmission, the practice of good handwashing, the use of adequate aseptic technique in all procedures, and the importance of general skin care for all hospitalized patients.

BOX 12-6

CONTROL AND PREVENTION OF BACTEREMIA FROM AN IV DEVICE

- Wash hands before inserting an IV cannula and before manipulating the cannula or line.
- Wear gloves and use strict aseptic technique for cannula insertion.
- Place sterile dressings over cannula insertion sites.
- Record the date of insertion in the medical record and where it can be easily found, such as on the dressing or tape at the IV site.
- Evaluate patients with IV devices at least every 8 hours.
- Inspect and care for peripheral IV sites often.
- Pain or tenderness at the IV site requires removal of the dressing and inspection of the site.
- Change IV administration tubing every 72 hours.

PREVENTION AND CONTROL

The first recommendations regarding hospital-acquired infections were developed by the American Hospital Association and published in 1958 (American Hospital Association, 1979). Since that time, the Joint Commission on Accreditation of Healthcare Organizations (JCAHO), the CDC, the Department of Health and Human Services, and various state licensing laws have established standards for infection control in hospitals. The general recommendations made by these organizations include (1) the establishment of an active hospital-wide infection control program, (2) the establishment of a multidisciplinary committee that is responsible for monitoring the infection control program, (3) the development of specific written infection control policies and procedures for all services in the hospital, and (4) the development of a practical system for reporting and evaluating infections among patients and personnel.

Infection Control Committee

The primary function of the infection contol committee is to establish and implement hospital policy relating to the investigation, control, and prevention of infections within hospitals. Standards of care must be developed that reduce the risk of hospital-associated infections among both patients and personnel. It is the responsibility of the committee to establish mechansims for effective nosocomial infection surveillance, institute control measures such as isolation techniques and aseptic procedures, review bacteriologic services, monitor antibiotic therapy, provide educational programs, and establish techniques for discovering infections that are not manifest until after discharge of the patient (Centers for Disease Control, 1982a; Joint Commission on Accreditation of Healthcare Organizations, 1995).

The composition of infection control committees varies with individual hospitals. However, membership should include the hospital epidemiologist, physician representatives of the major clinical departments, the infection control practitioner, a hospital administrator, a pathologist, a nursing service representative, and representatives from other departments of the hospital as appropriate for the individual facility. A representative from the local health department is often invited to become a member. The 1995 JCAHO standards do not require an infection control committe, but most hospitals are opting to maintain the committee to ensure active, ongoing infection control programs (Joint Commission on Accreditation of Healthcare Organizations, 1995).

Infection Control Practitioner

The infection control practitioner is the member of the infection control team who is primarily responsible for the development, coordination, and supervision of the entire infection control program within the hospital. Most infection control practitioners are nurses, although some are medical technologists, public health professionals, or members of other allied healthcare disciplines. Regardless of their background, most infection control practitioners belong to the Association for Professionals in Infection Control and Epidemiology (APIC). The organization provides its members guidance and leadership through materials and programs that include an annual educational conference, an official journal, and published guidelines for various aspects of practice.

One function of the infection control practitioner is to collect, analyze, and report data regarding nosocomial infections. This activity is called **surveillance.** Other functions of the infection control practitioner include monitoring patient care activities, developing and updating specific prevention and control policies, participating in education programs, conducting special studies, and collaborating with all disciplines and departments in the facility. Probably the most important attributes of an effective infection control practitioner are having an understanding of human nature and having the ability to develop effective interpersonal relationships. The APIC and CDC have recommended that there be one infection control practitioner for every 250 beds in an acute-care facility and one for every 500 beds in a long-term–healthcare facility.

Surveillance

The purpose of a surveillance program is to detect, record, and report hospital-associated infections in a systematic fashion so that effective and practical control measures can be instituted. In the past, surveillance centered on reports from the bacteriology laboratory and observations made by nursing personnel or house staff, whose time was devoted primarily to the care of patients. As a result, underreporting of nosocomial infection was a serious problem. No single surveillance system provides complete information on the occurrence of hospital-associated infections. Therefore a combination of techniques appropriate for the individual institution are used.

Laboratory reports remain an important source of information. Urine, chemistry, culture, and postmortem reports are checked. The criteria to identify nosocomial infections at various body sites must be established by the infection control committee. The patient's medical records is reviewed to determine if a nosocomial infection is present. Radiology report summaries, especially those involving the respiratory and gastrointestinal tracts, may provide evidence of infection. If the surveillance system includes the identification of all community-acquired infections for control purposes, patients who are admitted with known infections or suggestive symptoms should be investigated.

Most of the data can be gathered through daily rounds on patient units. The nursing staff, physicians, and others often offer information that can provide clues to possible nosocomial infections or identify possible sources of infection. Observing individual patient nursing care plans may provide clues that indicate that a patient may be at high risk for developing a nosocomial infection. Patients who have one of the risk factors are noted, and their charts are reviewed.

Two areas that are often neglected when surveying for nosocomial infections are infections that appear in hospital personnel and discharged patients. Physicians should be encouraged to notify the infection control practitioner when infections develop after a patient's discharge from the hospital. Employees with communicable diseases such as upper respiratory tract infection, open or draining skin infections, or enteric disease should not be allowed to handle food, equipment, or other objects that come in direct contact with patients, and they should not be allowed to participate in patient care. Employees who develop hospital-associated infections should be monitored.

NURSE ALERT

Employees with communicable infectious diseases should not be allowed to participate in patient care.

Knowing the usual prevalence, or **endemic,** rate of infection in a hospital allows the infection control practitioner to identify areas that require investigation, to institute more specific control measures, or to detect epidemics should they occur. Surveillance information can also be used for staff education, the evaluation of new control measures, or the establishment of goals to reduce nosocomial infections.

Not all hospital-associated infections can be prevented. The patient's underlying disease, condition, or therapy may increase his or her vulnerability to both exogenous and endogenous microorganisms. Hospitals with well-developed surveillance systems have demonstrated that after an initial reduction of nosocomial infection rates (presumably as a result of the impact of surveillance activities) a relatively stable endemic level of infection remains.

Preventive Policies and Procedures

The best basic way to prevent and control infectious diseases is to use general sanitary practices and aseptic techniques. *Prevention* refers to the elimination of the occurrence of an infectious process, whereas **control** pertains to restricting the spread of an infectious process. The single most important technique in both prevention and control is proper handwashing.

Handwashing

Every person has a relatively stable resident bacteria population on the skin. New bacteria may be added and, unless removed, may become part of the resident populations and be spread to other persons. Nurses constantly come into contact with contaminated equipment and material. In providing nursing care, they often move from patient to patient and may unconsciously transfer pathogenic organisms from one patient to another and even endanger their own health. The safest way for nurses to protect themselves and their patients is through thorough and careful handwashing.

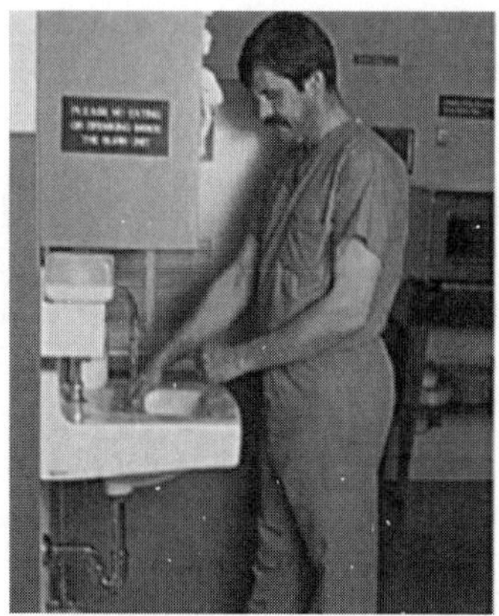

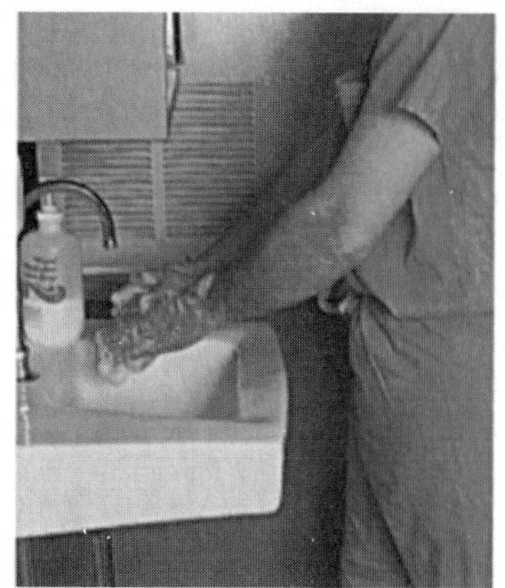

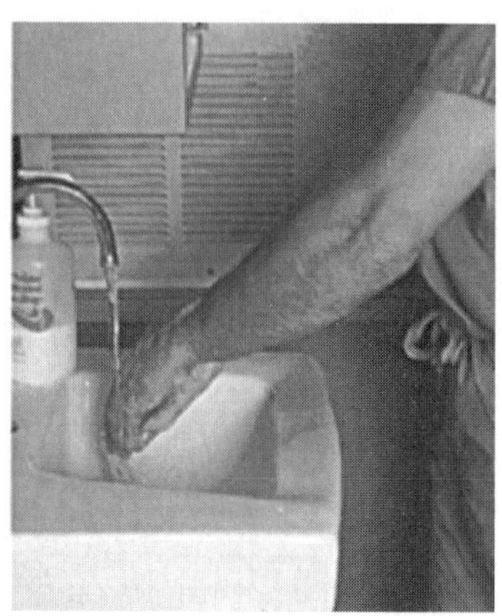

Figure 12-1 Good handwashing procedure involves a combination of soap, running water, friction, and time. Note that hands are kept in a downward position until dried. (From Perry AG, Potter PA: *Clinical nursing skills and techniques,* ed 3, St Louis, 1994, Mosby.)

NURSE ALERT

Handwashing is the single most important technique in the control and prevention of any nosocomial infection.

Ideal facilities for proper handwashing include a sink with knee or foot controls, hot and cold running water, soap, and paper towels. Antiseptic agents should be used for handwashing when the nurse is participating in an invasive procedure. Handwashing should be done between all patient contacts, even if gloves have been worn (Figure 12-1). The combination of soap, running water, friction, and time is the essential factor in good handwashing procedure. Fingernails and areas between the fingers should receive special attention. Hands should be thoroughly rinsed and kept in a downward position to prevent water from running up the arms, draining back again, and contaminating the hands. The hands should then be thoroughly dried. A dry paper towel should be used to turn off the faucets to prevent recontamination of the hands. The times at which handwashing should be performed are included in Box 12-7. The failure of hospital personnel to wash hands is a common cause of hospital-acquired infections.

BOX 12-7

WHEN TO WASH HANDS

- Before and after the workday
- After the direct care of any patient
- After handling any equipment
- Before performing invasive procedures, even if sterile gloves have been worn
- Before and after contact with any wound
- Before contact with a patient at high risk for infection
- After contact with a source likely to be contaminated with virulent microorganisms, such as secretions or excretions
- Between contact with different patients in special care units
- After removal of gloves

Sterilization and disinfection

Sterilization and disinfection procedures are crucial in the prevention of nosocomial infections. Inanimate objects used in the care of patients must be sterilized or disinfected between patients. **Sterilization** is the complete elimination or destruction of all microbial life, including large numbers of bacterial **spores.** Sterilization is accomplished by steam under pressure (autoclave), ethylene oxide (gas), dry heat, or the use of liquid chemicals. **Disinfection** eliminates many or all pathogenic organisms, with the exception of bacterial spores. Liquid chemicals are used for disinfection. Whether a device should be sterilized or disinfected between patients is determined by the degree of risk of infection. Four categories of medical devices have been defined: (1) critical instruments or devices, (2) semicritical instruments or devices, (3) noncritical instruments or devices, and (4) environmental surfaces (Adal and others, 1994; Favero, Bond, 1991).

A substantial risk of infection exists if critical instruments or devices are contaminated with any microorganism. Critical instruments enter the bloodstream or normally sterile body areas. Therefore they should be sterile. Examples of such devices include surgical instruments, cardiac catheters, implants, needles, and

ETHICAL DILEMMA

You have noticed that a colleague of yours often goes from patient room to patient room without washing her hands. When you try to talk to her about it, she replies that she is very busy and in a hurry so she can get all her work done. She asks, "What's the big deal?" From an ethical perspective, how do you explain to her what the "big deal" is?

transfer forceps. Biopsy forceps that penetrate mucosa barriers also fall into this category.

Semicritical instruments or devices are those that come in contact with mucous membranes or nonintact skin. Such instruments include flexible fiberoptic endoscopes, endotracheal tubes, bronchoscopes, respiratory therapy equipment, anesthesia breathing circuits, ophthalmic devices, and vaginal speculums. Items in this category must be manually and meticulously cleaned and submitted to a disinfection process that eradicates all microorganisms, with the exception of high numbers of bacterial spores.

Noncritical instruments or devices have contact only with nonbroken skin. Examples of these devices include blood pressure cuffs, face masks, most neurologic and cardiac diagnostic electrodes, and bedpans. Sterility of these items is not critical.

As described by Favero and Bond (1991), environmental surfaces include medical equipment surfaces such as adjustment knobs on dialysis machines, ventilators, x-ray machines, and IV pumps. A second group of environmental surfaces includes housekeeping surfaces such as floors, walls, tabletops, and curtains. Although items in this category are not usually in direct contact with patients, hand contact with these surfaces may lead to cross-contamination among patients. Cleaning these surfaces with a detergent or hospital-grade disinfectant detergent is adequate for environmental surfaces.

The disinfectant process has been divided into three levels of germicidal actions: (1) high-level, (2) intermediate-level, and (3) low-level. High-level disinfection (HLD) destroys all microorganisms, with the exception of bacterial spores. All semicritical medical devices should be subjected to HLD. HLD may be accomplished with glutaraldehyde, chlorine dioxide, 6% hydrogen peroxide, or peracetic-acid–based formulations. These same agents can also be used to achieve sterilization. The single most important variable in the achievement of sterilization and HLD is contact time.

Intermediate-level disinfection (ILD) destroys *Mycobacterium tuberculosis*, vegetative bacteria, most viruses, and most fungi but not necessarily bacterial spores. Examples of agents used for ILD include alcohol (70% to 90% ethyl or isopropyl), chlorine compounds (sodium or calcium hypochlorite, chlorine dioxide), certain phenolics, and certain iodophor preparations. Sodium hypochlorite (bleach) in a concentration of 0.5% has broad germicidal activity and is the most common disinfectant used worldwide.

Small nonlipid viruses, such as the enterovirus and rhinovirus, may be more resistant to germicides. However, medium and large lipid viruses, including Adenoviridae, the human immunodeficiency virus (HIV), and the hepatitis B virus (HBV), are more sensitive to germicides. HBV and non-A, non-B hepatitis are difficult to test in the laboratory because they are not cultured. However, no evidence exists that these viruses are unusually resistant to disinfectants. HIV is relatively unstable in the environment. The presence or absence of an Environmental Protection Agency label for HIV activity should not be a major criterion in the selection of a germicide.

Low-level disinfection (LLD) destroys vegetative forms of most bacteria and fungi, as well as medium to large lipid-containing viruses. LLD does not destroy bacterial endospores, mycobacteria, small nonlipid viruses, or some fungi. Low-level disinfectants include the quaternary ammonium compounds, certain iodophors, and certain phenolics.

A number of factors must be considered when using disinfectants. One of these factors is the length of time for the process. Medical items with smooth, nonporous, and cleanable surfaces are the easiest to disinfect. Instruments with crevices, joints, and pores in the surfaces represent potential barriers against cleaning and subsequent penetration of the germicide. Even sterilization methods can fail if organisms are trapped in organic materials. When medical devices are evaluated for purchase, the manufacturer's recommendations for cleaning and disinfection should be reviewed. Manufacturer guidelines should be consistent with the disinfection level required for that category of equipment. The type and level of microbial decontamination influences the effectiveness of the disinfectant, and the number of microorgansims present also influences the time necessary to achieve disinfection. For example, it takes much longer to kill 1000 bacterial spores than to kill 1 million cells of *S. aureus* (Favero, 1991). The amount of serum, blood, mucus, pus, or feces present on the device is a significant factor. Some disinfectants such as chlorine and iodine are inactivated in the presence of organic material. Therefore precleaning is required before disinfection.

Most disinfectants do not act quickly. Generally the greater the concentration of the germicide, the shorter the time required to kill the microorganism. The longer the time of exposure, the greater the effectiveness of the disinfectant process. For example, glutaraldehydes achieve high-level disinfection in 20 minutes of exposure but can achieve sterilization if the exposure time is extended to between 10 and 12 hours. All surfaces of the equipment being disinfected must have contact for the entire exposure time. Temperature, pH, water hardness, and the presence of other chemicals such as soaps may also affect disinfectant activity. Because of these variables, it is essential that the directions for the use of the disinfectant are read and followed.

Antisepsis

Antiseptics are nonirritating preparations that are used on the skin to inhibit or destroy microorganisms. The antimicrobial ingredient may be alcohol, chlorhexidine, hexachlorophene, iodine/iodophors, chloroxylenol (PCMX), or triclosan. Some of these ingredients are also found in disinfectants. However, because the formulations are usually different, it is crucial that product directions for use be strictly followed. Antiseptics are used for personal handwashing, surgical scrubs, and skin preparation for surgery or the insertion of invasive devices. A complete guideline for specific uses of various antiseptic agents has been published by the APIC (Larson, 1988).

Personnel and equipment

Hospital policies should be established to help prevent the transmission of infectious organisms. Personnel in charge of direct patient care should be free of infection and responsible for maintaining personal hygiene and grooming. All hospital personnel should maintain their immunization levels, report and treat all illnesses promptly, and refrain from patient care when they are ill. Employee health services are available and must be consulted for work-related injuries, illnesses, or exposures.

All patients should be assessed for infection when admitted, and attempts should be made to ensure that visitors are free of infection or disease. The hospital environment should be kept as free of pathogenic microorganisms as possible. All patient areas should be cleaned daily, and provisions should be made for adequate ventilation. Equipment and supplies should be sterilized or disinfected, and aseptic technique must be maintained.

High-risk areas

Delivery, operating, and recovery rooms; intensive care units; and other specialized units, such as the hemodialysis unit, are considered high-risk areas. Patients in these areas are usually considered compromised hosts and are therefore highly susceptible to infection or disease.

Patients who are identified as being at high risk for infection should have protective measures implemented as part of their care. Attempts should be made to decrease patient contact with infectious agents. Catheters and tubes that bypass normal defense mechanisms should be used judiciously. Special instructions should be given to the patient and family regarding health maintenance and the avoidance of contact with other infected persons. Thorough handwashing must be practiced between each patient contact.

Control Policies and Procedures

Isolation

The nursing care of a patient with an infectious disease involves two basic principles of medical asepsis: (1) confining all pathogens to a given area, which prevents their spread from an infected patient to others; and (2) protecting susceptible people from pathogens that are present in the environment or carried by others. **Isolation** is a means of interrupting the transmission of infectious organisms, because sources of infections and susceptible hosts are more difficult to control. The procedure establishes a barrier around the patient in an attempt to prevent the spread of infection either to or from the patient. Nurses assigned to the care of a patient in isolation should have a basic knowledge of the infectivity of the disease and its mode of transmission, as well as an understanding of the high-risk factors involved with susceptible patients.

The *CDC Guidelines for Isolation Precautions in Hospitals* (1983) recommends one of two different systems for isolation precautions: category-specific or disease-specific. Infection control committee members in each hospital determine which system best meets the needs of their hospital (Garner, Simmons, 1983). New CDC guidelines are expected late in 1995. These proposed guidelines are discussed on page 319.

Category-specific isolation precautions

Seven isolation categories have been defined and are derived by grouping diseases for which similar isolation precautions are indicated. A category ending with the term *isolation* requires a private room. A category ending with the term *precautions* indicates that a private room is not necessary.

Strict isolation prevents the transmission of highly contagious or virulent infections that may spread by both air and contact routes. A common disease requiring strict isolation is chickenpox. *Contact isolation* prevents the transmission of highly transmissible or epidemiologically important infections that do not warrant strict isolation. Multiple-resistant bacterial infections or colonizations; pediculosis; pneumonia caused by *S. aureus* or group A *Streptococcus;* scabies;

and major skin, wound, or burn infections are examples of diseases or conditions that require contact isolation. *Respiratory isolation* prevents the transmission of infectious diseases primarily over short distances through the air (droplet transmission). Measles, *H. influenzae* meningitis, meningococcal meningitis or pneumonia, and mumps are some of the diseases that require respiratory isolation.

Acid-fast bacilli (AFB) isolation is implemented for patients with suspected or known pulmonary or laryngeal tuberculosis (TB). Patients with a positive sputum smear for acid-fast organisms or a chest x-ray film that suggests active TB should be placed in AFB isolation. A private room is indicated, and ventilation is exhausted to the outside. Masks are required for all persons who enter the room. In general, infants and young children with pulmonary TB do not require isolation because they rarely cough, and their bronchial secretions excrete few AFB. To protect the patient's privacy, this category is referred to as AFB isolation rather than TB isolation. Because of the increased number of cases of TB and especially cases of drug-resistant TB, the CDC has recently updated its recommendations for isolation of the patient with TB or suspected TB. Room requirements include that the room be under negative air pressure in relation to the corridor, have six air exchanges per hour, and exhaust to the outside (Centers for Disease Control, 1990; Centers for Disease Control and Prevention, 1994b). The use of HEPA (high-efficiency particulate air) filters and ultraviolet light may be applied in some areas. The Occupational Safety and Health Administration (OSHA) (1993) has mandated the use of particulate respirators with HEPA filters as the minimum respiratory protection for those providing direct care to infectious TB patients. The need for a level of protection this extreme is controversial, because epidemiologic data do not exist to demonstrate its effectiveness. Data show that hospitals with programs for early detection and isolation of patients in properly ventilated rooms have not had nosocomial transmission of TB (Adal and others, 1994).

Enteric precautions prevent infections that are transmitted by direct or indirect contact with feces. Transmission usually requires ingestion of the infective agent. Amebic dysentery, hepatitis A, and gastroenteritis caused by *Campylobacter* organisms, *Cryptosporidium* organisms, salmonellae, and shigellae are examples of diseases that require enteric precautions. *Drainage/secretion precautions* prevent the spread of infections that are transmitted by direct or indirect contact with purulent material or with drainage from an infected body site. Minor skin, wound, or burn infections; minor **abscesses;** and conjunctivitis are included in this category. *Blood/body fluid precautions* prevent infections that are transmitted by direct or indirect contact with infective blood or body fluids. Diseases included in this category are Creutzfeldt-Jakob disease, hepatitis B, malaria, and HIV infection. Although still used in some hospitals, the implementation of **universal precautions** was intended to eliminate the need for them.

Instruction cards have been designed to give concise information about category-specific isolation precautions. The appropriate card should be posted where it is visible to all personnel who are providing care to the patient (Boxes 12-8 to 12-14).

BOX 12-8

STRICT ISOLATION

VISITORS—REPORT TO NURSE'S STATION BEFORE ENTERING ROOM

1 Masks are indicated for all persons entering room.
2 Gowns are indicated for all persons entering room.
3 Gloves are indicated for all persons entering room.
4 HANDS MUST BE WASHED AFTER TOUCHING THE PATIENT OR POTENTIALLY CONTAMINATED ARTICLES AND BEFORE TAKING CARE OF ANOTHER PATIENT.
5 Articles contaminated with infective material should be discarded or bagged and labeled before being sent for decontamination and reprocessing.

DISEASES REQUIRING STRICT ISOLATION*

Diphtheria, pharyngeal
Lassa fever and other viral hemorrhagic fevers, such as Marburg virus disease†
Plague, pneumonic
Smallpox†
Varicella-zoster (chickenpox), localized in immunocompromised patient, or disseminated

From Centers for Disease Control: Guidelines, Infection Control, MMWR 4(4): 284-290, 1983.
*A private room is indicated for strict isolation; in general, however, patients infected with the same organism may share a room. See *Draft Guidelines for Isolation Precautions in Hospitals* (CDC, 1994a) for details and for how long to apply precautions.
†A private room with special ventilation is indicated.

BOX 12-9

RESPIRATORY ISOLATION

VISITORS—REPORT TO NURSE'S STATION BEFORE ENTERING ROOM

1 Masks are indicated for all persons entering room.
2 Gowns are indicated for all persons entering room.
3 Gloves are indicated for all persons entering room.
4 HANDS MUST BE WASHED AFTER TOUCHING THE PATIENT OR POTENTIALLY CONTAMINATED ARTICLES AND BEFORE TAKING CARE OF ANOTHER PATIENT.
5 Articles contaminated with infective material should be discarded or bagged and labeled before being sent for decontamination and reprocessing.

DISEASES REQUIRING ISOLATION*

Epiglottitis, *Haemophilus influenzae*
Erythema infectiosum
Measles
Meningitis
  Bacterial, etiology unknown
  Haemophilus influenzae, known or suspected
  Meningococcal, known or suspected
Meningococcal pneumonia
Meningococcemia
Mumps
Pertussis (whooping cough)
Pneumonia, *Haemophilus influenzae,* in children (any age)

From Centers for Disease Control Guidelines, Infection Control, MMWR 4(4):284-290, 1983.
*A private room is indicated for respiratory isolation; in general, however, patients infected with the same organism may share a room. See *Draft Guidelines for Isolation Precautions in Hospitals* (CDC, 1994a) for details and for how long to apply precautions.

BOX 12-10

CONTACT ISOLATION

VISITORS—REPORT TO NURSE'S STATION BEFORE ENTERING ROOM

1 Masks are indicated for those who come close to patient.
2 Gowns are indicated if soiling is likely.
3 Gloves are indicated for touching infective material.
4 HANDS MUST BE WASHED AFTER TOUCHING THE PATIENT OR POTENTIALLY CONTAMINATED ARTICLES AND BEFORE TAKING CARE OF ANOTHER PATIENT.
5 Articles contaminated with infective material should be discarded or bagged and labeled before being sent for decontamination and reprocessing.

DISEASES REQUIRING CONTACT ISOLATION*

Acute respiratory tract infections in infants and young children, including croup, colds, bronchitis, and bronchiolitis caused by respiratory syncytial virus, adenovirus, coronavirus, influenza viruses, parainfluenza viruses, and rhinovirus
Conjunctivitis, gonococcal, in newborns
Diphtheria, cutaneous
Endometritis, group A Streptococcus
Furunculosis, staphylococcal, in newborns
Herpes simplex, disseminated, severe primary or neonatal
Impetigo
Influenza, in infants and young children
Multiple-resistant bacterial, infection or colonization (any site) with any of the following:

1 Gram-negative bacilli resistant to all aminoglycosides that are tested (in general, such organisms should be resistant to gentamicin, tobramycin, and amikacin for these special precautions to be indicated)
2 *Staphylococcus aureus* resistant to methicillin (or nafcillin or oxacillin if they are used instead of methicillin for testing)
3 Pneumococci resistant to penicillin
4 *Haemophilus influenzae* resistant to ampicillin (β-lactamase positive) and chloramphenicol
5 Other resistant bacteria if they are judged by the infection control team to be of special clinical and epidemiologic significance

Pediculosis
Pharyngitis, infectious, in infants and young children
Pneumonia, viral, in infants and young children
Pneumonia, *Staphylococcus aureus* or group A *Streptococcus*
Rabies
Rubella, congenital and other
Scabies
Scalded skin syndrome (Ritter's disease)
Skin, wound, or burn infection; major draining and not covered by a dressing or dressing does not adequately contain the purulent material; includes those infected with *Streptococcus*
Vaccinia (generalized and progressive eczema vaccinatum)

From Centers for Disease Control: Guidelines, Infection Control, MMWR 4(4):284-290, 1983.
*A private room is indicated for contact isolation; in general, however, patients infected with the same organism may share a room. During outbreaks, infants and young children with the same clinical syndrome may share a room. See *Draft Guidelines for Isolation Precautions in Hospitals* (CDC, 1994a) for details and for how long to apply precautions.

BOX 12-11

DRAINAGE/SECRETION PRECAUTIONS

VISITORS—REPORT TO NURSE'S STATION BEFORE ENTERING ROOM

1 Masks are not indicated.
2 Gowns are indicated if soiling is likely.
3 Gloves are indicated for touching infective material.
4 HANDS MUST BE WASHED AFTER TOUCHING THE PATIENT OR POTENTIALLY CONTAMINATED ARTICLES AND BEFORE TAKING CARE OF ANOTHER PATIENT.
5 Articles contaminated with infective material should be discarded or bagged and labeled before being sent for decontamination and reprocessing.

DISEASE REQUIRING DRAINAGE/SECRETION PRECAUTIONS*

Infectious diseases included in this category are those that result in production of infective purulent material, drainage, or secretions, unless the disease is included in another isolation category that requires more rigorous precautions. (If you have questions about a specific disease, see the listing ofinfectious diseases in *CDC Guideline for Isolation Precautions in Hospitals,* Table A, Disease-Specific Isolation Precautions.)

The following infections are examples of those included in this category provided they are not (1) caused by multiple-resistant microorganisms, (2) major (draining and not covered by a dressing or dressing does not adequately contain the drainage) skin wound, or burn infections, including those caused by *Staphylococcus aureus* or group A *Streptococcus,* or (3) gonococcal eye infections in newborns. See Contact Isolation if the infection is one of these three.

Abscess, minor or limited
Burn infection, minor or limited
Conjunctivitis
Decubitus ulcer, infected, minor or limited
Skin infection, minor or limited
Wound infection, minor or limited

From Centers for Disease Control: Guidelines, Infection Control, MMWR 4(4):284-290, 1983.
*A private room is usually not indicated for Drainage/Secretion Precautions. See *Draft Guidelines for Isolation Precautions in Hospitals* (CDC, 1994a) for details and for how long to apply precautions.

BOX 12-12

ENTERIC PRECAUTIONS

VISITORS—REPORT TO NURSE'S STATION BEFORE ENTERING ROOM

1 Masks are not indicated.
2 Gowns are indicated if soiling is likely.
3 Gloves are indicated for touching infective material.
4 HANDS MUST BE WASHED AFTER TOUCHING THE PATIENT OR POTENTIALLY CONTAMINATED ARTICLES AND BEFORE TAKING CARE OF ANOTHER PATIENT.
5 Articles contaminated with infective material should be discarded or bagged and labeled before being sent for decontamination and reprocessing.

DISEASES REQUIRING ENTERIC PRECAUTIONS*

Amebic dysentery
Cholera
Coxsackievirus disease
Diarrhea, acute illness with suspected infectious etiology
Echovirus disease
Encephalitis (unless known not to be caused by enteroviruses)
Enterocolitis caused by *Clostridium difficile* or *Staphylococcus aureus*
Enteroviral infection
Gastroenteritis caused by
  Campylobacter species
  Cryptosporidium species
  Dientamoeba fragilis
  Escherichia coli (enterotoxic, enteropathogenic, or enteroinvasive)
  Giardia lamblia
  Salmonella species
  Shigella species
  Vibrio parahaemolyticus
  Viruses - including Norwalk agent and rotavirus
  Yersinia enterocolitica
  Unknown etiology but presumed to be an infectious agent
Hand, foot, and mouth disease
Hepatitis, viral, type A
Herpangina
Meningitis, viral (unless known not to be caused by enteroviruses)
Necrotizing enterocolitis
Pleurodynia
Poliomyelitis
Typhoid fever *(Salmonella typhi)*
Viral pericarditis, myocarditis, or meningitis (unless known not to be caused by enteroviruses)

From Centers for Disease Control: Guidelines, Infection Control, MMWR 4(4):284-290, 1983.
*A private room is indicated for Enteric Precautions if patient hygiene is poor. A patient with poor hygiene does not wash hands after touching infective material, contaminates the environment with infective material, or shares contaminated articles with other patients. In general, patients infected with the same organism may share a room. See *Draft Guidelines for Isolation Precautions in Hospitals* (CDC, 1994a) for details and for how long to apply precautions.

BOX 12-13

AFB (TUBERCULOSIS) ISOLATION

VISITORS—REPORT TO NURSE'S STATION BEFORE ENTERING ROOM

1 Masks are indicated only when patient is coughing and does not reliably cover mouth.
2 Gowns are indicated only if needed to prevent gross contamination of clothing.
3 Gloves are not indicated.
4 HANDS MUST BE WASHED AFTER TOUCHING THE PATIENT OR POTENTIALLY CONTAMINATED ARTICLES AND BEFORE TAKING CARE OF ANOTHER PATIENT.
5 Articles should be discarded, cleaned, or sent for decontamination and reprocessing.

DISEASES REQUIRING AFB ISOLATION*

This isolation category is for patients with current pulmonary TB who have a positive sputum smear or a chest x-ray appearance that strongly suggests current (active) TB.

Laryngeal TB is also included in this category.

In general, infants and young children with pulmonary TB do not require isolation precautions because they rarely cough and their bronchial secretions contain few AFB compared with adults with pulmonary TB. To protect the patient's privacy, this instruction card is labeled AFB (acid-fast bacilli) isolation rather than tuberculosis isolation.

From Centers for Disease Control: Guidelines, Infection Control, MMWR 4(4):284-290, 1983.
*A private room with special ventilation is indicated for AFB isolation. In general, patients infected with the same organism may share a room. See *Draft Guidelines for Isolation Precautions in Hospitals* (CDC, 1994a) for details and for how long to apply precautions.

BOX 12-14

BLOOD/BODY FLUID PRECAUTIONS

VISITORS—REPORT TO NURSES' STATION BEFORE ENTERING ROOM

1 Masks are not indicated.
2 Gowns are indicated if soiling with blood or body fluids is likely.
3 Gloves are indicated for touching blood or body fluids.
4 HANDS SHOULD BE WASHED IMMEDIATELY IF THEY ARE POTENTIALLY CONTAMINATED WITH BLOOD OR BODY FLUIDS AND BEFORE TAKING CARE OF ANOTHER PATIENT.
5 Articles contaminated with blood or body fluids should be discarded or bagged and labeled before being sent for decontamination and reprocessing.
6 Care should be taken to avoid needle-stick injuries. Used needles should not be recapped or bent; they should be placed in a prominently labeled, puncture-resistant container designated specifically for such disposal.
7 Blood spills should be cleaned up promptly with a solution of 5.25% sodium hypochlorite diluted 1:10 with water.

DISEASES REQUIRING BLOOD/BODY FLUID PRECAUTIONS*

Acquired immunodeficiency syndrome (AIDS)
Arthropodborne viral fevers (for example, dengue, yellow fever, and Colorado tick fever)
Babesiosis
Creutzfeldt-Jakob disease
Hepatitis B (including HBsAg antigen carrier)
Hepatitis, non-A, non-B
Leptospirosis
Malaria
Rat-bite fever
Relapsing fever
Syphilis, primary and secondary with skin and mucous membrane lesions

From Centers for Disease Control Guidelines, Infection Control, *MMWR* 4(4): 284-290, 1983.
*A private room is indicated for blood-body fluid precautions if patient hygiene is poor. A patient with poor hygiene does not wash hands after touching infective material, contaminates the enviromental with infective material, or shares contaminated articles with other patients. In general, patients infected with the same organism may share a room. See *Draft Guidelines for Isolation Precautions in Hospitals* (CDC, 1994a) for details and for how long to apply precautions.

Disease-specific isolation precautions

Disease-specific precautions are an alternative to the category system of isolation. With this system, each infectious disease is considered individually. Most common infectious agents and diseases and the specifications for the required precautions (e.g., private room, mask, gown, and gloves) are listed in Garner and Simmons' *CDC Guidelines for Isolation Precautions in Hospitals* (1983). An instruction card is prepared and displayed near the patient.

Gowns should be worn whenever clothing might be soiled by infective materials. Gowns should be worn once, changed whenever wet, and discarded aseptically. Masks help prevent the spread of microorganisms that are transmitted through the air or by droplets. Masks should cover the nose and mouth, be used only once, and be changed periodically (Figure 12-2). Handwashing before and after each contact with the patient is the single most important way to prevent transmission of infection. Gloves should be used when handling fluids and body secretions and should be used once and discarded.

Contaminated equipment that was brought into the room should be sterilized or disinfected. Linens and other contaminated objects that are taken from the room should be bagged in leak-proof bags.

Many hospitals modify these guidelines to meet their specific requirements. Precautions may sometimes be required even if the patient does not fully meet the criteria for any type of isolation. For example, patients with UTIs who are catheterized can serve as reservoirs of infection for other catheterized patients in the same room. Practices must occasionally be modified for an infected patient who needs constant care or emergency therapy. Isolation procedures should be revised as each patient's disease resolves or progresses. When the patient poses no risk to others, isolation should be terminated.

Universal precautions

In August 1987, the CDC published a new set of recommendations for the prevention of HIV transmission in healthcare settings. The recommendations are referred to as universal blood and body fluid precautions, or universal precautions. Because it is impossible to recognize or be aware of all patients who are infected with bloodborne pathogens when giving care, universal precautions need to be implemented for all patients who are undergoing medical care. Universal precautions include the following:

1 All healthcare workers should routinely use appropriate barrier precautions to prevent skin and mucous membrane exposure when contact with a patient's blood or body fluids is anticipated. Gloves should be worn for touching blood and body fluids, mucous membranes, or nonintact skin of all patients; for handling items or surfaces that are soiled with bloody or body fluids; and for performing venipuncture and other vascular access procedures. Gloves should be changed after contact with each patient. To prevent exposure of mucous membranes of the mouth, nose, and eyes, masks and protective eyewear or face shields should be worn during procedures that are likely to generate droplets of blood or other body fluids (Figure 12-3). Gowns or aprons should be worn during procedures that are likely to generate splashes of blood or other body fluids.
2 Hands and other skin surfaces should be washed immediately and thoroughly if contaminated with blood or other body fluids. Hands should be washed immediately after gloves are removed.
3 All healthcare workers should take precautions to prevent injuries during the use of needles, scalpels, and other sharp instruments; during disposal of used needles; and when handling sharp instruments after procedures. To prevent needlestick injuries, needles should not be recapped, purposely bent or broken by hand, removed from disposable syringes, or otherwise manipulated by hand. After they are used, disposable syringes and needles, scalpel blades, and other sharp items should be placed in puncture-resistant containers for disposal. The puncture-resistant containers should be located as close to the area of use as is practical. Large-bore reusable needles should be placed in a puncture-resistant container for transport to the processing area.
4 Although saliva has not been implicated in HIV transmission, the potential exists. However, this

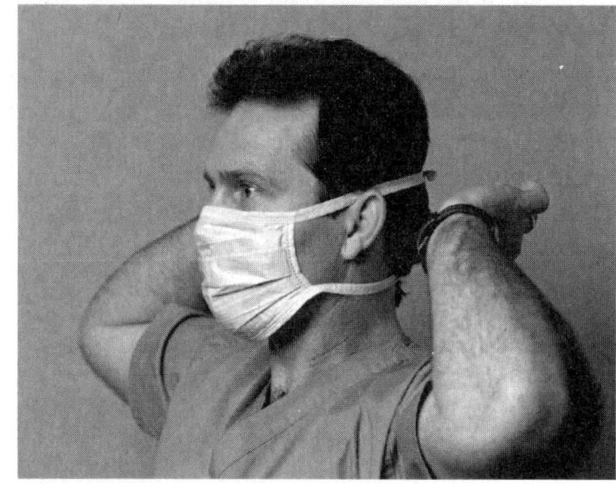

Figure 12-2 Masks should cover the nose and mouth and be used only once.

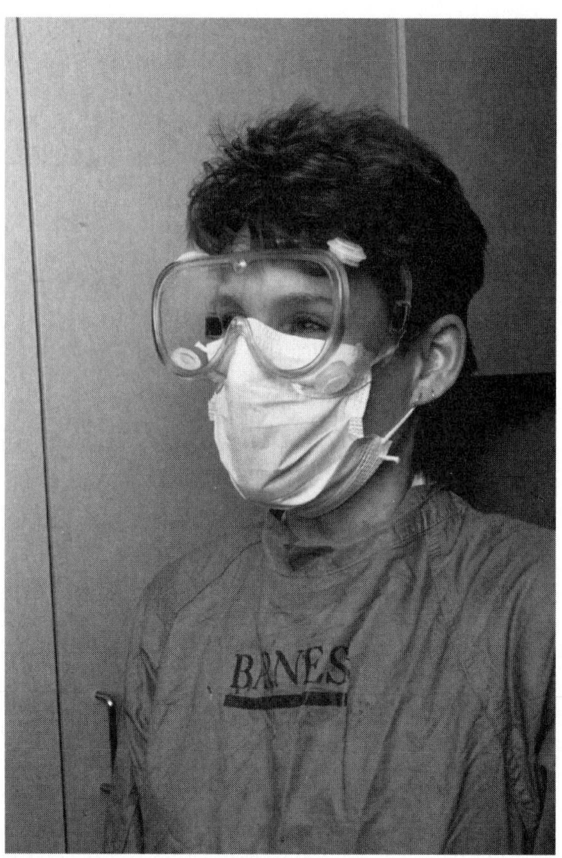

Figure 12-3 Protective goggles should be worn during procedures that generate droplets of blood or body fluids.

potential has not been scientifically documented. Mouthpieces, resuscitation bags, or other ventilation devices should be available for use in areas where the need for resuscitation is predictable, which minimizes the need for emergency mouth-to-mouth resuscitation.

5 Healthcare workers who have exudative lesions or weeping dermatitis should refrain from all direct patient care and from handling patient-care equipment until the condition resolves.

6 Pregnant healthcare workers are not known to be at a greater risk of contracting HIV infection. However, if a healthcare worker develops an HIV infection during pregnancy, the infant is at risk for HIV infection as a result of perinatal transmission. Because of this risk, pregnancy healthcare workers should be especially familiar with and strictly adhere to precautions to minimize the risk of HIV transmission.

7 All healthcare workers who have the potential to be exposed to blood or body fluids should receive a hepatitis B vaccine.

The body fluids to which universal precautions should apply include blood, semen, vaginal secretions, cerebral spinal fluid (CSF), synovial fluid, and amniotic fluid. Universal precautions do not apply to feces, nasal secretions, sputum, sweat, tears, urine, or vomitus unless they contain visible blood. As written, universal precautions are designed to protect healthcare workers from exposure to bloodborne pathogens, but they do not address the prevention of cross-contamination between patients (Centers for Disease Control, 1986, 1987). Implementation of universal precautions makes the use of blood/body fluids precautions unnecessary. Whether to use the blood/body fluid precaution card to identify patients known to be infected is currently controversial.

Healthcare employers are now being regulated by OSHA and are being charged with providing a safe working environment for all healthcare workers. OSHA issued regulations in 1991 that obligated hospitals to implement universal precautions in the care of all patients. In addition to requiring universal precautions, the regulations also make it obligatory for healthcare employers to provide a hepatitis B vaccine to employees who are often exposed to blood and potentially infectious materials, to provide postexposure evaluation and medical follow-up, to train all employees in the use of universal precautions, and to maintain records of training and occupational exposures (Rutala and others, 1981).

Body substance isolation

A system of isolation proposed by Lynch and others (1987) departs from the standard CDC isolation systems. This system is referred to as body substance isolation (BSI) and is used for all patients. Gloves are worn for any anticipated contact with blood or body fluids. Gloves are changed between all patients, and handwashing after patient contact is indicated. Gowns, aprons, masks, or goggles are worn when blood or body fluids are likely to touch the clothing, skin, or face. Private rooms may be necessary for those patients with airborne infections or for patients who soil the environment with body substances.

Under this system of isolation, a BSI card is placed in all patient rooms. A separate "stop sign alert" card with instructions is placed outside the rooms of patients who have airborne infections, and masks are worn for these particular patients. Other forms of isolation are not used under this system. BSI is intended to prevent the exposure of healthcare workers and cross-contamination between patients.

No standard system of isolation is appropriate for all hospitals. Each hospital must evaluate its own patient population and the attitudes of its employees. Many hospitals are now using a combination of the category-specific isolation system and universal precautions. All of these systems of isolation need analy-

BOX 12-15

SUMMARY OF STANDARD PRECAUTIONS AND TRANSMISSION-DRIVEN PRECAUTIONS (PROPOSED, 1994)

STANDARD PRECAUTIONS
- Used for the care of all patients regardless of diagnosis or presumed infection status
- Apply to blood, all body fluids, secretions, excretions, nonintact skin, and mucous membranes regardless of whether they contain visible blood
- Includes handwashing and the use of gloves, masks, eye protection, and gowns where splashing or soiling is likely to occur
- Combines universal precautions and BSI

AIRBORNE PRECAUTIONS
- Used for patients known or suspected to have serious illnesses that are transmitted by airborne nuclei, such as measles, varicella, and TB
- Incorporates AFB (TB) isolation
- Includes a negative-pressure isolation room with at least six air exchanges per hour

DROPLET PRECAUTIONS
- Used for patients who are known or suspected to have serious illnesses that are transmitted by large-particle droplets, such as invasive *H. influenzae* type b, invasive *Neisseria meningitidis,* invasive multidrug-resistant *S. pneumoniae,* and other serious bacterial and viral respiratory infections that are spread by droplet transmission
- Includes placing the patient in a private room and wearing a mask when working within 3 feet of the patient
- Incorporates respiratory precautions

CONTACT PRECAUTIONS
- Used for patients known or suspected to have serious illnesses that are easily transmitted by direct contact or by contact with the environment, such as gastrointestinal, respiratory, skin, or wound infections or colonization with multidrug-resistant bacteria; also includes enteric infections with a low infectious dose such as *Clostridium difficile,* respiratory syncytial virus, highly contagious skin infections, and conjunctivitis
- Includes placing the patient in a private room
- Incorporates aspects of contact isolation, respiratory isolation, drainage/secretion precautions, and enteric precautions

Modified from Centers for Disease Control and Prevention: *Draft Guidelines for Isolation Precautions in Hospitals,* Federal Register 59, November 7, 1994 (CDC, 1994).

sis to determine which best meets the objective of diminishing the transmission of infection (Larson, 1988).

A draft of new comprehensive isolation guidelines was published in October 1994. The revised system uses a new 2-tiered patient isolation system composed of standard precautions and transmission-driven precautions. Standard precautions incorporate the elements of universal precautions and BSI. Transmission-driven precautions include airborne precautions, droplet precautions, and contact precautions (Box 12-15) (Centers for Disease Control and Prevention, 1994a).

EMOTIONAL SUPPORT

Hospital-acquired infections cannot help but evoke feelings of anxiety, frustration, and hostility in the patient and family. Through no fault of his or her own, the patient has acquired an infection that may mean additional hospital days, increased hospital costs, time away from work, or disruption of home life. Isolation procedures are time consuming and costly and may discourage personnel from spending extra time with the patient. The solitude that usually accompanies isolation deprives the patient of normal social relationships, and emotional reactions are likely to occur.

A wide range of emotional reactions can be seen in isolation patients. They may exhibit overt abusive or aggressive behavior or show signs of withdrawal and depression. The excessive demands made by some patients can be extremely frustrating to nursing personnel. Family members may fear the possibility of developing the infection themselves and may therefore avoid contact with the patient. The procedures of gowning, masking, and proper handwashing may convey feelings of rejection.

Every patient in isolation should have a basic understanding of what to expect. Both the patient and family should be given a thorough explanation of the way in which the infection is transmitted and the procedures of isolation that tend to interrupt transmission. When they realize the significance of isolation and their roles in preventing further transmission, cooperation and acceptance can be achieved. Much can be done to relieve the patient's anxiety by maintaining a friendly, understanding, sympathetic, and reassuring manner.

Nursing Care Plan

PATIENT WITH A NOSOCOMIAL INFECTION

Mr. Jackson is a 48-year-old male who has been admitted from the emergency room with severe abdominal pain, abdominal rigidity, and nausea and vomiting. He has been experiencing vague abdominal discomfort for 3 days. However, the pain became increasingly severe over the 6 hours before admission. An abdominal x-ray examination indicated free air in the peritoneum, and an emergency exploratory laparotomy was done. He was found to have a ruptured diverticulum, and a temporary colostomy was performed.

Mr. Jackson develops a wound infection 3 days after surgery as evidenced by purulent drainage from the inferior aspect of the incision with erythema and warmth surrounding the incision, which is confirmed by a wound culture. The staples were removed from the inferior portion of the incision, the wound was irrigated, and dressing changes have been prescribed every 8 hours.

Past Medical History

No known allergies to food or drugs

Two pack-a-day smoker for 20 years

Hypertension for approximately 5 years; reports that it is well controlled with medications

Diverticulitis, hospitalized 2 years ago for an acute episode; has had difficulty following prescribed dietary changes as a result of his lifestyle; work requires meals on the road; dislikes fruits and vegetables.

Psychosocial Data

Married for 22 years; has 3 children ages 10, 13, and 16; wife is very supportive and has been trying to make dietary changes without much success

Wife is a homemaker and in excellent health

Employed as an advertising executive in a large firm; enjoys his work, but recently work environment has become tense and stressful as a result of layoffs and restructuring of departments

Works 12- to 14-hour days

Exercise is minimal

Involved in children's activities on the weekends

Watches television every evening

Assessment Data

Height 5′9″, weight 245 lb

Vital signs: T 100.9, P 96, R 22, BP 152/88

Alert and oriented × 3; appears stated age

Skin: Warm, dry, and intact (other than incision)

Eye ear nose throat: Mucous membranes moist; teeth in good repair; lips pink

Respiratory: Rate 22 to 26/minute, shallow, symmetrical; diminished breath sounds; bilateral bases; scattered rhonchi and crackles; occasional loose productive cough of white sputum; using incentive spirometer, approximately 1000 ml inspiratory volume

Abdominal: Protruberant, soft abdomen; hypoactive bowel sounds; colostomy patient draining scant serosanguinous drainage; no stool output yet; started on sips of CL today; vertical abdominal incision; superior portion of incision with staples intact and well-approximated; slight erythema around staple insertion site; inferior portion approximately 6 cm open with moderate amount of serosanguinous and purulent drainage; erythema around wound margin

Cardiovascular: AP 96 and regular; peripheral pulses strong bilaterally; no peripheral edema

Laboratory data

RBC 3.8, Hgb 11.4, Hct 36, WBC 14,000, Na 132, K 4.1, C1 96, CO_2 26

Blood gases: pH 7.37, PCO_2 45, PO_2 88, HCO_3 26, O_2 sat 91%

ECG: Normal sinus rhythm

Chest x-ray: Atelectesis bilateral lower lobes

Urinalysis: Within normal limits

Wound culture: S. aureus

Medications

meperidine (Demerol) 75-100 mg; hydroxyzine (Vistaril) 25-50 mg IM q 3-4 hr prn pain

enalapril (Vasotec) 10 mg bid

cefazolin (Ancef) 1 g IV q 6 hr

D5 ½ NS with 20 mEq KCl at 100 ml/hr

Oxygen 2 L/min nasal cannula

NURSING DIAGNOSIS

Risk for infection related to ruptured diverticulum, invasive procedure, obesity, inadequate nutrition as evidenced by wound culture, purulent wound drainage, and elevated temperature

NURSING INTERVENTIONS	EVALUATION OF EXPECTED OUTCOMES
Assess wound q 8 hr for evidence of healing, drainage, erythema, and warmth. Monitor vital signs q 4 hr. Monitor laboratory values, especially WBC. Maintain aseptic technique in dressing changes. Change dressing q 8 hr; dampen dressing with sterile normal saline. Administer antibiotics as prescribed. Discuss nutritional concerns with physician if patient does not advance diet in 1 to 2 days. Instruct patient and family on signs and symptoms of infection and current treatment. Make referral to infection control nurse if indicated.	Afebrile; vital signs within normal limits for patient Absence of purulent drainage from wound Wound shows evidence of healing

NURSING DIAGNOSIS

Ineffective breathing pattern related to smoking history, pain, immobility, and sedation for analgesics

NURSING INTERVENTIONS	EVALUATION OF EXPECTED OUTCOMES
Assess respiratory rate, depth, and breathing pattern q 8 hr. Assess for dyspnea at rest and with exertion. Auscultate breath sounds q 8 hr. Monitor for changes in orientation, increased restlessness, and anxiety. Monitor sputum for quantity, color, and consistency. Maintain patient in a position that supports optimal breathing with head of bed elevated. Maintain oxygen at 2 L/min nasal cannula; monitor O_2 sats as indicated. Encourage coughing and deep breathing and/or incentive spirometry q 2 hr. Provide a dose of analgesic that controls pain but does not oversedate. Encourage out-of-bed activity, sitting in chair tid for one hour and ambulating in hall qid. Instruct on the splinting of the abdominal incision with coughing, deep breathing, and activity.	Respiratory rate 20-24/min without oxygen Breath sounds clear Pink skin color and nailbeds Able to perform incentive spirometry to 1500 ml inspiratory volume No evidence of dyspnea or respiratory distress

continued

NURSING DIAGNOSIS

Pain related to surgical incision as evidenced by verbal complaints and pain behavior with movement

NURSING INTERVENTIONS	EVALUATION OF EXPECTED OUTCOMES
Assess pain characteristics q 4 hr and prn. Monitor vital signs. Administer analgesics as prescribed; evaluate effectiveness. Promote activity 30 minutes after analgesic is administered. Teach diversion, relaxation, splinting, and guided imagery. Help patient assume a comfortable position, and provide comfort measures.	Verbalizes pain relief Able to perform respiratory exercises and activity without severe pain Uses alternative pain control measures

NURSING DIAGNOSIS

Knowledge deficit related to necessary lifestyle changes, new ostomy as evidenced by numerous questions and verbalized difficulty with following previous dietary recommendations

NURSING INTERVENTIONS	EVALUATION OF EXPECTED OUTCOMES
Determine patient's understanding of the disease process. Review cause of disease and factors that may aggravate condition. Instruct patient on the purpose and care of ostomy; obtain an enterostomal therapy consult. Include wife in all teaching. Allow for return demonstrations and provide appropriate positive feedback. Provide dietary instruction (e.g., importance of adequate fluids, moderate use of high-fiber foods, and foods that cause flatus). Discuss effect of ostomy on body image and sexuality. Identify appropriate community resources (e.g., local ostomy support group, VNA, medical supply company).	Patient and wife verbalize understanding of disease, surgery, and treatment Able to care for ostomy Verbalizes available community resources

KEY CONCEPTS

- A nosocomial infection is a clinically active infection that occurs in a hospitalized patient and was not present or incubating at the time of admission to the healthcare facility.
- A reservoir is the location where microorganisms that cause infections are usually found, such as patients, healthcare personnel, healthcare devices, and the environment.
- The rates of nosocomial infection range from 3% to 15% of all patients admitted to hospitals.
- The urinary tract is the most common site for nosocomial infections and is followed by the lower respiratory tract and surgical wound infections.
- Exogenous infections are acquired from sources outside the patient, or from the environment.
- Endogenous infections occur when potentially virulent microorganisms that normally reside within the patient begin to multiply, which causes a pathologic condition within the patient.
- Microorganisms are transmitted to a susceptible host by contact, airborne, vehicle, and vectorborne routes.
- Primary nosocomial bacteremia associated with intravascular devices is an increasing problem in healthcare facilities.
- The infection control committee establishes and implements hospital policy relating to the investigation, control, and prevention of infections within heathcare facilities.
- The infection control practitioner is primarily responsible for the development, coordination, and supervision of the entire infection control program throughout the healthcare facility.
- Surveillance programs detect, record, and report hospital-associated infections in a systematic fashion so that effective and practical control measures can be instituted.
- The single most important technique in both prevention and control is proper handwashing.
- Sterilization and disinfection procedures are crucial to the control and prevention of nosocomial infections.
- Principles of medical asepsis include (1) confining all pathogens to a given area, which prevents their spread from an infected person to others; and (2) protecting susceptible people from pathogens that are present in the environment or are carried by other persons.
- Isolation may produce a wide range of emotional reactions in patients.

CRITICAL THINKING EXERCISES

1. Why are elderly hospitalized patients considered to be at high risk for nosocomial infections?
2. Outline a plan for prevention of UTIs, surgical wound infections, pneumonia, and bacteremia in acute and long-term care settings.
3. How can the staff nurse assist the infection control practitioner in surveillance for infections?
4. What is the rationale underlying the proposed changes in precaution for isolation of patients with infections?

REFERENCES AND ADDITIONAL READINGS

Adal K and others: The use of high-efficiency particulate air-filter respirators to protect hospital workers from tuberculosis, *New Engl J Med* 331(3):169-173, 1994.

American College of Surgeons: *Manual on control of infection in surgical patients,* ed 2, Philadelphia, 1984, JB Lippincott.

American Hospital Association: Infection control in the hospital, ed 4, Chicago, 1979, The Association.

Bennet JV, Brachman S: *Hospital infections,* Boston, 1986, Little, Brown.

Castle M: *Hospital infection control: principles and practice,* New York, 1987, John Wiley & Sons.

Centers for Disease Control: *Guidelines for the prevention of nosocomial infections,* Atlanta, 1982a, US Department of Health and Human Services.

Centers for Disease Control: *Guidelines for the prevention of nosocomial pneumonia,* Atlanta, 1982b, US Department of Health and Human Services.

Centers for Disease Control: *Guidelines for the prevention of surgical wound infections,* Atlanta, 1985, US Department of Health and Human Services.

Centers for Disease Control: *National nosocomial infections study report, annual summary—1984,* Atlanta, 1986, US Department of Health and Human Services.

Centers for Disease Control: *Recommendations for prevention of HIV transmission in health-care settings, MMWR* 36 (suppl 25):1S-18S 1987.

Centers for Disease Control: Update: universal precautions for prevention of transmission of human immunodeficiency virus, hepatitis B virus, and other bloodborne pathogens in health-care settings. *MMWR* 37(24):377-388, 1988.

Centers for Disease Control: Guidelines for preventing the transmission of tuberculosis in health-care settings, with special focus on HIV-related issues, *MMWR CDC Surveill Summ* 39 (No RR-17):1-29, 1990.

Centers for Disease Control: Nosocomial infection rates for interhospital comparison: limitations and possible solutions, *Infect Control Hosp Epidemiol* 12(10):609-621, 1991.

Centers for Disease Control and Prevention: *Draft guidelines for isolation precautions in hospitals,* Federal Register 59, November 7, 1994a.

Centers for Disease Control and Prevention: *Draft guidelines for preventing the transmission of mycobacterium tuberculosis in health-care facilities,* Federal Register 59, October 28, 1994b.

Cruse PJE, Foord R: The epidemiology of wound infection: a ten year prospective study of 62,939 wounds. *Surg Clin North Am* 60:27-40, 1980.

Favero MS, Bond WW: Chemical disinfection of medical and surgical materials. In Block SS editor: *Disinfection, sterilization, and preservation,* ed 4, Philadelphia, 1991, Lea & Febiger.

Garner JS, Simmons BP: *CDC guideline for isolation precautions in hospitals,* Atlanta, 1983, US Department of Health and Human Services.

Haley RW: Managing hospital infection control for cost effectiveness, Chicago, 1986, American Hospital Publishing.

Haley RW and others: Identifying patients at high risk of surgical wound infection: a simple multivariate index of patient susceptibility and wound contamination, *Am J Epidemiol* 121(2):206-215, 1985a.

Haley RW and others: The nationwide nosocomial infection rate, *Am J Epidemiol* 121(2):159-167, 1985b.

Joint Commission on Accreditation of Healthcare Organizations: *Accreditation Manual for Hospitals,* Chicago, 1985, The Commission.

Larson E: APIC Guideline for use of topical antimicrobial agents, *Am J Infect Control* 16(6):253-266, 1988.

Lynch P and others: Rethinking the role of isolation practices in the prevention of nosocomial infections, *Ann Intern Med,* 107(2):243-246, 1987.

Mandell G, Douglas G, Bennett J: Principles and practices of infectious diseases, ed 3, New York, 1990, Churchill Livingstone.

Occupational Safety and Health Administration: Enforcement policy and procedures for occupational exposure to tuberculosis, October 18, 1993, The Administration.

Rutala WA and others: Serratia marcescens nosocomial infections of the urinary tract associated with urine measuring containers and urinometers, *Am J Med* 70:659-663, 1981.

US Department of Labor: Occupational exposure to bloodborne pathogens, Federal Register 58, December 6, 1991.

Wenzel RP: Prevention and control of nosocomial infections, ed 2, Baltimore, 1993, Williams & Wilkins.

CHAPTER 13

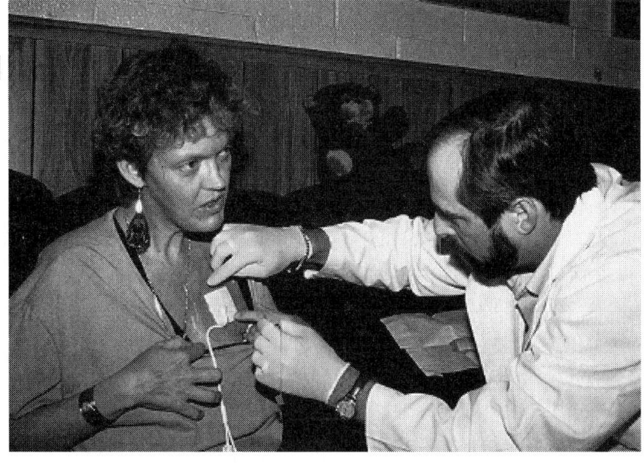

HIV Infection and AIDS

CHAPTER OBJECTIVES

1. Define acquired immunodeficiency syndrome (AIDS).
2. List three primary modes of transmission for human immunodeficiency virus (HIV).
3. Discuss the role of the CD4 T cell in the immune system.
4. Identify the major opportunistic infections seen in AIDS.
5. List the protective equipment necessary for practicing universal precautions.
6. Discuss how a nurse can prevent burnout when caring for an AIDS patient.
7. Identify nursing intervention for a patient with AIDS.
8. List the major medical interventions in the treatment of a person with AIDS.

KEY WORDS

acquired immunodeficiency syndrome (AIDS)
AIDS-related complex
Americans with Disabilities Act
burnout
candidiasis
CD4 cell count (T4 count)
condom
cotton-wool spots/patches
cytomegalovirus
enzyme-linked immunoabsorbent assay
HIV antibody
HIV infections
human immunodeficiency virus (HIV)
immunofluorescence assay
incubation period
Kaposi's sarcoma
Mycobacterium avium intracellulare
Mycobacterium avium complex
Mycobacterium tuberculosis
opportunistic infections
Pneumocystis carinii pneumonia
quality of life
Ryan White Act (Comprehensive AIDS Resources Emergency Act)
universal precautions
western blot

ACQUIRED IMMUNODEFICIENCY SYNDROME

The disease now called the **acquired immunodeficiency syndrome (AIDS)** is, as the name implies, an acquired, or secondary immune-system disorder. Presently an incurable and often fatal disease, AIDS is caused by the **human immunodeficiency virus,** type 1 **(HIV).** AIDS, the final and most serious stage of HIV infection, can be distinguished from HIV infection by its advanced position on the wide clinical spectrum of opportunistic infections.

Originally thought to be a disease of homosexual males, AIDS and HIV infections are now known to affect women and men of all sexual orientations, just as they affect infants, children, adolescents various races, and many ethnic and cultural groups. The World Health Organization (WHO) predicts that by the year 2000, 30 million to 40 million people in the world will be infected with HIV. Women, due to their biological makeup, may be the primary victims. The WHO also believes that by the year 2000, AIDS will be the third leading cause of death in the United States (U.S. Department of Health and Human Services, 1994).

The cost of AIDS and HIV is a tremendous burden on the healthcare system. In the United States alone, when the final figures are in, the medical cost of caring for these patients is expected to top $10 million for 1994 (Bartlett, 1993). This disease also creates extreme psychologic and emotional burdens as families and individuals attempt to cope. All healthcare providers will be affected by the increased diversion of resources to care for patients with AIDS. Knowledge of basic epidemiology, clinical presentations, drug therapy, and the use of the nursing process in planning care is important to all nurses who assist persons with HIV or AIDS.

Transmission

HIV has three primary modes of transmission: (1) sexual contact through anal or vaginal intercourse with an infected individual; (2) direct exposure to infected blood or blood product, often through needle-sharing among intravenous drug users; and (3) prenatal transmission from an infected woman to her fetus. Additionally, several cases of AIDS can be traced to HIV-contaminated blood supplied to patients before the **HIV antibody** test became available in 1985. Fortunately, the number of transfusion-related cases has begun to decline, and for the most part, the blood supply in the United States is considered safe (Centers for Disease Control, 1990).

It is important to the healthcare worker to prevent transmission of HIV through accidental contact. Accidental contact refers to needlesticks or direct contact with open lesions, mucous membranes, or breaks in the skin. To prevent accidental contact healthcare workers must practice universal precautions, or barrier protection, and be extremely careful when handling needles or sharp instruments. All patients must be considered infectious, and care must be taken with all blood and body fluids.

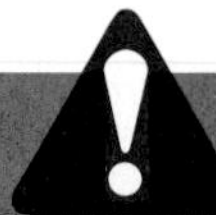

NURSE ALERT

There may be a long interval—up to 15 years—between the initial infection with HIV and the development of AIDS. A person who is HIV positive can transmit the virus to others at any time, even if he or she does not exhibit any symptoms.

The retrovirus that causes AIDS has the characteristics of a "slow" virus, meaning that the **incubation period** is months or years. The course of the resulting disease is relentless, progressive, and usually fatal. The virus can be recovered through most stages of the disease. However, it may take from 6 to 12 weeks for a person to manufacture enough antibodies to test positive for HIV (HIV+). The HIV+ diagnosis is made with a series of blood tests, starting with **enzyme-linked immunoabsorbent assay (ELISA),** followed by the **western blot,** and/or the immunofluorescence assay (IFA) are found to be positive.

The presence of HIV antibodies does not necessarily mean that a person has AIDS. It is only after the development of severe symptoms of immunodeficiency—AIDS dementia, opportunistic infections, or malignancies—that the AIDS diagnosis is made (Box 13-1). Additional diagnosis can be made by a blood test that evaluates a client's **CD4 cell counts.** It has been estimated that more than 1.5 million Americans have been infected with the virus (Centers for Disease Control, 1990). Although many people have no symptoms, they can transmit the disease.

Basic Immunology and HIV Infections

AIDS is classified as a secondary immune-system deficit. This means that immune responses are acquired rather than congenital. Both the humoral response (B lymphoctyes) and the cell-mediated response (T lymphocytes) are affected by the HIV virus, but the benchmark laboratory finding in AIDS is the depression of the cell-mediated response.

The agent known to cause AIDS is the immunodeficiency virus type 1 (HIV-1). The major target cell for HIV-1 is the CD4 T helper/inducer lymphocyte. These cells are responsible for a variety of special effects on both humoral and cell-mediated immune responses. The virus invades the CD4 T cell (Figure 13-1) and directs the cell to manufacture viral genetic products and proteins (Figure 13-2). This results in a decrease in helper T-cell number and function (Figure 13-3). Be-

BOX 13-1

CDC LIST OF CONDITIONS INCLUDED IN THE 1993 AIDS SURVEILLANCE CASE DEFINITION

- Candidiasis of bronchi, trachea, or lungs
- Candidiasis, esophageal
- Cervical cancer, invasive
- Coccidioidomycosis, disseminated or extrapulmonary
- Cryptococcosis, extrapulmonary
- Cryptosporidiosis, chronic intestinal (>1 month's duration)
- Cytomegalovirus disease (other than liver, spleen, or nodes)
- Cytomegalovirus retinities (with loss of vision)
- Encephalopathy, HIV-related
- Herpes simplex: chronic ulcer(s) (<1 month's duration); or bronchitis, pneumonitis, or esophagitis
- Histoplasmosis, disseminated or extrapulmonary
- Isosporiasis, chronic intestinal (>1 month's duration)
- Kaposi's sarcoma
- Lymphoma, Burkitt's (or equivalent term)
- Lymphoma, immunoblastic (or equivalent term)
- Lymphoma, primary, of brain
- *Mycobacterium avium* complex or *M. kansasii,* disseminated or extrapulmonary
- *Mycobacterium tuberculosis,* any site, (pulmonary or extrapulmonary)
- Mycobacterium, other species or unidentified species, disseminated or extrapulmonary
- *Pneumocystis carinii* pneumonia
- Pneumonia, recurrent
- Progressive multifocal leukoencephalopathy
- Salmonella septicemia, recurrent
- Toxoplasmosis of brain
- Wasting syndrome due to HIV

From Centers for Disease Control and Prevention: 1993 revised classification systems for HIV infection and expanded surveillance case definition for AIDS among adolescents and adults, *MMWR* 41(RR-17):1-19, 1992.

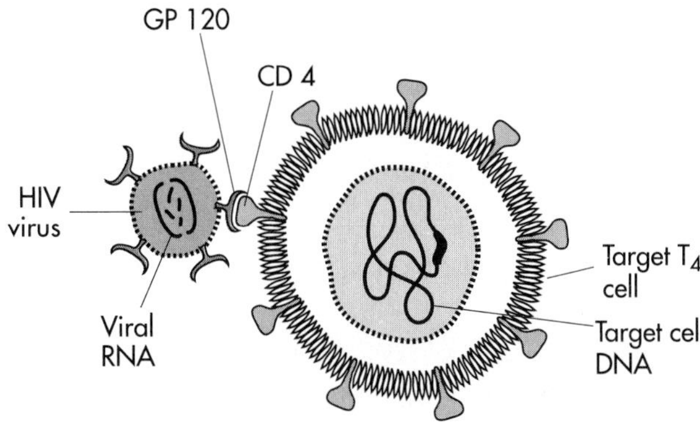

Figure 13-1 Binding of an HIV virus particle to a molecule on the target T-cell membrane.

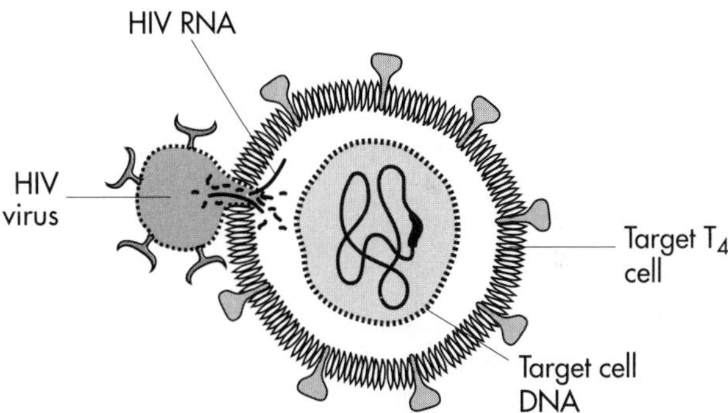

Figure 13-2 HIV ribonucleic acid (RNA) enters the target cell, causing changes in the nucleus.

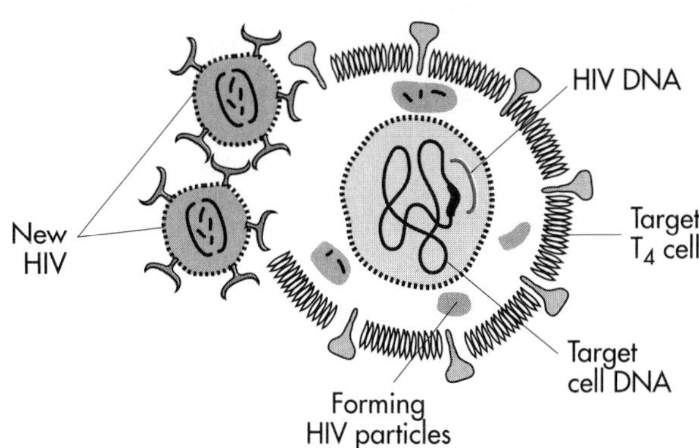

Figure 13-3 The HIV-infected cell can manufacture new HIV virus particles that are released into the environment when the cell dies or can enter a latent stage that can be activated at a later time.

cause the helper T cell plays a role in both humoral (B-cell) and cellular (T-cell) immunity, this virus causes an impairment in antibody production and in T-cell immunity; therefore AIDS virtually cripples the normal protective immune response of the body. For this reason, the evaluation and monitoring of CD4 cells is essential in the management of persons with HIV infections. In 1993, CDC expanded its case definition of AIDS to include CD4 counts of less than 200 cells/mm^3 (Table 13-1) (Centers for Disease Control and Prevention, 1992).

Disease Classification

The Centers for Disease Control and Prevention (CDC) has developed a classification system for the accurate staging of clients with HIV. This guides therapeutic decisions and provides prognostic information (Table 13-1). The new CD4-cell case definition and the 1993 list of conditions in HIV/AIDS surveillance and definition have resulted in a dramatic increase in the number of AIDS cases reported in the United States. For example, the CDC estimated that 85,000 to 90,000 new cases of AIDS would be reported in 1993, with 30,000 to 40,000 cases as a result of the new definitions (Centers for Disease Control and Prevention, 1993a).

CLINICAL MANIFESTATIONS

It usually takes between 6 and 12 weeks for antibodies against HIV to develop after the initial infection

TABLE 13-1

1993 Revised Classification System for HIV Infection and Expanded AIDS Surveillance Case Definition for Adolescents and Adults

	Clinical Categories*		
CD4 Cell Categories	**(A) Asymptomatic or PGL**	**(B) Symptomatic, Not (A) or (C) Conditions**	**(C) AIDS-Indicator Conditions**
>500/mm^3	A1	B1	C1
200-499/mm^3	A2	B2	C2
<200/mm^3 AIDS-indicator cell count	A3	B3	C3

Centers for Disease Control and Prevention: Impact of the expanded AIDS surveillance case definition on AIDS case reporting–US first quarter, 1993, *MMWR* 42(16):308-310, 1993a.

***Description of Clinical Categories**

A: One or more of the conditions listed below with documented HIV infection. Conditions listed in categories B and C must not have occurred.
- –asymptomatic HIV infection
- –persistent generalized lymphadenopathy (PGL)
- –acute (primary) HIV infection with accompanying illness or history of acute infection

B: Symptomatic conditions that meet at least one of the following criteria: (a) the conditions are attributed to HIV infection and/or are indicative of a defect in cell-mediated immunity; or (b) the conditions are considered by physicians to have a clinical course or management that is complicated by HIV infection. Examples of conditions in clinical category B include, but are not limited to:
- –bacterial endocarditis, meningitis, pneumonia, or sepsis
- –candidiasis, vulvovaginal that is persistent (greater than one month duration) or poorly responsive to therapy
- –candidiasis, oropharyngeal (thrush)
- –cervical dysplasia, severe; or carcinoma
- –constitutional symptoms, such as fever (38.4° C) or diarrhea lasting more than one month
- –hairy leukoplakia, oral
- –herpes zoster (shingles), involving at least two distinct episodes or more than one dermatome
- –idiopathic thrombocytopenic purpura
- –listeriosis
- –*Mycobacterium tuberculosis,* pulmonary
- –nocardiosis
- –pelvic inflammatory disease
- –peripheral neuropathy

C: Any condition listed in the 1993 surveillance case definition for AIDS (Box 13-1). The conditions in clinical category C are strongly associated with severe immumodeficiency, occur frequently in HIV-infected individuals, and cause serious morbidity or mortality.

takes place, but it may take up to 1 year. During that time the patient may or may not have symptoms that indicate infection. Some individuals experience flulike symptoms similar to those seen in mononucleosis. During the variable incubation period between infection and the development of AIDS (1 to 15 years), most patients have persistent and generalized lymphadenopathy. This may be accompanied by night sweats, fever, diarrhea, fatigue, weight loss, and unusual infections such as oral candidiasis. These symptoms are sometimes called **AIDS-related complex (ARC).** In a few infected persons the virus directly attacks the central nervous system, producing headaches, forgetfulness, and inability to concentrate. Studies suggest that dementia sometimes occurs before AIDS is diagnosed. Most of these infected individuals eventually develop AIDS within the next 15 years. For most persons there is a long interval, rather than a shorter one, between acquiring the initial infection and developing fullblown AIDS. Living with this phenomenon stimulates many concerns regarding the **quality of life.**

Because of their severely impaired cellular immunity, AIDS patients are susceptible to multiple opportunistic infections and unusual malignancies. Infections are difficult to control and can recur despite what appear to be good responses to treatment. Many of these HIV-related illnesses appear to be more severe than in patients without HIV. They can be spread easily, and they are rarely curable. A few of the characteristic opportunistic infections are discussed in this section.

Pneumocystic carinii pneumonia (PCP) is the most common opportunistic infection seen in AIDS. Clients may have nonspecific signs or symptoms such as nonproductive cough or malaise for several weeks, or they could have severe symptoms such as dyspnea and fevers. The chest x-ray shows a progression from normal to diffuse interstitial infiltration. Diagnosis is made by recovering the organism by bronchoscopy or by lung biopsy. Nurses should assess, by auscultation, breath sounds for rales, wheezes, and rhonci. History should include length and type of cough (Ungvarski, 1991).

The most common drug therapies used to treat PCP are timethoprim/sulfamethoxazole (TMP/SMX) and atovaquone (Division of AIDS, 1991). Before administering TMP/SMX, nurses should determine whether the client is allergic to sulfa, and after administration they should observe for rash, fever, or jaundice. Atovaquone, though less toxic, should be given with food because gastrointestinal upsets can occur. Another approved treatment for PCP is intravenous or aerosolizic pentamidine. Because aerosolized pentamidine treatments pose a risk for transmission of TB, the CDC now recommends that these treatments be administered in a contained area. Appropriate containment would be a special booth or a negative-airflow room, with the nurse or respiratory therapist wearing a high-filtration mask (Centers for Disease Control and Prevention, 1993b). Nurses should be familiar with dose levels and side effects of drugs commonly used in treating patients with HIV/AIDS (Table 13-2).

Kaposi's sarcoma (KS) was a relatively rare malignancy in the United States before the advent of AIDS. Before that time, it had been seen occasionally in older males living in the Mediterranean countries. It usually appears as pink-to-purple lesions on the skin (Figure 13-4) and is rarely painful but can be very disfiguring. KS also can involve the lungs, lymph nodes, brain, and gastrointestinal tract. Radiation therapy is beneficial for controlling obstructive lesions. Cytotoxia therapy has been used but is not effective in clients whose immune systems are already compromised. Patients should be assessed for nausea, vomiting, and potential reaction to treatments. Dietary concerns and skin care should be important when planning care.

Mucocutaneous **candidiasis,** the most commonly seen fungal infection in HIV patients, can appear as oral thrush, esophagitis, or vaginitis. Nurses may observe a whitish coating on the tongue, gums, or other mucous membranes when assessing patients. Nystatin and clotrimazole are topical therapies commonly used. Fluconazole can be given orally, but most oral agents are unsuccessful because decreased absorption occurs in many AIDS patients.

Cytomegalovirus (CMV) is commonly seen as retinitis in AIDS cases. This infection usually represents a reactivation of latent disease. The disease is progressive, usually beginning as floaters or **cotton-wool spots,** and advancing to blindness. Ganciclovir and foscarnet are drugs approved for CMV retinitis (Ungvarski, 1992). Both drugs are virustatic, not virucidal, so relapses occur if therapy is not continued. Nurses should instruct patients in the importance of continuing their therapy.

Cryptococcosis, a fungal infection often seen in AIDS patients, is acquired through the respiratory tract and primarily focuses on the lungs. It is also the major cause of meningitis in patients with AIDS. The most common symptoms are headache, fever, and stiff neck. Antifungal drugs such as oral fluconazole or intravenous amphotericin B may be ordered as treatment for cryptococcus infections (Saag, Powderly, Cloud and others, 1992). Nurses should note that amphotericin B may cause nausea, and therapy at or before mealtime should be avoided.

Toxoplasmosis is a common life-threatening infection of the central nervous system. It is caused by a

TABLE 13-2

Pharmacology of Drugs in HIV Infection and AIDS

Drug (Generic and Trade Name); Route and Dosage	Action/Indication	Common Side Effects and Nursing Considerations
ACYCLOVIR (Zovirax) **ROUTE:** PO, topical, IV (rare) **DOSAGE:** For genital herpes 200 mg q 4 h × 5 times a day × 10 days; for herpes zoster 800 mg q 4 h × 5 times a day × 7-10 days; for chickenpox (pediatric and adult); 20 mg/kg (not to exceed 800 mg/dose) qid × 5 days	Antiviral used in the prophylaxis and management of genital herpes and herpes zoster; also used for chickenpox	Dizziness, headache, diarrhea, nausea, vomiting, pain, and phlebitis; dose must be adjusted in renal impairment
AMPHOTERICIN B (Fungizone) **ROUTE:** IV and topical **DOSAGE:** Give initial test dose of 1.0 mg and observe for reaction; continue dose of 0.25 mg/kg slowly; increase daily doses slowly to 0.5 mg/kg (can give up to 1.0 mg/kg or 1.5 mg/kg every other day); topical 2-4 times daily	Antifungal used to treat active, progressive, potentially fatal fungal infections	Headache, hypotension, hypokalemia, nausea, vomiting, nephrotoxicity, fever and chills; use with caution in renal impairment and electrolyte abnormalities; drug is very irritating to tissues, and site must be monitored closely and patient assessed for febrile reaction
CLARITHROMYCIN (Biaxin) **ROUTE:** PO **DOSAGE:** 250-500 mg q 12 hr	Antiinfective used for some upper respiratory tract infections and lower respiratory tract infections including bronchitis and pneumonia	No major side effects; use with caution in severe liver and renal impairment
DAPSONE (Avlosulfon) **ROUTE:** PO **DOSAGE:** 50 to 100 mg/day	Antiinfective traditionally used for leprosy and malaria; now also used for prophylaxis against opportunistic infections in AIDS	Anorexia, pallor, skin rash, back or leg pain; hemolysis common at doses above 100 mg/day; cautious use in renal, anemia, or liver disease; recommend adequate fluid intake
FLUCONAZOLE (Diflucan) **ROUTE:** PO, IV **DOSAGE:** 100-400 mg/day PO and IV	Antifungal used for prophylaxis and treatment of multiple fungal infections in HIV/AIDS	Hepatotoxicity and exfoliative skin disorders; increased incidence of adverse reactions in AIDS; use with caution in renal and liver impairment
INTERFERON ALFA-2A (Roferon-A) **ROUTE:** IM, SQ **DOSAGE:** 36 million IU/day for 10-12 weeks; reduce dosage if severe adverse reactions occur	Antineoplastic used in treatment of AIDS-associated Kaposi's sarcoma	Fatigue, nausea, anorexia, diarrhea, vomiting, dry mouth, altered taste, rash, pruritis, anemia, leukopenia, myalgia, thrombocytopenia, flulike syndrome, fever, chills, and weight loss; use with caution in cardiac, renal, hepatic disease or decreased bone marrow

TABLE 13-2

Pharmacology of Drugs in HIV Infection and AIDS—cont'd

Drug (Generic and Trade Name); Route and Dosage	Action/Indication	Common Side Effects and Nursing Considerations
ISONIAZID **ROUTE:** PO, IM **DOSAGE:** PO and IM 5-10 mg/kg/day (usually 300 mg) or 15 mg/kg 2-3 times weekly after 2 mo at 300 mg/day	Antitubercular used as a first-line drug in combination with other agents in treatment of active TB; used for prevention of TB in patients exposed to the disease	Peripheral neuropathy; use with caution in liver or renal disease, malnourishment, diabetics, or chronic alcoholics; there are wide drug interactions and food interactions with tyramine
ITRACONAZOLE (Sporanox) **ROUTE:** PO **DOSAGE:** 200 mg tid for the first 3 days, then 200-400 mg/day	Antifungal used in treatment of histoplasmosis	Nausea; use with caution in hepatic impairment; food increases absorption
KETOCONAZOLE (Nizoral) **ROUTE:** PO, topical, shampoo **DOSAGE:** 200-400 mg/day; topical 2% 1-2 times daily	Antifungal used in treatment of candidiasis, histoplasmosis, and multiple dermatologic infections	Nausea and vomiting; use with caution in liver disease
LEUCOVORIN CALCIUM (folinic acid) **ROUTE:** PO, IM, IV **DOSAGE:** Up to 1 mg/day	Used in combination with Bactrim or dapsone mixed with pyrimethamine in treatment of HIV/AIDS patients who test positive for the toxoplasma antibody	Use with caution in renal failure; watch for thrombocytosis and allergic reactions
NYSTATIN (Mycostatin) **ROUTE:** PO **DOSAGE:** Oral suspension 400,000-600,000 units 4 times daily; usually swish and swallow	Antifungal used in the local treatment of Candida infections such as thrush	Increased irritation of mucous membranes may indicate need to discontinue treatment
PENTAMIDINE, AEROSOLIZED PENTAMIDINE **ROUTE:** IV, inhaler **DOSAGE:** IV 4 mg/kg once daily for 14-21 days (longer treatment may be required); inhaler via nebulizer 300 mg q 4 weeks	Antiinfective, antiprotozoal used in treatment and prophylaxis of *Pneumocystis carinii* (PCP)	Anxiety, headache, bronchospasm, cough, hypotension, nephrotoxicity, hypoglycemia, leukopenia, thrombocytopenia, anemia, and chills; use with caution in hypotension, hypertension, hypoglycemia, hyperglycemia, leukopenia, thrombocytopenia, anemia, diabetes mellitus, and in renal, liver, cardiovascular, or bone marrow disease
PYRIDOXINE (vitamin B_6) **ROUTE:** PO, IM, IV **DOSAGE:** PO, IM, IV 50-200 mg/day for 3 weeks, then 25-100 mg/day	Water-soluble vitamin used for treatment and prevention of INH-induced neuropathy	Use with caution in Parkinson's disease

continued

TABLE 13-2

Pharmacology of Drugs in HIV Infection and AIDS—cont'd

Drug (Generic and Trade Name); Route and Dosage	Action/Indication	Common Side Effects and Nursing Considerations
PYRIMETHAMINE (Daraprim) **ROUTE:** PO **DOSAGE:** 75 mg single dose used in combination with other agents	Antimalarial, antiprotozoal; used in combination with a sulfonamide to treat toxoplasmosis and *Pneumocystis carinii* pneumonia	Atrophic glossitis and megaloblastic anemia; use with caution in history of seizures, underlying anemia, bone marrow suppression, or impaired liver function
RIFABUTIN (Mycobutin) **ROUTE:** PO **DOSAGE:** 300 mg once daily; if gastrointestinal upset occurs, may give as 150 mg twice daily with food	Antimycrobacterial used to prevent *Mycobacterium avium* complex (MAC) disease in patients with advanced HIV infection	Brown-orange discoloration of tears, saliva, urine, and other body fluids; contraindicated in active TB
RIFAMPIN (Rifadin) **ROUTE:** PO, IV **DOSAGE:** PO, IV 10 mg/day (usual dose 600 mg/day); may also be given twice weekly	Antitubercular used in combination with other agents in management of active TB	Nausea, vomiting, heartburn, abdominal pain, flatulence, diarrhea, and red discoloration of all body fluids; contraindicated in hypertension; use with caution in liver disease
TRIMETHOPRIM AND SULFAMETHOXAZOLE (TMP/SMX) (Bactrim) **ROUTE:** PO, IV **DOSAGE:** PO 160 mg q 12 hr or daily; IV 8-20 mg/kg daily in divided doses q 6-12 hr	Anti-infective used in treatment and prevention of *Pneumocystis carinii* pneumonia	Nausea, vomiting, rashes, and phlebitis at IV site; use with caution in impaired renal and hepatic infection; increased incidence of adverse reactions in HIV
VINCRISTINE (Oncovin) **ROUTE:** IV **DOSAGE:** 10-30 μg/kg, may repeat weekly (not to exceed 2 mg each dose)	Antineoplastic agent used in treatment of Kaposi's sarcoma	Nausea, vomiting, alopecia, plebitis at IV site, and neurotoxicity; use with caution in hepatic disease and decreased bone marrow function
ZIDOVUDINE (Retrovir, AZT) **ROUTE:** PO, IV **DOSAGE:** PO, 100 mg q 4 hr; IV, 1-2 mg/kg infused over 1 hr q 4 hours; change to oral therapy as soon as possible	Antiviral used in management of HIV and AIDS	Headache, weakness, nausea, abdominal pain, diarrhea, anemia, and granulocytopenia; use with caution in decreased bone marrow, severe hepatic or renal disease; high degree of adverse reactions in HIV/AIDS

protozoan parasite, and disease may occur by ingestion of undercooked meat from infected animals. Cats can excrete the organism, so HIV patients should be instructed to wear gloves and wash hands when cleaning litter boxes. Pyrimethamine and sulfadiazine are the drugs of choice for toxoplasmosis, and patients receiving the drugs should be observed for rash or other signs of sulfa allergies.

Mycobacterium infections, especially ***Mycobacterium avium intracellulare*** **(MAI)** and ***Mycobacterium tuberculosis*** **(MTB),** are commonly seen in patients with AIDS. MAI is a bacillus commonly found in the environment and is not contagious. Unfortunately, it does spread throughout the body and is a major complication in late-stage HIV infections. Symptoms of infected patients include fever, night sweats, weight loss, and

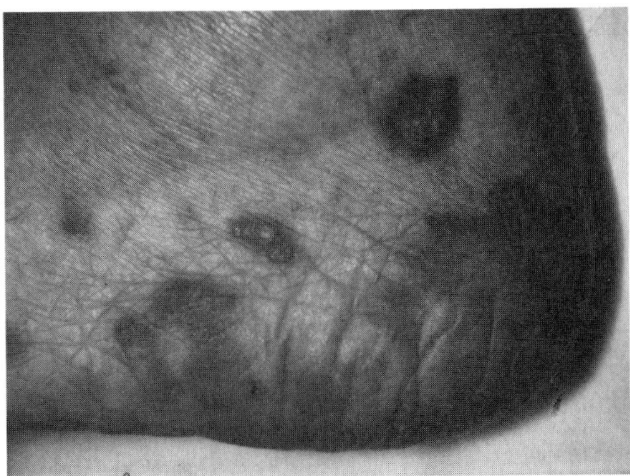

Figure 13-4 Violaceous plaques, purplish in color, of Kaposi's sarcoma on the heel and lateral foot.

OLDER ADULT CONSIDERATIONS

- Approximately 4% of all AIDS cases are among those aged 65 or older.
- Older adults engage in sexual activity.
- The reduction in mental acquity sometimes associated with the aging processes may complicate the diagnosis of dementia due to AIDS.
- For any diagnosis of immunosuppression, HIV infection should be considered as one of the possibilities in differential diagnosis.
- Previous infections may be reactivated as a result of HIV infection.
- Older adults may demonstrate different, enhanced, or delayed reactions to drug therapy.

diarrhea. The organism usually can be recovered from blood or stool. Multidrug regimens similar to those used to treat other *Mycobacterium* infections can be used (Benenson, 1990).

Mycobacterium tuberculosis, especially the drug-resistant strains, has been reported in the literature as a major cause of death in HIV patients. For this reason, TB screening upon initial entry into any healthcare setting is especially important for individuals known to be HIV positive. Pulmonary tuberculosis was added to the 1993 CDC classification of diseases seen in AIDS. A four-drug regimen is recommended for patients suspected of having or known to have TB. Isoniazid, rifampin, ethambutol, pyrazinamide, and streptomycin are a few of the drugs known to be effective in treating TB (Centers for Disease Control and Prevention 1993b). Nurses should instruct their patients on the importance of taking medication as prescribed. Because of the communicability of TB, nurses should make sure the patient with TB is properly isolated in a negative-flow, acid-fast-bacillus (AFB) isolation room. Nurses entering an AFB isolation room should wear a special high-filtration mask (Centers for Disease Control and Prevention, 1993b) (see Chapter 11 for futher discussion of TB).

There are many infectious complications seen in patients with HIV, such as herpes simplex, herpes zoster, salmonella, shigella, and other bacterial or viral infections. Coccidiomycosis and histoplasmosis are seen in their respective endemic areas. Cryptosporidiosis is a common cause of diarrhea and gastrointestinal disorders. The nurse must be aware that patients with AIDS may have many opportunistic infections. Nurses should be aware of current therapies and nursing responsibilities in giving medication and in instructing patients and families.

NURSING PROCESS

Assessment of Clients With HIV Infections and AIDS

The assessment component of the nursing process is a systematic method of obtaining information about the individual's needs, status, and perception of health. The nurse must be able to assess through conversation, physical examination, observation and record review, problem identification, collaboration with other caregivers, and observation and understanding of the coping skills of the patient and family.

The health history is the beginning point of the assessment, with specific questions aimed at obtaining information about the HIV infection. If a health history has already been obtained by another healthcare professional, the nurse should review it before the interview with the patient. A health history should cover unexplained weight loss, fever, loss of appetite, shortness of breath, skin lesions, cough, night sweats, swollen lymph nodes, diarrhea, history of sexually transmitted diseases, and central nervous system changes such as headaches, seizures, or changes in mental status.

It is important to assess the patient's risk factor for the disease. Important clues can come from sexual or drug histories and from reports of previous blood transfusions. Many times, however, patients are reluctant to discuss this information during the initial interview.

The nurse should be aware of the physical characteristics of the disease (Table 13-3), and a complete inspection of the patient should be performed by the nurse.

It is essential that the nurse determine the client's psychologic state and ability to cope with the disease.

TABLE 13-3

Physical Signs of HIV Infections

Area of Inspection	Signs/Symptoms	Possible Etiology
Central nervous system	Forgetfulness Loss of concentration Ataxia Headache Personality changes	HIV dementia
Eyes	Cotton-wool spots	CMV retinitis
Mouth	Whitish coating on tongue, gums, roof of mouth Purple spots or lesions Ridges on tongue Lesions inside/outside mouth	Oral candidiasis Kaposi's sarcoma Hairy leukoplakia Herpes simplex
Neck	Swollen, painful lymph nodes Stiff neck	Lymphadenopathy Cryptococcosis
Skin	Purple spots/lesions Rashes Lesions	Kaposi's sarcoma Syphilis Herpes simplex or zoster
Chest/lungs	Rales, rhonchi, wheezes Productive cough Cough longer than 2 weeks with/without hemophilus	PCP Bacterial pneumonia Tuberculosis
Gastrointestinal	Weight loss/wasting syndrome Diarrhea, longer than 1 month	MAI or MTB Cryptosporidiosis Salmonella
Genitourinary/rectal	Lesions Cervical dysplasia	Herpes simplex Cervical CA

The nurse should explore the patient's knowledge of AIDS and perceptions of outcomes of the disease. What changes in body image are perceived by the client? Are there outward expressions of fear, denial, grief, or loss? Does the patient have an adequate support system? What about family and friends? What coping strategies seem to work for the individual? Is there a real or perceived financial problem?

The nurse should ask open-ended questions and include, to the degree possible, family or significant others. From this assessment, a nursing diagnosis can be formed (Box 13-2).

Nursing Diagnosis

Individuals with HIV infection and AIDS can have a variety of symptoms, problems, and perceived needs (Kim, McFarland, McLane, 1993). Evaluation should be based on objective and subjective data gathered through the assessment process. Because many of the opportunistic infections can be life threatening, the first focus should be on measures to relieve symptoms. For example, if a patient has pneumonia, the nursing diagnosis "Airway clearance, ineffective" should be used. Due to the nature of the disease, all patients with AIDS could be diagnosed as "Infection, high risk for." When dealing with patients and their families, the diagnosis "Self-care deficits" should be considered. As much as possible, self-care measures should be stressed and taught. This will give patients with AIDS some control over their own care. Because at this time AIDS is considered a fatal disease, many of the psychosocial diagnoses such as "Coping, ineffective," "Denial," "Decisional conflict," and "Powerlessness" can be made. Some of the most common diagnoses can be found in Box 13-3.

Interventions

Treatment of AIDS remains largely supportive. There is no cure for AIDS, and mortality is high. However, the U.S. Food and Drug Administration (FDA) has approved three antiviral therapies for HIV infections: zidovudine (AZT), zalcitabine (ddC), and di-

BOX 13-2

Nursing Process

AIDS PATIENT

ASSESSMENT

General appearance
Signs and symptoms of infection
Knowledge of disease, transmission, and complications
Nutritional status (weight, serum albumin, stomatitis)
Coping mechanisms
Social support
Tolerance to activity
Respiratory status
Oral mucosa for lesions or ulcers
Musculoskeletal system for muscle wasting, weakness

NURSING DIAGNOSES

Powerlessness related to poor prognosis and perceived lack of control
Risk for infection related to inadequate immune system
Social isolation related to stigma attached to AIDS diagnosis
Altered nutrition: less than body requirements related to loss of appetite, oral discomfort, or high metabolic needs
Activity intolerance related to weakness, fatigue, and malnutrition
Knowledge deficit related to new condition

NURSING INTERVENTIONS

Reduce stigma of isolation by respecting the patient's dignity; encourage the patient to express feelings of isolation; provide feedback and support.
Assure the patient and significant others that AIDS does not spread by ordinary physical contact; encourage casual interactions.
Assess and chart behaviors indicative of social isolation; confer with other experts to establish a plan to decrease social isolation; specify plan; make local and national support groups or hot lines available to the patient (AIDS information number: 1-800-342-AIDS).
Explain rationale for protective isolation to patient and family; encourage telephone contact with significant others.
Monitor and document food intake; confer with the healthcare provider about the need for supplements, tube feedings, and total parenteral nutrition; develop the meal plan with the patient: meal schedules, eating environment, likes, dislikes, food temperature; encourage high-protein and high-carbohydrate foods.
Assess oral mucous membranes every 8 hours and provide appropriate interventions to decrease pain.
Weigh the patient qod.
Provide for periods of rest by scheduling treatments, minimizing room noise, and limiting visitors.
Instruct the patient on energy-saving techniques and improving nutritional status to increase activity tolerance; encourage progressive activity as tolerated; assess pulse, respiration, blood pressure, presence of dyspnea, cyanosis, and pain as indicators of overactivity.
Assist the patient with hygiene as needed.

EVALUATION OF EXPECTED OUTCOMES

Is free of opportunistic infections
Verbalizes factors that may increase risk of infection
Verbalizes a decrease in loneliness and sense of isolation
Maintains relationships with significant others
Maintains weight at _____ lbs
Tolerates prescribed diet
Exhibits healthy gums and oral mucous membranes
Demonstrates ability to alternate activity with appropriate rest periods
Verbalizes increased comfort while performing activities

danosine (ddI). All these drugs act by blocking viral replication (Figure 13-5). In 1990, the FDA approved zidovudine for all HIV-infected patients with CD4 counts of 500 cells/mm or less.

Zidovudine is well tolerated in most clients and has prolonged the survival of persons with AIDS. For this reason, AZT is the drug of choice. Some of the major side effects, occurring in about 5% of patients, are anemia and granulocytopenia. The FDA now approves ddI as a single-drug therapy for individuals who cannot tolerate AZT. Zalcitabine is approved for use in combination with AZT or ddI in patients who are de-

BOX 13-3

NURSING DIAGNOSES COMMONLY SEEN IN PATIENTS WITH HIV INFECTIONS

- Activity intolerance
- Adjustment, impaired
- Body image disturbance
- Body temperature, altered, risk for
- Breathing pattern, ineffective
- Coping, ineffective
- Decisional conflict
- Denial, ineffective
- Diarrhea
- Fatigue
- Gas exchange, impaired
- Grieving
- Hopelessness
- Infection, risk for
- Oral mucous membrane, altered
- Powerlessness
- Self-care deficit
- Self-esteem
- Sexuality patterns, altered
- Social isolation
- Violence, risk for: self-directed

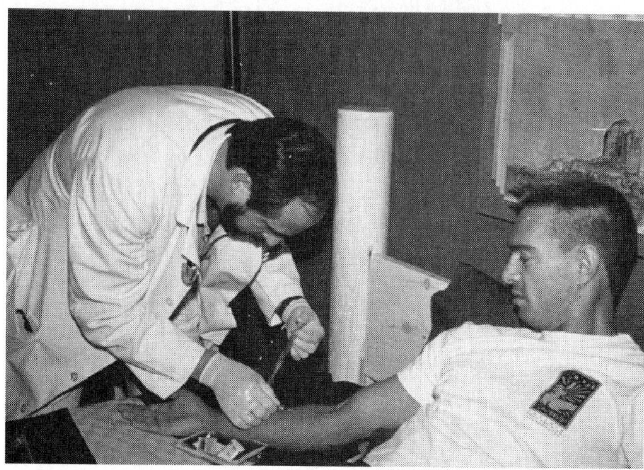

Figure 13-5 Viral replication is blocked by drugs such as zidovudine (AZT). (Courtesy Michael Clement, MD, Mesa, Ariz.)

teriorating on monotherapy (Meng, Fischl, and Boota, 1992). Nurses should instruct patients that if AZT upsets the stomach, they should take the medication with a light, low-fat meal (Vaccariello, Funesti, Laverty, Vasquez and Curran, 1993).

AIDS may affect every system of the body and every facet of a person's life. The nurse has a large role in assessing the many needs of these patients and in designing appropriate plans for care. The role of the nurse is supportive and is focused on minimizing distress from the numerous manifestations of the disease. Providing psychologic support is essential because the essence of nursing care is to assist the patient and his or her family through an enormous assault on the human spirit (Figure 13-6). As the wasting and the mental-status changes associated with progressing disease take hold, body-image changes become frightening. Fear of having transmitted the disease to loved ones and the experience of ostracism can be overwhelming. Physical symptoms such as the drenching sweats that occur daily are managed with frequent linen changes, bathing, and special skin care. Pressure sores may be prevented by use of protective devices on the bed and by frequent turning.

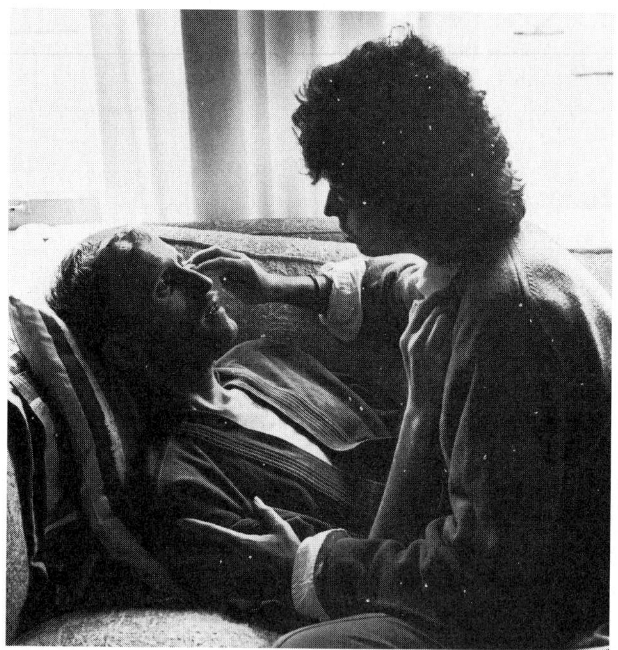

Figure 13-6 Compassionate support from the nursing staff can minimize distress from the numerous manifestations of AIDS.

Interventions should be based on goals agreed upon by the patient, the family, and the nurse. Individuals with HIV infections should be able to establish some boundaries of control over their plan of care. As much as possible, self-care goals should be used. Participation in care by the patient and/or family should be encouraged, and the nurse should devote as much time as possible to patient teaching. It is important to help the patient maintain independence while conserving energy. This can be accomplished by balancing activity with frequent rest periods. Encouraging the patient to perform consistent, frequent oral care will relieve the discomfort of a *Candida* infection. Sitz baths to relieve impaired perirectal mucosal integrity are offered three or four times a day. Maintaining safety is important for the confused, demented patient. It involves keeping bedside rails up, assisting with walking, ensuring a safe environment, and providing frequent reality orientation.

Educating the patient and family in the management of AIDS is extremely important. Informing the patient and the family about the ways in which the virus can be transmitted is essential to halting the spread of the disease. Patients should be informed that the virus is spread through semen and blood and that sexual intercourse should be avoided if the person is infected. Latex **condoms** have been recommended as a means to prevent spread. Abstaining from both anal and genital sex is recommended. Infected persons should not share toothbrushes or razors. Women partners of infected persons and women engaging in high-risk activities should prevent pregnancy, because the virus can be transmitted to the fetus. Persons who have a positive antibody test should notify their partners and should inform healthcare personnel before receiving treatment. They should never donate blood, organs, tissue, plasma, or sperm and should never share needles or syringes if they abuse drugs.

In the hospital, the nurse prevents the spread of HIV by following universal precautions and infection-control recommendations. When the patient is capable of performing self-care activities, the nurse needs to wear only gloves when handling blood and other specimen collections. The CDC guidelines for universal precautions to prevent transmission of HIV (Centers for Disease Control, 1988) are listed in Box 13-4. Other isolation procedures should be initiated if the patient has a communicable opportunistic infection. The major risk for healthcare workers has been associated with handling sharp objects. From a single needlestick with a needle that has been in contact with infected blood, the infection rate is estimated to be approximately 0.5%, or 1 in 200. Precautions to prevent needlestick injury by the nurse must be adhered to strictly.

The nurse should be well informed about this dread disease, which is epidemic among high-risk groups and in many areas of the world. It is essential that the nurse avoid the hysteria associated with AIDS and maintain a professional demeanor. This involves correcting misinformation, providing accurate information, and above all, protecting the patient's basic human right to privacy. The diagnosis should be kept confidential, and patient records should be guarded against invasion by others who may engage in unethical practices. Quality of care can be achieved only when that care is ethically based.

PATIENT/FAMILY TEACHING

Topics
- HIV/AIDS transmission and disease prevention
- HIV/AIDS signs and symptoms
- Wellness techniques such as nutrition and protection against communicable disease
- Medication and side effects
- Development of coping strategies
- Available resources
- Support groups
- Self-care strategies
- Infection-control practices

Focus
- Teach deep breathing techniques, splinting, use of spirometers, and possibly postural drainage.
- Teach use of trapeze when changing positions.
- Teach importance of hydration to promote liquefaction of secretions.
- Teach 24-hour care plan that incorporates short activities with rest periods.

PRECAUTIONS TO PREVENT TRANSMISSION OF HIV

Because medical history and examination cannot reliably identify all patients infected with HIV or other blood-borne pathogens, blood and body-fluid precautions should be used consistently for all patients. This approach, previously recommended by CDC and referred to as "universal blood and body-fluid precautions" or **universal precautions,** should be used in the care of all patients, especially those in emergency care settings, where the risk of blood exposure is increased and the infection status of the patient usually is unknown (Box 13-4).

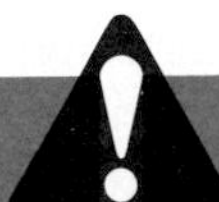

NURSE ALERT

Universal (standard) precautions should be used while caring for all patients in any setting.

BOX 13-4

UNIVERSAL PRECAUTIONS

Universal precautions apply to blood or other potentially infectious material such as the following body fluids: semen, vaginal secretions, cerebrospinal fluid, synovial fluid, saliva in dental procedures, any body fluid that is visibly contaminated with blood, and all body-fluid situations where it is difficult or impossible to differentiate between body fluids.

Hands must be washed after gloves are removed or if there has been potential contamination with blood or other infectious material.

Gloves shall be worn when one can reasonably anticipate contact with blood or other potentially infectious materials, mucous membranes, non-intact skin, or other such conditions when performing vascular access procedures.

Gloves should be replaced if contaminated, torn, punctured, or when their ability to function as a barrier is compromised.

Gloves should be changed between contact with different patients.

Masks, eye protection, and face shields shall be worn whenever splashes, spray, splatter, or droplets of blood or other infectious material may be generated and when eye, nose, or mouth contamination can be reasonably anticipated.

Gowns, aprons, and other protective body clothing shall be worn in occupational exposure situations. Type depends on task and degree of exposure.

Surgical caps or hoods and/or shoe covers or boots shall be worn in instances when gross contamination can be reasonably anticipated.

Contaminated needles and other contaminated sharps shall not be bent or sheared. Recapping is prohibited unless there is no other alternative; then a recapping device or one-handed technique may be used.

Immediately after use, contaminated needles or sharps shall be placed in puncture-resistant, leakproof containers as close to the site of use as possible.

Specimens shall be placed in a leakproof container. Care is taken to avoid contaminating outside of containers.

HIV/AIDS LEGAL ISSUES

Since the first reported cases of AIDS in the United States, there has been much controversy over the laws and regulations that govern HIV-infected persons. It is often difficult to protect the rights of the public without infringing on the right of the person with AIDS. For example, certain sexually transmitted diseases have been designated as reportable diseases by the U.S. Health Department. Although there is no agreement on the reporting of HIV infections, all states require the reporting of AIDS cases. Under the new definition of AIDS, characterized by CD4 T-cell counts below 200 and the increase in the list of opportunistic infections and cancers, the number of persons reported with AIDS has increased. Also, under the Ryan White Act, physicians and hospitals may also be required to notify first responders, emergency rescue personnel, and mortuaries of their contact with persons diagnosed with certain contagious diseases (Centers for Disease Control and Prevention, 1994).

Both state and federal laws address healthcare issues for persons infected with HIV. The duty to treat, the requirement or permission to test for a contagious disease, and the duty to contact those who have been exposed is addressed in all states. Additionally, since AIDS is considered a handicap, the Federal Rehabilitation Act and the Americans with Disabilities Act apply to HIV-infected persons.

State laws vary regarding the serologic screening for HIV, but all stress the importance of maintaining the patient's rights. Most states require the following: an explanation of the HIV test procedures, consent for testing, disclosure of test results by properly trained personnel, confidentiality that limits release of results to only those designated by law as eligible to know, and use of universal precautions to reduce exposure to healthcare workers.

What about HIV-infected healthcare workers? Their rights are subject to the same laws that safeguard everyone else who may be discriminated against in the workplace because of a handicap. The CDC estimates that 5.5% of all HIV-positive persons are employed in the healthcare field. The CDC recommends that certain surgical procedures not be performed by a surgeon who is HIV positive (Centers for Disease Control, 1991).

Healthcare workers who become infected with HIV on the job may have a claim under state workers compensation acts. Employers have to provide a safe working environment under the Occupational Safety and Health Act (OSHA). OSHA standards dealing with HIV exposures in the workplace are covered in regulations, and OSHA monitors and inspects the use of universal precautions as recommended by the CDC (*AIDS-Alert*, 1992).

Nurses have the responsibility of knowing the current HIV laws and regulations in the state where they are employed. Protecting the rights of both the patient and the public is an essential requirement for today's nurse.

ETHICAL DILEMMA

You have heard that a nurse you work with in the neonatal intensive care unit (NICU) is HIV positive. You are aware that universal precautions are not closely followed in the NICU, and you are therefore concerned about patient safety. However, you are also concerned about loyalty to your nurse colleague and about confidentiality regarding this coworker's medical condition. What should you do?

BURNOUT

As caregivers at the bedside, many nurses are experiencing emotional exhaustion and distress or burnout when working with HIV-infected patients (Driedger, Cox, 1991). Emotional exhaustion is an outcome of particular concern when nurse-patient interaction requires considerable involvement. Nurses need to be comfortable with AIDS problems such as mortality, issues of sexuality and drug use, watching young people die, and fear of contagion (Meisenhelder, LaCharite, 1989). It is important to be able to recognize issues that cause discomfort and to develop coping strategies that maintain a sense of control when dealing with uncomfortable situations. The first step is to identify the sources of stress when dealing with AIDS patients.

As human beings, nurses must deal with feelings toward death and dying. This is particularly important because they seem less able to deal with death among young people. Because of religious or philosophic outlooks, many feel that death is a part of the life process, but everyone has difficulty dealing with loss. Nurses need to be able to grieve when a patient dies and to evaluate their feelings toward death.

Appropriate methods for dealing with mortality issues would include talking with peers or discussion groups. Attending funerals, writing cards, or expressing sympathy to family members also can assist with working through a feeling of sadness.

Many nurses must address their own attitudes toward homosexuality when caring for patients with AIDS. In the United States the majority of persons with AIDS are gay or bisexual men. Nurses cannot identify "who is or who is not," and this uncertainty may raise their stress levels. Research has shown that nurses may be more nonjudgmental of homosexuals if they have a friend or relative who is gay.

The incidence of drug use in the United States is staggering. To many in healthcare, drug abuse is viewed as a crime rather than a disease. They feel frustrated when patients appear to be literally killing themselves with illegal substances. Drug users are often seen as weak people who chose their own lifestyle. Nurses should stay informed regarding drug addiction as a disease process and should view this as a treatable condition.

Nurses can overcome their fear of contagion by keeping themselves educated about HIV infection. By understanding the disease process and universal precautions, nurses can protect themselves from the disease.

There are several steps in preventing or reducing burnout. First, nurses need to recognize the stress they are encountering, step back, set priorities, and try to balance the workload. Second, nurses are encouraged to discuss their feelings with peers or join a support discussion group (Stein, Wade, Smith, 1991). Third, nurses must take care of their physical needs through exercise and good nutrition. Fourth, nurses benefit from learning to relax, developing a sense of humor, and participating in non–work-related activities. The nurse should be optimistic. Maintaining hope for new therapies and treatments enables the nurse to feel hopeful for the future of patients with AIDS.

Nursing Care Plan

PATIENT WITH ACQUIRED IMMUNODEFICIENCY SYNDROME (AIDS)

The patient is a 37-year-old male who reenters the medical unit after having been discharged 3 months ago. He is diagnosed as having AIDS and has been receiving outpatient therapy for chronic symptoms, including fever, night sweats, diarrhea, fatigue, and weight loss. He is experiencing dyspnea, shortness of breath (SOB), and cough, which began 2 days ago. The SOB has intensified, causing him to become anxious and at times confused. *Pneumocystis carinii* is confirmed by assessments, x-ray studies, and cultures. He is admitted for further evaluation, nursing care, and treatment. He has no known food or drug allergies, does not smoke or tolerate secondhand smoke, and denies use of alcohol or drugs.

Past Medical History	Psychosocial Data	Assessment Data
Generally healthy until 1 year ago, when he developed generalized lymphadenopathy; sought medical advice immediately Blood test confirmed the presence of HIV antibodies; started on zidovudine (AZT) and Bactrim DS on an outpatient basis Progress monitored by a private medical doctor 50-lb weight loss in 6 months Depression for 3 months; receiving psychotherapy on a weekly basis Homosexual activity began at 18	Has significant other (SO) partner with whom he has had a 6-year relationship; partner unwilling to be tested for AIDS at this time; supportive relationship with lover Both parents well, in their early 60s, live out of state and plan to retire soon from professional careers; said to be adjusting to son's homosexual disclosure and illness; have been to visit twice; patient considers significant other as the present family One brother age 35, and a sister age 30; both well; no family history of hypertension, diabetes, or renal disease; cancer history in both sets of grandparents (now deceased) Self-employed as a dentist; has been unable to maintain practice and is in process of selling practice and applying for disability benefits under Social Security Issue of confidentiality requested by client; believes that "giving up" license to practice denotes surrendering to illness Owns own home; easy entrance access Has private medical insurance through group practice; anxious over continuing coverage once illness progresses *Religion:* Protestant; attends services only on holidays; has discussed illness with minister. *Hobbies:* Likes listening to classical music; follows sports on TV; interested in antique cars	Frail, thin male who appears much older than his stated age Flat affect with very little verbal exchange; responds to questions but offers no extra information; some eye contact Height 5 ft 10 in; weight 130 lb Oriented × 3 (time, place, and person), color pale *Vital signs:* T 100.6, P 92, R 38, BP 140/70 *Skin:* Warm, dry, and intact; no signs of rashes, bruises, or decubiti *Eye, ear, nose, throat:* Mucous membranes moist; no mouth lesions; extraocular motions intact; both nares patent; prominent cheek bones from apparent weight loss; generalized lymphadenopathy: cervical, postauricular, and axillary nodes enlarged bilaterally *Respiratory:* Rate 36-40; labored with increased use of accessory muscles; dyspnea on exertion (DOE); bilateral wheezes heard in both lower lobes, greater on expiration than inspirtion; adventitious sounds heard in all lung fields; "guarding" chest while coughing; productive cough *Abdominal:* Wasted appearance, decreased tone; hypotonic bowel sounds heard in all four quadrants *Musculoskeletal:* Range of motion in all joints, with some obvious degree of discomfort; unsteady gait; positive peripheral pulses; No edema in ankles or feet ***Laboratory data:*** RBC 3.09, Hgb 8.1, Hct 29, WBC 18,000, cholesterol 105

Nursing Care Plan

PATIENT WITH ACQUIRED IMMUNODEFICIENCY SYNDROME (AIDS)—cont'd

Past Medical History	Psychosocial Data	Assessment Data
		Platelets 300,000; Electrolytes: Na 145, K. 4.2 Chloride 108, CO_2 24 *Blood gases:* pH 7.36, pCO_2 47, HCO_3 28, Po_2 78, O_2 sat. 82% *ECG:* Within normal limits Chest x-ray examination shows infiltration, both lungs *Urinalysis:* Within normal limits *Stool culture:* Positive for *Giardia lamblia* ***Medications*** zidovudine (Retrovir) 100 mg PO four times a day metronidazole (Flagyl) 400 mg IVPB q 6 hr (infuse over 1 hr) trimethoprim/sulfamethoxazole (Bactrim DS) 2 tabs PO q 8 hr diazepam (Valium) 5 mg PO q 4-6 hr prn anxiety 1000 ml D5W with 10 mEq KCl q 8 hr Oxygen at 6 L via nasal cannula *Universal precautions maintained*

NURSING DIAGNOSIS

Ineffective airway clearance related to *Pneumocystis carinii* pneumonia as indicated by dyspnea, cough, and increased respiration

NURSING INTERVENTIONS

Monitor vital signs q 4 hr and prn.
Assess breath sounds.
Have patient turn, cough, deep breathe q 4 hr.
Demonstrate and assist with splinting technique during coughing and deep breathing.
Offer cough medication q 4 hr (not prn); not to be given with meals.
Encourage use of cough drops and tea with lemon and honey.
Offer warm saline mouthwash and gargle for sore throat.
Provide 2.5 liters of fluids per day for adequate hydration; offer 8-12 oz of fluids q 4 hr during waking hours (likes ginger ale and apple juice); monitor I & O.
Encourage use of assistance devices such as trapeze, wheelchair, and walker.
Assist patient and family in planning care to conserve energy, such as shower chair while bathing, sitting down while dressing.

EVALUATION OF EXPECTED OUTCOMES

Vital signs and breath sounds within normal limits
Verbalizes improved respiratory functioning
Patient and family able to demonstrate use of pillow as splint during coughing
Regulates own medication
Has decreased cough symptoms
Does not have a sore throat
Identifies preferred fluids, maintains intake at 2.5 L, keeps self-record of intake at bedside
Able to use assistance devices to conserve energy
Patient and family able to plan 24 hours of care

continued

NURSING DIAGNOSIS

Anticipatory grieving related to advancement of illness as evidenced by behavior manifestations

NURSING INTERVENTIONS	EVALUATION OF EXPECTED OUTCOMES
Help patient to understand the grieving process and to accept his feelings as normal. Emphasize patient's identified strengths; provide positive reinforcement for effective coping behaviors. Inform him of existing support groups in the facility/community; offer to contact clergy of his choice; accept his way of responding to the illness; provide privacy, dignified care, and acceptance on a daily basis. Help patient discuss his fears by establishing a trusting relationship. Plan time during each shift to sit with and actively listen to him. Give private time with friend and his family.	Uses healthy coping mechanisms Contacts support group within 2 weeks of hospitalization Shares his feelings with his significant other, family, friends, and clergy Expresses his feelings about his illness Communicates his understanding about the stages of grief Accepts feelings and behavior brought on by the potential loss

NURSING DIAGNOSIS

Decisional conflict related to surrender of dental practice and license as evidenced by delayed decision making and vacillation between choices

NURSING INTERVENTIONS	EVALUATION OF EXPECTED OUTCOMES
Acknowledge patient's feelings; be supportive and use a nonjudgmental approach. Help him to identify available options and their possible consequences. Help patient make decisions about daily activities; keep him oriented to reality. Encourage visits with family, friends, clergy, and peers. Demonstrate respect for his right to choose decisions based on values and beliefs.	Openly expresses feelings about necessary decisions that he faces Describes conflicts related to illness, disclosure, and treatment Identifies consequences of potential choices Makes at least two care-related decisions daily Expresses increased comfort in dealing with conflicts

NURSING DIAGNOSIS

Powerlessness related to chronic illness as evidenced by sadness, crying, and passivity

NURSING INTERVENTIONS	EVALUATION OF EXPECTED OUTCOMES
Encourage patient to express feelings; set aside time for discussion; allow silence; listen for clues of expression. Accept patient's feelings of powerlessness as normal; try to be present during situations when feelings of powerlessness are likely to be greatest, to help him cope in a positive way. Identify and develop patient's coping mechanisms, strengths, and resources. Discuss situations that provoke feelings of anger, anxiety, or powerlessness. Encourage participation in self-care as much as possible.	Verbalizes both positive and negative feelings about current situation Describes strategies for reducing anxiety Demonstrates control by participating in decision making related to care Actively plans and executes aspects of decision making regarding future of dental practice Includes friend in a discussion of his feelings and needs Identifies the potential for appointing a "power of attorney" as his illness progresses Being a part of that decision leads to increased feelings of dignity

NURSING INTERVENTIONS	EVALUATION OF EXPECTED OUTCOMES
Provide as many opportunities as possible for patient to make decisions regarding care (positioning, rest, choosing an IV site, visiting, fluid and food choices). Modify the environment when available to meet his self-care needs (commode, lounge chair). Encourage family and friend to support patient without taking control. Reinforce patient's rights as stated in Patient Bill of Rights. Identify and arrange to accommodate his spiritual needs.	

KEY CONCEPTS

- HIV infection presently is an incurable and often fatal disease. The most severe form of the infection is AIDS.
- HIV infection is transmitted by sexual contact with an infected individual, by direct exposure to infected blood or blood products, and by prenatal exposure from an infected woman to her fetus.
- Healthcare workers are at risk for transmission through accidental contact with open lesions, mucous membranes, or breaks in the skin (needlesticks).
- Infected persons can transmit HIV at any time during the course of the infection.
- HIV is a retrovirus with an incubation period of months or years. It usually takes 6 to 12 weeks for a person to create enough antibodies to test positive for HIV.
- Diagnostic tests for HIV infection include the enzyme-linked immunoabsorbent assay (ELISA), the western blot, and/or the immunofluorescence assay (IFA).
- The HIV particle attaches to CD4 receptor sites on body cells, usually the T cell of the immune system. The result is either cell death or disruption of cell function.
- The Centers for Disease Control and Prevention (CDC) has developed a classification system for the accurate staging of persons with HIV infection.
- Because of the progressive deterioration of the immune system, opportunistic infections can occur. These include *Pneumocystis carinii* pneumonia, Kaposi's sarcoma, mucocutaneous candidiasis and other fungal infections, and mycobacterium infections including tuberculosis.
- Intervention for HIV infection and AIDS remains largely supportive, although three antiviral therapies have been approved by the Food and Drug Administration: zidovudine (AZT), zalcitabine (ddC), and didanosine (ddI).
- Nursing care involves providing supportive activities and minimizing distress from the numerous manifestations of the disease. Psychologic support is essential.
- Universal (standard) precautions are very important for the care of all patients in all settings.
- Many legal and ethical issues surround HIV and AIDS. It is difficult to protect the rights of the public without infringing on the rights of the person with HIV/AIDS.

CRITICAL THINKING EXERCISES

1. Outline a plan to prevent HIV infection among sexually active adolescents.
2. Compare and contrast primary (acute) HIV infection, asymptomatic HIV infection, mild symptomatic HIV disease, and advanced HIV infection.
3. Relate the clinical manifestations of AIDS to the underlying pathology.
4. Identify the patient care needs that should be included in a plan of care for an AIDS patient.
5. For the patient and for the family, what are the likely psychologic reactions to the diagnosis of HIV infection?

REFERENCES AND ADDITIONAL READINGS

Bartlett J: *Care and management of patients with HIV infections,* 1993, Glaxo.

Benenson A: *Control of communicable diseases in man,* ed 15, Washington, DC, 1990, American Public Health Association.

Centers for Disease Control: Update: Universal precautions for prevention of transmission of human immunodeficiency virus, hepatitis B virus, and other blood borne pathogens in health care settings, *MMWR* 37(24):377-382; 387-388, 1988.

Centers for Disease Control: Surveillance for HIV2 infections in blood donors—United States 1987-1989, *MMWR* 39(46):829-831, 1990.

Centers for Disease Control: Recommendations for preventing transmission of human immunodeficiency virus and hepatitis B virus to patient during exposure-prone invasive procedures, *MMWR* 49(RR8):1-9, 1991.

Centers for Disease Control and Prevention: 1993 revised classification systems for HIV infection and expanded surveillance case definition for AIDS among adolescents and adults. *MMWR* 41(RR-17):1-19, 1992.

Centers for Disease Control and Prevention: Impact of the expanded AIDS surveillance case definition on AIDS case reporting—U.S. first quarter, 1993, *MMWR* 42(16):308-310, 1993a.

Centers for Disease Control and Prevention: Draft guidelines for preventing the transmission of tuberculosis in health-care facilities, ed 2, *Fed Regis,* October 12, 1993b.

Centers for Disease Control and Prevention: Implementation of provisions of the Ryan White comprehensive AIDS resource emergency act regarding emergency response envelope, *Fed Regis* 59(4):13418-13428, 1994.

Division of AIDS: *Important information on the prevention of recurrent Pneumocystic carinii pneumonia in persons with AIDS,* National Institute of Allergies and Infectious Diseases, NIH, October 11, 1991.

Driedger S, Cox D: Burnout in nurses who care for PWAS, *AIDS Patient Care* 5(4):197-203, 1991.

HIV-infected nurse wins $5.37 million: *AIDS Alert* 7(10), 149-152, 1992.

Kim M, McFarland G, McLane A: *Nursing diagnosis,* ed 5, St Louis, 1993, Mosby.

Meisenhelder J, La Charite C: Fear of contagion: a stress response to acquired immunodeficiency syndrome, *Adv Nurs Sci* 11(2):29-38, 1989.

Meng T, and others: Combination therapy with zidovudine and dideoxyctidine in patients with advanced human immuno deficiency virus. *Ann Int Med* 116:13-20, 1992.

Saag M and others: Comparison of Amphotericin B with Fluconazole in the treatment of acute AIDS-associated cryptococcal meningitis, *N Engl J Med* 326(2):83-89, 1992.

Stein E, Wade K, Smith D: Clinical support groups that work for nurses who care for patients with AIDS. *JANAC* 2(2):29-36, 1991.

Ungvarski P: Nursing care of the client with infection due to pneumocystis carinii, *JANAC* 2(2):15-28, 1991.

Ungvarski P: Nursing care of the adult client with AIDS and cytomegalovirus infections, *JANAC* 3(11);9-18, 1992.

U.S.Department of Health and Human Services: *Evaluation and management of early HIV infections,* Rockville, Md, January 1994 (AHCPR Publication No 94-0572).

Vaccariello J and others: The administration of didanosine (ddI) in the adult: a nursing perspective, *JANAC* 4(1):23-33, 1993.

CHAPTER 14

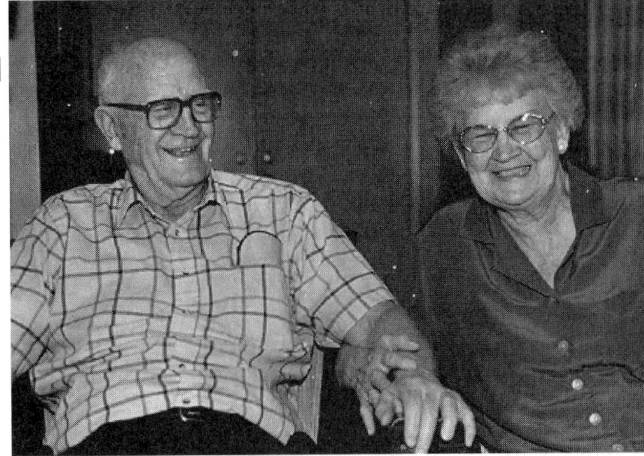

The Older Adult

CHAPTER OBJECTIVES

1 Differentiate between *geriatrics* and *gerontology.*
2 Discuss the effects of the increasing number of persons over age 65 on the healthcare system in the United States.
3 Discuss socioeconomic and cultural factors that affect persons over age 65.
4 Identify biologic, psychologic, and social changes related to aging.
5 Identify the adjustments usually required of the aging person.
6 Discuss the factors involved in maintaining mental health for the person over age 65.
7 Discuss current theories of the causes of aging.
8 Discuss the effects of aging on intelligence and memory.
9 Identify the physiologic changes that occur with aging.
10 Identify assessment techniques used to evaluate the physiologic changes of aging.
11 Identify nursing interventions related to physiologic changes that occur with aging.
12 Discuss nursing measures that help prevent injury and promote function for the aged person.
13 Describe the modifications in diet required by those over age 65.
14 Identify factors that contribute to sexual satisfaction in the elderly person.
15 Discuss the ways in which age-related pathophysiologic changes affect drug action and toxicity.
16 Discuss the reaction of the elderly to central nervous system depressants and stimulants.
17 Explain the need for reducing dosages of most drugs prescribed for the elderly.
18 Identify alternatives to institutional care for the aged person.

KEY WORDS

Alzheimer's disease
delirium
dementia
depression
Mini-Mental-Status Examination (MMSE)
geriatrics
gerontology
home care
Medicare
nursing home
reality orientation
reminiscing
remotivation
retirement
senescence
sexuality

The term **geriatrics** is defined by Webster's as the branch of medicine that deals with the diseases and problems of old age and aging people (Webster's, 1986). It is derived from the Greek word *geras*, meaning old age. **Gerontology** is the scientific study of the process of aging and its effects (Webster's, 1986). The science of gerontology is multidisciplinary and includes the social, biologic, spiritual, and psychologic aspects of aging. **Senescence** is the final stage in the life cycle. It denotes a time of gradual physical decline that is preceded by a period of attaining maturity. Senescence is not a pathologic condition but a normal biologic process (Figure 14-1).

DEMOGRAPHICS

The need for nurses to educate themselves regarding the health needs of older persons is a necessity. In the next several decades, the number of older persons, particularly those over age 85, will increase rapidly. While the number of persons over the age of 65 will more than double from about 32 million today to more than 67 million by the year 2040 (United States Census Bureau, 1991), the number of persons over the age of 85 is expected to quadruple. With this dramatic increase in the "old old" population will come an increased number of people with chronic health problems such as hypertension, chronic lung disease, sensory impairments, and memory deficits. In 1900 only 4% of the population was 65 years of age or older. In 1991 13.5% were age 65 or over. By the year 2030, a predicted 50 million people will be age 65 or over and will make up 17% of the total population. A white female at age 65 is expected to have another 20 years of life, and men will have nearly 16 more years (Social Security Administration, 1988).

As the number and proportion of older adults increases, the proportion of working adults (ages 18 to 64) decreases. This means that there are fewer persons contributing to the national economy and fewer family members to provide support for the elderly, both financially and in times of crises. Adult daughters, who traditionally have been the caregivers of the older generation, are now more likely to be working in paid employment outside the home. In view of such social and economic changes, the government may have to assume a greater role in providing these services to the older population (Esberger, Hughes, 1989).

Since the turn of the century, life expectancy has increased greatly, from an average of 47.3 years in 1900 to 75 years for the person born in 1984. In general, women live longer than men. Among the most common causes of death for those aged 75 and over, pneumonia and flu are the only infectious disease categories remaining (Table 14-1). To a large extent, the increase in life expectancy has been brought about by reducing the number of deaths from infectious diseases and acute illnesses. However, this has resulted in an increase in the death rate from chronic illnesses such as cancer and heart disease. Persons suffering from chronic illnesses require more healthcare and nursing services to remain functional. This may place additional demands on the healthcare system as the population continues to age and the number of older persons continues to grow.

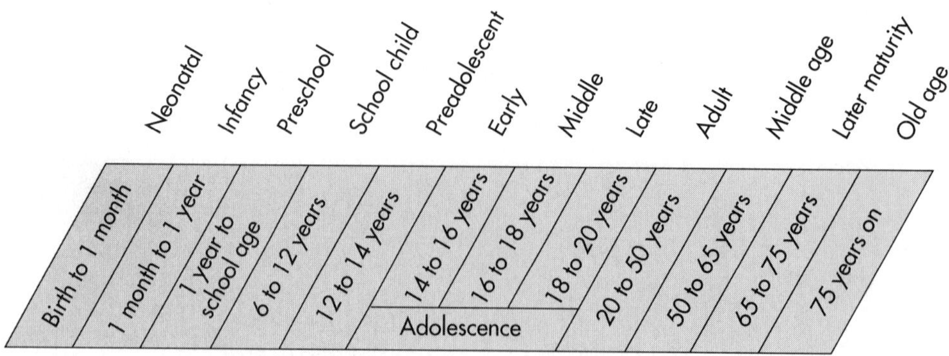

Figure 14-1 Life span is continuous but has been divided into stages, each presenting different needs. The geriatric patient is near the end of the continuum and has his or her own special needs.

TABLE 14-1

Nine Most Common Causes of Death Among Persons 75 Years to 84 Years and Older by Frequency of Occurrence per 100,000 Population of That Age Group

	Men	Women	Men	Women
	75-84		85 and Older	
Heart disease	3239	2122	7830	6810
Malignancies	1861	982	2528	1292
Cerebrovascular accident (CVA)	603	523	1625	1738
Chronic obstructive pulmonary disease (COPD)	504	197	777	245
Pneumonia and flu	352	199	1428	1006
Accidents	143	84	375	225
Diabetes	127	123	229	219
Suicide	57	7	60	5
Liver disease	44	25	34	14

From U.S. Bureau of the Census: *Statistical abstract of the United States,* 111th ed, Washington, DC, 1991, US Government Printing Office. From Ebersole P, Hess P: *Toward healthy aging: human needs and nursing response,* ed 4, St Louis, 1994, Mosby.

The social support system of the elderly person also is changing. Of those over age 75, about 20% of men and 50% of women live alone. Of those who live alone, about 50% see their adult children at least once a week. The others either have no children or are separated geographically from their children and see them less often. Concerns exist for those older persons who require some form of care that is essential to their survival or to maintaining a high quality of life. It can be predicted with reasonable accuracy that this trend will continue for many decades. The increase in life expectancy does mean that some older people will be healthier as they move into their later years. This group will need information and guidance regarding health promotion and maintenance to keep them in a healthy state.

However, for the "old-old" population, the demand for long-term care will increase. The 7 million elderly persons needing some long-term care assistance represent 24% of the total elderly population. Most require assistance with activities of daily living (ADLs) and personal care. About 78% of older people receiving long-term care live in the community, and the remaining 22% live in nursing homes. Nurses have long provided healthcare and illness care to the elderly and will continue to be needed long into the foreseeable future.

PROGRESS AND RESEARCH

Since 1961, when the first White House Conference on Aging was held, there has been an awakening to the needs of the elderly. One of the most important recommendations submitted to this conference eventually led to enactment of legislation establishing **Medicare** and the Older Americans Act.

Benefits under Medicare became available July 1, 1966. Although changes have been made in the original act, millions of older Americans continue to receive hospital and medical care under its provisions. However beneficial it may be, Medicare does not cover all medical expenses for all elderly persons. For example, it does not cover outpatient drug expenses, there is a deductible charge for hospitalization, and only about 80% of outpatient services are reimbursed. The older person must pay these expenses out of pocket or purchase additional insurance to close this gap.

The Older Americans Act became law in 1965, and since then it too has undergone numerous changes. Parts of the act are administered by the federal government through the Department of Health and Human Services, and other parts are implemented by state and local agencies. The act covers a wide range of services to the elderly, and special emphasis has been placed on meeting nutritional needs of elderly persons. Programs funded under various parts of the Older Americans Act include homemaker services, home health aides, foster grandparents program, employment referrals, housing, health screening, research and demonstration programs, and training programs in the field of aging.

The Social Security Act as revised in 1965 and its subsequent amendments provide monthly benefits for elderly persons. Periodic increases in benefits have been granted to cover increased living costs. As the Social Security benefit has been increased, the ceiling on earned income has been raised without loss of the monthly benefit. This makes it possible for elderly persons to continue part-time work. In addition to the financial emphasis of Social Security, efforts to improve the aged person's quality of life also have been approached from the research perspective. Many universities and medical centers have opened research centers to study the biologic and psychologic factors related to aging.

Although tremendous strides have been made to provide a better life for millions of elderly Americans in the United States, not all are receiving these benefits. Many communities have active, ongoing programs, whereas other communities lag far behind and have little interest in improving the life of the elderly.

FACTORS AFFECTING AGING

Cultural and Ethnic Factors

Many variations exist in the cultural patterns of different groups of people. In early oriental cultures the older members of society were revered and called the "wise ones." In primitive cultures the elderly persons were the source for information and knowledge. They always knew where to find food and water, and they traveled with the tribe. When they became too feeble to travel and could not be cared for, they accepted death. In the early culture of the United States the older citizens also were important sources of information. They were consulted about the political and educational affairs of the community. They were respected because of the knowledge that they had acquired during their lives. Present day American culture is youth oriented, and the elderly occupy a lower position and endure lower prestige. They may look back with feelings of nostalgia to a time when there was solidarity of the family unit and young people showed respect and devotion to the aged members of the family. The social system imposes retirement and forces the individual to find new roles at a time when it is more difficult to make decisions than it was at an earlier age. Limited financial resources affect many elderly as inflation reduces the buying power of a fixed income from pensions or Social Security payments. Refer to Chapter 4 for a complete discussion on the importance of considering cultural factors when delivering nursing care.

Socioeconomic Factors

Housing is a pressing problem. Most elderly wish to remain in their own homes, in familiar surroundings. However, this may be difficult or impossible when there are financial or health problems. Some older people have found themselves to be victims of urban renewal. They may have lived in areas within the city that have recently become popular with the young urban working crowd and may have found their apartments being sold as condominiums or their rents raised drastically. This has resulted in an increase in the number of older persons who find themselves homeless. Other older people with health deficits find they are no longer able to care for a large home with rising taxes and maintenance costs that have become a burden. When the adult children are all working outside of the home and/or residing in other cities, it may be difficult for frail older persons to care for themselves, and they may be forced to leave their home. Whether they move in with one of their children or enter an extended-care facility, an adjustment is necessary and often difficult. Abrupt changes often are made without consideration for individual differences and needs. Lifetime patterns are not easily changed and must be evaluated in terms of what they mean to the individual.

Under the Federal Housing Act, funds have been made available for construction of housing units for the aged. High-rise apartment complexes for the elderly are found in many urban and suburban areas. Although they may solve the problem of housing, many of these complexes provide no health services or cannot meet all the healthcare needs of the residents. For example, residents who are physically frail may need to have vital signs monitored and have their conditions assessed on a regular basis to prevent a health crisis and the resulting hospitalization. Support services such as visiting nurses, housekeeping, transportation, Meals on Wheels, and adult day care may supplement the services delivered in senior citizen

CASE STUDY

Mrs. Smith, an 83-year-old widow, lived in two small basement rooms of a house in a textile mill village. One day she fell and broke her wrist while carrying groceries down the stairs to her apartment. Mrs. Smith's daughter was afraid she would fall again and insisted that her mother give up her apartment and move in with her and her family on the other side of town. Mrs. Smith didn't want to leave her neighbors and give up her independence, but she didn't want to offend her daughter, so she sadly said "yes" and agreed to the move. Even after a 6 month adjustment period, Mrs. Smith seemed withdrawn and spent most of her time alone in her room.

housing and may allow some frail older persons to remain independent in their own apartments.

Ambulatory services can be used to supplement housing and institutional services to keep older persons from becoming permanent residents of long-term care facilities (Figure 14-2). Nurses play a pivotal role in this process by becoming involved in the linkage process and providing information, participating in discharge planning, working as case managers, and participating in multidisciplinary geriatric assessment teams.

Although many elderly persons are forced to leave their homes because of urban renewal and must readjust their lifelong patterns of living, not all elderly persons are confronted with this problem. Those with adequate health and financial resources are able to maintain their desired lifestyles, but some of the elderly need assistance through community services. It is important to remember that the vast majority of elderly persons (95%) live independently in the community, with varying levels of assistance from family and friends. However, successful aging and retirement take planning and preparation, both of which should begin in middle age.

Retirement and Aging

During the early history of the United States the economy was rural and agricultural and there was little concern about retirement. Individuals worked well into their later years, and when they were even more advanced in years, chores kept the elders occupied and provided an opportunity for them to make a contribution to society. Today's society remains essentially work oriented, but the older worker is pressured into retirement to provide jobs for the young.

Mandatory retirement was abolished for most people in the late 1970s, although many people continue to retire between ages 62 and 65. **Retirement** is thought of as a positive reward for labor, a special time free from worry, but many persons facing retirement have difficulty coping with this abrupt change in lifestyle. Many retired persons become bored with their lifestyles and inactivity after a brief "honeymoon" period. The increased number of women in today's labor force makes retirement a concern for men and women alike, but women usually adjust to retirement more easily than men do because they often have many social ties, continuing homemaker responsibilities, and ongoing family responsibilities.

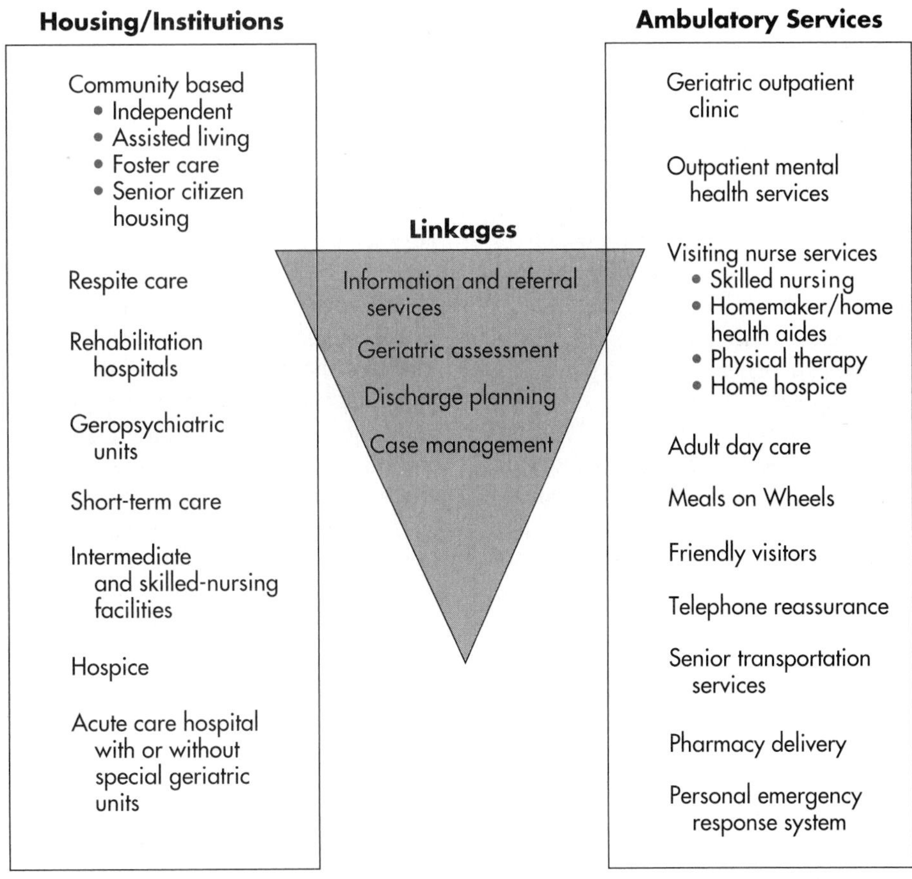

Figure 14-2 The long-term care continuum of services for older adults.

CASE STUDY

Mrs. Clay had lived for 46 years in the home that had belonged to her parents. However, when urban renewal came, Mrs. Clay had to move. When asked about her new home, Mrs. Clay said, "I like it quite well, but it's very inconvenient. You see, I was right there in town. Out here I have to call a taxi every time I want to go to the store, and I don't always have the money."

In retirement, sustained activity is no longer required. The absence of social roles for the elderly makes a work substitute difficult to find. Enforced inactivity over an extended period can be harmful to the health of the retired person. Add to this the effect of bereavement for a spouse, friends, and even children, and there may be a tendency for the individual to give up and withdraw.

The basic needs of the retired older worker are to feel financially secure, to be useful, to form new associations and interact with people, to maintain a sense of dignity and self-respect, and to feel needed and wanted in society. Many older retirees now can take free courses at community colleges and can serve as volunteers in a variety of programs including Foster Grandparents, Vista, the Peace Corps, Elderhostel, Retired Senior Executive Corps, and numerous other opportunities. Society has begun to recognize that the skills and experiences gained over a lifetime are valuable resources that can improve the situation of others while allowing older people an opportunity to feel helpful and involved with life.

Biopsychosocial Factors

The biology of aging

The biologic process of aging causes physiologic changes in the total human organism. Changes usually develop slowly, and most older persons consider themselves to be in good or excellent health. Scientists continue to investigate the cause of aging, not only to extend life but also to achieve a life free of degenerative disease. Some believe that the aging process is programmed by genes, whereas others theorize that it is related to a chemical blockage of thyroxine. The most recent evidence relates the aging process to the immune system. It has been found that a type of white blood cell, the T cell, provides resistance to cancer cells, viruses, bacteria, and fungi, but it loses its effectiveness with age, and the host therefore loses immunity to disease. It is believed that these cells become less effective because the thymus gland shrinks with age, and it is the thymus gland that secretes chemicals that stimulate the bone marrow cells to produce T cells.

CASE STUDY

John, who had worked for 45 years in the electronics industry, was asked to take early retirement at the age of 62, when his company became less profitable. He was offered a financial retirement package that prompted him to accept the offer. However, John was bothered by the idea that people would think of him as "over the hill." After 3 months of retirement, he became bored with golf and television. His wife, who still worked part time in the town library, urged him to take up a new hobby or look for a part-time job. She was worried because John just didn't seem like himself.

Experiments have been conducted in which T cells removed from animals were frozen for as long as 15 years and then reinjected. The T cells maintained their youthful immune powers while frozen and were perfectly normal when thawed. When the frozen cells were reintroduced into the aging host, the immune system returned to the potency found in young adulthood. Scientists believe that this dwindling immunity may be responsible for the degenerative diseases of aging such as cancer, arthritis, diabetes, and kidney disease, and for an increase in susceptibility to infection. The prospect of controlling the degeneration that accompanies old age is, indeed, an extremely exciting one.

However, it is important to remember that lifestyle choices greatly affect the aging process and function in old age. Bad habits undertaken in youth and middle age, such as cigarette smoking, high-fat diets, lack of exercise, and chronic sun exposure, often can cause problems for the older person. Certainly genes influence aging, and family history of certain diseases may cause threats to health, but lifestyle choices impact equally or even more significantly upon health (Schoenfeld, 1994). It is never too late to try to influence the formation of good habits, even in our older patients. Good health is very important to most older people. They fear becoming a burden to their spouse or children, and they realize that health is precious and should not be taken for granted.

Mental health

It is generally believed that individuals who are well adjusted and able to meet problems and make adaptations during their younger years are better prepared to face problems in advancing years. Erikson identified this stage of life as that of ego integrity versus despair. Erikson (1950) defines ego integrity as acceptance of one's own unique life cycle and the people who have become significant to it. He emphasizes that this life cycle and its significant people are something that must be and that, by necessity, allows no substitutions. Achieving integrity means that the individual accepts past events, experiences, and lifestyle, including the mistakes made along the way. The person who does not achieve ego integrity feels despair or disgust about the course of his or her life and may blame circumstances on someone or something else. He or she experiences regret that it is too late to start over or change that life.

The older person may be confronted with fears of illness, physical suffering, helplessness, and death. Chronic death or illness results in low morale, but when meaningful friendships exist, even when health is poor, the individual is less likely to suffer from low morale. At these times a caring nurse or a referral to a mental health clinic can provide emotional support and give the individual a feeling of friendship, warmth, and a sense of personal worth.

Some elderly persons depend on others for part or all of their care. Dependency can result in loss of dignity, diminished self-esteem, and lowered morale. When disease and illness are superimposed on normal aging changes, adaptation is difficult for the individual. The dependency that elderly persons experience may give rise to feelings of resentment toward family, friends, or those trying to help. The dependent older person may become demanding, tend to magnify normal aches and pains, and complain of loss of sleep and of various digestive disturbances. However, vague symptoms can be indications of underlying pathologic conditions. It must be remembered that older persons have many adjustments to make during a period of their lives when they tolerate stressful situations poorly. Adjustments that older persons may have to make include the death of a spouse or friends, retirement and reduced income, identification with an older age group, and adjustment to chronic illness and a gradually changing body.

Depression often goes unrecognized and untreated in the older population. Older people are less likely to complain of sadness or "feeling blue," but they may instead complain of weight loss, feelings of fatigue, memory loss and difficulty in concentration, anxiety, constipation, or other symptoms that are general in nature. Physical conditions associated with depression include cerebrovascular accident (CVA), thyroid disease, Parkinson's disease, and other chronic illnesses. Some of the medications known to cause depression in older persons include beta blockers taken for hypertension and some sleeping pills and tranquilizers. A depression scale is available for differential assessment of dementia, depression, and delerium. Nurses often administer these scales.

Older persons diagnosed with depression may be treated with counseling and/or antidepressant medications. The success rate of treatment of depression in the older person is equal to the success rate for treatment of middle-aged and young adults. Some of the newer antidepression medications work very well with elderly persons and do not cause the harmful side effects that have been associated with the older medications of the past. Some hospitals and long-term care facilities specialize in mental health problems of the elderly and accept patients for short-term stays (under 2 weeks) to begin treatment and stabilize the patient on medications. These units are called geropsychiatric units.

Most elderly persons become aware of the shortness of time. They become concerned about changes in their bodies and their loss of strength or the presence of disease. The grief after the loss of a spouse or close friend may cause the person to question continued existence. The individual may progress to a state of depression and prefer self-destruction to continuation of life. With the increased incidence of geriatric suicide, the nurse caring for elderly patients should be alert to warning signs. The person who expresses a desire to die or makes threats of suicide should be taken seriously. The elderly are at the highest risk for successful suicides. It is during such periods of crisis that the individual needs emotional support. Each community has access to emergency mental health services, and the nurse should become familiar with the reporting process before a crisis occurs. An older person who speaks of death should be questioned carefully to see if they have a plan for their death and a means to carry it out. If so, emergency services must be mobilized immediately to prevent the person from harming himself or herself.

CASE STUDY

Mr. Jones is a retired 72-year-old man who has gradually lost the ability to walk because of Parkinson's disease. The visiting nurse noticed one day when providing care to Mr. Jones that there was a gun in the hall closet. When questioned about the gun, Mr. Jones said, "Yes, it's loaded, and I keep that gun close to me because one day I will use it to end it all." The nurse immediately called her supervisor and obtained emergency mental health services for Mr. Jones.

Many of the concepts concerning psychosocial factors in old age have never been proven and are now being questioned. It can no longer be assumed that all older people are lonely, depressed, not interested in sex, fixated on their aches and pains, and happy to sit in a rocking chair all day. It is only recently that research, although limited, has enabled society to learn some of the factors that affect the social life and attitudes of elderly persons. It has been stated that chronologic age may be unrelated to old age. Elderly people are individuals, and all 70-year olds are not alike, just as all 20-year olds are not alike. It has been suggested that older persons represent a "subculture." Society has fostered such a culture through community programs that tend to segregate older persons, such as senior citizen centers, golden age groups, and adult day-care centers. These programs take older persons out of the mainstream of society and provide little opportunity for interaction with younger persons. New programs that encourage interactions and socialization with all age groups are needed.

The success of a mental health program for the elderly depends on a social consciousness within the community that is oriented toward mental health. The nurse can be an innovator of new ideas and can be a source of inspiration, not only to individuals but also to the community, in developing an ongoing mental health program for its elderly population.

Maintaining mental health does not mean doing *for* the older person; it means doing *with* the older person. A large number of elderly citizens want something to do and want to feel that they are useful. Many are ambulatory and able to remain in their own homes, where they are happier. For some, however, this is not possible. Older persons face many social and economic problems in later life, and these problems can have a profound impact on their lives. A community counseling service should be available where the person can have privacy, quiet, and an unhurried atmosphere to talk over problems. Community groups of elderly persons can be formed to develop social contacts. With the help of a group leader, the members of the group assist each other in devising methods to handle problems faced in the community.

Aging and Intelligence

It is a myth that intelligence decreases with age. Although the elderly will achieve lower scores on intelligence tests, this is usually because their reaction times are slower and they need more time to complete the examination. The lower scores are not associated with a deficit in the ability to think. The elderly replace speed with accuracy, and research shows that they often do better than younger persons when the time limit is removed. Leading an active life that includes mastery of new knowledge and skills is considered essential to maintaining intelligence in the elderly.

Aging and Memory

It is common in our society to blame advancing age when a person experiences any lapse in memory. Scientific tests have shown that depression, not aging, is more often the cause of memory lapse (White, 1986).

The elderly are sometimes described as rigid in their approach to problem solving. The tendency to persist in a particular approach to a problem despite additional information suggesting a change is believed to be associated not with the age of the individual but with the level of education achieved. It has been demonstrated that the greater the number of years that have elapsed since the individual was involved in formal schooling, the more likely it is that the individual will solve problems by applying relevant knowledge from his or her stored experience. Analyzing a problem and employing a new solution depend on recent exposure to this type of thinking, which is commonly found in the educational setting. All of these facts point to the importance of continued lifelong learning in the maintenance of mental functioning.

Every older person who complains of memory loss should have a formal mental status assessment. A mental status assessment examines cognitive functions such as the ability to think and make decisions. In addition to establishing important baseline information about the older patient, the mental status assessment can be used to chart the progression of a cognitive deficit if it is present, and document the effect of treatment and nursing interventions.

The **Folstein Mini-Mental Status Examination (MMSE)** (Folstein and others, 1975) is used widely in the clinical setting. It assesses orientation, short-term memory, ability to attend to tasks (attention), calculation, recall (memory), and language. Each area provides neurologic information and may assist in identifying the cognition problem and its extent. Out of a possible score of 30, a score of 20 to 29 indicates a moderate cognitive deficit, and a score of 19 or below reflects a more serious deficit.

At first, the nurse may be uncomfortable using the MMSE. There are ways to become comfortable with this technique, such as trying out the MMSE on family and friends, watching geriatric nursing experts who use the examination often, and explaining to patients that the examination gives valuable information and helps ensure high quality nursing care. If the patient misses answers, the nurse should move on to the next question and not dwell on failures. The nurse should be certain the older person is physically comfortable, can see the nurse, and can hear the instructions. When charting the results of the MMSE, the nurse should note the total score and where the patient had deficits (memory, orientation, or language). This information is vital to the nursing care plan.

PHYSIOLOGY OF AGING

When a person has reached maturity, a gradual aging of all body tissues and organs begins. Loss of cells and loss of physiologic reserves may be the major way in which the body ages. By the time a person has reached 70 years of age, the aging process may be well advanced. The rate and extent of aging vary among individuals, and the rate at which various organs age may also vary. Among the various physiologic changes seen in elderly persons, some begin when people are in their thirties (Table 14-2).

When normal aging progresses without the presence of disease, the end result is a loss of organ reserve. This means that normal function of the body continues as before, but the body is less likely to respond to stress in a positive manner. This may be why newspapers often carry a report of an older person suffering a heart attack while shoveling the driveway during the first snowstorm of winter. The older heart, which functions well under normal conditions, may not be able to respond to the sudden demand for increased oxygen needed by the muscles during vigorous exercise. The zone of adaptation is smaller for an older person because of loss of organ reserve, presence of underlying chronic illnesses, and the effects of some drugs that many older persons take to control symptoms of illness (Figure 14-3).

Although normal aging varies among individuals, some elderly persons complain of physical symptoms that should be given medical attention. Many older people—and the physicians and nurses who care for them—think that fatigue, incontinence, falls, and confusion are normal parts of aging and therefore not worth mentioning to anyone. Because of negative stereotypes of aging, many older people suffer needlessly with conditions that can be treated. Older persons who seek medical help and offer various complaints about their health should have a complete investigation into the cause of the complaint.

Cardiovascular System

The heart size usually remains the same, but it may increase as a result of decreased activity or longstanding hypertension. With an enlarged heart the heart rate is slower in response to demand and cardiac output is reduced. As a result, there is less rapid movement of blood carrying oxygen and nutrients to all the organs and tissues in the body. This in turn affects the function of these organs. In the presence of stress, either physical or psychologic, reduced cardiac output means that there is less oxygen to meet the increased need caused by the stress. The heart needs more rest between beats; therefore tachycardia easily results in heart failure. Arteriosclerotic changes are common in the elderly, and these changes make the blood vessels less elastic and more resistant to blood flow, which results in elevated blood pressure. Exercise can increase cardiac output, and daily exercise such as walking is excellent for the elderly.

Assessment

Assessment of the cardiovascular system should begin with noting the rate, rhythm, and character of the pulse for 1 full minute in a resting state. Pulses are checked bilaterally for symmetry because older people may have arterial insufficiency. Blood pressure is taken first with the person lying down and then standing. Orthostatic hypotension is common in the elderly. The medications the person is taking should be assessed for their effect on blood pressure. The presence or absence of pedal edema is evaluated when palpating pedal pulses. The temperature of the hands and feet is noted. Cool, dry extremities reflect a decrease in peripheral circulation. Family history of heart disease, if any, should be obtained. The individual's lifestyle, including smoking, diet and obesity, exercise, and stress, should be assessed.

Common pathologic conditions

Cardiovascular problems are among the most common diseases of the elderly. Some recent studies support the theory that lifestyle is the cause of many cardiovascular pathologic conditions. The effects of the aging process do, however, contribute to the progress of pathologic conditions.

Hypertension. Hypertension is commonly found among the elderly and is defined as blood pressure that is consistently above what is considered normal. A person is considered hypertensive with a systolic blood pressure greater than 140 mm Hg and/or a diastolic pressure greater than 90 mm Hg. The diastolic reading is as important as the systolic pressure because the diastolic reading indicates the pressure in the cardiovascular system when the heart is at rest between beats, and the systolic reading indicates the maximum pressure on the system when the heart pumps. See Chapter 21 for a complete discussion of the pathophysiology, assessment, and intervention of hypertension.

Arteriosclerosis and atherosclerosis. The changes that occur in the heart and vascular system begin early in life and progress over the years. Arteriosclerosis, a condition in which the blood vessels lose their elasticity, is also known as hardening of the arteries. Atherosclerosis is a form of arteriosclerosis, and it results from fatty deposits (plaque) that form in the intima of the blood vessels. These changes make it increasingly difficult for blood to flow through the vascular system. The flow of blood to the kidneys, brain, and lower extremities is often affected. The condition may become severe enough to cause serious disease of the heart,

TABLE 14-2

Physiologic Changes of Aging

Body System	Physiologic Changes*	Results*
Cardiovascular	↑ Number of heartbeat irregularities	↓ Oxygenation
	↓ Cardiac output	↑ Chance of heart failure
	↓ Heart rate	↑ Blood pressure
	↑ Atherosclerosis	↓ Blood supply to peripheral areas
Sensory	↓ Accommodation	↓ Light to retina
	↓ Diameter of pupil	↓ Night vision
	↑ Opacity of lens	↑ Sensitivity to glare
		↓ Peripheral vision
	↓ Sense of smell	↓ Color vision
	↓ Number of taste buds	↓ High-frequency sounds
	↓ Functioning of middle and inner ear	↓ Balance
Integumentary	↓ Sebaceous secretions	↑ Dry skin
	↓ Subcutaneous fat	↑ Wrinkling
	↓ Thickness of epidermis	↑ Susceptibility to heat and cold
		↑ Thickness of nails
		↓ Hair color and distribution
Musculoskeletal	↓ Bone calcium	↑ Curvature of spine—osteoporosis
	↓ Water of intervertebral disks	↓ Height
	↓ Blood supply	↓ Mobility
	↓ Elastic tissue	↑ Risk of falls and fractures
	↓ Muscle mass	
Nervous	↓ Brain cells	↓ Reflexes
	↓ Nerve fibers	↓ Short-term memory
	↓ Touch receptors	↓ Pain recognition
Digestive	↓ Gastric secretions	↑ Constipation
	↓ Peristalsis	↓ Appetite
	↓ Sensory receptors	↓ Ability to taste
	↓ Number of teeth	↓ Ability to chew
		↓ Nutritional status
Urinary	↓ Blood supply	↓ Urine concentration
	↓ Nephrons	↓ Bladder capacity
	↓ Muscle tone	↑ Residual urine
	♂ ↑ Size of prostate	↑ Chance of infection
		♂ ↓ Urinary stream
Respiratory	↓ Elasticity	↓ Gas exchange
	↑ Thickness of capillaries	↓ Vital capacity
	↓ Number of capillaries	↑ Risk of disease
		↓ Cough efficiency
Reproductive	♀ ↓ Estrogen	♀ ↓ Epithelial cells of vulva
	♂ ↓ Testosterone	♀ ↓ Vaginal secretions
		♀ ↓ Breast size
		♀ ↓ Ovary and uterus size
		♂ ↓ Ejaculation
		♂ ↑ Time to achieve erection

*↑, increased; ↓, decreased; ♀, female; ♂, male.

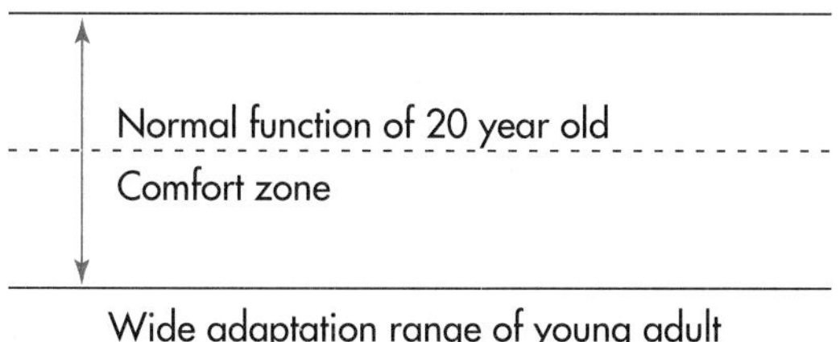

Wide adaptation range of young adult

Normal function of 80 year old

Comfort zone

Adaptation range of older adult

Causes of narrowing of adaptation range

- Loss of organ reserve
- Underlying chronic illness
- Possible drug response

Threats to adaptation

- Illness (acute/chronic)
- Stress
- Social isolation
- Malnutrition/dehydration
- Depression/mental status change

Figure 14-3 The physiology of aging and narrowing of the adaptation range.

CASE STUDY

Mary, an 82-year-old widow, always felt tired and slept most of the day. She had been told that at her age that was normal. However, Mary knew that until a few months ago, she had had plenty of energy, played bridge socially, and enjoyed brisk walks in good weather. Finally, Mary called her physician, who performed a physical examination and some blood tests. He found that Mary's thyroid gland was not producing enough of a hormone (H_4) needed for her normal function. A thyroid-replacement hormone was started (levothyroxine [Synthroid]), and now Mary is again enjoying a more active life.

such as coronary artery disease, myocardial infarction, or congestive heart failure. There is a direct link between atherosclerosis and arterial occlusive disease. See Chapter 21 for coverage of these conditions.

Cerebrovascular accident. Cerebrovascular accident (CVA or stroke) is one of the leading causes of death in the elderly and is the result of an interruption of circulation in the brain. Hypertension is a major factor in the occurrence of a stroke. See Chapter 16 for pathophysiology and intervention for CVA.

Nursing interventions

The most important nursing intervention relating to the cardiovascular system is the prevention and management of cardiovascular disease. Promoting a healthy lifestyle in all individuals will decrease the incidence of cardiovascular pathologic conditions in the elderly. The importance of a good diet cannot be overemphasized. The nurse should encourage and help the elderly to decrease their intake of salt, saturated fats, and alcohol, and to increase their intake of grains, fresh fruits, and vegetables. A regular program of exercise tailored to the individual is very important. Smokers should be encouraged to quit. Nursing interventions for individuals with cardiovascular problems include monitoring and evaluating the effects of the medical therapies. The nurse will need to teach the patient about the medications prescribed by the physician, their side effects, and the importance of continuing the medications. Careful monitoring of the patient for side effects is important because the patient who stops medication because of fatigue, impotence, dizziness, or other complaints will be at risk for increased blood pressure, cardiac enlargement, or possible CVA. With the newer classes of antihypertension medication, most older people can attain adequate control of their blood pressure without suffering ill effects from their medication.

Sensory System

The status of the individual's sensory system affects the way in which the individual reacts to the environment and the people in it. Deficits in hearing or vision have the effect of isolating an individual from what is going on around him or her.

Vision

With aging there is a gradual decrease in visual accommodation. This means that the elderly require more time to focus when looking from one object to the other. Night vision is reduced, and more time is needed for the eyes to adjust to the dark. Increased lens opacity causes light to scatter and makes the elderly person more sensitive to glare. These changes cause many older people to discontinue driving at night. Senile miosis, a condition that decreases the size of the pupils, results in a reduction in the amount of light reaching the retina, so the elderly need more light to work, read, and walk safely. Peripheral vision, the ability to distinguish objects at the edges of the visual field, is reduced. Sometimes the elderly do not communicate with people sitting beside them simply because they do not see them. The lens yellows with age, causing the elderly difficulty in discriminating colors. Blues and greens tend to fade and are easily confused. Reds, oranges, and yellows can be seen best.

Assessment. The patient should be asked about visual problems such as double vision, blurring, tunnel vision, or any other visual disturbance. Headaches or pain in or around the eye should be noted. Vision can be assessed by using an eye chart or by determining whether the person can recognize the number of fingers held up by the examiner at 2 feet and 10 feet away. Newspaper headlines also can be used to check vision. Peripheral vision can be gauged by wiggling the fingers while slowly bringing them toward the patient's center of vision. Color discrimination can be checked by using a color chart, colored paper, or colors in the environment.

Common pathologic conditions. The most common visual problems of the elderly are cataracts, glaucoma, senile macular degeneration, and diabetic retinopathy. These problems are covered in Chapter 29.

Nursing interventions. Nurses should be aware of visual changes that occur with aging so that they can help elderly patients adapt to these changes. When moving back and forth between brightly lit and darker areas, such as coming indoors on a sunny day or coming out of a darkened theatre into the daylight, elderly individuals should pause to allow the eyes to accommodate to the change. Sunglasses help to reduce glare in bright daylight. Elderly persons who drive at night can be advised to use lighted and divided highways to reduce the glare from oncoming cars. Indoors, lamps and windows should be shaded to allow adequate light but reduce glare. Supplemental light should be provided for tasks such as reading or sewing. Adequate lighting of stairs is essential. Stair edges should be marked with contrasting color. Night lights will help the elderly when they need to arise during the night. Older patients who have decreased peripheral vision should be approached from the front, and objects should be placed directly in front of them.

Hearing

Hearing impairment is common and is first demonstrated by an inability to hear the higher frequencies. This affects the individual's ability to discriminate words, and there will be certain words that the individual will not hear or will confuse with other words. Peripheral conversation (background words) is not heard fully; this results in reduced sensory stimulation and may lead to withdrawal and social isolation. Changes in the middle ear and inner ear may result in some loss of balance. Ear wax becomes drier and may accumulate in the ear, causing further loss of hearing acuity.

Assessment. Hearing should be assessed by an examiner standing behind the individual, first covering one ear and then the other. The examiner, speaking in a normal voice, should ask the person to respond to questions or repeat a series of words. Both ears should be checked.

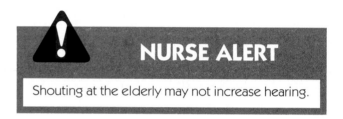

Shouting at the elderly may not increase hearing.

Nursing interventions. When caring for the elderly, the nurse should stand face to face with the individual and then speak clearly and at a moderate rate. It is important not to overarticulate, shout, or mumble. Shouting may not help the person hear better. It may make hearing more difficult because when most persons increase the volume of their voice, they also raise the pitch, and higher pitched sounds are more difficult for the elderly to hear. Hearing aids can help with some types of hearing loss. However, some individuals may refuse to wear a hearing aid because of vanity or because hearing aids often amplify background noise as well as conversation and can be very difficult to adjust to.

Taste and smell

It has been generally thought that the senses of taste and smell decrease with age. The sense of smell begins to decline in middle age, and it often continues to diminish during the later years (Knapp, 1989). The number of taste buds declines with age, and as a result many older persons choose salty and sugary foods in an attempt to enhance flavor (Pettigrew, 1989). Smoking and medications also can negatively affect taste and smell.

Nursing interventions. When caring for the elderly, the nurse should encourage them to use a variety of spices in cooking to increase taste. Dried or fresh herbs such as parsley, basil, or garlic can make a dish look attractive and taste better. Older persons with deficits in smell should be medically evaluated for medication toxicity and for overall health status. Older persons who lack a sense of smell should seek the help of others to make sure food has not spoiled in the refrigerator, and they should have smoke detectors to alert them in case of fire.

Touch

Like the other senses, the sense of touch is generally thought to decrease with age. There is some evidence that a person's ability to detect temperature extremes or pain is affected by age, but more and better research is needed in this area. Individuals with an impaired sense of touch may be unable to determine whether a surface, such as a coffee pot, or water is hot enough to cause injury. With a decreased sense of pain a person may not realize the extent of an injury such as a broken hip following a fall. The nurse can assess the individual's sensitivity to temperature by using containers of hot and cold water. Pain sensitivity can be checked by using the ends of a Q-tip. Those whose sense of touch is diminished can be counseled to be particularly vigilant to prevent injury. Patients with diabetes may be at special risk because of diabetic neuropathies and slow healing time after injury occurs.

Integumentary System

The signs of aging are perhaps most visible in the skin and hair. The epidermis and dermis become thinner, although there may be some thickening in areas exposed to sunlight. Decreased vascularity in the dermis leads to increased fragility of the skin. This results in easier bruising and greater susceptibility to skin problems such as decubiti. There is less secretion of the sebaceous glands, which causes the skin to become dry. Wrinkling of the skin is caused by loss of subcutaneous fat and by a decrease in the skin's water content. The nails become hard and brittle, leading to cracking and splitting. Hair becomes lighter and thinner. About half of the population over age 50 has at least 50% gray body hair. The elderly are more susceptible to heat and cold, so heat applications must be at a reduced temperature to avoid burns. Since reduced activity results in reduced heat production, elderly persons will often feel cold when others are comfortable.

NURSE ALERT
Never use a heating pad setting above medium.

Assessment

Examination of the skin should be done by exposing all areas under good lighting. Pressure areas need to be checked for signs of redness or open lesions. Skin folds should be parted to check for irritation or signs of infection. Note the moisture of the skin and the size and location of any skin lesions. Older persons bruise easily and may have reddened areas called senile purpura.

Common pathologic conditions

The most common skin disorders among the elderly are skin cancers, keratoses, pigmentary disturbances, psoriasis, dermatitis, and urticaria (Matteson, McConnell, 1988). The immobile elderly are more likely to develop pressure sores. See Chapter 31 for discussion of these conditions. Dryness and itching (pruritus) are very common among the elderly. In most cases, dry skin is the cause of pruritus. However, other systemic problems should be ruled out in the case of severe pruritus. Conditions that may aggravate dry skin and itching include dry heat and air conditioning, daily hot baths or showers, and use of harsh or deodorant soaps.

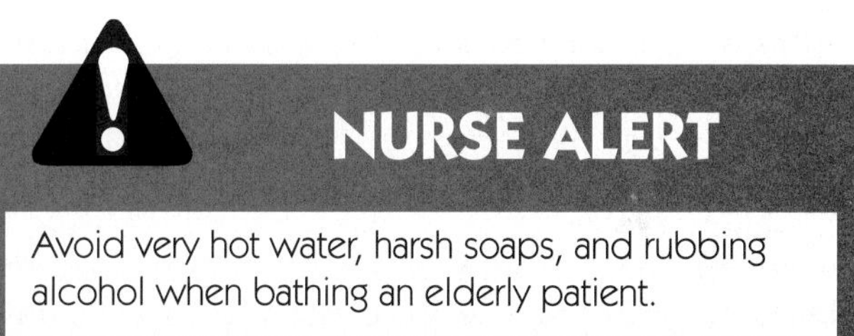
NURSE ALERT
Avoid very hot water, harsh soaps, and rubbing alcohol when bathing an elderly patient.

Nursing interventions

The goal of nursing should be to maintain the integrity of the skin. Because the skin of the older person is more fragile, it should be given more gentle care. The use of very hot water, harsh or deodorant soaps, and rubbing alcohol should be avoided. A complete bath two or three times a week is sufficient when supplemented with partial baths. When bathing the elderly, the nurse should use gentle and superfatted soaps and should pat the skin dry rather than rub it. The nurse should use creams and lotions while the skin is still slightly damp. Bath oil must not be used in the water, because this makes the bathtub slippery and increases the likelihood of falling. The nurse should use cornstarch rather than talcum powder in skin folds. Talcum tends to cake and irritate when it becomes moist. Skin should be examined frequently for early signs of irritation or pathologic conditions. Proper humidity in the heated or air-conditioned environment should be maintained. Nutrition greatly influences skin condition, and older people should be taught the importance of a sound and healthy diet.

Musculoskeletal System

Aging of the musculoskeletal system affects bones, joints, muscles, and muscle attachments. There is a decrease in bone mass and a thinning of the intervertebral discs of the spinal column that results in a shortening of the trunk. This, along with a general flexion of the joints, results in a decrease in height, forward projection of the head and neck, and kyphosis (dowager's hump). Loss of bone mass and postural changes increase the risk of fractures and falling. Fear of falling frequently leads to reduced mobilization which then decreases bone mass. There is a decrease in muscle fiber as muscle regeneration slows. Muscles atrophy and are replaced by fibrous tissue. These changes result in decreased muscle strength. Subcutaneous tissue is redistributed, with a decrease in the face and extremities and an increase around the abdomen and hips. Changes occur in the cartilage of the joints, especially the weight-bearing joints such as knees and hips, causing stiffness. These changes can be aggravated by joint stress, obesity, and decrease in ambulation. While the decreased muscle strength and increased joint stiffness cannot be halted, they can be significantly slowed with exercise.

Assessment

Assessment of the musculoskeletal system is done by first noting the curvature of the spine. The nurse should ask the individual to bend forward, sideways, and slightly backward to check the range of motion of the spine. The nurse should next ask the person to sit. This routine assesses the spinal muscles and hip muscles. The nurse should assess the upper extremities, symmetrically checking each joint in active and passive range of motion. The nurse should palpate the joints, noting deformities, tenderness, or areas of warmth. To check the lower extremities, the individual's gait should be observed. The nurse should examine the joints as with the upper extremities but should note carefully the internal and external rotation of the hips.

Common pathologic conditions

The most common problems affecting the musculoskeletal system in the elderly include arthritis, osteoarthritis, gout, and fractures (see Chapter 32). Osteoporosis is a condition characterized by decreased bone density, resulting in weakness and brittleness of the bone. The bones become very fragile and fracture easily, often following only slight trauma. The sites most affected are the vertebrae, the hip, and the wrist. The kyphosis seen in many older women is caused by collapse fractures of the thoracic vertebrae. Osteoporosis results from the aging of the bone-remodeling process. Before age 45 or so, bone formation, or absorption, is greater than bone loss, or resorption. After age 45 the process reverses, and bone mass is lost. Risk factors that appear to increase the occurrence of osteoporosis include cigarette smoking, high caffeine intake, excessive alcohol intake, a high-protein diet, a history of low dietary calcium, low vitamin D, a slender body build with little body fat, and a sedentary lifestyle. Bone loss increases significantly after menopause, which puts women at greater risk. Treatment of osteoporosis is aimed at prevention. There is no way to replace bone already lost, but there are ways of slowing the loss. Ideally, prevention begins in the early years of life. Building up the bones throughout childhood and early adulthood by adequate calcium intake provides for greater bone mass. When bone loss begins later in life, there is a greater percentage of bone mass remaining. Prevention of osteoporosis in mature persons includes exercise, calcium, and estrogen replacement. Weight-bearing exercise such as walking, jogging, bicycling, and dancing stimulates bone formation and retards bone-mass reduction (Goodman, 1987). Older adults should increase their intake of dietary calcium to the equivalent of 3 or 4 glasses of skim milk per day. Alternate sources of calcium include cheese, yogurt, canned salmon (with the bones), and calcium supplements. Calcium carbonate is more easily absorbed from the gastrointestinal tract and is recommended. Estrogen-replacement therapy after menopause may be recommended for those at high risk of osteoporosis.

Nursing interventions

A person's sense of self is directly affected by his or her ability to be independently mobile. Likewise, a healthy mental attitude will stimulate the individual to take measures to maintain motor function. Nurses can assist the older adult to assume a positive mental attitude and outlook on life. Exercise is extremely important in maintaining motor function. Every older adult will benefit from exercise, but it must be appropriate to the capabilities of the individual. Walking, swimming, dancing, jogging, stretching, and aerobics are all beneficial in maintaining muscle strength and joint movement. Pain management for elderly persons who have muscle and joint pain is essential in maintaining mobility (Matteson, McConnell, 1988). Good nutrition is important in supplying the energy, vitamins, and minerals needed to maintain a healthy state. Safety is of primary concern in preserving motor function. The nurse should assess the person's environment and recommend measures such as appropriate lighting and the use of grab bars, canes, or walkers when appropriate. Area rugs and other obstructions that could cause falls and injuries should be removed.

Neurologic System

Changes occurring in the nervous system of the aging adult include a decrease in the number of functioning neurons. This is a gradual change, becoming more pronounced over age 70. The loss of neurons means the loss of neuronal interconnections, which results in slower conduction of nerve impulses. For this reason, it is more difficult for the elderly to maintain body homeostasis. Recovery from stress is slower and incomplete. The elderly are at risk for hypothermia and hyperthermia that may become life threatening. Reaction time is also decreased among the elderly. Reflexes are diminished, and motor activity is slower. Tremors are common, especially in the head, face, and hands. The sense of pain is also diminished, and the elderly may be free of pain in such acute disorders as myocardial infarction or pneumonia. Older adults take longer to fall asleep, have shorter periods of deep sleep, and awaken more frequently during the night (Hamby, Turnbull, Clark, Lancaster, 1994; Matteson, McConnell, 1988).

Assessment

Assessment of the nervous system is a complex process, but several simple techniques can provide valuable information. Careful observation of the person's gait will reveal the ability to coordinate muscle movements. The reflexes may be slowed but should be equal bilaterally. Sometimes severe arthritis can depress the knee-jerk reflex. Sensory testing can be done by using a cotton wisp for light touch and a Q-tip for deep touch. The nurse should touch the skin at different places bilaterally, from head to toe, while the person's eyes are closed. The person is asked to say when the wisp is felt. Deep touch is assessed in the same way, using a broken Q-tip, first the point, and then the head. The person is asked to identify "sharp" and "dull."

Common pathologic conditions

The most common pathologic conditions of the neurological system in older adults are **delirium** and **dementia.** Delirium (acute confusional states) is usually a temporary, reversible condition frequently associated with physical or mental illness in older adults (Hamby, Turnbull, Clark, Lancaster, 1994; Matteson, McConnell, 1988). Dementia (chronic brain syndrome) is a progressive decline in an individual's intellectual function.

Delirium is associated with metabolic changes and disruptions. It can be caused by cardiovascular changes such as cerebral vascular accident, decreased blood supply, congestive heart failure, or infection, as well as by metabolic disturbances such as hypokalemia, hyperkalemia, hypoglycemia, hyperglycemia, acidosis, or alkalosis. Psychologic disturbances such as depression, grief, fatigue, or severe emotional stress, and environmental factors such as sensory deprivation or sensory overload can also be responsible for a state of delirium. Symptoms include sudden onset of confusion, disorientation, hallucinations, incoherent speech, anger, apathy, or changes in psychomotor activity. The delirium state is usually temporary and can be reversed by identifying and correcting the underlying condition that is causing it.

Dementia is a group of pathologic conditions characterized by a gradual decline in intellectual function with symptoms such as loss of memory for recent and remote events, impaired ability to problem solve or to make judgments, and personality changes. The most common of the dementias is Alzheimer's disease.

Alzheimer's Disease

Alzheimer's disease is a chronic, degenerative, and irreversible disease. It is more common in women. No genetic links have been found; however, it does have familial tendencies. The disease results in characteristic changes in the brain that can be identified only on autopsy: cerebral atrophy, senile plaques, and neurofibrillary tangles. The cause of Alzheimer's disease remains unknown. There is a great deal of research being conducted to isolate a cause, and there are many theories including environmental factors such as aluminum, head trauma, infection, immunologic factors, and genetic factors (Drachman and others, 1991). While aluminum is found in the damaged cells, some believe it enters the cell only as a result of the damage, not as the cause. There is no cure, and death usually occurs in an average of 5 to 8 years, although some Alzheimer's victims have been known to live for 15 to 20 years after contracting the disease.

Alzheimer's is classified into three stages. The *first stage,* the forgetful or mild stage, is characterized by short-term memory loss, mild disorientation for time and date, difficulty in completing mathematical calculations, and subtle behavioral changes such as a decreased interest in work, family, or recreation (Matteson, McConnell, 1988). The *second stage* is the confused stage, and symptoms include extreme confusion, suspiciousness and paranoia, and difficulty with daily living activities such as driving, money management, and home maintenance. Patients are easily lost even in familiar places and will wander off, especially at night. They have difficulty functioning in environments other than home. During this stage patients neglect personal hygiene and withdraw from social groups. Individuals may become extremely depressed if they are aware of what is happening (Goodman, 1987; Lawton, Brody, 1969). The *third stage* is the dementia or terminal stage, in which people have flat affect and no longer ambulate. They do not recognize family or friends, are unable to communicate, and have no interaction with the environment. They become malnourished, emaciated, and are incontinent (Hall, 1988; Matteson, McConnell, 1988). This last stage may progress to a condition known as "chronic vegetative state," where the patient becomes unresponsive, even to pain, and lies in the fetal position. These patients are completely dependent on the nurse to maintain their skin integrity, nutritional status, and personal hygiene, and to prevent injury.

Assessment

There are no definitive tests to confirm a diagnosis of Alzheimer's disease. Only by examination of the brain on autopsy can the diagnosis be confirmed. Diagnosis is made on the basis of cognitive and behavioral symptoms and by ruling out other physiologic and psychologic disorders. A complete history and physical examination are needed, and laboratory testing should include a complete blood count, blood chemistries, thyroid function tests, and folate and B_{12} levels. A CAT scan of the head may also be needed. Careful review of all prescription and over-the-counter medications is imperative. A differential assessment for dementia, depression, and delirium (Table 14-3) should be performed, and experts in geriatric evaluation should be consulted to perform the examination and interpret the findings. Since the goal of nursing care will be to keep the individual functioning at his or her highest possible level, the nurse will need to assess the patient's abilities on an ongoing basis. Those areas that should be assessed include level of consciousness, reality orientation, memory, ability to reason, ability to carry out activities of daily living, interaction with others, and response to environmental stimuli (Folstein and others, 1975).

Nursing interventions

There is no known cure for Alzheimer's disease. Medications may be used to decrease agitation or depression, but the use of drugs is controversial. The focus of nursing care for Alzheimer's patients is to maintain the highest possible level of functioning for each person. Most Alzheimer's patients are cared for at home during the early stages of the disease and are institutionalized when the resources of the caregivers are exhausted. As the disease progresses, care becomes more and more difficult for family members. They need reassurance and help with developing and maintaining an ever-changing plan of care. Community resources for families of Alzheimer's patients often are lacking, but the nurse can assist by working through the political and social systems to provide this desperately needed support. The Alzheimer's Association has many local chapters that conduct caregiver support groups and information sessions. Caregivers should be encouraged to attend these meetings. Care of the Alzheimer's patient, at home or in an institution, should establish effective verbal and nonverbal communication, provide a safe and structured environment, maintain normal daily living patterns, maintain mobility and exercise as much as possible, provide cognitive stimulation in the environment, maintain optimal nutritional status, and maintain bowel and bladder continence as long as possible (Box 14-1) (Matteson, McConnell, 1988).

Digestive System

Most of the problems associated with the gastrointestinal system of the elderly are the result of pathologic conditions and are not part of the normal aging process. The loss of teeth commonly attributed to aging is preventable if there has been good dental hygiene earlier in life. There is a slight decrease in gastric secretion and a slowing of peristalsis in the bowel. This may lead to various complaints, one of the most frequent being constipation and its complications, colon flatus, and fecal impaction. Some older adults become lactose intolerant and find that eating or drinking milk products causes bloating and diarrhea. Avoiding foods high in lactose may alleviate this problem. Pathologic conditions in the older adult are the same as those seen in all adults. Chapter 23 discusses problems associated with the gastrointestinal system.

Constipation

Constipation is a common complaint among the elderly. It is most important to determine the person's definition of constipation. Many people subscribe to the theory that daily bowel movements are necessary and that less frequent movements indicate constipation. They spend a great deal of time and money attempting to induce daily movements, and many become laxative dependent. The nurse can help to reeducate these elderly people about good bowel hygiene. Laxatives should be taken only under the direction of a physician.

TABLE 14-3

Differential Assessment of Dementia, Depression, and Delirium

	Normal Aging	Dementia	Depression	Delirium
Onset		Insidious	Acute	Rapid onset
Duration		Months to years	Weeks to months	Hours to days
Behavior	Less physical; activity less and slower	Shuffling; restlessness; pacing	Slower; retarded movements	Increased or decreased activity level; change in level of consciousness
Mood	Appropriate to situation; normal, has energy	Normal; labile; sad	Sad; negative	Fear and suspicion may be prominent
Speech	Normal; may concentrate on past history, separation, and death; it is goal directed and has information	Confabulate; vague; focused on past	Negative; clear; repetitive; demanding	Slurred and incoherent
Thinking	Normal; intact	Illusions; old memories; suspicious	Distorted self and body image; distortion of other's motives; overpersonalized	Sensory misinterpretations; visual, auditory and tactile hallucinations may be florid
Memory	Slowing in memory storage, but easy access to information	Loss of recent memory; denies loss; conceals deficits	May be decreased by preoccupation; exaggerates loss; "I don't know" answers	Impaired by poor attention
Intelligence	Intact	Impaired; cannot recall previous learning	Intact; may be slow but will be accurate	Fluctuation of problem solving ability
Orientation (time, place, person)	O.K.	First loses times, then place, and lastly orientation to person	Intact	Disoriented
Judgment (ability to evaluate a situation)	O.K.; perhaps better due to life experience	Impaired; decreased creativity; cannot use experience; cannot generalize	Intact except for evaluation of self	Fluctuation

BOX 14-1 **Nursing Process**

ALZHEIMER'S DISEASE

ASSESSMENT

Mobility impairment
Presence of impulsive behavior
Cognitive impairment
Orientation to time, place, person
Self-care ability and routine
Patterns of elimination
Coping mechanisms of patient and family
Environment for safety

NURSING DIAGNOSES

Risk for injury/trauma related to inability to recognize danger, deterioration, or weakness
Altered thought processes related to loss of memory
Self-care deficit related to impaired cognition, memory, or judgment
Risk for total incontinence related to lack of sensation to void
Risk for bowel incontinence related to impaired cognition
Anticipatory grieving related to change in behavior
Dysfunctional grieving related to perception in loss of loved one
Caregiver role strain related to multiple demands, inadequate resources, or difficult situation

NURSING INTERVENTIONS

Eliminate identified hazards in the environment.
Redirect attention when the patient is agitated.
Provide an identification bracelet for the patient.
Avoid use of restraints.
Approach in a calm manner.
Speak in a low, slow voice.
Use simple words and statements.
Avoid negative criticism or confrontations.
Provide a safe home environment.
Explore possibilities of a home-security device to decrease wandering.
Make useful activities of repetitive activities (dusting, sweeping floor, collecting junk mail).
Administer medications as prescribed.
Provide assistance with self-care activities; encourage independence.
Maintain routine.
Encourage regular intervals for toileting.
Encourage adequate fluids but limit them after 6 PM.
Use protective clothing or incontinence pads as needed.
Identify support systems and support groups.
Encourage the care provider to set aside time for herself or himself.

EVALUATION OF EXPECTED OUTCOMES

Experiences no injury
Participates in self-care activities
Continent of bowel and bladder
Caregiver competent and confident in care
Caregiver identifies resources and support
Family expresses concerns and discusses loss

Assessment

Assessment of the elderly digestive tract includes a good oral examination. The condition of the mucous membrane should be noted. The nurse should examine the teeth for the presence or absence of caries and good hygiene. If dentures are in place, the individual should remove them so the nurse can inspect the gums. The nurse should question the older patient about fluid intake, because many older persons restrict fluids or take dehydrating diuretics, both of which contribute to dry, hard stool and constipation. A stethoscope can be set lightly on the abdomen to listen for bowel sounds. It may take up to 1 minute to hear sounds in any one area. Increased sounds can mean a hyperactive intestine as in diarrhea, and decreased sounds can be a sign of a paralytic ileus or an obstruction. A rectal examination will provide information about anal sphincter tone. Fecal impaction may be present if large amounts of hard stool are in the rectum. The stool should be tested for signs of occult blood.

Nursing interventions

Nursing interventions for the gastrointestinal system will focus on providing for and maintaining a healthy state of functioning in the patient. Good mouth care and attention to dental problems are essential. Teaching about and providing a healthy diet are important. It is not easy for older adults to change lifelong eating habits, so this may present a challenge to the nurse. Healthy bowel habits are necessary to prevent constipation. These include a sufficient intake of high fiber foods and raw fruits and vegetables, 6 to 8 glasses of water daily, a regular program of exercise, and a regular, unhurried time for bowel movements. Use of laxatives and enemas should be discouraged unless prescribed by a physician. Institutionalized elderly will need more assistance in assuming the above habits for healthy bowel management. The use of laxatives, cathartics, and enemas should not be routine in institutions that care for the elderly.

Urinary System

With aging there is a decrease in the number of nephrons in the kidneys and a decrease in the blood supply that together adversely affect the functioning of the urinary system. The kidneys become less efficient in concentrating or diluting urine. The renal threshold for glucose is elevated, and individuals tested for high blood glucose will not show elevated levels in the urine. Excretion of drugs is altered, and the elderly must be closely observed for signs of drug toxicity. The smooth muscle and elastic tissue of the bladder are replaced with fibrous connective tissue. This results in decreased bladder capacity and increased frequency of urination. The elderly also experience more nocturia. There is a decrease in the force of the stream, and some may experience stress incontinence. For these reasons many elderly may limit their appearance in public or avoid long trips. Some decrease their fluid intake to avoid embarrassment. Bladder outlet changes may cause obstruction in the male and incontinence in the female (Matteson, McConnell, 1988).

Assessment

Assessment of the urinary system is done indirectly by asking the elderly patient about his or her urinary habits. The kidneys themselves are rarely palpated. If there is a severe kidney infection, the individual can have flank tenderness. The amount, color, and odor of urine is one way to assess the urinary system. The external meatus of both men and women should be inspected and kept clean to prevent infections. If the urinary bladder is overfilled with urine, it can be palpated above the pubic bone.

Common pathologic conditions

Decrease in the function of the urinary system causes certain pathologic conditions to be seen regularly among the elderly. The diminished efficiency of the kidneys may result in acute and chronic renal failure (see Chapter 24). Bladder problems such as urinary retention, urinary tract infections, and cancer of the bladder appear (see Chaper 24). Urinary incontinence is especially troublesome in women, while benign prostatic hypertrophy and prostate cancer are major problems for men (see Chapters 25 and 26).

Nursing interventions

The elderly may feel uncomfortable talking about a genitourinary problem and may live with the problem rather than face the embarrassment of mentioning it. The understanding nurse will appreciate these feelings and will provide a private, gentle, and sensitive environment for this discussion. Nursing interventions should be focused on maintaining normal function of the urinary system. Mobility and activity promote normal urinary function, so the nurse should encourage the elderly to remain as active as possible. Older adults should be aware of their patterns of elimination and should plan their schedules accordingly. Medications that affect elimination, such as diuretics, should be taken in the morning so that they do not interfere with sleep. When away from home the elderly should locate the washroom in any public place before it is needed. Clothing can be modified to permit ease and speed in its removal. The environment also should be modified to accommodate individual needs, which might require providing unobstructed pathways to the bathroom, using night lights, and having hand rails alongside the toilet to assist in getting up and down. Maintaining adequate fluid intake is essential for bladder functioning, and good personal hygiene is important in preventing infection and controlling odor. Urine should be examined for indication of a urinary tract infection, and the patient should be treated if one is present. Women with dry, friable vaginal tissue will benefit from topical estrogen cream. Exercises can be taught to decrease stress incontinence (Kegel exercises). These exercises involve tightening the muscles of the pelvic floor in a regular, scheduled pattern (see Chapter 15).

Respiratory System

The function of the pulmonary system decreases with age, and the loss reduces the reserve that is necessary during stress. These losses are not great enough, however, to interfere with ordinary activity (Matteson, McConnell, 1988). Skeletal changes reduce the flexibility of the rib cage, and it tends to remain expanded. The respiratory muscles weaken, resulting in reduced ability of the thoracic cavity to enlarge with inspiration and to recoil with expiration. Smoking, immobility, and obesity can further compromise lung function. Because the lungs are less elastic, more air remains in the lungs, and less air is exchanged. Thickened and decreased capillaries reduce the exchange of oxygen and carbon dioxide in the lungs. The elderly become short of breath more readily and have greater difficulty recovering from respiratory diseases.

Assessment

Assess the respiratory system by first looking at the shape of the chest. Note the condition of the skin and whether the accessory muscles are used for breathing. Breathing should be unstrained and symmetrical. Auscultation of the lungs is done posteriorly first and then anteriorly, going side to side, top to bottom. The individual is asked to take a deep breath through the mouth while the stethoscope is placed on the chest. The nurse should observe the person carefully for signs of hyperventilation during this examination. Breath sounds may be distant but should be clear. Soft or loud crackles or wheezes are considered abnormal sounds.

Common pathologic conditions

The most common respiratory diseases among the elderly include chronic obstructive pulmonary disease (COPD), emphysema, chronic bronchitis, asthma, tuberculosis, and lung cancer. These are not problems brought on by aging of the lungs but are the result of lifestyle and environmental factors, including smoking and air pollutants. Pneumonia is also common in older adults. Several factors contribute to the increased incidence of pneumonia among the elderly: weakened immune system, immobility, chronic illness, and debility. Institutionalized elderly persons are more vulnerable. These respiratory diseases are discussed in Chapter 20.

Nursing interventions

As with other systems, mobility and exercise play an important role in maintaining a healthy respiratory system. Exercise will help to reduce the effects of aging on the lungs and will increase the muscle tone of the chest and the individual's ability to fight off infection. The elderly who smoke should be encouraged and helped to quit. For those older adults who have lung problems, the nurse can assist in adapting the environment to reduce irritants. This might mean using filters, humidifiers or dehumidifiers, and air conditioning. Older persons at risk for lung diseases should have flu vaccines yearly in the fall. Pneumococcal vaccine should be administered once in a lifetime for the prevention of pneumonia. Colds and other respiratory infections should be attended to promptly (Matteson, McConnell, 1988).

Reproductive System

After menopause women experience a decrease in estrogens, tissue changes in the vulva and vagina, thinning of the epithelial cells, and loss of normal vaginal acidity. The elderly woman is more susceptible to vaginitis because of these changes. The breasts, uterus, and ovaries begin to atrophy. Men will experience a reduction in seminal fluid. The prostate may enlarge, and the testes may become smaller and less firm.

Assessment

Assessment of the breast tissue in elderly women is important because cancer is a concern. The breasts are inspected for symmetry, nipple discharge, or dimpled skin. Circular palpation is done from the axilla, gradually working toward the nipple. A pelvic examination for the elderly woman can be helpful in determining pelvic muscle tone and a possible cystocele, rectocele, or uterine prolapse. These are all factors that can contribute to incontinence. Some of these conditions can be noted with careful external inspection. A pelvic examination should be conducted by a physician or nurse practitioner. The elderly man is examined externally for signs of phimosis (tight foreskin), testicular swelling, hydrocele, or herniations. A physician or nurse practitioner should evaluate the status of the prostate gland by rectal examination.

Common pathologic conditions

Problems of the reproductive system in elderly females include relaxation of the pelvic musculature (cystocele, rectocele, and uterine prolapse) and cancer of the reproductive organs. Breast cancer is the most common form. In elderly males benign prostatic hypertrophy and cancer of the prostate are often seen (see Chapter 26).

Nursing interventions

The focus of nursing interventions should be education. Many elderly feel embarrassed about discussing problems related to their reproductive organs. The nurse needs to be sensitive to their embarrassment and provide an environment in which they can more easily discuss this subject. Adults should be taught breast self-examination or testicular self-examination and encouraged to practice it monthly. Annual mammograms are recommended for women over age 50. Regular physical examinations are recommended for both sexes, including Pap smears for women and digital rectal examinations for men.

NURSING THE ELDERLY

The process of aging does not necessarily mean a process of decline. Although the elderly are more susceptible to illness, aging does not mean sickness. Physical changes do occur, but physical debility is not a normal part of the aging process. Nursing care of the aging individual requires respecting each as a unique and valued person. This includes the manner in which the person is addressed. Every adult person should be asked what he or she would like to be called. Use of an elderly person's first name by a much younger person is considered by many as a breach of etiquette. To address an older adult as "Grandma" or "Gramps" or "dear" is inappropriate and degrading. Care of the elderly includes procedures designed to maintain and improve functional ability and quality of life, protect against injury, recognize individuality, meet nutritional needs, maintain personal hygiene, and prevent complications from drug therapy.

Maintaining and Improving Functional Ability

A functional assessment identifies the person's level of independence, focusing on abilities rather than disabilities. Each person's ability to perform activities of daily living is assessed using a numeric scale.

Both physical activities of daily living (ADLs) and instrumental activities of daily living (IADLs) need to be assessed. Physical ADLs include bathing, dressing, eating, ambulating, grooming, managing assistive devices, and using the toilet. IADLs involve balancing a checkbook, housekeeping, going to the store, doing laundry, using the telephone, and managing medications.

CASE STUDY

Mrs. Taylor is an 84-year-old woman who lives in a senior high-rise housing complex. She recently stopped bathing because she had difficulty getting out of the bathtub and was fearful of falling. However, she missed her baths very much and did not feel clean when just washing at the sink. Her nurse assessed her ability to rise from a sitting position and found her quadriceps muscles to be weak. She also noticed that the safety bath mat used by Mrs. Taylor in her tub was old and tended to slip. Mrs. Taylor and her nurse agreed to start a plan that eventually would allow her to bathe again. The plan was to strengthen her leg muscles by walking and exercising and to prevent injury by purchasing a new bath mat. In the meantime, Mrs. Taylor agreed not to bathe in the tub unless her daughter was present to help her should she have trouble getting out of the tub.

Assessment of functional ability allows the members of the healthcare team to design a care plan that considers the patient's ability to care for himself or herself independently. The assessment forms the basis from which goals and nursing interventions will be developed. The patient should be involved in the plan of care and can assist in the goalsetting process. Each step can be discussed and a plan agreed upon.

The nurse may involve other members of the healthcare system who can assist in reaching functional goals. Physical therapy, occupational therapy, speech therapy, dieticians, social workers, and many others have skills that may improve the functional ability of the older person. The best care delivered to older people is multidisciplinary in nature. The nurse often plays the role of coordinator because nursing has a holistic focus.

The functional assessment also serves as a means of evaluation. Through periodic assessment, it can be determined whether abilities have improved or remained stable. In assessing functional status, each function may be evaluated numerically on a scale. As abilities change, the numbers change. The choice of a functional assessment instrument depends on the facility. Some instruments used in clinical practice include the Katz Index of ADL (Katz and others, 1963), the Barthel Index (Mahoney, Barthel, 1965), the PULSES Profile (Moskowitz, McCann, 1957), the Rapid Disability Scale (Lin, Linn, 1982), and the Scale for Instrumental Activities of Daily Living (Lawton, Brody, 1969).

Maintaining and Improving Quality of Life

Most older persons wish to live a life that involves autonomy, security, and the freedom to establish and maintain interpersonal relationships. Although defining **quality of life** is difficult, these concepts, among others, constitute what many older people would call a good life (Grossman, Weiner, 1988). Gerontology focuses on improving the quality of life for older persons because focusing only on length of life may not be adequate in many circumstances. Many older persons prefer to live "a few good years" rather than many years of disability, pain, loneliness, and isolation.

Quality of life is of concern to nursing because the emphasis is on caring and on the well-being of the whole person. Nurses often intervene to improve the quality of life of an older person. Certainly, control of pain and improvement of function can improve the quality of a person's life, but this is just the beginning. Opportunities for growth and development, leisure activities, and privacy are necessary for most older people. Many of the concepts already discussed under the mental health section apply here.

CASE STUDY

Mrs. Kline, age 84, recently returned home after hospitalization for a broken hip. Because she had to limit her activities until fully recuperated, Mrs. Kline could not go to the senior center. The home care nurse found her bored and angry. "I don't want to live like an invalid. I'm bored." The nurse realized that Mrs. Kline was fearful of isolation and that this negatively affected her quality of life. The nurse was able to arrange transportation so that Mrs. Carter, Mrs. Kline's best friend, could visit daily. The nurse also helped her contact the local library for home delivery of books. Although Mrs. Kline continued to be impatient for a full recovery, her feelings of boredom and isolation were lessened, and she greatly enjoyed Mrs. Carter's visits and reading her favorite library books.

Quality of life can be measured by asking older persons to reflect on their day-to-day lives and to state their level of satisfaction with their life circumstances. Although the nurse may not be able to improve many things in an older person's life, many areas may be addressed by the healthcare team.

Physical well-being, psychologic well being, and quality of life are all closely correlated in the elderly patient. Nurses should make sure that the nursing care plan includes interventions designed to maintain and improve quality of life for the elderly.

Group Work With the Elderly

Working with the aged in groups can be effective in meeting psychosocial needs. Group work of this nature is not to be confused with group psychotherapy, which deals with people who have psychiatric problems. Group work has been used to treat and prevent psychosocial problems in the elderly and to maintain mental health. Groups have been conducted for reality orientation, remotivation, reminiscing, and health teaching. In some instances the family also is involved with the group.

Reality orientation groups are used with regressed aged persons, especially those with chronic brain syndrome. A small group of four or five persons meets daily with their leader, who emphasizes time, day, month, weather conditions, and the like, which are then posted on a board for all to see throughout the day. **Remotivation** groups are the next step in progression after reality orientation. The leader must have specialized training to conduct these groups.

Reminiscing groups have been pioneered by Ebersole, a psychiatric nurse (Ebersole, Hess, 1994). **Reminiscing** is an adaptive response to aging and can be used effectively to preserve and rebuild self-concept and maintain social integrity. It will help elderly persons to remember who they are and thus stimulate self-esteem.

Nurses should be encouraged to investigate possibilities of working with groups, seek whatever training is required, and implement or assist in group work with the elderly when opportunities arise. Group work requires the support and cooperation of everyone in the agency if it is to be successful.

Helping the Older Person Prepare for Death

Many older persons wish to establish a living will, name a healthcare proxy or durable power of attorney, or leave advance directives regarding their healthcare with a close friend or relative. These concepts are fully discussed in Chapter 5. Although nurses may feel uncomfortable discussing these issues with essentially healthy older people, it should be remembered that preparation for death is one of the normal developmental tasks of aging. When and if a time comes when a person cannot make decisions for himself or herself, it is important that someone be able to communicate the wishes of the patient. Although each individual is different, many older people have seen friends or loved ones die while on ventilators or in the critical care units of hospitals and may wish to die a more "natural death." Natural death occurs when declining organ function becomes insufficient to sustain life (Fries, Crapo, 1981).

Individuals who have lived a long life and survived many threats of illness and accident may die a death in extreme old age without any obvious cause whatsoever. It is estimated that about one third of all deaths of elderly people are "natural deaths" that occur in the final stages of senescence (Fries, Crapo, 1981).

CASE STUDY

Mr. Watson, age 87, lives alone in his apartment near his son and daughter-in-law. His family notices that he is gradually failing, yet his doctor can find nothing wrong. For the next 6 months, he is just not himself and doesn't have his usual zest for life. One night he dies quietly in his sleep, and even after an autopsy no obvious cause of death can be found.

Preventing Injury

Injuries resulting from accidents are a major and largely preventable cause of death and illness in the elderly. A great many accidental deaths are the result of complications following falls.

Because most falls occur in the home, precautions should be taken to protect elderly persons. Scatter rugs should not be used unless they are secured by rubber mats beneath them. Toys left on the floor and furniture moved to unfamiliar places may be responsible for a fall. Rubber mats should be placed in bathtubs, and support should be provided to assist persons stepping from the tub (Figure 14-4).

Night-lights and lights in bathrooms and on stairs should be left on at night, and increased illumination should be provided in the evening. Elderly persons are susceptible to accidents on streets and highways at dusk or in the evening. To avoid such accidents, an elderly person should be accompanied, should carry a flashlight, and should have reflective material attached to his or her clothing.

Recognizing Individuality

With aging comes increased diversity. Individual preferences and abilities become unique to each person with the aging process. Society tends to stereotype the elderly as a group with members very like one another. In books, on television, and in most advertising, the elderly often are depicted as needing assistance, forgetful, and asexual. Sometimes nurses and physicians have the most negative stereotypes about aging because healthcare providers work mostly with sick older persons, many of whom have cognitive deficits. There are, however, great differences among older persons. It is unfair for healthcare providers to limit an

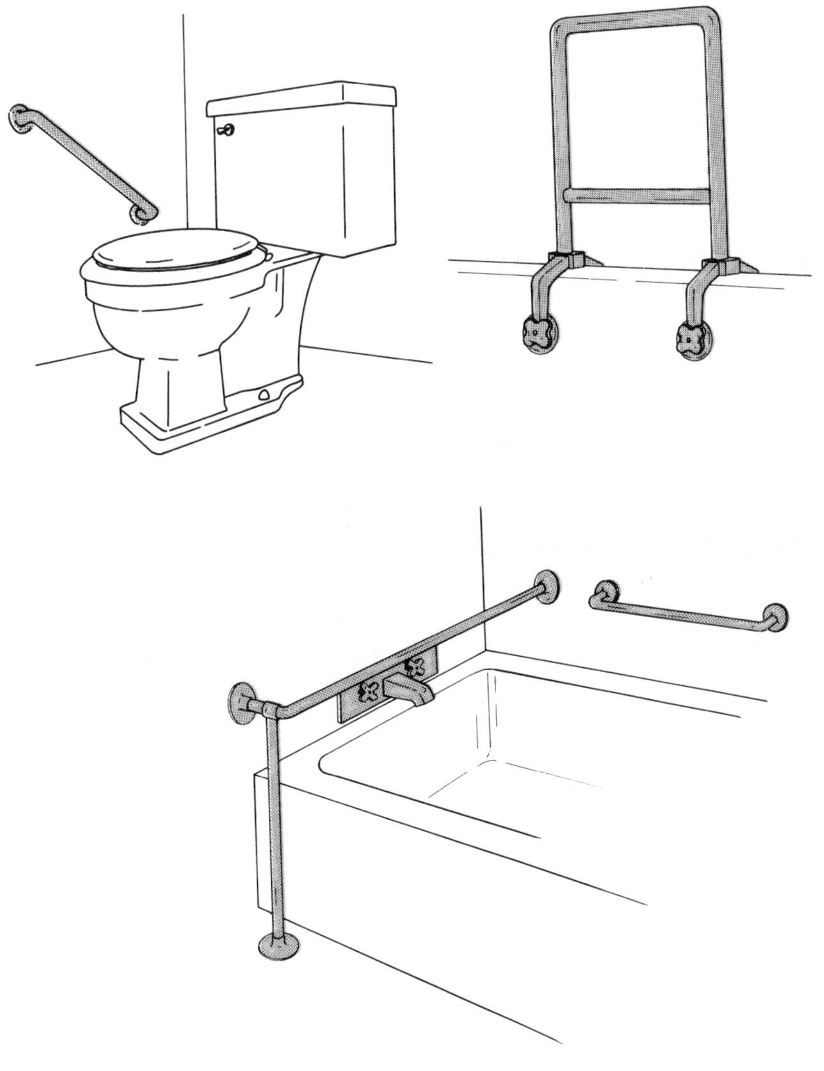

Figure 14-4 Hand bars placed on bathtubs and beside toilets provide support for patient and prevent falls from loss of balance.

older person's choices and opportunities for rehabilitation because they assume that most older people are hard of hearing, dislike spicy food, care little about sexual relationships, and enjoy a sedentary lifestyle without new experiences.

NURSE ALERT

Individual preferences and abilities of the elderly must be carefully assessed and incorporated into their nursing care plan.

Society has held the stereotyped belief that sexual desires and activity begin to diminish in the mid-forties and cease completely sometime in the later years and that this is appropriate. Sexually active elderly persons are considered perverse or, at best, to be lying about their activities. Open expressions of **sexuality** between elderly partners are often met with the disapproval of grown children because they believe that sex is not appropriate for this age group. The work of Kinsey, Masters and Johnson, and recent studies conducted at Duke University are proving quite the opposite.

Although Kinsey's work did not deal with a large sample of elderly persons, it did show that most men over age 60 were capable of sexual intercourse (Kinsey and others, 1948) and that sexual activity in women varied more with marital status than it did with age (Kinsey and others, 1953). Masters and Johnson devoted a great deal of their study to the sexual responses of aged persons. They found that physically, men over age 60 are slower to respond sexually and the physiologic response of women diminishes somewhat, but both are capable of orgasm, especially those who are often exposed to effective stimulation (Masters, Johnson, 1970). Studies continue to add to the evidence that sex continues to play an important role in the lives of many elderly persons. These studies, along with the work of Masters and Johnson, lead to some overall conclusions that are quite different from the stereotype held by society, namely that there is no specific age when sexual activity will and should cease. Frequency of sexual activity is related to the availability of a socially sanctioned partner rather than to age. An individual who has frequent sexual experiences earlier in life will continue to have more frequent sexual experiences later in life than will the person who is less active in early years. Good physical health affects sexual functioning and will affect the quality and quantity of sexual activity in the elderly.

These current findings should be considered by the nurse working with the elderly. Nurses must become comfortable with the idea that the elderly have or desire to have an active sex life. The elderly do receive pleasure from sex, and sexual problems may, in turn, trouble older persons. The nurse must educate others in this area and try to remove prejudices. The nurse must consider each elderly person as an individual in the area of sexuality, as well as in other human needs. The elderly person's sexual needs will be affected by his or her present and previous lifestyle rather than by some concrete standard of performance. Again, the best gerontologic care is provided by a multidisciplinary team, and nurses can consult with other healthcare providers to set realistic goals for the older patient that are consistent with the individual's needs and strengths.

CASE STUDY

Mr. Jackson, age 69, recently had a stroke that left him paralyzed on his right side and unable to talk. He uses a wheelchair but is able to walk short distances with the assistance of a cane. Mrs. Jackson visits her husband each day in the rehabilitation unit of the hospital. Mrs. Jackson asked one of the evening nurses when she and Mr. Jackson could resume their sexual relationship, which she described as very intimate and satisfying to both of them. The nurse blushed with embarrassment and said, "I don't know. You'd better ask the doctor." Mrs. Jackson felt that she had said the wrong thing to the nurse and did not mention anything about sex again during the remainder of her husband's rehabilitation.

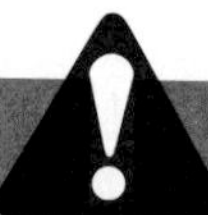

NURSE ALERT

Prejudices of the nurse have no place in providing care to the elderly.

Meeting Nutritional Needs

As a group, elderly people appear to be highly susceptible to malnutrition. In senescence, the metabolic processes decrease by 10% to 30%, physical activity decreases, and the individual needs fewer calories. However, if appetite fails, the individual will become malnourished. Some elderly persons are obese and continue to follow dietary patterns of overeating, particularly rich foods. They, too, may be undernourished, not in calories but in dietary essentials (Box 14-2).

The diet should include all of the nutritional requirements, that is, carbohydrates, fats, proteins, vitamins, minerals, and water. Because of reduced physical activity and a decline in metabolic activity, elderly persons need fewer calories than when they were younger. Caloric needs must be evaluated individually. Men may require more calories than women, and some persons will require more calories than others because they are more active and expend more energy. It has been suggested that calories should be reduced by 7% to 8% every 10 years after a person has reached age 25.

The diet should include the five basic food groups: (1) breads, cereals, pasta, and rice; (2) fruits; (3) vegetables; (4) milk and cheese; (5) meat, fish, poultry, eggs, dry beans, and nuts. The basic food groups apply to all persons regardless of age, with the calories adjusted through smaller or larger servings. There is some evidence that proper use of food in the body requires that all nutrients be present at approximately the same time. Although the "basic five" diet provides a simple, systematic guide to food selection, it does not regulate intake of salt, cholesterol, and saturated fat. Additional information must be provided to guide the elderly in selecting a diet that is well balanced and at the same time low in salt, cholesterol, and saturated fat (Ebersole, Hess, 1994). The frequency and amount of food served is also important, and it is recommended that the daily food requirement be divided into six small meals. Vitamin and mineral supplements should be used only on the advice of the physician. Whenever possible, the individual should eat with the family, and food should be prepared the way the person likes it and then served attractively. The elderly should be allowed to participate in food selection and preparation if they are able, and guidance in including all essential foods in the diet should be provided as necessary. For those frail elderly who live at home and need assistance with meal preparation, home-delivered meals for the elderly (Meals on Wheels) may be appropriate. Many community senior citizen centers sponsor daily lunch programs at minimal cost for those elderly persons who attend activities at the center. In addition to a good meal, socialization and recreational activities may benefit the older person.

BOX 14-2

FACTORS AFFECTING SOME DIETARY PATTERNS OF THE ELDERLY

1. Reduced income
2. Inadequacy of cooking facilities
3. Loneliness and having to eat alone
4. Physical inability to prepare food
5. Loss of teeth or poorly fitting dentures
6. Lack of transportation or delivery service
7. Side effects of multiple medications that may affect the taste of food

Maintaining Personal Hygiene

Daily baths result in excessive dryness and scaling of the skin, often accompanied by itching. Inadequate rinsing may cause a dermatitis, producing a great deal of discomfort from burning and itching of the affected parts. Complete baths should be reduced to two or three a week, with careful rinsing and drying. However, attention should be given to the perineal area on a daily basis. Bath oils may be added to the water, but extra caution must be taken to prevent falls, since these oils may make the tub more slippery. Showers, taken with a hand-held shower head in a stall that has a seat or is large enough for a bath chair, provide for thorough rinsing and are easier to maneuver in and out of than are bathtubs. An elderly person should not be alone in a locked bathroom. However, it is important to ensure privacy, which can be accomplished by a sign on the door or hanging from the doorknob to tell others than the room is occupied. Because of diminished activity of oil glands, the hair should be shampooed less frequently and shampoos containing alcohol should be avoided because of their drying effect.

Cold weather and dry furnace heat can aggravate the problem of dry skin. Older people who spend the winter in cold climates should take extra precautions to prevent skin problems. Wearing soft clothing and using skin lotions can help prevent dryness.

Care of the feet is also important. Warm soaks with thorough drying, particularly between the toes, followed by massage with baby oil or lanolin will prevent excessive drying. A member of the family or the nurse should trim the nails. If financial resources permit, the individual may be taken to a podiatrist for foot care. Visits may be scheduled at 4- to 6-week intervals. Corns, calluses, and infections require special care.

Many elderly people will have partial or full dentures. Some will have teeth missing. The loss of teeth, dental caries, and poorly fitting dentures can affect the person's general health by interfering with dietary needs. Normal shrinking of the gums exposes the soft parts of the tooth structure, which are more sensitive to injury. Improperly fitting dentures may cause the gums to become sore. Regular gum massage will stimulate circulation and help to keep gums healthy. For those who have their own teeth, regular visits to the dentist are necessary. Teeth should be brushed after meals with a mild dentifrice and a soft-bristle brush, and dentures also should be brushed after each meal.

Sluggishness of the bowel, which may accompany aging, is primarily the result of inactivity and faulty diet. When it occurs, it is not unusual for the person to resort to the use of a laxative that was seen advertised or one that a well-meaning friend or neighbor has suggested. Laxatives, like any other medication, should be prescribed by the physician. Regular bowel habits should be encouraged and, when possible, diet should include some soft bulk to facilitate bowel evacuation. Simple measures such as prune juice at night or a glass of warm water with a little lemon juice before breakfast may be all that is required.

Decreased muscle tone and reduced capacity of the bladder may cause urinary incontinence. This may result in embarrassment for the individual. A medical examination should be done to rule out infection or other pathologic condition. Clothing should be changed as often as necessary to prevent odor and skin excoriation. If there is no pathologic condition, incontinence can be prevented by planning frequent use of the bathroom, commode, or bedpan during the day and by limiting fluids after the evening meal.

The individual should be encouraged to maintain good personal hygiene and good personal appearance, particularly with reference to hair and clothing. For many elderly persons some member of the family will have to help with or supervise daily care. The same principles of personal hygiene apply to the individual who may be hospitalized or in a nursing home.

Preventing Complications From Drug Use

Twenty-five percent of all medications are taken by the 10% of the population who are over age 65. For this reason, and because of the physiologic effects of aging on drug action, drug use in the elderly must be carefully examined.

It is said that 85% of all prescriptions written by a physician are based on what the patient says. When an older patient complains of sleep problems, lack of energy, feelings of sadness or chronic pain, a busy physician may be tempted to write a prescription for a medicine to solve the problem rather than get a full history relating to the problem. In other words, sometimes older people are treated for symptoms of physical problems without an adequate exploration of the cause of the problem. This approach sometimes makes the patient's problem worse because many medications may cause side effects and further decrease the patient's functional ability. These potential problems make it particularly important that older patients know about their drugs, understand their actions, and keep their physicians informed. It is equally important for the nurse to be aware of age-related factors that affect drug action and increase toxicity in this age group.

The age-related factors that account for changes in drug action and increased toxicity are numerous. Gastric emptying time is slowed in the older person, and the motility of the gastrointestinal tract is slower. Intestinal blood flow is reduced, and absorption by the cells also is reduced. For these reasons, drugs taken orally and absorbed in the gastrointestinal tract are absorbed more slowly than they would be in a younger person. Metabolism slows with age, and any drug that affects or is affected by metabolism will be needed in lower doses. For example, dosage of antibiotics should be reduced because an elderly person retains antibiotics in the body longer than a younger person. The absorption and distribution of a drug changes with age. Passage across the blood-brain barrier, however, is always good, which means that the drug will manage to get to the brain, even though it may not be supplied as well to other parts of the body. This accounts for the fact that confusion frequently is an early sign of drug toxicity in the elderly. Excretion is another factor affecting drug action. The nephrons in the kidney are reduced by 50% to 60% with aging, and liver function decreases, both of which slow the rate at which drugs are excreted from the body. Cumulative actions can be a problem if doses are not reduced to account for the aging process.

When evaluating drug dosages ordered for the elderly, one must remember that recommended drug dosages are tested on 25-year-old, healthy men weighing approximately 150 pounds. One commonly used drug, diazepam (Valium), has a recommended adult dosage of 15 to 50 mg per day, usually given in three or four doses. In the elderly it is found that 5 to 15 mg diazepam per day is the maximum that should be given and that 2 mg per dose or 6 mg per day is probably the most beneficial. Diazepam is commonly ordered for the elderly, but at 5 or 10 mg three times a day. Like diazepam, all tranquilizers and antidepressants should be administered in reduced dosages. Dosages ordered for elderly patients, as well as the symptoms they are exhibiting, should be examined. If a patient is showing confusion, it could be because these drugs are being excreted slowly by the body and are crossing the blood-brain barrier in toxic levels. Confusion may be one of the earliest signs of toxicity. When older persons act confused, they are often labeled senile, but medications should be checked to see whether the confusion is, in fact, drug induced.

Sedatives and other nervous system depressants have an intensified effect on the elderly, so only small doses of the drugs should be given. Elderly persons may exhibit bizarre behavior when given a sedative or hypnotic. Memory loss, disorientation, falls, and incontinence commonly occur.

Barbiturates include in their action an ability to slow the heart rate. For this reason, it is best to avoid the use of barbiturates for the elderly, and some authorities believe that they should not be used by anyone. Any elderly patient who is taking a barbiturate should be watched for signs of reduced heart action, and extreme care should be exercised if that patient has a heart problem. The nurse should be sure to report these symptoms to the main provider immediately so that the medication order might be reconsidered.

In drug idiosyncrasies, known to be common in the elderly, the action obtained from the drug is just the opposite of the intended action. For example, if a sleeping pill is given and the individual has an idiosyncrasy to that particular drug, sleeplessness rather than sleep will result.

Drug interactions are a problem not only for the elderly but for all individuals taking drugs. Drugs interact with foods and with other drugs in ways that may affect the action of the drug. The dangers of giving aspirin with anticoagulants and causing an increase in bleeding are well known. Antacids are not to be given with an antibiotic because they tie up the antibiotic and reduce its effectiveness. There are literally hundreds and hundreds of possible drug interactions, and the nurse should consult drug references to identify the possible interactions for each drug the patient is taking.

It is important that all drugs taken by the elderly be identified. This includes not only those prescribed by all providers but also the over-the-counter drugs that the elderly may not even consider as drugs or medications. A very careful history must be taken to identify every drug that the elderly person is taking to avoid interactions and possible toxic effects. The route and method of administration must be as clearly understood by elderly persons as by younger persons taking medications. If the drug is to be taken under the tongue or taken without chewing, it is important that the person understand those directions to achieve therapeutic effect.

An elderly person with dementia may resist taking medications. Some will very aggressively refuse. It is necessary to see the patient swallow the drug and to be sure that the patient has not hidden the drug under the tongue, in the buccal cavity, in the hand or bed linen, or in any other number of places. The nurse should stay with the patient while he or she takes the drug and ensure that it is gone from the mouth. It may even be necessary to check the mouth after the person supposedly has taken the drug to be sure that it has been swallowed and that he or she does not aspirate. Preventing complications from drug therapy is one of the major nursing goals in the care of the elderly (Box 14-3).

CARE OF THE HOSPITALIZED ELDERLY PATIENT

Nursing elderly patients with acute mental or surgical conditions is different in many respects from nursing younger persons. The normal changes of aging produce physiologic and psychologic patterns that would not be observed in younger persons. Nursing care probably will require more time because the elderly person is slower to move and act. More assistance may be required in performing activities of daily living. A gentle touch is also important, since the older person is susceptible to injury to skin, bones, and connective tissue. The assistance of other nursing personnel may be necessary to aid in turning, lifting, and ambulating the older patient and to prevent injury.

Mental Status and Vital Signs

The level of orientation, memory, and level of consciousness of older persons may change when they are acutely ill. The acute confusional state is called delirium and has been discussed previously. When delirium occurs, the nurse should conduct a careful search for the cause. This would include a complete examination of all medications, review of bowel function and vital signs, and inspection of the physical environment surrounding the patient. While protecting the patient from injury, the nurse and other members of the healthcare team can attempt to correct the cause of the delirium.

Elderly patients often do not tolerate sedative drugs as well as do younger patients, and after surgery they

BOX 14-3

CARE OF THE ELDERLY

MAJOR NURSING GOALS

- Maintain and improve functional ability
- Maintain and improve quality of life
- Protect from injury
- Recognize individuality
- Meet nutritional needs
- Maintain personal hygiene
- Prevent complications from drug therapy

usually require smaller amounts of narcotics. Changing the patient's position, giving a warm drink, or sitting with an anxious patient often will be of greater value than administering a drug. When a hypnotic is administered to an elderly person at bedtime, it is important for the nurse to check on the patient frequently. Often the patient may become confused, try to get out of bed, and fall, causing serious injury. When administering any medication to elderly persons, it is advisable not to use the term "drugs," since many of them associate drugs with addiction.

Blood pressure is influenced by age, but the range of systolic pressure may be rather wide; however, the diastolic range is less wide. Any significant change in blood pressure should always be reported. The blood pressure of elderly persons may be affected by chronic disease or the stress of illness. In the elderly person, a small change in blood pressure may be more important than it would be in a younger person, and the rate of the pulse may be less significant than its volume and rhythm. The rate must be considered together with other symptoms and the patient's condition. It is not uncommon for the pulse in an elderly person to be intermittent, and patients who are receiving digitalis often exhibit changes in the normal rate and rhythm of the pulse. Most people over 70 years of age have premature beats, which occur sooner than expected in the rhythmic pattern. The nurse should develop a sensitivity to what is felt and be able to report it accurately.

Intake and Output and Nutritional Needs

Total fluid intake, including that contained in foods, should be sufficient to produce 1500 ml of urine in 24 hours. Since many older persons are dehydrated, fluids often will be retained until a physiologic balance has been established. A severely dehydrated patient may retain and absorb solution administered as an enema. Persuading an individual to take oral fluids is often a frustrating experience, and small amounts at frequent intervals often will be better accepted than will a large amount at one time. When fluids are restricted because of a cardiac or other condition, the nurse should understand the amount permitted and calculate it carefully.

In some conditions and postoperatively, the physician may order the administration of solutions intravenously. An important factor in the administration of intravenous fluids to elderly persons is the rate of flow. Severe cardiac disturbance may result if fluids are administered too rapidly. Unless ordered otherwise by the physician, 1000 ml of fluid should not be administered in less than 4 hours. Frequently, elderly persons do not tolerate blood transfusions well. The blood should be administered slowly, and the patient should be carefully observed during the procedure. Careful records of intake and output should be maintained and accurate measurements should be made.

Nutrition for the hospitalized elder may be difficult because many older patients may not wish to eat on a hospital schedule or may dislike the quality and variety of foods served. If allowed, family members may wish to bring in favorite foods from home that the patient may enjoy. Food not eaten at mealtime can be labeled and stored in the refrigerator for a snack at bedtime. Liquid protein drinks can be given between meals to boost caloric intake and protein ingestion. Older patients who select their own daily menu should be urged to choose a wide variety of foods representing a balanced diet and extra protein choices to speed the healing process after surgery.

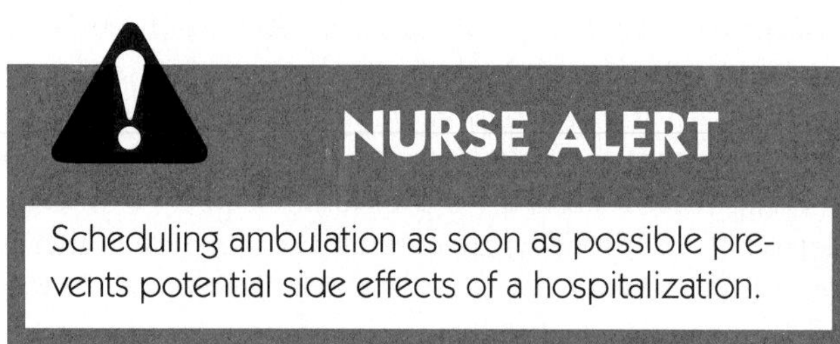

Scheduling ambulation as soon as possible prevents potential side effects of a hospitalization.

Ambulation and Rehabilitation

Recovery from acute illness is often accompanied by chronic disease, which may affect the rate of recovery. Older people require longer periods for recovery than do younger persons, and their progress is slower. The elderly should be out of bed as much as their condition permits to prevent complications of bedrest. The process of ambulation should be slow and progressive, beginning with elevating the patient in bed. The next steps are to have the patient sit on the side of the bed, then sit up in a chair for 15 to 20 minutes beside the bed, then take a few steps, then gradually lengthen the time up and the extent of walking. The patient should be observed for color, respiration, and pulse rate, and if faintness or dizziness occurs the patient should be returned to bed. An elderly person out of bed for the first time should not be left alone.

The older patient recovering from surgery or serious illness may become anxious and frustrated because of the slow rate of recovery and long convalescence. The nurse should recognize that these emotions can affect the patient's desire to participate in care and continue with prescribed activities. A caring attitude, encouragement, and support are important aspects of care.

When caring for elderly patients in the hospital or in the home, the nurse should speak clearly and distinctly and be sure that the patient understands. This is especially important when giving medications or treatments, since the patient may respond to a name that is not his or her own. When working with elderly patients in the hospital or in the home, the nurse should not expect to make requests and secure a quick response. The patient may respond with "all right" or "in a minute." Directions should be given slowly, making certain that the patient understands. The patient may indicate that he or she understands, but action may be slow. The older person should not be hurried, since this may create confusion and render the patient unable to respond appropriately (Box 14-4).

NURSING HOMES

Only 5% of the elderly population live in institutions, but of these, most are in **nursing homes.** Many of those residing in nursing homes could be cared for in their own homes. There is a move to provide additional services to families to make home care feasible, but nursing homes remain an important provider of healthcare. Nursing homes may provide sheltered care for the ambulatory patient, intermediate care, or skilled care for the patient requiring extensive nursing services. A home may provide only one or all three of these levels of care, and the home is chosen according to the nursing needs of the prospective resident.

Nursing homes approved for Medicare require that the personnel maintain nursing care plans for each patient. Plans should be based on the immediate and long-term needs of the patient. Like plans prepared in the general hospital, they should reflect the thinking of the entire nursing staff.

The average nursing home resident differs little from most other persons of the same chronologic age. In addition to the normal degenerative changes, many nursing home residents have chronic diseases and may be malnourished and debilitated. The nursing care must be individualized according to the individual's particular needs. Some patients are ambulatory and can provide much of their own care, others need assistance with personal hygiene, and some must have total care. The patient's psychologic needs should be met. They should be reassured of their personal worth and should be helped to maintain a sense of dignity and self-respect. Chapter 16 discusses in more depth the problems related to caring for elderly residents in nursing homes.

BOX 14-4

CARE OF THE HOSPITALIZED ELDERLY PATIENT

NURSING INTERVENTIONS

Recognize changes in vital signs and mental status.
Maintain adequate fluid and nutritional intake.
Assist with ambulation and rehabilitation.
Prevent injury and complications.
Provide individualized care based on the patient's strengths and abilities.
Be aware of side effects and toxic effects of all medications administered.

ALTERNATIVES TO INSTITUTIONAL CARE

Home Care

If the patient is to be cared for in his or her own home, the family and the community must provide the necessary services. Most elderly persons prefer to remain in their own homes and are happier when they can do so. Each person must be carefully evaluated medically and socially for **home care.** When the person's potential for self-care has been determined, an individualized program is planned. There may be a need for services available under the Older Americans Act, such as meals, transportation to physicians or clinics, home health aides, and homemaker service. Visits by the public health nurse or visiting nurse may also be needed. "Home care can preserve the elderly person's independence, dignity, and identity—precious human qualities that are often lost when the elderly person is placed in an institution" (Hewner, 1986) (see Chapter 16).

With the introduction of the prospective payment system and **diagnosis related groups,** the incentive to provide alternatives to hospitalization is greater. Home care programs and preventive programs are expanding in an effort to keep elderly individuals from being hospitalized. Health maintenance organizations have become more involved in providing Medicare benefits to the elderly. This involvement has created greater use of alternate care services such as home care, day care, and preventive programs.

Day Hospital

Experimental programs for daytime care of the aged are being tried in both the United States and Canada. The objective is to prevent or delay admission to an institution and to promote independence. Individuals must be ambulatory, but they may be permitted to use a walker or cane. Emergency care is available if needed. A kitchen may be available for retraining and motivation. Transportation is provided, and a noon meal is provided in a cafeteria. Each person is encouraged to participate in group activities and in various crafts. A team approach is used, with the team usually consisting of a physician, nurse, dietitian, psychiatrist, and occupational therapist. The progress of each patient is evaluated, and some of those who become sufficiently independent to maintain themselves at home may leave the program as others are admitted.

Foster Home

Care of the elderly in foster homes has had limited success. The concept that an elderly person will be happier in a home environment and be able to share in family relationships has been difficult to implement in many communities. Disadvantages have centered around the lack of medical care and the fact that the foster home is being operated for profit.

Other Services

The extended-care facility provides short-term, intermediate, and convalescent care. It may be operated as part of a general hospital or as an independent institution. Its function is to provide care after an acute illness until the person is able to return home.

A variety of community outpatient services is available in many communities. These include mental health clinics, physical therapy, dental clinics, speech clinics, and numerous social services.

ETHICAL DILEMMA

You are caring for Mr. Black, an 84-year-old man who was admitted to the intensive care unit (ICU) with a diagnosis of chronic obstructive pulmonary disease (COPD). You overhear a discussion among some of the physicians about making Mr. Black a "No code" because he is so old and his care is costing Medicare (and therefore all of us) a fortune. How would you evaluate this discussion and the physician's reasoning from an ethical perspective?

KEY CONCEPTS

- Senescence, or biologic aging, is a normal process.
- The number of elderly persons is increasing, and one result is the increasing demand on the healthcare system.
- Medicare benefits pay only part of the healthcare costs of the elderly.
- Cultural, ethnic, and socioeconomic factors affect the aging process.
- Retirement is a major transition in an older person's life, and it requires preparation and planning for success.
- Biologic aging is a slow, progressive process that affects all organ systems of the body.
- Mental health in old age involves coping with numerous losses, accepting changes within the body, and staying involved with society.
- Normal aging does not include senility or loss of intelligence.
- Cardiovascular problems are among the most common diseases of the elderly and are associated with the changes of aging and the effects of lifestyle.
- The senses of vision, hearing, touch, taste and smell all tend to decline in old age.
- With aging, the skin becomes thinner, drier, and more prone to injury.
- Changes in the musculoskeletal system increase the older person's risk of falling and injury from falls.
- Changes in the nervous system result in decreased reaction times, slowed reflexes, and diminished pain responses.
- Alzheimer's disease is a slow, progressive, irreversible dementia that requires careful evaluation by a multidisciplinary team of healthcare professionals.
- The changes in the aging digestive system require attention to oral hygiene, a balanced high-fiber diet, and 6 to 8 glasses of fluid per day.
- The kidneys become less efficient with aging. This may affect how older persons metabolize drugs.
- Changes in the respiratory system may place the older person at risk for infection and pneumonia.
- The male and female reproductive systems change with aging, but satisfying sexual relationships are possible in the healthy older adult.
- Goals of nursing care for the elderly person involve maintaining and improving functional ability, maintaining and improving quality of life, helping the older person prepare for death, preventing injury, recognizing individuality, meeting nutritional needs, maintaining personal hygiene, and preventing complications from drug use.
- Caring for the hospitalized elderly person requires careful monitoring of mental status and vital signs.
- Long-term care may be provided in nursing homes, patients' homes, day hospitals, foster homes, or in a variety of community-based settings.

CRITICAL THINKING EXERCISES

1 Today's elderly were born before 1925. Discuss the social, scientific, and political events that have taken place during their lifetimes. How might these events affect their lives and health?

2 Discuss ways of increasing activity for the institutionalized elderly. Consider those who are ambulatory and those who are not.

3 Develop a nursing care plan for the home care of a patient in the second stage of Alzheimer's disease.

REFERENCES AND ADDITIONAL READINGS

Agency for Health Care Policy and Research: *Pressure ulcers in adults; prediction and prevention. Clinical Practice Guideline, Number 3,* Rockville, Md, 1992. US Department of Health and Human Services, AHCPR Publication No 92-0048.

Agency for Health Care Policy and Research: *Urinary incontinence in adults: clinical practice guideline,* Rockville, Md, 1992. US Department of Health and Human Services, AHCPR Publication No 92-0038.

Burnside IM: *Nursing and the aged: a self-care approach,* ed 3, New York, 1988, McGraw-Hill.

Carnevali DL, Patrick M: *Nursing management for the elderly,* ed 2, New York, 1986, JB Lippincott.

Drachman D and others: Alzheimer's disease: diagnosis, *Patient Care* 25(18):13-43, 1991.

Ebersole P, Hess P: *Toward healthy aging: human needs and nursing response,* ed 4, St Louis, 1994, Mosby.

Erikson EH: *Identity and the life cycle: psychologic issues,* New York, 1950, International Universities Press.

Esberger KK, Hughes ST Jr: *Nursing care of the aged,* Norwalk, Conn, 1989, Appleton & Lange.

Ferri R: *Care planning for the older adult,* Philadelphia, 1994, WB Saunders.

Folstein M and others: Mini mental state, *J Psych Res* 12(3): 189-198, 1975.

Fries J, Crapo L: *Vitality and aging,* San Francisco, 1981, W.H. Freeman.

Goodman CE: Osteoporosis and physical activity. *AAOHN J* 35(12):539-542, 1987.

Grossman H, Weiner A: Quality of life: the institutional culture defined by administrative and resident values, *J Appl Gerontol* 7(3):390-405, 1988.

Hamby R, Turnbull J, Clark W, Lancaster N: *Alzheimer's disease: a handbook for caretakers,* St Louis, 1994, Mosby.

Hall GR: Care of the patient with Alzheimer's disease living at home, *Nurs Clin North Am* 23(1):31-46, 1988.

Hewner SJ: Bringing home the health care, *J Gerontol Nurs* 12(2):29-30, 32-35, 1986.

Huey, FL: What teaching nursing homes are teaching us, *Am J Nurs* 85(6):678-683, 1985.

Kane RL, Ouslander JG, Abrass IB: *Essentials of clinical geriatrics,* New York, 1994, McGraw-Hill.

Katz S and others: Studies of illness in the aged. The index of ADL: a standardized measure of biological and psychosocial function, *JAMA* 185(21):914-919, 1963.

Kinsey AC and others: *Sexual behavior in the human male,* Philadelphia, 1948, WB Saunders.

Kinsey AC and others: *Sexual behavior in the human female,* Philadelphia, 1953, WB Saunders.

Kirkpatrick M: A self care model for osteoporosis, *AAOHN J* 35(12):531-535, 1987.

Knapp M: A rose is still a rose, *Geriatric Nurs* 10(6):290-291, 1989.

Lawton HP, Brody EM: Assessment of older people: self-maintaining and instrumental activities of daily living, *Gerontologist* 9(3):179, 1969.

Lin MW, Linn BSW: The rapid disability rating scale-2, *J Am Geriatr Soc* 30(6):378-382, 1982.

Madson S: How to reduce the risk of postmenopausal osteoporosis, *J Gerontol Nurs* 15(9):20-24, 1989.

Mahoney F, Barthel D: Functional evaluation: the Barthel index, *Maryland State Med J* 14:61-65, February 1965.

Masters WH, Johnson VE: *Human sexuality inadequacy,* Boston, 1970, Little Brown.

Matteson MA, McConnell ES: *Gerontological nursing: concepts and practice,* Philadelphia, 1988, WB Saunders Company.

Miller C: *Nursing care of older adults: therapy and practice,* Philadelphia, 1995, JB Lippincott.

Moskowitz E, McCann C: Classification of disability in the chronically ill and aging, *J Chronic Dis* 5:342-346, 1957.

Ouslander J, Osterweil D, Morley J: *Medical care in the nursing home,* New York, 1991, McGraw-Hill.

Parsons CL: Group reminiscence therapy and levels of depression in the elderly, *Nurs Pract* 11(3):68-76, 1986.

Pettigrew D: Investing in mouth care, *Geriatr Nurs* 10(1): 22-24, 1989.

Profile of older Americans: 1990, Washington, DC, 1990. Program resources department, AARP, and Administration on Aging, US Department of Health and Human Services.

Roberts B, Dunkle R, Haug M: Physical, psychological and social resources as moderators of the relationship of stress to mental health in the very old, *J Gerontol* 49(1):535-543, 1994.

Schoenfeld D and others: Self-rated health and mortality in the high-functioning elderly, *J Gerontol* 49(3):109-115, 1994.

Social Security Administration: *Year 2000: a strategic plan*. Baltimore, Md, Jan, 1988. Office of Strategic Planning, Social Security Administration.

Stolley J: When your patient has Alzheimer's disease, *Am J Nurs* 94(8):34-40, 1994.

US Bureau of the Census: *Current population reports*, Washington, DC, March 1991, US Government Printing Office.

Wallace M: Management of sexual relationships among elderly residents in long-term care facilities, *Geriatr Nurs* 13(6): 308-314, 1992.

Webster's medical desk dictionary, Springfield, Mass, 1986, Merriam-Webster.

White JE: Osteoporosis: strategies for prevention, *Nurs Pract* 11(9):36-51, 1986.

Yurick AG and others: *The aged person and the nursing process*, ed 3, Norwalk, Conn, 1989, Appleton & Lange.

Part IV

15 Rehabilitation
16 Long-Term Care
17 Home Healthcare
18 Care of the Surgical Patient
19 Emergency and Trauma Care

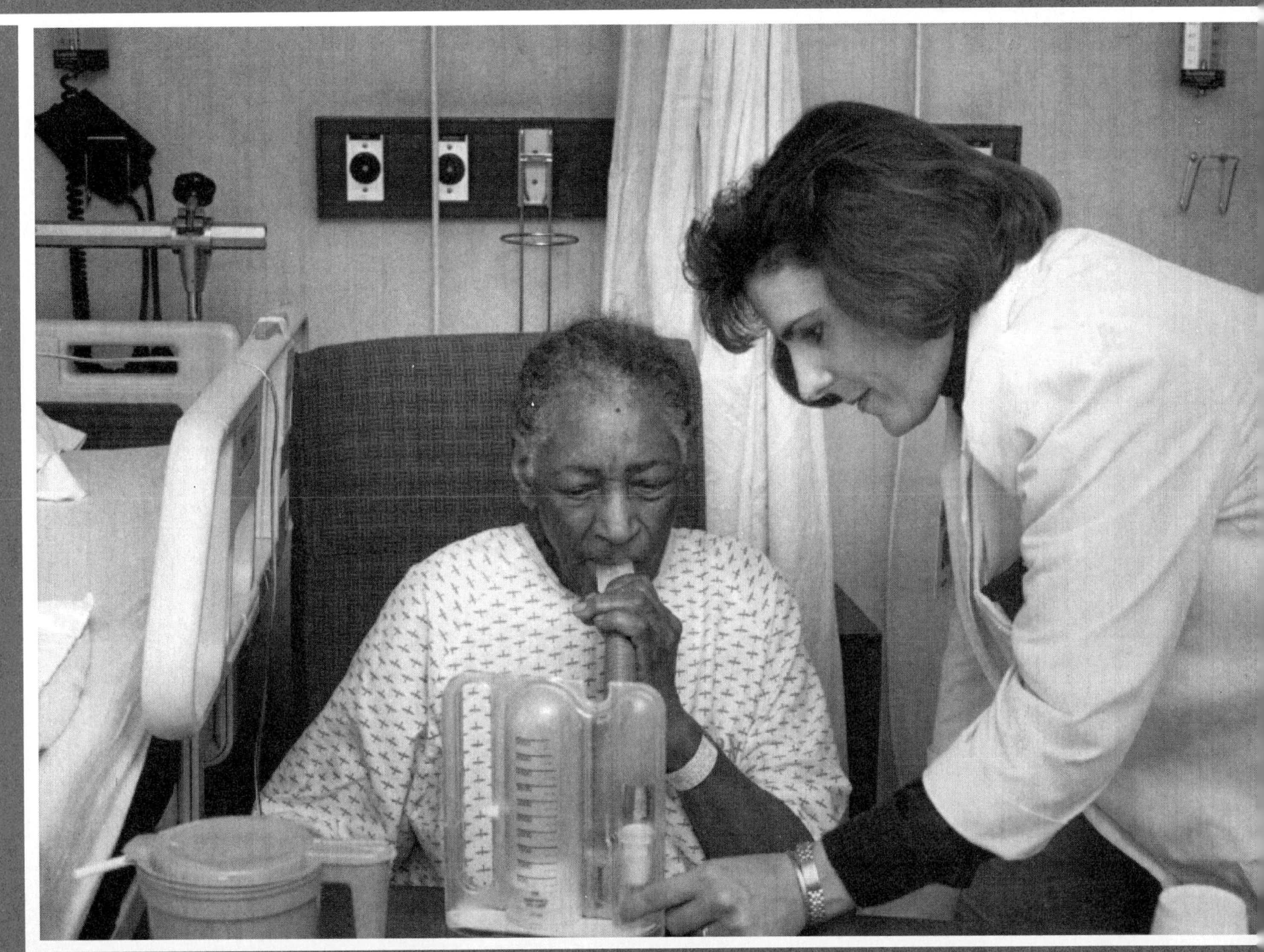

SPECIAL CARE SETTINGS

CHAPTER 15

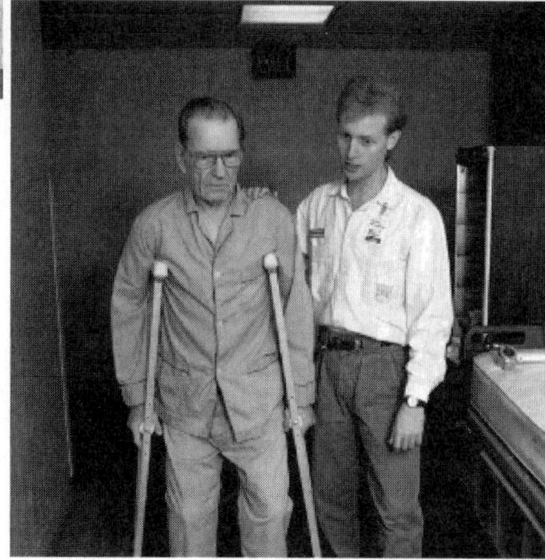

Rehabilitation

CHAPTER OBJECTIVES

1 Identify the goals of rehabilitation.
2 Describe the application of rehabilitation principles to the practice of nursing.
3 Define disability and theoretical models of disability.
4 Discuss the concept of a rehabilitation team, its members, and their roles.
5 Identify types of facilities and agencies that provide rehabilitation services.
6 Discuss the rehabilitative aspects of each phase of patient care: primary, secondary, and tertiary.
7 Identify the emotional responses to disability and discuss related nursing interventions.
8 Identify nursing activities that promote mobility and movement: range-of-joint motion, positioning, transfers, and participation in self-care.
9 Discuss nursing interventions for incontinence, skin breakdown, and impaired swallowing.
10 Discuss the role of the rehabilitation nurse as a motivator and teacher.
11 Discuss the use of prostheses, braces, and crutches.
12 Give examples of assistive and adaptive devices for disabled persons.

KEY WORDS

activities of daily living (ADLs)
adaptation
body image
braces
continuity
contracture
crutches
disability
dysphagia
functional assessment
functional limitation
impairment
motivation
prosthesis
range-of-motion
rehabilitation
rehabilitation nursing

The concept of **rehabilitation** is a fundamental process in providing total patient care. Many definitions and interpretations of rehabilitation exist, but all share a common meaning. Basically, rehabilitation is the process of assisting individuals with disability or chronic illness in recovering to the highest possible level of independence and well-being. The need for rehabilitation occurs when a person's previous way of life is changed by illness or injury. Depending on the type of disability, the physical, mental, vocational, social, and economic aspects of a person's life may be altered. Some disabling events may be minor and the need for rehabilitation limited. Others may require extensive rehabilitation that involves many facets of a person's life (Box 15-1).

An important concept of rehabilitation is that individuals be restored to the fullest ability of which they are capable in all areas. The rehabilitation process helps the individual to live the most productive life possible. Instead of the classic emphasis on disease, diagnosis, and therapeutic procedure, rehabilitation stresses restoration of normal function, prevention of complications, education of patient and family, and adaptation.

Adaptation is the process of adjusting to life changes that occur with disability. Adapting to the changes imposed by illness or injury may be difficult for some patients and seem relatively stress-free for others. Patients need to make some degree of adaptation, or rehabilitation will be incomplete or unsuccessful. The personal styles of indivdiduals adapting to disability are wide-ranging. Some patients may respond with anger and rage, while others use humor to cope with the changes in their lives. Some disabled individuals may totally deny their experience while still participating in an active rehabilitation program.

BOX 15-1

FOCUS OF REHABILITATION

- Physical
- Emotional
- Social
- Educational
- Vocational

DEFINITION OF DISABILITY

There are a variety of terms used to describe individuals who have lost independent functioning. It is important to be clear about these terms because of the stigma often associated with such terms as *handicapped* or *crippled*. Over the past 25 years conceptual models of disability have been developed that help to define these terms. The two main theorists of disability models are Saad Nagi and Philip Wood (Kelly-Hayes, 1995).

Nagi describes three potential consequences of pathology or disease: an **impairment** or physiologic alteration; **functional limitations,** which are limitations in the ability to perform activities such as walking and dressing; and **disability,** which is a limitation in the ability to perform social roles and activities such as work, family life, and independent living (Nagi, 1965).

Philip Wood continued the work of Nagi and developed a model that included the concept of a handicap

CASE STUDY

Mr. Jones is a 35-year-old married father of five. One day while at work he was driving his pickup truck along a rain-slicked expressway when, without warning, a large truck crossed the highway and crashed into his vehicle. Mr. Jones was rushed by ambulance to the hospital, where his condition was considered serious. Both of his legs were so badly injured that above-knee amputations were necessary. Soon thereafter, Mr. Jones was admitted to a rehabilitation hospital. After being evaluated by the nursing, therapy, social service, and medical staff, Mr. Jones' rehabilitation began. He participated in therapy, was fitted with artificial limbs, and learned how to walk with them. He and his family were taught about care of his amputation sites and care of the prostheses. They also had the opportunity to discuss how the accident affected their lives and their expectations for the future. Plans were made for Mr. Jones to train for a new kind of work. He is now at home and in an outpatient rehabilitation program. He is anxious to progress with his rehabilitation. At times he is fearful and sad, yet ready to proceed with his training. He is looking forward to complete independence and being able to care for his family.

for The World Health Organization International Classification of Impairments, Disabilities, and Handicaps. A handicap was described as a disadvantage for a given individual, resulting from an impairment or disability, that limits or prevents the fulfillment of a role that is normal for that individual (World Health Organization, 1980). Handicap in this model is similar to Nagi's use of the term *disability*. However, because of the stigma associated with the term *handicap*, the Nagi model is the one most often utilized by rehabilitation professionals, and the term *handicap* is discouraged.

The Americans with Disabilities Act (ADA) definition of disability requires an individual to meet at least one of three criteria. An individual must (1) have a physical or mental impairment that substantially limits one or more major life activities; (2) have a record of such an impairment; or (3) be regarded as having such an impairment. The ADA goes on to define *physical* or *mental impairment* as the following:

- Any physiologic disorder or condition, cosmetic disfigurement, or anatomic loss affecting one or more of the body systems
- Any mental or psychologic disorder, such as mental retardation, organic brain syndrome, or emotional or mental illness
- A specific learning disability (Americans with Disability Act, 1992).

REHABILITATION NURSING

Rehabilitation may be viewed as an underlying theme of all nursing care. Regardless of the care setting—acute-care hospital, long-term care facility, rehabilitation facility, or the community—nurses use patient-care practices and techniques that aim at restoration of function and prevention of complications. These approaches form some of the basic tenets of nursing practice. For example, the nurse caring for the bed-bound patient uses methods to position the patient in bed and provide movement and exercise to prevent skin breakdown, respiratory complications, and joint deformity. As the patient improves, the nurse uses a range of techniques. Methods to improve mobility through transfer training, strengthening exercises, and ambulation are planned in coordination with the physical therapist. Improved ability of the patient to participate in **activities of daily living (ADLs)** such as bathing, grooming, dressing, feeding, walking, and toileting are emphasized. And, if needed, methods to assess and correct such problems as poor nutritional intake and incontinence, are utilized.

Although principles of rehabilitation are integral to all nursing practice, **rehabilitation nursing** is viewed as a specialty within nursing. In 1988, the Association of Rehabilitation Nurses in cooperation with the American Nurses Association defined rehabilitation nursing and stated its goals as follows:

> Rehabilitation nursing is a specialty practice area within the scope of professional nursing practice. Rehabilitation nursing is the diagnosis and treatment of human responses of individuals and groups to actual or potential health problems stemming from altered functional ability and altered lifestyle. The goal of rehabilitation nursing is to assist the individual with disability and chronic illness in the restoration and maintenance of maximal health. The rehabilitation nurse should be skilled at treating alterations in functional ability and lifestyle resulting from physical disability and chronic illness (American Nurses Association and Association of Rehabilitation Nurses, 1988, p.4).

Rehabilitation nurses care for patients with a wide range of disabling conditions such as stroke, spinal cord injury, brain injury, amputation, cancer, congenital deficits, and problems of addiction. In addition to providing nursing care that is based on the rehabilitation philosophy of maximizing function and preventing complications, rehabilitation nurses understand the impact of these conditions on the patient and are knowledgeable about specific nursing interventions that these patients need. For example, in caring for the person with a brain injury, the nurse must have the ability to assess behavioral and communication problems occurring as a result of the injury. In caring for the person with a spinal cord injury, the nurse needs to develop specialized approaches to bowel and bladder care.

In this chapter some of the basic techniques of rehabilitation nursing are described. For a more detailed description of rehabilitation nursing care of patients with specific disabilities, the nurse should consult a rehabilitation nursing textbook (Dittmar, 1989; Hoeman, 1995).

REHABILITATION IN EACH PHASE OF HEALTHCARE

Healthcare may be divided into three phases or stages: *primary health care* refers to preventive efforts, *secondary health care* deals with the period of acute illness, and *tertiary health care* involves recovery and rehabilitation from illness or accident. Rehabilitation philosophy and practices are part of all aspects of healthcare and are integral to each phase of nursing care.

Primary Healthcare

In the primary phase of healthcare, emphasis is placed on *prevention* of disease and accidents. One aspect is the protection of all susceptible individuals against diseases for which immunizing agents are available. The crippling conditions of poliomyelitis have been nearly eliminated by the administration of the polio vaccine. Another aspect involves early assessment and education about chronic conditions to decrease long-term disability. Hypertension, when detected early, can be managed through a variety of approaches including dietary management, smoking cessation, exercise, meditation, and, when needed, medications. If carefully managed, the long-term risks associated with hypertension—heart disease, renal disease, and stroke—can be reduced. Another focus is injury prevention. Methods to promote safety in the workplace, enhanced driving safety through reduced speed and use of seat belts, and reduction of pollutants in the environment are examples of these preventive health practices. Nurses working in primary care and in all other healthcare settings have the opportunity to educate individuals and groups in many preventive health practices. These include the importance of regular health and dental evaluation, well-balanced nutrition, exercise, smoking cessation, approaches to management of chronic disease, and appropriate use of therapeutics, including medications. The goal of these practices is to keep the individual at a maximum level of health and well-being. From this perspective, these practices can be said to be rehabilitative in focus.

Secondary Healthcare

Rehabilitation nursing concepts are essential aspects in caring for acutely ill patients. During the patient's acute-care hospital stay, the nurse must recognize the potential impact of illness and disability on physical function and emotional state. With ongoing nursing assessment, the extent of the patients' functional limitation—limitation in the ability to care for themselves, level of mobility, and continence status—can be determined and interventions planned to support and maintain recovery of these functions. Even at the earliest stages of illness and disability, the nurse and patient should establish realistic short- and long-term goals that reflect the patient's potential for participation in a rehabilitation program. The nurse should use these goals to plan daily care.

By planning with the physician and other members of the healthcare team, the nurse helps the patient to participate in a program of increased activity. The nurse needs to continually assess the effects of this increased activity on the patient. For the elderly, fatigue may have a greater impact on recovery and increased activity than it does for younger patients. As a result, activity tolerance must be carefully assessed in an acutely ill older person. Measuring vital signs; observing respiratory and skin color changes during activity; and determining endurance for participation in sitting, transferring, and walking are a few of these assessment parameters (Mol, Baker, 1991).

Of great importance during this time is the prevention of *secondary complications* such as pressure sores or contracture formations that may occur as a result of the patient's immobility and altered physical status. The goal is to keep the patient as mobile and well-nourished as possible. Maintaining body alignment, providing range-of-motion exercises, preventing excessive pressure against the patient's skin, and getting the patient out of bed and mobile as soon as possible will help reduce the incidence of secondary problems.

Tertiary Healthcare

Tertiary healthcare is provided outside the acute-care hospital. The period of recovery is one of convalescence, which is a gradual process that may extend over a considerable period and may be punctuated with one or more relapses.

Rehabilitation practices should be part of all nursing care, whether the illness is acute or chronic, temporary or permanent, disabling or nondisabling. However, as soon as the acute phase of illness has passed, a careful evaluation of the patient's need for continued care should be made. If needed, an appropriate rehabilitation setting should be identified. Rehabilitation programs are based in a variety of settings—within acute-care hospitals, in free-standing facilities, within long-term care facilities, and in the community. Centers are operated by for-profit and not-for-profit organizations, state vocational agencies, insurance companies, private agencies, and a variety of community agencies. The selection of setting depends on the severity of the patient's disability, the limitations on his or her ability to care for himself or herself, and the potential for some level of recovery.

Of particular importance during the transition period between acute hospital care and teritary setting is communication between acute hospital and rehabilitation staff. A copy of the acute hospital record and clearly written and detailed referral information are necessary for the patient's smooth transition into the new setting. Nursing data are essential components of this information and should include the patient's level of independence, nutrition, sleep patterns, continence, and medication regimen, as well as specific nursing interventions that are needed. This information is necessary to the nurses in the new setting to safely begin care of the patient.

A patient in need of an intense, comprehensive rehabilitation program may be admitted to an inpatient rehabilitation unit within an acute-care hospital or to an inpatient free-standing rehabilitation hospital. These programs tend to provide a multitude of comprehensive services. In addition, they require the patient to be able to participate in an active rehabilitation program, which usually includes 2 or 3 hours of therapy each day. This requires a number of things of the patient. He or she must be able to comprehend the instructions and teachings that are part of the therapy. The patient must also have the endurance to be out of bed sitting for at least 1 hour at a time and have no medical problems that would be contraindicated by the level of physical activity (Box 15-2). Following assessment by members of the interdisciplinary team, the team, the patient, and the family are involved in setting goals and planning for discharge.

Rehabilitation programs are also offered in skilled-nursing facilities. Some of these programs are as comprehensive as inpatient programs, whereas others are less intense. Often these programs are designed for the more elderly, frail patient. Rehabilitation of the aged and chronically ill can be a long process. The short-term and long-term goals have to be adjusted to fit the individual's potential. It may take longer for an older person to attain certain skills. Fatigue and decreased endurance and stamina may be more of a factor for an older person than for a younger one. Dependency and low self-esteem may cause the aged person to reject participation in rehabilitation (Hesse, Campion, 1983). However, recent studies have documented the impact of exercise and increased activity on strength and endurance in the elderly. (Fiatarone and others, 1994; Fiatarone, 1993; Lowman, Klinger, 1969)

More recently, rehabilitation programs that are provided in the patient's home have been developed. A full range of services are available and provided on a regular basis. Staff have the benefit of observing the patient in the home setting and may be able to better determine what is needed for independence in that setting. Also, a patient's desire to be in the home and out of the hospital makes rehabilitation efforts more successful in the home setting. Safety factors such as fall prevention are important considerations in this type of program (Box 15-3). For home rehabilitation to be effective, there needs to be sufficient support of family and friends. Home rehabilitation programs lack the shared experience with other patients and families with similar disabilities that is a benefit of inpatient programs.

Some patients are able to obtain rehabilitation services in an outpatient setting. Patients who participate in this type of program are usually more independent and need the services of fewer rehabilitation profes-

BOX 15-2

CRITERIA FOR PATIENT ADMISSION TO INPATIENT REHABILITATION

- Sufficient endurance to tolerate 2 to 3 hours of therapy each day
- Ability to comprehend instruction and teaching
- No medical problems that would contraindicate the level of physical activity required

NURSE ALERT

Rehabilitation programs require a team of experts from many areas according to the restorative needs of the patient.

BOX 15-3 **Guidelines for Care of Patients At Risk of Falling**

Patients at risk of falling may demonstrate some of the following characteristics:

- Altered mobility; difficulty with transfers; problems with sitting, standing, and balance; and decreased coordination
- Altered self-care ability
- Cognitive changes resulting in confusion and disorientation
- Perceptual deficits, which alter spatial appreciation and comprehension
- Elimination problems, which may cause the patient to try to get out of bed or a chair without assistance; urine on the floor, which may lead to slips and falls
- Communication problems, which prevent the patient from being able to explain needs

Interventions to reduce the incidence of patient falls include the following:

- Identification of the patient at risk
- Development of unit-based programs to prevent slips and falls
- Interdisciplinary collaborative approach to prevent falls
- Patient and family education
- Technologic approaches to fall prevention (e.g., specialized seat cushions and alarm systems)

sionals. Having necessary transportation and the support of family and friends are important aspects of participation in outpatient rehabilitation services.

For some disabled or chronically ill individuals, full participation in the level of activity that a rehabilitation program requires may be diminished by physical, cognitive, and emotional limitations. It may not be possible to restore all patients to the level of independence they desire; severe disability may limit the potential for total independence. Options for living situations may be limited by care requirements, financial constraints, and lack of family support. When this occurs, the continued guidance and support of the interdisciplinary team is needed. The services of the entire team are needed to identify approaches in finding a supportive and safe environment for the patient in the community or in a long-term care facility.

If a patient becmes acutely ill while participating in a rehabilitation program, returning the patient to the acute-care hospital may be necessary. Most inpatient rehabilitation programs, skilled-nursing facilities, and home services do not have the diagnostic and treatment capabilities of the acute-care hospital. Acute cardiac, respiratory, and infectious processes need to be treated in the acute-care hospital. If the acute illness is protracted, the disabled person may lose the gains made in a rehabilitation program. Communication among referring agencies is particularly important in attempting to maintain those gains.

THE REHABILITATION TEAM

Any comprehensive program in rehabilitation requires a group of experts in various areas of restorative care because no single profession can provide all the necessary services. This group, or interdisciplinary team, meets regularly to establish patient goals, evaluate progress, and revise the treatment plan (Figure 15-1). In the more comprehensive rehabilitation programs, a full spectrum of rehabilitation professionals may be available; whereas in the less intense programs, there may be limited rehabilitation staff.

Patient

The most important member of the rehabilitation team is the patient. Success in a rehabilitation program can only occur if the patient has an understanding of his or her disability, is involved in setting goals, and participates in the plan of care. Because of the stress of adapting to all the life changes imposed by the disability, the patient may have lost motivation for this level of participation. Involvement of family and significant others is often pivotal in helping the patient become motivated. Family and friends often can provide the impetus for participation that the patient is unable to find on his or her own. Meetings with the patient, family, and members of the team provide the information necessary for a more successful outcome. Such meetings should occur during the early part of the program to aid the patient in adjustment, then on a regular basis and in preparation for discharge.

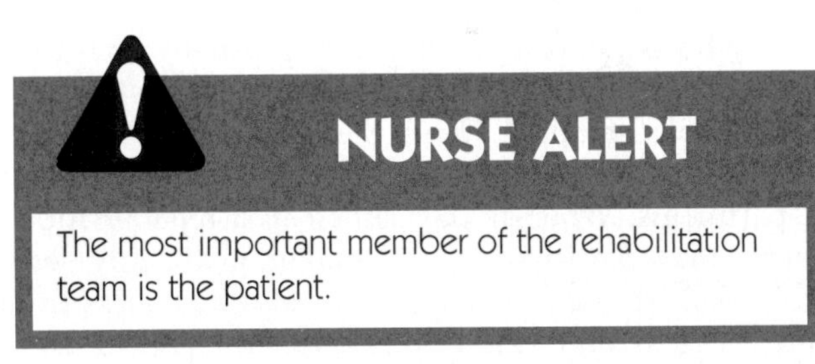

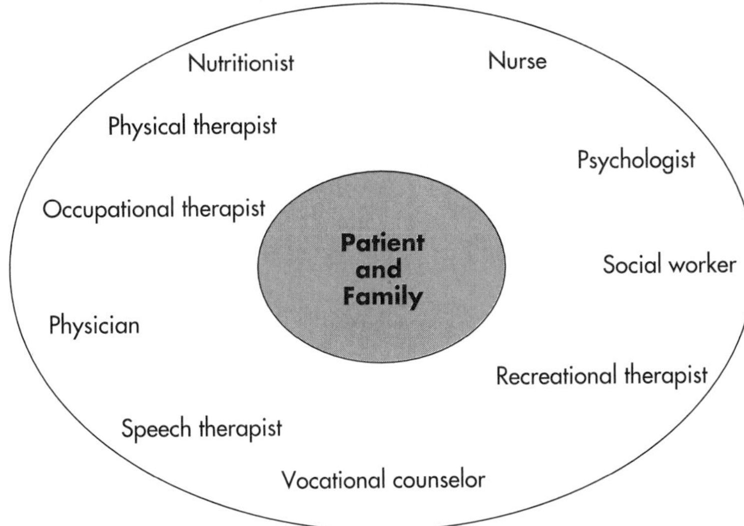

Figure 15-1 The interdisciplinary team.

Nurse

The role of the nurse in a rehabilitation setting is diverse. Nurses function as caregivers, teachers, coordinators, evaluators, and facilitators for patients and family members. The nursing staff spends the most time with the patient, being present 24 hours a day. This affords the opportunity for nurses to observe, assess, teach, reinforce, and evaluate the effects of the total rehabilitation program. Nurses use assessment criteria to determine the patient's level of disability, stage of adaptation and adjustment, and learning needs. Nursing care is based on these findings. In some settings, the nurse coordinates the interdisciplinary team meetings. The nurse, as well as other members of the team, contribute pertinent information that provides a clear picture of the patient's progress. Assessment and documentation of patient progress are important aspects of rehabilitation.

Outside of established rehabilitation programs, the team may consist of physician, nurse, patient, and family. The nurse who has a basic understanding of rehabilitation and whose philosophy includes the whole patient is key within the team approach. In the acute-care setting, it is often the responsibility of the nurse to plan and coordinate the patient's rehabilitation program and initiate early interventions. When caring for patients in extended-care facilities, it is usually the nurse who helps the patient perform activities or exercises prescribed by physical therapists. The patient who is cared for at home may benefit from the services of a physical therapist, speech therapist, or occupational therapist. These therapists may be provided either through private agencies or public health departments. Whereas the patient in a rehabilitation center may participate in rehabilitation therapy sessions daily, those at home may receive visits less frequently. It is often the community-based nurse's responsibility to supervise and conduct therapy as prescribed by each therapist and to report the patient's progress.

Physician

The physician member of the team may be a psychiatrist trained in physical rehabilitation. However, in some settings, the physician may be a member of another medical specialty such as neurology, orthopedics, oncology, cardiology, medicine, or pediatrics. Physicians trained in these areas who choose to practice in a rehabilitation setting often have a special interest in this phase of care. The physician assesses the medical status of the patient and prescribes various evaluative procedures, medications, consultations, and therapies as needed and provides important information about the patient's status to other members of the team, the patient, and the family.

Occupational Therapist

The occupational therapist (OT) evaluates the impact of the disability on the patient's physical and cognitive abilities in a variety of domains. An occupational therapist assesses (1) the patient's ability to perform a variety of ADLs such as bathing, dressing, and eating; (2) the patient's cognitive ability to perceive and understand the environment in order to function in a safe and meaningful way; and (3) movement problems. With the nurse, physician, and speech therapist, the OT may assist with the evaluation and treatment of chewing and swallowing problems. An OT's treatment approach may include exercise regimens; modalities such as heat, cold, or vibration; and craft activities to strengthen muscles and improve coordination and balance. Methods to improve concentration and the prescription of assistance devices such as splints, adapted eating utensils, and dressing aids may also be included. The OT may also be involved in patient driving evaluations and return-to-work planning.

Physical Therapist

The physical therapist (PT) deals with problems of mobility, muscle strength, and exercise. After an initial assessment of such functions as muscle strength and tone, joint range of motion, sitting and standing balance, gait, stability of gait, and endurance, the therapist implements exercises and therapeutic techniques. Ongoing assessment and evaluation are reported to the interdisciplinary team, together with specific approaches that work well for the patient. The PT also implements prescriptions for splints, braces, prostheses, and wheelchairs, and is an excellent resource for the nurse when problems arise with this equipment.

Social Worker

The social worker addresses the stresses of adapting to the disability experienced by the patient, family, and friends. The problems of family relationships, housing, finances, and transportation are concerns of the social worker as well. This team member is often the link between the institution and the community, assisting the patient and family in solving the problems of transition, the need for placement in another setting, or the need for home supports.

Speech Therapist

Patients who have experienced brain damage from conditions such as stroke, brain injury, tumor, and progressive neurologic disease may develop problems with language and communication. The speech therapist assesses patients with communication deficits and develops therapeutic interventions to return as much communication ability as possible. The speech therapist works with other members of the team and the family to identify the best approach to communication with the patient. The speech therapist may also assist with the evaluation and treatment of the patient with swallowing problems.

Psychologist

Emotional problems are bound to occur in a crisis situation such as sudden disability. Disruptions of lifestyle, family structure, and body image may result in profound psychologic stress. The psychologist may use specific testing as well as interviews with the patient and family to identify problems. In addition the psychologist works with the patient and family in developing coping mechanisms and approaches for adjusting to the disability. Advising other team members on how to deal with patients undergoing emotional distress is an important role of the psychologist.

Recreational Therapist

Recreation and play are as important to patient care as physical and emotional support. The recreational therapist assesses interests and provides for involvement in games, sports, hobbies, music, and other forms of diversion. Structured programs within the institution are implemented to meet patient needs. Trips outside the facility to movies, shops, restaurants, and plays, as well as other activities, assist the individual in applying some adaptation skills learned in the rehabilitation process.

Vocational Counselor

The vocational counselor or therapist assesses the patient's job skills, educational needs, interests, and motivation. If the disability results in the need to change occupation, the vocational therapist counsels the patient about opportunities and arrangements for return to work.

Other Team Members

Often the rehabilitation team includes a dietitian, an orthopedist, a dentist, a teacher, the clergy, and members of other professions, depending on the type of disability.

The Work of the Interdisciplinary Team

The interdisciplinary team approach to patient care is an important concept of rehabilitation (Figure 15-2). The expertise of many professionals often is needed to care for a disabled person, and the team approach is a method to coordinate this care. On admission to a rehabilitation program, a patient is assessed by each member of the team, and plans of care are developed. The interdisciplinary team meets on a regular basis to discuss patients being cared for by that team. Newly admitted patients are discussed. The team shares assessment data; defines short- and long-term goals; outlines interventions; and identifies emotional, social, and educational needs. For patients already enrolled in the program, the team discusses progress toward goals, adaptation to disability, and discharge planning.

Soon after admission, members of the interdisciplinary team may meet with the patient and family to discuss the rehabilitation plan, expected length of stay, discharge plan, and need for follow-up care. The team also addresses any concerns of the patient and family. These meetings may be held at additional times during the patient's stay and in preparation for discharge (Glennon, Smith, 1990).

REHABILITATION LEGISLATION

An increase in personal disabilities as a result of World War II emphasized the need to establish programs and centers for rehabilitation treatment. Over the past 40 years there has been a rapid growth in such programs. During this same period, federal legislation affecting services to disabled persons was established.

In 1954 the Vocational Rehabilitation Act was passed by the U.S. Congress. This law provided funds to state agencies for improvement and expansion of rehabilitation services. The act was updated in 1973 and amended in 1978 to include a comprehensive definition of independent living as well as an improved de-

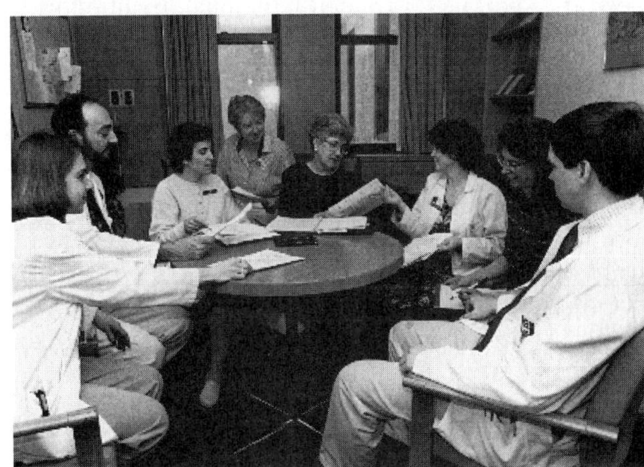

Figure 15-2 Rehabilitation team participating in interdisciplinary team conference. (Courtesy Beth Israel Hospital, Boston.)

finition of funding for disabled persons. The amendment mandated that any institution receiving federal funds must make its facilities open and accessible to the disabled. This included not only government buildings, but institutions of higher learning, medical facilities, public schools, national parks and recreation areas, as well as local programs funded by the federal government.

In July 1990 Congress passed the American with Disabilities Act, Public Law 101-336. This law was passed to provide uniform protection against discrimination for the disabled throughout the United States. This law prohibits discrimination on the basis of disability in employment, activities of state and local governments, public and private transportation, and telecommunications. It is much broader than the Rehabilitation Act of 1973. The law requires that all persons with disabilities be allowed to participate in all services and programs in an integrated way. As an example, in the past, public school systems operated special classes for children with disabilities, and there were schools established for children with specific disabilities. With the passage of this act, public schools are now mandated to integrate children with disabilities into the regular classroom (Americans with Disability Act, 1992).

The primary objective of the Social and Rehabilitation Service (formerly called the Vocational Rehabilitation Department) is the education and training of persons for employment. Many disabled persons, through participation in rehabilitation, can become employed and economically independent and self-sufficient. The services under the Social and Rehabilitation Service have been expanded to cover many more types of disabilities. The developmental disabilities program now extends services to persons afflicted by mental retardation, cerebral palsy, convulsive disorders, and other neurologic disorders. A problem has been the shortage of trained personnel. In an effort to overcome this problem, the Social and Rehabilitation Service has provided grants to universities and certain institutions to train individuals in vocational rehabilitation. Medicare, administered by the Social Security Administration, now includes rehabilitative services for both hospitalized patients and those recuperating elsewhere. The Veterans Administration provides rehabilitation services for veterans.

Other areas of concern are being discussed at both the local and federal levels, such as chronic alcoholism and drug addition. Centers, public and private, are available to treat and rehabilitate addicted persons. Also, federal and state governments are developing programs for research in mental retardation and mental illness. It is not only important to learn more about the causes of these conditions, but also to learn how many individuals with these conditions can be rehabilitated to lead productive lives in the community.

Physical, psychologic, and developmental disabilities are not the only areas in which rehabilitative services are needed. There is a growing awareness of other factors that can lead to disability in our society: poverty, health problems of the poor (migrant workers, the poor elderly, etc.), violent crime, and the lack of supports for women and children. Some rehabilitative efforts are being made in these areas, but much remains to be done.

EMOTIONAL RESPONSE TO DISABILITY

A disabling event often creates a period of crisis for the patient. With loss of body function, loss of ability to work, or loss of ability to function independently, feelings of self-worth may be changed for a limited period or for a long time. The individual's **body image,** or personal view of his or her body, may undergo significant changes. The person with a new disability may gradually realize that he or she is different and that life will probably be changed forever. The individual may wonder how family, friends, and colleagues will accept him or her. Fear, worry, anxiety, and apprehension are increased. The person may enter a period of shock and dismay. Discouragement and depression are common during this early time.

Many factors can influence a person's ability to cope with a disabling event. Some of these include age, type and severity of disability, and the meaning of the loss to the person. The age at onset of disability and the needs at certain periods of life may have an impact on how well the person copes. As an example, a person born with a physical disability may adjust to the limitations in life but experience difficulty at certain times. Adolescence may be such a time. The adolescent goal of independence from family may be limited by physical care needs. The disabled adolescent may refuse to participate in long-established care routines as a form of seeking independence. Another example of the impact of age on the reaction to disability may be seen in the elderly disabled person. He or she may experience difficulty in accepting the rationale for participation in the difficult work of recovery, feeling that he or she is just "too old" for such an effort.

The person who becomes disabled from a traumatic event may experience an acute emotional reaction to the loss and changes that occur. The reaction may be severe enough to limit the person's participation in rehabilitation. Individuals with chronic progressive disease may adapt to the gradual changes in function but may experience emotional distress if acute medical problems require hospitalization or when supports cannot meet their needs. When patients with chronic progressive disease reach a point in the course of their disease when independent living is no longer possible, the need for placement in an extended-care facility may create great distress.

The meaning of a loss of function will vary with every person. Loss of an arm may affect a professional pianist or carpenter more severely than a school teacher or chemist. Much depends on how the loss affects the patient's everyday life. Personality problems that develop after a disability may occur as a result of the patient's personality before the injury. A person who could easily be made to feel inadequate before the injury may have these feelings compounded by the emotional stress of the injury.

The initial reaction to a physical injury may be *shock.* The patient experiences disbelief, anxiety, and fear, which are considered part of the mourning process. *Loss* of anything that is meaningful to the patient may produce a period of grief (Strauss, Glaser 1984; Werner-Beland, 1980). The patient may be unable to face the change, attempting to deny its existence. Gradually the patient will begin to talk about the change, and nurses are often the first to be questioned about the disability. The patient may ask to see the disabled part and may seem both fascinated and revolted.

During this stage of adjustment, depression and anger may be present. Eventually the patient may realize that life cannot be as it was before and will begin to examine the values placed on conventional "normality." He or she may realize that the disability need not alter his or her entire life and may begin to react more openly with others. Time is essential for this process of adaptation and adjustment. Similar reactions occur with patients facing surgery or progressively deteriorating diseases. The surgical patient usually has time to adapt before surgery. Patients with chronic illnesses have to adjust to each stage of their illness.

An initial nursing assessment of the patient's and family's coping abilities is important. A psychosocial history obtained on admission and updated over time will help the nurse plan therapeutic interventions geared to the specific patient and family.

Motivation

Motivation is an important aspect of rehabilitation. In order for a disabled person to gain independence, he or she must possess the desire to participate in the difficult work of recovery. Motivation is the force, the desire, and the drive necessary for this participation. The work of rehabilitation is not only physically demanding, but it is also emotionally and spiritually stressful. Nurses are with the patient 24 hours each day, and therapy treatments are often long. During the length of hospitalization that some disabilities require, the nurses, therapists, patients, and family members often develop strong relationships that are a vital part of rehabilitation. Nurses and therapists can use their relationships with patients to help patients create a desire for self-sufficiency and independence (Banja, 1990). Emphasizing capabilities and improvements can be of great value at a time when patients are discouraged and lacking in self-confidence (Learman and others, 1990).

ETHICAL DILEMMA

Daniel P. is a paraplegic as a result of an automobile accident. The members of the healthcare team believe they have accomplished all they can for him in the acute care setting and are ready to move him to the rehabilitation unit. However, Daniel says, "No way. My life is ruined anyway, and I just want to get out of here. Leave me alone."

Analyze the ethical issues present in this case.

Patients may experience periods of regression as they move toward independence. When patients are unsuccessful in efforts at learning new skills or tasks, they may think "What's the use?" Frustration and depression may result. It is then that the nurse's gentle reminder of what has been accomplished—no matter how small—and encouragement to talk about frustrations and fears can be of great value. Acknowledging that rehabilitation is hard work expresses compassion to the patient.

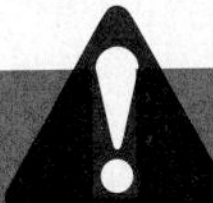

NURSE ALERT

Motivation is the force, the desire, and the drive to participate in the difficult work of recovery.

Some patients may receive maximum benefit from rehabilitation but only achieve partial recovery. An understanding approach to these patients is extremely important because they may be resentful, angry, and depressed. Conveying acceptance, along with a positive attitude stressing what the patient can do, may help eliminate the feeling of rejection and antagonism.

The nurse who is constantly alert to the patient's emotional stress and pain and who encourages the expression of feelings may help relieve some of the pressure the patient feels. Stress may become so great that the patient is unable to find the energy to participate in rehabilitation. In this case, the entire interdisciplinary team must discuss how to assist the patient through this period. Psychiatric counseling is often beneficial to the patient to identify ways of coping and adapting. Group counseling consisting of patients with similar disabilities and group leaders (e.g., psychiatric therapists, social workers, nurses, and occupational or physical therapists) can be very helpful. Some patients may need the assistance of psychotropic medications to deal with the depression and hopelessness they feel as a result of their illnesses and disabilities.

The Patient's Family

A family's response to a patient's illness and loss of function is based on many factors. The relationships of the individuals involved, methods of family coping, role of the patient in the family, and economic issues may all have an impact. During the acute phase of care, the family will suffer from anxiety, apprehension, and fear. The family should be given emotional support, comfort, and all the information possible during this critical period. If the patient is the primary wage earner, the spouse may be distressed about how medical and hospital bills will be paid or how to provide for the family. A serious disability may mean social isolation for the family, as well as for the patient. This isolation may lead to loneliness and depression. As soon as a prognosis can be made, long-term goals should be established for the patient. The family should be given information about sources of help in rehabilitation and economic assistance. A social worker may help the family with plans, but if a social worker is unavailable, nurses should be familiar with appropriate community agencies and organizations. Specific support groups are available for families of disabled persons. For example, the National Head Injury Foundation* provides information, education, resources, and peer support for patients and their families.

When considering the total patient and the family, the area of sexuality must be addressed. To discuss this with patients, nurses need an understanding of their own feelings about sexuality and be knowledgeable about the effects of disability on sexual function. The patient may be hesitant to ask questions or bring up the subject of sex, but if the nurse lets it be known that it is an appropriate topic, the patient may discuss it. Experts in this field, often disabled persons themselves, are available for referral, and literature is available in nursing journals, from rehabilitation hospitals, and from state rehabilitation departments.

If the nurse feels unqualified or uncomfortable with the topic of sexuality, the patient should be told that it is an appropriate topic to raise but that another team member could better address these concerns. In a rehabilitation setting, there is often a team member who is an expert in the area of sexuality and sexual counseling who can assist the patient or help others on the team counsel the patient. In other settings, the sexual concerns of patients are not always discussed. Across the country, there are many training programs to help health professionals become more knowledgeable in this important area of health.

*National Head Injury Foundation, 33 Turnpike Road, Southborough, MA 01772

NURSING APPROACHES TO REHABILITATION CARE

The nurse, as a member of the rehabilitation team, must assume a share of the responsibility for guiding the disabled patient toward health and independence. In some situations, the nurse will work with the physician without the services of other persons who contribute to a comprehensive rehabilitation program. Therefore it is increasingly important for the nurse to be familiar with the local and state agencies that can provide rehabilitation services, as well as agencies, societies, and foundations that provide educational materials and information about specific disabilities.

Assessment

Nursing care begins with an assessment of the patient. During the initial assessment the nurse should gather information about the patient to establish goals of care and plan interventions. Many institutions and agencies have established admission nursing assessment guidelines. Ongoing assessment occurs with every interaction between the nurse and patient. In the rehabilitation setting, there is usually an interdisciplinary approach to assessment, and there are a variety of assessment tools available to document patient status. Some of the tools specific to rehabilitation measure functional status or the patient's ability to perform basic ADLs, while others measure more complex activities such as shopping and money management or emotional state or quality of life. A **functional assessment** determines physical functional status, documents the need for interventions, aids in planning treatment, and helps measure progress (Kelly-Hayes, 1995).

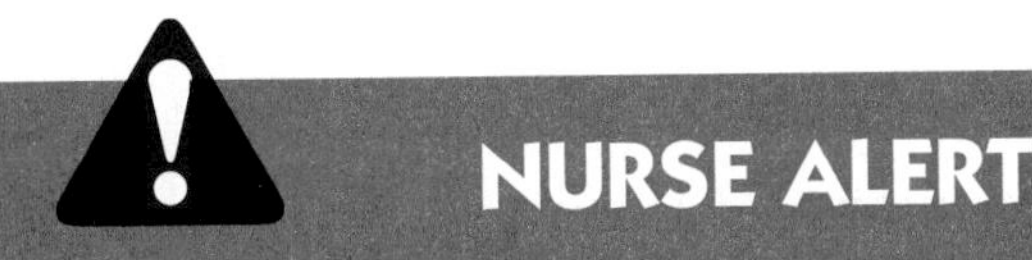

All patients need a thorough physical, emotional, and social assessment before establishing an individualized rehabilitation program.

Nurses may use these assessment tools as part of their own practice or as part of the work of the interdisciplinary team. The information obtained may assist the nurse in providing a baseline measure of the patient's status, communicating the patients' status to other caregivers, assessing the patient's need for rehabilitation, identifying the need for supportive services in the home, and measuring outcomes of care. In some settings, functional assessment may be included as a measure of the intensity of nursing care needed on a nursing unit.

Functional data are obtained by observing the patient in self-care activities. The two functional assessment tools commonly used in the rehabilitation setting are the Barthel Index and the Functional Independent Measure (FIM). The Barthel Index measures performance in mobility, self-care, and continence (Mahoney, 1965). The FIM measures function in feeding, grooming, bathing, dressing the upper body, dressing the lower body, toileting, bladder and bowel management, transfer ability, locomotion, communication, and social cognition (Figure 15-3) (Guide for the Uniform Data Set for Medical Rehabilitation, 1993; Kelly-Hayes, 1995).

LEVELS	Functional Independence Measure (FIM)	
	7 Complete independence (timely, safely) **6** Modified independence (device)	NO HELPER
	Modified dependence **5** Supervision **4** Minimal assist (Subject=75%+) **3** Moderate assist (Subject=50%+) **Complete dependence** **2** Maximal assist (Subject=25%+) **1** Total assist (Subject=0%+)	HELPER

	ADMIT	DISCHG	FOL-UP
Self-care			
A. Feeding	___	___	___
B. Grooming	___	___	___
C. Bathing	___	___	___
D. Dressing–upper body	___	___	___
E. Dressing–lower body	___	___	___
F. Toileting	___	___	___
Sphincter control			
G. Bladder management	___	___	___
H. Bowel management	___	___	___
Mobility			
Transfer:			
I. Bed, chair, w/chair	___	___	___
J. Toilet	___	___	___
K. Tub, shower	___	___	___
Locomotion			
L. Walk/wheelchair	w___ c___ ___	w___ c___ ___	w___ c___ ___
M. Stairs	___	___	___
Communication			
N. Comprehension	a___ v___ ___	a___ v___ ___	a___ v___ ___
O. Expression	v___ n___ ___	v___ n___ ___	v___ n___ ___
Social cognition			
P. Social interaction	___	___	___
Q. Problem solving	___	___	___
R. Memory	___	___	___
TOTAL	☐	☐	☐

Figure 15-3 The Functional Independence Measure (From *Guide for the Uniform Data Set for Medical Rehabilitation (Adult FIM)*, Version 4.0, Buffalo, NY, 1993, State University of New York at Buffalo. Reprinted with permission.)

Nursing Interventions

In caring for patients, particularly those who are immobile, the nurse needs to use rehabilitation techniques to promote maximum functioning and to prevent secondary complications. These techniques include (1) methods to improve movement and mobility (range-of-motion, positioning and transferring of the patient, and encouraging patient participation in self-care); (2) approaches to prevention of complications (bladder and bowel care, skin care, care of the patient with swallowing difficulty); and (3) use of adaptive equipment, mobility aids, and prosthetic equipment. Teaching the patient the implications of the diagnosis, reinforcing aspects of self-care, and providing for continuity of care are underlying themes of nursing the disabled (Box 15-4).

Methods to improve mobility

Range-of-motion. Each joint of the human body has a potential range of motion that is normal for that joint. For movement to be maintained, the limbs of the body must be moved to stretch the muscles, ligaments, and tendons that surround and support each joint. This stretching occurs with normal daily activity. However, when illness or injury limits normal movement, there is a potential to lose movement in joints and strength in muscles. Without the stretching associated with normal movement, the muscles, tendons, and ligaments surrounding joints can become shortened, limiting the amount of possible movement. When this occurs, a **contracture,** or fixed movement, of the joint may develop. With loss of muscle strength or with paralysis, the development of a contracture can

BOX 15-4 **Nursing Process**

REHABILITATION OF THE IMMOBILE PATIENT

ASSESSMENT

Mobility deficits
ROM
Ability to perform ADL
Skin integrity
Nutritional status
Respiratory status
For complications: thrombophlebitis, constipation
Coping mechanisms
Laboratory studies: albumin, transferrin, hemoglobin, hematocrit

NURSING DIAGNOSES

Impaired physical mobility related to musculoskeletal or neuromuscular impairment, weakness, or pain
Constipation related to immobility
Self-care deficit related to physical impairment or weakness
Impaired skin integrity related to immobility, incontinence, or poor nutritional status
Powerlessness related to dependence on others

NURSING INTERVENTIONS

Perform or assist with active/passive ROM to all extremities 3 to 4 times a day.
Reposition every 2 hours, maintaining proper body alignment.
Support feet with foot board or firm pillows to prevent footdrop.
Encourage/assist with early mobilization.
Assist with transfer using appropriate devices and assistance.
Allow patient to perform tasks at own rate.
Encourage participation in self-care activities.
Obtain pressure-relieving bed/chair cushions as indicated.
Avoid pressure to heels with pillows, splints, or boots.
Keep skin clean and dry. Lubricate skin as necessary.
Encourage optimal nutrition.
Encourage coughing and deep breathing.
Encourage fluid intake to 2000 ml every 24 hours (if not contraindicated)
Encourage verbalization of feelings and frustrations.
Emphasize ability vs. disability.

EVALUATION OF EXPECTED OUTCOMES

Able to perform physical activities with assistive devices as needed
No evidence of complications of immobility
Skin integrity intact
No sign/symptoms of thrombophlebitis
Bowel pattern returns to previous level of functioning

occur within a relatively short period. Spasticity, an excessive amount of tone within a muscle, can also cause a contracture to develop quickly. A contracture can limit function in a joint and cause secondary complications. For example, a foot contracted in a position of foot drop may not be able to support the leg for walking. Or an elbow severely contracted in the flexed position may cause skin breakdown in the antecubital space because of pressure and maceration of the skin.

When a patient is unable to move, nurses need to provide the movement necessary to keep joints as mobile as possible. This type of movement regimen, **range-of-motion** (ROM), needs to be provided several times a day to each joint of the body to prevent stiffness and contracture formation. Joints that should be exercised include the neck, shoulders, elbows, wrists, fingers, hips, knees, ankles, and toes. For patients unable to move, the exercises will be passive, and the nurse will exercise the joints without assistance from the patient. Passive exercises help keep joints mobile, promote venous return and lymphatic flow, and help prevent excess demineralization in the bone that is exacerbated by inactivity. If the patient is able to move, he or she can perform active range of motion by taking the limbs through all the potential degrees of movement.

Areas of assessment that the nurse should consider before initiating ROM include muscle strength of the involved limbs; muscle tone; degree of possible joint movement; and presence of pain, stiffness, bony deformities, or edema.

Normal ROM for joints include the following (Figure 15-4):

- **Neck** The neck is able to rotate from side to side, flex toward the chest and extend toward the back, and extend away from the flex toward the shoulders on each side.
- **Shoulders** The shoulders are able to rotate (with arms moving in a circular motion), flex forward, extend backward, move away from the body (abduction), and move toward the body (adduction).

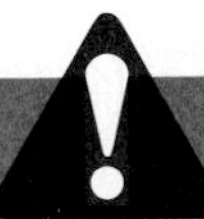

NURSE ALERT

Prevention of contractures through range-of-motion exercises is fundamental to rehabilitation programs.

- **Elbows** The elbows are able to flex toward the upper arm and extend away from the upper arm.
- **Hips** The hips are able to rotate in a circular motion, flex toward the body, extend and hyperextend away from the body, and move toward the body (adduction) and away from the body (abduction).
- **Knees** The knees are able to bend (flex) and straighten (extend).

When providing ROM exercises, the nurse should never push or stretch the joint beyond the point of stiffness, pain, or discomfort (Box 15-5). A physical or occupational therapist can assist with the care of tight and painful joints. When providing such exercises, the nurse should support the limb and the joints involved. For example, if a nurse is flexing a patient's hip, the patient's leg should be cradled in the nurse's arm at the knee. The nurse should gently hold the hip down with the other hand to prevent the hip from lifting up. Use of the principles of body mechanics is important while lifting or moving the patient during ROM exercises (Box 15-6). The nurse should stand as close as possible to the patient, with the height of the bed adjusted to prevent the nurse having back, shoulder, or arm strain. The patient's family can also be taught the exercises. Having the family perform ROM exercises is often an initial approach to include the family in the patient's care.

If the patient has weakness or paralysis in one limb or on one side of the body and has normal strength on the other side, the patient can be taught self-ROM exercises. The nurse or therapist can instruct the patient to cradle and lift the weaker limb with the strong limb. A stroke patient can use the strong arm to lift and exercise the weak arm and can use the strong foot and leg by pushing it under the weak leg and lifting. In acute-care hospitals, nursing homes, rehabilitation hospitals, and adult day care programs in the community, nurses and therapists organize patients to participate in group exercise programs. Some of these programs incorporate self-ROM and active ROM exercises as part of the program. These programs have been found to have additional benefits such as increased activity tolerance and socialization. (Paillard, Nowak, Klinger, 1985) Recent evidence suggests that resistance exercises are effective in increasing strength, even in the oldest old, those in their 90s (Fiatarone, and others, 1994; Fiatarone and others, 1993; Lowman, Klinger, 1969).

Positioning

In addition to ROM exercises, proper positioning of the immobile patient in a lying or sitting position is necessary to prevent joint deformities and skin breakdown, as well as to promote respiratory function. Continued nursing assessment is a necessary aspect of de-

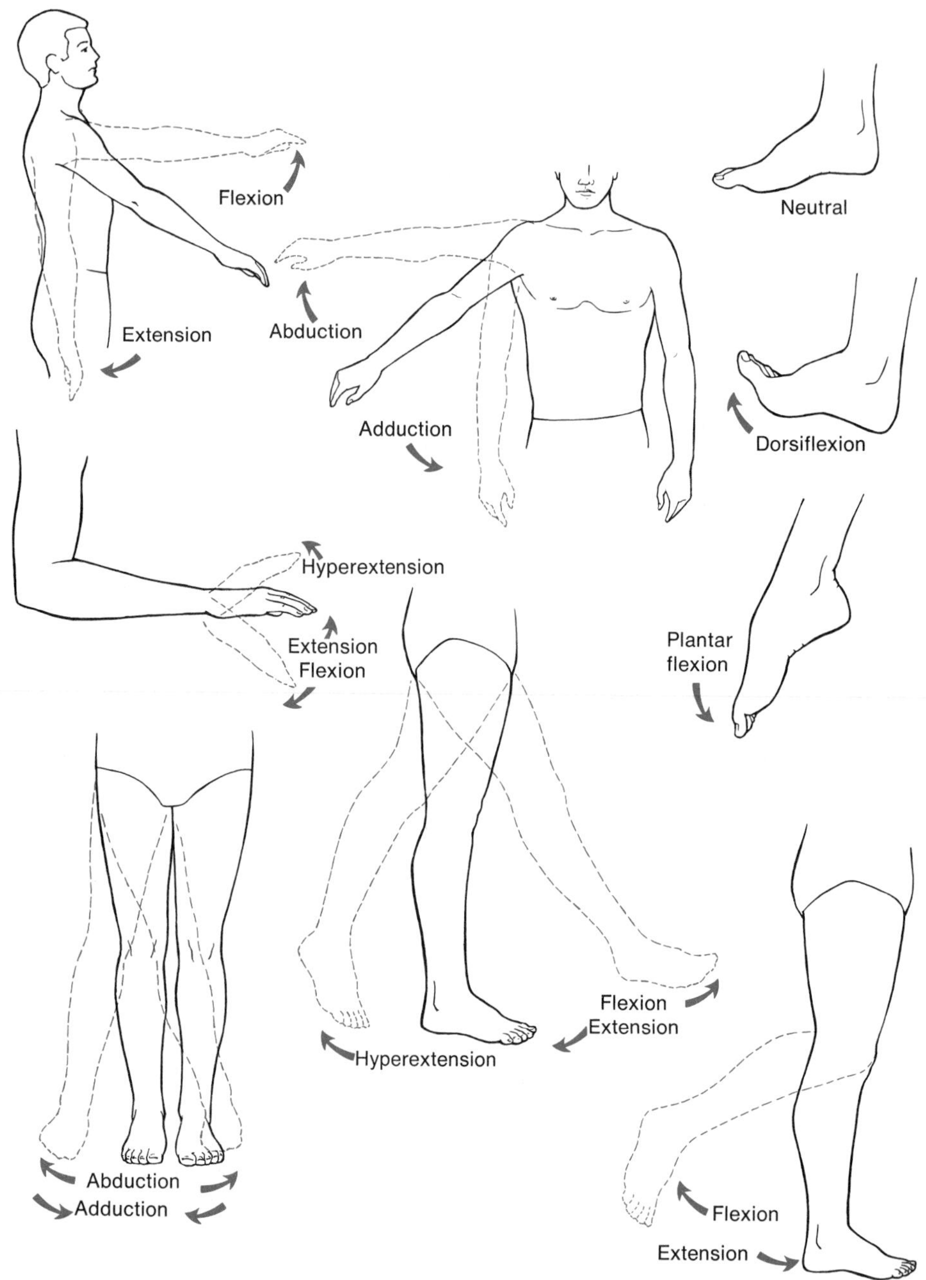

Figure 15-4 Range of motion. Methods of exercising joints to prevent contractures and to stimulate circulation.

BOX 15-5 Guidelines of Care In Providing Range-of-Motion Exercises

- Maintain body mechanics.
- Stand as close to the patient as possible.
- Provide support to the limb and joints involved.
- Assess for pain, resistance, and fatigue.
- Never push or stretch the joint beyond the point of pain or resistance.
- For the immobile patient, range each joint through full motion five times, three to four times each day.
- Teach the patient and family how to perform the exercises.

BOX 15-6

PRINCIPLES OF BODY MECHANICS WHEN MOVING A PATIENT

- Communicate your plan to the patient.
- Decide if you are able to move the patient by yourself or if you need assistance.
- Give yourself a broad base of support and good balance by keeping your feet apart.
- Get as close to the patient as possible.
- Keep your back straight and bend at the knees.
- Turn your body in the direction you are moving the patient.
- Straighten your legs as you lift.
- Do not twist your back or shift your feet or the direction of your body as you turn.
- Lift smoothly and in coordination with others helping you.
- Push and pull the patient on a draw sheet rather than lift the patient.

termining the patient's positioning needs. The presence of pressure sores, paralysis or weakness, edema, pain, restricted respiratory status, joint deformity, an unstable fracture, or an acute medical problem such as cardiopulmonary distress may restrict the possible positions available as well as influence the timing of position changes.

The scheduling of position changes depends on the needs of the patient. A patient in severe pain or a patient with very fragile skin may have to be turned every hour or more often. Patients who are totally unable to move because of paralysis, coma, edema, or loss of sensation may have to be turned every 2 hours. The patient who has some degree of movement may not have to be turned as frequently (Agency for Health Care Policy and Research, 1992a). Determining priorities of care is another factor in planning a turning schedule. As an example, waking the sleep-deprived patient for turning should be carefully considered. The nurse needs to determine if the priority of care for this patient is the need to be repositioned or the need for sleep.

Assessment areas the nurse may consider in planning a position schedule include (1) examination of bony prominences for signs of redness and discoloration; (2) examination of edematous extremities for indentations of the skin and weeping of fluid through the skin; (3) development of tightness around joints or a contracted position that is difficult to correct; and (4) patient complaints of pain, stiffness, or soreness. Contraindications for specific positions include the presence of an unstable fracture, increased intracranial pressure or poor cerebral perfusion, and cardiac or pulmonary restrictions.

NURSE ALERT

Proper scheduling of position changes depends on a thorough assessment of need.

The following are guidelines for placing patients in various positions:

In the supine or back-lying position:

- A small pillow should be placed under the head, neck, and shoulders. A large pillow under the head will place the head in an excessively flexed position.
- Arms and hands should be positioned to provide support and comfort. A neutral position with the arms at the sides of the body may be comfortable for some patients, whereas the presence of edema or pain may require supporting the arms and hands on pillows. Hand rolls can be used to maintain a functional position of the hand and prevent wrist-drop if paralysis is present. In some situations, the occupational therapist may be of assistance in selecting the type of hand roll needed. Patients with spasticity of the hand muscles may require a firm hand roll because the use of a roll made of soft material is thought to increase spasticity (Jamison, 1980).
- Excessive hip flexion and outward rotation of the hips and legs should be avoided. A firm mattress will reduce hip flexion. Immobile patients who use a soft bed surface or who have had an above-the-knee amputation and who lay for long periods in a supine position are at risk for a hip flexion contracture that can severely limit ambulation and mobility. A sagging bed makes it difficult to maintain body alignment, and a bed board placed between the box spring and mattress will help provide firmness. To prevent outward rotation of the hip and leg, the nurse should place a rolled towel or trochanter roll along the side of the body between the hip and knee (Figure 15-5).
- Legs and feet should be kept in line with the torso of the body. An adjustable footboard that extends above the toes can be used to help prevent foot-drop and keep covers off the feet. Heels should be kept free from pressure through use of pillows, splints, or protective boots (Agency for Health Care Policy and Research, 1992a). If the mattress has removable sections, the foot section can be removed to reduce pressure over the heels.

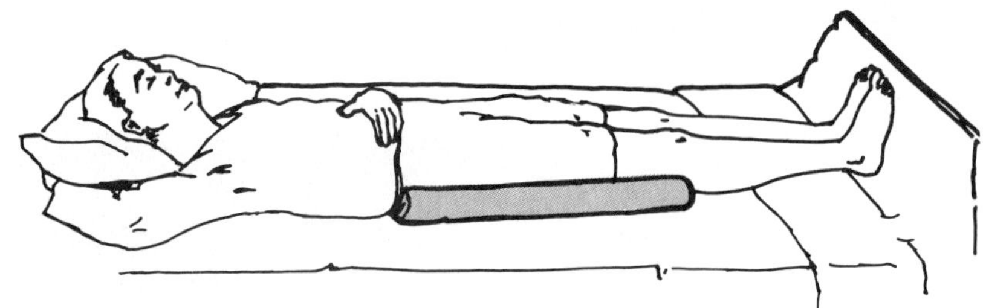

Figure 15-5 Trochanter roll is placed against patient's body between hip and knee to prevent external rotation of hip and excessive pressure against hip and side of ankle.

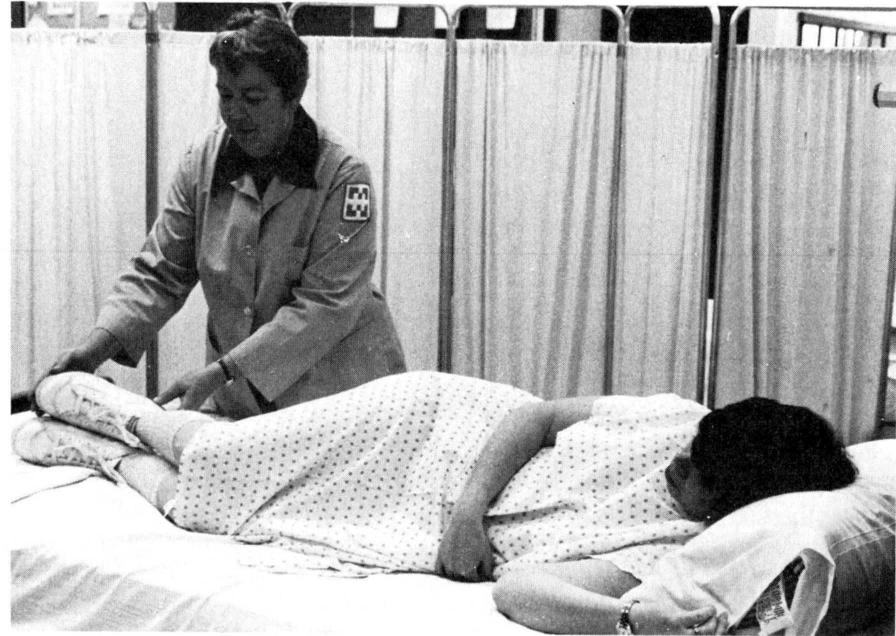

Figure 15-6 High-topped canvas shoes maintain foot alignment regardless of patient's position in bed. Shoes are worn with socks for 3 hours, removed for 1 hour, and reapplied. (Courtesy William Rainey Harper College, Palatine, Ill.)

- The feet should be kept at right angles to the legs. High-topped tennis shoes with socks or foot splints can be used intermittently (3 hours on, 1 hour off) to prevent footdrop (Figure 15-6). Unlike a footboard, these shoes and splints maintain proper alignment when the patient is positioned on either side. The bony prominences of the foot should be inspected when these devices are removed to ensure that they do not cause excessive pressure and potential skin breakdown.

In the lateral or side-lying position:

- The nurse should support the patient in a side-lying position by placing a pillow along the back.
- A pillow should be placed under the head.
- The downward arm should lie along the side of body, and the arm on the upward side should be supported by pillows.
- The upward leg may be flexed, brought forward, and supported by pillows to prevent pressure on the downward leg (Figure 15-7).

In the prone position:

- The head should be turned to one side and a small pillow placed under the head for support
- Pillows may be placed under the chest and thighs to provide comfort and support to the legs.
- A pillow under the lower legs may keep the feet at right angles to the legs, or the patient may be positioned lower in the bed so that the feet can be placed over the bottom edge of the bed.

In positioning in a chair:

- Placement is dependent on the patient's height, weight, posture, sitting balance, strength, and muscle tone.

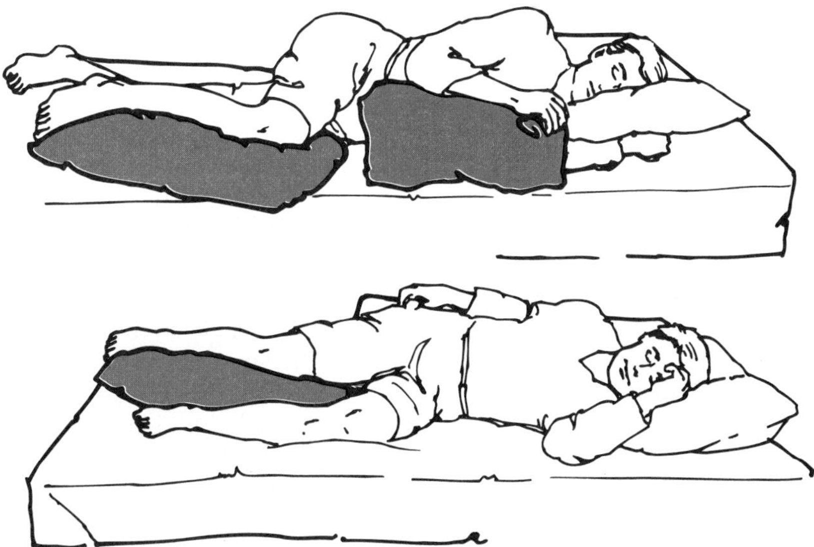

Figure 15-7 In side-lying position, arm and leg should be supported with pillows. The patient's trunk and limbs can be positioned toward front of body or toward back.

- The chair must be checked for safety, support, mobility, and independence. The patient should sit in the middle of seat, with buttocks against the back of the chair, arms supported, feet supported without excessive pressure placed on knees and hips, and knees and hips at 90 degrees.

Patient transfers. The patient's level of independence in transferring should be assessed by the physical therapist and nurse (Box 15-7). During recovery, as a patient's strength and endurance increase, the ability to lift out of bed into a chair or commode also increases. Patients with severe disabilities may be totally dependent in this area or in need of moderate to minimum assistance. Safety is of prime importance when transferring a patient. The prevention of injury to the patient and nurse must be considered before the patient is moved. Assessment areas include (1) ability to comprehend instructions, (2) weight and height, (3) ability to stand, (4) ability to bear own weight, (5) presence of medical or orthopedic instability, and (6) the presence of orthostatic hypotension. Carefully planning the transfer and describing each step to the patient and other caregivers helps decrease the possibility of injury. If the patient is totally dependent and several staff members are involved in the transfer activity, one staff person should be designated the leader and direct all steps of the transfer. Transfer activity may be described as between bed and chair; to wheelchair, toilet, bath, or shower; or between wheelchair and car.

BOX 15-7

PATIENT ASSESSMENT AREAS FOR TRANSFER ABILITY

- Ability to comprehend instructions
- Weight and height
- Ability to stand and bear own weight
- Presence of medical or orthopedic instability
- Presence of orthostatic hypotension

Use of a transfer belt may make transferring safer and easier. Transfer belts are strong and made of leather or nylon with sturdy loops on the sides and back. In preparation for transfer, the belt is placed securely around the patient's waist and then closed. The nurse bends down at the knees and places hands through the side loops and holds onto the back loop. This allows the nurse to have a secure hold on the patient as the patient stands. As the patient comes into a standing position, the nurse brings the patient as close as possible. This allows for a more stable transfer because the patient's center of gravity is close to the nurse's center of gravity. The nurse then guides the patient into a chair.

Types of transfers include the following (Box 15-8):

Dependent transfer. The patient is unable to assist with any aspect of this activity. Moving the patient may require that nursing staff lift the patient through a total lift or pivot transfer or use a lift sheet, a transfer board, or a hydraulic lift.

Lifts for the totally dependent patient include the following:

The A-P (anterior-posterior) transfer. The nurse should place the chair at right angles to the bed and lock the chair brakes. Using a sheet, the nurse should turn the patient across the bed so that his or her back is to the chair. Next the nurse should slide the patient into the chair. This procedure should be reversed to return the patient to bed.

The total lift. At least two nurses need to involved in this lift. One nurse should stand behind the patient with arms placed under the patient's arms and around the chest and hands gripped together. The second nurse should face the patient with arms placed under the patient's knees. Together the nurses lift the patient up into the bed or chair.

Pivot transfer. This transfer requires one or two persons to assist the patient. In a one-person pivot transfer, the patient should be placed in a sitting position on the side of the bed. The nurse should stand in front of the patient while bending the knees to lower the body and the center of gravity for greater stability and safety. The nurse's arms should be placed under the patient's arms and around the back. At the same time, the patient's arms should be placed around the nurse's shoulders. Through a gentle rocking motion, the nurse should lift the patient to a standing position, pull the patient forward, and slowly turn the patient toward the chair and lower into the chair.

A two-person pivot transfer should be used for a more debilitated patient. The patient should be placed in a sitting position in bed. Each nurse should face the patient, one on each side of the patient's body. The nurses should then bend their knees, lowering their bodies and their centers of gravity. One nurse should place an arm under the patient's arm and around the back. The second nurse should do the same on the other side. Through a rocking motion, they should bring the patient to a standing position and turn and lower the patient into the chair.

Hydraulic lifts. This lift uses a one- or two-piece sling placed under the patient and attached to the lift. By pumping the lift, the patient is raised off the bed and can be easily moved. Contraindications for use of such devices include excessive weight or height; agitation; or medical or orthopedic instability.

Partially dependent transfer. The patient is able to assist the nurse to some degree with this activity (Dittmar, 1989).

Hemiplegic transfer. The wheelchair should be placed at the side of the bed on the patient's unaffected side of the body. The nurse should then remove the armrest and lock the brakes. Next the patient should be helped to sit on the side of the bed, then to stand, turn, and back up to the chair. The nurse may need to assist the patient to move the hemiplegic leg by placing a foot at right angles to the patient's involved foot and bracing a knee against the patient's involved knee. The patient should place the strong arm on the wheelchair arm, while sitting back into chair.

BOX 15-8

TYPES OF TRANSFERS

- Dependent
  Total, pivot, A-P, hydraulic lift
- Partially dependent
  Hemiplegic, amputee, sliding board

Paraplegic or bilateral amputee transfer. This is the same as the A-P transfer described previously, except that the patient should have enough arm strength to hold himself or herself up in bed and scoot back into the chair.

Sliding board transfer. The nurse should place the wheelchair at the side of the bed, lock the brakes, and remove the armrest of the chair. The height of the bed should be the same height as the chair seat. The nurse should assist the patient to sit on the side of the bed. One end of the sliding board should be placed under the patient's buttocks and the other end placed on the chair seat. The patient should reach for the arm of the wheelchair and pull across the board into the chair.

Not all patients are able to sit in a wheelchair. The very debilitated patient may need a recliner chair for comfort, support, and safety, particularly the style of chair that can be fitted with a tray. Recliner-style chairs are used widely across the country, yet the chair design makes patient transfers most difficult and, with some patients, unsafe. It is important to be sure that the chair is in good working order. If the brakes are not operational, the chair should be placed against a wall. Most of these chairs do not have removable arms, and nurses need to assist the patient over the arm and into the chair. For a frail patient, two nurses assisting with a two-person pivot transfer may be needed. However, if the patient has difficulty bearing weight or is confused, it is safer to use the A-P transfer, a total lift with a sheet, or a hydraulic lift.

Patient participation in self-care. The nurse can promote activity, mobility, and exercise by encouraging the patient to participate in his or her own care. For the patient who has been acutely ill, this activity may be limited. Turning independently in bed and balancing oneself while sitting on the side of the bed may increase strength, endurance, and balance.

While the patient sits on the side of the bed or sits in a chair, the nurse should have the patient raise one leg for a few seconds, lower that leg, and raise the other. This simple exercise helps to strengthen the quadriceps muscles, a major muscle group involved in standing and walking (Lewis, 1989). Brushing one's own hair or teeth may promote upper-extremity strength and trunk balance. Gradually the patient should engage in increased activity. The nurse and the physical therapist need to work together to reinforce patient independence in transfers in and out of bed, standing, and walking. As the patient increases activity level, strength and endurance will increase. Recent studies on the impact of exercise and the very elderly indicate that resistance exercise, with use of weights, is the most effective means of increasing strength. Patients in their 90s made improvements through participation in regular resistance training (Fiatarone and others, 1994; Payton, Poland, 1983)

Preventive approaches to care

Skin breakdown. Prevention of skin breakdown is another aspect of care of the immobile or disabled person. Skin breakdown, or formation of a pressure sore, occurs when there is excessive pressure from bed or chair surfaces against the bony prominences of the body (Figure 15-8). The common names for this problem (bedsore or decubitus ulcer) are inaccurate terms. *Decubitus* comes from the Latin word meaning "lying down." The source of the problem is not solely from lying down or being in bed. The real culprit is pressure. Pressure that is excessive and of a long duration occludes capillary blood flow to the tissue overlaying the bony prominences of the body, depriving the tissue of needed oxygen. This hypoxic tissue cannot survive, and a wound forms. The size and depth of the wound depends on the intensity of pressure and the length of time the pressure is unrelieved. Healthy people can feel discomfort from sitting in one position for too long, and they simply change their position. A person who is unable to move or who cannot feel painful sensations cannot relieve the pressure on his or her own, and the risk for the development of this problem is much greater.

Other factors play an important role in this outcome: nutritional status, mobility, sensory ability, medical status, continence, and circulatory status. Aging-associated changes in the skin make the older patient more susceptible to skin breakdown. The skin of the older person has less elasticity, is drier, and has less subcutaneous tissue. On admission, the nurse needs to identify the patient at risk for the development of pressure sores. The national practice guidelines for the prevention of pressure sores recommends the use of a risk assessment tool to identify patients at risk for pressure sore development (Agency for Health Care Policy and Research, 1992a). Two tools recommended in this guide are the Braden Scale (Figure 15-9) and the Norton Scale (Table 15-1) (Bergstram and others, 1987; Braden, Bergstrom, 1989; Norton, McLaren, Exton-Smith, 1962).

If a patient is identified as at risk, multiple nursing interventions should be instituted to avoid development of a pressure sore. Pressure relief is obtained by placing the patient on a turning schedule as needed;

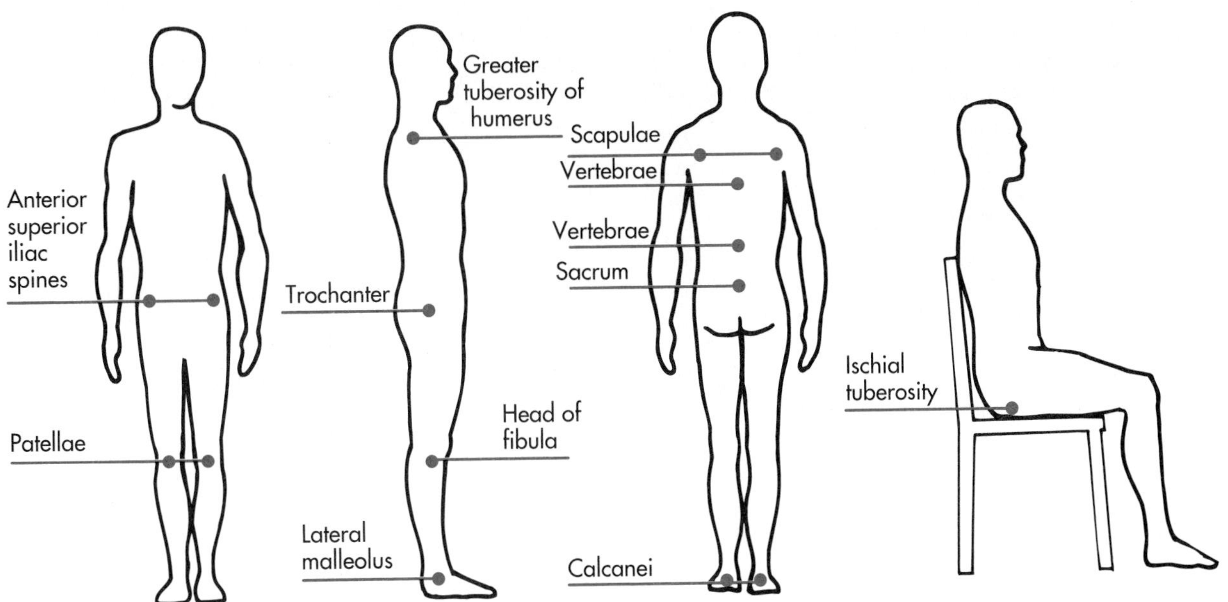

Figure 15-8 Bony prominences of the body.

Note: Bed- and chairbound individuals or those with impaired ability to reposition should be assessed upon admission for their risk of developing pressure ulcers. Patients with established pressure ulcers should be reassessed periodically.

PATIENT NAME ____________

ROOM NUMBER ________ DATE ________

Sensory perception Ability to respond meaningfully to pressure-related discomfort	**1. Completely limited:** Unresponsive (does not moan, flinch, or gasp) to painful stimuli, due to diminished level of consciousness or sedation **Or** Limited ability to feel pain over most of body surface	**2. Very limited:** Responds only to painful stimuli; cannot communicate discomfort except by moaning or restlessness **Or** Has a sensory impairment that limits the ability to feel pain or discomfort over ½ of body	**3. Slightly limited:** Responds to verbal commands but cannot always communicate discomfort or need to be turned **Or** Has some sensory impairment that limits ability to feel pain or discomfort in one or two extremities	**4. No impairment:** Responds to verbal commands; has no sensory deficit that would limit ability to feel or voice pain or discomfort	(Indicate appropriate score)
Moisture Degree to which skin is exposed to moisture	**1. Constantly moist:** Skin is kept moist almost constantly by perspiration, urine, etc.; dampness is detected every time patient is moved or turned	**2. Very moist:** Skin is often, but not always, moist; linen must be changed at least once a shift	**3. Occasionally moist:** Skin is occasionally moist, requiring an extra linen change approximately once a day	**4. Rarely moist:** Skin is usually dry; linen only requires changing at routine intervals	
Activity Degree of physical activity	**1. Bedfast:** Confined to bed	**2. Chairfast:** Ability to walk severely limited or nonexistent; cannot bear own weight and/or must be assisted into chair or wheelchair	**3. Walks occasionally:** Walks occasionally during day, but for very short distances, with or without assistance; spends majority of each shift in bed or chair	**4. Walks frequently:** Walks outside the room at least twice a day and inside room at least once every 2 hours during waking hours	
Mobility Ability to change and control body position	**1. Completely immobile:** Does not make even slight changes in body or extremity position without assistance	**2. Very limited:** Makes occasional slight changes in body or extremity position but unable to make frequent or significant changes independently	**3. Slightly limited:** Makes frequent though slight changes in body or extremity position independently	**4. No limitations:** Makes major and frequent changes in position without assistance	
Nutrition Usual food intake pattern	**1. Very poor:** Never eats a complete meal; rarely eats more than ⅓ of any food offered; eats two servings or less of protein (meat or dairy products) per day; takes fluids poorly; does not take a liquid dietary supplement **Or** Is NPO and/or maintained on clear liquids or IVs for more than 5 days	**2. Probably inadequate:** Rarely eats a complete meal or generally eats only about ½ of any food offered; protein intake includes only three servings of meat or dairy products per day; occasionally will take a dietary supplement **Or** Receives less than optimum amount of liquid diet or tube feeding	**3. Adequate:** Eats over half of most meals; eats a total of four servings of protein (meat, dairy products) each day; occasionally will refuse a meal, but will usually take a supplement if offered **Or** Is on a tube feeding or TPN regimen which probably meets most of nutritional needs	**4. Excellent:** Eats most of every meal; never refuses a meal; usually eats a total of four or more servings of meat and dairy products; occasionally eats between meals; does not require supplementation	
Friction and shear	**1. Problem:** Requires moderate to maximum assistance in moving; complete lifting without sliding against sheets is impossible; frequently slides down in bed or chair, requiring frequent repositioning with maximum assistance; spasticity, contractures, or agitation lead to almost constant friction	**2. Potential problem:** Moves freely or requires minimum assistance; during a move, skin probably slides to some extent against sheets, chair, restraints, or other devices; maintains relatively good position in chair or bed most of the time but occasionally slides down	**3. No apparent problem:** Moves in bed and in chair independently and has sufficient muscle strength to lift up completely during move; maintains good position in bed or chair at all times		
Note: patients with a total score of 16 or less are considered to be at risk of developing pressure ulcers. (15 or 16 = low risk, 13 or 14 = moderate risk, 12 or less = high risk).				**Total score**	

Figure 15-9 Braden Risk Assessment Scale. (Copyright 1988 Barbara Braden and Nancy Bergstrom. Reprinted with permission.)

TABLE 15-1

Norton Scale

		Physical Condition		Mental Condition		Activity		Mobility		Incontinent		Total Score
		Good	4	Alert	4	Ambulant	4	Full	4	Not	4	
		Fair	3	Apathetic	3	Walk/help	3	Slightly limited	3	Occasionally	3	
		Poor	2	Confused	2	Chairbound	2	Very limited	2	Usually/ urine	2	
		Very bad	1	Stupor	1	Bed	1	Immobile	1	Doubly	1	
Name	Date											

From Centre for Policy on Ageing, London, England. Reprinted with permission.

obtaining pressure-reducing bed and chair surfaces; or protecting the heels through pillows, splints, or boots or removable heel blocks (Agency for Health Care Policy and Research, 1992a). The at-risk patient needs careful attention to nutritional and fluid intake. Obtaining and monitoring laboratory values that indicate the patient's nutritional and medical status are necessary. Albumin and transferrin levels provide data on the visceral protein stores available to the patient to promote tissue integrity and wound healing. Total lymphocyte count, hematocrit, hemoglobin, and body chemistries need to be monitored, as these values are reflective of the patient's health. Vitamin and mineral levels are important, as these elements serve a vital role in healing.

Nutritional consultation is needed for the malnourished patient at risk of developing a pressure sore. It is necessary to cleanse the skin and pay close attention to the condition of the skin. If the skin is too dry, lubricating creams and ointments should be applied. If the skin is too moist, a light application of a drying powder may be beneficial. A bladder and bowel program should be planned for the incontinent person to prevent skin maceration.

The patient who sits in a wheelchair or other chair should be protected from pressure on the sitting surfaces of the body through the use of a wheelchair cushion. A bed pillow does not provide adequate pressure relief. A 4-inch foam cushion may be fine for most patients, whereas a more therapeutic cushion may be required by patients who are unable to move or who have poor sensation.

For the patient who has already developed a pressure sore, many of the above interventions need to be initiated. The treatment of a pressure sore is based on the size and depth of the wound. Many hospitals have developed protocols for care of pressure sores. Based on the size and depth of the wound and the appearance of the wound bed, cleaning agents, dressings for the wounds, and bed surface selection are recommended (Phipps, Bauman, 1984). The Agency for Health Care Policy and Research has developed national guidelines for the treatment of pressure sores.

Some pressure sores extend down to bone and can place the patient at risk of death because of infection and sepsis. Pressure sores are, for the most part, a preventable problem. If there is no pressure, an ulcer does not form. Scrupulous attention must be paid to the patient at risk to prevent the formation of pressure sores. In the patient who has no pressure relief, a pressure sore can develop within a few hours. All at-risk patients should be out of bed as much as possible. This is especially true of older patients. In addition to providing pressure relief, moving from bed to chair provides activity for muscles that otherwise receive little exercise. It also provides for better ventilation of the lungs by helping to prevent the accumulation of fluid at the base of the lung (Box 15-9).

Urinary incontinence. Urinary incontinence is a major healthcare problem. The impact of this problem is felt not only in financial terms, which are great, but also in the disruption of the incontinent person's social and personal life. It has been estimated that 15% to 30% of noninstitutionalized adults over the age of 60 and as many as half of the 1.5 million Americans in long-term care facilities experience urinary incontinence. In the elderly, urinary incontinence is one of the three major causes of long-term care placement. Urinary incontinence can also lead to secondary problems such as skin breakdown or falls from slipping in urine.

BOX 15-9

Nursing Process

PRESSURE SORE

ASSESSMENT

General condition of skin
Skin over body prominences
Awareness of pressure sensation
Ability to move
Nutritional status
Urinary or fecal incontinence
Amount of shear and friction on skin
Pressure ulcer staging: color, odor, presence of necrotic tissue, exudate, and condition of surrounding skin
Vital signs: temperature
Laboratory values: albumin, ferritin, wound culture, WBC
Family's ability to provide associated care

NURSING DIAGNOSES

Impaired skin integrity related to friction, shear, or pressure
Risk for infection related to open pressure sore and/or poor nutritional status
Impaired home maintenance management related to long-term therapy
Risk for caregiver role strain related to long-term therapy
Altered nutrition: less than body requirements related to chronic illness

NURSING INTERVENTIONS

Maintain preventive measures including pressure reduction/relief.
Maintain nutritional needs and management of incontinence.
Provide aseptic local wound care as ordered.
Maintain no pressure on pressure sore until healed.
Provide perineal hygiene after incontinence.
Encourage high-protein, high-calorie diet (if not contraindicated).
Administer antibiotics as prescribed.
Refer to social worker to assist with discharge planning needs.
Discuss possible need for respite care.

EVALUATION OF EXPECTED OUTCOMES

Pressure ulcer shows evidence of healing
No evidence of local or systemic infection
Verbalizes necessary home-care measures
Verbalizes available resources

Care of the incontinent patient involves assessment of the underlying cause of the incontinence and development of approaches to improve the condition. The nurse must work closely with the patient and family, the physician, and other healthcare team members to find methods to improve the patient's incontinence or, if needed, to determine alternative safe and convenient interventions (Box 15-10). Of particular importance in caring for the elderly incontinent patient is recognizing that urinary incontinence is not normal in old age but is an abnormal development that often has multiple identifiable causes. Urinary incontinence is a symptom, not a disease or a condition.

There are a variety of ways to describe urinary incontinence. One of the most useful approaches is to categorize incontinence as either a transient condition that can be corrected or as an established or fixed condition that cannot be corrected. Nursing assessment and interventions are important aspects of the care of patients with either type of urinary incontinence. The Agency for Health Care Policy and Research has developed a national practice guideline, *Urinary Incontinence in Adults* (Agency for Health Care Policy and Research, 1992b). The goals of this guideline are to develop national recognition of the scope of the problem of urinary incontinence and to offer research-based approaches to interventions.

Transient or temporary incontinence has been described as an uncontrolled leakage of urine that may be reversible once the underlying causes are corrected. Recognized causes of temporary incontinence include confusion, infection, medication side effects, immobility that may limit the patient's access to toilet facilities, constipation, depression, inadequate fluid intake, and medical conditions that lead to excessive urine production. Elderly women may develop urinary incontinence because of cellular changes that occur in the lower urinary tract following menopause. This condition, *atrophic urethritis,* may be corrected with medicated creams.

Often patients will have a combination of factors that lead to temporary urinary incontinence. For example, elderly patients admitted to acute-care hospitals for pneumonia or a hip fracture may develop

BOX 15-10 **Nursing Process**

REHABILITATION OF THE INCONTINENT PATIENT

ASSESSMENT

Episodes and frequency of incontinence
Pain or burning with urination
Ability to manage clothes
Ability to get to the bathroom
Mental status
Fluid volume status
Bladder distention

NURSING DIAGNOSES

Altered urinary elimination: incontinence related to trauma, musculoskeletal, neurologic injury, infection, injury to urinary system, or impaired cognition
Body image disturbance related to incontinence
Impaired skin integrity related to incontinence
Self-care deficit: toileting related to neuromuscular or musculoskeletal disorder or cognitive impairment

NURSING INTERVENTIONS

Offer bedpan or urinal, or assist to bathroom every 2 to 3 hours. Gradually lengthen time interval.
Assist with normal position for voiding.
Instruct to perform perineal exercises.
Space fluid intake throughout the day.
Limit oral intake in the evening.
Instruct to avoid caffeinated beverages.
Use behavior modification as indicated.
Administer medications as prescribed.

EVALUATION OF EXPECTED OUTCOMES

Remains continent of urine
Verbalizes management strategies

fever, decreased fluid intake, confusion, immobility, and constipation. Urinary incontinence may be an outcome of these multiple factors. Once the medical problems are corrected, the incontinence usually improves.

Fixed urinary incontinence is not reversible. However, like temporary incontinence, it may have multiple causes. Pathologic, physiologic, or anatomic changes within the urinary tract and its supporting structures or within the nervous system pathways that integrate bladder function lead to this problem. Some neurologic disorders, such as multiple sclerosis or spinal cord injury, leave the patient with fixed urinary incontinence. The care of patients with fixed incontinence requires medical assessment to identify the cause and to define the specific type. The physician and nurse work closely with the patient and family to plan the best method to manage the incontinence. The medical evaluation may include specific procedures to describe the type of fixed urinary incontinence, such as cystometrogram and urine flow studies.

The Agency for Health Care Policy and Research practice guideline describes three types of incontinence: urge, stress, and overflow (Box 15-11). Urge incontinence is the involuntary loss of urine associated with an abrupt and strong desire to void (Agency for Health Care Policy and Research, 1992b). If there is no associated neurologic disorder, this condition may be defined as detrusor instability. The detrusor is the muscle mass that forms the urinary bladder. If the patient has a neurologic disorder, this type of bladder dysfunction may be classified as detrusor hyperreflexia. Stress incontinence is the involuntary loss of urine during coughing, sneezing, laughing, or other activites that increase abdominal pressure (Wells, 1988). Overflow incontinence occurs when there is overdistension of the bladder. There are multiple causes of both stress and overflow incontinence. The importance of a complete and thorough medical evaluation for any type of urinary incontinence cannot be overemphasized because in many situations it is a treatable condition.

BOX 15-11

TYPES OF URINARY INCONTINENCE

- Urge incontinence
- Stress incontinence
- Overflow incontinence

The nursing assessment of the patient with urinary incontinence involves obtaining a patient history and performing a physical assessment. Interviewing the patient and family about the incontinence may provide important and helpful information. The nurse might ask specific questions of the patient and family, such as the following:

- What problems are you having with urination?
- Can you feel when your bladder is full?

INCONTINENCE RECORD

Patient's name ______________________

Room number ______________________

Date:		Date:		Date:	
Time	Wet or dry	Time	Wet or dry	Time	Wet or dry
8 am		8 am		8 am	
10 am		10 am		10 am	
12 N		12 N		12 N	
2 pm		2 pm		2 pm	
4 pm		4 pm		4 pm	
6 pm		6 pm		6 pm	
8 pm		8 pm		8 pm	
10 pm		10 pm		10 pm	
12 MN		12 MN		12 MN	
2 am		2 am		2 am	
4 am		4 am		4 am	
6 am		6 am		6 am	

Figure 15-10 Example of 48-hour incontinence record.

- How long can you wait to get to the bathroom after you feel the need to empty your bladder?
- Do you need to get out of bed at night to urinate?
- Do you have any dribbling of urine when you laugh, cough, or sneeze?
- Do you have pain or burning with urination?
- Have you noticed a change in the color or odor of your urine?

The nurse may need to assess the patient's mental status because confusion can lead to incontinence. A limited mental status assessment includes an examination of the patient's orientation to person, place, and time, as well as the patient's long- and short-term memory. If possible, the nurse should assess the patient's ability to get in and out of bed, to get in and out of the toilet facility, and to manage clothing and toilet tissue. For the bed-bound patient, the nurse may assess the patient's ability to manipulate a urinal or bedpan.

A 48-hour record of the patient's fluid intake and urinary output is helpful in determining fluid balance. A 48-hour history of urinary incontinence is best recorded with the use of an incontinence chart that indicates the patient's condition, wet or dry, at 2-hour intervals (Figure 15-10). Keeping this chart may help the nurse detect a possible pattern of urinary incontinence.

The physician and nurse together should assess the patient's physical status to determine bladder fullness or distention and to determine if the bowel is impacted. A neurologic examination, including an evaluation of reflex activity needed for normal blader function, may be useful. The patient's medical record should be reviewed to identify important factors that could be relevant to bladder problems, such as a medical diagnosis, medications, laboratory values, or previous surgeries.

Once this information is collected and documented, the nurse and other members of the healthcare team should plan specific interventions. All reversible causes of incontinence need to be identified. Once such factors as confusion, fever, constipation, dehydration, immobility, and decreased fluid intake are corrected, incontinence may diminish. If incontinence persists or is unrelated to these factors, the assessment should continue and a plan for intervention should be developed.

Interventions for urinary incontinence include medication, surgery, or behavioral approaches (Box 15-12). The first two interventions are beyond the scope of this chapter, but extensive literature on these subjects is available (Agency for Health Care Policy and Re-

BOX 15-12

INTERVENTIONS FOR URINARY INCONTINENCE

- Bladder training
- Habit training
- Prompted voiding
- Kegel exercises

search, 1992b; Wells, 1988). Behavioral approaches are often the domain of the nurse and include bladder training (retraining), habit training (timed voiding), prompted voiding, and pelvic floor exercises.

Bladder training is based on clear patterns of communication between staff and patients to regulate fluid intake and develop a pattern or schedule of urinary elimination. The patient's past voiding history, fluid intake record, and incontinence chart should be reviewed to establish the schedule. If no pattern of incontinence can be identified from the incontinence chart, the nurse should establish a bladder-emptying schedule. The voiding schedule should also include a plan to progressively increase the time between scheduled voidings. The patient's schedule and expected outcome should be clearly documented and understood by all staff, as well as the patient and family. The patient's response to the bladder program must be documented and communicated to all involved.

A bladder program developed for a patient who is consistently incontinent after meals may include the following:

Fluid intake

2000 to 3000 ml/day: 200 ml every 2 hours beginning at 6 AM and ending at 8 PM. Fluids are restricted at night. A variety of fluids preferred by the patient should be offered.

Voiding routine

On arising, ½ hour after each meal, ½ hour before going to bed.

If the patient is incontinent between voiding times, the times and surrounding event should be noted. The time between voiding should be gradually increased, and the patient should be encouraged to delay voiding.

Habit training is generally used for the patient who has no clear pattern of incontinence. A bladder program might include a similar fluid regimen but a planned voiding routine of 2-hour toileting, or whatever time interval allows the patient to remain dry. When the patient attempts to void, the immediate environment should be private, and the patient should be in a comfortable position.

Prompted voiding is often used with cognitively impaired patients. This type of program involves monitoring the patient's state of dryness, prompting the person to use the toilet, and using praise when he or she is continent (Wells, 1988). Success in bladder training depends on patient cooperation. Prompted voiding is a form of behavior modification used to motivate patients to cooperate with the program. Behavior modification is a therapeutic program that involves rewards or positive reinforcements for desired behavior. The likes and dislikes of each patient will vary. An action or reward that is positive for one patient may be negative for another. The desired behavior, in this case, continence, is more likely to be repeated if the patient experiences some reward for that behavior. The reward may be a material object or may be in the form of praise, but it must be seen as a reward by the patient if it is to be effective. The patient is checked every 2 hours. If dry, a reward is given. If incontinent, no reward is given. Appropriate use of the toilet or commode is also rewarded. The short-term goal of staying dry or using the commode appropriately will lead to the long-term goal of continence and independent use of bathroom facilities. The entire staff must fully understand the program and its methods and implement it appropriately.

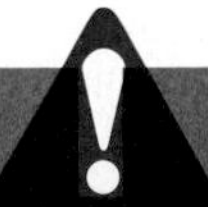

NURSE ALERT

Behavioral approaches to urinary incontinence are often the domain of the nurse. These include bladder training, habit training, prompted voiding, and pelvic floor exercises.

The goal of pelvic floor exercises, or Kegel exercises, is to strengthen the muscles that aid in urethral closing. This is accomplished through contraction and relaxation of the perivaginal muscles (Box 15-13) (Wells, 1988).

An indwelling catheter should be avoided as a method to treat incontinence because the patient with an indwelling catheter has a high probability of developing a urinary tract infection. Some estimates indicate that 70% of patients develop a urinary tract infection within 72 hours of catheter insertion. However, an indwelling catheter is necessary for some individuals, such as a patient with an acute illness, following surgery, an incontinent patient in such severe pain that linen change is difficult, or a patient who cannot urinate. Bladder training of the patient with an indwelling catheter is controversial. If the patient has a urinary tract infection, the physician may decide to

BOX 15-13

PELVIC FLOOR (KEGEL) EXERCISES

INTRODUCTION

Kegel, or pelvic floor, exercises are designed for men and women to strengthen the muscles, ligaments, and tendons of the pelvic floor that support the bladder and lower bowel. By strengthening and toning these muscles, symptoms of stress urinary incontinence (i.e., involuntary loss of urine when sneezing, coughing, laughing) may be decreased or relieved.

The nurse should review the following points with the patient.

IDENTIFYING THE CORRECT MUSCLES

1 To find the muscle, place your finger inside your vagina or rectum. Try to squeeze around your finger. That's the muscle you want to exercise. This is the same muscle you use to hold back a bowel movement or gas.
2 Never use your stomach, leg, or buttocks muscles. The most common mistake is using too many muscles. To find out if you are contracting your stomach muscles, place your hand on your abdomen while you squeeze your pelvic floor muscles. If you feel your abdomen move, you are also using these muscles.
3 These exercises can be practiced anytime, in any place. Because the muscle is internal, no one can see you exercising these muscles.

PERFORMING THE EXERCISE

1 Squeeze the muscle that you identified earlier and hold for a count of 10, or for 10 seconds. Then relax for a count of 10. Remember, it is as important to relax as it is to contract the muscle.
2 Choose one of the following schedules:
   - Do 15 exercises in the morning, 15 in the afternoon, and 15 at night.
   - Exercise for 10 minutes, three times a day

You may notice a change in about 2 weeks of consistent daily exercises. In 1 month you may notice an even bigger change.

treat the infection with medication. Another approach is to simply remove the catheter as the source of infection rather than treating the patient with medication. There is also some disagreement regarding the benefit gained by clamping and unclamping the indwelling catheter before removal. Some authorities believe that it is necessary to clamp the catheter periodically to increase bladder capacity and sensation; however, others believe that clamping has no impact on outcome (Gross, 1990). Whether the catheter is clamped or removed abruptly, the patient's attention should be directed to the sensation caused by the expansion of the bladder as it fills and the contraction of the bladder as it empties.

Behavioral techniques may help patients with either temporary or fixed incontinence. However, other approaches may be necessary because of the extent and type of bladder dysfunction. If the patient has no sensation of bladder fullness and no ability to empty the bladder, a program of intermittent catheterization may be initiated. The scheduling of this program is based on fluid intake and volume of catheterized urine. Initially the patient is catheterized every 4 hours, and then this schedule is decreased to every 6 to 8 hours while the patient is awake. Depending on the type of bladder dysfunction, this program may eventually allow for reflex bladder emptying without catheterization. For some patients, intermittent catheterization becomes the only method of urinary elimination, and the patient may be taught self-catheterization. A clean, rather than sterile, technique may be used by the patient doing self-catheterization in the home. This technique allows the patient to reuse catheters after washing them with soap and water. Sterile techniques should be used for self-catheterization in the hospital.

Some individuals may need to use an indwelling catheter on a long-term basis. Urinary tract infection is a constant threat with long-term catheterization. Individuals should be monitored by a healthcare professional if they have been sent home with the catheter. Adequate fluid intake, care of the catheter and collecting bags, and attention to skin care must become part of the patient's daily routine.

Urine-collecting devices are another means of managing incontinence. A condom-collecting system may be beneficial to some men. The condom should be changed daily, with close attention given to skin care and cleaning. Several urine-collecting devices are available for women. These products fit over the perineum and are connected to a drainage bag. Proper fit is a problem for many women. If the fit is not tight, urine will leak. Close attention to skin care is also essential with these devices.

Diapering may be the method chosen by some individuals to manage their urinary incontinence, particularly if soiling of clothing or slipping in urine is a problem. However, a complete assessment and all other treatment interventions should be evaluated before adopting this method. Preventing skin problems due to wet diapers becomes an important aspect of care. Many diapering products are available and should be selected based on the individual's specific needs. In the bedbound patient, diapers must be changed when wet because of the high potential for skin breakdown. Some disposable diapers are made to keep the layer next to the skin dry while absorbing the urine in other layers.

Altered bowel function. The patient with altered bowel function requires an in-depth nursing assessment before interventions are initiated. The patient's history should be taken and should include any medical condition that would lead to altered bowel function, the pattern of elimination, dietary habits, difficulty with bowel elimination, review of medications, abdominal surgical procedures, problems with dentition that would limit dietary intake, and mobility problems.

Altered bowel function may be seen as constipation, diarrhea, or fecal incontinence. It is beyond the scope of this chapter to review all the factors that can lead to the development of these problems. However, disabled persons may develop altered bowel function and may need specialized approaches to bowel care. The bowel pattern may need to be "retrained" because of the consequences of neurologic disease, immobility, altered nutritional intake, medication, and altered mobility. This training involves developing a pattern of scheduled elimination.

Bowel function is aided by the addition of high-residue foods to the diet. Whole-grain breads, bran cereal, prune juice, and fresh fruits have been found to be very effective in stimulating bowel function. Adequate fluid intake and exercise are essential to normal bowel function. Medication may be prescribed to soften the stool and/or increase peristalsis. Harsh laxatives and enemas should not be used to regulate bowel function. Dietary restrictions and other physician orders should be considered, and the physician should be consulted when planning a retraining program for the incontinent patient.

A bowel program is an individualized approach to schedule elimination (Venn and others, 1992). Some points to remember are found in Box 15-14. When a patient begins a bowel program, fecal impaction can become a problem but can usually be corrected by adjusting fluid intake. In some cases stronger laxatives or enemas may be necessary. A 3- or 4-day trial of any pharmacologic agent is necessary to determine its effect. A routine can be established that prevents accidental elimination. Patients with certain neurologic disorders may require digital stimulation for an evacuation to occur. This requires placing a gloved and lubricated finger into the rectum and moving the finger in a circular motion to stimulate the anal sphincter to relax. Some patients are able to do this independently or with an adaptive device.

Impaired swallowing ability. Dysphagia describes disorders of swallowing mechanisms due to anatomic impairment or neurologic disorders (Kohler, 1991). Early assessment and identification of impaired ability to swallow is necessary for the prevention of aspira-

BOX 15-14 Guidelines of Care for Patient Establishing a Bowel Program

- A bowel program should begin without the presence of fecal impaction. If impaction is present, a Fleet's enema or soapsuds enema may be necessary.
- If possible, the patient should eat a high-fiber diet and, if medically possible, take in at least 2000 ml of fluid per day.
- Consider bowel medications if indicated. A mild laxative increases peristaltic activity. It takes about 8 hours for this medication to take effect, so plan the dose accordingly. If the elimination is scheduled for the morning, the laxative should be given the evening before. A mild suppository stimulates the rectum. It must be placed into the rectum, beyond the anal sphincter, against the rectal wall. Suppositories require about 15 to 30 minutes to take effect.
- If possible, get the patient out of bed and sitting on a toilet or commode, because the squatting position is the most effective for evacuation. The abdominal muscles contract when the thighs are flexed against the abdomen and increase intraabdominal pressure, which aids in expelling feces. If the toilet seat is too high to allow this position, a footstool or sturdy box should be placed under the patient's feet. The patient who cannot assume this squatting position will have more difficulty in establishing regular bowel patterns. Exercises that strengthen the abdominal muscles will aid evacuation, and the contraction and relaxation of perineal muscles will assist in the control of bowel evacuation.
- A regular time for evacuation should be established. The gastrocolic reflex, the increase in intestinal peristaltic activity that occurs when food enters the stomach, reaches its maximum effect 30 minutes after eating. For some patients, the most effective evacuation time is 30 minutes after breakfast. However, this is not true for everyone, and the time for evacuation is best scheduled on the previous elimination pattern.
- Privacy must be provided, and the patient should feel relaxed.

BOX 15-15

CONSEQUENCES OF DYSPHAGIA

- Aspiration pneumonia
- Malnutrition and dehydration

BOX 15-16

STAGES OF SWALLOWING

- Oral preparatory
- Oral
- Pharyngeal
- Esophageal

tion and malnutrition (Box 15-15). Aspiration has been described as the entry of material into the airway below the true vocal cords (Logemann, 1986). This can lead to the development of pneumonia and sepsis. Malnutrition may result from the patient's inability to take in sufficient nutrients to support metabolic needs.

The act of swallowing can be divided into four stages (Box 15-16). The first two are under voluntary control. During the oral preparatory stage, food is chewed and then formed into a bolus by the action of the tongue. The lips are closed tightly to keep the food and fluid in the mouth. The tongue then moves the bolus to the back of the mouth. In the oral stage the tongue squeezes the bolus against the hard palate and into the pharynx. During the pharygneal stage the reflexive, involuntary phase of swallowing begins. Pharyngeal peristalsis propels the bolus toward the esophagus, while laryngeal elevation and vocal cord closure protect the airway from aspiration. This occurs within a few seconds. In the esophageal stage, peristaltic activity allows the bolus to pass from the pharynx and enter the stomach via the cardiac sphincter. Problems wth swallowing can occur in any one of these four stages.

NURSE ALERT

Prevention of aspiration is essential in the rehabilitation of a dysphagic patient.

The patient may overtly demonstrate difficulty with swallowing by the following symptoms: dribbling food out of the mouth, holding food in the mouth for a long time without swallowing, pocketing food in one side of the mouth, little appetite, food draining from the nose, coughing or choking while eating (Phipps, 1991b) (Box 15-17). However, the patient may not demonstrate any symptoms. Swallowing difficulty may first be identified when the patient develops an aspiration pneumonia, diagnosed by a particular pattern seen on the chest x-ray film. This lack of symptoms is referred to as *silent aspiration* (Horner, Massey, 1988). The medical diagnosis may be the only indication that the patient is at risk for silent aspiration. Patients at risk include those with stroke, multiple sclerosis, Parkinson's disease, brain tumor, dementia, cranial nerve damage, or structural or anatomic changes of the swallowing mechanisms. Elderly, debilitated patients are also considered at risk, with one author suggesting that as many as 74% of nursing home patients experience eating difficulties (Kohler, 1991)

BOX 15-17

SIGNS AND SYMPTOMS OF DYSPHAGIA

Any of the following symptoms or combination of symptoms may indicate a problem with swallowing:

- Decreased appetite
- Loss of taste
- Nasal burning and dripping
- Burning or itching at back of throat
- Coughing after taking food or fluids
- Holding food in mouth
- Gurgly, wet voice
- Nasal-sounding voice
- Pocketing in affected cheek
- Drooling; asymmetry of face
- Loss of oral secretions
- Untouched food
- Eating very quickly/slowly
- Unpleasant taste in mouth

OLDER ADULT CONSIDERATIONS

Swallowing Problems of the Elderly

- Changes in muscles and ligaments involved in swallowing
- Poor dentition
- Atrophy of tongue muscles
- Diseases associated with aging
- Anatomic changes
- Neurologic disease that impairs swallowing

BOX 15-18 Guidelines for Assessing the Patient at Risk for Dysphagia

Facial-muscle testing
Ask patient to clench teeth. Palpate masseter muscle function on both sides of the face.
Ask patient to smile, frown, and whistle. Observe for bilateral function.
Tongue function
Ask patient to stick out tongue and move it to the left and to the right.
Ask patient to stick out tongue and resist pressure of tongue blade on lateral movements of the tongue.
Cough reflex
Ask patient to cough two times in rapid succession.
Swallowing reflex
Gently place thumb and forefinger on laryngeal protuberance. Ask patient to swallow. Feel for laryngeal elevation.
Gag reflex
Do not test unless cough/swallow reflexes are intact
With throat swab, gently stroke the posterior pharyngeal wall on each side observing for gag. Traditionally the gag reflex has been used as the sole initial assessment of swallowing ability. However the gag reflex is only one aspect of the process. It is the swallowing reflex that is the most protective mechanism in the swallowing process.
Quality of patient's voice
Dysphonia
Wet/hoarse
Changes in speech fluency while eating
Oral motor/sensory problems, apraxia, and perceptual problems, such as visual neglect, which have an impact on eating
Condition of the mouth and teeth

Early assessment of dysphagia, early initiation of interventions to prevent aspiration, and utilization of therapeutic techniques and feeding methods designed to fit the specific deficit in swallowing are essential aspects of care (Box 15-18).

Other assessment factors may include observing the condition of the mouth and teeth and looking into the patients' mouth for the presence of food or medication after he or she has swallowed (DiIorio, Price, 1990; Phipps, 1991).

If a patient demonstrates any difficulty during the initial assessment or is considered to be at risk of aspiration pneumonia because of a medical condition, a more detailed swallowing evaluation should be taken. The use of videofluoroscopy, using the modified barium swallow method developed by Logemann, is recommended for assessment of swallowing ability and the identification of aspiration (Chen and others, 1990; Horner, Massey, 1988; Horner and others, 1988; Logemann, 1986). The patient needs to be able to sit in a chair and to cooperate with instructions for this examination to proceed. The patient is given barium-enhanced liquid and foods of different consistencies. Swallowing is then observed and recorded through videofluoroscopy.

There is a wide variety of interventions for dysphagia and methods to prevent aspiration described in the literature (Boxes 15-19 and 15-20). If a patient is suspected of having a swallowing problem, suctioning equipment should be available during meals. Mouth care before and after eating may enhance the ability to eat. Some nursing approaches include the following:

- **Positioning**
  Ensuring that the patient is out of bed and sitting up straight in a chair
  Positioning the patient's head so that it tilts forward to enlarge the vallecular space
  Identifing the required food consistency, temperature, and texture (some patients are more successful with a thicker consistency)
- **Eating techniques**
  Feeding the patient in smaller bolus amounts
  Identifying the most effective method of feeding the patient (e.g., a teaspoon may be better than a fork)
  Teaching the patient to cough and clear before inhaling after swallowing
  Teaching the patient to swallow again after swallowing food ("the double-swallow technique")
- **Group dysphagia program** (Emick-Herring, Wood, 1990)
  Using a feeding program in a group with close supervision that includes proper positioning, patient teaching and assessment, monitoring of eating ability, and teaching about adaptive equipment
- **Patient/family education**
  Describing dysphagia and its causes
  Discussing complications of dysphagia
  Explaining approaches to feeding

Adaptive equipment

Adaptive equipment and assistive devices are selected for patients who need the support of a piece of equipment or a device to perform ADLs (Boxes 15-21 and 15-22). In settings in which there is an interdisciplinary team available to make such decisions, the physical therapist, occupational therapist, prosthetist, and orthotist assist the nurse in assessing and teaching the patient in how to use the equipment or device. In some areas of the country, there may not be such a wealth of rehabilitation professionals, and the nurse plays a more central role in teaching the patient.

The patient's functional level and level of adaptation to the disability and the architecture of his or her living environment need to be considered when selecting equipment. If they are not considered, ordered equipment may be unnecessary or may be inadequate to meet the patient's needs. Equipment selected without consultation with the patient and family may be left unused or discarded. Much of this equipment is expensive, and the insurance coverage and patient's financial situation need to be considered before a decision is made to purchase (Lowman, Klinger, 1969).

Prostheses. A **prosthesis** is an artificial substitute for some part of the body. The most common types of prostheses are artificial legs, arms, eyes, and breasts. Prostheses for amputees must be fitted for and adapted to the weight and size of the individual patient. They are made of various types of materials; however, those made of plastic are light in weight, easy to keep clean, and do not absorb body odors. Prostheses for legs are held in place by pelvic belts, waistbands, or suction cups.

Depending on the condition of the patient, temporary prostheses for above- and below-the-knee amputations can be fitted immediately following surgery. This is not always possible in the severely debilitated or medically unstable patient. These prosthesis are made of casting materials contoured to the amputation stump and provide a rigid dressing that helps to control bleeding and swelling postoperatively. A temporary peg, or pylon, and foot are attached to the cast, which allows the patient to dangle and stand with aid within a few days after surgery. There are many advantages to this procedure. The patient is more active, muscle activity and circulation are stimulated, and the process of physical rehabilitation begins immediately. An upright position soon after surgery encourages the patient and helps in adjusting to an altered body image. Application of this device at the time of surgery

BOX 15-19

NURSING INTERVENTIONS FOR DYSPHAGIA

- Positioning of the patient
- Quiet environment
- Food consistency and temperature
- Bolus size
- Swallowing techniques
- Individual therapeutic interventions
- Group therapeutic interventions
- Patient and family education

BOX 15-20 Nursing Process

REHABILITATION OF THE DYSPHAGIC PATIENT

ASSESSMENT

Gag reflex
Facial muscle strength, tongue function, ability to swallow
Residual food in mouth after eating
Choking/coughing with eating and drinking
Respiratory status
Condition of mouth and teeth

NURSING DIAGNOSES

Impaired swallowing related to neuromuscular or mechanical factor, fatigue, or decreased cognition
Risk for aspiration related to depressed cough and gag reflex and impaired swallowing

NURSING INTERVENTIONS

Maintain suction equipment at bedside.
Maintain quiet environment for meals.
Position in upright position, preferably in a chair.
Provide thick consistency of foods.
Encourage only small amounts of food at one time.
Instruct not to talk while eating.
Encourage thorough chewing and double swallowing.
Supervise all meals and fluid intake.

EVALUATION OF EXPECTED OUTCOMES

Maintains stable weight
Presents no evidence of aspiration
Verbalizes techniques that prevent choking
Demonstrates emergency measures

may decrease phantom pain, which is an unpleasant, painful sensation arising from the area of the amputated limb. This first prosthesis is temporary. Fitting of the permanent prosthesis is postponed until stump shrinkage subsides.

The amputee is confronted not only with a physical problem, but also with social, vocational, and psychological problems that require the services of the entire rehabilitation team including a skilled prosthetist, the designer and maker of the prosthesis. When healing is underway, the stump must be molded to a conical shape to fit into the prosthesis. Compression bandages are generally used for this purpose, and wrapping the stump to achieve this shape becomes part of daily care. Elastic stump-shrinking socks are also used for this purpose. Careful washing of the stump is important, and bandages should be removed and rewrapped several times a day. The skin should be completely dry before the bandages are reapplied; this prevents maceration of the suture line.

There is a wider variety of prostheses available for the patient with lower-extremity amputation than for the patient with upper-extremity amputation. The function of the arm and hand makes it more difficult to develop an upper-extremity prosthesis that is both cosmetically acceptable and functional. The hook-type is most frequently used, and cosmetic hands are available

BOX 15-21

EXAMPLES OF ASSISTIVE PRODUCTS AND DEVICES

- Sponge instead of washcloth for bathing
- Sponge attached to a long handle with a pocket for soap
- Loose clothing with large armholes
- Clothing with front closing and grippers rather than buttons
- Neckties already tied
- Elastic shoelaces and long-handled shoehorns
- Suction cups or sponge rubber mats for dishes Runways and ramps for wheelchairs
- Hand rails
- Wheelchair or ordinary chair with seat cut to fit over toilet
- Lavatories, sinks, appliances, and electrical outlets placed at a height easily reached by the patient
- Special eating utensils such as silverware with padded or curved handles, glass holders, and place guards (Figures 15-11 and 15-12)
- Food arranged clockwise on the plate and tray for the visually impaired patient (Figure 15-13)

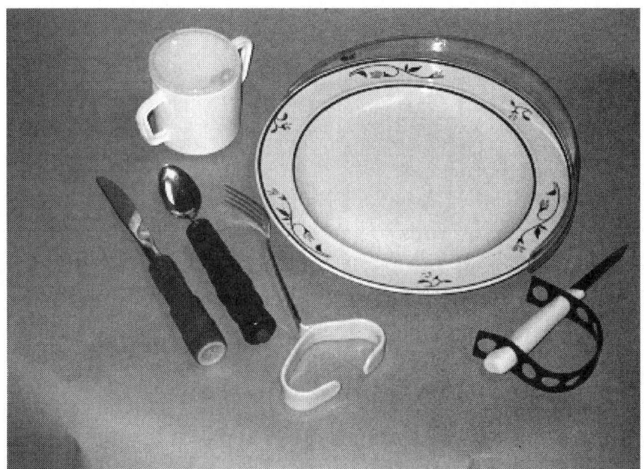

Figure 15-11 Special eating utensils. (From Elkin M and others: *Nursing interventions and clinical skills,* St Louis, 1996, Mosby.)

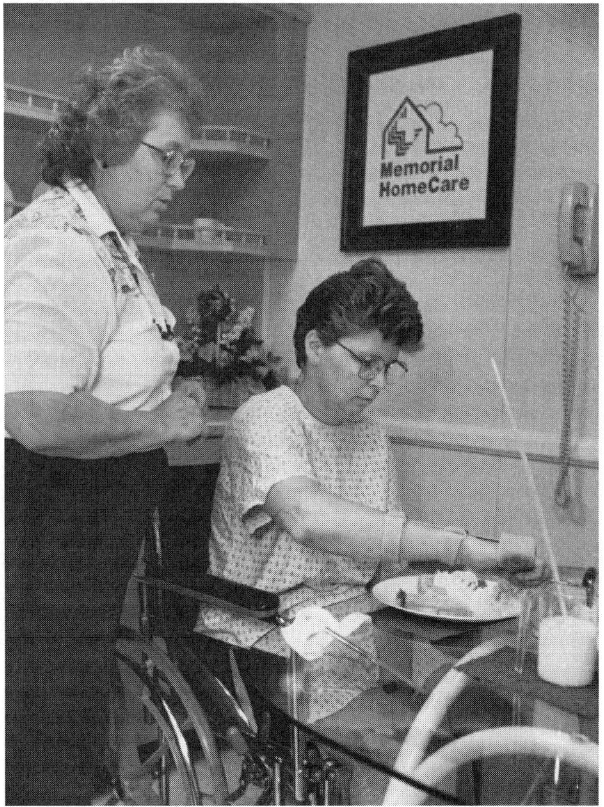

Figure 15-12 Assistive devices foster independence for those persons with handicaps.

BOX 15-22

ASSISTIVE DEVICES

EATING DEVICES

- Built-up handles on utensils for weak or incomplete grasp
- Universal cuff placed on utensils for weak or incomplete grasp
- Rocking knife for one-handed cutting
- Nonskid mats to stabilize plate for eating with one hand
- Plate guards or scoop dishes for scooping food off of plate when there is weakness or incoordination in the arm/hand
- Cuff-type holder to assist with lifting a cup
- Specially designed cups to hold liquid in the upper part of the cup to prevent excessive tilting back of the head when drinking; for patients who are at risk of aspiration because of swallowing difficulty

BATHING AND GROOMING DEVICES

- Long-handled sponge for limited reach
- Washcloth or sponge mitt for decreased grasp
- Toothbrush, hairbrush, and comb with built-up handle or universal cuff for decreased or weakened grasp
- Adapted shaving equipment
- Handheld shower nozzle
- Long-handled mirror for inspection of skin; for patients who have reaching and turning limitations and are at risk for skin breakdown

TUB AND SHOWER TRANSFER EQUIPMENT

- Nonskid mats placed in tub or shower to prevent slipping and falling
- Grab bars for use in tub or shower, if possible
- Shower and tub seats designed for decreased ability to stand in shower or sit in tub
- Shower and tub transfer seats for difficulty transferring and remaining in shower or tub
- Shower chairs that can be pushed into wheelchair-accessible shower for inability to transfer or stand while showering
- Hydraulic and motorized tub lifts for inability to get in to or out of tub, depending on architecture of bathroom

DRESSING EQUIPMENT

- Velcro closures for one-handed dressing
- Button hooks, zipper pulls, elastized shoestrings for one-handed dressing
- Long-handled reachers to pull up clothing for limited reaching ability
- Long-handled shoehorn for limited reach (Figure 15-14)

WALKING DEVICES

- Canes to provide a single point of contact with the floor and to improve stability of gait when lower extremity muscles are minimally or moderately involved. A cane should be fit to the patient, and the patient should be instructed in its use. The cane should be equipped with a rubber tip to provide traction and safety.
- Tripod or quad canes to provide three or four points of contact with the ground. These canes provide greater stability than a regular cane but are bulkier to handle.
- Walkers which differ according to structure and purpose (Ditmar, 1989): (1) adjustable, pick-up walkers are used for patients who are able to lift walker and maintain balance; (2) reciprocal walkers are designed for patients who might lose their balance when lifting a regular walker; and (3) rolling walkers increase energy-efficient walking. These walkers can be too unstable for some patients.

WHEELCHAIRS

- May be selected for the disabled patient unable to walk because of the severity of motor deficits or because of fatigue, medical complications, or other functional problems
- Selection may be a joint decision of the interdisciplinary team with direction from physical and occupational therapy.
- Selection based on the patient's dimensions, need for modifications, wheelchair weight requirements, and the patient's need for safety, comfort, and maneuverability.

WHEELCHAIR CUSHIONS

- Should be used by any patient who spends time sitting in wheelchair, particularly for comfort and prevention of skin breakdown.
- Selection based on the patient's mobility status, body build, nutrition, and skin care status.

TRANSFER DEVICES

- Transfer boards, plastic or wooden boards for the patient who cannot stand, to perform sliding transfer from bed to wheelchair or wheelchair to and from car
- Hydraulic lifts for bed-to-chair, chair-to-tub, or chair-to-car transfers; for patients unable to stand to transfer
- Hydraulic or electric stair lifts; for patients unable to climb stairs
- Chairs with seats that raise electrically or mechanically; for patients unable to lift out of seat

to fit over the hook on some models. This prosthesis is very difficult to master. The myoelectric prosthesis is more acceptable cosmetically and has capabilities not previously available. It is capable of gross hand motion, index finger-thumb opposition, grasp, and wrist pronation and supination. It does not, however, provide fine movements of the fingers and hand. It is most effective when the lost extremity is on the nondominant side. The right-handed person who loses his left arm will not require as much fine movement in the prosthesis. When the prosthesis arrives and the patient begins to wear it, the patient and the family should be instructed in care of the stump and the prosthesis. Not all patients are suitable candidates for an artificial extremity, and numerous factors, with careful examination of the individual patients, have to be considered.

In teaching a patient to care for a prosthesis, a number of areas should be addressed. Cleanliness is important to prevent skin problems. The socket of the prosthesis should be washed, rinsed, and dried daily. Lint and dirt should be removed and joints lightly oiled once a week. Joints should be inspected for loose or worn parts and replacements made promptly by a prosthetist. Any problems or changes in the fit (as occur normally when the stump shrinks) should be reported as well. The skin beneath the prosthesis is prone to irritation and breakdown if not carefully cared for and inspected. Daily hygiene is essential. Soap and water followed by a thorough rinsing is adequate. The patient should avoid creams or preparations containing alcohol. When a stump sock is used, it must fit well and be free of wrinkles and mended areas. The sock is also washed daily in cool water and mild soap. A lower-extremity stump will shrink over time, requiring adjustments to the socket of the prosthesis. The patient should be warned against padding the stump or socket with cotton or washcloths, because the uneven pressure distribution that results will cause pressure areas on the skin and possible infection. A change in stump size requires a visit to the prosthetist for adjustment. Also, if the patient has a change in weight, the fit of the prosthesis can be affected.

An artificial eye is made of glass or plastic and is painted by a skilled artist to match the patient's other eye. Eyes made of glass are heavier than those made of plastic and are easily broken if dropped. Those made of plastic, although lighter, are less durable and may be scratched unless care is taken. The prosthesis may be used as soon as the socket is healed, which may be from 3 to 6 weeks after surgery.

When the artificial eye is removed for cleaning, it can be removed by pulling down on the lower eyelid and letting the prosthesis slip out of the eye socket. The prosthesis can be washed with soap and water and stored in a clean piece of gauze or a labeled enve-

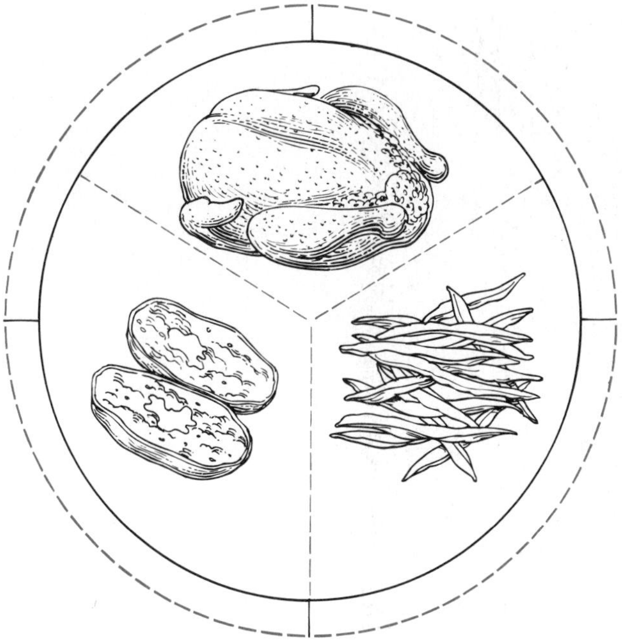

Figure 15-13 Clockwise arrangement of food for visually impaired. (From Elkin M and others: *Nursing interventions and clinical skills,* St Louis, 1996, Mosby.)

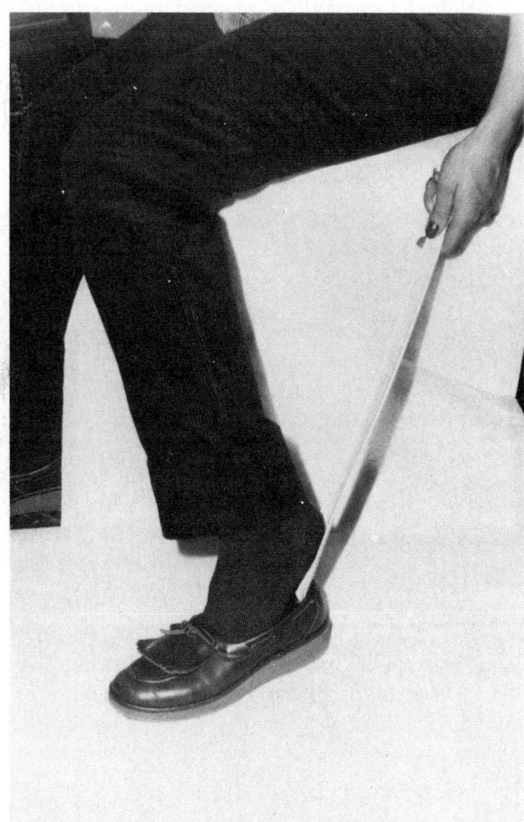

Figure 15-14 Long-handled shoehorn. (From Phipps M and others: *Medical-surgical nursing,* ed 5, St Louis, 1995, Mosby.

lope. It will need to be moistened before it is reinserted; sterile saline is generally used for this. To replace the prosthesis, the nurse should pull down on the lower eyelid, slip the artificial eye into the eye socket, lift up the upper lid, and position the prosthesis in place. The patient must be taught how to remove and insert the prosthesis. The patient may be nervous at first but will soon master the technique and develop skill and confidence. When a patient with an eye prosthesis is admitted to the hospital, the nurse should realize that the patient has a special method of caring for the eye and should supply whatever equipment needed. The nurse should not try to change the person's methods.

Braces. The overall purpose of using **braces** is to improve patient mobility. Specifically, braces may be used to support the body weight, limit involuntary movement of the body, and prevent and correct deformities. Leg braces may be of the short-leg or long-leg type and may have attachments, depending on the purpose for which they are used. Braces usually consist of a steel frame with joints, hinges, and straps. Belts are used to secure them in place. Braces are generally attached to the heel of the shoe. An inside lining on the straps protects the body from friction.

The patient should be taught proper care of the brace. All locks should be opened regularly, and lint and dirt should be removed. A drop of machine oil should be placed in each joint and the excess wiped away because any oil left on leather causes deterioration. The leather parts may be washed with warm water and saddle soap, then dried and polished. Shoes should be kept in good repair and should have rubber heels. If knees pads are part of the brace, they should be worn with it. The skin under the brace should be inspected daily for discoloration, bruises, abrasions, or evidence of friction.

Children who wear braces during their growth periods should be checked at intervals. Any changes indicated should be made promptly. A brace that is too small for a growing child may do more harm than good. Braces may be used to support the torso and should be applied with the patient lying down with the body in good alignment. A cotton shirt worn beneath a back brace helps absorb perspiration and body odors and contributes to comfort.

The patient needs to be prepared for the use of a brace. Range-of-motion exercises and other prescribed exercises should be taught to the patient and done regularly before the brace is applied. The patient needs to be instructed on the proper position to assume when applying the brace. A back brace is more easily applied while the patient is in bed. To be prepared psychologically, the patient should understand why the braces are necessary, how they will help, and how to care for them. Unless the patient is prepared, he or she may resent it and develop a negative attitude, in which case its value may be minimized. Young persons may be concerned with the cosmetic effect and must be given the chance to express their feelings.

Crutches. **Crutches** are assistive walking devices (Figure 15-15). They may be used temporarily or per-

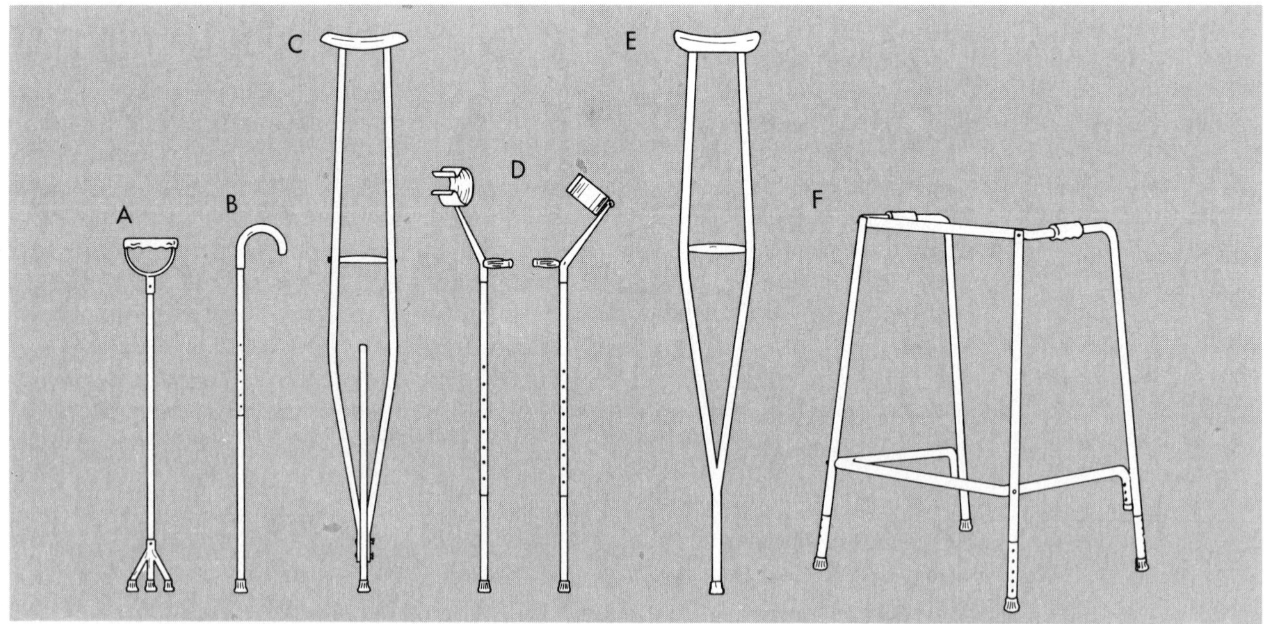

Figure 15-15 Types of crutches and canes. **A,** Quadripod cane. **B,** Adjustable aluminum cane. **C,** Adjustable aluminum crutch. **D,** Adjustable aluminum Canadian crutch. **E,** Nonadjustable wooden crutch available in various lengths, **F,** Walker.

BOX 15-23 Guidelines of Care for Patient Using Crutch Walking

1 The patient should be measured for crutches so that they will be the right length. Crutches should be adjustable and have heavy rubber tips.
2 Padding of the axillary bar is generally discouraged because it encourages the patient to place weight or lean on it. By doing so, the patient may develop a paralysis of the radial nerve (crutch paralysis). Crutches that are too long or too short may also cause crutch paralysis. Crutch length should be adjustable so that the patient bears *no* weight in the axilla.
3 The patient should be taught from the beginning to maintain good posture. The head should be held high and straight, with the pelvis over the feet (see Figure 15-16).
4 Crutch walking must be taught. Several short lessons a day are of more value to the patient than one long session, which can result in fatigue.
5 When ambulation is begun, it is desirable to have an attendant in front of the patient and one behind; however, they should not touch the patient.
6 Whether the patient is able to bear weight or shift weight will depend on the disability and the physician's order. Some patients, especially elderly ones, may learn to use a walker before using crutches.

manently, but in either case both the nurse and the physical therapist have important roles in helping to prepare the patient for crutch walking (Box 15-23). If the patient is on bed rest, exercises can begin in bed to strengthen the muscle groups involved in the use of crutches. These include the muscles of the neck, arms, shoulders, chest, and back. Resistance exercises with the use of weights are the most effective way to increase strength. Weights can be attached to the overhead trapeze or a rope fastened to a pulley at the foot of the bed. The patient can be taught how to do push-ups by placing his or her palms flat on the bed, or sawed-off crutches can be used. The ability to stand and the status of standing balance are important areas to consider prior to initiating crutch training. Older patients may have a poor sense of balance and coordination. They may be fearful and find it difficult to strengthen muscles before walking. Ideally, parallel bars should be used in helping the patient stand and achieve balance before crutch walking is attempted. The physical therapist usually fits the patient with crutches and assists the patient with standing and balance during initial attempts to walk with crutches. In many places it is the responsibility of the physician and the nurse (Figure 15-16).

There are several types of crutch walking or crutch gait. The type used depends on the disability. The most common types of crutch gait include four-point gait, two-point gait, and swing-to or swing-through gait (Figure 15-17). In four-point gait the patient bears weight on both legs, one at each step. There are always three points of contact with the floor—the crutch tips and one foot. This type of gait requires constant shifting. In two-point gait there are two points of contact with the floor. This method is similar to the four-point gait, but it is faster. In swing-to gait the patient places the crutches ahead, then lifts his or her weight on the crutches and swings the body to the crutches. Swing-through gait is similar, except the patient lifts his or her weight and swings beyond the crutches. In three-point gait, weight is placed on the crutches and the unaffected leg. It may be used when partial weight bearing is permitted.

A patient who has been taught to use crutches should have mastered sufficient daily care activities to be independent when leaving the hospital. The patient should also have been taught how to get up and down steps and into and out of cars.

PATIENT TEACHING IN REHABILITATION

The nurse assumes a major role in teaching the patient and family. For a patient participating in a rehabilitation program this teaching might include the following:

- Reinforcement of skills taught in therapy sessions, such as self-care activities, transfers, and crutch walking
- A description of the illness or disability and a description of the expected course of the disease process
- Health practices that the patient needs to incorporate into daily living to stay healthy
- Symptoms that indicate a health problem has developed and further healthcare is needed
- Methods to find healthcare when needed
- A description of the rationale for medications and potential side effects

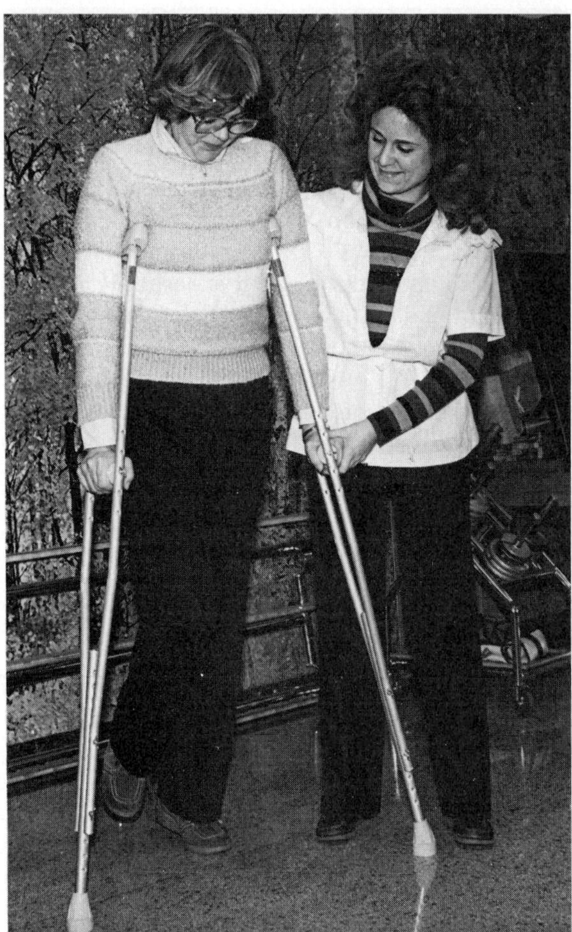

Figure 15-16 In assessing patient using crutches, nurse observes fit, posture, and gait. (Courtesy Copley Memorial Hospital, Aurora, Ill.)

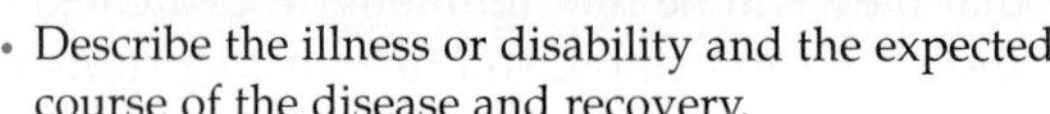

PATIENT/FAMILY TEACHING

- Describe the illness or disability and the expected course of the disease and recovery.
- The patient and family should be involved with rehabilitation efforts and discharge planning.
- Education should be ongoing as the patient progresses toward discharge.
- Assess the learning needs and abilities of the patient and family members.
- Provide an environment conducive to learning.
- Review educational materials before giving them to the patient and family.
- Progress from the simple to the complex.
- Treat the patient and family as adults.
- Provide time for practice, discussion, and feedback.
- Evaluate the need for a group-teaching program.
- Evaluate the impact of teaching.
- Reinforce skills taught in therapy sessions, such as self-care activities, transfers, and crutch walking.
- Review health practices that the patient needs to incorporate into daily living to stay healthy.
- Staff should continually assess the patient's and family's understanding of the information provided.
- List symptoms that indicate a health problem has developed and further healthcare is needed.
- Go over methods to find healthcare when needed.
- Describe the rationale for medications and potential side effects.
- Medication changes should be reviewed as they are made.
- Offer approaches to locating home supports when needed.
- Teach approaches to instructing others in how to care for the patient.
- Families should be urged to continue participation in family-education programs.
- Families should be provided as much information as possible about rehabilitation programs and services.
- Follow-up appointments with physicians and therapists should be scheduled prior to discharge.
- Visiting nurse and discharge summaries should be prepared for the patient's discharge.

- Approaches to locating home supports when needed

The nurse should assess the learning needs and abilities of the patient before establishing a teaching plan. An important question to ask is, "What does the patient and family need to know to have an easier transition at discharge?" When teaching a patient an activity or providing some important information, the environment should be as conducive to learning as possible. Teaching during a nonstressful time of day, in a quiet place, and without any sense of haste is important. This is especially true for the elderly, who do not have difficulty learning new material in general but have difficulty learning new skills in a limited period of time (Katzman, Terry, 1983). Finding a quiet environment in an acute-care hospital may be difficult, but with planning, it is not impossible. Some patients will tire easily and will need frequent rest periods.

Along with teaching, the nurse should provide educational materials. The stress of learning new information may decrease retention. Having reference materials available to reinforce new information may help the patient and family in understanding and applying new ideas. Not all educational materials contain correct information or are appropriate to the needs of all patients. In some hospitals or agencies, nurses participate in patient-education committees. One task of this committee is to review patient-education materials for

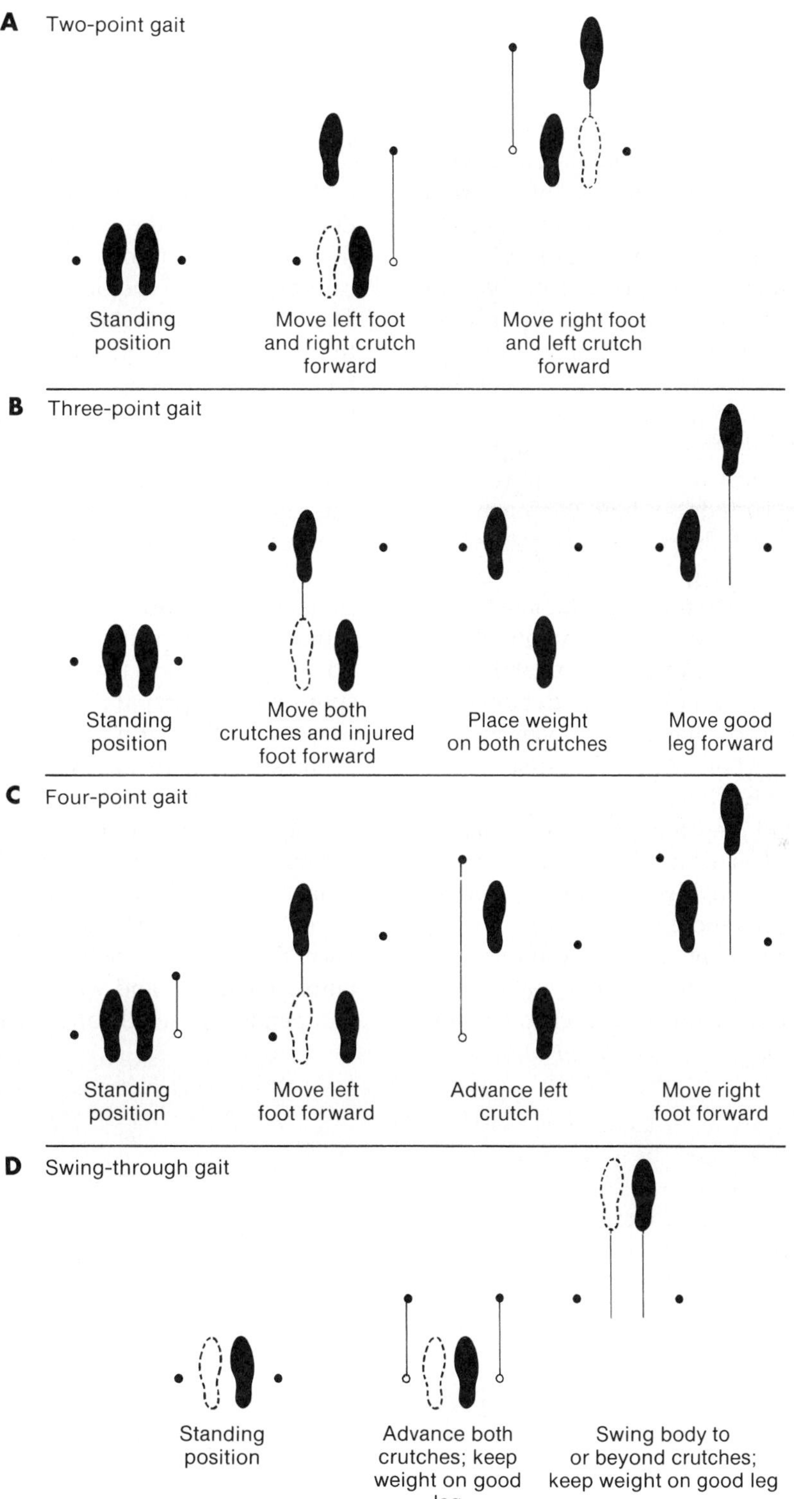

Figure 15-17 Crutch walking. **A,** Two-point gait. **B,** Three-point gait. **C,** Four-point gait. **D,** Swing-through gait.

acceptability, readability, and accuracy.

A basic principle of teaching and learning is to progress from the simple to the complex. Simple activities should be taught first and each mastered before a new one is begun. The patient may become discouraged and need encouragement. Even the slightest progress should be noted. The patient needs to be treated as an adult and never belittled or demeaned if unable to master a new skill or retain new information. Patience will need to be learned by those who become frustrated and overwhelmed by the amount of detail needed to complete some skills. Some patients may never develop this degree of patience, and participation in rehabilitation will remain a difficult task. The nurse also needs to demonstrate a keen understanding and patience when assisting patients.

Providing a patient with the opportunity to practice a task or to discuss information is also important. In teaching the patient to be independent, the nurse may need to sit back and watch the patient struggle with a new task. After demonstrating the task and giving the patient an opportunity to return the demonstration and practice, the nurse must let the patient do the work or task alone. Nurses working in rehabilitation have to learn to "hold their hands behind their backs," and let the patients do for themselves, even if it involves discomfort for the patient and the nurse.

Another approach to teaching new skills or new information is the use of group-teaching sessions for both patients and families. Bringing together patients with similar disabilities provides the opportunity for the nurse to reach a larger audience and for patients to share their insights, questions, and frustrations with each other. Within these group situations, patients often develop close relationships with each other and can learn new ways of coping. Laughter, one of the most important coping skills, often becomes an important part of these group activities (Schmitt, 1990). Group-teaching programs for families can also provide information, support, and coping strategies.

CONTINUITY OF CARE

There must be continuity between the care the patient receives in the hospital and the care received in the home. In addition, there must be continuity in the care given by all members of the rehabilitation team. The patient must be taught one way to perform an activity and practice on a single method. If the patient is taught different ways, he or she will become confused, frustrated, and discouraged. The nurse can assist each therapist who works with the patient by observing and reporting progress or lack of progress. The nurse can report to the therapist any significant problems in connection with the activities the patient practices. If the patient must leave the ward for therapy, it is important that the nurse see that the appointment is kept promptly and that the patient is in presentable condition. As progress is made, the patient may be held responsible for preparation and for keeping appointments with little or no help from the nurse.

Participation in a rehabilitation program is a tremendous challenge for the patient and family. Through this process, disabled persons and those with chronic illnesses are assisted in achieving the maximum level of independence possible. With knowledge, skill, understanding, patience, and perseverance, the nurse can help the disabled person and the family recognize and work toward the possibilities of independence, health, and well-being.

Nursing Care Plan*

CARE OF THE STROKE PATIENT

Mr. Roberts, a 64-year-old retired salesman, was admitted to the emergency room of an acute-care hospital with hemiplegia, paralysis of the arm, trunk, and leg, on the right side of his body. He was also unable to speak. He has a long history of hypertension and had been a diabetic for the past 16 years. He also has a long history of smoking and is significantly overweight. He was diagnosed as having a stroke and was transferred to the stroke unit.

During the first 24 hours on this unit, Mr. Roberts was carefully assessed by the nursing staff. Vital signs and neurologic evaluation were completed every 2 hours. His cardiac status was monitored via telemetry. He was placed on bed rest and made NPO. He was given fluids intravenously. An MRI performed that day revealed that Mr. Roberts had not sustained a hemorrhagic stroke. He was diagnosed as having a thrombotic stroke, caused by the narrowing of his internal carotid artery.

The nurse's assessment indicated that Mr. Roberts had difficulty swallowing, so the head of his bed was raised 30 degrees to prevent aspiration. Occupational, physical, swallowing, and speech therapy consultation were requested. The social services department was notified of this patient's arrival.

On the second day in the hospital, Mr. Roberts was evaluated by all members of the interdisciplinary team, and the team met to plan his care. He was found to have a severe paralysis of his right arm, with some improvement in the movement of his right leg. He was dependent in self-care activities. He was able to begin making some speech, although it was rather garbled. The swallowing therapist felt that Mr. Roberts had some problems with swallowing because of weakness in the muscles of his face and some delay in initiating swallowing. The nurse related that Mr. Roberts was extremely fearful and his wife and children were very anxious and worried. Mr. Roberts had been incontinent and had problems sitting up straight in bed. The social worker made plans to meet with the patient and family. The team identified the need to educate the Roberts family about stroke and the consequences of stroke, as well as describe the rehabilitation services in the community.

Over the next few days Mr. Roberts made remarkable progress. He was able to sit on the edge of the bed and with the assistance of the therapist and nurse, stand and turn to sit in a chair. He was able to assist with his bath but not with dressing. He tired easily but was able to sit up in a wheelchair. He was started on a soft solid diet, taken with the supervision of the nurse. He did well with this and did not appear to aspirate or choke. His speech became more clear, and his urinary incontinence cleared. He was screened and accepted by a local rehabilitation hospital.

The nurse discussed the outcome of stroke with the patient and family. They were given materials to read, and the nurse talked with them about approaches to prevent another stroke. His medications were reviewed, and the nurse stressed the importance of blood pressure control, careful monitoring of his diabetes, weight loss, and smoking cessation.

After 6 days in the acute-care hospital, Mr. Roberts was transferred to the rehabilitation hospital.

NURSING DIAGNOSIS

Impaired physical mobility related to neurologic impairment
Self-care deficit related to impaired mobility
Impaired verbal communication related to neurologic impairment
Altered urinary elimination pattern related to neurologic impairment
Altered bowel elimination, related to neurologic impairment
Risk for injury: falling related to impaired mobility
Risk for impaired skin integrity related to impaired mobility
Impaired swallowing related to neurologic impairment
Risk for activity intolerance related to impaired mobility
Body image disturbance related to neurologic deficits

*This style of care plan is common in rehabilitation hospitals. This care plan is based on a critical pathway for evaluation of the progress of a stroke patient.

continued

Nursing Care Plan

CARE OF THE STROKE PATIENT—CONT'D

Days 1-2

Assessment Data	Nursing Interventions	Patient and Family Teaching
• *Neurologic:* Motor, sensory, and cognitive assessment swallowing assessment • *Cardiovascular and respiratory:* Vital sign monitoring every 2-4 hours; ECG monitoring; cardiac telemetry; monitoring of cardiac enzymes; respiratory rate and rhythm; breath sounds; ability to handle secretions • Laboratory studies • *Volume status:* I&O measurement; daily weight • Consultations to be made within the first 24 hours include social services, physical therapy, and occupational therapy • Additional consultations to be made within the first 24 hours based on neurologic findings include swallowing therapy, speech therapy, nutrition, and neuropsychology • Monitoring for presence of deep vein thrombosis • *Nutrition:* Swallowing and eating ability; weight and height; diet history and dietary requirements; baseline laboratory measures of nutritional status • *Medical history:* Previous stroke, TIA, hypertension, diabetes, cardiac or pulmonary disease, history of smoking, excessive alcohol intake • Medication history, medication compliance • Functional status prior to admission, living arrangements prior to admission • Assessment of family and social support • *Beginning fall risk assessment:* History of falls prior to admission	• Notify physician of any changes in neurologic, cardiac, or pulmonary status, or of any abnormal laboratory findings. • Maintain optimum pulmonary function. Turn every 2 to 4 hours, encourage deep breathing and coughing to clear airway, chest physiotherapy as needed, oxygen therapy as needed. • Monitor blood pressure control within physician-designated parameters. • Continue to monitor fluid and volume status. • Monitor patient activity. The patient is typically on bed rest for the first 24 hours. Bed rest is maintained to rule out myocardial infarction and/or to provide adequate cerebral perfusion. The patient is turned and repositioned every 2 hours, with bony prominences and skin assessed with repositioning. Affected limbs should be positioned to protect joint mobility and prevent injury. The patient is carefully moved in bed to prevent injury to paretic limbs; a pull sheet is used to prevent pulling on hemiparetic limbs. Range-of-motion is provided to involved limbs to promote movement and prevent joint contracture formation. Splints are used as needed; splints are removed and skin is inspected frequently. Bed mobility is encouraged by having the patient assist with turning and moving in bed. Fall prevention strategies are initiated (e.g., bed alarms and toileting schedule). • Institute measures to prevent deep vein thrombosis. • Monitor medications. • Prepare patient and family for evaluative procedures (e.g., CT scan, MRI, Holter monitor, echo cardiography).	• Patient and family education about stroke begins on admission. • Interdisciplinary team members collaborate and provide the family with initial information about stroke; the impact of stroke; and the rationale for initial medical, nursing, and therapeutic interventions. • Evaluative procedures and the experience of acute-care hospitalization are discussed. • The family is provided with reading materials about stroke and invited to stroke-education forums.

Nursing Care Plan

CARE OF THE STROKE PATIENT—CONT'D

Nursing Assessment	Days 3-4 Nursing Interventions	Patient and Family Teaching
• Assessment is ongoing and dependent upon the severity and complications of the stroke. • Neurologic assessment • *Cardiovascular and respiratory assessment:* As the patient's activity level is increased, endurance should be monitored through frequent vital-sign measurements and assessing patient's appearance and complaints of fatigue. • *Functional assessment:* Levels of functional ability such as bed mobility, sitting balance, transfer ability, standing balance, and walking ability should be evaluated. Orthostatic hypotension is evaluated prior to getting the patient out of bed. Self-care ability should be evaluated and include bathing, grooming, feeding, dressing, and toileting • Continued swallowing and nutritional assessment • *Bladder and bowel assessment:* Indwelling catheters should be removed as soon as possible. For continued urinary incontinence, review additional factors such as history of incontinence, physical examination, urinalysis, functional ability, mental status, presence of urinary tract infection, and gynecologic or prostatic problems. Obtain a 24-hour incontinence record. Identify type of bowel dysfunction and evaluate cause: immobility and inactivity, inadequate fluid or nutritional intake, infection, cognitive deficit, impaired mobility. • Continued fall risk assessment: If the patient's activity is increased, the patient's balance and stability while sitting and walking should be evaluated. Mental status evaluation and perceptual evaluation are other factors to consider.	• The level of nursing intervention depends on the severity of the patient's stroke, the resultant functional and cognitive deficits, and the medical condition. Many of these interventions are initiated in the acute-care setting and continued in the rehabilitation setting or home. Interdisciplinary collaboration is an integral aspect of planning interventions. • Continue cardiac monitoring. Cardiac telemetry will most likely be continued if arrhythmias are present. Otherwise telemetry will generally be discontinued. • Continue to monitor pertinent laboratory results. • Continue respiratory monitoring. • Continue to monitor patient activity. The patient should be out of bed and sitting in chair as soon as medically and neurologically possible. The patient's level of activity is determined by cardiac and respiratory status and level of endurance. The initiation of rehabilitation therapies—physical, occupational, speech, and swallowing—should begin as soon as possible. The patient should be encouraged to participate in as much self-care as possible. • *Approaches to swallowing:* Identify needed changes in positioning: position of trunk and position of head. Identify the need for changes in food consistency, temperature, and bolus size. Identify environmental factors: need for decreased distractions and quiet and privacy during eating. • *Approaches to urinary incontinence:* Involves early removal of indwelling urinary catheter and determination of postvoid residuals through catheterization. If residual is greater than 100 ml, determine need for intermittent catheterization. Place patient on scheduled program of toileting, with schedule based on 24-hour incontinence record. Ensure protection of	• Patients and families will need continued support and education. At this time, teaching should center on assessing the family's ability to be involved in the patient's care. Once the family's level of involvement is determined, learning needs can be better established. During this time of great stress, explanations may require frequent repetition. Results of tests and procedures may be available and need to be shared with the patient and/or family. Further investigation of the patient's living situation and potential discharge plans should begin to be addressed. The social worker will be informed of the needs and involved in the planning. Discussion of the need for rehabilitation and the type of needed setting are initiated.

continued

Nursing Care Plan

CARE OF THE STROKE PATIENT—CONT'D

Days 3-4

Nursing Assessment	Nursing Interventions	Patient and Family Teaching
• *Language assessment:* Speech therapy should be consulted if there is any indication that the patient is having difficulty with the production or comprehension of language; reading, writing, or using gestures; or moving the lips, tongue, and mouth in a coordinated fashion to produce speech. • *Perceptual assessment:* Occupational therapy should assist the nurse in identifying the presence of any perceptual deficits. Examples of some patient cues include lack of acknowledgement of one side of the environment; inability to recognize function of object by shape and/or touch; denial of one side of the body; denial of illness.	skin through cleaning and use of skin barriers. When necessary, maintain containment of urine through condom drainage system for men. • *Approaches to bowel care:* Establish a bowel program based on previous bowel pattern. Begin a high-fiber diet if possible. Encourage adequate fluid intake. Establish an elimination schedule. If necessary, use a stool softener and suppository regime, but enforce judicious use of laxatives. • *Approaches to language disturbance:* Collaborate with speech therapist in planning communication strategies. Keep communication with patient simple. Attempt to limit patient's frustrations with limitations in communication ability. • *Approaches to perceptual deficits:* Collaborate with occupational therapist and all members of the interdisciplinary team in planning strategies of care. • Identify methods to promote patient safety. Identify environmental factors that may enhance perceptual ability.	

Days 4-7, Through Discharge

Nursing Assessment	Nursing Interventions
• The focus of nursing assessment is shifted toward assessment of rehabilitation needs and discharge planning. Patient and family coping will be continually addressed as well. Nursing assessment should continue to include all the previously discussed areas with particular emphasis on neurological and functional status and ongoing assessment of the patient's ability to swallow and nutritional status if a problem has been identified in these areas. Cardiac telemetry will be discontinued if the patient has remained stable hemodynamically. Otherwise, it will continue until any problems have been addressed. Monitoring of laboratory results will continue throughout the hospitalization, particularly if the patient is being anticoagulated or has an ongoing medical problem.	• The patient's functional status and available family and community supports determine the need for continued rehabilitation services. Discharge planning is the major focus at this time. Members of the interdisciplinary team are actively involved in identifying the need for continued rehabilitation and the selection of the best type of facility or agency to provide those needed services.

KEY CONCEPTS

- Rehabilitation is the process of assisting individuals with disability or chronic illness to the highest possible level of independence and well-being.
- Rehabilitation programs are designed to restore an individual's ability to function physically, emotionally, socially, educationally, and vocationally.
- Rehabilitation stresses restoration of normal function, prevention of complications, education of patient and family, and adaptation.
- Short- and long-term care plans are developed with the patient in consideration of his or her values, beliefs, lifestyle choices, and culture.
- Application of all the components of the nursing process are an integral part of rehabilitation programs.
- Communication with the rehabilitation team is essential during all levels of health service.
- An individual's body image may undergo significant changes as a result of disability or chronic illness.
- The success of rehabilitation programs depends on the individual's motivation.
- Plans that incorporate range-of-motion are integral activities for the nurse and patient during all phases of care.
- Pressure sores are preventable through a disciplined plan of movement, frequent positioning, and selected equipment.
- Urinary incontinence can be reduced or prevented through bladder and habit training, prompt voiding, and Kegel exercises.
- Aspiration can be reduced or prevented by positioning the patient properly while eating, adjusting the consistency of food, and applying different eating techniques.
- Adaptive equipment is chosen in an individual basis, in consideration of need, cost, and usefulness in different settings.
- Aspects of patient education are incorporated into the rehabilitation program.

CRITICAL THINKING EXERCISES

1. Why is it important to consider the whole patient (incuding family and community) in attempts to restore an individual to a productive life?
2. What factors make rehabilitation of the elderly and chronically ill more difficult than other patient groups?
3. How do race and culture affect the individual's plan of care?

REFERENCES AND ADDITIONAL READINGS

Agency for Health Care Policy and Research: *Pressure sores in adults: prediction and prevention,* Rockville, Md, 1992a. Public Health Service, Department of Health and Human Service, Publication No 92-0047.

Agency for Health Care Policy and Research: *Urinary incontinence in the adult,* Rockville, Md, 1992b. Public Health Service, US Department of Health and Human Service Publication No 92-0038.

American Nurses Association and Association of Rehabilitation Nurses: *Rehabilitation Nursing,* Kansas City, Mo. 1988, The Association.

Americans with Disability Act: *A guide to provisions affecting persons with seizure disorders,* Landover, Md, 1992, Epilepsy Foundation of America.

Banja JD: Rehabilitation and empowerment, *Archives of Phys Med Rehab* 71(8):614-615, 1990.

Bergstrom, N, et al: The Braden Scale for predicting pressure sore risk, *Nurs Res* 36(4):205-210, 1987.

Braden B, Bergstrom N: Clinical utility of the Braden Scale for predicting pressure sore risk, *Decubitus* 2(3):44-51, 1989.

Chen M and others: Oropharynx in patients with cerebrovascular disease: evaluation with videofluoroscopy, *Rad* 176(3):641-643, 1990.

DiIorio C, Price M: Swallowing: an assessment guide, *Am J Nurs* 90(7):42-46, 1990.

Dittmar S, editor: *Rehabilitation Nursing,* St Louis, 1989, Mosby.

Emick-Herring B, Wood P: A team approach to neurologically based swallowing disorders, *Rehab Nurs* 15(3):126-131, 1990.

Fiatarone M and others: Exercise training and nutritional supplementation for physical frailty in elderly people, *N*

Engl J Med 330(25):1769-1775, 1994.

Fiatarone M and others: The Boston FICSIT study: the effects of resistance training and nutritional supplementation on physical frailty in the oldest old, *J Am Geriatr Soc* 41(2):333-337, 1993.

Glennon TP, Smith BS: Questions asked by patients and their support groups during family conferences on inpatient rehabilitation units, *Archives of Phys Med Rehab* 71(8):699-702, 1990.

Gross J: Bladder dysfunction after stroke, *J Gerontol Nurs* 16(4):20-25, 1990.

Guide for the Uniform Data Set for Medical Rehabilitation (Adult FIM), Version 4.0. Buffalo, 1993, State University of New York at Buffalo.

Hesse K, Campion E: Motivating the geriatric patient for rehabilitation, *J Am Geriatr Soc* 31(10):586-589, 1983.

Hoeman S, editor: *Rehabilitation nursing*, ed 2, St Louis, 1995, Mosby.

Horner J, Massey E: Silent aspiration following stroke, *Neurology* 38(2):317-319, 1988.

Horner J and others: Aspiration following stroke: clinical correlates and outcomes, *Neurology* 38(6):1359-1362, 1988.

Jamison S: A handheld positioning device to reduce wrist and finger hypertonicity, *Nurs Res* 29(5):285-289, 1980.

Jette A (ed): Functional disability and rehabilitation of the aged, *Top Geriatr Rehab* 1(3):1-9, 1986.

Katzman R, Terry R: *The neurology of aging.* Philadelphia, 1983, FA Davis.

Kelly-Hayes M: A preventive approach to stroke, *Nurs Clin North Am* 26(4):931-943, 1991.

Kohler E: A dysphagia model for rural elderly, *Phys Occup Ther Geriatr* 10(1):81-95, 1991.

Learman LA and others: Pygmalion in the nursing home: the effect of caregiver expectations on patient outcome, *J Am Geriatr Soc* 38(7):797-803, 1990.

Lewis C: *Improving mobility in older patients,* Rockville, Md, 1989, Aspen Publications.

Logemann J: Treatment for aspiration related to dysphagia: an overview, *Dysphagia,* 1:34-38, 1986.

Lowman E, Klinger J: *Aids to independent living,* NY, 1969, McGraw-Hill.

Mahoney FI: Functional evaluation: the Barthel Index, *Maryland State Med J* 14:56-61, 1965.

McCourt A, editor: *The specialty practice of rehabilitation nursing: a core curriculum* (3 ed), Skokie, Ill, 1993, Rehabilitation Nursing Foundation.

Mol V, Baker C: Activity intolerance in the elderly stroke patient, *Rehab Nurs* 16(6):337-343, 1991.

Nagi S: Disability concepts revisited. In *Sociology and rehabilitation,* Washington, DC, 1965, American Sociological Association.

Norton D, McLaren R, Exton-Smith: *An investigation of geriatric nursing problems in the hospital,* London, 1962, National Corporation for the Care of Old People (now the Centre for Policy on Ageing).

Paillard M, Nowak K: Use of exercise to help older adults, *J Gerontol Nurs* 11(7):36-39, 1985.

Payton O, Poland J: Aging process: implications for clinical practice, *Phys Therapy* 63(1):41-47, 1983.

Phipps M, Kelly-Hayes M: Rehabilitation of Older Adults. In *Perspectives in Gerontological Nursing,* Newbury Park, Calif, 1991, Safe Publications.

Phipps M: Assessment of neurologic deficits in stroke: acute-care and rehabilitation implications, *Nurs Clin North Am* 26(4):957-971, 1991.

Phipps M, Bauman B: Staging care for pressure sores, *Am J Nurs* 84(8):999-1003, 1984.

Schmitt N: Patients perception of laughter in a rehabilitation hospital, *Rehab Nurs* 15(3):143-147, 1990.

Smith E, editor: Exercise and aging, *Top Geriatr Rehab* 1(1):1-88, 1985.

Strauss A, Glaser B: *Chronic illness and the quality of life,* ed 2, St Louis, 1984, Mosby.

Sudarsky L: Geriatrics: gait disorders in the elderly, *N Engl J Med* 322(20):1441-1446, 1990.

Venn R and others: The influence of timing and suppository use on efficiency and effectiveness of bowel training after stroke, *Rehab Nurs* 17(3):116-120, 1992.

Wells T: Additional treatments for urinary incontinence, *Top Geriatr Rehab* 3(2):48-58, 1988.

Werner-Beland J: *Grief responses to long-term illness and disability,* Reston, Va, 1980, Reston Publishing.

World Health Organization: *International classification of impairments, disabilities, and handicaps: a manual of classification relating to the consequences of disease,* Geneva, 1980, The Organization.

CHAPTER 16

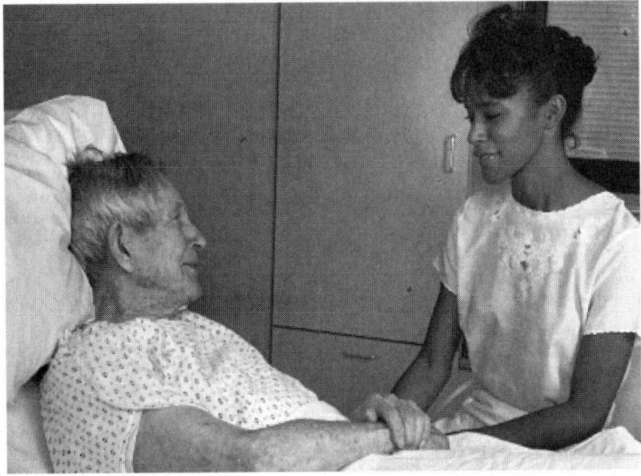

Long-Term Care

CHAPTER OBJECTIVES

1 Explain the relationship of a nursing home to long-term care.
2 Explain how the concepts of autonomy, independence, and maintenance or improvement of function guide the care of the nursing home resident.
3 Define medical ethics.
4 Explain differences between life-sustaining measures and "do not resuscitate" orders.
5 Discuss general areas important for a nursing assessment of the older person.
6 Discuss risk factors and preventive measures for falls among the elderly nursing home resident.
7 Discuss problems associated with the use of restraints and identify alternatives.
8 Discuss assessments and interventions for the nursing home resident with urinary incontinence.
9 Discuss assessment of the nursing home resident with constipation.
10 Explain risk factors for preventive measures and interventions for skin breakdown among nursing home residents.
11 Discuss possible interventions for the confused nursing home resident.

KEY WORDS

autonomy
chemical restraints
delirium
dementia
depression
DNR (do not resuscitate)
ethical dilemma
functional assessment
long-term care
mental status assessment
minimum data sets (MDS)
physical restraints

At one time, the words **long-term care** or *nursing home* might have conjured up images of very old, confused people living out their last days in sadness and neglect. Today long-term care encompasses a variety of services within the healthcare system that enables people in all stages of chronic illness and all levels of ability to live as fully and independently as possible. In the near future, more people age 65 and older will need a variety of long-term care services, and new models of healthcare are being developed to accommodate this expected increase. For a complete discussion of the long-term care continuum, see Chapter 17.

The nursing home is only one of many types of long-term care available today. The older person who moves into a nursing home generally cannot live independently. This does not mean that the person is totally dependent, but the person has deficits in functional ability when compared with older people living independently. Approximately 50% of all nursing home residents have impairment of six activities of daily living (ADLs) (Matteson, 1988). These residents may need assistance with eating, transferring, toileting, dressing, bathing, or mobility. The source of their deficit may be the result of a physical or cognitive impairment. About 50% of all nursing home residents are diagnosed with Alzheimer's disease or some other cognitive impairment.

The typical nursing home resident is about 84 years old, white, female, widowed, and has few financial resources. In addition, the resident has age-related physiologic changes and multiple chronic diseases that require a wide variety of medications and health services. The older person in a nursing home may require complex healthcare to meet all of his or her needs. When families are choosing a nursing home, the nurse may be consulted for advice. The family should be urged to look carefully for an institution that best meets the needs of the older loved one. Some area agencies on aging publish comprehensive guides to local nursing homes, including those offering special Alzheimer's units. Additional information may be found at a local branch of the Alzheimer's Association, a community visiting nurse association, and a geriatric program at a local hospital. In general, when choosing a nursing home, a convenient location is important, as most families prefer to make more frequent short visits rather than extended visits. Families should be encouraged to also consider the following:

1. *Physical environment.* Is the home clean? What is the noise level? Are there unpleasant odors? Are there lounges and places for residents to gather? Are the meals served in a pleasant dining room? Is the food palatable?
2. *Daily activities.* Are the residents up and dressed? Are residents "parked around the nurses' station" with nothing to do? Are the residents treated respectfully by staff? Is there an activities program appropriate to the needs and likes of the loved one?
3. *Staff qualifications.* Are the units staffed by licensed nursing personnel? What are the qualifications of the medical director? Are consultants available, such as podiatrists, dietitians, dentists, social workers, and pharmacists?
4. *Policies and procedures.* What is the policy of the nursing home toward resident privacy, use of physical restraints, wandering, and use of sedative or hypnotic drugs?

Many families feel strongly about the care their family member will receive. They should be urged to communicate their preferences clearly before placing their loved one in the nursing facility. Families may have preferences regarding where meals are served, the time residents are put to bed, the policy toward the use of physical and chemical restraints, and policies guiding the use of outside consultants such as dentists, podiatrists, and mental health professionals.

Most nursing homes welcome visits from families of potential residents. These visits should be planned at various times of the day to get an accurate picture of the lifestyle offered by each facility.

Caring for the resident of a nursing home is one of the most rewarding and challenging areas of nursing practice. The nurse in long-term care has the opportunity to be creative and independent, acting as a case manager and promoting multidisciplinary care. Additionally, the nurse has the opportunity to really get to know the patients and their families. Unlike acute-care hospitals where the length of stay is often very short, the residents in an extended care facility often develop close relationships with their caregivers. When successes are achieved and a resident's condition improves or stabilizes, most nurses share in the joy with the resident and family.

There are three related concepts that guide the care of the nursing home resident: autonomy, promotion of independence, and maintenance or improvement of function. **Autonomy** can be defined simply as self-governance, or not being controlled by outside forces or individuals. An autonomous person makes decisions about his or her care, chooses activities and organizes care according to his or her preferences, and generally takes charge of any situations that arise. Although complete autonomy is not always possible, each nursing plan of care must be established with the input of the resident and the family, as appropriate. It is important for the nurse to remember that the older person is a special type of survivor who is usually quite capable of decision making if given the chance. If the nurse promotes autonomy and independence, then maintenance or improvement of function is likely to follow.

By recognizing the need for autonomy in the nursing home resident, including those with cognitive impairment, the nurse often serves as an advocate. Many nursing home residents feel as though they have lost control of their lives and can no longer make decisions for themselves. The nurse may be tempted to "do for" the resident rather than teach, encourage, and arrange things so that the resident can do things for himself or herself. It may take longer to assist a frail resident with dressing, but the resident will feel tremendous satisfaction from choosing the appropriate clothing, working at his or her own pace, and dressing himself or herself. Increasing self-care ability helps the older resident feel a sense of autonomy.

CASE STUDY

Mrs. Allen had been a resident in the nursing home for several months and had been known as a "good eater." Her weight had been stable at about 126 lbs since her admission. However, a few weeks ago she stopped eating well and began to "pick at her food." The chart documented a 4 lb loss in a 2-week period, and Mrs. Allen's daughter was very concerned. The nurse, after watching Mrs. Allen eat, carefully checked the fit of her dentures and noted an area of ulceration on the lower gum. A dentist was consulted, and the dentures were adjusted for a better fit. A few days later, Mrs. Allen began eating as well as she had before. Mrs. Allen's daughter called the nurse to thank her and nicknamed her "Nurse Sherlock Holmes" because she had solved the mystery.

CASE STUDY

Mrs. Kitt is an 84-year-old nursing home resident with a diagnosis of hypertension and Alzheimer's disease. Although she usually enjoys going to exercise class, today she is refusing to attend. The nurse senses that Mrs. Kitt is upset because of the recent hospitalization of her roommate. Rather than insisting that she attend exercise class, the nurse asks Mrs. Kitt if she would prefer to read a magazine. Mrs. Kitt seems pleased to stay quietly in her room.

ETHICAL DILEMMAS IN LONG-TERM CARE

When promoting autonomy, ethical issues will arise. Ethics is a philosophic discipline, and medical ethics is a unique field within ethics. Medical ethics explores grounds for deciding moral actions. Medical ethics asks questions such as, "What is informed consent?" "When is a person considered informed?" "What is quality of life?" "When is it morally right to make decisions for someone else?"

There are, of course, no absolute answers to these and other ethical questions. The purpose of asking questions is to clarify thoughts and values, specify the dilemma, and identify information needed to make decisions. An **ethical dilemma** occurs when there are conflicting values and answers to questions.

Ethical dilemmas typically arise when the resident's competence is diminished and there is a conflict between protecting safety and preserving autonomy

ETHICAL DILEMMA

Mr. Macy, an 84-year-old man, is your patient in the nursing home in which you work. His recent history includes a long hospitalization for a hip fracture following a fall in his home. He also has a 3-year history of Parkinson's disease, is being treated with medication, and has had several falls in that 3-year period.

After several weeks in the nursing home, he becomes depressed about being in the nursing home and about his increasing dependency. Most upsetting to him is the use of physical restraints, which are applied when he goes to bed at night and when he is sitting in a chair. He cries when he describes his inability to move in bed and to get comfortable. He appears to understand the risk of falling but claims that he wants to be able to move in bed and to walk around during the day. His wife is worried about him falling and breaking his hip again and wants the use of restraints to be continued.

How would you, his nurse, analyze the ethical problems in this case?

(Freeman, 1990). Nurses, like others in the healthcare system, often have erred on the side of excessive safety. For instance, it is not possible to prevent all falls in the nursing home, unless each resident is restrained 24 hours a day and not permitted to walk at all. Policies and nursing interventions that attempt to find a balance between safety and autonomy should be developed, even if there is some risk.

The Patient Self-Determination Act requires the development of advance directives at the time of a hospital admission. Its purpose is to involve patients in the care they receive. Some older people discuss these issues with their caregivers and families, and others do not. Nurses need to assess if there has been any discussion about life-sustaining measures. Often little or no information is available. Many times the **do not resuscitate (DNR)** order has been written but there is no mention of other life-sustaining measures. Cardiopulmonary resuscitation (CPR) is only one of many life-sustaining measures and generally has an unfavorable outcome in the elderly nursing home resident. The very frail; those with serious illness such as pneumonia, cancer, or renal failure; and those with severe functional disabilities have a very poor survival rate of 5% or less (Eisenberg, 1990). Often frail older people who receive CPR suffer broken ribs, cognitive deficits from hypoxia to the brain, and subsequent cardiac arrhythmias that are life-threatening.

Other life-sustaining measures in the nursing home include artificial feedings (gastric and nasogastric feedings), ventilators, antibiotics, and even transfer to an acute care hospital for an acute illness. Many nursing homes have checklists that state the residents' and families' preferences for each intervention. These decisions are best made in nonemergency situations, when the resident and family have the opportunity to ask questions, receive accurate information regarding the various interventions, and weigh the risks and benefits of each decision. All long-term care facilities need specific policies and procedures relating to all aspects of life-sustaining measures.

CASE STUDY

Mr. Jackson has always had a fear of becoming a burden on his children. When he was diagnosed with Alzheimer's disease, he asked his son to "let me go when my time comes." He specifically asked that no tubes or ventilators be used because he had a fear of choking. Mr. Jackson's son, his designated healthcare proxy, communicated these wishes to the nursing home staff and medical director when Mr. Jackson was admitted to the Alzheimer's unit. The nurse in charge sensed the relief in Mr. Jackson's son when all the appropriate paperwork was completed and the notations made in his chart. He had honored his father's request for a natural death.

While end-of-life decision-making is of major importance, it is not the only decision to be made in long-term care. Although independence and decision-making abilities in the older patient are valued by healthcare professionals, the patient is commonly excluded from decisions about treatment and care. It is often assumed that the older person is cognitively impaired or should be spared difficult decisions. Involvement in discussions about goals and interventions promotes feelings of self-determination. The older person values independence, as does the healthcare professional.

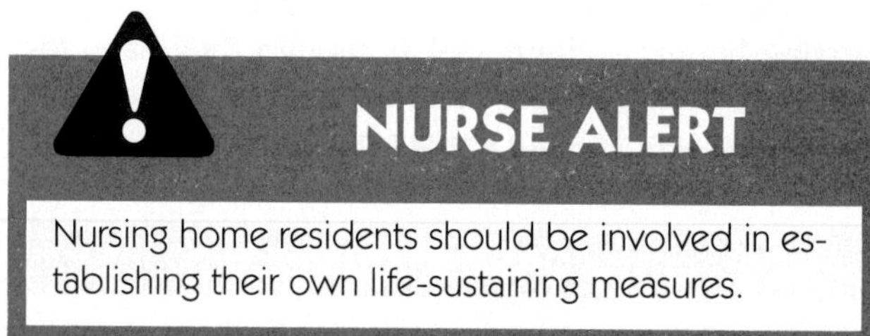

NURSE ALERT
Nursing home residents should be involved in establishing their own life-sustaining measures.

GENERAL ASSESSMENT GUIDELINES

Nursing assessments are crucial for identifying barriers to autonomy, independence, and functional abilities. The combination of changes in physiology, multiple chronic illnesses, multiple medications, and years of life experience makes assessment difficult. Signs and symptoms of acute illness are often vague or seem unrelated to a particular illness. Because of this, the initial nursing assessment must be complete so that even subtle changes will be recognized.

Each nursing home completes a holistic assessment of new residents called the **Minimum Data Set (MDS).** This assessment includes information on health practices, activities, exercise, elimination patterns, coping styles, nutrition, sleep patterns, sexuality, support systems (including family and friends), cognition/perception, spirituality, and self-concept. When gathering this data, the nurse must remember that the person admitted to the nursing home has had an average of 84 years of experience. It is important to find out what the person was like as a youth, young adult, adult, and older person. Questions about childhood activities, family relationships, household responsibilities, education, leisure activities, activities with family and friends, occupation, and roles and relationships all add to the understanding of who the person is today. Previous behavior patterns, learning styles, interaction styles, and coping styles will continue in some form.

Using this information, nursing interventions can be creative and individualized to maintain the resident's autonomy as much as possible.

In addition to a general assessment, specific assessment data regarding functional status, mental status, and depression must be gathered on each nursing home resident.

Functional Assessment

A **functional assessment** identifies the person's level of independence, focusing on abilities rather than disabilities. Each person's ability to perform ADLs is often assessed upon admission and periodically thereafter. An accurate representation of each resident's functional ability allows the nurse to devise a nursing care plan consistent with the resident's abilities. Abrupt changes in functional status may also be a key indicator when a cognitively impaired resident becomes ill. Residents who usually walk with minimal assistance and then suddenly become unable to walk may be injured or constipated, have the beginnings of pneumonia or another infection, or have suffered a cerebrovascular accident (CVA) or heart attack. Functional status is the chief indicator of a resident's health in the nursing home and requires careful assessment. Refer to Chapter 15 for a more complete discussion of instruments and measures of functional assessment.

Both physical ADLs and instrumental ADLs need to be assessed. Physical ADLs are bathing, dressing, eating, ambulating, managing a wheelchair, and using the toilet. Instrumental ADLs involve balancing a checkbook, housekeeping, going to the store, doing laundry, answering the telephone, and managing medications. Most often, physical ADLs are assessed in the nursing home, as the staff performs instrumental ADLs.

The nurse may identify other members of the healthcare team who can assist the resident in reaching goals. The resident and healthcare team may then establish a contract that clearly outlines the strategies to be used in achieving those goals. For instance, a person may need to improve muscle strength. The nurse or physical therapist may design an individualized exercise program that the resident can perform independently on a routine basis. In this way, both the healthcare provider and the patient play a role in improving functional status.

Instrumental ADLs provide insights into abilities. The resident can be encouraged to continue activities according to abilities and goals within the constraints of the facility. It may be possible for the resident to keep some medications at the bedside. Nursing interventions may also include encouraging the person to make decisions, keep plants in the room, make his or her own bed, or rearrange his or her room. There are a number of creative approaches to the care of the older person that can be developed using the functional assessment as a base.

Mental Status Assessment

Every person entering a nursing home needs a **mental status assessment.** A mental status assessment examines cognitive functions such as the ability to think and make decisions. In addition to this admission assessment, it is important to ascertain previous mental status and mental status after 3 months of institutionalization. Many times the nursing home resident is first admitted to an acute-care hospital, treated for an acute illness, and then transferred to the long-term care facility.

Before the acute episode, the person may have had no problems with mental status. But the acute episode and the change in environment may cause changes in mental status that have not resolved on admission to the nursing home. Knowledge of past function helps identify recent changes and give direction for care. Often when the person adjusts to the new environment, intact mental status will return. A mental status assessment is also performed any time the nurse feels that there has been a change in cognitive function. It is best to avoid labeling someone as "confused," because this is a general term that gives little information. When describing someone with deficits in mental status, it is important that the nurse be as specific as possible. For instance, the notation may read: "Mr. Jones has deficits in short-term memory but is oriented to time, place, and person." Or, "Mrs. Lawry has intact long- and short-term memory but exhibits deficits in ability to perform calculations and abstract thinking."

The mental status assessment serves three purposes. The first is to give baseline information about the person's cognitive state so that changes can be identified. The second is to screen for problems or potential problems. And the third is to identify areas of strength and weakness and areas in need of additional evaluation.

There are a number of mental status questionnaires useful in long-term care. Because altered mental status can involve many parts of the central nervous system, the mental status assessment uses a variety of questions aimed at identifying specific areas of dysfunction. Thus assessment of mental status is more than an examination of orientation. Refer to Chapter 14 for a complete discussion of instruments and scoring of mental status.

Depression Assessment

Because **depression** affects many older people, but is often not diagnosed or treated, all nursing assessments should include a measure of depression. See Chapter

14 for a discussion of instruments and ways to measure depression in the elderly. Rates of depression are highest in physically ill older adults and those in long-term care facilities, in which 40% to 50% of residents are found to be depressed (Cornacchione, Slusser, 1994). Depression in the nursing home is found to be related to physical illness, medication, and psychosocial losses. Physical illnesses linked to depression include liver disease, diabetes, chronic obstructive pulmonary disease, CVA, Alzheimer's disease, congestive heart failure, and anemia. Signs and symptoms of these diseases include decreased energy, anorexia, sleep disturbances, and other somatic symptoms that mimic depression. The relationship between physical illness and depression is unknown, but it is difficult to enjoy life when symptoms of physical illness exist. Improvement of physical status may relieve some of the symptoms of depression.

Research indicates that depression and **dementia** coexist in approximately 23% of cognitively impaired older adults (Cornacchione, Slusser, 1994). Many older people with Alzheimer's disease realize they are losing their ability to function and feel great sadness and loss over their state of health and their prognosis. The nurse should take time to talk with the depressed resident and his or her family, listen carefully for clues of depression, and address any concerns promptly. The multidisciplinary team can assist in evaluating the presence of depression and in planning care. Medications, psychotherapy, support groups, and involvement in social activities may all be appropriate interventions.

Medications associated with depression in the elderly include antihypertensives (especially beta-blockers), narcotic analgesics, antiparkinson drugs, sedatives, and alcohol. A careful assessment of all prescription and nonprescription drugs should be obtained from all residents on admission to the nursing home. If the onset of depression is associated with a new medication, the physician should be notified so that new medications can be substituted.

Psychosocial losses can contribute to depression in the nursing home. Lack of contact with family and friends, isolation from pleasurable activities, and changes in health status often are associated with nursing home admission. Despite everyone's best efforts to provide a loving, homelike environment in the nursing home, it is never quite the same as living independently in one's own home. It may be especially difficult around the holidays, when residents think back to the days when they were younger, healthier, and surrounded by family and friends. Many elderly people have little time to grieve between losses. The following is part of an account written by Anna Mae Halgrim Seaver, an 84-year-old nursing home resident (Seaver, 1994).

> This is my world now. It's all I have left. You see, I'm old. And, I'm not as healthy as I used to be. I'm not necessarily happy with it, but I accept it. Occasionally, a member of my family will stop in to see me. He or she will bring me some flowers or a little present. Maybe a set of slippers—I've got eight pair. We'll visit for awhile and then they will return to the outside world and I'll be alone again. . . .

RISK AND SPECIFIC CARE ISSUES

Falls

Falls and associated morbidity and mortality represent a major problem for the elderly. Sequelae include fractures, decreased mobility, loss of confidence, psychologic distress, and self-imposed isolation due to fear of falling. Resulting disability leads to loss of function and independence. Autonomy is threatened.

There are both intrinsic and extrinsic risk factors for falls (Figure 16-1). Intrinsic factors involve age-related changes such as altered gait and balance, visual and hearing changes, osteoporosis, loss of muscle mass, and degenerative joint disease. These factors may be the result of aging, the presence of acute or chronic disease, and/or the side effects of medications or treatments.

Extrinsic factors include hazards in the environment, including scatter rugs, poorly fitting slippers, waxed floors, dimly lit hallways, and dangling electric cords. Many nursing homes are bustling with activity and movement, and residents, staff, and families congregate around the nurses' station. It may be difficult for residents with walkers, wheelchairs, and poor vision or hearing to pass up and down the corridor safely. The nurse should always be alert for hazards such as congested areas, wet spots on the floor, lightbulbs needing replacement, and other extrinsic factors that could be dangerous for residents. If a resident should fall, the nurse should carefully examine the area where the fall occurred to assess for environmental hazards. Such information will be helpful when deciding on what changes, if any, should be made in the nursing care plan.

Gait and balance

Elderly persons at risk for falls may have a gait that is slow, with short, irregular shuffling steps, and they may place their feet widely apart. A change in gait produces a less secure base of support and an inability to recover from a change in balance. Balance is a function of vision, proprioception, stabilizing muscles, and vibratory senses. Problems may be caused by vestibular (inner ear) alterations resulting in vertigo and dizziness. Proprioception is knowing where extremities are in space. Changes in proprioception result in errors in placing the feet.

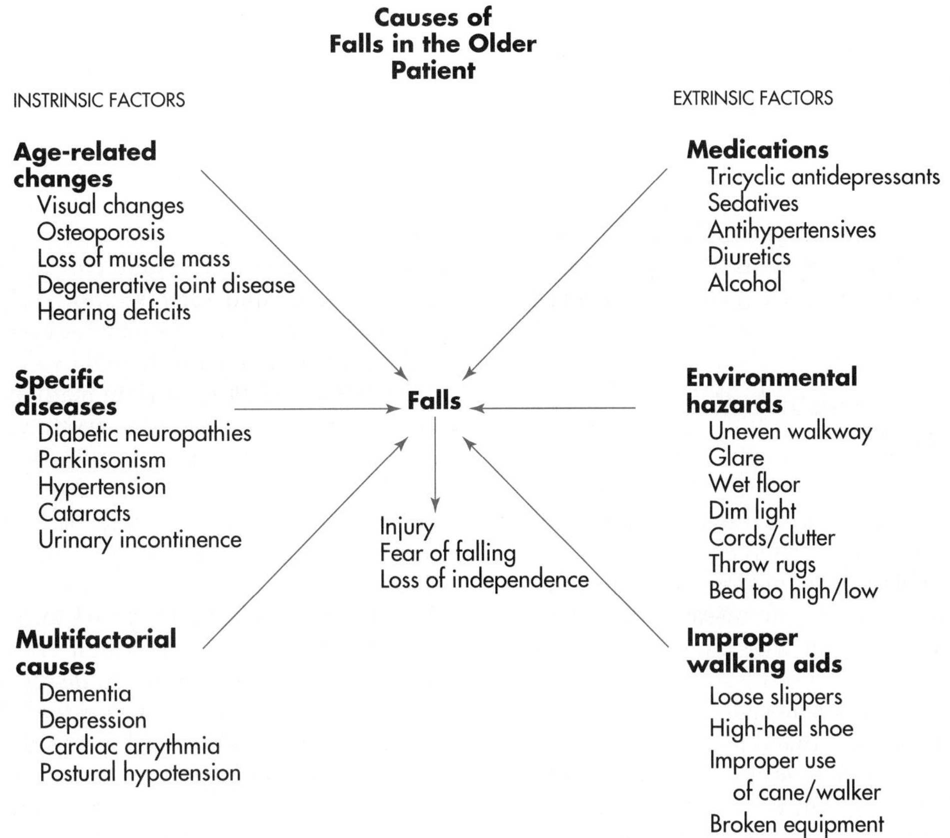

Figure 16-1 Causes of falls in older adults.

Muscle strength

Muscle strength may also put the elderly person at risk of falling. It was once thought that muscle weakness and atrophy were "normal" consequences of aging. Biology-of-aging researchers find, however, that the person who exercises regularly does not lose strength and endurance. In addition, older people who have not exercised but who begin a regular exercise program have increased strength and endurance.

Aging muscle that is not exercised loses lean mass, strength, and endurance, particularly in the essential weight-bearing muscles of the legs. Immobility produces progressive loss of muscle tone and weakness and may be associated with psychogenic vertigo and dizziness. Immobility also contributes to loss of calcium from the long bones, resulting in an increased risk of fractures.

Balance, gait, and muscle strength are probably the most important risk factors for falls. However, there are numerous contributory factors that must also be assessed.

Sensory changes

Sensory changes in vision and hearing in the older person contribute to altered depth perception. Visual acuity decreases, and the ability to distinguish blues and greens diminishes. Glare, especially from highly waxed floors, disturbs depth perception and may actually "blind" the person, so perception of surroundings becomes difficult, if not impossible. Glaucoma alters peripheral vision. Cataracts, dirty or out-of-date prescription glasses, and dim lighting alter direct vision. Impaired hearing places the older person at risk because he or she may not hear approaching food carts, the warnings of other residents, or the approach of other environmental hazards.

Medications

Medications produce a variety of risk factors including orthostatic hypotension, dizziness, and confusion. Each medication must be evaluated by the pharmacist for possible interaction with other drugs being taken and the physiologic state of the resident. Diuretics tend to dehydrate older persons and place them at risk for orthostatic hypotension. Beta-blockers suppress cardiac output and can induce heart failure. Sedative hypnotics tend to impair balance and make the older person less attentive to the environment. Careful assessment of vital signs, a complete medication history, and discontinuation of all nonessential medications are appropriate nursing measures for the older person at risk for falling in the nursing home.

Incontinence

Incontinence is another major risk factor for falls. The older person may attempt to get to the bathroom in a hurry and fall or may dribble urine and slip and fall. Placing a commode by the bedside and assessing and treating urinary incontinence may reduce the risk of falling.

Age and gender and history of falls and confusion

Age and gender are associated with falls. The older the person, the higher the risk. Women are more likely to fall than men. This gender difference reflects the fact that there are more older women than older men, that older women have more chronic diseases than older men, and that older women take more medications than older men.

Previous history of falls represents yet another important risk factor. An assessment must include information on incidents of falling at home or in the nursing home. Residents who fall tend to fall again. Impaired cognitive status also places the person at risk for falls and tends to form a dangerous combination with all risk factors.

The risk of falling is complex and requires careful evaluation. Table 16-1 lists risk factors that should be part of the nursing assessment and used to explore additional assessments and/or plan interventions.

Interventions

Examining the list of risk factors associated with falls helps identify possible interventions. A change in environment, stressful life events, or a change in medications all place the person at risk. Additional orientation to the new facility and extra supervision and observation, particularly at night, will decrease the risk. Evaluation of mental status and depression helps identify the extent of the problem. Taking time to listen to concerns and offer support helps the person gain an understanding of events. Autonomy and independence should be encouraged.

Medications are the culprit in many problems of old age. Blood pressure should be taken when the person is reclining and again upon standing to identify orthostatic hypotension. Periods of dizziness, disorientation, or change in mental status should be observed and related to routine medications or medications taken as needed.

The resident should be referred to physical and occupational therapy for a thorough evaluation of function, with an emphasis on potential for falls. The treatment plan should address individual risk factors for falls. Group and individual exercises should be encouraged. Even the person in a wheelchair can benefit from regular exercise. The nurse should ensure that lighting is adequate and that glare is kept to a minimum. Bright colors for bedspreads and walls help perceptual problems.

Records of incontinence and bladder and bowel patterns help identify when the person should be taken to the bathroom. A common time for falls is at night when the person tries to climb over the side rails of the

TABLE 16-1

Assessment of Risk Factors for Falls

Risk Factor	Yes	No	Risk Factor	Yes	No
Admission (within 2 weeks)			Incontinent (urine)		
Transfer to unit or room change			Hearing deficit		
Medication change (within 30 days)			Visual deficit		
Cardiac medications			Confusion		
Antihypertensives			Head injury		
Diuretics			CVA		
Tranquilizers			Amputee		
Sleeping medications			Diabetic		
Pain medication			Metastatic disease		
More than 5 medications			Degenerative neuromuscular disease		
			Previous falls		
			Proper use of cane/walker		
			Environmental hazards		
			Safe shoes/footwear		

bed to get to the bathroom. If used at all, half side rails are best. These assist the person in moving in bed and provide a means of stabilization when the person sits up on the edge of the bed.

One of the most common, but incorrect, methods of preventing falls is **physical restraints.** Interestingly, a high percentage of falls occur when restraints are in place and side rails are up (Mion and others, 1994). Physical restraints are defined as any manual method or physical device that the resident cannot remove; that restricts the resident's physical activity; and that is not a usual and customary part of a medical, diagnostic, or treatment procedure. Further, a physical restraint does not serve to promote the resident's independent functioning (Strumpf, Evans, 1988). Vest restraints, waist restraints, seat belts, and geri-chairs are all types of physical restraints. Cognitively impaired residents often untie or attempt to slide out of the restraints and become entangled, choke, fall, or seriously injure themselves. Morbidity and mortality risks associated with physical restraints include nerve injury, pressure sores, pneumonia, incontinence, increased confusion, inappropriate drug use, strangulation, and asphyxiation (Evans, Strumpf, 1987). When a person with a cognitive impairment is put to bed with side rails up, they often attempt to climb over them, becoming entangled and causing injury. Of all possible interventions, restraints are the most harmful to the person's sense of autonomy, independence, function, and self-esteem. Federal regulations under the Omnibus Reconciliation Act (OBRA 87) mandate against using restraints that are (1) used for discipline or convenience of the staff, (2) used without a trial of less-restrictive measures, or used without the consent of the resident or his or her legal representative. Residents who are restrained should be released, exercised, toileted, and checked for skin redness every 2 hours. The need for the restraint should be reevaluated periodically. It is the responsibility of the medical director and nursing home administrators with the input of nursing staff to develop policies and procedures for the appropriate use of restraints. This ensures the highest quality of life and promotes autonomy of the residents.

Many nurses and long-term care administrators are concerned because they fear they will be held liable for injuries from a fall. While the move to restraint-free environments is relatively new in the United States, it is not new in England and other European countries. In England and the Scandinavian countries, restraints are not used at all. In the United States, pilot projects have shown that the number of falls and injuries from falls has not increased when restraints are removed (Evans, Strumpf, 1987). Careful environmental assessment, reduced psychotropic drug use, and supervision of the frequent faller are all effective in reducing the risk of falls and avoiding restraints.

OBRA 87 also sets standards for the use of **chemical restraints,** which are defined as sedative and antipsychotic drugs. Studies done in the 1980s in nursing homes revealed that there had been excessive, often inappropriate use of these drugs and that they were associated with significant risk for injury (Rader, Donius, 1991). Conditions that are considered inappropriate for antipsychotic drug treatment include wandering, anxiety, fidgeting, nervousness, agitation, and anxiety. Use of antipsychotic drugs is limited to specific conditions such as psychotic mood disorder and schizophrenia. Behaviors that make the resident a danger to himself or herself or others, as well as behaviors that make the delivery of nursing care impossible, are considered justifiable reasons for the use of psychotropic drugs. If these drugs are used, the nurse should carefully document the need for the medication, using a 24-hour behavior log. Once the medication is administered, the behavior log should reflect an improvement in the troublesome behaviors. If not, the medication should be discontinued. Regulations further state that trial dose reductions and discontinuation of these drugs should be instituted on a regular basis.

Identifying alternatives to physical and chemical restraints should occur after exploring the need for restraints. If the reason is the potential for falls, an evaluation of the risk factors and the measures to correct them can provide the nurse with alternatives. Exercise programs, activity programs, lower bed height, and relocation closer to the nurses' station are possible interventions to permit the removal of restraints. Bed monitors signal the nurses' station when a frequent faller arises from bed and may need supervision. Nonskid mats placed on the path to the bathroom keep the floor dry for incontinent patients. Behavioral interventions are suggested for dealing with the cognitively impaired resident who refuses care, exhibits symptoms of agitation, or presents a danger to himself or herself or others (Box 16-1) (Besdine and others, 1991).

Urinary Incontinence

Urinary incontinence, the involuntary loss of urine, is a problem for at least 10 million noninstitutionalized American adults and accounts for approximately $10 billion spent on products to manage the problem. Urinary incontinence causes significant disability and dependency and is a leading cause of institutionalization.

It is often assumed that urinary incontinence is a consequence of aging, that there is no treatment, and that therefore one must learn to live with it. There is a large market for incontinence pads and adult diapers.

BOX 16-1

GUIDELINES FOR DEALING WITH THE COGNITIVELY IMPAIRED NURSING HOME RESIDENT

Prevention is the most effective approach for reducing behavior problems. Be aware of the person's history, strengths, and weaknesses. There may be a better time to approach the resident. Don't force a confrontation.

Be objective when assessing problems. If the problem is more an inconvenience to caregivers than the resident, no intervention may be necessary.

Determine the reason for the behavior. If the resident is not cooperating with care, is it the way he or she was approached? Is the resident overwhelmed with sensory stimulation? Is the resident ill, constipated, or fatigued? Is it the time of the day?

Assess problems as a team. Seek input from all involved, including other nurses, therapists, social workers, activities therapists, families, and nurses aides. Remember that others see the resident from a different perspective and that all information is helpful.

Do not blame the resident for the behavior. Cognitively impaired residents have a disease that inhibits their ability to think clearly. It is the responsibility of nurses to devise the best environment that supports maximum function. Sleep, appetite, bowel function, and personality are all affected by the degenerative brain changes that occur in Alzheimer's disease.

Be creative in your approach. Use calming music (Tabloski and others, 1995), pictures of family members, favorite foods, and a flexible approach to bathing, sleeping, and eating routines. Your efforts will be well worth it, and the older person's dignity will be respected. When you find something that works, share it with others. You'll be a role model for others, and the resident will benefit from a consistent approach.

Urinary incontinence, however, is a symptom rather than a disease, and it is not a normal part of the aging process. Unfortunately, the evaluation and treatment of urinary incontinence is often neglected by healthcare professionals. When treated appropriately, however, mobility, function, and independence improve significantly.

In long-term care, 50% or more of the residents probably will have urinary problems. Urinary incontinence is complex, with multiple causative factors. There are three main types: stress incontinence, urge incontinence, and overflow incontinence. Although there are three distinct types, older people may have two or three at the same time. The nurse plays a vital role in the treatment of urinary incontinence that begins with a complete assessment, which includes a mental status examination, functional assessment, documentation of the pattern of incontinence, and assessment aimed at identifying the type of incontinence. Table 16-2 illustrates important diagnostic criteria for the three types of incontinence.

CASE STUDY

Mr. Alcott is a 78-year-old nursing home resident with Alzheimer's disease. He often attempts to strike the nurses when he receives his weekly bath. The nurses and aides are frightened of him and approach him with fear. Ms. Bradley, the new staff nurse, suggests the following approach: (1) Mr. Alcott seems to like one nurse better than the others. Therefore she should arrange for his bath. (2) Mr. Alcott seems more calm in the early morning rather than the afternoon. His bath time should be rescheduled to the morning. (3) Mrs. Alcott should be asked to bring in a tape recording of some of Mr. Alcott's favorite music to play in the background during the bath. These measures greatly reduce Mr. Alcott's fear, and he becomes less combative during bathtime.

Stress incontinence

Stress incontinence, the involuntary leakage of small amounts of urine usually in response to increased intraabdominal pressure, accounts for about 35% of incontinence in older people. The person complains of losing small amounts of urine, usually during the day, when coughing, laughing, sneezing, bending, or changing position. Stress incontinence occurs primarily in women who have had multiple pregnancies or significant weight gain. Additional assessment may reveal the presence of a cystocele, rectocele, uterine prolapse, urethral prolapse, atrophic vaginitis due to lack of estrogen, obesity, or use of certain antihypertensive medications. The person with stress incontinence is able to completely empty the bladder, and little residual volume remains after voiding.

Urge incontinence

Urge incontinence is the involuntary loss of large amounts of urine associated with a strong desire to void. It accounts for 60% to 70% of urinary inconti-

TABLE 16-2

Urinary Incontinence Analysis

Data obtained from history and/or incontinence assessment tool	Type of Incontinence		
	Stress	**Urge**	**Overflow**
Amount of leakage	+ Small squirts	+ Large	+ Dribbling
Time of day of leakage	+ Day	+ Day and night	+ Day
Associated events	+ Coughing; laughing; sneezing; bending; changing position	+ Strong urge to void; unable to hold it until toilet reached	+ None
Stream of urine	Normal	Normal	+ Hesitancy; interruption; weak
Awareness of urge to void at time of incontinent episode	–	+	–
Feeling of incomplete emptying after void	–	–	+
Physical findings			
Fecal impaction or incontinence	–	–	+
Enlarged prostate	–	–	+
Palpable bladder postvoid	–	–	+
Cystocele, rectocele, uterine prolapse, urethral prolapse	+	–	–
Atrophic vaginitis	+	+	–
Leakage of urine after cough (full bladder)	+ Immediate	+ 3-5 seconds after cough	–
Catheter for residual	< 100 ml	< 100 ml	> 100 ml
Obesity	+	–	–
Presence of girdle	+	–	–

nence in older people. The person complains of losing large amounts of urine day or night and of having a strong desire to void but being unable to hold urine until reaching the bathroom. The person will experience leaking urine 3 to 5 seconds after coughing, rather than with coughing as with stress incontinence. Additional assessment may reveal moderate to high caffeine intake (coffee, tea, cola), atrophic vaginitis, diabetes, infections, degenerative neurologic conditions such as a CVA or Parkinson's disease, alcoholism, or use of certain medications such as sedatives and diuretics. As with stress incontinence, little residual volume remains in the bladder after voiding.

Overflow incontinence

Overflow incontinence, the involuntary dribbling of urine due to an obstruction of the bladder outlet, accounts for 10% to 15% of urinary incontinence in older people. The person complains of dribbling without warning during the day. When voiding, there is a hesitancy and interruption in the stream of urine and the feeling of incomplete emptying of the bladder. If catheterized, there would be more than 100 ml of residual urine present in the bladder. Additional assessment may reveal a fecal impaction, enlarged prostate, diabetes, a spinal cord injury or disk disease, or use of certain drugs such as alcohol, antihistamines, decongestants, phenothiazines, and muscle relaxants.

The person with urinary incontinence requires a thorough evaluation by the healthcare team. In addition to the causes identified for each type of incontinence, there are multiple environmental factors to assess. Immobility or being unable to get to the bathroom, commode, or bedpan; unfamiliar surroundings; inadequate lighting; dehydration causing concentration of urine, which may irritate the mucosa; and irritation of the bladder wall are all correctable factors that should be considered.

Voiding record

There are a variety of methods to record voiding patterns (Wells, 1988). The purpose of the record is to identify the pattern of incontinence in terms of frequency, amount, and conditions surrounding the incontinent episode. It can be kept by the resident, family, or nursing staff. The record requires cooperation by everyone because it encompasses at least one 24-hour period. The resident is observed on an hourly basis to determine whether he or she was incontinent, dry, or voided normally. The amount of urine is documented. If the person was incontinent, the following is noted: the approximate amount of urine, awareness of the urge to eliminate, associated conditions (coughing, sneezing, impaction or urge to defecate, walking, or changing position), and the availability of appropriate facilities. In addition, an accurate record of the amount, type, and time of fluid intake is kept. Analyzing this record will help determine the person's normal patterns of elimination and assist in the development of nursing interventions.

Urinary incontinence is complex. A thorough assessment will help identify the type of urinary incontinence, enabling the healthcare team to determine appropriate interventions.

Intervention

Intervention for urinary incontinence depends on the type of incontinence and, whenever possible, the cause. The goal of all treatment is to promote independence and improve function. For stress incontinence, Kegel exercises aim at strengthening the pelvic floor and can be taught by the nurse. The person is taught to find the pelvic floor muscle by trying to stop a stream of urine. The muscle that is pulled is the muscle to be exercised. The person is instructed to tighten the muscle, hold it for a count of 10, and relax for a count of 10. This is repeated 10 to 15 times in the morning, afternoon, and evening. The exercise can be done anytime, anyplace. When teaching the exercise, the nurse needs to emphasize the importance of relaxation as well as tightening. Also, the nurse needs to be sure the person does not use the abdomen, legs (or crossing legs), or buttocks, and that the person does not hold his or her breath while exercising. Posting a schedule for the person to mark off when completing the exercise places responsibility on the person and serves as a reminder.

Additional interventions for stress incontinence include oral or topical estrogen for atrophic vaginitis, development of a weight-loss program, use of loose garments, evaluation of medications (particularly antihypertensive medications), possible use of anticholinergic medications, surgery, and habit training.

The purpose of habit training is to avoid large amounts of urine in the bladder. It begins by examining the voiding record to identify normal frequency patterns. A regular, rigid voiding schedule is then established. The person is taken to the bathroom every 2 hours regardless of whether there is a desire to void and regardless of incontinence.

There are multiple interventions for urge incontinence that can be initiated by the nurse in cooperation with the healthcare team. First, the nurse assesses the environment to be sure it facilitates normal voiding. This includes ensuring that the bathroom, commode, bedpan, and urinal are accessible and assistive devices needed for independence are close at hand. Obstacles are removed, and lighting is checked to ensure that it is adequate. It may be necessary to have the resident's eyes examined and vision corrected. The person's mobility may be improved with physical therapy. The occupational therapy department may help design easy-to-open clothing.

Bladder training and habit training for urge incontinence are also useful. The goal of bladder training is to increase to 4 hours the interval between voiding. The person is taught to inhibit the urge to void and increase bladder capacity, thus increasing the interval between voiding. Relaxation exercises often help the person overcome the urge to void. The nurse works with the resident, encouraging slow, deep breathing until the urge disappears. The resident is encouraged to wait 5 minutes and then void. If an accident occurs before 5 minutes, the waiting time is shortened to 3 minutes. When it becomes easy to wait 3 minutes, the time can be increased to 4 or 5 minutes. The waiting time is gradually increased. To have a successful bladder-training program, the person must maintain adequate intake of fluids, usually between 2000 and 2500 ml per day. Natural diuretics such as coffee, tea,

OLDER ADULT CONSIDERATIONS

When assessing elimination patterns of older people, the nurse should ask questions that help identify the type of incontinence. Questions such as, "Do you ever lose urine when you don't want to?" "Do you lose urine when you sneeze, laugh, or cough?" "Do you have trouble getting to the bathroom on time?" "Do you wear something to keep you dry during the day and/or night?" will elicit a great deal of important information.

cocoa, cola, and grapefruit juice should be avoided. An evaluation of medications that could cause incontinence should also be performed.

Overflow incontinence is often neurogenic in etiology. The resident and family can be taught measures to assist in voiding. The person should sit on the toilet or commode. Deep breathing, blowing through a straw while leaning forward, and the Crede maneuver (manual pressure on the bladder) may help initiate voiding. Each technique may be successful at different times. Because one does not work once does not mean that it will not work another time. Successful management depends on patience and a willingness to try various methods.

Another treatment of choice for overflow incontinence is intermittent catheterization. Treatment of incontinence in many healthcare settings involves the placement of an indwelling catheter, which in turn places the person at risk for infection, decreases independence and mobility, increases the risk of trauma, and increases the need for medical supervision. Sterile intermittent catheterization by a nurse or clean technique taught to a cognitively intact person, simulates normal voiding patterns and decreases the risk of infection. In addition, intermittent catheterization promotes independence and functional abilities.

The first intervention for incontinence associated with outlet obstruction is to relieve the obstruction. This may involve removal of the fecal impaction or surgery for an enlarged prostate. Next, medications are evaluated to identify those that tighten sphincters or contribute to urinary retention.

Care of the person with urinary incontinence represents a challenge to the nurse and requires thorough assessment and creative problem-solving with the resident, the family, and the healthcare team.

Constipation

As with all problems encountered in the long-term care setting, constipation has multiple causative factors. The elderly use more over-the-counter preparations to promote bowel elimination than any other age group. Persistent use of laxatives tends to inhibit normal patterns, thereby creating an impression of constipation that stimulates perpetual use of laxatives. Also, in a misguided attempt to prevent incontinence, the older person may decrease fluid intake, thereby increasing the tendency toward constipation. Diets lacking in roughage and fruit, medications, inhibitory practices (ignoring the bowel reflex as well as using laxatives), and lack of exercise all contribute to constipation. Added to this are cultural beliefs about the importance of regular—often translated as *daily*—bowel movements.

Assessment

An accurate assessment of constipation is essential for planning appropriate interventions. The assessment should include the following:

- *Time:* What are the usual days and times of bowel movements?
- *Frequency:* Do bowel movements occur daily, three times a week, twice a week, or weekly?
- *Consistency:* Is the stool formed, hard, soft, or loose?
- *Fluid intake:* What is the amount of daily fluid intake and the type of fluid?
- *Nutrition:* A 24-hour recall is helpful for a variety of assessment areas, including elimination. Ask specific questions regarding foods and amounts consumed at meals, snacks, and bedtime. Note amounts of cereals, fresh fruit, vegetables, and breads.
- *Stimulants:* What does the person use to stimulate bowel movements? This could include coffee, prunes, bran, and other natural laxatives, plus medications, enemas, suppositories, and digital stimulation.
- *Habits associated with elimination:* What is the usual place for elimination? Are activities such as reading or smoking done during bowel evacuation?
- *Medications:* What medications does the person take? Certain medications cause constipation, such as anticholinergic drugs, aluminum or calcium antacids, and high doses of aspirin.
- *Exercise:* How much and how often does the person exercise? What type of exercise does he or she do?
- *Physical assessment:* A rectal examination to check for impaction, bowel sounds, and skin turgor (dehydration), and a palpation of the abdomen for masses should be performed. Note chronic medical conditions.

Intervention

If constipation and impaction are present, the bowel must be cleansed before a bowel program can be successful. Laxatives and enemas should be used as needed to clean the bowel. Then, the assessment data can be used to identify normal patterns and begin a reeducation of the bowel. When developing a bowel program, it is usually easier to reestablish old patterns than to develop new ones. If the person usually has a bowel movement at bedtime, retraining should begin at this time using the natural cues that the person finds effective. Nutritional stimulants such as bran may be added to the morning or afternoon meals, prunes or other dried fruits may be served, and fresh fruit or bran cereal can be suggested as a snack.

If no bowel movement occurs within the first 48 hours, a gentle stimulant such as a glycerine suppository at the time the person normally has a bowel movement may be needed. Whenever using artificial bowel stimulants, the nurse should start with the most natural and work up to the more irritating.

The person should be encouraged to respond to the urge to evacuate the bowel. The environment should be conducive to having a bowel movement. The nurse can provide privacy and ensure that the bathroom, commode, or bedpan is accessible. No bowel program will work immediately. Each intervention should be given approximately 2 weeks to be effective. The person will usually respond to encouragement and support. Punishing words or actions place an unnecessary barrier to success. For most people, it is unnatural to be dependent on others for toileting. Whenever possible, the nurse should facilitate independence.

Pressure Sores

As a person ages, changes in the skin contribute to the potential for skin breakdown. With aging, there is a decrease in vascularity, subcutaneous fat, elasticity, hair follicles, and temperature and touch receptors. The result is skin that is fragile, easily injured, and slow to heal.

In addition to aging, risk factors for skin breakdown include immobility, diabetes, incontinence, poor nutrition, inadequate fluid intake, and edema. An assessment of the skin of the older person must consider all factors, plus an accurate description of the altered skin. Pressure sores, in the past called *decubitus ulcers*, are the most common form of alteration in skin integrity, caused by continued unrelieved pressure. They develop over bony prominences where the pressure causes occlusion of capillaries and local inflammation from inadequate nutrient exchange (Agency for Health Care Policy and Research, 1992a; White and others, 1994).

Assessment

Pressure sores should be assessed and described using a standard classification system. Identification of stages helps determine interventions (Figure 16-2; Box 16-2). Refer to Chapters 15 and 31 for further information on pressure sores.

It is extremely useful to photograph pressure sores, including a tape measure in the photograph to indicate

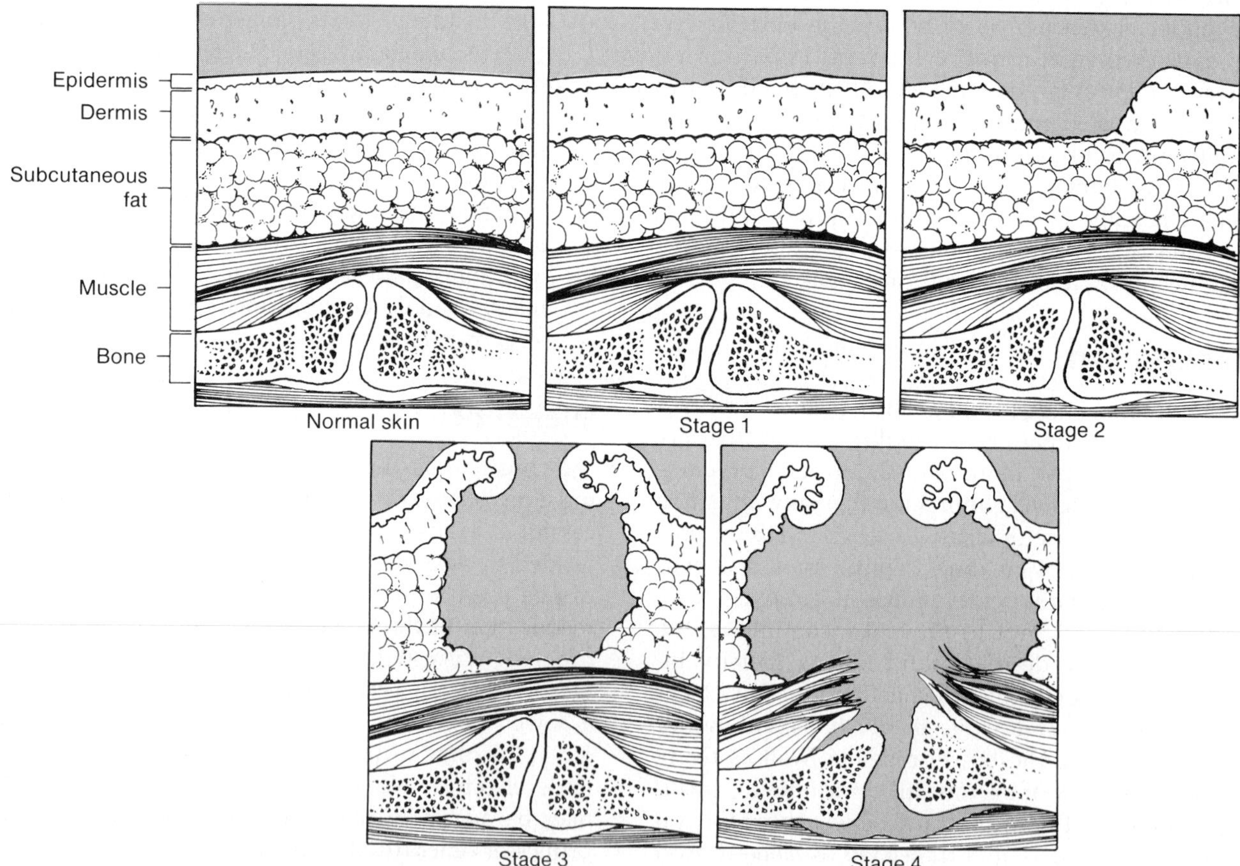

Figure 16-2 Normal skin and pressure sore formation.

BOX 16-2

PRESSURE SORE STAGES

Stage 1: Inflammatory response (redness, swelling, and heat), with or without a break in the skin.
Stage 2: Shallow ulcer with distinct edges and drainage, surrounded by an area of redness, heat, and swelling. The dermis is involved.
Stage 3: Irregular ulceration involving subcutaneous fat. Drainage may be copious.
Stage 4: Deep ulceration that extends into the muscle tissue with visualization of ligaments and bone. The wound and drainage from the wound are foul smelling, and the borders are thick and pigmented.

size. The photograph serves as both a means to assess the extent of the problem and to evaluate the effectiveness of treatment. Before photographing the pressure sore, permission from the patient or family must be obtained. The picture with the date and location of the wound, along with the treatment plan, are then placed in the record. Pictures should be taken weekly until the lesion is healed.

Intervention

A key factor to healing pressure sores is a consistent approach by all who care for the person. The proposed treatment must be given time to work. All long-term care facilities need to develop a skin protocol that fits their facility and residents. The protocol outlines assessment, identification of the person at risk, preventive measures, and, when pressure sores develop, a protocol for intervention. The treatment protocol requires collaboration with the physician, but the nurse plays a primary role in the care of pressure sores (Box 16-3).

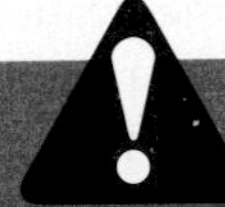

NURSE ALERT

Pressure sores can be prevented by systematic assessment and management as part of the overall plan of care.

Initial interventions aim at identifying the person at risk, as well as prevention. Once pressure sores begin to develop, interventions are designed according to the extent of the lesions and center around the relief of pressure. Basic nursing interventions include a routine of turning every 2 hours; special mattresses such as a waterbed mattress, a circulating air mattress, or an egg crate mattress; special cushions for the wheelchair; range-of-motion exercises; ambulation; and special skin care. For additional information regarding pressure sores, see Chapter 31.

In addition, residents and families can be taught how to prevent pressure sores and encouraged to take part in the treatment plan. Residents who sit in chairs for extended periods should be taught to change position frequently. They can push up on the arms of their chairs to relieve the pressure. Isometric flexion exercises of the buttocks increase circulation and relieve pressure. The nurse may need to remind residents to follow their treatment plans.

There are numerous products for the management of pressure sores. Treatment must begin as soon as redness develops. Once the skin breaks, the wound should be cleansed with an isotonic solution (normal saline). These solutions are not toxic and do not damage healthy skin cells surrounding the ulcer. Wounds that look infected should be cultured. Antiseptics are appropriate for "dirty" wounds only (Thomason, 1989). Synthetic dressings such as the hydrocolloids (Duoderm; Comfeel), moisture vapor permeable transparent dressings (Opsite; Tegaderm), and absorption dressings (Bard; Debrisman) are useful for Stage 2 and some Stage 3 pressure sores if they are not infected. Deeper wounds, and wounds with a great deal of drainage, require dressings such as Sorbsan. Karaya powder absorbs the exudate without drying the wound.

When necrotic tissue is present, the pressure sore must be debrided. Noninvasive wet-to-dry dressings are often the treatment of choice. However, this debridement process does take time to be effective. Other measures include use of a scalpel and scissors to remove necrotic tissue, followed by enzyme ointments such as Elase to continue debridement. The appearance of pink granulation tissue heralds the end of the debridement process.

Povidone iodine kills bacteria, spores, fungi, and viruses. However it inhibits the formation of granulation tissue (Thomason, 1989). It is recommended that povidone iodine be used only on dirty wounds and in a dilution of no more than 1%. Hydrogen peroxide helps debride wounds but can damage healthy tissue. It is best used only at the start of wound care for cleansing and debridement. For infected wounds, especially in the presence of diabetes, the physician should be contacted for advice regarding use of systemic antibiotics.

In addition to the physician, other members of the healthcare team need to be involved in the treatment plan. An in-depth nutritional assessment and treatment plan needs to be instituted. When a pressure sore drains, the person loses albumin, a necessary factor in

BOX 16-3

Nursing Process

PRESSURE SORES

ASSESSMENT

General condition of skin
Skin over bony prominences
Awareness of pressure sensation
Ability to move
Nutritional status
Urinary or fecal incontinence
Amount of shear and friction on skin
Pressure ulcer staging: color, odor, presence of necrotic tissue, exudate, condition of surrounding skin
Vital signs and temperature
Laboratory values: albumin, ferriten, wound culture, white blood cells
Family's ability to provide associated care

NURSING DIAGNOSES

Impaired skin integrity related to friction, shear, or pressure
Risk for infection related to open pressure ulcer and/or poor nutritional status
Impaired home maintenance management related to long-term therapy
Risk for caregiver role strain related to long-term therapy
Altered nutrition: less than body requirements related to chronic illness

NURSING INTERVENTIONS

Maintain preventive measures, including pressure reduction/relief.
Maintain nutritional needs and management of incontinence.
Provide aseptic local wound care as ordered.
Maintain no pressure on pressure ulcer until it has healed.
Provide perineal hygiene after incontinence.
Encourage a high protein, high caloric diet, if not contraindicated.
Administer antibiotics as prescribed.
Refer patient to social worker to assist with discharge planning needs.
Discuss possible need for respite care.

EVALUATION OF EXPECTED OUTCOMES

Pressure ulcer shows evidence of healing
No evidence of local or systemic infection
Verbalizes necessary home care measures
Verbalizes available resources

healing. Nutritional interventions include an increase in protein, either at mealtime or by the use of supplements. Periodic albumin levels are needed to monitor nutritional sufficiency. Physical and occupational therapy may help in the development of an activity plan. Special cushions for the wheelchair or assistive devices will help the person move more independently.

Pressure sores severely limit independence and threaten functional ability. Prevention and treatment decisions often rest on the nurse. Resident, family, and staff teaching are important aspects of practice in addition to coordination of care with the interdisciplinary team.

NURSE ALERT

The primary cause of cognitive decline is medication.

Decline in Mental Status

A decline in mental status in the elderly is poorly understood and evaluated. Unfortunately, memory loss is often considered a consequence of aging by both the older person and the healthcare professional. However, a decline in mental status is a symptom rather than a disease and may actually be the symptom of any number of underlying conditions. The primary cause of cognitive decline among the elderly is medication. In the nursing home, multiple medications are often used, doses may be too high, and medications may be given after the underlying problem is resolved, making the medication inappropriate. Periodic reevaluation of all medications should occur on a regular basis.

Other causes of cognitive decline include infections (e.g., respiratory or urinary tract infections), metabolic problems (e.g., diabetes, thyroid conditions), poor nutrition, sensory disturbances, tumors, anemia, atherosclerosis, alcohol abuse, trauma, and environmental factors. Confusion is not a simple phenomenon. The person with confusion often requires an extensive evaluation to determine the cause.

There are three *D*'s associated with confusion in the elderly: **delirium, depression,** and **dementia.** Although discussed separately, the confused older person commonly has two and often three of the conditions at the same time. See Chapter 14 for a more complete discussion of delirium, depression, and dementia.

Delirium

Delirium is a common, nonspecific presentation of illness in the elderly. It is often the first sign of underlying disease. And it is a symptom in need of evaluation. *Delirium* and *acute confusional state* may be terms used interchangeably to describe the same syndrome. *Delirium* replaces terminology once used to include acute organic brain syndrome, acute dementia, and toxic confusional state. Delirium is a global cognitive impairment of memory and organization of thought. Its onset is sudden and is characterized by uncooperative behavior, drowsiness and/or hyperactivity, mood swings, inappropriate language, delusions, hallucinations, and confused visual-spacial relationships. Symptoms are more severe at night. The mental status assessment will show an inability to attend to tasks and an altered level of consciousness.

Depression

Another common cause of confusion is depression. Again, confusion may be the presenting symptom. Depression often goes unrecognized and untreated in the older population, yet the elderly are at highest risk for successful suicides. It is likely that between 30% and 50% of the residents in long-term care have some type of depression. In addition to confusion, the depressed older person will have a variety of somatic complaints. They are commonly labeled hypochondriacs.

Conditions often associated with depression include thyroid and adrenal abnormalities, Parkinson's disease, CVA, medications, and other psychiatric syndromes. The mental status assessment will reveal only mild, if any, impairment. Interviews with the person will be difficult with many "I don't know" answers. The score on the Geriatric Depression Scale (short form) will indicate depression with a score of 5 or higher.

Dementia

Dementia, once called *organic brain syndrome,* is a term used to describe a global cognitive dysfunction with impairment in short- and long-term memory, orientation, abstract thinking, and judgment, as well as personality changes. Disturbances in cortical function that cause aphasia (language disorders), apraxia (inability to carry out motor function), and agnosia (failure to recognize objects and people that are familiar) are also included. The mental status assessment will show a global cognitive impairment, but depending on the stage of the illness, the person may be able to attend to tasks and perform calculations (Besdine and others, 1991). There are many different types of dementia. The most common is dementia of the Alzheimer's type (DAT). Unlike delirium, the onset of DAT is slow and insidious, and the disease is progressive and irreversible. The disease process continues for many years and places considerable burden on the family. Families will report that the person is not quite the same but may have trouble describing the exact problem. Getting lost while walking or driving or forgetting to turn off the burners on the stove are common behaviors that bring the family to a healthcare provider.

When assessing the person with dementia, the nurse will note many "near miss" answers to questions and an attempt to conceal problems. The person may also be unsociable, uncooperative, hostile, and confused and disoriented. Because confusion is one of the presenting symptoms and there is no differential diagnosis for dementia, there needs to be a complete evaluation that includes laboratory tests, x-ray examinations, computed tomography scans, magnetic resonance imagery, and psychiatric and neurologic testing.

Intervention

Caring for the person who has an alteration in thought processes is difficult. The person with delirium needs a consistent, quiet, and calm approach to care. The environment should be organized to avoid extremes and excessive sensory input. The room should be quiet with familiar people to provide care, changes in personnel and routines should be avoided, and lighting should be decreased at night. Orientation to person, time, and place may be helpful. Once the underlying condition is corrected, the delirium will clear. Mental status will become normal providing there is no other cognitive problem.

Depression should be treated with both medications and therapy. There may be a resistance to therapy from the healthcare workers and the older person. Beneath the resistance is the belief that therapy for the older person is not cost effective and is of little use. The older person, however, will benefit and regain independence and function, as well as have an improved mental status. Reminiscence, life review, and support groups are useful and beneficial interventions that can be initiated by the nurse.

The nursing home resident with dementia needs structure and consistency. Routines are helpful. Because wandering may be a problem, warning devices that let the nurse know that the person is out of bed or opening a door should be used. They allow the person freedom of movement, independence, and functioning ability while maintaining a safe environment. The person can also be seated close to the nurses' station for closer observation.

Of primary importance when caring for the person with dementia is care of the family. Placement of the loved one in a long-term care facility was probably a difficult decision. Watching the slow deterioration and not being recognized are difficult adjustments for any family member. The nurse who reassures the family, offers support, and provides information will help their anticipatory grieving process.

KEY CONCEPTS

- The nursing home is only a part of the long-term continuum of services.
- Care of the nursing home resident is challenging and rewarding.
- Caring for nursing home residents requires the promotion of autonomy, independence, and improvement of function.
- Ethical dilemmas arise when there is tension between promoting autonomy and protecting the safety of the resident.
- Providing appropriate care at the end of life requires input and attention from the nursing staff.
- A complete assessment of the resident's function, mental status, and level of depression is necessary upon admission to the nursing home and on a routine basis thereafter.
- Falls, a significant problem in the nursing home, can be influenced by the resident's gait and balance, muscle strength, sensory changes, and medications.
- Physical and chemical restraints in the nursing home may increase injuries and harm the autonomy of the resident.
- Behavioral approaches are the best way to deal with troublesome behaviors in the resident with dementia.
- Urinary incontinence of the nursing home resident should be carefully assessed and treated.
- Constipation can be treated by changes in diet, fluid intake, and exercise, rather than dependence on laxatives.
- Pressure sores can usually be prevented by careful attention to position, skin care, hygiene, and nutrition.

CRITICAL THINKING EXERCISES

1. Describe your personal feelings about the use of life-sustaining methods in the critically ill.
2. Discuss the risk factors and preventive measures for falls among elderly nursing home residents.
3. Describe your feelings about life as a resident in a nursing home.
4. Discuss the pros and cons of using restraints to prevent falls.

REFERENCES AND ADDITIONAL READINGS

Agency for Health Care Policy and Research: *Pressure ulcers in adults: prediction and prevention: clinical practice guideline.* Rockville, Md, 1992a, US Department of Health and Human Services AHCPR Publication no 92-0048.

Agency for Health Care Policy and Research: *Urinary incontinence in adults: clinical practice guideline.* Rockville, Md, 1992b. US Department of Health and Human Services AHCPR Publication no 92-0038.

Besdine R and others: Managing advanced Alzheimer's disease, *Patient Care* 25(18):75-100, 1991.

Cornacchione M, Slusser M: Depression in the long-term-care setting, *Nurs Home Med* 2(2):24-36, 1994.

Eisenberg MS and others: Cardiopulmonary resuscitation in the elderly, *Ann Intern Med* 113:408-409, 1990.

Evans LK, Strumpf NE: Patterns of restraint: a cross-cultural view, *Gerontologist* 12:272, 1987.

Freeman I: Developing systems that promote autonomy: policy considerations. In Kane R, Caplan A, (editors): *Everyday ethics: resolving dilemmas in nursing home life,* New York, 1990, Springer.

Matteson MA, McConnell A: *Gerontological nursing: concepts*

and practice, New York, 1988, WB Saunders.
Mion L and others: Use of physical restraints in the hospital setting: implications for the nurse, *Geriatr Nurs* 15(3):127-132, 1994.
Neugarten B: *Middle age and aging,* Chicago, 1968, University of Chicago Press.
Rader J, Donius M: Leveling off restraints, *Geriatr Nurs* 12(2):71-73, 1991.
Seaver AMH: My world now, *Newsweek,* p11, June 27, 1994.
Semla T and others: Effect of the Omnibus Reconciliation Act 1987 on antipsychotic prescribing in nursing home residents, *J Am Geriatr Soc* 42:648-652, 1994.
Strumpf NE, Evans L: Physical restraints of hospitalized elderly: perceptions of patients and nurses, *Nurs Res* 37:132, 1988.
Tabloski PA and others: Effects of calming music on the level of agitation in cognitively impaired nursing home residents, *Am J Alzheimer Care Res* 10(1):10-15, 1995.
Thomason S: Frontline antiseptics, *Geriatr Nurs* 10(5): 235-236, 1989.
Wells T, editor: The rehabilitation management of urinary incontinence, *Top Geriatr Rehab* 3:1-77, 1988.
White M and others: Skin tears in frail elders: a practical approach to prevention, *Geriatr Nursing,* 15(2):95-99, 1994.

CHAPTER 17

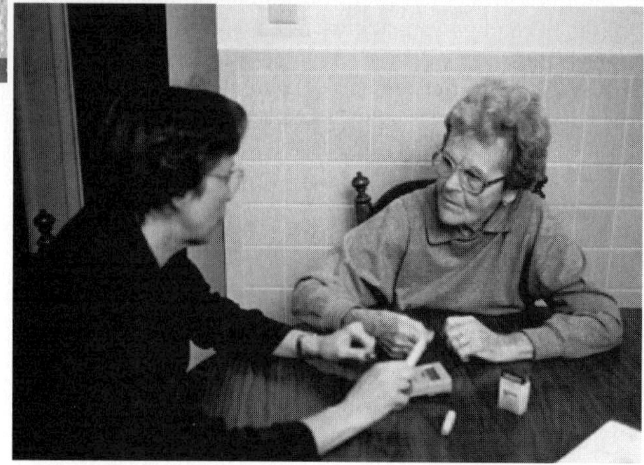

Home Healthcare

CHAPTER OBJECTIVES

1 Identify the concept of home healthcare.
2 Describe the historic development of home healthcare.
3 Identify the types of home health agencies.
4 Identify the services provided by home health agencies.
5 Discuss the concept of the team in home healthcare.
6 Discuss the role of and the activities provided by the nurse in the home setting.
7 Identify the sources of reimbursement for home health services.
8 Identify trends and future directions in home healthcare.
9 Discuss the relationship of long-term care to home healthcare.
10 Give examples of the rewards and opportunities in home healthcare.

KEY WORDS

diagnosis-related groups (DRGs)
environment
populations
reimbursement
socioeconomic

Home healthcare is provided in the home to maintain or restore a person's health and well-being. The concept of home healthcare has grown out of a rich tradition in the history of nursing. It has evolved in response to the needs of patients and families in community settings. Home health services have been a dynamic and energetic force in healthcare since the early part of the twentieth century, when nurses began to work in the urban slums of the nation.

Home healthcare in the United States began in the late nineteenth century as "visiting" or "district" nursing. In many communities, interested and benevolent citizens formed associations, raised funds, and hired nurses to visit the "sick and poor" in their homes. These developments occurred when urban areas in America were undergoing expansion. Immigration was at its peak, and thousands of foreign-born people thronged the cities. Epidemics of influenza, cholera, and other highly contagious diseases were rampant. Physicians were in short supply, and it was the nurse who stepped in to help family members care for their sick. The development of district nursing was a response to the needs of this population.

In many cities, the first of these organizations was the visiting nurse associations and district nurse associations. In 1893 Lilian Wald and Mary Brewster established one of the first visiting nurse programs at the Henry Street Settlement in New York City (Freeman, 1963). These organizations were formed as charitable entities to provide nursing services to those who could not afford to pay for nursing care. Early organizations developed in such cities as Buffalo, New York, Boston, and Philadelphia (Figure 17-1). The focus of these services was not only to provide nursing care as needed but also to teach family members the principles of good hygiene and cleanliness (Freeman, 1963). These concepts of teaching and prevention continue to be a part of home healthcare.

Because care occurs in the home setting, the family is the unit of service and plays a major role in the delivery of service. Because service occurs in the community setting, the **socioeconomic,** cultural, political, and **environmental** characteristics of the community influence the practice of home healthcare. Therefore, the visiting nurse associations responded to the growing needs of the population, and many municipalities and government agencies began to assume responsibility for community health services. Their role emphasized controlling outbreaks of communicable diseases. As the health problems of the nation changed from tuberculosis to heart disease, cancer, and stroke, the programs of those official agencies who provided public health nursing also changed (Gardner, 1987).

Visiting nursing has evolved into public health nursing, community health nursing, and home healthcare nursing. Public health nursing is usually delivered by a town, city, or state governmental agency. The goal of the public health model is to prevent disease and educate large **populations** who are at risk for

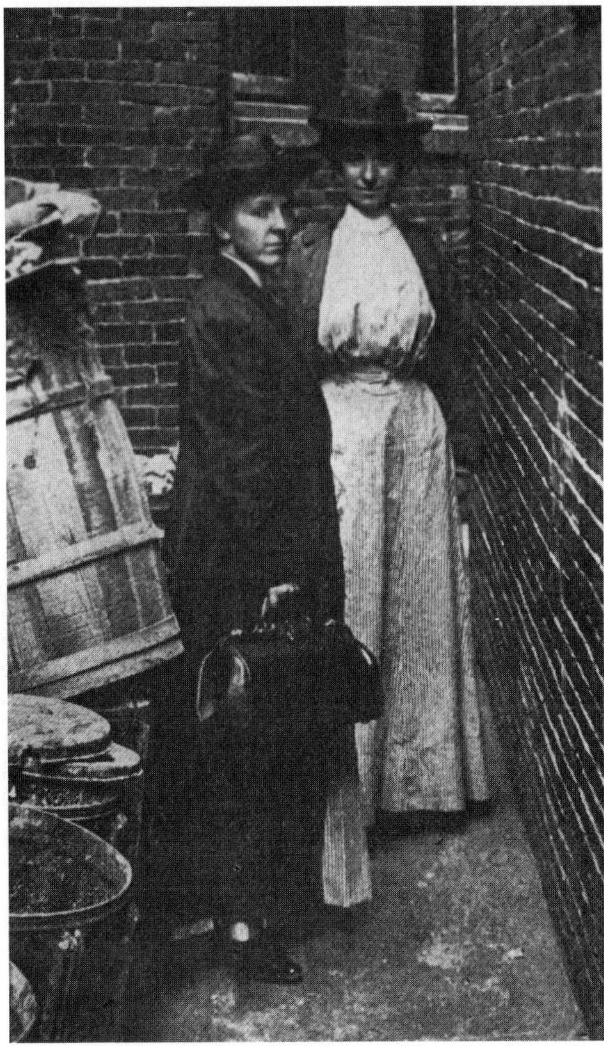

Figure 17-1 Two visiting nurses in Boston's North End, 1909. (Courtesy Boston Visiting Nurse Association, Boston; Nursing Archives, Mugar Memorial Library, Boston University.)

certain diseases. Home health nursing integrates prevention and education into its model of services, which is the care of acutely ill and chronically ill persons at home (Janczak, 1985). These services are usually provided by a freestanding or hospital-based home health agency. The National Association for Home Care estimates that there are 3000 home health agencies nationwide (McNiff, 1986). The following types of organizations deliver home health services:

- *Voluntary agency*—a nonprofit organization with a volunteer board of directors (e.g., visiting nurse associations [VNAs])
- *Official agency*—a tax-supported unit of a governmental or municipal organization (e.g., a health department of a town or city)
- *Proprietary agency*—a for-profit organization that delivers home health services (e.g., investor-owned national chains such as Medical Personnel Pool, Upjohn)
- *Hospital-based agency*—a unit or department of a hospital that delivers services to persons who have left the hospital but still need nursing care in their homes

HOME HEALTH SERVICES

Most home health agencies offer a range of services. These services usually include skilled nursing, home health aides, rehabilitation services, medical social work, and specialty care.

Skilled Nursing

Skilled nursing care involves assessing patient needs and establishing and carrying out the plan of care. Skilled nursing in the home setting may be provided by nurses who have had 1 to 2 years of acute care nursing experience. Skilled care in the home setting includes, but is not limited to, assessing and teaching the medication and dietary regimens, dressing care, catheter care, injections, and other therapeutic treatments.

Home Health Aide

Services provided by the home health aide include personal care, assistance with the activities of daily living, meal preparation, and bowel and bladder management. The services provided by the home health aide are determined and supervised by a registered nurse (RN).

Rehabilitation Services

Physical therapy, occupational therapy, and speech therapy are forms of rehabilitation. These services are provided by a registered therapist and include evaluating and assessing the patient's status, developing a rehabilitation program, and implementing the treatment plan. Rehabilitation can include range-of-motion exercises, strengthening exercises, and assistance with ambulation and mobility. Patients who benefit from rehabilitation services are those who have had cerebrovascular accidents, those with neurologic injuries or diseases, and those with orthopedic conditions such as total hip or knee replacements. The goal is to restore function, develop maximum independence, and provide ways in which patients may cope with a long-term disability (Figure 17-2).

Medical Social Work

Social work services include counseling, support for patients and their families, help with coping with the problems of illness and disease, and assistance in learning to use community resources. Patients may also be advised about and provided assistance with financial problems such as budgeting and applying for financial aid.

Specialty Care

Home health services now encompass many areas that were traditionally provided in the hospital setting. These include administration of medications through heparin locks, parenteral/enteral therapy, ostomy care, ventilator care, and respiratory therapy. It is also possible to have a full array of laboratory services available to patients at home, including electrocardiographic monitoring, pneumograms, and x-ray films (Kraus, 1994).

Other Services

The home health services available to special populations include pediatric care; hospice care; psychiatric care; and cardiac, enterostomal, and gerontologic community health nursing services.

Supplies and Equipment

The home health agency can supply directly or make arrangements for items such as dressings, intravenous (IV) or oxygen equipment, catheters, walkers, wheelchairs, and hospital beds. The ability to provide this service allows patients to be cared for in their homes and in an environment that mimics the hospital setting (Stanhope, Lancaster 1992).

SUPPORTIVE SERVICES IN THE COMMUNITY

Other supportive services in the community augment professional services and family support and enable patients to remain at home. The following services may be provided directly by the home healthcare agency or arranged for by the nurse in the organization (McNiff, 1986):

- *Day care*—offers supervised activities and meals at a specific site, such as a senior center or long-term–care facility (e.g., chronic disease/rehabilitation hospital, extended-care facility)
- *Telephone reassurance*—provides contact by phone and offers support to those who are homebound and alone
- *Friendly visitors*—volunteers visit those who are unable to get out of their homes themselves; workers provide socialization and companionship and occasionally do errands
- *Meals on Wheels*—a service provided to the geriatric population either in their homes or in a group residential setting; purpose is to assist with meal preparation and to provide older people with a well-balanced diet
- *Homemakers*—homemakers assist with meal preparation, housekeeping, laundry, or food shopping
- *Personal Emergency Response Systems*—a system available to persons who live alone at home; electronic devices are connected by telephone to a central location that alerts relatives and emergency services in the event of a fall or accident (Brickner, 1994)

THE HOME HEALTHCARE TEAM

The team concept is essential for delivering services to persons in their own home. In addition to the RN, who serves as the coordinator and case manager, other nursing roles contribute to the care of patients at home, including the licensed practical nurse (LPN) and the *certified home health aide.* Both of these workers help care for patients in the home setting and function in collaboration with the RN. The RN supervises the home health aide in carrying out the plan of care. The *physician* is also a member of the team and authorizes the medical orders in the care plan. The social worker acts on the physician's medical orders, provides support and counseling, and focuses on helping the patient and family or significant other cope with the socioeconomic consequences of the disease, illness, or disability. Others brought into the home as needed include the physical therapist, occupational therapist, and speech pathologist. A nutritionist may help patients remain at home by providing nutrition counseling and teaching about special and therapeutic diets.

NURSING IN THE HOME SETTING

Nursing is the core service in the delivery of home healthcare. The nurse is the case manager and works within the framework of a team that includes the pa-

A

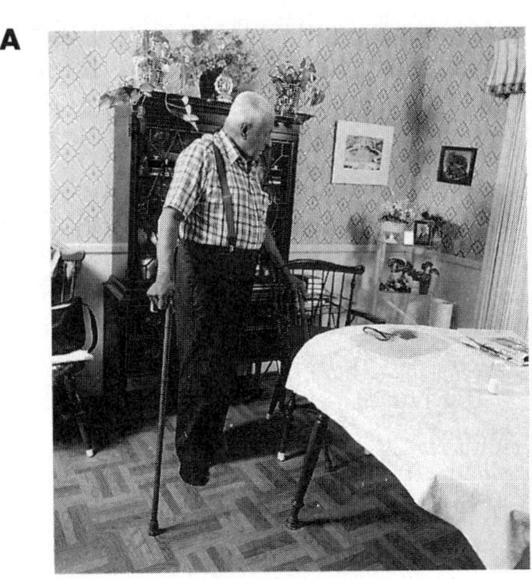

B

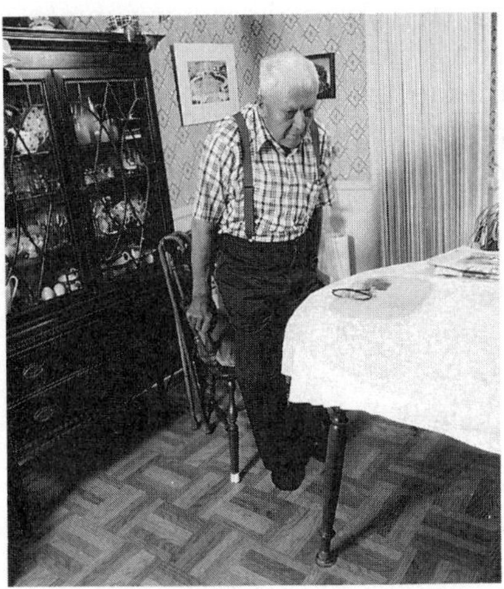

Figure 17-2 Assessment of activities of daily living are an important nursing responsibility. **A,** An elderly man demonstrates his method of walking with the use of two canes. **B,** He demonstrates his method of lowering himself into and lifting himself up from his chair. (From Barkauskas VH and others: *Health and physical assessment,* St Louis, 1994, Mosby.

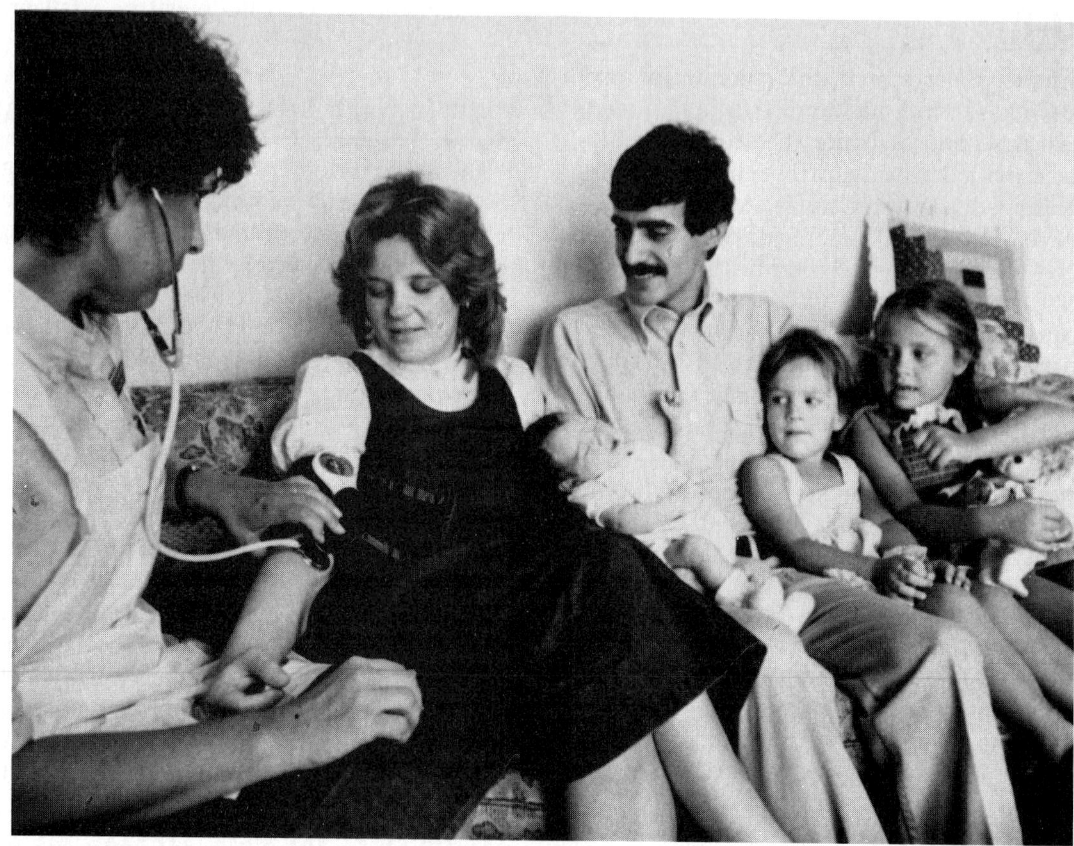

Figure 17-3 During a home visit, nurses determine the health status of all family members and assess family dynamics. (From Clemen-Stone S, Eigsti DG, McGuire SL: *Comprehensive community health nursing,* ed 4, St Louis, 1995, Mosby.

tient, family, physician, and others. The nurse is responsible for assessing the patient; developing, implementing, and evaluating the care plan; and evaluating its outcome. Using the nursing process, the nurse tries to minimize the symptoms of illness, disease, and disability and to promote health within the context of home and community (Figure 17-3).

The nurse in the home setting not only works with the team but also arranges for other programs and services to be made available to the patient and family at home. The nurse may use other community resources to allow the patient to remain at home, such as Meals on Wheels and temporary homemakers. A major responsibility of the nurse is to link patients and their families to available community resources such as welfare programs, counseling resources, and rehabilitation services (Stanhope, Lancaster, 1992).

General Versus Specialty Care

The nurse practicing in the home setting has been viewed historically as a generalist who provides care to patients and families of all age groups and with all health problems, diseases, or disabilities. The nurse cares for patients with cardiac problems, diabetes, cancer, pulmonary disease, and other problems. In caring for patients, the nurse integrates the principles of patient teaching and learning in the plan of care. The focus is on teaching the patient and family the necessary care and techniques to allow the patient to remain at home and prevent costly hospitalization (Kraus, 1994).

As the technology of healthcare has changed, many specialized services have been developed and provided by home health agencies. Specially prepared nurses offer services directly to patients and offer collaboration consultation to others who are providing services. The specialty areas now available include pediatric, ostomy, oncologic, hospice, and geriatric care, as well as psychiatric–mental health services. Technology that was once available only in the institutional setting has become more readily adaptable to the home setting. Along with providing home care in the traditional sense, nurses now provide home care to patients who require infusion therapy, parenteral/enteral nutrition, oxygen, mechanical ventilation, and respiratory therapy (Figure 17-4).

CASE STUDY

Mr. Smith is a 48-year-old married man and is a self-employed carpenter. His wife works part time in a local grocery store, and he has two children, a 15-year-old boy and a 12-year-old girl. Up until the time he was seen in the emergency department of the local hospital, he had been very healthy and had not seen a physician for many years.

Mr. Smith was seen in the emergency department after experiencing an acute onset of chest pain while scraping paint from a house. Tests and a physical examination confirmed an acute evolving myocardial infarction. During his hospital stay, he was diagnosed with a severe anterior wall myocardial infarction with continuing hypertension. While in the hospital, Mr. Smith appeared to be ambivalent about instructions concerning his condition, diet, medications, and activity restrictions. He also verbalized anxiety regarding his finances. His blood pressure was unstable, and he was receiving antihypertensive agents.

Because Mr. Smith would soon be discharged from the hospital to conform to his insurance guidelines, he was referred to the local home health agency for follow-up teaching and monitoring of compliance with his medical regimen.

A nurse from the local visiting nurse and home health agency visited Mr. Smith in his home the day after his discharge. The nurse explained to him and his wife that the physician had requested visits to assess his condition and teach him about his medications, which now included warfarin (Coumadin) and methyldopa (Aldomet), and to assist with his recovery at home. During the visit, Mr. Smith expressed concern regarding his finances. Although he was ambulatory, he was unable to return to his previous level of activity as a carpenter. During the nursing assessment visit, it became apparent that Mr. Smith was denying the extent of his disability.

Using the nursing process, the visiting nurse collected objective and subjective data to provide a baseline patient assessment. This assessment established the database needed to identify existing and potential patient health concerns that would require nursing interventions (Gordon, 1995). The nursing assessment included a cardiopulmonary evaluation—blood pressure readings, measurement of pulse rates, oral temperature, and auscultation of the lungs. Mr. Smith denied complaints of chest pain. Mr. Smith was not able to verbalize an understanding of the need to continue to take his medications even if he did not have any symptoms or felt sick.

Using the nursing process to develop the plan of care, the visiting nurse established a patient care plan that included the family and incorporated the medical orders. Arrangements were made for Mr. Smith and his family to be seen by the home health agency social worker, who would assist in getting the family the necessary financial assistance. The nurse collaborated with the social worker to focus on Mr. Smith's and his family's adjustment to the illness, as well as on his denial of the illness.

A 4 g sodium diet had been prescribed by the physician. Therefore the visiting nurse began teaching Mr. Smith and his family how to develop a diet plan that included food sources low in sodium, how to read food labels, and how to avoid prepackaged processed foods.

The nurse told the family that she would return the next day, and she continued to visit three times per week for 1 week to provide support, encouragement, teaching, and assessment of Mr. Smith's status. Through the help of the social worker, the family was eligible to receive financial assistance, which helped reduce Mr. Smith's anxiety level and made him more willing to learn about his disease, its signs and symptoms, and the limitations imposed by his diagnosis. He also began to understand the importance of taking his medications. The nurse continued to see Mr. Smith one time per week for 3 weeks to assess and teach the dietary restrictions with his family and to provide an overall assessment of his status. Through counseling with the social worker, Mr. Smith began preparing to enter a job retraining program in which he would learn new skills and find employment in a less strenuous job.

The visiting nurse was in contact, both verbally and in writing, with Mr. Smith's physician throughout the home care program. The visiting nurse provided feedback and clinical information regarding his status, which was reviewed with the physician. When Mr. Smith and his wife were independent in all aspects of care, the nurse informed the physician of her intent to discharge him from the program.

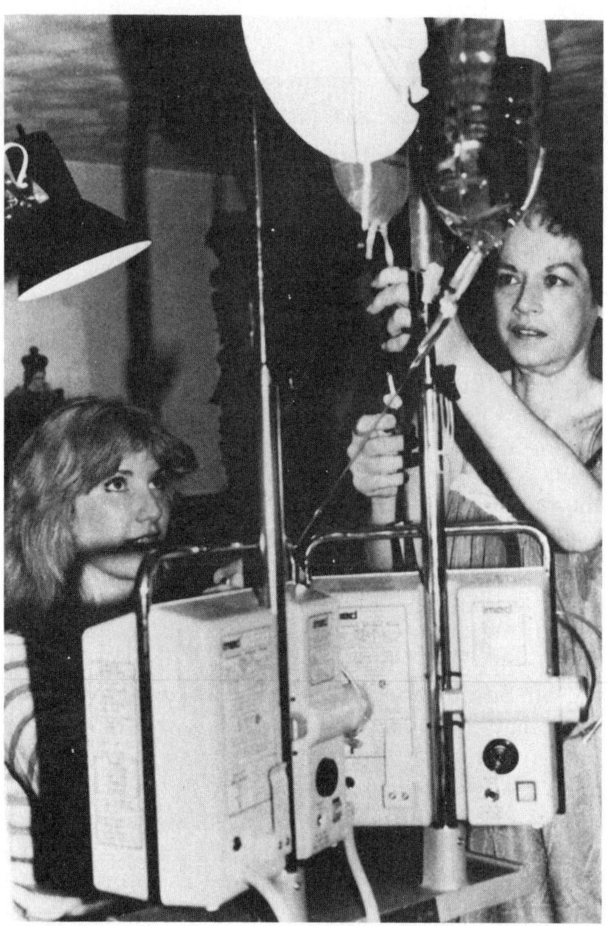

Figure 17-4 A patient learns to care for an infusion pump with the assistance of a nurse from the home health agency. (Courtesy Boston Visiting Nurse Association, Boston; Nursing Archives, Mugar Memorial Library, Boston University.

Reimbursement

Home health services are **reimbursed** through a variety of third-party payers. Major support comes from Medicare and, in most states, Medicaid. Private insurance coverage for home health services is currently limited but is growing as insurance companies compare the higher cost of hospital care to home care. A growing market in health maintenance organizations (HMOs) has led to the provision of home health services to the subscribers of these types of insurance plans. HMOs view home health services as one way to substitute for the more expensive types of care (McNiff, 1986). Voluntary agencies typically charge for services on a "sliding-scale" basis, which establishes the amount of payment that a patient should pay for services on the basis of income level.

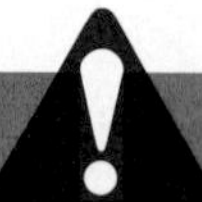

NURSE ALERT

For the agency to be reimbursed under Medicare, the patient must be homebound and have a physician's approval for the care plan.

Impact of Reimbursement on Delivery of Services

The most significant impact on the development and growth of home healthcare came more than 20 years ago with the initiation of Title XVIII (Medicare) and Title XIX (Medicaid) of the Social Security Act. Under the Medicare legislation, the Home Health Benefit was created, and home health services were developed for older Americans. What had been known as community health nursing gradually began to evolve into home healthcare. The traditional visiting nurse association has become known as the certified home health agency. The titles and names of many organizations were amended to reflect these changes (e.g., Visiting Nurse and Home Health Agency). Under the regulations of the Medicare program, agencies must provide skilled nursing and one other service such as physical therapy, occupational therapy, or speech therapy. Many agencies provide these services plus other programs such as home health aides. Agencies must meet federally defined standards known as the "Conditions of Participation" to be eligible for reimbursement. When Medicare legislation passed in 1966, states were also eligible to receive federal funding for health services for those entitled because of income levels. This program, known as Medicaid, also provided support for home health services in most states. These two pieces of legislation had sweeping effects on the delivery of home health services in the United States and led to the growth and proliferation of many types of home health services. What had once been a socially benevolent service that was provided through district nursing in the framework of public health and community nursing was now a distinct component of the healthcare system that had come of age (Gardner, 1987).

To be eligible for reimbursement under Title XVIII and Title XIX for home health services, agencies must be surveyed each year to evaluate their compliance with the "Conditions of Participation." This evaluation is usually carried out by the public health department in each state. Over the years this process has mandated that home health agencies develop practices, programs, and procedures that meet certain standards.

The standards are related to the administrative, program, and quality assurance structure of the home health agency. These governmental mandates have affected the delivery of services and have required agencies to develop comprehensive programs and more sophisticated administrative systems. The mandates have not only led to a more consumer-oriented philosophy but also have increased the costs of services. What had been provided free or for a minimum charge in the early days of visiting nursing is now more expensive. However, compared with the costs of hospital care or other types of institutional care, home healthcare is much less expensive and often more humane and desirable.

The Older Americans Act of 1972 made possible the payment of a broad range of supportive and social services that allow elderly persons to remain at home. These federally supported programs include homemaker services, home health aide services, and home-delivered meals (Gardner, 1987).

Trends

Recent changes in the methods by which the federal government and other payers reimburse hospitals for services have had an impact on home health services. More patients who a short time ago would have been cared for in the acute care setting of the hospital are now being cared for at home. This is because of the **diagnosis-related group (DRG)** system. Hospitals who care for Medicare beneficiaries are reimbursed at a fixed rate by the prospective payment system on the basis of the DRG system. Hospitals are reimbursed according to the patient's diagnosis, and a specified number of hospital days is allowed for each diagnosis (Iglehark, 1993). This system has given hospitals an incentive to discharge patients earlier from the hospital than ever before. Therefore these home health patients are more acutely ill, have more intense needs for services, and require more care. This trend is similar to the historic tradition of caring for the sick at home. Long before the development of hospitals and other healthcare institutions, ill persons were cared for in their homes by family members or neighbors. Products are being developed that allow patients to remain at home safely, including portable ventilators; cardiac monitors; and pumps for administering nutrients, antibiotics, and pain medications. In addition, the home setting can be adapted easily to meet the needs of patients. Psychologically, patients do well and can recover faster at home. They can sleep in their own beds, eat the food they like, and maintain more control over their own lives.

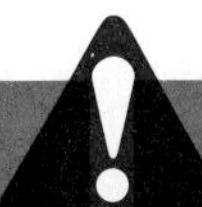

NURSE ALERT

Cultural competency is required by all members of the home care team.

To work in the home setting, a nurse must be able to provide care to a variety of populations and in many different settings. The nurse needs to be sensitive to the ethnic, socioeconomic, and cultural differences of patients. Working in the home setting increases one's sensitivity to the differences in persons and groups and requires an understanding of the cultural and socioeconomic issues that offset health status and affect how a person copes with illness.

Working in the home setting also demands a different focus than working in the institutional setting. The home environment requires creativity, flexibility, adaptability, and the capacity to improvise in a variety of settings. The ability to communicate with other team members in the community and with other healthcare providers is also very important. Because the physician or social worker is usually not physically present in the home, other measures must be used to communicate and collaborate.

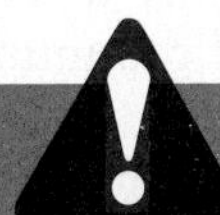

NURSE ALERT

Wisdom and ingenuity are major characteristics needed by the home care nurse.

HEALTHCARE REFORM

The need for healthcare reform may have a major impact on the delivery of care in the home and on other community-based services. Of the many proposals that will be debated, each will illustrate an increased need for disease prevention and health promotion. Health promotion has been a significant focus for professional nursing, but until recently did not generate payment for service and thus was often omitted. Any reform, whether enacted by the federal or by state governments, should have a strong emphasis on disease-prevention methods. See Chapter 1 for a discussion of *Healthy People 2000*.

ETHICAL DILEMMA

Mrs. Peters, an 82-year-old widow with no children, lives by herself on the fourth floor of an apartment in a deteriorating neighborhood. She is increasingly confused, and her eyesight is worsening. Her home health team believes she needs 24-hour-a-day care because she is unable to care for her daily activities of living, let alone the problems resulting from her diabetes. Medicaid will not pay for around-the-clock care, so the case worker suggests that she go into a nursing home, where she will be in a safe environment and have someone to care for her 24 hours a day. Mrs. Peters adamantly refuses to consider this alternative and states that she has a right to stay in the home where she has lived for 35 years.

What ethical principles are involved, and what actions would you take?

LONG-TERM CARE AND HOME HEALTHCARE

As the elderly population continues to increase through the year 2000, the need for services for this group will grow proportionately, including the needs for supportive, maintenance, and chronic care. Nursing is the pivotal profession in the delivery of long-term care, and there is increasing support to have long-term care delivered in the home and community setting (Brickner, 1994).

The largest single-age group served by home health agencies consists of those persons over 65 years of age. However, Medicare does not pay for custodial care or long-term care of elderly persons in the home. Coverage is available only for acute episodes of illness as evidenced by documented skilled care. The Medicare term *skilled nursing* describes the administration of tasks such as catheterization, injection, and dressings that require a nurse's care. The needs of those who require long-term care, disabled older adults, usually do not fall within this narrow designation. Disabled older adults need supportive and custodial services. These services allow them to remain in the community and include assistance with the activities of daily living, such as bathing, routine assessment of medications, teaching, reinforcement of health practices, diet, exercise, and hygiene. Currently these services are not reimbursed. In many states, Medicaid pays for the cost of these services for those who are eligible because of income levels. However, for many Americans, there are significant gaps in coverage for long-term care (Freeman, 1963). The United States must soon deal with these issues to ensure that its citizens are not caught in a "no-care zone." It must also formulate policies for the future to ensure that the growing long-term care needs of the disabled elderly population will be met and financed appropriately (Brickner, 1994) (see Chapter 16).

Home healthcare is a challenging and rewarding experience and is one of the fastest growing systems of healthcare delivery. Practitioners draw on a variety of resources to coordinate a total program of services that allows patients to remain at home. Older patients are the heaviest users of home health services. They also benefit from supportive services such as homemakers, volunteer visitors, and Meals on Wheels. With future trends anticipating extraordinary growth in the elderly population, there is certain to be a subsequent surge in providers of home healthcare. Home healthcare has been identified by many as the future of nursing.

Home healthcare also provides many special opportunities and rewards to the clinician, who must use ingenuity and creativity to deliver care in a variety of environments. Working with other members of the team in carrying out the plan of care can provide quality patient care. The opportunity to learn and understand the aspects of care that are unique to the home and community setting are stimulants to the practitioner. The psychosocial impact of illness and disability on the patient and family are more readily apparent in the home setting than in the institution. These factors affect the services provided and cannot be separated from the medical and other health needs of the patient. Because care is provided in the home, the patient maintains control and mastery over the environment. The home health nurse is viewed as a guest and helper in the delivery of expert care in collaboration with the patient and family.

KEY CONCEPTS

- Home healthcare requires the provision of skilled nursing care and may incorporate other services.
- Home healthcare has a long and distinguished history, including district nursing, public health nursing, and visiting nurses.
- The home health nurse is the leader of a team of other professionals who are concerned with the delivery of care in the home.
- Most technical services are now available to the patient in the home setting.
- Significant barriers exist for the reimbursement of services for the chronically ill.
- The plan for home care is designed to meet individual values, beliefs, and customs.

CRITICAL THINKING EXERCISES

1 What are the factors that influence healthcare in the home setting?
2 Discuss the concept of the family as the unit of service.
3 What is the single most important challenge for home healthcare delivery in the future?

REFERENCES AND ADDITIONAL READINGS

Brickner P: The fate of the homebound aged, *Caring* 13(3):8-9, 1994.

D'Arrigio T: Taking control of cardiovascular care, *Caring* 12(2):14-21, 1994.

Freeman RB: *Public health nursing practice,* Philadelphia, 1963, WB Saunders.

Gardner M: *Public health nursing,* New York, 1987, Macmillan Publishing.

Gordon M: *Nursing diagnosis: process and application,* ed 4, St Louis, 1995, Mosby.

Iglehark JK: The American health care system, *New Engl J Med* 328(21):896-900, 1993.

Janczak DF: Changes in rural public health nursing program: a community profile, *Home Health Nurse,* 3(5):28-34, 1985.

Kraus C: Easing the transition to high-tech home care, *Caring* 13(2):5, 1994

McNiff ML: HMOs and home care: a VNA's experience, *Caring* 5(5):30-33, 1986.

Stanhope M, Lancaster J: *Community health nursing,* ed 3, St Louis, 1992, Mosby.

CHAPTER 18

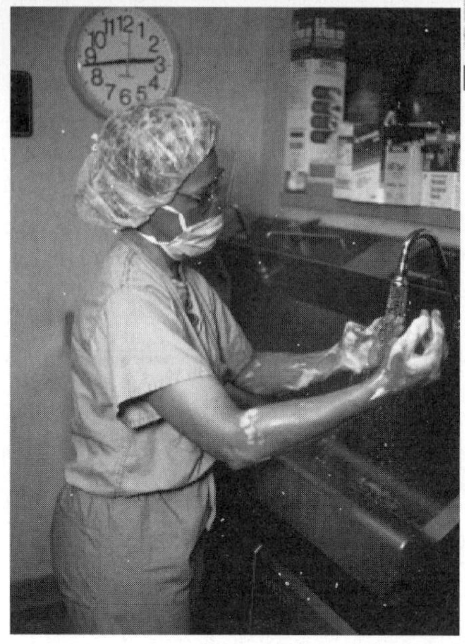

Care of the Surgical Patient

CHAPTER OBJECTIVES

1 Identify four reasons for undergoing surgery.
2 Discuss four negative effects of surgery.
3 Describe the criteria for and the advantages of outpatient surgery.
4 State the major goal of preoperative preparation.
5 Describe the general preoperative preparation of the surgical patient.
6 Identify special considerations for the surgical patient who is obese or older or who has diabetes.
7 Explain surgical asepsis.
8 Describe the roles of the perioperative team.
9 List the common types of anesthesia techniques and their uses.
10 Discuss nursing responsibilities in patient care immediately after surgery.
11 Identify nursing measures that can be used to decrease postoperative discomfort.
12 Explain nursing responsibilities when dealing with the major complications of surgical intervention.
13 Discuss discharge planning for the surgical patient.

KEY WORDS

airway
ambulation
anesthesia
asepsis
atelectasis
autoclave
body image
dehiscence
embolism
evisceration
hemorrhage
hypothermia
laser surgery
pain management
postanesthesia care unit
recovery room
sterilization
surgical procedure
thrombosis
wound healing
wound infection

THE SURGICAL EXPERIENCE

Modern surgery has alleviated many diseases that in past generations had crippled or killed people. Surgery is a planned alteration of physiologic processes within the body in an attempt to arrest or eliminate disease or illness. Surgical procedures are also used for the purposes of examination and reconstruction (Box 18-1). The meaning of surgery varies with each individual, but it is generally a frightening experience to even the most prepared person. Surgery invades one's most intimate privacy. Therefore confidence in the physician, the nurse, and other healthcare workers is an important aspect of helping the patient cope during this time of need.

Surgical procedures may be classified in several ways. A surgical procedure may be done as an emergency or may be scheduled in advance. It may be necessary to save a life or it may be an optional (elective) procedure that is intended to improve health. Elective surgery can be scheduled in advance, which allows the individual to prepare for it physically and psychologically. Knowing the purpose and anticipated outcomes of various surgical procedures can help the nurse to educate and support the patient more effectively.

BOX 18-1

TYPES OF SURGERY

- **Diagnostic** or **exploratory** surgery, which is performed to determine the cause and/or extent of a disease process
- **Curative** surgery, such as an appendectomy, which attempts to remove diseased organs or tissues
- **Palliative** surgery, such as a local sympathectomy for pain control, which lessens the symptoms of a disease without curing it
- **Restorative** or **cosmetic** surgery, such as repair of a fracture or skin grafting for burns, which attempts to restore or improve function or appearance

Negative Effects of Surgery

Stress

The stress response describes a complex physiologic and psychologic reaction to any external or internal threat to the body's equilibrium. This response can result in profound neurochemical changes in the body. These changes initially help the body cope with the invasive reality of surgery, but if the stress response is too severe or prolonged, the body's defenses become depleted and the immune response is suppressed. Organ failure, infection, and life-threatening electrolyte imbalance can occur. The nurse can minimize the potential for these negative effects of stress by identifying factors (other than the surgical experience) that may be contributing to the patient's concern. Careful preoperative preparation and teaching by the nurse greatly lessens the patient's anxiety. During the preoperative period, the surgeon and the anesthetist carefully evaluate any other physical conditions that may increase the risk related to surgery. Some of these risks include electrolyte imbalance, diabetes, liver or renal disease, anemia, lung and heart disorders, malnutrition, obesity, and emotional instability.

Increased susceptibility to infection

Intact skin is the body's first line of defense against bacterial invasion. When the skin is surgically incised, the risk of a local infection greatly increases. Suppression of the immune system caused by stress and breaks in skin integrity make infection a real possibility for every surgical patient. Antibiotic therapy may be prescribed prophylactically, but meticulous surgical and postsurgical aseptic techniques are the keys to preventing infection.

Potential body image changes

Body image, or subjective feelings about personal appearance, is formed early in life. A surgical procedure may significantly alter this self-perception. Operations that cause a visible change in an individual, such as amputation of a body part, involve not only a physical but also a psychologic loss. The removal of organs that have an emotional and social importance, such as the uterus or testicles, may also profoundly affect a patient despite the fact that there is no visible evidence of change. In some cases, such as cosmetic and reconstructive surgeries, these changes are positive and are desired by the patient. The nurse can help a patient who is undergoing a surgical procedure that may affect body image by encouraging him or her to express his or her concerns. A number of community support groups exist, such as ostomy clubs, as well as branches of Reach to Recovery for women who have had mastectomies.

BOX 18-2

CRITERIA FOR OUTPATIENT SURGERY

Patient	Procedure
Accepts the idea of outpatient surgery	Is elective and does not produce severe alterations in physiologic status
Can follow postoperative discharge instructions	Does not require acute or intensive postoperative care such as transfusions or intensive monitoring
Has a home environment and support system that fosters early postoperative recovery at home	Generally causes only minimal pain that can be managed by oral analgesics
Has no other medical conditions that pose a serious risk for home recovery	

Disruption of lifestyle

Every person who undergoes a major surgical procedure experiences at least a temporary change in lifestyle. A person's career, job security, and social activities may be jeopardized if rehabilitation is prolonged or if normal function has been permanently altered. The nurse can often help the patient identify these potential changes and develop coping strategies and can give referrals to appropriate agencies and resources.

Spiritual distress

Spirituality is a uniquely human characteristic. It is a broad concept that represents an individual's search for the meaning of life and death, and it should be considered by nurses when caring for patients who are about to have surgery. Often these issues are not confronted until a patient faces serious illness and the possibility of death. Although some patients may be quite open in expressing their beliefs in a higher power and may find strength and support in this practice, many others exhibit only subtle clues to their states of spiritual need. Patients may ask the nurse to describe personal beliefs about an afterlife, or they may ask if there is a chaplain in the hospital. It is important to allow patients to discuss these issues and to determine if spiritual support would be useful. To do this comfortably, nurses need to examine their own spirituality. Some nurses may offer to pray with patients or to pray privately for them at a later time. It is most important to support the patient and facilitate personal expressions of spirituality.

Objectives of Surgical Nursing

The objective of surgical nursing is to prepare the patient mentally and physically for surgery and to assist in full recovery in the shortest time possible and with the least discomfort. The nursing care of surgical patients is a step-by-step process that begins before the patient is admitted to the hospital and ends when recovery is complete and the patient returns to an optimal personal state of health. The nurse who cares for surgical patients needs to have a broad understanding of individual reactions to the surgical procedure. Most surgical patients experience fear and anxiety, and the nurse must be able to recognize the verbal and nonverbal expressions of these emotions and respond in a helping manner. Open communication must be maintained among the nurse, patient, family, and surgeon. The nurse can assist the patient and family by reporting appropriate concerns and questions to the surgeon as they arise or by encouraging the patient to do so. The nurse must possess a wide range of technical skills and keen sense of critical observation. The line between safety and danger in the care of many surgical patients, especially older patients, may be narrow. The alert nurse must recognize early signs of impending complications and report them so that preventive measures may be taken.

Outpatient Surgery

In the past, a patient needing elective surgery that could not be done in the physician's office was admitted to the hospital for preoperative testing and preparation 1 or more days before the surgery. Many of these surgical procedures are now performed with the patient being admitted, treated, and discharged on the same day. These outpatient (same-day) surgeries have the following advantages:

1 Reduced stress because the patient is not hospitalized and because the atmosphere in these units is generally informal and relaxed
2 Lower costs, which benefit the individual and healthcare insurers, including industry and government

However, not all surgeries can be done on an outpatient basis (Box 18-2). Although outpatient surgical procedures may not be as extensive as those that take place in the traditional surgical setting, the role and responsibilities of the nurse remain challenging. The nurse still needs to assess and teach the patient and plan for the patient's discharge. All of these objectives must be accomplished in a short span of time. Ideally patient assessment and teaching can occur several days before the procedure when the patient comes to the hospital or freestanding surgical clinic for preoperative diagnostic testing. A telephone interview and written assessment and discharge planning forms also help make the outpatient surgical experience safe and satisfactory for the patient.

ADMISSION OF THE PATIENT

Surgical patients who are admitted to the hospital in emergency situations may be suffering from traumatic injuries received in an accident or from conditions that require immediate surgery, such as acute appendicitis. In these instances, patients may be taken to the operating room with limited preparation. In the absence of an emergency, patients are usually admitted on the morning of surgery according to prearranged plans made by the surgeon. Many patients are admitted for only a few hours to the outpatient unit. The necessary presurgery testing is completed before admission to the hospital. If diagnostic studies or specialized care is required, the patient may be admitted several days before surgery.

The nurse should be ready to receive the patient at the time of admission, and a friendly, interested, and unhurried attitude helps the patient feel secure. The physical condition of the patient should be assessed, and the patient should be given a complete orientation to the unit. The nurse should be alert to any fears or apprehensions expressed by the patient and should transmit such information to the surgeon. The patient and family should be encouraged to communicate freely with the physician.

A complete history, including previous illnesses; accidents; surgeries; and the present illness and its symptoms, duration, and related information are obtained from the patient by both the nurse and the physician (Box 18-3). The nursing assessment includes a psychosocial, spiritual, and educational history of the patient. With children and older adults, members of the patient's family may be helpful in supplying information. The physician examines the patient. Often a number of laboratory examinations may be completed before admission, including urinalysis; a complete blood cell count; and determination of hemoglobin value, bleeding time, clotting time, and hematocrit level. A blood chemistry is ordered, and the nurse should particularly note the preoperative serum potassium level. In some cases a blood glucose test and electrocardiogram may be ordered. Many hospitals automatically require a chest x-ray examination of each patient admitted.

BOX 18-3

PATIENT HISTORY

Information collected for the patient history should include the following:

- Past surgical experiences, problems, or complications
  Other illnesses or chronic conditions that the patient has that increase surgical risk, such as diabetes, liver disease, obesity, and cardiorespiratory deficiencies
- The potential for postoperative activity
- All medications the patient is taking, as well as allergies or intolerance to medications because many medications interact with perioperative agents and drugs and can affect recovery
- Habits such as smoking, excessive alcohol use, or a sedentary lifestyle that could impede recovery
- Support systems available to the patient and any potential problems for recovery in the home environment

The physician evaluates the patient's nutritional status for dehydration and malnutrition. When severe vomiting and diarrhea have occurred, there may be an electrolyte imbalance and a protein and vitamin deficiency, which can result in decreased resistance to infection and delayed wound healing. To prevent such complications and to improve nutritional status, the patient may be given total parenteral nutrition, also called hyperalimentation, for several days before surgery (see Chapter 23).

If a **hemorrhage** or slow bleeding has occurred, there may be a decrease in hemoglobin value and red blood cells. It may be necessary to transfuse the patient with whole blood or packed cells or to administer fluids, electrolytes, and vitamins intravenously before surgery. If the patient's blood count is normal and loss of blood during surgery is anticipated, many patients and physicians prefer autologous (self) predonation of blood or the selection of their own donors. This technique is seen as an additional precaution against exposure to bloodborne diseases such as acquired immunodeficiency syndrome (AIDS) and hepatitis.

INFORMED CONSENT

A written statement giving consent to have a surgical procedure performed is required before surgery. This statement is signed by the patient in the presence of an authorized witness. It protects the patient from unsanctioned surgery and protects the surgical team from claims that unauthorized surgery was performed. The statement also implies informed consent, which means that the physician has provided the patient with an explanation of the surgical procedure, the possible consequences of the procedure, and what to expect during the postoperative period.

Patients sign their own operative permits if they are of legal age and mentally capable. A responsible family member may sign the permit if the patient is a minor or if the patient is unconscious or judged to be incapable of understanding his or her actions. Refusal to have the operation is the patient's privilege. The operative permit, when signed, becomes part of the patient's chart.

PREOPERATIVE PREPARATION

The preparation and care of the patient before surgery has one major goal—to promote the best possible physical and psychologic state of the patient before surgical therapy. To achieve this goal, the patient's individual needs must be ascertained, and his or her strengths and limitations must be evaluated. A plan of care can be developed to help the patient adjust to the surgical experience, both physically and emotionally.

Nursing Assessment

Before any surgery, the nurse must assess the patient for the following:

1. Knowledge and understanding of the surgical procedure and the recovery phase
2. Physiologic status
3. Psychologic status
4. Cultural needs

Preoperative patient and family teaching

One of the nurse's most important responsibilities during the preoperative period is to teach the patient and family about the upcoming surgery and the postoperative strategies that will speed recovery. The nurse must first find out what the patient already knows, what explanations the physician has already given, and how much the patient needs and wants to know. Excessive and detailed descriptions of the surgical experience may actually increase preoperative anxiety.

ETHICAL DILEMMA

When Mrs. Murphy checks in at the outpatient surgical center at 6:00 AM for her surgery, it becomes clear to you that she does not fully understand all the aspects of the consent form that she has signed. That is, she apparently has not given a truly informed consent. From an ethical perspective, what is necessary for informed consent to be fully autonomous?

Physiologic status

The patient's physiologic status is explored by both the physician and the nurse in separate admission histories and examinations. Often the nurse can elicit information that the patient may have neglected to mention to the physician. This information may be important for a successful surgery or may require canceling the surgery.

Individuals vary greatly in physiologic status and needs. Older patients, obese patients, and patients with diabetes require special assessments (Boxes 18-4 and 18-5) (Hogstel, 1994; Saltiel-Berzin, 1992). With shorter and less invasive surgical techniques, many older adults are now considered good surgical candidates if they receive careful preoperative planning and good postoperative care. Ambulatory or outpatient surgery, when possible, is often desirable because it is less disruptive, lower in cost, and allows for more contact with family and friends.

Psychologic status

An evaluation of the patient's psychologic status and readiness for surgery is also essential. The surgeon should be informed if the patient is extremely anxious or convinced that the surgery will be fatal. If further explanation by the surgeon does not alleviate excessive anxiety, surgery is often postponed or canceled. The nurse should assess the following:

1. The level of anxiety and specific concerns about surgery
2. Coping patterns of the patient
3. Support systems, which may include family, friends, and religious beliefs and practices
4. Factors that may increase stress levels, such as marital or family discord and financial problems

Cultural needs

Cultural sensitivity involves the acceptance of diversity among people. Nurses must examine their own feelings regarding people whose culture differs from theirs, and they must convey respect for the beliefs and customs of all patients. If a patient does not speak

English, an interpreter should be called to help with preoperative explanations. The nurse must attempt to find out how the patient feels about surgery, the use of blood transfusions, the disposal of body parts, and personal privacy. Such beliefs are only a few of the many differences among cultures. The status and role of the nurse also differs among cultures, and the patient's feelings about nurses affect the nurse-patient relationship. Younger members of the patient's family who have been exposed to American culture since childhood are often a great help in language interpretation and cultural clues that help the nurse provide sensitive care to the patient before and after the surgical experience.

BOX 18-4

Guidelines for Care of the Obese Patient

Areas of Concern	Assessments and Interventions
Additional demands on a cardiovascular system that is already overburdened may lead to rapid heart rate and hypertension with exertion. Fatty tissue reduces circulation, so blood clots more easily.	Assess vital signs before and after activity. Pace activities but be sure that the patient is on a consistent schedule of increasing activity, particularly early ambulation.
Obese people have more difficulty expanding their chest and moving and walking easily, so respiratory congestion is more likely in the postoperative period.	Assess lung sounds every shift. Ensure that the patient does deep breathing exercises and uses an incentive spirometer, if ordered, every hour when awake. Check the position of abdominal binders often and position them low on the abdomen to enhance chest expansion.
Fatty tissue is less vascular, so wound healing is poor. Wound separation, infection, and incisional hernias are more common.	Assess the incision every shift and document any redness or drainage. Use sterile technique in giving wound care. Because infections often do not occur until after discharge, teach the patient to assess and care for the incision.
Extreme obesity is not acceptable in the U.S. culture, and many people react negatively to the overweight person.	Avoid judgmental behaviors. Anticipate that the patient may need extra assistance with personal hygiene and postoperative activities but may be unwilling to ask. Find gowns, chairs, and other materials that are large enough for the patient's comfort.

BOX 18-5

Guidelines for Care of the Surgical Patient With Diabetes

Preoperative Period:

Assess type of diabetes, current medications, electrolytes (especially potassium), and blood sugar.

Maintain metabolic control, with blood sugar levels between 80 and 180 mg/dl.

Monitor stress response, presence of infection, and increased blood sugar levels.

Assess for renal, cardiovascular, and peripheral vascular disease.

Intraoperative Period:

Anticipate the possible need for intravenous (IV) insulin during the procedure.

Monitor for symptoms of hypoglycemia.

Postoperative Period:

Test blood glucose often.

Check for hypokalemia (see Chapter 8).

With Type II diabetics, resume oral hypoglycemic when blood glucose is stable.

Advise patients to check blood glucose more often at home during convalescence.

Planning and Interventions

Preoperative instruction

Preoperative instructions can help relieve some of the patient's anxiety. Nursing personnel must know what information has been given to the patient and family regarding the surgery. Questioning the patient about what he or she has been told enables the nurse to clarify and reinforce knowledge. The patient's anxieties, needs, and resources must be considered because they vary considerably from patient to patient. The nurse usually informs the patient and family about the hospital routines surrounding the surgical experience in a manner that is sensitive to their individual needs. It is not appropriate for the nurse to discuss the diagnosis and prognosis of the patient. These matters should be referred to the physician.

The nurse should be able to explain the purposes of and the preparation for diagnostic tests, x-ray procedures, laboratory tests, medications, and nursing procedures. The surgical procedure and postoperative expectations often can be discussed with the patient. Preoperative instruction should be planned so that the patient has time to assimilate the information and to ask questions. Various studies regarding preoperative instruction have indicated that a well-prepared patient recuperates more rapidly, needs medication less often, and develops fewer complications after surgery. In addition, the time of hospitalization is often shortened.

OLDER ADULT CONSIDERATIONS

Areas of Concern	Assessments and Interventions
Perioperative period	
Aging body systems	Organ systems, including nutritional and hydration status, must be carefully and totally assessed. Preoperative medications are not well absorbed and may have extra side effects.
Learning needs	The patient may have hearing or vision problems. Older adults learn well, but more slowly. Ensure that teaching sessions are unhurried and are paced to meet the patient's needs.
Evaluation of other health problems	Cardiovascular, renal, and respiratory systems are compromised by age and pose increased surgical risks. Assess, document, and inform the surgeon of any problems.
Medical history	In addition to prescription drugs, question the patient carefully about over-the-counter drugs such as aspirin, which can increase bleeding.
Intraoperative period	
Hypothermia	Keep the patient covered as much as possible and monitor temperature during surgery.
Physical trauma	Careful positioning and gentle transfer are needed to prevent bone, joint, and skin injury.
Postoperative period	
Increased danger of aspiration, atelectasis, and airway obstruction because of weakened respiratory muscles	Avoid the supine position. Use narcotics with caution and evaluate respiratory status often.
Increased risk of myocardial infarction, kidney failure, and fluid and electrolyte imbalance as a result of cardiovascular and renal aging	Avoid Valsalva's maneuver. Careful monitoring of intake and output is needed. Be alert for dehydration, overhydration, congestive heart failure, clotting problems, and urinary retention. Avoid catheterization if possible because of the increased risk of infection.
Confusion, sensory deficits	Alert staff if vision or hearing loss exists. Give clear explanations of postoperative events. Provide a safe environment and assign the same nurses to the patient as often as possible.
Pain control	Give the lowest effective dose of analgesics. Use nonchemical pain strategies such as relaxation techniques, backrubs, and other comfort measures.
Slower gastrointestinal motility, constipation	Stool softeners are often needed. Encourage fluids, ambulation, and, if permitted, remedies such as prunes and juices that the patient can take at home to achieve regularity.

Specific patient instructions are often given concerning deep breathing and coughing, turning and moving, medications, and special equipment that may be used postoperatively. Patients should be taught how to take a deep breath and exhale slowly in a sitting position. Such breathing provides good ventilation of the lungs and oxygenation of the blood. After practicing this several times, the patient should take a short breath and cough deeply if congestion is present. Coughing helps remove secretions from the bronchi and the lungs. The patient can be taught to splint an abdominal or thoracic incision by interlacing the fingers and placing the palms over the incision site. A towel or small pillow can also be used. Splinting lessens the muscular strain around the incision when the patient coughs.

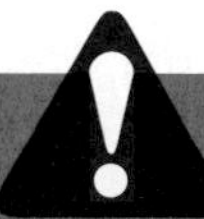

NURSE ALERT

Vigorous coughing is discouraged after some types of surgeries, such as hernia repair and brain or eye surgery, in which increased intracranial pressure must be avoided.

Postoperative positions should be explained to the patient. Position should be changed often after surgery to improve circulation, increase respiratory function, and prevent venous stasis. Leg exercises are taught if it is anticipated that the patient will not be ambulatory within a day after surgery. These exercises include extension and flexion of the knee and hip joints and circular rotation of the foot. Other exercises may be recommended according to the patient's specific surgical procedure.

Psychologic preparation

Preparation for surgery should begin as soon as the patient is told that an operation is necessary. The anticipation of any surgical procedure results in an emotional reaction. Much can be done to alleviate fears before and during hospitalization. The patient's reaction depends on many factors, including personality structure and the pattern of reaction to stressful events in the past.

A surgical operation is a stressful situation in which the patient may believe that there is danger of acute pain, serious damage, disability, and death. There is also a fear of the unknown, which can be complicated by fear of anesthesia or fear of separation from activities, family, and friends. Many patients worry about financial problems, family responsibilities, and employment status. Anxiety often increases as the time for surgery draws near.

Reassuring the patient that medications will be available postoperatively to control discomfort helps lower the patient's anxiety. Any special equipment such as drainage tubes and equipment, intravenous (IV) therapy, or an assistive breathing apparatus should be explained to the patient before surgery. A knowledge of this special equipment helps decrease postoperative anxiety. Many patients are placed in intensive care units after extensive surgical procedures. Electronic monitoring equipment may frighten the patient and family if they are not informed of how it contributes to patient care. The patient's family may believe that the patient is in a critical condition when placed in the intensive care unit. The family and the patient should receive the same information. Explanations concerning the patient's care can often be given when the family is present.

The nurse can help the patient, family, and surgical personnel by listening and helping the patient verbalize any fears. Often the patient wants only the opportunity to express fears to a caring, understanding, and accepting person. Members of the patient's family are often not able to listen to or empathize with the patient because of their own feelings and stress.

Patients are more willing to express their feelings if they have established a good relationship with a member of the nursing team. Therefore nurses should try to establish an atmosphere of acceptance and understanding. No attempt should be made to minimize a patient's fears by dismissing them as "normal." A thorough discussion of the patient's concerns and the appropriate explanations or referrals to the physician should be carried out by the nurse. Denial may be one of the major defense mechanisms that the patient uses to deal with stress, and the nurse should not attempt to give detailed descriptions or instructions to a patient who is unable to hear them because he or she has not fully accepted the fact that surgery is needed. The nurse can help dispel any misconceptions and assure the patient that the nurse and physician are available to discuss concerns. Occasionally it is helpful to have the patient talk with other people who have undergone a similar surgery. The patient's family should be included in any discussions or explanations whenever possible and should be encouraged to understand the anxiety the patient faces and to visit often.

Preoperative Orders

The physician writes the preoperative orders for the patient. Hospitals and physicians vary in the type of preoperative preparation desired, but certain routine procedures are fairly common.

Diet

It is essential that the patient be optimally nourished before surgery. Usually nothing by mouth (NPO) is allowed from midnight until surgery the next morning. However, if the planned surgery is not scheduled until late in the day or will be done using local anesthesia, the patient may be allowed to eat up until 6 to 8 hours before surgery. Withholding food and fluids minimizes the chances of vomiting and of aspirating vomitus into the lungs during or immediately after surgery. Instructions concerning the elimination of food and fluid must be given to the patient before surgery. Accidentally ingesting food or water usually delays surgery, which increases the hospital stay and expense. The nurse is responsible for removing water from the hospitalized patient's room and for communicating the patient's NPO status to everyone involved in his or her care.

Elimination

For some types of surgery, the physician may request that an indwelling catheter be inserted to keep the bladder empty. A distended bladder can complicate surgical procedures on the lower abdomen and increase the chances of bladder trauma during surgery. If the patient is not catheterized, the patient should void before surgery.

Many surgical patients are given a preoperative enema, which may consist of soapsuds, saline, or tap water (Box 18-6). Commercially prepared enemas, which are more comfortable for the patient, are being used more often.

Bisacodyl (Dulcolax) suppositories and tablets or other commercially prepared laxative solutions may be ordered instead of enemas. When bowel surgery is to be performed, "enemas until clear" may be ordered, which means that enemas must be given until no fecal matter returns with the solution. The nurse should be sure that all enema solution is returned, and failure to achieve the proper results should be reported to the physician. Solutions such as Go-Lyte are often ordered in place of enemas. To stimulate elimination the day before surgery, the patient drinks one cup of the solution every 15 minutes for 3 hours. A clear liquid diet may be ordered for the 3 or 4 days preceding the surgery to facilitate bowel cleansing. The administration of enemas or laxatives and the manipulation of the intestines during some surgeries leads to a delay in the return of normal elimination patterns for several days after surgery.

BOX 18-6

REASONS FOR ADMINISTERING A PREOPERATIVE ENEMA

- To remove feces from the intestine before surgery that involves the gastrointestinal tract
- To relieve the patient of postoperative pain that might be caused by straining to have a bowel movement after abdominal surgery
- To avoid a postoperative impaction
- To avoid exertion or the tendency to strain after certain types of surgery, such as eye surgery

Skin preparation

It used to be customary for the nurse to shave the patient on the night before surgery. However, recent research shows that this practice is 10 times more likely to cause wound infection than shaving the incisional area just before surgery. For this reason, the current practice is to avoid shaving the patient if the hair does not interfere with the surgical site.

If shaving must occur, hair is removed from the area with a sharp, disposable razor. Strokes should be with the grain of the hair shaft to prevent nicking or scraping the skin because such cuts may become sites of infection. If the skin is injured, the surgeon may refuse to perform the surgery. Caution must be used in shaving around moles or warts, and any skin eruptions must be reported. In shaving areas such as the axilla and pubic area, the nurse may clip the long hair first to make shaving easier. Care should be taken not to expose or embarrass the patient, who should be left dry and comfortable after the procedure. Scrubbing the surgical site with an antiseptic such as povidone-iodine the night before or the morning of surgery has also been found to decrease wound infections.

Sedation

The physician usually orders a sedative for the hospitalized patient. The sedative is given at bedtime the evening before surgery to ensure that the patient gets adequate sleep and rest. After administration of the sedative, the patient should be instructed to remain in bed because he or she may experience dizziness or confusion. Siderails should be used with elderly persons, and patients should be observed at frequent intervals. The call light should always be placed within easy reach, and the patient should be taught how to use it properly. Because the majority of patients are not admitted on the morning of surgery, they may not have had adequate rest or may have awakened earlier than usual.

DAY OF SURGERY

Visitors

On the day of surgery, the patient should be allowed to rest and should be kept as quiet as possible. Close family members should be advised to arrive at least 1 to 2 hours before the scheduled time of surgery. Time should be allowed for personal hygiene such as bathing, oral care, and shaving. The nurse should allow time in both the inpatient and outpatient settings to make the families and friends of patients comfortable and to deal with their questions and concerns.

Assessment

The vital signs (temperature, pulse, respiration, and blood pressure) are checked and recorded. Any temperature elevation must be reported immediately. The skin surface in the surgical area should be assessed for cuts or abrasions if an earlier shave has been done.

The nurse should check the chart carefully to ensure that all data, such as laboratory reports of blood and urine, have been recorded and that a signed operative permit is attached to the chart. Operative permits must be signed before the administration of medications because a patient who has been sedated is not considered legally competent to sign a permit. All preoperative medications and procedures should be accurately charted before the patient goes to the operating room. The nurse documents the preoperative baseline status of the patient, including physical, psychosocial, and spiritual assessments. Charge vouchers and special forms should be included in the patient's chart (Figure 18-1; Box 18-7).

Prostheses

Just before transportation to surgery, dentures and removable bridges should be removed and placed in a container that is marked with the patient's name. The container should be put in a safe place to prevent loss or damage. Contact lenses and any prostheses such as hearing aids, glasses, and wigs should be removed and stored or sent to the postoperative recovery unit.

Makeup

Procedures vary among anesthesiologists, but often anesthetists prefer that all makeup be removed before the patient goes to surgery because any reduction of oxygen to the tissues may be observed in the lips, face, and nailbeds or may be detected by the color of the blood at the operative site. Polish must generally be removed from at least one fingernail for the proper use of a pulse oximetry finger monitor, which is a current standard of care during surgery.

Valuables

Valuables such as money and jewelry should be removed and itemized in the patient's presence, sealed in an envelope, and locked up or given to a responsible member of the family. Patients who are being admitted for elective surgery should leave all valuables at home. The nurse should be familiar with hospital policy concerning the care of valuables and should use every precaution to protect the patient's personal property. Often considerable sentiment is attached to a wedding ring, and the patient may be allowed to wear it, but it should be anchored securely with tape to prevent losing it.

Preoperative Orders

The patient is given a hospital gown that ties in the back, and all personal articles of clothing are removed. The patient's hair may be covered with a surgical cap. Depending on the type of surgery and the patient's age and condition, the physician may order a retention catheter, which is inserted into the urinary bladder before surgery. The physician may also order intravenous fluids or the insertion of a gastric tube before surgery. The surgeon may request that midthigh or kneehigh elastic stockings be applied or that the patient's legs be wrapped with elastic bandages to help prevent thrombophlebitis. If elastic stockings are ordered, the nurse should follow the manufacturer's directions for measuring and applying them. If elastic bandages are ordered, 4-, 5-, or 6-inch bandages should be used to wrap the patient's legs from the metatarsals to midthigh, and the bandages should be fastened securely. Sequential compression devices, if ordered, should be placed correctly on the patient's legs.

Preoperative medications, which are ordered by the anesthesiologist, are usually administered intramuscularly or orally. The purpose of preoperative medications is to reduce the patient's anxiety about anesthesia and to provide for a smoother induction. Some medications also reduce secretions, and others reduce postoperative nausea (Table 18-1). Preoperative medications are ordered individually for each patient, and consideration is given to the patient's age and general condition, the presence of other diseases that require medications, and the anesthetizing agent to be administered.

The medication is ordered to be administered on call or at a specific hour, and it is important that the

NORTHWEST COMMUNITY HOSPITAL
ARLINGTON HEIGHTS, ILLINOIS 60005
PREOPERATIVE CHECKLIST

Date: ____________

PATIENT ASSESSMENT

☐ ID bracelet attached ☐ Allergy bracelet on

Allergies: ____________

Time pt. ate or drank ____ Last menses ________

Time: T____ P____ R____ B/P ______

Height ____________ Scaled weight ______

Check for following and remove:

☐ Jewlery/Watch ☐ Hearing aid(s)
☐ Rings taped ☐ Makeup off
☐ Rings removed ☐ Nail polish
☐ Dentures ☐ Wig
☐ Glasses ☐ Prosthesis
☐ Contact lenses ☐ Other__________

Initials: ______

Medication taken at home today: ____________

Preop meds & Dose:	Rte.	Time	Init.

IV start Time____ Solution ______Gauge ______

Site ______ Rate ______ By ______

Preps:

☐ Enema given ☐ Foley in situ
☐ Douche given ☐ Ted hose on
☐ Hospital gown only ☐ Antiembolism device on
☐ Side rails up ☐ NG tube in situ

Shave prep done by: ____ Site checked by: ______

Voiding time: ________ Time to OR: ________

CHART Initial

Consent complete ☐ ____
History & physical complete ☐ ____
Old records on chart ☐ ____

Test results:

ECG (age 35 & up – within 1 mo) ☐ ____
Chest x-ray (within 3 mo) ☐ ____

☐ on chart ☐ in x-ray dept. ☐ brought own x-rays

Labs drawn/on chart:

CBC ☐ ____ IVY bleeding time ☐ ____
UA ☐ ____ PT/PTT ☐ ____
Chem. pro. (age 14 & up) ☐ ___ Coag. pro. ☐ ____
RPR ☐ ____ Preg. test (under 45) ☐ ____

Additional labs: ____________

Abnormal labs:	Anes. notified	MD notified	Comments	Init.

Blood Orders:

Type and screened ☐ ____
Type and crossmatched ☐ ____
No. units ordered ______
Autologous blood available ______
Directed donor blood available ______
Consent for transfusion signed ☐ ____

Comments:

Initials	Signature	Initials	Signature

Figure 18-1 Preoperative check list. (Permission authorized by Central Healthcare and Affiliates, October 1994.)

BOX 18-7 **Nursing Process**

PREOPERATIVE PREPARATION

ASSESSMENT

Organ system baselines
Understanding of and readiness for surgery
Cultural background and language barriers
Anxiety, coping ability, and support systems
Nutritional status, obesity, malnourishment, dehydration
History of diabetes or cardiac, respiratory, or renal disease
Medications and allergies
Laboratory values, particularly serum potassium, complete blood count, clotting time

NURSING DIAGNOSES

Anxiety related to unknown outcomes and unknown environment
Sleep pattern disturbance related to anxiety and unfamiliar surroundings
Risk for injury related to premedication sedation
Knowledge deficit, postoperative exercise, and activity related to lack of exposure to surgery and the hospital environment

NURSING INTERVENTIONS

General
Provide a restful environment.
Explain the operative process.
Provide patient with the opportunity to verbalize fears.
Demonstrate and practice deep breathing and coughing.
Explain postoperative positioning.
Explain special procedures and equipment and demonstrate when possible.
Demonstrate and encourage pertinent exercises.
Explain dietary restrictions, such as nothing by mouth after midnight.
Prepare skin as ordered.
Explain and administer medications.
Provide for spiritual needs.

Immediate
Check that identification band is in place and legible.
Remove and store hairpins, dentures, jewelry, contact lenses, and prostheses.
Store valuables.
Give patient a hospital gown.
Have patient void; chart time and amount.
Administer and chart medications.
Instruct the patient to remain in bed; put the bedrails up.
Complete patient's chart, including the following:
- Operative permit signed
- Laboratory data complete
- Order sheets, progress notes, history, patient status, and response to medication included in chart

EVALUATION OF EXPECTED OUTCOMES

Demonstrates optimal physical and psychologic status
Behavior indicates adjustment to the surgical experience
Postoperative complications avoided

nurse give the medication on time so that its maximum effect is reached during the induction of **anesthesia.** If for any reason the medication is not administered as directed, the anesthesiologist should be notified so that the necessary adjustments may be made. Identification should be attached to the patient's wrist, including such information as the patient's name, room number, medication given, and hour and site of administration, as well as the signature of the nurse.

Just before being medicated, the patient should be requested to void, and the amount and time should be noted. A patient's inability to void should be reported to the physician. Vital signs should be taken and recorded. The nurse should advise the patient to stay in bed after the medication has been given and should put the bedrails up.

Transport

The patient may be transferred to the operating room in his or her own bed or by stretcher, and the patient should be moved carefully and with as little confusion as possible. The nurse should protect the patient from drafts and exposure by applying cotton blankets and should make him or her comfortable with a pillow. The nurse or transport personnel accompany the patient and remain until relieved by a member of the operating room staff. The patient's record is given to the operating room nurse, who is also advised verbally of the pa-

TABLE 18-1

Pharmacology of Drugs Used for the Surgical Patient

Drug (Generic and Trade Name); Route and Dosage	Action/Indication	Common Side Effects and Nursing Considerations
DIAZEPAM (Valium) **ROUTE:** PO, IM, IV **DOSAGE:** Skeletal muscle relaxation, PO, 2-10 mg 3-4 times daily, 2-2.5 mg in elderly or debilitated; IM, IV, 5-10 mg (2-5 mg in debilitated patients) and may repeat in 2-4 hr	Benzodiazepine sedative/hypnotic used for the management of anxiety; for preoperative sedation, light anesthesia, and amnesia; as a skeletal muscle relaxant; for status epilepticus; and for the management of symptoms of alcohol withdrawal	Dizziness, drowsiness, and lethargy; contraindicated in comatose patients, preexisting CNS depression, uncontrolled severe pain, and glaucoma; use cautiously in hepatic and severe renal disease, suicidal, addicted, elderly, or debilitated
DROPERIDOL (Inapsine) **ROUTE:** IM, IV **DOSAGE:** Preoperative, IM 2.5-10 mg ½ hr before surgery; induction, IV 2.5 mg/20-25 lb given with analgesic or general anesthetic; maintain general anesthesia, IV 1.25-2.5 mg	Neuroleptic used for premedication for surgery, induction of anesthesia, and the maintenance of general anesthesia	Laryngospasm, bronchospasm, dystonia, akathisia, flexion of arms, fine tremors, dizziness, anxiety, drowsiness, restlessness, hallucinations, depression, tachycardia, hypotension, chills, facial swelling, shivering; assess vital signs soon after first dose
FENTANYL CITRATE (Sublimaze) **ROUTE:** IM, IV **DOSAGE:** Anesthetic, IV, 0.05-0.1 mg q 2-3 min prn; preoperatively, IM, 0.05-0.1 mg q 30-60 min before surgery; postoperatively, IM 0.05-0.1 mg q 1-2 hr prn	Narcotic analgesic used preoperatively and postoperatively and as an adjunct to general anesthesia when combined with droperidol	Bradycardia, cardiac arrest, respiratory depression, respiratory arrest, and laryngospasm; contraindicated in hypersensitivity to opiates and myasthenia gravis; use with caution in elderly, respiratory depression, increased intracranial pressure, seizure disorders, and cardiac arrhythmias
GLYCOPYRROLATE (Robinul) **ROUTE:** PO, IM, IV **DOSAGE:** Preoperatively, IM, 0.002 mg/lb ½-1 hr before surgery; reversal of neuromuscular blockage, IV, 0.2 mg for each 1 mg of neostigmine or 5 mg IV of pyridostigmine simultaneously; GI disorders, PO, 1-2 mg bid-tid, IM, IV, 0.1-0.2 mg tid-qid, titrated to patient response	Cholinergic blocker used to decrease secretions before surgery, and for the reversal of neuromuscular blockade, peptic ulcer disease, and irritable bowel syndrome	Dryness of mouth and constipation; contraindicated in glaucoma, myasthenia gravis, gastrointestinal or genitourinary obstruction, tachycardia, hepatic disease, ulcerative colitis, and toxic megacolon
HALOTHANE (Fluothane, Somnothane) **ROUTE:** Inhaled anesthetic **DOSAGE:** Minimal alveolar concentration 0.7% in O_2	CNS depressant anesthetic that causes complete anesthesia	Hypotension, cardiovascular depression, lowered body temperature, respiratory depression, malignant hyperthermia, emergence shivering, trembling, confusion, hallucinations, nervousness, and increased excitability; may cause hepatic dysfunction
ISOFLURANE (Forane) **ROUTE:** Inhaled anesthetic **DOSAGE:** Minimal alveolar concentration 1.15% in O_2	CNS depressant anesthetic that causes complete anesthesia	Same as above, except no hepatic complications; exhaled largely unchanged

TABLE 18-1

Pharmacology of Drugs Used for the Surgical Patient—cont'd

Drug (Generic and Trade Name); Route and Dosage	Action/Indication	Common Side Effects and Nursing Considerations
LIDOCAINE (Xylocaine) **ROUTE:** SC **DOSAGE:** Usual adult dosage depends on site and length of surgical procedure	Subcutaneously injected local anesthetic with intermediate duration (1-3 hr)	Most common side effects such as headache, dizziness, convulsions, hypotension, and bradycardia, not present because SC dose is so small; watch for hypersensitivity and persistent loss of sensation at site
MEPERIDINE (Demerol) **ROUTE:** IM, IV, PO **DOSAGE:** Preoperatively, IM, 50-100 mg 30-90 min before surgery, IV dose should be reduced; sometimes may be given PO	Narcotic analgesic used preoperatively and for moderate to severe pain	Increased intracranial pressure and respiratory depression; contraindicated if hypersensitive or previously addicted; use with caution in addictive personality, heart disease, respiratory depression, hepatic or renal disease
MIDAZOLAM (Versed) **ROUTE:** IM, IV **DOSAGE:** Preoperative sedation, IM 0.07-0.08 mg/kg ½-1 hr before general anesthesia; induction of general anesthesia, 1-10 mg IV	General anesthetic used for preoperative sedation, general anesthesia induction, and other sedation indications	Apnea, bronchospasm, laryngospasm, nausea and vomiting; contraindicated in shock, coma, alcohol intoxication, and glaucoma; use with caution in chronic obstructive pulmonary disease, congestive heart failure, chronic renal failure, chills, the elderly, and the debilitated; has less duration than valium; is a better anesthetic
MORPHINE (Morphine) **ROUTE:** PO, IM, IV **DOSAGE:** IM, 4-15 mg q 4 hr prn; PO, 10-30 mg q 4 hr prn; IV, 4-10 mg diluted in 4-5 ml H_2O for injection over 5 min	Narcotic analgesic used preoperatively and for severe pain	Respiratory depression; contraindicated in the addicted and with hemorrhage, bronchial asthma, and increased intracranial pressure; use with caution in addictive personality, severe heart disease, and hepatic and renal disease
NALOXONE (Narcan) **ROUTE:** IC, SC, IM **DOSAGE:** Narcotic-induced respiratory depression, IV, SC, IM, 0.4-2 mg, and repeat q 2-3 min if needed; postoperative respiratory depression, IV, 0.1-0.2 mg q 2-3 min prn	Narcotic antagonist used to reverse respiratory depression caused by narcotics, pentazocine, and propoxyphene	Rapid overdosage could predispose to pulmonary edema; almost immediate onset
NITROUS OXIDE **ROUTE:** Inhaled anesthetic **DOSAGE:** 50-70%	Incomplete, "weak" anesthetic	Weak anesthetic with no muscle relaxation. Must be administered with 20% oxygen to avoid hypoxia; may cause bowel distention and may contribute to postoperative nausea and vomiting

continued

TABLE 18-1

Pharmacology of Drugs Used for the Surgical Patient—cont'd

Drug (Generic and Trade Name); Route and Dosage	Action/Indication	Common Side Effects and Nursing Considerations
PANCURONIUM (Pavulon) **ROUTE:** IV **DOSAGE:** 0.1 mg/kg	Nondepolarizing skeletal muscle relaxant (neuromuscular block)	Muscle relaxant anesthetic has a duration of 45-60 min; is reversible with anticholinesterase agents; no histamine release; slow increase in pulse rate initially
PROCAINE (Novocain) **ROUTE:** Varies by route of anesthesia **DOSAGE:** 14 mg/kg at one time	Local anesthetic used for spinal anesthesia, epidural, peripheral nerve block, perineum, lower extremities, and infiltration	Convulsions, decreased level of consciousness, myocardial depression, cardiac arrest, arrhythmias, status asthmaticus, respiratory depression, and anaphylaxis; contraindicated in severe liver disease; use with caution in elderly and severe drug allergies
PROMETHAZINE (Phenergan) **ROUTE:** PO, IM, IV **DOSAGE:** Sedation, preoperative/postoperative, PO, IM, IV, 25-50 mg	Antihistamine H1-receptor antagonist used for motion sickness, rhinitis, allergy symptoms, sedation, nausea, and pre- and postoperative sedation	Dizziness, drowsiness, respiratory depression and hypotension; watch for thrombocytopenia with chronic usage; contraindicated in acute asthma attack and lower respiratory disease; use with caution in increased intraocular pressure, renal and cardiac disease, hypertension, bronchial asthma, seizure disorder, peptic ulcers, hyperthyroidism, and benign prostatic hypertrophy
SCOPOLAMINE **ROUTE:** SC **DOSAGE:** 0.4-0.6 mg	Cholinergic blocker used to reduce secretions before surgery, to calm delirium, and for motion sickness	Dryness of mouth, constipation, and paralytic ileus; contraindicated in glaucoma, myasthenia gravis, and hypersensitivity to belladonna and barbiturates; use with caution in elderly, benign prostatic hypertrophy, congestive heart failure, hypertension, dysrhythmias, and gastric ulcers
SUCCINYLCHOLINE (Anectine, Quelicin, Sucostrin) **ROUTE:** IV, IM **DOSAGE:** IV, 25-75 mg, then 2.5 mg/min as needed; IM, 2.5 mg/kg, not to exceed 150 mg	Neuromuscular blocker used for the facilitation of intubation and skeletal muscle relaxation, especially during orthopedic manipulations	Sinus arrest, arrhythmias, prolonged apnea, bronchospasm, cyanosis, respiratory depression, and myoglobulinemia; contraindicated in malignant hyperthermia, penetrating eye injuries, and glaucoma; use with caution in cardiac disease, severe burns, electrolyte imbalances, dehydration, neuromuscular diseases, respiratory diseases, collagen diseases, glaucoma, the elderly, and the debilitated

TABLE 18-1

Pharmacology of Drugs Used for the Surgical Patient—cont'd

Drug (Generic and Trade Name); Route and Dosage	Action/Indication	Common Side Effects and Nursing Considerations
THIOPENTAL SODIUM (Pentothal) **ROUTE:** IV **DOSAGE:** Induction, 210-280 mg or 3-5 ml/kg; general anesthetic, 50-75 mg given at 20-40 sec intervals; sedation, 12-20 mg/lb	Barbiturate general anesthetic used in short general anesthesia and induction anesthesia before other anesthetics	Respiratory depression, bronchospasm, myocardial depression, arrhythmias, and shivering; contraindicated in status asthmaticus; use with caution in severe cardiac disease, renal disease, liver disease, hypotension, myxedema, myasthenia gravis, asthma, and increased intracranial pressure
TUBOCURARINE CHLORIDE, CURARE (Tubocurarine) **ROUTE:** IV **DOSAGE:** IV bolus 0.4-0.5 mg/kg, then 0.08-0.10 mg/kg 20-45 min after first dose if needed for prolonged procedures	Neuromuscular blocker used for the facilitation of endotracheal intubation, skeletal muscle relaxation during mechanical ventilation, surgery, or general anesthesia	Prolonged apnea, bronchospasm, cyanosis, and respiratory depression; use with caution in cardiac disease, electrolyte imbalances, dehydration, and neuromuscular or respiratory disease
VECURONIUM (Norcuron) **ROUTE:** IV **DOSAGE:** IV bolus 0.08-0.10 mg/kg, then 0.010-0.015 mg/kg for prolonged procedures	Neuromuscular blocker used for the facilitation of endotracheal intubation, skeletal muscle relaxation during mechanical ventilation, surgery, and general anesthesia	Prolonged apnea and possible respiratory paralysis; use with caution in cardiac disease, electrolyte imbalances, dehydration, and neuromuscular or respiratory disease

tient's name and any significant problem that currently exists. Family members should be told where to wait during the surgery.

INTRAOPERATIVE CARE

In the past decade, modern surgery has become increasingly sophisticated with the use of new techniques and tools. The common use of endoscopic techniques for surgery has reduced the length of stay and the convalescent period for patients. **Laser surgery,** which uses a high energy beam of light to cut and cauterize tissue, has improved surgical techniques and patient safety (Gallagher, Kahn, 1990). However, the conscientious use of aseptic practices remains the primary element of safe surgery.

Aseptic surgery began around 1867 with the work of Joseph Lister, an English surgeon. At that time wound infection complicated most surgeries, and puerperal infection was common in obstetric wards. Lister observed the process of wound infection and concluded that it was caused by microbes. On the basis of this belief, Lister began using a solution of carbolic acid in the operating room and also began saturating dressings over wounds. These measures resulted in a remarkable decrease in the incidence of wound infection.

Surgical Asepsis

Although modern science has progressed since Lister, the basic definition of surgical **asepsis** remains unchanged. Surgical asepsis is a condition in which there is a complete absence of germs. It is absolute. There is no compromise or modification. Many situations on the clinical unit require surgical aseptic techniques, such as catheterization or surgical dressing changes. The slightest error may mean prolonged illness or hospitalization for the patient. The nurse should know the methods used to achieve asepsis and the variables that determine the effectiveness or ineffectiveness, whatever method is used.

Surgical asepsis prevents organisms from entering the body. Surgical aseptic techniques are used whenever the skin or mucous membranes are perforated or incised. To prevent contaminants from entering the area of operation or any wound, any object that comes in contact with a wound must be absolutely free of pathogenic organisms. Procedures in operating rooms are carried out under strict surgical asepsis and require preparation of the patient's skin and sterilization of all instruments, linens, dressings, or other materials that come in contact with the wound. Surgical asepsis includes special attire for the surgeon and assistants, properly cleaning and disinfecting all inanimate objects in the room, and maintaining proper temperature and humidity. Laminar air flow systems may be used to reduce the number of airborne organisms. Other terms for surgical asepsis are sterile technique and aseptic technique.

Sterilization

Sterilization is a process by which all forms of living microorganisms are completely destroyed, including spores and viruses. The sterilization of materials usually occurs in the central processing department of the hospital or surgical area. The method of sterilization is determined by the supplies and equipment that are to be used. In surgical asepsis all supplies and equipment are sterilized before use and are handled only with sterile equipment. Two factors are important in determining the type of sterilization to be used:

1. The type of microorganism, because some pathogens are easily destroyed by ordinary methods of disinfection, whereas others are extremely resistant
2. The degree of contamination, because the greater the amount of contamination, the longer it takes to ensure complete destruction of pathogenic organisms

Heat is one of the most effective and convenient methods of destroying microorganisms. *Boiling,* a form of moist heat, is one of the oldest methods of sterilization. It is commonly used in the home and is adequate under most conditions. Equipment that is to be sterilized by boiling must be completely immersed in the water, and timing begins when the water starts to boil. Most vegetative forms of bacteria are killed if boiled for 10 to 20 minutes.

Steam under pressure is the most dependable method of sterilizing because it rapidly destroys all forms of microorganisms. This method of sterilizing is called autoclaving. Steam enters the **autoclave** under pressure, which increases the temperature of the steam. During the sterilizing process, the temperature is maintained at approximately 250° F (121° C) and at 15 to 17 pounds of pressure for a specified time. At the completion of the process, the pressure is reduced to zero, and the load is allowed to dry.

Dry heat sterilization circulates hot air, which is provided by an electric oven sterilizer. This method may be compared to an ordinary baking oven. Dry heat sterilization penetrates many different materials, such as oils and closed containers that are not affected by steam. The type of materials, their packaging, and the loading of the oven determines the time necessary for sterilization. Generally hot air sterilization requires between 1 and 6 hours and in some cases may be longer.

Ethylene oxide is a chemical that is found as both a liquid and a vapor. If the liquid form comes into contact with the skin, it causes blisters. Inhaling the gas causes nausea, vomiting, dizziness, and irritation of the mucous membranes. Research has demonstrated that exposure to ethylene oxide gas kills all forms of vegetative bacteria, including spore-forming types, and viruses. Its use has increased in sterilizing equipment that cannot be subjected to other methods of sterilizing, such as instruments with lenses (cystoscope and bronchoscope) and plastic equipment such as infant incubators and the artificial kidney dialyzer. Polyethylene tubing and some rubber products are usually sterilized with ethylene oxide.

The use of ethylene oxide gas requires special types of sterilizers. The process of sterilization is complex and involves several factors, including temperature, time, moisture, concentration of the gas, and proper packaging of materials. The actual sterilizing time varies from 1 to 4 hours, but all the residual gas must be allowed to dissipate before the supplies or equipment can be used. Therefore materials exposed to ethylene oxide are not used for 24 to 36 hours.

The Operative Team

Those giving care to the patient during the intraoperative period are generally prepared to be sterile or nonsterile members of the surgical team. Sterile members of the team include the surgeon, who may be assisted by another physician, and the scrub nurse or technician. Nonsterile personnel include the anesthesiologist (a physician) or anesthetist (a nurse), the circulating nurse, and various technicians. To best serve the needs of the patient at a critical time, team members must work efficiently as a unit.

Scrub nurse or technician

As the sterile nursing member of the operative team, the primary role of the scrub nurse or technician is to anticipate the needs of the surgeon and to assist at the operative site. This nurse prepares the instruments and materials to be used by the surgeon and may assist with the surgical procedure (Figure 18-2). The scrub nurse or technician must have a thorough knowledge of aseptic

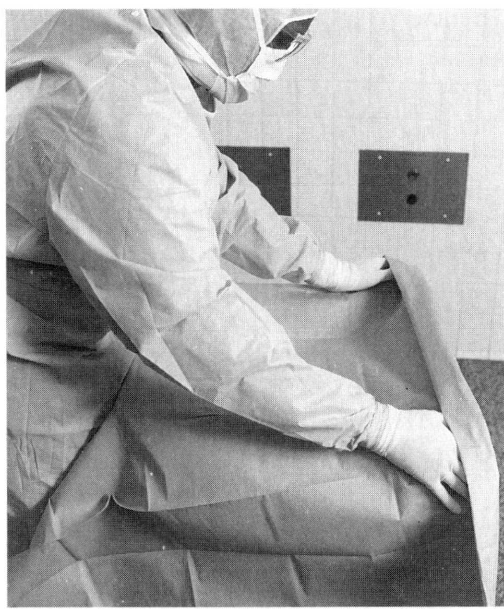

Figure 18-2 Scrub nurse protects gloves with cuff of drape when opening inner wrapper of pack, which serves as a sterile table cover. (From Meeker MH, Rothrock JC: *Alexander's care of the patient in surgery,* ed 10, St Louis, 1995, Mosby.)

technique and the ability and stamina to work efficiently under pressure (Figure 18-3). Manual dexterity and good organizational skills are also important.

Circulating nurse

The circulating nurse must be a registered nurse and has a major role in managing the operating room. This nonsterile team member must have an overall picture of the needs of the patient and of the other team members. The duties of the circulating nurse include the following:

1. Maintaining a safe environment for the patient by observing breaks in sterile technique, providing for safe use of complex equipment, and keeping the patient and staff free from hazards
2. Anticipating the need for and obtaining supplies and equipment for the sterile team
3. Communicating information about the patient's status to other members of the health team and to the patient's significant others

Anesthesia

Anesthesia means "the absence of pain." Most patients have some fear of anesthesia. They may worry about going to sleep and not waking up, or they may fear the unknown. Some patients may fear waking up and experiencing pain during surgery, acting strangely when anesthetized, or experiencing uncomfortable aftereffects such as nausea and vomiting.

Most fears can be allayed if the patient is well informed about the anesthetic chosen and the effects it will produce. The type of anesthetic medication and technique are selected for the individual patient on the basis of his or her physical condition; age; preference; and the type, site, and length of the operation to be performed (Figure 18-4). An anesthesiologist, a physician who specializes in the selection and administration of anesthetics, chooses the anesthetic medication and techniques following a preoperative visit. During the visit, the anesthesiologist assesses the patient's physical and emotional state, discusses individual preferences, explains the procedure of inducing anesthesia, answers questions, and generally promotes confidence and helps relieve anxiety.

Anesthesia is induced by a physician-anesthesiologist or a certified nurse anesthetist. A nurse anesthetist is a professional nurse who has received postgraduate education in the administration of anesthetics and generally functions under the supervision of an anesthesiologist.

The anesthesia team continually monitors the patient's oxygenation vital signs, organ function, and fluid status during the surgery and the immediate postsurgical period. It should be remembered that the patient is sedated and in a strange and sometimes frightening environment. There should be no bright lights or unnecessary noise and talking. Hearing is the last sense to respond to anesthetic agents and the first to return after the effects of the anesthetic wear off. Therefore unnecessary noise, conversation, joking, or inappropriate comments must be avoided by staff members.

The type of anesthetic administered may affect the postoperative condition and the return to consciousness. An understanding of anesthetizing agents helps the nurse assess the patient's condition and anticipate postoperative needs.

Types

Anesthesia is classified as *general* or *regional.* When the surgeon wishes all sensations in the entire body to be suspended temporarily, the patient is given a general anesthetic. When only a part of the body is involved, the patient may be given a regional anesthetic. General anesthetics include drugs that are administered by inhalation or by injection into the bloodstream (Table 18-2).

General anesthesia

Inhalation anesthesia. Drugs used in inhalation anesthesia may be liquids that vaporize, with the patient inhaling the vapor. Examples of such drugs in-

A 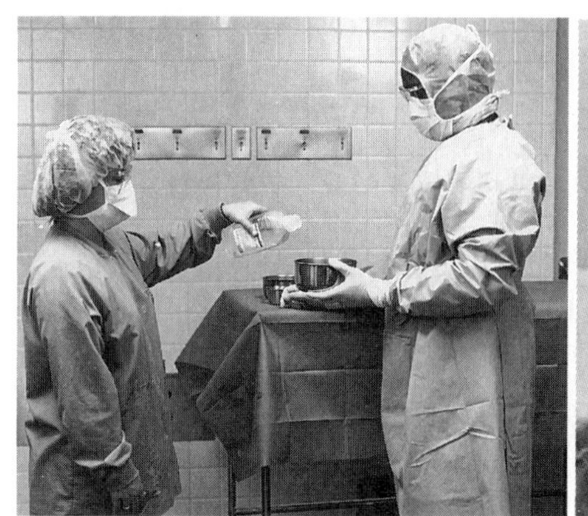

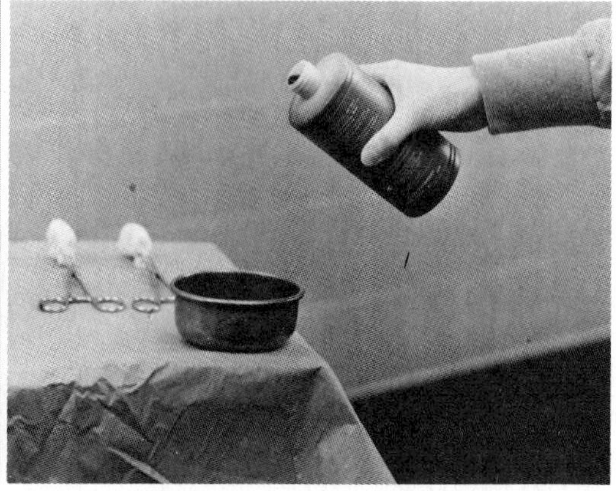 B

Figure 18-3 **A,** When pouring solution into receptacle held by scrub nurse, the circulating nurse maintains a safe margin of space to avoid contamination of sterile surfaces. **B,** Care must be used when pouring solution into a receptacle that is on a sterile field to avoid splashing fluids onto sterile field. Placing a receptacle near the edge of the table permits the circulating nurse to pour the solution without reaching over any portion of sterile field. (From Meeker MH, Rothrock JC: *Alexander's care of the patient in surgery,* ed 10, St Louis, 1995, Mosby.)

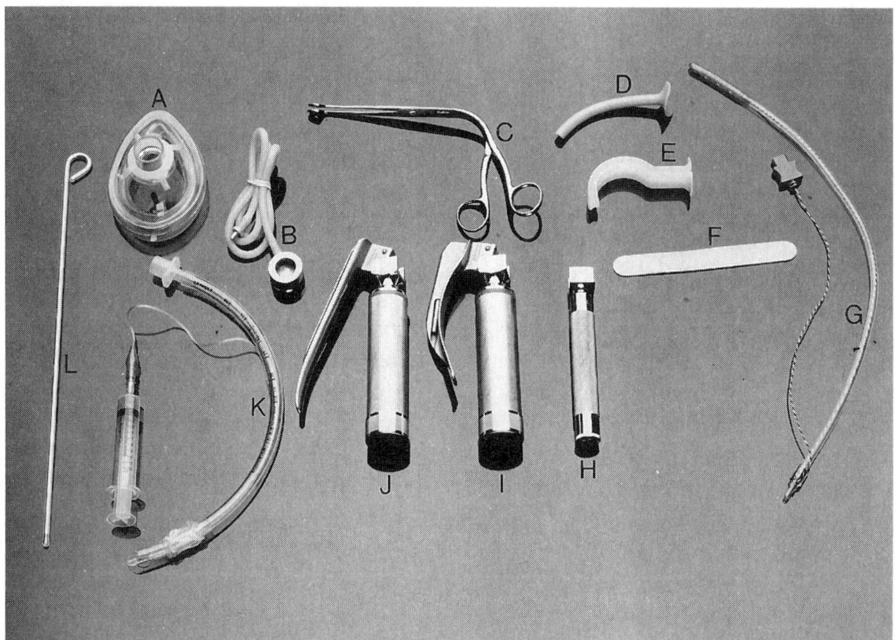

Figure 18-4 Commonly used anesthesia equipment. **A,** Mask. **B,** Precordial stethoscope. **C,** McGill forceps. **D,** Nasal airway. **E,** Oral airway. **F,** Tongue blade. **G,** Esophageal stethoscope with esophageal temperature monitor. **H,** Pediatric laryngoscope handle. Fiberoptic laryngoscope blades and handles: **I,** MacIntosh; **J,** Miller. **K,** Endotracheal tube. **L,** Intubating stylet for endotracheal tube.

clude isoflurane (Forane) and halothane (Fluothane). Inhalation drugs are also in the form of gases, such as nitrous oxide (Table 18-2). Inhalation anesthetics render the patient unconscious, and therefore awareness of pain and anxiety are eliminated. They also provide muscle relaxation. Inhalation anesthetics are administered in combination with oxygen or air through a mask or through a tube that is inserted into the trachea.

Endotracheal intubation ensures that the airway remains open and that the lungs can be aerated even when the chest wall is entered. The endotracheal tube is held in place by a balloon that is inflated after it is in-

TABLE 18-2

Selected General Anesthetics

Drug	Characteristics	Nursing considerations
Inhalant agents		
isoflurane (Forane)	Volatile liquid; provides good muscle relaxation; rapid induction, and recovery; potentiates muscle relaxants significantly	All inhalants depress respirations. Monitor rate and quality of respirations closely. Agent may cause immediate postoperative coughing and laryngospasm.
halothane (Fluothane)	Volatile liquid; rapid induction but poor degree of muscle relaxation; evidence suggests that liver damage may be a side effect; shivering commonly occurs as patient awakens	Anesthesiologist should be informed if patient has any history of liver disease, alcoholism, or gallbladder disease. Keep patient warm postoperatively. Monitor patient closely for cardiac arrhythmias.
enflurane (Ethrane)	Volatile liquid; slow acting but fairly good muscle relaxation, and analgesia can be achieved; can cause fatal arrhythmias, particularly in presence of epinephrine-like drugs	Monitor vital signs closely and provide for safety during what is often a prolonged (45-minute) wake-up period. Blood pressure may fall, and the pulse rate may rise.
nitrous oxide	Gas; very popular, weak agent used in combination with oxygen and other anesthetic agents; nonexplosive; may create hypoxia	Monitor for hypoxia and be prepared to administer oxygen.
Intravenous agents		
Short-acting barbiturates: methohexital (Brevital), thiamylal (Surital), thiopental (Pentothal)	Thiopental sodium is most popular of this group; given at onset of surgery to provide rapid and smooth induction; may cause laryngospasm, respiratory depression, and sudden hypotension	Assess postoperative respiratory status closely. Patient may be sedated but may still be in pain and require additional medication.
Narcotic and nonnarcotic analgesics: morphine, meperidine, droperidol (Innovar), fentanyl	Used with other anesthetic agents to provide effective analgesia during surgery; major side effect is respiratory depression	Monitor respirations closely. Keep naloxone (Narcan) on hand to reverse narcotic effect. Use narcotics sparingly or in decreased doses during the first 12 hours after surgery.
ketamine (Ketalar, Ketaject)	Dissociative agent used for short procedures; provides analgesia and loss of memory of procedure; often used in pediatric surgery	Protect patients from additional stimuli (noises, touching) during waking period; in adults, may cause confusion and excitement for 24 hours after surgery; assess for hypertension and respiratory depression

serted (Figure 18-5). The balloon and the pressure it exerts on the walls of the trachea cause some irritation of the mucosa. Occasionally it can cause postoperative edema in the area, resulting in respiratory difficulty. Therefore when an endotracheal tube has been used, the patient must be watched carefully for symptoms of respiratory obstruction.

Intravenous drugs. Barbiturates, narcotics, and other drugs are administered with inhalation anesthetics and reduce the amount of the inhalation anesthetics required (see Table 18-2). Short-acting barbiturates produce unconsciousness in 30 seconds. The most commonly used intravenous drugs are thiopental (Pentothal) and thiamylal (Surital). When large amounts of these drugs have been given, the patient does not return to consciousness quickly. The patient must be watched carefully for laryngeal spasm, which may be indicated by retraction of the soft tissues around the neck muscles; crowing respirations, air hunger, and restlessness. A pulse oximeter is a simple and essential tool for accurate and ongoing assessment of the patient's blood oxygen levels.

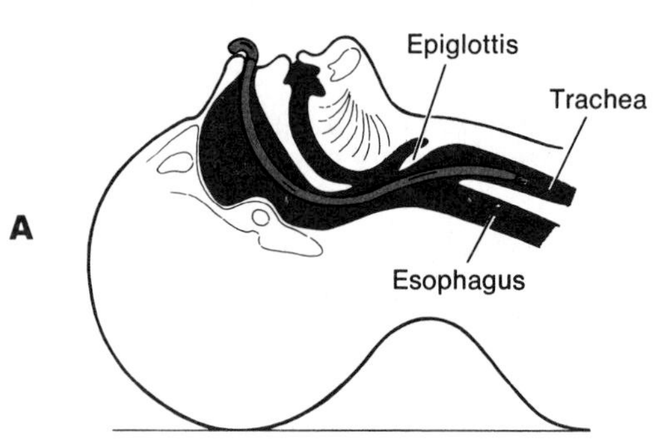

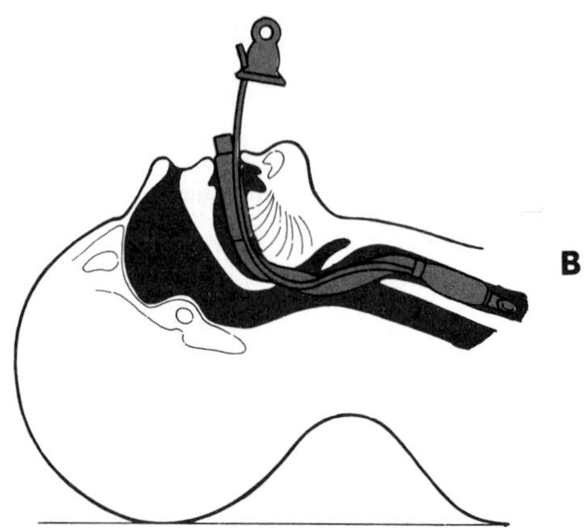

Figure 18-5 **A,** Intranasal intubation. Note adapter at proximal end of tube that can be used to attach anesthetic equipment. **B,** Oral intubation. Note inflated cuff.

TABLE 18-3

Selected Regional Anesthetics

Drug	Characteristics	Nursing Considerations
procaine (Novocain)	Used for infiltration, spinal nerve block; widely used in dentistry; available with or without epinephrine	Observe for allergic reaction. May cause poor local circulation if combined with epinephrine for use on injured fingers or toes.
benzocaine (Solarcaine)	Use topically and available commercially	Avoid use near eyes. May cause skin irritation.
lidocaine (Xylocaine)	Used topically and for infiltration nerve block, such as epidural, caudal, and spinal; rapid action and medium duration; also used to treat cardiac arrhythmias; comes with and without epinephrine	Monitor for changes in vital signs, excitability, and seizures if used systemically.
tetracaine (Pontocaine)	Used topically and for infiltration nerve block, such as spinal and caudal; more potent and has more toxicity and longer duration than other agents	Protect patient from injury and burns during the period when no sensation is present.
bupivacaine (Marcaine)	Used for infiltration nerve blocks; spinal; long acting	Observe for allergic or toxic reactions. Monitor and protect patient.

Other intravenous agents such as morphine, meperidine (Demerol) and fentanyl (Sublimaze) are commonly used to maintain anesthesia throughout the surgical procedure and to provide pain relief in the early postoperative period. These are often used in conjunction with nitrous oxide and are referred to as nitrous-narcotic anesthetics. Ketamine (Ketalar) is a dissociative anesthesia that leaves the patient awake in a trancelike state with no pain or memory of the surgery.

Muscle relaxants. Curare and succinylcholine (Anectine) are powerful depolarizing muscle relaxants that may be administered to increase the relaxation of the abdominal muscles during surgery or to facilitate endotracheal intubation. Pancuronium (Pavulon) is a synthetic neuromuscular blocking agent that is used primarily to produce skeletal muscle relaxation during surgery after general anesthesia has been induced. It is compatible with all the general anesthetics currently in use. Depolarizing drugs may cause respiratory difficulty by suppressing muscle function. All patients must be monitored carefully.

Regional anesthetics. Regional anesthetics use narcotics or local anesthetics to inhibit nerve impulses to various parts of the body (Table 18-3). A local anesthetic drug is injected in and around nerves, which results in anesthesia of the area that is supplied by the particular nerves. Several different drugs may be used, including procaine (Novocain), tetracaine (Pontocaine), and lidocaine (Xylocaine). Regional anesthetics may be divided into the categories of spinal, epidural, nerve block, infiltration, and local.

Spinal anesthesia. To induce spinal anesthesia, a solution of a local anesthetic may be injected into the subarachnoid space, which contains cerebrospinal fluid. The drug anesthetizes nerves as they leave the spinal cord. The method of injection is the same as that for any spinal puncture (Figure 18-6). This type of anesthesia is used for surgery that involves the abdomen, perineum, and lower extremities. Use of this method on the upper part of the body or inadvertent migration of medication to the upper spinal canal paralyzes the respiratory muscles and the diaphragm.

The patient may remain awake under spinal anestheia. Therefore it is necessary that the surgical team avoid any careless conversation that could be misinterpreted by the patient. During the operation the patient may be aware of pressure or pulling sensations but no pain. After spinal anesthesia, the patient generally is kept flat in bed for several hours. Vital signs, especially blood pressure, should be watched because hypotension may occur. Sensations to the anesthetized part do not return immediately, and careful positioning of the patient is important to prevent later discomfort or pressure injury. The patient may have a severe headache, which is thought to be caused by spinal fluid leaking from the puncture site. The headache often lasts for several days, but analgesics plus an increased oral intake help alleviate the discomfort. Measures taken by the anesthesiologist to reduce the incidence of headache include the use of fine-gauge needles and the placement of a "blood patch" at the insertion site to prevent the leakage of spinal fluid.

Epidural anesthesia. Epidural anesthesia involves the injection of a local agent into the extradural space outside the spinal canal. Examples of epidural anesthetics are the sacral and caudal blocks, which are used to anesthetize the perineum during deliveries.

Peripheral nerve block. A peripheral nerve block is used to provide anesthesia or freedom from pain in body structures that are innervated by selected nerve systems. Examples include the brachial, femoral, and sciatic nerves.

Infiltration anesthesia. Infiltration anesthesia is achieved by injecting a local anesthetic drug directly into the tissues. This type of anesthetic is used for minor operations in which tissue is incised, or it may be used to provide pain control after major operations.

Because all drugs used for local anesthesia are potentially toxic or may cause an allergic response, the patient should be carefully observed for signs of itching, twitching, convulsions, cyanosis, nausea, and vomiting. The patient's blood pressure, pulse, and respirations should also be carefully checked. The patient is conscious but may be drowsy if a sedative has been administered before the surgical procedure.

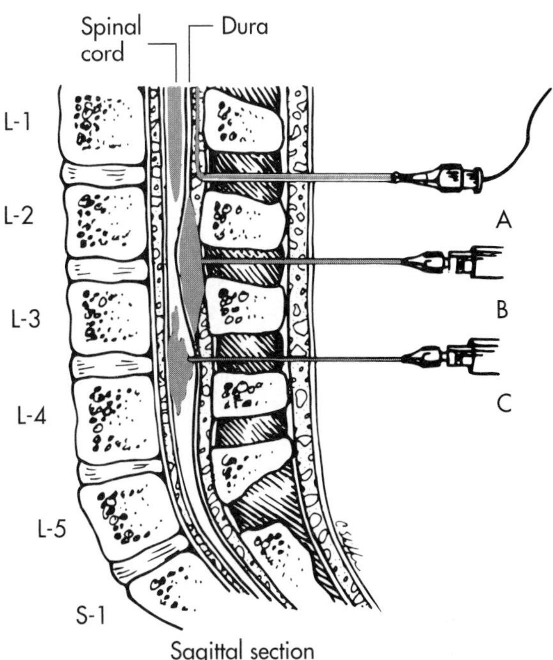

Figure 18-6 Location of needle point and injected anesthetic relative to dura. **A,** Epidural catheter. **B,** Single injection epidural. **C,** Spinal anesthesia. (Interspaces most commonly used are L4-5, L3-4, and L2-3.) (From Meeker MH, Rothrock JC: *Alexander's care of the patient in surgery,* ed 10, St Louis, 1995, Mosby.)

Topical anesthesia. Drops, sprays, lotions, and ointments are types of topical anesthetics. They are applied directly to the skin or mucosa for temporary anesthesia before a simple procedure or for pain relief. Many of these products are sold over the counter in pharmacies.

Alternative forms of anesthesia

Such methods as hypnosis and acupuncture do have the advantage of causing none of the side effects of chemical anesthetics, but these techniques are not widely used or well regarded by many physicians in this country. Acupuncture is an ancient Oriental method in which fine metal needles are inserted beneath the skin at particular body points to provide anesthesia. There is no clear explanation as to why it is effective, but the technique has been successfully used, particularly for minor procedures. The power of the mind over the body forms the basis for hypnosis as an anesthetic practice. With hypnosis, pain is controlled by the power of suggestion.

Intraoperative complications

Malignant hyperthermia. Malignant hyperthermia is a rapid rise in body temperature that can be triggered by the anesthetic agents or muscle relaxants used during surgery. Its exact pathophysiology is not known, but it is related to a defect in cellular metabolism that results in hypercalcemia. Early warning signs of this potentially fatal complication are tachycardia, muscle rigidity, and a rapid rise in temperature (as much as 1° C every 5 minutes). Treatment consists of cardiopulmonary support during which efforts are made to stabilize vital signs, cool the patient with ice, and reduce muscle spasms with dantrolene (Dantrium). Because this condition is hereditary, the nurse who is preparing the patient for surgery should ask if there has been any family history of this condition or of sudden death during surgery. Patients known to have experienced this complication should be advised to wear a Medic Alert bracelet that identifies this problem.

Potential hypothermia. It is not uncommon for patients to experience a significant drop in body temperature (95° F or lower) during surgery as a result of low room temperature, incisional exposure of body cavities to the environment, and lowered metabolism. Warm blankets and increased room temperature can limit heat loss.

Patient injury. Because patients cannot protect themselves during surgery and anesthesia, the surgical staff must be aware of the potential for harm. Poor positioning may cause skin or nerve damage, as well as respiratory complications. A break in aseptic technique may cause postoperative infection. There are many electrical and equipment hazards because of the increased use of modern equipment. Laser surgery involves special precautions for both patient and staff.

POSTOPERATIVE ASSESSMENT AND INTERVENTIONS

Postanesthesia Care

Patients recovering from anesthesia must be closely monitored until their airway reflexes return, their breathing is satisfactory, and their vital signs are stable. Most hospitals maintain facilities for the immediate postoperative care of the patient, and the patient is transferred from the operating room to the postanesthesia recovery unit on a specially designed bed or stretcher. The recovery area, which may be designated as PACU (**Postanesthesia Care Unit**) or PAR (Postanesthesia Recovery) is generally located near the operating room and is equipped with the necessary supplies, drugs, and equipment to care for any emergency that might arise. The **recovery room** is considered a part of the surgical suite and is supervised by the anesthesiologist (Figure 18-7).

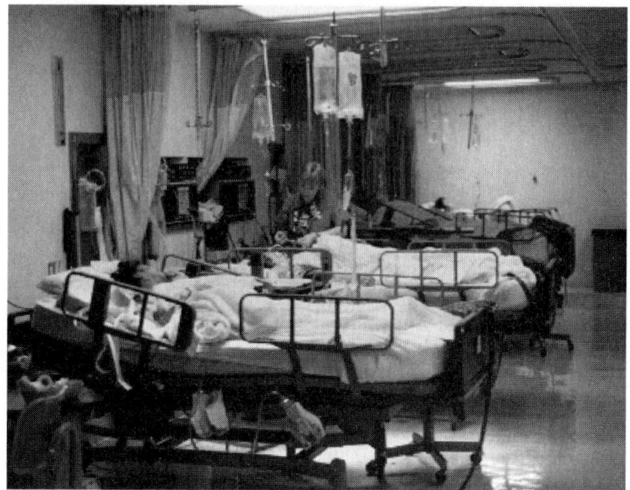

Figure 18-7 A recovery room or postanesthesia care unit facilitates close observation of the patient during recovery from anesthesia. (From Potter PA, Perry, AG: *Basic nursing,* ed 3, St Louis, 1995, Mosby.)

The anesthetist or anesthesiologist accompanies the patient from the operating room to the recovery room and advises the nurses of the patient's condition and any special problems that require care or attention. The anesthetist or anesthesiologist ensures that the patient's airway is clear and that his or her vital signs are satisfactory. Before leaving the patient, the anesthesiologist informs the recovery room nurse of the patient's condition, and the postoperative vital signs are taken. The patient should be protected by siderails on the bed, which may be padded to prevent injury to a particularly restless patient. The patient should be moved as carefully as possible. Anesthetics are stored in the body during surgery, and until they are metabolized, every movement of the patient (e.g., moving from operating table to stretcher or bed, riding in elevators, or wheeling around corners in corridors) may affect vital signs. Regardless of the type of surgery that the patient has undergone, immediate postoperative care should include the maintenance of privacy and warmth, proper body alignment, and **pain management.**

Airway

The immediate responsibility of the nurse is to ensure that the **airway** is clear and remains clear. If increased secretions obstruct the respiratory passages, they are aspirated with a catheter that has been attached to suction. The catheter must be inserted without suction (suction port open) to prevent damage to the mucous membranes. If secretions have been removed but evidence of respiratory difficulty is still

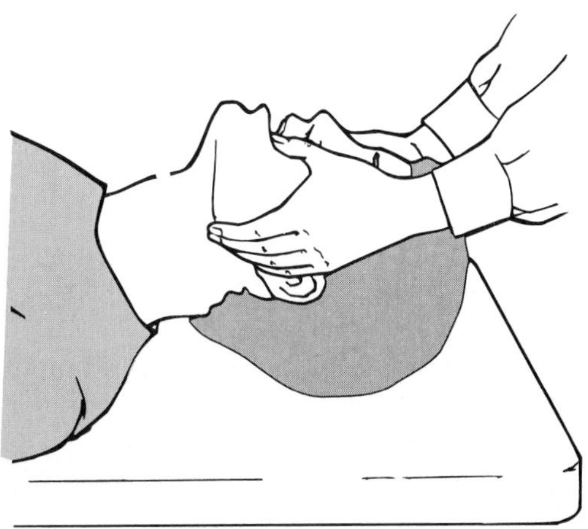

Figure 18-8 Method of pushing jaw forward to relieve respiratory difficulty.

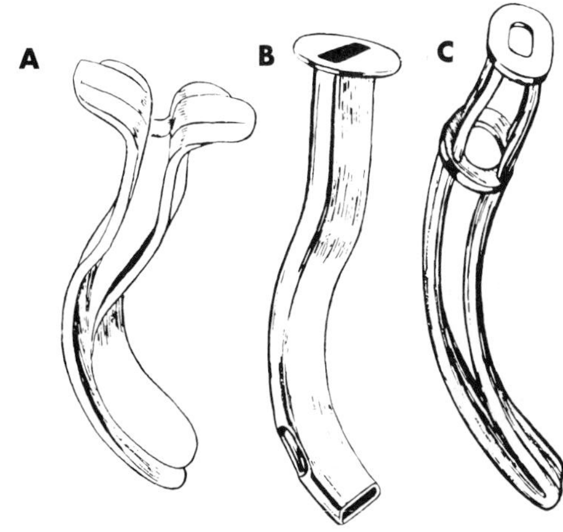

Figure 18-9 Artificial airways. **A,** Plastic. **B,** Rubber. **C,** Metal.

present, the nurse's thumbs and fingers should be placed at the angle of the patient's jaw on both sides, and the jaw should be pushed forward (Figure 18-8). The tongue is the most common cause of airway obstruction and may be grasped with a piece of gauze and pulled forward. If these measures do not open the airway, the nurse may insert an oral or nasal airway or call the anesthesiologist. Often the anesthesiologist leaves an airway in place until the patient shows signs of regaining consciousness (Figure 18-9).

Breathing

The patient's respiratory rate should be checked often. Oversedation; shallow, quiet, and slow respirations; noisy respirations; and restlessness may be early signs of respiratory depression. The movement of air into and out of the lungs can be felt by holding a hand near the patient's mouth. Respiratory rates of 30 or above or below 12 per minute should alert the nurse to respiratory difficulty (Box 18-8).

Many anesthetics and anesthetic adjuncts depress the respiratory mechanism. Narcotic anesthetics, sedatives, and neuromuscular blockers all have a negative effect on respiratory activity. The recovery room nurse must be aware of the types of agents used during the surgery and of the time of their administration. The patient who has had a neuromuscular block (curare, succinylcholine) is often requested to lift the head or in some other way demonstrate the return of muscle control before the airway is removed (McConnell, Lawler, 1991).

Patients whose respirations are below 12 per minute as a result of narcotic anesthesia may be medicated with a narcotic antagonist such as naloxone (Narcan) or levallorphan (Lorfan). These drugs, given parenterally, work rapidly to reverse narcotic-induced respiratory depression.

Circulation

The patient's blood pressure and pulse should be taken as ordered or more often as the patient's condition indicates. The patient's preoperative blood pressure should be known so that comparisons can be made. A falling systolic pressure or cardiac arrhythmias should be reported immediately. A critical systolic pressure must be determined for each patient individually and on the basis of preoperative readings. A drop in blood pressure may occur after the administration of certain types of anesthetics, muscle-relaxing drugs, or some tranquilizing drugs. It may also occur as the result of moving the patient or of unrelieved pain. The pulse should be checked for rate, rhythm, and volume. A drop in blood pressure and a weak, rapid, thready pulse with cool, moist skin may indicate severe bleeding or shock, and the physician should be notified immediately. Treatment is based on the cause, and the physician orders the appropriate procedures.

Drainage

All drainage tubes are connected to the appropriate type of drainage and should be properly connected and patent. Gastric tubes are connected to suction, and urinary drainage tubes are connected to the proper drainage container. Dressings should be checked for blood or secretions and constriction, and wound drainage units should be checked for patency. The physician must be notified if bright red bleeding is increasing.

BOX 18-8

SYMPTOMS OF RESPIRATORY DISTRESS/HYPOXIA

- Slow, sighing respirations
- Rapid, shallow breathing
- Noisy respirations
- Dyspnea
- Rapid, thready pulse
- Apprehension
- Restlessness
- Pallor
- Cyanosis

Intravenous therapy

The nurse should check and carry out the physician's orders for any procedures or medications, such as administration of IV fluids or blood. It is the nurse's responsibility to carefully observe a patient who is receiving IV fluids. The rate of flow is ordered, and the number of milliliters per hour must be regulated. The infusion site should be watched for swelling, tenderness, and redness. Blood should appear in the tubing when the nurse aspirates the line with a syringe. If blood does not appear, the IV fluid has infiltrated. Infiltration can also be verified by observing *continued* flow after the vein is compressed with a tourniquet, which is applied above the infusion site. Flow will stop if the needle is still in the vein. The patient's complaint of burning pain at the intravenous site is often the first sign of inflammation or infiltration. When these symptoms occur, the IV infusion should be removed and restarted in another area. Nurses should be continuously alert for possible complications such as respiratory difficulty, circulatory overload, and thrombophlebitis (see Chapter 8).

Relief of pain

The awakening patient may complain of pain. Before giving pain-relieving drugs, the nurse should consider the length of time since the preoperative sedatives were administered, the type and action of the anesthetizing agent, the status of vital signs, and the age of the patient. The physician should be consulted whenever any question arises concerning the administration of a narcotic. The patient should be closely monitored for signs of respiratory depression and hypotension.

Voiding

The patient may need to void while still in the recovery room and should be encouraged to do so in the outpatient unit before discharge. With the return to full consciousness and the awareness of pain, the patient becomes tense, and voiding may become difficult. The nurse should encourage the patient to void before painful stimuli cause tension or after the pain has been relieved by analgesics. If the patient has an indwelling catheter, the nurse should position the collection unit for optimum drainage. An accurate record of urinary output should be maintained.

Transfer to Patient's Room or Special Unit

The length of time the patient remains in the recovery room is determined by the immediate postoperative condition. When the vital signs are stabilized and consciousness has been regained, the patient may be transferred from the recovery room. An alert patient can demonstrate orientation to person, place, and time. At the time of transfer the recovery room nurse gives a report about the patient's condition, including any problems that occurred during the immediate postoperative period, to the nurse who will next care for that patient. If the patient needs continued close monitoring, transfer to a special unit may be necessary.

Intensive Care Unit

The evolution of the intensive care unit (ICU) began in the early 1960s, and almost all units were in large metropolitan hospitals. Now even small rural hospitals have a few beds set aside for the care of critically ill patients. The nurse-to-patient ratio is low, and the nurses have additional education to provide expert nursing care and to meet any emergency that might arise. The number of beds has increased, and the numbers and types of patients admitted to the ICU have also increased. A patient is admitted to the ICU because of the need for intensive nursing and medical care, which it is assumed cannot be given in the regular clinical units.

The increasing number of patients whose lives may be saved cannot always be cared for adequately in a single unit. Separate ICUs for specific types of patients exist in most large hospitals and include burn units, shock units, coronary care units, respiratory care units, surgical units, neonatal and pediatric care units, and renal care units. Nurses assigned to these units have participated in special courses and are considered experts in intensive care nursing.

Continuing Postoperative Care

The continued postoperative care of the patient is directed toward the prevention of complications, rehabilitation, and a return to normal living. Family members should be encouraged to see the patient and in some instances may be allowed to remain with the patient beyond visiting hours.

Comfort and safety measures

Postoperative patients should be protected by raising the siderails on the bed. A pillow may be placed under the patient's head, and the head of the bed may be slightly elevated. Because the patient is sensitive to temperature changes, care should be taken to prevent exposure to drafts to avoid chilling. The patient may feel cool to the touch and may complain of being cold because of the cooler temperatures in operating and recovery rooms, as well as the normal circulatory response to stress. The patient may be covered with a blanket until the skin is warm and dry, after which the blanket should be removed to prevent overheating. The patient who becomes too warm becomes restless, and excessive perspiration results in the loss of body fluids and important electrolytes. Oral and back care should be given, and the patient's face and hands should be washed. The patient is turned to the side in Sims' position, with a pillow placed to the back and between the legs to give support. If water intake is not permitted, the lips should be moistened with cool water at intervals. The room should be well ventilated and free from unnecessary noise. The patient should be turned from side to side every 2 hours unless the type of surgery performed limits positioning. Turning is essential to prevent respiratory complications and thrombus formation.

NURSE ALERT

If the patient's extremities are still cool several hours after surgery, monitor vital signs closely. A failure to "warm up" may be a sign of compensated shock caused by internal bleeding.

Coughing and deep breathing

The purposes of having the patient breathe deeply and cough are to remove mucus and other secretions that accumulate in the respiratory passages during anesthesia and to facilitate expansion of the lungs. Research suggests that forceful expulsive coughing may compromise respiratory recovery by collapsing the alveoli. Coughing exercises therefore are generally done only for patients who have secretions and mucus in the bronchial passageways. When the patient has been taught these exercises before surgery and understands their importance, coughing and deep breathing are accomplished more readily and thoroughly.

Many hospitals use techniques such as encouragement of the patient to yawn, use of the incentive spirometer, and specific respiratory therapies such as intermittent positive pressure breathing. All of these techniques stimulate deep breathing. If coughing is indicated, it is encouraged after deep breathing, should be deep, and should result in expectorating the mass of mucus from the respiratory passages. Better results may be obtained if the patient is placed in a sitting position and if the nurse helps relieve the strain by splinting the incision with a folded towel or pillow. Pain medication that is administered approximately 1 hour before coughing and deep breathing benefits the patient who is experiencing discomfort. If the patient is unable to cough up the mucus and secretions that have accumulated in the respiratory passages, the secretions may need to be removed by suctioning. Patients who have had surgery of the brain, spinal cord, or eyes should not be permitted to cough because coughing increases intracranial pressure. Lung sounds should be evaluated regularly (i.e., at least once each shift) to assess the lungs for secretions or diminished breath sounds.

Voiding

Unless an indwelling catheter is in place, the postoperative patient should void within 8 to 10 hours after surgery. The combination of anesthesia, surgery, pain, and apprehension can result in a patient's inability to urinate. A distended bladder can be palpated by examining for fullness above the symphysis pubis. Often the patient is uncomfortable and may void often and only in small amounts.

If the patient's condition permits, the bathroom may be used with the nurse's assistance. Providing adequate hydration through IV fluids or taking increased fluids by mouth when permitted facilitates voiding. Running water while the patient is attempting to void, placing the patient's hands in warm water, or pouring warm water over the genital area may also help. The patient should be catheterized only as a last resort and only when the bladder is distended and palpable above the pubis and the patient complains of distress.

If the patient has an indwelling urinary catheter, the nurse should monitor the output every 2 hours for the first 24 hours. Care should be taken to position the collecting unit below the patient to facilitate gravity drainage. Routine catheter care should be followed to minimize the possibility of bladder infection. Records should be maintained of all output.

Bowel function

After surgery of the gastrointestinal tract, peristalsis is temporarily absent and usually does not return for approximately 48 hours. The patient's expulsion of flatus or spontaneous movement of the bowels indicates that normal peristalsis has returned. Bowel sounds should be checked once each shift in all four quadrants of the abdomen with a stethoscope, and the nurse should question the patient concerning the passing of gas. Cathartics are not usually administered to surgical patients, and patients should be reassured that usual elimination patterns may not occur for several days. Patients who are accustomed to having a daily bowel movement often become worried. Frequent **ambulation** and extra fluids should be encouraged, and stool softeners may be prescribed.

Diet

Many surgical patients are not given food until peristalsis returns because eating may result in nausea, vomiting, and gas formation. They may be allowed sips of cool water (ice chips moisten the mucous membranes and may help prevent nausea), and they are usually given IV fluids. Before administering oral fluids after surgery, the nurse should check the physician's orders and the patient's ability to swallow. Fluids should initially be given slowly, a few sips at a time. Patients having surgery in an area other than the gastrointestinal tract may be allowed a soft or regular diet soon after surgery. Liquids such as fruit juices, tea, and water are generally desired by the patient and may be better tolerated than solids during the early postoperative period.

Tubes

When the patient has a retention catheter in the urinary bladder or a nasogastric tube, the nurse must check it often to ensure that it is draining properly. Irrigations or special procedures that may have been ordered by the physician should be carried out regularly. All drainage should be measured, observed, described, and recorded on the patient's chart.

Dressings

The nurse must check dressings, wound drainage units, and bed linens beneath the patient often for evidence of excessive drainage or bleeding. If bright red blood appears, the dressing should be observed again within a short period. The surgeon should be notified if there is any increase in bleeding. Dressings should also be checked for constriction of local circulation.

If drainage soaks through the dressing, it may be reinforced with additional dressings until an order has been secured for changing. All wound dressing changes must be carried out under strict surgical asepsis to promote wound healing. Most hospitals have approved procedures for dressing wounds, and these procedures, including the types of dressings and equipment used, vary among hospitals and surgeons. Some types of dressings, such as those used for severe burns or plastic surgery, may be changed only by the surgeon, and the patient may be given narcotic analgesics and a light anesthetic for the procedure. Abdominal binders may be worn to support the incision while the patient is ambulating. By the time the patient leaves the hospital, no dressing may be required.

Wound drains are commonly used after any surgery in which leakage of fluids around the surgical site is anticipated. Closed drainage systems with the drain exiting the skin through a small stab wound separate from the incision are most common and reduce the risk of incisional disruption and infection (Figure 18-10). These drains empty into a closed reservoir.

Open drainage systems such as the Penrose drain function through capillary action (Figure 18-11). Fluid from the surgical site is drawn to the body surface and into a dressing. Penrose drains are not used as often now because of the advantages presented by closed drainage systems. If open drainage systems are used, the nurse should change the dressing often, because damp dressings encourage bacterial growth. These dressings are often held in place with Montgomery straps to avoid the repeated use of tape on the skin (Figure 18-12).

Exercises

Unless contraindicated, exercises should be started as soon after surgery as possible or by the end of the first postoperative day. Starting exercises soon after surgery is especially important if early ambulation is to be delayed. Exercises stimulate circulation; prevent venous stasis, contractures, and loss of function; and facilitate recovery. The patient should be encouraged to exercise the fingers, hands, arms, feet, and legs. Leg exercises are particularly important to prevent thrombus formation. The patient can alternately flex and ex-

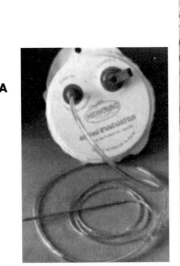

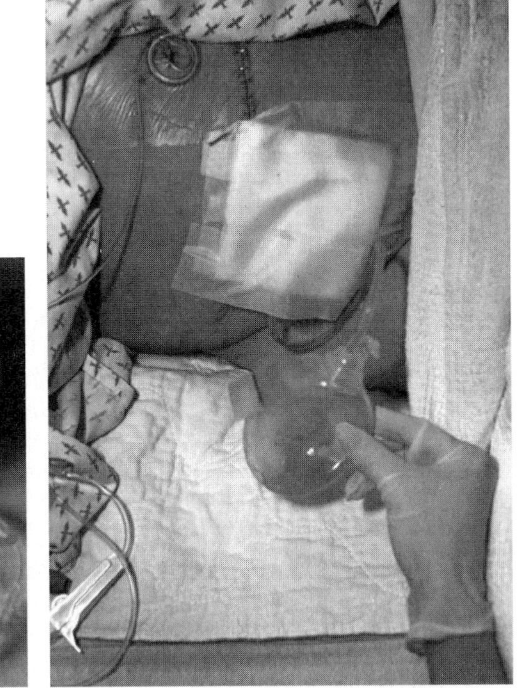

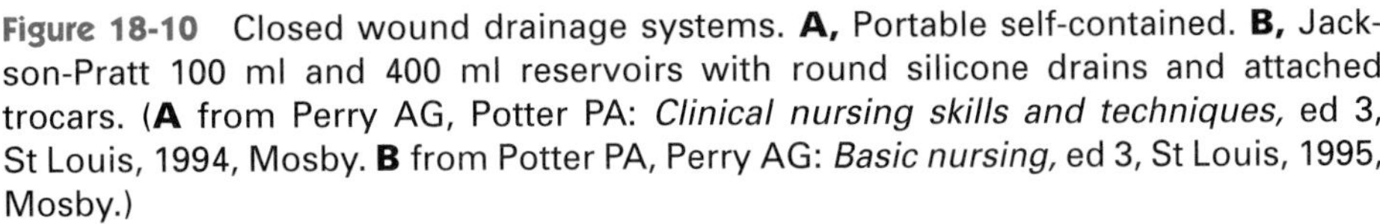

Figure 18-10 Closed wound drainage systems. **A,** Portable self-contained. **B,** Jackson-Pratt 100 ml and 400 ml reservoirs with round silicone drains and attached trocars. (**A** from Perry AG, Potter PA: *Clinical nursing skills and techniques,* ed 3, St Louis, 1994, Mosby. **B** from Potter PA, Perry AG: *Basic nursing,* ed 3, St Louis, 1995, Mosby.)

tend the legs by bending the knees and straightening the legs while lying in bed. Reminding the patient to perform these exercises encourages the patient to actively participate in his or her recovery.

Pillows should not be placed under the patient's knees, and the knee gatch of the bed should not be elevated. The patient should not sit on the side of the bed or be up in a chair with the legs dependent for extended periods of time. These positions cause pressure on the veins and engorgement of blood in the lower limbs and contribute to clot formation.

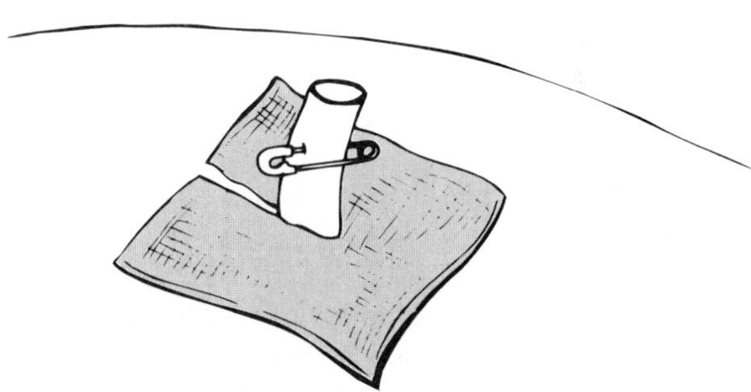

Figure 18-11 Penrose drain. (From Perry AG, Potter PA: *Clinical nursing skills and techniques,* ed 3, St Louis 1994, Mosby.)

Wound healing

Wound healing occurs by primary or secondary intention. Most surgical wounds are sutured closely at the time of surgery and heal by primary intention and generally with a minimum of scarring. If a wound is large and has edges that cannot be approximated, it must be allowed to heal by secondary intention, which is the filling of the area from the bottom with scar tissue. Open wounds are far more susceptible to infection. Frequent dressing changes are needed and may include packing these wounds with antiseptic gauze or applying moist dressings. Montgomery straps may be used to avoid tape injuries to the skin when dressings must be changed often.

Ambulation

Early **ambulation** facilitates the normal functioning of all body organs and systems and therefore reduces the danger of postoperative complications. Erect posture and activity encourage deep breathing and help

A

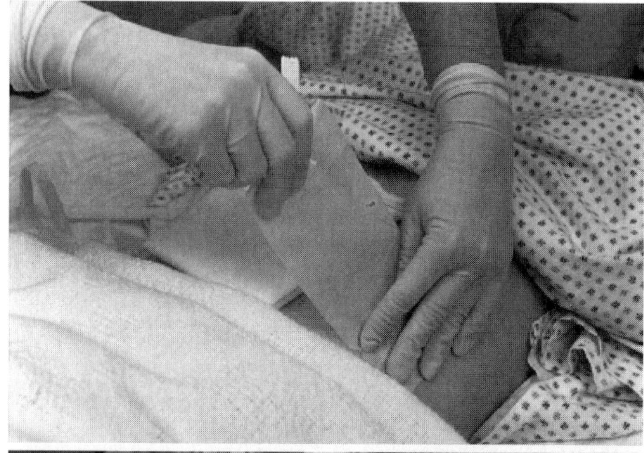

B

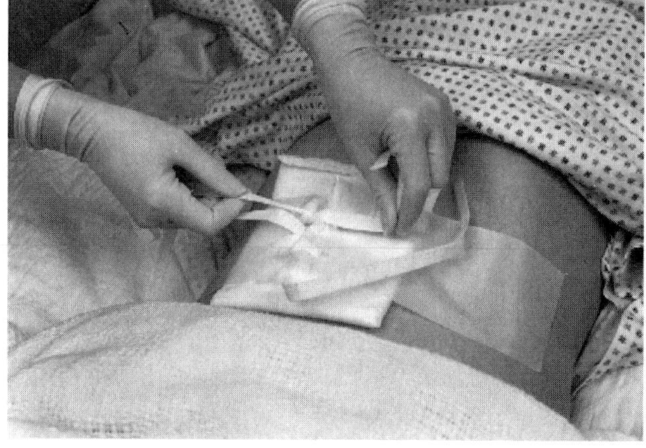

Figure 18-12 Montgomery straps may be used when frequent dressing changes are anticipated. (From Potter PA, Perry AG: *Basic nursing,* ed 3, St Louis, 1995, Mosby.)

prevent lung congestion. Walking stimulates the venous circulation and helps prevent thrombosis. Urinary retention and constipation occur less often in patients who ambulate early in the postoperative period.

Patients are allowed out of bed on the day of most major surgeries. Care should be taken while helping a patient get up. If at any time faintness or nausea is experienced, the patient should return to the last previous comfortable position and remain there for a few minutes before trying to rise again. Getting out of bed and walking soon after a surgical experience may cause apprehension and a fear of pain. The benefits of early ambulation should be well explained before surgery if possible. The type of surgery and the condition of the patient determines when ambulation may be started and the extent of walking permitted. Ambulation means walking, not sitting in a chair, but it should be a gradual process and should not exhaust the patient. The bed should be elevated to a sitting position before a patient is allowed out of bed. When allowed out of bed, the patient should be assisted by the nurse. A few steps may be sufficient at first. Ambulation permits the patient to be independent, self-sufficient, and able to carry out most self-care activities. It decreases feelings of helplessness, shortens the hospital stay, and enables the patient to regain strength more readily (Box 18-9).

POSTOPERATIVE COMPLAINTS AND COMPLICATIONS

Complaints

Pain

Pain is a subjective symptom that indicates physical or emotional distress. The expression of pain varies widely among individuals and cultures. The nurse should remember that pain is always real to the person experiencing it and that efforts should be made toward its relief.

The patient may verbally complain of discomfort, or the pain may be manifested in other ways. Facial expressions such as clenched teeth, a wrinkled forehead, widely open or tightly shut eyes, and grimacing are excellent indications of pain. Often a patient groans, cries, gasps, or cries out. Body movements such as muscle tension, immobilization of some or all of the body, kicking, tossing, turning, and rubbing can also indicate the presence of pain. Observing these symptoms can help the nurse and physician assess the level of pain and provide adequate relief. Patients may be unaware that they are permitted to have a pain medication, or they may be reluctant to ask for an analgesic.

The patient's first complaints of pain occur early in the postoperative period. One of the primary responsibilities of the nurse is to evaluate the patient's need for pain medication. When a patient complains of pain, the nurse should note the location of the pain and ask the patient whether it is a constant, intermittent, sharp, dull, or burning sensation. This information should be recorded on the patient's chart. The early administration of a pain-relieving drug such as morphine or meperidine (Demerol) often provides relief for several hours and permits restful, quiet sleep. Pain resulting from the surgical procedure should diminish after the first 24 to 48 hours, after which new orders are often written for pain management. Pain may be the result of other causes, such as abdominal distention, urinary retention, and casts that are too tight and are pressing on a nerve. A headache sometimes results from spinal anesthesia, and patients recovering from abdominal surgery experience pain when coughing deeply. The apprehensive and nervous patient may complain of more pain than the calm, passive individual. Older adults may be able to tolerate

BOX 18-9 **Nursing Process**

POSTOPERATIVE CARE

ASSESSMENT

Immediate
Airway and breathing
Cardiovascular status
Incision, dressings, drains, IVs
Level of consciousness, return of voluntary muscle control
Pain status
Vital signs
Skin, nailbed, and lip color

Continuing
Ability to cough and deep breathe
Respiratory status
Response to pain interventions
Incisional healing
Postoperative complications
Fluid volume status
Ability to perform self-ADLs
Nutrition and elimination patterns
Support systems postdischarge
Ability to understand follow-up care

NURSING DIAGNOSES

Risk for fluid deficit/excess related to fluid loss, fluid shift (third spacing), and fluid therapy
Pain, acute related to tissue trauma, pressure, or spasms
Risk for infection related to broken skin and traumatized tissue
Risk for injury: electrolyte loss, shock, falling related to surgical intervention
Impaired physical mobility related to activity restrictions
Urinary retention related to surgical intervention, anesthesia, analgesia
Impaired gas exchange related to anesthesia and reduced lung expansion
Altered nutrition: less than body requirements related to inadequate nutritional replacement or decreased oral intake
Self-care deficit related to impaired physical mobility or pain
Knowledge deficit related to new diagnosis, condition, home care

NURSING INTERVENTIONS

Immediate
Maintain patent airway.
Observe for signs of hypoxia.
Suction secretions from respiratory passageways as necessary.
Check vital signs often.
Check dressing often.
Observe for early signs of shock.
Maintain proper drainage and/or suction of tubes.
Provide for pain relief.
Regulate and observe infusion of IV fluids.
Evaluate level of consciousness.

Continuing
Encourage deep breathing and coughing.
Turn and position patient often.
Evaluate the need for pain medication.
Position the patient for comfort.
Encourage voiding.
Check for flatus or bowel sounds.
Maintain patency of drainage tubes.
Measure and record intake and output.
Care for the wound using aseptic technique.
Observe for bleeding and drainage.
Encourage exercises and ambulation.
Apply antiembolism stockings as ordered. Remove for 1 hour every 8 hours.
Assist with ADLs as needed.
Observe for postoperative complications.

EVALUATION OF EXPECTED OUTCOMES

Returns to normal activity and function
Follows postoperative instructions
Complications avoided

more pain than younger persons. Obese persons and those who abuse drugs and alcohol often need larger amounts of drugs to relieve pain.

Whatever the cause of pain, the nurse should make every effort to relieve it and to make the patient comfortable. Changing the patient's position, washing his or her face and hands, giving the patient a backrub, applying a cold cloth to his or her forehead, or just sitting with the patient may provide relief and decrease the need for drugs. Drugs such as morphine depress respirations and should not be given when respirations are compromised, when the blood pressure is below what has been established as normal for the patient, or when blood pressure is unstable because shock may result. Narcotics should be given 1 hour before postoperative activities such as ambulation. Nursing care should be given when the patient is receiving the most benefit from the medication. The patient should be told that the medication is for pain. The psychologic effect of knowing that something is being done relieves anxiety and tension, which contributes to the effectiveness of the drug. When a narcotic has been given to an older adult, the nurse must be particularly observant of the patient because the drug may cause restlessness or disorientation.

Patient-controlled analgesia (PCA pump) Pain medication is now commonly administered intravenously with a PCA (patient-controlled analgesia) pump. Morphine or meperidine cartridges are attached to IV fluid tubing in a mechanical pump. The patient controls the flow of the medication by pushing a button and is instructed to push the button when any discomfort is present. Overdose is prevented by programming the machine to allow infusion at a predetermined interval. The amount of drug administered is also controlled by settings on the machine. This method gives the patient the ability to control pain and to maintain a consistent level of medication in the blood, which makes pain tolerable. When using a PCA pump, less medication is required than with the traditional method of allowing pain to return before medication is given.

Nausea and vomiting

Postoperative nausea and vomiting result from any one of several causes, including the anesthetic, sensitivity to drugs, surgical manipulation, or serious postoperative complications. Patients who have experienced considerable preoperative vomiting and who fear vomiting postoperatively may be more prone to vomit. A nasogastric tube attached to suction siphonage may be left in place for 24 to 48 hours to keep the stomach empty and to reduce the incidence of nausea and vomiting. Nausea and vomiting that result from anesthesia may last 24 or more hours. Analgesics may also cause nausea and vomiting. When vomiting appears to be the result of drugs, the physician usually changes the medication order. Most postoperative vomiting is mild and self-limiting and requires little treatment. However, several drugs belonging to the group known as phenothiazines may have an antiemetic effect for some patients and are often ordered by the physician. Some of these include prochlorperazine (Compazine), thiethylperazine (Torecan), promazine (Sparine), and promethazine (Phenergan). H_2 receptor antagonists such as cimetidine (Tagamet), ranitidine (Zantac), and famotidine (Pepcid) also reduce postoperative nausea and gastrointestinal distress. If the patient is permitted to have fluids by mouth, sips of ginger ale or cola drinks may be given to relieve nausea. Persistent vomiting results in a loss of body fluids and electrolytes and may be serious.

Retention of urine

An overdistended bladder may cause the patient considerable discomfort and actual pain. Patients who have had surgery of the rectum, pelvis, or lower abdomen commonly have difficulty voiding. Catheterization using sterilization technique is indicated when the nurse has exhausted all measures designed to help the patient void. Because a continued inability to void results in overdistention and loss of bladder tone, the physician may order a retention catheter to be inserted until the patient's condition improves (see Chapter 24).

Abdominal distention

Abdominal distention occurs when gas accumulates in the stomach and intestines. Most surgical patients have "gas pains" as a result of temporary loss of peristalsis. Gas is not moved through the intestinal tract, and it accumulates in the greatest amount in the large intestine. The cause of gas accumulation in the intestinal tract is not clearly understood. Severe abdominal distention may interfere with respiratory function. Measures to provide relief include the use of a well-lubricated rectal tube, which should be inserted just past the internal sphincter. The tube should not be left in for longer than 30 minutes because spasms of the sphincter may occur. However, the tube may be used every 3 to 4 hours if it provides relief. The surgeon may order a nasogastric tube that is inserted through the nose, into the stomach, and attached to suction to prevent the stomach from becoming dilated with gas and to prevent paralysis of the intestines (paralytic ileus). Drugs that stimulate peristalsis, such as neostigmine (Prostigmin) or metoclopramide (Reglan), are sometimes ordered. Early ambulation can prevent or reduce the amount of distention and can promote the return of peristalsis.

Complications

The incidence of postoperative complications has been reduced through more careful preoperative preparation for surgery, improved surgical procedures, early postoperative activity, and adequate pain control. However, several postoperative complications continue to occur and probably always will to some extent. The most serious postoperative complications are hemorrhage, surgical shock, respiratory disorders, thrombosis, embolism, wound infection, dehiscence, and evisceration.

Hemorrhage and shock

Blood loss may occur during the surgical procedure or after the surgery has been completed and the patient has been returned to his or her room. The surgeon evaluates the amount of blood lost during surgery and, if the loss has been great enough, orders a transfusion of whole blood. A secondary **hemorrhage** may result from an untied blood vessel or from the slipping of a ligature. It may involve a capillary, vein, or artery and may be external or internal (into a body cavity or organ). All types of hemorrhage create an emergency situation and require immediate steps be taken to control bleeding and to restore blood volume.

Early detection is important to prevent damage to the cells and vital organs and, in some cases, death. The nurse should be conscientious about inspecting the dressing for evidence of bleeding from the wound. A small amount of oozing may be controlled by placing a sterile dressing over the site and applying a pressure bandage. If an extremity is involved, the part may be elevated. When bleeding is internal, the patient is returned to the operating room so that the wound can be opened. The nurse should be alert to the symptoms that may indicate internal bleeding.

Symptoms of hemorrhage are essentially those of hypovolemic shock. Early signs include cool extremities, restlessness, apprehension, an increasing pulse rate, and oliguria. Later the skin becomes pale, moist, and cool; the respiratory and pulse rates increase; the temperature becomes subnormal; and the blood pressure falls. In addition to blood on dressings, external evidence of hemorrhage may be observed, such as blood in vomitus, in urine, or from the lungs (hemoptysis). Patients who are receiving anticoagulant drugs should always be watched for bleeding into the skin or from a body orifice. If a patient shows signs of hemorrhage, the nurse should check the oxyhemoglobin saturation with the pulse oximeter, remain calm, and reassure the patient while carrying out emergency measures until the surgeon arrives (see Chapter 8).

Other causes of postoperative shock are sepsis, cardiac failure, drug reactions (including anesthetic drugs), transfusion reactions, pulmonary embolism, adrenal failure, and sepsis. Each cause results in a pathologic process that ultimately produces cardiovascular collapse and poor oxygenation of all body tissues. The symptoms of each type of shock are essentially the same as those of hypovolemic shock. Treatment depends on the cause of shock, but oxygen and IV solutions are always administered. The patient is kept flat and warm, and vital signs are checked at frequent intervals and recorded (see Chapter 8).

Respiratory disorders

Many respiratory complications can be prevented through careful postoperative care. Patients who have a respiratory disease before surgery are most likely to develop complications after surgery. Before surgery, the nurse should observe the patient for congestion, coughing, or sneezing and report such symptoms to the physician. The most common complications are bronchopneumonia, hypostatic pneumonia, bronchitis, pleurisy, and **atelectasis** (see Chapter 20). Maintaining a clear airway, instructing the patient to breathe deeply and to cough, turning the patient regularly, placing the patient in Fowler's position, and encouraging early ambulation are nursing interventions that are designed to prevent respiratory complications.

Thrombosis and embolism

Several factors contribute to the formation of a blood clot, or thrombus, in the vein. This complication, called thrombosis, is most common in persons who are required to maintain a schedule of bed rest. Other predisposing factors include tight abdominal binders; injury or pressure to veins, which occurs in the operating room at the time of surgery; decreased respiration and blood pressure; or any condition that results in the decreased flow of blood through the veins. **Embolism** occurs when a blood clot breaks away from a vessel and enters the circulation. Emboli that originate from thrombi in veins usually follow the normal circulatory pathways until the next capillary system is reached, which is that of the lungs. Pulmonary embolism is a

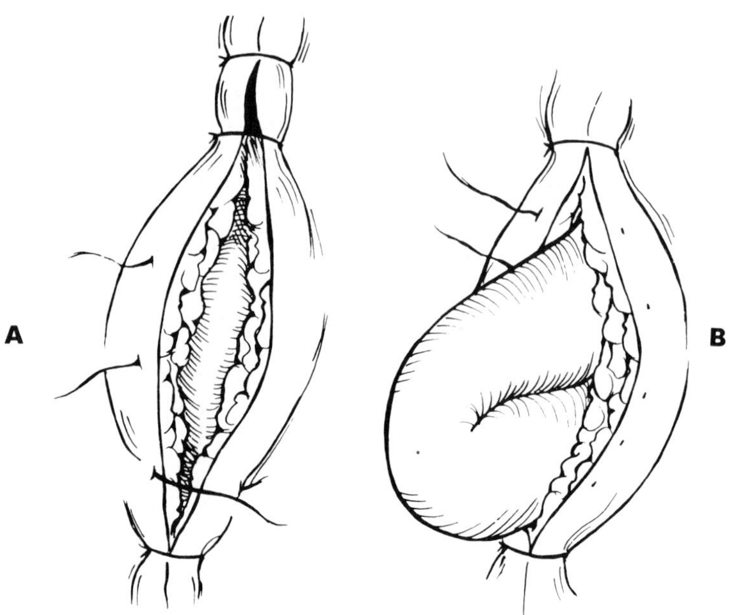

Figure 18-13 **A,** Wound dehiscence. **B,** Evisceration. (From Meeker MH, Rothrock JC: *Alexander's care of the patient in surgery,* ed 10, St Louis, 1995, Mosby.)

serious complication of surgery (see Chapter 20). Postoperative exercises, early ambulation, and frequent position changes are nursing interventions that help prevent these complications. TED hose (elastic support stockings) and pneumatic leg wrappings (sequential compression devices [SCDs]) "squeeze" the legs upward in a sequential manner, which promotes venous blood return. TED hose and SCDs may also be ordered to prevent venous pooling in the legs.

Wound infection

Surgical **wound infections** usually are manifest by the fifth postoperative day. The organism most often involved is *Staphylococcus aureus,* but *Escherichia coli, Proteus vulgaris, Aerobacter aerogenes,* and *Pseudomonas aeruginosa* are also involved. A postoperative wound infection is classified as a hospital-acquired, or nosocomial, infection (see Chapter 12). Factors such as preexisting illness, obesity, advanced age, complicated surgery, and forms of therapy such as radiation and chemotherapy predispose the patient to postoperative infections. A break in surgical asepsis and a failure to use an aseptic technique during wound care can also result in infection. Infected wounds are cleaned and irrigated by the physician, and often a drain is placed in the incision. The drainage is cultured, and appropriate antibiotic drugs are administered. Clean incised wounds should heal without infection if they are uncontaminated. Infection may also be caused by contaminated IV and bladder catheters.

Dehiscence and evisceration

Dehiscence and **evisceration** may result from infection, abdominal distention, coughing, and poor nutrition. These conditions occur more often in a chronically ill or obese patient and usually on the sixth to seventh postoperative day, which is usually when the patient is back home. Both conditions are caused by the sloughing of sutures or staples before healing takes place. In dehiscence some or all of the sutures may give way, which causes the edges of the skin to separate. When evisceration occurs, the incision suddenly opens up and the intestines are released to the outside (Figure 18-13). The patient describes feeling as if something has given way, and inspection of the dressing reveals a clear, pink drainage. Any pink drainage from the wound of a postoperative patient should be investigated immediately. The wound should be covered with a sterile dressing or a sterile towel and held loosely in place with a binder. The surgeon should be notified immediately. The nurse should remain calm and should reassure the patient while checking vital signs. The patient should be placed in a low Fowler's position, and food or fluids should be withheld until the patient is seen by the physician. Generally the patient is returned to surgery, and the wound is resutured.

PATIENT AND FAMILY TEACHING AND PLANNING FOR DISCHARGE

Careful planning for the transition from the postoperative unit to the home setting or extended-care facility is essential for optimum recovery. This planning is done by the patient, family, nurse, and other appropriate members of the healthcare team. Postoperative hospital stays have decreased in length dramatically in the past decade, which has increased the need for teaching the patient and family numerous procedures and therapies that were once only carried out in the hospital setting. Nowhere is the need more evident than in the outpatient surgery setting. Postoperative patients may be discharged with dressings and urinary and surgical drains still in place and even with ongoing intravenous infusions.

The nurse should collaborate with the physician in determining what care the patient and family can provide at home, as well as what community resources and home nursing care agencies may be necessary. If dressing changes or other procedures will be done at home, the nurse should not only teach the patient and family how to perform them but should also provide a small supply of equipment, written instructions, and the location in the community where additional supplies can be obtained. Patients being discharged should also know the time of their appointment for follow-up care with the physician. If the patient is being discharged to an extended-care facility, a written summary of the medical regimen and nursing care plan should be completed by the physician and nurse and should accompany the patient. If the patient is being discharged from the day-surgery or outpatient unit, the nurse telephones him or her within 24 hours to follow up on the condition and to answer any questions (Box 18-10).

BOX 18-10

DISCHARGE CRITERIA OR OUTCOMES FOR THE POSTSURGICAL PATIENT

INPATIENT AND OUTPATIENT

- The incision is clean and dry and approximated.
- The vital signs are within preoperative normal levels.
- The patient is voiding without difficulty and in adequate amounts.
- The patient has only mild to moderate pain, which is managed by oral analgesics.
- Family or friends are available to transport the patient home and be available.
- The patient has no signs and symptoms of complications, and the patient and family verbalize a knowledge of signs and symptoms of postoperative complications.
- The patient is tolerating the prescribed diet and can describe any dietary or activity changes that are necessitated by the surgery.
- The patient or a family member demonstrates an ability to care for the incision, take medications, or do any procedures needed for continuing convalescence.
- The patient can describe the schedule of follow-up care with the physician.
- The patient verbalizes a knowledge of community resources and support groups that may be useful in promoting recovery.

ADDITIONAL INPATIENT CRITERIA

- The patient is able to carry out activities of daily living without significant increase in pain and fatigue.
- Elimination patterns have been reestablished.
- The patient is able to correctly perform breathing exercises and shows no evidence of respiratory distress.

KEY CONCEPTS

- The nurse can minimize the potential for the negative effects of stress by identifying factors (other than the surgical experience) that may be contributing to the patient's concern.
- Stress and breaks in the skin, such as a surgical incision, make infection a real possibility for every surgical patient. Antibiotic therapy may be prescribed prophylactically, but meticulous surgical and postsurgical aseptic techniques are the keys to preventing infection.
- The surgical procedure may alter the patient's perception of body image and always causes a temporary or permanent disruption of lifestyle.
- Issues of spirituality, the broad concept that represents an individual's search for the meaning of life and death, are often not confronted until a time of serious illness and the possibility of death. Therefore in preparing the patient for surgery, it is important to support the patient and facilitate his or her personal expressions of spirituality.

KEY CONCEPTS

- The objective of surgical nursing is to prepare the patient mentally and physically for surgery and to assist in full recovery in the shortest time possible and with the least discomfort.
- Informed consent means that the physician has provided the patient with an explanation of the surgical procedure, the possible consequences of the surgery, and what to expect during the postoperative period.
- The goal of preoperative preparation and care of the patient is to promote the best possible physical and psychologic state of the patient before surgical therapy.
- Preoperative instruction usually includes deep breathing and coughing, turning and moving, medications, and special equipment that may be used postoperatively. Vigorous coughing is discouraged in cases in which increased intracranial pressure must be avoided.
- During the immediate postanesthesia period, the nurse is responsible for ensuring that the airway remains clear, that normal respirations are maintained, and that signs of hemorrhage are treated. The patient's temperature, respiratory rate, blood pressure, and pulse must be monitored; the dressings must be checked; and the drainage tubes and intravenous therapy must be maintained.
- Discharge planning must begin before surgery and involves the patient, family, nurse, and other members of the healthcare team. Resources for the specific needs of each patient must be identified.

CRITICAL THINKING EXERCISES

1 Mr. Burns is admitted to the hospital for elective surgery. The day before surgery, he is given preoperative care. He is taught how to cough and breathe deeply, turn in bed, and perform leg exercises. In reviewing Mr. Burns' chart, the nurse sees that the consent for surgery has been signed and that all necessary laboratory work is on the chart. However, on the morning of surgery, the nurse enters Mr. Burns' room to assist him with morning care and sees him sitting in his chair fully clothed. When the nurse asks Mr. Burns about this, he states, "I've changed my mind, and I've decided to go home." How would you, as the nurse, respond to this situation? What are some fears that Mr. Burns may have concerning his surgery?

2 Mrs. Hops is admitted to the hospital for removal of her gallbladder. Mrs. Hops is 36 years of age, is 5 feet 4 inches tall, and weighs 194 lbs. She tells the nurse that she has been in the hospital three times, when she delivered her children, but has never had surgery. When she had her last child 4 years ago, she had a blood clot in her leg and had to remain in the hospital for 6 additional days.

Why are deep breathing and leg exercises especially important for Mrs. Hops to learn? What complications must the nurse be alert for in caring for Mrs. Hops after her surgery? Why will the postoperative orders for Mrs. Hops probably include applying an abdominal binder when she is out of bed?

REFERENCES AND ADDITIONAL READINGS

Beare P, Myers J: *Adult health nursing,* ed 2, St Louis, 1994, Mosby.

Black J, Matassarin-Jacobs E: *Luckman and Sorensen's medical-surgical nursing,* ed 4, Philadelphia, 1993, WB Saunders.

Gallagher M, Kahn C: Lasers: scalpels of light, *RN* 53(5):46-53, May 1990.

Good M: Relaxation techniques for surgical patients, *Am J Nurs* 95(5):39-43, 1995.

Hogstel M, editor: *Nursing care of the older adult,* ed 3, Albany, 1994, Delmar.

Keep N: Identifying pulmonary embolism, *Am J Nurs* 95(4):52, 1995.

Long B, Phipps W, Cassmeyer V: *Medical-surgical nursing: a nursing process approach,* ed 3, St Louis, 1993, Mosby.

McConnell E, Lawler M: Preventing postop complications, *Nurs* 21(11):33-47, 1991.

Nicholson C and others: Are you ready for video thoroscopy, *Am J Nurs* 93(3):54-57, March 1993.

Rocuronium Z: A safer fast muscle relaxant? *Am J Nurs* 95(3):56-57, 1995.

Saltiel-Berzin R: Managing a surgical patient who has diabetes, *Nursing* 22(4):34-42, April 1992

CHAPTER 19

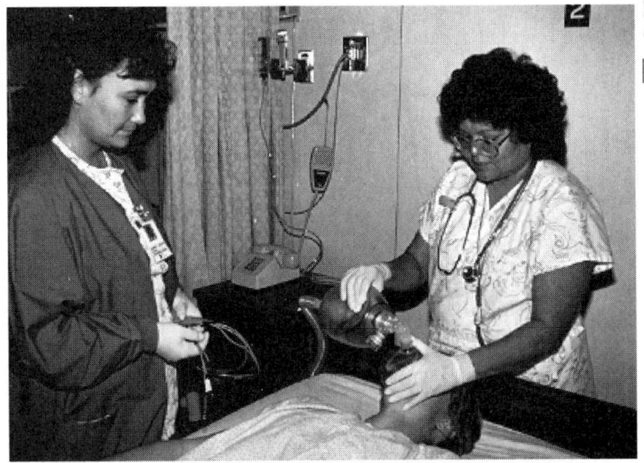

Emergency and Trauma Care

CHAPTER OBJECTIVES

1 Define the four goals of emergency care.
2 Discuss legislation related to emergency departments.
3 List the characteristics unique to emergency nursing practice.
4 Define the difference between hospital triage and disaster triage.
5 Discuss basic life support and airway obstruction.
6 Identify the three assessments done on all emergency patients and identify injuries for each assessment area.
7 Identify three life-threatening traumatic injuries affecting airway, breathing, and circulation.
8 Discuss the signs and symptoms of shock and the initial interventions and outcomes.
9 Discuss the precautions to take when administering intravenous conscious sedation.
10 Identify a brief neurologic examination and discuss how it relates to patients with head injuries, environmental emergencies, and psychiatric emergencies.
11 Discuss why violence is a problem.
12 Discuss the four types of maltreatment/abuse and the five areas of maltreatment. Identify the nurse's legal role.
13 Identify three behaviors a psychiatric patient may exhibit during the initial examination in the emergency department.
14 Discuss care of the patient who has overdosed and the patient who is suicidal.
15 Discuss specific selected areas related to emergency care: heat/cold emergencies, head injured patient, and anaphylaxis.
16 Identify how to help a family who has just experienced sudden death.
17 List the components of critical incidence stress debriefing and discuss what occurs in each component.

KEY WORDS

agitation
blood alcohol concentration (BAC)
cardiopulmonary resuscitation (CPR)
chain of custody
child maltreatment/abuse
Consolidated Omnibus Reconciliation Act (COBRA)
cricothyroidotomy
domestic violence
high-efficiency particulate air (HEPA) respirator
hyperthermia
hypothermia
prioritization
resuscitation
sexual assault
stabilization
triage

EMERGENCY DEPARTMENT

It has been estimated that emergency departments (EDs) see approximately 100 million patients a year. Before 1970 the general public had little awareness of emergency care. The emergency room was seen as the back door to the hospital until legislation was enacted that developed prehospital care, and criteria were set for hospital trauma designation (Table 19-1; Box 19-1).

This legislation resulted in the development of improved emergency services and EDs through the establishment of prehospital care and goals for the ED. The ED is now seen as the front door to the hospital, giving patients their first impression of the institution.

Goals of the Emergency Department

The goals of EDs are to stabilize and resuscitate reduce suffering, provide emotional support, and educate the public on how to care for themselves once they leave the ED. These goals are obtained through the collaborative efforts of the healthcare team.

Emergency Care Team

The emergency care team includes many members. The physician, emergency nurse, respiratory therapists, chaplain, social services, patient care representatives, nurses extenders, and x-ray and laboratory technicians all allow the patient coming to the ED to obtain the most complete care (Figure 19-1). The emergency nurse is a key component of this team. The nurse's responsibilities vary with each situation, the number of emergencies, the available professional personnel, and the policies of the individual institution.

TABLE 19-1

Legislation Affecting Prehospital and Emergency Care

Year	Legislation	
1966	Highway Safety Act	Federal government established protocols and standards for prehospital care by developing the Emergency Medical System (EMS).
1973	Emergency Medical Services Systems Act	Funds allocated to communities for the regionalization of the EMS. These funds provided dollars for the education of emergency medical technicians (EMTs) and paramedics. Communities were able to purchase equipment to provide prehospital care such as transport vehicles, telemetry/defibrillation monitors, and medications.
1976	Trauma System Designation	The American College of Surgeons published an article discussing levels of care for the trauma patient. These recommendations were recognized by the Joint Commission for Accreditation of Health Organizations (JCAHO), and hospitals were voluntarily able to be classified by these trauma standards.
1986/1990	**Consolidated Omnibus Budget Reconciliation Act (COBRA)**	Enacted to prevent "patient dumping," COBRA stated that all hospitals receiving Medicare dollars must perform an initial screening to any person who arrives at an emergency department to see if a medical emergency exists. Stabilization of the person must occur. If the patient is transferred, a physician at the receiving hospital must accept the person. All medical records including x-ray films must be transferred with the person. This act is constantly under revision (Emergency Nurses Association, 1993).

BOX 19-1

LEVELS OF TRAUMA CENTER DESIGNATION

LEVEL I

Level I trauma centers are regional resource hospitals that provide total care for every aspect of injury. This hospital helps with research and injury prevention. Available resources include 24-hour capability for computerized tomography, angiograms, and surgery. Designated specialties can be available within 30 minutes. Patients taken routinely to Level I trauma centers by paramedics are those who do not have spontaneous eye opening; have penetrating injuries to the head, neck, or abdomen; have fallen from a height of greater than 15 feet; or live patients who have been in the same car involving a fatality.

LEVEL II

Level II hospitals have the ability to administer 24-hour emergency care by a qualified emergency physician. A surgeon needs to be available on call within 20 to 30 minutes. The hospital needs to have prearranged transfer agreements for critical specialty injuries. Examples of these injuries are burns, spinal cord injuries, acute head trauma, and reimplantation of amputated body parts.

LEVEL III

Level III hospitals need to have an emergency physician on call 24 hours a day and available within 30 minutes. They need not have 24-hour capability for computed tomography (CT) or the ability to perform surgery 24 hours a day. These hospitals are seen in rural settings.

RURAL HOSPITALS

Rural hospitals are institutions where life-saving measures may be initiated. The patient is stabilized and transferred to the nearest qualified facility. (American College of Surgeons, 1990)

EMERGENCY NURSING

Emergency nursing as defined by the Emergency Nurses Association (ENA) is the practice of emergency care by a registered professional nurse. Emergency nurses work in a variety of settings: hospitals, urgent-care centers, industrial plants, schools, and nonacute clinics. The emergency nurse has a role in the prehospital care of patients and in the education of prehospital providers.

Emergency nursing has been recognized as a nursing specialty since 1970, when the ENA was established. Standards for practice in emergency nursing are established through the ENA. Time is critical when

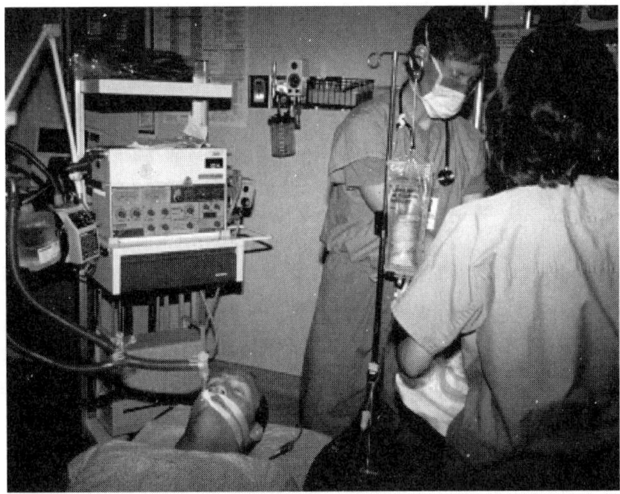

Figure 19-1 Members of the emergency care team. (Courtesy Michael Clement, MD, Mesa, Ariz.)

using the nursing processes of assessment and analysis, which include *triage* and *prioritization* and intervention. Emergency nurses manage patients of all ages who require **stabilization** and/or **resuscitation** for life- or limb-saving measures. They also intervene in crisis intervention. The ED nurse must provide care in an unpredictable and uncontrolled environment (Dains and others, 1991).

Characteristics of the Emergency Nurse

Emergency nurses must have the ability to work quickly and efficiently, to continuously prioritize patient care; to be flexible and energetic; and to communicate effectively. The nurse must be able to intervene with families in grief, perform crisis intervention, diffuse volatile situations, and teach patients and families expectations of care. Most activities of the nurse include procedures learned in basic and medical-surgical nursing courses. Additional education required includes electrocardiogram interpretation and basics of trauma care. The nurse may carry out various procedures including administration of medications, catheterization, lavage, and oxygen therapy. The emergency nurse must be able to work as a team member but have the self-confidence to practice autonomously with collaboration of the physician and healthcare team. The nurse must have good technical skills and be knowledgeable regarding the rapid changes in this highly critical area. Hospitals have developed standards of care and protocols to allow for quicker response to patient illness. The nurse is a patient advocate, who communicates the plan of care and keeps the patient informed as care progresses.

Role of the Emergency Nurse

The emergency nurse has many roles as the direct caregiver of patients in the emergency department. These roles include triage nurse, primary nurse, and associate primary nurse. Two advanced-practice emergency nursing roles that are developing for the masters-prepared registered nurse are the clinical nurse specialist (CNS) and the emergency nurse practitioner (NP). Emergency nurses practicing in the prehospital setting include the mobile intensive care nurse (MICN), the field registered nurse (RN), and the flight nurse (FN). Finally, the importance of the ED nurse manager cannot be overlooked.

Triage nurse

The triage nurse is the nurse who first assesses patients when they enter the emergency department. For more information about triage, see the triage section.

Primary nurse

The primary nurse is the main nursing caregiver for the patient. A complete secondary and focused survey is performed and the findings communicated to the physician. The primary nurse must be able to give a quick but accurate report to the emergency physician so that a plan of care can be determined. The nurse may order specific tests or x-ray examinations or initiate care according to the policy standards in the ED.

Associate primary nurse

The associate primary nurse may be a licensed practical nurse (LPN), who accepts tasks delegated after the complete assessment of the patient has been completed.

Emergency nurse manager

Because the ED is the front door to the hospital, it is constantly under scrutiny. The nurse manager must be fiscally responsible for the unit, supportive of the ED staff, and have good public relations and communications skills. The manager must be able to handle patient comments as well as be proactive in instituting change.

PATIENT ARRIVAL/CONSENT

Patients may arrive at the ED in an EMS unit (ambulance) from home, work, or an accident scene. They may arrive on their own or be brought by family or friends. They may arrive by helicopter from an accident scene or as a transfer from another facility. No matter how a patient arrives, the care is determined by a systematic approach. All patients receive a screening to see if an emergency exists. The triage nurse usually provides this initial screening. Consent for treatment in the ED must be obtained. This consent is either expressed, implied, or involuntary (Box 19-2).

BOX 19-2

TYPES OF CONSENT FOR TREATMENT

Expressed—The person comes and asks for care. If the person is under the age of 18, consent should be obtained from the parent or legal guardian. If an emergency does exist, the emergency physician can sign for consent for treatment until formal consent is obtained from the parent or guardian.

Implied—The patient comes in by ambulance and is in need of life-saving measures. It is implied that care is being sought. Consent for care should be obtained from a family member, if possible.

Involuntary—The patient refuses treatment but is judged to be incompetent, so care is performed. These patients include intoxicated patients, overdose patients, and suicidal patients (Klein and others, 1994).

It is important that ED nurses know basic first aid and cardiopulmonary resuscitation (CPR). The American Red Cross offers courses in basic first aid. When a patient arrives at the ED, care should be started immediately to prevent complications. However, the nurse's safety should never be jeopardized when administering care.

Infectious Disease Precautions

When preparing to care for any patient, it is imperative that the emergency team is ready to protect itself against infection from the human immunodeficiency virus (HIV), hepatitis B, and tuberculosis (TB). The emergency team should follow infection-control guidelines as indicated by the Centers for Disease Control and Prevention (CDC). Current federal Occupational Safety and Health Administration (OSHA) published guidelines have been developed to protect the healthcare worker from contracting TB. The guidelines state that healthcare workers need to wear a **high-efficiency particulate air (HEPA) respirator** for high-risk activities such as suctioning and intubation. Although this is required, the two HEPA respirators currently on the market have only been tested for industrial use. There have not been studies to prove they are efficient in decreasing the chance of exposure from a TB patient (Hays, 1994).

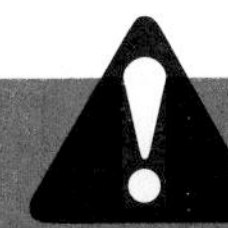

NURSE ALERT

Hands should always be washed after any contact with a patient, even if gloves were worn. This decreases the chance of transmission of diseases.

TRIAGE

The patient is triaged for determination of treatment. **Triage** was originally used during World War II to sort out battlefield casualties. The military triage system selected those most likely to live and gave them priority in care and evacuation to medical facilities. This type of triage is still used today during disasters. In contrast, triage used by hospital EDs classifies patients by prioritizing those who are most serious and need the most immediate attention. This is done through the identification of a chief complaint and a brief assessment. The patient is then classified as emergent, urgent, or nonurgent. During a disaster, *expectant* is also used as a classification. (Box 19-3).

Role of Triage During a Disaster

The role of triage during a disaster changes to field triage. A temporary satellite health facility is set up at the scene of the disaster. Prehospital triage is initiated by the EMS. EMTs are taught to assume the leadership role at the scene of a disaster in deciding the prioritization of patient care and the organized transport of the victims to hospitals. In-hospital triage begins when the patient is received from the ambulance or walks into the ED. Each system depends on the immediate assessment of the patient's status and the identification and immediate treatment of those victims seriously compromised. A tag securely attached to the patient is used to identify the victim instead of the normal chart because of the great influx of patients. The tag includes space for identification of the patient, allergies or current medications, vital signs, medications, treatments, x-ray films, and any significant history. The "expectant" patient who has massive injuries is transported to the hospital after the "emergent" and "urgent" patients have already been treated.

BOX 19-3

TRIAGE CLASSIFICATIONS

Emergent refers to a life-threatening problem. If the patient is not seen immediately, he or she will die or lose sight or a limb. Some of these patients are in cardiac arrest, have uncontrolled bleeding, have taken a drug overdose, are experiencing sudden loss of vision, have received chemical or electrical burns, or are in respiratory distress.

Urgent implies that care can be delayed from 20 minutes to 2 hours without significant mortality or increased disability to the patient. These include patients who have open fractures or are experiencing moderate to severe pain. These patients need to be reassessed every 15 minutes to monitor changes in their conditions.

Nonurgent implies that care can be delayed more than 2 hours. These patients have simple rib fractures, sprains, fractures without neurovascular compromise, earaches, or simple lacerations.

Expectant is a classification used during a disaster that indicates that the patient will die shortly from his or her injuries. These patients may have experienced an acute head injury with protruding brain matter or extensive burns (Sheehy, 1992).

Telephone Triage

According to ENA's position statement written in conjunction with the position statement by the American College of Emergency Physicians, **a diagnosis should never be given over the telephone.** The nurse should encourage the caller to come to the ED for care or to see his or her physician. If the patient tells the triage nurse of a situation that could be life-threatening, the nurse should inform the person to call the paramedics and provide whatever information is needed to save the patient's life while waiting for help. (Emergency Nurses Association, 1991)

Triage Assessment

A brief primary survey is conducted to investigate the patient's complaint (Box 19-4). The patient's actual or stated weight is obtained, and for female patients, the last menstrual cycle is documented.

Examination After Triage Assessment

The patient is assigned to an area where a more thorough history and examination can be performed.

BOX 19-4

TRIAGE HISTORY

Allergies
Medications
Past medical history
Last meal
Events

BOX 19-5

PQRST PAIN ASSESSMENT

Pain
Quality/Quantity
Radiation/Region
Severity
Timing

Obtaining a thorough history from a patient allows the healthcare team to identify problems and determine the degree of concern of the patient's condition. It is imperative to identify and recognize the severity of a patient's condition to allow for an optimal outcome. One question to ask is: "What is the mechanism of injury?"

Mechanism of injury, or how an injury occurred, is a significant factor in determining the extent of potential impairment. It may suggest the likelihood of the development of further problems during the hospital stay. Some sample questions to ask to determine the mechanism of injury include the following:

- Was a seat belt worn?
- Was a helmet worn?
- Was the patient injured at a high or low rate of speed?
- How far did the person fall, and what caused the fall?
- What instrument was used to cause the injury (gun, knife)?
- Who inflicted the injury (male or female; size of assailant)?

Other questions can include: How long have the symptoms existed? Where is the pain? What makes the pain worse or better? (Box 19-5)

This history should augment the history already obtained by the triage nurse or the EMT. The severity of the complaint or condition of the patient will determine who performs the initial examination. The primary nurse conducts the secondary assessment unless the patient is critically ill or injured. In this case it is not uncommon to have a physician and other members of the healthcare team work aggressively together to stabilize the patient.

PHYSICAL ASSESSMENT

The physical assessment should include the areas of inspection, auscultation, and palpation. These areas are evaluated during the primary, secondary, and focused surveys or assessments (Tables 19-2 and 19-3).

Primary Assessment

Airway, **B**reathing, and **C**irculation (ABCs) are the key components of the first assessment of any patient. The goal of the primary assessment is to identify all life-threatening problems and intervene with resuscitative measures. This is a quick but thorough assessment of the patency of the airway, stability of the cervical spine, ability to breathe, and circulatory status. These are the ABCs of emergency care.

Primary assessment of the airway/cervical spine

Is there a patent airway? An airway may be partially or completely obstructed (Figure 19-2). If the airway is partially obstructed, the patient will exchange air. If the air exchange is good, the patient can cough forcefully, dislodging the obstruction. Sometimes the air exchange is good initially but becomes poor. If the air exchange is poor, the patient's cough will be ineffective. There will be a high-pitched noise with inhalations called stridor, a violent respiratory effort using abdominal and intercostal muscles, and even cyanosis.

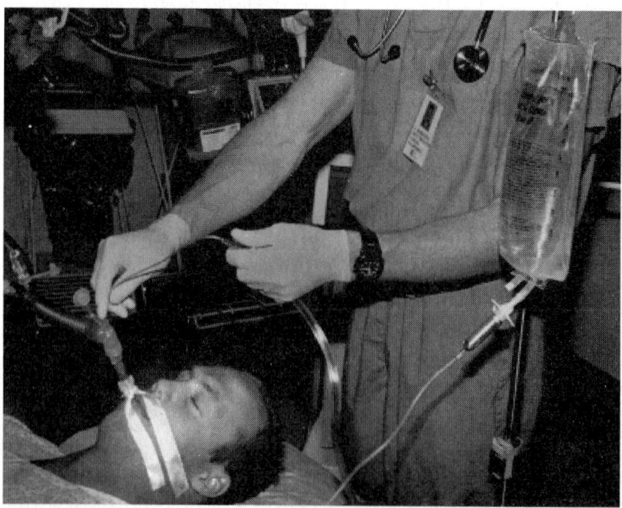

Figure 19-2 Patient is intubated to maintain airway. (Courtesy Michael Clement, MD, Mesa, Ariz.)

TABLE 19-2

Emergency Physical Examination

Primary Assessment (ABCDE)	Assessment	Intervention
Airway/cervical spine	Obstructed	Perform jaw thrust or chin lift. Remove debris: teeth, emesis. Insert oral/nasal airway. Prepare for intubation or a cricothyroidotomy.
	Patent	Immobilize cervical spine if this is a trauma patient.
Breathing	Absent	Bag/valve/mask at 15 L. Prepare for intubation. Prepare for positive pressure ventilation.
	Present	Administer oxygen if needed (see Figure 19-2).
Circulation	Absent	Begin CPR.
	Present	Assess location, quality, rate of pulse. Assess blood pressure, skin color, temperature, and capillary refill. Identify source of bleeding. Initiate intravenous access. Send type and cross match.
Disability (Neurologic)	Responsive	Assess level of consciousness. Assess response to stimuli (verbal, pain). Assess pupils for symmetry and response.
	Unresponsive	Prepare to protect patient from harm (secure an endotracheal airway to prevent aspiration; position the patient).
Expose		Completely undress patient. Cover patient to prevent heat loss.

With complete airway obstruction the patient cannot speak, breathe (no air movement), or cough, and he or she may clutch the neck (Figure 19-3). This is the universal choking sign.

Obstructed airway. The nurse should ask the patient to speak. If the patient cannot speak, the nurse should attempt to clear the airway. The nurse should stand behind the patient, wrapping the arms around the patient's waist (Figure 19-4). Making a fist with one hand and placing the thumbside against the patient's abdominal midline slightly above the naval and well below the xiphoid process, the nurse should grasp the fist with the other hand. The nurse should then press the patient's abdomen with quick upward thrusts. This process is commonly called the Heimlich maneuver, named for Dr. Harry J. Heimlich, who developed it. Each thrust should be distinct and delivered with the intent of relieving the airway obstruction. The thrusts should be repeated until either the foreign body is expelled or the patient becomes unconscious.

If the patient lapses into unconsciousness, the nurse

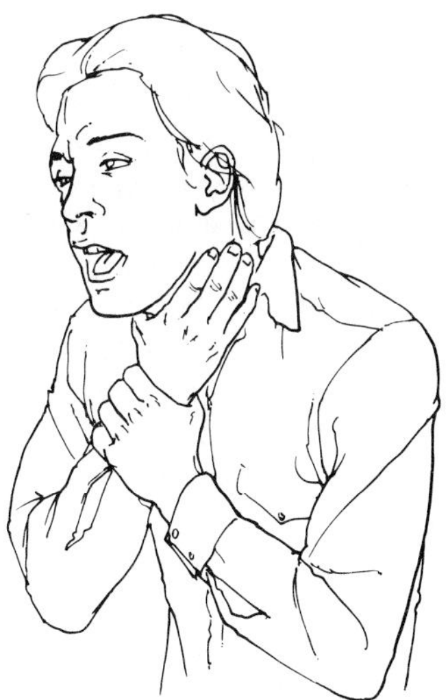

Figure 19-3 Universal distress signal for choking. (From *Standards and guidelines for cardiopulmonary resuscitation and emergency cardiac care, part 2,* 255:2915-2932.)

TABLE 19-3

Emergency Physical Examination—Secondary Assessment

Area of Assessment	Mode of Assessment
Head	**Inspect** for any bleeding, depressions of the skull, lacerations, avulsions, embedded foreign bodies, puncture wounds, swelling, and ecchymosis. Look at symmetry of face. **Palpate** for tenderness and bony deformities.
Eyes	**Inspect** for bruising around eyes and redness in eyes. Check for contact lenses. Assess gross vision. Is patient able to see from either eye? Assess pupillary response, size of pupils, and symmetry. Assess movement of eyes.
Ears	**Inspect** for drainage from ears. Note color of drainage. **Inspect** for bruising behind ears. Check for lacerations.
Nose	**Inspect** for drainage from nose. Note color of drainage. **Palpate** for tenderness and bony deformities.
Neck	**Inspect** for penetrating objects, tracheal deviation, neck vein distention, swelling, and bruising. **Palpate** for tenderness, tracheal deviation, and subcutaneous emphysema.
Chest	**Inspect** for penetrating objects, lacerations, avulsions, embedded foreign bodies, puncture wounds, swelling, and ecchymosis. Look at symmetry and expansion of chest wall. Observe rate of respirations, depth, and use of accessory muscles. **Palpate** for tenderness, bony deformities, and subcutaneous emphysema. **Auscultate** for breath sounds and heart sounds.
Abdomen	**Inspect** for penetrating objects, lacerations, avulsions, embedded foreign bodies, puncture wounds, swelling, and ecchymosis. Inspect for protruding abdominal contents and and distention. **Palpate** for tenderness or rigidity.
Pelvis/genitalia	**Inspect** for deformity of pelvis and blood at the urinary meatus or rectum. Check rectal sphincter tone. Observe for priapism. **Palpate** for tenderness or pain.
Extremities	**Inspect** for deformities, lacerations, missing fingers and toes, swelling, and bruising. Assess circulation to area, sensation, and ability to move. **Palpate** for tenderness, pain, and pulses.
Back	**Inspect** for deformities, lacerations, and bruising. **Palpate** for tenderness of the spine and costovertebral angle. **Auscultate** for posterior breath sounds.

should position the patient on his or her back and open the airway by performing a chin-lift or jaw-thrust maneuver, which pulls the tongue away from the posterior pharynx. To open the airway using the chin-lift maneuver, the nurse should open the mouth by grasping both the tongue and lower jaw between the thumb and fingers, lifting the mandible forward (Figure 19-5). The jaw is supported and helps tilt the head back. This method should not be used in a suspected cervical spine trauma patient because the neck hyperextends (Box 19-6). In the jaw-thrust maneuver, the nurse should place fingers at the angle of the jaw and push the mandible forward, keeping the patient's head in a neutral position (Figure 19-6).

Using a finger, the nurse should sweep deeply into the mouth to remove any foreign material such as blood, teeth, or emesis. The nurse should then attempt to ventilate the patient by using one of the above methods. If the airway is still obstructed, the nurse should straddle the patient's thighs and place the heel of one hand against the abdomen, midline above the naval and well below the xiphoid (Figure 19-7). The nurse should place the second hand directly on top of the first hand and press into the abdomen with five quick, upward thrusts. The nurse should check the patient's mouth again for foreign material by sweeping a finger deeply into the mouth, reposition the head, and attempt to ventilate. If the airway is still

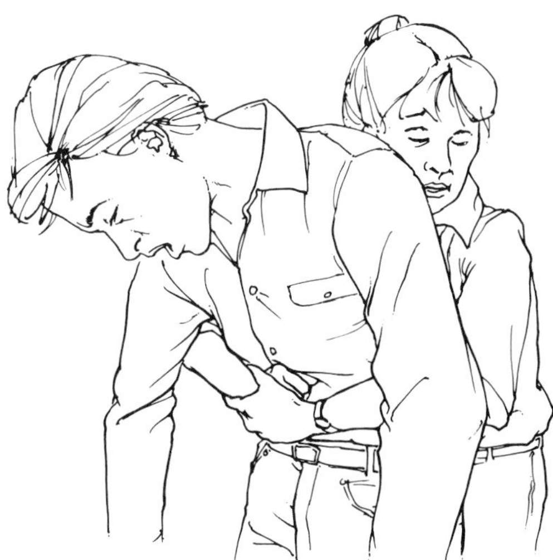

Figure 19-4 Heimlich maneuver. Conscious victim with foreign-body airway obstruction. (From *Standards and guidelines for cardiopulmonary resuscitation and emergency cardiac care, part 2,* 255:2915-2932.)

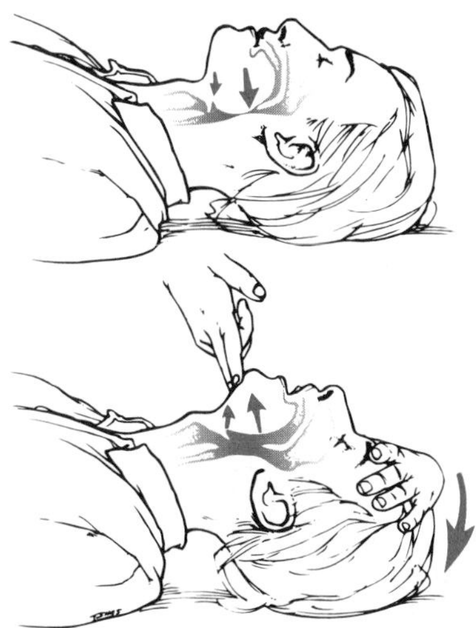

Figure 19-5 Head-tilt/chin-lift method of opening airway. (From *Standards and guidelines for cardiopulmonary resuscitation and emergency cardiac care, part 2,* 255:2915-2932).

BOX 19-6

CERVICAL SPINE PRECAUTIONS IN THE TRAUMA VICTIM

The cervical spine should not be hyperextended in a trauma patient because of the potential for a cervical spine injury (JAMA, 1992; Sheehy, 1992). Caution should be taken with all patients with trauma above the clavicles because they may have a cervical spine fracture. The cervical spine should be immobilized until x-ray films have been taken to show that there is no fracture through C7. A trauma patient should be immobilized on a backboard with a cervical collar and paracervical immobilization. If the patient cannot lay flat because of injury and a threatened impairment of breathing, it is necessary to stabilize the cervical spine as best as possible and quickly assess the patient.

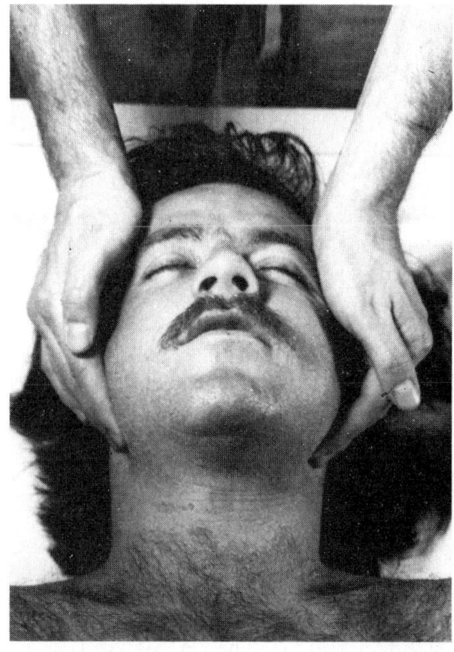

Figure 19-6 Jaw-thrust maneuver. (From Sheehy SB and others: *Manual of clinical trauma care: the first hour,* ed 2, St Louis, 1994, Mosby.)

obstructed, the nurse should straddle the patient's thighs again and repeat the process until the airway is clear. Foreign matter should be removed, and patency of the airway should be determined. If the patient is not breathing, an oral or nasal endotracheal tube should be placed, and rescue breathing should begin.

If a head injury is suspected, a nasotracheal tube should not be used because of a possible basilar skull fracture. A patient with facial fractures or a fractured larynx may have a complete airway obstruction. A laryngeal fracture should be suspected if there are bruises on the neck or if subcutaneous emphysema is observed and palpated in the neck area. Air is forced into the subcutaneous tissue when the larynx is damaged. The patient may exhibit hoarseness, coughing, or hemoptysis. Emergently, the patient would need a procedure called a **cricothyroidotomy.** This is when an incision is placed in the cricothyroid membrane of the trachea to secure an emergency airway. A tra-

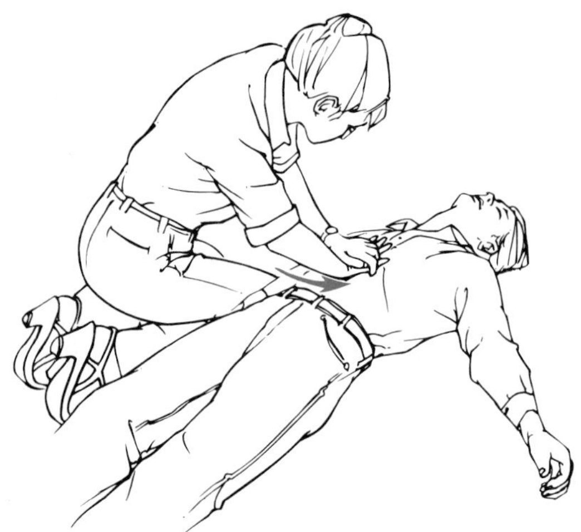

Figure 19-7 Heimlich maneuver. Unconscious victim with foreign body airway obstruction. (From *Standards and guidelines for cardiopulmonary resuscitation and emergency cardiac care, part 2,* 255:2915-2932.)

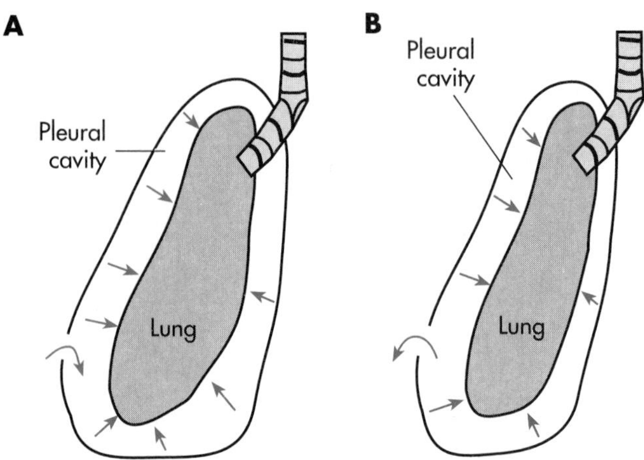

Figure 19-9 Open pneumothorax. **A,** Air enters pleural cavity during inspiration. **B,** Air exits pleural cavity during expiration. (Modified from Sheehy SB: *Emergency nursing: principles and practice,* ed 3, St Louis, 1992, Mosby.)

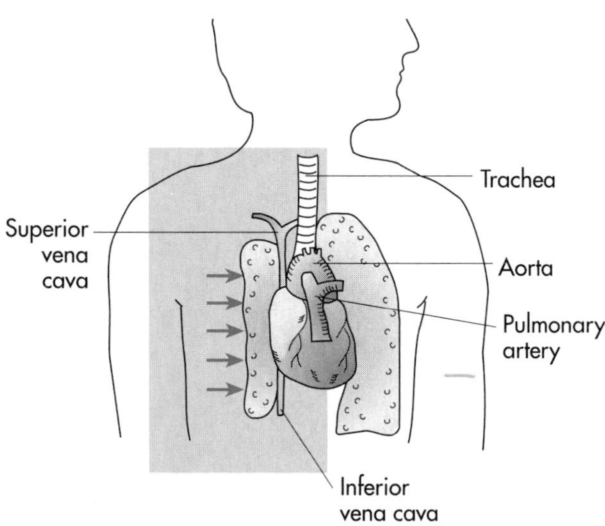

Figure 19-8 Tension pneumothorax. (From Sheehy SB: *Emergency nursing: principles and practice,* ed 3, St Louis, 1992, Mosby.)

cheostomy will need to be performed later in the operating room to better maintain the patient's airway for a long period. An emergency tracheotomy is usually not performed in the ED because of the potential for uncontrolled bleeding during the procedure.

The abdominal thrust should never be practiced on an individual who is not experiencing airway obstruction. Nurses should seek complete training in first aid and **cardiopulmonary resuscitation (CPR)** for obstruction of the airway with a foreign body through the American Red Cross or the American Heart Association. Thousands of lives could be saved each year if more people were trained in these rescue maneuvers.

Primary assessment of breathing

The assessment of breathing includes rate of respirations, quality of breaths, air movement, and use of accessory muscles or intercostal muscles. Signs and symptoms of ineffective breathing include asymmetry of chest-wall expansion, cyanosis, altered level of consciousness, distended neck veins, or tracheal shift. If noted, a life-threatening problem exists and intervention needs to be immediate. *All patients with breathing impairment need oxygen.* Determining the type of oxygen needed is the next step. For more information about oxygen therapy, see Chapter 20.

Life-threatening breathing problems.

Tension pneumothorax. One of the easiest life-threatening breathing problems in which to intervene is a tension pneumothorax (Figure 19-8). It is usually caused by blunt chest trauma but can also occur in patients with chronic obstructive lung disease or lung cancer. A tension pneumothorax is a condition in which air gets in between the parietal and visceral pleurae of the lung but cannot get out. Air gets trapped in this space, compressing the lung tissue. The lung tissue then shifts to the opposite side, compressing the heart and the great vessels. This causes a decrease in cardiac output. If not relieved immediately, the patient will die. Signs and symptoms include severe respiratory distress, tracheal shift to the unaffected side, absent breath sounds on the injured side, distended neck veins, and hyperresonance to percussion. Hyperresonance is a tympanic sound, like the sound of a kettle drum. Treatment should not wait for a chest x-ray examination. Immediate treatment is a needle thoracostomy. A 16-gauge needle is placed in the second-to-third intercostal space at the midclavicular line on the side of the chest that has no breath sounds. Pressure should be relieved, and marked improvement of the patient should be noted. Until a chest tube can be inserted by a physician, an intravenous (IV) tubing can be attached to the hub of the catheter and the tubing lowered into a bottle of saline to make a water seal. For more information, see Chapter 20.

Open pneumothorax. An open pneumothorax (Figure 19-9) or "sucking chest wound" is usually caused by a penetrating injury such as a gunshot wound or knife injury. The result is that air can enter into the pleural cavity through the chest wall. This especially occurs if the diameter of the hole is greater than two-thirds of the tracheal opening. Signs and symptoms are severe respiratory distress, gurgling, sucking chest sounds, tachypnea, and grunting. Initial treatment includes placing a Vaseline gauze over the penetrating injury opening during forceful expiration. The dressing should be taped on three sides to allow air to escape. If air collects in the pleural space after the dressing is applied, a tension pneumothorax could result. The patient will exhibit signs of increasing respiratory distress. The dressing should be loosened or removed to allow the air to escape. The patient will need a chest tube. The patient with a large, open pneumothorax will need to be intubated and ventilated with positive pressure and will need to go to the operating room to have the defect repaired (see Chapter 18).

Flail chest. The third condition that poses a life-threatening ventilation problem is a flail chest (Figure 19-10). This is usually caused by a blunt chest trauma such as a fall or a kick to the chest. It also can be the result of compressions during CPR. A flail chest occurs when three or more adjacent ribs are fractured in two or more places, or when the sternum is detached. This allows for a paradoxical (or opposite) movement of that chest segment. On inspiration, when the rest of the rib cage moves outward, the flail segment sinks inward. On expiration, when the rib cage moves inward, the flail segment bulges outward. Because pressure within the chest is decreased as a result of this paradoxical movement, movement of air is decreased. Signs and symptoms are a paradoxical chest movement of the flail segment, respiratory distress, cyanosis, and hypoxia. Treatment involves intubating the patient and placing him or her on a ventilator.

Hemothorax. A final complication of breathing is a hemothorax, which is a collection of blood in the pleural cavity. Enough blood could collect to cause symptoms of shock to develop. Signs and symptoms are difficulty breathing, cyanosis, dyspnea, use of in-

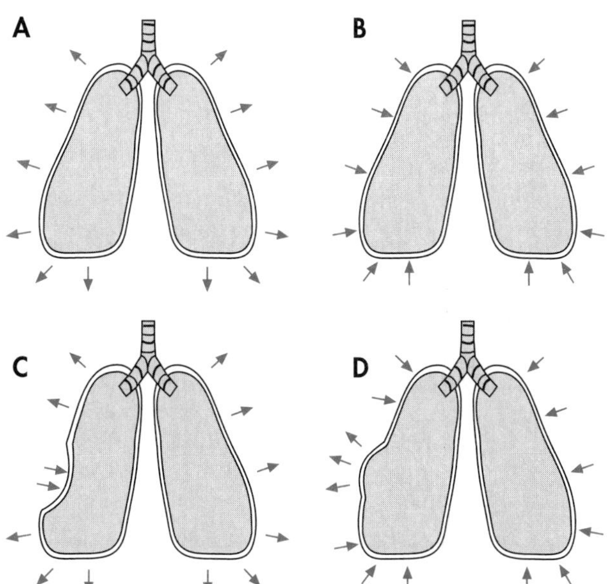

Figure 19-10 Flail chest. **A,** Normal lungs during inspiration. **B,** Normal lungs during expiration. **C,** Flail chest during inspiration. **D,** Flail chest during expiration. (Modified from Sheehy SB: *Emergency nursing: principles and practice,* ed 3, St Louis, 1992, Mosby.)

tercostal muscles, dullness with percussion to the area, and signs of shock (tachycardia; hypotension; cool, clammy skin; and decreased urine output). Treatment to improve the patient's breathing is to administer oxygen and prepare for chest-tube insertion. If the patient is bleeding profusely into the hemothorax, autotransfusion may be necessary (Box 19-7).

Primary assessment of circulation

Circulatory status and the identification of a shock state should be assessed. Hypovolemic shock is the most commonly occurring type of shock seen in trauma patients (for more information, see Chapter 8). The objective assessment includes location, quality, and rate of pulse. Where a pulse can be palpated gives an estimate of the patient's blood pressure (Table 19-4). If no carotid pulse is palpated, CPR is initiated.

Basic cardiac life support. Two organizations are primarily responsible for basic cardiac life-support standards in the United States: the American Heart Association and the American Red Cross. These standards are taught to healthcare providers and the general public by certified instructors across the nation. Once lost, cardiac function must be restored as quickly as possible to avoid cerebral damage. All nurses should be prepared in CPR.

The American Red Cross offers courses in basic first aid. CPR is taught in most hospitals or community

BOX 19-7

TREATMENT FOR HEMOTHORAX

CHEST TUBE INSERTION SITES

The chest tube is placed on the affected side, fifth intercostal space, midaxillary line, if fluid is to be relieved. If the tube is to relieve air from the pleural cavity, it is placed in the second intercostal space, midclavicular line (see Chapter 20).

AUTOTRANSFUSION

The purpose of autotransfusion is to reinfuse the patient's own blood into the intravascular space. It is performed only from clean areas such as chest trauma from a hemothorax or perioperatively during hip surgery. It is never done from a contaminated area such as the abdomen.

TABLE 19-4

Pulse and Blood Pressure

Pulse site	Estimated Blood Pressure
Carotid only	60 mm Hg
Femoral	70 mm Hg
Radial	80 mm Hg

If a radial pulse is present, the systolic blood pressure is at least 80 mm Hg. If a radial pulse is absent but a femoral pulse is present, the estimated systolic blood pressure is 70 mm Hg.

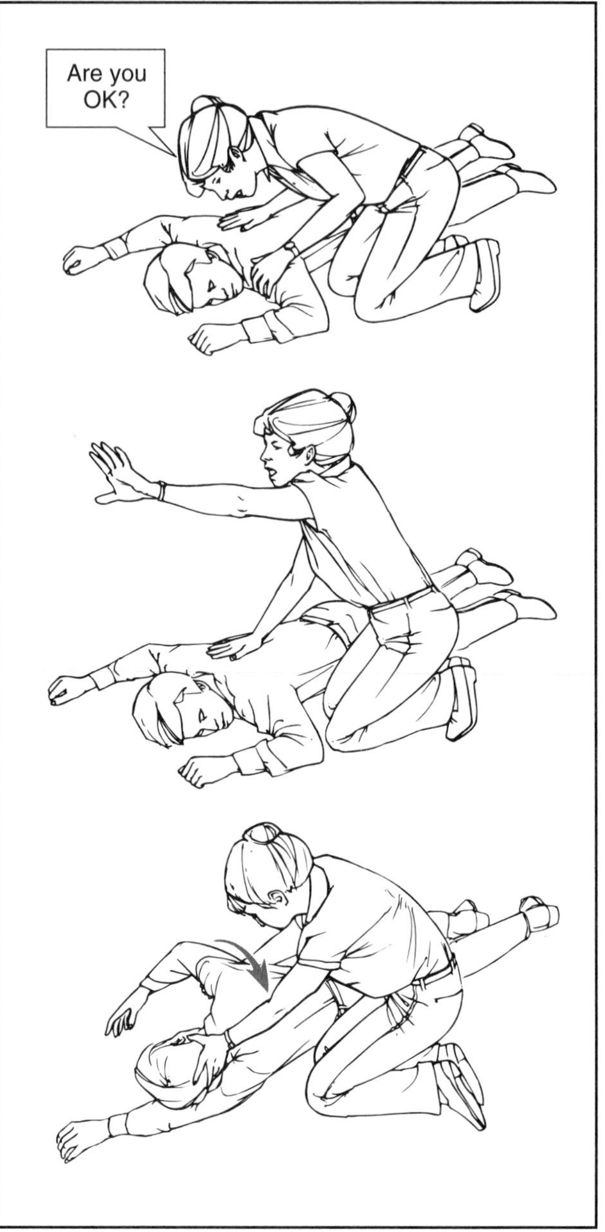

Figure 19-11 Initial steps in cardiopulmonary resuscitation. *Top,* Determining unresponsiveness. *Center,* calling for help. *Bottom,* correct positioning. (From *Standards and guidelines for cardiopulmonary resuscitation and emergency cardiac care, part 2,* 255:2915-2932.)

colleges. Care should be started immediately to prevent complications. The nurse's safety should never be jeopardized when administering care.

Before starting basic life support, it must first be determined that the patient is unresponsive. This is accomplished by gently tapping the patient's shoulder and asking, "Are you OK?" If the patient does not respond, help should be called. This may mean briefly leaving the patient to get additional help. 9-1-1 is the telephone number used in many areas to activate the EMS. Calling for help will allow for access to advanced cardiac life support treatments such as defibrillation, oxygenation, and medications. Next the patient should be assessed for the presence or absence of respirations by turning the patient on his or her back (Figure 19-11; Box 19-8).

The airway is opened using the chin lift or jaw thrust (see Figure 19-5 and Figure 19-6). Without muscle tone, the tongue and epiglottis will obstruct the pharynx and larynx.

Breathlessness should be determined by placing an ear over the patient's mouth and nose while maintaining an open airway. The patient's chest should be observed to see if it rises and falls. In addition, air rushing during exhalation should be listened for, and airflow should be felt (Figure 19-12).

Rescue breathing should begin by sealing the mouth and nose. Two slow breaths of $1\frac{1}{2}$-2 seconds each should be delivered. An observation of the chest should be made to see if it rises and falls, and then movement of air should be listened and felt for. If the patient is unable to ventilate, the head should be repositioned and rescue breathing repeated. If the patient

BOX 19-8

ROLE OF FIRST RESPONDER

Many times the nurse will be the first responder to an emergency scene or the first person in a patient's room when an emergency is occurring. The first response has three steps:

1 Check
The nurse must **check** the patient and recognize an emergency exists.
2 Call
Decide to act. Then **call** for help.
3 Care
(Newell and others, 1993)

cannot be ventilated after repositioning the head, the procedure for airway obstruction previously mentioned should begin.

Circulation should be assessed. The carotid artery should be palpatated for 5 to 10 seconds because it is the strongest palpable pulse. If the pulse is present, rescue breathing should continue at 10 to 12 breaths per minute or 1 breath every 5 to 6 seconds. If the pulse is absent, external compressions should begin. It is important to take time to adequately check for a pulse because external compressions are dangerous to a beating heart.

External compressions should be performed in the following manner: While kneeling by the patient's shoulders, the palm of a hand should be placed on the sternum, with two fingers above the xiphoid process (Figure 19-13). A second hand should be placed on top of the first. The sternum should be compressed $1\frac{1}{2}$ to 2 inches for adults. Compressions should be equal. Hands should remain on the sternum during upstroke, when the chest should relax completely. The compression rate should be 15 to 18 in 15 seconds to maintain a rate of 80 to 100 beats per minute for an adult. Two breaths should then be administered. Four cycles of 15 to 18 compressions and two ventilations should be completed before rechecking the carotid pulse. If the pulse returns, cardiac compressions should be stopped. Once spontaneous respirations begin, the patient will need assessment of the respiratory system. CPR should be performed until the patient regains his or her own pulse or all resuscitative measures have been exhausted (JAMA, 1992).

Any death of a patient in the ED or less than 24 hours after admission needs to be reported to the medical examiner. The medical examiner will decide if an autopsy needs to be performed. The Uniform Anatomical Gift Act recognizes the right of a person to donate organs and tissues. The next of kin can make the decision for the deceased if intent is unknown. It is up to the healthcare professional to address donation with the family.

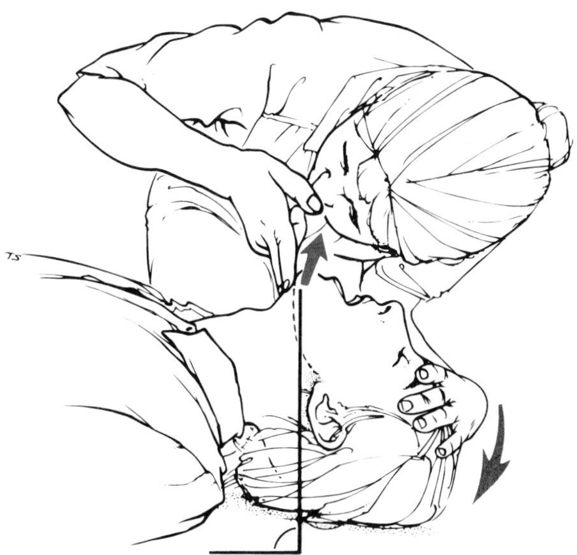

Figure 19-12 Determination of breathlessness. (From *Standards and guidelines for cardiopulmonary resuscitation and emergency cardiac care, part 2,* 255:2915-2932.)

The consent for donation or refusal must be documented in the medical record. This is the law (Emergency Nurses Association, 1992).

All patients with impaired circulatory function should be placed on cardiac monitoring, administered oxygen, and have an intravenous catheter with a solution of 0.9% normal saline or Ringer's Lactate established. Further cardiac assessment should include capillary refill. However, this may not be an adequate assessment tool if the patient has Raynaud's disease or circulatory problems. Skin color and temperature should be noted, as should any signs of bleeding. The level of consciousness should also be assessed.

Signs and symptoms of hypovolemic shock are decreased level of consciousness; uncontrolled bleeding; tachycardia; hypotension; prolonged capillary refill; and cool, pale skin. The patient in hypovolemic shock has flat neck veins. The patient with a condition that mimics shock, such as cardiac tamponade, would have distended neck veins and distant (more muffled or quieter) heart sounds.

Life-threatening circulatory problems.

Uncontrolled external or internal bleeding. Uncontrolled external or internal bleeding is a life-threatening condition. External bleeding could be an arterial laceration or venous laceration that has not had pressure applied to stop the bleeding. Ways to control external bleeding are direct pressure, elevation, or use of pressure points. When using pressure points, the nurse should first identify the artery that supplies the area of uncontrolled bleeding. The nurse should compress the artery against the bone that lays behind it to occlude

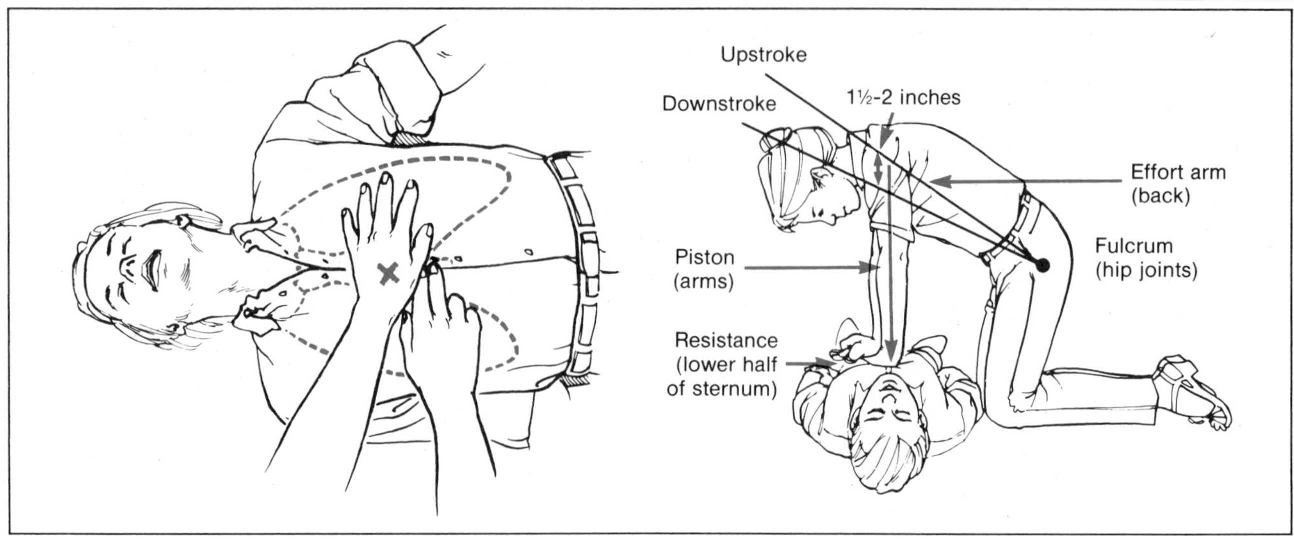

Figure 19-13 External chest compression. (From *Standards and guidelines for cardiopulmonary resuscitation and emergency cardiac care, part 2,* 255:2915-2932.)

the flow of blood to the bleeding area (Figure 19-14). The nurse must remember that a tourniquet is a last resort and may result in loss of distal limb. Internal bleeding could be from a lacerated spleen or liver or another internal injury such as an acute gastrointestinal bleed. The patient would need a blood sample sent for a type and cross match, and surgery may be required to control the bleeding.

NURSE ALERT

Only red blood cells have hemoglobin, which is necessary to carry oxygen throughout the body.

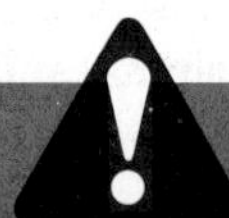

NURSE ALERT

All blood products must be administered in an intravenous solution of 0.9% normal saline.

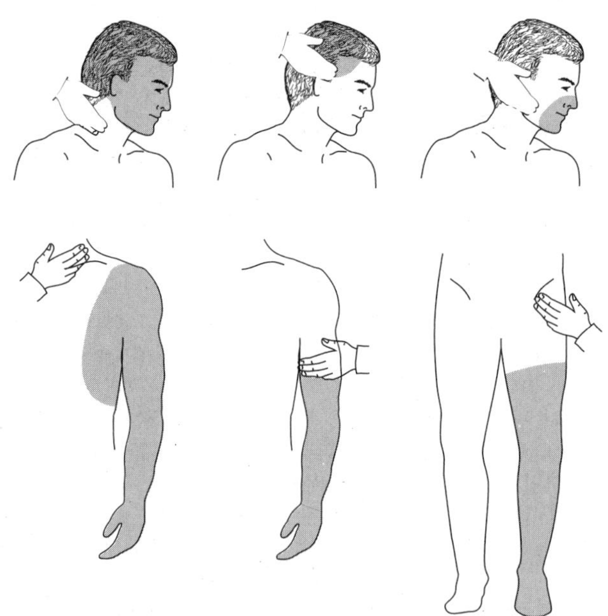

Figure 19-14 Common pressure point locations to control bleeding. Firm pressure should be applied to the area compressing the artery against the underlying bone. Elevation of the extremity will also help decrease the blood flow to the area to help stop the bleeding

MAST pants. Military AntiShock Trousers or a Pneumatic AntiShock Garment (MAST or PASG) may be applied if the patient exhibits signs of shock in the prehospital setting. These garments apply pressure to the lower extremities and abdomen to help increase the blood return to the vital organs and decrease the blood in the lower extremities. They are used to keep the systolic blood pressure greater than 80 mm Hg. They are contraindicated in patients with severe head injury, congestive heart failure, or an intrathoracic bleed. When the garment is inflated, the pulses in the lower extremities must be checked. The garment should never obscure the pulse. Once the blood volume has been restored with fluids and blood products, the garment can be removed by deflating the area over the abdomen first and then one leg at a time. If the blood pressure drops more than 5 mm Hg, the deflation is stopped until the blood pressure returns to the previous reading. Many times these garments are removed in the operating room. The operating room staff should be advised not to remove the garment with scissors.

Cardiac tamponade. This condition involves the accumulation of blood or fluid in the pericardial sac from blunt chest trauma or from a disease process such as an infection or cancer. Approximately 60 to 100 ml of fluid accumulating in the pericardial sac can impede the heart's ability to pump. Signs and symptoms of cardiac tamponade are distended neck veins, distant heart sounds, and hypotension. Treatment for a pericardial tamponade is a pericardiocentesis. The purpose of this procedure is to remove fluid from the pericardial sac. A needle is placed to the left of the xiphoid process toward the ipsilateral (same side) shoulder. When the needle enters the pericardial sac, fluid is removed. Touching the heart muscle could send the patient into ventricular fibrillation or produce a myocardial laceration.

Aortic or great vessel injury. If there is trauma to a great vessel such as the aorta or superior/inferior vena cava, the patient is usually dead at the scene of the accident. If the patient makes it to the hospital alive, he or she usually dies within the first 24 hours. A patient may also come to the hospital with excruciating pain from a dissecting aortic or abdominal aneurysm. This is a condition that occurs when there is increased stress on the aorta, causing damage to the middle layer of the blood vessel. This condition is seen in patients with uncontrolled hypertension, arteriosclerosis, and infection. Signs and symptoms include hypovolemic shock, marked variation of blood pressure between the right and left arms, chest wall ecchymosis (if seen in a trauma patient), decreased pedal pulses, widened mediastinum (this is seen on a chest x-ray film and is interpreted by the physician or radiologist), or a bulging pulsatile abdominal mass. The patient needs to go to the operating room to have these extensive injuries repaired.

Lacerated liver. Traumatic lacerations to the liver are common because of the size of the liver and its location. A ruptured diaphragm may accompany this injury. Fractured ribs on the right side could lacerate the liver. Signs and symptoms of a lacerated liver are hypovolemic shock (caused by hemorrhage), abdominal guarding, right upper-abdominal pain, and positive peritoneal lavage. A positive peritoneal lavage indicates intraabdominal trauma when peritoneal fluid contains a RBC count of greater than 100,000/μl. Many hospitals now do a CT scan of the abdomen instead of a peritoneal lavage to see if any other abdominal injuries exist. Treatment involves surgery to explore the injury and control the bleeding.

Ruptured spleen. The patient with a ruptured spleen initially exhibits blunt abdominal trauma to the left side of the abdomen and may have fractured lower ribs. Signs and symptoms are hypovolemic shock; Kerr's sign, which is pain under the left scapula; guarding of the abdomen; and absent bowel sounds. The shock symptoms are treated as the patient is prepared for surgery.

Life-threatening airway, breathing, and circulation problem.

Anaphylaxis. Anaphylactic shock is a life-threatening medical emergency. Anaphylactic shock is a systemic response to a type I hypersensitivity reaction. It is potentially fatal and can appear in minutes in people who have been previously sensitized to the allergen.

Immunoglobulin (IgE) antibody formation produces the anaphylactic response after a series of exposures. These trigger agents are caused by injection of vaccines, insect venoms, inhalation and absorption from use of latex, and ingestion of food products such as nuts, eggs, or antibiotics. Nonmediated IgE formation means the person can have an anaphylactic reaction without ever being presensitized to the trigger agent. These non-IgE reactions can occur from nonsteroidal antiinflammatory drugs, Amphotericin B and other antibiotics, exercise, or can have no particular cause.

Pathophysiology. Anaphylactic shock results from an abnormal antigen-antibody response. The IgE antibody produced causes the release of histamine from mast cells and basophils. The release of histamine results in arterial and venous dilation and increased capillary permeability. Vasodilation and decreased cardiac output cause a decrease in systolic and diastolic blood pressure. Plasma leaks through the vascular bed into the interstitial space, leading to circulatory collapse. Histamine contracts the smooth muscle of the bronchi, causing bronchospasm, asthma, and panting. The bronchioles constrict and contribute to hypoxemia.

Assessment. Initial symptoms of anaphylaxis are edema, itching of the eyes and ears and/or at the site of injection, sneezing, and apprehension. In seconds or minutes, edema of the face, hands, and other parts of the body occur. Respiratory distress from bronchospasm, sneezing and coughing, wheezing, dyspnea, and cyanosis follows. Edema of the larynx and laryngospasm may lead to death. Gastrointestinal symptoms such as nausea and vomiting, abdominal pain, and diarrhea may be present. Cardiovascular signs such as arrhythmia, tachycardia, or bradycardia may be followed by circulatory collapse, which is indicated by a falling blood pressure, pallor, and loss of consciousness. In extreme cases death may occur in 5 to 10 minutes after onset of the reaction (Box 19-9) (Hollingsworth, 1992).

Patient teaching should include instructions on how to obtain a medical alert bracelet, a warning to avoid the known antigen, a demonstration of procedures to treat an anaphylactic response (use of an epi pen to self-administer epinephrine), and an explanation of other desensitizing measures (allergy shots).

After airway, breathing, and circulation are assessed, an assessment for disability or a brief neurologic examination is performed.

Neurologic examination Glasgow Coma Scale. The Glasgow Coma Scale is a reliable tool used to assess levels of consciousness. The coma scale includes a rank or rating assigned to the patient's best effort at eye opening, verbal response, and motor response. Each is rated, and the total equals from 3 to 15 points. The higher the point value, the better the neurologic examination (Table 19-5). Also included in the brief neurologic examination is an assessment of pupil size and response.

Exposure

The final step in the primary assessment is to make sure the patient is fully exposed. A cover should be placed to prevent hypothermia. Interventions after the primary examination include inserting an oral/nasogastric tube to decrease abdominal distention, which can impair breathing. An indwelling urinary catheter is inserted to obtain an accurate recording of urine output, which is a valuable indicator of kidney perfusion and hydration. Blood should be drawn for a type and crossmatch, hemoglobin/hematocrit, electrolytes, bleeding studies, and a toxicology screen. Other laboratory examinations ordered would be determined by the nature of the injury. The first hemoglobin and hematocrit are drawn as baseline data because they take hours to show a drop as a result of blood loss. If the mechanism of injury indicates a potential cervical spine injury, cervical spine x-ray films should be obtained before proceeding with further care. **Blood alcohol concentration (BAC)** is routinely obtained if the patient's condition warrants the test. An altered level of consciousness, seizure activity, trauma, or patients

BOX 19-9 **Nursing Process**

EMERGENCY CARE OF INDIVIDUALS IN ANAPHYLACTIC SHOCK

ASSESSMENT

Rapid, shallow breathing
Bronchospasms
Dyspnea
Cyanosis
Restlessness
"Sense of doom"
Irritability
Laryngeal edema
Hypotension
Rapid, thready pulse
Edema and itching at site of injection or insect bite

NURSING DIAGNOSIS

Risk for injury related to anaphylactic shock

NURSING INTERVENTIONS

Prepare for oropharyngeal intubation or surgical insertion of tracheotomy; oxygen therapy per order.

Prepare for administration of antihistamines such as Benadryl 50 mg IV over 3 minutes or Aminophylline IV drip. Administer corticosteriods to decrease inflammation, as ordered.

Have patient in supine position to increase blood flow to the brain. Administer 0.2-0.5 ml 1 : 1000 epinephrine solution SC or IM into upper arm and massage site to hasten absorption. Prepare an epinephrine drip for continuous infusion or prepare to administer vasopressor drugs such as levarterenol bitarate and high-dose dopamine. Monitor pulse and blood pressure every 3-5 minutes until stable.

Remove the bee stinger or stop the infusion causing the reaction.

Place a tourniquet above the site of the antigen. Remove tourniquet every 10 to 15 minutes or until reaction is under control. Apply ice.

EVALUATION OF EXPECTED OUTCOMES

Maintains patent airway.
Demonstrates effective breathing pattern.
Maintains hemodynamic stability as evidenced by blood pressure and pulse in normal range.
Reduces systemic absorption of the antigen.

PATIENT/FAMILY TEACHING

Allergic Reaction

Explain that an allergic reaction is caused by an increased sensitivity to a medication, sting, or food product.

Tell the patient, "You experienced an allergic reaction today," and explain the following:

- Take the medication (Benadryl/Atarax) as prescribed. It will cause sleepiness, so do not drive while on the medication. Take it for at least 3 days. If Tagamet has been ordered, do not drink alcohol with the medication. Tagamet will not cause drowsiness.
- Avoid scratching.
- Avoid hot baths/showers. Tepid or cool compresses may help with itching.
- Return to the ED if experiencing difficulty breathing, lightheadness, or difficulty swallowing.
- See physician if signs of infection or no resolution of rash occurs.
- Apply for a Medic Alert tag to indicate allergies.
- Avoid the substances that caused the allergic reaction.

who have taken an overdose, are a few examples of when a BAC would be obtained.

BAC is a test that measures the concentration of alcohol in a person's blood. It is expressed in a blood alcohol concentration percentage. An alcohol blood level of 0.10 is considered legal intoxication. Some mental impairment and physical impairment is noticed at this level (Newell and others, 1993). A patient may be brought to the ED under police custody to obtain a BAC. The patient has the right to refuse the test. If the patient is violent or injury to the patient could occur from the drawing of the sample, someone other than a healthcare provider should obtain the sample.

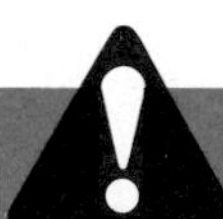

NURSE ALERT

A patient using alcohol or drugs may not respond properly, which suggests a head injury or an altered response to shock.

TABLE 19-5

Glasgow Coma Scale

Finding	Score
Eye opening	
Spontaneous	4
To voice	3
To pain	2
None	1
Best verbal response	
Oriented	5
Confused	4
Inappropriate words	3
Incomprehensible sounds	2
None	1
Best motor response	
Obeys commands	6
Purposeful movement	5
Withdraw	4
Flexion	3
Extension	2
None	1

Scoring is from 3 to 15. The higher the score the better the neurologic findings. Motor movement is assessed with painful stimuli (pressing on nailbed or sternal rub) (Klein and others, 1994; Sheehy, 1992).

Secondary Assessment

A secondary assessment is a brief survey to assess and set priorities on all injuries and problems. A full set of vital signs—blood pressure, pulse, respirations, and temperature—is obtained. A complete head-to-toe assessment is performed with a repeat neurologic examination. This assessment is done on an emergency patient to determine what is causing the patient's complaint. Obtaining a thorough history is important to identify and treat the problem. Subjective data (what is said) is as important as objective data (what can be seen and measured). Nurses should look to see if the patient has a Medic Alert tag. If a life-threatening problem occurs during any of the assessments, it must be treated before resuming definitive care. Additional laboratory tests and x-ray examinations are ordered. If the patient is stable, a complete history is obtained.

Focused Assessment/Intervention

Finally a focused assessment is performed. During the focused assessment, interventions may be performed for the specific identified injuries or problem. This is when definitive treatment is completed, which may include interventions such as administering pain medication to make the patient more comfortable or applying a cast to a fracture.

Immunization

Diphtheria tetanus toxoid (dT) 0.5 ml is administered intramuscularly to all patients who had their last immunization more than 10 years ago and have a break in the skin. This includes fractures, abrasions, animal bites, and burns. For individuals who have never received a dT immunization, they also receive 250 units of tetanus immunoglobulin (TIG) along with the start of a dT series and repeat injections of dT 1 month and 6 months after receiving the first immunization.

Removal of foreign bodies from the eye

Many patients come to the ED with complaints of pain in or drainage from the eye. They also may complain of acute vision loss. The emergency caregiver needs to determine the cause of the patient's problem (see Chapter 29). A foreign body in the eye causes pain, often as a result of a corneal abrasion. A corneal abrasion is a scratch to the outer surface of the eye. The objective in removing a foreign body from the eye is to prevent injury to the cornea and conjunctiva (Figure 19-15). If the foreign body is under the lower lid, the lid should be pulled down and the foreign body removed with a cotton swab. If a foreign body is suspected under the upper lid, there are four steps to evert the eyelid to examine the eye. First the patient should close his or her eyelid. Next a cotton swab should be placed at the medial corner of the upper eyelid (eyelashes should be pulled down and back over the swab). Then the eyelid should be everted over the swab. Finally the inside of the eyelid and the eye should be examined to see if any injury is present. Treatment for a corneal abrasion includes applying prescribed antibiotic eye drops to prevent infection and patching the eyelid closed. Patching the eyelid closed allows for decreased movement of the eyelid over the abraded area. This decreased irritation allows the eye to heal. Pain medications are prescribed, and the patient is instructed to rest while the eye is patched. The patient should not drive with the eye patched or open the eye underneath the patch.

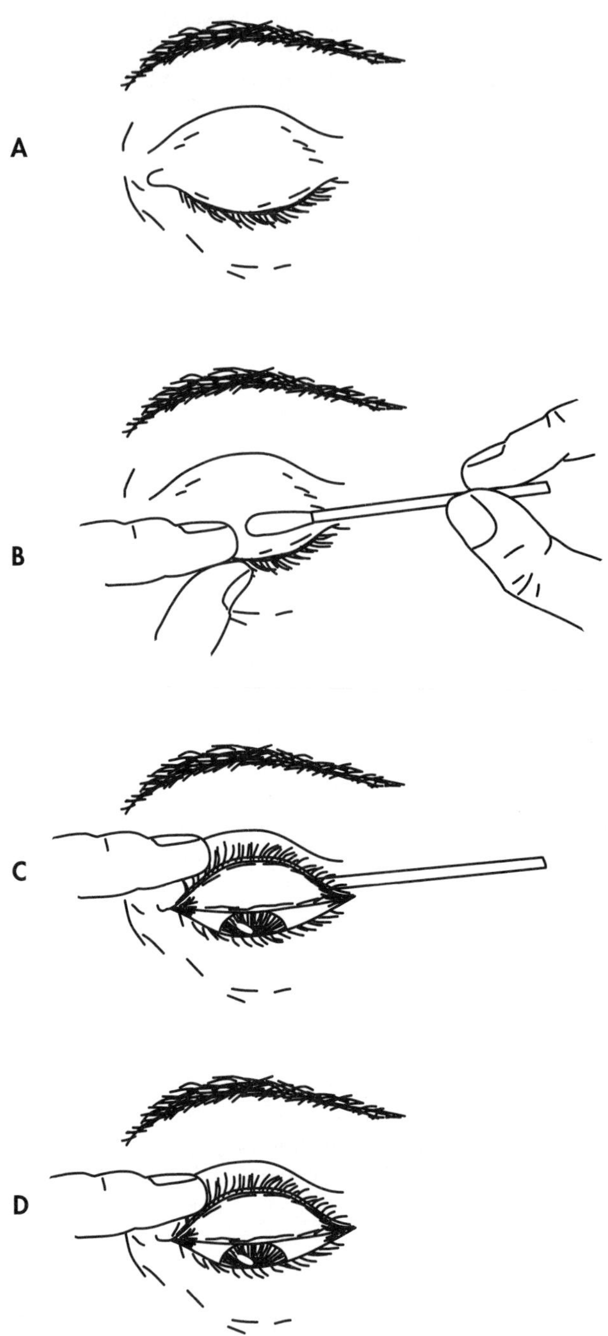

Figure 19-15 Steps in everting eyelid. **A,** Eyelid. **B,** Placement of cotton swab (eyelashes are pulled down and back over swab). **C,** Eyelid everted over swab. **D,** Examination of inside of eyelid and eye. (From Sheehy SB: *Emergency nursing: principles and practice,* ed 3, St Louis, 1992, Mosby.)

Wound care

The objectives for the care of a patient with surface trauma are to stop the bleeding, prevent infection, and preserve function. The dT immunization should be administered if needed.

Abrasions/Lacerations. The first step in treating abrasions and lacerations is to stop the bleeding. This is done either by direct pressure, elevation, or pressure points. The area should be cleaned with soap and water, removing any foreign bodies such as glass or gravel. Definitive treatment for lacerations is to suture

PATIENT/FAMILY TEACHING

Wound Care

Keep area clean and dry.
Apply antibiotic ointment; cover with bandage.
Elevate extremity.
Make an appointment for suture removal.
Suture removal for the face is 5 days, other areas 7 to 10 days, and over joints 10 to 14 days.
Watch for signs of infection and notify doctor if any of the following occur:

- Redness or red streaks
- Purulent drainage
- Increased swelling
- Fever
- Increased warmth to area

if it is a full thickness wound, or Steri-strip if the wound is partial thickness. An antibiotic ointment such as Bacitracin should be applied, and the wound should be covered with a sterile dressing.

Puncture wounds. Puncture wounds should be soaked in a Betadine solution for 20 minutes, and the physician determines if a prophylactic antibiotic is needed. An x-ray examination may be ordered depending on the object that caused the injury.

NURSE ALERT

Never remove an impaled object. Secure the object. Removal should be done in the operating room.

Amputation. The ideal treatment for an amputation is to save the amputated part. The amputated part should be placed in a moist but not wet, clean dressing, in a sterile container, and on ice. The amputated tissue should not be frozen. Saline dressing should be placed on the cleansed portion of the remaining body part. Reimplantation may be accomplished, so both parts must be brought for treatment. Both the extremity and the amputated part need x-ray examination. The patient should be prepared for transport to the operating room or a reimplantation center, if appropriate.

Bites. In the case of a bite the nurse needs to try to determine the type of bite, assess the area of the bite, and determine if the bite affects underlying tissue. A hand bite usually affects the tendon sheath of the hand. The age of the injury should be determined, and the nurse should look for signs of infection. Treatment requires a 10-minute scrub with soap and water. The decision to close the bite is determined by the location and the age of the bite. If the bite is caused by a raccoon or skunk, rabies protocol should be initiated. The area should be loosely dressed. Antibiotics may be started, if appropriate. Animal bites are commonly reported to law-enforcement agencies.

Contusions (bruises). A contusion is a tissue injury that does not break the skin. The injury leads to swelling and discoloration as a result of the release of blood and fluids from damaged cells and capillaries.

The nurse should assess a contusion in the same manner as an abrasion and check for underlying fractures. Treatment includes applying ice and elevating the area. If the area is muscular and if increasing leakage of fluids in the muscle could occur, a compression wrap may be applied with an Ace bandage. Discoloration from a contusion can take 2 to 3 weeks to clear.

Crush injuries. With crush injuries, the nurse should assess patients for neurocompromise, including loss of function, sensation, capillary refill, and pulse. The nurse should also check for compartment syndrome (see Chapter 32). Treatment for crush injuries is ice, elevation, and immobilization.

Fractures and dislocations

Initial treatment for a patient with a fracture includes removing jewelry from the extremity and checking the pulse before and after immobilization (splinting) of the fracture. Immobilization can be done with an armboard or many types of splints. Pelvic fractures may be immobilized with the MAST suit. The nurse should always apply the splint above and below the joint to give the maximum immobilization. It is important to check the neurovascular integrity of the extremity. This includes the five P's: pain, pallor (capillary refill, skin temperature, color), pulses, paresthesia, and paralysis. If a bone has protruded through the skin, a saline or Betadine dressing should be applied to the area. The nurse should never try to relocate the fracture. If no pulse is felt, the physician should be notified immediately. Ice should be applied to the injured area, and the extremity should be elevated higher than the heart. For more information on fractures and dislocations, see Chapter 32.

Administering pain medication to these patients is important. It is sometimes easier to obtain an order for an intravenous solution of 0.9% normal saline to be started so that pain medications can be given intravenously for an acute fracture. The IV also may be used to administer medications if re-

BOX 19-10 Guidelines for Conscious Sedation

The purpose of conscious sedation is to depress the level of consciousness but allow the patient to maintain independent airway management and be able to respond with physical and verbal stimulation.

Equipment needed for conscious sedation includes oxygen, suction, ambu bag/mask, oral/nasal airways and endotracheal tubes, pulse oximeter, sphygmomanometer or noninvasive blood pressure cuff, and cardiac monitoring.

A registered nurse needs to be with the patient during the entire procedure and may not leave to do other tasks. The nurse must be CPR-recognized, have knowledge of the drugs to be given, and be able to monitor arrhythmias and airway. Emergency equipment and personnel should be easily accessible. The steps the nurse should take are as follows:

- Establish an IV.
- Prepare the patient with all the monitoring equipment.
- Receive an order for sedation medication and have the physician in the room while the medication is administered. Commonly used medications for sedation are midazolam or diazepam along with a pain medication such as meperidine, hydromorphone, fentanyl, or morphine sulfate.
- Monitor for signs of hypoventilation (the pulse oximetry reading will drop) continuously and blood pressure and pulse every 15 minutes.
- Observe for arrhythmia on the cardiac monitor.
- Assess arousability and level of consciousness.
- Assess skin condition.
- Document medications given and patient's response (*Penn Nurse,* 1992).

duction of a fracture is necessary or antibiotics need to be given.

Conscious sedation is now being performed in the ED to aid in reducing dislocations and repositioning of closed fractures before casting (Box 19-10). Conscious sedation requires prudent monitoring of the patient.

Rib fractures. A rib fracture is a common injury and usually affects one rib. The nurse should encourage the patient to take deep breaths to prevent pneumonia. Analgesics are prescribed for pain. A rib fracture can be a life-threatening problem if the fracture involves the lower ribs, which could lacerate the liver or spleen, or if a flail segment is present.

PATIENT/FAMILY TEACHING

Cast Care

The purpose of a cast is to immobilize the injured bone to allow it to heal.

It takes 48 hours for a plaster cast to dry. Do not use a blow dryer to aid in this process. Be careful when touching the cast during this time because pressure areas could form under the cast.

Do not get the cast wet.

Do not sit in the sun for long periods, because perspiration will soften the cast.

Do not remove any of the casting material or place any object into the cast.

Keep the cast clean. It is porous and needs to breathe.

Elevate the extremity as instructed.

Exercise fingers or toes every hour.

Call the physician immediately if experiencing any of the following: increased pain, tightness or swelling, numbness in fingertips or toes, or discolored or blue of tips of fingers or toes.

If cast gets broken or has foul odor, notify physician.

Burns

In the case of a burn, the nurse should treat the trauma first—assessing airway, breathing, and circulation—then treat the burn.

The immediate action and intervention of a burn patient is to stop the burning process. This is done prior to the patient coming to the ED. The area should be cooled with water. Then the extent of the burn, the location, and other possible complications such as smoke inhalation with respiratory involvement should be determined. Debridement of any blistered area that would impede function may be done with a physician's order. The nurse should then cover the burn with a sterile dressing and apply an antibiotic ointment such as bacitracin or Silvadene (see Chapter 31).

Head injuries

Head injuries affect a significant number of people each year. They are caused by motor vehicle accidents, sports injuries, assaults, and falls. Patients arriving at the ED with symptoms or a complaint of head injury with a loss of consciousness receive a CT scan of the head to look for any signs of cerebral bleeding (see Chapter 28).

It is important for the nurse to instruct the patient and family of symptoms that indicate the need to return to the ED after a head injury.

In the ED, if a change in the neurologic examination indicates increased intracranial pressure (ICP), the physician may decide to place burr holes into the patient's skull to help relieve the pressure until neurosurgery can be performed. Therefore a patient with an altered level of consciousness should be taken, if possible, to a Level I trauma center, where emergency neurosurgery is quickly available. For more information about ICP, see Chapter 28.

Cerebral hematomas. There are three types of cerebral hematomas: epidural, subdural, and intracerebral (Figure 19-16). Bleeding causes a hematoma to form. The location of the hematoma determines the symptoms a patient will exhibit.

Epidural hematoma. An epidural hematoma involves rapid bleeding between the skull and the dura due to laceration of the meningeal artery and vein. The patient has a history of head trauma with a loss of consciousness, followed by a lucid period and a rapid decrease in level of consciousness. The pupils become fixed and dilated on the side of the injury (ipsilateral), and paralysis occurs on the opposite side of the injury (contralateral).

Subdural hematoma. A subdural hematoma involves bleeding under the dura. This bleeding can accumulate quickly (acute) within 48 hours or slowly (chronic) within weeks. Patients more prone to chronic subdural hematomas are alcoholics, the elderly, or those on anticoagulants. Symptoms are headache, drowsiness, and confusion. As the symptoms become more severe, ipsilateral pupil dilation and contralateral paralysis occur. Symptoms for a chronic subdural hematoma are the same, but symptoms evolve slowly.

Treatment for both the subdural and epidural hematomas is to decrease intracranial pressure and surgically remove the hematoma.

Intracerebral hematoma. An intracerebral hematoma is the result of a large contusion to any area of the brain, with small vessel damage. These have high mortality rates because evacuating the hematoma is not as easy as with the two other hematomas. A rapid deterioration occurs (Aumick, 1991; Salluzzo and others, 1992).

PATIENT/FAMILY TEACHING

When to Return to the ED After a Head Injury

A return to the ED is necessary if symptoms of increased intracranial pressure arise, including the following:

- Change in level of consciousness, such as confusion, loss of memory, or unusual behavior
- Increased drowsiness or inability to be aroused
- Persistent headache or stiff neck
- Change in pupil size or in equality of pupils
- Projectile or uncontrolled vomiting

VIOLENCE

Recent studies have shown that the fear of violence has replaced economic issues as a national concern. The CDC has termed violence an epidemic health problem. In 1990 injuries from firearms exceeded injuries from motor vehicle accidents in six states. There has been an increasing number of hospital assaults. The assaults usually occurred in the ED, and the nurse was the person most at risk. The growing number of handguns has led to increased accidental shootings. In the past, a playground disagreement would usually end with a black eye. Now it is not uncommon for it to end with a child being shot. Violence is not only in the streets but in homes as well and includes child and elder maltreatment, spousal abuse, and sexual assault.

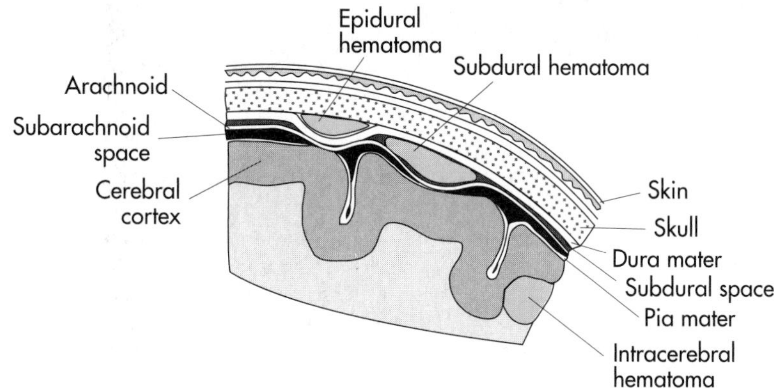

Figure 19-16 Location of cerebral hematomas.

Causes of increased violence are poverty, racism, denial of educational opportunities, low self-esteem, disregard for human life, disintegration of the family, and a lack of positive role models.

No family is immune to the effects that violence has on our society. Prevention is the key to solving this problem, and emergency nurses and physicians are trying to intervene. After they continued to see the devastating effects on children, hospitals such as Children's Memorial Hospital in Chicago have developed programs called HELP to educate families about handgun violence. There is also a national organization called STOP. This organization is working to prevent firearm injuries by educating parents and the community about the risks of keeping handguns in the home (Campbell, 1994).

Emergency Department Violence

The ED is predisposed to violence as a result of its 24-hour accessibility, long waiting times, overcrowding, availability of drugs and hostages, staff shortages, and its utilization by psychiatric patients and patients with drug and alcohol problems. The ENA has a position statement regarding violence in the emergency setting.

It is important for the emergency nurse to stop violence before it starts. First, potentially violent patients must be identified (Box 19-11). It is imperative that the nurse be aware of signs of increasing aggression so that interventions can occur before the patient or staff gets injured. Signs of increasing verbal aggression are loud talking, rapid speech, increasing verbal threats, or angry tone of voice. Signs of physical agitation or aggression are an inability to stay seated, grinding or clenched teeth, tense posture, or pacing.

Before approaching an angry patient, the nurse needs to ensure that safety measures are taken. Pens in pockets, earrings, and stethoscopes should be removed. The person should be taken to a quiet environment that is safe. Help to control the patient should be readily available. The nurse should not get trapped between the patient and a wall. An exit should always be available.

Communication should be tried first to deescalate the aggression. The nurse should be confident. The patient should be addressed by his or her complete name (Ms. Smith) and allowed to verbalize his or her feelings. The nurse should listen to the patient's response and watch the patient's behavior. Explanations for long delays should be offered.

Second, rapid tranquilization should be tried to control the violent patient. Medications often used are lorazepam (Ativan) combined with thiothixene (Navane) or haloperidol (Haldol).

The nurse should be proactive, restraining the patient if necessary, especially if a painful or uncomfortable procedure is to be performed. It is best to have five people to restrain a violent person. This allows for one person at each extremity and one person at the head.

Nurses need to be involved in the development of security and safety issues in the ED. Panic buttons and panic watches should be available to get help immediately (Dubin, Tardiff, Maier, 1992; Kinkle, 1993).

Family Violence

Family violence is violence that occurs in a setting where people live together. It includes child and elder maltreatment, spousal abuse, and sexual assault (Box 19-12).

BOX 19-11

POTENTIALLY VIOLENT PATIENTS

- Patients with a known history of violent acts or drug or alcohol abuse
- Male gender under the age of 30
- Patients involved in accidents including their families
- Patients brought in by police
- Medical reason for violence, such as the hypoglycemic, head injured, overdose, or postictal (awakening from a seizure) patient
- Patients with psychiatric problems: acute psychosis or mania, alcohol or drug withdrawal, or personality disorders

BOX 19-12

TYPES OF MALTREATMENT

Physical abuse involves intentional injury inflicted on the survivor. Some examples are kicking, slapping, biting, shaking, or burning.

Emotional abuse involves behavior is that is degrading, terrorizing, isolating, or rejecting.

Sexual assault/abuse refers to sexual contact to the survivor without consent, by either coercion, persuasion, or force.

Neglect includes acts of omission and failure to meet the patient's needs, such as not obtaining medical care when needed or failure to provide food, clothing, and a safe place to live.

Exploitation involves the elderly and includes the improper or illegal use of the patient's resources by a caregiver.

History

An accurate history and assessment are essential for any patient who comes to the ED as the result of a violent act. The documentation from the emergency visit may be subpoenaed for court. The nurse should approach the survivor in a professional, nonjudgmental, and nonaccusatory manner. The survivor/patient and significant family must be interviewed separately. Open-ended questions and language the patient can understand should be used. The information must be kept confidential. If a child or elder states that a parent/caregiver inflicted the injury, relating this to them could put the patient at risk for further harm. The nurse should listen to responses and compare information for discrepancies. Exact quotes of what the patient stated should be documented, as well as the history of where the injuries happened, the date and time, and whether anyone else was present. The nurse and physician should perform the history and assessment together. If sexual assault is suspected, a person who has special training in this area should do the history and examination. Some nurses have undergone special training to become a sexual assault nurse examiner (SANE). These nurses are called to the ED when a sexual assault survivor is present. This allows for increased accuracy of obtaining evidence and the complete attention of one nurse to the patient's needs.

Assessment examination

The patient should fully undress. If it is a child older than 8, consent to perform the physical examination must be granted. Young children may want to stay on a parent's lap for the examination. Other physical signs of injury should be observed. All injuries should be documented using a body map. If bruising is noted, it is important to document the colors of the bruises because this indicates the stage of the healing process. Photographs should be taken of all injuries, and they should be documented. X-ray films should also be obtained for all injuries.

Child Maltreatment

In 1991 2.7 million cases of child maltreatment were reported to child protection agencies in the United States. This does not reflect all the cases that go unreported. **Child maltreatment/abuse** is any threat to a child's health or welfare. It is required by law in all states that all cases of suspected and actual child maltreatment be reported by emergency personnel to protection agencies. Reporting in good faith and protecting the child from a dangerous situation guarantees immunity from civil or criminal liability. The law does not protect the healthcare worker who fails to report suspicions.

Persons likely to cause maltreatment can be parents, relatives, close friends, teachers, or babysitters. Maltreatment occurs within every economic class, every religion, and every race.

People who may potentially maltreat a child are those who have drug or alcohol problems, have been maltreated themselves, have a chronic illness, are in crisis and under extreme stress, or have unrealistic expectations of the child. Children who are at risk for potential maltreatment are those with developmental problems or retardation, those of multiple births, or those who were premature.

If the child is in threat of harm or reprisal because emergency treatment has been sought, the ED child protection team should be notified, and the child should be placed in protective custody. This initially means the child will be admitted to the hospital until a judge can determine what is best for the child (Devlin and Reynolds, 1994; Klein and others, 1994).

Indicators of physical child maltreatment

Head injury is the leading cause of death in the maltreated child under the age of 1. Early recognition of signs and symptoms of ICP is necessary. "Shaken baby syndrome" occurs when a child is shaken with intense force without the head being supported. The neck is able to hyperextend and hyperflex, causing a whiplash-type injury. There is no outward sign of physical trauma, but the patient has an unexplained loss of consciousness, increased irritability, bulging fontanels, or seizure activity. The child may appear lethargic and have the inability to suck or feed. Medical problems such as sepsis or meningitis need to be ruled out. A CT scan of the head usually shows a subdural hematoma.

Other physical indicators of maltreatment are obvious traumas unrelated to the age of the child. Indicators include fractures in multiple stages of healing; ecchymosis or abrasions on wrists or ankles, indicating use of restraints; or bite marks. Burns are of concern if they are circumferential, which indicates immersion injuries, or if they involve the entire buttocks or both hands and wrists. Well-demarcated burned areas suggest the use of a cigarette or a hot instrument, and the shape may identify the instrument used.

The second leading cause of death as a result of child maltreatment is an abdominal injury. Bruising may be minimal or absent as a result of the elasticity of the child's abdomen. When signs of peritonitis or shock occur, it may be too late to help the child.

Indicators of emotional child maltreatment

Emotional maltreatment may be harder to identify. Symptoms may include speech disorders, failure to thrive, delayed development, or physical problems such as asthma, headaches, ulcers, or allergies. The nurse should watch how the caregiver interacts with the child. Does he or she push the child away or ignore the child when the child is asking for comfort? It is more difficult for the ED staff to recognize this type of maltreatment because of the short interaction they have with the child and caregiver.

Indicators of neglect

Neglect may be suspected if the child is inappropriately dressed, is emaciated, has lice, or has medical needs that go unattended. If the problem is that the caregiver does not have the financial ability to provide these things for the child, the family should be referred to a social agency for assistance.

Sexual abuse

Sexual abuse is usually committed by a male family member or male family friend who has gained the child's trust. This person may have been abused as a child.

Certain physical findings may suggest sexual abuse. The nurse should look for bruising or bleeding from the external genitalia, frequent urinary tract infections, pregnancy in adolescents, vaginal or rectal pain or itching, sexually transmitted diseases, or an inability to control urination or defecation in a child who is of an age that control should be obtained. Behavioral findings include sexual promiscuity, age-inappropriate sexual behavior, eating or sleeping disorders, suicide attempts in adolescents, school difficulties, and chronic withdrawal or depression.

Elder Maltreatment

One million elderly persons are victims of abuse, neglect, or exploitation each year. These numbers have increased because the elderly are living longer and need to turn to their families more for assistance. Many times the family does not know how to respond to the increasing demands placed on them. Individual states have set their own guidelines for reporting elder abuse. Only the states of Wisconsin, Colorado, and New York have voluntary reporting of elder abuse. All other states have mandatory reporting. Protection for reporting suspected abuse is the same as in child abuse.

Victims of elder or geriatric abuse are usually dependent on their abusers. The geriatric patient usually gives up his or her independence to the abuser because of physical health problems such as a cerebral vascular accident or because of a deterioration in mental health. Perpetrators of the abuse are usually dependent on their victims for financial support and may have a problem with mental illness, chronic disease, or drug or alcohol problems. The abuser may be the spouse, child, or grandchild of the victim.

The victim may be in denial that the abuse is occurring because of embarrassment, dependence on the caregiver, and the fear of public scrutiny. The abused also may not want to pursue filing a complaint against the perpetrator due to fear for his or her life.

Elder abuse is on the rise in the United States. It is up to medical personnel to recognize and report these incidences for the protection of the elderly (Stewart, Stewart, Weissberg, 1991).

ETHICAL DILEMMA

A child is brought to the emergency room with a number of injuries. A nurse suspects child abuse, but the physician gives instructions not to report it because nothing will change.

What should the nurse do?

Battered Patients

Three to four million women are beaten in their homes each year by their husbands or partners. Women make up 94% to 95% of the victims of domestic violence. Domestic violence is sometimes seen by law enforcement agencies as a personal family problem. **Domestic violence** is the abuse of power in an intimate relationship. Domestic violence is also called spousal abuse. There is no mandatory reporting to law enforcement agencies regarding victims of spousal abuse. The ED reports any acts of violence. Domestic violence falls into this category, and these cases are reported to document that an attack has occurred. The victim/survivor has the right to refuse to sign a complaint with the law enforcement agency because the survivors of these attacks are adults and are competent to make their own decisions regarding their care. The current term of *survivor* is used instead of *victim* to communicate that the person can take control of these acts of violence.

It is not uncommon for a domestic violence survivor to be seen in an ED many times before he or she is able to decide that this treatment cannot continue. Police officers are sometimes reluctant to pursue complaints in domestic violence cases because many feel it is a family issue. The violence occurs many times before the survivor breaks the cycle. Battering has an effect on the entire family. The person doing the battering to the spouse may also abuse the children in the family. The episodes of violence usually increase in frequency and severity. Forty percent of the women murdered in this country are killed by their husbands or partners. Many women arriving in EDs may have injuries related to being battered (Box 19-13). A police report should be completed even if the patient does not press formal charges of assault and battery.

BOX 19-13

SIGNALS OF DOMESTIC VIOLENCE

Suspicion should be heightened regarding potential domestic violence when the following occurs:

- Bruising and swelling is noted around the eyes or face
- Injuries are bilateral
- Multiple injuries are noted
- History does not correlate with findings
- Defense injuries are noted on hands or arms
- The patient does not answer questions, but the significant other does the explaining

Treatment Goals for Survivors of Violent Attacks

The goal of treatment for any survivor of a violent attack is to help the survivor regain control of his or her life. This is done by allowing the survivor to verbalize feelings and make decisions and by supporting those decisions. The person's confidence needs to be regained. The nurse can help by giving the survivor phone numbers of support groups and social agencies. Safety for the survivor and the children should be encouraged. If needed, the nurse can help make arrangements to find a safe place to stay.

All survivors need their physical injuries cared for with follow up as needed for the specific injuries (Salber, Blair, 1992).

Sexual Assault

Sexual assault includes all forms of sexual activity performed on another person without that person's consent. *Rape* is the legal term for sexual assault. It is an act of forced sexual penetration against a man or woman. Sexual assault is a violent crime, and the survivor fears for his or her life. Treatment of sexual assault patients in the ED is usually lengthy, and information obtained through history, physical examination, and gathered evidence will likely be subpoenaed for the criminal court case if the survivor presses charges.

Treatment goals for sexual assault survivors

The goal of treatment for the sexual assault patient is to provide medical and psychosocial care in a humane, tactful, and nonjudgmental manner while complying with the law regarding collection of evidence.

When the survivor initially comes to the ED, a one-to-one nurse-patient relationship should be established. The patient should be placed in a private room, and a sexual assault counselor should be notified. The sexual assault counselor will act as a resource after the patient leaves the ED. It is mandated by law that law enforcement agencies be notified of sexual assaults. The patient should not use the bathroom, change clothes, or eat or drink anything until after the physical examination. The ED staff should attend to the patient as quickly as possible. When a law enforcement officer questions the patient, a counselor or nurse should be in the room. When the physical examination is performed, the officer should be outside the room. Medical information and evidence cannot be released without the patient's consent. The patient is given a choice if he or she wishes to file a police report, but the hospital must notify the police of the attack.

Documentation

Documentation of sexual assault should reflect a brief subjective account of the survivor's description of the incident. Physical evidence, objective findings, chain of custody of evidence, medications, discharge instructions, pamphlets, and follow up should also be documented.

All procedures should be explained before the physical examination. The examination entails first treating any life-threatening problems: assessing airway, breathing, and circulation. It is not uncommon for these survivors to have injuries caused by choking. Physical injuries should be documented and photographed, and a pelvic examination of the female patient should be performed.

Chain of custody

Obtaining evidence and maintaining the chain of custody are very important. **Chain of custody** of evidence is the ability to trace the evidence collected to the point at which it was first obtained. The evidence should stay with the person collecting it until it is sealed and turned over to the next person in the chain. The nurse obtains the samples, seals them, and turns the evidence over to the police only if the patient consents. Specimens should remain unaltered. When collecting evidence for a sexual assault survivor, it is important to have him or her place all clothing in the evidence bags, which are made out of paper. The patient should undress over a sheet so that falling debris can be saved. Evidence kits include equipment necessary to obtain the specimens. Specimens include clothing, pubic hair, head hair, saliva, blood samples, fingernail scrapings, vaginal swabs, and rectal swabs. Laboratory tests obtained are rapid plasma reagin (RPR); cultures of affected areas; HIV; urine for sperm, trichomonas, and fungus; and a serum pregnancy test.

Treatment

Treatment for medical injuries resulting from the sexual assault is then performed. Treatment to prevent sexually transmitted diseases (gonorrhea and *Chlamydia*) and to prevent pregnancy is initiated in the ED. A concern today is the risk of contracting HIV. The patient should be counseled regarding this. A patient is tested initially for HIV to make sure he or she did not have the disease before the attack. As a follow up, patients are tested at 6 months and 1 year to see if they have converted to HIV-positive. It is thought that the likelihood of HIV is rare if conversion has not occurred within the first year.

Medication treatment is ceftriaxone 250 mg intramuscularly, spectinomycin 2 g intramuscularly, or ciprofloxacin 500 mg orally once followed by a 7-day dosage of another antibiotic: tetracycline, doxycycline, or erythromycin. Treatment to prevent pregnancy is controversial, but this should be discussed with the survivor. The medication most likely to prevent pregnancy is ethinyl estradiol/norgestrel (Ovral). Two pills are given immediately, and two more pills are taken 12 hours later.

The psychologic effects, referred to as "rape trauma syndrome," can last for a long time. These symptoms include reliving the rape, crying outbursts, fear, anger, inability to sleep, angry outbursts, trouble concentrating, and an inability to remember parts of the event.

The ED should make arrangements for counseling follow-up. Having the sexual assault advocate meet the patient in the ED allows the survivor to develop a rapport with the advocate and gives the survivor a link to help once he or she leaves the ED. Written information regarding all aspects of sexual-assault care should be given to the survivor before leaving the ED (Blair, Warner, 1992).

PSYCHIATRIC EMERGENCIES

The ED is often the clearinghouse for psychiatric patients. It is their first port of entry into a structured healthcare setting. These patients often arrive in police custody, by paramedics, or by family or friends as a result of a change in the patient's mental status. There are three behaviors the emergency psychiatric patient may exhibit: agitation, confusion, or depression.

Goal of Psychiatric Care in the Emergency Department

The goal of care for the psychiatric patient in the ED is to keep the patient and staff safe. This is done by providing a safe environment and having the patient observed until definitive care is decided or until the patient is admitted to a psychiatric facility. The patient may need to be chemically sedated with medication or physically restrained to maintain a safe environment. Commonly seen in psychiatric patients are suicidal gestures, acute psychosis, and drug and alcohol problems.

Agitation

Symptoms of **agitation** are pacing, wringing of hands, tachycardia, hyperactivity, and incessant talking. These patients are at risk of hurting themselves. The symptoms may be caused by drug or alcohol problems, an inability to cope with a crisis, anxiety, or organic brain disease. Interventions need to be performed so the agitated patient does not harm himself or herself. Interventions include talking in a calm, quiet voice. A sedative may be prescribed to calm the behavior. The patient may need to be restrained to avoid injury to the patient or the staff caring for the patient.

Confusion

Symptoms of confusion are a disheveled appearance, a dazed expression, an inability to follow instructions, and/or an inability to communicate basic needs. Causes of confusion are manic-depressive disease; alcohol or drug withdrawal or intoxication; or a medical problem such as Alzheimer's disease, acute head trauma, seizure disorder, or hypoglycemia. Medical problems need to be ruled out before determining that the cause is psychiatric. Interventions for the confused patient are aimed at protecting the patient because he or she is unable to care for himself or herself. A safe environment should be provided. Stimuli should be decreased by dimming the lights, placing the patient in a quiet room, and speaking softly. The patient should be reoriented to the surroundings. For more information about caring for the patient who is confused, see Chapter 28.

Depression

Symptoms of depression include being tired all the time, having no appetite, having the inability to sleep, maintaining poor eye contact, and having a loss of interest in life and surroundings. These patients may be a suicide risk. Interventions for the depressed patient include allowing the patient to verbalize feelings. The nurse should try to identify if a suicide attempt is imminent and should protect the patient from harming himself or herself.

Suicidal Emergencies

Suicidal patients are seen in the ED before receiving psychiatric care. They are often patients who are depressed, have experienced a life crisis, have family problems, or abuse drugs or alcohol. Suicide is the eighth leading cause of death in elderly white males. Adolescent suicide has been increasing. Twenty percent of attempted suicides involve alcohol.

Patients who have a history of suicide attempts usually have an underlying psychiatric problem such as depression or a personality disorder. Suicidal patients who have lost their will to live, have experienced or witnessed a violent attack such as rape, or are under the influence of alcohol or drugs are more likely to follow through with their threats. The nurse should question the patient openly about suicidal thoughts and intentions (Box 19-14). If a plan of how to commit suicide is already thought out, the patient is more likely to attempt suicide again.

Suicidal patients must be kept from harm. A security person or sitter should have direct sight of the patient at all times. The room should be free from anything that the patient could get to harm himself or herself (e.g., instruments, oxygen tubing, glass). The patient should be completely undressed, and belongings should be stored in a safe place.

Restraints may be necessary to control behavior that could harm the patient or someone else. Once restraints are determined to be necessary, they should be applied. They are not to be used as a threat or a bargaining tool. If restraints are used, the patient should have his or her extremities checked every 15 minutes for circulation, sensation, and mobility. The patient's position should be changed every hour, and the patient should be offered bathroom facilities every 2 hours. Frequent assessments of the patient's psychologic status should be made. If the patient remains violent, chemical sedation should be given. Drugs commonly used are haloperidol (either orally or intramuscularly) or lorazepam intramuscularly until the violent behavior has subsided. Careful monitoring of the respiratory status of suicidal patients is necessary after chemical sedation. The physician, with input from the psychiatric consultant, determines if hospitalization is necessary.

BOX 19-14

QUESTIONS TO ASK THE SUICIDAL PATIENT

Ask direct questions such as:

Were you trying to kill yourself?
Have you ever done this before?
How do you feel about being alive?

OVERDOSE EMERGENCY MANAGEMENT

A patient can come to the ED with an accidental or intentional overdose. It is estimated that 5 million overdoses occur annually. An accidental overdose usually involves only one substance. Intentional overdoses usually involve more than one substance. The substances taken should be identified as quickly as possible so that known antidotes can be given. Treatment should never wait until the substance has been identified. Many times the patient arrives with an unknown polydrug ingestion. For any potential emergency patient, the basics must be assessed first. The nurse should evaluate and intervene on any life-threatening problem affecting the ABCs. Many times these patients need to be intubated because they are unable to protect their airway and their breathing is inadequate. The patient also will need an IV access to be prepared for potential problems and to administer naloxone (Narcan), thiamine, and 50% dextrose. Dextrose is given to patients in case their symptoms are caused by hypoglycemia. A dextrose stick may be obtained before administration of dextrose.

After life-saving measures are instituted, the nurse should obtain a history and complete physical (secondary survey). The patient should be asked what drugs were taken, when they were taken, how many, and why. If paramedics bring the patient to the ED, they will bring any containers of medications found at the prehospital scene. Measures are then instituted to decrease the absorption of the substance.

Definitive measures are performed to help the body eliminate the toxic substances with the least detrimental effects. These procedures are gastric lavage and administering activated charcoal, a cathartic, and any known antidotes for the ingested substances. If the patient does not respond favorably to these treatments, he or she may need to be dialyzed.

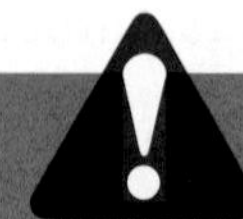

NURSE ALERT

Restrain the patient before initiating noxious (painful or uncomfortable) procedures to protect the patient and staff from injury.

Gastric Emptying

Ipecac syrup may be used to help accomplish gastric emptying. Emergency physicians do not like to give this medication because of the effects of retching. If the patient is retching, he or she will be unable to take activated charcoal until the effects of the ipecac have worn off. In addition the patient may be at risk for aspiration if he or she experiences a change in level of consciousness or has seizure activity as a result of the medications ingested before the effects of ipecac end.

Gastric lavage is used to empty any remaining substances from the stomach. An oral or nasal gastric tube is placed. The patient is then positioned on the left side in Trendelenburg's position. Five liters of tap water are instilled. The amount of water instilled should be the same amount of water returned. A closed gastric lavage system should be used to decrease the chance of exposure to infections. Universal precautions should be followed, including wearing a mask and protective eye wear. Gastric lavage is contraindicated in patients who have ingested hydrocarbons or caustic ingestion. Care should be taken to prevent hypothermia from the administration of the irrigating solution.

Activated Charcoal

Activated charcoal is used to decrease the absorption rate of the ingested substance. If an oral/nasal gastric tube is in place, the patient should have the charcoal administered through the tube before the tube is removed. The medication also can be taken orally. The usual dose is 1 g/kg, and the total usual adult dose is 50 g. If the patient is to swallow the medication, it can be combined with the cathartic.

Cathartics

A cathartic such as sorbital 50 ml or magnesium citrate 4 ml/kg up to 300 ml/kg is given to aid in the elimination of the charcoal. The patient will usually get diarrhea, and the stool will be black. Sorbital should not be administered to children because studies have shown it can cause retinal hemorrhages.

Antidotes

The known antidote for the known toxic substance is given after the preceding treatments are completed. A commonly ingested substance is acetaminophen, and the antidote is acetylcysteine (Mucomyst).

Laboratory Tests

A serum and urine toxicology screen, complete blood count, electrolytes, alcohol level, and arterial blood gases are all laboratory tests that should be ordered for the overdose patient. Specific drug levels will be ordered when the ingested drug is known, such as acetaminophen, aspirin, or digoxin.

Diagnostic Tests

Cardiac monitoring with an electrocardiogram, pulse oximetry with supplemental oxygen, and a chest x-ray examination are ordered. A CT scan of the head may be ordered for altered mental status.

Psychiatric Examination

A psychiatric evaluation should be done on all intentional or suspicious accidental toxic ingestions. The patient should be protected from harm and have close observation (Weinman, 1993; Klein and others, 1994).

POISONINGS

One to two million poisonings occur each year in the United States. Ninety percent of all poisonings take place at home. There are four routes for a poison to enter the body: inhalation, absorption, ingestion, and injection. Many poisonings can be prevented by educating people about the dangers of products and medications they have at home. Preventing poisonings is the best solution. This is done through patient teaching. Some guidelines to prevent accidental poisonings include the following:

- Keep all medications out of the reach of children. Use containers with childproof covers. Close medications tightly after every use.
- Tell children when they are taking medication and never refer to it as candy.
- Never place dangerous liquids such as paint thin-

ner or gasoline into drinking cups or bottles.

- Read labels before taking any medication.
- Keep all medications and household products in locked cabinets.
- Work in a well-ventilated room when painting or using products that emit fumes.
- Dress appropriately when working outside or hiking. This includes wearing gloves when gardening, and shoes, socks, and long pants when hiking.

Basic First Aid for Poisoning

For ingestion poisonings the nature of the substance will indicate whether vomiting should be induced. If the substance is a petroleum product such as kerosene, gasoline, or lighter fluid, or if it is a corrosive acid or alkali, vomiting should not be induced because it will further damage the gastrointestinal tract on its return. Toilet bowel cleaners are usually acidic, and drain cleaners and nonphosphate detergents are usually alkaline. Vomiting should never be induced in an unconscious or convulsing patient because of the risk of aspiration. It may be possible to neutralize a corrosive acid or alkali to protect the mucosa of the gastrointestinal tract if the patient is able to swallow. Milk or milk of magnesia will neutralize an acid, and milk, water, or olive oil will neutralize an alkali. Products today have basic first aid instructions on the label. A person involved in a poisoning should contact a poison control center for first aid instructions and the need for follow-up. Many EDs have a poison control index to look up the name of the poison and the advice for first aid. The advice for a triage call is to offer the caller initial first aid instructions and to tell the caller to see a physician or go to an emergency department for further care. If a patient is unresponsive or is having problems breathing, the EMS should be activated.

For injection poisonings such as bites or stings, the stinger should be removed by scraping it with a credit card. The stinger should never be squeezed, because this can inject more toxin into the bloodstream. Medical help should be sought.

For inhalation poisonings such as chlorine gas or carbon monoxide, the patient should be taken out of the area and given fresh air. Clothing should be loosened to assist with respirations. Help should be called.

For absorption poisonings, the chemical should be brushed off the skin, and the area should be washed with soap and water. Medical help should be sought if there is continued irritation or any sign of respiratory distress (Newell and others, 1993).

ENVIRONMENTAL EMERGENCIES

Environmental emergencies can be related to extreme heat or cold. They can affect anyone, but the elderly and young, as well as people with chronic conditions such as alcoholism, HIV, or cancer, are extremely vulnerable. The body tries to maintain a core temperature of approximately 100° F (37.8° C).

Heat Emergencies

Hyperthermia is an abnormally high body temperature. As the body temperature rises, the hypothalamus is stimulated and the body tries to compensate for the increase in temperature by first causing peripheral vasodilation. This allows for the heat to dissipate. Then sweat is produced to help the body cool. If the temperature continues to rise, the body will increase heart rate and cardiac output. The kidney will reserve sodium and water. If the temperature is still uncontrollable, the patient will begin to exhibit symptoms of heat emergencies: heat cramps, heat syncope, heat exhaustion, and heatstroke.

Heatstroke

Mortality for heatstroke can be as high as 80%. The body's thermoregulation system is overwhelmed and shuts down. Core body temperature usually goes above 104° F (40° C). Heatstroke is more likely to occur when the temperature and humidity are high. Symptoms include marked confusion, psychotic behavior, and seizures. Skin is hot, dry, and ashen. Heart rate may be very weak and rapid. Signs of dehydration include no urine output, hypotension, tachypnea, and tachycardia. The cells of the brain are injured by the high temperature, and the patient will die if treatment is not initiated to reduce the temperature before the patient is transported to the hospital. The patient should be moved to a cool place, and ice compresses should be applied. Alcohol should never be used to sponge the patient. It can be absorbed through the skin, and the patient can become toxic. An ambulance should be called, and the patient should be transported to the hospital. Interventions begin with the ABCs. Oxygen should be applied, and the patient should be prepped for intubation. Two large-gauge IVs should be established, and vasopressor agents such as Dopamine should be administered if the patient does not respond to IV hydration. A nasogastric tube and Foley catheter should be inserted. The patient should be cooled with a cooling mattress, and the nurse should continuously monitor body temperature. The patient should be on a cardiac monitor so that arrhythmia can be detected. Prevention of shivering is accomplished by administering medica-

OLDER ADULT CONSIDERATIONS

Hypothermia and Hyperthermia

Administer fluids cautiously while monitoring the respiratory status of the elderly. The elderly are more likely to have pulmonary edema as a complication of overhydration. It is important to listen to breath sounds while hydrating to determine if rales are present. Monitor urine output to assess hydration.

Also monitor body temperature closely because the elderly become hypothermic and hyperthermic more easily.

tions such as chlorpromazine 10 to 50 mg IV. Seizures are controlled with antineuroleptic medications phenytoin (Dilantin) or diazepam.

Heat cramps

Heat cramps usually occur in athletes after exercise. The person sweats, and electrolytes become imbalanced. They affect large muscles such as the abdomen, thighs, and calves. The person has lost potassium and sodium through sweat. Electrolytes are further diluted if the person drank water instead of a sports drink containing sodium and potassium.

The treatment for heat cramps begins by getting the patient in a cool environment. Fluids should be replaced with an electrolyte-balanced drink, or IV fluids may be necessary. Salt tablets *should not* be given, because they irritate the stomach mucosa and cause hypernatremia. When the electrolyte imbalance is corrected, the symptoms resolve.

Heat syncope

Heat syncope can occur during exercise. The patient's temperature rises, and the body's blood vessels dilate. This shunt of fluid to the skin can cause symptoms of postural lightheadness, dizziness, or actual loss of consciousness. Treatment is to get the person into a cool place and rest. The symptoms usually resolve quickly.

Heat exhaustion

The patient suffering heat exhaustion exhibits signs of flulike symptoms such as nausea, vomiting, and headache. The skin can be cool and dry, and the patient may have an altered level of consciousness. The body temperature may elevate to 100.4° F (38° C). This person needs IV hydration. The initial IV fluid used is normal saline. The patient should be kept in a cool environment and be given nothing by mouth (Stewart, 1993).

Cold Emergencies

Hypothermia

Hypothermia is defined as a core temperature less than 95° F (35° C). The body is unable to produce enough heat to maintain its temperature. In mild hypothermia (93° F to 95° F or 34° to 35° C) the patient is conscious and alert and demonstrates tachycardia, tachypnea, cutaneous vasoconstriction, and shivering. With moderate hypothermia (86° to 93° F; 30° to 34° C) symptoms include difficulty speaking, decreased sensorium, and hyperglycemia from decreased utilization of glucose. Shivering has stopped. With severe hypothermia, the nurse will see unconsiousness, deterioration of vital signs, shallow respirations, and cardiac arrhythmias. If no pulse is present, the nurse should begin CPR. The patient should be gradually rewarmed 1 to 2 degrees every hour. The patient should have dry clothes. The worse the hypothermia, the more aggressive the warming techniques. In mild hypothermia the patient's clothes are dry, so warming can be done passively with warm blankets and warmed oral fluids. In severe hypothermia the patient is actively rewarmed with IV fluids, gastric lavage, peritoneal lavage, and oxygen. Pronouncing a patient dead after being hypothermic does not occur until the patient has been rewarmed, which leads to long resuscitative measures.

NURSE ALERT

Hypothermia is a life-threatening medical emergency.

Patient teaching should include education on layering clothing to stay warm, avoiding alcohol and caffeine when out in the cold, and seeking shelter during a snowstorm or severe weather.

Frostbite

The skin responds to cold with vasoconstriction, resulting in decreased blood flow and decreased oxygen to the tissue. Severe cold or extended exposure to cold results in damage to vessel walls and leakage of plasma into the interstitial spaces. The blood remaining in the vessel is therefore more concentrated and, together with the narrowed lumen caused by vasoconstriction, results in the formation of small clots that block the small vessels. The pressure from the obstruction causes the arteriovenous shunts to open, and blood bypasses the area. The tissue is essentially without a blood supply. The tissues are cooled to the point that ice crystals form in the extracellular spaces, and the extracellular fluid becomes hypertonic and draws fluid from the cells. If one third of the cells' fluid is lost, dehydration and disruption of enzymatic processes result in injury to the cells. The skin will change to white and will not redden when pressure is applied.

Frostbite most often involves the feet or toes, hands, ears, chin, cheeks, or nose. It is divided into superficial or partial freezing of the skin, or deep, full thickness freezing involving the skin, subcutaneous tissue, and deep tissue.

The frozen tissue looks red and is painful, or it is waxy in appearance, blue or black. The tissue may blister. Treatment involves rapidly rewarming the area. Before starting rewarming, the nurse needs to make sure that there is no chance for refreezing to occur. The temperature of the water for rewarming should be maintained between 100° F and 105° F (37.8° C and 40.5° C). The tissue should not be rubbed. Rubbing will cause increased cellular damage. The extent of the injury will not be known for at least 24 hours. The frozen area is treated like a burn. Antibiotic ointment should be applied, and the area should be covered with a sterile dressing. The area must be kept from refreezing. If the frostbite is severe and involves tissue beneath the outer layers of the skin, it may permanently remain red and tender, and the affected area will always be very sensitive to cold.

Patient teaching includes information about protecting body parts from further cold injuries, wearing protective clothing, and monitoring the frostbitten areas for signs of infection (Schneider, 1992; Klein and others, 1994).

DISASTER PREPAREDNESS

Disasters do not occur every day in local communities, but when they do occur, the ED is the unit of the hospital that decides the acuity of the patient and the definitive treatment. A disaster is any situation that causes a large number of victims to seek medical care. It can be caused by natural forces such as hurricane, flood, or tornado. It can be caused by an explosion in an industrial site, or it can be the result of an accident or terrorist/hostage activities. This influx of victims overloads the existing emergency care structure, and an alternative method of deciding treatment for these victims needs to be established. Hospitals now have practice drills to test their disaster plans so that when a disaster occurs, everyone is familiar with his or her role.

Types of Injuries

Most casualties from a disaster are surgical in nature, and nursing care is largely the same as that given to any surgical patient. Disaster injuries usually include contusions, lacerations, fractures, crush injuries, burns, and severe hemorrhage from wounds. Many patients suffer from shock, and uninjured persons suffer psychologic stress. In addition, a large group of curious onlookers who feel they must know what is going on is always present.

Disaster nursing differs from emergency nursing only in the number of persons who must be seen. Every effort should be made to protect the individual from further injury and infection, but in the case of mass casualties, the precise techniques that the nurse has learned may require considerable modification. For more information about triage, see the beginning of this chapter.

Community Services

Two agencies available to provide services are the Federal Emergency Management Agency (FEMA) and the National Disaster Medical System (NDMS). FEMA activates the government response to secure the disaster area. NDMS coordinates the medical system response.

Community agencies often involved include the fire and police departments, the American Red Cross, Salvation Army, Department of Children and Family Services, Public Health Department, hospitals, clinics, and other agencies. In many disasters the local hospital and medical facilities are adequate for the emergency. However, emergency first-aid centers may be established in schools or churches to care for those with minor injuries and to refer those suffering from more serious injuries to the hospital. If the disaster has caused many deaths, a temporary morgue may need to be set up.

The nurse may assist in various community activities when a disaster occurs. Centers are often set up to immunize large numbers of people when water supplies have been contaminated. Temporary shelters need the assistance of a nurse to help with dealing with families in crisis. The nurse must work with the other disaster team members to help the disaster victims.

Psychologic Reactions to Disaster

It is normal for the disaster victim to show some signs of disturbance. The victim may tremble or perspire and feel weak and nauseated. After the victim recovers from the first impact of the experience, he or she usually regains composure fairly quickly. Others will panic and seem to lose all ability to make judgments and attempt to escape the situation by fleeing from the site. This reaction can excite others, so it is important to keep a calm manner and reassure persons so they are able to regain control.

It is important that nurses know their own limitations in order to handle these persons in crisis. Sedatives are usually not prescribed because they can add to the victim's confusion and delay handling of the real problem.

Family and friends can help a disaster victim with support and assistance. The emotional care of the survivor is as important as the physical care. The nurse must convey a feeling of caring if the patient and family are to feel comfortable enough to express feelings. It is important to provide a place for family members to express themselves freely.

Psychologic support for the healthcare team is also important, and critical incidence stress debriefing or management is now an important part of caring *for the caregiver* after a disaster (Box 19-15).

SUDDEN DEATH

The ED often deals with sudden death. Sudden death of an infant, a death from a violent attack or car crash, or a natural death from a cardiac arrest or other medical problem all lead to stress for the family of the deceased as well as for the ED staff.

There is limited time for healthcare professionals to develop a rapport with families before breaking the news of the death. The grief process begins after the family is told of the death. Each family member's response to the death will vary depending on the person's culture, the closeness of the person to the deceased, the person's learned response to dealing with death, and the circumstances of the death.

BOX 19-15

CRITICAL INCIDENCE STRESS DEBRIEFING

Every case of sudden death is different and has a different effect on the healthcare staff. Critical Incidence Stress Debriefing (CISD) is a support session that occurs after a traumatic event to allow the staff to express feelings. This session usually is best performed 24 to 72 hours after the incident. CISD has shown that if people talk about their feelings, they are better able to resolve them. Unresolved feelings can lead to increased stress.

COMPONENTS OF DEBRIEFING

The debriefing session is held with the group moderator—a social worker, chaplain, or someone trained in debriefing. The session usually lasts 1 hour, and the group size should be no more than 10 people. There are seven components to the debriefing session: introduction, facts, thoughts, reactions, symptoms, teaching, and closure:

1. *Introduction:* The group members introduce themselves.
2. *Facts:* The group starts talking about the facts of the incident. For example: Allen, a local paramedic was brought here by his friends—fellow paramedics—after falling during a routine response drill. He was looking backward and stumbled, hitting his head. He was pronounced brain dead 3 hours after coming to the ED, and life support measures were stopped after organ donation.
3. *Thoughts:* The group members discuss how they feel, as well as their reactions to the incident. Continuing the example, many members state that they feel vulnerable because the accident was so sudden. Discussion also centers around caring for a co-worker in a time of emergency.
4. *Reaction:* Two questions are answered: How did you feel at the time, and how do you feel now? This is probably the hardest component of the debriefing. Often tears are shed at this point, and physical support with hugs is appreciated by members.
5. *Symptoms:* The group is asked if it is experiencing any signs or symptoms related to increased stress. It is not uncommon to have nightmares after a traumatic event. Signs of increased stress are physical symptoms: headaches, fatigue, muscle soreness, chest pains, gastrointestinal complaints, inability to concentrate, insomnia, and change of eating habits.
6. *Teaching:* The group is reminded of the normal response to crisis. It is reeducated regarding the symptoms of increased stress.
7. *Closure/Reentry:* Finally the group members share how they can help each other better deal with the incident. The example group members decide to get a plaque for the department honoring the deceased coworker (Klein and others, 1994).

Not all members of the staff will participate in these sessions. It is voluntary, but the staff who attend the sessions view the response from the session as positive.

On arrival to the ED, the family should be escorted to a quiet room with a phone. It sometimes helps to prepare them by having a healthcare member (usually the nurse who will be available for the family members while they are in the ED) talk to the family prior to the actual discussion regarding the death. When addressing the family, the nurse should make introductions and find out who is being addressed. Proper names should be used when speaking to the family of the deceased. The nurse should empathize. The nurse should sit and talk to the family, find out what is already known, and add unknown information. The word *dead* should be used, so that there is no question regarding the condition of the deceased. The significant others should be encouraged to express themselves. The deceased person can be viewed by the family. This may help to overcome the denial process. It is the family's option to view the deceased. The family should not be rushed into leaving. Some cultures will bring their entire family to the ED. If this is the case, move the deceased to a room where the family can have some privacy. Before family members leave the ED, it is important for the nurse to give them a name and number to contact if they have any questions. The funeral home is the usually the contact that helps once the family has left the ED.

DISCHARGE AND TEACHING

The ENA's Standards of Practice emphasize the importance of teaching to help patients and their significant others prevent illness and injury as well as understand prescribed treatments (Dains and others, 1991). This is accomplished by the constant teaching emergency nurses do on a daily basis. From the moment patients arrive at the ED, teaching is started regarding what care they will receive, the time frame of test results, and test results. This is a collaborative process that is shared by the healthcare team. Every patient leaving the hospital is given formal discharge instructions that explain how to care for the illness or injury and who to contact later if there is a problem.

Many emergency nurses are involved in educating the public by presenting programs regarding health issues. One organization is ENCARE, Emergency Nurses Cancel Alcohol-Related Emergencies. This organization encourages emergency nurses to speak to high school students regarding the problem of drinking and driving. As stated previously, organizations such as STOP and HELP use nurses to educate the public regarding handgun violence. Nurses also speak at rotary clubs and other meetings about when to use the ED.

Nurses who work in emergency nursing understand that prevention is the key to decreasing accidental injuries.

TRENDS

As managed-care groups treat patients with minor illnesses, the majority of patients admitted to the ED will continue to be more acutely ill. With a decrease in the length of stay of hospital patients, the discharged patients need more care at home. Sometimes these patients return to the ED in less than 24 hours and need to be readmitted for the same problem as their original admission. To meet the needs of these patients, the ED will become even more high tech. Fast-track systems have been established to separate the critically ill from patients with minor illnesses. Patients who are admitted to observation areas will need the skill of critical care technology. Critical pathways are now being developed to help streamline patient care. The ED will be the first entry level in these critical pathways. Emergency nursing is constantly changing to meet the needs of the diverse population it treats.

Nursing Care Plan

PATIENT WITH A HEAT-RELATED EMERGENCY

Marc Stevens is a 26-year-old male who is brought to the ED by a friend. The friend states "My friend is barely moving and not acting right." When helping Mr. Stevens out of the car it is noted that he has no breathing impairment, is disoriented, responds to verbal stimuli, and is unable to walk.

The friend reports that they rode bicycles 30 miles before experiencing any problems. The outside temperature is 95°F, but they drank some fluids during the ride. Normally they ride on long trips two to three times per week.

Past Medical History	Psychosocial Data	Assessment Data
No known allergies Takes no medications No significant past medical history	Unknown	Height 6 ft 1 in, weight 176 lbs Well nourished, muscular appearance Alert and oriented × 2, disoriented to time Answers some questions inappropriately *Vital signs:* Temperature 100° F, pulse 120, respirations 24, blood pressure 100/60, PERRL *Respiratory:* Lungs clear; no dyspnea; respirations deep symmetrical *Abdomen:* Soft; nontender; nondistended; hypoactive bowel sounds. *Skin:* Pale in color; cool and dry; no diaphoresis; no surface trauma head to toe *Cardiovascular:* Apical pulse 124 and regular; orthostatic hypotension; strong peripheral pulses ***Laboratory data*** Hct 40, Hgb 14.2 g/100 ml, RBC 4.8, BUN 33 mg/100 ml, Cr 1.3 mg/100 ml, Na 130 mg/100 ml, K 3.0 mEq/L, Cl 90 mEq/L ***Medications*** Normal saline IV wide open rate Oxygen 2 L/min nasal cannula Cardiac monitor Cooling of patient with air conditioner

NURSING DIAGNOSIS

Hyperthermia related to environmental factors

NURSING INTERVENTIONS	EVALUATION OF EXPECTED OUTCOMES
Monitor rectal temperature, skin temperature, and overall color. Maintain cool environment. Remove excess clothing and covers. Administer antipyretic medications, if prescribed. Assess for shivering. If it occurs, administer diazepam or lorazepam as ordered. Monitor level of consciousness. Assess for nausea and vomiting.	Rectal temperature 99.6° F Skin warm and dry Normal skin color Alert and oriented × 3 No agitation Nausea and vomiting subsided No shivering

NURSING DIAGNOSIS

Risk for ineffective airway clearance related to decreased level of consciousness

NURSING INTERVENTIONS	EVALUATION OF EXPECTED OUTCOMES
Provide airway management as indicated. Administer supplemental oxygen. Monitor respiratory status continuously until stable (O_2 sat, breath sounds, rate, depth). Assess for decreased level of consciousness. Position for optimal respiratory effort.	Airway remains patent Pulse oximetry > 95% Respiratory rate 16-20 min Lungs clear bilaterally Awake, alert, and oriented × 3

NURSING DIAGNOSIS

Fluid volume deficit related to peripheral vasodilation, inadequate intake

NURSING INTERVENTIONS	EVALUATION OF EXPECTED OUTCOMES
Administer IV fluids as ordered, normal saline at fast rate until stable. Monitor vital signs, urine output, skin turgor, capillary refill. Monitor for orthostatic hypotension if indicated. Monitor cardiac status with telemetry.	Normal vital signs without orthostatic changes Normal sinus rhythm without ectopy Urine output 15-30 ml/hr No evidence of dehydration

NURSING DIAGNOSIS

Knowledge deficit related to prevention of subsequent heat illness

NURSING INTERVENTIONS	EVALUATION OF EXPECTED OUTCOMES
Assess level of knowledge related to heat illness, discussing early signs and symptoms. Discuss predisposing factors to heat illness (outside temperature, increased activity, lack of hydration). Teach importance of hydration and cooling. Provide written discharge instructions.	Verbalizes understanding of information Identifies early signs of heat illness and measures to prevent heat illness

KEY CONCEPTS

- The goal of emergency care is to resuscitate and stabilize patients, reduce suffering, provide for emotional needs, and educate regarding discharge instructions and prevention.
- Emergency care involves a collaborative approach.
- Legislation affecting emergency care includes COBRA, mandatory reporting of violent acts, and trauma center designations.
- Unique characteristics of emergency practice are assessment, analysis/diagnosis, and treatment of emergent, urgent, and nonurgent individuals of all ages; triage and prioritization; disaster preparedness; stabilization and resuscitation; and crisis intervention.
- Priorities differ between daily triage and disaster triage. In daily triage the most critical patient is treated first. In disaster triage the most salvageable patient is treated first. An "expectant" category is added to disaster triage.
- Disaster triage starts at the disaster scene. The patients arriving at the hospital have already had their care prioritized at least once.
- History, including mechanism of injury, is vital for a thorough assessment and plan of care for the patient.
- Primary assessment includes airway, breathing, circulation, and a brief neurologic exam. Intervention is for any life-threatening problem.
- Secondary survey identifies all injuries.
- Focused survey assesses each area identified in the secondary survey. It includes definitive care and patient teaching.
- All patients who have impaired skin integrity from an injury receive tetanus (dT) immunization if last booster was given more than 10 years ago and there is no contraindication.
- A cervical spine injury should be suspected for any trauma above the level of the clavicle.
- When administering IV conscious sedation, resuscitative equipment and medication reversal should be ready.
- Changes in the neurologic signs of a head-injured patient indicate the need for immediate intervention.
- No family is immune from the effects of violence.
- It is mandatory to report any acts of violence to a law enforcement agency.
- Safety is the goal for any psychiatric patient.
- Anaphylaxis is a life-threatening emergency. After the critical event patients need to be educated on how to avoid a recurrence and measures to take if contact with the allergen occurs.
- Eighty percent of all patients who experience heatstroke die.
- Frostbitten areas should never be rubbed.
- Hypothermic patients are never dead until they are warm and dead. This leads to prolonged resuscitative measures of the hypothermic patient.
- A patient with hypothermia should have his or her temperature raised only 1 to 2 degrees an hour.
- The emergency nurse needs to be aware of legal and ethical problems that can arise.
- If a patient with a head injury has signs of hypovolemic shock, the nurse should look for other injuries that cause bleeding.
- The nurse needs to be empathic to families who have just experienced a death. Every family will deal with death differently.
- When a traumatic event occurs in the ED, a debriefing session should occur between 24 to 72 hours to allow the staff to express feelings and aid in the resolution of those feelings.

CRITICAL THINKING EXERCISES

1 Identify the most important signs and symptoms you would assess in the chest injured patient.
2 What would you do if one of your fellow nurses began to exhibit signs of inability to sleep, weight loss, and increased agitation after caring for a burn victim?
3 Identify five types of maltreatment seen in situations of family violence. Give examples of each.
4 In suporting a grieving family member, how would your approach differ if the death was sudden?

REFERENCES AND ADDITIONAL READINGS

Aumick J: Head trauma guidelines for care, *RN* 58(4):27-31, 1991.

Blair TMH, Warner CG: Sexual assault, *Top Emerg Med* 14(4): 58-77, 1992.

Bone LB, Chapman MW: Initial management of the patient with multiple injuries, *Instructional Course Lectures,* 39: 557-563, 1990.

Campbell JC: Violence and our nation's health, *Healthcare Trends and Transition* 5(4):10-39, 1994.

Carrol P: Speed the essential response to anaphylaxis, *RN* 57(6):26-31, 1994.

Chez N: Helping the victim of domestic violence, *Am J Nurs* 94(7):33-37, 1994.

Dains J and others: *Standards of emergency nursing practice,* ed 2, St Louis, 1991, Mosby.

Devlin BK, Reynolds E: Child abuse: how to recognize it, how to intervene, *AJN* 94(4): 26-32, 1994.

Dubin WR, Tardiff K, Maier G: Overcoming danger with violent patients: guidelines for safe and effective management, *Emerg Med Rep* 13(14):105-112, 1992.

Dwyer B, Weissberg MP, Rund DA: Strategies for recognizing and managing suicidal patients, *Emerg Med Rep* 14(11): 91-98, 1993.

Emergency Nurses Association: *Orientation to emergency nursing: diversity in practice,* Chicago, 1993, The Association.

Emergency Nurses Association: Role of the emergency nurse in tissue and organ procurement, *Emergency Nurses Association position statement,* Chicago, 1992, The Association.

American College of Surgeons: *Resources for optimal care of the injured patient,* Philadelphia, 1990, The College.

Emergency Nurses Association: Telephone advice: *Emergency Nurses Association position statement,* Chicago, 1991, The Association.

Emergency Nurses Assocation: *Violence in the emergency setting, Emergency Nurses Association position statement,* Chicago, 1991, The Association.

Guidelines for cardiopulmonary resuscitation and emergency care, *JAMA* 268(16): 2185-2193, 1992.

Hays NK: What is a HEPA respirator and what does it mean to me? *JEMS* 19(1):74-76, 1994.

Hollingsworth HM and others: Anaphylaxis, *Emerg Med* 24(12):142-154, 1992.

IV conscious sedation guidelines published, *Penn Nurse* 47(5):7, 1992.

Jackson L: Quick response to hypothermia and frostbite, *Am J Nurs,* 95(3):52, March 1995.

Kinkle SL: Violence in the ED: how to stop it before it starts, *AJN* 93(7):22-24, 1993.

Klein AR and others: *Emergency nursing core curriculum,* ed 4, Philadelphia, 1994, WB Saunders.

Malestic S: Fight violence with forensic evidence, *RN* 58(1): 30-33, 1995.

Newell L and others: *Community first aid and safety,* St Louis, 1993, Mosby.

Parker V: Battered, *RN* 58(1):26-29, 1995.

Salber PS, Blair TMH: Battered women, *Top Emerg Med* 14(4): 78-84, 1992.

Salluzzo RF and others: Looking at your options: how to manage the head-injured patient, *Emerg Med Rep* 13(9):54-64, 1992.

Schneider SM: Hypothermia: from recognition to rewarming, *Emerg Med Rep* 13(1):1-10, 1992.

Sheehy SB: *Emergency nursing: principles and practice,* ed 3, St Louis, 1992, Mosby.

Somerson S, Justed C, Sicilia M: Insights into conscious sedation, *Am J Nurs* 95(6):26-33, 1995.

Stewart C: Acute hyperthermia: the spectrum of heat emergencies, *Emerg Med Rep* 14(16):133-144, 1993.

Stewart CH, Stewart CA, Weissberg M: Confronting the grim realities of elder abuse and neglect, *Emerg Med Rep* 12(20):179-186, 1991.

Trunkey D: Initial treatment of patients with extensive trauma, *N Engl J Med* 324(18):1259-1263, 1991.

Wainscott MP, Morgan DL, Shrestha M: Management of the difficult family in the emergency department, *Top Emerg Med* 14(4):1-11, 1992.

Weinman S: Emergency management of drug overdose, *Critical Care Nurs* 13(6):45-51, 1993.

Part V

20 Respiration
21 Circulation
22 Blood
23 Gastrointestinal Function
24 Urinary Function
25 Women's Reproductive Health
26 Men's Reproductive Health
27 Endocrine Function
28 Neurologic Function
29 Vision
30 Hearing
31 Skin Integrity
32 Mobility

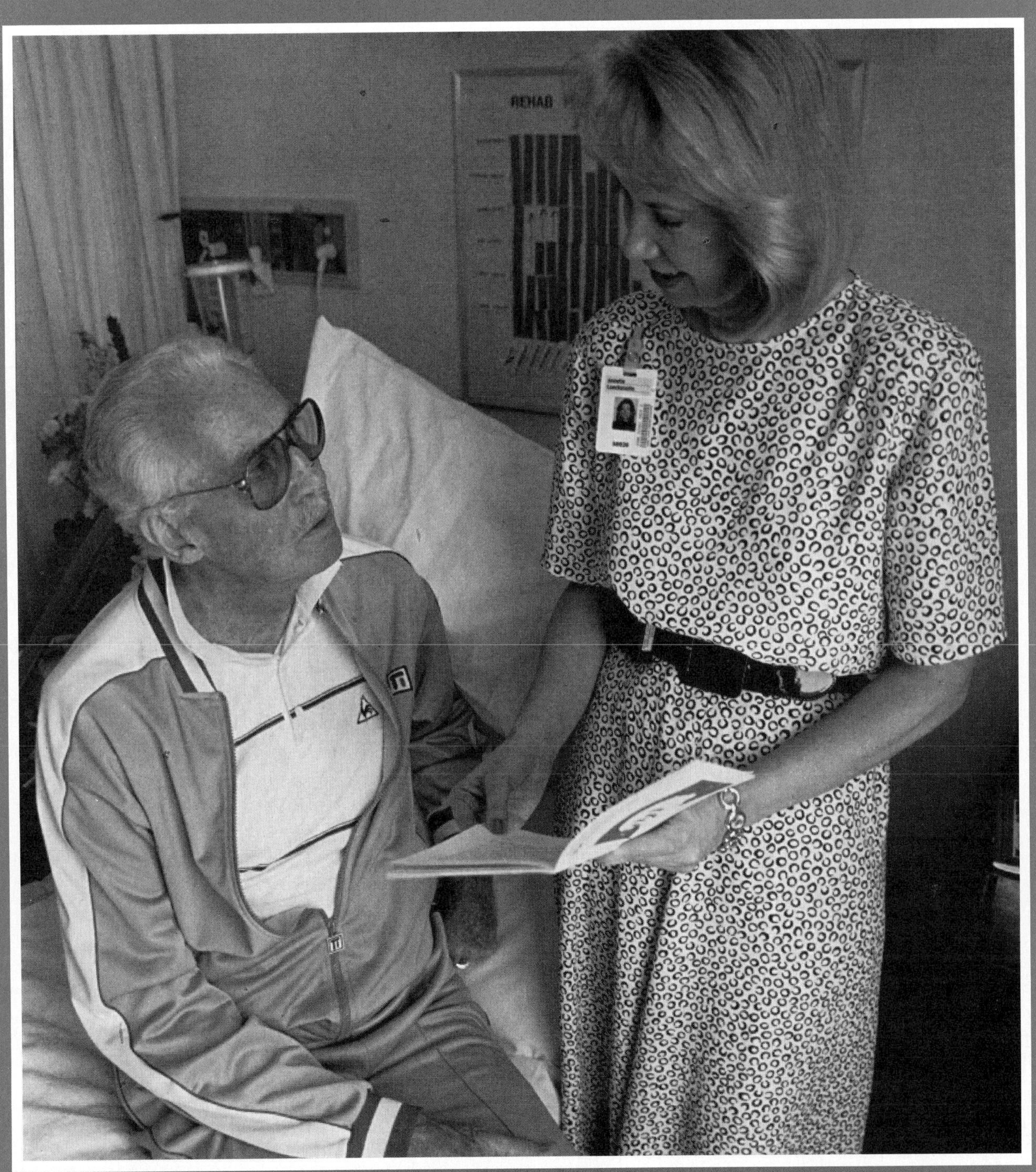

MEDICAL-SURGICAL PROBLEMS

CHAPTER 20

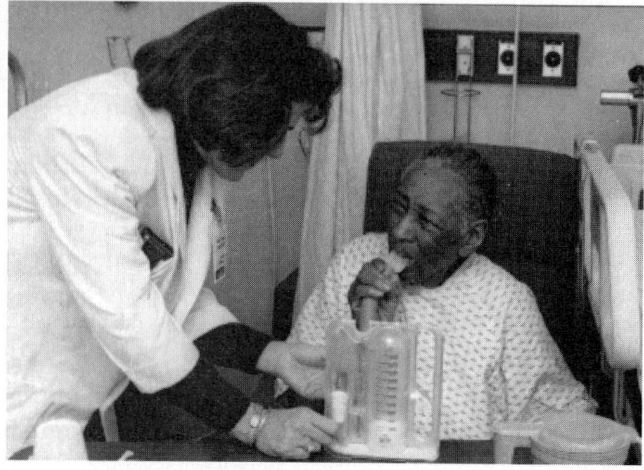

Respiration

CHAPTER OBJECTIVES

1 Describe the normal passage of oxygen and carbon dioxide through the respiratory system.
2 Describe how to obtain relevant subjective information from a patient who is experiencing alterations in respiratory function.
3 Discuss the elements to include when performing a physical examination of the respiratory system.
4 Describe the preparation and care of a patient who is undergoing diagnostic testing to evaluate the respiratory system.
5 Identify at least four nursing interventions that assist patients in reducing retained secretions in the tracheobronchial tree.
6 Describe nursing responsibilities involved when caring for a patient who is receiving oxygen therapy.
7 List at least three nursing observations that relate to the care of a patient with closed chest drainage.
8 Describe the significance of preoperative nursing assessment and patient teaching for a patient who is undergoing thoracic surgery.
9 Identify three actions the nurse can use to teach patients how to decrease the spread of respiratory tract infections.
10 Discuss patient education following a total laryngectomy.
11 Discuss the nursing care for patients with chronic obstructive pulmonary disease (COPD), including patient education.
12 Develop a nursing care plan for the patient with pneumonia.
13 Identify risk factors for the development of pulmonary embolism, and determine appropriate deep vein thrombosis prophylaxis given patient risk.
14 Discuss ways to prevent the development of atelectasis in the postoperative patient.
15 Describe types of chest trauma and nursing management for each.

KEY WORDS

adult respiratory distress syndrome (ARDS)
asthma
atelectasis
bronchitis
cyanosis
dyspnea
emphysema
epistaxis
hemoptysis
laryngectomy
lobectomy
pleurisy
pneumonectomy
pneumonia
pneumothorax
pulmonary embolism
thoracotomy
tonsillectomy
tracheostomy
tracheotomy
tuberculosis
ventilation

STRUCTURE AND FUNCTION OF THE RESPIRATORY SYSTEM

The primary function of the respiratory system is to provide oxygen to meet metabolic needs and to remove carbon dioxide, which is an end product of cellular metabolism. The structures of the upper respiratory system include the nose, pharynx, larynx, and trachea (Figure 20-1). The nose serves as a passageway for air to pass to and from the lungs. Impurities are trapped by nasal hair and moist mucous membranes, and air is humidified and warmed as it is inhaled into the lungs. The pharynx, or throat, is a tubelike structure with two main functions. It serves as a common pathway for air to enter the trachea and food to enter the esophagus, and it also plays an important role in the formation of sound, particularly vowel sounds. The pharynx connects the nasal and oral cavities to the larynx, which is commonly referred to as the "voice box." Air enters the larynx through the opened epiglottis, a flap of cartilage that covers the opening of the larynx during swallowing. The larynx contains the vocal cords and is located at the upper end of the trachea. The trachea is a 4- to 5-inch-long and 1-inch-wide tube composed of smooth muscle that is supported by regluarly spaced rings of cartilage and maintains an open passageway for airflow. At its lower end (the carina), the trachea divides into the right and left primary bronchi. The right main bronchus is shorter, more vertical, and has a larger diameter than the left bronchus. Because of these charac-

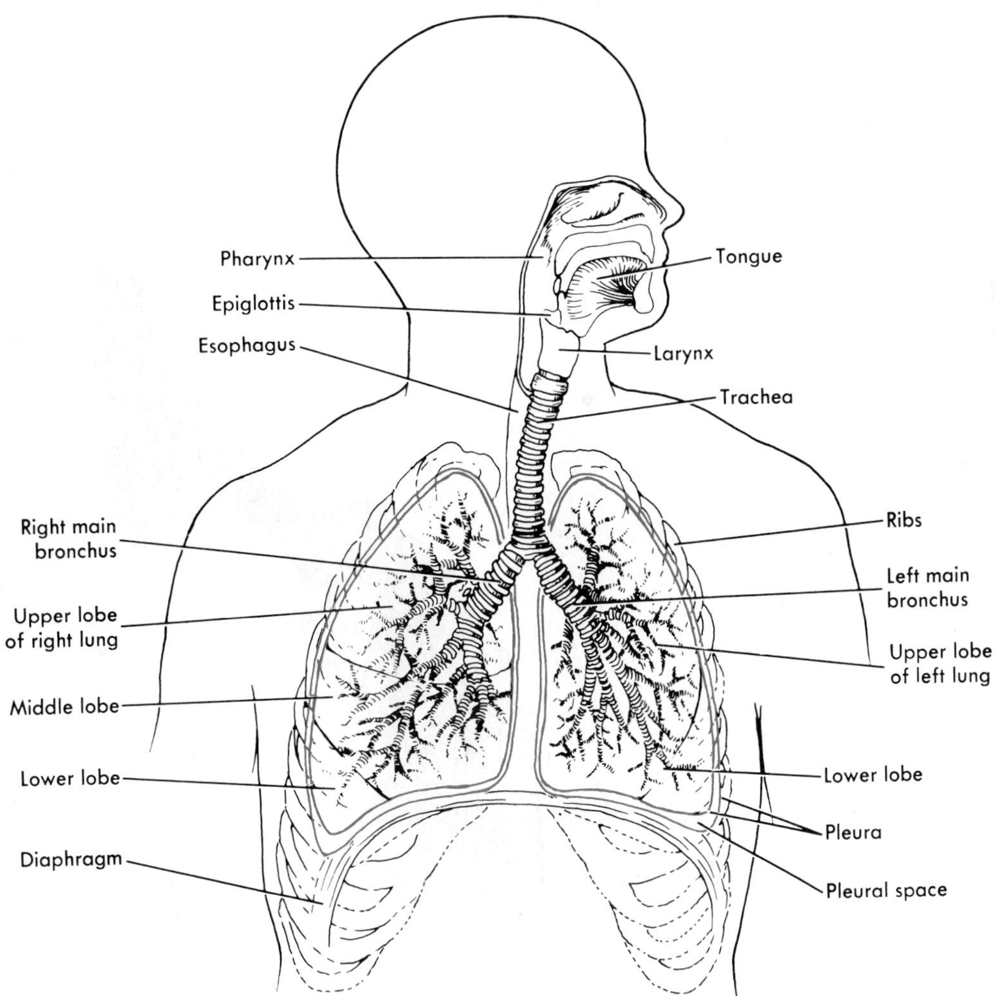

Figure 20-1 Anatomy of the thorax and lungs. (From Phipps WJ and others: *Medical surgical nursing: concepts and clinical practice,* ed 5, St Louis, 1995, Mosby.)

teristics, aspirated foreign bodies often lodge in the right lung (Sexton, 1990). Mucous membranes line the entire upper respiratory tract, and many of its cells contain fine hairlike projections called *cilia.* Mucus and impurities continually sweep toward the pharynx, where they are expectorated or swallowed.

The right and left bronchi, their subdivisions, and the lungs form the lower respiratory system (see Figure 20-1). The bronchi are similar in structure to the trachea and are lined with ciliated columnar epithelium. Each bronchus enters a lung, where it divides and branches to form bronchioles. This structure resembles an inverted tree. Further branching produces microscopic alveolar ducts, which end in alveolar sacs called *alveoli* (Figure 20-2). Inside each lung, 300 million alveoli are interlaced in a network of capillaries, where oxygen is transferred to the blood and carbon dioxide is removed from the blood and eliminated from the body. Some of the cells in the alveoli secrete a liquid called *surfactant,* which serves to increase lung compliance (ease of inflation) and to keep alveoli evenly inflated and dry (Porth, 1990).

The lungs are cone-shaped organs that are separated from each other by the mediastinum. The uppermost portion of the lung is called the apex, which extends approximately 1½ inches above the clavicle. The lower part of each lung is called the base. The left lung consists of two lobes, an upper and lower. The right lung has an upper, middle, and lower lobe. Each lobe is further divided into two to five segments that are separated by fissures and are extensions of the pleura (see Figure 20-2).

The lower part of the respiratory system and part of the trachea are enclosed in a bony framework known as the *thoracic cage.* The thoracic cage is separated from the abdominal cavity by the diaphragm, which contracts to create a partial vacuum during inspiration and relaxes during expiration, permitting abdominal organs to push upward and help force air from the lungs. The thoracic cavity is lined with a serous membrane, the *parietal pleura,* and each lung is enclosed in a saclike structure of serous membrane, the *visceral pleura.* A potential space exists between the layers of the parietal and visceral pleura. This space is lubricated by a small amount of pleural fluid, which allows the layers of the pleura to glide over each other during breathing. This pleural space can become inflamed and fill with air or fluid, causing a disruption in the negative pressure of the pleural cavity. This loss of normal negative pressure causes the lung to contract and eventually collapse.

Control of Breathing

Respiration is controlled primarily by the respiratory center in the medulla oblongata of the brain.

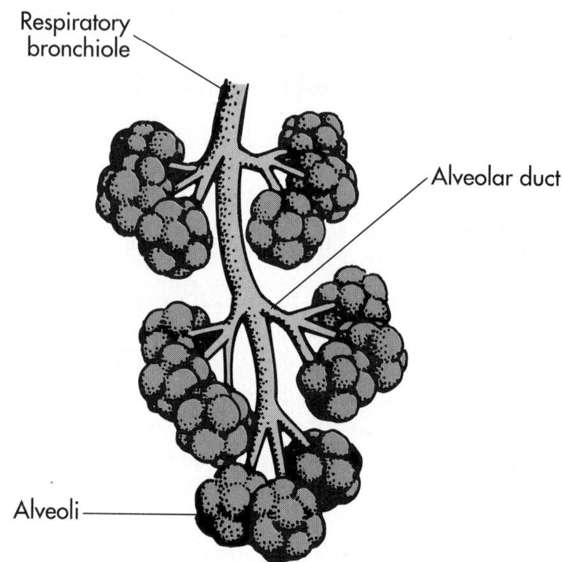

Figure 20-2 Microscopic illustration of alveolar sacs, where oxygen is transferred to blood and carbon dioxide is removed for elimination through the respiratory tract. (From Phipps WJ and others: *Medical-surgical nursing: concepts and clinical practice,* ed 5, St Louis, 1995, Mosby.)

The phrenic, glossopharyngeal, and vagus nerves innervate the diaphragm, larynx, tracheobronchial tree, and lungs, as well as transmit impulses to and from the respiratory center. Chemoreceptors also play a role in controlling breathing. A central chemoreceptor located in the medulla is sensitive to increases in the concentration of carbon dioxide and hydrogen in the cerebrospinal fluid. Additional chemoreceptors located in the aortic arch (aortic bodies) and at the carotid bifurcation (carotid bodies) respond to decreases in oxygen and pH and increases in carbon dioxide (Porth, 1990).

Ventilation

The function of the respiratory system is to exchange gases, which is accomplished through the process of respiration. Respiration is both external and internal. External respiration **(ventilation)** consists of the movement of oxygen into the lungs (inhalation) and the removal of carbon dioxide out of the lungs (exhalation). During the inhalation phase, oxygen from inspired air passes through the permeable membranes of the alveoli and capillaries and reaches the blood. Oxygen combines with hemoglobin in the red blood cells and is transported by the circulatory system to the body cells. Internal respiration is the process by which oxygen is transferred from blood to body cells and carbon dioxide is passed from body cells to blood to be eliminated from the body.

OLDER ADULT CONSIDERATIONS

Physiologic changes in the respiratory system

At all times during the life cycle, the respiratory system is vulnerable to injuries caused by infections, environmental pollutants, and allergic reactions. These are often far more damaging to the system than the decline in function that is a normal component of aging.

Age-related changes include an increased susceptibility to infection because of a decline in the protection normally provided by the intact mucous barrier, a decrease in the effectiveness of the bronchial cilia, and changes in the composition of the connective tissues of the lungs and chest. Elderly persons rely far more on the diaphragm for inspiration, and breathing requires more effort, especially when lying down. Vital capacity declines with age, and it takes longer to inspire or expire air because of the decline in the elastic recoil of the lungs and an increase in the stiffness of the chest wall. Although total lung volume does not change significantly, residual volume increases; and although the alveolar partial pressure of oxygen usually does not change, the alveolar-capillary gradient does increase slightly.

From Beare PG, Myers JL: *Principles and practice of adult health nursing,* ed 2, St Louis, 1994, Mosby.

BOX 20-1

DYSPNEA DESCRIPTORS

TIMING
Chronic or acute
Episodic or paroxysmal
Onset
Duration
Frequency

CHARACTERISTICS
Perceived severity
Phase of respiratory cycle
- Inspiratory
- Expiratory
- Throughout entire cycle

Other symptoms related to dyspnea
Associated factors
- Time of day
- Seasonal or weather changes
- Environmental irritants
- Anxiety
- Body position
  - Paroxysmal nocturnal dyspnea (PND): sudden onset while sleeping in recumbent position
  - Orthopnea: breathlessness upon assuming recumbent position

From Phipps WJ and others: *Medical-surgical nursing: concepts and clinical practice,* ed 5, St Louis, 1995, Mosby.

ASSESSMENT OF SIGNS AND SYMPTOMS OF RESPIRATORY DISEASE

The signs and symptoms most closely associated with respiratory disease are dyspnea, chest pain, cough, sputum production, wheezing, hemoptysis, and cyanosis.

Dyspnea

When breathing becomes difficult or labored and requires considerable exertion, patients are said to have **dyspnea,** which is a highly subjective symptom of respiratory difficulty that involves both a physiologic and a cognitive component (Box 20-1) (Gift, 1990). It may result from pain, pulmonary disease, anemia, heart failure, obstruction such as from a pulmonary embolism, or emotional factors. When patients are unable to breathe except in a sitting position, they are said to have orthopnea. Orthopnea may occur in individuals with chronic obstructive pulmonary disease (COPD) and heart disease. Dyspnea is one of the most frightening symptoms for patients and their families. Patients often feel their lives are threatened, and as they become more anxious, their dyspnea may increase. The nurse caring for a patient with dyspnea should be calm, reassuring, and confident and should attempt to determine the underlying cause of the problem. Relief may be achieved by elevating the person's head. Supplemental oxygen may be necessary if dyspnea continues or worsens.

Chest Pain

Chest pain of a pulmonary origin may result from a variety of conditions such as pulmonary embolism, pneumonia, pleurisy, and lung cancer (Beare, Meyers, 1994; Smeltzer, Bare, 1992). The pain may be described as sharp, stabbing, dull, aching, diffuse, or localized (Table 20-1). It is important to determine not only the location of the pain but also its onset, duration, quality, quantity, and the setting in which it occurs. The nurse should also be alert to the alleviation of the pain and what aggravates it.

Cough

An irritation of mucous membranes anywhere in the respiratory tract can produce a cough. Coughing pro-

TABLE 20-1

Thoracic-pulmonary chest pain

Origin	Characteristics	Possible Cause
Chest wall	Well-localized constant ache increasing with movement	Trauma; cough; herpes zoster
Pleura	Sharp, abrupt onset increasing with inspiration or with sudden ventilatory effect (cough, sneeze), unilateral	Pleural inflammation (pleurisy); pulmonary infarction; pneumothorax; tumors
Lung parenchyma	Dull, constant ache, poorly localized	Benign pulmonary tumors; carcinoma; pneumothorax

From Phipps WJ and others: *Medical-surgical nursing: concepts and clinical practice,* ed 5, St Louis, 1995, Mosby.

tects the lungs against the accumulation of secretions in the bronchi and bronchioles. It is often stimulated by an infectious process or by irritants present in the air, such as smoke (Beare, Meyers, 1994; Patrick and others, 1991; Smeltzer, Bare, 1992). Coughing may also indicate pulmonary disease (Kersten, 1989). It is important to consider when the cough began (onset). A cough of recent onset is often seen with an acute infectious process.

The quality of the cough is also important. Is the cough productive, nonproductive, dry, moist, brassy, barking, hoarse, or hacking? The nurse should ask the patient whether he or she has noticed if the quality of the cough has changed over time. A severe or changing cough may be associated with bronchogenic carcinoma. The nurse should note at what time of the day the cough occurs and if it is brought on by specific activities, body positions, or movements.

Coughing at night may be associated with failure on the left side of the heart. Coughing during eating may indicate aspiration of ingested materials into the tracheobronchial tree. Individuals with bronchitis may complain of a productive cough, especially in the morning (Beare, Meyers, 1994; Phipps, 1995; Smeltzer, Bare; 1992).

Sputum Production

The goblet cells and mucous glands of the lung secrete mucus that coats the interior lung surface. The lung cilia propel mucus upward toward the pharynx. Sputum production is the reaction of the lungs to any continual irritant.

To evaluate and visually inspect sputum production, have the patient cough into a white tissue or clean cup with a white interior surface (Kersten, 1989). Sputum is evaluated for color, amount, and consistency. The color and consistency of the sputum may point to specific diseases. For example, creamy yellow sputum often occurs with staphylococcal pneumonia, and pink frothy sputum occurs with pulmonary edema. Any change in sputum color should be investigated. The change may be from the normal anticipated sputum color or from the patient's baseline color.

Wheezing

Wheezing is often found in patients who have bronchoconstriction, or airway narrowing. Wheezes are further assessed during the physical examination of the respiratory system when the breath sounds are evaluated.

Hemoptysis

Hemoptysis is the coughing up of blood from the respiratory tract. The most common causes of hemoptysis are pulmonary infection, lung cancer, abnormalities of the heart or blood vessels, pulmonary embolism and infarction, and pulmonary artery or vein abnormalities (Beare, Meyers, 1994; Smeltzer, Bare, 1992).

A good history and physical examination help diagnose any underlying respiratory disease, and a diagnostic evaluation often includes blood testing, chest x-ray examinations, and bronchoscopy. Additional studies may need to be performed to identify the source of the bleeding because the bleeding may be coming from the gums, upper respiratory tract, lungs and adjacent structures, or the stomach.

True hemoptysis usually contains some frothy portions of bright red blood and is followed by blood-tinged sputum for several days as the site of injury in the lung heals. The pH is alkaline (> 7). Hematemesis refers to the vomiting of blood from the stomach. If hematemesis is suspected rather than hemoptysis, consider the patient's history, which usually is that of gastric problems, liver disease, or alcoholism. (Phipps, 1995). Food particles may be evident in the vomitus; the blood is dark red, never frothy; and the pH is acidic (< 7).

Cyanosis

Cyanosis is characterized by a bluish discoloration of the skin and mucous membranes. Peripheral cyanosis may be observed at the earlobes, the tip of the nose, or the fingertips. Because peripheral cyanosis may be caused by vasoconstriction as a result of cold or nervousness, it is not a reliable indicator of inadequate oxygenation. Central cyanosis may be evident at the lips, tongue, or inside the mouth, where the tissue is usually warm. For cyanosis to appear here, at least 5 g/dl of reduced hemoglobin must be present. This level approximates the oxygen saturation of venous blood (Smeltzer, 1992). Although the presence of cyanosis should be identified, it must be noted that the absence of it does not guarantee adequate arterial oxygenation. The overall status of the patient must be considered, and the conditions that influence oxygenation must be identified (Hudak, Gallo, Benz, 1990; Kersten, 1989).

NURSING ASSESSMENT OF THE PATIENT WITH A RESPIRATORY PROBLEM

History

Individuals with altered respiratory function may seek healthcare for a variety of complaints, including dyspnea, chest pain, coughing, sputum production, hemoptysis, or cyanosis. When obtaining a respiratory history, it is important to determine why the patient is seeking healthcare. Any complaint should be explored, and the symptom should be evaluated for onset, duration, location, quality, quantity, setting, precipitating factors, aggravating and alleviating factors, and associated signs and symptoms. It is also important to consider smoking habits, exercise tolerance, allergens, environmental pollutants, recent respiratory tract infections, exposure to others with respiratory tract infections, medications, and occupational respiratory hazards.

Physical Examination

Following the history, a systematic physical assessment of the patient is performed. An assessment of the lungs and thorax involves the techniques of inspection, palpation, percussion, and auscultation.

Inspection

The first step in respiratory tract assessment is *inspection*. Both the anterior and posterior sides of the chest are observed for lesions, scars, skin color, and any deformities (Figures 20-3 and 20-4). Normally the ratio of the anterior-posterior diameter to the lateral diameter is 1:2. An increased diameter results in a barrel chest, which is a sign of COPD (Figure 20-5). Other

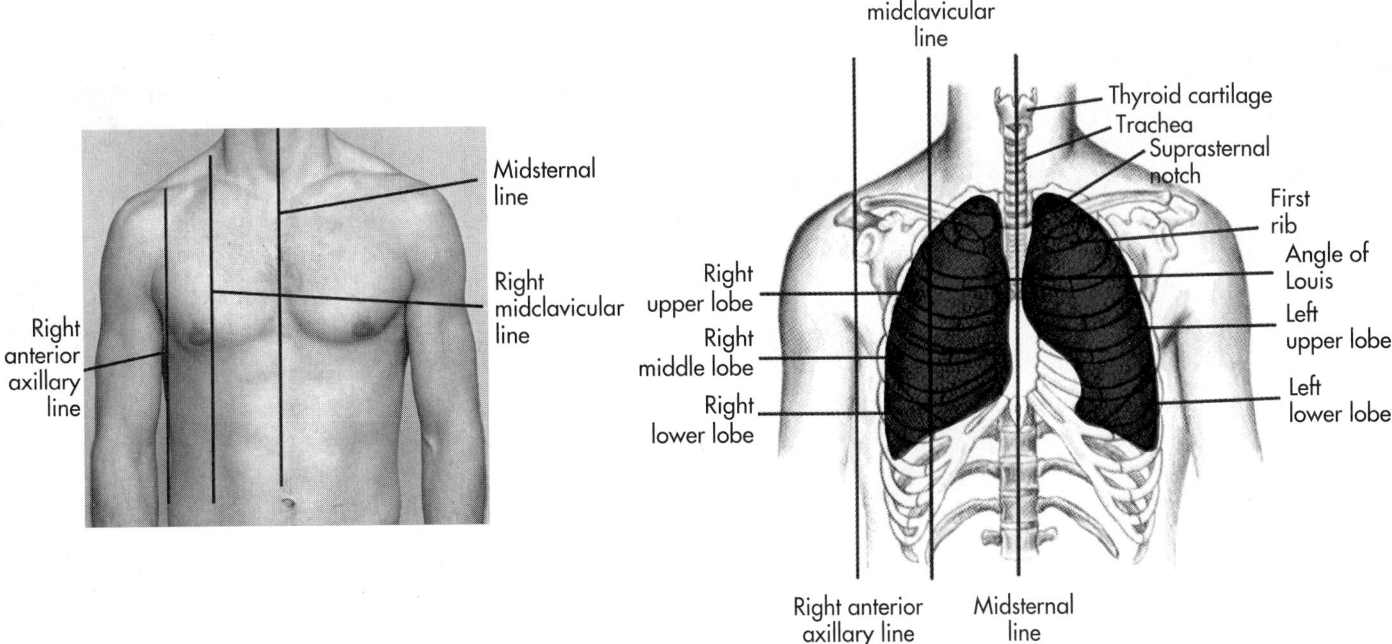

Figure 20-3 Anterior thorax landmarks. (From Seidel HM and others: *Mosby's guide to physical examination*, ed 3, St Louis, 1995, Mosby.)

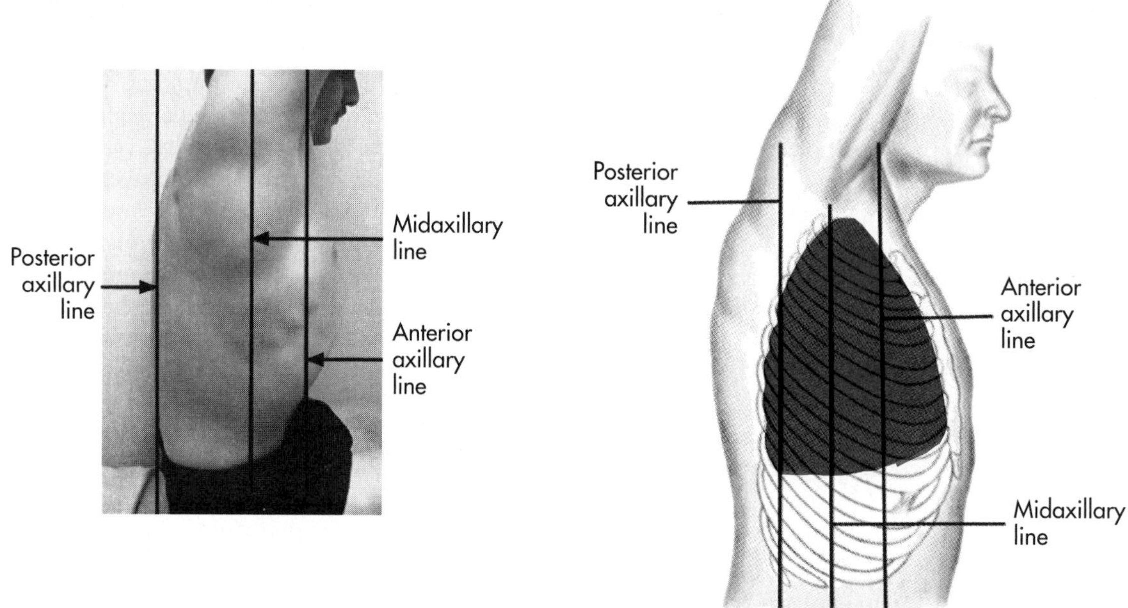

Figure 20-4 Right lateral thorax landmarks. (From Seidel HM and others: *Mosby's guide to physical examination,* ed 3, St Louis, 1995, Mosby.)

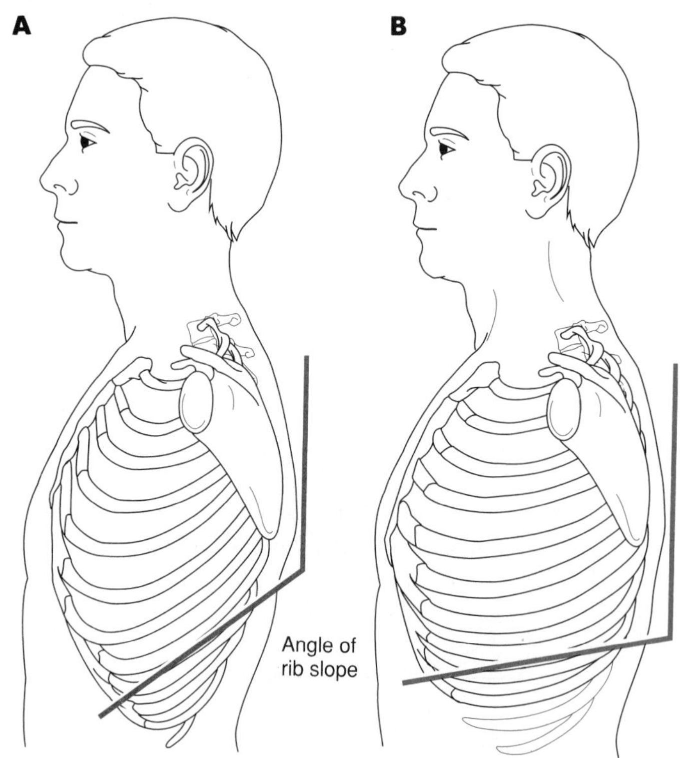

Figure 20-5 **A,** Patient with normal thoracic configuration. **B,** Patient with an increased anteroposterior diameter. Note contrast in the angle of the slope of the ribs. (From Barkauskas VH and others: *Health and physical assessment,* St Louis, 1994, Mosby.)

chest deformities associated with respiratory disease that might be evident are pigeon chest, funnel chest, and kyphoscoliosis. In kyphoscoliosis there is a progressive musculoskeletal deformity characterized by lateral and posterior angulations of the spine, similar to the deformities that occur with osteoporosis or skeletal disorders (Kersten, 1989).

The rate, depth, type, and quality of respirations are assessed (Table 20-2). The nurse should consider the following questions during the examination (Malasanos, Barkauskas, Stoltenberg-Allen, 1990; Siedel and others, 1991):

- Is the breathing regular or irregular?
- Are the respirations deep or shallow?
- Do both sides of the chest expand equally?
- Is the patient experiencing intercostal retractions?
- Is cyanosis of nailbeds, lips, and mucous membranes present?
- Is the breathing pattern abdominal, thoracic, or paradoxic?

Palpation

The second step in the physical examination is *palpation.* The patient should be in a sitting position, although a supine position is acceptable if the patient is unable to sit up. The nurse places warmed hands side by side, with the thumbs close together and the fingers spread out over the anterior chest wall. The patient takes several deep breaths, and the respiratory move-

TABLE 20-2

Characteristics of Commonly Observed Respiratory Patterns

Type of Respiration	Diagram	Discussion
Normal		2-20 respirations/min in adults; regular in rhythm; ratio of respiratory rate to pulse rate is 1:4
Hyperventilation or Kussmaul's respiration		Increase in both rate and depth; hyperpnea is an increase in depth only
Periodic respiration		Alternating hyperpnea, shallow respiration, and apnea; sometimes called Cheyne-Stokes respiration; often occurs in the severely ill
Sighing respiration		Deep and audible; audible portion sounds like a sigh
Air trapping		Present in obstructive pulmonary diseases; air is trapped in the lungs; respiratory level rises, and breathing becomes shallow
Biot's breathing		Shallow breathing interrupted by apnea; seen in some CNS disorders and in healthy persons

From Barkauskas VH and others: *Health and physical assessment,* St Louis, 1994, Mosby.

ments of both sides of the chest are compared. The nurse's thumbs should move apart at the same time and be equally distant. The patterns of expansion and contraction are noted, as well as equal or unequal expansion, depression of the chest wall during inspiration, degree of expansion, and diaphragmatic excursion. The nurse palpates the chest for any painful areas, swelling, masses, or crepitation. The trachea is palpated for position. It should be vertical and stretch downward on inspiration. The nurse repeats the procedure on the posterior chest wall (Malasanos, Barkauskas, Stoltenberg-Allen, 1990; Siedel and others, 1991).

Assessment of fremitus. A useful technique for palpation is tactile fremitus. This technique requires practice but can support other assessment findings. Vocal, or tactile, fremitus is the palpation of the vibrations of the thoracic wall that are produced by the normal spoken word. The nurse places the hand palm-down on the chest wall, has the patient repeat the phrase "ninety-nine" or "blue moon," and compares the transmission of the vibration on both sides of the chest (Figure 20-6). An increase in fremitus occurs with secretions or consolidation in the lung, as in pneumonia or atelectasis. Bronchial obstruction or the presence of air or fluid in the pleural space causes a decrease in or an absence of fremitus (Table 20-3).

Percussion

The third step in the respiratory assessment is *percussion* (Figure 20-7). Tapping the surface of the chest wall with the fingers produces sounds that may indicate changes in lung density:

- *Resonance* is the normal sound; it is hollow, low pitched, nonmusical, and loudest where the chest is thinnest.

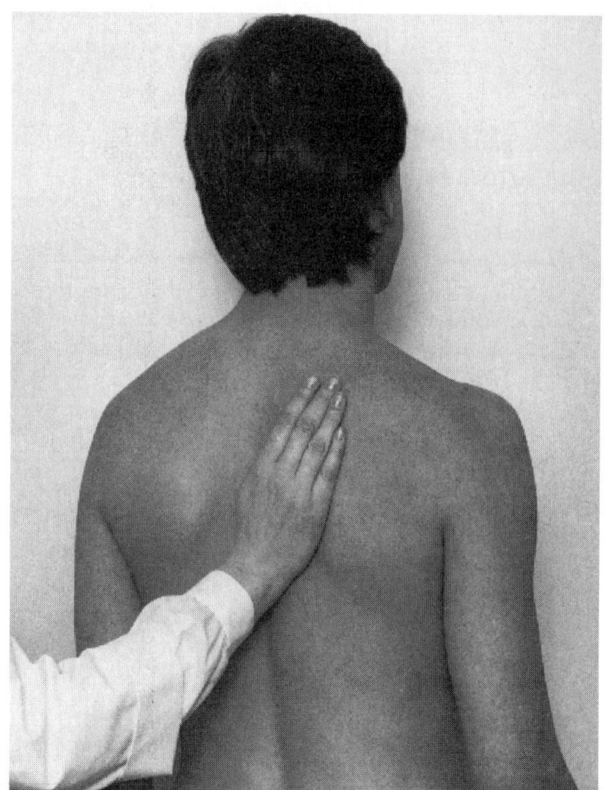

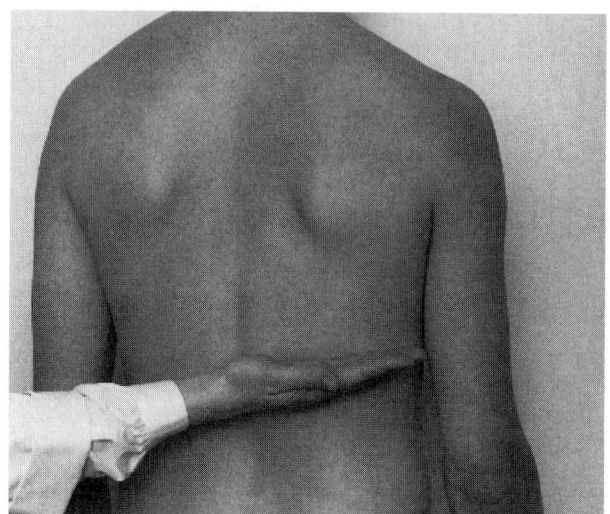

Figure 20-6 Palpitation for assessment of vocal fremitus. (From Barkauskas VH and others: *Health and physical assessment,* St Louis, 1994, Mosby.)

TABLE 20-3

Characteristics of Normal and Abnormal Tactile Fremitus

Type of fremitus	Characteristics
Normal (moderate) fremitus	Varies greatly from person to person and depends on the intensity and pitch of the voice, the position and distance of the bronchi in relation to the chest wall, and the thickness of the chest wall; fremitus is most intense in the second intercostal spaces at the sternal border near the area of bronchial bifurcation
Increased tactile fremitus	May occur in pneumonia, compressed lung, lung tumor, or pulmonary fibrosis; a solid medium of uniform structure conducts vibrations with greater intensity than a porous medium
Decreased or absent tactile fremitus	Occurs when there is diminished production of sounds, a diminished transmission of sounds, or the addition of a medium through which sounds must pass before reaching the thoracic wall, such as in pleural effusion, pleural thickening, pneumothorax, bronchial obstruction, or emphysema
Pleural friction rub	Vibration produced by inflamed pleural surfaces rubbing together; felt as a grating, is synchronous with respiratory movements, and is more commonly felt on inspiration
Rhonchial fremitus	Coarse vibrations produced by the passage of air through thick exudates in the large air passages; can be cleared or altered by coughing

Modified from Barkauskas V and others: *Health and physical assessment,* St Louis, 1994, Mosby.

- *Dullness* is heard normally over the scapulae and heavy shoulder muscles and over solid organs such as the heart and liver. An area of consolidation, which can occur in pneumonia, produces a dull sound.
- A *tympanic* sound may be heard over an area where air is trapped, such as in the hyperinflated lung of a patient with emphysema. The tympanic sound is louder, longer, higher pitched, and drumlike.

OLDER ADULT CONSIDERATIONS

Respiratory Assessment

GENERAL APPROACH

- Allow more time than for a younger adult.
- Articulate clearly; the elderly patient may be hearing impaired.
- Provide clear, concise instructions.

HISTORY COLLECTION

- Use fewer open-ended questions and provide some choices as needed, such as "Is your chest pain dull, sharp, aching, or stabbing?"
- Repeat questions as needed.
- Be alert for answers that do not appear appropriate. The patient may not have understood the question correctly because of impaired hearing or impaired comprehension.

PHYSICAL ASSESSMENT

- The physical examination itself is not different, but the approach may need to be altered so that the appropriate information is assessed without undue discomfort or embarrassment for the patient.
- Provide an environment with minimal noise, distraction, and interruption.
- Require as few position changes as possible.
- Kyphosis is associated with aging.
- Chest expansion may be decreased.
- Breathing may be more shallow.
- Crackles may be present in the bases in the absence of respiratory or cardiovascular disease secondary to atelectasis or fibrotic lung changes.

Modified from Beare PG, Myers JL: *Principles and practice of adult health nursing,* ed 2, St Louis, 1994, Mosby.

Auscultation

The final step in the assessment procedure is *auscultation* (see Figure 20-7). The patient is instructed to maintain a sitting position and to take slow, deep breaths through the mouth. The surroundings should be calm and quiet, and the room temperature should be comfortable. The diaphragm of the stethoscope is placed firmly against the chest wall to decrease the sounds produced by skin or hair rubbing against it. A systematic approach is used, starting at the right scapular area and comparing the sounds heard there with the sounds heard in the left scapular area. The nurse continues down both sides of the posterior side of the chest to the base of the lungs. The procedure is repeated on the anterior side of the chest, and both sides are compared. The nurse should listen through several respiratory cycles over each area.

Breath sounds reveal important data about a patient's condition. The sounds should be evaluated for location, pitch, quality, intensity, and duration of inspiration and expiration. The nurse should distinguish between three normal types of breath sounds. *Vesicular breath sounds* are heard over most of the normal lung as air passes into the alveoli. They are soft, low-pitched, breezy sounds with an inspiratory phase greater than the expiratory phase. *Bronchial breath sounds* are normally heard over the trachea. If heard elsewhere, they are abnormal and indicate areas of consolidation. Bronchial sounds are loud, high pitched, and hollow with an expiratory phase greater than the inspiratory phase. *Bronchovesicular breath sounds* are heard anteriorly over the mainstem bronchi on either side of the sternum in the first and second intercostal space. They are heard posteriorly between the scapulae. If heard elsewhere, they are abnormal. Bronchovesicular sounds are a mixture of vesicular and bronchial sounds and are softer and slightly lower-pitched than bronchial sounds, and their inspiratory and expiratory phases are nearly equal (Tables 20-4 and 20-5). Decreased or absent breath sounds may occur with shallow breathing, obesity, barrel chest, or fluid in the lung tissue.

Abnormal breath sounds, called *adventitious sounds,* may be superimposed over normal breath sounds and include crackles, rhonchi, wheezes, and pleural friction rubs. When describing adventitious breath sounds, the nurse should include the type, location, and timing of the sound (Kersten, 1989; Siedel and others, 1991).

Crackles (rales) are caused by the passage of air through moisture or secretions in the alveoli and small airways and are described as fine, medium, or coarse (Dossey, Guzzetta, Kenner, 1990; Malasanos, Barkauskas, Stoltenberg-Allen, 1990). Crackles resemble the sound of a cellophane wrapper being gently crinkled and can also be simulated by rubbing pieces of hair together between the fingers. They usually are heard only on inspiration. *Rhonchi* and *wheezes* are caused by air passing through the larger airways that have been narrowed by the accumulation of fluids and secretions, by mucosal edema, or by smooth muscle spasms. Rhonchi usually are heard more often on expiration and are described as musical, bubbling, or snoring sounds. Wheezes may be expiratory, inspiratory, or both. *Pleural friction rubs* are caused by the inflamed pleural linings rubbing together. They produce a grating, squeaking sound, such as that produced when two pieces of leather are rubbed together. The absence of normal breath sounds in their proper locations should also be considered abnormal.

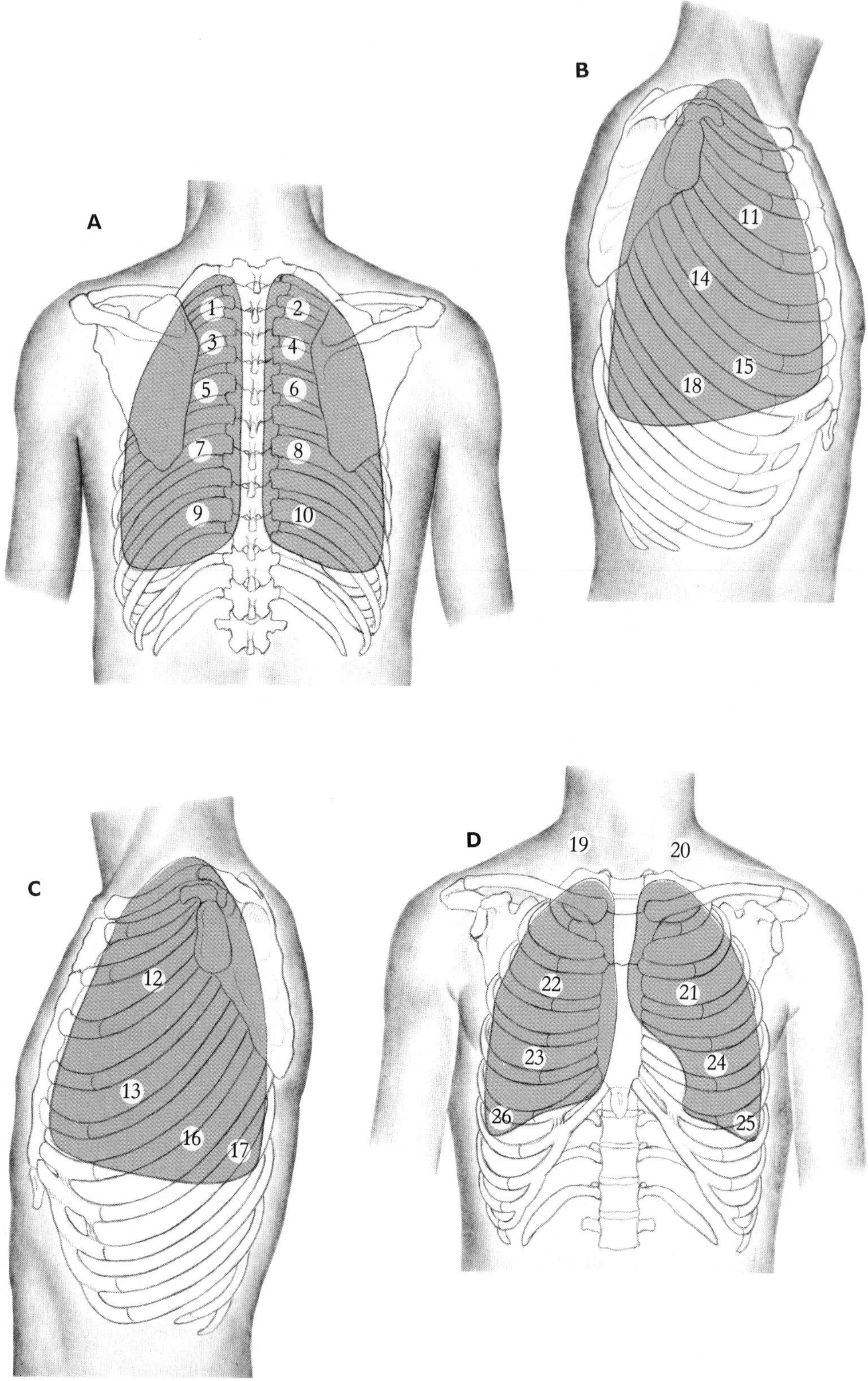

Figure 20-7 Suggested sequence for systematic percussion and auscultation of the thorax. **A,** Posterior thorax. **B,** Right lateral thorax. **C,** Left lateral thorax. **D,** Anterior thorax. (From Seidel HM and others: *Mosby's guide to physical examination,* ed 3, St Louis, 1995, Mosby.)

TABLE 20-4

Characteristics of Breath Sounds

Sound	Duration of Inspiration and Expiration	Diagram of Sound	Pitch	Intensity	Normal Location	Abnormal Location
Vesicular	Inspiration > expiration 2.5:1		Low	Soft	Peripheral lung	Not applicable
Bronchovesicular	Inspiration = expiration 1:1		Medium	Medium	First and second intercostal spaces at sternal border anteriorly; posteriorly at T4 medial to scapulae	Peripheral lung
Bronchial (tubular)	Inspiration < expiration 1:2		High	Loud	Over trachea	Lung area

From Barkauskas VH and others: *Health and physical assessment,* St Louis, 1994, Mosby

TABLE 20-5

Origin and Characteristics of Adventitious Sounds

Sound	Diagram of Sound	Origin	Characteristics
Crackles*—fine to medium		Air passing through moisture in small air passages and alveoli	Discrete, discontinuous; inspiratory; have a dry or wet crackling quality; not cleared by coughing; sound is simulated by rolling a lock of hair near the ear
Crackles*—medium to coarse		Air passing through moisture in the bronchioles, bronchi, and trachea	As above; louder than fine crackles
Wheezes—sonorous		Air passing through air passages narrowed by secretions, swelling, tumors, and so on	Continuous sounds; originate in large air passages; may be inspiratory and expiratory but usually predominate in expiration; low-pitched, moaning or snoring quality; coughing may alter sounds
Wheezes—sibilant		Same as sonorous wheezes	Continuous sounds; originate in the small air passages; may be inspiratory and expiratory but usually predominated in expiration; high-pitched, wheezing sounds
Friction rubs		Rubbing together of inflamed and roughened pleural surfaces	Creaking or grating quality; superficial sounding; inspiratory and expiratory; heard most often in the lower anterolateral chest (area of greatest thoracic expansion); coughing has no effect

From Barkauskas VH and others: *Health and physical assessment,* St Louis, 1994, Mosby.
*Crackles are also called rales or crepitations.

LABORATORY DIAGNOSTIC EVALUATION

Blood Examinations

Routine blood examinations are usually ordered for patients with respiratory disease and may include a red blood cell count, white blood cell count, and hemoglobin determination. Abnormal increases in the number of white blood cells may indicate the mobilization of the body's defenses against a respiratory tract infection, whereas significant decreases in red blood cells and hemoglobin decrease the oxygen-carrying capacity of the blood. Depending on the specific diagnosis of respiratory disease, additional blood studies may be required.

Arterial Blood Gas Studies

Blood gas analysis provides important information that is necessary in the diagnosis and treatment of patients with acute and chronic lung diseases. The values obtained assess the ability of the lungs to provide adequate oxygen and remove carbon dioxide and the ability of the kidneys to excrete or reabsorb bicarbonate ions to maintain normal body pH (Kischbach, 1992; Kersten, 1989; Smeltzer, Bare 1992).

The partial pressure of oxygen (Pao_2) indicates the degree of oxygenation of the blood. The oxygen saturation (Sao_2) reflects the percentage of hemoglobin bound with oxygen. The partial pressure of carbon dioxide ($Paco_2$) indicates the adequacy of alveolar ventilation. The pH and plasma bicarbonate concentration (HCO_3) reflect acid-base balance (Table 20-6).

Sputum Examination

The examination of sputum is done by persons trained in laboratory methods, but the collection of the specimen is usually a nursing responsibility. Sputum consists of material that is expectorated from the lungs, and it may contain pathogenic and nonpathogenic organisms. If sputum is to be used for diagnosis, it must be collected correctly. Specimens should be collected early in the morning, when sputum production usually is greatest. Before collection, patients should rinse their mouths with clear water, after which they should be encouraged to cough deeply and expectorate into a sterile container.

If an adequate specimen is not obtained, sputum may be obtained by inducing coughing with aerosolized mist inhalations or nasotracheal suctioning. The physician may also obtain a transtracheal aspirate through the cricothyroid membrane via a needle puncture and the introduction of a fine catheter through the needle and into the trachea. The catheter is left in place, and sterile saline is injected into the catheter to loosen secretions and promote coughing. The material is aspirated back through the catheter into a syringe (Smeltzer, Bare, 1992).

If the patient is intubated, tracheal aspiration is accomplished by attaching a mucous trap to the suction source during routine suctioning of sputum. The specimen should be properly labeled and sent immediately to the laboratory.

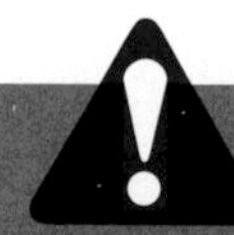

NURSE ALERT

The first sputum coughed up in the morning usually contains the most organisms.

The general appearance of sputum depends on the types of substances and pathogenic organisms it contains. Normally sputum is odorless, but in suppurative conditions of the lungs, such as a lung abscess, it may have a foul odor. Sputum examination using Papanicolaou's (Pap) smear technique may be useful in detecting the presence of cancer cells. The amount, odor, and appearance of all sputum should be recorded on the patient's record.

Pulmonary Function Tests

Pulmonary function tests (PFTs) evaluate lung function and may indicate the existence of some impairment or the necessity for additional investigation. They also are used to monitor the patient's respiratory status when disease is present and to evaluate the effectiveness of the therapy instituted. PFTs are useful in evaluating individuals scheduled for upper abdominal or thoracic procedures who have preexisting pulmonary risk factors, including smoking, obesity, dyspnea, cough, or COPD (Huddleston, 1990; Kersten, 1989).

The most common pulmonary function tests are performed by spirometry, which measures lung volumes and capacities and flow rates (Kischbach, 1992). Lung volumes and capacities are measured to determine the amount of air that can be inhaled and exhaled. Flow-rate measurements are used to evaluate the ability of the individual to move air into and out of the lungs. Flow-rate determinations are helpful in identifying whether altered respiratory muscle strength, lung and chest wall compliance, or airway and lung tissue resistance have affected lung function (Kersten, 1989). Essentially, test values are flow rates during forced breathing maneuvers, usually forced exhalation.

TABLE 20-6

Normal Blood Gas Values of Arterial Blood*

$Paco_2$: Partial pressure of carbon dioxide in arterial blood; gives information about the adequacy of ventilation	34-45 mm Hg
Pao_2: Partial pressure of oxygen; the amount of oxygen dissolved in arterial blood	80-100 mm Hg
Sao_2: Percent saturation of hemoglobin with oxygen in arterial blood	97%-100%
pH: Hydrogen ion concentration in the blood; acidity/alkalinity of blood sample	7.35-7.45
HCO_3: Plasma bicarbonate concentration; a measurement of the nonrespiratory contribution to acid-base balance	24-30 mEq/L

*Arterial blood should be obtained through either a puncture of an artery, such as the femoral or radial, with a small needle or from a catheter previously placed into the artery. All air is expelled after the sample is obtained, and the sample is placed on ice and sent immediately to the laboratory for analysis. If an artery was entered to obtain the sample, direct pressure is applied for at least 5 minutes. If the radial artery is to be used to obtain the arterial sample, the Allen's test should be performed, which evaluates the patency of the radial and ulnar arteries. With the Allen's test, the patient is asked to make a fist. The radial and ulnar arteries are then simultaneously compressed, which causes the hand to blanch. The patient is asked to open the fist, and the pressure on the ulnar artery is released while pressure on the radial artery is maintained. The hand turns pink if the ulnar artery is patent. (Malasanos, Barkauskas, Stotlenberg-Allen, 1990, Siedel and others, 1991).

During spirometry, the patient sits upright with a noseclip in place. All tight clothing is loosened, and the patient breathes into a mouthpiece connected to a spirometer. A graphic recording (spirogram) is produced. Test results are interpreted on the basis of age, height, weight, and gender. Patient results are compared to normal values that have been established (Box 20-2).

Although nurses usually do not perform the PFT, they should relieve any apprehension that patients may have by explaining the purpose of the procedure because patient cooperation is important for accurate results. When PFTs are performed preoperatively, the information obtained may allow the nurse to plan preoperative teaching and postoperative interventions, which may include coughing and deep breathing, use of the incentive spirometer, medication education, and information on smoking cessation.

Radiographic Examination

The chest x-ray examination is one of the most common of all radiographic procedures. It is useful in detecting disease of the chest or in monitoring change over time. Many hospitals require routine chest x-ray films of all admitted patients.

Because normal pulmonary tissue is radiolucent (allows the x-ray beam to pass through it), densities produced by tumors, foreign bodies, or other conditions may be detected on an x-ray film (Smeltzer, Bare, 1992). A routine chest film consists of posteroanterior (PA) and lateral views. Individuals are usually instructed to take a deep breath and hold it. Once the film is obtained, they are instructed to exhale.

Patient preparation

When chest x-ray films are prescribed, the nurse should see that the patient wears a hospital gown that is tied in the back. All metal objects above the waist are removed, because the presence of metal produces a shadow over the film. Patients are transported to the x-ray department by stretcher or wheelchair and should be accompanied by an attendant. If the patient is too ill to be taken to the x-ray department, a portable x-ray machine may be taken to the patient's bedside. However, the preparation of the patient is the same.

Lung tomography provides clearly focused radiographic images of sections of the lungs at different planes within the thorax. It is useful in further evaluating chest lesions. The nurse should inform the patient that the test takes approximately 30 to 60 minutes and requires that he or she remain as still as possible within the x-ray machine. All jewelry and any metal objects should be removed. No restriction of food or fluids is necessary (Smeltzer, Bare, 1992).

Computed tomography (CT) is a method in which the lungs are scanned in successive cross-sections by a narrow x-ray beam. It adds computer technology to tomography techniques (Patrick and others, 1991). The test may be performed with or without the injection of a radiopaque contrast medium. The results are subsequently analyzed by computer to identify small nodules, tumors, or other abnormalities that may not be visible on conventional x-ray films. The nurse should inform the patient that the test allows for visualization of structures within the chest, usually takes 45 to 60 minutes to perform, and requires that one lie very still inside the x-ray machine. The nurse should ensure that jewelry and any metal objects are removed. If the scan

BOX 20-2

VOLUME, CAPACITIES, AND FLOW RATES

PFTs that are abnormal and indicate disease are generally classified into three patterns: obstructive, restrictive, or mixed.

Obstructive disorders are those that narrow airway passages, which creates an increased resistance to air flow, especially on exhalation. Examples are emphysema, chronic bronchitis, bronchiectasis, and cystic fibrosis. Lung volumes are usually normal or increased. Air trapping occurs, and there is difficulty expelling air via the narrowed airways. Residual volume (RV) is often increased as is functional residual capacity (FRC). Total lung capacity (TLC) may also increase, and vital capacity (VC) may decrease in severe obstruction. Forced expiratory values are usually reduced as a result of air trapping.

In *restrictive disorders* lung expansion is compromised. Therefore volumes and capacities tend to be decreased, but RV and TLC will be normal. Examples of restrictive conditions are pulmonary edema, pneumonia, and kyphoscoliosis. Flow rates may be reduced, normal, or increased.

In patients with more than one disorder, both obstructive and restrictive patterns may be seen. The VC is reduced in *mixed disorders,* and flow rates are reduced out of proportion to the reduced VC (Kersten, 1989; Smeltzer, Bare, 1992).

LUNG CAPACITIES AND VOLUMES

Total lung capacity—Total volume of air that lungs can contain when fully inflated

Vital capacity—Maximum amount of air that can be exhaled after maximum inspiration

Inspiratory capacity (IC)—Maximum volume of air inspired after a normal exhalation

Functional residual capacity (FRC)—Volume of air remaining in lungs after a normal expiration

Tidal volume (V_T)—Maximum volume of air that can be moved in and out of the lung during quiet breathing (usually 10% of vital capacity)

Inspiratory reserve volume (IRV)—Maximum volume of air that can be inhaled beyond normal inspiration

Expiratory reserve volume (ERV)—Maximum volume of air that can be exhaled beyond normal exhalation

Residual volume (RV)—Amount of air remaining in lungs after maximum expiration

FLOW RATES

FVC—Forced vital capacity

FEV_1—Forced expiratory volume in 1 second

FEV_1/FVC—Ratio of forced expiratory volume in 1 second to the forced vital capacity

FEF 25%-75%—Forced expiratory flow over the midportion of the forced vital capacity

MVV—Maximal voluntary ventilation.

Modified from Beare PG, Myers JL: *Principles and practice of adult health nursing,* ed 2, St Louis, 1994, Mosby.

will be performed using contrast, the patient's sensitivity to iodine-based preparations should be determined. The nurse should inform the patient that because contrast is being used, he or she will be allowed nothing by mouth for at least 4 hours before the test. The patient should be prepared for the sensation of warmth or flushing that he or she may feel with dye injection. If no contrast is being used, food and fluid restrictions are not necessary (Kischbach, 1992; Smeltzer, Bare, 1992).

Pulmonary angiography is a test in which radiopaque dye is injected into the pulmonary circulation, after which a series of x-ray films are taken. This test evaluates the circulation in the pulmonary vasculature and is used to identify thromboembolic disease of the lungs and congenital abnormalities of the pulmonary tree. Ventilation/perfusion lung scans are radiologic tests that are performed to detect pulmonary emboli. Lung scans are used to determine areas of the lung that are being ventilated but not perfused as a result of the presence of an obstruction or clot (pulmonary emboli) in the pulmonary circulation.

Endoscopy Procedures

Bronchoscopy

In the past, visualization of the trachea and bronchi was limited by the large, rigid, metal bronchoscope. With the advent of smaller, flexible, fiberoptic bronchoscopes, a more accurate picture of the airway can now be transmitted. The fiberoptic bronchoscope also allows easier passage through the nasal or oral route. After a topical anesthetic has been administered, the bronchoscope is passed through the mouth and into the trachea and major bronchi. The room is darkened, and visualization of the bronchial tree is possible when light is reflected through the instrument. The examination is used to remove foreign bodies that have lodged in the bronchi, to suction secretions for laboratory examination, to observe the respiratory passageways for disease, and to obtain biopsy specimens.

Patient preparation. The emotional preparation for bronchoscopy is important. The procedure causes a certain amount of discomfort, and an apprehensive, fearful patient may cooperate poorly. Explaining to pa-

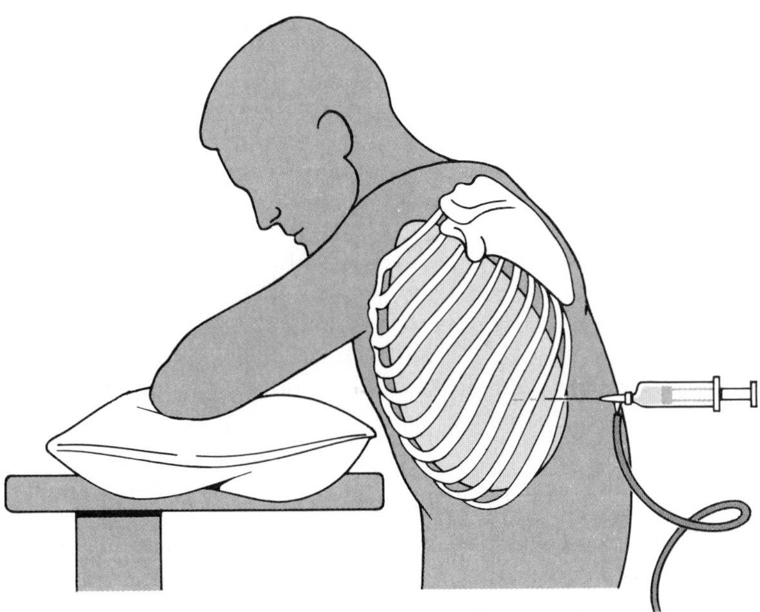

Figure 20-8 A thoracentesis is performed to obtain a sample of pleural fluid or pleura, to remove accumulated pleural fluid, or to instill medication. (From Beare PG, Myers JL: *Principles and practice of adult health nursing,* ed 2, St Louis, 1994, Mosby.)

tients what to expect and teaching them how to breathe and relax during the procedure provides a greater feeling of security and helps relieve their anxiety.

Before a bronchoscopy, no food or fluid by mouth is allowed after midnight. Postural drainage may be ordered in the morning to remove any secretions that may have drained into the trachea or bronchi during the night. Special mouth care should be given after postural drainage, and dentures, bridges, contact lenses, and glasses should be removed. A sedative may be ordered to relieve anxiety. An anticholinergic agent, such as atropine, is also ordered to alleviate symptoms of bradycardia, arrhythmia, and hypotension; to suppress the cough reflex; and to inhibit secretions. If the procedure is performed in the operating room, the usual preoperative nursing measures are required.

Postprocedure care. When the patients return to their rooms, they should be properly positioned on either side and usually in a semi-Fowler's position to allow for easier removal of secretions. No food or fluids should be given until the gag reflex returns, and vital signs are monitored according to protocol. Patients should be watched carefully for respiratory difficulties, including bronchospasms and laryngospasms. If a biopsy has been done, sputum may be tinged with blood for several days. However, the nurse should be alert for any unusual bleeding, and the primary provider should be notified immediately if it occurs. If throat soreness and discomfort are prolonged, a mild analgesic such as aspirin may be ordered. Persistent throat soreness and a hoarse voice should be evaluated because injury to the trachea or larynx can occur during the procedure.

Thoracentesis

A thoracentesis is performed to obtain pleural fluid for diagnostic purposes, to biopsy the pleura, to remove pleural fluid for therapeutic purposes, or to instill medication (Phipps, 1995). The procedure usually is performed in the patient's room. The patient is in a sitting position with head and arms resting on a pillow that has been placed on the overbed table (Figure 20-8). Using aseptic technique, the skin is cleansed, generally in the area of the eighth or ninth rib interspace, and a local anesthetic is injected into the tissues. The patient must be cautioned not to move while the needle is being inserted to prevent damage to the lung or pleura. The pulse and respiration should be checked several times, and the patient should be observed for diaphoresis or for any change in skin color (Box 20-3).

Pulse Oximetry

Pulse oximetry provides continuous, noninvasive monitoring of arterial oxygen saturation (SaO_2), the amount of hemoglobin-carrying oxygen in relation to its total carrying capacity. Pulse oximetry can be used

BOX 20-3 Guidelines for Care of the Patient Undergoing Thoracentesis

1. Explain the procedure to the patient. Emphasize the importance of not moving, of breathing quietly, and of not coughing during the procedure to avoid injury to the pleura. Although a local anesthetic is used, the patient may feel some discomfort as the needle enters the pleura.
2. Obtain baseline vital signs, including blood pressure, heart rate, and respiratory rate. Compare subsequent readings to baseline.
3. Help the patient obtain the optimal position for performance of the test. If possible, the patient sits on the edge of the bed with the feet supported. Using an elevated overbed table, the patient can maintain a position with the head resting on folded arms (Figure 20-6). Patients who are unable to sit up may be turned onto the unaffected side with the head of the bed elevated approximately 30 degrees.
4. Provide support and reassurance to the patient as needed.
5. Monitor vital signs; general appearance; and respiratory rate, depth, and effort throughout the procedure. No more than 1500 ml of pleural fluid should be removed within a 30-minute period because of the risk of intravascular fluid shift with resultant pulmonary edema.
6. Apply a sterile occlusive dressing over the insertion site after the needle is removed.
7. After the procedure is completed, position the patient on the unaffected side with the insertion site up. A chest x-ray film is obtained to assess for **pneumothorax.**
8. Monitor respiratory status, vital signs, and puncture site after the procedure. Observe for the following complications:
   - Intravascular shift: shortness of breath, hypotension, increased pulse rate
   - Lung trauma: bloody sputum, tracheal deviation, and uncontrollable coughing

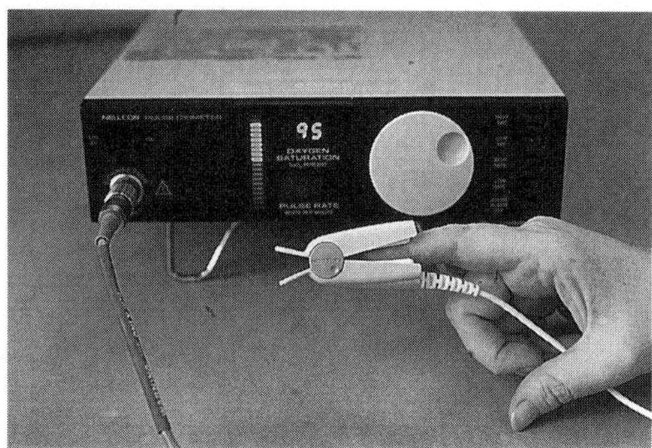

Figure 20-9 Oximeter probe that attaches to a finger or an ear. (From Perry AG, Potter PA: *Clinical nursing skills and techniques,* ed 3, St Louis, 1994, Mosby.)

to regulate oxygen therapy in a variety of patients and is useful in evaluating sleep disorders (Patrick and others, 1991; Spyr, Preach 1990). Oximetry technology allows the nurse to assess minute-to-minute changes in saturation, intervene before hypoxemia produces serious symptoms, and evaluate a patient's response to therapy.

The oximeter consists of two light-emitting diodes (LEDs) and may be applied to any site that has a pulsating vascular bed, such as the finger, toe, or earlobe (Figure 20-9). The device transmits wavelengths of light through the site and measures infrared and red light absorption through the skin. The signals are returned to the device and displayed on a monitor. A computer within the oximeter calculates oxyhemoglobin saturation on the basis of the fact that red light is more easily transmitted through oxygenated than deoxygenated blood. The value obtained corresponds to the arterial hemoglobin saturation. Oximetry readings and measurements taken from arterial blood have been shown to correlate within a range of 2% (Patrick and others, 1991; Spyr, Preach, 1990).

The device depends on pulsations from the vascular bed to confirm the presence of a level of blood flow known to be associated with accurate saturation readings. Therefore any condition that alters perfusion (e.g., hypovolemia, hypotension, hypothermia, vasoconstrictive drugs) may cause no reading to be obtained. This phenomenon is a limitation of oximetry (Patrick and others, 1991; Spyr, Preach, 1990). Patient movement may also create artifacts that make interpretation difficult. Despite its limitations, oximetry is useful, and low values often indicate that a patient needs additional interventions.

NURSING STRATEGIES FOR COMMON RESPIRATORY PROBLEMS

A variety of treatment modalities are used when caring for a patient who has an alteration in respiratory function. The modalities selected are based on the dis-

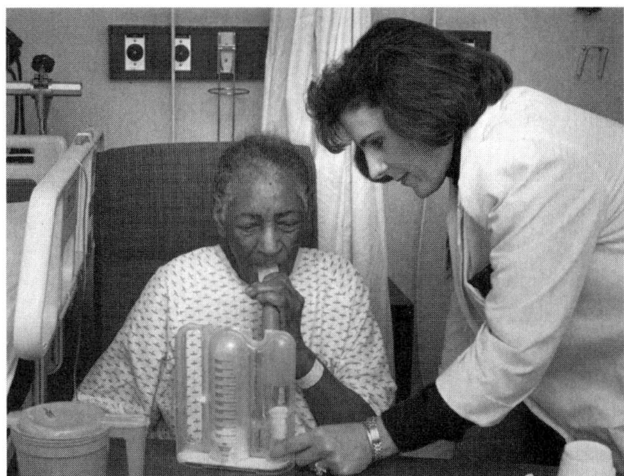

Figure 20-10 An incentive spirometer device used by patients to stimulate deep breathing. This procedure facilitates increased expansion of the lungs, which reduces pulmonary complications.

PATIENT/FAMILY TEACHING 

Using the incentive spirometer

Sit as upright as possible.
Seal lips around the mouthpiece.
Inhale as slowly and deeply as possible, and watch the spirometer indicator rise.
Hold the deep breath for a count of "3," if possible.
Remove the mouthpiece from the mouth, and breathe out slowly.
Aim for a higher number with each successive breath.
Repeat this process for 10 breaths, and cough after the last breath.
Follow the cough with an additional deep breath.
Use the spirometer every hour while awake, especially during the first 2 to 3 days after surgery.

order and include incentive spirometry, coughing and deep breathing, and suctioning.

Incentive Spirometry

The incentive spirometer (IS) is the device most commonly used to assess an individual's ability to take a deep breath (Figure 20-10). The IS is available in several models and consists of one or more small plastic balls on closed chambers that are connected to tubing and a mouthpiece. The patient is instructed to inhale slowly through the tubing, which creates a vacuum and raises the ball(s).

Early studies of IS therapy demonstrated best results when patients used the device often (Bartlett, 1982; Bartlett, Gazzaniqa, Geraghty, 1973). Holding the breath at the end of inspiration for 3 to 5 seconds is important to promote air distribution throughout the lung and allow inflation of even the smallest, most distant alveoli. Use of the IS may be taught to patients preoperatively and its use continued postoperatively. It is especially useful to patients who are undergoing upper abdominal and thoracic surgery.

Coughing and Deep Breathing

Coughing is used to remove secretions and to provide adequate ventilation in the lungs by maintaining a clear airway. For some patients, their own deep productive coughing may be sufficient. For others, the nurse may be responsible for clearing the airway. When possible, the patient should be placed in a sitting position with the feet supported on the floor. If coughing is painful, the nurse should help the patient by splinting the chest. In addition, analgesics may need to be given before coughing to reduce discomfort. Sputum should be collected in tissues and placed in paper bags at the bedside or kept in a sterile container to assess 24-hour sputum production. The patient should be taught to take a deep breath, hold it for 1 second, and cough on expiration. Persistent shallow coughing is of no value and only tires the patient. Tissues should be folded and placed in the patient's cupped hand. Nurses who handle sputum should wear gloves and wash their hands thoroughly after each encounter.

Many cough medicines are available on the market. Some may be purchased over-the-counter in drugstores, but others require a prescription. Cough medicines may be narcotic or nonnarcotic antitussives and are classified as demulcents, expectorants, or sedatives. The type of cough remedy prescribed depends on the condition for which it is needed and the result desired. Demulcents are protective and may be expected to relieve irritation of the throat by providing a soothing effect and protecting the mucous membranes from the air. Demulcents often are found in gargles, lozenges, and syrups that contain various flavoring agents such as wild cherry. Some lozenges contain an analgesic that adds little, if anything, to its effectiveness. Expectorants act to increase or modify mucous secretions in the respiratory tract, making mucus less thick and more easily expectorated. The expectorant drug used is glycerol guaiacolate (Robitussin TG) and iodide preparations (Saturated solution of potassium iodide [SSKI]. Sedative agents reduce coughing by depressing the cough reflex. They may contain a narcotic or a barbiturate, which depress the respiratory center. Their use usually is limited to disorders that involve extremely painful coughing. If an allergic factor is involved, an antihistamine may be prescribed. In an acute infection, nasal congestion often contributes to the patient's discomfort. Phenylephrine (Neo-Synephrine), ephedrine, or any of the numerous sprays and drops available may be prescribed.

Suctioning

If a patient is unable to clear secretions with coughing, the secretions may be removed by suctioning. Suctioning is also used to obtain a sputum specimen when the patient is unable to produce a sample by coughing.

When a patient is in respiratory distress because of an obstructed airway, the nurse may observe the following signs: gurgling, increased pulse and respiratory rates, a harsh respiratory sound, restlessness, anxiety, pallor with cyanosis around the mouth, or generalized cyanosis. If the distress is caused by mucus that is obstructing the airway, the patient should be suctioned immediately, carefully, and thoroughly to relieve the symptoms and to restore a patent airway. The suction catheter is passed through an artificial airway if one is in place. Otherwise, the catheter is inserted through the nose and into the trachea.

The procedure used to suction a patient involves attaching a whistle-tip catheter to tubing and a continuous suction device. The whistle-tip catheter provides the nurse fingertip control of the suctioning. During suctioning, sterile gloves are worn, and sterile catheters are used to prevent contamination of the respiratory tract. When aspirating secretions, the nurse should maintain strict aseptic technique to prevent serious complications. Separate catheters must be used for nasal and tracheobronchial secretions. The nurse should use caution to avoid injuring the mucous membranes. The procedure should be fully explained to the patient before the procedure is started.

The patient should be hyperventilated and hyperoxygenated before and after suctioning because both air and secretions are removed during suctioning. Several methods may be used to hyperoxygenate patients: (1) if they are able, the nurse should instruct patients to deep breathe for 1 minute; (2) the nurse should have patients use a face mask and rebreathing bags with oxygen attached; (3) if patients are on mechanical ventilation, the oxygen should be increased to 100% for 1 minute and manually depress the sigh-cycle button two or three times; or (4) patients should be manually ventilated with an Ambu bag that has been adapted to deliver 100% oxygen. Suction should not be applied until after the catheter has been inserted and is being withdrawn. The whistle-tip catheter is rotated while it is being withdrawn, and suction should be made intermittent by removing and replacing the finger to the tube valve during the withdrawal of the catheter. If possible, patients should be placed in Fowler's position before beginning the procedure. Each suction should not exceed 10 seconds, and an interval of 3 minutes should elapse before repeating the procedure. During this interval, oxygen is administered, and the patient is reconnected to the mechanical ventilator. When suctioning through an airway or an endotracheal or tracheostomy tube, the catheter should be inserted until resistance is felt (the carina).

During suctioning, the tip may come into contact with the carina, which stimulates the patient's cough reflex. Although this helps the patient expectorate secretions, the coughing could be violent enough to expel the tracheostomy or endotracheal tube, which is very uncomfortable for the patient. Therefore the nurse should ensure that the tube is secured before suctioning. The patient should be informed that suctioning may cause coughing, and the suction catheter tip should be withdrawn from the carina to reduce further cough stimulation. The closed tracheal suctioning catheter system (CTSS) is a new technique for suctioning airway secretions in a patient who is receiving mechanical ventilation. The CTSS is composed of a suction catheter that is enclosed within a plastic sleeve, which can be directed into the endotracheal or tracheostomy tube. The CTSS attaches directly to the ventilator tubing circuit, and ventilator function is not disrupted when it is used. The catheter set-up is usually changed once a day.

Postural Drainage

Postural drainage is used to drain excessive secretions from the lungs (including pus from lung abscesses). Drainage is facilitated by placing the patient in a position that allows gravity to aid in the procedure. The position of the patient should be determined by the area of the lung to be drained. The upper lobes of the lung can best be drained in the sitting position, and the lower lobes are best drained in a lying position (Figure 20-11). However, positions vary according to the patient's condition, strength, and respiratory function. Gravity drainage of the lungs can be accomplished in several ways. In most cases younger patients tolerate lowering the head better than older or debilitated patients. If possible, the mouth should be approximately 20 inches lower than the base of the lungs. Special beds and tables are available, but the patient's own bed may also be used. During the procedure, patients should be encouraged to cough deeply, and after returning to bed they may be expected to cough and expectorate large amounts of sputum.

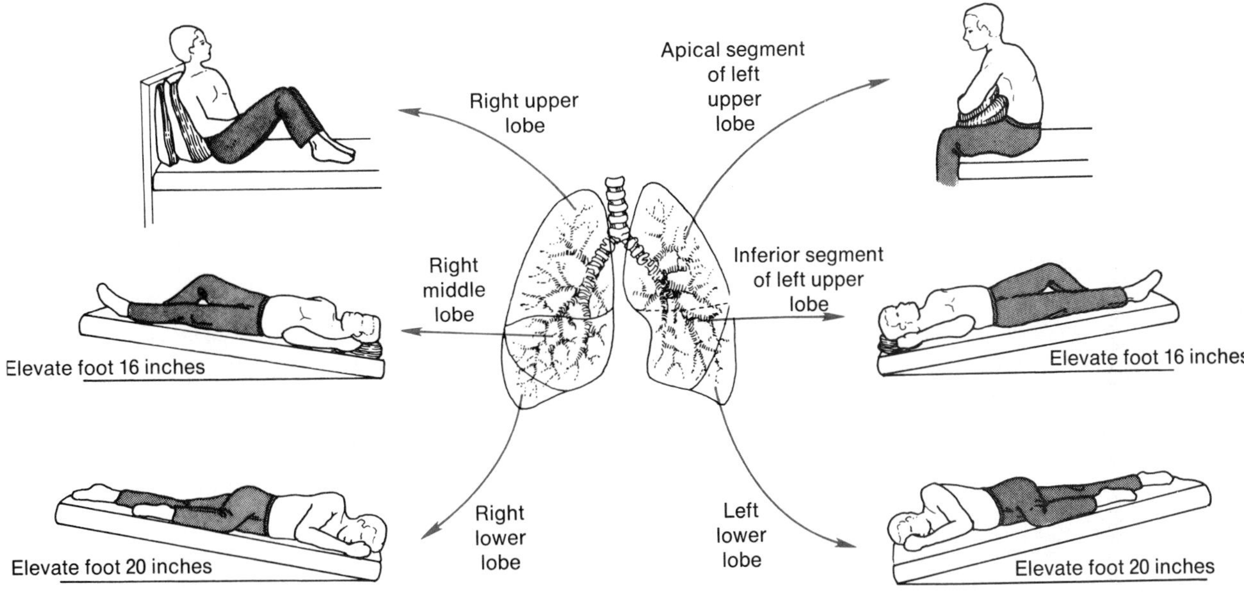

Figure 20-11 Postural drainage positions for draining various portions of the lung.

Older adults with hypertrophic arthritis may be unable to bend their bodies over the bed for postural drainage, but fairly satisfactory results may be obtained by elevating the foot of the bed. Postural drainage often is fatiguing for debilitated patients, and they may be able to remain in the position for only a few minutes. However, with each effort they experience less discomfort. The procedure should be supervised by the nurse and is best carried out midway between meals to prevent nausea and vomiting. The patient's teeth should be brushed after the procedure, and an antiseptic mouthwash may be used if desired. The patient should be protected from chilling during the procedure and should be allowed to rest after returning to bed.

If the drainage is to be measured, it should be collected in a receptacle that is suitable for measuring. The color, amount, and consistency of the drainage should be recorded on the patient's chart.

Percussion/Vibration

Percussion may be provided during postural drainage. During percussion, the hands are cupped so that an air pocket is created within the palm of the hand. The caregiver rhythmically and alternatively claps the chest wall over the involved area to help loosen mucous plugs and move them into the bronchi, where they may be drained out or expectorated (Figure 20-12) (Beare, Meyers, 1994; Kersten, 1989; Malasanos, Barkauskas, Stoltenberg, Allen, 1990). Vibration is performed by placing the hands against the chest wall and gently "quivering" them as the patient exhales. Clapping and vibrating are not used when there is a danger of hemorrhage or if the patient complains of pain. The procedure should be performed by a nurse or therapist who has been trained in the technique. Also available are automatic mechanical percussors that strap to the chest or are handheld. They may be used in the hospital setting or by the patient at home (Kersten, 1989).

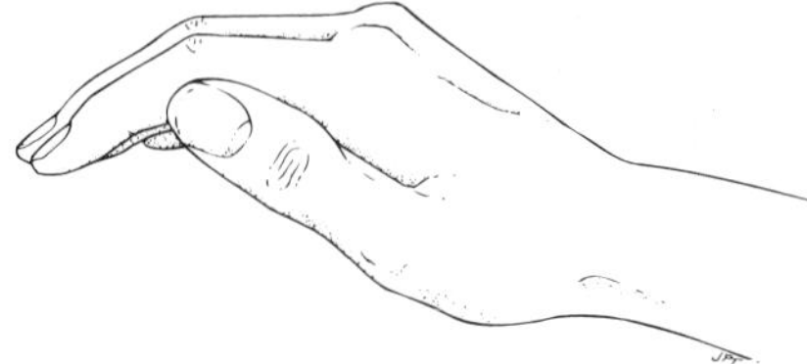

Figure 20-12 The nurse uses a cupped hand position for chest percussion. (From Beare PG, Myers JL: *Principles and practice of adult health nursing,* ed 2, St Louis, 1994, Mosby.)

Throat Irrigations, Humidifications, and Aerosol Therapy

Persons suffering from nasopharyngeal and bronchial infections often secure relief with warm throat irrigations. A physiologic saline solution at a temperature of 120° F (49° C) is usually used, and irrigations may be used several times a day. The application of heat to the irritated membranes promotes drainage of secretions; stimulates circulation; and re-

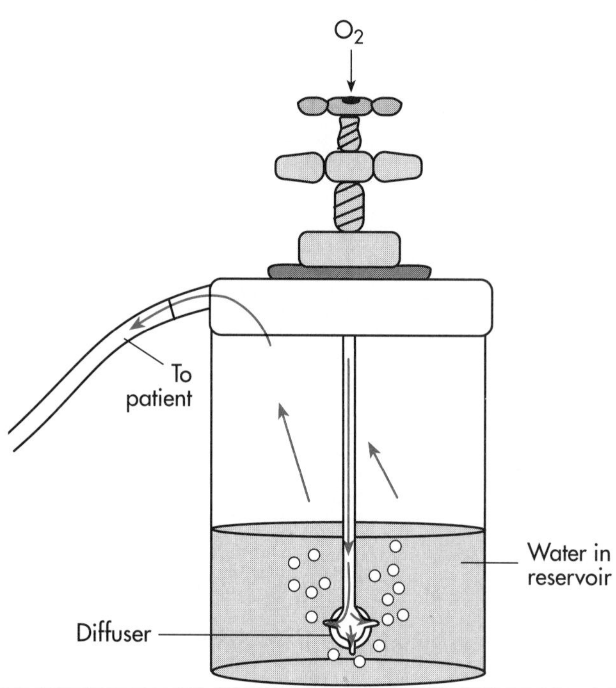

Figure 20-13 Bubble humidifier. Gas is directed below the surface of the water and bubbles back to the top. (From Beare PG, Myers JL: *Principles and practice of adult health nursing,* ed 2, St Louis, 1994, Mosby.)

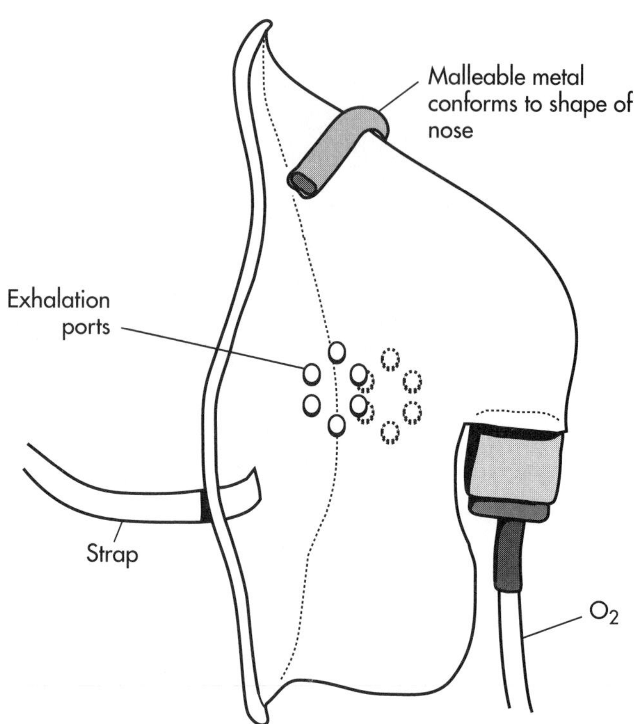

Figure 20-14 Simple face mask.

lieves pain, swelling, and muscle spasms. The nurse may assist the patient with the procedure, or the patient may be taught to carry out the procedure under professional supervision.

Normally air is heated and humidified in the upper airway as it is inhaled. Humidifiers or nebulizers are used when the upper airway is bypassed or when added water vapor is desired to improve patient comfort, to maximize secretion mobility, or to deliver inhaled medications (Figure 20-13). Humidifiers add water vapor to inhaled air and are used primarily to moisten dry mucous membranes when a patient receives oxygen therapy. Cool humidifiers provide additional water vapor in the inspired air and usually are adequate if the patient is breathing through the upper airway. However, if the upper airway is bypassed with a tracheostomy, the water vapor must be heated to provide sufficient humidification and to prevent drying of mucous membranes and retention of thick secretions.

Nebulizers add water or medication particles to inhaled air by breaking it up into small particles, which produces a mist therapy. The medication is inhaled as a fine mist of droplets suspended in air. The smaller the particle size, the deeper into the lung it can be inhaled. Nebulizers are effective in administering highly humidified air or oxygen to patients with respiratory problems. The administration of bronchodilators and mucolytic agents by nebulization is a common part of the therapeutic regimen. A handheld nebulizer can be used, or the medication can be administered with oxygen under pressure. When oxygen is forced through a nebulizer that contains the medication, it carries fine particles of the medication deep into the respiratory tract. The patient breathes slowly and deeply, holds his or her breath for 3 or 4 seconds after an inspiration, and exhales through pursed lips. The procedure is repeated until all the medication has been inhaled as ordered. The teeth should be brushed and the mouth rinsed after the procedure to prevent soreness. Nearly all forms of respiratory therapy include some form of humidity or aerosol (Kersten, 1989).

Oxygen Therapy

Oxygen therapy is used for patients who suffer from hypoxemia (low arterial oxygen tension). The many devices available for oxygen therapy are divided into two groups: low-flow and high-flow systems (Bolgiano, Bunting, and Shoenberger, 1990). Low-flow systems contribute partially to the inspired gas the patient breathes (i.e., part of each breath contains room air). Low-flow systems do not provide a constant or known concentration of inspired oxygen. As the patient's breathing patterns change, the amount of oxygen inspired also changes. Examples of low-flow sys-

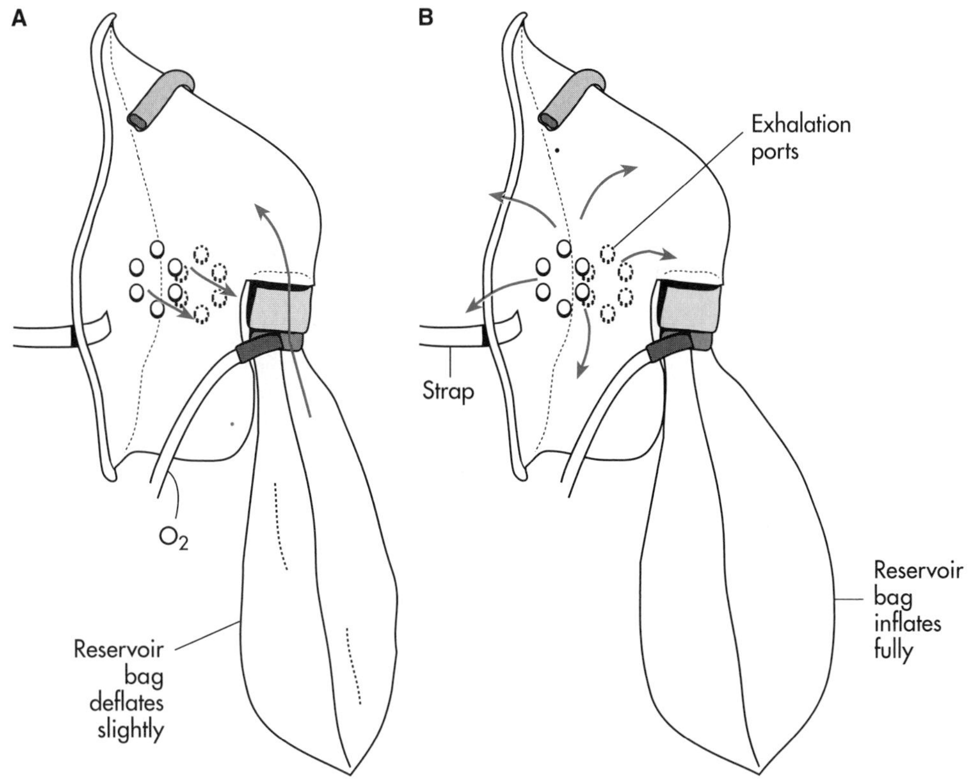

Figure 20-15 Partial rebreathing mask. **A,** Inhalation. **B,** Exhalation. Note direction of gas movement indicated by the arrows.

tems include the nasal cannula, simple oxygen mask, partial rebreathing mask, and nonrebreathing mask (Figures 20-14, 20-15, and 20-16). High-flow systems provide the total amount of inspired gas. A specific percentage of oxygen is delivered independent of the patient's breathing pattern. Examples of high-flow systems include Venturi masks (Figure 20-17).

The decision to administer oxygen, the amount to deliver, and the method to be used depend on the purpose for which it is being administered (Dossey, Guzzetta, Kenner, 1990; Kersten, 1989). The effectiveness of oxygen in the treatment of the patient depends on the pathologic process present. The physician indicates the method by which oxygen is to be given and the number of liters per minute. The nurse responsible for carrying out the directive should act promptly and remember that although oxygen may be beneficial, it may also be dangerous. Therefore the nurse should carefully observe any patient who is receiving oxygen.

Oxygen by nasal cannula

The nasal cannula is useful when an extremely low concentration of oxygen is needed. The oxygen cannula is made of plastic and consists of two prongs, which are placed in the nostrils, and either a strap around the head or a plastic bow similar to the bow on glasses, which fits over the ears. The flow meter should be set at the prescribed number of liters with the oxygen flowing through the cannula before its insertion because the patient may otherwise receive a blast of oxygen that is meant to flush the system. Oxygen concentrations from 24% to 44% may be delivered. At a flow rate of 6 L/min, the nasal cannula delivers a concentration of 44% oxygen. This is the maximum rate a cannula should deliver. The nasal cannula works on the same principle as the Venturi mask, except that the work of mixing oxygen and air is done in the nasopharynx and oropharynx. Therefore whether a patient breathes through the nose or mouth does not matter because oxygen and atmospheric air are mixed before they enter the trachea and lungs. Proper placement of the prongs is important to prevent a direct stream of oxygen against the nasal mucosa. Even with correct positioning of the prongs, a greater degree of nasal drying occurs with this method. When the flow rate is more than 4 L/min, humidification of the oxygen is necessary. If the patient's nasal mucosa becomes dry and irritated, a water-based lubricant may be used to moisten the nostrils.

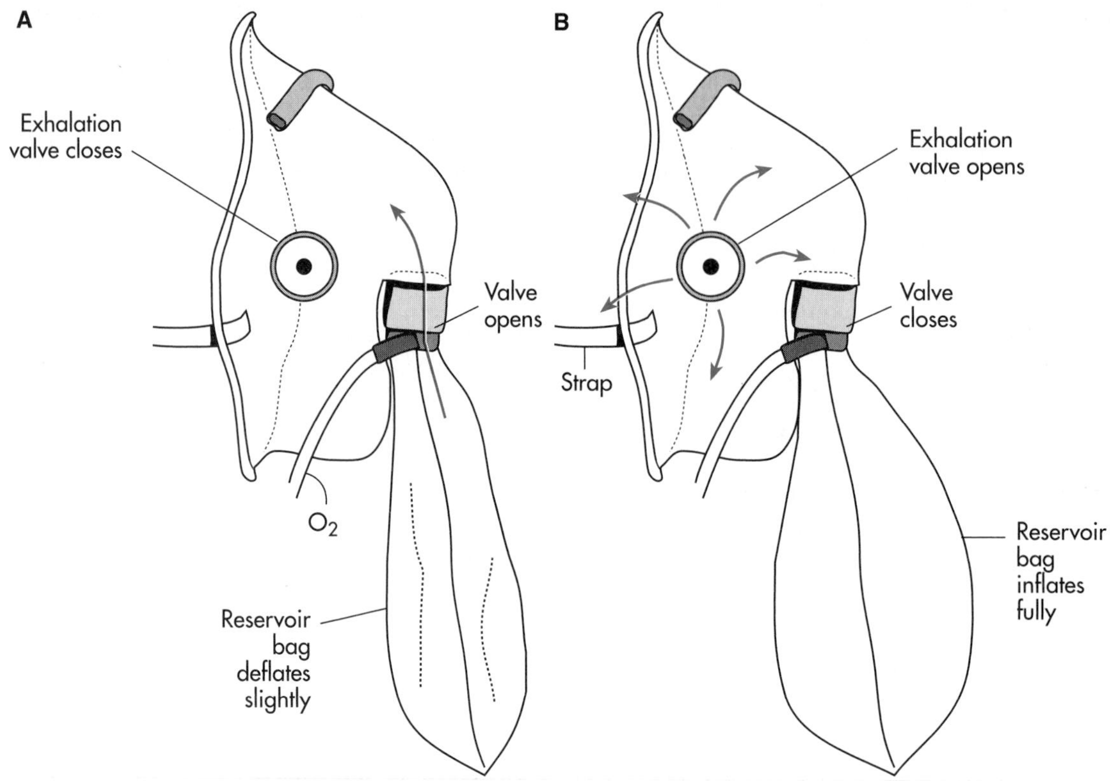

Figure 20-16 Nonrebreathing mask. **A,** Inhalation. **B,** Exhalation. Arrows indicate the direction of gas movement.

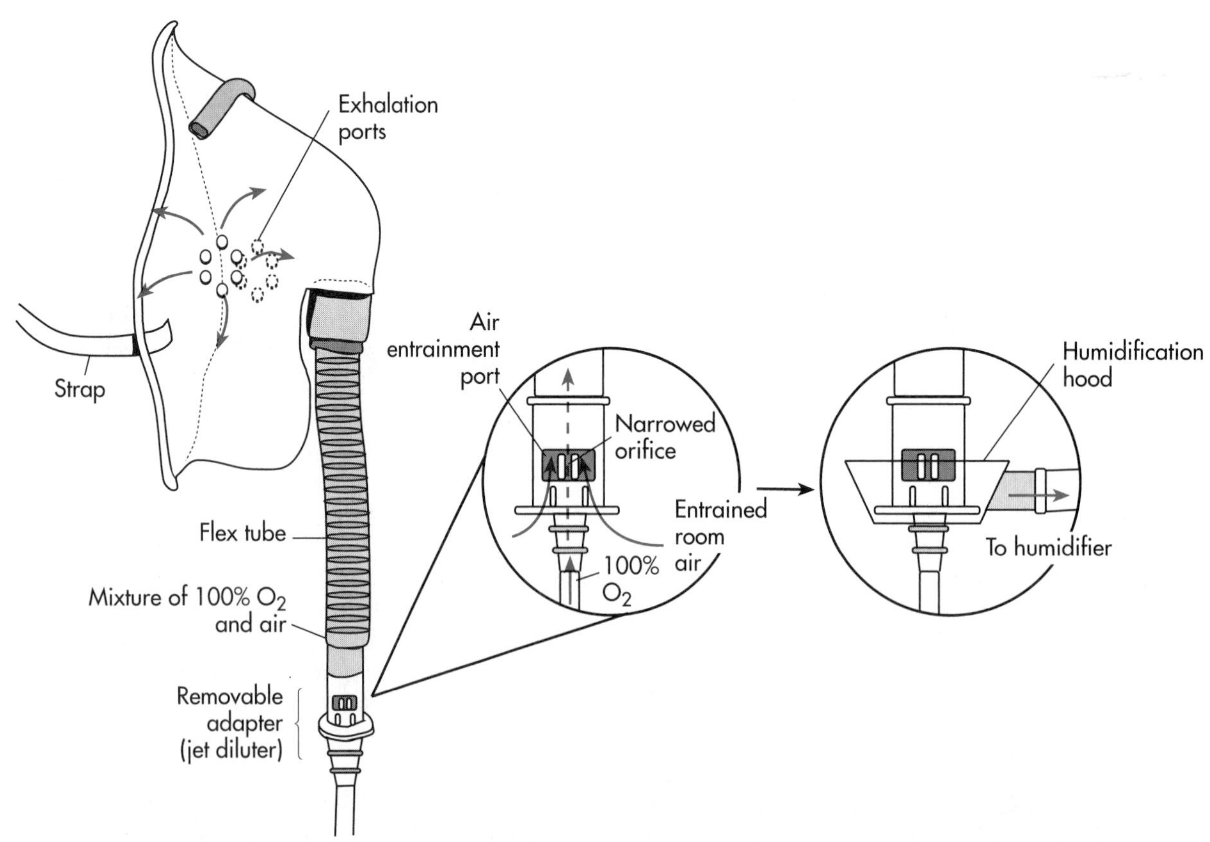

Figure 20-17 Venturi mask. A hood has been added to provide humidification and to protect the air ports.

Oxygen by mask

Oxygen masks are comfortable and are used when higher concentrations of oxygen than can be delivered by nasal cannula are desired. A simple oxygen mask provides concentrations of oxygen from 40% to 60%, depending on the patient's ventilatory pattern. As the patient inspires, room air is drawn in through the holes in the mask and around the edges and mixes with the oxygen. Flow rates of 5 to 8 L/min are normally required.

Venturi masks, partial rebreather masks, aerosol masks, and nonrebreathing masks are other types of masks that may be used for the patient. Venturi masks are high-flow systems that can deliver oxygen concentrations from 24% to 40%. This system is particularly useful in individuals with COPD, who may lose their hypoxic respiratory drive at higher concentrations of oxygen. Aerosol masks are used with nebulizers and can be adjusted to deliver oxygen concentrations from 22% to 100%. Partial rebreather masks consist of a face mask and a reservoir bag. They can deliver between 35% to 60% oxygen concentration. Nonrebreather masks consist of a mask and reservoir that are separated by a one-way valve that prevents expired air from mixing with supplemental oxygen. Exhaled air is directed out of the mask through exhalation ports. If the mask conforms tightly to the face, 100% oxygen concentration can be delivered (Table 20-7).

All patients do not tolerate oxygen by mask equally well. The head strap should be adjusted to a position that is most comfortable for the patient. The patient who is apprehensive or who has acute dyspnea may have a feeling of suffocation. Depending on the patient's condition, the mask should be removed and the face bathed and dried. The mask must be removed and replaced with a nasal cannula during meals. The minimum flow for any type of mask should be 5 L/min. Because moisture tends to collect in the mask, it should be wiped dry regularly.

Hyperbaric oxygen

Hyperbaric oxygenation is achieved by exposing the patient to pressure greater than normal atmospheric pressure. As a result, the amount of oxygen dissolved in the plasma is increased, which causes an increase in oxygen levels in the tissues of the body. Therapy is carried out in either small or large steel chambers that the patient enters alone or with staff members. All personnel involved are subjected to rigid physical examination and training.

The use of hyperbaric oxygen in the treatment of disease is still in the experimental stage. Although not all authorities agree on its value, most agree that it may serve as an adjunct to other therapies. Approximately 50 different conditions are reportedly being

TABLE 20-7

Standard Oxygen Delivery Devices With Oxygen Concentration

Oxygen Delivery Device	Flow Rate (L/min)	Oxygen Concentration (percentage)
Low-flow systems		
Nasal cannula	1	24
	2	28
	3	32
	4	36
	5	40
	6	44
Simple face mask	5-6	40
	6-7	50
	7-10	60
Partial-rebreather mask	6-10	35-60
Non-rebreather mask	6-10	60-100
High-flow systems		
Venturi mask	4	24
	4	28
	6	31
	8	35
	8	40
	10	50

Modified from Kersten LD: *Comprehensive respiratory nursing: a decision making approach,* Philadelphia, 1989, WB Saunders.

treated with hyperbaric oxygen, including cancer, in which it has been used as an adjunct to radiation therapy. Researchers also have determined that there is a danger of severe side effects from hyperbaric oxygen.

Oxygen precautions

Regardless of what method of oxygen administration is used, certain precautions must be adhered to when a patient is receiving oxygen. Smoking is not permitted because oxygen supports combustion and causes anything that is burning in its presence to burn brighter and faster. When oxygen tanks are being used, they should be secured in such a way that they will not tip over. They should not be placed near lamps, radiators, or other heating devices.

THE PATIENT WHO REQUIRES AIRWAY MANAGEMENT

Endotracheal Intubation

In endotracheal intubation, a tube is passed through the nose or mouth into the patient's trachea. Like a tracheostomy tube, it has an inflatable cuff that must be inflated and managed in the same manner. The endotracheal tube is often placed during an emergency to facilitate a patient's breathing, and the patient receives mechanical ventilation. If continued ventilatory support is required for more than 2 to 3 weeks, a tracheotomy is usually performed.

Tracheotomy

A **tracheotomy** is a surgical procedure during which an artificial opening in the anterior wall of the trachea is created to establish an airway. After the procedure is completed, a **tracheostomy** tube of the proper size is inserted. Patients who have had laryngectomy surgery have permanent tracheostomies. A tracheotomy may be an elective procedure or may be performed in an emergency. If at all possible, it should be done in the operating room under strict aseptic technique. The following signs may indicate the need for a trachestomy:

1. Prolonged intubation—many surgeons consider a tracheotomy after 2 weeks of mechanical ventilation. The tracheotomy permits ventilation-dependent patients oral alimentation, verbal communication, and greater patient comfort
2. Airway obstruction secondary to a tumor, an edema, or an infection
3. Preliminary tracheotomy in patients who are undergoing head and neck surgery because of anticipated swelling and edema
4. Laryngeal dysfunction (e.g., bilateral vocal cord paralysis.)
5. Trauma with facial fractures, especially mandibular
6. Clearance of respiratory secretions in individuals with a depressed cough, neuromuscular disorders, or aspiration.

After the surgical procedure, a tracheostomy tube is inserted into the opening and securely tied around the patient's neck with cotton tape. Velcro devices are also available to secure the tracheostomy tube. A sterile gauze dressing (unfilled) covers the surgical wound around the tube. (Figure 20-18). The tracheostomy tube may consist of two or three pieces: the outer cannula, the inner cannula, and the obturator, or simply a single cannula and an obturator (Fig. 20-19). In double-cannula tubes, the obturator is used to guide the outer cannula through the surgical opening into the trachea, after which it is removed and the inner cannula inserted into the outer cannula and locked in place. Single-cannula tubes usually are used because newer materials and adequate humidification have eliminated the need for a removable inner cannula.

Generally two types of tracheostomy tubes, cuffed and cuffless, may be used. Cuffed tubes are used when ventilatory support is needed or sometimes to reduce aspiration. These tubes are made of plastic material and have a cuff surrounding the middle portion of the tube that can be inflated with air (Figure 20-20). The cuff prevents air from leaking around the sides of the tube and holds the tube in place. Although the newer low-pressure, high-volume cuffs minimize irritation to the tracheal mucosa, the cuff pressure should be measured at least every 8 hours. The pressure should be kept at 18 to 21 mm Hg to allow for adequate capillary blood flow. If increased cuff pressures are required, the physician should be notified and the tube changed to a larger size.

The nurse should remember that patients with cuffed tracheostomy tubes in place are not able to speak because air does not pass directly through the larynx. These patients should be assured that they will be able to speak normally again when the cuffed tracheostomy tube is removed. Cuffless tubes are used when ventilatory support is not needed and serve to maintain the patency of the tracheotomy tube. These tubes may be plastic or metal.

A primary nursing responsibility is the maintenance of a patent airway. A patient who has a newly formed tracheotomy needs suctioning often. If a form of mechanical ventilation is not used, a nebulizer may be used to keep secretions moist. A mid-Fowler's position provides comfort and facilitates breathing. Provisions

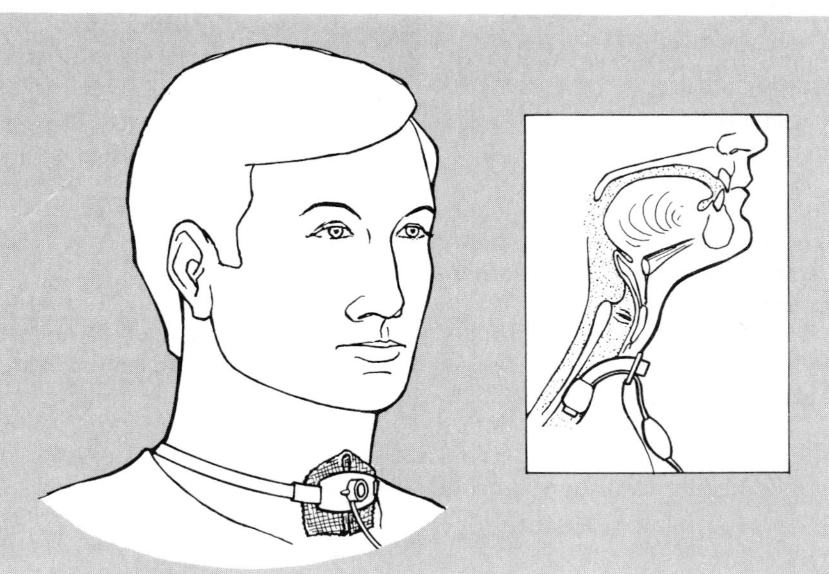

Figure 20-18 Cuffed tracheostomy tube is in place and tied around the patient's neck. The wound is protected with a sterile dressing.

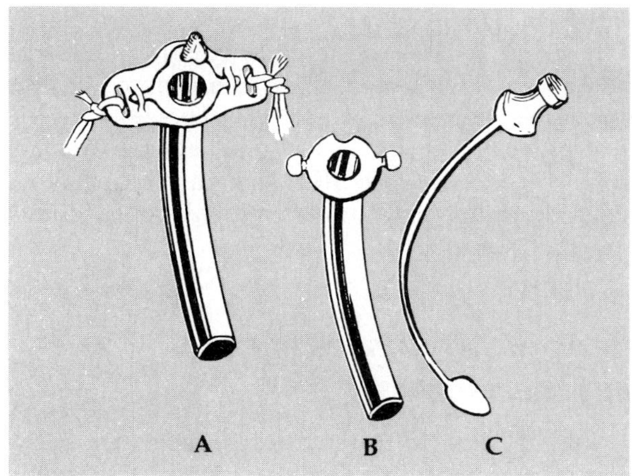

Figure 20-19 Tracheostomy tube. **A,** Outer cannula. **B,** Inner cannula. **C,** Obturator.

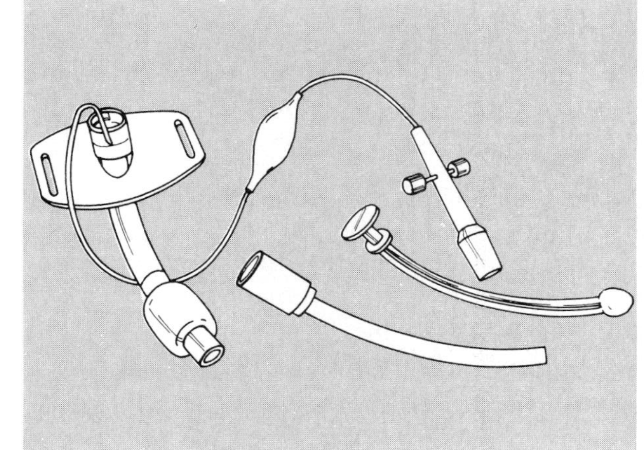

Figure 20-20 Cuffed tracheostomy tube.

must be made for the patient to communicate because he or she may be unable to speak. Patients are usually apprehensive and fear choking. The nurse must observe the patient for complications, which may include apnea, cyanosis, shortness of breath, bleeding from the wound, and hypotension. Blood pressure measurements should be taken before the surgical procedure and at intervals after the surgery. An extra sterile tracheostomy set of the same size and a tracheostomy insertion tray should be kept at the patient's bedside for emergency use if the tube becomes displaced. Any patient who has undergone a tracheotomy should be closely monitored during the first 24 hours after insertion of the tube.

If the patient is discharged with a tracheostomy tube, he or she must be taught how to care for it (Wilson, Malley, 1990). Suction equipment should be available at home. Persons who have a permanent tracheostomy must be instructed not to swim and to use caution when bathing so that water is not aspirated. Scarfs or collars worn around the tracheostomy opening should be made of porous materials.

Mechanical Ventilation

Pulmonary ventilation is the process of taking oxygen into the lungs and releasing carbon dioxide in the exhaled gas. Under certain conditions the patient is unable to maintain optimum levels of arterial oxygen, carbon dioxide, or both. When this occurs, the patient's survival depends on mechanical ventilation. Several conditions exist for which the patient may need ventilatory assistance. Among these disorders are drug overdoses, respiratory failure, certain neuromuscular disorders, cardiac arrest, and pulmonary edema caused by ventricular failure.

When mechanical ventilation is used, the patient must usually be intubated with an artificial airway and connected to an artificial ventilator. The natural airway is bypassed, which necessitates some form of humidification to prevent drying of mucous membranes and thickening of respiratory secretions. Patients receiving mechanical ventilation therapy require close and careful monitoring. The nurse must be familiar with the ventilator and its connecting tubing. Ventilator settings are prescribed by the physician and should include tidal volume, respiratory rate, frequency of sighs, and percentage of oxygen. Most ventilators have several modes or types of ventilatory support to choose from. Each requires a different contribution or effort by the patient to support breathing. These modes include control, assist/control (A/C), intermittent mandatory ventilation (IMV), and continuous positive airway pressure (CPAP). The mode should be ordered according to the severity and type of breathing problem. Positive-end expiratory pressure (PEEP) is often used with patients who are receiving mechanical ventilation to improve the oxygen transfer across the lung. The nurse should monitor patients' exhaled tidal volume, respiratory rate, inspired oxygen level, and peak pressure (pressure required to deliver the tidal volume into the patient's lungs) while they are receiving mechanical ventilation. The heart rate and rhythm, blood pressure level, and skin color should be observed carefully. Blood gas studies are obtained often to evaluate and optimize ventilatory support. Often an arterial catheter is placed to avoid frequent arterial punctures.

The nursing care of patients receiving ventilation therapy includes the following:

- Monitoring all vital signs
- Positioning to provide optimum ventilation
- Frequent turning
- Performing passive range-of-motion exercises
- Recording fluid intake and output
- Assessing airway maintenance and determining the need for suctioning at least every 2 hours
- Maintaining adequate nutrition and fluid balance

If bronchodilating drugs are administered, the patient should be observed for side effects. The nurse should provide emotional support and explain procedures and equipment if the patient is conscious. When conscious, patients may be anxious and require sedation. Before administering sedatives or narcotics, the blood pressure, pulse, and ventilator parameters should be checked (Dossey, 1990).

THE PATIENT UNDERGOING THORACIC SURGERY

Surgery of the chest is performed to cure or to relieve disease conditions such as bronchiectasis, lung abscesses, lung cancer, cysts, and benign tumors. The type of operative procedure used depends on the purpose for which it is to be done. An exploratory thoracotomy is done to confirm a diagnosis of lung or chest disease. A thoracotomy refers to a surgical opening into the thoracic cavity. Often a biopsy is done and the chest is closed, with the possibility of future operations to treat the disease process. In some conditions only a small portion or segment of lung tissue may be removed. This procedure is called segmental resection of the lung. Removal of an entire lobe of one lung is a **lobectomy,** whereas removal of an entire lung is a **pneumonectomy** (Figure 20-21). The latter is done most often for treatment of bronchogenic carcinoma. Many patients are cared for in intensive care units or in cardiopulmonary units immediately following surgery.

Preoperative Assessment and Intervention

Patients being considered for a lobectomy or pneumonectomy are screened carefully by the surgeon because not all patients are eligible for these types of surgery. Many patients are seen in the surgeon's office, and tests and examinations are performed on an outpatient basis. Some patients are admitted to the hospital for their preoperative preparation, which is both psychologic and physical. Patients may have been chronically ill for a long time, and therefore their physical condition may have been affected. Emotional reactions to the proposed surgery may also be affected by poor physical status. While efforts are being directed toward improving the physical condition, efforts should also be made to identify and discuss the patient's fears. The nurse should encourage the patient to communicate feelings to the team of caretakers. During this period, the team must initiate efforts toward

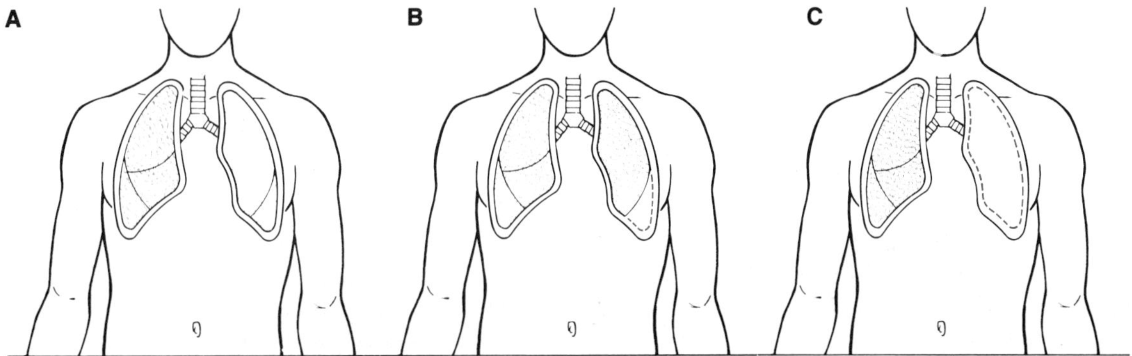

Figure 20-21 Lobectomy and pneumonectomy. **A,** Normal lung. **B,** Lobectomy with lower lobe of left lung removed. **C,** Pneumonectomy with entire left lung removed.

addressing any condition that might affect the outcome of surgery.

Preoperative Preparation

The patient should know that several examinations and tests will be performed. A bronchoscopic examination, an electrocardiogram (ECG), a chest x-ray examination, and a sputum examination may be performed. Tests of pulmonary function and a number of blood tests may be done. Patients may receive blood transfusions before surgery, and antibiotic drugs are often administered. Drugs by nebulization may also be ordered. Mouth hygiene is extremely important, and the nurse should ensure that the teeth are brushed in the morning, after each meal, and at bedtime. Postural drainage is done several times daily, first when the patient is awakened in the morning and last at bedtime. The patient should be encouraged to cough deeply and to expectorate as much mucus as possible during postural drainage. The diet should be nourishing, and the patient should be weighed at specified intervals. Unless contraindicated, the patient should be ambulatory during the preoperative preparation to maintain muscle tone. The patient should be given an explanation concerning the nursing procedures to be carried out after surgery. The patient should be told that he or she will be admitted to the intensive care unit for 1 to 2 days postoperatively, that there may be pain because the nerves between the ribs have been cut, that blood and other fluids will be received, that oxygen will be administered, and that vital signs will be checked often for several hours. If a chest tube will be used after surgery, the patient should be told that it will drain the fluid and air that normally accumulate after chest surgery. The patient should be taught incentive spirometry with coughing and deep breathing techniques and how to do arm and shoulder exercises.

Postoperative Preparation

The intensive care unit is prepared for the patient's return from surgery and is equipped for any emergency that might arise. Oxygen, ventilators, monitors, infusion pumps, a thoracentesis tray, a tracheotomy tray and tubes, chest drainage tubes, and closed drainage systems are needed. A wall suction source with catheters for oral and nasal suctioning may also be required.

Postoperative Assessment and Management

After surgery, the blood pressure, pulse, and respiration rates are checked according to institutional protocols. Oxygen is administered by a mechanical ventilator, nasal cannula, or mask for as long as necessary. Because a reduction in lung capacity requires a period of physiologic adjustment, fluids may be at a low hourly rate, unless prescribed by the surgeon. This procedure prevents overloading the circulation and precipitating pulmonary edema and is especially important in older patients. Fluids by mouth are allowed early in the postoperative period.

When the patient is conscious and the vital signs have been stabilized, the head of the bed may be elevated to an angle of approximately 30 to 45 degrees. Directions concerning the positioning of the patient should be received. The patient with a pneumonectomy usually is turned every hour from the back to the affected side and should not be completely turned to the unoperated side. This type of turning allows the fluid left in the space to consolidate and prevents the remaining lung and the heart from shifting toward the operative side (mediastinal shift). The patient with a lobectomy may be turned to either side, and the patient with a segmental resection usually is not turned onto the affected side unless this position is prescribed by the surgeon.

Medication for pain is needed for several days and must be planned for the individual patient. Coughing and incentive spirometry is painful, and better cooperation is secured from the patient if the pain-relieving medication is administered before he or she is instructed to cough. Coughing must be deep enough to bring up secretions, and the nurse should splint the chest when the patient coughs (Figure 20-22). Both the anterior and the posterior side of the chest must be splinted. The nurse's forearms or palms or a towel that is placed around the chest and held tightly may be used. If the mucus is thick and the patient has difficulty bringing it up, respiratory treatments with aerosol may be prescribed. The surgeon should be notified if efforts to cough and bring up mucus fail.

Exercises are begun early in the postoperative period to facilitate lung ventilation and to maintain normal muscle tension in the shoulder and trunk. At first the exercises are performed passively by the nurse, but they are performed actively by the patient as soon as he or she is ambulatory or able to sit on the side of the bed and stand. The physical therapist assists with the exercises, but in the absence of the physical therapist, the nurse must be able to teach and to help the patient with the exercises.

The nurse must be constantly on the alert for signs indicating serious complications. Cyanosis, dyspnea, and acute chest pain may indicate atelectasis and should be reported immediately. Pallor, an increase in pulse rate, and any significant drop in blood pressure may indicate an internal hemorrhage. Dressings should be checked often for the presence of bright red blood, which may indicate an external hemorrhage. Mobilization of the patient with chest surgery may begin the first or second postoperative day. Initially the patient is allowed to sit on the side of the bed or to stand beside the bed. Ambulation depends on progress made by the individual patient.

Chest Drainage

When the pleura is entered during surgery, atmospheric air enters the pleural space and the involved lung collapses. Therefore after thoracic surgery, the patient usually has one or more chest tubes placed in the pleural cavity, which permit the escape of air so that the lung will expand and allow for drainage of fluid from the pleural space. One tube may be placed in the upper chest to remove air, and another tube in a lower position to remove fluids. The chest tubes are then attached to a closed drainage system.

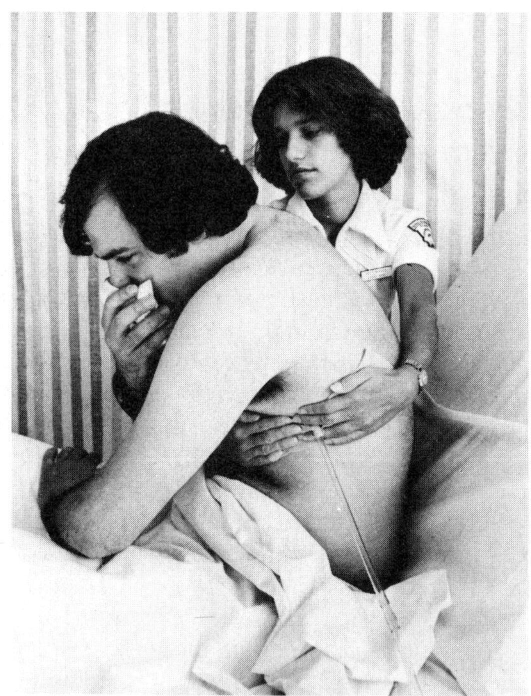

Figure 20-22 Nurse uses her hands to provide firm support while splinting the patient's incision. This technique lessens muscle stress and reduces discomfort when the patient coughs. Note that the nurse keeps her head behind the patient while he coughs and that the patient is using a tissue to cover his mouth. (From Phipps WJ: *Medical-surgical nursing: concepts and clinical practice,* ed 5, St Louis, 1995, Mosby.)

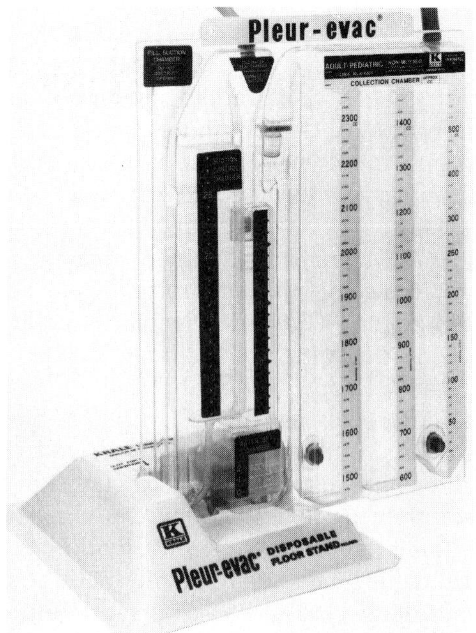

Figure 20-23 Adult-pediatric nonmetered Pleur-Evac. (Courtesy Deknatel, Inc., Queens Village, NY.)

A chest drainage system must be capable of removing whatever accumulates in the pleural space so that a normal pleural space may be restored and maintained. Commercially available systems are the most common modalities to provide water-seal drainage (Figure 20-23). The chest tube is attached to the drainage system. Drainage accumulates in the first chamber, and water in the second chamber acts as a seal. It allows air to be removed from the chest but does not allow it to reenter the chest. Suction may be applied to the second chamber to create negative pressure, which facilitates the removal of fluid and air from the pleural cavity. The addition of suction creates constant bubbling in the third chamber.

The use of the bottle systems has decreased with the availability of self-contained, disposable commercial units. Figure 20-24 depicts chest tube placement, three types of mechanical drainage systems, and the Pleur-Evac system.

In a single-bottle water seal system the end of the drainage tube from the patient's chest is covered by a layer of water, which allows air and fluid to exit the pleural space but does not allow it to return. Drainage depends on gravity and varies with respirations. As the fluid level in the bottle increases, removing air and fluid from the pleural space becomes more difficult, and suction may need to be applied (Smeltzer, Bare, 1992). A two-bottle system consists of the same water-seal chamber just described, plus a fluid collection bottle. When fluid drains in this system, the water seal is not affected by the amount of drainage. In a three-bottle system a third bottle is added to the two bottles previously described to control the amount of suction applied (Figure 20-25). The amount of suction is deter-

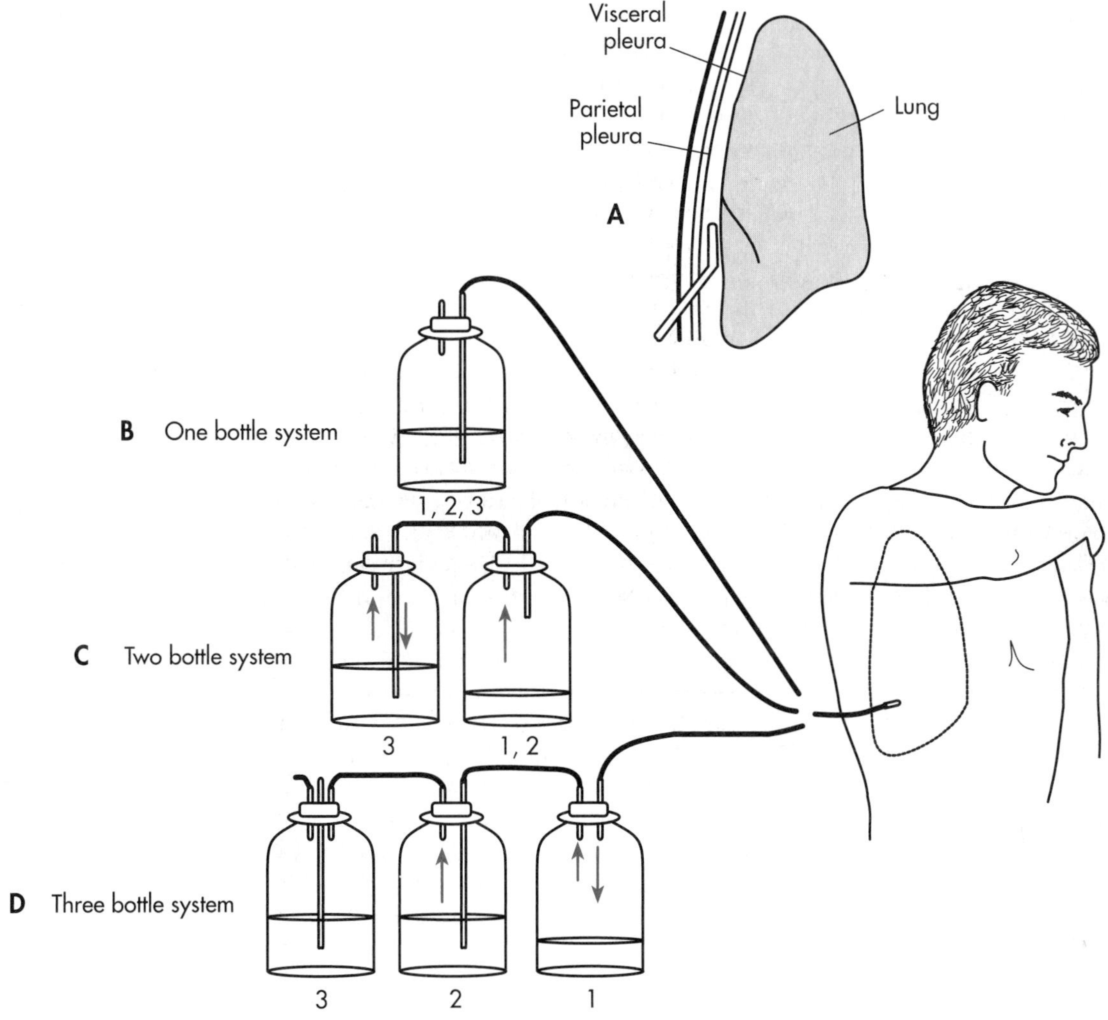

Figure 20-24 Chest drainage system. **A,** Chest catheter is placed in the pleural space of the chest cavity. **B,** One bottle drainage system. **C,** Two bottle drainage system. **D,** Three bottle drainage system.

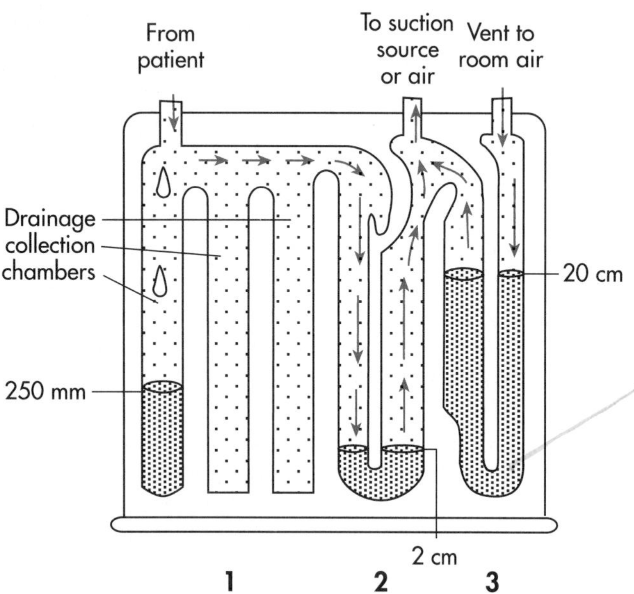

Figure 20-25 The Pleur-Evac is a single unit with all three bottles identified as chambers. *1.* Collection chamber; *2.* Water seal chamber; *3.* Suction control chamber.

mined by the depth to which the tip of the venting glass tube is submerged in water. The usual depth is 20 cm, which means that 20 cm of water suction is being applied to the chest wall of the patient (Smeltzer, Bare, 1992). In the three-bottle system, drainage depends on gravity or the amount of suction applied. The suction apparatus creates and maintains negative pressure throughout the entire closed drainage system. If the vacuum in the system becomes greater than the depth to which the tube is submerged, outside air can enter the system. The result is constant bubbling in the pressure-regulator bottle, which indicates that the system is functioning properly.

It is important to assess the respiratory status of the patient and to maintain and monitor the chest drainage system. Monitoring the drainage system includes identifying an air leak (Erickson, 1989a; Erickson, 1989b). An air leak is indicated by constant bubbling in the water-seal chamber. Maintaining the drainage system becomes especially important if an air leak is present because as the patient inhales, air is taken into the lungs, and small amounts of air may be released from a leak that escapes into the pleural cavity.

If no escape route exists for the air (the chest drainage system), the patient may develop a tension pneumothorax that could be life threatening.Therefore the practice of clamping chest tubes is discouraged. Signs of a tension pneumothorax include an increase in respiratory rate, an increase in heart rate, and cyanosis. The nurse should monitor for a mediastinal shift, which can occur as the lung, heart, and other structures shift away from the pneumothorax (Hudak, Gallo, Benz, 1990).

Frequent inspection is necessary to ascertain that the system remains airtight, that it is working correctly, and that the tubing does not become kinked when the patient is lying on his or her side. A small pillow, folded towel, or rubber ring placed under the chest when the patient is in a side-lying position helps prevent obstruction of the tube. If the chest tube accidentally falls out, the nurse should have the patient exhale and should apply an occlusive dressing at the insertion site. The nurse should monitor the patient closely for signs and symptoms of respiratory distress and should notify the physician if they occur. If the chest tube comes apart, the nurse should clean the ends with alcohol if it is readily available and should reconnect the tube. If necessary, the nurse should use a bottle of sterile water to act as a temporary water seal (Erickson, 1989a; Erickson, 1989b).

The Heimlich chest drainage valve does not use a water-sealed unit. It is a sterile, disposable flutter valve that is attached between the chest drainage catheter and a drainage collection bag. The flutter valve allows fluid and air to pass through it but prevents any reflux of fluids and air. With it in place, the patient can be more mobile because it works in any position.

A chest tube may be temporarily clamped to locate the source of leaks in the system and to replace drainage bottles. If continuous bubbling is noted in the water-seal chamber or the Pleur-Evac unit, the nurse starts clamping close to the chest and works down to the drainage unit. When the tube is clamped between the air leak and the drainage unit, the bubbling stops. If the cause is a loose connection, it is reconnected, and if the drainage unit is cracked, it is replaced. If the air leak is into the patient's pleural space, the physician should be notified immediately. The nurse must remember to assess the reasons why the patient has a chest tube. If a new air leak develops, it must be investigated immediately.

The nurse should be familiar with the purpose for which the drainage system is being used and the type of drainage to expect. If the drainage contains excessive amounts of blood, the physician should be notified. Blood clots may form in the tubing and cause an obstruction. To prevent this from happening, the physician may prescribe the tubing to be milked. Milking should be done carefully to avoid generating significant amounts of pressure in the chest. Stripping a chest tube is avoided because it can generate negative suction pressures in excess of −200 mm Hg (Duncan, Erickson, 1982). Fragile blood vessels, lung tissue, and fresh sutures can be "sucked" through the holes of the chest tube (Box 20-4).

BOX 20-4 Guidelines for Care of the Patient With Water-Seal Chest Drainage

1 Fill the water-seal chamber with sterile water to the 2 cm water level via the latex suction tubing.
2 If suction is required, fill the suction control chamber with sterile water through the atmospheric vent to the level prescribed. This level is usually 20 cm.
3 Attach the drainage catheter (chest tube) coming from the patient to the latex tubing that is attached to the collection chamber of the Pleur-Evac. Tape this connection securely with adhesive tape.
4 If suction is required, connect the suction control chamber tubing to the suction unit. Turn on the suction unit and increase the pressure until gentle bubbling is produced in the suction control chamber.
5 Ensure that the latex tubing is not looping or kinking.
6 Maintain the tubing and drainage system below the patient's chest at all times to allow gravity drainage and to prevent fluid backup.
7 Monitor the amount of drainage in the collection chamber as ordered. It is calibrated in 2 to 5 ml increments and has a surface on which to mark the time and date of drainage.
8 Help the patient achieve a comfortable position. Use pillows to maintain good body alignment.
9 Medicate the patient with analgesics as needed and document their effectiveness.
10 Encourage movement of the arm and shoulder on the affected side.
11 Gently milk the tubing in the direction of the collection chamber every 2 hours or according to institutional policy.
12 Monitor the water-seal chamber for fluctuations (tidaling), which indicate that the closed-drainage system is patent.
13 Fluctuations in the water-seal chamber stop when (a) the lung has reexpanded, (b) the tubing is obstructed, (c) A dependent loop develops, or (d) the suction control apparatus is not working properly.
14 Monitor the patient for an air leak as indicated by constant bubbling in the water-seal chamber.
15 Use techniques of respiratory assessment and note the patient's respiratory rate, depth, and effort, as well as his or her ease of respirations. Monitor breath sounds and note any adventitious sounds.
16 Encourage the patient to cough and to deep breathe at frequent intervals, and use analgesics as needed to promote comfort.
17 When assisting with chest tube removal, instruct the patient to inhale all the way and perform Valsalva's maneuver as the tube is removed smoothly and quickly.
18 An occlusive dressing with Vaseline gauze is applied immediately to prevent atmospheric air from entering the pleural space. The occlusive dressing may be removed in 24 to 48 hours and changed according to institutional policies.

Patient/family education focuses on methods to improve gas exchange, including use of the IS, deep breathing, and coughing. The patient is taught how to splint the incision, and exercises are taught to improve mobility of the shoulder and arm.

THE PATIENT WITH DISEASES AND DISORDERS OF THE RESPIRATORY SYSTEM

Diseases of the respiratory system may result from many different causes, including infections, benign or malignant tumors, physical or chemical agents, allergies, senescence, and emotional factors. Specific symptoms vary with the particular disease. However, dyspnea, chest pain, a cough with or without sputum production, wheezing, hemoptysis, and cyanosis are characteristics of many diseases. Respiratory diseases are discussed under two broad headings: conditions of the upper respiratory system and conditions of the chest and lower respiratory system.

Conditions of the Upper Respiratory System

Infectious respiratory conditions—upper airway infections

A large number of diseases of the respiratory tract are infectious. Many of these bacterial or viral diseases find their way into the respiratory tract when an individual inhales air that is saturated with the disease organism. Many infections follow a pattern, beginning with what appears to be a common cold but gradually

Nursing Care Plan

PATIENT FOLLOWING THORACOTOMY

Mr. Scott is a 71-year-old man who is scheduled for a right lower lobe lobectomy for lung cancer. He has undergone an extensive preoperative evaluation as an outpatient, including routine blood work, an arterial blood gas analysis, a chest x-ray examination, sputum cultures, pulmonary function testing, and a chest CT scan.

Past Medical History	Psychosocial Data	Assessment Data
Denies cardiac disease, hypertension, emphysema, and non–insulin-dependent diabetes mellitus Has smoked two packs of cigarettes per day for 50 years Denies alcohol consumption	Widowed; wife died 2 years ago One son, one daughter, six grandchildren Retired engineer Practicing Catholic Active social life, many friends Owns own home *Hobbies:* fishing, chess, crossword puzzles	Alert and oriented × 3 (time, place, and person) Afebrile, 98.4° F *Cardiovascular:* Pulse 84, regular rate without murmurs; skin warm and dry; peripheral pulses palpable bilaterally *Respiratory:* Respirations 20, not labored, moist cough productive of thin/thick white sputum; scattered rhonchi throughout lung fields; decreased breath sounds right middle and lower lobes; complaining of dyspnea and shortness of breath with exertion *Abdominal:* Soft, nontender, nondistended; bowel sounds in all four quadrants; bowel movement morning of admission *Skin:* No breakdown noted; no rashes Electrolytes within normal limits Complete Blood Count within normal limits *Pulmonary function tests:* Ordered *Arterial blood gases:* 7.45/35/94/98% *Chest x-ray examination:* Consistent with lesion in right lower lobe of lung Patient to be NPO after midnight IV to be started Permit for surgery needs to be signed and witnessed cefazolin (Ancef) on call to the OR Anesthesia visit this evening to discuss patient surgical plan

NURSING DIAGNOSIS

Ineffective airway clearance related to lung impairment, pain, and general anesthesia as evidenced by secretions, abnormal breath sounds, and increased respiratory rate

NURSING INTERVENTIONS	EVALUATION OF EXPECTED OUTCOMES
Maintain a patent airway. While patient is on a ventilator, provide endotracheal suctioning to remove secretions until patient able to cough and deep breathe. Teach patient how to use the IS and encourage its use every hour while awake. Administer humidification and respiratory treatments as indicated. Monitor amount, color, and consistency of sputum.	Airway is patent Breath sounds clear Effective cough demonstrated with expectoration of sputum if present Splints incision when coughing and seeks analgesic medication before coughing if it has not been given

NURSING INTERVENTIONS—cont'd	EVALUATION OF EXPECTED OUTCOMES—cont'd
Assist with postural drainage and chest percussion/vibration as needed. Do not percuss or vibrate over the operative site. Auscultate breath sounds as ordered or as patient condition warrants. Teach splinting of incision and medicate before coughing and deep breathing to allow for increased comfort.	

NURSING DIAGNOSIS

Pain related to surgical procedure and resulting thoracotomy incision

NURSING INTERVENTIONS	EVALUATION OF EXPECTED OUTCOMES
Determine location, onset, quality, and quantity of pain. Use pain assessment tools that are available in several textbooks or at healthcare institutions. Provide analgesics as ordered and determine their effectiveness. Attempt to obtain a new or different analgesic order if ineffective pain relief is obtained. Instruct patient on nonpharmacologic measures to reduce pain if patient is willing to use them (e.g., relaxation, distraction). Turn and position for comfort at least every 2 hours. Monitor incision line for healing and identify any signs and symptoms of possible wound infection, including redness, swelling, drainage, and an increase in wound pain.	Asks for pain medication when needed Uses nonpharmacologic modalities to reduce discomfort Verbalizes acceptable pain score (usually < 3 on 0-10 scale) No signs of wound infection

NURSING DIAGNOSIS

Anxiety related to outcomes of surgery, use of many invasive lines/tubes, pain

NURSING INTERVENTIONS	EVALUATION OF EXPECTED OUTCOMES
Explain all procedures in simple terms. If working with patient preoperatively, review preoperative preparation and how patient can help with his or her own recovery. During the postoperative period, limit noise as much as possible and turn down lights to promote rest and sleep. Encourage and support patient and provide opportunities for expression of fears and concerns. Involve family in care and mobilize additional resources (e.g., social work, clinical nurse specialist, clergy) to help patient cope with the diagnosis and outcomes of surgery	States that anxiety is within a manageable level for him or her Participates in preoperative plan of care Uses appropriate coping skills Uses additional resources if needed

continued

NURSING DIAGNOSIS

Impaired physical mobility of the upper extremities related to thoracic surgery

NURSING INTERVENTIONS	EVALUATION OF EXPECTED OUTCOMES
Assist patient with normal range of motion and function of upper body (arms, shoulder): • Teach breathing exercises to mobilize thorax. • Teach and encourage exercises that promote shoulder abduction. • Help patient to turn and position self in bed, and have patient out of bed to chair and ambulating as condition permits. • Involve physical therapy in care if patient condition warrants.	Demonstrates arm and shoulder exercises and verbalizes importance of performing them Participates in progressive ambulation program

NURSING DIAGNOSIS

Knowledge deficit related to postoperative recovery and follow-up care needed

NURSING INTERVENTIONS	EVALUATION OF EXPECTED OUTCOMES
Instruct patient in the following regarding home care: • Avoid heavy lifting (greater than 5 lb) until incision is healed. • Take analgesics as prescribed to relieve surgical discomfort, especially before increases in activity. • Use nonpharmacologic measures to promote comfort (e.g., relaxation). • Alternate activities with rest periods; don't try to do too much all at once. • Perform arm exercises and shoulder exercises 3 to 5 times daily. • Practice breathing exercises several times a day. • Avoid bronchial irritants. • Prevent colds or lung infections. • Stop smoking. • Keep follow-up appointment with physician.	Verbalizes the importance of avoiding heavylifting until incision is well healed, analgesic use to promote comfort, nonpharmacologic measures to relieve discomfort, arm and breathing exercises to regain function, avoidance of bronchial irritants, preventing colds or lung infection, stopping smoking, and keeping follow-up appointments

involving all parts of the respiratory tract. A large number of infections of the lower respiratory tract begin as upper respiratory infections.

Invasion of the upper respiratory system by pathogenic microorganisms, usually viral, causes inflammation and edema of the mucous membranes. The mucus-secreting glands become hyperactive and produce large amounts of serous-to-mucopurulent exudate. The cervical lymph nodes enlarge and are tender. Air passages become occluded, which causes impaired pulmonary ventilation. Respiratory rates increase in an effort to get more air to the lungs, and the heart works harder to supply the body's tissues with oxygen. The body mobilizes its forces to combat the invading pathogen, and leukocytosis occurs. The inflammatory condition of the mucous membranes causes the throat to become red, sore, and dry; the voice becomes hoarse; and a dry painful cough develops. The pathogen may invade the contiguous mucous membranes of the sinuses and the ears.

Acute coryza (common cold). Acute coryza may be caused by one or several viruses. The causative virus is believed to be present constantly in the upper respiratory tract. A person's susceptibility to the virus increases periodically from a wide variety of factors. Symptoms usually appear within 24 to 48 hours after exposure and may be transmitted to others several hours afterward. Symptoms include a chilly sensation and sneezing. The nasal membranes feel hot, dry, and congested. A slight throat irritation may occur, which is followed by a thin, serous nasal discharge. Nasal congestion causes pressure, which results in headache and tenderness of cervical lymph nodes. If the infection remains uncomplicated, it generally subsides in approximately 1 week. If nasal discharge becomes purulent, it is an indication that the infection is complicated by a bacterial invasion. Symptomatic treatment is appropriate, and the use of antibiotics provides no scientific benefit for viral infections.

Acute pharyngitis. Bacteria or viruses from acute coryza may extend to the pharynx, or pharyngitis may occur without prior evidence of a cold. The throat becomes inflamed and red, the tonsils and cervical lymph nodes become tender, and a sensation of rawness and a dry cough may occur. Chronic pharyngitis may result from a chronic infection of the sinuses or nasal mucosa and may not produce any significant symptoms. Acute pharyngitis usually responds to symptomatic treatment, with recovery occurring in approximately 1 week. If the condition is caused by one of several bacteria, such as the hemolytic streptococcus, *Staphylococcus aureus,* or *Haemophilus influenzae,* symptoms may be more serious and complications may occur.

Acute laryngitis. Acute laryngitis generally is secondary to other upper respiratory tract infections. The mucous membrane that lines the larynx becomes inflamed, and the vocal cords become swollen. The disease is characterized by hoarseness or loss of voice and a cough. Although rare, a tracheotomy may be required in some cases. If it remains uncomplicated, acute laryngitis usually clears in a few days.

Tonsillitis. Acute follicular tonsillitis is an inflammation of the tonsils and is often caused by streptococcus or staphylococcus bacteria. The throat is sore and painful; swallowing is difficult; and generalized muscle aches, chills, and a temperature elevation occur. If tonsillitis is caused by the hemolytic *Streptococcus,* the symptoms may be more severe, with nausea and vomiting and an increased leukocyte count. The primary concern is the prevention of complications such as rheumatic fever and nephritis. Repeated attacks of tonsillitis may require surgical removal of the tonsils, or a **tonsillectomy.** Care of a patient who is undergoing a tonsillectomy is discussed later in this chapter.

Sinusitis. Sinusitis may be acute or chronic and usually occurs as the result of other upper respiratory tract infections. Because mucous membranes of the nasal cavities are contiguous with the sinuses, infection may be spread easily to the sinuses. Inflammation of the sinuses may occur from obstructions such as nasal polyps or from a deviated septum that blocks the drainage from the sinuses. Sinusitis may also be a complication of influenza or pneumonia. If an acute sinusitis is left untreated, it may become chronic or may lead to more serious conditions such as meningitis, brain abscess, osteomyelitis, and septicemia.

The primary symptom of sinusitis is pain, and its location is related to the sinus involved. When the maxillary sinus is affected, the pain occurs over the cheeks and may radiate downward to the teeth. A frontal sinus infection causes pain in and above the eyes. The bone over the affected sinus usually is sensitive to slight pressure, and puffiness over the area may be observed (Loch and others, 1990). Depending on the extent of the infection and the particular microorganism involved, the patient may have an elevated temperature, nausea, and loss of appetite. When a continuous postnasal dripping into the back of the throat occurs, coughing and soreness of the throat may result. Acute sinusitis causes discomfort and often results in lost work time and an inability to perform other activities of daily living.

Influenza. Influenza is an acute disease of the respiratory tract and is accompanied by fever and systemic symptoms. It is caused by a virus that has been identified and classified as type A, B, or C. Type D is now known as parainfluenza 1, and strains of A are known as A prime, or A_1 and A_2. In 1968, 1969, and 1974, various parts of the world, including the United States, experienced a fairly mild form of influenza caused by a new strain of the A_2 virus, which was called *A_2 Hong Kong influenza.*

The first symptoms of influenza occur with rapidity, and the typical picture is one of chills; a temperature of 102° F to 104° F (39° C to 40° C); severe aching of the back, head, and extremities; sore throat; cough; considerable prostration; sneezing; coated tongue; and weakness. If the infection is uncomplicated, the acute period usually lasts from 3 to 5 days. Some cases do not follow the typical pattern but begin with gastrointestinal symptoms, bronchopneumonia, pleurisy, or sinusitis (Box 20-5). Influenza is especially hazardous for older persons, and the mortality from influenza-pneumonia generally rises sharply during an influenza epidemic.

Interventions in upper airway infections. The treatment of upper airway infections is directed toward relieving the discomfort of symptoms and preventing complications. Precautionary measures should be taken to prevent the spread of the infection to others. Nasal sprays, moist inhalations, warm saline gargles, throat irrigations, and acetaminophen (Tylenol) provide symptomatic relief and promote comfort. Fluid intake should be increased to provide systemic hydration.

BOX 20-5

Nursing Process

INFLUENZA

ASSESSMENT

Vital signs (fever)
Cervical lymph nodes
Respiratory status
Fluid volume status
Anorexia, chills, malaise, sore throat

NURSING DIAGNOSES

Ineffective airway clearance related to bronchial secretions
Risk for fluid volume deficit related to hyperthermia and decreased intake
Activity intolerance related to weakness

NURSING INTERVENTIONS

Position for optimal breathing (head of bed elevated).
Encourage bedrest for 2 or 3 days.
Encourage position changes.
Provide cool mist humidification, if indicated.
Administer decongestants, as prescribed.
Encourage liberal fluid intake (2 L/day) unless contraindicated.
Plan and encourage rest periods between activities.
Provide progressive increases in activity as tolerated.
Encourage high risk persons to get influenza vaccines yearly before the "flu" season.

EVALUATION OF EXPECTED OUTCOMES

Clear breath sounds
No evidence of dehydration
Able to perform ADLs without fatigue
Afebrile
Verbalizes understanding of treatment regimen

When pharyngitis or laryngitis accompanies acute coryza, relief may be obtained by cool mist vaporizers, which loosen secretions and reduce inflammation of the mucous membranes. If coughing is disturbing, an analgesic cough mixture or a mild sedative for rest at night may be ordered. When severe pharyngitis is present, the nurse should be alert to the possibility of complications. Temperature, pulse rates, and respiration rates should be checked every 4 hours unless otherwise ordered. The diet may need to be liquid or soft, with fluids forced. The patient may be encouraged to drink 2 to 3 liters of fluid per day. If the infection is caused by bacteria such as streptococci, the patient should be observed for a skin rash, which might indicate scarlet fever. Blood cultures, a white blood cell count, and a urinalysis may be prescribed. In bacterial infections, an elevation of the white blood cell count may be seen. When the larynx is involved, talking should be avoided or reduced. Antibiotic drugs may be ordered when the infection is caused by bacteria.

Most patients with respiratory tract infections are more comfortable when placed in a low (15 degrees) Fowler's position, which provides for better drainage of secretions. A cool (68° F to 70° F [20° C to 21° C]), well-ventilated, draft-free, and high-humidity room provides a greater degree of comfort than an overheated room.

Patient/family teaching. The prevention of most upper airway infections is difficult because there are many possible causes. The nurse instructs the patient about the following measures that support the host's defenses and thereby reduce one's susceptibility to respiratory infections:

- Live healthy; eat a nutritious diet, get adequate rest and sleep, and exercise.
- Avoid excesses in alcohol, smoke, and irritants.
- Ensure adequate home humidification, especially during the cold months.
- Avoid irritants (tobacco, smoke, chemicals) and allergens whenever possible.
- Obtain an influenza vaccine, especially if recommended by a healthcare provider. (A flu vaccine may be recommended for persons who are over 65 years, have a chronic disease, or are employed in a healthcare setting.)
- Avoid crowds during the flu season.
- Maintain good dental hygiene.
- Practice good handwashing.

Obstruction and trauma of the upper airway

Epistaxis. A nosebleed is rarely fatal or even serious, but it may cause the patient considerable anxiety. A number of causes of **epistaxis** exist. The nasal cavities are supplied by a fine network of blood capillaries, and anything that congests the nasal membrane may rupture a small capillary and result in bleeding. The condition may occur in persons with hypertension, cardiovascular disease, blood dyscrasias, and some communicable diseases. Epistaxis may also be caused by injury to the nose, picking, or forceful blowing.

Assessment. The cause should be determined by careful examination and assessment. Data to be obtained include history, frequency, and duration of bleeding episodes; precipitating factors; signs of upper respiratory tract infections or allergic conditions; present medications that might influence clotting; history of physical abuse to the face; and measures used to try to stop the bleeding. The patient should also be observed for site, color, and amount of bleeding; signs of respiratory difficulty; and signs of progressing hemorrhage. The primary provider may request laboratory tests to determine the extent and possible cause of the bleeding.

Intervention. Nursing procedures include placing the patient in a Fowler's position with the head forward. The patient should be encouraged to let the blood drain from the nose, to breathe through the mouth, and to avoid swallowing the blood because it may cause nausea and vomiting. The nostrils should be compressed tightly below the bone and held for at least 10 minutes. This procedure controls most cases of epistaxis. Ice packs applied to the area may help control bleeding by causing reflex vasoconstriction of the capillaries.

Topical administration of vasoconstricting agents may also be performed. These drugs decrease blood supply to the area and control bleeding. A cotton ball or nasal pack is saturated with a 1:1000 solution of phenylephrine and inserted into the nostril. Pressure is applied for several minutes. The cotton ball is removed, and any bleeding is monitored (Patrick and others, 1991; Smeltzer, Bare, 1992).

If bleeding cannot be controlled, packing the nose may be necessary. Hemostatic agents such as an absorbable gelatin sponge (Gelfoam), packing saturated with a 1:1000 solution of epinephrine, petroleum gauze, and oxidized cellulose (Oxycel) often are used. A gauze pad can be placed under the nostrils to absorb any drainage or blood. The patient with the nasal packing in place should be monitored for signs and symptoms of infection. Respiratory status should be monitored, and airway patency should be assessed because hypoxemia can result if the packing slips out of position and obstructs the airway. In rare cases, cauterizing the bleeding vessel may be necessary.

Patient/family teaching. Patients should be taught proper positioning to facilitate the drainage of blood and the proper application of pressure to the area to control bleeding. Ice packs may also be applied. If bleeding continues, the physician should be notified and the origin of the bleeding determined (Smeltzer, Bare, 1992).

Deviated septum and nasal polyps. The nasal septum divides the two nasal cavities. Most people have some irregularity of the septum but are unaware of the condition unless it is great enough to obstruct breathing. During childhood, injuries to the nose, including fractures, can occur. If not cared for, these injuries may result in a bending of the septum to one side or the other. If the deviation is severe, it causes a partial blocking of the respiratory passageway on one side. When obstruction occurs, surgical correction is necessary.

A polyp is a small tumor that is attached to the mucous membranes of the nose. It may have been caused by prolonged inflammation of the sinuses, and because it obstructs free drainage of secretions, the inflammatory condition may be aggravated. Surgical removal may be necessary to relieve the inflammatory condition.

Respiratory obstruction from a deviated septum or nasal polyps may be corrected by a surgical procedure called *submucous resection.* The procedure is performed after administration of preoperative sedation and while the patient is under local anesthesia. After the procedure, the nose is packed for approximately 12 to 24 hours. Generally the packing is soaked in liquid petrolatum to facilitate its removal. The patient is placed in a Fowler's position, and analgesics are administered to relieve pain. Because breathing will be through the mouth, the patient may be given chipped ice to help keep the mouth moist. Petroleum jelly may be applied to the lips, and iced compresses may be applied over the nose. The patient should be observed for hemorrhage, which is indicated by expectoration of bright red blood, frequent swallowing, or an increased flow of bright red blood through the packing. After removal of the packing, the patient is allowed a diet as desired and bathroom privileges. The patient should be told to expect a loss of the sense of smell for approximately 1 week.

Enlarged tonsils and adenoids. The pharyngeal tonsils (adenoids) are a mass of lymphoid tissue located at the back of the nose in the upper pharynx. The palatine tonsils, also composed of lymphoid tissue, are located on each side of the soft palate in the throat. These tissues are normally larger in childhood, and under normal conditions removal is not considered necessary unless they become infected with bacteria and do not respond to conservative treatment. The tonsils also may obstruct the eustachian tube opening in the back of the throat and may cause some loss of hearing. Removing these lymphoid structures surgically may be necessary to restore normal breathing and hearing.

Intervention. A tonsillectomy may be performed using a local anesthetic. On return from surgery, the patient is placed in a Fowler's position. When a general anesthetic has been given, the patient may be placed on his or her side. Vital signs should be checked, just as for any postoperative patient. An ice collar is applied to the throat to relieve discomfort. The patient should be instructed not to cough or clear the throat, and talking should be discouraged for several hours. The patient should always be observed for postoperative hemorrhaging, and care is directed toward its prevention. The patient should not be allowed to gargle before healing begins because it may dislodge a clot and produce bleeding. If nausea is not present and if no bleeding develops, water or chipped ice may be given. If a temperature elevation occurs, the surgeon should be notified. A trace of blood is to be anticipated, but any unusual amount of bright red blood should be reported immediately. Suction equipment and packing should be available for emergencies.

Patient/family teaching. After returning home, patients need to get enough rest, eat soft foods, drink fluids, and gradually resume activity. Because delayed hemorrhaging may occur, bleeding is reported promptly to the physician.

Foreign bodies. If foreign materials become lodged in the throat or trachea, emergency treatment must be instituted. If the object cannot be dislodged by the finger, the nurse should stand behind the choking individual, hold the individual below the rib cage, and quickly squeeze (similar to a bear hug). This action, called the Heimlich maneuver, forces residual air and the foreign object out of the respiratory tract.

Aspirated foreign bodies are more likely to enter the right main bronchus, which is larger and in a more vertical position. If the object is small, coughing occurs and slight dyspnea develops. Aspiration of a foreign body often creates an acute emergency and necessitates prompt removal with a laryngoscope or bronchoscope. Occasionally a tracheotomy may be required to establish an airway. The nurse needs to approach the situation with calmness and carry out emergency orders with efficiency. When foreign bodies are removed from the bronchus or lung, steam inhalations may be prescribed along with sedative or analgesic drugs to relieve discomfort.

Tumors of the Respiratory System

Benign or malignant tumors may occur in any part of the respiratory system. Malignant tumors of the upper respiratory system are less common than are tumors in other parts of the body.

Cancer of the larynx accounts for a small percentage of neoplasms. As with malignant tumors in other parts of the body, the cause of carcinoma of the larynx is unknown. However, persons with laryngeal cancer are often heavy smokers. When the condition is diagnosed early, a cure is possible. The disease is most common in men over 45 years of age.

Assessment

The first symptom of laryngeal cancer that may be observed is hoarseness of the voice, which becomes progressively worse without treatment. If this symptom is neglected, metastasis to other structures occurs, and pain on swallowing or pain in the vicinity of the "Adam's apple" radiates to the ear. Ultimately the airway becomes obstructed and dyspnea occurs. Carcinoma of the larynx is diagnosed by obtaining a history and by visually examining the larynx with a laryngoscope. Mobility of the vocal cords is assessed. A biopsy is done for laboratory confirmation of the clinical findings. Depending on the location of the tumor and the extent of involvement, a partial or a total **laryngectomy** is performed.

Intervention

Treatment varies with the extent of the malignancy and may include radiation therapy, partial laryngectomy, supraglottic laryngectomy, or total laryngectomy (Table 20-8).

When a total laryngectomy is performed, the larynx, vocal cords, thyroid cartilage, and epiglottis are removed surgically. The trachea is sutured to the anterior surface of the neck as a permanent tracheostomy (Figure 20-26). Because the patient no longer breathes through the nose, he or she has little sense of smell. The patient must be prepared emotionally for the loss of normal speech and the change in normal breathing.

Before the surgery, the patient should be given an explanation of the operation by discussing the way in which normal speech is produced and how the operation will affect the production of normal speech. The patient should also be given information about speech therapy and informed that these resources will be available postoperatively.

After surgery the patient may be placed in the intensive care unit because continuous nursing care should be provided for the first 48 hours, or longer if necessary. If the patient is admitted directly to the surgical unit, it should be prepared to receive the patient after surgery. Heated nebulizers are used to humidify the air. Equipment for caring for and cleaning a tracheostomy tube should be available, as well as suction, tissues, and a pencil and paper or slate. Some surgeons do not insert a tracheostomy tube because the method of suturing keeps the wound open. If a tube is inserted, it is a laryngeal (laryngectomy) tube, which is slightly larger in diameter and shorter than the ordi-

TABLE 20-8

Laryngectomy Surgery for Cancer

Type	Description	Voice Result
Partial laryngectomy; laryngofissure	Opening into larynx through thyroid cartilage with removal of diseased vocal cord	Husky but acceptable
Hemilaryngectomy	Same approach as for laryngofissure with removal of diseased false cord, arytenoid, and one side of thyroid cartilage	Hoarse voice
Supraglottic partial laryngectomy	Horizontal incision passes above true cords (left intact) with removal of epiglottis and diseased tissue	Normal voice
Total laryngectomy	Removal of epiglottis, thyroid cartilage, and 3 or 4 tracheal rings; closure of pharynx with trachea; permanent tracheostomy	No voice

From Phipps WJ and others: *Medical-surgical nursing: concepts and clinical practice,* ed 5, St Louis, 1995, Mosby.

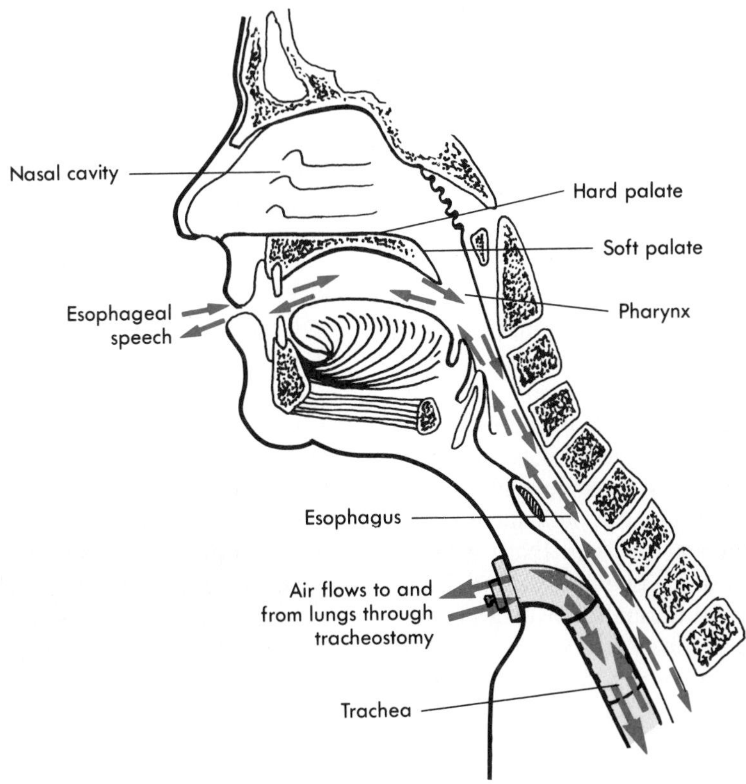

Figure 20-26 Permanent tracheostomy. Note that there is no connection between the trachea and esophagus. (From Phipps WJ: *Medical-surgical nursing: concepts and clinical practice,* ed 5, St Louis, 1995, Mosby.)

nary tracheostomy (Figure 20-27). If a tube is inserted, a sterile set the same size as the one inserted should be available at the bedside for emergency use if the first tube comes out.

The most important function of the nurse is to keep the airway clear. The nurse must be available to wipe or suction secretions when the patient coughs. In the beginning, suctioning may be necessary as often as every 5 minutes. The suction catheter should not be inserted more than the length of the tube, and the physician should be notified if the secretions cannot be removed. Efforts should be made to prevent wound in-

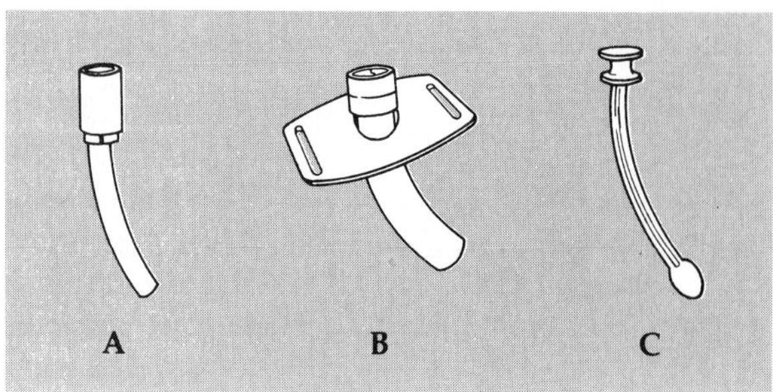

Figure 20-27 Laryngectomy tube. **A,** Inner cannula. **B,** Outer cannula. **C,** Obturator.

fection by maintaining aseptic technique. Oxygen may be administered for 1 to 2 days.

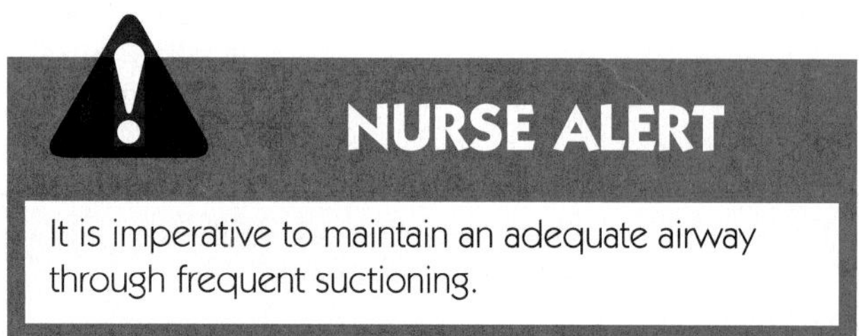

It is imperative to maintain an adequate airway through frequent suctioning.

The character of respirations must be observed for any rate increase, wheezing, or crowing sounds, which indicates airway obstruction. Secretions may be tinged with blood for 1 or 2 days, but any continued bleeding may be from an internal hemorrhage and should be reported. Meticulous mouth care with an antiseptic mouthwash should be given often. If intravenous fluids are given, they should not be placed in the arm that the patient uses for writing if possible. The patient may not be allowed anything by mouth for a week. Feedings are given by means of a tube that is passed through the patient's nose. When the patient is allowed food by mouth, the food should be soft until healing is complete. Some surgeons do not order tube feedings but allow patients to eat soft food and drink liquids if they feel well enough. A patient with a laryngectomy usually is most comfortable in a 45-degree Fowler's position, which makes breathing easier. The lips should be kept moist, and crusts should not be allowed to form around the nares.

As patients improve, they should be taught how to care for their own tracheostomy, and if they are unable to do so, some member of the family should be taught (Feinstein, 1987). When a tube is used, it may be left in place for approximately 6 weeks. As soon as the neck wounds have healed, the therapist may begin speech training. Esophageal speech is the means of communication used after a laryngectomy. If esophageal speech cannot be learned, a vibrator or an electronic artificial larynx can be used. Much assistance can be obtained from local chapters of the American Cancer Society, including information on a Lost Cord Club or a New Voice Club. Most patients with total laryngectomies are able to return to normal roles in life, but they should be cautioned about occupational hazards such as dust and fumes and should seek to protect themselves against respiratory tract infections.

Conditions of the Chest and Lower Respiratory System

Chronic obstructive pulmonary disease or chronic airflow limitation

Diseases that interfere with ventilation cause psychologic, physical, and social problems for the individual. Fear, tension, frustration, and panic accompany these diseases. One of the most important aspects of medical and nursing care is the relief of anxiety. Inadequate ventilation disturbs the homeostasis of the body. Electrolyte balance is affected, changes occur in the extracellular fluid, and serious cardiac complications may occur. The constant shortness of breath, fatigue, and limitation of activity may cause retirement from employment, limitation of social activities, and feelings of social isolation and depression. COPDs include emphysema, chronic bronchitis, bronchiectasis, and asthma, each of which may result in varying degrees of incapacitation for the individual (Box 20-6).

Pulmonary emphysema. Pulmonary **emphysema** affects persons of all socioeconomic levels. An estimated 10 million persons in the United States have emphysema, and one out of every four wage earners over age 45 is disabled because of the disease. The disease is more common in men than in women, and reports indicate that most men over age 70 have destructive emphysema. The cause of emphysema is unknown, but chronic bronchitis and asthma are often associated with emphysema. Research has indicated that cigarette smoking is the largest factor in the development of pulmonary emphysema. Air pollution, temperature changes, and humidity appear to have an adverse effect on the disease.

Pathophysiology. In pulmonary emphysema the alveolar walls and capillaries are destroyed, which decreases the area available for gas exchange between the bloodstream and the air. Chronic irritation to the bronchi, bronchioles, and alveoli causes inflammation with swelling and secretions. The lumen of the bronchioles narrows, especially during expiration, and air becomes trapped in the alveoli. The alveoli become distended and rupture or become scarred and thickened with a loss of elasticity. Infections hasten the process.

PATIENT/FAMILY TEACHING

Laryngectomy and Radical Neck Dissection

GENERAL HYGIENE

- Clean teeth and mouth 3 times daily, because the ability to detect mouth odor is lessened; use mouthwash frequently.
- Wear a protective cover over the tracheostomy when taking a shower.
- Wear a protective cover over the stoma while shaving or having a haircut to prevent hair and dust particles from entering.

STOMA CARE

- Observe the stoma daily for signs of redness, secretions, or swelling; observe also for fever.
- To prevent infection, always wash hands before touching the stoma.
- Clean the stoma twice daily using a clean, damp washcloth; the use of soaps should be avoided because they irritate the skin; tissues may obstruct the airway.
- Apply petrolatum around the exterior of the stoma, if ordered, taking care not to allow any to enter.
- Cover the stoma with a bib (a piece of cotton cloth) to aid in warming and filtering inspired air; a variety of clothing and accessories can be worn by men and women to cover the bib; high-neck sweaters, turtlenecks, and scarves work well; there should always be easy access to the stoma for inserting a handkerchief or for emergency actions.

EMERGENCY CARE

- Wear a Medic Alert bracelet or carry a card indicating that a laryngectomy has been done and containing instructions regarding first aid should the stoma become obstructed or a cardiopulmonary arrest occur.
- Swimming may be possible with new commercial covers, but be aware that drowning could easily occur without getting the head wet; other people who have been instructed in first aid measures should be present during swimming.

STOMAL HYDRATION

- Additional hydration is needed for airway; use of commercial humidifiers or a pan of water on the stove or radiator will greatly add to comfort.
- When taking a bath or shower, allow water to accumulate 4 to 6 inches while sitting in the tub or standing in the shower stall on a nonslip mat; a well-wrung towel can be draped around the neck for added moisture and to prevent perspiration from dripping into the stoma.

OTHER HEALTHFUL BEHAVIORS

- Moderation is the key rule in all normal activities; move slowly, control emotions, and exercise with moderation to avoid fatigue.
- When coughing, remember to cover stoma instead of mouth; moisture and secretions can be expelled onto clothing.
- Report persistent coughing to the primary provider.
- If there is a history of alcohol intake, moderation or abstinence must be practiced; smokers should stop and should seek assistance to do so.
- Use available community resources for support and speech rehabilitation as needed (American Cancer Society, Lost Cord Club).

From Beare PG, Myers JL: *Principles and practice of adult health nursing,* ed 2, St Louis, 1994, Mosby.

Expiration of air depends on the elasticity of the lungs, but because of lost elasticity and obstructed bronchioles, all of the inspired air cannot be forced out of the lungs. Increased pressure in the alveoli causes them to collapse. Distended air sacs (blebs) occurring on the surface of the lung may rupture and allow air to enter the pleural cavity, causing a spontaneous pneumothorax. The pathologic changes cause a decrease in vital capacity and an increase in the residual volume of air retained in the lungs. Oxygenation of the arterial blood is decreased, and carbon dioxide tension of the arterial blood is increased. The retention of carbon dioxide in the blood may result in respiratory acidosis or carbon dioxide narcosis, stupor, and coma.

Assessment. Emphysema has an insidious onset, with dyspnea being the predominant symptom. As the disease progresses, the dyspnea is not only experienced on exertion but also at rest. Any emotional upset, exertion, or excitement increases the dyspnea and respiratory distress. Other manifestations of the disease include hypoxia, coughing with copious amounts of mucopurulent sputum, a barrel-shaped chest, the use of accessory muscles of respiration, wheezing, grunting on expiration, peripheral cyanosis, digital clubbing, chronic respiratory acidosis, chronic weight loss, anorexia, and malaise. Auscultation of the lung fields reveal diminished breath sounds with rhonchi and prolonged expiration. Percussion yields hyperres-

BOX 20-6 **Nursing Process**

CHRONIC OBSTRUCTIVE PULMONARY DISEASE

ASSESSMENT

Dyspnea
Hypoxemia
Productive cough with mucopurulent sputum; barrel-shaped chest
Use of accessory muscles
Wheezing; diminished breath sounds with rhonchi and prolonged expiration
Peripheral cyanosis
Chronic weight loss
Anorexia

NURSING DIAGNOSES

Impaired gas exchange related to inequality between ventilation-perfusion
Ineffective airway clearance related to bronchoconstriction, increased mucus production, ineffective cough, and infection
Ineffective breathing pattern related to shortness of breath, mucus production, bronchoconstriction
Self-care deficit related to fatigue that is promoted by increase in work of breathing
Activity intolerance related to hypoxemia and fatigue
Ineffective individual coping related to effects of illness on lifestyle
Anxiety related to respiratory difficulty

NURSING INTERVENTIONS

Administer bronchodilators as prescribed.
Evaluate effectiveness of respiratory treatments.
Administer oxygen only if ordered and in low concentrations (flow rate of 1 to 2 L/min).
Teach and demonstrate diaphragmatic breathing and coughing.
Give patient 6 to 8 glasses of fluids every day unless cor pulmonale is present.
Provide a diet consisting of several small meals each day.
Perform postural drainage with percussion and vibration as prescribed.
Monitor for signs and symptoms of respiratory infections, including change in sputum amount, color, or consistency; shortness of breath; increased coughing.
Maintain activity level within patient's abilities; encourage alternating activity with rest periods.
Assist patient in developing a regular activity program to recondition and strengthen muscles; work with other disciplines (e.g., physical therapy) as needed.
Observe for complications such as cor pulmonale or congestive heart failure.

EVALUATION OF EXPECTED OUTCOMES

Verbalizes the need for bronchodilators and for taking them at specified times
Demonstrates the ability to use and care for the specific respiratory equipment being used
Uses oxygen when appropriate and verbalizes safe handling of oxygen
Demonstrates diaphragmatic breathing/coughing
Verbalizes the need to consume 6 to 8 glasses of fluid each day
Discusses diet and the need to consume several small meals each day
Performs postural drainage correctly
Identifies signs of early infection (e.g., sputum, shortness of breath, increased coughing)
Verbalizes that pollens, fumes, gases, dusts and extremes of temperature and humidity are irritants to be avoided
Verbalizes the importance of maintaining regular activity; understands the need for rest periods and pacing of activities
Participates in discharge plan
Explores resources available in community

onance and a decrease in fremitus (Kersten, 1989).

Intervention. The most important factor in the treatment of patients with emphysema is prevention. The patient should be protected from respiratory tract infections and must be treated at the earliest signs of infection. Laboratory examination of sputum should be performed to determine the specific bacteria present. A broad-spectrum antibiotic is usually given. The patient should be encouraged to secure an influenza vaccine in early autumn. Because cigarette smoking is hazardous, every effort should be made to persuade the patient to discontinue the habit. The patient should avoid drafts and changes of temperature. Windows should be kept closed, and air conditioning is desir-

OLDER ADULT CONSIDERATIONS

Bronchodilator therapy for COPD

Age-related changes in pharmacokinetics and the presence of other chronic health problems increase the older adult's risk for side effects associated with bronchodilator drugs used to treat COPD. For theophylline preparations the older adult should have drug levels monitored at more frequent intervals than the young adult.

Side effects associated with anticholinergic bronchodilators, such as urinary retention and blurred vision, may be particularly troublesome for the older adult. Ipratropium bromide administered by inhalation will provide therapeutic benefit with fewer systemic side effects. The older adult should exercise caution in using over-the-counter bronchodilators. These drugs usually contain alpha and beta agonists (epinephrine and ephedrine) that can aggravate preexisting health problems such as hypertension or diabetes.

Although metered-dose inhalers may produce fewer side effects, the older adult may have difficulty learning to coordinate drug administration with respiratory activity. Decreased motor function and range of motion in the hands may render the older adult less able to use the device effectively.

From Beare PG, Myers JL: *Principles and practice of adult health nursing,* ed 2, St Louis, 1994, Mosby.

able. The patient should have a sleeping room and bath on the first floor if indicated. Treatment is palliative and is directed toward making breathing as easy as possible. Some patients do better in moderate climates with minimum temperature changes.

Coughing is the emphysema patient's first defense. Deep breathing, incentive spirometry, and aerosolized bronchodilators help loosen secretions and optimize ventilation. Producing low, small, grunting coughs after deep breaths while supporting the abdominal muscles usually yields the best results. The patient may be taught to inhale by using the stomach muscles and exhale by blowing gently through pursed lips. Chest physical therapy such as percussion, vibration, and postural drainage are often effective in removing secretions from affected lungs (Kersten, 1989).

Bronchodilators are prescribed to dilate the airways. Because they influence edema of the bronchial mucosa and relieve muscle spasm, they improve gas exchange and reduce airway obstruction. Bronchodilators include isoproterenol (Isuprel), isoetharine (Bronkosol), or metaproterenol (Alupent) (Table 20-9).

If the bronchodilating drugs become ineffective, corticosteroids may be added. Usually 5 to 10 mg of prednisone given orally once a day is ordered. If steroid therapy is continued, the patient must have an increased intake of potassium and be monitored for side effects, including gastrointestinal upset and increased appetite. When steroids are being discontinued, a steroid taper is performed.

Because of the constant high level of carbon dioxide in the blood and tissues of the emphysema patient, the body begins to rely on low levels of oxygen as the main stimulus for respiration. Therefore administering high concentrations of oxygen to such patients may depress their respirations. If prescribed, oxygen should not be administered with a flow rate greater than 2 to 3 L/min. In severe emphysema, oxygen may be administered at least 16 hr/day, with 24 hours often required. Oxygen should be started slowly, and the patient should be observed for restlessness, apprehension, flushed skin, shallow respirations, and stupor. The patient should also be observed for signs of right ventricular failure (cor pulmonale). Because the capillaries in the lungs have been destroyed by the disease process, the heart must work harder to pump blood through the diseased lungs. Edema of the feet and legs and distended neck veins may indicate the onset of right ventricular failure. Gastric ulcers also tend to occur in patients with emphysema, although the specific cause is unknown.

Physical therapy should be part of every patient's therapy program. Its purpose is to recondition and strengthen muscles that have become soft and flabby and have lost their tone because of inactivity. Patients should be encouraged to follow a graded program of daily exercise. Patients with emphysema usually breathe most easily when sitting up and may feel less well in the morning because secretions have collected in the lungs and bronchi during the night. A hot drink may help loosen tenacious sputum so that it may be coughed up. By the end of the day, patients may feel completely exhausted. They should be encouraged to care for themselves within the limits of their ability. The diet should be nourishing, and gas-forming foods should be eliminated. The appetite may be poor, and several small, attractive meals a day may be better than large meals. Fluids should be encouraged, if appropriate, to avoid the tendency toward dehydration. The nose and mouth should be kept clean, and all nursing care should be adapted to the needs of the individual patient. These needs change as the disease progresses, and the physician, nurse, patient, and family must work together to plan a way of life for the patient.

Chronic bronchitis. Chronic bronchitis often occurs with pulmonary emphysema. In pulmonary em-

TABLE 20-9

Pharmacology of Drugs Used in Respiration

Drug (Generic and Trade Name); Route and Dosage	Action/Indication	Common Side Effects and Nursing Considerations
ACETYLCYSTEINE (Mucocil) **ROUTE:** Nebulization via face mask, instillation via tracheostomy tube, or oral **DOSAGE:** Usual dose is 6-10 ml 10% solution 3-4 times/day	Decreases the viscosity or thickness of mucus and secretions in patients who are debilitated or unable to cough and maintain a patent airway	Nausea, vomiting, rhinorrhea, stomatitis, fever, tracheal and bronchial irritation, chest tightness, and bronchospasm; cautious use in bronchial asthma, debilitated persons with respiratory disease
CODEINE (used in many cough/cold preparations) **ROUTE:** PO, liquid **DOSAGE:** Usually 120 mg maximum over 24 hr; varies with product	Narcotic antitussive used in suppression of nonproductive coughing and relief of mild-to-moderate pain	Lightheadedness, dizziness, sedation, sweating, and nausea; cautious use in asthma or other pulmonary diseases; contraindicated with known or suspected narcotic addiction
DEXTROMETHORPHAN (Comtrex, Dimetane-DX, Humidid-DM, Rondec-DM, Tylenol Cold Medication). **ROUTE:** PO, chewable pieces, liquid, lozenges, syrup **DOSAGE:** 10-20 mg PO q 4 hr or 30 mg q 6-8 hr; controlled-release liquid (60 MG bid)	Nonnarcotic antitussive (cough suppressant), used for nonproductive cough only	Dizziness, GI distress, and drowsiness; contraindicated with MAO inhibitors
GUAIFENESIN (Robitussin) **ROUTE:** PO liquid, tablets, capsules. **DOSAGE:** 100-400 mg q 3-6 hr; maximum 2.4 g/day	Expectorant used for symptomatic relief of dry, unproductive cough; associated with common respiratory disorders such as colds and bronchitis	Nausea, vomiting, GI distress, and drowsiness, cautious use with persistent cough, high fever, persistent headache, or rash; may decrease platelets and cause bleeding
IPRATROPIUM (Atrovent) **ROUTE:** Inhaler **DOSAGE:** Two inhalations 4 times/day, to a maximum of 12 inhalations within 24 hr	Anticholinergic bronchodilator used in the treatment of bronchospasm associated with asthma, chronic bronchitis, or emyphysema	Coughing, dryness of oropharynx, gastric upset, and nervousness; cautious use in glaucoma, prostatic hypertrophy, and bladder obstruction; contraindicated in treatment of acute bronchospastic episodes
THEOPHYLLINE ETHYLENEDIAMINE (Aminophylline; closely related to theophylline, slophyllin, theo-dur, uniphyl, slo-bid) **ROUTE:** PO liquids, tablets, capsules, injection, rectal **DOSAGE:** Highly individualized and adjusted on the basis of serum theophylline levels (optimal range 10-20 g/ml)	Symptomatic relief from or prevention of bronchial asthma and bronchospasm associated with chronic bronchitis, emphysema, and other obstructive pulmonary diseases	GI upset, nausea, nervousness, and urinary frequency; cautious use in elderly with circulatory impairment, renal or hepatic disease, peptic ulcer, hyperthyroidism, and diabetes; contraindicated in hypersensitivity to caffeine, severe gastritis, peptic ulcer disease, and myocardial stimulation

TABLE 20-9

Pharmacology of Drugs Used in Respiration—cont'd

Drug (Generic and Trade Name); Route and Dosage	Action/Indication	Common Side Effects and Nursing Considerations
TRIAMCINOLONE (Azmacort) **ROUTE:** Inhaler **DOSAGE:** 2 inhalations 3-4 times/day; maximum 16 inhalations/day	An inhaled corticosteroid used in treatment of bronchial asthma	Euphoria, insomnia, and peptic ulcer; bronchodilator inhalers should be taken before corticosteroid inhalers; overuse of inhalers may be harmful; sudden withdrawal of this inhaler could be fatal; corticosteroid inhalers should be terminated gradually if discontinued
Antitubular Agents		
ETHAMBUTOL (Myambutol) **ROUTE:** PO **DOSAGE:** 15-25 mg/kg/day	Antitubercular used in combination with at least one other drug in the treatment of active tuberculosis or other mycobacterial diseases	Optic neuritis; use with caution in renal and severe hepatic impairment
ISONIAZID (INH) (Isoniazid) **ROUTE:** PO, IM **DOSAGE:** PO, IM, 5-10 mg/kg/day (usually 300 mg) or 15 mg/kg 2-3 times weekly after 2 mo at 300 mg/day	Antitubercular used as a first-line drug in combination with other agents in the treatment of the active disease; also used for prevention of tuberculosis in patients exposed to active disease	Peripheral neuropathy; contraindicated in acute liver disease and previous hepatitis from INH; use with caution in history of liver damage, chronic alcohol ingestion, severe renal impairment, malnourished patients, and diabetics; possible additive CNS toxicity with other antituberculars; severe reactions may occur with ingestion of foods containing high concentrations of tyramine
RIFABUTIN (Mycobutin) **ROUTE:** PO **DOSAGE:** 300 mg once daily; if GI upset occurs, may give as 150 mg twice daily with food	Antimycobacterial used to prevent disseminated *Mycobacterium avium complex* (MAC) disease in patients with advanced HIV infection and used in the treatment of most strains of *Mycobacterium tuberculosis*	Brown-orange discoloration of tears, saliva, urine, and body fluids; cross-sensitivity with other rifamycins (Rifampin) may occur
RIFAMPIN (Rifadin, Rimactane) **ROUTE:** PO, IV **DOSAGE:** PO, IV, 10 mg/kg/day (usual dose 600 mg/day) single dose; may also be given twice weekly	Antitubercular used in combination with other agents in the management of active TB	Nausea, vomiting, heartburn, abdominal pain, flatulence, diarrhea, and red discoloration of all body fluids; use with caution in history of liver disease or concurrent use of other hepatotoxic agents
STREPTOMYCIN (Streptomycin) **ROUTE:** IM **DOSAGE:** 15 mg/kg/day (not to exceed 1 g) or 25-30 mg/kg (not to exceed 1.5 g) 2-3 times weekly	Antiinfective, antitubercular used in combination therapy for active TB and for streptococcal or enterococcal endocarditis	Ototoxicity and nephrotoxicity; use with caution in renal impairment, neuromuscular diseases, and in the elderly

physema it is possible to define the pathologic changes in the lungs. However, in chronic bronchitis, the changes are functional and cannot be observed on x-ray film. Physiologic findings in obstructive chronic bronchitis are similar to pulmonary emphysema. The incidence of chronic bronchitis is greater among persons who smoke cigarettes, and cigarette smoking is considered to be the primary etiologic factor. Other inhalants may be contributing factors. For example, severe air pollution has been found to aggravate the disorder and cause respiratory failure.

Pathophysiology. In chronic bronchitis, an abnormal increase in the mucus-secreting cells of the bronchial epithelium and trachea occurs. The goblet cells (so named because of their shape) of the surface epithelium are increased. The bronchi become thickened, and fibrosis of the bronchioles with infiltration by inflammatory cells may occur. Chronic infection of the mucous membranes usually is present, and the sputum may contain a variety of pathogenic microorganisms. The normal function of the cilia is impaired, and they are unable to move secretions upward, where they may be coughed up. Therefore mucus secretions may form plugs in small bronchi, where they become a media for infection.

Assessment. The most common physiologic response in chronic bronchitis is a persistent cough with large amounts of sticky but fairly thin liquid mucus. The cough lasts 3 months a year for 2 consecutive years, thus making it chronic. In the presence of shortness of breath, the vital capacity is reduced, and dyspnea, cyanosis, and wheezing occur. Severely debilitated patients may be unable to cough and clear the respiratory passages, and respiratory function is compromised.

Intervention. Treatment of chronic bronchitis consists primarily of the patient adopting a healthy lifestyle. Patients should get adequate sleep and rest, eat a well-balanced diet, and participate in some form of recreational activity. They should be cautioned to avoid exposure to respiratory tract infections, dust, and other irritants. Work that requires being outside during cold or wet weather should be avoided. If a change of employment is necessary, the patient may be referred to the Social and Rehabilitation Service.

The most effective factor in treatment is to encourage the patient to stop smoking. Most methods of treatment, including bronchodilators, nebulized agents, and oral medications, have been shown to have a limited effect on chronic bronchitis. However, some patients may think that they do provide some relief. Although antibiotics often are administered to prevent infection, the time to begin such therapy is debatable. When chronic bronchitis with airway obstruction has existed over a long period, the patient may develop respiratory failure and right ventricular failure (Box 20-7).

Bronchiectasis. Bronchiectasis is characterized by a permanent dilation of one or more of the bronchi as a result of repeated infections. A single lobe of one lung or more or more lobes in both lungs may be affected. The left lung tends to be involved more often than the right lung, although both lungs are involved in approximately 50% of all patients. The cause of the disease is unknown, and although some cases are believed to be congenital, most appear to result from chronic bronchitis and severe attacks of infectious respiratory diseases. Bronchiectasis is primarily a disease of the young and often affects persons 20 years of age or younger.

Assessment. In the early stages of bronchiectasis, no symptoms may be present, but as the disease progresses, the most characteristic symptom is a productive cough. The cough is worse in the morning, and any change in position may produce paroxysms of coughing. The cough produces large amounts of purulent sputum, which may be tinged with blood. Hemoptysis occurs in a large number of cases, although it usually is not serious. As the disease gradually worsens, fever, chills, fatigue, weight loss, clubbing of the fingers, and a loss of appetite may occur. The diagnosis is made by x-ray examination and bronchoscopy. The only cure is surgical removal of the affected area (lobectomy). However, each patient must be carefully evaluated in relation to pulmonary function and prognosis because all patients are not suitable candidates for such surgery.

Intervention. Palliative treatment consists of measures to improve the general health, such as adequate diet, rest, and prevention of respiratory tract infections. Smoking, alcohol, and excessive exercise should be avoided. Irritants from air pollution may contribute to recurrent episodes of acute respiratory tract infections. Sputum cultures often indicate the presence of specific microorganisms, and antibiotic therapy for the particular pathogen is administered. Postural drainage should be part of the patient's daily routine, and moist inhalations may make it easier to produce thin, tenacious sputum. Many patients are treated on an outpatient basis, but in severe exacerbation the patient is admitted to the hospital. The nurse should encourage and reassure the patient and assist with postural drainage or other chest therapy. Mouth care must be given several times a day, and the use of an antiseptic mouthwash before meals may be desirable. The patient should be constantly on the alert for airway obstruction from large plugs of mucus (Box 20-8).

Patient/Family Education. Patients are taught diaphragmatic breathing and postural drainage. They are encouraged to avoid pulmonary irritants such as smoke; to monitor sputum for any changes in amount,

BOX 20-7 **Nursing Process**

CHRONIC BRONCHITIS

ASSESSMENT

Vital signs
Respiratory status (e.g., work of breathing, breath sounds, sputum, cough, cyanosis)
Restlessness, confusion
Nutritional status
Level of anxiety
Tolerance of activity
Sputum culture and sensitivity

NURSING DIAGNOSES

Ineffective airway clearance related to bronchial secretions
Impaired gas exchange related to inadequate oxygenation
Altered nutrition: less than body requirements related to dyspnea and fatigue
Activity intolerance related to fatigue, work of breathing
Risk for infection related to decreased pulmonary function, ineffective airway clearance, and stasis of secretions
Anxiety related to changes in health, hypoxia

NURSING INTERVENTIONS

Encourage coughing and deep breathing.
Position patient for optimal breathing.
Assist with position changes.
Provide room/oxygen humidification.
Administer expectorants, bronchodilators, corticosteroids, and antibiotics as prescribed.
Encourage fluid intake of 1½ to 2 L/day, unless contraindicated.
Administer oxygen as prescribed.
Provide small, frequent feedings.
Provide a high-protein, low carbohydrate diet.
Avoid gas-forming foods.
Plan rest periods.
Provide a progressive increase in activity as tolerated.
Encourage discussion of feelings, fears, concerns.
Remain with patient during anxious periods.

EVALUATION OF EXPECTED OUTCOMES

Clear breath sounds
No evidence of hypoxia
$Pa_{O_2} > 60$ mm Hg
Stable weight
Afebrile
Acknowledges anxiety
Demonstrates knowledge of disease process with home care management

color, or consistency; and to obtain an influenza and pneumococcal vaccine if recommended by their healthcare providers.

Asthma. Asthma can be classified as *extrinsic asthma,* which means that it is caused by substances, or antigens, outside of the body to which the individual is hypersensitive. Approximately half of all persons with asthma fall into this category. When it is impossible to determine any extrinsic factor, the disease is considered to be *intrinsic asthma,* or asthma that results from internal causes. Intrinsic asthma is most often caused by chronic recurrent respiratory tract infections. Attacks may be precipitated by emotional stress, irritating fumes, changes in temperature and humidity, and increased physical activity. No cure for asthma is available. Approximately one out of every four persons who develop the disease in childhood has a spontaneous recovery, and an equal number become progressively worse. Few adults with asthma have spontaneous recoveries. Instead they become progressively worse, with attacks lasting longer, becoming more frequent, and gradually becoming chronic (Kersten, 1989).

Pathophysiology. In acute attacks of asthma, the lumina of the small bronchi become narrow and edematous. Spasm of the bronchial muscles occurs. The mucus-secreting glands of the bronchi secrete a thick, tenacious mucus, which obstructs the narrowed passages of the bronchi. Inspiration and expiration become difficult, and in an effort to get more air, the patient uses the accessory muscles of respiration. More air is forced into the lungs than can be expelled, which causes the lungs to increase in size. The vital capacity is decreased, but an increase in the residual volume of air occurs. Cyanosis occurs because of inadequate ventilation. The heart is not affected, and the respiratory rate remains almost normal. After the acute attack subsides, the narrow lumen widens, and the patient is able to cough and produce large amounts of thick,

BOX 20-8

Nursing Process

BRONCHIECTASIS

ASSESSMENT

Vital signs
Respiratory status (breath sounds, cough, sputum)
Breathing patterns
Hemoptysis
Chest x-ray films
Sputum culture and sensitivity

NURSING DIAGNOSES

Ineffective airway clearance related to bronchial secretions
Ineffective breathing pattern related to bronchial obstruction and inflammatory process
Altered nutrition: less than body requirements related to anorexia and dyspnea
Activity intolerance related to weakness and dyspnea
Fear related to hemoptysis

NURSING INTERVENTIONS

Position with head of bed elevated.
Encourage deep breathing and coughing.
Avoid vigorous coughing.
Assist with position changes.
Administer oxygen as prescribed.
Increase room humidification.
Administer mucolytic agents, bronchodilators, antibiotics as prescribed.
Encourage fluid intake to 1½ to 2 L/day, unless contraindicated.
Provide oral hygiene before meals.
Provide for small, frequent meals.
Provide soft or liquid high-protein diet.
Plan rest periods.
Encourage adaptive breathing with activity.
Provide progressive increase in activity.
Validate sources of fear.
Encourage discussion of feelings toward illness.

EVALUATION OF EXPECTED OUTCOMES

Breath sounds clear
Vital capacity optimal for patient
No evidence of dyspnea
Tolerating diet without dyspnea
Stable weight
Able to express fear

stringy sputum. Although the lungs return to their normal size after an attack, continued episodes lead to permanent impairment and emphysema.

Assessment. The characteristic physiologic symptoms of asthma are shortness of breath accompanied by wheezing and coughing. Severe symptoms indicate a severe attack. Pronounced wheezing that progresses to absent breath sounds is an ominous sign and indicates the need for immediate intervention. Results of arterial blood gas studies vary depending on severity and duration of the attack. In asthma, as in chronic bronchitis and emphysema, exhaling is more difficult than inhaling. Patients can reduce dyspnea markedly by sitting up and tilting their head forward during exhalation. After the normal exhalation, the patient should gradually contract the abdominal muscles until no more air can be expelled from the lungs and then inhale. This procedure reduces the effort required for exhaling. As a result of the ventilation difficulty, the patient may become cyanotic, and asphyxiation and death may occur during prolonged attacks if the patient is not treated with appropriate interventions, including mechanical ventilation. The patient generally perspires freely, may have a weak pulse, and may complain of pain in the chest caused by the respiratory effort. Nausea and diarrhea may occur in children. The cough of persons with asthma usually is tight and dry in the beginning, but as the attack continues, the thin, mucus secretion becomes copious, thick, and stringy and is expectorated with difficulty.

Intervention. Treatment and care of asthma is directed toward three factors: (1) relief of the immediate attack, (2) control of causal factors, and (3) general care of the patient. Adults may be given 0.3 to 0.5 ml of a 1:1000 solution of epinephrine subcutaneously. Other drugs used in the treatment of an asthma attack include giving terbutaline and aminophylline parenterally, combined with an aerosolized medication such as isoproterenol, isoetharine, or metaproterenol (see Table 20-9). These medications in various forms may be continued as part of the patient's long-term therapeutic regimen along with corticosteroids and cromolym sodium to prevent recurrent attacks.

During an acute attack of asthma, the patient should be placed in a sitting position and made as comfortable as possible. Humidification of inspired air helps loosen secretions so that they can be expectorated more easily. Dietary orders should be carried out, and the patient should be encouraged to drink adequate

BOX 20-9

Nursing Process

ASTHMA

ASSESSMENT

Personal history of asthma
Current medications
Respiratory status (breath sounds, breathing patterns, sputum)
Evidence of respiratory distress
Level of anxiety
Vital signs
Pulmonary function tests

NURSING DIAGNOSES

Ineffective breathing pattern related to anxiety and decreased lung expansion
Ineffective airway clearance related to secretions and bronchospasm
Activity intolerance related to imbalance between oxygen supply and demand
Risk for infection related to steroid therapy and stasis of airway secretions
Anxiety related to difficulty breathing

NURSING INTERVENTIONS

Assist with positions for optimal breathing (head of bed elevated).
Administer oxygen as prescribed.
Assist with relaxation techniques.
Increase room humidification.
Encourage fluid intake to 1½ to 2 L/day, unless contraindicated.
Plan rest periods.
Provide progressive increase in activity as tolerated.
Assist with nebulizer respiratory therapy and physiotherapy.
Encourage oral hygiene after aerated corticosteroids.
Encourage optimal nutrition.
Assist with identifying coping skills.
Encourage questions and discussion of feelings.
Provide accurate information about asthma.
Provide comfort measures.
Stay with patient during acute attack.

EVALUATION OF EXPECTED OUTCOMES

Vital capacity measurements optimal for patient
Clear breath sounds
Able to perform ADLs
Afebrile
No evidence of anxiety
Demonstrates knowledge of disease process and home care management

amounts of fluids. If the fluid intake is inadequate, intravenous fluids may be ordered. Most attacks subside in 30 to 60 minutes, although they may continue for days or weeks. The patient who has frequent asthma attacks may eventually become resistant to all forms of treatment and may develop what is called *status asthmaticus,* in which acute symptoms continue and a prolonged attack can cause exhaustion and require mechanical ventilation. Severe asthma attacks are frightening, and the patient and family need reassurance and support.

The control of asthma depends on finding and eliminating the cause. If the disease is caused by extrinsic factors (allergy), identification of the offending allergen may be made through skin tests, and the patient can be desensitized. If intrinsic factors are suspected, a thorough physical examination should be made to determine a source of infection, specific organisms, or other physical factors (Box 20-9).

Patient/Family Education Patients with asthma should be advised against smoking and should avoid exposure to cold, wet weather. A program of personal hygiene, with sleep, rest, and breathing exercises, should be instituted.

RESPIRATORY INFECTIONS

Acute Bronchitis

Bronchitis is caused by inflammation of the bronchial tree and the trachea. It is secondary to infection in the upper respiratory tract but may also result from bronchial irritation caused by exposure to chemical agents or as a complication of communicable diseases such as measles. Acute bronchitis usually begins with hoarseness and cough, a slight elevation in temperature, muscular aching, and a headache. The cough may be dry and painful but gradually becomes productive. Bedrest is indicated as long as the temperature is elevated. Treatments should be directed toward preventing the extension of the infection. Both plain and medicated cool mist vaporizers soothe irritated respiratory passages. Aerosol therapy may be given, and antibiotics may be ordered. Sedative or expectorant drugs may be ordered for the cough. If no complications occur, recovery may be expected in a week to 10 days.

Pneumonia

Pneumonia is a disease of the lungs and is caused by bacteria, viruses, fungi, and mycobacteria. It may occur in comatose or oversedated patients and in those whose pulmonary ventilation is inadequate. It may result from aspiration of infected secretions from the upper respiratory or gastrointestinal tracts; may complicate certain viral diseases such as measles or influenza; and may cause complications, including empyema, septicemia, meningitis, and endocarditis. Most community-acquired pneumonia is caused by *Streptococcus pneumoniae* (pneumococcus) and occurs in the very young and older adults.

Hospital-acquired nosocomial pneumonias are most often related to bacterial invasion of the lower respiratory tract by *Pseudomonas aeruginosna, Klebsiella pneumoniae,* and *S. aureus* (Figure 20-28). Nosocomial pneumonias account for 16% of all hospital-acquired infections. Patient morbidity and mortality is related to the etiologic agent and to the overall status of the patient (Smeltzer, Bare, 1992).

Legionnaires' disease is an acute bacterial bronchopneumonia that is caused by a gram-negative bacillus. It derived its name from the 1976 American Legion convention in Philadelphia, during which the disease affected 180 people and caused 29 deaths. The bacteria is airborne and has an affinity for stagnant water such as that found in air-conditioning and cooling systems. Therefore it tends to affect people who work together in one building or who come together in large groups, such as at conventions. It tends to occur epidemically, particularly during the summer, with a severity that ranges from a mild pneumonitis to a multilobar pneumonia with a 10% to 15% mortality. The symptoms are similar to bacterial pneumonia, but the cough may be nonproductive at first and signs of gastrointestinal upset are more likely to be present.

Pneumonia caused by a virus usually appears as a patchy infection throughout the lung (see Figure 20-28). The onset is slower and is characterized by chills, fever, profuse sweating, aching, and a painful cough. The sputum is mucopurulent and may contain

OLDER ADULT CONSIDERATIONS

Pneumonia

Pneumonia is the fourth leading cause of death among people over 65 years of age. Older adults living in nursing homes are at highest risk. Because the older adult may have other chronic health problems, morbidity and mortality from pneumonia are higher than in younger adults. Several factors contribute to the older adult's increased risk: age-related changes in immune function, decreased cough reflex, decreased functional reserve, and decreased mobility. The bedridden older adult is at increased risk for aspiration pneumonia.

Pneumonia is overlooked in the older adult because the symptoms do not present a typical clinical picture. Instead of fever and pulmonary symptoms, pneumonia in the older adult may be manifested by lethargy, confusion, tachypnea, and dehydration.

From Beare PG, Myers JL: *Principles and practice of adult health nursing,* ed 2, St Louis, 1994, Mosby.

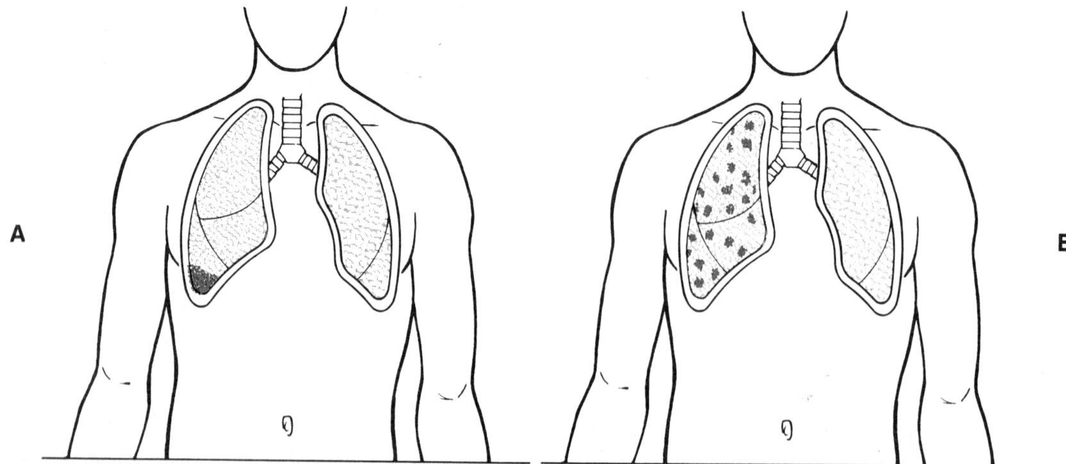

Figure 20-28 **A,** Bacterial pneumonia may affect one or more lobes of the lung. **B,** Viral pneumonia appears as a patchy distribution throughout the lung.

blood. The white blood cell count is normal. The temperature elevation generally runs an irregular course, varies even during the day, and may continue for as long as 3 weeks. Viral pneumonia rarely is fatal, and although the patient is extremely uncomfortable, it is less serious than bacterial pneumonia. However, patients with viral pneumonia may require a longer period of convalescence.

Cytomegalovirus is the most common cause of viral pneumonia in immunosuppressed persons. It may occur in patients with organ transplants or acquired immunodeficiency syndrome (AIDS) and in those taking antineoplastic drugs. Cytomegalovirus produces a severe pneumonia with high mortality rates. *Pneumocystis carinii* pneumonia has the greatest incidence in patients with AIDS and in patients who are receiving immunosuppressive therapy. It is thought to be caused by a unicellular protozoan, but recent evidence suggests that it may be a fungus (Smeltzer, Bare, 1992).

Pathophysiology

Infected secretions from the upper respiratory tract drain into the alveoli, where the normal defense mechanisms, such as ciliary action and coughing, are unable to remove them. An inflammatory process begins, and increased amounts of fluid are released in the area. The serous fluid moves easily into additional alveoli and bronchioles. As the process continues, less surface area is available for the absorption of oxygen and the release of carbon dioxide. Leukocytes and a few erythrocytes begin to accumulate in the affected alveoli, and they increase in number until they completely fill each alveolus, which results in consolidation. Phagocytosis begins in the consolidated alveolus, and the area is finally cleared. In the beginning, only one lobe of the lung may be involved, but the infected fluid may spread to the bronchial tree of another lobe and begin another infection process.

Assessment

Symptoms may vary with the individual. However, the onset of bacterial pneumonia usually is sudden and accompanied by severe chills and chest pain. These symptoms are followed by a temperature elevation, which may be as high as 105° F (40.5° C), and an increase in pulse and respiratory rates. The patient develops a cough that may be painful and constant. Initially the sputum may be clear or tinged with blood, but within 48 hours it develops a characteristic rusty appearance. The sputum is thick and tenacious and may be expectorated with difficulty. Suction should be available if needed to help clear the airway. Leukocytosis is present, with the number of white blood cells ranging from 20,000 to 30,000; the skin is hot and moist; the lips are dry; and the tongue is parched. Nausea, vomiting, diarrhea, and jaundice occasionally appear. Fever blisters (herpes simplex) may appear on the lips and nose, and sores may cover the tongue. Restlessness and delirium may accompany pneumonia.

Intervention

Nursing care of patients with pneumonia is a major factor in the progress and prognosis of the illness. Pneumonia is debilitating and exhausting. Treatment and care involve keeping the patient as comfortable as possible, planning care to avoid any unnecessary expenditure of energy, and using antibiotic and sulfonamide agents to help the body's defenses overcome the infection. The type of antibiotic used depends on the particular organism present and whether the organism remains sensitive to the drug. Sputum cultures should be obtained before treatment with the antibiotic is started. Analgesics may be used to relieve pain, and nonpharmacologic measures may also be used to promote comfort. The patient may also be encouraged to deep breathe and cough if secretions are present. Cough analgesics and increased humidity tend to relieve coughing. Oxygen may be prescribed if the patient has cyanosis, dyspnea, or shortness of breath.

The patient's room should be well ventilated, have a temperature between 68° F and 70° F (20° C to 21° C), and be free from drafts. A restful, quiet environment should be provided. The patient should be positioned to allow for the greatest comfort and may be placed in a high, 90-degree Fowler's position or on the affected side. The position should be changed often. The nursing care plan should be made to provide nursing care with periods of uninterrupted rest. Visiting should be limited during the acute phase of the disease. Blood pressure and temperature, pulse, and respiratory rates are checked every 4 hours or as the patient's condition indicates. The diet usually consists of liquids, and the total fluid intake may be increased to 2000 or 3000 ml/day. The patient may need to be encouraged to take food or fluids. If pneumonia occurs in a patient with cardiac disease, the nurse should determine if fluids and sodium are to be restricted. Intake and output records should be maintained. Intravenous fluids designed to maintain electrolyte balance may be ordered. Special mouth care must be given several times each day. A lubricant should be applied to the lips and should be used to soften any crusts on the nares. Fever blisters should be kept dry.

Tuberculosis

Tuberculosis (TB) continues to be a public health problem in the United States, with over 20,000 cases reported annually. Since 1984, there has not been the

Nursing Care Plan

PATIENT WITH PNEUMONIA

Mr. Jenkins is a 61-year-old male who comes to the emergency department with a complaint of shortness of breath, chills, fatigue, and "feeling terrible." He states that he has not been well for 1 week, has a loss of appetite, has muscle aches, and feels "very drawn."

Past Medical History	Psychosocial Data	Assessment Data
Denies COPD, cardiac disease, hypertension, and diabetes mellitus Has a history of smoking one pack per day (PPD) of cigarettes since the age of 13 (48 pack years) Denies alcohol consumption Has good health behaviors as evidenced by yearly physicals Involved in physical sports until 4 years ago; now his activity level is sedentary	Married 40 years; supportive, caring wife Three adult daughters, all with young children, live locally and visit often Full-time truck driver (retired as a limousine driver) Practices Catholic religion Active social life, with many friends Owns home Insured through private medical insurance *Hobbies:* Gardening and fixing cars	Alert and oriented × 3 (time, place, and person) Febrile to 101° F-103° F; Respirations 24 to 26, regular but labored; some use of accessory muscles; painful cough with small amount of sputum (thick, tenacious, yellowish mucoid); oxygen at 3 L *Respiratory:* Bilateral scattered crackles throughout entire lung fields *Cardiovascular:* Pulse 86 to 90, regular rate; no murmurs; brachial, radial, femoral, popliteal, and pedal pulses palpable bilaterally *Abdominal:* Soft, nontender, nondistended, with bowel sounds heard in all four quadrants; bowel movement on day of admission *Skin:* Clean and intact; no broken skin areas, no pressure ulcers or rashes ***Laboratory Data*** WBC 18,000, Hgb 12.2, Hct 39, Electrolytes WNL Purified protein derivative placed Sputum sent for culture and acid-fast bacillus (AFB) *Urinalysis:* WNL *Chest x-ray:* Consistent with pneumonia bilateral lower lobes ***Medications*** IV-D5 ½ N/S at 100 ml/hr cefazolin (Ancef) 1 g in 50 ml D5W over 20 minutes q 6 hr acetaminophen (Tylenol) tabs prn for discomfort

NURSING DIAGNOSIS

Ineffective airway clearance related to tracheobronchial secretions as evidenced by abnormal breath sounds (crackles) and labored breathing

NURSING INTERVENTIONS	EVALUATION OF EXPECTED OUTCOMES
Help the patient cough productively. Teach effective coughing and deep breathing exercises; have patient sit or lie on side with knees flexed. Splint patient's chest when coughing or straining. Administer analgesic before having patient cough. Use nonpharmacologic measures to reduce pleuritic pain (relaxation, distraction). Humidify air to loosen secretions and promote ventilation.	Demonstrates effective coughing techniques Verbalizes importance of drinking enough fluid to liquify secretions Verbalizes minimal pain and uses measures to reduce pain Airway is free of secretions Verbalizes need to take antibiotics at prescribed times Maintains oxygen saturation (Sao_2) at a predetermined level

NURSING INTERVENTIONS—cont'd	EVALUATION OF EXPECTED OUTCOMES—cont'd
Encourage fluids 2000-3000 ml daily unless contraindicated. Perform postural drainage, percussion, and vibration to mobilize secretions. Administer prescribed antibiotics at correct time intervals. Provide oxygen as ordered for dyspnea, hypoxemia, or confusion; monitor pulse oximetry to determine effectiveness of oxygen therapy. Monitor patient's response to therapy. Assess vital signs q 4 hr or as indicated, including blood pressure, pulse, respirations, and temperature. Auscultate chest q 4 hr or as indicated, identifying crackles (rales) or signs of consolidation (decreased breath sounds, dullness on percussion).	Blood pressure within patient's normal range Temperature normal Pulse and respiratory rate within normal range Breath sounds clear without evidence of crackles, rhonchi, or decreased breath sounds

NURSING DIAGNOSIS

Anxiety related to respiratory difficulties

NURSING INTERVENTIONS	EVALUATION OF EXPECTED OUTCOMES
Teach relaxation techniques. Use a caring approach; provide time to actively listen. Encourage participation in care as tolerated. Discuss physical feelings and relate them to the compromised lung status. Help patient compare and contrast behaviors of progress.	Demonstrates decreased anxiety through facial expressions and body language Participates in own care Discusses fears and feelings and identifies behaviors of progress

NURSING DIAGNOSIS

Activity intolerance related to imbalance between oxygen supply and demand as evidenced by shortness of breath (SOB) and increased respiratory rate with activity.

NURSING INTERVENTIONS	EVALUATION OF EXPECTED OUTCOMES
Provide environment conducive to rest; turn down lights when resting; monitor for noise level. Help patient assume and maintain a comfortable position. Plan nursing care to include uninterrupted rest periods. Encourage patient to help plan activity progression.	Lists factors that cause fatigue and shows increasing tolerance with activity level after periods of rest Assumes optimal position for adequate rest and breathing Participates in plans for activities of daily living (ADLs)

continued

NURSING DIAGNOSIS

Knowledge deficit related to course of illness and health risk behaviors (smoking) as evidenced by verbal questioning

NURSING INTERVENTIONS	EVALUATION OF EXPECTED OUTCOMES
Explain the rationale for rest, increased fluids, and activity monitoring because they maintain the body's natural defenses.	States factors that contributed to the illness
Discuss behaviors that suggest the need for modification of ADLs; initiate a discussion on smoking.	Identifies behaviors of progress and discusses the rationale for rest, increased fluids, and ADL monitoring
Ask if patient is motivated to stop smoking; discuss any previous attempts to quit, and identify the rationale for previous failures; cite statistics related to the risks of smoking, including cardiovascular and pulmonary problems; recommend self-help groups for support.	Identifies the risks involved in smoking, and cites motivational level to quit; plans to attend a self-help smoking cessation group
Discuss the importance of obtaining an influenza vaccine and pneumococcal vaccine at specified intervals.	Plans to obtain vaccinations
Discuss importance of follow-up examinations after discharge.	Makes an appointment for follow-up care

decline in TB morbidity that health officials would have expected (see Chapter 11). In fact, there have been substantial increases in TB in areas with a high prevalence of human immunodeficiency virus (HIV) infection (see Chapter 13).

The hazard associated with TB has increased as multiple–drug-resistant strains of tuberculosis (MDR-TB) have developed. With effective treatment being delayed as healthcare providers search for an appropriate drug therapy, individuals remain in an infectious state for longer periods of time, which increases the risk of infecting those with whom they come in contact (Center for Prevention Services, 1991).

Pulmonary TB is caused by an acid-fast bacterium, the *tubercle bacillus (Mycobacterium tuberculosis).* It is carried through the air in infectious droplet nuclei, which are produced when the infected person sneezes, coughs, speaks, or sings. When persons breathe air that has been contaminated by an infectious patient, they may become infected with the TB organism. Individuals at the greatest risk for developing TB include those who are immunocompromised, such as in HIV infection; those living in close or crowded conditions such as homeless shelters, nursing homes, and prisons; and persons who use intravenous drugs and alcohol. The elderly and the malnourished are also at risk.

When the bacillus enters the lung, the body responds by surrounding it with monocytes, which fuse together to form giant cells. Fibrous tissue grows around the area, and the central portion of this growth of cells becomes necrotic. The entire inflammatory process is called granulomatous inflammation. If the number of organisms entering the lung is small and the resistance of the body is high, healing occurs by scarring. If a large number of organisms are inhaled into the lung, the inflammation overwhelms the body's defenses, and a more extensive destruction of lung tissue occurs, which results in lung cavities. TB can be a primary or secondary disorder. Secondary TB usually occurs late in life or when individuals are immunocompromised.

Assessment

Symptoms vary from patient to patient depending on the extent of the disease. The most common symptom of pulmonary TB is a cough. Initially the cough is nonproductive, but if left untreated it becomes productive with mucoid or mucopurulent sputum. Hemoptysis may eventually develop. Patients may complain of pleuritic chest pain and systemic effects, including weight loss, night sweats, fever, malaise, anorexia, and fatigue. TB is detected with skin testing, acid-fast stained sputum specimens, and chest x-ray examinations.

BOX 20-10 **Nursing Process**

ACTIVE TUBERCULOSIS

ASSESSMENT

Respiratory status (breath sounds, cough, breathing pattern)
Weight loss, anorexia, night sweats, chest pains
Previous exposure to TB
Vital signs (temperature q 4 hr)
Sputum culture (AFB)
ABGs, if indicated

NURSING DIAGNOSES

Ineffective breathing pattern related to sputum production
Risk for infection related to active pulmonary TB
Diversional activity deficit related to isolation
Ineffective management of therapeutic regimen related to long-term therapy
Knowledge deficit related to new diagnosis and treatment
Altered nutrition: less than body requirements related to fatigue, malaise

NURSING INTERVENTIONS

Administer oxygen as prescribed.
Position for optimal breathing (head of bed elevated).
Encourage fluids.
Maintain respiratory isolation.
Keep tissues at bedside and teach proper disposal of secretions.
Administer medications as prescribed.
Encourage expression of feelings.
Encourage diversional activities.
Discuss importance of following medical treatment.
Encourage optimal nutrition.

EVALUATION OF EXPECTED OUTCOMES

Clear breath sounds
Negative sputum culture
Stable weight
Participates in satisfying activities
Adheres to treatment regimen
Verbalizes knowledge of TB medications and follow-up therapy

Treatment

Treatment usually requires more than one drug. Triple therapy in the form of streptomycin, isoniazid (INH), and rifampin is prescribed. The Centers for Disease Control and Prevention recommend a minimum of 6 months of therapy with isoniazid, rifampin, and pyrazinamide for the first 2 months, followed by 4 months of isoniazid and rifampin. A 9-month treatment regimen is also acceptable and includes isoniazid and rifampin (see Table 20-9) (Center for Prevention Services, 1991). The best way to measure the effectiveness of therapy for pulmonary TB is to monitor sputum specimens at least every month. In patients with negative sputum before treatment, follow-up treatment focuses on chest x-ray examinations and clinical evaluation of symptoms.

The only acceptable method for administration of the TB test is the Mantoux method of purified protein derivative (PPD). The patient receives an intradermal injection of 0.1 ml of polysorbate- (Tween) stabilized PPD containing 5 tuberculin units into the volar surface of the forearm. The test is interpreted between 48 and 72 hours after administration. The presence and measurement of induration is used as the basis for reading a test as positive. The amount of induration at the test site is measured (in millimeters) and recorded (Box 20-10).

Patient/family education

Patients and family members need to be aware that not treating TB can lead to potentially serious consequences. Education needs to be individualized to meet the needs of the patient and family and should focus on the following objectives:

- Disease process and transmission
- Medication education (understanding of regimen)
- Medication action, dosage, and side effects
- Hand washing
- Use of tissues and proper disposal
- Treatment regimen
- Reporting for sputum monitoring
- Smoking cessation, if indicated
- Encouraging close contacts (family, friends) to report for examination

OLDER ADULT CONSIDERATIONS

Tuberculosis

Many factors contribute to the increased incidence of tuberculosis among older adults. Normal age-related changes in immune function and the presence of chronic health problems increase their susceptibility. Many older adults were exposed to tuberculosis when younger because of its former prevalence. The occurrence of tuberculosis in the older adult may represent reactivation of a dormant infection. The decreased immune function limits the usefulness of skin tests in diagnosing the disorder. A chest x-ray film or sputum culture is more accurate.

The classic symptoms may not be present. Instead the older adult may only have weight loss or anorexia as a clinical manifestation. Drug therapy for tuberculosis is effective in the older adult, but more frequent monitoring for side effects is an important part of nursing management.

From Beare PG, Myers JL: *Principles and practice of adult health nursing,* ed 2, St Louis, 1994, Mosby.

- Attending follow-up appointments
- Importance of compliance of therapy
- Taking medications as prescribed
- Signs and symptoms of relapse

Acquired Immunodeficiency Syndrome

Patients with AIDS are at great risk for pulmonary infection, particularly pneumonia caused by *P. carinii.* Patients with AIDS also are at risk for development of TB and legionnaire's disease (see Chapter 13).

PLEURAL CONDITIONS

Pleurisy and Empyema

Pleurisy results from inflammation of any part of the pleura. Several forms of the disease exist, which are referred to as dry pleurisy, wet pleurisy, or pleurisy with effusion. Empyema is characterized by pus formation. Although the disease may occur spontaneously, it is more likely to be a complication of pneumonia or TB. The disease has been less common since the development of antibiotic therapy.

Assessment

The first symptom may be a severe knifelike pain on inspiration, which may be referred to the shoulder or to the abdomen on the affected side. This pain occurs when the inflamed pleurae rub together during respiration. Coughing, dyspnea, and vomiting may occur, and the patient may hold the abdomen with a boardlike rigidity.

Pleurisy with effusion is less dramatic than dry pleurisy, and the first symptom may be dyspnea, which occurs when the accumulation of fluid in the pleural cavity has become large enough to compress the lung. The acuteness of the dyspnea depends on the size of the effusion. Other symptoms are related to the cause and may include a temperature elevation. If the fluid becomes purulent and empyema develops, the temperature may reach 105° F (40.5° C), with chills, profuse perspiration, and prostration.

Intervention

The treatment of pleurisy depends on the type and stage of the disease and is directed toward removing the underlying cause through the administration of the appropriate antibiotic to combat the infection. If fluid is present in the pleural cavity, a thoracentesis may be performed and the fluid aspirated, followed by the instillation of an antibiotic. If the pleural fluid has become purulent and empyema has developed, adequate drainage and specific antibiotics must be provided. With antibiotic therapy, the need for an open **thoracotomy** has been almost eliminated. Patients with pleurisy usually are apprehensive and worried. A quiet environment and a nurse's sympathetic and understanding approach to patients and their conditions help their recovery. Patients are more comfortable if they lie on the affected side and turn toward this side when coughing. Pain should be relieved, and generally the use of acetaminophen is sufficient. Oxygen may be administered if dyspnea is severe. Because pleurisy often follows a debilitating disease, an adequate diet is important. The diet should be high in protein, calories, vitamins, and minerals, and supplemental feedings may be helpful.

Atelectasis

Atelectasis is a common postoperative complication that can occur when the patient breathes rapidly and shallowly to prevent pain at the surgical site. The supine position, respiratory depression from narcotics and relaxants, and abdominal distention increase the risk for atelectasis. It may also be seen in smokers, obese individuals who are on prolonged bedrest, and patients with respiratory tract infections or chronic obstructive pulmonary disease (COPD).

Pathophysiology

Atelectasis occurs from the blockage of air to a portion of the lung. It may result from pressure against the lung as a result of air or fluid in the pleural cavity, tumors, an enlarged heart, or any abdominal condition that pushes the diaphragm upward. It may also result from an obstruction within one of the bronchi. A foreign body or a thick plug of mucus may completely occlude a bronchus and shut off all air to a portion of the lung. As the air in the isolated part of the lung is absorbed by the capillaries and new air no longer enters, the part involved collapses.

Assessment

The severity of the symptoms depends on the degree of alveolar tissue involved, the rate at which the obstruction develops, and the presence of a secondary infection. Patients who develop atelectasis usually have dyspnea, anxiety, cyanosis, tachypnea, tachycardia, decreased blood pressure, elevated temperature, and pain on the affected side. Crackles and decreased breath sounds may be auscultated in the affected areas.

Intervention

The key to the treatment of atelectasis is prevention. Postoperative and other high risk patients should be taught how to cough and breathe deeply. Mobility should be encouraged, and bedridden patients should be turned and repositioned every 1 to 2 hours. IS may be used to promote deep inspiration and to improve ventilation and bronchial drainage. Chest percussion and postural drainage help with expectoration of bronchial secretions. Suctioning, oxygen, and administration of aerosols and humidity are also used.

Pulmonary Embolism and Infarction

In the United States today, deep vein thrombosis (DVT) and **pulmonary embolism** (PE) constitute major health problems that result in significant morbidity and mortality. It is estimated that DVT and PE are associated with 300,000 to 600,000 hospitalizations each year, and as many as 100,000 hospitalized persons die each year as a result of PE (Consensus Conference, 1986).

Pulmonary embolism may occur as a postoperative complication following orthopedic surgery; certain types of general surgery; and gynecologic, obstetric, urologic, or neurosurgical procedures. Patients with various types of medical disease, usually chronic, are also at high risk for thrombotic events (Hull, Moser, Salzman, 1989). Risk factors include conditions or events that predispose the individual to venous stasis, vessel wall injury (injury to the innermost lining of the vein), and hypercoagulability (Box 20-11). These three factors are most associated with the development of DVT and subsequent PE (Currie, 1990).

A PE is a thrombus (clot) or foreign substance that travels through the systemic circulation and into the pulmonary circulation, which causes a complete or partial obstruction of the pulmonary artery or one of its branches. Generally 90% to 95% of all PEs arise from the deep veins of the leg. Other causes of PE include air embolism, fat embolism, septic emboli, tumor emboli, and clots originating from the right atrium or ventricle (Currie, 1990).

BOX 20-11

PULMONARY EMBOLISM RISK FACTORS

VENOUS STASIS
- Heart diseases
  - Congestive heart failure
  - Myocardial infarction
  - Cardiomyopathy
  - Constrictive pericarditis
- Anasarca
- Dehydration
- Immobility (bedrest > 72°, long travel)
- Incompetent venous valves
- Obesity (>20% ideal body weight (IBW))
- Pregnancy

VESSEL WALL INJURY
- Trauma
- Fracture
- Extensive burns
- Infection
- Venipuncture
- Intravenous infusion of irritant solutions
- History of previous major surgery

HYPERCOAGULABILITY
- Blood dyscrasias
- Antithrombin II deficiency
- Protein deficiency
- Polycythemia vera
- Anemias
- Trauma/surgery
- Advanced malignant disease
- Estrogen therapy
- Smoking
- Systemic infection

Once an embolus lodges, pulmonary blood flow is interrupted, which results in a ventilation-perfusion mismatch. Although a portion of the lung is still being ventilated, no blood is flowing to pick up oxygen and remove carbon dioxide. To maintain adequate gas exchange, ventilation increases in uninvolved lung areas, and bronchoconstriction occurs to reduce wasted ventilation. The airways distal to the embolus constrict, and the alveoli shrink and collapse. Ventilation is shifted away from areas of poor perfusion. Atelectasis may follow.

Assessment

The symptoms of PE vary with the severity of the condition, but the most common are pleuritic chest pain, tachypnea, dyspnea, and apprehension. Other signs and symptoms include crackles (rales), hemoptysis, tachycardia, cyanosis (in severe cases), and shock. Diagnostic evaluation includes chest x-ray examinations, electrocardiograms (ECG), ventilation-perfusion (V/Q) scanning, and pulmonary angiography. The chest x-ray film may be normal, and the ECG often shows tachycardia. The arterial blood gas shows hypoxemia with a decrease in PaO_2. PaO_2 also decreases as a result of tachypnea. With a decrease in PaO_2 and $PaCO_2$, the pH increases. The V/Q scan demonstrates areas of ventilation without perfusion. If there is V/Q mismatch, a high probability of PE exists. If a DVT is suspected, evaluation may also include doppler ultrasonography, duplex scanning, impedence plethysmography, and venography. These tests serve to evaluate lower extremity circulation and determine any obstruction resulting from a thrombus.

Intervention

The patient must be immediately stabilized, and further assessments must be performed. Continued nursing care focuses on the improvement of gas exchange, the maintenance of optimal cardiac output, the reduction of anxiety, and the relief of pain. When anticoagulation is initiated, the nurse also maintains anticoagulation, monitors for bleeding, and educates the patient regarding the anticoagulant(s) being administered. Nursing measures include the following (Currie, 1990):

1 Initial stabilization and further assessment
  - a Initiate bedrest.
  - b Provide oxygen via nasal cannula or face mask.
  - c Help patient assume a semi-Fowler's position.
  - d Evaluate respirations, noting rate, rhythm, depth, and effort.
  - e Arrange for arterial blood gases (ABGs).
  - f Obtain intravenous access.
  - g Arrange for chest x-ray examinations.
  - h Reassess for increased signs of hypoxia, such as pallor, cyanosis, restlessness, nasal flaring, retraction of intercostal spaces, gasping respirations, and the use of accessory muscles.
  - i Encourage patient to breathe normally.
  - j Be prepared to use mechanical ventilation if patient respiratory distress is severe.

2 Improvement of gas exchange
  - a Reassess for signs of hypoxemia.
  - b Monitor ABGs.
  - c Provide oxygen as needed.
  - d Position patient to achieve an optimal V/Q relationship.

3 Maintenance of optimal cardiac output
  - a Monitor vital signs every 30 minutes to 1 hour.
  - b Monitor for cardiac arrhythmias.
  - c Maintain IV line patency.
  - d Be prepared to administer fluids and medications to maintain cardiac output.

4 Reduction of anxiety and relief of pain
  - a Provide pain medication as ordered.
  - b Provide assurance, approach patient calmly, and maintain as stable an environment as possible (quiet).
  - c Position patient for comfort and to optimize V/Q relationship.

5 Maintenance of therapeutic anticoagulation and prevention of bleeding
  - a Initiate anticoagulation medications as ordered.
  - b Monitor prothrombin times (PT) and partial thromboplastin times (PTT).
  - c Monitor for signs and symptoms of bleeding.
  - d Keep anticoagulant antagonist available.

6 Recognize the hazards of immobility

7 Provide education

The treatment of PE may include anticoagulation therapy, thrombolytic therapy, or surgery. Intravenous heparin is often the initial treatment. It can be initiated when the patient is being evaluated and before all diagnostic testing has been completed, especially if there is a strong suspicion of a pulmonary embolus or if the patient is unstable. Heparin is used to prevent the extension and propagation of a thrombus and the development of new thrombi. The patient is usually given a loading bolus of 5000 to 10,000 units, and a continuous infusion is begun. The goal is to maintain the PTT at 1.5 to 2 times normal. Heparin therapy is usually maintained for 7 to 10 days (Currie, 1990). Warfarin (Coumadin) administration is usually started while the heparin therapy is being maintained (over-

BOX 20-12 **Nursing Process**

PULMONARY EMBOLISM

ASSESSMENT

Respiratory status (breath sounds, breathing patterns)
Evidence of respiratory distress, apprehension, confusion)
Evidence of thrombophlebitis
Evidence of bleeding if on anticoagulants (skin, stools, urine, sputum)
Complaints of chest pain
Skin temperature, peripheral pulses
Vital signs
Level of consciousness
Laboratory studies: ABGs, CBC, PT, PTT

NURSING DIAGNOSES

Impaired gas exchange related to alteration in ventilation/perfusion
Ineffective breathing pattern related to substernal chest pain, anxiety, hypoxia
Risk for injury: bleeding related to anticoagulant therapy
Anxiety related to hypoxia, dyspnea, and sudden change in health
Risk for decreased cardiac output related to pulmonary hypertension
Pain related to acute inflammatory process in lungs
Knowledge deficit related to new medical condition and treatment

NURSING INTERVENTIONS

Administer oxygen as prescribed.
Anticipate the need for intubation.
Position for optimal breathing (head of bed elevated).
Administer anticoagulants as prescribed.
Monitor IV delivery system.
Maintain bedrest during acute episode.
Assist with position changes q 2 hr.
Administer IV fluids.
Administer analgesics as prescribed.
Monitor pulse oximetry continuously during acute episode.
Provide rest periods.
Encourage discussion of feelings.
Provide emotional support.

EVALUATION OF EXPECTED OUTCOMES

ABGs WNL for patient
Clear breath sounds
No evidence of respiratory distress
No pain with respiratory effort
No evidence of bleeding
Verbalizes decreased or absent anxiety

lapping of therapies) and continues for 3 to 6 months following a PE. Warfarin works on vitamin K–dependent clotting factors, which are synthesized by the liver (factors II, VII, IX, X). Because the half-lives of these factors range from 6 hours to 90 minutes, it may take 3 to 5 days for the PT to become therapeutic (Box 20-12).

The PT is maintained at approximately 1.5 times the control. Anticoagulation therapy is contraindicated in patients who are at risk for bleeding, and bleeding must be watched for when a patient is receiving heparin or warfarin. Bleeding may be seen in the form of hematemesis, hematuria, or ecchymosis. Before initiating anticoagulation, a baseline PT/PTT should be obtained; and the hemoglobin, hematocrit, and platelet count should be monitored at intervals before and during anticoagulation therapy.

Thrombolytic therapy (urokinase, streptokinase) may also be used in treatment. These agents result in a more rapid resolution of the thrombi or emboli as they dissolve the existing clot. Because bleeding is a significant side effect, thrombolytics are reserved for those with massive PE or those with severe DVT that affects the thigh or pelvis because the likelihood of the clot embolizing in these patients is greater (Smeltzer, Bare 1992).

Before thrombolytic therapy is initiated, thrombin time (TT), PTT, PT, hematocrit level, and platelet counts are obtained. During therapy, all but absolutely essential invasive procedures are avoided. If necessary, blood products are used to reverse the bleeding tendency (e.g., fresh frozen plasma). Surgical intervention may be indicated if the patient has persistent hypotension, shock, and respiratory distress. An embolectomy may be performed if the pulmonary artery pressure is greatly elevated and if arteriography shows obstruction in a significant portion of the pulmonary vasculature (Smeltzer, Bare, 1992).

Vena caval interruption is used to prevent recurrent PE by interrupting the venous flow. Vena caval interruption may also be indicated for those in whom anticoagulation therapy is contraindicated, in those who have had recurrent PE despite adequate anticoagulation, or in very high risk patients with complex diseases. The procedure is carried out through a transvenous approach to the inferior vena cava through the femoral or jugular vein. The procedure requires local anesthesia and sedation and is relatively minor. The effectiveness in preventing PE appears equal to that of ligation or vena cava clip insertion (Brewster, 1984). Figure 20-29 illustrates the use of an umbrella filter, which is implanted into the inferior vena cava to prevent pulmonary embolism.

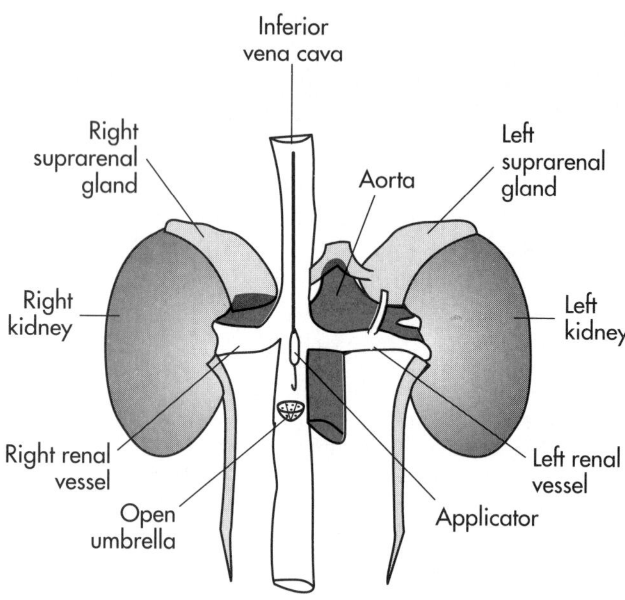

Figure 20-29 Insertion of an umbrella filter into the inferior vena cava is a procedure performed to prevent pulmonary embolism. A filter is compressed within an applicator and is inserted into the right internal jugular vein through an incision. After release, the filter expands and attaches to the wall of the inferior vena cava, and the applicator is withdrawn.

Patient/family education

Patient/family education focuses on teaching the patient about the anticoagulant he or she is taking. This information can be provided to patients when Coumadin therapy is instituted. Patients should also be taught how to decrease their risk of developing a DVT or PE (Box 20-13).

Measures to prevent DVT and subsequent PE

Nurses have an important responsibility in teaching patients how to prevent DVT and PE (see Box 20-13). Identifying patients at risk for DVT and PE is important, followed by taking action to prevent thrombus formation. These actions include pharmacologic and mechanical (nonpharmacologic) modalities. In 1986 the National Heart, Lung, and Blood Institute and the NIH Office of Medical Applications of Research discussed and agreed on particular prophylactic measures, which take into consideration patient age, health history, risk factors, and the surgery being performed, as well as the efficacy and safety of these measures.

Pharmacologic measures include low-dose subcutaneous heparin usually given as 5000 units two or three times a day until the patient is discharged. It can be used in moderate or high risk patients and may also be combined with other mechanical measures. Coumadin may also be used in high risk patients such as candidates for hip replacement and those with hip fractures. When receiving these agents, patients need to be monitored for any bleeding.

Mechanical (nonpharmacologic) measures include graduated compression stockings, which may be used in very low risk patients, and intermittent pneumatic compression (IPC). With IPC, a pair of inflatable sleeves are applied to the patient's lower legs. The sleeves are connected via air tubes to a pump compression unit that rapidly inflates them to a pressure between 40 and 50 mm Hg, maintains the pressure for 10 to 12 seconds, and deflates. IPC is well suited for patients who cannot tolerate anticoagulant therapy because of bleeding risks and can be used in low, moderate, and high risk patients. IPC can also be combined with anticoagulant therapy if indicated.

TUMORS OF THE LUNG

Tumors of the lung may be benign or malignant. A malignant chest tumor can be primary and arise from within the lung or mediastinum, or it may represent a metastasis from a primary tumor site somewhere else in the body. Because the bloodstream transports free cancer cells from primary cancers elsewhere in the body, metastatic tumors of the lung often occur and may invade the alveoli and the bronchi (Smeltzer, Bare, 1992).

Many tumors of the lung arise from bronchial epithelium. Bronchial adenomas are slow-growing and usually benign but are also very vascular and therefore produce symptoms of bronchial obstruction and bleeding. Bronchogenic carcinoma is a malignant tumor that arises from the bronchus. Such a tumor is epidermoid and is usually located in the larger bronchi, or it is an adenocarcinoma and arises farther out in the lung. Several intermediate or undifferentiated types of lung cancer also exist and are identified by cell type.

PATIENT/FAMILY TEACHING

Coumadin Therapy

Coumadin is an anticoagulant and is sometimes called a blood "thinner." Coumadin lengthens the time it takes the blood to clot and helps prevent clots from forming in the bloodstream. You and your healthcare provider (physician or nurse) are partners in your care.

A blood test must be done to check your body's response to Coumadin. The test is called a "Prothrombin time" or "Protime." This test is performed every day while you are in the hospital and at scheduled times after you go home.

The following guidelines can add to the success of your treatment:

1 Inform your healthcare provider and dentist that you take Coumadin.
2 Do not take any medicines, especially aspirin, ibuprofen, cold tablets, and vitamin K without checking with your provider. These medicines can affect your Protime.
3 Limit your intake of alcohol.
4 Eat a well-balanced diet. Do not eat large amounts of food that are high in vitamin K, such as liver, dark green leafy vegetables, cauliflower, tomatoes, bananas, fish, cheese, egg yolks, and beef fat.
5 Take your Coumadin at the same time each day according to directions given to you. If you forget to take a pill, call your provider. Do not take another pill to catch up.
6 Obtain your protime blood test as instructed. Your provider will talk with you about where to go (laboratory or hospital) for the test.
7 Notify your provider if you notice any sign of bleeding:
   a Black or bloody bowel movements
   b Blood in the urine
   c Bleeding gums
   d Nosebleeds that do not stop
   e Bad headaches or dizziness
   f Abdominal pain or vomiting of liquid that looks like "coffee grounds"
   g Easy bruising

Do Not stop taking Coumadin on your own. Instead talk with your healthcare provider about any concerns or problems you may have.

Safety Measures:

1 Use a soft toothbrush.
2 Use an electric razor.
3 Do not go barefoot.
4 Talk with your healthcare provider before beginning any contact sports.
5 Carry a card in your wallet or purse to let people know that you take Coumadin.

BOX 20-13

Guidelines for Nursing Care to Prevent Deep Vein Thrombosis Pulmonary Embolism

1 Prevention is the key.
2 Identify the risk factors that predispose the patient to the development of a DVT.
3 Implement appropriately prescribed prophylactic regimens.
4 Document patient tolerance of prophylactic measures.
5 Assess lower extremities each shift and monitor for signs and symptoms of DVT, including swelling, tenderness, warmth, and redness. Remember to investigate risk factors because the patient may be without symptoms.
6 Encourage early ambulation and leg exercises every hour while the patient is awake.
7 Perform passive range-of-motion exercises if the patient is immobile.
8 Avoid placing pillows directly under the knees.
9 Encourage fluid intake to avoid dehydration and monitor input and output (I&O).
10 Monitor laboratory values as ordered.
11 Educate patient regarding anticoagulant therapy.

The incidence of malignant tumors (bronchogenic carcinoma) of the lung has been increasing. It is more common in men than in women, but the incidence in women is steadily climbing. It is also more common in smokers than in nonsmokers and is related to the duration and the amount (intensity) of smoking. Additional risk factors include occupational exposure to asbestos, radioactive dusts, arsenic, and particular plastics, either alone or in combination with tobacco smoke.

Assessment

Depending on the location and size of the tumor, the patient may or may not experience symptoms. Usually a cough and dyspnea are the only signs, and the tumors may have been present for some time before they are detected. The cough may begin as a hacking, nonproductive cough and may later progress to a point where the sputum becomes thick and purulent. Therefore a cough that changes in character should warrant further investigation (Kersten, 1989; Smeltzer, Bare, 1992). A wheeze may be present if a bronchus becomes partially obstructed, and blood-tinged sputum may also be noted, especially in the morning. Pain is usually a late symptom and may be related to bone metastasis. If the tumor spreads to adjacent structures and lymph nodes, symptoms may occur as a result of obstruction or of pressure on structures. These symptoms include chest pain and tightness, hoarseness, dysphagia, head and neck edema, and pleural or pericardial effusion (Beare, Myers, 1994).

Diagnostic evaluation includes many of the tests previously discussed, including a chest x-ray examination, sputum examination, bronchoscopy, and CT scanning. Preoperative evaluation of the patient is important and includes information already presented on page 554.

Intervention

Treatment depends on cell type, stage of the disease, and the general health status of the patient. It may involve surgery, radiation therapy, and chemotherapy, which may be used alone or in combination. Nursing interventions focus on ways to maintain airway patency, including coughing when indicated, use of the IS, and deep breathing. Oxygen therapy may be used with pulse oximetry and monitored at specified intervals.

The psychologic aspects of caring for the patient with lung cancer are extremely important. The patient may be faced with many decisions and must choose among treatment options. Providing an atmosphere in which the patient can share his or her feelings and concerns is essential. Depending on the particular patient situation, resources to help the individual adjust and cope with the diagnosis are available in the hospital or community and include advanced practice nurses in oncology and mental health, as well as nurses in hospice settings.

CHEST WOUNDS

Chest trauma accounts for approximately 25% of all trauma-related deaths in the United States. Injuries to the chest are serious surgical emergencies and may involve the thoracic cage, pleura, lungs, heart, diaphragm, and abdominal organs. The care of the patient is determined by the extent of the injury. Patients with chest wounds are often apprehensive, and the nurse should explain procedures that are done to or with the patient (Beare, Myers, 1994; Carrere, Wayne, 1989).

When treating chest trauma, time is of the essence. Patient history focuses on the time the event occurred and on identifying the mechanism of injury. Blood loss is estimated, and, if the patient is responsive, the use of alcohol or drugs is determined.

The physical examination includes assessment of the airway, breathing pattern, vital signs, and skin color. The position of the trachea is assessed, and breath sounds are auscultated. Initial laboratory tests include electrolytes, complete blood count (CBC), type and crossmatch, chest x-ray examinations, urinalysis, ECG, and arterial blood gases. The patient's level of consciousness is also assessed. Agitation and confusion are signs of decreased blood flow and delivery of oxygen to the brain. Initial management involves maintaining the airway via whatever means possible, including mechanical ventilation. Any pneumothorax or hemothorax is managed, usually via insertion of a chest tube that is connected to water-seal drainage. Hypovolemia is corrected using colloid (e.g., blood products, albumin) and crystalloid, such as dextrose and normal saline or lactated Ringer's solution administered intravenously.

Rib fractures are the most common type of chest trauma. The fifth through the ninth ribs are those most commonly injured. The patient experiences severe pain and muscle spasm at the site of the fracture. Pain is exacerbated by movement, deep breathing, and coughing. Management focuses on pain control. Sedation is used to relieve pain and to allow for deep breathing and coughing. A chest binder may decrease pain on movement. Caution must be taken to relieve pain but not compromise respiratory function. Pain usually shows improvement in 5 to 7 days, at which time nonnarcotic analgesics may be used. Most fractures heal in 3 to 6 weeks.

Multiple adjacent rib fractures can result in a free-floating segment of the rib cage (flail chest). When this occurs, the free segment loses continuity with the rest of the chest wall and moves paradoxically. Therefore on inspiration, when the rest of the rib cage is moving outward, the flail segment sinks inward. On expiration, when the rib cage is moving inward, the flail segment bulges outward. Because pressure within the chest is decreased as a result of this paradoxical movement, movement of air is decreased. Previously all patients with flail chest were treated with mechanical ventilation, but now mechanical ventilation is avoided unless absolutely necessary. Patients are given analgesics to help decrease pain and to facilitate deep breathing and coughing. The patient should be encouraged to cough and breathe deeply and should be ambulatory as soon as the condition permits.

Penetrating wounds may be caused by any foreign object. Knife and bullet wounds may penetrate the lungs and cause an air leak. When this occurs, the air may compress the lung and cause a pneumothorax, or bleeding into the pleural cavity may occur and cause the lung to collapse. Both phenomena are serious because they may lead to cardiac or respiratory arrest unless immediate emergency treatment is given. The patient should be observed for dyspnea, and the blood pressure, pulse, and respiratory rates should be checked at frequent intervals. Oxygen may be administered, and a chest tube may be inserted and connected to closed drainage to remove air and blood. If the injury is such that surgical repair is necessary, a thoracotomy is later performed. An antibiotic and tetanus toxoid injection generally is administered. A tracheotomy may be required to provide for adequate ventilation in cases in which respiration is severely compromised.

ADULT RESPIRATORY DISTRESS SYNDROME

Adult respiratory distress syndrome (ARDS) (referred to as shock lung, wet lung, stiff lung, and congestive lung syndrome) is a combination of symptoms that result from direct or indirect injury to the lung. Many factors contribute to the development of ARDS, including viral and bacterial pneumonia, chest trauma, head injury, surgery, any form of shock, oxygen toxicity, smoke inhalation, aspiration of toxic irritants, near drowning, drug overdose, fat or air emboli, sepsis, disseminated intravascular coagulation, massive blood transfusions, renal failure, pancreatitis, and radiation injury to the lung.

Pathophysiology

In ARDS an alteration in the alveolar capillary membrane occurs, and the increased capillary permeability causes fluids to leak into the interstitial spaces, small airways, and eventually the alveoli. The lungs become edematous, and hypoxemia occurs. The fluid affects the activity of surfactant (the lipoprotein that helps maintain the elasticity of the alveolar tissue), and the alveoli collapse, which leads to shunting of blood through the fluid-filled or collapsed alveoli and interferes with oxygen transport. Plasma and red blood cells escape from the damaged capillaries and cause hemorrhage.

Assessment

Symptoms of ARDS may occur within hours of the lung injury or may not appear for several days. Initially the patient experiences rapid, shallow breathing and dyspnea. The dyspnea and tachypnea rapidly become more severe, and hypoxia, intercostal retractions, cyanosis, crackles, rhonchi, and tachycardia appear. Hypoxia and cyanosis respond poorly to oxygen therapy. As the ventilation-perfusion imbalance worsens, the hypoxia becomes overwhelming and results in hypotension and signs and symptoms of respiratory and metabolic acidosis.

Intervention

Treatment of ARDS is aimed at maintaining adequate alveolar ventilation and tissue oxygenation and at correcting the underlying cause. Many of the respiratory modalities discussed earlier in this chapter are instituted. High concentrations of oxygen are administered through a tightly fitting mask, which allows for the use of continuous positive air pressure. Often, the patient requires intubation with mechanical ventilatory support and PEEP. PEEP improves ventilation and perfusion by stretching the stiff lung tissue and keeping the alveoli from collapsing. High-frequency jet ventilation may be required in some cases. This method of ventilator therapy allows for the delivery of high levels of PEEP without raising peak mean-airway

ETHICAL DILEMMA

Mr. Huxley, a 59-year-old man with amyotrophic lateral sclerosis, has been a patient in the ICU for 10 days in an attempt to wean him from the ventilator, which has been used to treat a respiratory infection. He has been totally paralyzed for several years and is dependent on his family for care.

After several unsuccessful attempts to wean him from the ventilator, he has asked his physician to remove the ventilator and allow him to die. He is "tired of fighting this demon disease." He is not afraid to die but does fear the possible pain and feelings of suffocation.

How would you analyze the ethical issues in this case?

BOX 20-14 **Nursing Process**

ADULT RESPIRATORY DISTRESS SYNDROME

ASSESSMENT

Respiratory status (breath sounds, breathing pattern, sputum)
Vital signs
Hemodynamic pressures, if indicated (cardiac output)
Ventilator settings; endotracheal tube (ET) position
Signs of barotrauma q 1 hr, if on mechanical ventilation
Urine output
Skin and nailbed color; temperature; and quality of peripheral pulses
Level of consciousness
ABGs, electrolytes, complete blood count (CBC)
Chest x-ray examination

NURSING DIAGNOSES

Impaired gas exchange related to alveolar-capillary membrane changes
Ineffective breathing pattern related to decreased lung compliance, fatigue, and decreased energy
Ineffective airway clearance related to pulmonary and interstitial edema
Risk for decreased cardiac output related to positive pressure ventilation
Fear related to difficulty breathing, mechanical ventilation, and inability to communicate
Risk for infection related to decreased pulmonary function
Risk for injury: barotrauma related to positive pressure ventilation and decreased pulmonary compliance
Risk for impaired skin integrity related to prolonged bed rest/immobility
Impaired physical mobility related to mechanical ventilation, acute respiratory failure
Inability to sustain spontaneous ventilation related to acute respiratory failure
Impaired verbal communication related to endotracheal intubation

NURSING INTERVENTIONS

Maintain oxygen delivery system as prescribed, for O_2 saturation > 90%
Provide reassurance.
Keep healthcare provider informed of respiratory status.
Anticipate need for intubation and mechanical ventilation.
Prevent dislodgement of ET tube with restraints to extremities, as needed.
Provide nursing care related to ET tube.
Provide nonverbal means of communication.
Use pulse oximetry for continuous monitoring of O_2 saturation.
Combine nursing actions to conserve patient energy.
Turn and position q 2 hr.
Aseptic suctioning prn, as prescribed.
Turn and position q 2 hr.
Administer medications as prescribed.
Administer IV fluids as prescribed.
Anticipate need for chest tube placement, if barotrauma occurs.
Maintain limbs in proper body alignment.
Perform range-of-motion exercises.
Initiate activity increases as condition improves.
Maintain skin integrity.

EVALUATION OF EXPECTED OUTCOMES

Maintenance of optimal breathing with assistance as indicated
O_2 saturation > 90%
ABGs WNL for patient
Breath sounds clear or improved
Alert mentation
Urine output > 30 ml/hr
Strong peripheral pulses
No evidence of barotrauma
No evidence of skin breakdown

pressure to the extent required by conventional ventilators. It ventilates the patient with small tidal volumes and high respiratory rates (Smith, 1988).

Nursing care consists of continued support of the patient's respiratory function and of detection and prevention of complications. Vital signs, breath sounds, intake and output, arterial blood gases, and serum electrolytes should be assessed often. Airway patency should be maintained by suctioning using a sterile technique. Ventilator settings are checked often. The patient's position should be changed often, and passive range of motion should be performed. The environment must be quiet and relaxed, and adequate rest periods must be planned. As always, the nurse collaborates with the physician and respiratory therapist and notes respiratory changes promptly (Box 20-14).

KEY CONCEPTS

- The primary function of the respiratory system is to provide oxygen to meet metabolic needs and to remove carbon dioxide.
- The signs and symptoms most closely associated with respiratory disease are dyspnea, chest pain, cough, sputum production, wheezing, hemoptysis, and cyanosis.
- Nursing assessment of the patient with respiratory problems begins with the patient history.
- Physical assessment of the lungs and thorax includes inspection, palpation, percussion, and auscultation.
- Arterial blood gases assess (1) the ability of the lungs to provide adequate oxygen and remove carbon dioxide, and (2) the ability of the kidneys to excrete or reabsorb bicarbonate ions to maintain normal body pH.
- Pulmonary function tests evaluate lung function. The most common tests are performed by spirometry, which measures lung volumes and capacities and flow rates.
- Bronchoscopy allows for visual examination of the lungs.
- Thoracentesis is performed to obtain pleural fluid for diagnostic purposes, to remove pleural fluid for therapeutic purposes, to biopsy the pleura, or to instill medication.
- Nursing strategies for common respiratory problems include incentive spirometry, coughing and deep breathing, suctioning, postural drainage, percussion, and vibration.
- Precautions are important when oxygen is being used because it supports combustion.
- The primary nursing responsibility in caring for a patient with a tracheostomy tube is to maintain airway patency. Tracheal suctioning is often required, and secretions should be kept moist. Monitoring for cyanosis, shortness of breath, bleeding from the wound, and hypotension is essential.
- The nursing care of patients who are receiving mechanical ventilation includes monitoring vital signs, positioning to provide optimum ventilation, turning, performing active and passive range-of-motion exercises, assessing airway maintenance, determining the need for suctioning, recording intake and output, maintaining adequate nutrition and hydration, and providing emotional support.
- Following thoracic surgery, postoperative care focuses on maintaining the closed drainage system; positioning; encouraging frequent coughing, deep breathing, and use of the incentive spirometer; maintaining patient comfort using medications and techniques such as relaxation; observing for complications; and teaching and reinforcing postoperative arm exercises and activity progression.
- Invasion of the upper respiratory system by microorganisms, usually viral, may cause inflammation and edema of the mucous membranes; cervical lymph node enlargement; dryness, redness, and soreness of the mucous membranes of the throat; voice hoarseness with painful cough; and leukocytosis to combat infection. Interventions are directed toward preventing complications, preventing the spread of infection, and relieving discomfort from symptoms.
- Hoarseness is often the first symptom of laryngeal cancer. Interventions include radiation therapy and partial, supraglottic, or total laryngectomies. Preoperative preparation, especially psychologic, is important. As the patient improves, the goals are self-care and speech training. Patient teaching focuses on good hygiene, stoma care, emergency care, stomal hydration, and overall healthy behaviors.
- COPD causes psychologic, physical, and social problems for the patient. COPDs include emphysema, chronic bronchitis, bronchiectasis, and asthma. Nursing interventions include administration of bronchodilators, evaluation of the effectiveness of respiratory treatments, administration of bronchodilators, evaluation of the effectiveness of respiratory treatments, administration of oxygen, instruction on diaphragmatic breathing, maintenance of adequate hydration and nutrition, performance of postural drainage with percussion and vibration if needed, maintenance of activity level, and development of a regular activity program.
- Pneumonia is caused by bacteria, viruses, fungi, and mycobacteria. Most community-acquired pneumonia is caused by *Pneumococcus* and occurs in the very young and in older adults. Interventions are aimed at keeping the patient comfortable, avoiding unnecessary expenditures of energy, and using antibiotic and sulfonamide agents to help the body's defenses overcome the infection.

KEY CONCEPTS

- Tuberculosis is caused by acid-fast bacterium. Signs and symptoms of TB include cough, hemoptysis, pleuritic chest pain, weight loss, night sweats, fever, malaise, anorexia, and fatigue. TB is detected through skin testing, examinations of sputum for AFB, and chest x-ray examinations. Treatment requires more than one drug for 6 to 9 months. Patient education includes teaching the patient about the medication regimen and encouraging him or her to remain in close contact with the healthcare provider so that progress can be monitored.
- Atelectasis occurs from the blockage of air to a portion of the lung, which causes collapse. It may be a postoperative complication or may be caused by tumors, an enlarged heart, or obstruction of bronchus by a foreign body or mucous plug. Interventions include deep breathing, incentive spirometry, chest percussion and vibration, and postural drainage. Suctioning, oxygen, administration of aerosols, and humidity are also used.
- Pulmonary embolism and infarction are blood clots or other foreign material that originate in the venous system and are carried to the lung. PEs can cause death of lung tissue and infarction. Nursing interventions focus on the initial stabilization of the patient, improvement of gas exchange, maintenance of optimal cardiac function, reduction of anxiety, and relief of pain.
- Prevention of deep vein thrombosis is important because 90% to 95% of all pulmonary emboli originate from the deep veins of the leg. Measures can be pharmacologic, nonpharmacologic, or a combination of the two.
- Lung cancer is more common in men than women and is more common in smokers than in nonsmokers. Treatment depends on the cell type, stage of the disease, and general health status of the patient. Treatment may involve surgery, radiation therapy, and chemotherapy, either used alone or in combination.
- Chest wounds represent serious medical or surgical emergencies. Patient care is determined by the extent of the injury. Patient history focuses on the time the event occurred, the mechanism of the injury, the estimation of blood loss, and whether alcohol or drugs were used. Physical examination includes the assessment of respiratory and neurologic function.
- ARDS has a combination of symptoms that result from direct or indirect injury to lung and changes that occur in the alveolar capillary membrane. Interventions include oxygen therapy, suctioning, percussion, vibration, and postural drainage. Intubation and mechanical ventilation are often required.

CRITICAL THINKING EXERCISES

1 What are the difficulties in administering oxygen therapy to a patient with emphysema?
2 Explain the dynamics of closed chest drainage for a patient with pneumothorax.
3 Design a plan to prevent the development of a DVT and subsequent PE in a patient with advanced cancer.
4 Outline the preoperative assessment for a patient with a lung tumor who is undergoing a lobectomy.

REFERENCES AND ADDITIONAL READINGS

Barkauskas VH and others: *Health and physical assessment*, St Louis, 1994, Mosby.

Bartlett RH: Postoperative pulmonary prophylaxis: breathe deeply and read carefully, *Chest* 81(1):1-2, 1982.

Bartlett RH, Gazzaniga AB, Geraghty TR: Respiratory maneuvers to prevent postoperative pulmonary complications, *JAMA* 224(7):1017-1021, 1973.

Beare PG, Myers JL: *Principles and practice of adult health nursing*, ed 2, St Louis, 1994, Mosby.

Bolgiano CS, Bunting K, Shoenberger M: Administering oxygen therapy: what you need to know, *Nurs 90* 20(6): 47-51, 1990.

Brewster DC: Introduction to symposium on transvenous vena cava interruption, *J Vas Surgery* 1(3):487-490, 1984.

Carrere R, Wayne M: Chest trauma, *Emerg Clin North Am* 7(2):389-418, 1989.

Center for Prevention Services, Division of Tuberculosis Elimination and the American Thoracic Society, *Core Curriculum on Tuberculosis*, ed 2, Atlanta, 1991, US Department of Health and Human Services, Public Health Service, Centers for Disease Control.

Consensus conference: Prevention of venous thrombosis and pulmonary emboli, *JAMA* 256:744-749, 1986.

Currie DL: Pulmonary embolism: diagnosis and management, *Crit Care Nurs Quart* 13(2):41-49, 1990.

Dossey BM, Guzzetta CE, Kenner CV: *Essentials of critical care nursing: body-mind-spirit,* Philadelphia, 1990, JB Lippincott.

Duncan C, Erickson R: Pressure associated with chest tube stripping, *Heart Lung* 11(2):166-171, 1982.

Erickson RS: Mastering the ins and outs of chest drainage, Part 1, *Nurs 89* 19(5):37-44, 1989a.

Erickson RS: Mastering the ins and outs of chest drainage, Part 2, *Nurs 89* 19(6):46-50, 1989b.

Feinstein D: What to teach the patient who's had a total laryngectomy, *RN* 50(4):53-57, 1987.

Gift AG: Dyspnea, *Nurs Clin North Am* 25(4):955-965, 1990.

Hudak CM, Gallo BM, Benz JJ: *Critical care nursing: a holistic approach,* ed 5, Philadelphia, 1990, JB Lippincott.

Huddleston VB: Pulmonary problems, *Crit Care Nurs Clin North Am* 2(4):527-536, 1990.

Hull RD, Moser KM, Salzman EW: Preventing pulmonary embolism, *Patient Care* 23 (4): 63-66; 71-72; 75-76:2-11, 1989.

Kersten LD: *Comprehensive respiratory nursing: a decision making approach,* Philadelphia, 1989, WB Saunders.

Kischbach F: *A manual of laboratory and diagnostic tests,* ed 4, Philadelphia, 1992, JB Lippincott.

Loch WE and others: Sinusitis, *Primary Care* 17(2):323-334, 1990.

Malasanos L, Barkauskas V, Stoltenberg-Allen K: *Health assessment,* ed 4, St Louis, 1990, Mosby.

Patrick ML and others: *Medical-surgical nursing: pathophysiological concepts,* ed 2, Philadelphia, 1991, JB Lippincott.

Phipps WJ and others: *Medical-surgical nursing: concepts and clinical practice,* ed 5, St Louis, 1995, Mosby.

Porth CM: *Pathophysiology: concepts of altered health states,* ed 3, Philadelphia, 1990, JB Lippincott.

Sexton DL: *Nursing care of the respiratory patient,* Norwalk, Conn, 1990, Appleton & Lange.

Siedel HM and others: *Mosby's guide to physical examination,* ed 2, St Louis, 1991, Mosby.

Smeltzer SC, Bare BG: *Brunner and Suddarth's textbook of medical-surgical nursing,* ed 7, Philadelphia, 1992, JB Lippincott.

Smith S: High-frequency jet ventilation in the treatment of idiopathic pulmonary fibrosis complicating ARDS: a nursing challenge, *Crit Care Nurse Quart* 11(3):29-35, 1988.

Spyr J, Preach MA: Pulse oximetry: understanding the concept, knowing the limits, *RN* 53(5):38-43, 1990.

Wilson EB, Malley N: Discharge planning for the patient with a new tracheostomy, *Crit Care Nurs* 10(7):73-79, 1990.

CHAPTER 21

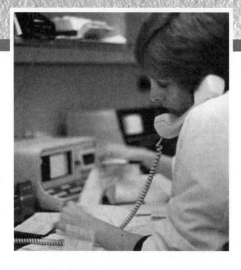

Circulation

CHAPTER OBJECTIVES

1. Describe the normal flow of blood through the heart and circulatory system.
2. Trace the normal electric conduction through the heart.
3. Identify common cardiac arrhythmias and their effects on cardiac output.
4. Describe the assessment of a patient with a cardiac disorder.
5. Describe the nursing responsibilities associated with diagnostic testing of patients with cardiovascular disorders.
6. Describe the major risk factors for cardiovascular diseases.
7. Compare the nursing assessment and interventions indicated for a patient who has angina pectoris with the assessment and interventions indicated for a patient convalescing from a myocardial infarction.
8. Compare nursing assessment and interventions indicated for a patient who has acute pulmonary edema with the assessment and interventions indicated for a patient with congestive heart failure.
9. Describe those items that should be included in a patient-education program on hypertension.
10. Identify nursing assessment and interventions related to the postoperative care of a patient with a vein ligation and stripping.
11. List at least three precautions the nurse should teach to patients with permanent pacemakers.
12. Describe nursing responsibilities related to the preoperative and postoperative phases for a patient undergoing cardiac surgery.
13. List steps of basic cardiac life support.
14. Describe the sequence of events to care for a patient with an obstructed airway.

KEY WORDS

aneurysm
angina pectoris
angioplasty
arrhythmia
arteriosclerosis
ascites
atherosclerosis
atrial fibrillation
bacterial endocarditis
cardiac output
cardiogenic shock
central venous pressure
cholesterol
defibrillation
diuretics
depolarization
electrocardiogram
embolectomy
hypertension
ischemic heart disease
isoenzyme
lymphangitis
myocardial infarction
pacemaker
plaques
pulmonary edema
risk factors
sinoatrial node
sinus bradycardia
sinus tachycardia
stenosis
thrombophlebitis
varicosities
ventricular fibrillation
ventricular tachycardia

CARDIOVASCULAR STRUCTURE AND FUNCTION

Cardiac Anatomy

The heart, a hollow muscular organ, pumps blood through the cardiovascular system. It is located behind the sternum, within the mediastinum, between the lungs, and above the diaphragm. The base of the heart is located just below the second rib. The lower part of the heart, the apex, is pointed downward and to the left. It is located just below the left, fifth rib. The heart is protected anteriorly by the rib cage and sternum and posteriorly by the rib cage and vertebral column.

Heart chambers

The heart is made up of four chambers (Figure 21-1). The upper chambers are the *right atrium* and *left atrium.* The lower chambers, the *right ventricle* and *left ventricle,* are thick, muscle-walled chambers. The right and left side of the heart are separated by a *septum.*

The right atrium receives venous blood from all body tissues except the lung. The right ventricle pumps venous blood through the pulmonary artery to the lungs, where carbon dioxide is exchanged for oxygen. Oxygenated blood from the lungs is received in the left atrium. The left ventricle pumps blood through the aorta to all parts of the body.

Heart muscle

There are three distinct layers of the heart muscle. The outer layer, the *epicardium,* is a thin, transparent covering layer commonly infiltrated with fat. The *myocardium,* the middle layer, consists of striated cardiac muscle fibers that permit the heart to contract. The inner layer of the heart muscle, the *endocardium,* is a thin layer of endothelial tissue that lines the inner cavity of the heart and covers the valves of the heart and the chordae tendineae, which are tendons that hold the cardiac valves open. The endocardium is contiguous with the inner lining of the vessels. Inflammation of the endocardium is called *endocarditis* and may be caused by microorganisms. These microorganisms in-

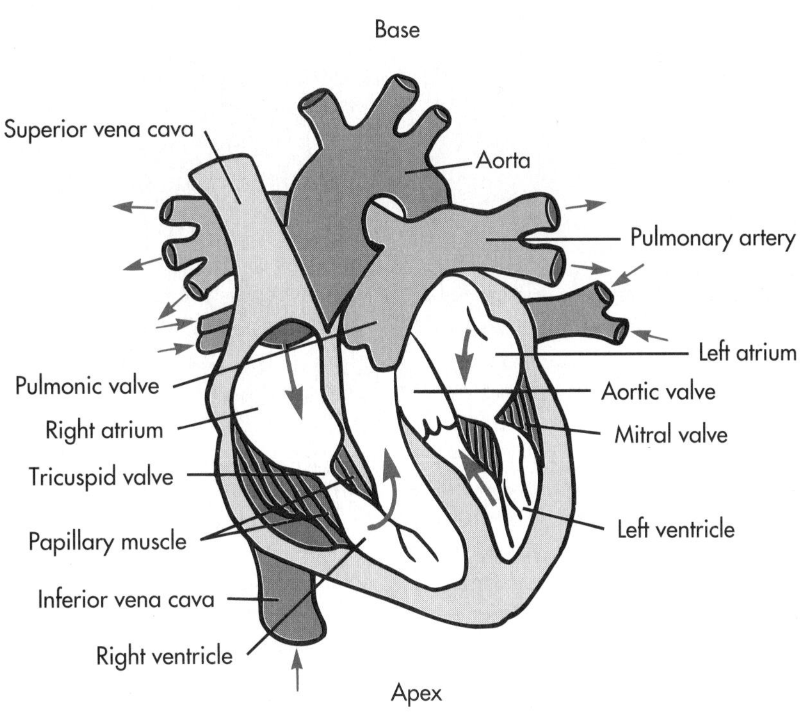

Figure 21-1 Blood flow through heart.

clude bacteria, fungi, rickettsiae, and, rarely, viruses and parasites.

The heart is surrounded by a fibroserous sac called the *pericardium.* The pericardium consists of an external fibrous layer and an internal serous layer that adheres to the heart and to the epicardium. The serous layer is further divided into two layers containing a thin film of pericardial fluid between the layers. This serous fluid lubricates the two layers with each heartbeat. Inflammation of the pericardium is called *pericarditis.* The cause is often idiopathic but may also result from a viral or bacterial infection. Noninfectious causes include uremia, myocardial infarction, tumors, radiation, and certain pharmaceutical agents (Lilly, 1993).

Heart valves

The forward flow of blood through the heart is controlled by a series of one-way valves that prevent backflow within the heart. Heart valves are nonmuscular tissue. The *tricuspid valve,* between the right atrium and right ventricle, and the *mitral valve,* between the left atrium and left ventricle, are often called atrioventricular valves because they direct the blood flow between the atria and the ventricles. The valve between the right ventricle and the pulmonary artery is the *pulmonic valve,* and the *aortic valve* is between the left ventricle and the aorta. These valves are called *semilunar valves.*

The heart, like other organ systems, has its own blood supply. The coronary arteries are the first branches from the aorta. They surround the heart and provide blood to all portions of the myocardium and the heart's electrical conduction system. Coronary veins return deoxygenated blood to the right atrium.

Vascular System

Blood vessels

Blood vessels are a network of arteries, arterioles, capillaries, venules, and veins that circulate blood to and from the heart. The major divisions of this network are the *systemic circulation* and the *pulmonary circulation.* The portal circulation of the liver and the lymphatic circulation are also important components of the circulatory status of the body. The circulatory system transports nutrients and oxygen to body cells and carries waste products to the appropriate organs of the body to be eliminated. All systemic arteries branch from the aorta. Blood in veins of the systemic circulation flows into the *superior vena cava* or into the *inferior vena cava,* both of which flow into the right atrium.

Pulmonary circulation carries blood from the right ventricle to the lungs and back to the left atrium. The right and left pulmonary arteries arise from the right ventricle and immediately subdivide into a series of short branches, ending in capillaries that encircle the lungs' air sacs (alveoli), pick up oxygen, and release the waste product, carbon dioxide. The capillaries gradually come together to form pulmonary veins that carry oxygenated blood from the lungs to the left atrium.

Blood and blood components

Blood volume makes up about 8% of a person's total body weight. This percentage varies with environmental temperature, altitude, individual weight, sex, age, nutrition, and pregnancy (Ganong, 1993). During a normal pregnancy the blood volume increases to about 50% above nonpregnant levels (Douglas, 1993; Chandrasoma, Taylor, 1991). Approximately 40% of blood is composed of circulating cells, and the other 60% is plasma (Guyton, 1990). Red blood cells transport hemoglobin, which has the unique property of binding and releasing oxygen. The percentage of red blood cells in the whole blood volume is measured as a hematocrit value. White blood cells are the body's first enzymes and chemicals needed for the inflammation process and for coagulation of blood. Plasma, which is similar to tissue (interstitial) fluid but contains three times more proteins, contributes to cardiovascular function by maintaining blood volume, blood viscosity, and osmotic pressure. Each side of the heart, left and right, accomodates (holds) about 4% of the total circulating blood volume. The remaining blood volume is distributed within the vasculature, with approximately 4% in the capillaries, 16% in the arterial vessels and 64% in the venous vessels (Porth, 1994).

Lymphatic Circulation

Lymphatic fluid is excess tissue (interstitial) fluid that has accumulated around body cells. Lymphatic drainage maintains equilibrium of the fluid surrounding body cells. Lymphatic vessels begin as tiny lymphatic capillaries similar to blood capillaries. These unite and form large vessels (thoracic duct and right lymphatic duct) that empty into veins. Lymph moves as a result of skeletal muscle contraction, negative intrathoracic pressure, and the suction effect of blood flow in the veins. The lymphatic fluid flow depends on venous pressure and on the condition of venous vessels. Distributed along the lymphatic vessel system are small, round bodies, called lymph nodes, that serve as filters to remove proteins. Lymph node function is related to the immune system (see Chapter 7). Venous vessel obstruction or elevated venous pressure can affect interstitial fluid volume and capillary exchange.

Cardiac Cycle

Blood circulation throughout the cardiovascular system is regulated by the cardiac cycle, which coordinates activities of the heart. The cardiac cycle consists of two phases: *systole* (contraction) and *diastole* (relaxation). The cardiac cycle is less than 0.8 seconds long and includes systole, when atrial and ventricular muscular contractions are propelling blood forward, and diastole, when the heart muscle relaxes and is refilled with blood.

Heart sounds

The opening and closing of the heart valves produces the sounds made by the heart. S_1 and S_2 are the normal heart sounds. S_3 and S_4 are considered abnormal heart sounds unless proven otherwise.

The first heart sound, S_1, corresponds to the onset of ventricular contraction and is produced by the closing of the mitral valve and the tricuspid valve. The second heart sound, S_2, occurs at the end of ventricular contraction and coincides with the onset of ventricular diastole. Relaxation of the ventricles results in closing of the aortic and pulmonic valves, which produces the S_2 sound (Lilly, 1993).

The third heart sound (S_3), if present, occurs early in diastole, just after the S_2. The S_3 sound, which results from vibrations produced by rapid ventricular filling, is transmitted by the ventricular muscle. The third heart sound is not an unusual finding in children and young adults, but in mature adults it suggests altered cardiac function such as chronic heart failure. When S_1, S_2, and S_3 are heard with a stethoscope, the sound they produce has a rhythm similar to the word *Kentucky*.

The fourth heart sound, S_4, occurs during ventricular diastole after atrial contraction and immediately before S_1. The S_4 sound results because the ventricle is dilated but resists filling. This is common in patients with **hypertension.** When S_1, S_2, and S_4 are heard with a stethoscope, the sound they produce has a rhythm similar to the word *Tennessee.*

Normal electrical cardiac conduction

The heart beats in an orderly sequence: the atria contract first, contraction of the ventricles follows immediately, then all four chambers relax during diastole. Myocardial cells have a special ability to contract together with minimal electrical resistance. This is known as a syncytium. The heart has its own electric conduction system to initiate the cardiac cycle and maintain the regularity of the cycle (Figure 21-2). The conduction system is composed of the *sinus node, atrioventricular (AV) junctional tissue, the bundle of His,* and the *His-Purkinje system.* The sinus node, also called the **sinoatrial node** or SA node, is located near the junction of the superior vena cava and right atrium. It is the sinus node that initiates the electrical impulse and is therefore known as the heart's normal pacemaker. The impulse spreads over both atria, and contraction results. The impulse is then sent through highly specialized conduction tissue called the *AV node.* The AV node is situated in the right posterior portion of the interatrial septum, behind the tricuspid valve. The AV node delays the electrical impulse transmission from the atria to the ventricles. This delay permits maximum filling of the right and left ventricles before the electrical impulse reaches them. After passing through the AV node, the electrical impulse stimulates the bundle of His. The impulse is carried along the bundle of His and its right and left bundle branches. It then subdivides further into the *Purkinje fibers,* where the impulse causes the ventricles to contract.

The electrical conduction system is extremely complex and is located under the endocardial surface of the heart. That is why the conduction system is highly susceptible to disease and lack of blood supply. When

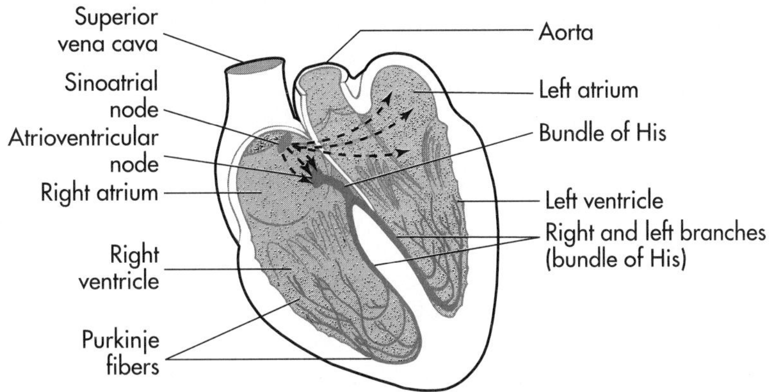

Figure 21-2 Conduction system of heart.

the conduction system is damaged, the normal pacemaker function of the SA node may be altered. In this case other components of the conduction system would assume the SA node's pacemaker function. This is called an ectopic pacemaker. The different parts of the conduction system have inherently different rates of contraction. The SA node beats at about 60 to 100 times per minute and is the normal pacemaker of the heart. If the AV node is forced to assume pacemaker functions, a rhythmic but slower rate of 40 to 60 beats per minute results (Grauer, 1992).

Neurohumoral Controls of the Heart

Many physiologic entities can control the heart. Some of these controls are the sympathetic (stimulating) nervous system and the parasympathetic (inhibitory) nervous system.

Alpha-, $beta_1$-, and $beta_2$-adrenergic receptors

Stimulation of alpha receptors raises blood pressure by constricting peripheral vascular arterioles. Stimulation of $beta_1$-receptors affects the conduction system. Stimulation of $beta_2$-receptors causes dilation of peripheral vessels and relaxation of constricted bronchial muscles.

Baroreceptors

Baroreceptors are located in the carotid sinuses and aortic arch. They are receptors that are sensitive to changes in blood pressure. For example, if blood pressure increases suddenly, baroreceptors are stimulated, which causes the cardiac control center in the brain to slow the heart rate and lower blood pressure.

Chemoreceptors

Chemoreceptors in the carotid arteries and the aorta detect increased carbon dioxide levels or oxygen deficiencies. The heart rate is increased, and arterioles and venous reservoirs constrict. (Berne, Levy, 1990).

Temperature

An increase in body temperature increases the metabolism rate of the SA node, which causes it to discharge impulses faster. Conversely, a lowered body temperature will decrease the heart rate by slowing the SA node's metabolism and discharge rates.

Electrolytes and hormones

Epinephrine stimulates the sympathetic nervous system, which causes the heart rate to increase. Insulin has a positive inotropic effect on the heart (Berne, Levy, 1990), which means, essentially, that it causes the heart to work harder by moving more blood per beat. Positive inotropes affect myocardial contractility by increasing the velocity and stroke volume of the contraction. Other positive inotropes are epinephrine, norepinephrine, dopamine, calcium salt infusion, and excess thyroid hormone. Negative inotropes work the opposite way, decreasing myocardial contraction velocity and stroke volume. Negative inotropes include alcohol, procainamide, quinidine, and propranolol (McKance, Heuther, 1994). Thyroid hormone deficiency results in a slower heart rate and decreased cardiac output.

Excess potassium within the heart muscle causes the heart to become dilated and flaccid, which decreases the heart rate. Excess potassium also can impede conduction of electrical impulses from the atria to the ventricles. Low potassium levels tend to reduce responsiveness of muscles to nerve stimulation, and arrhythmias, or abnormal cardiac rhythms, may occur.

NURSING ASSESSMENT OF THE PATIENT WITH A CARDIOVASCULAR PROBLEM

Nursing assessment begins with a comprehensive history of the patient's problem. This includes a review of seven dimensions of a patient problem, which ensures that no detail of the problem is overlooked. These seven dimensions are location, quality, quantity, chronology (the timetable of events), aggravating/alleviating factors, associated symptoms, and any treatment sought and its effect.

When assessing the cardiovascular system it is also important to identify risk factors that, if present, indicate an increased chance of developing a cardiovascular problem. **Risk factors** are conditions that have been identified through research as contributing to cardiovascular problems (Table 21-1).

After obtaining the patient's cardiovascular history, the nurse should conduct a systematic physical examination of the heart. The objective of this partial examination is to gain information about the muscular movement of the patient's heart. The four techniques of physical assessment are *inspection, palpation, percussion,* and *auscultation.* The physical assessment is performed with the patient in three positions: sitting, supine, and lying on the left side.

Inspection

Inspection includes visual assessment of the shape of the patient's chest and observation of the heart area for visible pulsations (Figure 21-3). Abnormal shapes can influence cardiac function. Normally, no pulsation will be visible unless the patient is very thin, in which case a slight pulsation may be detected. The finding of an abnormal pulsation requires further assessment.

Palpation

Palpation is used to detect pulsation or vibration (thrills) that may not have been identified with inspection or to further assess pulsations that were identified during inspection. The same areas of the chest are assessed (Figure 21-3). The best palpation technique for detecting vibrations is to use the palmar bases of the fingers of the right hand to locate a vibration and then use the pads of the middle and index fingers to make finer assessments. Detection of vibrations suggests the presence of a pathologic condition and requires further assessment. Special attention should be given to finding the point of maximum impulse (PMI). This is the most lateral pulsation of the left ventricle, detected over the apex of the heart. Normally this apical impulse is located approximately 7.5 to 9 cm from the midsternal line. A displaced apical impulse or one that has abnormal vibration indicates cardiovascular disease. An abnormal vibration is classified as a *lift* if it is a slightly more sustained thrust than normal. A *heave* is an impulse whose force pushes out against the palpating hand.

TABLE 21-1

Cardiac Risk Factors

Nonmodifiable	Potentially Modifiable
Gender (male) Age (increased) Family history of heart disease	Hypertension Diabetes mellitus Smoking history Hypercholesteremia Obesity Sedentary lifestyle Stressful behavior

Percussion

Percussion is an assessment technique that produces sound by tapping a body part, thus indicating the size, density, and location of an underlying structure or fluid/air space. Percussion may be used to identify cardiac borders, but x-ray examination and fluoroscopy are more accurate diagnostic measures and are more commonly used. Usually there are midsternal shifts to the left in pregnant women and in patients with liver cirrhosis.

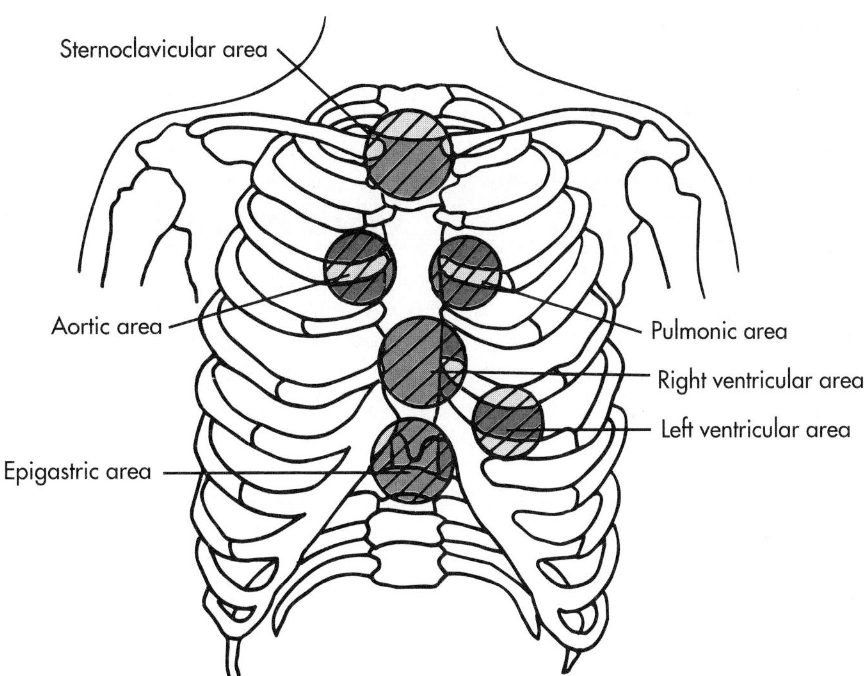

Figure 21-3 Areas of inspection and palpation for cardiac assessment.

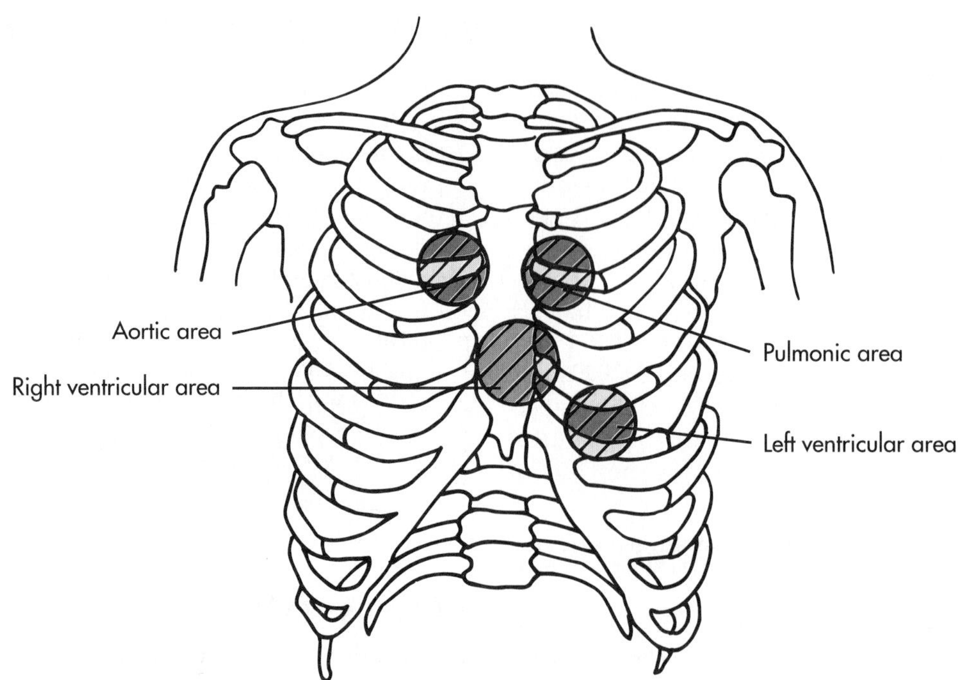

Figure 21-4 Areas of cardiac auscultation.

Auscultation

Auscultation is the perception and interpretation of sound through a stethoscope (Figure 21-4). It is the most difficult technique because the ear of the nurse must be trained to identify normal sounds and recognize specific characteristics of abnormal sounds. Variations in sounds are described by the sound, location, time, intensity, and pitch. Specific heart sounds include the vibrations produced by all activity occurring in the heart. These sounds are influenced by the viscosity and velocity of blood, elasticity of the heart valves, and distention of the cardiac chambers. Normally the heart has two distinct sounds: S_1 and S_2. Additional sounds, S_3 and S_4, may be present, as may heart murmurs.

The nurse listens systematically in all areas surrounding the heart, first with the diaphragm of the stethoscope and then with its bell. The diaphragm picks up high-pitched sounds, and the bell picks up low-pitched sounds. It is vital for the nurse to have confidence in hearing and recognizing S_1 and S_2 before expecting to identify S_3, S_4, or murmurs (Table 21-2).

Murmurs are vascular sounds that produce vibrations within the heart or great blood vessels (i.e., aorta, pulmonary vein) and are most often associated with **stenosis** or regurgitation. Stenosis is the result of thickened valvular leaflets that cause narrowed passage and restricted blood flow. Regurgitation is the backward flow of blood through valve leaflets that have lost their ability to close snugly. Murmurs may be considered a normal finding if no other signs or symptoms of cardiovascular disease are found.

Additional heart sounds that may be heard are an *ejection click* (the opening of pulmonic and aortic valves), an *opening snap* (opening of the mitral and tricuspid valves), or the *splitting* of either S_1 or S_2 (single sound perceived as two sounds). Splitting may be physiologic (occurring with respirations) or pathologic (related to a cardiovascular problem).

Blood Pressure

Assessment of the cardiovascular system includes measurement of blood pressure. Systolic blood pressure reflects stroke volume and pressure exerted against the interior walls of the aorta, whereas diastolic blood pressure indicates the resistance of the blood vessels. To ensure an accurate reading, the blood pressure cuff is placed directly on the skin and must fit adequately around the patient's arm. Because blood pressure sounds are low pitched, they are best heard with the bell of the stethoscope, although the diaphragm can be used for this reading. The audible vibrations within an artery are called *Korotkoff's sounds.* Blood pressure readings vary with age, and adults are seen with lower limits of 90/60 mm Hg and upper limits of 140/90 mm Hg. Systolic pressure may vary by 5 to 10 mm Hg between one arm and the other. The

TABLE 21-2

Characteristics of the Four Heart Sounds

	S_1	S_2	S_3	S_4
Sound	Lubb	Dubb	Ken-tuck-y S_1, S_2, S_3	Tenn-ess-ee S_1, S_2, S_4
Location	Mitral tricuspid valve	Aortic-pulmonic area	Apex	Medial to apex
Time	Systolic, longer than S_2	Diastolic, shorter than S_1	Early diastole	Late diastole, presystole
Intensity	Louder at apex	Louder at base	Dull	Higher than S_3
Pitch	Low	Higher than S_1	Low pitch	Duller than crisp S_1
Clinical interpretation	Normal	Normal	Normal in children or after exercise; may be sign of congestive heart failure or mitral regurgitation	Normally not heard; associated with hypertension, aortic or pulmonic stenosis

pulse pressure is the difference between the systolic and diastolic measurements and is usually between 30 to 40 mm Hg.

A blood pressure measurement usually is taken with the patient sitting. If possible it is helpful also to measure the patient's blood pressure while he or she is lying or standing. Normally the blood pressure measurement should remain the same in any position. A decrease in systolic measurement of more than 10 mm Hg or a decrease in diastolic measurement of more than 5 mm Hg suggests postural hypotension, possibly caused by antihypertensive medication, prolonged bed rest, or low fluid volume.

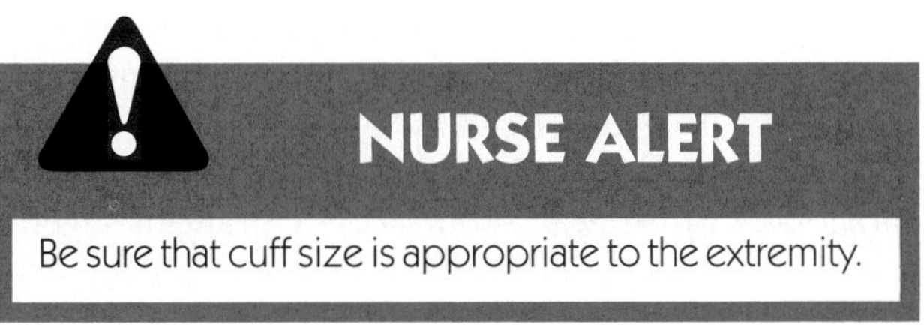
NURSE ALERT
Be sure that cuff size is appropriate to the extremity.

Anxiety raises blood pressure. The nurse should try to have the patient relax if possible. If the patient is very obese and there is difficulty with the standard cuff fit, the nurse can secure an oversized cuff or use the standard cuff on the forearm and listen over the radial artery (Bates, 1987). Even scrupulous adherence to blood-pressure–taking technique may be compromised with conditions such as cardiac arrhythmias, aortic regurgitation, and venous congestion. When cardiac irregularities persist, it may be necessary to take an average of several pressures and record it as such. To minimize venous congestion, the nurse should try to avoid repeated, slow inflations of the cuff.

Arterial Pulses

In addition to determining the cardiac rate, the nurse should evaluate the quality of the peripheral circulation by examining the pulses. If the rhythm is irregular, it is better to auscultate the cardiac rate because it is possible to miss early or ectopic beats. It is important to compare vessels on both the right and left sides. The carotid, radial, brachial, femoral, popliteal, dorsalis pedis, and posterior tibial blood vessels are the ones most commonly assessed. Of these, the carotids are easily accessable, but caution is needed. The carotids should be palpated only one side at a time because excess pressure on this sensitive area may slow the pulse or drop the blood pressure. The most distal vessels usually are palpated in the extremities. Hands and feet that are cool and pale suggest ar-

OLDER ADULT CONSIDERATIONS

Some common complaints from older adult patients with cardiovascular disease include confusion, syncope, palpitations, coughs and wheezing, shortness of breath, hemoptysis, fatigue, chest pains, and leg edema. The apical pulse may be more difficult to auscultate because of the change in the anteroposterior diameter of the chest. Listen for a *carotid bruit* (a humming sound of vascular origin) to detect arterial narrowing. Orthostatic (postural) hypotension is fairly common in older adults. Causes include prescription drugs, depleted blood volume, prolonged bedrest, and conditions affecting the autonomic nervous system, such as diabetes mellitus.

terial vessel involvement, whereas warm, cyanotic extremities indicate venous problems.

Peripheral Veins

Thrombosis, varicose veins, and edema are signs of venous insufficiency. Tenderness, thickening, or redness over a superficial vein may indicate thrombophlebitis. The nurse should assess all the extremities for the presence of these conditions.

Venous measurement

Inspection of the jugular venous pulse is a good indicator of hemodynamics (forces resulting in blood circulation) of the right side of the heart and central venous pressure. Jugular pulsations reflect atrial contractions (Figure 21-5). The internal jugular veins give a more accurate pressure measurement than do the external jugular veins, which are more visible. When a patient is sitting upright, the jugular veins are not visibly distended. As the patient gradually assumes a supine position, the veins' fill-level should become visible approximately 1 to 2 cm above the level of the manubrium (upper portion of the sternum). With the patient flat, the jugular veins will pulsate at the top of their length as they transit the neck. To measure the jugular venous pressure, the head of the bed should be raised to a 45-degree angle, and the nurse should observe pulsations of the internal jugular vein. If pulsations of the internal jugular veins still cannot be seen, the head of the bed should be lowered until pulsations are visible. The nurse should hold a short ruler on a horizontal plane next to the neck of the patient where the jugular pulsations are. The nurse should place another ruler on the sternal angle (the angle of Louis, a bony ridge between the manubrium and the sternum at the level of the second intercostal space) and should extend the ruler vertically. The nurse should measure in centimeters the point where the horizontal ruler crosses the vertical ruler. A change in the jugular venous pressure is most significant when compared with previous jugular venous pressure readings. Increased readings suggest hypervolemia, and decreased readings suggest hypovolemia. If the patient's pulse is greater than 90 beats/min, the value of this assessment is questionable. Record the height of the venous pressure in centimeters above the sternal angle as well as the elevation of the patient's head. Values exceeding 4 to 6 cm are considered abnormal.

Lymph node

Lymph node evaluation is part of the peripheral vascular assessment. Normally lymph nodes should not be felt on palpation. Disruption of the normal balance between the hydrostatic and osmotic pressures governing the fluids in the body will affect the lymphatic circulation. The most common result is edema.

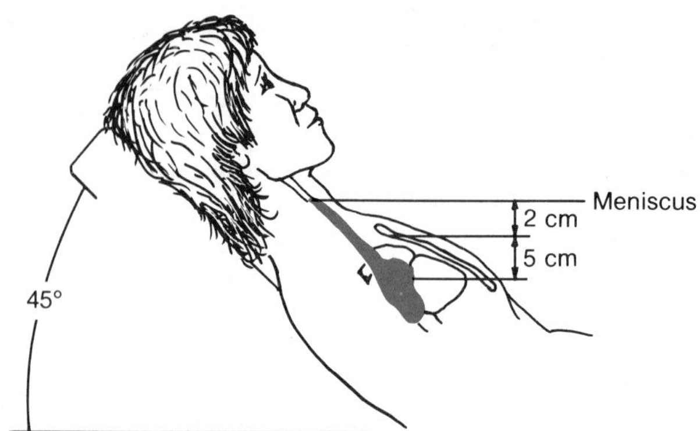

Figure 21-5 Jugular venous pressure.

Edema

Edema is the accumulation of excess interstitial fluid. Systemic causes include congestive heart failure and kidney disease. Local causes may be venous or lymphatic stasis. Edema is most commonly found in the lower extremities and may also appear in the sacral area of patients in the supine position. Edema is not a normal finding and is suggestive of chronic heart failure. It may also be a sign of venous disease, arterial occlusion, or lymphatic obstruction. Edema of one extremity suggests a local cause, whereas bilateral edema indicates a systemic cause. Edema may be described as *pitting edema* if indentation of the edematous area persists after finger pressure is withdrawn. The severity of pitting edema is described by the depth of the indentation, measured in millimeters or centimeters. Some practitioners use a four-point scale to grade its severity, but the scale lacks standardization (Bates, 1987).

ELECTROCARDIOGRAPHY

Heart muscle contraction results from an electrochemical process when electrically charged particles (sodium, calcium, and potassium) on the outer and inner surface of the cell membrane move into and out of the cell. When the myocardial cells are stimulated and change the permeability of their cell membrane (action potential), the surface electrical charges are altered. This electrical activation of the heart muscle is called *depolarization* and results in heart muscle contraction. The process of reversing to its previous state is known as repolarization and results in relaxation of the heart muscle. One of the unique properties of cardiac muscle is its action potential. It is much longer in

1.3 cm

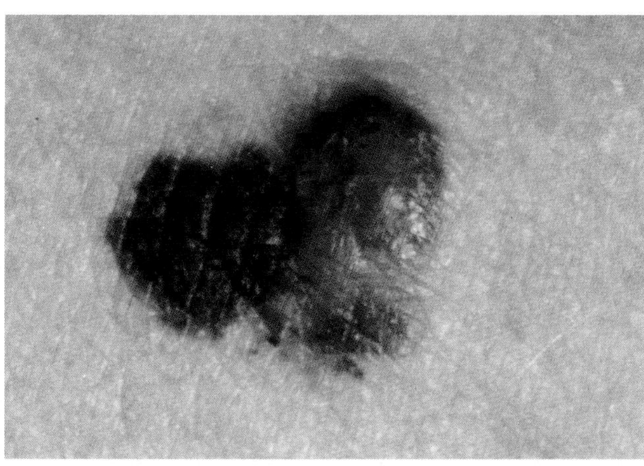

3 cm

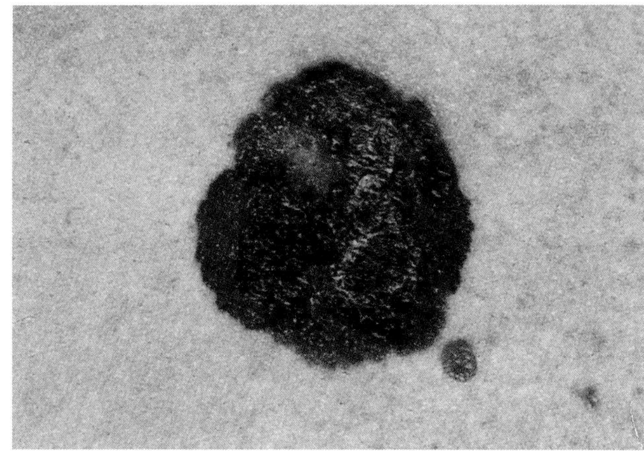

Figure 1 Superficial spreading melanomas. (From Habif TP: *Clinical dermatology,* ed 2, St Louis, 1990, Mosby.)

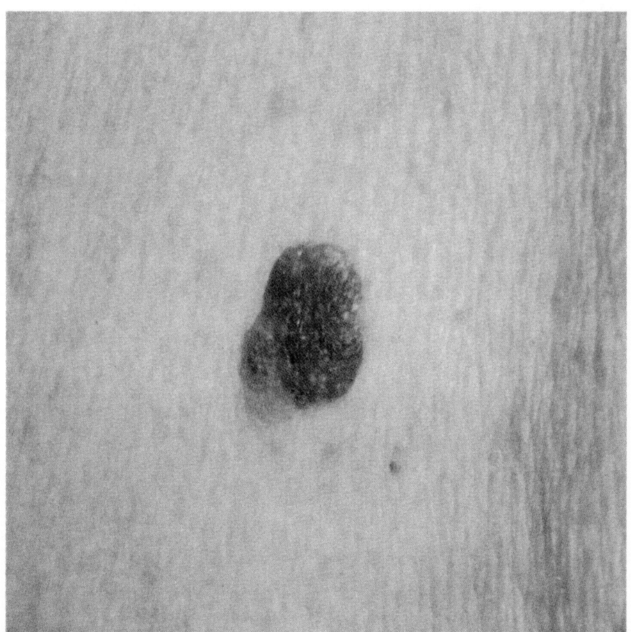

Figure 2 Seborrheic keratosis. (From Barkauskas VH and others: *Health and physical assessment,* St Louis, 1994, Mosby.)

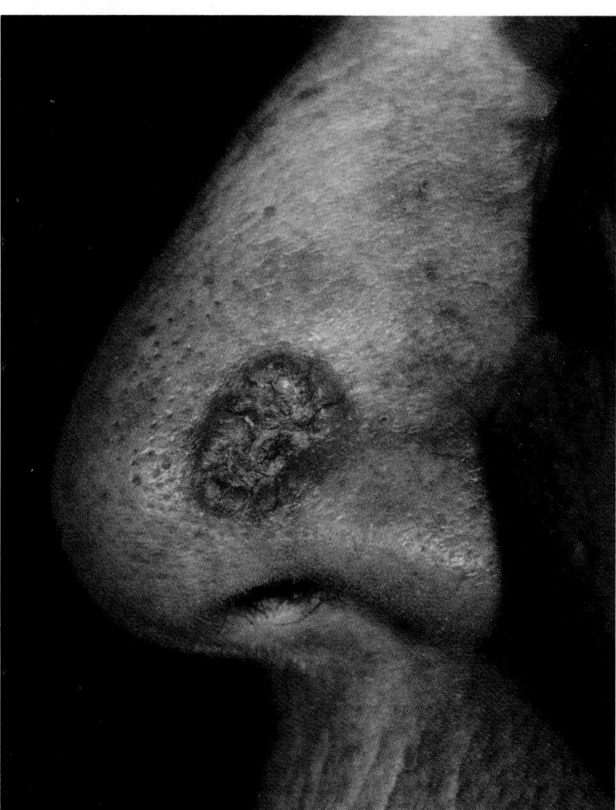

Figure 3 Squamous cell carcinoma. (From Habif TP: *Clinical dermatology,* ed 2, St Louis, 1990, Mosby.)

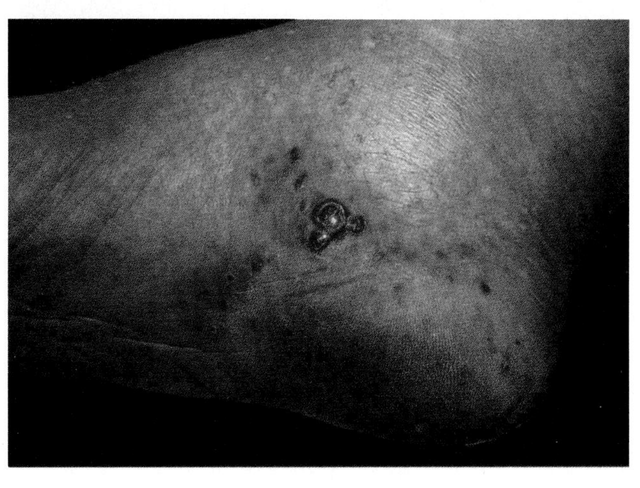

Figure 4 Kaposi's sarcoma. (From Habif TP: *Clinical dermatology,* ed 2, St Louis, 1990, Mosby.)

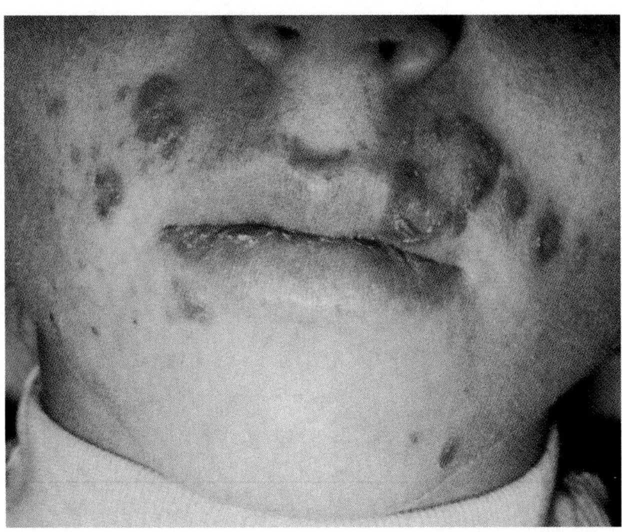

Figure 5 Impetigo (bullous). (Courtesy American Academy of Dermatology and Institute for Dermatologic Communication and Education, Schaumburg, Illinois.)

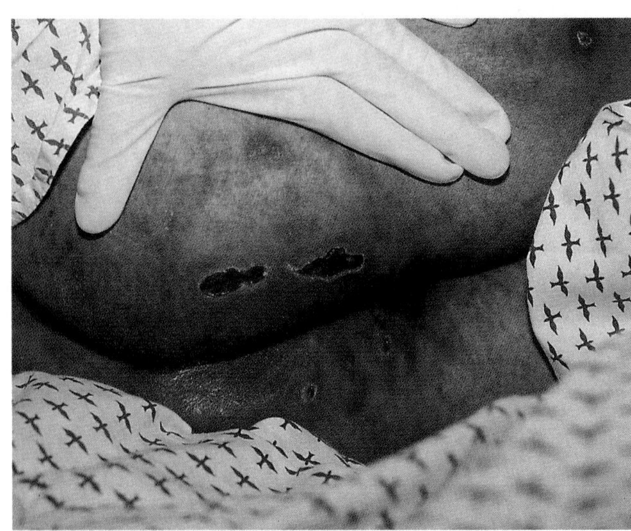

Figure 6 Pressure ulcers. (From Potter PA, Perry AG: *Fundamentals of nursing,* ed 3, St Louis, 1993, Mosby.)

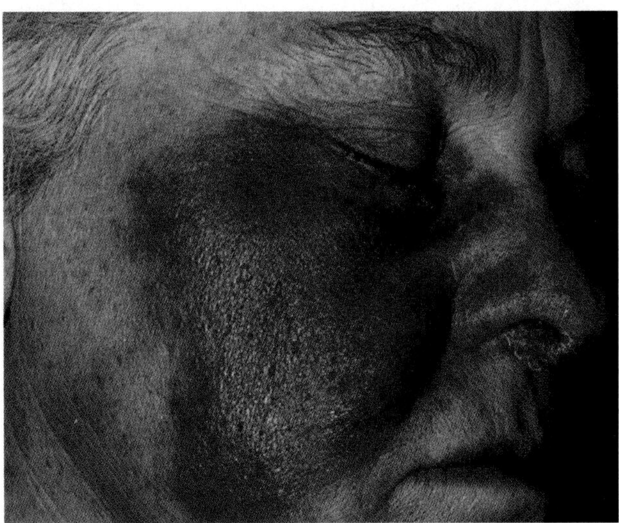

Figure 7 Streptococcal cellulitis—acute phase with intense erythema (erysipelas). (From Habif TP: *Clinical dermatology,* ed 2, St Louis, 1990, Mosby.)

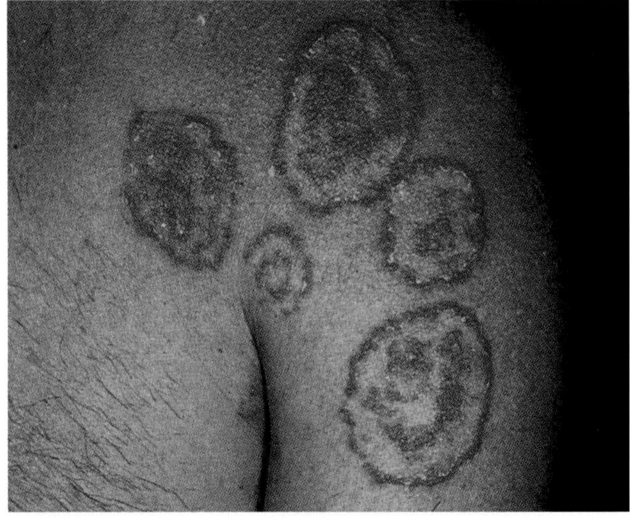

Figure 8 Tinea corporis. (From Habif TP: *Clinical dermatology,* ed 2, St Louis, 1990, Mosby.)

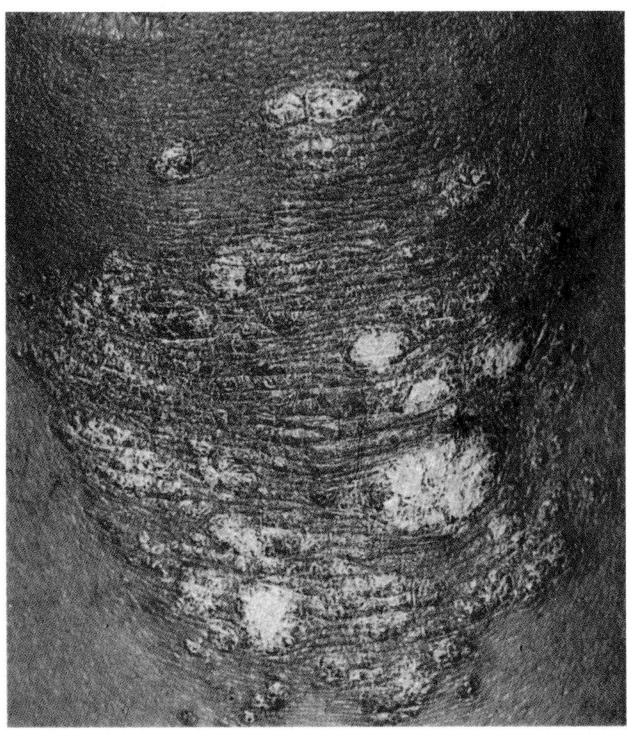

Figure 9 Psoriasis. Note characteristic silvery scaling. (From Habif TP: *Clinical dermatology,* ed 2, St Louis, 1990, Mosby.)

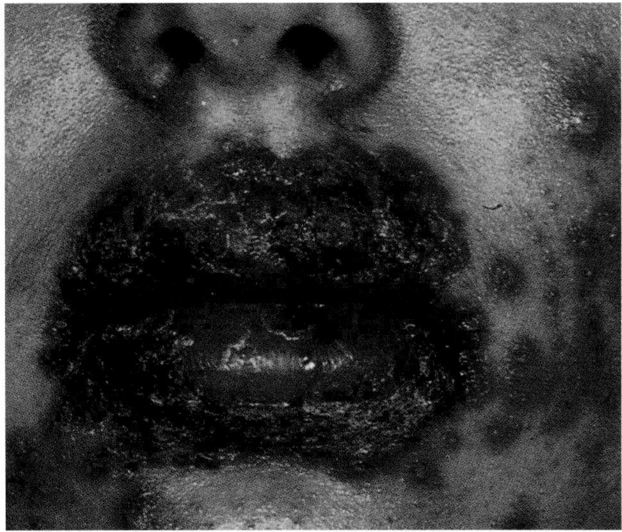

Figure 10 Oral herpes simplex. (From Habif TP: *Clinical dermatology,* ed 2, St Louis, 1990, Mosby.)

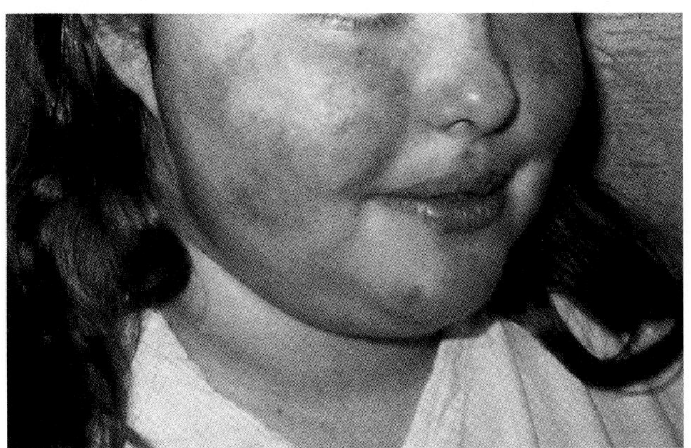

Figure 11 Butterfly rash of systemic lupus erythematosus. Note butterfly-shaped rash over malar surfaces and bridge of nose. Either a blush with swelling or scaly, red, maculopapular lesions may be present. (Courtesy Walter Tunnessen, MD, The University of Pennsylvania School of Medicine, Philadelphia. From Seidel HM and others: *Mosby's guide to physical examination,* ed 3, St Louis, 1994, Mosby.)

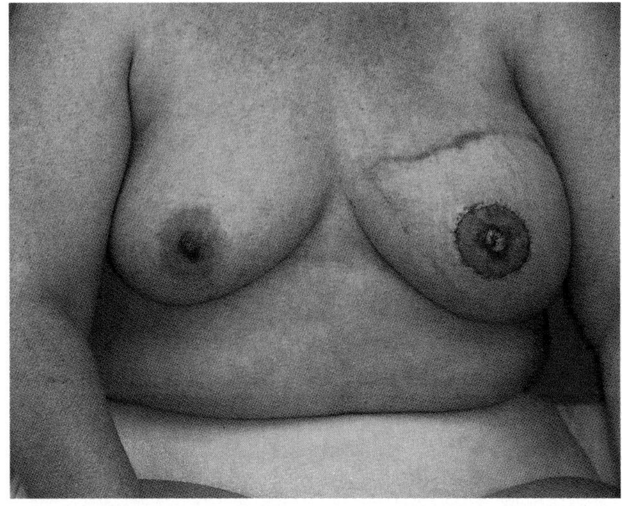

Figure 12 Reconstructed breast, nipple, and areola. (Courtesy Michael A Epstein, MD, Elk Grove Village, Ill.)

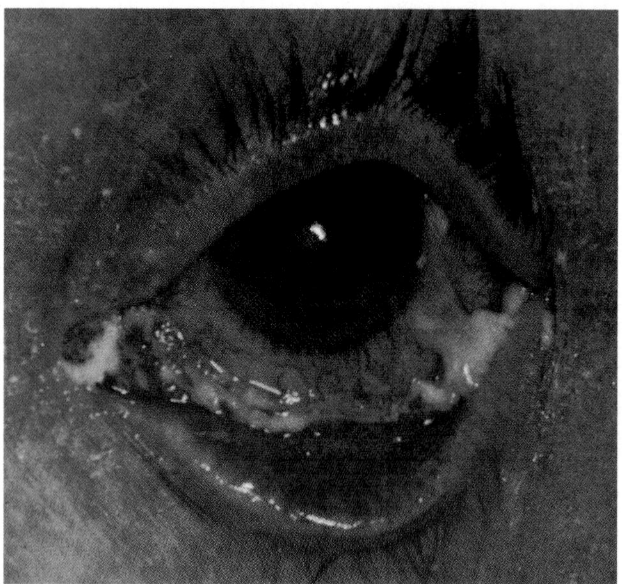

Figure 13 Acute purulent conjunctivitis. (From Newell FW: *Ophthalmology: principles and concepts,* ed 6, St Louis, 1986, Mosby.)

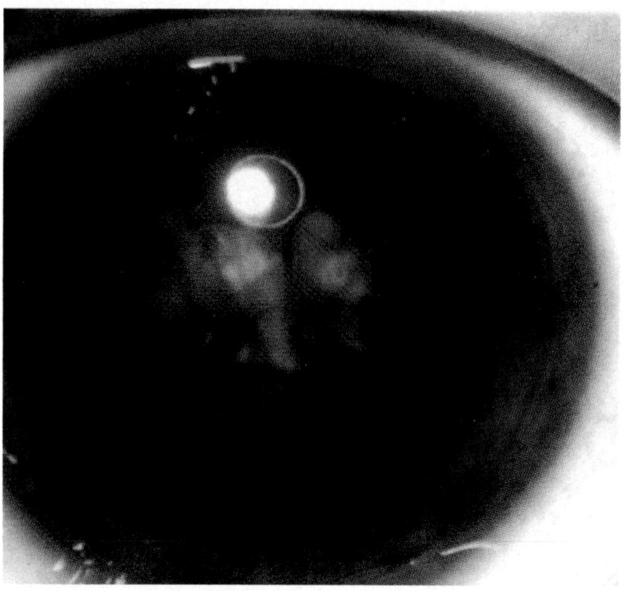

Figure 14 Snowflake cataract of diabetes. (From Donaldson DD: *Atlas of diseases of the anterior segment of the eye,* vol 5, *The crystalline lens,* St Louis, 1976, Mosby. In Seidel HM and others: *Mosby's guide to physical examination,* ed 3, St Louis, 1994, Mosby.)

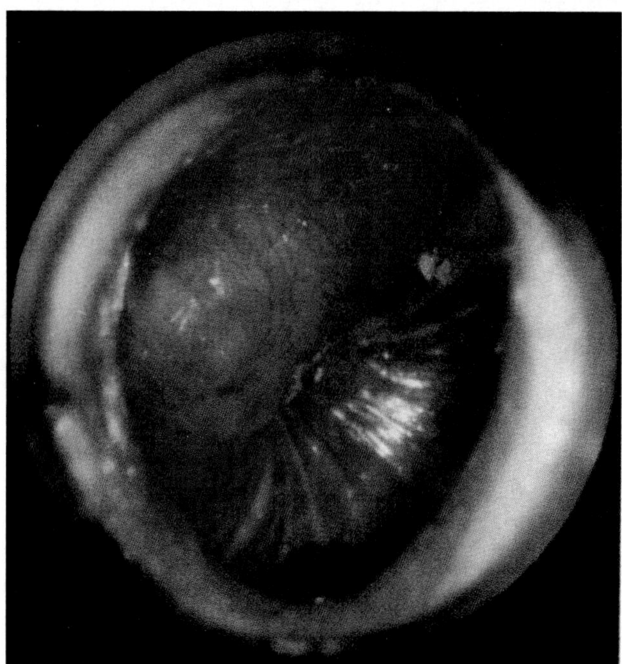

Figure 15 Acute otitis media—red, nonmobile tympanic membrane with loss of bony landmarks and light reflex. (Courtesy Dr. Richard A Buckingham, Clinical Professor, Otolaryngology, Abraham Lincoln School of Medicine, University of Illinois, Chicago, Ill. In Barkauskas VH and others: *Health and physical assessment,* St Louis, 1994, Mosby.)

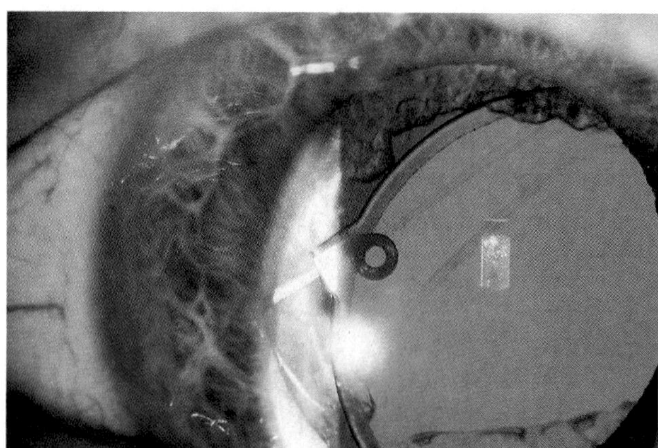

Figure 16 Intraocular lens implant following cataract extraction. (Courtesy Dr. RJ Epstein, Chicago, Ill.)

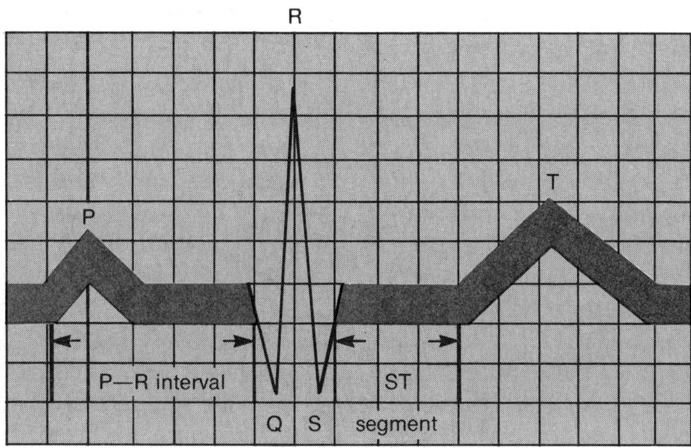

Figure 21-6 ECG of one heartbeat.

duration than that for skeletal muscle. Under normal circumstances this permits the ventricles to empty and refill prior to the next contraction (Lilly, 1993). The electrical events can be visualized with electrocardiograph machines. These machines measure the electrical current generated by the heart muscle contraction and display a continuous picture of the electrical current on an oscilloscope. An **electrocardiogram** (ECG) is the written output of an electrocardiograph machine and appears on graph paper. Time intervals are measured horizontally, and amplitude or force is measured vertically.

To obtain an ECG, positive and negative electrodes are placed on specific areas of the chest wall and limbs, with the heart always between a positive and a negative electrode. This procedure provides different views (leads) of the heart's electrical activity. The up or down direction (deflection) of the waveforms on the graph paper depends on whether the electrical wave is moving toward the positive electrode or the negative electrode or in a line between the two electrodes.

Heart monitoring is useful for identification of normal and *abnormal heart rhythms* **(arrhythmias).** Detection of arrhythmias permits immediate pharmacologic or mechanical (**defibrillation**/cardioversion) intervention. This intervention can prevent other serious problems.

BOX 21-1

FIVE STEPS TO ECG INTERPRETATION

1 Determine rate (the number of counted heart beats per minute)
2 Determine rhythm (the regularity with which the heart beats)
3 Determine the presence or absence of P waves
4 Determine the length of the PR interval
5 Determine the configuration of the QRS complex

Electrocardiogram Interpretation

Each heart muscle contraction should produce a P, Q, R, S, and T wave on the ECG graph paper (Figure 21-6). The first positive deflection occurring above the isoelectric line (baseline) is the P wave, which represents the firing of SA node and depolarization of the atria. The QRS complex, or waves, is a series of negative-positive-negative deflections that demonstrate the depolarization of the ventricles. The positive deflection after the QRS complex is the T wave and represents the repolarization of the ventricle. During this period, the heart will not accept an impulse from the SA node, and this allows the electrical charges to realign on either side of the cell membrane.

The spaces between the waves are also important when studying cardiac activity. The PR interval is the space between the beginning of the P and the beginning of the QRS complex. This represents the time the impulse travels from the atria and through the AV node. Between the QRS complex and the T wave lies the ST segment, which represents the completion of the ventricle contraction and the repolarization period. The angle at the point where the ST segment begins and the QRS wave ends is known as the J point. With changes in the ST segment, the J point may deviate from the isoelectric line.

Every ECG strip should be interpreted by following five basic steps (Box 21-1). Following these steps will foster a systematic approach to ECG strip interpretation and reduce confusion.

Rate

The ventricular rate is usually considered the heart rate. It can be felt in the radial pulse and is the counted beats per minute. When reviewing an ECG, the ventricular rate can be estimated by counting the number of R waves in a 6-second strip and then multiplying by 10. (If the rhythm is irregular, an exact rate cannot be determined by this method.) The atrial rate can be calculated by counting the P waves in a similar fashion. In some abnormal conditions, there is a difference between the atrial rate and the ventricular rate, so it is important to determine both. Quality of the pulse is another attribute to consider. A weak pulse feels small and may indicate hypovolemia or heart failure. Conversely, a bounding pulse is caused by increased stroke volume as seen in fever, anemia, or some heart conditions (Bates, 1987).

Rhythm

The rhythm reveals whether the patient's heart is beating regularly or irregularly. The atrial and ventricular rhythms should be identified. The atrial rhythm is determined by measuring the distance between two consecutive P waves. Calipers for marking the point on paper at each consecutive P wave will accomplish this measurement. The two dot points should then be aligned with the next two P waves (moving left to right). If the distance is equal between all the P waves, the rhythm is regular; if it is unequal, the rhythm is irregular. The ventricular rhythm is determined by the same method, except that it is the R-wave intervals that are measured.

P wave

The P wave is a result of atrial depolarization. All P waves should point in the same direction. The direction should be appropriate for the lead being recorded. There should be one P wave for every QRS complex, and the distance between them should be regular. All P waves should be similar in shape and size. A difference indicates irritation in the atrial tissue or damage near the SA node.

PR interval

The PR interval measures the AV conduction time. It is measured from the onset of the P wave to the beginning of the QRS complex. The normal PR interval is 0.12 to 0.2 seconds. A shorter PR interval means that the impulse originated in an area other than the SA node. A longer PR interval signifies a delay in the impulse as it passes through the AV node.

Configuration and location

Evaluating the configuration and location of the P, Q, R, S, and T waves on a rhythm strip reveals information about the location and extent of myocardial damage. Each wave should be evaluated systematically. P waves should precede QRS complexes. The QRS complexes should be reviewed for shape, size, direction, and location in relation to the T wave. QRS complexes close to the preceding T wave mean the ventricles are contracting prematurely. The T wave represents ventricular relaxation. The closer the QRS is to the T wave, the greater the risk is for serious ventricular arrhythmia.

The ST segment can be slightly elevated above the baseline but should not be depressed. It then curves very slightly into the start of the T wave. An abnormality of the ST segment is an early sign of myocardial infarction. T waves should also be observed for size and shape and should deflect in the same direction as the QRS complex. T waves should follow the QRS. Elevated or "tented" T waves can be a sign of elevated potassium levels.

DISORDERS OF RATE AND RHYTHM OF THE HEART

The pulse is one of the most sensitive indices for assessing heart function. Nurses should develop a keen sensitivity to what they feel when obtaining a peripheral pulse. When the heart is functioning normally, the pulse is felt as smooth, regular, equally spaced beats of equal strength and volume that occur from 60 to 100 times per minute. Under certain conditions, changes occur in the pulse rate, its rhythm, and volume. Some of these conditions are called cardiac arrhythmias.

Arrhythmia

Cardiac arrhythmia

Cardiac **arrhythmias** occur in well persons and in those with cardiovascular disease. Any deviation from normal sinus rhythm is defined as an arrhythmia. Arrhythmias may result from an abnormal rate, a site of impulse formation other than the SA node, or from abnormal conduction within the system. Arrhythmias are categorized by site of origin, which may be sinus, atrial, nodal (junctional), or ventricular. The nurse may be the first person to detect changes in the patient's pulse.

Sinus arrhythmia

The SA node is the source of all sinus rhythms, but the frequency of its discharge varies. The heart rate in-

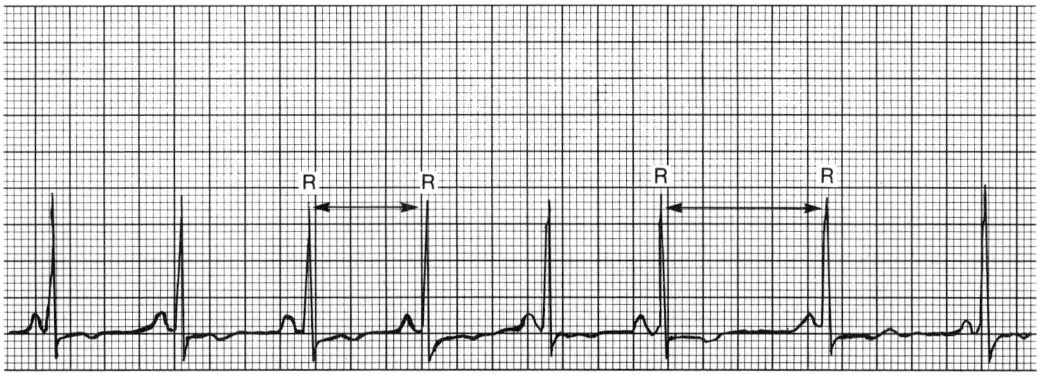

Figure 21-7 Sinus arrhythmia.

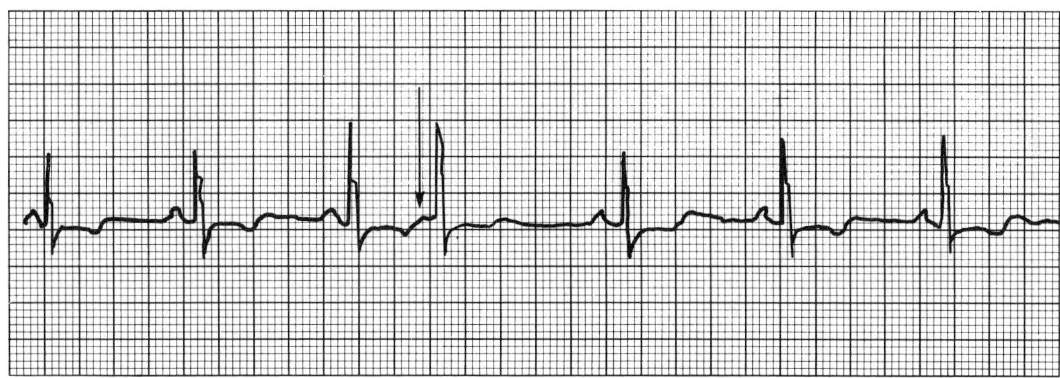

Figure 21-8 Premature atrial contraction (PAC).

creases and decreases as the SA node fires prematurely or late (Figure 21-7). Normally, the SA node discharges at a rate of 60 to 100 times/min. If the rate falls below 60 times/min, the process is termed **sinus bradycardia.** If, however, the rate is greater than 100 times/min, it is termed **sinus tachycardia.** In healthy young individuals, the rate may vary with respiration asymptomatically. Sick sinus syndrome occurs when marked bradycardia and/or tachycardia accompanies dizziness and syncope.

Atrium

Premature atrial contraction

Normally the SA node originates the impulse to begin the cardiac cycle. Sometimes, however, an impulse will arise from another area of the atrium before the SA node fires; such an impulse is called a premature atrial contraction (PAC). This impulse usually occurs earlier than expected and is represented by a P wave that has a configuration different from that of P waves representing impulses that begin in the SA node. The QRS complex of the PAC usually is normal, but it may have a different configuration because the path of conduction is different (Flynn, Bruce, 1993) . This is called aberrancy. A short pause usually is present between the T wave and the next P wave (Figure 21-8).

PACs are a common arrhythmia. In normal individuals they result from factors such as caffeine, nicotine, or strong emotions. In patients they may be associated with myocardial infarctions, digitalis toxicity, low potassium levels, hypoxia, rheumatic heart disease, or hyperthyroidism (Lilly, 1993). In many patients no treatment is indicated. Patients with symptoms may receive a mild sedative. If underlying heart disease is thought to be the cause of the PACs, drugs such as quinidine, digitalis, disopyramide, or propranolol may be prescribed.

Atrial flutter

Atrial flutter is an atrial rhythm occurring at a rate of 250 to 350 beats/min (Figure 21-9). The impulse does not originate from the SA node. The ectopic atrial focus becomes the pacemaker that originates all of these impulses. The regular, rapid atrial rate results in a "saw-tooth" flutter wave on an ECG tracing. QRS complexes do not follow each flutter because the AV

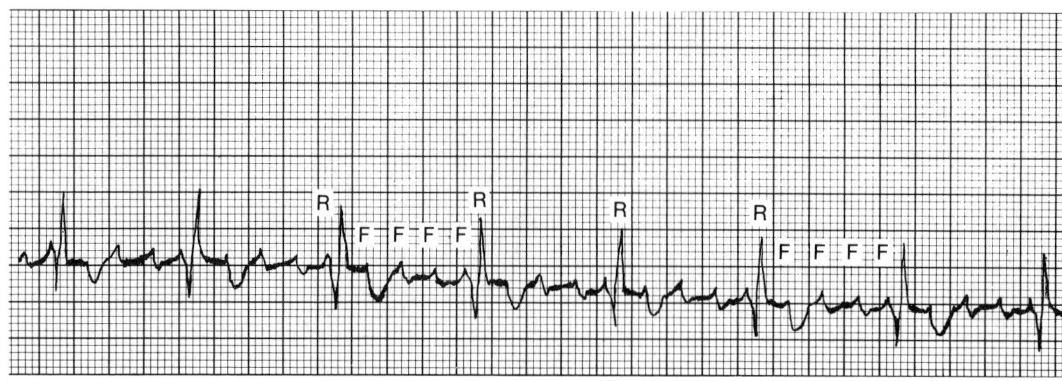

Figure 21-9 Atrial flutter. *R,* R wave. *F,* flutter wave.

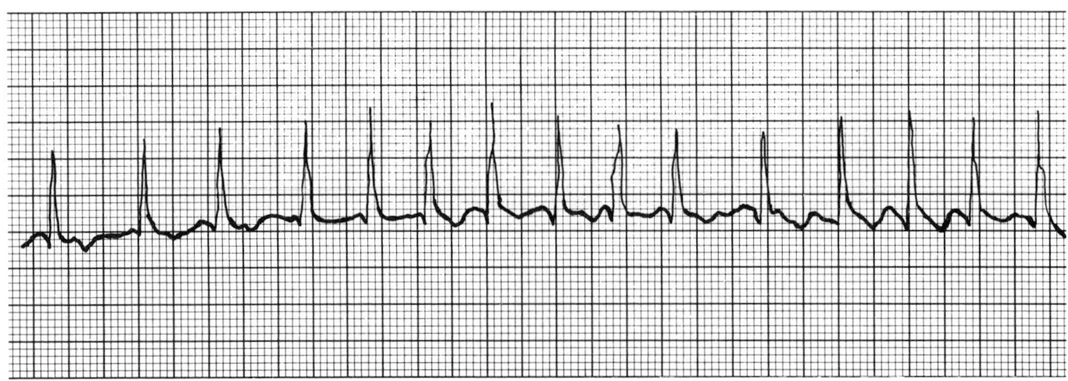

Figure 21-10 Rapid atrial fibrillation.

node does not transmit each impulse. Usually a 2:1 ratio of impulses is conducted through the system to the ventricles. This means that the ventricles cannot respond as rapidly as the atria, and the ventricular rate is less than the atrial rate, often approximately half the atrial rate. The QRS complex will appear normal unless an aberrant conduction is present. Cardiovascular problems such as coronary artery disease, rheumatic heart disease, or cor pulmonale usually are present in patients with atrial flutter.

Cardiac output will remain within normal limits as long as the ventricular rate is within normal limits. If allowed to persist, atrial flutter usually converts to atrial fibrillation. Treatment is indicated when the ventricular rate is so rapid that the ventricles cannot fill. The goal of treatment is to slow the ventricular rate or change the rhythm to a sinus-node–initiated impulse. Pharmacologic treatment is directed at slowing the flutter rate while controlling conduction ratio with Class I antiarrhythmics and digitalis. In severe situations, cardioversion is used (Wilson and others, 1991). *Cardioversion* is a procedure that gives the heart external electrical stimulation. The external electrical stimulation will interrupt the irregular conduction pattern of the heart and restore it to normal sinus rhythm. The patient's heart rhythm is monitored and the synchronized electric shock is delivered during ventricular contraction. Delivery of electric shock at any other time could cause severe, life-threatening arrhythmia. Cardioversion is performed by a physician with a patient's written consent. The nurse monitors the patient's heart rate, rhythm, blood pressure, and respirations throughout the procedure.

Atrial fibrillation

Atrial fibrillation is a chaotic atrial rhythm with a rapid atrial rate of 400 to 600 beats/min and a variable ventricular rate from as low as 50 beats/min in some patients to as high as 170 beats/min in others. The ventricular rate varies because the AV node cannot conduct every atrial impulse (Figure 21-10). P waves are absent, and the ECG tracing has classic fibrillation waves. QRS complexes are normal or reflect aberrant (deviant) conduction. In healthy young people, atrial fibrillation may be a transient arrhythmia. Continuous atrial fibrillation, however, is associated with heart disease. PACs usually precede atrial fibrillation. Cardiac

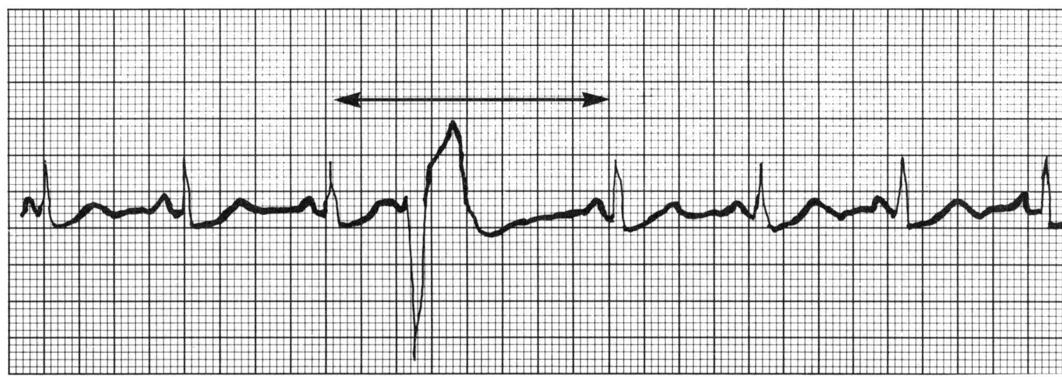

Figure 21-11 Isolated premature ventricular contraction (PVC).

output decreases, and there is a risk of thromboembolization to the brain, lungs, or other organs. The radial pulse is slower than the apical pulse because some systolic contractions are weaker and cannot be palpated in the arteries.

Treatment depends on cardiac output. If cardiac output remains adequate, digitalis is used to increase AV node blocking and to allow more time for the ventricles to fill. Quinidine may help in regaining a sinus rhythm. The patient's pulse should be checked for a slow rate (<60 beats/min) before giving digitalis or quinidine. If it is slow, the drug may need to be withheld and the physician notified to safeguard against the possible complications of digitalis toxicity (Walthall and others, 1993). Digitalis toxicity is common because there is a small difference between the therapeutic and toxic concentration levels of the drug (Lilly, 1993). Signs and symptoms of digitalis toxicity are palpitations, arrhythmias, nausea, dizziness, syncope, and visual disturbances (Opie, 1991). If cardiac output falls, cardioversion is the treatment of choice to return the heart rate and rhythm to normal.

Ventricle

Premature ventricular contractions

Premature ventricular contractions (PVCs) are ventricular contractions that do not originate from the normal SA-node-to-AV-node pathway (Figure 21-11). PVCs result from an impulse site in the Purkinje's fibers and occurs earlier than a sinus beat. The P wave does not precede the QRS complex. Instead an inverted P wave may follow the PVC. This happens because the impulse is conducted retrograde (backward) and depolarizes the atria (Lipman, Cascio 1994). The QRS complex is widened, often notched, and may be of greater amplitude (dimension) than normal. The T-wave deflection is in the opposite direction of the QRS complex. A "compensatory" pause usually follows the PVC as the heart waits for another normal SA node impulse. This pause occurs because the heart is refractory (resistant to stimulation) at the time of the P wave immediately following the PVC, so the pause is not conducted. PVCs are the most common arrhythmias. They may occur in people with or without heart disease. PVCs may be expected in patients after a myocardial infarction or cardiac surgery or in patients with myocardial irritability.

Rare PVCs are not treated. Frequent PVCs, two (couplet) or three (ventricular tachycardia) consecutive PVCs, PVCs that occur every other (bigeminy) or every third (trigeminy) beat, or PVCs that occur close to the T wave of the previous beat demand attention. Those PVCs occurring on or close to the T wave (R-on-T phenomenon) may start a lethal ventricular arrhythmia. PVC treatment varies by institution. Most are treated with antiarrhythmic drugs such as lidocaine, procainamide, quinidine, and propranolol. If the cause of PVCs is hypokalemia, potassium chloride replacements are given; if the cause is digitalis toxicity, the digitalis is discontinued.

Ventricular tachycardia

Ventricular tachycardia is a serious arrhythmia that results from a series of rapid, regular impulses originating in a ventricular ectopic focus (Figure 21-12). Ventricular contraction does not follow atrial contraction, and the ventricular rate ranges from 100 to 220 beats/min. P waves are rarely seen. The QRS complex is widened and often notched with greater amplitude. The T wave may be buried in the QRS complex, and if it is visible, it will deflect in the direction opposite that of the QRS. Ventricular tachycardia is a complication of digitalis toxicity or myocardial infarction, and it must be terminated promptly. Treatment consists of

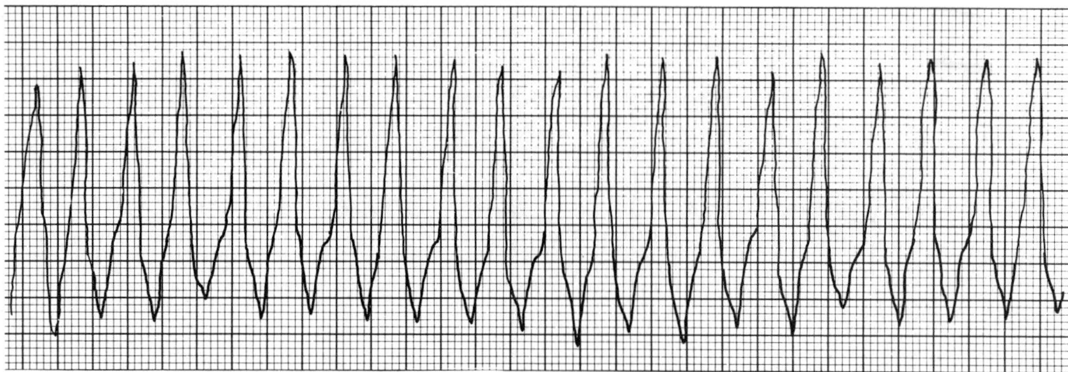

Figure 21-12 Ventricular tachycardia (rapid).

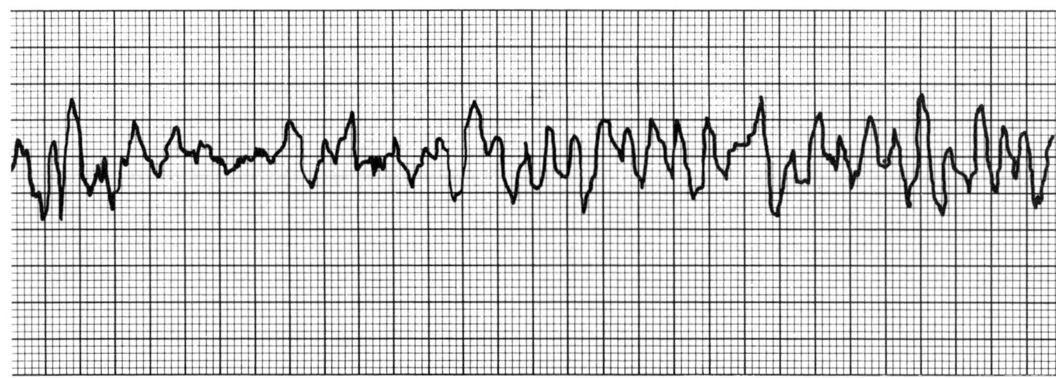

Figure 21-13 Ventricular fibrillation.

drug therapy such as lidocaine, procainamide, or bretylium. If digitalis toxicity is the cause, the digitalis should be discontinued and potassium levels corrected as necessary. Hypokalemia enhances the toxicity of digitalis by inhibiting the sodium-potassium pump within the cell. Electrical countershock is usually effective.

Ventricular fibrillation

Ventricular fibrillation is rapid, irregular "twitching" of the ventricles, demonstrated by a wavering baseline and bizarre waveform (Figure 21-13). Ventricular fibrillation may result from myocardial infarction, digitalis and quinidine toxicity, or a PVC occurring at the apex of the preceding T wave (R-on-T phenomenon). During ventricular fibrillation, the ventricles cannot deliver blood to the body. If left untreated, death will occur. Immediate treatment is defibrillation with direct-current countershock. Ventricular fibrillation can often be avoided by aggressive treatment of PVCs that are encroaching on the T wave or occurring in multiples.

Heart Block

Heart block results from a disturbance in the conduction system, specifically at the AV junction. Heart block is categorized as first-degree, second-degree, or third-degree block. First-degree AV block is identified by a PR interval greater than 0.2 second. The impulse originates in the SA node and travels normally through the atria. The conduction is abnormally delayed at the AV junction, but it does pass through, and the ventricles respond normally. Reversible first-degree block may result from transient ischemia or from therapy with digitalis, beta-blockers, or calcium channel blockers. Structural causes include myocardial infarction or degenerative changes in the conduction system. Usually no treatment is necessary.

There are two types of second-degree heart block. Mobitz type I (sometimes called Wenckebach) block results from the same conduction defect as first-degree block. However, with each beat the conduction delay through the AV junction increases progressively until the sinus impulse is completely blocked and no QRS complex occurs. This arrhythmia is often seen in patients with inferior myocardial infarction and digitalis toxicity. The treatment is to discontinue the digitalis if the condition is drug related. Atropine may also be used to alleviate symptoms.

Mobitz type II block is demonstrated by conduction of some sinus impulses through the AV junction without a prolonged PR interval; however, other sinus impulses are blocked completely. The result is that the ventricular rate is a fraction of the atrial rate. This is a more serious arrhythmia, is usually seen in acute anterior myocardial infarction, and indicates damage to the ventricular septum. Treatment may include isoproterenol and epinephrine infusion or transvenous pacing.

Third-degree (complete) block occurs when none of the sinus impulses are conducted through the AV junction. The atria and ventricles act independently of one another. The atrial rate is usually regular and of normal frequency. Without stimuli from the SA node, the ventricles beat at their own intrinsic rate, usually 30 to 45 beats/min. The QRS complex will be widened if the ventricular impulse originates in the bundle branch system. Complete heart block may be a result of digitalis toxicity, age, myocarditis, acute myocardial infarction, or cardiac surgery. Isoproterenol is used to treat third-degree (complete) block. Permanent cardiac pacing is almost always recommended.

Bundle-branch block is a defect of intraventricular conduction resulting in a conduction delay through the right or left branches of the bundle of His. The PR interval is normal, and the QRS complex is prolonged by at least 0.12 second and may be notched and widened. Myocardial infarction, hypertension, and cardiomyopathy are common causes of bundle-branch block. It also can be drug induced by procainamide or quinidine or caused by hyperkalemia. Treatment is focused on the underlying problem.

Electronic Cardiac Pacemakers

Electronic cardiac pacing is indicated for any condition in which the heart's SA node fails to initiate or conduct the impulse at the rate needed to obtain good cardiac output. Pacemakers may be internal or external and may provide a fixed rate (asynchronous) pacing or a demand (synchronous) pacing of the ventricles.

The **pacemaker** is an electrically operated mechanical device that enables the ventricle to contract normally. It may be used in an emergency or for a temporary period, or it can be implanted permanently in the patient's chest. Several approaches are possible in initiating the use of the pacemaker. If it is to be temporary, a catheter may be inserted through a vein, often the jugular or subclavian vein, and it is attached to an external pacemaker. Patients with an occasional blockage of the electric impulses in the heart, such as after heart surgery or a myocardial infarction, may need this temporary type of pacemaker. Usually it is inserted while the patient is in the operating room or in a cardiac catheterization laboratory, where fluoroscopy is used to guide the catheter directly into the right ventricle.

Permanent pacemakers are necessary if the patient has irreversible damage to the conductive nerve pathways of the heart. A permanent pacemaker also is inserted through a vein, but the battery box is permanently implanted within the subcutaneous tissue of the patient's chest or abdomen. Occasionally the patient's chest is opened, and the electrodes are sutured onto the ventricle. The energy source for most internal pacemakers is a lithium-powered battery, which lasts 7 to 10 years. Nuclear-powered pacemakers are no longer produced (Dossey, Guzzetta, Kenner, 1992).

Another device available for treating arrhythmias is the automatic implantable cardioverter-defibrillator (AICD or ICD). This type of cardiac-rhythm-sensing device provides an electrical discharge to the myocardium (shock) when a tachycardia rate goes above a preset limit. Increasing sophistication of these devices will allow them to analyze the heart's electrical signal and provide pacemaker regulation (Stewart and others, 1993).

Assessment and intervention

The nursing care of the patient is determined by the procedure used. In any case, the patient will have a wound that must be protected from infection. If a catheter is inserted into a vein, care must be taken to prevent its displacement. When a temporary pacemaker is in use, all electric equipment in the room must be grounded, and only one machine may be connected to any electric outlet. Any exposed electrodes should be insulated. The nurse should remember that the implanted pacemaker is a foreign object, and the patient should be observed for any elevation of temperature that might indicate trouble. The nurse also should be certain that an infusion set and a defibrillator are at the bedside for emergency use. Patients with implanted pacemakers often are apprehensive and fearful. The primary responsibilities of nurses include helping the patient to accept the instrument and relieving fear and apprehension. Every patient must be taught the technique of counting his or her pulse for a full 60 seconds while at rest. While it is not always necessary for patients to monitor their pulse rates daily, it is often a source of reassurance to them. Most patients with lithium-powered pacemakers can check their pulses weekly or when symptoms arise (Dossey, Guzzetta, Kenner, 1992). Patients should know the rate

BOX 21-2 **Nursing Process**

PATIENT UNDERGOING PERMANENT PACEMAKER PLACEMENT

ASSESSMENT

Cardiac status: vital signs, cardiac rhythm, edema
Neurologic signs: fatigue, syncope, level of consciousness
Respiratory status: cyanosis, breathing, crackles
Renal status: urinary output, laboratory values
Mental status: anxiety, perception of illness, self-concept
Pain

NURSING DIAGNOSES

Decreased cardiac output, potential or real related to arrhythmia
Anxiety related to procedure
Risk for fluid volume excess related to arrhythmia
Risk for fluid volume deficit related to arrhythmia
Risk for impaired gas exchange related to arrhythmia
Risk for infection related to procedure
Pain related to procedure
Knowledge deficit related to pacemaker

NURSING INTERVENTIONS

Monitor the patient for systolic blood pressure below 90 mm Hg.
Evaluate the patient's cardiac rhythm on the ECG monitor.
Monitor the patient and the device for signs of pacemaker failure.
Check to see that the patient maintains urinary output of no less than 30 ml per hour
Notify the physician of changes in vital signs.
Have emergency drugs available (atropine, digitalis, lidocaine).
Monitor the patient for signs and symptoms of wound infection.
Check temperature every 4 hours for 24 hours.
Encourage the patient to cough often, turn often, and breathe deeply.
Monitor for shortness of breath, cyanosis, and absence of breath sounds over the affected area.
Have oxygen support available.
Provide reassurance to the patient and the family that the device is functioning properly.
Provide adequate pain control.
Teach the patient self-monitoring of pulse and symptoms of pacemaker failure.

EVALUATION OF EXPECTED OUTCOMES

Quick response to potential hemodynamic instability
Normal pacemaker and adequate cardiac function
Adequate fluid balance
Wound healing without infection
Absence of respiratory complications
Absence of high-anxiety states
Acceptance of realistic lifestyle and cooperation with treatment plan

at which the pacemaker is set. Any irregularities or a pulse rate below that at which the pacemaker is set may be an indication of intrinsic beats or pacemaker malfunction. These problems should be reported to the patients' healthcare providers, and patients themselves should be taught the symptoms and meaning of battery failure (Box 21-2). Patients also will benefit from knowing that replacing the power source is not as difficult a procedure as the initial placement of the pacemaker.

All patients with pacemakers should carry identification/alert cards containing information about the manufacturer and the type, model, and milliamperage at which their pacers are set. Newer models of pacemakers usually have metal shielding to protect them from external interference. Most electrical devices can be used safely. Microwave ovens now have special shields and usually will not affect the pacemaker. Arc-welding equipment and power transmitters should be avoided. Therapeutic devices such as transcutaneous nerve stimulaters (TENS) and magnetic resonance imagers (MRIs) may create interference. Patients should be taught to inform their therapists about their pacemakers and to use caution near the antitheft devices in some stores. Airport metal detectors may be triggered, so the patient may need to provide a pacemaker identification card.

CORONARY CARE UNIT

The coronary care unit (CCU) or the cardiopulmonary unit is a specially designed unit of the hospital. The unit is equipped with all supplies and equipment, including emergency drugs, to meet the needs of each patient admitted to the unit. It provides continuous monitoring of the patient's cardiac function.

The overall objective of the CCU is to save lives. During the early development of these units, emphasis was placed on prompt treatment of patients with cardiac arrest. With increased knowledge and understanding of coronary artery disease, the emphasis is now placed on preventing cardiac arrest. If not identified, treated, and controlled, minor disorders of rhythm may lead to serious arrhythmias, heart failure, and death. It cannot be expected that all patients admitted to the unit will survive, but mortality has been significantly reduced.

Large medical centers have specially designed, separate CCUs, but some community hospitals care for coronary disease patients in intensive care units (ICUs) with other seriously ill patients. There are definite disadvantages to this combined ICU system, especially when the ICU is a ward rather than a private-room complex. However, the environmental location of the patient is not always what is most important—the quality of nursing care often is. Nurses are the key to the success of the CCU. They are the first to offer basic life support and to start treatment of life-threatening arrhythmias. Nurses are with the patient 24 hours a day and are in a position to assess and detect the first sign of trouble. Their immediate assessment of the problem and appropriate emergency action may be lifesaving. The CCU, with its effective monitoring system and trained personnel, has effectively reduced in-hospital death from heart attacks.

Patients in a CCU may experience extreme emotional and physical stress. They are anxious about loss of function, helplessness, finances, family, and the possibility of death. The CCU environment is foreign and frightening. Coronary care nurses must have the technical proficiency and sensitivity to care for CCU patients and their families in crisis. Much can be done to reassure patients and families by supplying information that will relieve anxiety, by listening carefully to the patient, and by treating the patient with respect. The caring and empathy on which nursing was founded is demonstrated during the patient's most serious crises.

Nurses in the CCU are often responsible for keen assessment of the patient's physiologic changes and for taking ECGs, observing and recording cardiac monitor readings, maintaining oxygen therapy, and observing and regulating intravenous fluids. They should also be prepared to provide basic cardiac life support, defibrillation, and intravenous infusions.

Laboratory Examinations

It is usually important to conduct several laboratory studies to establish an accurate diagnosis or to follow the course of the cardiovascular disease.

Complete blood count

The routine laboratory examination comprises a count of red and white blood cells, an estimate of hemoglobin, and a differential count, which includes many different cells that are usually few in number. An increase in the number of white blood cells indicates that an inflammatory condition or tissue destruction is present. Determination of red blood cell count and hemoglobin level helps to determine how well the blood is being oxygenated.

Acute phase reactants

The erythrocyte sedimentation rate (ESR) and the C-reactive protein (CRP) are nonspecific tests to confirm the presence of an inflammatory process. The sedimentation rate is elevated in many conditions, including rheumatic fever and myocardial infarction. It is useful both in diagnosing rheumatic fever and in following the course of the disease.

Blood cultures

When **bacterial endocarditis** is suspected, the diagnosis may be established by finding the causative organism in the blood. Often several blood cultures may be necessary before a positive diagnosis can be made.

Serum enzyme tests

Enzymes are proteins that are present in all body cells. Certain enzymes are specific to particular tissues and are present in high concentrations in these tissues, such as the heart, liver, and kidneys. When damage occurs to these tissues, significant amounts of the enzymes are released into the bloodstream.

Cardiac **isoenzymes** are specific to heart muscle tissue and are useful in diagnosing acute myocardial infarction. One isoenzyme is lactic dehydrogenase (LDH), numbered 1 to 5. Within 48 hours after a myocardial infarction, 80% of patients will have an increased LDH. Another isoenzyme contributing to the diagnosis of myocardial infarction is the CPK (creatine phosphokinase). There are three classes of these enzymes: CPK-MM, CPK-BB, and CPK-MB. The CPK-MB is specific to myocardial tissue and increases within 4 to 8 hours after the onset of cellular insult and peaks at 24 hours. Blood samples are drawn and analyzed every 3 to 6 hours after the onset of symptoms so that the pattern of isoenzyme can be established. Recent developments in rapid assays of this isoenzyme have made it possible to rule out a myocardial infarction within the first 6 hours after the onset of symptoms (Puleo and others, 1994).

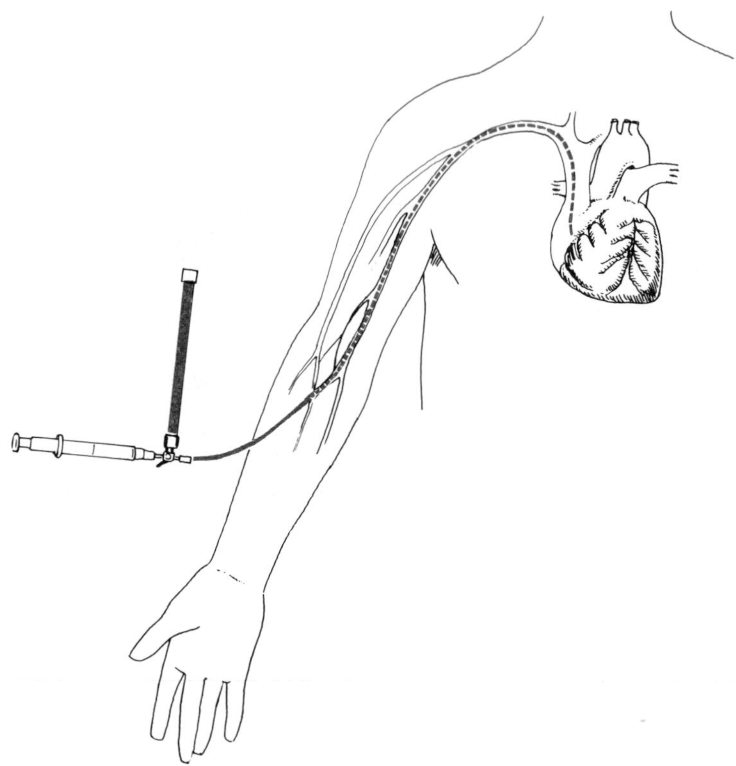

Figure 21-14 Central venous pressure.

Blood chemistries

The mechanisms controlling metabolic balance are often disturbed during serious illness. Assessment of serum electrolytes is important in determining the status of sodium, potassium, chloride, carbon dioxide, bilirubin, calcium, creatinine, glucose, magnesium, phosphorus, alkaline phosphatase, urea nitrogen, and uric acid levels in CCU patients.

Cholesterol

Cholesterol is one of the lipid, or fat-like, substances in blood. Increased levels of lipids (hyperlipidemia) have been found to be a risk factor for coronary artery disease. It is thought that the lipids accumulate within the inner lining of blood vessels, decreasing the blood vessel diameter. This is called **atherosclerosis.** The narrowed blood vessels decrease the circulation efficiency of the blood, which is laden with oxygen and nutrients. If the heart muscle does not receive enough oxygen, a person experiences chest pain, which is a symptom of impending damage to the myocardial muscle. Studies show that blood cholesterol levels can be lowered by decreasing the dietary intake of foods high in saturated fat and cholesterol.

Blood gases

Arterial blood gases help to determine the status of the patient's oxygenation and acid-base balance.

Coagulation studies

Because many of the patients in CCUs have had a thrombolic insult, the use of anticoagulation therapies is not unusual. In addition, current emphasis on reperfusion of the at-risk myocardium with thrombolytic therapies means that many patients will be receiving anticoagulant therapy. Coagulation studies include platelet counts, prothrombin time counts, partial thromboplastin time (PPT) and activated partial thromboplastin time (APTT) counts, activated clotting time counts, fibrinogen level studies, thrombin time counts, and recalcification time counts.

Diagnostic and Imaging Tests

Central venous pressure

Central venous pressure (CVP) provides information about circulating blood volume (Figure 21-14). It is a direct reflection of right atrial pressure (RAP) and an indirect reflection of the preload of the right ventricle. Preload refers to the amount of stretch in the ventricular muscle just before contraction. Preload is defined as the pressure generated at the end of diastole (Guyton, 1990; McKance, Heuther, 1994).

The CVP measurement gives some indication of the heart's ability to pump blood. A physician introduces a catheter into a peripheral or central vein and then into the vena cava or right atrium. The catheter is secured and attached to an intravenous solution with a manometer attached (see Figure 21-14). Placement is verified by a chest x-ray examination. A sterile, occlusive dressing covers the site. The tubing and dressing should be changed according to hospital policy, at which time the site should be observed for any sign of redness, swelling, and drainage. These signs or any complaints of pain from the patient should be documented and reported to the physician.

The pressure is measured in centimeters of water. The normal range of CVP measurement is 4 to 10 cm. An increase in CVP indicates decreased contractility of the myocardium, vasoconstriction, or increased circulating blood volume. Conversely, a decreased CVP reading indicates increased myocardial contractility, vasodilation, or hypovolemia.

Pulmonary artery and pulmonary artery wedge pressures

Because the CVP does not provide an accurate reading of pressure in the left side of the heart, patients who are critically ill often receive pulmonary artery (PA) catheters. During diastole, an open column of blood extends from the pulmonary artery through the lungs and into the heart to the open mitral valve. This permits measurement of left ventricular preload because the catheter is placed in the pulmonary artery and the measurement there reflects the value within the left ventricle. This is one of several measurements used to determine cardiac performance.

The physician inserts the PA catheter into a central vein (subclavian or jugular). It is also possible to use the femoral or brachial veins. The multilumen catheter is advanced into the right ventricle and from there into the pulmonary artery (Figure 21-15). The catheter is attached to a pressure transducer and intravenous solution. Placement is verified by a chest x-ray examination. Measurement is done with an electronic monitor. The PA catheter has a distal balloon that, with inflation, can provide the pulmonary artery wedge pressure that indicates function of the left side of the heart. In addition to providing these measurements, an additional lumen within the catheter ends in a thermistor (a device for measuring very small changes in temperature) port and permits measurement of cardiac output. A small bolus of solution is injected into the catheter, and the thermistor senses the temperature difference of the injectate. A formula is then used to compute the cardiac output.

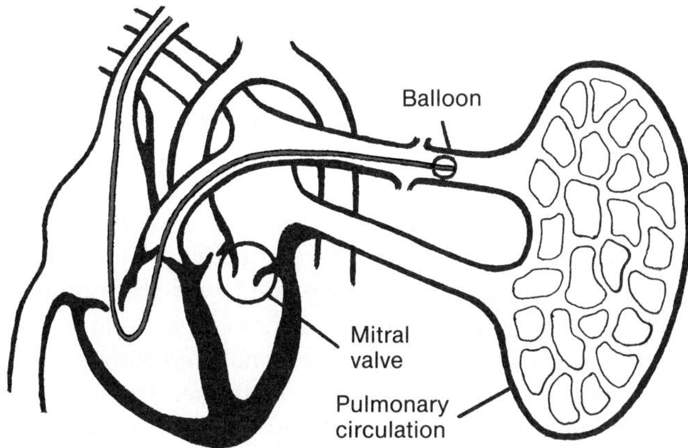

Figure 21-15 Pulmonary artery catheter in wedge position during diastole.

Complications associated with placement of a PA catheter include infection, pulmonary artery rupture, pulmonary thromboembolism, catheter kinking, arrhythmias, and air embolism. If the catheter becomes kinked within the heart, severe valvular damage may occur with its removal. On rare occasions, surgical intervention may be necessary. Many of these complications occur during the placement or removal of the catheter. These procedures and manipulation of the catheter in place should only be done by a nurse practitioner with special training or by a physician.

Exercise tolerance test

An exercise tolerance test (ETT) is valuable in diagnosing ischemic heart disease. The patient's ECG is continuously monitored while he or she is subjected to a gradually increasing level of exercise on a motorized treadmill or bicycle. A depression in the ST segment of the ECG indicates lack of oxygen to the heart muscle. The ETT is also used to diagnose arrhythmias and to evaluate the patient's cardiac tolerance of exercise. The patient needs to understand what the test includes because his or her cooperation is necessary. The patient should also know that the test will be stopped if any pain, dyspnea, or extreme fatigue occur. The patient is advised to avoid smoking, to have nothing by mouth except water for several hours before the test, and to wear clothing suitable for exercise. Medications that affect the heart may be withheld.

Ambulatory electrocardiography

Ambulatory electrocardiography is made possible by a special monitor designed in the 1930s by Dr. Norman J. Holter. New technology has permitted its redesign into a compact, battery-operated tape recorder that is worn by the patient. The Holter monitor records cardiac events occurring in the normal conduct of patients' lives: work, sleep, stress, or activity. Three skin electrodes are attached to the patient, with the monitor worn on the belt or shoulder harness for a 24-hour period. The tape recording is then analyzed for any abnormalities. Patients should be instructed to keep the electrodes dry and to record any symptoms, medications, or activity in the event diary provided with the monitor.

Echocardiogram, phonocardiogram, and vectorcardiogram

The echocardiogram, phonocardiogram, and vectorcardiogram are noninvasive tests that pose no risk or discomfort to the patient. Before testing, the patient should be informed that the procedures are painless and that he or she must lie quietly for approximately 30 minutes.

The echocardiogram uses high-frequency ultrasonic waves bounced off the heart to locate and record the motion of cardiac structures. The data are transmitted through an oscilloscope and recorded on photographic paper or film. An echocardiogram is useful in determining the function of the left ventricle and the cardiac valves, especially the mitral valve. It also indicates the presence of cardiac tumors, pericardial effusion, and congenital heart defects.

The phonocardiogram expands the limits of heart sounds that may be heard with a stethoscope. Microphones are placed on the surface of the body, and a graphic recording is made of sounds that originate in the heart and the great vessels. An ECG, or echocardiogram, is sometimes taken at the same time.

The vectorcardiogram is a continuous-loop tracing, in two-dimensions, of the heart's electric conduction performance. The vectorcardiogram is extremely useful in detecting inferior-wall myocardial infarctions, and in analyzing Q waves and abnormal intraventricular conduction (Wilson, 1991). The patient preparation is the same as for an ECG.

X-ray Examination and Fluoroscopy

X-ray films

X-ray examination is one of the most valuable tools available for appraising the size and shape of the heart. The heart is opaque to x-rays, but contour can be readily outlined, and the thoracic aorta can be seen. Fluoroscopic examination allows visualization of the heart in motion. The outline of the heart may be traced on the fluoroscope screen and copied on paper for further study, a procedure called *orthodiagraphy*. The lungs can be evaluated at the same time, and this should be done because lung congestion occurs early in heart failure and may be the first sign of heart failure.

Angiography

Examination of the chambers of the heart, valves, and blood vessels is made by injecting a contrast medium into a vein or artery. X-ray films called *angiograms* are then taken. Selective angiography uses a smaller amount of the contrast medium and injects it in or near the area to be studied. This method has proved more satisfactory than injecting the contrast medium into the vein. Selective angiography makes it possible to study any part of the vascular system. Patients undergoing this procedure should be questioned carefully about allergies because some persons are sensitive to the dye. Preceding the examination, food usually is withheld from the patient to avoid nausea and vomiting, and a mild sedative may be given. These patients are usually fearful and apprehensive and need a great deal of education and reassurance. After the procedure, the patient should be monitored for bleeding from the site of the injection, and blood pressure should be monitored.

Cardiac Catheterization

Cardiac catheterization requires a team of well-trained physicians and nurses and usually is done only in medical centers where facilities exist for open heart surgery. The purposes of cardiac catheterization are to measure the pressure in the heart chambers and pulmonary arteries, to obtain blood samples from the heart and vessels so that analysis can determine the amount of oxygen and carbon dioxide present, and to detect congenital or acquired defects. The catheterization may be done on either the right side or the left side of the heart. A cutdown is made over a vein in the arm or leg, and a small catheter is introduced into the vein. It is slowly passed through the vein to the heart with the aid of the fluoroscope, and x-ray films are taken along the route. The examination permits a more precise diagnosis. The left side of the heart may be catheterized in a similar way by inserting a catheter into the femoral artery and passing it up the aorta and into the heart. If atrial stenosis is present, a needle can be passed into the heart by means of a special bronchoscope, or the heart may be entered directly through the chest wall. Before the catheterization, the procedure is explained to the

BOX 21-3

POSTCATHETERIZATION NURSING INTERVENTION

1 Direct the patient to remain in bed, flat for 6 hours.
2 Monitor vital signs every 30 minutes for 2 hours, then every hour for 4 hours or until stable.
3 Check the insertion site every 15 minutes for the first hour and every ½ hour to 1 hour for the next 4 hours for bleeding, hematoma, and swelling. Place a sandbag over the insertion site for 4 to 6 hours.
4 Check pulses and signs of circulatory compromise in the limb of insertion every 15 minutes for the first hour and every ½ hour to 1 hour for the next 4 hours.
5 Encourage the patient to wait 12 hours before flexing or hyperextending the leg or arm in which the catheter was inserted.

patient and a signed consent is obtained. After the catheterization, the nurse should monitor vital signs, examine the insertion site, and help the patient to resume precatheterization status (Box 21-3).

Electrophysiology Studies

Another invasive test that assists in arrythmia diagnosis is the electrophysiology study (EPS). With this test, specific areas of the heart can be tested to see if they are responsible for causing arrhythmias. In a technique similar to cardiac catheterization, special electrophysiology catheters with pacing abilities are advanced into the patient. The electrophysiologist stimulates different areas of the myocardium through the catheters, searching for the abnormal site by deliberately provoking an arrhythmia under controlled conditions. The arrhythmia is then reversed to normal sinus rhythm by pacing, medication, or cardioversion/defibrillation. Therapy such as medication or catheter-accessed ablation (removal) of the site can then be prescribed for the patient.

THE PATIENT WITH DISEASES AND DISORDERS OF THE CARDIOVASCULAR SYSTEM

The leading cause of death in the United States is cardiovascular disease. Since the initiation of a massive campaign to educate people about risk factors in 1968, mortality has been declining steadily (Thelan and others, 1994; Vitello-Cicciu, Morrissey, 1993). Each year complications from cardiovascular disease account for more than 900,000 deaths. More than half of these deaths—about one half million people a year—are from acute myocardial infarctions. Reducing morbidity and mortality from heart disease is a primary concern of healthcare providers. The nurse needs to be aware of the risk factors and should encourage patients to modify habits that predispose them to heart disease.

Arteriosclerosis and Atherosclerosis

Arteriosclerosis is a process of degeneration and decreased elasticity of the artery walls caused by chronic inflammation and scarring. This degenerative process weakens the vessel walls, predisposing them to hemorrhage, thrombosis, and hypertension. It is also related to the aging process. Atherosclerosis is a type of arteriosclerosis related to fatty deposits. It affects the large arteries, such as the aorta and its major branches, the coronary arteries, and the large arteries of the brain. It is very serious because it is the underlying cause of most heart and brain infarcts.

Pathophysiology

Atherosclerosis is characterized by deposits of fat (usually cholesterol) within the inner lining of the arteries. These deposits initiate a low-grade inflammatory reaction and healing process, which eventually results in hard, irregular, multicolored **plaques.** These plaques form fibrous tissue and calcify within the inner lining of the arteries (Figure 21-16). This process weakens and narrows the walls of the major arteries, and partial or complete obstruction can occur. Whenever obstruction occurs, the tissue beyond the obstruction is deprived of its blood supply, and death of the tissue may result. The deprivation of blood to the heart is referred to as **ischemic heart disease,** and the pathologic condition involves the coronary arteries.

Intervention

There is no effective treatment or cure for arteriosclerosis and atherosclerosis. The process probably begins early in life and develops gradually over the years. Earlier sections of this chapter discuss factors that increase the risk of heart disease. Surgical procedures have been developed that will remove plaques from certain areas and increase the circulation beyond. To decrease the risk of ischemic heart disease, however, the individual must establish good health habits

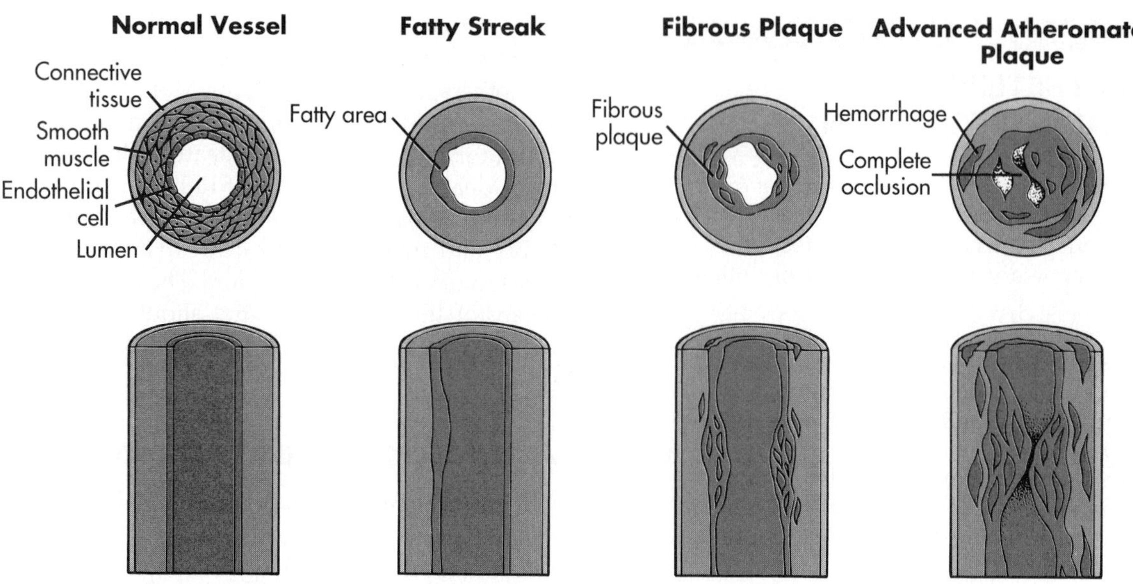

Figure 21-16 Progression of atherosclerosis shown in both the longitudinal and the cross-sectional views. **A,** Normal vessel. **B,** First stage, fatty streaks. **C,** Second stage, fibrous plaque development. **D,** Third stage, advanced (complicated) lesions. (From Thelan LA, Davie JK, Urden LD: *Textbook of critical care nursing, diagnosis and management,* ed 2, St Louis, 1994, Mosby.)

during the early years of life. It is believed that the disease process can be slowed by modifications in daily living. A reduction of dietary cholesterol usually will cause a decrease of the serum cholesterol. Most cholesterol in the diet comes from animal fats. Foods that should be eliminated from the diet include whole milk, butter, eggs, organ meats, and other animal fats (Box 21-4). Use of polyunsaturated oils, skim milk, and low-fat cheese and the addition of complex carbohydrates to the diet should be considered. The nurse should encourage young persons to not smoke or to stop smoking and to establish good dietary patterns. Exercise also has been shown to be effective in controlling and preventing high levels of cholesterol.

BOX 21-4

FOODS HIGH IN SATURATED FAT AND CHOLESTEROL

- Whole milk
- Dairy cream and substitutes made from tropical oils
- Cheese
- Butter
- Red meat, heavily marbled or fatty
- Prime cuts
- Sausage
- Bacon
- Ribs
- Ground meat with high fat percentages
- Cold cuts
- Lard
- Meat fat
- Poultry skin
- Coconut or palm oil
- Hydrogenated vegetable shortening

Hypertension and Hypertensive Heart Disease

Hypertension refers to an elevation of blood pressure to a level higher than would normally be expected for the individual's age, weight, and sex. Secondary hypertension, which affects 5% to 10% of all people with hypertension, can be attributed to a specific cause, and when the underlying pathologic condition is treated, the blood pressure returns to normal. When an abnormally high blood pressure occurs without any known cause, it is called essential or primary hypertension, and it is this type that affects 80% to 90% of hypertensive individuals.

A common feature of hypertension is elevation of both blood pressure parameters: systolic and diastolic. In some patients, however, the systolic blood pressure is elevated without a corresponding elevation of the diastolic blood pressure. This is often seen in older adult patients and in patients with hyperthyroidism or aortic insufficiency.

The normal values for blood pressure, and the criteria for defining hypertension, were set by a national commission, with the following recommendations: If, on at least three consecutive visits to a health provider, two or more diastolic pressures exceed 90mm Hg, or if systolic pressures exceed 140 mm Hg consistently, hypertension can be confirmed in adults over age eighteen (Bates, 1987).

The course of this disease is insidious. Some people who are hypertensive remain untreated for years. If the disease is left untreated, severe organ damage can occur, and the result can be myocardial infarction, cerebral vascular accidents, heart failure, renal failure, and sometimes death.

Three major systems of control that have an interdependent effect on blood pressure are (1) sodium and extracellular fluid volume, (2) the sympathetic nervous system, and (3) the renin-angiotensin system.

Sodium

Normally when a person consumes salt, physiologic responses are triggered that result in the excretion of salt. However, a person with hypertension has an altered response to sodium and requires higher filtration pressures in the kidneys to remove the sodium.

Sympathetic nervous system

Increased levels of plasma norepinephrine have been found in some hypertensive individuals, which suggests higher levels of sympathetic activity, especially in people with borderline hypertension, high cardiac output, and a rapid heart rate.

Renin-angiotensin system

Renin is a hormone that limits the formation of the potent vasopressor angiotensin II. Angiotensin II raises blood pressure directly through vasoconstriction and increased sympathetic nervous system activity. It also raises blood pressure indirectly through increased aldosterone, increased antidiuretic hormone, and increased thirst.

Whatever the cause, pathologic changes in the arterioles lead to constriction and increased peripheral resistance. As hypertension progresses, the deterioration in the blood vessels affects vital organs such as the retina, brain, kidney, and heart. As blood flows from arteries into capillaries and veins and meets resistance, blood from the heart is pumped at an increased pressure to compensate for this resistance and to maintain the circulatory flow. Gradually the walls of the left ventricle and the arteries become thickened. The left ventricle is enlarged because it works harder and harder to force the blood out into the body. Eventually the heart cannot function efficiently, and congestive heart failure ensues.

Assessment

Hypertension has been termed the "silent killer" because individuals often remain asymptomatic until signs of vital organ damage begin to appear. The patient may complain of headache, fatigue, dyspnea on exertion, blurred vision or dizziness, and faintness, but the only true indices of hypertension involve the blood pressure. One blood pressure reading is not diagnostic. Several readings should be made at weekly intervals for the outpatient and hourly or daily for the hospitalized patient. The blood pressure of some patients is higher during office visits than at home. The blood pressure reading also can be affected by the technique for obtaining the reading, such as whether the blood pressure cuff is the correct size for the patient's arm. Blood pressure should be measured in both arms while the patient is supine, sitting, and standing. The patient's arm should be at the level of the heart and should be supported, and the patient should not wear constrictive clothing.

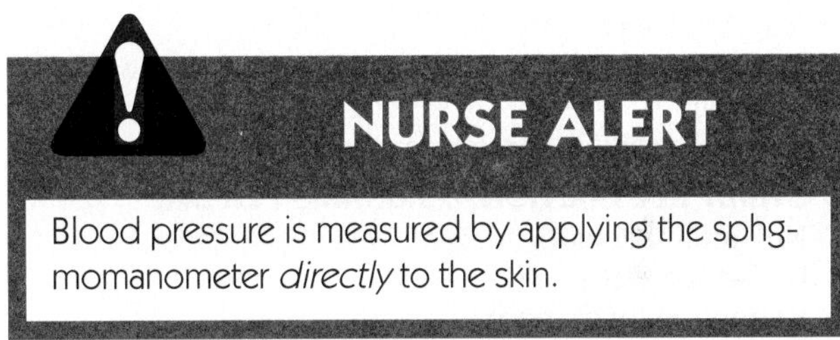

NURSE ALERT
Blood pressure is measured by applying the sphygmomanometer *directly* to the skin.

A thorough personal and social history should be obtained and should include stress factors in the patient's life and dietary and exercise habits. The patient's knowledge of hypertension and willingness to comply with the medication regimen should be evaluated.

Intervention

There is no agreement on the best treatment method for essential hypertension. There is agreement, however, that several factors need to be considered, such as age, sex, family history, living habits, and whether vascular changes have occurred. The value of the diastolic blood pressure is more important than the value of the systolic pressure because risks of cardiovascular complications drop when the diastolic readings are maintained below 90 mm Hg (Kaplan, 1994). The goal of treatment is to maintain the patient's blood pressure as close to an individual normal as possible.

It is important to set realistic treatment goals for the patient's blood pressure, weight, and diet. The nurse

BOX 21-5

LIFESTYLE TREATMENT OF HYPERTENSION

Weight control
Dietary sodium restriction, for "salt-sensitive" patients
Alcohol restriction
Caffeine restriction
Exercise: avoid isometric, emphasize aerobic
Smoking cessation

BOX 21-6

SODIUM-RESTRICTED DIETS

MILD RESTRICTION: 2 TO 3 GRAMS PER DAY
Salt *lightly* in cooking
No added salt
Restrict consumption of pickles, olives, bacon, ham, chips, and heavily salted processed foods

MODERATE RESTRICTION: 1 GRAM PER DAY
No salt in cooking
No added salt
Salt-free substitutions for canned or packaged foods
Meat and milk in moderate portions

STRICT RESTRICTION: 0.5 GRAMS PER DAY
No salt in cooking
No added salt
Salt-free substitutions
Meat, milk, and eggs in small portions

should recognize that lifestyle and habits are difficult to change, and there may be some initial resistance to changes such as the sodium-restricted diets that are often recommended (Boxes 21-5 and 21-6). The mean arterial pressure (MAP) is used for establishing blood pressure goals. The ideal MAP is equal to or less than 100 mm Hg. It is calculated by using the following formula:

MAP = diastolic blood pressure + one third of the pulse pressure. Pulse pressure is systolic blood pressure minus the diastolic blood pressure

Treatment of hypertension is multifaceted, and many considerations must be given to antihypertensive therapy. The stepped-care approach is one plan of treatment (Box 21-7). Nonpharmacologic approaches are used first. These include stress relief, weight reduction, sodium and alcohol restriction, cessation of smoking, and maintenance of a regular exercise regimen. The nurse has a pivotal role in assisting patients to learn these lifestyle adjustments. If the patient is unable to show gains in reducing blood pressure levels, pharmacologic treatment is started. Low doses of medication, whenever possible, are generally considered to be best. This reduces drug side effects, increases tolerance, and improves compliance. The less often the medication must be taken, the better the rate of compliance. Consideration also needs to be given to the physiologic changes in older adults and to characteristics such as race and sex. Studies show that young patients with more norepinephrine do well with beta-blockers. Black patients do well with diuretics. Angiotensin-converting enzyme inhibitors are effective in people with renal vascular hypertension and in patients who do not tolerate diuretics. If blood pressure control is not satisfactory, the drug that is being used is reevaluated, and factors such as compliance and duration of drug action are taken into account. Another goal of treatment is to preserve the quality of the patient's life. Offering the patient several treatment options increases his or her participation and takes advantage of the opportunity to make choices.

BOX 21-7

STEPPED-CARE TREATMENT OF HYPERTENSION

1 Nonpharmacologic approaches.
2 Partial dose: If blood pressure remains high, give partial doses:
Diuretic—Chlorothiazide (Diuril), hydrochlorothiazide (HydroDIURIL), chlorthalidone (Hygroton)
Beta-blocker—propranolol (Inderal), atenolol (Tenormin), metoprolol (Lopressor)
Calcium antagonist—nifedipine (Adalat, Procardia)
Angiotensin converting enzyme (ACE)—captopril (Capoten), enalapril (Vasotec)
3 If blood pressure remains high, doses are adjusted. Substitution is made to an ACE inhibitor or calcium antagonist.
4 If blood pressure remains high, a vasodilator—minoxidil (Loniten) is added. The substitution outlined in step 3 may be reserved for this step.
5 If blood pressure remains high, a third or fourth drug may be added.

Rheumatic Heart Disease

Rheumatic heart disease is a term applied to the long-term consequences of the scarring and damage done to cardiac structures by rheumatic fever. Rheumatic fever has no specific set of symptoms because the signs vary with the age of the individual. A diagnosis is established through careful laboratory examinations and observation of the patient. Approximately 10% of patients with rheumatic fever develop rheumatic heart disease. Rheumatic fever may be recurring, and each new attack further damages the heart. Patients undergoing a rheumatic fever attack with heart involvement develop an inflammation of the heart (carditis) that invades all three layers, particularly the endocardium, including the valves and their attachments. This results in valvular scarring and loss of elasticity. The formation of scar tissue in the heart may cause the valves to leak, which results in insufficiency, or a narrowing of the valve may occur, resulting in stenosis. The mitral and aortic valves are the ones most often affected, but the other valves may be involved. Extensive damage to the heart muscle from a severe attack of rheumatic fever may result in heart failure and death at the time of the illness. However, the disease is more likely to become chronic and to result in death many years later. Some individuals recover with no heart damage, but careful healthcare supervision over a long period is necessary to eliminate the possibility of heart involvement.

Mitral stenosis and aortic stenosis are the most serious complications of repeated attacks of rheumatic fever, although mitral insufficiency, mitral valve prolapse, and aortic insufficiency also can occur. Valves may become thickened and fused together, which causes heart failure. Symptoms include dyspnea on exertion and **pulmonary edema,** which is a direct result of failure of the left side of the heart.

Treatment varies with the severity of the condition. Conservative treatment involves limiting activity, reducing sodium intake, and administering digitalis and diuretics. If the patient becomes increasingly incapacitated while undergoing this therapy, surgery may be necessary. Mitral stenosis can be treated surgically by performing a mitral commissurotomy. In this procedure, the surgeon makes an incision into the left atrium and inserts the finger, a knife, or a dilator through the valve and breaks apart the stenosed tissue. Mitral valve replacement is another treatment option. Aortic stenosis is treated by replacing the aortic valve with a mechanical or biologic substitute during open heart surgery assisted by the heart-lung machine.

Bacterial Endocarditis

The endocardium is the serous membrane that lines the inside of the heart and covers the flaps of the valves. Bacterial endocarditis is an inflammation of this lining caused by bacteria, and it may be acute or subacute.

Subacute bacterial endocarditis

Subacute bacterial endocarditis may occur in persons who have had rheumatic fever that damaged the heart valves or in persons with congenital defects of the valves. This type of inflammation is believed to result from a hospital-acquired infection after various types of surgery, including open heart surgery. It also may occur after a dental extraction or tonsillectomy. Usually the causative organism belongs to the *Streptococcus viridans* group of organisms. The organism is present in the bloodstream and directly invades the heart. The valves usually are involved and become inflamed and covered with bacterial growth. The healing process may result in scarring, which will gradually reduce the effectiveness of the heart.

Assessment

The classic findings in the patient with endocarditis include fever, anemia, and a heart murmur. The onset is generally insidious over a period of several weeks, and the symptoms, which may be numerous, gradually become more serious. There may be weight loss, cough, headache, and joint pains. Tachycardia is common. One of the most characteristic symptoms is the appearance of petechiae, which are small hemorrhages from capillaries. These hemorrhages often occur in the mouth and on the conjunctiva and legs. Small nodes, called Osler's nodes, occur on the tips of the fingers and toes, and clubbing of the fingers is common. The tendency to hemorrhage gives rise to menstrual disorders, and hematuria may occur. Emboli from the vegetative lesions on the heart valves may be carried to the lungs, spleen, or kidneys. Confirmed diagnosis usually is made when the organism is found in blood cultures. Observation of the patient for petechiae, location of pain, vomiting, speech difficulty, paralysis, visual disturbances, hematuria, and changes in vital signs is an important assessment responsibility for the nurse.

Intervention

Long-term parenteral administration of antibiotics that are effective against the causative organism is the usual plan of therapy for the patient with endocarditis. Patients may be hospitalized until acute symptoms subside, and bedrest is indicated. Some may be candidates for home intravenous therapy. A penicillin that is effective against susceptible streptococci is the drug of choice. If the patient is allergic to penicillin, alternative therapy is a first-generation cephalosporin or vancomycin. The duration of antibiotic therapy is long because the microorganisms are protected by the dense platelet-fibrin vegetation that surrounds them. A diet

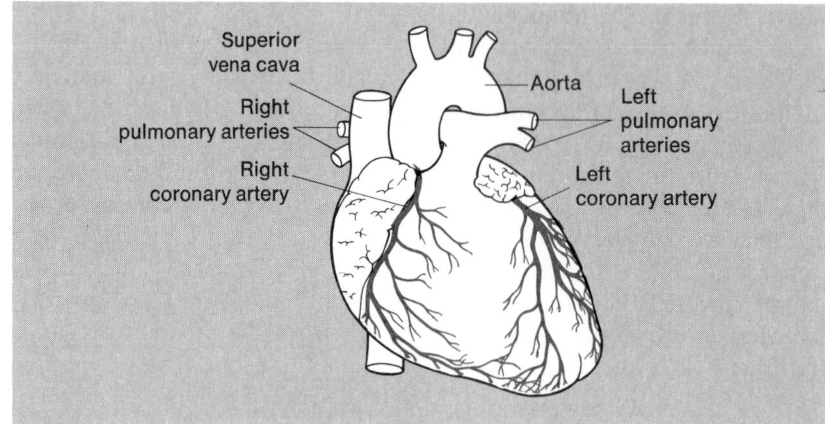

Figure 21-17 Coronary arteries arise from aorta just above heart, one on left side and one on right side.

high in calories is often indicated, so the patient may need creative nursing encouragement to overcome loss of appetite.

Coronary Artery and Heart Disease

The two coronary arteries, right and left, arise from the aorta just above the aortic semilunar valve, at the point where the ascending aorta begins. They are the first blood vessels to branch off from the aorta. Each coronary artery fans out over the myocardium and subdivides into smaller branches that supply the myocardium with oxygen and nutrients (Figure 21-17).

Symptoms of disease occur when obstruction of one of the coronary arteries or its branches is severe enough to deprive the heart of its oxygen supply. When the oxygen supply is cut off from any part of the heart muscle, the affected tissue dies. Angina pectoris and myocardial infarction are the most common diseases that result from coronary obstruction.

Angina pectoris (anginal syndrome)

Angina pectoris is a condition reflecting a change in the normal balance between myocardial oxygen supply and demand. One of the causes of angina pectoris is arterial spasm resulting in decreased blood flow through the coronary arteries, which results in less oxygen reaching the myocardium. The disease usually is the result of atherosclerosis but conditions such as hypertension, diabetes mellitus, syphilis, or rheumatic heart disease can predispose a patient to the disorder.

Assessment

The characteristic symptom of angina pectoris is a sudden, agonizing pain in the substernal region of the chest and the pain may be severe enough to completely immobilize the person. The pain may radiate to the jaw or to the left shoulder and down the inner side of the arm into one or more of the fingers (Figure 21-18). The pain is inconsistent, and the patient is often unable to describe it because of its many variations. At times it may appear only as a digestive upset. During an acute episode the patient's face may have an ashen appearance, and the patient may be covered with cold, clammy perspiration and may be unable to speak. The pulse rate may remain normal, the pulse volume does not change, and the blood pressure shows little or no change. The patient may be extremely apprehensive, and the great physical and mental pain may trigger thoughts of death.

Any one of several factors may precipitate an attack of angina, including exposure to cold, emotional upsets, an unusually heavy meal, particularly at night, or any activity that will increase the work of the heart or decrease the supply of blood to the heart muscle.

Intervention

The treatment of angina pectoris requires the treatment of the individual as a whole rather than treatment of the disease only. The patient needs to understand the nature of the pain and what can cause it. The nurse can help the patient learn to maintain a daily plan of living that reduces or eliminates the attacks of pain. The patient should be protected from the cold by wearing warm clothing in cold weather. The use of tea, coffee, and tobacco should be discouraged, and meals should be regular and of moderate proportion. If the patient is overweight, plans should be made for a gradual reduction to a range that is nearly normal for the patient's age and height. Rest and relaxation are essential elements of treatment. Adjustments should be made when necessary to relieve the individual of tension and emotional strain. Treatment of angina is directed toward re-

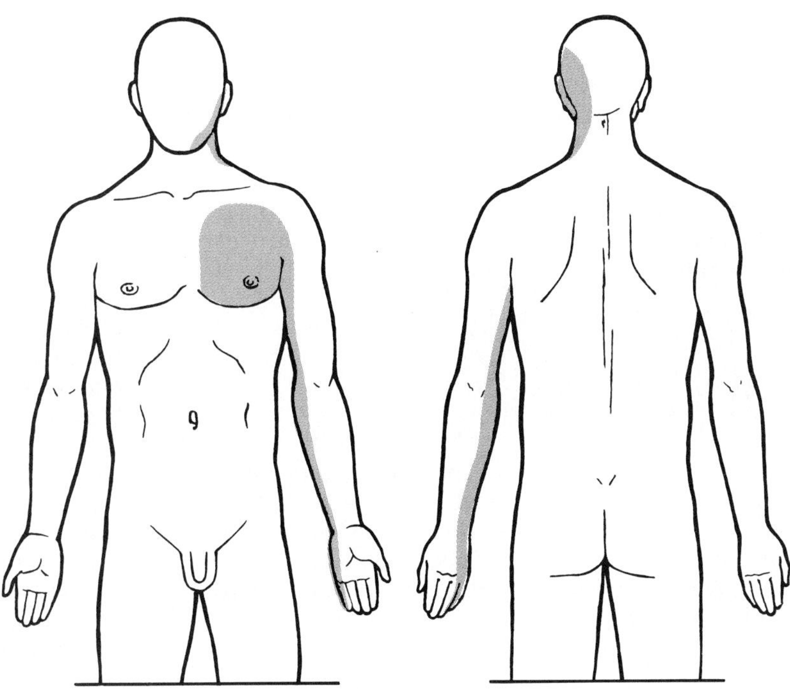

Figure 21-18 Area to which pain radiates in angina pectoris.

lieving the attack and decreasing the frequency and severity of attacks. The sublingual administration of nitroglycerin, 0.32 to 0.65 mg, or isosorbide (Isordil), 5 to 10 mg, to relieve the immediate attack may be ordered (Table 21-3). Transdermal preparations, permitting timed release of the active drug, are often used for prophylaxis while the patients are monitored for development of tolerance. If tolerance is evident, intermittent long-acting preparations may be substituted (Opie, 1991). These medications dilate the arteriole system and increase the blood flow to the heart muscle. All nitrate preparations may cause flushing of the skin and an increase in pulse and respirations, and a headache may occur. Patients with angina pectoris should always carry a nitroglycerin preparation with them and may use it freely. Propranolol (Inderal) also is often used on a daily schedule with a nitrate preparation to reduce cardiac muscle work and oxygen need. These medications are given on a schedule that is designed to cause maximum vasodilation at the times when the patient is most active. Therefore the patient must be educated about the specific times to take the medications and about the actions, uses, and side effects of the drugs (Guzetta, Dossey, 1992).

A major aspect of nursing care is to relieve the patient's anxiety. This is particularly important if attacks occur at night. The nurse must rely on the patient for information about the quality, intensity, and duration of pain, and medication should be given promptly. The patient may be raised to a sitting position and made comfortable. The patient also needs support and reassurance, and these can best be provided if the nurse is calm, has a well-modulated voice, and is firm yet provides care with gentleness, understanding, sympathy, and efficiency. The nurse must be able to differentiate between dyspnea as a subjective complaint and dyspnea resulting from congestive failure, when the respiration is wheezy and the patient is cyanotic (Drew, 1994).

Myocardial Infarction

Myocardial infarction (MI) occurs when one of the coronary arteries or its branches suddenly becomes occluded (see Figure 21-16). The cause may be a coronary thrombosis, in which a blood clot forms and interrupts the blood supply. Blockage from other causes, such as vasoconstriction of the arteries or sudden atherosclerotic changes, is referred to as a coronary occlusion. The part of the heart supplied by the blocked vessel is deprived of its blood supply and, as a result, dies. The area becomes soft and necrotic (infarct). It is gradually replaced by fibrous tissue, and collateral circulation is established.

Men in middle life who generally consider themselves to be in robust health are often the persons who have MI. They usually have some degree of atherosclerosis and may or may not have hypertension. In some cases the condition may develop slowly, and often the individual believes the condition to be mild indigestion. The diagnosis may be difficult to establish at this stage.

TABLE 21-3

Pharmacology of Drugs Used for Circulation

Drug (Generic and Trade Name); Route and Dosage	Action/Indication	Common Side Effects and Nursing Considerations
ATENOLOL (Tenormin) **ROUTE:** PO, IV **DOSAGE:** PO, 50-150 mg once daily (up to 200 mg/day); IV, 5 mg initially, wait 10 min then give another 5 mg	Antihypertensive, selective beta-blocker used in the treatment of hypertension, angina pectoris and in prevention of myocardial infarction	Fatigue, weakness, bradycardia, CHF, and pulmonary edema; contraindicated in uncompensated CHF, pulmonary edema, cardiogenic shock, bradycardia, and heart block; use with caution in thyrotoxicosis, diabetes mellitus, and renal impairment; monitor closely with IV administration
CAPTOPRIL (Capoten) **ROUTE:** PO **DOSAGE:** Hypertension, 12.5 mg 2-3 × daily; may increase to 50 mg bid-tid at 1-2 wk intervals; usual range: 25-150 mg bid-tid; max: 450 mg; CHF, 12.5 mg 2-3 × daily given with diuretic; may increase to 50 mg bid-tid; after 14 days, may increase to 150 mg tid if needed	Antihypertensive, angiotensin-converting enzyme (ACE) inhibitor used for hypertension and heart failure not responsive to conventional therapy	Hypotension, loss of taste perception, proteinuria, and rashes; use with caution in renal impairment and aortic stenosis; use extreme caution with family history of hereditary angiodema
DIGOXIN (Lanoxin, Lanoxicaps) **ROUTE:** PO, IV **DOSAGE:** PO, 8-12 μg/kg (6-10 μg/kg for inotrophic effect, 10-15 μg/kg for atrial arrhythmias); give half of this initially, remainder at 4-8 hr intervals based on response; maintenance dose: 15%-25% of loading dose (usual adult oral dose 0.1-0.25 mg/day); IV, 8-12 μg/kg initially in several divided doses given q 4-8 hr; maintenance dose: 25%-35% of initial dose given as single daily dose	Cardiac glycoside, inotropic agent, and antiarrhythmic used in the treatment of congestive heart failure, to slow the ventricular rate of tachyarrhythmias, and to terminate paroxysmal atrial tachycardia	Fatigue, arrhythmias, bradycardia, nausea, vomiting, and anorexia; contraindicated in uncontrolled ventricular arrhythmias, AV block, idiopathic hypertrophic aortic stenosis, constrictive pericarditis, and known alcohol intolerance; use with caution in electrolyte abnormalities, especially hypokalemia, hypercalcemia, and hypomagnesemia; dose should be based on body weight; therapeutic dose range is very narrow and should be monitored closely
CHOLESTYRAMINE (Questran) **ROUTE:** PO **DOSAGE:** 4 g 1-6 times daily.	Lipid-lowering agent used as an adjunct in the management of primary hypercholesterolemia and in the relief of pruritis associated with elevated levels of bile acids	Nausea, constipation, and abdominal discomfort; contraindicated in complete biliary obstruction; use with caution with history of constipation
DILTIAZEM (Cardizem, Cardizem SR, Cardizem CD, Dilacor XR) **ROUTE:** PO, IV **DOSAGE:** PO, 30-120 mg 3-4 times daily, or 60-120 mg twice daily as SR capsules, or 180-240 mg once daily as CD or XR capsules (up to 360 mg/day); IV, 0.25 mg/kg and may repeat in 15 min with 0.35 mg/kg; may follow with continuous infusion at 10 mg/hr (range 5-15 mg/hr) for up to 24 hr	Calcium channel blocker, antianginal, coronary vasodilator used for angina pectoris, hypertension, and conversion of atrial arrhythmias, including atrial fibrillation, flutter, and PSVT	Headache, fatigue, arrhythmias, edema, hypotension, constipation, and rash; contraindicated in sick sinus syndrome, severe hypotension, and second- and third-degree heart block; use with caution in severe hepatic disease and CHF; monitor vitals and ECG closely during IV administration

TABLE 21-3

Pharmacology of Drugs Used for Circulation—cont'd

Drug (Generic and Trade Name); Route and Dosage	Action/Indication	Common Side Effects and Nursing Considerations
DIPYRIDAMOLE (Persantine) **ROUTE:** PO **DOSAGE:** 75-100 mg 4 times daily in divided doses	Antiplatelet agent and coronary vasodilator used in the prevention of thromboembolism in patients with prosthetic heart valves, to maintain patency of grafts after surgical bypass, and as a diagnostic agent in lieu of exercise during thallium myocardial imaging	Headache, dizziness, hypotension, and nausea; use with caution in hypotensive patients and patients with platelet defects
ENALAPRIL (Vasotec) **ROUTE:** PO, IV **DOSAGE:** PO, hypertension, initial dose 5 mg/day, increased as required by response (usual range 10-40 mg/day in 1-2 divided doses); CHF, initial dose 2.5 mg 1-2 times daily, increased as required by response (usual range 5-20 mg/day in 1-2 divided doses); IV, 0.626-1.25 mg q 6 hr	Antihypertensive, angiotensin-converting enzyme (ACE) inhibitor used in the management of hypertension and CHF	Headache, dizziness, fatigue, hypotension, and angioedema; use with caution in renal impairment, hypotension, and aortic stenosis
GEMFIBROZIL (Lopid) **ROUTE:** PO **DOSAGE:** 600 mg twice daily 30 min before breakfast and dinner	Lipid-lowering agent used as adjunct therapy in the management of hyperlipidemias associated with high triglyceride levels	Abdominal pain, epigastric pain, and diarrhea; contraindicated in primary biliary cirrhosis; use with caution in gall bladder, liver, and renal disease; check liver function tests periodically
HEPARIN (Hep-Lock) **ROUTE:** SC, IV **DOSAGE:** SC, 5000 U IV, followed by initial SC dose of 10,000-20,000 U, then 8,000-10,000 U q 8 hr, or 15,000-20,000 U q 12 hr; IV bolus, 10,000 U, followed by 5,000-10,000 U q 4-6 hr, IV infusion, 5,000 U, followed by 20,000-40,000 U infused over 24 hr (approximately 1000 U/hr)	Anticoagulant used in the prophylaxis and treatment of multiple thromboembolic disorders, including pulmonary emboli and venous thromboembolism; used in small doses to maintain patency of IV catheters	Bleeding and thrombocytopenia; contraindicated in uncontrolled bleeding and in severe liver or kidney disease; use with caution with ulcers, spinal cord or brain injury, untreated hypertension; must monitor therapeutic dose range closely with partial thromboplastin time, partial prothrombin time, and blood studies.
METOPROLOL (Lopressor) **ROUTE:** PO, IV **DOSAGE:** PO, 100-450 mg/day as single dose or bid; extended-release tablets (Toprol XL) are given once daily; acute treatment myocardial infarction prophylaxis, 5 mg q 2 min IV for 3 doses; then 15 min after last IV dose, start 50 mg PO q 6 hr for 48 hr, then 100 mg bid	Antihypertensive, antianginal, selective beta blocker used for hypertension, angina pectoris, and treatment of myocardial infarction; also used for prophylaxis and treatment of arrhythmias, hypertrophic cardiomyopathy, and in the prevention of vascular headaches	Fatigue, weakness, depression, bradycardia, CHF, and pulmonary edema; contraindicated in uncompensated CHF, pulmonary edema, bradycardia, and heart block; use with caution in hyperthyroidism and diabetes mellitus; monitor vitals and ECG closely with IV administration; administer atropine if HR drops to < 40

continued

TABLE 21-3

Pharmacology of Drugs Used for Circulation—cont'd

Drug (Generic and Trade Name); Route and Dosage	Action/Indication	Common Side Effects and Nursing Considerations
NIFEDIPINE (Adalat, Procardia, Procardia XL) **ROUTE:** PO, SL **DOSAGE:** PO, 10-30 mg 3 times daily (not to exceed 180 mg/day) or 30-90 mg once daily as sustained-release form (not to exceed 90-120 mg/day); SL, 10 mg, repeated in 15 min	Calcium channel blocker, antianginal, coronary vasodilator, antihypertensive used in the management of angina pectoris, vasospasm, and hypertension	Dizziness, lightheadedness, giddiness, headache, nervousness, nasal congestion, sore throat, dyspnea, cough, wheezing, nausea, flushing, and warmth; contraindicated in severe hypotension; use with caution in severe hepatic disease, CHF, edema, and aortic stenosis
NITROGLYCERIN (Nitrostat, NitroBid, Nitrolingual Spray, Nitro Ointment, Nitro-Dur Patches) **ROUTE:** PO, IV, SL, topical **DOSAGE:** PO, 2.5-9 mg q 8-12 hr as extended-release capsules or 1.3-6.5 mg q 8-12 hr as extended release tablet, up to 26 mg 4 times daily, IV, 5 μg/min to 20 μg/min, then increase by 10-20 μg/min q 3-5 min (dosing determined by hemodynamic and BP parameters); SL, 0.15-0.6 mg, may repeat q 5 min for 15 min for acute anginal attack; lingual spray, 0.4 mg/spray, 1-2 sprays, may repeat q 5 min for 15 min; topical, ointment 1-2 in (1 inch = 15 mg) q 8 hr (up to 5 in q 4 hr), transdermal patch, 0.1-0.6 mg/hr, up to 0.8 mg/hr; patch should be worn ONLY 12-14 hr/day	Vasodilator, antianginal, coronary vasodilator used for angina pectoris, adjunct treatment of myocardial infarction and CHF and for maintenance of controlled blood pressure	Headache, dizziness, hypotension, and tachycardia; contraindicated in severe anemia, pericardial tamponade, constrictive pericarditis, and idiopathic hypertrophic subaortic stenosis; use with caution in hypotension, head or cerebral trauma, glaucoma, severe liver impairment, and hypovolemia; some patients extremely sensitive to nitroglycerine and will experience sudden hypotension
PROPANOLOL (Inderal) **ROUTE:** PO, IV **DOSAGE:** Arrhythmias, PO 10-30 mg tid-qid, IV bolus 0.5-3.0 mg at 1 mg/min, and may repeat in 2 min; hypertension, PO, 40 mg bid or 80 mg/day initially, usual dose 120-240 mg/day bid-tid or 120-160 mg/day; angina, PO 80-320 mg in divided doses bid-qid or 80 mg/day (usual dose 160 mg/day), MI, PO, 180-240 mg/day tid-qid; migraine, PO, 80 mg/day in divided doses, may increase to 160-240 mg/day in divided doses	Antihypertensive, antianginal, nonselective beta blocker used for chronic stable angina pectoris, hypertension, supraventricular arrhythmias, migraine, prophylaxis, and MI	Bronchospasm, bradycardia, hypotension, agranulocytosis, and thrombocytopenia; contraindicated in cardiac failure, 2nd or 3rd degree heart block, bronchospastic disease, sinus bradycardia, and CHF; use with caution in diabetes mellitus, renal and hepatic disease, hyperthyroidism, COPD, myasthenia gravis, peripheral vascular disease, hypotension, and CHF; monitor vitals and ECG during IV administration

TABLE 21-3

Pharmacology of Drugs Used for Circulation—cont'd

Drug (Generic and Trade Name); Route and Dosage	Action/Indication	Common Side Effects and Nursing Considerations
QUINIDINE, QUINIDINE GLUCONATE, QUINIDINE SULFATE, QUINIDINE POLYGALACTURONATE (Quinora, Quiniglute Dura-Tabs, Cardioquin, Quinidex Extentabs) **ROUTE:** PO, IV **DOSAGE:** Quinidine gluconate (62% quinidine), PO, 324-660 q 6-12 hr as extended-release tablets, IV, infuse at 16 mg/min; quinidine polygalacturonate (60% quinidine), PO, 275-825 mg q 3-4 hr for 3-4 doses then may increase by 137.5-275 mg and repeat 3-4 times until arrhythmia is controlled; quinidine sulfate (83% quinidine), PO, 200-300 mg q 6-8 hr or 300-600 mg of extended-release preparation q 8-12 hr maintenance (not to exceed 4 g/day)	Antiarrhythmic used in the management of a wide variety of atrial and ventricular arrhythmias.	Diarrhea, nausea, cramping, and anorexia; contraindicated in cardiac glycoside toxicity—increases serum digoxin levels; use with caution in CHF or severe liver disease; toxicity may cause widening of QRS; milk with medication administration may decrease gastric distress
WARFARIN (Coumadin) **ROUTE:** PO **DOSAGE:** 10 mg/day for 2-4 days, then adjust daily dose by results of prothrombin time (range 2-10 mg/day); initiate therapy with lower doses in elderly or debilitated patients	Anticoagulant used in the prophylaxis and treatment of venous thrombosis, pulmonary embolism, atrial fibrillation with embolization, adjunct in the treatment of coronary occlusion, and in the prevention of thrombus formation and embolization after prosthetic valve replacement.	Bleeding; contraindicated in uncontrolled bleeding, active ulcer disease, malignancy, recent brain, eye, or spinal cord injury or surgery, severe liver disease, or hypertension; ingestion of large quantities of food high in vitamin K content may antagonize the anticoagulant effect of warfarin; medication requires 3-5 days to reach therapeutic levels

Assessment

The typical symptoms of acute MI include a sudden and severe pressure-like pain in the area of the midsternum and upper abdomen. The pain may increase in severity and radiate to the shoulders and down the arms or to the jaw. The left shoulder and the left arm are more often affected. The pulse becomes rapid, weak, and irregular. Vomiting may occur, and the patient is covered with cold, clammy perspiration. In massive infarcts the blood pressure may fall, and all the signs of **cardiogenic shock** are present. Most patients are acutely aware of their condition and are extremely apprehensive. In a few hours the temperature rises, but it rarely exceeds 101° F (38.3° C). Both the leukocyte count and the sedimentation rate are increased. An electrocardiogram is obtained when the patient is admitted to the hospital and it is repeated at intervals to monitor the patient's progress. An x-ray examination of the chest is also done.

Three laboratory tests have proved to be valuable in assessing damage to the heart. All three tests are based on the fact that when cardiac muscle dies, intracellular enzymes are released into the bloodstream. These enzymes are also present in tissue other than heart muscle, but their elevation indicates that damage of tissue has occurred. This rise in enzyme levels, plus ECG changes and the presence of typical symptoms, leads to a firm diagnosis of myocardial infarction. The serum glutamic-oxaloacetic transaminase (SGOT) level may rise as early as 4 to 6 hours after the infarct. It peaks in

1 or 2 days and returns to normal in approximately 4 days. The lactic dehydrogenase (LDH) level becomes elevated within a day after cardiac damage, peaks in 3 days, and returns to normal within 1 or 2 weeks. The CPK-MB level is often elevated within 3 to 5 hours after the initial symptoms, peaks in approximately 24 to 36 hours, and returns to normal in 3 days if no further damage has occurred (Chandrasoma, Taylor, 1991).

Intervention

Most patients with MIs are taken to the CCU or ICU. The goal of intensive therapy is to stabilize and prevent further increase of the infarct size or complications. The first 6 hours are extremely important. If aggressive therapy is started within hours after the onset of symptoms, the myocardial damage may be reduced or prevented through reperfusion techniques. These techniques include medications to dissolve the occluding clot or emergency surgery to reopen the blocked vessel.

The relief of pain is of primary importance, and morphine or meperidine (Demerol) is usually given intravenously. Oxygen is administered by nasal cannula or mask. Intravenous infusions are started immediately, usually in the emergency department. Because the injured tissue may affect the conduction pathways, any arrhythmias are closely monitored and treated. Cardiovascular shock and consequent collapse of the vessels are a potential threat, and a vein should be kept open for the administration of emergency drugs.

Vasopressor drugs may be ordered and infused slowly. The drip rate is regulated by the blood pressure, which is taken, with the pulse, at frequent intervals (e.g., every 5 to 15 minutes). The nurse caring for a patient receiving vasopressor medications (e.g. dopamine, norepinephrine) should remember that they are dangerous drugs, and extreme caution must be used while they are being administered. The patient's temperature is taken every 4 to 6 hours. Fever may develop from the inflammatory changes that are occurring within the heart. Although the use of anticoagulant therapy in the management of patients with MIs is controversial, an anticoagulant drug such as heparin sodium usually is given to prevent venous thrombosis or pulmonary embolism (Rippe, 1989), and no difference in mortality rates has been shown in patients so treated (Bongard, Sue, 1994; Rippe, 1989). Patients who are at high risk for systemic embolism because of atrial fibrillation or congestive heart failure may receive a full dose of anticoagulation medication. This may be delivered as a form of heparin or as an oral anticoagulant drug. The prothrombin time (PT) is closely monitored while the patient is receiving anticoagulant therapy. The optimal range of PT for a patient is 1½ to 2 times the control time (Opie, 1991). The patient should be observed for signs of bleeding during anticoagulant therapy. Bleeding may occur from the gums or from sites of injections. All emesis, urine, and stools should be tested for occult blood. Any sudden signs of dyspnea and changes in rate, rhythm, or volume of the pulse should be reported at once.

Thrombolytic therapy as an attempt to recannulize the obstructed coronary arteries by dissolving the clot—as compared to anticoagulants that prevent formation of clots—has become routine for patients who are treated within a short time (ideally, less than 6 hours) of the infarct. Currently there are three agents capable of dissolving the thrombus; urokinase (Abbokinase), streptokinase (Kabikinase, Streptase), and tissue plasminogen activator (TPA) (Opie, 1991; Underhill and others, 1990). Additional criteria may apply before a patient is selected for this therapy. Thrombolytic therapy is not used if the patient's history includes significant gastrointestinal bleeding or cerebral vascular disease, cardiopulmonary resuscitation within the previous two weeks, major surgery within the previous month, pregnancy, or a bleeding disorder. However, limitations on thrombolytic therapy for patients over the age of 75, are growing controversial (Box 21-8) (Bongard, Sue, 1994).

The patient with MI must be assured of maximum rest from the moment of the attack. Procedures should be planned to allow long periods of undisturbed rest. During the acute phase only close members of the patient's family and/or significant others are permitted to visit at times that do not interfere with rest. Complete bedrest is the usual way to provide maximum rest. However, studies indicate that the work demanded of the heart may be lessened if the patient is in an upright position, and some physicians will permit the patient to sit in an armchair for short periods several times a day. Most patients do have bedside commode privileges. The patient should be assessed closely for any cardiovascular changes. ECG readings and serum cardiac isoenzyme levels are used as a guide for gradually increasing the patient's activity schedule.

The diet prescribed depends on the patient's condition and may be liquid, soft, or regular. Foods known to be gas producing should be avoided. Bowel elimination may be regulated by mild laxatives and stool softeners. The patient should not strain.

Early mobilization of MI patients is now routine in most settings. The need for limited movement and exercise was recognized as early as the eighteenth century, but in the 1950s and 1960s it was common practice to keep patients on strict, hospitalized bedrest for 6 weeks. In the late 1960s, however, early mobilization of acute MI patients began to show positive results

BOX 21-8 **Guidelines for Care of the Person Receiving Anticoagulant or Thrombolytic Therapy**

1 Monitor the infusion accurately; maintain desired therapeutic rate of units per minute or hour.
2 Assess skin for signs of bleeding: bleeding gums, nosebleeds, petechiae (pinpoint red areas on skin), ecchymosis (bruising), hematoma formation, and venipuncture sites.
3 Monitor urine, stool, emesis, and gastric secretions for blood.
4 Avoid administration of medications by intramuscular route to prevent bleeding.
5 Avoid unnecessary bleeding.
   a Use a soft toothbrush and brush teeth gently.
   b Use an electric razor rather than razor blade for shaving.
   c Avoid use of rectal thermometers (may cause mucosal bleeding).
6 Special care with *anticoagulant therapy:*
   a Give heparin by deep subcutaneous injection; use a fine-gauge needle at a 90-degree angle; do not aspirate nor massage site after injection (can result in bleeding); rotate sites on a regular basis.
   b Administer protamine sulfate, if necessary, as a heparin antagonist to reverse anticoagulant effects.
   c Hold pressure for 3 to 5 minutes on venipuncture sites.
   d Monitor results of blood work: a partial thromboplastin time should be 2 to 3 times normal level (normal APTT is 33 to 45 seconds); a prothrombin time (PT) should be 1.2 to 1.5 times normal level (normal PT is 11 to 12 seconds).
   e Avoid use of aspirin; aspirin inhibits platelet adhesion, thus having an anticoagulant effect.
7 Special care with *thrombolytic therapy:*
   a Assess patient for signs of intracranial bleeding—headache, vomiting, disorientation, mental confusion.
   b Assess patient for signs of retroperitoneal bleeding—low back pain, muscle weakness, or numbness in lower extremity.
   c Assess patient for allergic reaction—chills, bronchospasm, rash, malaise; an IV steroid may be given to counteract potential allergic reaction.
   d Avoid insertion of unnecessary venous and arterial lines; insert before initiation of therapy if necessary.
   e Hold pressure on all venipuncture and other bleeding sites for 20 to 30 minutes to allow blood to clot.
   f Give medication to avoid gastrointestinal ulceration or bleeding.

From Phipps WJ and others: *Medical-surgical nursing: concepts and clinical practice,* ed 5, St Louis, 1995, Mosby.

(Hudak, Gallo, Benz, 1990). Now cardiac rehabilitation programs are available in most large hospitals. Patients are permitted limited, planned progression in activity as soon as they are stabilized in CCUs. (For further discussion, refer to the section on cardiac rehabilitation, p. 635.)

As the heart heals, collateral circulation develops and the necrotic tissue in the myocardium heals with fibrotic scar formation. The first 2 weeks after an MI are considered the most dangerous, and the patient's condition must be watched closely for 4 weeks. Healing usually occurs in 6 weeks, although convalescence takes 2 to 3 months. Gradually the patient will be able to return to a normal or nearly normal life.

The management and care of the patient with MI must be individualized according to the severity of the attack, complications, and progress. Cardiac monitoring equipment has made it possible to detect cardiac disturbances that otherwise would have been missed. Nurses should realize that machines can contribute much to the care of the patient, but they may also increase the patient's fear, anxiety, and apprehension unless he or she understands their contribution to care. Above all, it should be remembered that machines cannot provide emotional support or the intelligent, empathetic understanding essential to the patient's progress (Box 21-9).

THE PATIENT WITH OPERATIVE CONDITIONS OF THE CARDIOVASCULAR SYSTEM

Surgery of the cardiovascular system is one of the most significant accomplishments of medical science in the twentieth century. It now saves lives and provides lifetimes of health free from crippling cardiac conditions.

Heart surgery requires a vast array of equipment and a staff of highly trained, efficient professionals. In no other aspect of medical-surgical care is the team

BOX 21-9

Nursing Process

MYOCARDIAL INFARCTION

ASSESSMENT

Pain: presence, location, quality
Pulse: quality, rate, rhythm
Respirations: rate, rhythm, dyspnea
Skin: color, temperature, moisture
Mood and mental status
Knowledge of event and status

NURSING DIAGNOSES

Decreased cardiac output related to decreased cardiac perfusion
Altered tissue perfusion related to interruption of arterial blood flow
Pain related to poor cardiac perfusion
Self-care deficit related to weakness
Anxiety related to inability to control illness
Impaired physical mobility related to discomfort and activity intolerance
Risk for fluid volume excess related to cardiac failure
Risk for ineffective breathing pattern related to discomfort and pulmonary vascular congestion
Risk for ineffective individual coping related to effect of illness on lifestyle
Risk for impaired gas exchange related to pulmonary vascular congestion
Risk for fear of death related to knowledge of or misperceptions about condition

NURSING INTERVENTIONS

Check vital signs often.
Maintain complete bedrest in the first stage of recovery; transfer the patient to a chair as ordered, and increase activity gradually.
Observe for signs and symptoms of cardiogenic shock, pulmonary edema, cardiac arrhythmia, and congestive heart failure.
Allow for long periods of undisturbed rest.
Restrict visitors, and space visits so they do not interfere with rest periods.
Administer pain medication as needed.
Administer oxygen as needed.
Regulate bowel elimination with laxatives and diet; do not permit straining at defecation.
Alleviate anxiety or apprehension of the patient and the family.
Restrict sodium and cholesterol intake; provide a well-balanced diet.
Orient the patient to his or her surroundings and to any therapeutic devices in use; teach activity restrictions and support the patient's understanding of cardiac rehabilitation principles.

EVALUATION OF EXPECTED OUTCOMES

Vital signs within normal limits
Free of cardiorespiratory complications
Dietary restrictions on sodium and cholesterol being followed
Purposes of prescribed medications understood
Knowledge of what myocardial infarction is and identification of risk factors
Exercise rehabilitation plan being followed and activity limitations acknowledged
Adjustments to health problem and any changes necessary in lifestyle being made

concept of greater importance than in operative procedures involving the heart. Judgment, technical competence, and skill in observation are demanded of the nurse, and an ability to understand the feelings and emotional responses of the patient is of equal importance. The nurse's responsibility begins with diagnosis, continues long after the surgery has been completed, and ends only when convalescence and rehabilitation have returned the patient to his or her optimum condition. Because almost all cardiac surgery is performed in large medical centers, patients may be away from their families and friends. They are in an unfamiliar environment and may be fearful of what is happening to them. The warm, friendly attitude of the nurse contributes to the patient's feeling of security and may lead the patient to verbalize fears, anxiety, and other related problems.

Cardiovascular surgery may be performed to correct congenital or acquired conditions. It may be performed inside the heart (open heart surgery), or it may be done to relieve or correct some condition outside the heart (closed heart surgery). It may involve the valves of the heart, the heart muscle or its covering, or the great blood vessels of the body. The surgical re-

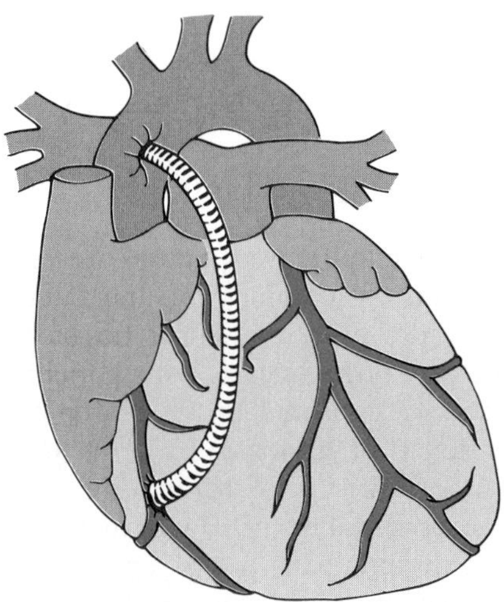

Figure 21-19 Aortocoronary artery saphenous vein bypass graft. (From Kinney MR and others: *AACN's clinical reference for critical care nursing,* St Louis, 1993, Mosby.)

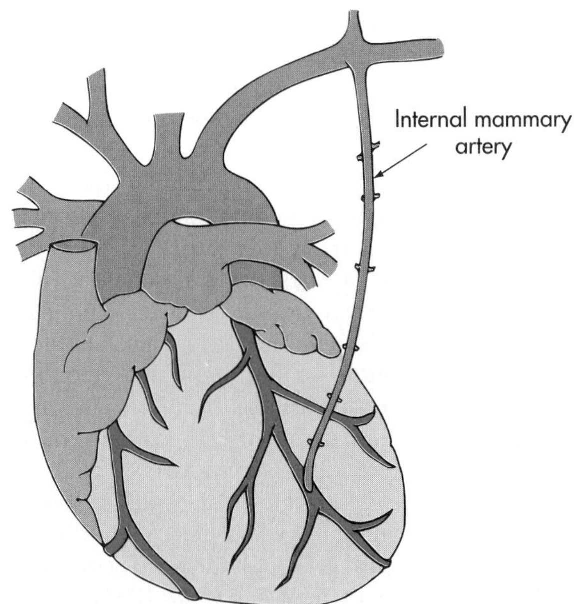

Figure 21-20 Internal mammary artery coronary artery bypass graft. (From Kinney MR and others: *AACN's clinical reference for critical care nursing,* St Louis, 1993, Mosby.)

moval of a patient's diseased heart and its replacement with a normal heart (heart transplant) has become fairly routine in some large medical centers.

Surgery is also used to treat coronary artery disease, and the coronary artery bypass is one of the most commonly performed heart operations in the United States. To create the bypass, the surgeon removes one of the patient's veins (usually from the leg or chest) and sutures one end to a new opening in the aorta near the junction of the coronary arteries. The other end is connected to the coronary artery beyond the diseased area (Figures 21-19 and 21-20). This procedure bypasses the obstruction that is limiting blood flow and immediately increases the oxygen supply to the heart muscle. The operation does not "cure" the process of atherosclerosis, which is the primary cause of coronary artery disease. The patient must maintain a low-fat, low-cholesterol diet and follow recommendations designed to prevent the progression of the atherosclerosis. If the patient does not follow the recommendations, the bypass arteries may also become occluded. Open heart surgery can be performed only with the use of a heart-lung machine. Although there are many models, all machines provide gas exchange of oxygen and carbon dioxide, which normally occurs in the lungs, and then pump oxygenated blood to the body tissues, which duplicates the action of the heart. This process is called a cardiopulmonary bypass. In addition, the patient's body temperature is lowered during surgery to slow metabolic processes.

Cardiac surgery may be performed on very young infants, middle-aged persons, and selected older persons. Not all persons who need surgery are suitable candidates for cardiac surgery, and not all of those who do have surgery will be completely cured. Sometimes damage already done cannot be corrected, but further damage can be prevented. Controversy exists about whether older adult patients should be made to endure the surgery, since their life expectancy is not increased. The physician may recommend surgery to the patient, but the final decision is always the patient's. In the case of a young child the parent must make the decision, which is not always easy because there is some risk involved and sometimes, even when the child may be helped, there is no possibility of complete cure.

Cardiac Surgery

Preoperative care

The patient is admitted to the hospital a day before surgery or may already have been admitted as an emergency following a myocardial infarction. In either event, the patient is often very apprehensive. Before elective surgery, the patient receives detailed examinations, including laboratory studies and special tests outlined earlier in this chapter. The physician will plan for a conference with the patient and family to give them information about the surgery. The nurse should participate in the conference so that information can be repeated and reinforced at a later time.

Before surgery, the patient's weight and vital signs are recorded to establish a normal baseline. The patient continues with a sodium-restricted diet and current medication regimen. Unless there is a reason to restrict activity, the patient should be up and walking about to maintain strength and muscle tone.

The surgeon and nurse will review with the patient the details of the postoperative care. The patient should be taught how to breathe deeply and cough and may practice this procedure under supervision because it will be essential after surgery. The patient should be informed that chest tubes, nasogastric tubes, an endotracheal tube, a urinary catheter, and intravenous lines may be used. The patient also should be assured that vital signs will be monitored frequently and that pain medication will be available. The physical preparation is similar to that for most surgical patients. The skin preparation usually covers a wide area from chin to ankles. A sedative for sleep and rest is recommended the evening before surgery, with fluids restricted after midnight. Although the fear is not always verbalized, the patient may expect to die, and may have made necessary material preparation. On the day of surgery members of the family and a religious counselor should be permitted to visit the patient.

Early postoperative care

The first 48 hours after heart surgery are the most critical for the patient. The patient is transferred to an ICU for close assessment and for sophisticated hemodynamic monitoring. Potential for volume disorders and coagulopathies is great because of the nature of the surgical insult and the contact the systemic blood has had with the extracorporeal oxygenator. A mediastinal tube is often placed for bloody drainage. Excess drainage may be collected in a special autotransfusion device and returned to the patient. Mild systolic hypertension (MAP > 95mm Hg) associated with increased plasma renin and catecholamine levels is not uncommon. Hypovolemia may occur as a result of the bypass procedure itself or as a result of the diuretics given when the procedure is completed. The myocardium may be irritable, and the potential for arrhythmias is strong. Epicardial pacemaker wires permit simple and immediate treatment of atrial arrhythmias, and medication controls ventricular ectopy when indicated.

Less common complications arise in the pulmonary and renal systems. Chest catheters may be used to provide closed drainage for both the right and left pleural cavities or for one side only. They are attached to a water-sealed drainage system and must be kept free of clots and kinks (see Chapter 20). Drainage should be observed for excessive amounts of blood. The amount of drainage in 24 hours will depend on the type of surgery and may vary from 400 to 1200 ml in some patients. Absence of drainage must be reported promptly because fluid may be accumulating in the chest cavity, an event that results in serious cardiac complication. When turning the patient, the nurse should provide for adequate slack in the tubing to prevent disconnection or displacement of the chest catheters.

Late postoperative care

Vital signs. Hemodynamic values are very closely monitored while the patient is in the intensive care unit. Once stabilized, the patient is transferred to an intermediate care unit. Although the patient is stable, the nurse should continue to assess the vital signs for any evidence of abnormality. The apical-radial pulse, blood pressure, and respiration are checked and recorded at frequent intervals ranging from 2 to 4 hours. The rhythm, rate, and strength of the pulse should be observed, and the nurse should constantly observe for arrhythmias. The physician should indicate the lowest level of systolic pressure that the patient can tolerate without harmful effects. If the surgery has involved coronary arteries, systolic pressure must be watched more closely. Any elevation of temperature to more than 102° F (39° C) should be reported because temperature elevation increases the work of the heart.

Respiratory assistance. For the first few hours after surgery, the patient is given controlled or assisted ventilation and oxygen. This procedure decreases the possibility of hypoxia and the resulting arrhythmias. Oxygen administration may continue for several days after the patient is extubated. Patients may suffer enough discomfort in their surgical sites to prohibit their full respiratory excursion. They are encouraged to cough and breathe deeply every 2 hours. Some patients may be placed in a semi-Fowler's position and turned from side to side every 2 hours, others may be turned to one side only, and patients undergoing some types of surgery must remain flat and may not be turned. One purpose of deep breathing and coughing is to bring up secretions and maintain a clear airway. The nurse may assist the patient by supporting the chest and upper abdomen with a pillow. Deep coughing is often a problem because the patient fears pain, so coughing and deep breathing are most effective approximately 30 minutes after receiving pain medication.

Other interventions. A nasogastric tube is inserted and connected to suction to keep the stomach empty. Although most patients are allowed fluids by mouth as soon as nausea and vomiting have ceased, intravenous infusions are maintained for a few days. Occasionally, fluid intake is restricted, and an accurate measurement of intake and output must be maintained. A sodium-restricted diet is usually given to the patient as tolerated. Potassium replacement is usually necessary. Blood samples are taken daily for several days to monitor serum electrolyte values. Activity is increased as the patient's recovery permits. Patients usually sit in a chair 24 hours after surgery and ambulate short distances 24 to 48 hours after surgery. The patient then begins a prescribed exercise program. Patients report the most pain during the first 48 hours because of rib retraction during surgery. Meperidine or morphine sulfate usually is required.

Prevention of complications

Antibiotics are routinely given to all patients to prevent infection. X-ray examinations of the chest and ECGs are usually done within the first 24 hours after surgery. Dressings should be checked often for evidence of any unusual bleeding. Any numbness, tingling, pain, or loss of motion in the extremities should be reported. Assessments for shock, hemorrhage, pneumothorax, pulmonary edema, and congestive heart failure are made at regular intervals. Disorientation is common after heart surgery, but it should always be noted and reported. The patient may have profuse sweating, and the bed should be kept dry.

Ambulation

The type of surgery and the condition and progress of the patient will determine how soon the patient returns to ambulatory activity. The process should be a gradual one, and early attempts at walking may consist of only a few steps. Length of stay within hospitals varies greatly, and the trend is toward earlier discharge for all types of patients. Most coronary artery bypass graft (CABG) patients are discharged within the first week after surgery (Box 21-10).

Percutaneous Transluminal Coronary Angioplasty

Percutaneous transluminal coronary angioplasty (PTCA) offers patients with symptomatic coronary artery disease a treatment option other than coronary artery bypass grafting (CABG). PTCA provides favorable results in terms of risks, success rate, cost, and physical capacity after the procedure. However, restenosis (recurrence of stenosis) data differ greatly between these two options. The rate of restenosis within 6 months following PTCA is 30% (Halfman-Franey, Levine, 1989; Lilly, 1993; Vitello-Cicciu, Morrissey, 1993). With CABG, the long-term patency is reported to be better with an internal mammary artery graft (88.5% at one year; 84.1% at ten years) as compared to a saphenous vein graft (76% at one year; 52% at ten years) (Stewart and others, 1993).

The **angioplasty** procedure (PTCA) involves dilating the stenosed coronary arteries with a double-lumen balloon catheter (Figure 21-21). The procedure is performed with local anesthesia in the cardiac catheterization laboratory. The coronary artery usually is accessed through the femoral percutaneous approach, but the brachial percutaneous approach or a cutdown also can be used.

Nursing care of patients undergoing angioplasty is similar to a patient undergoing surgery. The patient and the family need to be knowledgeable about the angioplasty procedure to reduce anxiety and establish trust and cooperation. During the procedure, the nurse instructs the patient to report sensations of chest pain. The nurse will also continuously monitor the patient's blood pressure, heart rate, and rhythm.

Immediately after the angioplasty procedure, the patient is transferred to the CCU or the unit that ensures close hemodynamic monitoring. The patient is then monitored for excessive bleeding at the catheter insertion site, chest pain, or arrhythmia, which could indicate that the newly dilated artery is closing.

Patient education after the procedure should focus on modifying risk factors by changing nutritional and dietary patterns. Diets low in cholesterol, saturated fats, sodium, and often calories, are the norm. Other lifestyle modifications such as regular exercise and discontinuing tobacco are recommended. The patient's length of stay is usually 3 days or less.

Additional techniques using a percutaneous approach are directional coronary atherectomy (DCA), laser angioplasty, and procedures using intracoronary stents. DCA was first performed on humans in 1986 to overcome the problem of restenosis following PCTA. The reasoning suggests that removal of the plaque is better than compressing it against the arterial wall. In this technique, a special catheter with a rotating blade is introduced into the occluded artery and the plaque is reduced in size by the rotations of the cutting blade. It is often used instead of or in combination with the traditional PTCA. Excimer laser angioplasty (ELA) is a similar conceptual technique. In this procedure, a laser is used to vaporize the occluding plaque instead of cutting it away as is done in the DCA procedure. Endovascular stents are devices anchored within the occluded vessel and expanded over the area of the plaque to mechanically hold the vessel open. Many different types of stents are under investigation to determine the most suitable design and material for their use in diseased vessels.

Embolectomy

Throughout this text, stress is placed on prevention of venous stasis and clot formation. The surgical removal of an embolus from an artery or, infrequently, a vein is called an **embolectomy.** Arterial occlusion usually occurs as a result of decreased blood flow in narrowed vessels. This can be due to hypovolemia, de-

Nursing Process

CARDIAC SURGERY

...y tolerance
- Discomfort/chest pain
- Knowledge of procedure and therapeutic plan
- Mental status
- Plans for postdischarge care, including diet and exercise

Postoperative
- Cardiac rate, rhythm, and hemodynamic values (early postoperative phase)
- Respiratory rate, volume, adventitious sounds, arterial gas levels
- Fluid volume and electrolyte status: intake/output/third spacing
- Core temperature
- Pain
- Surgical wound drainage
- Activity tolerance
- Level of consciousness, disorientation, and motor/sensory deficits

NURSING DIAGNOSES

- Ineffective breathing pattern related to discomfort and musculoskeletal impairment related to chest surgery
- Pain related to surgical intervention
- Anxiety related to inability to control illness
- Impaired physical mobility related to discomfort and activity intolerance
- Self-care deficit related to discomfort and activity intolerance
- Fear of death related to knowledge of and perception about condition
- Risk for decreased cardiac output associated with decreased cardiac function
- Risk for altered tissue perfusion related to interruption of arterial blood flow
- Risk for impaired gas exchange associated with possible decrease in cardiac function
- Risk for fluid volume deficit or excess related to altered cardiac function

NURSING INTERVENTIONS

Preoperative phase
- Explain laboratory tests to the patient.
- Monitor apical-radial pulses and blood pressure.
- Weigh the patient daily.
- Continue sodium-restricted diet, diuretics, and digitalis preparations as prescribed.
- Provide activity as tolerated.
- Teach deep-breathing and coughing exercises.
- Explain postoperative care and equipment to the patient.
- Provide emotional support and anticipate patient needs.
- Observe for signs and symptoms of cardiorespiratory complications.

Immediate postoperative phase
- Check vital signs every 15 minutes until they are stable and then hourly for 24 hours.
- Observe for cardiac arrhythmia.
- Monitor pressures within the heart.
- Report any temperature elevation above 102° F (39° C).
- Administer oxygen and assisted ventilation as ordered.
- Assist patient to cough and breathe deeply every hour.
- Maintain patency of closed chest drainage; observe for excessive drainage.
- Administer intravenous infusions as ordered.
- Maintain the patency of nasogastric tube; give good oral and nasal hygiene.
- Observe for signs of electrolyte imbalance and fluid retention.
- Encourage progressive activity as tolerated and ordered.
- Maintain the patency of the indwelling urethral catheter.
- Measure and record hourly urine output; report if it is less than 30 ml per hour.
- Check and record the specific gravity of the urine every hour.
- Administer pain medication as needed.
- Observe for complications: shock, hemorrhage, pneumothorax, pulmonary edema, cyanosis, and congestive heart failure.
- Check dressings often for amount and type of drainage.
- Observe for disorientation or psychosis.
- Provide frequent rest periods.

EVALUATION OF EXPECTED OUTCOMES

- Vital signs within normal ranges
- Deep breathe and cough exercise performed every hour
- Normal fluid and electrolyte balance achieved
- Relief from pain obtained
- Proper rest and sleep obtained
- Postoperative or cardiorespiratory complications absent

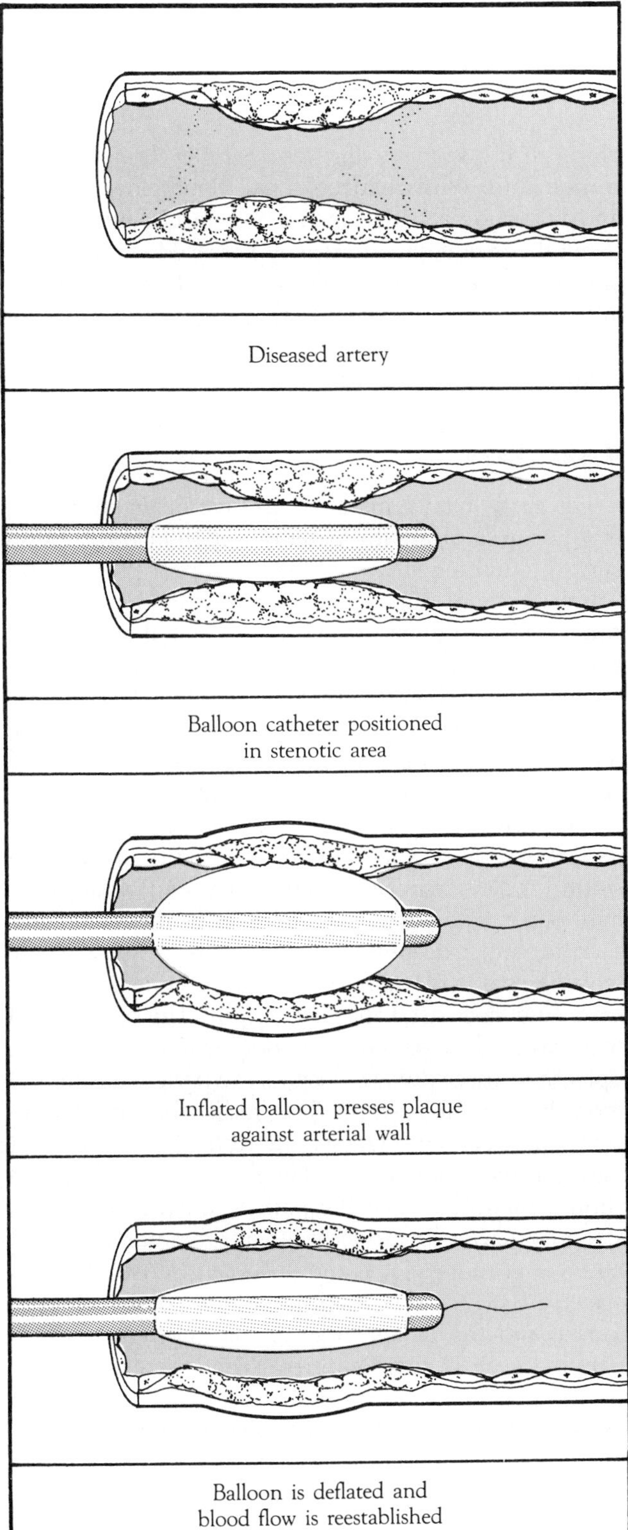

Diseased artery
Balloon catheter positioned in stenotic area
Inflated balloon presses plaque against arterial wall
Balloon is deflated and blood flow is reestablished

Figure 21-21 Coronary angioplasty procedure. (From Thompson JM and others: *Mosby's clinical nursing,* ed 3, St Louis, 1993, Mosby.)

creased cardiac output, or atherosclerotically diseased vessels. An embolus may lodge in an artery and completely shut off blood flow to the part supplied by that artery. Symptoms are pain, changes in sensation, and discoloration of the affected body part. Emergency surgery is often required to correct the problem. When an embolectomy has been performed, the extremity must be protected from injury. No external heat or cold should be applied. Anticoagulant drugs are given to prevent clot formation, and antibiotics are given to prevent infection. Vital signs are observed as they are in all surgical procedures.

CARDIAC REHABILITATION

Cardiac rehabilitation is designed to maintain or restore the cardiac patient to his or her optimum level of physiologic, psychologic, educational, and social function (Box 21-11). It includes educational and exercise programs, counseling, and social networking for patients who have undergone cardiac surgery and for those with myocardial infarction, chronic angina, and cardiomyopathy. Cardiac rehabilitation usually includes four phases (Box 21-12).

BOX 21-11

CARDIAC REHABILITATION GOALS

Prevent or delay complications
Improve participation in activities of daily living
Resume work
Attain a positive psychologic adjustment
Reduce cardiovascular risk factors

BOX 21-12

FOUR PHASES OF CARDIAC REHABILITATION

PHASE I
In-patient (CCU): ambulation and range of motion achieved (when patient is considered stable)

PHASE II
Remainder of hospitalization: gradual increase in exercise with stair climbing

PHASE III
Convalescence at home: expanded moderate-intensity exercises

PHASE IV
Long-term (lifelong) conditioning: exercise prescribed by exercise specialist nurse in conjunction with cardiologist

COMPLICATIONS OF MYOCARDIAL INFARCTION

Cardiogenic shock, congestive heart failure, pulmonary edema, and arrhythmia (p. 606), can occur as complications of a myocardial infarction.

Cardiogenic shock

Cardiogenic shock occurs when the heart fails to pump an adequate amount of blood to the vital organs. Whenever a portion of the heart muscle dies, that area can no longer contract and do its share of the work required to pump the blood through the circulatory system. Therefore the cardiac output will decrease and less blood will be available to supply oxygen and nutrients to the body tissues.

The signs and symptoms of cardiogenic shock occur in stages. At first the cardiovascular system tries to compensate by increasing pulse and trying to maintain blood pressure. The patient feels cool as peripheral vessels constrict. As the compensatory mechanisms fail, other symptoms appear: restlessness, agitation, pallor, tachycardia, and decline in blood pressure. As compensation falls behind even farther, urine production decreases and mental status declines. The patient exhibits cold, clammy, and moist skin; a weak, thready, irregular, and rapid pulse; and shallow, rapid respirations. Loss of organ perfusion results in progressive, irreversible damage and death. It is important to recognize early signs of preshock, because cardiogenic shock has a high mortality rate (Rippe, 1989).

Congestive Heart Failure

Congestive heart failure occurs when the **cardiac output** (the volume of blood ejected by the heart each minute) can no longer meet the needs of the body tissues. It may be the result of arteriosclerosis, hypertension, myocardial infarction, bacterial endocarditis, damage from rheumatic fever, syphilitic heart disease, or congenital heart disease. It may also occur from other disorders, including chronic obstructive pulmonary disease and blood transfusions. It may affect the right or the left side of the heart, but ultimately both sides are affected.

Pathophysiology

When the heart fails to pump enough blood to meet the needs of the body, all body organs and tissues are affected. The pulmonary vascular system becomes congested because it is no longer emptied sufficiently by the left atrium and ventricle. As the pressure in the heart chambers increases, the blood begins to back up in the atria and the large veins. Blood returning to the heart cannot be pumped rapidly enough into the congested pulmonary vessels, and the venous system becomes engorged. As the pressure in the venous system rises, other organs of the body become congested. The decreased cardiac output causes a diminished flow of blood to the kidneys and reduces the glomerular filtration rate. With reduced renal blood flow, sodium and water are retained in the body and contribute to generalized edema. Because of increased venous pressure and stasis, fluid is pushed out of the capillaries and venules. The liver and other organs become congested, and fluid escapes into the abdominal cavity, a condition termed **ascites.**

Assessment

The early symptoms of congestive heart failure are (1) shortness of breath, usually apparent on exertion such as climbing stairs or walking rapidly, (2) a slight cough, more of a hacking type, (3) a tendency to become easily fatigued, (4) slight abdominal discomfort, and (5) swelling of the feet and ankles. The edema of the feet and ankles subsides at night when the person is in a supine position. As the disease becomes advanced, the dyspnea may be of a panting type and may be so severe that the person must remain in an upright position (orthopnea) even when sleeping. Some patients may use several pillows to maintain a partially upright position for sleeping. The cough is dry, and hemoptysis may occur. The edema may extend to the face, neck, sacrum, and extremities and is a pitting type. There may be cyanosis, enlargement and tenderness of the liver, and decreased urinary output. The edema that worsens during the daylight hours when the patient is upright reduces during sleep as the patient assumes a more horizontal position. This redistribution of fluid promotes renal perfusion and diuresis. The patient may complain of nocturia. The lungs are affected in a similar manner. When the patient is awakened from sleep by severe breathlessness approximately 2 or 3 hours after retiring, it is known as *paroxysmal nocturnal dyspnea* (PND). Abnormalities of the pulse may be found, and the patient may or may not complain of pain in the chest and abdomen. When there is left ventricular failure, acute pulmonary edema may occur. Dyspnea is increased, cyanosis occurs, and a productive cough is present. This is always a serious emergency, and immediate treatment is necessary.

When right ventricular failure occurs, there may be excessive weight gain because of the fluid retention. As the venous pressure increases, the patient complains of pain in the upper abdomen as the liver capsule is stretched and the gastrointestinal tract becomes edematous. The patient is weak and experiences loss

BOX 21-13 **Nursing Process**

CONGESTIVE HEART FAILURE

ASSESSMENT

Respirations: rate, quality, dyspnea, shortness of breath, orthopnea, paroxysmal nocturnal dyspnea, hemoptysis
Pulse: quality, rate, rhythm, including peripheral pulses
Weakness, energy level
Pain: presence, location, quality
Skin: edema, color, temperature, moisture
Appetite
Mood and mental status
Knowledge of condition, diet, medication regimen

NURSING DIAGNOSES

Decreased cardiac output related to cardiac failure
Ineffective breathing pattern related to pulmonary vascular congestion
Impaired gas exchange related to pulmonary vascular congestion
Impaired physical mobility related to weakness
Anxiety related to inability to control illness and ineffective breathing patterns
Altered nutrition: less than body requirements related to inability to digest large meals and abdominal discomfort
Self-care deficit related to weakness
Fluid volume excess related to decreased renal blood flow
Risk for fear of death related to severity of illness
Risk for ineffective individual coping mechanisms related to effect of illness on lifestyle
Risk for altered thought processes related to poor tissue perfusion

NURSING INTERVENTIONS

Position the patient in Fowler's position, with back, arms, and legs supported for optimum respiratory ventilation.
Observe for signs of fluid excess: pitting edema, dyspnea, cough, pulmonary edema, distended neck veins, and tachycardia.
Check vital signs often.
Observe for signs of disorientation or mental confusion.
Observe for signs of hypokalemia.
Administer digitalis preparation as ordered and observe for signs of toxicity.
Administer diuretics as ordered.
Administer oxygen as needed.
Turn the patient every 2 hours.
Provide a quiet, restful environment.
Allow for periods of rest after activity.
Provide small, frequent feedings with easily digested items that the patient likes.
Restrict sodium intake as ordered.
Weigh the patient daily.
Explain the therapeutic and side effects of medications, dosing regimen, and diet.

EVALUATION OF EXPECTED OUTCOMES

Optimum respiratory ventilation achieved
Vital signs within normal limits
Few or no signs of fluid excess exhibited
Proper rest and sleep achieved
Purposes of sodium-restricted diet and prescribed medications understood

of appetite, excessive perspiration, and nocturnal diuresis. Pitting edema occurs, particularly in the lower extremities. The central venous pressure is elevated but will decrease gradually with effective treatment. (Box 21-13).

Intervention

In addition to finding and treating the cause, the treatment of congestive heart failure also seeks to decrease the oxygen requirements and edema and to enhance cardiac performance. To accomplish these objectives, three approaches are usually taken: rest to reduce the oxygen requirements; medications to reduce the edema, with digitalis to improve the cardiac output; and proper diet to reduce sodium intake and increase potassium.

Rest

The patient with congestive heart failure must be treated on an individual basis. Many patients with mild or moderate failure can avoid serious complications such as venous stasis or pulmonary embolism if they are out of bed and leading a relatively normal life. Because the benefits of mobility are well recognized, many physicians do not confine such persons to long periods of bedrest. If the condition is severe, bedrest is often necessary, and the length of rest is determined for the individual patient. The hospital environment should be quiet and restful. The nurse needs to be aware that emotional exertion, like physical exertion, increases the metabolic activity and increases oxygen needs. The nurse should be alert to signs that indicate anxiety, frustration, and fear. The patient may fear immediate danger of complications and a prolonged helplessness and loss of independence. The patient may express these feelings verbally or may show them by hostility or failure to cooperate. The patient may feel safe only when someone is nearby, and arrangements may need to be made for a member of the family or others to stay near the patient. Reassuring the patient often may be accomplished by a calm, cheerful attitude and efficient, confident administration of care. However, listening to the patient's expressions of concern and providing explanations of procedures and care updates can go a long way toward reducing anxiety.

Drugs

The goal of drug therapy is to reduce cardiac workload and increase cardiac output and cardiac reserve. **Diuretics** are drugs administered for the purpose of removing excess water that has been retained by the body. In the presence of the diuretic, urinary output is increased, edema and ascites are relieved, and breathing is made easier. All diuretics produce similar effects: excretion of sodium chloride and water. Because potassium also is lost, the patient must have his or her potassium level checked daily and supplemented as necessary. Potassium also may be increased by adding foods rich in potassium to the diet (Box 21-14). When severe ascites is present, the patient may require an abdominal paracentesis, or if fluid has accumulated in the chest cavity, a thoracentesis may be done.

The physician often orders an inotropic agent, usually digitalis in some form, to slow the heart rate and increase the force of the beat, thereby improving cardiac output. A therapeutic level of the inotropic agent can be obtained quickly by starting with several large doses. This loading-dose treatment is called *digitalization.* During this time the patient must be carefully monitored for toxic symptoms such as nausea, vomiting, irregular pulse, diarrhea, anorexia, and visual disturbances. If any of these symptoms occur, the drug should be withheld and the physician notified. As soon as the maximum effect has been obtained, the patient is given a maintenance dose. The nurse should remember to count the pulse before giving digitalis. It has been the traditional practice of nurses to routinely withhold digitalis preparations from patients with pulse rates below 60 beats/minute. Digitalis has only a minor affect on slowing the SA node. It has a greater affect on the AV node, where it delays conduction and slows the ventricles. Therefore, in patients who have normal sinus rhythm, routinely withholding their dose *may* contribute to reducing their therapeutic level of the drug. Appropriate nursing action is to withhold digitalis from patients with atrial flutter and atrial fibrillation and to seek further assistance in examining clinical parameters for its proper administration. These would include assessment of signs and symptoms of digitalis toxicity and laboratory assessment of therapeutic plasma levels (Walthall, 1993).

Hypokalemia predisposes patients to digitalis toxicity. Many patients receiving diuretic therapy are at risk for low potassium levels. Frequent electrolyte values are necessary (Walthall and others, 1993).

A mild sedative may be needed for sleep and rest at night. Meperidine (Demerol) or morphine sulfate may be ordered to relieve pain. However, nursing measures such as changing the patient's position and keeping the patient informed of his or her progress may relieve the need for sedation. A mild laxative or stool softener is given to avoid straining while defecating. When dyspnea or cyanosis is present, oxygen may be administered.

BOX 21-14

FOODS RICH IN POTASSIUM

Almonds
Apricots
Bananas
Beet greens
Bran flakes
Broccoli
Brussels sprouts
Buttermilk
Citrus fruits and juices
Dates
Fish
Garlic
Lima beans
Molasses
Mushrooms
Oats
Parsnips
Peanuts
Poultry
Potatoes
Seafood
Swiss chard
Walnuts
Yeast

Diet

Patients with congestive heart failure, as well as patients with other heart diseases, are prescribed a sodium-restricted diet. The body requires a certain amount of sodium, and any excess normally is excreted by the kidneys. In patients with congestive heart failure, in which water is retained in the tissues, sodium is retained as well. Sodium contributes to water retention, but when sodium is absent, water is excreted. The sodium-restricted diet is often misunderstood and is misinterpreted by the patient to mean no consumption of salt. The selection of foods that are low in natural sodium is most important. Foods high in potassium should be encouraged to compensate for potential potassium loss.

Meals for patients should be small to keep the diaphragm low and allow expansion of the lungs. The patient's fluid intake and output must be monitored carefully.

Other interventions

The patient should be placed in a position that affords the greatest amount of comfort and rest. Most patients are comfortable in a high Fowler's position, with the back, arms, and knees supported with pillows. A small pillow may be placed at the back of the head and one in the small of the back. This position allows for maximum lung expansion for best ventilation and slows the venous blood return to the heart.

A patient on complete bedrest is predisposed to venous stasis. If the patient is unable to move his or her legs, the nurse should provide passive exercise every 2 to 4 hours by flexing the extremities. Often therapeutic elastic stockings are applied to promote venous return. Complete bed baths may be too fatiguing for the patient, and partial baths, with special care of the skin and all bony prominences, may be adequate. Because of poor circulation, the patient is susceptible to stasis and pressure ulcers, and frequent inspection and massage are required for their prevention. Accurate intake and output records are necessary, and the patient should be weighed daily. Loss of fluid will cause a marked decrease in weight. The patient should be assisted on and off the bedpan, and an orthopedic pan may facilitate the procedure with less strain on the patient. Some patients may be permitted to use a bedside commode.

The patient should be observed for any change in skin color or in the rate, rhythm, or volume of the pulse. The nurse also should observe for dyspnea, increase or decrease of edema, and any evidence of mental confusion or psychoses. During the acute stage of congestive heart failure, visitors should be limited to immediate members of the family and significant others, who should not tire the patient with lengthy conversations or disturbing affairs. As the patient improves, the activity level is gradually increased.

Acute Pulmonary Edema

Acute pulmonary edema occurs when there is an excess of fluid in the interstitium and alveolar spaces of the lung. It can follow a myocardial infarction or complicate chronic cardiac heart failure. Although it is caused by cardiac failure, it is the pulmonary system that is affected. Because the left side of the heart cannot adequately pump blood to the body, excessive amounts of blood collect in the left side of the heart, the pulmonary veins, and the pulmonary capillaries. The increased pressure in the capillaries causes the serous portion of the blood to be pushed through the capillaries into the alveoli. Fluid rapidly reaches the bronchioles, and the patient begins to suffocate in his or her own secretions. This acute condition can also complicate renal failure or excessive and rapid administration of intravenous fluids. It is a dramatic and terrifying experience for the patient and constitutes a life-threatening emergency situation.

Assessment

The patient with pulmonary edema becomes hypoxic and dyspneic. The pulse is weak and rapid, and respirations become wheezy and sound moist with gurgling. The patient is unable to breathe without sitting up and may develop a productive cough with frothy, pink-tinged sputum. The patient may be restless, apprehensive, and covered with cold, clammy perspiration.

Intervention

Objectives of care for the patient in acute pulmonary edema are to achieve physical and mental rest, relieve hypoxia, decrease the venous return to the heart, and improve the function of the heart. The nurse should remain with the patient. The patient should be placed in a high Fowler's position or be allowed to remain in any position of comfort. Physical and mental relaxation is most important. Morphine sulfate may be given to relieve anxiety and apprehension and to help achieve muscular relaxation. Because morphine is a respiratory depressant, any patient who receives it must be carefully observed. It is rarely given to patients with obstructive pulmonary disease. Oxygen is administered through a nonrebreathing mask or nasal cannula. A rapid-acting intravenous diuretic is also given to help reduce ventricular preload. Other phar-

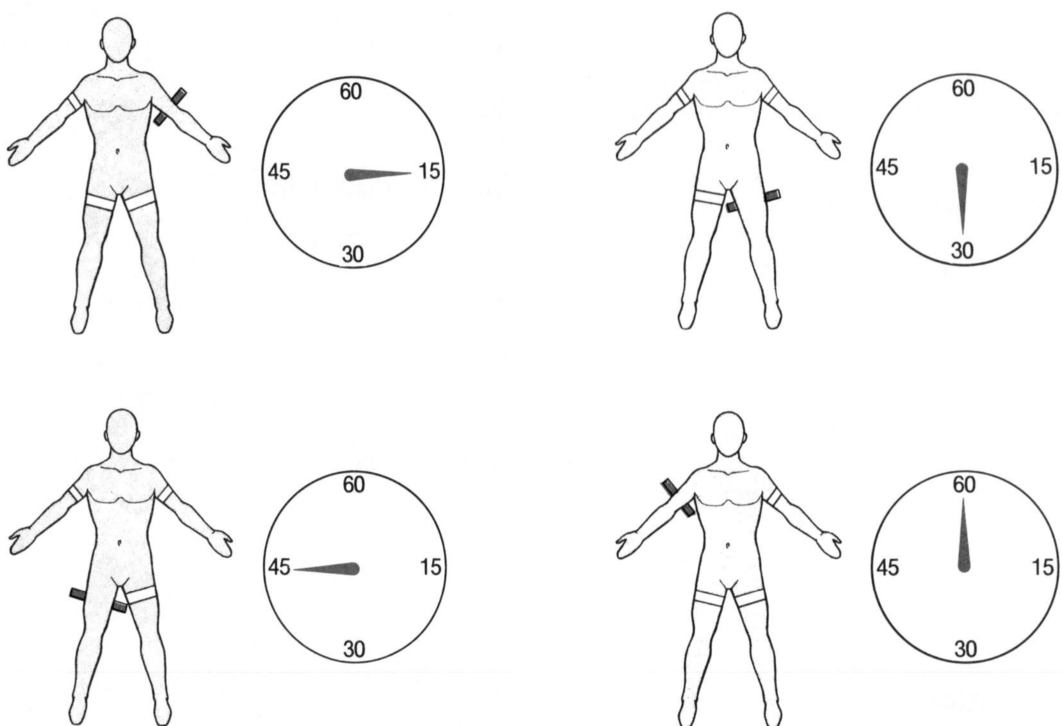

Figure 21-22 Procedure for rotating tourniquets to reduce pulmonary edema. Note that tourniquets are rotated clockwise every 15 minutes and that one extremity remains free.

macologic agents given include drugs to strengthen cardiac function (inotropes).

Rotating tourniquets may be ordered to reduce the venous pressure and the venous return of blood to the right side of the heart. This allows more blood to be pooled temporarily in the extremities and slows its return to the heart. The physician orders the procedure and specifies the interval for rotation and the time that the procedure is to be continued. It then becomes the responsibility of the nurse to understand the technique of compression and release of the tourniquets and to recognize any complications should they occur.

When rotating tourniquets are ordered, either of the following methods may be used: (1) four blood pressure cuffs or (2) the commercial automatic rotating tourniquet machine that is supplied with four pneumatic cuffs. The tourniquets are placed on the proximal third of the arm between the elbow and the shoulder and on the proximal third of the thigh between the knee and the hip. One extremity is always left free. Moving clockwise or counterclockwise, the nurse removes one tourniquet at the prescribed interval, usually 15 minutes. The fourth tourniquet is applied first, and then one is removed so that tourniquets are on three extremities at one time. The procedure continues for the time specified by the physician. When the tourniquets are discontinued, they are removed one at a time, observing the same order and interval until all have been removed (Figure 21-22). The nurse should maintain a time schedule at the bedside so that the procedure may be carried out in the proper order. If the patient is conscious, the procedure and its purpose should be explained. The blood pressure should be taken before beginning the procedure and at intervals during the procedure. The pulse should be taken after the application of each tourniquet. The tourniquet must be tight enough to occlude the venous flow but must not occlude the arterial flow. If the arterial flow is occluded, it may cause pulmonary embolism or phlebothrombosis. Special attention must be paid to color and warmth of the skin, and peripheral pulses should be monitored. When the procedure has been completed, the nurse should complete the patient's record with the following information: (1) the time the procedure was begun and ended, (2) the interval of rotation, (3) blood pressure and pulse readings, (4) any medications given, (5) urinary output, and (6) the patient's response to the procedure. During the procedure, the nurse should observe the patient for hypotension, quality of peripheral pulses, and any decreased urinary output. Deterioration in any of these factors should be reported immediately.

• • •

Patients report that while they were hospitalized their greatest source of information and care was the nurse. Patients and their families should have all available information about their physical condition, their treatment plan, and the hospital environment.

The population of the United States is increasing, and every year more people are reaching the age when heart disease most often manifests itself and takes it greatest toll. Diseases of the heart and blood vessels cost the country approximately $20 billion annually, with atherosclerotic coronary artery disease accounting for most of the money spent. The intangible costs are deprivation of the family, physical and mental suffering, and loss to society when the individual is unable to function as a social being. However, research has provided guidelines for preventing some kinds of heart disease. Moreover, adequate medical care and evaluation, followed by sound programs of rehabilitation, have made it possible for many heart patients to become contributing members of society.

HEART DISEASE COMPLICATED BY PREGNANCY

Pregnancy produces changes in normal women that mimic the symptoms of cardiovascular disease in others: fatigue, hyperventilation and dyspnea on exertion, lightheadedness, and peripheral edema. The pregnancy can provoke maternal disorders that were not present before the pregnancy. Such disorders include toxemia, systemic hypertension, peripartum cardiomyopathy, and pulmonary hypertension. The first two are common and, fortunately, the others are rare. Pregnancy-associated cardiac disease has declined largely because of the decrease in rheumatic fever and its long-term complications. The woman is often unaware that she has heart disease until she visits an obstetrician for antepartum care. Treatment is designed to prevent congestive heart failure, and the obstetrician may consult a cardiologist to assist with the management of the patient (Douglas, 1993).

Assessment

With the trend toward increased age of pregnant women, the known risk factors for cardiovascular disease are important: cigarette smoking, hyperlipidemia, family history, and sedentary lifestyle. Recreational drugs such as cocaine are associated with acute myocardial infarction, and their use should also be assessed. The health history often includes rheumatic fever, chorea, congenital heart disease, and heart murmur. A careful evaluation of any existing cardiac problem is made, and the patient's activity is planned according to the cardiac findings. Activities requiring the greatest amount of energy output should be reduced or eliminated. The patient is advised to get adequate rest at night and to have several rest periods during the day. She is cautioned against exposure to respiratory tract infections such as colds and sore throats. The third trimester of pregnancy places the greatest burden on the heart. At this time the patient should be carefully observed for increased dyspnea, cough, hemoptysis, peripheral edema, anemia, or increased pulse rate. The patient may be hospitalized, have fluids restricted, undergo digitalization, and be placed on a sodium-restricted diet.

Intervention

The nurse providing prenatal care has the opportunity to observe the patient carefully on each visit and to report any noticeable symptoms to the primary provider. The patient will usually be required to visit her provider more often, usually every 2 weeks.

The patient's respiratory and cardiac status are monitored carefully during labor. Dyspnea may be relieved by placing the patient in a semirecumbent position. The pulse and respiratory rates should be taken frequently, and emergency equipment and supplies should be available for any emergency. During the postpartum period, the patient should not become fatigued. Rest periods and moderation in activities should be continued after discharge.

DISEASES AND DISORDERS OF THE ARTERIES, VEINS, AND LYMPHATICS

Aneurysm

When the wall of an artery becomes weakened from disease or from injury, it may become distended at the weakened place. The distended part is called an **aneurysm.** Aneurysms can be classified as congenital or acquired. The acquired aneurysm is the most common, and it is caused by arteriosclerosis, trauma, infections, or syphilis (Sabiston, 1991). Almost all aneurysms involve the aorta, and most of them are in the arch of the aorta. However, they may occur in arteries located elsewhere in the body. A fusiform aneurysm affects the entire circumference of the artery and is similar to a partially blown up, long balloon (Figure 21-23). A saccular aneurysm involves only a portion of the artery wall and forms an outpouching on the side of an otherwise normal artery (Figure 21-24). The distended part fills with blood and gradu-

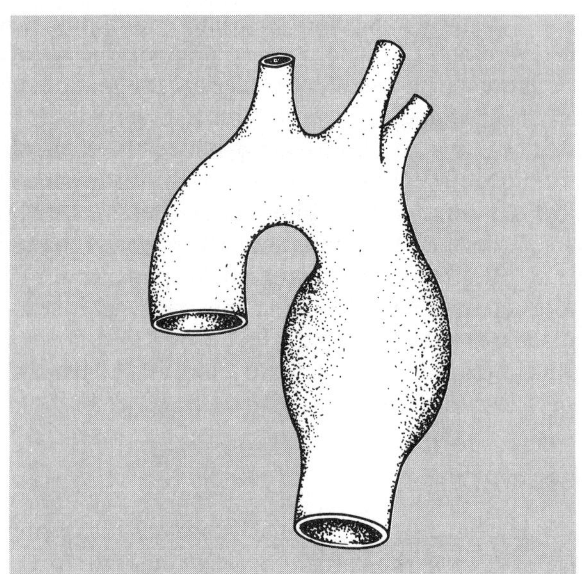

Figure 21-23 Fusiform aneurysm.

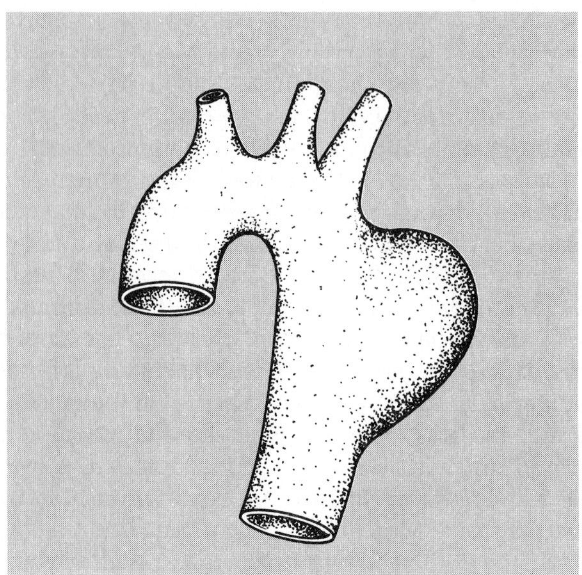

Figure 21-24 Saccular aneurysm.

ally becomes larger and larger, until it has the appearance of a pulsating tumor.

Assessment

The symptoms of aneurysm are related to the structures, bones, or nerves that are compressed by the aneurysm. Most aneurysms are below the diaphragm in the abdominal aorta, and a common symptom is back pain. Aneurysms are diagnosed through imaging techniques such as x-ray, CT, or ultrasound examinations.

Intervention

Treatment consists of decreased physical activity to reduce the work of the heart and to decrease the arterial pressure. Many aneurysms are corrected or improved through surgical techniques. A fusiform aneurysm can be removed and replaced with a graft of synthetic fiber such as Dacron or Teflon or with a vessel taken from another region of the patient's body. Saccular aneurysms can be removed and the vessel sutured, or a patch graft can be used to replace the deformity. For patients who are not suitable candidates for surgery, treatment and nursing care are based on their symptoms. The prognosis is poor.

Arterial Occlusive Disease

Arterial occlusive disease has been directly linked to atherosclerosis. The buildup of plaques in the intimal layer of the arteries leads to narrowing and obstructions, which decrease the blood flow in the main arteries. Smoking, high-cholesterol diets, obesity, a family history of occlusive disease, hypertension, and diabetes may all be considered predisposing factors. The disease is more common in men than women. Any of the major arteries may be affected, and the prognosis depends on the location and severity of the occlusion.

Assessment

A health history should include information on risk factors and health habits. Signs indicating diminished flow of blood and oxygen to the affected tissues include diminished or absent peripheral pulses, pallor, coldness of extremities, tingling or numbness, and muscle cramping while at rest or after exercise. Diagnostic tests such as arteriography are done to determine the location of the occlusion and the extent of the decreased blood flow.

Intervention

Treatment for arterial occlusive disease is aimed at improving circulation and preventing ischemia, and it depends on the location, cause, and size of the obstruction. General care measures include encouraging the patient to follow a moderate exercise program that includes walking. Chilling and cold environments should be avoided, and meticulous foot care should be performed daily. Any position that causes legs to be crossed or hips and knees to be flexed for long periods should be discouraged. Restrictive clothing such as garters or tight shoes should be avoided. Treatment may include the use of vasodilators or anticoagulants. Surgery may be necessary to restore circulation and may include bypass grafts, endarterectomy, patch grafting, or a sympathectomy. A sympathectomy is a removal of a portion of the sympathetic nervous system's autonomic division and may include a nerve, nerve plexus, and one or more ganglia.

Raynaud's Disease

Raynaud's disease is a chronic peripheral vascular disorder that often affects women. Attacks are often triggered by cold or emotional stress. Vasospasm of the arteries of the hands or feet leads to blanching of the fingers or toes. This is accompanied by a sensation of coldness and numbness followed by throbbing pain, tingling, and swelling (Wilson and others, 1991). The patient should be reassured that the disease is unlikely to lead to serious disability and that the symptoms will be more a matter of inconvenience. The patient should keep the extremities warm and avoid contact with cold objects. Stressful situations that precipitate the attacks should be identified and dealt with accordingly. Care should be taken to prevent injury or infection to the affected extremities, and smoking should be discouraged. Vasodilators are rarely prescribed unless the symptoms are severe. A sympathectomy may be helpful for patients who have not obtained relief by any other method. Although the surgery has been somewhat controversial, the resulting vasodilation has been helpful in some patients.

Buerger's Disease

Buerger's disease (thromboangiitis obliterans) is an acute inflammation of the arteries and veins of the lower extremities that leads to development of lesions that eventually cause thrombus formation. This results in decreased blood flow to the legs and feet. Leg ulcers and gangrene are frequent complications. The incidence is highest among young men who are heavy smokers. Intermittent claudication—muscle cramping occurring after exercise but relieved by rest—is a common symptom. Peripheral pulses may be absent or diminished, and the lower extremities may be cold, numb, tingly, red, or cyanotic. Smoking is known to have a negative influence on the course of the disease, so the patient should be advised to stop smoking. Skin and foot care to prevent infections is vital, and exposure to cold and trauma should be avoided. Vasodilators may be used, and a sympathectomy may be performed.

Thrombophlebitis

Simple phlebitis is the inflammation of the wall of a vein, whereas **thrombophlebitis** is inflammation accompanied by a blood clot in the vein. A classic triad (Virchow's) is responsible for predisposition to the formation of venous clots: stasis of venous circulation, hypercoagulability, and vessel damage (McKance, Heuther, 1994). Thrombophlebitis may occur easily in older persons who have sclerotic changes in the veins that cause the blood to flow slowly (Box 21-15).

BOX 21-15

RISK FACTORS FOR THROMBOPHLEBITIS

Age
History of varicose veins or deep venous thrombosis
Obesity
Prolonged abdominal or pelvic surgery
Cardiac failure
Hypercoagulability states:
- Cancer of pancreas, lung, stomach, breast, or genitourinary tract
- Systemic lupus erythematosus

Injury to the extremities
Prolonged bedrest
Dehydration
Pregnancy
Estrogen use
Venous injury

The nurse can contribute much toward preventing thrombophlebitis by carrying out several nursing procedures. Active exercise while the patient is in bed, including dorsiflexion (bending backward) and plantar flexion (bending forward) of the toes, should be done several times each hour or for 3 minutes each hour while the patient is awake. This simple exercise will do more to stimulate circulation than will telling the patient to move his or her legs. Fluid intake should be encouraged to prevent dehydration, and accurate intake and output records should be maintained.

NURSE ALERT

Avoid placing pillows under the patient's knees.

Elevating the knees by changing the position of the Gatch bed and placing pillows under the knees should be avoided because these procedures will compress the undersurface of the knee and cause a pooling of blood and increased pressure in the veins of the calf of the leg. The same situation occurs when the patient is sitting in a chair, which permits the calf of the leg and the knee to be compressed. Placing the patient's feet on a stool will avoid pressure on veins under the knee. Tight abdominal binders and dressings and drugs that depress respiration should be avoided after surgery.

Assessment

The veins of the lower extremities usually are the ones affected by thrombophlebitis. The patient may complain of pain or cramps in the calf of the leg, and these pains may follow the course of the vein. Tenderness and abnormal distention of the vein may be noted. There is often an increase in temperature, and the sedimentation rate also is elevated. The most serious complication of thrombophlebitis is pulmonary embolism, which may lead to a pulmonary infarction.

Intervention

Prevention is the primary objective of treatment for thrombophlebitis, and all measures to avoid or reduce the risk factors should be considered. Treatment of the patient with thrombophlebitis depends on whether superficial veins or deep vessels are involved and on the extent of involvement. If the phlebitis involves only the superficial veins, anticoagulant therapy may not be required. Bedrest with continuous hot, moist packs is usually prescribed, and as soon as the acute condition has subsided, the patient may be allowed out of bed. If the phlebitis involves the deep veins, anticoagulant therapy with heparin is usually ordered. An ultrasound or other noninvasive imaging test will determine the exact site and extent of the involvement. A surgical procedure known as *thrombectomy* (removal of a thrombus from the vein) may be done. Hot compresses or an Aquamatic-K pad may also be used. Antiembolic (elastic/sequential) stockings may be used for patients preoperatively for routine abdominal and pelvic surgery. Alternatively, compression pneumatic stockings are used intraoperatively and postoperatively while the patient remains on bedrest. Postoperative use of antiembolic stockings is also a routine. The stockings should be put on before the patient gets out of bed and removed several times during the day for inspection of the leg. Elastic stockings should not be rolled at the top.

Patients with deep vein thrombosis are at very high risk for pulmonary embolism. The nurse should carefully watch for the early signs and symptoms of respiratory difficulty or circulatory collapse: chest pain, sudden onset of dyspnea, tachypnea, changes in mentation or levels of consciousness, apprehension, syncope, and diaphoresis.

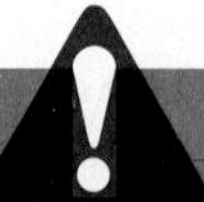

NURSE ALERT

For patients at high risk for pulmonary embolism, careful and frequent assessment is required.

Varicose Veins

Varicose veins develop when blood flow in the legs becomes permanently sluggish and the veins permanently dilate. Other forms of venous **varicosities** are hemorrhoids and varicocele (varicose veins of the spermatic cord). Several factors contribute to the cause of varicose veins. The underlying cause may be a congenital weakness in the walls of the vein, an abnormal placement of the valves in the vein, or a defect of the valves. The immediate causes include severe physical strain such as that produced by prolonged standing and heavy lifting. Pressure on pelvic veins from the enlarging uterus during pregnancy, pelvic tumors that may press on the veins, obesity, and wearing tight round garters also contribute to the development of varicose veins (Figure 21-25).

Assessment

Varicose veins develop insidiously, beginning in young adults and gradually increasing in severity with increasing age. At first there may be no symptoms, but the patient eventually may complain of pain in the feet and ankles accompanied by a tired, heavy feeling in the legs. Swelling that may occur in the feet usually subsides during the night and reappears as soon as the patient is up on his or her feet again. Pigmented areas with eczema-like lesions may appear on the skin above the ankles. These lesions eventually may break down, and ulcers may occur. Rupture of the varicose vein through one of these ulcers may cause considerable blood loss.

Intervention

Treatment of patients with varicose veins includes bedrest and elevation of the extremity, use of an elastic stocking or elastic bandage, or the surgical removal of the vein (vein stripping). When small veins are involved, the physician may inject a solution into the vein that causes it to sclerose but does not provide a permanent cure.

Vein ligation and stripping

Ligation and stripping is one of the most common types of surgery performed on the veins. Before

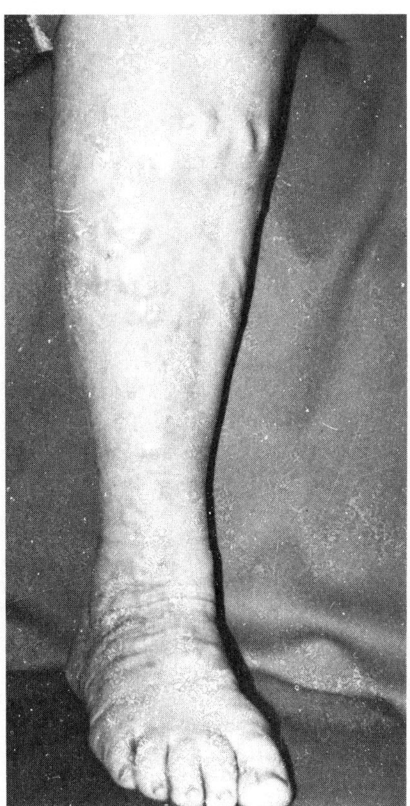

Figure 21-25 Varicose veins on lower leg with nodular bulges. (From Bowers AC, Thompson JM: *Clinical manual of health assessment,* ed 4, St Louis, 1992, Mosby.)

surgery, the physician determines whether the deep veins of the extremity are open. Not all patients with varicose veins need to have them surgically removed, but when there is edema and pigmentation that may lead to ulceration, surgery is usually advised. Sometimes veins are so distended that they become unsightly, and surgery may be done for cosmetic reasons. The physician usually sees the patient before surgery and marks the route of the veins that are to be removed. The long saphenous vein, which branches from the groin and extends to the ankle, is often the one removed. One or both extremities may be involved. The entire leg and pubis are shaved, with special attention given to the groin area, which will be the site of ligation. Other preparation is the same as that for other surgical patients. The remainder of the preoperative preparation is consistent with that for all patients undergoing local anesthesia. If the procedure is predicted to be long and painful, the patient is usually given a general anesthetic.

Postoperative intervention

When the patient returns from surgery, the extremity will be wrapped with elastic bandages. Small, sterile dressings will cover the areas in which veins were ligated. These dressings should be checked often for evidence of bleeding. Bandages should be removed only on the physician's direction. The knee section of the Gatch bed should not be raised, but the foot of the bed may be elevated about 8 inches to facilitate the return of venous blood. The foot and toes should be observed for skin color and edema, and the patient should be encouraged to move them as soon as possible. The patient may have some pain for several days after surgery. Meperidine may be prescribed while the patient is in the hospital, and percocet may be prescribed after discharge. Patients remain hospitalized for 24 hours and are ambulatory as soon as they have recovered from anesthesia. Patients should be encouraged to walk and discouraged from sitting and standing. An elastic stocking is worn for several weeks. Patients should be advised not to use depilatory cream on the legs, especially where the skin may be thin. They should avoid scratching and bruising the legs. They should not sit with their legs crossed and are advised to avoid wearing panty girdles that may compress veins in the groin and thighs.

Lymphedema

The lymphatic vessels function in the drainage of interstitial fluid and with infections. Lymphedema is a condition in which the lymphatic structures become obstructed. This condition is considered primary if the lymph channels are absent or malformed. Secondary lymphedema is a result of damage to the lymph vessels from infection, direct trauma, or obstruction. When the lymph channels cannot drain the interstitial fluid adequately, the fluid accumulates within the tissues. The resulting swelling may be pitting edema. If it is painful, there is an inflammatory process present as well. It may be debilitating to patients who suffer cosmetic and functional losses. Progressive attacks of lymphedema with fibrosis of the subcutaneous tissues is known as elephantiasis.

Lymphangitis

Lymphangitis is an acute inflammation of the lymph vessels caused by the invasion of bacteria such as the streptococcus organism. It is characterized by red streaks that follow the course of the vessel involved. The patient may experience an elevated temperature and chills. In some patients, the lymph nodes along the course of the vessel may be swollen and tender. Usually, however, the inflammatory condition terminates at the first lymph node. The condition may be serious if the causative organism reaches the bloodstream because septicemia may occur.

Treatment of lymphangitis is based on controlling the underlying cause. Warm, moist dressings may need to be applied over the affected vessels. Skin care should be scrupulous, and all abrasions should be given immediate attention. The affected part is elevated, and sulfonamide or antibiotic therapy is prescribed. The condition usually responds quickly to therapy. Any abscesses that form may require incision and drainage.

BASIC CARDIAC LIFE SUPPORT

Two organizations are primarily responsible for basic cardiac life-support (BCLS) standards in the United States: the American Heart Association and the American Red Cross. These standards are taught throughout the nation by certified instructors who conduct classes for healthcare providers and for the general public. In most institutions, nurses are required to be prepared and current in CPR. Basic life support is described in the following paragraphs.

Before starting basic life support, it must first be determined that the patient is unresponsive. This is accomplished by gently tapping the person's shoulder and asking "Are you OK?" If the person does not respond, call for help. Do not leave the person. Next, assess the person for the presence or absence of respirations by turning the patient on his or her back (Figure 21-26).

Open the person's airway. Without muscle tone, the tongue and epiglottis will obstruct the pharynx and larynx. The head tilt/chin lift technique is an effective method for opening the airway. To accomplish the head tilt, place one hand on the person's forehead and use the palm of your hand to apply firm, backward pressure to tilt the head back. Place the fingers of the other hand under the lower jaw near the chin, and lift to bring the chin forward. The jaw is supported and helps to tilt the head back (Figure 21-27). This procedure should not be attempted on persons with suspected cervical or head injuries.

Determine breathlessness by placing your ear over the person's mouth and nose while maintaining an open airway. Watch the person's chest to see if it rises and falls, and listen for air rushing during exhalation, and feel for airflow (Figure 21-28).

Begin rescue breathing by sealing the mouth and nose. Deliver two breaths of 1 to 1½ seconds each. Observe chest rise and fall (a sign of adequate ventilation) and then listen and feel for movement of air. If the patient is unable to ventilate, reposition the head and repeat rescue breathing. If the person cannot be ventilated after repositioning the head, begin the procedure for airway obstruction. Assess for circulation. Palpate the carotid artery (5 to 10 seconds) because it is the strongest palpable pulse. If the pulse is absent, begin external cardiac compressions. It is important to take time to adequately check for a pulse, because external cardiac compressions are dangerous to a beating heart.

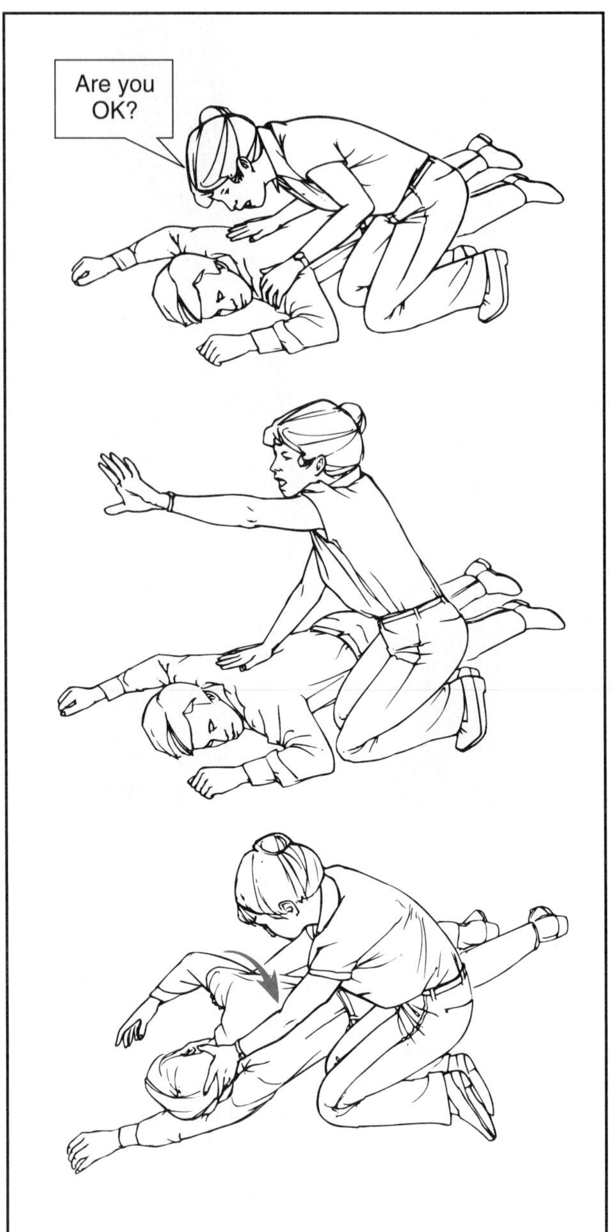

Figure 21-26 Initial steps in cardiopulmonary resuscitation. *Top,* Determining unresponsiveness; *center,* calling for help; *bottom,* correct positioning. (From *Standards and guidelines for cardiopulmonary resuscitation and emergency cardiac care, part 2,* 255:2915-2932.)

Kneel by the person's shoulders, placing the palm of one hand on the sternum and two fingers above the xiphoid process (Figure 21-29). Place your second hand on top of the first. Compress the sternum 1½ to 2 inches for adults. Compressions should be equal. Hands remain on the sternum during upstroke, when the chest should relax completely. The compression-

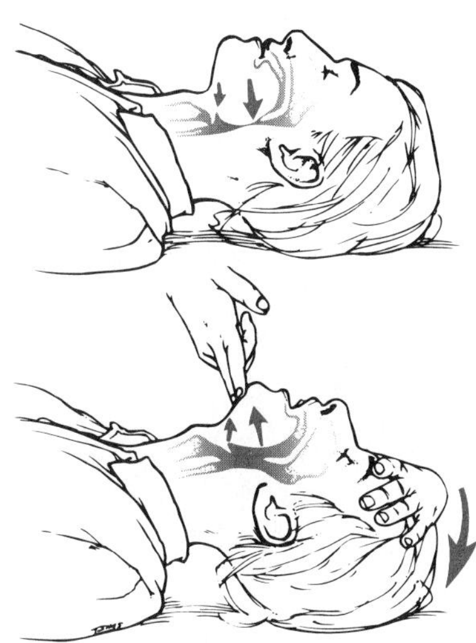

Figure 21-27 Head tilt/chin lift method of opening airway. (From *Standards and guidelines for cardiopulmonary resuscitation and emergency cardiac care, part 2,* 255:2915-2932.)

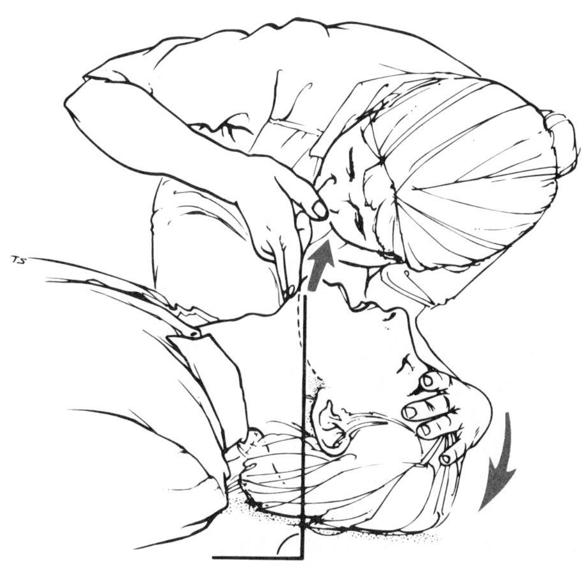

Figure 21-28 Determination of breathlessness. (From *Standards and guidelines for cardiopulmonary resuscitation and emergency cardiac care, part 2,* 255:2915-2932.)

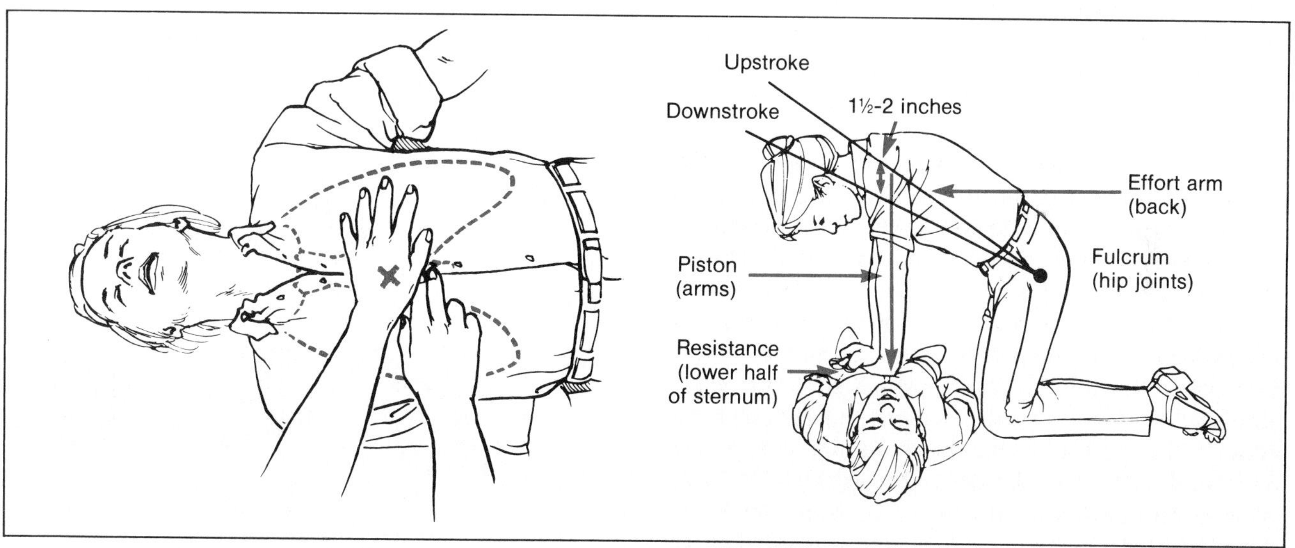

Figure 21-29 External chest compression. (From *Standards and guidelines for cardiopulmonary resuscitation and emergency cardiac care, part 2,* 255:2915-2932.)

breathing sequence should be 15 compressions followed by 2 breaths, with compressions at a rate of 80 to 100 compressions per minute for adults and children, 100 compressions per minute for infants. After the 15 compressions, go back to the head of the patient, position the head, and administer two breaths. Complete four cycles of 15 compressions and two ventilations before rechecking for a carotid pulse. If the pulse returns, stop cardiac compressions. Once spontaneous respirations begin, mouth-to-mouth resuscitation can be stopped.

ADVANCED CARDIAC LIFE SUPPORT

Advanced cardiac life support (ACLS) is a protocol for emergency life support activities that includes defibrillation, oxygen therapy, airway and ventilation support, and medications. It represents the next phase in the resuscitation of individuals unrecovered with basic life support, or it supercedes BCLS in hospitals or controlled environments. Like BCLS certification, ACLS certification requires a special training program.

AIRWAY OBSTRUCTION

An airway may be partially or completely obstructed. If the airway is partially obstructed, the person will exchange air. If air exchange is good, the person can cough forcefully enough to dislodge the obstruction. Sometimes the air exchange is good initially but becomes poor. If the air exchange is poor, the person's cough will be ineffective. There is a high-pitched noise with inhalations and there may be cyanosis. With complete airway obstruction the person cannot speak, breathe, or cough and may clutch the throat (Figure 21-30). This is the universal choking sign.

The procedure is known as the *Heimlich maneuver* and includes the following actions. Ask the person to speak. If the person cannot, attempt to clear the person's airway. Stand behind the person, wrapping your arms around the victim's waist (Figure 21-31). Make a fist with one hand and place the thumb side against the person's abdomen, in the midline, slightly above the naval and well below the tip of the xiphoid process. Grasp your fist with the other hand. Press the person's abdomen with quick upward thrusts. Each thrust should be distinct and delivered with the intent of relieving the airway obstruction. Repeat thrusts until the foreign body is expelled or the person becomes unconscious.

If the person lapses into unconsciousness, position the person on his or her back, open the mouth by grasping both the tongue and lower jaw between the thumb and fingers, and lift the mandible. This is the tongue-jaw lift. Using your finger, sweep deeply into the mouth to remove any foreign material. Attempt to ventilate the person by using the tongue-jaw lift to open the mouth. If the airway is still obstructed, straddle the person's thighs, place the heel of one hand against the person's abdomen, midline above the naval and well below the xiphoid (Figure 21-32). Place your second hand directly on top of your first hand. Press into the abdomen with quick, upward thrusts, six to ten times. Check the person's mouth again for foreign material by sweeping a finger deeply into the mouth. Reposition the patient's head and try to ventilate. If the airway is still obstructed, straddle the person's thighs again and repeat the process until the airway is clear. If the person does not breathe spontaneously after a foreign body is removed, ventilate the person and check for a pulse. If no pulse is present, begin cardiac compressions.

The abdominal thrust should not be practiced on an individual who is not experiencing airway obstruction. Nurses are expected to be prepared in the Heimlich maneuver upon graduation, and periodic refresher courses may be available through the American Red Cross and the American Heart Association. Thousands of lives are saved each year because professionals and the public are prepared in these rescue maneuvers.

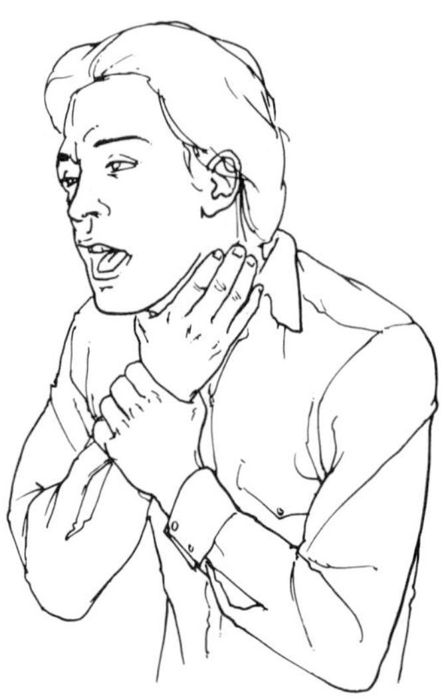

Figure 21-30 Universal distress signal for choking. (From *Standards and guidelines for cardiopulmonary resuscitation and emergency cardiac care, part 2,* 255:2915-2932.)

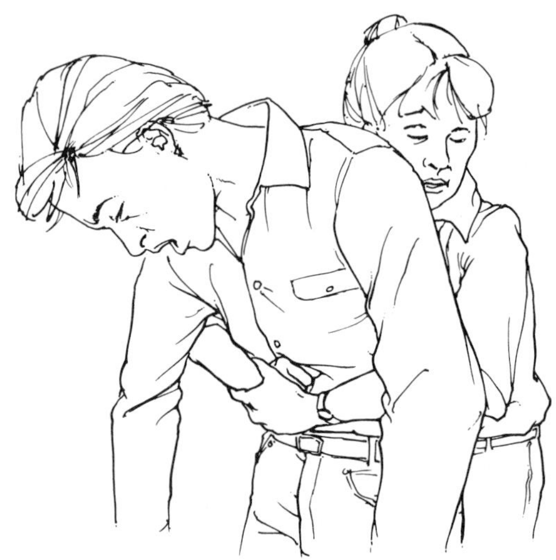

Figure 21-31 Heimlich maneuver. Conscious victim with foreign-body airway obstruction. (From *Standards and guidelines for cardiopulmonary resuscitation and emergency cardiac care, part 2,* 255:2915-2932.)

If the airway is obstructed by secretions, it must be cleared by suction or by gravity drainage. The patient with multiple injuries must not be turned on the side to drain secretions because there is always the possi-

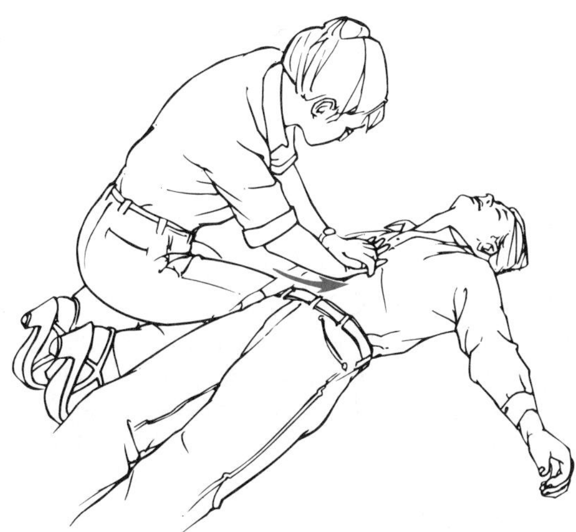

Figure 21-32 Heimlich maneuver. Unconscious victim with foreign-body airway obstruction. (From *Standards and guidelines for cardiopulmonary resuscitation and emergency cardiac care, part 2,* 255:2915-2932.)

bility of spinal cord injury. If a vertebral fracture is suspected, the patient's neck should not be hyperextended to open the airway. The nurse places one hand on each side of the patient's head, holding it in a fixed, neutral position. The mandible is pushed forward with the index fingers without tilting the head backward. Two fingers can then be inserted into the patient's mouth to remove foreign bodies or secretions if suction equipment is not available. If the patient is breathing, respirations should be assessed. The force of expiration, the presence of noise or retractions, and the patient's skin color will warn of inadequate oxygenation. It is also important to note whether the chest wall is intact and the chest movements symmetric. The patient with a flail chest moves the chest in a direction opposite to the rest of the thorax during respirations. The patient will be cyanotic, respirations will be noisy, and the patient will have a deathlike pallor.

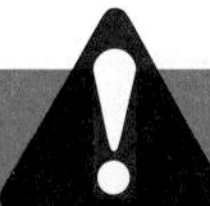

NURSE ALERT

Do not hyperextend the patient's neck to establish an airway.

Another life-threatening condition is tension pneumothorax. The pleural space of the affected side becomes filled with air, which causes lung collapse. Decreased breath sounds are heard on the affected side, and the trachea shifts to the unaffected side. The neck veins become distended, and there are changes in the level of consciousness. A fracture of the larynx will obstruct the airway completely. A laryngeal fracture should be suspected if there are bruises on the neck or if subcutaneous emphysema is observed in the neck area. Air is forced into the subcutaneous tissues when the larynx is damaged. The patient may also exhibit hoarseness, coughing, and hemoptysis. These conditions usually require a tracheostomy to maintain a patent airway.

ETHICAL DILEMMA

Mrs. Wagner is an 89-year-old widow who lives alone in her apartment. She suffers from frequent bouts of angina that are not always adequately controlled by nitroglycerin. She is very frightened by these attacks. Except for these attacks, her health is good. She lives an active life with family and friends. She plays bridge four to six times a week, goes on social outings, and does her own food shopping and preparation. Her physician has told her that the only solution to the angina is coronary arterial bypass surgery. She is uncertain about what to do.

What ethical issues are involved in helping her to make a decision?

Nursing Care Plan

PATIENT WITH CONGESTIVE HEART FAILURE AND OLIGURIA

The patient is a 68-year-old woman with morbid obesity who was admitted directly from her physician's office to the emergency department with a medical diagnosis of oliguria and congestive heart failure. She has been on continuous oxygen at home because of chronic hypoxia, sleep apnea, and now with increasing dyspnea. She has noticed increasing generalized edema and now has a dry, hacking cough that interferes with sleep. She complains of mild abdominal pain unrelated to eating or defecating.

She was cardioverted in the emergency department for atrial fibrillation. An echocardiogram done at that time showed a mural thrombus, and she was given anticoagulants. Lasix and Metalazone were administered to increase urinary output. Verapamil (Calan) was given to dilate the coronary arteries and decrease oxygen demand. Procan was given as an antiarrhythmic. She was admitted to the coronary care unit for 5 days and then transferred to a medical unit.

Past Medical History

- Hospitalized as a child for a fractured femur from a bicycle accident
- Pregnancies complicated by excess weight, preeclampsia, and gestational diabetes
- C-sectioned × 3 with viable infants; all infants weighed over 10 lbs
- Abdominal hysterectomy 12 years ago because of excessive bleeding and fibroid tumors; uterus removed along with both ovaries and tubes
- Maintained on estrogen therapy until age 60
- States she has always been "heavy"
- Diabetes mellitus type II, (noninsulin dependent), (NIDDM) × 25 years
- Hypertension for 20 years; has been on various antihypertensive meds with moderately good response; quality compliance to drug therapy
- COPD-chronic hypoxia and difficulty with activities of daily living (ADLs); uses oxygen at home via nasal cannula
- Biventricular congestive heart failure for past 2 years

Psychosocial Data

- Married, supportive husband; three adult children, two live out of state; six grandchildren; one granddaughter in college lives in the home and gives some assistance to her grandmother
- Jewish religion, husband cantor in temple
- Retired from lighting supply company as cashier (sedentary activity)
- Has private health insurance plus Medicare
- Owns home, one level, few stairs; wheelchair ramp being built onto side of house
- Has never smoked; denies overuse of alcohol or drugs
- No known food allergies; allergic to sulfa drugs, questionable allergy to some tapes

Assessment Data

Oriented × 3 (time, place, and person)
Vital signs: T 97 rectally, P 62, R 20, BP 162/78.
Weight on admission: 362 lb. (bed scale)
Current weight: 351 lbs (6 days later)
Height: 5 ft 1 in

Skin: Multiple open weepy blisters on left thigh and right arm, both draining clear fluid; many open areas on back of thighs and buttocks; evidence of irritation from scratching; blister on right great toe, covered with bandage.

Respiratory: Decreased breath sounds in lower lobes bilaterally; bibasilar crackles (rales) heard; upper lobes clear to ascultation.

Cardiovascular: Apical pulse 68, regular rhythm; neck veins distended.

Abdominal: Pendulous abdomen with many fatty indentations; difficult to hear bowel sounds because of depth of adipose tissue; girth 64 to 68 inches; abdomen nontender, soft on palpation; Midline scars from previous surgeries

Musculoskeletal: Grossly edematous extremities, 3 + pitting edema; negative pedal, posterior tibial, popliteal pulses; positive femoral pulses felt bilaterally

Urinary: Foley catheter draining cloudy urine, specific gravity 1.024

Laboratory data

Hgb 9.1, Hct 29, blood sugar 212
BUN 63 (normal 5-20)
Creatinine clearance 3.7 (normal 0.8-1.4 mg/dl)
K 5.2, Na 136
O_2 sat 94-97 on oxygen at 2 L, drops to 78-80 when off oxygen

Medications

40 units NPH insulin daily in morning

Nursing Care Plan

PATIENT WITH CONGESTIVE HEART FAILURE AND OLIGURIA—CONT'D

Past Medical History	Psychosocial Data	Assessment Data
Sleep apnea, prefers to sleep in recliner Chronic renal failure, requires diuretics daily Atrial fibrillation in past, responded to meds; cardioversion in the emergency department—first time needed		4 units regular insulin/coverage if blood sugar over 160 prednisone 15 mg PO daily verapamil (Calan) SR 240 mg PO daily procainamide (Procan) SR 500 mg PO tid digitalis 0.125 mg PO bid docusate sodium (Colace) 100 mg PO bid Ducolax 10 mg × 1 prn constipation (rectally) Diet: 1800-calorie ADA diet, with 800 ml fluid restriction

NURSING DIAGNOSIS

Decreased cardiac output related to cardiac failure, as evidenced by increasing shortness of breath and inability to perform activities of daily living (ADLs)

NURSING INTERVENTIONS	EVALUATION OF EXPECTED OUTCOMES
Monitor BP, pulse, cardiac rhythm, temperature, and breath sounds every 4 hours. Record and report changes from baseline. Take temperature rectally if dyspnea present. Carefully monitor I & O and specific gravity every 4 hours. Monitor BUN, creatinine, electrolytes, Hgb, and Hct. Discuss patient's food preferences, and plan according to dietary restrictions. Assist her with meal planning. Provide mouth care every 4 hours. Keep her mucous membranes moist with a water-soluble lubricant. Keep on oxygen at 2 L via nasal cannula. Explain the rationale for not increasing the oxygen above 2 L at home. Support patient with positive feedback about adherences to restrictions. Give skin care every 4 hours. Examine skin daily for signs of breakdown/infection. Change patient's position at least every 2 hours. Elevate edematous extremities. Maintain on bedrest while dyspnea present. Teach patient to conserve energy. Increase her level of activity as tolerated. Ambulate with assistance until patient's strength improves. Apply antiembolism stockings to increase venous return. Remove for 1 hour every 8 hours. Teach patient foods that are rich in potassium (bananas, all citrus fruits and juices, broccoli, bran flakes, raw carrots, prunes).	Patient has less shortness of breath; gradually shows improvement in her ability to perform ADLs without undue fatigue BP will remain within normal range; signs of hyperkalemia, (peaked or elevated T waves, prolonged P-R intervals, widened QRS complexes or depressed ST segments) do not appear on ECG Patient's I&O remain within established limits: intake of no more than 800 ml daily and output no less than 25 ml per hour Skin remains free of infection and shows signs of healing, with no new blisters apparent Patient identifies the signs and symptoms to report to her physician Urine specific gravity remains between 1.010 and 1.020 Hct stays above 30 BUN, creatinine, sodium, and potassium stay within acceptable levels Patient participates in passive exercises every 1 to 2 hours when awake Patient demonstrates her skill in selecting permitted food

continued

NURSING DIAGNOSIS

Fluid volume excess related to congestive heart failure

NURSING INTERVENTIONS	EVALUATION OF EXPECTED OUTCOMES
Weigh daily before breakfast. Check for signs of further dependent edema, such as sacral edema, increasing pitting edema, and increased ascites. Monitor fluid restriction of 800 ml; help patient to make a schedule for timed amounts. Provide sour hard candy to decrease thirst and improve taste. Explain the reasons for fluid and dietary restrictions. Assess skin turgor for signs of dehydration. Measure abdominal girth daily; compare to previous measurements. Provide sodium-restricted diet; teach foods low in sodium. Administer diuretics as ordered; monitor for increased output as response. Assess for peripheral edema; measure girths to check for decreases. Explain the cause for fluid volume excess. Provide information regarding congestive heart failure, the relationship of diet, medications, activity, and followup care. Ask patient to repeat back teachings; check for any misinformation.	Body weight will decrease by 2 to 3 lbs daily; hemodynamic status will be restored to normal range Pulmonary status will be restored to an acceptable range Patient reports less dyspnea and experiences more comfort Urine specific gravity will decrease as urine output increases Electrolyte levels, BUN, and creatinine will return to as nearly normal a range as possible Patient plans a 24-hour-intake schedule Patient and family demonstrate adequate knowledge of how excess fluid volume affects congestive heart failure Patient states the rationales for restricted fluids, medications, and the need for compliance to orders Complications of excess fluid do not remain

NURSING DIAGNOSIS

Self-care deficit related to shortness of breath, morbid obesity, and fatigue, as evidenced by her inability to carry out aspects of self-care such as bathing and personal hygiene

NURSING INTERVENTIONS	EVALUATION OF EXPECTED OUTCOMES
Identify patient's optimum time to attempt self-care (morning, after a period of rest after breakfast). Provide privacy. Encourage a discussion of feelings related to body size and overall edema. Provide dignity to nursing care by showing feelings of acceptance. Place all articles of self-care within her reach. Praise patient for any attempts of self-care. Allow ample time to perform tasks. Rewarm the bath water if cold. Monitor for fatigue. Encourage her to plan rest periods before moving on to new tasks. Assist her when necessary. Check her color and overall adaptations. Provide constructive feedback.	Patient grows in her ability to perform some self-care needs Demonstrates the use of assistive devices Performs some parts of the tasks of bathing and personal hygiene Discusses and shows signs of acceptance of her body image Grows in her ability to accept constructive feedback, and plans ways to incorporate new learnings after discharge

NURSING DIAGNOSIS

Constipation related to immobility and diet, as evidenced by hard, formed stool and painful defecation

NURSING INTERVENTIONS	EVALUATION OF EXPECTED OUTCOMES
Assess bowel sounds and bowel habits daily. Consult with dietician for use of prune juice as a fruit exchange. Administer docusate sodium (Colace) or Dulcolax as needed. Encourage as much movement as possible when awake. Progressive ambulation is best once dyspnea decreases. Discuss foods that are high in bulk and roughage. Provide commode at bedside. Maintain privacy. Allow time for evacuation. Keep toilet articles within reach. Instruct patient to avoid straining if possible. Tell patient that abdominal massage may relieve discomfort and promote defecation.	Patient has less pain on defecation Bowel pattern returns to a more normal pattern for her Patient identifies the relationships among inactivity, diet, and bowel habits Patient uses the dietician as a resource person to discuss food exchanges and foods high in fiber and bulk

KEY CONCEPTS

- Assessment, palpation, percussion, and auscultation are essential components of a physical examination.
- Arrhythmias can be detected by the nurse when taking a radial pulse.
- Ventricular tachycardia requires immediate intervention.
- When a patient is to receive a mechanical stimulator such as a pacemaker, complete teaching and gentle reassurance by the nurse is essential.
- Nonpharmacologic and pharmacologic measures are used to treat hypertension.
- Relieving anxiety in the patient who has had a heart attack is a significant responsibility for nurses.
- When nurses, physicians, and laypersons perform CPR and the Heimlich maneuver in emergency situations, countless lives are saved.

CRITICAL THINKING EXERCISES

1. Describe how the risk factors for development of coronary artery disease differ between men and women.
2. Discuss why patients with hypertension have difficulty complying with prescribed lifestyle and medication therapies.
3. Why would blood in the right atrium be darker than blood in the left atrium?
4. What symptoms exhibited by a patient would cause you to withhold a dose of digitalis?

REFERENCES AND ADDITIONAL READINGS

Barden C and others: Balloon aortic valvuloplasty: nursing care implications, *Crit Care Nurs* 10(6):22-30, 1990.

Berne RM, Levy MN: *Principles of physiology,* 1990, St Louis, Mosby.

Bongard RS, Sue DY: *Current critical care diagnosis and treatment,* Norwalk, Conn, 1994, Appleton and Lange.

Bowers AC, Thompson JM: *Clinical Manual of Health Assessment,* ed 4, St Louis, 1992, Mosby.

Brewer C, Markis J: Streptokinase and tissue plasminogen activator in acute myocardial infarction, *Heart Lung* 15(6): 552-568, 1986.

Budny J, Anderson-Drevs K: IV inotropic agents: dopamine, dobutamine, and amrinone. *Crit Care Nurse* 10(2):54-62, 1990.

Chandrasoma P, Taylor CR: *Concise pathology,* Norwalk, Conn, 1991, Appleton & Lange.

Conover MB: *Understanding electrocardiology,* ed 6, St Louis, 1992, Mosby.

Cuny J, Enger EL: Management of chronic heart failure, *Crit Care Nurs Clin N Am,* 5(4):573-587, 1993.

Dossey BM, Guzzetta CE, Kenner CV: *Critical care nursing: body-mind-spirit,* ed 3, Philadelphia, 1992, JB Lippincott.

Douglas PS: *Cardiovascular health and disease in women,* Philadelphia, 1993, WB Saunders.

Drew B: Cardiac electrophysiology, *Crit Care Nurs Clin N Am,* 6(1):xv, 1994.

Flynn JM, Bruce NP: *Introduction to critical care skills,* St Louis, 1993, Mosby.

Ganong WF: *Review of medical physiology,* ed 16, Norwalk, Conn, 1993, Appleton & Lange.

Goodkind J, Coombs V, Golobic RA: Excimer laser angioplasty, *Heart Lung* 22(1):26-35, 1993.

Grauer K: *A practical guide to ECG interpretation,* St Louis, 1992, Mosby.

Guyton AC: *Textbook of medical physiology,* ed 8, Philadelphia, 1990, WB Saunders.

Guzetta CE, Dossey BM: *Cardiovascular nursing: holistic practice,* St Louis, 1992, Mosby.

Halfman-Franey M, Levine S: Intracoronary stents, *Crit Care Nurs Clin N Am* 1(2):327-337, 1989.

Huang SH and others: Cardiac rehabilitation of the myocardial infarction patient. In Huang SH and others, editors: *Coronary care nursing,* Philadelphia, 1989, WB Saunders.

Hudak CM, Gallo BM, Benz JJ: *Critical care nursing,* Philadelphia, 1990, JB Lippincott.

Hurst JW: *Cardiovascular diagnosis: the initial exam,* St Louis, 1993, Mosby.

Kaplan N: *Clinical hypertension,* ed 6, Baltimore, 1994, Williams & Wilkins.

Kinney MR, Packa DR, Dunbar SB: *AACN's Clinical reference for critical-care nursing,* St Louis, 1993, Mosby.

Lilly LS: *Pathophysiology of heart disease,* Malvern, Pa, 1993, Lea & Febiger.

Lipman BC, Cascio T: *ECG: assessment and interpretation,* Philadelphia, 1994, FA Davis.

McKance KL, Heuther SE: *Pathophysiology: the biologic basis for disease in adults and children,* St Louis, 1994, Mosby.

Opie LH: *Drugs for the heart,* ed 3, Philadelphia, 1991, WB Saunders.

Perloff D: Hypertension in women. In Douglas PS, Brest AN, editors: *Heart disease in women,* Philadelphia, 1989, FA Davis.

Porth CM: *Pathophysiology: concepts of altered health states,* ed 4, Philadelphia, 1994, JB Lippincott.

Puleo PR and others: Use of a rapid assay of subforms of creatine kinase MB to diagnose or rule out acute myocardial infarction, *N Engl J Med* 331(9):561-566, 1994.

Purcell JA: Cardiac electrical activity. In Kinney MR, Packa DR, Dunbar SB: *AACN's clinical reference for critical-care nursing,* St Louis, 1993, Mosby.

Rippe, JM: *Manual of intensive care medicine,* ed 2, Boston, 1989, Little, Brown.

Sabiston, DC: *Textbook of surgery,* ed 14, Philadelphia, 1991, WB Saunders.

Seidel HM and others: *Mosby's guide to physical examination,* ed 3, St Louis, 1995, Mosby.

Standards and guidelines for cardiopulmonary resuscitation (CPR) and emergency cardiac care (ECC), *JAMA* 255:2905-2984, 1986.

Stewart SL and others: Cardiac surgery. In Kinney MR, Packa DR, Dunbar, SB: *AACN's Clinical reference for critical-care nursing,* St Louis, 1993, Mosby.

Thelan LA and others: *Critical care nursing: diagnosis and management,* St Louis, 1994, Mosby.

Thompson JM and others: *Mosby's clinical nursing,* ed 3, St Louis, 1993, Mosby.

Toscone NC and others: Discharge teaching for the directional coronary atherectomy patient, *Dimens Crit Care Nurs* 13(4):208-217, 1994.

Underhill SL and others: *Cardiac nursing,* ed 2, Philadelphia, 1989, JB Lippincott.

Underhill SL and others: *Cardiovascular medications for cardiac nursing,* Philadelphia, 1990, JB Lippincott.

Vitello-Cicciu J, Morrissey AM: Coronary artery disease. In Kinney MR, Packa DR, Dunbar, SB: *AACN's Clinical reference for critical-care nursing,* St Louis, 1993, Mosby.

Walthall SA and others: Routine withholding of digitalis for heart rate below 60 beats per minute: widespread misconceptions, *Heart Lung,* 22(6):472-476, 1993.

Wilson JD and others: *Harrison's principles of internal medicine,* ed 12, New York, 1991, McGraw-Hill.

CHAPTER 22

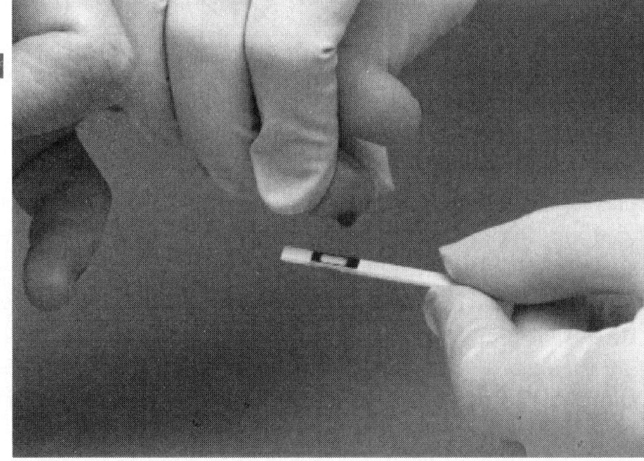

Blood

CHAPTER OBJECTIVES

1 Discuss the importance of the blood components as a measure of health and illness.
2 Describe the common diagnostic tests for blood disorders.
3 Differentiate among hemorrhagic, iron-deficiency, pernicious, sickle cell, and aplastic anemias according to their pathophysiologic features and nursing assessment and intervention.
4 Discuss the significance of leukocytosis and leukopenia as indicators of illness.
5 Discuss the nursing care plan for the patient with leukemia and anemia.
6 Discuss the pathophysiology, assessment, and nursing interventions in caring for patients with hemorrhagic disorders.

KEY WORDS

anemia
autologous blood transfusion
blood dyscrasias
cryoprecipitate
ecchymoses
erythrocytes
erythropoiesis
erythropoietin
granulocytes
granulocytopenia
hemoglobin electrophoresis
hemophilia
Hodgkin's disease
homeostasis
leukapheresis
leukemia
leukocytes
leukocytosis
leukopenia
molecule
petechiae
phlebotomy
plasma pheresis
polycythemia
purpura
sickle cell anemia
splenomegaly
thrombocytes
viscosity

FUNCTION OF BLOOD

The circulatory system is the transportation system of the body. Through its vast network of vessels, blood carries oxygen to the cells and returns carbon dioxide to the lungs to be eliminated. It transports food to nourish the cells so that they may carry on their normal functions and carries away waste products of cell metabolism. Water, electrolytes, hormones, and enzymes, all of which have important functions in keeping the body in a state of equilibrium **(homeostasis),** are transported by the blood. Heat is carried by the blood, thereby regulating body temperature. Immune cells and antibodies that help to prevent disease are also important parts of the blood. Through a complex system, the blood provides clotting factors and prevents serious loss of fluids in case of injury. It also prevents clot formation in blood vessels, which would seriously interfere with the oxygen supply to the cells. Any disease or condition that affects the blood or its transport system may pose a serious threat to the individual.

STRUCTURE OF BLOOD

The blood is slightly sticky and has a characteristic odor and a faint salty taste. It is bright red in the arteries because it is carrying oxygen; it is dark red in the veins because the cells have taken up the oxygen and the blood is carrying carbon dioxide to be eliminated by the respiratory system. The blood is composed of two parts: the liquid part, called *plasma,* which constitutes slightly more than half of the total volume; and the formed elements, or cells. The cells have been divided into several groups: (1) **erythrocytes,** or red blood cells; (2) **leukocytes,** or white blood cells; and (3) **thrombocytes,** or platelets.

Blood volume remains fairly constant in one person, but there are variations among individuals. Factors such as age, sex, size of the body frame, and the amount of adipose tissue may affect the volume of circulating blood.

Plasma

Plasma contains no cells and is estimated to be approximately 90% water. It is a clear, straw-colored fluid with a large number of substances dissolved in it. Among the most important of these substances are the *plasma proteins,* which include *serum albumin, serum globulin,* and *fibrinogen* (Figure 22-1). The proteins have some individual functions, but all of them are important in nutrition and regulation of blood volume through osmotic pressure. Serum albumin, in particular, influences blood volume because it comprises more than half of the total proteins. Serum globulins are divided into α-(alpha), β-(beta), and γ-(gamma) globulins. The γ-globulins are significant in the immune response because they are the body's antibodies. Fibrinogen contributes to blood coagulation through its role in the formation of fibrin. Other substances dissolved in plasma include urea, uric acid, glucose, respiratory gases, hormones, and electrolytes. Minute amounts of other substances essential to the body are also found in plasma. Plasma can be separated from the formed elements, and because it contains the proteins that assist in the clotting of blood, it may be administered for several bleeding disorders.

Erythrocytes

Formation

Erythrocytes are formed in the red bone marrow, which develops in the pelvis, vertebrae, ribs, skull, and proximal ends of the femur and humerus (Beare, Myers, 1994). Before birth the production is carried on by the liver and the spleen. The production of erythrocytes, **erythropoiesis,** is a continuous process, and in the absence of disease, the number remains relatively constant.

Number

The number of erythrocytes is usually slightly higher in men (4.5 to 6 million/mm^3 blood) than in women (4.3 to 5.5 million/mm^3 blood). In the newborn infant the number may be increased (5 to 7 million/mm^3 blood), but it gradually decreases to adult levels by 15 years of age. Recent discovery of substances called hematopoietic growth factors has contributed to an understanding of erythrocyte homeostasis. **Erythropoietin** is one of the growth factors that stimulates marrow production of red blood cells. It is thought that the kidney produces erythropoietin in response to low tissue oxygen levels. In addition to the growth factors, effective erythropoiesis requires healthy bone marrow with normal stem cell populations and adequate supplies of folic acid, vitamin B_{12}, and iron.

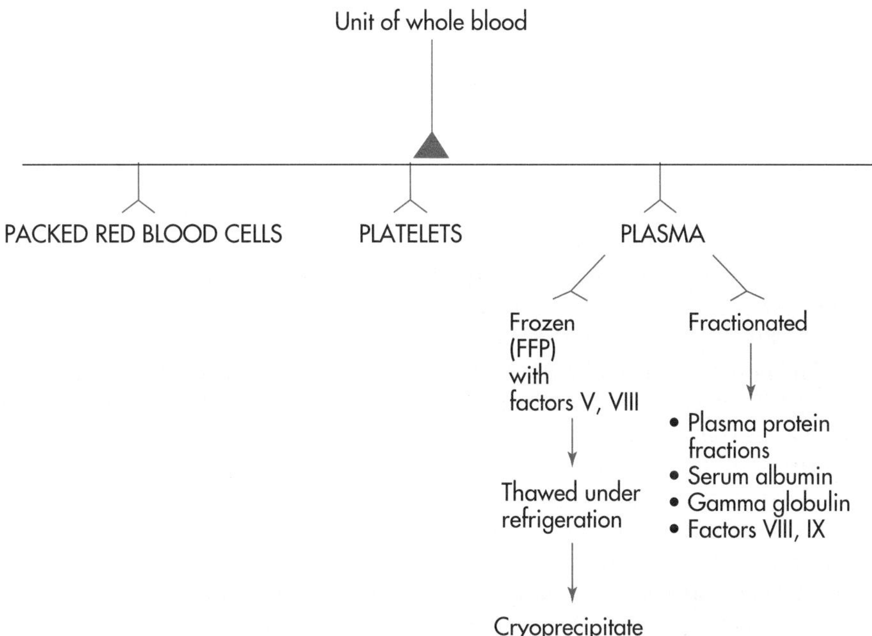

Figure 22-1 Reduction of unit of whole blood into fractions.

Hemoglobin

The main ingredient of the erythrocyte is hemoglobin. Within each red blood cell there are millions of molecules of hemoglobin. The amount of hemoglobin in the red blood cell depends on adequate iron storage, which is essential for the synthesis of hemoglobin and for the oxygen-carrying ability of the hemoglobin **molecule.** Hemoglobin carries oxygen to the cells of the body, and thus the amount of oxygen available to the cells depends on the amount of hemoglobin in the blood. Hemoglobin is measured in grams per deciliter of blood, whereas red blood cells are measured in millions per cubic millimeter of blood.

Blood loss

Loss of blood through hemorrhage causes a decrease in the amount of circulating fluid, the number of red blood cells, the amount of hemoglobin, and, in turn, the amount of iron. Because the oxygen-carrying power of the blood has been decreased, the heart must work harder to supply the cells with oxygen. Thus a person suffering from loss of blood may be expected to have an increased pulse rate. There will also be an increase in the respiration rate as the body attempts to provide more oxygen for circulation.

Chronic blood loss also causes anemia, although the blood volume in the vascular system is stabilized more readily. Certain diseases of the blood and blood-forming organs may affect the production of erythrocytes so that the number is decreased or their structure is immature. In some genetic diseases, the erythrocytes may have an abnormal shape. In contrast to the disease states mentioned that cause anemia, some disorders cause an overproduction of erythrocytes. Having too many red blood cells in the circulation is undesirable and may at times be life threatening.

Leukocytes

Formation

Leukocytes, in a manner similar to that of erythrocytes and thrombocytes, arise from stem cells in bone marrow. Disorders of white blood cells can result from overproduction, underproduction, or abnormal maturation of any one or all leukocyte cell lines.

Number

Leukocytes, or white blood cells, are not as numerous as the erythrocytes, or red blood cells. The number of white blood cells in 1 mm^3 of blood varies between 5000 and 10,000. The number is essentially the same for men and women. When there is an increase of more than 10,000 white blood cells, it may indicate the presence of some pathologic condition. Such an increase is called **leukocytosis.** Under some conditions, there may be a decrease in the number of leukocytes, which is called **leukopenia.** ***Granulocytopenia*** is a term that is used interchangeably with leukopenia but refers specifically to a low number of circulating granulocytes or neutrophils.

Classification

Leukocytes are classified as granular or nongranular, depending on the color of their cytoplasm and the shape of their nuclei. Granular leukocytes are called **granulocytes,** and approximately 50% to 75% of leukocytes are granulocytes. Approximately 50% of the mature granulocytes released from the bone marrow into the circulation adhere to the walls of small blood vessels. The remainder pass from the circulation into the tissues to perform their specific functions. The granulocytes are divided into three types: *neutrophils, basophils,* and *eosinophils.* The nongranular leukocytes, or *agranulocytes,* comprise less than one third of the cells and include the *lymphocytes* and *monocytes.*

Granulocytes. The primary function of the *neutrophils* is *phagocytosis,* the ingestion and digestion of debris and foreign material throughout the body. They are the first cells to arrive at the scene when an inflammatory reaction is stimulated. Neutrophils are attracted to the foreign substance in response to chemicals that are released from inflamed tissue. Neutrophils are also referred to as myelocytes, "polys," and granulocytes.

The *basophils* do not phagocytize material but contain powerful chemicals such as histamine that can be released locally. They are important during the inflammatory process in modulating the formation of clots and their growth. The specific function of these cells is not completely understood.

The *eosinophils* appear to play a role in allergic or foreign protein reactions and are elevated in number in patients with allergies or parasitic infestations.

Agranulocytes. The monocytes become larger phagocytic cells when stimulated and play an important role in the inflammatory process. Lymphocytes are the primary cells concerned with the development of immunity. Although they arise from stem cells in the bone marrow, maturation occurs in the lymphatic or reticuloendothelial systems.

The leukocytes have many functions in the body, and their mobility allows them to protect the body from infection and to repair damaged tissue. A count of white blood cells is often an important aid to the physician in establishing a diagnosis. For example, in suspected acute appendicitis, an increase in the number of white blood cells, together with clinical symptoms, may indicate to the physician the need for an appendectomy (Thibodeau, Patton, 1993).

Differential count

A differential count is a measure of the total number of white blood cells and the percentage of each of the five classes. For many patients, one drop of blood obtained from a fingertip is sufficient for this test. After the specimen is placed on a slide, it is examined under a microscope, and each type of leukocyte is identified and counted. Each type of cell is reported as a percentage of all classes of white blood cells. In various diseases certain kinds of cells may be increased; for example, in some bacterial infections, the number of lymphocytes may increase.

Thrombocytes

Formation

Thrombocytes, or platelets, are tiny, fragile elements in the blood. They are formed in red bone marrow and are thought to be minute fragments of larger cells called *megakaryocytes.*

Number

The exact number of platelets is unknown, but various estimates have placed the number from 150,000 to 500,000/mm^3 of blood. In the hemorrhagic disorder called *thrombocytopenia,* a decrease in the number of platelets may cause serious bleeding, whereas in other diseases there may be an abnormally high number of platelets, called *thrombocytosis.*

Function

The primary function of platelets is to control bleeding. When an injury to a blood vessel occurs, the platelets concentrate at the site of the injury and control bleeding by forming thrombotic plugs and by releasing a substance, factor III, which is necessary for coagulation and the formation of fibrin. They continue their activity in helping to shrink the clots and bring together the margins of the damaged vessel.

THERAPEUTIC BLOOD FRACTIONS

Blood may be broken down into its component parts so that patients with certain conditions may be given specific blood fractions to meet their individual needs (Table 22-1; see Figure 22-1).

Blood Plasma

Plasma may be separated from whole blood that has been stored, or it may be separated from fresh blood taken from a donor and immediately frozen. The primary use of plasma is to treat conditions in which clotting of the blood is defective. When fresh blood plasma is used, it contains all of the factors essential for clotting, including the antihemophilic factor.

TABLE 22-1

Pharmacology of Drugs, Blood, and Blood By-Products

Drug (Generic and Trade Name); Route and Dosage	Action/Indication	Common Side Effects and Nursing Considerations
EPOETIN ALFA (Epogen) **ROUTE:** IV, subcutaneous **DOSAGE:** IV or SQ 50-100 units/kg 3 times weekly, then adjust dosage by increments of 25 units/kg to maintain hematocrit	Treatment of anemia associated with chronic renal failure and for anemia secondary to AZT in HIV-infected	Hypertension or seizures; use may increase need for heparin in dialysis
FOLIC ACID (folate, vitamin B_9) **ROUTE:** PO, IM, SQ, PO **DOSAGE:** 0.25 to 1.0 mg/day for anemia. 0.1 to 1.0 mg/day as dietary supplement	Used in treatment of anemia and given during pregnancy to promote normal fetal development	Use with caution in uncorrected pernicious anemia
IRON (FERROUS) SALTS **ROUTE:** PO, IV, IM **DOSAGE:** PO 200 mg/day; IM, IV total dose = 0.0476 × kg × (14.8 − patient hemoglobin) + 1 ml/5 kg up to 14 ml for iron stores	Treatment and prevention of iron deficiency anemias	Hypotension, staining at IM site, constipation, diarrhea, nausea, dark stools, epigastric pain, and staining of teeth in liquid preparations; use cautiously with peptic ulcer and inflammatory bowel disease
PHYTONADIONE (AquaMEPHYTON, Vitamin K_1) **ROUTE:** PO, IM, SQ **DOSAGE:** 2.5 to 10 mg, repeat PO in 12-48 hr if necessary; SQ or IM in neonates 0.5 to 1.0 mg within 1 hour of birth	Prevention and treatment of anemias; antidote for overdose of salicylates and oral anticoagulants; nutritional deficiencies and prolonged total parenteral nutrition; prevention of hemorrhagic disease in the newborn	Large doses counter the effects of oral anticoagulants; cautious use in liver disease
ALBUMIN **ROUTE:** IV in 5% solution: 250 ml and 500 ml; 25% solution: 50 ml and 100 ml **DOSAGE:** 5% solution infuse 1 to 10 ml/minute, or more rapidly if patient in shock; 25% solution infuse 0.2 to 0.4 ml/minute	Blood by-product used for acute liver failure, burns, and hemolytic disease of newborn, as well as volume expansion when crystalloid solutions are not adequate; shock and massive hemorrhage	Cross match not necessary; cannot be used as plasma substitute because albumin contains no clotting factors; watch for circulatory overload hypertension
CRYOPRECIPITATE AND FACTOR VIII **ROUTE:** IV 5 to 20 ml depending on preparation method **DOSAGE:** Rapidly 1 to 2 ml/min	Both are blood by-products; Cryo used to treat von Willebrand's disease, hypofibrinogenemia, or factor XIII deficiency; Factor VIII used for deficiencies, including hemophilia type A	ABO compatibility preferred; contraindicated in undefined coagulation deficiency; watch for infectious diseases and allergic reactions
FACTOR II, VII, IX, AND X COMPLEXES **ROUTE:** IV **DOSAGE:** Infuse 2 to 3 ml/min	Freeze-dried prepared blood by-product made from pooled plasma; used for hemophilia type B, congenital factor VII or X deficiency	Cross matching not necessary; use only with specific factor deficiency; watch for allergic reactions and infectious diseases

continued

TABLE 22-1

Pharmacology of Drugs, Blood, and Blood By-Products—cont'd

Drug (Generic and Trade Name); Route and Dosage	Action/Indication	Common Side Effects and Nursing Considerations
GRANULOCYTES **ROUTE:** IV, with platelets 200 to 400 ml; without platelets 100 to 200 ml **DOSAGE:** Very slowly, approximately 50 ml/hr, for up to 4 hours	Blood by-product used for antibiotic-resistant neutropenia or congenital WBC dysfunction; sometimes used as prophylaxis for infection when conventional therapies have failed	Cross matching not necessary, but must be ABO compatible; watch for circulatory overload and increased incidence of febrile, nonhemolytic reactions
PLASMA **ROUTE:** IV, 185 to 225 ml/bag **DOSAGE:** May be infused rapidly—10 ml to 20 ml over 3 minutes, or slowly if potential for circulatory overload exists	Blood by-product separated from RBC and frozen within 6 hours after collection; contains plasma proteins, fibrinogen, and factors V, VIII, and IX, as well as water, electrolytes, sugars, proteins, vitamins, minerals, hormones, and antibodies; used to increase levels of clotting factors when there is a deficiency	Cross matching not necessary and must be ABO compatible; not for nutritional supplementation or volume expansion; watch for infectious diseases, allergic reactions, circulatory overload, and hemolytic reactions
PLATELETS (platelet concentrate) **ROUTE:** IV, 50 to 70 ml **DOSAGE:** May be infused rapidly—1 unit in 10 minutes or less; must be infused within 4 hours	Platelets are blood by-products centrifuged from plasma; used for bleeding as a result of deficiency in platelet function or number	Cross matching not necessary, but ABO compatibility preferred; watch for infectious diseases and septic, toxic, allergic, or febrile reactions
RED BLOOD CELLS (packed RBCs) **ROUTE:** IV, 250 ml to 350 ml, depending on specific bag volume **DOSAGE:** Infuse up to 4 hours only	Blood by-product prepared by removing up to 90% of the plasma; used for blood loss and anemia	Cross matching and ABO compatibility necessary; watch for all hemolytic, febrile, and allergic reactions (including uticaria up to anaphylactic shock); also circulatory overload, hyperkalemia as a result of potassium release, hepatitis, HIV, CMV, and other infectious diseases; watch for reactions; especially with massive transfusion
WHOLE BLOOD **ROUTE:** IV, 400 to 500 ml **DOSAGE:** Infuse over no more than 4 hr	Whole blood consists of RBC, platelets, plasma, anticoagulant, and preservative; when stored, it loses clotting factors and releases potassium; used to treat acute, massive blood loss, but is not often given; instead crystalloid and colloid solutions, RBC, or other blood components are given	Cross matching and ABO compatibility is necessary; watch for all reactions as mentioned for RBC transfusion

Platelets

Platelets may be separated from whole blood and administered to patients with severe hematologic disorders, open heart surgery, and postoperative bleeding. The demand for platelets has increased, and it is now believed that patients who are bleeding from any site, internal or external, and whose platelet count is below 20,000/mm^3 of blood should receive platelets. The administration of platelets has been a lifesaving measure for many patients who are receiving chemotherapy for malignant disorders.

Platelets are administered most often in the form of a concentrate that has been separated from one or more units of whole blood. The advantage of the platelet concentrate is that it may be infused in only 50 ml of fluid. When long-term administration is required, it avoids overloading the circulatory system.

Pheresis

In **plasma pheresis,** pheresed platelets that are matched with human lymphocyte antigen (HLA) are preferred over pooled or random donor platelets for patients who are at risk for developing antibodies to donor platelet antigens. The life span and functional capacities of platelets are diminished when these antibodies develop. This also interferes with successful bone marrow transplantation. With the exception of hemolytic reactions, the patient receiving platelets may have reactions similar to those from whole blood transfusions. Therefore close observation of the patient is essential.

Plasma Protein Fractions

Plasma proteins may also be given as individual blood components.

γ-Globulin

The primary use of γ-globulin is in the prevention or modification of infectious disease. Immune human γ-globulins are fractions of blood obtained from persons with circulating antibodies against a specific disease. Such persons may have antibodies as a result of having had the disease or having been immunized against it. When administered to nonimmune persons, immune human γ-globulin prevents disease or complications of diseases such as tetanus, mumps, pertussis, or rubella.

Serum albumin

Purified human serum albumin may be administered to maintain **osmotic pressure** of the plasma. It is useful in any condition in which the albumin/globulin ratio has been lowered. It may be administered to burn patients, as well as to treat hypovolemic shock and liver disease.

Fibrinogen

Fibrinogen is an essential factor for clotting blood. A deficiency may be a congenital disorder or an acquired condition resulting from massive hemorrhage, prolonged active bleeding, or other hematologic conditions dependent on the clotting mechanism.

Cryoprecipitate

Cryoprecipitate, prepared by the thawing of fresh frozen plasma, contains an average of 150 mg of fibrinogen and is used to restore a patient's clotting factors to normal ranges (American Red Cross, 1994). Cryoprecipitate also contains factor VIII (the antihemophilic factor), factor XIII, and von Willebrand's factor. A deficiency in any one of these coagulation factors can result in severe bleeding. Cryoprecipitate may be used to correct the deficit. However, replacing the specific factor concentrate that is deficient is usually preferred (American Red Cross, 1994).

Packed Red Blood Cells

Packed red blood cells are red blood cells without the plasma. The cells and the plasma are separated by centrifugation of whole blood. In conditions in which the blood volume is normal but the number of red blood cells and amount of hemoglobin are decreased, packed red blood cells may be given to the patient. Because packed red blood cells are placed in only a small amount of fluid, the danger of overloading the circulatory system is avoided. The removal of plasma containing white blood cells and antibodies reduces the risk of allergic reaction. To provide safer transfusions to recipients, whole blood is rarely administered except when specifically indicated, as in the case of massive hemorrhage or total blood transfusions to newborns.

Leukocytes

Leukocytes may be obtained through a special process called **leukapheresis** (or granulocytapheresis). Because leukocytes cannot be obtained in sufficient amounts from a single unit of blood, it is necessary to obtain them from a single compatible donor by removing the leukocytes and replacing the blood. The procedure yields leukocytes that are predominantly granulocytes. Recipients of this component are those with life-threatening, low white blood cell counts who have infections that are unresponsive to antibiotic therapy; those with leukemia or immunosuppressive disorders; and those undergoing extensive field radiation therapy or intensive chemotherapy. Granulocytes have a short survival time and must be infused as soon as possible after collection, in less than 24 hours. The infusion must be given slowly, and the recipient should be observed closely for negative reactions. The long-term therapeutic benefit of granulocyte transfusion is still questionable and continues to be evaluated.

COLLECTION OF BLOOD

The collection and storage of blood began during World War II. Because of the progress of medical science, whole blood, plasma, and blood fractions have become essential to the practice of modern medicine. Along with the increased demand have come improved methods of collection, storage, and distribution. At present there are three main collection systems: the American Red Cross, hospitals, and commercial centers. The American Red Cross maintains regional centers for the collection of blood and mobile units that may be taken to communities, industrial plants, or college campuses. The arrival of the mobile unit is usually the culmination of drives for donors sponsored by local citizens. Most hospitals collect blood to meet their individual needs. Donors often are members of the patient's family, friends of the patient, or other persons interested in the patient. In an emergency, when large amounts of blood may be needed, the hospital may call on citizens of the community or the American Red Cross to help meet its needs. In most instances donors to hospitals and the American Red Cross do not receive payment for their blood. Commercial centers that offer a small fee to donors have come under attack and are being scrutinized. They often are banned by state governments.

Testing

Although all prospective donors are examined and interviewed, donors may be unwilling or unable to provide an accurate history about exposure to and incidence of blood-transmitted diseases, including acquired immunodeficiency syndrome (AIDS), hepatitis, syphilis, malaria, cytomegalovirus (CMV), or Epstein-Barr virus. Therefore the Federal Drug Administration (FDA) requires that all donated blood be tested for antibodies to human immunodeficiency virus (anti-HIV); hepatitis B surface antigen (HB_sAg); antibody to hepatitis B core antigen (anti-HB_c); antibody to hepatitis C virus (anti-HCV); antibody to human T-cell lymphotropic virus, type I (anti-HTLV-I); and syphilis. However, such donor screening and testing does not totally eliminate the risk of transmitting disease by transfusion (American Red Cross, 1994).

Autologous Blood

In many areas blood collection agencies can store autologous (one's own) blood for use in elective surgery. Recent technologic developments also allow the reinfusion of a patient's blood shed during and after surgical procedures. These developments contribute to the safer use of blood products but have limited application in high blood use groups.

NURSING RESPONSIBILITIES FOR DIAGNOSTIC TESTS

A large number of blood tests are done for diagnostic purposes, but some are useful in guiding the physician in the course and treatment of disease. Some tests are performed on capillary blood and require only a few drops, which is usually secured by pricking the finger or the earlobe. Blood for other tests requiring a larger amount of blood is secured from a vein with a needle and syringe. Some of the more common tests are reviewed here, and others are found in different sections of this book, according to their relation to specific diseases. Table 22-2 lists normal hematologic values for various diagnostic tests.

Complete Blood Count

The complete blood count (CBC) is the most common of all tests made on the blood. It consists of a count of the erythrocytes and leukocytes, measurement of hemoglobin and hematocrit, and a differential count of the leukocytes. A platelet count is often included. The physician orders the examination, which is made by persons trained in laboratory methods. However, it is often the responsibility of the nurse to execute the proper forms and notify the laboratory of the physician's request. Many hospitals require that routine blood counts be completed for all patients on admission, and some hospitals route the patient from the admission office to the laboratory for the examination before the patient is admitted to the clinical unit. Elevated red blood cell counts may indicate polycythemia or dehydration; lowered counts may suggest anemia. Elevated white blood cell counts may result from infection or leukemia, whereas decreased counts may suggest bone marrow depression from various causes.

Hemoglobin

Hemoglobin (Hgb) is the oxygen-carrying pigment of the red blood cells that gives blood its red color. Its

TABLE 22-2

Normal Values for Complete Blood Count Tests

Test	Normal Ranges	
White blood cells (leukocytes)	5000-10,000 mm^3	
	Absolute Values (mm^3)	**Relative Values (% of Total White Blood Cells)**
Differential white blood cell count		
Granulocytes		
Neutrophils	3000-7000	60%-70%
Eosinophils	50-400	1%-4%
Basophils	25-100	0.5%-1%
Agranulocytes		
Lymphocytes	1000-4000	20%-40%
Monocytes	100-600	2%-6%
Red blood cell count		
Men	4.5-5.4 million	
Women	3.6-5 million	
Red blood cell indices		
Mean corpuscular volume	84-99 μ^3/red blood cell	
Mean corpuscular hemoglobin	26-32 μ^3/red blood cell	
Mean corpuscular hemoglobin concentration	30%-36%	
Hematocrit values		
Men	40%-50%	
Women	37%-47%	
Hemoglobin values		
Men	14-16.5 g/dl	
Women	12-15 g/dl	
Platelet count	150,000-400,000 mm^3	
Normal values for coagulation tests		
Bleeding time		
Earlobe method	1-6 min	
Forearm method	1-9 min	
Prothrombin time	11-16 sec	
Partial thromboplastin time	30-45 sec	
Fibrinogen level	160-415 mg/dl	
Lee-White clotting time	5-10 min	

primary function is to transport oxygen from the lungs to the tissues of the body. Measurements of the total amount of hemoglobin in the peripheral blood are important in diagnosing different types of anemias. **Hemoglobin electrophoresis** is used to identify various abnormal hemoglobins in the blood. The most common abnormal hemoglobin is seen in sickle cell anemia.

Hematocrit

The test for hematocrit measures the relative volume of cells and plasma in the blood. In anemia after hemorrhage and in extracellular fluid excess, the hematocrit value is lowered; in dehydration it is increased. A microhematocrit test may be performed on capillary blood, which is secured by pricking the finger.

Coagulation Tests

Tests for coagulation measure the ability of the blood to clot, which may be affected by many factors. The criteria most commonly used to measure the clotting ability of blood are bleeding time, prothrombin time, and partial thromboplastin time (Phipps, Long, 1995).

Bleeding time

The bleeding time test measures the amount of time it takes for platelets to interact with the wall of the blood vessel to form a clot or hemostatic plug. A small stab wound is made in either the earlobe or forearm, and the time it takes for a clot to form is measured and recorded. The bleeding time test is most useful in detecting vascular abnormalities and has some value in detecting platelet abnormalities or deficiencies. Its principal use is in the diagnosis of von Willebrand's disease, a hereditary defect involving factor VII that causes excessive bleeding. It is considered a pseudohemophilia (Fischbach, 1992).

Prothrombin time

Prothrombin is converted to thrombin in the clotting process. When prothrombin time is increased, it indicates a longer time for clotting to occur. When greatly increased, the prothrombin time warns of a person at risk for bleeding or hemorrhage. The time may increase in the presence of some diseases or when the patient is receiving coumarin therapy. All patients receiving coumarin therapy should be tested often. A decreased prothrombin time may indicate intravascular clotting and suggest a patient at risk for thrombus formation.

Partial thromboplastin time

A more sensitive test than the prothrombin time is the partial thromboplastin time. The PTT, as it is commonly called, is affected by the reduction of even one of the clotting factors. Heparin dosage is often regulated by monitoring the PTT to maintain specific levels of therapy. When the PTT is greatly increased, the possibility of bleeding is also increased. Patients should be assessed for any sign of bleeding, such as ecchymoses, bleeding from gums or any body surface, tarry stools, or bloody urine. A low PTT may indicate a patient at risk for clot formation.

Sedimentation Rate

The test for sedimentation rate measures the time required for the red blood cells to settle to the bottom of a test tube, usually based on a duration of 1 hour. The test is most often used to observe the course of some diseases, such as rheumatic fever and rheumatoid arthritis.

Blood Gas Analysis

A blood gas analysis is used to measure the oxygen and carbon dioxide content of the blood and to determine the functional ability of the lungs to maintain adequate gas levels in the blood. Blood is secured from the radial or femoral artery. The test is used primarily in respiratory diseases and disorders and guides the physician in the administration of oxygen and/or medications (see Chapter 20).

Schilling Test

Intrinsic factor secreted by the gastric mucosa is necessary for the absorption of vitamin B_{12}. The Shilling test is used to diagnose pernicious anemia, in which the intrinsic factor is deficient and which results in a reduction of vitamin B_{12} absorption. Normally a person ingests and absorbs more vitamin B_{12} than needed, with the excess excreted in the urine. However, when vitamin B_{12} cannot be absorbed, it passes on through the gastrointestinal system without appearing in the urine. To perform the Schilling test, an injection of vitamin B_{12} is given to meet body needs, with subsequent administration of oral radioactive vitamin B_{12}. If absorption is unimpeded, the excess vitamin B_{12} should be found in the urine. All urine is collected for 24 hours, and the amount of radioactive vitamin B_{12} is measured. Little or no radioactive vitamin B_{12} in the urine indicates an absorption problem. The next step is to determine whether the malabsorption results from intrinsic factor deficiency or some other cause, such as intestinal disease. The Schilling test is repeated, and oral intrinsic factor is added. If the radioactive vitamin B_{12} in the urine now rises, it is clear that a intrinsic factor deficiency is the problem, which establishes a diagnosis of pernicious anemia. If radioactive vitamin B_{12} remains low, other malabsorption causes are implicated.

Bone Marrow Aspiration

Bone marrow is aspirated to obtain a specimen of cells for biopsy (Figure 22-2). Examination of the cells gives an indication of their reproductive ability and is useful in the diagnosis of certain blood dyscrasias. A local anesthetic is injected into the area surrounding the biopsy site. The most common site in adults and children over 18 months of age is the posterior iliac crest (Figure 22-3). The nurse's role is to reinforce the explanation of the procedure with the patient and to assist with positioning. Guided imagery techniques can be used to elicit patient cooperation and to minimize the pain associated with the procedure. Because of the risk of bleeding, pressure should be applied to the site for a full 5 minutes, and the patient should be closely observed (Luckmann, Sorenson, 1993). If the patient has a problem with prolonged bleeding, the puncture site should be assessed often for oozing or frank bleeding, and pressure should be applied if this occurs.

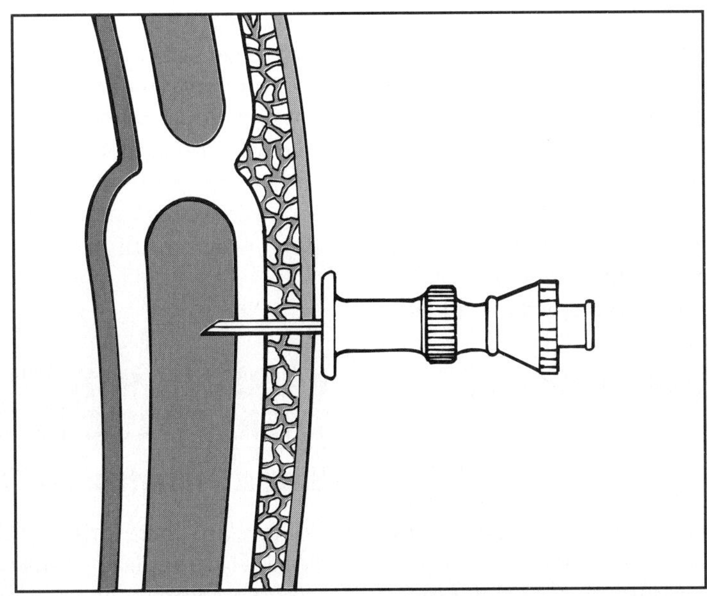

Figure 22-2 Bone marrow aspiration: penetration into marrow cavity. (From Powers LW: *Diagnostic hematology,* ed 1, St Louis, 1989, Mosby.)

A

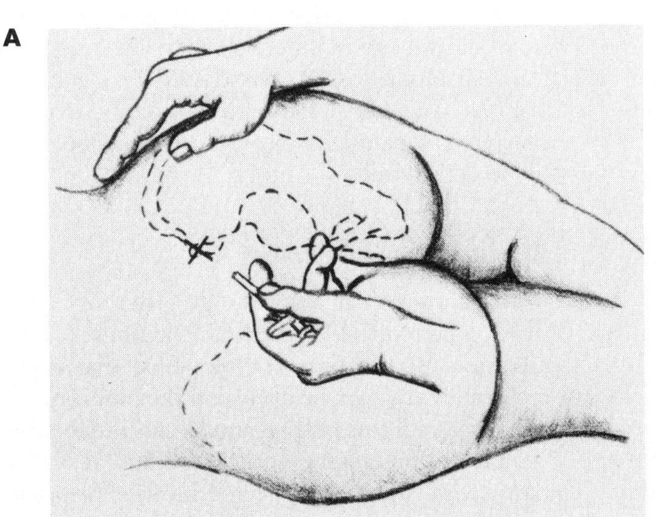

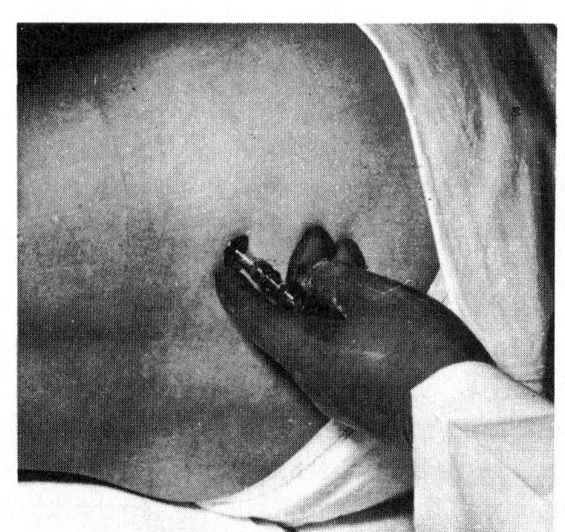

B

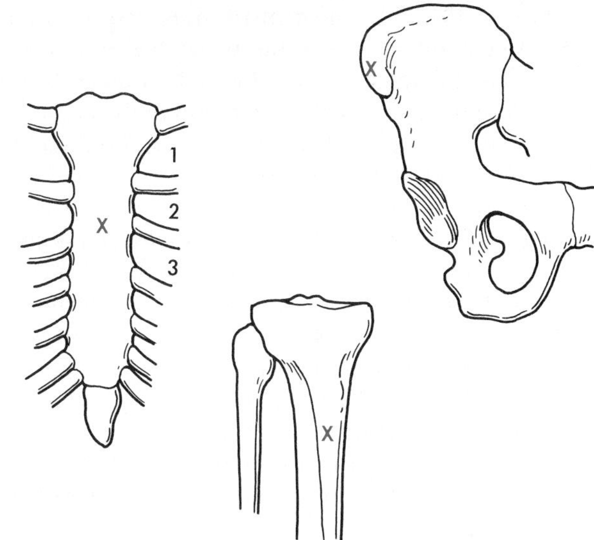

Figure 22-3 **A,** Bone marrow aspiration; posterior iliac crest. *Left,* Drawing of anatomic site. *Right,* Photograph of aspiration technique. **B,** Sites for bone marrow aspiration; sternum, iliac crest (most common), and tibia. (**A,** *left,* from Miale JB: *Laboratory medicine hematology,* ed 6, St Louis, 1982, Mosby; *right,* from Bauer JD: *Clinical laboratory methods,* ed 9, St Louis, 1982, Mosby; **B,** from Phipps WJ and others: *Medical surgical nursing,* ed 5, St Louis, 1995, Mosby.)

Blood Chemistry

The chemical analysis of blood involves a large number of tests, some of which are carried out on whole blood, a few on plasma, and others on blood serum. Many of these tests are related to the diagnosis of specific diseases and are discussed elsewhere. However, blood for chemical analysis is usually collected early in the morning, while the patient is in a fasting state. The patient may not be allowed anything by mouth after midnight, and breakfast may be withheld.

Blood Typing and Cross-matching

It is important for the blood of the donor and the blood of the recipient to be compatible. If they are not, the patient may suffer a severe or fatal reaction. There are many different systems for matching blood, and more than 100 different blood factors are known. However, the most familiar system classifies blood types as A, B, AB, and O (Table 22-3). It is always best to transfuse the patient with blood of his or her own type whenever possible. However, if the same type cannot be secured or if there is a delay in typing and cross-matching, the O type may be used in an emergency, but the patient must be watched carefully for indications of a reaction. Usually 500 ml of whole blood administered to a patient will elevate the number of red blood cells and the amount of hemoglobin by 15% in 24 hours. Plasma may be administered to people of all blood types, but because reactions to plasma may occur, the same precautions should be taken as for whole blood.

Rh Factor

In addition to the kinds of protein substances found in the four types of blood, some persons have an extra protein substance called the *Rh factor.* Approximately 85% of all persons have this protein and are said to be *Rh positive;* the remaining 15% are said to be *Rh negative.* It is just as important to determine the Rh factor in cross-matching blood for transfusion as it is to determine the blood type. If an Rh-negative person is transfused with Rh-positive blood, he or she may develop antibodies against the Rh-positive factor. If given further transfusions with Rh-positive blood, he or she may develop severe reactions. An Rh-positive fetus in utero may precipitate the formation of antibodies in an Rh-negative mother. If any of these antibodies reaches the fetal circulation, it may cause the infant to be stillborn or may result in the disease called *erythroblastosis fetalis.*

TABLE 22-3

ABO Blood Types

Recipient's Blood Type	Compatible Donor Type
A	A, O
B	B, O
AB	A, B, AB, O
O	O

NURSING RESPONSIBILITIES FOR THERAPEUTIC PROCEDURES

Blood Transfusion Therapy

There are three primary reasons for administering blood: (1) to replace or maintain blood volume, (2) to preserve the oxygen-carrying function of the blood, and (3) to increase or maintain the coagulation abilities of the blood. A transfusion introduces whole blood, or any of its components, from a donor into the bloodstream of the recipient. Whole blood is rarely used these days, even in an emergency. The only exception is when blood loss is massive (25% or more of total volume) and the patient needs volume expansion of plasma as well as the oxygen-carrying capacity of red blood cells (Harous, Antony, 1993).

Procedures

When the physician writes an order for blood transfusion, the request is sent to the laboratory along with a sample of the patient's blood so that typing and cross-matching can be done and the pints or units to be administered can be prepared. The nurse should assemble the necessary equipment and record the patient's vital signs. A registered nurse is responsible for the administration and handling of blood once it arrives on the unit. Most institutions require that two registered nurses check the blood before administration. The blood should be checked for expiration date, and the label indicating the patient's name, room number, and identification number should be compared to the patient's identification band. The patient's blood group and Rh status should be compared with the donor's blood group and Rh status. If any discrepancy is found, the blood is not given. Blood brought to the unit should be used immediately or returned to the blood bank. It is administered through an infusion set with a filter in the drip chamber that will remove any precipitates or clots that may form (Figure 22-4). The infusion line is primed and rinsed with saline because other solutions can cause hemolysis of the cells. The blood filter should not be used for more than 4 hours, and a unit of blood should not be transfused for more than 4 hours.

After the transfusion has begun, the nurse should carefully observe the patient while the first 50 ml is infused. Symptoms of severe reaction are usually seen during the first 50 ml of blood infusion. The infusion should be started slowly—at 5 ml/minute or less for the first 15 minutes. Vital signs should be taken before and 15 minutes after the transfusion is started and frequently during the transfusion. The patient should be observed for symptoms of potential complications.

Transfusion reactions

Transfusion reactions from contaminated blood, the presence of antibodies to donor cells, and allergic reactions can occur after only a small amount of blood has been given. If symptoms of a reaction occur (Table 22-4), the transfusion should be discontinued, the intravenous tubing changed, and the vein kept open with a slow saline solution drip. The blood should not be destroyed but should be saved for examination to determine the cause of the reaction.

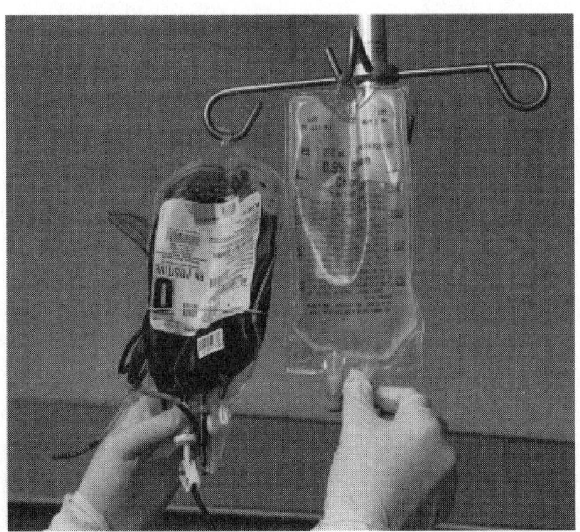

Figure 22-4 Blood is transfused through tubing that has a special filter. The tubing is flushed with normal saline before and after the blood is administered.

Circulation overload

Circulation overload is a complication that can result from too rapid fluid infusion. Cough, increasing pulse rate, dyspnea, and edema are symptoms of this complication. Packed cells rather than whole blood are indicated for patients who are susceptible to circulatory overload. This includes people with cardiac and renal impairment, as well as the elderly.

Air embolism

Air embolism is a rare but often fatal complication from a blood transfusion and is caused by air being allowed to enter the circulation. This is most likely to occur when blood is being given under pressure. Symptoms that indicate an air embolus include chest pain, acute shortness of breath, and shock. The patient should be turned immediately onto his or her left side, and his or her head should be lowered. Air embolism is a rare complication but requires immediate action if it occurs.

NURSE ALERT

When the patient is receiving blood, notify the physician of a drop in blood pressure, a rise in pulse, chills, or fever. Chest pain, shortness of breath, and shock indicate air embolism. Turn patient to his or her left side, stop the infusion, call for life support, and notify the physician.

TABLE 22-4

Blood Transfusion Reactions

Type of Reaction	Cause	Symptoms
Allergic reaction	Hypersensivity to antibodies in donor's blood	Urticaria, pruritus, fever, anaphylactic shock
Hemolytic reaction	Incompatibility	Nausea, vomiting, pain in lower back, hypotension, increase in pulse rate, decrease in urinary output, hematuria
Pyogenic febrile reaction (most common)	Antibodies to donor platelets or leukocytes, or contamination of blood	Fever, chills, nausea, headache, flushing, tachycardia, palpitations

ETHICAL DILEMMA

A Jehovah's Witness refuses a needed blood transfusion following a car accident. How would you analyze this dilemma? Would your analysis be different if the patient were a minor?

Interventions

Policies and procedures related to transfusion of blood or its components vary between institutions, but the care of the patient should always include strict adherence to universal precautions and measures to prevent transfusion reactions through proper identification of blood donor and recipient compatibility, and careful handling of the blood product to prevent contamination and hemolysis. The specific action the nurse takes varies with the type of reaction that is suspected. In general, vital signs should be monitored throughout the transfusion, and the patient should be assessed for signs and symptoms that indicate a reaction. When a hemolytic reaction is suspected, the nurse monitors the patient for shock, taking frequent blood pressure and pulse measurements, recording accurate intake and output, and obtaining a first-voided urine specimen. If the patient complains of itching and wheezes within the first few minutes of the transfusion, an allergic reaction should be suspected. Chills and fever occurring about 1 hour after the start of a transfusion indicate a pyogenic reaction. If the physician determines that these symptoms are not a result of hemolytic reaction or contaminated blood, the patient may be treated with antipyretics and steroids to alleviate the symptoms, and the transfusion is then continued.

THE PATIENT WITH BLOOD DYSCRASIAS

Blood dyscrasias are diseases or disorders of the blood and blood-forming organs. These include a wide range of conditions with varying prognoses. Lifestyle may predispose persons to certain disorders, whereas heredity may account for others. Often the cause is unknown. Similarly, treatment may cause a dramatic response or simply be palliative. Some diseases may be controlled, but a lifetime of compliance to treatment is required. Box 22-1 is a partial classification of diseases and disorders of the blood and the blood-forming organs. These include red blood cell, white blood cell, and hemorrhagic disorders.

BOX 22-1

BLOOD DYSCRASIAS

RED BLOOD CELL DISORDERS

Anemia
- Hemorrhagic
- Iron-deficiency or nutritional
- Pernicious
- Sickle cell
- Aplastic

Polycythemia

WHITE BLOOD CELL DISORDERS

Leukocytosis
Leukopenia
Infectious mononucleosis
Hodgkin's disease
Leukemia

HEMORRHAGIC DISORDERS

Hemophilia
Purpura
Splenomegaly

Disorders of Erythrocytes

Anemia is not a disease but a condition resulting from one or a combination of causes. It is defined as a lower than normal number of red blood cells and quantity of hemoglobin. The major manifestations of anemia, including pallor, decreased activity tolerance, and orthostatic hypotension, result from the body's attempts to provide adequate levels of oxygen to the brain and other vital organs. Vasoconstriction of peripheral blood vessels in the skin and blood vessels in the kidneys are the mechanisms that are responsible for the symptoms of anemia. It accompanies several diseases, and its development may be so insidious that an individual is unaware of the condition until symptoms appear. It may develop slowly when there is a slow bleeding from the intestinal tract, or it may develop quickly if there is a massive hemorrhage. Anemia is usually present in diseases in which there is destruction of red blood cells or when there is immature development of the red blood cells. Any condition that causes a decrease in red blood cells, in hemoglobin, and in iron will cause varying degrees of anemia.

Assessment of the patient with anemia

The nurse should examine the patient's skin for the texture and level of hydration and for the presence of any ulcerated areas. The nurse should also assess the eyes for pallor of the conjunctiva or a yellowish tinge to the sclera and for brightness or luster. The oral cavity is assessed for color, and the tongue is assessed for any evidence of sores or swelling. The patient should be asked about the presence of such symptoms as headaches, ringing in the ears, dizziness with position changes, difficulty concentrating, or difficulty swallowing. Other areas included in the assessment are the diet history and a past or present history of blood loss from the rectum, hemorrhoids, urine, vomitus, and prolonged or frequent menstrual bleeding. The nurse should inquire about a history of gastric ulcer, gastric or colon surgery, anemia, or a family history of anemia or blood disease.

Hemorrhagic anemia

Anemia resulting from loss of blood may be acute or chronic. Acute anemia or *hypovolemic shock* occurs when there has been a sudden loss of a large amount of blood. This may be caused by traumatic injury, *hemoptysis,* hemorrhage at childbirth, ulcerative lesions, and disorders of coagulation. Anemia may result from lesser degrees of hemorrhage or slow bleeding, such as that from a bleeding gastric ulcer or bleeding hemorrhoids.

Pathophysiology. The loss of blood decreases the amount of circulating fluid and hemoglobin and the amount of oxygen carried to the tissues of the body, which must have oxygen to survive. Blood loss may be classified as severe, moderate, or mild. The degree and rapidity of the blood loss are related to the severity and number of symptoms observed in the patient.

Severe blood loss may be caused by trauma if large blood vessels are ruptured or severed. Massive uterine hemorrhage may accompany childbirth, or it may result from cancer. A ruptured tubal pregnancy may release large amounts of blood into the peritoneal cavity. Severe blood loss can also occur when the number of platelets in the blood is low or when the coagulation process is abnormal.

Less severe blood loss occurs in many conditions, including prolonged or frequent menstrual periods, a bleeding gastric ulcer, or bleeding hemorrhoids.

Assessment. When blood loss is severe, the patient may experience hematogenic or hypovolemic shock. Symptoms include prostration, thirst, a rapid pulse rate, pallor, hypotension, clammy skin, or mental confusion because of decreased oxygen supply to the brain. When anemia is caused by slow bleeding, the symptoms are less dramatic. Fatigue is a primary symptom. The volume and rate of the pulse are normal. On exertion the blood pressure may drop, and tachycardia may occur. There is a tendency toward fainting and dizziness because of orthostatic hypotension. If bleeding continues for a prolonged period, pallor will develop, and shortness of breath on exertion, headache, drowsiness, and menstrual disturbances may occur.

PATIENT/FAMILY TEACHING 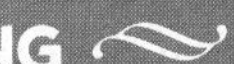

Administration of oral iron preparations

- Use a straw with liquid iron preparations to prevent staining of teeth.
- Take oral dose of iron with orange or other citrus juice to enhance absorption.
- Avoid milk, milk products, and antacids, which inhibit absorption.
- Take iron preparations with meals to reduce gastric irritation.
- Expect dark stools.

Intervention. In the case of massive hemorrhage, measures are taken to control the bleeding, treat for shock, and replace the volume of circulating fluid (see Chapter 8). Patients should be observed for evidence of further bleeding. They should lie flat and be kept warm, and vital signs should be taken at frequent intervals. Care should be taken to prevent injury to a restless or confused patient.

The immediate concern in chronic bleeding is to locate and remove the cause. This requires a carefully taken history and physical examination. Laboratory examination and x-ray studies may be required. Depending on the degree of anemia, blood transfusions may be given and iron therapy instituted.

The patient may or may not be given iron preparations. If any disorder of the intestinal tract makes the oral administration of iron undesirable, it may be given intramuscularly in the form of iron dextran (Imferon). It is given in the gluteal muscle in 1- to 5-ml injections daily or less often, and it may be continued until the hemoglobin returns to normal. Deep injection using the Z-tract method is necessary to avoid leakage into subcutaneous tissue, which stains skin.

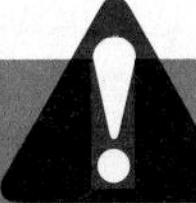

NURSE ALERT

When administering liquid iron preparations, have the patient use a straw to prevent staining of teeth. Take in citrus juice, with meals, but not with milk products for best absorption.

TABLE 22-5

Average Normal Daily Iron Requirements

Sex and Age Group	Amount
Men and postmenopausal women	10 mg
Women during childbearing period	18 mg
During pregnancy	15-35 mg
Infants	1.5 mg/kg of body weight (approximately 5-15 mg)
Children	10-18 mg
Adolescent boys	10-15 mg
Adolescent girls	10-25 mg

Iron-deficiency (hypochromic) anemia

Anemia caused by iron deficiency is the most common type of anemia. It is estimated that 90% of the iron-deficiency anemia in adults is found in women. It is the most common cause of anemia in infancy and childhood. The iron stored by the fetus in utero is depleted during the first 6 months after birth. Iron deficiency after 6 months is usually the result of inadequate iron in the diet. Average normal daily iron requirements are found in Table 22-5.

Approximately two thirds of all iron in the body is in the hemoglobin of the blood. For the most part this iron is used over and over, with essentially no excretion, and small reserves are available if needed. Reserves are stored in the bone marrow, spleen, liver, and muscle; in menstruating women almost all of the body's iron is stored in the red blood cells. Sources for storage include iron recycled from the destruction of old blood cells and dietary intake. Because iron is not lost through normal excretion, anemia caused by loss of iron must result from some other cause. In the adult, diet is a factor only if iron is being lost by some route other than normal excretion, including excessive menstrual bleeding, repeated pregnancies with blood loss and transfer of iron to the fetus in utero, and blood loss from the gastrointestinal tract, as might occur from carcinoma. In some cases, the body fails to assimilate and use iron.

Pathophysiology. Loss of blood is the most common cause of iron-deficiency anemia, which is characterized by a decrease in hemoglobin in the red blood cells. Although the red blood cell count may be within a normal range, the cells are small, microcytic, and poorly shaped and therefore are unable to carry their normal amount of hemoglobin. The body gradually exhausts its supply of stored iron, and the blood develops an abnormally low color index (hypochromia). Iron is an essential constituent of enzymes within the cells, and without it, the metabolism of the cell is affected. Eventually the entire body suffers.

Assessment. Iron-deficiency anemia develops gradually, and the individual may consult a physician because of fatigue and weakness. Sometimes during the early stages, the anemia may be found on a routine physical examination. Symptoms include pallor, dyspnea, palpitation, and loss of appetite. The nails become brittle and poorly shaped, the tongue is sore, and in some instances there may be difficulty in swallowing. The hemoglobin level will be found to be as low as 10 mg/dl of blood, and if the condition is severe it may be lower. The most reliable test for the diagnosis of iron-deficiency anemia is a bone marrow biopsy.

Intervention. In the absence of observed bleeding, a thorough examination should be made to locate any internal source of bleeding. Treatment for iron-deficiency anemia is the administration of iron and the identification and treatment of the cause. Commonly used iron preparations are found in Table 22-6. Iron is absorbed much more slowly when administered orally than it is when injected, and administration may have to be continued for several months. For varying reasons some patients cannot be given iron orally and must receive it intramuscularly. When iron is injected, the results are faster and the duration of therapy is shortened. However, it does carry some risk—fatal reactions have been reported but are rare.

Most patients with iron-deficiency anemia are cared for in the physician's office or the outpatient clinic. Patients should be evaluated for compliance with iron replacement regimens because of the drug's tendency to cause gastrointestinal problems. If the patient is experiencing side effects that prevent compliance, there are actions that can be taken to minimize the discomfort. When the problem is constipation, reducing the daily dose is helpful; for gastric distress the patient can be instructed to take the drug with meals. Another reason for noncompliance may be the cost of the drug. The nurse should consult the pharmacist for a less expensive preparation or should contact a social worker who

OLDER ADULT CONSIDERATIONS

Anemia is not a normal consequence of the aging process but is primarily a result of deficiencies commonly found in older populations. The elderly often lack the money or mobility to purchase and prepare foods. Others may lack interest in cooking or eating as a result of decreased sense of smell and taste, or from loneliness. Dentures, alcoholism, and chronic illness can also affect nutritional intake.

TABLE 22-6

Commonly Used Iron Preparations

Drug	Nursing Considerations
Oral administration	
Ferrous sulfate (Feosol) 300 mg (most common and least expensive) Ferrous gluconate (Fergon) 900 mg Ferrous fumurate (Ircon) 600-800 mg	• Do not administer with tetracyclines, antacids, eggs, milk, coffee, or tea, which inhibit absorption. • Take with meals to reduce gastric irriation. • Black and tarry or dark green stools or constipation may occur. • Eat foods high in iron.
Intramuscular/intravenous injection	
Iron dextran (Imferon) IM not to exceed 250 mg/day IV 100 mg/day as a bolus or dilute total dose and infuse over 1 to 6 hr (Valleraud, Deglin, 1994)	• Use Z-track method for IM injection. • Monitor blood pressure and heart rate. • Assess for signs and symptoms of anaphylaxis (rash, pruritus, edema, wheezing). • Monitor hemoglobin, hematocrit, and reticulocyte values.

PATIENT/FAMILY TEACHING

Iron deficiency anemia

- Patient education regarding iron therapy and proper diet is vital.
- Foods high in iron should be identified: eggs, organ meats, red kidney beans, dried raisins and apricots, yellow vegetables such as carrots and turnips, spinach, and whole wheat bread.
- Teenagers in particular need help with diet modification.

may be able to identify sources of financial assistance (Spratto, Woods, 1994). Replacement iron is usually given orally, 90–300 mg/day. Therapy continues for 2 to 4 months after the hemoglobin, hematocrit, and reticulocyte levels return to normal, indicating that the anemia is reversed. This could be a total of 6 months or more (Spratto, Woods, 1994).

Pernicious anemia (vitamin B_{12} deficiency anemia)

Until 1928 pernicious anemia was considered incurable, and the patient was subject to remissions, relapses, and ultimately death. Although the disease remains incurable, modern treatment has made it possible for the patient to have a normal life span. Patients with pernicious anemia who die usually do so from some other cause. The disease primarily affects middle-aged and older persons. Individuals who have had a total or partial gastrectomy will inevitably develop the disease because the gastric fundus (the source of the intrinsic factor) has been removed. Persons who are strict vegetarians and persons with a history of surgery or disease of the ileum are at risk for vitamin B_{12}–deficiency anemia. Pernicious anemia is not the same as iron-deficiency anemia; however, it is believed that iron-deficiency anemia of long duration may predispose an individual to pernicious anemia.

Pathophysiology. An intrinsic factor secreted by the fundus of the stomach is necessary for the absorption of vitamin B_{12} by the intestinal mucosa. Persons who have pernicious anemia lack this intrinsic factor and thus develop vitamin B_{12} deficiency. Vitamin B_{12} is a necessary element in the production of erythrocytes and nervous system function. The red blood cells in the bone marrow fail to mature, and their rate of destruction exceeds their rate of production. The erythrocytes that do reach the bloodstream may be few in number and abnormally large or megaloblastic. The red blood cell count may be low, and the hemoglobin is decreased. The skin may have a pale lemon-yellow color (mild jaundice) because of the excessive death rate of the red blood cells, which causes the bile pigments to be increased in the blood serum. There is little or no secretion of hydrochloric acid in the stomach.

Assessment. The onset of pernicious anemia is usually insidious, with symptoms of a slowly developing anemia. Pallor develops gradually, and there is a yellowish tint to the skin. There may be palpitation, nausea, vomiting, flatulence, indigestion, constipation, and often diarrhea. There is soreness and burning of the tongue, which appears smooth and red, with infection around the teeth and gums. Fever, weakness, anorexia, and difficulty in swallowing may also occur. Neurologic symptoms may develop, including tingling of the hands and feet and loss of sense of body position. Cerebral symptoms include loss of memory, mental confusion, and depression. Personality changes and behavior problems can occur.

Severe neurologic impairments can result from inappropriate treatment and inadequate diagnostic evaluation of vitamin B_{12} anemia. These impairments include partial or total paralysis, which results from destruction of the nerve fibers of the spinal cord. Peripheral nerve damage causes the paresthesia and lack of position sense seen in this disorder.

Intervention. Once the diagnosis has been established, the treatment consists of injections of hydroxocobalamin (vitamin B_{12}). If the anemia is severe, the patient may be transfused with packed red blood cells. The patient may also require treatment for coexisting conditions such as cardiovascular disorders. Injections of vitamin B_{12} must be continued throughout the person's lifetime. Treatment is individualized, but one injection every 2 months may keep the patient free of symptoms. The nursing care of the patient depends to some extent on the stage the disease had reached when it was discovered. While the patient is confined to the hospital, his or her vital signs should be checked daily and recorded. An increase in pulse and respiration is to be expected from the body's adjustment to transfer oxygen to the cells, especially with exertion, but any great change should be reported immediately. The mouth should be cleaned by the patient several times a day with a solution that is nonirritating to the mucous membrane.

Meals should be carefully planned to provide a diet high in protein, vitamins, and minerals. It is better to use complete proteins of a high order, such as meat, milk, eggs, and shellfish. Because the patient may have a poor appetite, considerable encouragement to eat may be needed. The attractive preparation and serving of food will often stimulate the patient's appetite. Unusually hot, acid, salty, and spicy foods should be avoided because of the soreness of the mouth. Constipation may be treated with mild laxatives prescribed by the physician.

Patients with pernicious anemia are especially sensitive to cold, and extra lightweight, warm blankets may be needed. Cotton flannel nightclothing, a warm bed jacket, and bed socks will make the patient more comfortable. Hot-water bottles and electric heating pads should be avoided because of the danger of burning the patient.

Nursing care of the patient with a vitamin B_{12}–deficiency anemia also includes evaluation of patient problems such as self-care deficits, fatigue, weakness, activity intolerance, and potential for injury. The goals of care are to conserve energy and prevent injury. Energy can be conserved by assisting the patient with physical care and balancing activities with rest periods. Passive exercises maintain bone and muscle mass that would otherwise be depleted during prolonged inactivity. As soon as they can be tolerated, active exercises such as progressive ambulation should be instituted. Loss of independence and altered self-image are common problems and must be considered in the plan of care. Maintenance of skin integrity is managed by frequent skin inspections, position changes, and the use of protective devices. Intensive and comprehensive rehabilitation programs are appropriate for individuals with severe neurologic deficits and can be instituted when the anemia is corrected.

Most patients with pernicious anemia are older than 40 years of age, and lifetime patterns have been established. Learning that they have an incurable disease may cause considerable emotional shock for some patients. The patient may reject the diagnosis and lose valuable time needed for therapy. The nurse may help the patient by stressing how regular treatment will help the patient feel well, be well, and live a happy, normal life. Persons who are economically depressed may need assistance from a community social agency and Medicaid, and elderly persons may be provided for through the Medicare program.

Sickle cell anemia

Sickle cell anemia is found almost exclusively in blacks, and its distribution is worldwide. The disease is a genetic hemolytic blood disorder affecting both men and women. Approximately one of every 10 black Americans carries the gene for the abnormal sickle hemoglobin and therefore has the sickle cell trait. The disease is diagnosed most often in children, often in infancy, and the mortality rate is high. Only half of these

PATIENT/FAMILY TEACHING

Pernicious anemia

- Daily mouth care and a high protein diet is important.
- Avoid hot, spicy foods.
- Keep warm.
- Pace activities.
- Assess daily for skin impairment.

patients live beyond 20 years of age, although survival rates are increasing with improved care.

Screening clinics have been established in many areas of the United States to identify persons with the trait. Although there is no preventive treatment or cure for the disease, counseling helps the person to avoid the factors that may predispose him or her to a serious exacerbation. Furthermore, couples who either have the trait or have sickle cell disease should be advised of the risks involved so they can make informed decisions about becoming parents. The risk of having a child with sickle cell anemia depends on the genetic characteristics of the prospective parents.

Pathophysiology. Sickle cell anemia is caused by an abnormal hemoglobin molecule (hemoglobin S). When the molecule is present in the red blood cell, it causes the cell to acquire a sickle or crescent shape when the oxygen supply is decreased. The sickle-shaped cell cannot move normally through the blood vessels and tends to block or clog small vessels. As tissue hypoxia worsens and as more oxygen is given up to the tissues, further sickling occurs, blood **viscosity** increases, hemolysis increases, and more clots form in the microcirculation. A sickle cell crisis ensues.

Assessment. The life of the sickled cell is short, and the production of new cells is not fast enough to keep oxygen supplied to the tissues of the body. The person may experience attacks of severe pain in various organs and in the bones. There may be fever, anemia, and thrombi in the lungs and spleen, and the spleen may be enlarged. Leg ulcers may occur. Because of red blood cell destruction, jaundice is often seen. Children develop abnormal growth patterns, and infections account for the high mortality in the very young. These persons are especially susceptible to osteomyelitis as a result of salmonella infections and to pneumonia caused by the pneumococcus bacterium. The rate of maternal complications in pregnancy, such as hemorrhage and eclamptic conditions, is reported to be high.

Intervention. Treatment is preventive and supportive. Children should be immunized against preventable diseases. Any activity that causes stress or requires strenuous exercise and would limit oxygen supply should be avoided. Good health habits, including rest, proper diet, avoidance of respiratory tract infections, and regular medical supervision should be encouraged. If an acute exacerbation (crisis) occurs, the patient is admitted to the hospital and placed on a regimen of bedrest. The patient may experience fever; severe pain in the chest, joints, and abdomen; edema; and leukocytosis. Routine administration of analgesics is indicated for pain during a crisis, as is assistance with activities of daily living and frequent rest periods. Because dehydration contributes to sickling, oral or intravenous administration of fluids is very important. Local applications of heat may be used to relieve pain, but cold applications should not be used because they promote sickling. Bacterial infection is a serious complication of sickle cell anemia, and immunization to prevent pneumococcal pneumonia in these patients is recommended. Death from sickle cell anemia usually results from the long-term effects of repeated tissue damage in major organs such as the heart, kidneys, and liver. The patient with sickle cell anemia and his or her parents need a great deal of encouragement and emotional support during the long course of chronic illness. Repeated hospitalizations that begin in early childhood often cause ineffective family and patient coping. The loss of independence can lead to depression and to noncompliance with crisis prevention approaches. The adolescent is particularly vulnerable to ineffective coping because many activities such as vigorous athletics must be avoided, as must situations where exposure to infection is a risk. It is very difficult to achieve the developmental tasks of childhood and adolescence while having to cope with a chronic and life-threatening illness. Early referral to resources such as the Sickle Cell Foundation can provide the patient and family with support. The nurse needs to maintain a sensitive awareness of the needs of each age group afflicted with sickle cell anemia. A common need is the presence of a trusting relationship with healthcare providers. An area of potential conflict in this relationship is that of pain management. In a sickle cell crisis, pain is severe. However, it is often ineffectively managed because of caregiver attitudes and lack of knowledge. When the patient seeks pain relief but cannot obtain it because of these problems, trust is threatened and the patient experiences alienation from the staff. If the patient uses strategies that exacerbate the alienation, a vicious cycle begins and the patient suffers needlessly. The nurse is in the best position to prevent this escalation of events through early recognition and confrontation.

NURSE ALERT

Do not use cold applications for pain of anemia because cold promotes sickling.

Aplastic anemia

Aplastic anemia results from bone marrow failure that is congenital or acquired; in approximately 50% of cases the cause is unknown (Monahan, Drake, Neighbors, 1994). It may be induced by radiation, chemicals, or drug therapy, especially with antineoplastic drugs

PATIENT/FAMILY TEACHING

Sickle cell anemia

- Avoid strenuous exercise.
- Encourage good health habits, proper rest, and diet.
- Adequate daily fluid intake.
- Avoid cold applications.
- Explore pain management techniques.

PATIENT/FAMILY TEACHING

Aplastic anemia

- Maintain meticulous skin care.
- Maintain proper mouth care.
- Provide rest periods and pace activities.
- Maintain regular bowel movements.
- Assess stools and urine for blood.
- Avoid injury/trauma to skin.

and chloramphenicol. This is a severe, life-threatening anemia with a poor prognosis and requires careful medical management and excellent nursing care.

Pathophysiology. In aplastic anemia, insufficient red blood cells are produced as a result of an interference with the stem cells in the bone marrow. In rare instances, only the red blood cells are affected, but usually there is depression of all the cells originating in the bone marrow. This depression of red blood cells (erythrocytes), white blood cells (leukocytes), and platelets (thrombocytes) is referred to as *pancytopenia.*

Assessment. The reduction of erythrocytes produces classic signs and symptoms of anemia: pallor, weakness, dyspnea, and hypoxia. The patient may be tired, lethargic, or confused because of the lack of oxygen to the brain. Infection poses a very real threat because of decreased white blood cells (leukopenia). Thrombocytopenia (reduced thrombocytes or platelets) increases the risk of bleeding. Even an intramuscular injection may produce a site for fatal bleeding.

Intervention. The cause of aplastic anemia must be identified promptly and removed or discontinued. Bone marrow suppression is expected with certain antineoplastic drugs or radiation therapy, and therefore laboratory values should be monitored often to maintain control. The margin for therapeutic treatment in such cases is exceedingly narrow. Supportive treatment includes transfusions of packed red blood cells and platelets as indicated.

Blood transfusions are avoided to prevent iron overloading and the development of antibodies to tissue antigens. Platelet transfusions that are HLA (human lymphocyte antigen) matched are used to treat serious bleeding in the thrombocytopenic patient. Cautious use of blood transfusion is necessary to minimize the risk of rejection for the bone marrow transplant candidate. Antibiotics are not given prophylactically but may be lifesaving when given for a specific infection (Brunner, Suddarth, 1992).

A splenectomy may be required in patients with hypersplenism when it is responsible for destruction of normal platelets or for marrow suppression of platelet production. Steroids and androgens are sometimes used in an attempt to stimulate the bone marrow. Antithymocyte globulin has recently become an important therapy for patients who are not candidates for bone marrow transplantation.

Bone marrow transplantation is the treatment of choice in patients under the age of 50 who have a compatible donor. Lectin separation of donor T lymphocytes offers hope for patients without a suitable donor. Bone marrow transplantation involves several processes: immunosuppression of the recipient with total lymph node irradiation and high-dose cyclophosphamide, followed by aspiration of donor marrow from the anterior and posterior iliac crests. Approximately 100 aspirates are taken. The bone marrow is then infused intravenously into the recipient and migrates to the bone marrow cavities. Establishment of the graft (engraftment), if it takes place, occurs in 10 to 30 days. During that period the patient is at enormous risk for severe and irreversible bleeding and infection.

The patient receives immunosuppressive therapy for approximately 6 months to prevent rejection and graft-vs-host disease. In 30% to 70% of patients graft-vs-host disease occurs with varying degrees of severity. The long-term physical problems include skin changes that cause contractures and muscular wasting, fluid and electrolyte abnormalities caused by chronic diarrhea, fatigue, and jaundice and pruritus caused by inflammation of the liver. Patients and families are confronted with numerous stressors, including prolonged hospitalization and isolation from friends and support systems, an altered patient self-concept as a result of physical changes and the inability to carry out role responsibilities, and the need to learn complex care regimens after discharge from the hospital.

Patients with aplastic anemia are highly susceptible to infection, and thus nursing care should be directed

BOX 22-2 **Nursing Process**

ANEMIAS

ASSESSMENT

Nutritional status and appetite
Oral mucosa and skin
Gastrointestinal system for nausea, abdominal distention, diarrhea, constipation, and enlarged spleen/liver
Tolerance to activity
Dyspnea at rest or with exertion, weakness, or fatigue
Vital signs
Bleeding tendency or active bleeding
Signs and symptoms of heart failure
Laboratory studies (hemoglobin, hematocrit, RBC indices, folate, B_{12})

NURSING DIAGNOSES

Altered nutrition: less than body requirements related to anorexia
Pain related to decreased oral mucous membrane integrity
Activity intolerance related to an imbalance between oxygen supply and demand
Risk for impaired skin integrity related to immobility
Risk for injury related to decreased hemoglobin
Risk for impaired gas exchange related to inadequate oxygen-carrying capacity
Risk for trauma (falling) related to weakness
Anxiety related to prescribed treatment plan
Altered family processes related to hospitalization
Knowledge deficit related to prescribed diet and medication therapy

NURSING INTERVENTIONS

Encourage small, frequent meals.
Provide a pleasant dining environment.
Provide oral hygiene before meals and prn.
Provide cool, bland foods if indicated.
Provide frequent rest periods.
Encourage patient to request assistance with activities.
Increase activity as tolerated.
Elevate head of bed as tolerated.
Prevent unnecessary exertion.
Prevent skin breakdown.
Provide an atmosphere of acceptance.
Provide positive reinforcement.
Encourage family to visit.
Prevent falls.
Keep environment free of clutter.

EVALUATION OF EXPECTED OUTCOMES

Tolerates prescribed diet
Describes foods high in specific dietary need (iron, B_{12}, folate)
Mucous membranes remain intact
Verbalizes pain relief
Participates in required activity
Verbalizes need for assistance
No evidence of respiratory distress
Vital signs are within normal limits for patient
Complete blood count is within normal range for patient
Verbalizes sources of anxiety
Family members participate in patient's care
Skin remains intact
Verbalizes signs and symptoms of anemia and reportable conditions

toward prevention. Strict aseptic technique must be adhered to for dressing changes and administration of intravenous fluids or medications. Meticulous care to prevent impaired skin and mucous membrane integrity includes avoiding intramuscular injections and the administration of rectal medications or the use of rectal thermometers. When bedrest is prescribed, the patient should be helped to change position often to prevent the development of decubitus ulcers caused by tissue hypoxia. Protective devices such as egg crate or water mattresses are indicated. Bowel movements must be kept soft and regular to prevent irritation to the mucous membrane, which could act as a site for infection. Rest periods and assistance will help alleviate shortness of breath and conserve energy. Thrombocytopenia should alert the nurse to any signs of bleeding, and even the slightest trauma must be prevented. The patient's urine and stool should be monitored for occult or gross bleeding. Assessment of the oral cavity includes noting the presence of bleeding gums or bleeding from mucosal areas. Medications should be given orally whenever possible. Although the prognosis is poor, careful medical and nursing management improves the chance of survival (Box 22-2).

Polycythemia

Polycythemia is a chronic disease that occurs most commonly in middle-aged men of Jewish ancestry.

Pathophysiology. The disease is caused by a proliferation of erythrocytes in the bone marrow. The red blood cell count may range from 7000 to 10 million/mm^3 of blood. The disease occurs in two forms: primary and secondary. The cause of primary polycythemia is unknown. In the absence of cardiorespiratory disease the oxygen content of the blood is normal, but the rate of flow is decreased and the viscosity is increased. The decreased rate of flow and increased viscosity may lead to thrombosis in small blood vessels. The leukocyte count is increased in true or primary polycythemia and may reach 25,000 to 50,000/mm^3. Increased numbers of platelets predispose the patient to intravascular thrombosis. The spleen and liver are enlarged, and bleeding in the form of ecchymosis occurs in mucous membranes and skin. The secondary form of the disease accompanies several other chronic disorders, including cardiac and pulmonary disease. This form has been associated with benign and malignant tumors, particularly malignant tumors of the kidney. In the absence of infection the leukocyte count is near normal. The causative factor in secondary polycythemia is decreased oxygen in the blood.

Assessment. Symptoms are caused by the effects of massive numbers of red blood cells, which result in hyperviscosity of the blood and hypervolemia. The patient appears plethoric with an appearance of fullness and may complain of headache, fatigue, night sweats, pruritus, paraesthesia, and dyspnea. The spleen and liver will be enlarged, and bruises may be seen on the skin and mucous membranes. These persons appear to be predisposed to gout and peptic ulcers.

Intervention. The objective of treatment of polycythemia is to suppress the bone marrow, reduce the blood cell mass, maintain the hematocrit value at or below 50%, and reduce the leukocyte and platelet count. **Phlebotomy** and the removal of up to 500 ml of blood at intervals may accomplish the objectives for some patients. Chemotherapeutic drugs may also be used, including melphalan (Alkeran), chlorambucil (Leukeran), and busulfan (Myleran). Radioactive phosphorus (^{32}P) may be administered intravenously. Combinations of phlebotomy with chemotherapy and/or radioactive phosphorus are used to provide sustained control of this disease.

The survival time is long, and patients will be required to continue receiving medication. Persons who survive for 10 years or longer often develop leukemia. The role of the nurse is supportive and directed at minimizing the symptoms. The patient should be encouraged to maintain good health habits and regular medical supervision.

Disorders of White Blood Cells

Leukocytosis

Leukocytosis is an increase in the number of white blood cells. It is both a protective and a destructive mechanism. In many diseases that are potentially dangerous, leukocytes are increased and play an important role in helping the body to overcome an infection. In some forms of leukemia, large numbers of immature leukocytes are produced, causing changes in the spleen, liver, and lymph nodes. Although the number of leukocytes is increased, the cells are immature and do not offer protection against infection.

Leukopenia

Leukopenia is a condition in which the number of leukocytes is greatly reduced. When the granulocytes are reduced, serious bacterial infection may occur. There are numerous conditions causing leukopenia, including chemical agents known to be toxic to the body. Among these are the antineoplastic drugs. Whenever leukopenia occurs, the patient should be protected from infection. Because the protective mechanism offered by the leukocytes has decreased, the patient's life could be in danger if infection should develop.

Infectious mononucleosis

Infectious mononucleosis is an acute infectious disease involving the white blood cells. The number of leukocytes may be increased from 10,000 to 25,000/mm.[3] The lymphocytes are also increased, some of which will be immature, although most will be mature. The clinical manifestations of the disease involve the lymphoid tissues of the body, particularly the lymph nodes and the spleen (see Chapter 11). The *Paul-Bunnell* (heterophil antibody) *test* is used to determine the presence or absence of antibodies to the Epstein-Barr virus, which causes infectious mononucleosis.

Hodgkin's disease

Hodgkin's disease is classified as a malignant lymphoma and involves the lymph nodes and lymphatic tissues. The disease occurs more often in men than in women and in those 15 to 34 and over 50 years of age. In the past, Hodgkin's disease was always fatal, but now many persons can be cured. Early diagnosis in stage I and treatment with radiation can offer a 90% to 100% cure.

Pathophysiology. The cause of Hodgkin's disease is unknown, although environmental, genetic, infectious, and immunologic causes have been studied.

Assessment. The first sign of the disease in two thirds of all cases is an asymptomatic enlargement of a lymph node in the neck. As the disease progresses, the deep lymph nodes in the mediastinum and the retroperitoneal cavity and adjacent tissues are involved.

When systemic symptoms such as loss of 10% of body weight, fever, and night sweats are present, the prognosis is less favorable, regardless of the stage of disease at diagnosis; this is denoted as "B" in the staging system (for example, stage IIB Hodgkin's disease). The spleen and liver become enlarged, and in about one fifth of cases the bone marrow is affected. Symptoms are associated with the extent of lymph node and organ involvement. Mediastinal lymph node involvement can compress the trachea and underlying lung tissue, causing dyspnea and difficulty in swallowing. Retroperitoneal involvement is associated with edema of the lower extremities and back pain. Jaundice and fatigue are symptoms of liver involvement. The diagnosis is usually established by biopsy of a lymph node and identification of large atypical cells called Reed-Sternberg cells.

Intervention. Hodgkin's disease is classified into stages according to pathologic findings and the probable prognosis. From stage I, each subsequent stage represents increased activity and progression of the disease. Depending on the stage, treatment may be curative or only palliative. In stages I and II, treatment consists of radiotherapy of the involved lymph nodes and the contiguous tissues with a view toward cure. In later stages a combination of radiotherapy and chemotherapy is used. When the disease becomes widespread, radiotherapy has little benefit, and chemotherapeutic drugs and steroids are administered in cycles. Although a cure may not be achieved in the late stage of the disease, remission extending over several years may occur (Brunner, Suddarth, 1992). Nursing management of the patient with Hodgkin's disease includes intervention to reduce the effects of problems such as dyspnea, pain, fatigue, pruritus, and impaired skin and mucous membrane integrity. The patient is especially susceptible to infection and should be protected against respiratory tract infections and skin infections, which may result from scratching. Treatment of Hodgkin's disease contributes to the severity of the patient's problems.

Leukemia

Leukemia is a neoplastic disorder resulting in widespread proliferation of white blood cells and their precursors throughout the body. It is a disease of the bone marrow, which is where leukocytes are formed. Specific causes of leukemia are unknown, but ionizing radiation, viruses, and genetic abnormalities have been linked to the disease.

Leukemia may be acute or chronic and is classified according to the type of cells involved, such as granulocytes, monocytes, and lymphocytes.

Acute lymphoblastic leukemia is the form most common in children, but chronic forms may also occur. Chronic leukemia is more common in persons older than 45 years of age, but acute leukemia may occur in adult persons of any age. Approximately 50% to 60% of all leukemia in the United States is classified as acute leukemia.

Acute leukemia. The acute leukemias are divided into lymphocytic leukemia (ALL), which originates from lymphocytes, and myelocytic leukemia (AML), which originates from granulocytes. ALL occurs primarily in children, and AML occurs primarily in adults. In children the disease usually affects those 2 to 4 years of age, with most deaths occurring in children under 2 years of age. Regardless of the type of the cells involved, whether in children or adults, the characteristics and progress of the disease are similar.

Pathophysiology. Abnormal growth of immature cells, or *blasts,* will occur. AML is diagnosed when bone marrow aspiration and biopsy show an overgrowth of very immature cells of the myeloblast. ALL is characterized by lymphoblasts, which are cells that are precursors of lymphocytes (Brunner, Suddarth, 1992).

Early in the course of acute lymphoblastic leukemia, lymphatic tissues are involved, including lymph nodes and the spleen. The enlarged lymph nodes may be the first signs of the disease in some persons. In all forms of acute leukemia, the leukemic cells multiply in the bone marrow. Their proliferation causes a decrease in the production of red blood cells and shortens their life. The platelets are also reduced. With the reduction of erythrocytes, anemia may develop, and the decreased platelets interfere with the blood clotting mechanism, which results in bleeding. During the course of the disease, almost all organs of the body become involved. With treatment, remissions may occur, during which blood cell production may return to nearly normal levels.

Assessment. The onset of the disease often begins with a slight cold or tonsillitis. The temperature may range from low to high grade. The child may complain of headache and abdominal pain; in the very young child, pain may be evidenced by crying, restlessness, and reluctance to move or be moved. In the adult the onset of the disease may be traced to a cold from which recovery was slow. This is followed by prostration, weakness, anemia, and anorexia. If the anemia is severe, there may be pallor. Ulcerations may occur around the mouth, skin, and rectum. Bleeding varies from ecchymosis and petechiae to purpura, which may become necrotic and ulcerative. Bone pain results from the rapid proliferation of cells in the marrow. Symptoms will vary widely as various organs or parts of the body are involved.

Intervention. Tremendous progress in the treatment of leukemia has been made during the last decade by using a complex combination of drug and radiation therapy (see Chapter 10). The survival of children with acute lymphoblastic leukemia has increased from an average of 3 months before modern therapy to the point where the majority of those treated have no evidence of the disease after 5 years. Acute nonlymphocytic (myelocytic) leukemia has shown less response to treatment. Only 50% of these patients respond to treatment.

Bone marrow transplantation may be selected as the treatment of choice in patients with suitable donors if initial remission of the acute leukemia has been induced. Before transplantation, the patient's bone marrow cells and leukemic cells must be killed by massive chemotherapy and total body irradiation. The patient may succumb to infection, hemorrhage, or graft-vs-host disease.

Many of the symptoms concurrent with leukemia are the result of treatment rather than the disease. Side effects of the chemotherapeutic drugs and reactions to radiation therapy should be noted (see Chapter 10). If the person receives blood transfusions, packed red blood cells, or platelets, he or she must be observed for transfusion reaction. When numerous transfusions are given, the danger of reaction is increased. Hematomas or hemorrhage may occur from any trauma to the skin. Infections and hemorrhage account for many complications of leukemia, and the nurse must be constantly alert to protect the patient from infection and to report immediately any severe bleeding or indication of infection (Box 22-3).

The child with acute leukemia may come into the hospital several times during the course of the disease. Examinations and treatment may be painful experiences for the child, and he or she may be fearful. The nurse should do everything possible to relieve the anxiety of both the child and the parents. Parents need tender, loving care at this time as much as, and perhaps more than, the child.

Chronic leukemia. Chronic leukemia is confined almost entirely to adults and develops slowly. The chronic leukemias are divided into lymphocytic (CLL) and myelogenous (CML) leukemia. The individual may be completely asymptomatic when the disorder is discovered by routine physical examination.

Pathophysiology. In chronic myelogenous leukemia, the spleen becomes enlarged to the extent that the patient can palpate it and is aware of a heavy feeling in the upper left abdomen. Chronic lymphocytic leukemia may progress slowly, or it may progress rapidly to a fatal termination. The leukocyte count is increased, and lymph nodes throughout the body are enlarged but are not painful. Chronic myelocytic leukemia is characterized by the presence of a chromosomal marker, the Philadelphia chromosome, and by a progressive fibrosing of the bone marrow (Beare, Myers, 1994).

Assessment. All forms of chronic leukemia are characterized by similar symptoms, including weakness, fever, bone pain, loss of appetite, loss of weight, anemia, enlargement of body organs, and hemorrhage.

Intervention. The objectives of treatment in chronic leukemia partially depend on the kind of cells that are involved. In chronic myelogenous leukemia, the purpose of treatment is to bring about a reduction in the number of leukocytes and thrombocytes and in spleen size. When the white blood cell count is kept at or near normal, other symptoms are modified. In chronic lymphocytic leukemia, the primary consideration is directed toward relief of the conditions that arise from the increased production of lymphocytes, such as enlarged and painful lymph nodes and spleen, anemia, and a decrease in the number of platelets. Drugs commonly used in chronic leukemia include chlorambucil (Leukeran), hydroxyurea, corticosteroids, and cyclophosphamide (Cytoxan). Irradiation of lymph nodes is often used, and blood transfusions may be given if the anemia is severe. Although drugs are not curative, they help to prolong life expectancy for patients with chronic leukemia. The median survival time for patients with chronic myelogenous leukemia is 3½ to 4 years, whereas that for patients with chronic lymphocytic leukemia is 6 years (Beare, Myers, 1994). The nursing care required during severe relapses is the same as that for patients with acute leukemia. When the patient is ambulatory in the hospital or in the home, regular daily rest periods should be observed to minimize fatigue and weakness.

OLDER ADULT CONSIDERATIONS

The symptoms of leukemia and the progression of the disease are more severe in the older adult. The older adult will have more difficulty tolerating chemotherapy and radiation, which are often the treatments of choice in leukocyte disorders. Reduced gastric motility results in decreased drug absorption, which increases the likelihood of side effects of chemotherapy (Monahan, Drake, Neighbors, 1994).

BOX 22-3 **Nursing Process**

LEUKEMIA

ASSESSMENT

Vital signs
Body sites for evidence of infection (oral cavity, skin, perineum, rectum)
Respiratory system for evidence of congestion
IV sites and bone marrow biopsy sites for evidence of bleeding
Signs and symptoms of bleeding (skin, urine, stool, emesis, sputum, nose, gums)
Dizziness with position changes and orthostatic hypotension
Tolerance to activity
Mental status for signs of restlessness, agitation, confusion
Lymphadenopathy, pallor, or fatigue
Laboratory studies (WBC, platelet count, hemoglobin, hematocrit)

NURSING DIAGNOSES

Risk for infection related to leukopenia
Risk for injury related to thrombocytopenia
Activity intolerance related to weakness and fatigue
Risk for ineffective coping related to loss of health and associated stress
Knowledge deficit related to diagnosis and treatment
Anticipatory grieving related to potential loss of life

NURSING INTERVENTIONS

Report abnormalities in vital signs.
Encourage optimal personal hygiene.
Provide frequent oral hygiene.
Wash hands before patient contact.
Reduce number of visitors.
Prevent patient contact with persons with respiratory infections, flu.
Administer antibiotic/antifungal medications on time, as ordered.
Encourage deep breathing and coughing.
Use protective devices (e.g., egg crate mattress) to prevent skin breakdown.
Assist with frequent position changes; provide skin care.
Report any bleeding or evidence of infection.
Avoid IM injections, indwelling urinary catheters, rectal thermometers, suppositories.
Apply pressure to venipuncture sites and bone marrow sites for 5 minutes.
Provide patient with a soft toothbrush.
Instruct patient to use an electric razor.
Provide patient with shoes/slippers when ambulating.
Have patient change position slowly and wait for assistance with ambulation.
Keep siderails up.
Provide frequent rest periods.
Assist with self-care activities.
Establish communication.
Assist patient/family with coping.
Provide referral for home care as needed.

EVALUATION OF EXPECTED OUTCOMES

Describes signs and symptoms of infection and preventive measures
Maintains adequate nutrition
Demonstrates no evidence of active bleeding
Laboratory values within normal range for patient
Avoids physical trauma
Verbalizes a need for assistance
Spaces activity throughout the day
Demonstrates progression with activity and endurance
Strives toward independence
Begins coping with lifestyle changes

Hemorrhagic Disorders

Hemophilia

Hemophilia is a general term that is applied to a group of diseases that have certain things in common. They are all hereditary bleeding diseases that have a prolonged bleeding time. They all exhibit a deficiency in one or more of the factors essential for coagulation of the blood.

Pathophysiology. The most common form of hemophilia is *classic hemophilia A.* This form appears only in males and is transmitted by the female. *Christmas disease* (hemophilia B) occurs in the same manner as hemophilia A but is a result of a deficiency of factor IX. A third form of the disease is *von Willebrand's disease* (hemophilia C, vascular hemophilia), which occurs in both men and women.

Assessment. Severe bleeding may occur in any

part of the body. Repeated hemorrhages into joints (hemarthrosis) such as ankles, knees, and elbows may damage them to the extent that mobility is difficult. Hemorrhage into muscles may lead to contractures. Bleeding occurs into soft tissues and throughout the gastrointestinal tract, and minor injuries such as cuts, lacerations, or bruises may lead to fatal bleeding. There may be hematomas and hematuria, and anemia is often present.

NURSE ALERT

When giving medication by injection to patients with leukemia or hemophilia, use the smallest gauge needle possible and apply firm pressure to the site for at least 1 minute after the injection.

PATIENT/FAMILY TEACHING

Hemophilia

- Assess level of knowledge about disease and treatment.
- Report signs of internal bleeding—pallor, weakness, restlessness.
- If a joint injury occurs, apply cold and immobilize the area.
- Avoid aspirin and other salicylates.
- Safety-proof the environment.
- Wear a Medic Alert bracelet.
- Carefully brush teeth and get regular flouride treatments to avoid tooth extractions.
- Encourage the use of condoms if positive for the human immunodeficiency virus (HIV).
- Refer to community services as needed.
- Evaluate the teaching response.

Intervention. Treatment is first preventive. The individual with hemophilia in any form must be guarded against injuries. Contact sports are contraindicated. Parents should receive instruction concerning activities for young children and should know when an injury is serious enough to call the physician. Genetic counseling should be available to the family. If there has been a severe hemorrhage, fresh whole blood may be given. At the present time cryoprecipitates or commercial concentrates of factor VIII are the treatment of choice for persons with hemophilia A. In hemophilia B, concentrates containing the deficient factor IX may be administered. In hemophilia C, cryoprecipitate is given. Mild to moderate hemophilia A and von Willebrand's type I may be treated with a synthetic analog of vasopressin. This has been shown to increase factor VIII levels and can reduce the risk of AIDS and hepatitis transmitted by blood transfusions. Nurses monitor the patient for side effects of the drug, which include fluid retention, tachycardia, hyponatremia, and hypokalemia. The blood pressure and pulse rate are measured often during the infusion, and fluids are usually restricted. Patients experiencing pain from joint or muscle complications may need analgesics to relieve pain. Analgesics containing aspirin or narcotics are usually avoided.

When injections are unavoidable, the nurse should use a small needle and apply firm pressure to the injection site for some time after the injection. The patient should be helped to remain quiet by the use of a recommended sedative, if necessary. The diet should be high in iron, vitamin C, and protein, and include high-protein drinks between meals. The application of cold compresses and pressure sometimes lessens the amount of bleeding into the tissues. Persons with hemophilia should inform physicians and dentists of this condition. Identification should be worn or carried, which indicates that the person has hemophilia and names the type.

Some psychosocial concerns are common to the hemophiliac and family and must be addressed. In hemophilia A and B, the gene is transmitted by the mother, who may experience guilt feelings and compensate by overprotecting the child. As in sickle cell anemia or in any chronic condition that requires extra attention for the affected child, sibling rivalry and jealousy may be exaggerated. The hemophilic child learns early that trauma is associated with bleeding and may use defense mechanisms such as denial to cope. In adolescence and young adulthood this can be manifested in risk-taking behavior. Other adaptations include stress-related spontaneous bleeding and passive reliance on others, neither of which is an effective coping response. The nurse can assist the patient and family by recognizing these responses and confronting them. Referral to the National Hemophilia Foundation may be helpful.

Vascular purpuras

Assessment. **Purpura** is a condition in which there are small, spontaneous hemorrhages into the skin or mucous membrane. Tiny hemorrhages appearing as pinpoint purplish spots are called **petechiae;** larger hemorrhages are called **ecchymoses.**

Pathophysiology. Purpura may be divided into two categories: those associated with the destruction of platelets and those caused by failure of the bone marrow to produce platelets. *Idiopathic* or *autoimmune thrombocytopenic purpura* (ITP) is caused by the destruction of the platelets in the blood. The destruction results in a greatly reduced number of platelets and leads to bleeding. The disorder occurs in an acute form in children and may progress to a chronic disorder. It also occurs as a chronic disorder, most commonly in young adult females. Destruction of the platelets is caused by an antiplatelet factor in the plasma. In the chronic form, it may occur as a complication of a primary disease or after the ingestion of certain drugs. In some forms the platelets are deposited in large numbers in the spleen, causing splenomegaly. The second form of the disease, *thrombocytopenic purpura,* is caused by a failure in the production of platelets, which may be the result of damage to the bone marrow. Drugs and chemicals or conditions that require massive blood transfusions may result in purpura.

Intervention. Treatment and care depend on discovering and eliminating the cause. If purpura is caused by the destruction of platelets, both the acute and chronic stages of the disorder are treated with steroids. In some situations removal of the spleen may be indicated. If purpura is caused by a drug, withdrawing the drug usually corrects the condition.

Splenomegaly

The spleen is located in the upper part of the abdominal cavity under the lower part of the rib cage. It has four major functions: removal of microorganisms from the blood, formation of red blood cells under abnormal conditions, removal of old red blood cells and platelets from the circulation, and storage of blood. In blood dyscrasias, in which blood cell production in the marrow is compromised, the spleen may assume the function of producing all the blood cells. Not all of the functions of the spleen are understood. Enlargement of the spleen occurs in several diseases and is called **splenomegaly.**

Pathophysiology. Chronic congestive splenomegaly is commonly associated with certain blood dyscrasias in which removal of the spleen, *splenectomy,* may be indicated. Various disorders affecting the spleen may also require its removal. Injury to the organ, especially a crushing type, is always a surgical emergency. Splenectomy is done only as a reluctant, final intervention in children.

Postoperative nursing intervention. The nursing care of the patient after a splenectomy is essentially the same as that for other patients after abdominal surgery (see Chapter 17). Because the spleen has a rich blood supply and the patient may have a blood dyscrasia, it is important that the patient be carefully observed for postoperative hemorrhage. The patient should be carefully monitored for the development of a subphrenic abscess in the dead space created by removal of the spleen.

Nursing Care Plan

PATIENT WITH APLASTIC ANEMIA

Mr. Edwards is a 40-year-old male on the medical unit with a diagnosis of aplastic anemia. He saw his private physician 2 weeks earlier with complaints of fatigue, epistaxis, easy bruising, and hematuria. Since admission, he has undergone multiple diagnostic studies and is currently being prepared to transfer to an oncology regional center as a potential candidate for a bone marrow transplant. Various members of his extended family are being considered as potential donors, but no one has been identified as a tissue match as yet.

Mr. Edwards states that he lost 20 lbs before admission, but he has regained 5 lbs since admission. He received 10 units of cryoprecipitate the second day of his hospital stay, 1 unit of fresh frozen plasma the third day, and 2 units of packed red blood cells (PRBCs) the fourth day. Implantation of a porta-cath into the right subclavian region was performed under local anesthetic.

Mr. Edwards has no known food or drug allergies. Aspirin and nonsteroidal antiinflammatory drugs (NSAIDs) are contraindicated because of his pathologic condition.

Past Medical History

No previous hospitalizations, history of occasional premature ventricular contractions (PVCs), noted on recent inoffice ECGs; has hypertension (HTN), which is under control with the atenolol (Tenormin), 50 mg daily

Spontaneous passing of a kidney stone (nephrolithasis), 1 year before current illness

As a Vietnam veteran was exposed to Agent Orange while on ground patrol in that country (prolonged exposure)

Health risk behaviors: Smoked 3 to 4 packs of cigarettes per day × 21 years; drinks 2 to 3 cans of beer per day × 15 years

Health strengths: Has yearly physical examinations; eats a low fat diet, exercises at least twice per week (plays tennis); works out at the gym when he feels that his weight is climbing

Family History

Father died at age 67 from myocardial infarction (MI)

Mother alive and well, age 65, only health problem is hypertension, which is under control with medication

Older brother Sam died 3 months ago from a motor vehicle accident

Younger brother Joe, age 38; excellent health; lives in Europe

Psychosocial Data

Married for 16 years; periods of separation × 2; states that the last visits to the marriage counselor have strengthened their communication skills and now they have a quality "understanding" relationship; one daughter Sally, age 14, who is currently being shielded from the knowledge of the gravity of her father's illness; large extended family on wife's side

Has worked at automotive factory for 22 years; has HMO-oriented health insurance plan

Religion: Protestant; goes to church sporadically

Hobbies: Bowling, fishing, some contact sports; likes TV, but dislikes reading

Assessment Data

Appears chronically ill; oriented × 3 (time, place, and person)

Height 6 ft, weight 195 lb

Skin: Pale, with evidence of multiple bruises in various stages of healing; bruises mostly on trunk and upper arms; no rashes, no evidence of skin breakdown

Anterior chest wall has two intact, sutured incisions with no dressings; very slight serosangineous drainage from lower incision; no redness or edema present in either incision

Hematoma 5 × 6 cm noted to the right of incisions; patient keeping ice over the swelling

Respiratory: Rate 16-20; regular depth and rhythm; clear to percussion and ascultation

Abdominal: Soft, nondistended; positive bowel sounds heard in all four quadrants

Cardiovascular: Apical pulse of 78; best heard over apex

Musculoskeletal: Full range of motion all joints

Laboratory Data

WBC 6,000
RBC 2.69
Hgb 7.3
Hct 23.4
} All low = pancytopenia

Platelets 114,000

Oxygen saturation level = 79-81 without additional oxygen; improves up to 95 with 4 L oxygen continuously

BUN, creatinine, chloride, and potassium within normal limits.

Nursing Care Plan

PATIENT WITH APLASTIC ANEMIA—cont'd

Past Medical History	Psychosocial Data	Assessment Data
Two sisters, ages 33 and 34, both in good health; supportive relationships; all said to be willing to be tested as a candidate for bone marrow transplant *Medications* atenolol (Tenormin) 50 mg po daily allopurinol 300 mg po bid phytonadione (aqua METHYTON) 15 mg po bid methylprednisolone (SoluMedrol) 20 mg po q 6 hr		Calcium high at 11.2 (nl = 8.5-10.4) Sodium (Na) high at 148 (nl = 135-145) Albumin low at 3.2 (nl = 3.3-5.0) PT high at 14.0 PTT high at 42.5 IV 1000 ml normal saline at 100 ml/hr; may discontinue if po intake adequate; convert to a heparin lock

NURSING DIAGNOSIS

Risk for infection related to pancytopenia and surgical incision

NURSING INTERVENTIONS	EVALUATION OF EXPECTED OUTCOMES
Monitor vital signs at least every 4 hours and report any deviations from the baseline. Minimize the risk of infection by careful handwashing. All personnel, family, visitors, and staff need to comply. Use strict aseptic technique when inserting IV lines, changing dressings, and providing wound care. Have patient cough and deep breathe every 4 hours to help remove secretions and prevent pulmonary complications. Help patient turn q 2 hr; provide skin care, especially to bony prominences to prevent venous stasis and skin breakdown. Ensure adequate nutritional intake. Patient needs 2000 calories daily. Offer high protein supplemental snacks; patient likes milkshakes if cold. Arrange for reverse isolation if WBC count falls low. Monitor flow and number of visitors. Explain rationale to patient and family. Educate patient and family about good handwashing techniques and/or any other factors that increase infection risks.	Temperature and vital signs remain within the normal range WBC and differential count remain within a normal range Cultures do not grow pathogens Demonstrates appropriate personal/oral hygiene Incision site (port-a-cath) remains clear and pink and free of purulent drainage IV sites do not show signs of inflammation; skin does not exhibit signs of breakdown Lists risk factors that contribute to infection; remains free of infection

NURSING DIAGNOSIS

Risk for injury or fatigue related to altered hemodynamics

continued

NURSING INTERVENTIONS	EVALUATION OF EXPECTED OUTCOMES
Monitor daily laboratory values and document findings; report any abnormal values immediately to the physician. Assess for excessive bleeding, fatigue, or new bruising; inspect skin daily during bath. Guiac all stools. Place patient on neurovital signs. Monitor for changes in level of consciousness (LOC) or any signs of confusion. Keep on oxygen at 4 L. Check oxygen saturation levels every 4 hours. Monitor for a fall of O_2 saturation level if off oxygen. Assess for hematuria, epistaxis, blood in the stool, or dyspnea. Maintain IV hydration as ordered. Monitor intake and output. Force fluids (at least 1000 ml per shift) while on the allopurinol. Maintain patient safety measures such as no aspirin or nonsteroidal antiinflammatory drug (NSAID) products. No intramuscular injections when platelet count is so low. Put pressure on any venipuncture sticks for 5 minutes. Assist patient in and out of bed; monitor for safety. Monitor administration of blood and blood products. Assess baseline vital signs before and during any procedure according to hospital protocol. Check laboratory values before and after treatments, and watch for adverse reactions during the administration of any blood or blood products (assess for rash, hives, fever, or generalized urticaria). Teach patient ways to conserve energy (e.g., alternate periods of rest). Inform patient of the adverse effects of smoking, and encourage him to stop.	Laboratory values improve after the infusion of platelets and packed RBCs Fatigue will be lessened, and patient identifies ways to conserve energy; bruising diminishes No signs of covert or overt bleeding Has no untoward reaction during transfusion therapy Clotting profile return profiles returns to normal limits Patient improves in his ability to carry out ADLs

NURSING DIAGNOSIS

Risk for anxiety related to diagnosis as evidenced by restlessness, insomnia, aggression toward staff and family, changes in communiction patterns, and verbalization of inability to cope and meet role expectations

NURSING INTERVENTIONS	EVALUATION OF EXPECTED OUTCOMES
Spend 10 minutes with patient twice each shift; convey a willingness to listen. Offer verbal reassurance such as, "I know you're frightened, I'll stay with you." Give patient concise explanation of anything that is about to occur.	Patient reports decreased restlessness and anxiety; has longer periods of uninterrupted sleep Patient and family have quality discussions on the projected effects of the illness and lifestyle changes that might be necessary Daughter is included in the family discussions, and the exclusion behaviors are eradicated

NURSING INTERVENTIONS—cont'd	EVALUATION OF EXPECTED OUTCOMES—cont'd
Avoid information overload, because an anxious patient cannot assimilate many details. Make no demands on patient. Identify and reduce as many environmental stressors as possible. Have patient state what types of activities promote feelings of comfort, and encourage him to perform them. Remain with patient during severe anxiety. Include him in decisions related to care when feasible. Support the family in coping with patient's anxious behavior. Allow extra visiting periods with his family if this seems to allay anxiety. Teach patient relaxation techniques to be performed at least every 4 hours, such as guided imagery, progressive muscle relaxation, and meditation. Praise patient for initiating discussion with daughter; encourage daughter to share feelings. Refer patient to community or professional mental health resources as needed.	Patient and wife identify their usual patterns of coping and relate these to the perceived illness threat; draw strength from one another Patient practices relaxation techniques on an ongoing basis

NURSING DIAGNOSIS

Knowledge deficit related to lack of information regarding treatment protocol as evidenced by questioning drugs, side effects, and infusion therapies

NURSING INTERVENTIONS	EVALUATION OF EXPECTED OUTCOMES
Establish an environment of mutual trust and respect to enhance learning. Ascertain what patient already knows; clarify any misinformation; negotiate with patient to develop goals for learning. Select teaching strategies, such as discussion of visual materials and demonstration. Answer patient's questions honestly. Refer him to physician on matters related to medical protocol. Give clear explanations on the drugs that the patient is taking. Explain the dose, time, and need for compliance. Teach the patient the skills that he must incorporate into his daily lifestyle (dressing changes). Have patient give a return demonstration. Provide emotional support if patient questions the overall prognosis. Discuss bone marrow transplantation after the concept is introduced to him. Encourage the patient to ask further questions. Reinforce the prevention of infection.	Expresses a desire for new knowledge related to his treatment protocol Demonstrates newly learned skills and health-related behaviors Develops realistic learning goals Can state each drug he is taking, the correct dosage, the rationale for use, and some common side effects Writes down any questions related to his medical regimen to further enhance his knowledge about his illness Indicates an openness to discuss the potential of bone marrow transplantation and the availability of a matched donor

KEY CONCEPTS

- Blood, through its network of vessels, carries oxygen to cells and returns carbon dioxide to the lungs to be eliminated.
- Blood is composed of a liquid component called plasma and formed elements or cells.
- Cells are divided into (1) erythrocytes, or red blood cells; (2) leukocytes, or white blood cells; and (3) thrombocytes, or platelets.
- Types of diagnostic tests for blood disorders include complete blood count (CBC), coagulation tests, blood gas analysis, Schilling test, bone marrow aspiration, blood typing and cross-matching, and Rh factor.
- Blood transfusion reactions include allergic, hemolytic, pyogenic, circulation overload, and air embolism.
- Hemorrhagic anemia results from a loss of blood, which decreases the amount of circulating fluid and hemoglobin and the amount of oxygen delivered to the tissues.
- Symptoms of acute hemorrhagic anemia include thirst, rapid pulse rate, pallor, hypotension, and clammy skin.
- Interventions for massive hemorrhage include controlling the bleeding, treatment for shock, and replacing circulating volume.
- Anemia caused by iron deficiency is the most common type of anemia.
- Loss of blood is the most common cause of iron-deficiency anemia.
- Symptoms of iron-deficiency anemia include pallor, dyspnea, palpitations, and loss of appetite.
- Pernicious anemia results from the lack of an intrinsic factor and the subsequent development of vitamin B_{12} deficiency.
- Symptoms of pernicious anemia include pallor, nausea, vomiting, indigestion, constipation, diarrhea, and anorexia.
- Treatment of pernicious anemia includes injections of vitamin B_{12}, a high-protein diet, warm comfortable clothing, and rest periods.
- Sickle cell anemia is caused by an abnormal hemoglobin molecule (hemoglobin S).
- Symptoms of sickle cell anemia include fever, anemia, enlarged spleen and lungs, jaundice, and leg ulcers.
- Treatment of sickle cell anemia includes avoidance of stress and strenuous exercise, analgesics for pain, fluid therapy, avoiding respiratory tract infections, and rest periods.
- In aplastic anemia, insufficient red blood cells are produced as a result of an interference with the stem cells in the bone marrow.
- Symptoms of aplastic anemia include pallor, weakness, dyspnea, hypoxia, lethargy, and fatigue.
- Treatment of aplastic anemia includes antineoplastic drugs and radiation, or bone marrow transplantation.
- Polycythemia is caused by a proliferation of erythrocytes in the bone marrow.
- Symptoms of polycythemia include complaints of headache, fatigue, night sweats, pruritus, and dyspnea.
- The main treatment of polycythemia is to suppress the bone marrow, reduce blood cell mass, maintain the hematocrit at or below 50%, and reduce the leukocyte and platelet count.
- Leukocytosis is an increase in the number of white blood cells. In some forms of leukemia, the number of leukocytes is increased; however, the cells are immature.
- Leukopenia is a condition in which the number of leukocytes is greatly reduced. Patients with leukopenia need to be protected against infection.
- Symptoms of Hodgkin's disease include enlarged lymph nodes in the neck, weight loss, fever, and night sweats.
- Hodgkin's disease is classified into stages according to pathologic findings and probable prognosis.
- Leukemia is a neoplastic disorder resulting in widespread proliferation of white blood cells and their precursors throughout the body.
- Leukemia may be acute or chronic and is classified according to the type of cells involved.
- Nursing care for the patient with leukemia includes monitoring vital signs, inspecting for skin impairment, conserving the patient's energy, frequent oral hygiene, preventing infection, and monitoring white blood cell counts.
- Hemophilia refers to hereditary bleeding diseases that have prolonged bleeding times. The forms are classic hemophilia A, Christmas disease (hemophilia B), and von Willebrand's disease (hemophilia C).
- Symptoms of hemophilia include repeated hemorrhages into joints, ankles, knees and elbows; hematomas; hematuria; and anemia.
- Intervention for hemophilia includes prevention of injury, genetic counseling, transfusion therapy, avoiding injections and aspirin, a high iron and protein diet, and analgesics for pain.

CRITICAL THINKING EXERCISES

1 List three priority nursing diagnoses for the patient with anemia.
2 Describe the nursing responsibilities before blood transfusion therapy.
3 How would you evaluate the effectiveness of your teaching plan for the patient with leukemia?

REFERENCES AND ADDITIONAL READINGS

American Red Cross: *Circular of information for the use of human blood and blood components,* 1994, The American Red Cross.

Beare P, Myers J: *Principles and practice of adult health nursing,* ed 2, St Louis, 1994, Mosby.

Burtis R, Evangelist J: Will universal precautions protect me? A look at staff nurse's attitudes, *Nurs Outlook* 40(3):133-138, 1992.

Brunner L, Suddarth D: *Textbook of medical-surgical nursing,* ed 7, Philadelphia, 1992, JB Lippincott.

Cerrato P: Does your patient need more iron? *RN* 53(7):63-66, 1990.

Cerrato P: Your patient's anemic—but the problem isn't iron, *RN* 54(7):61-64, 1991.

Deglin J, Vallerand A: *Davis's drug guide for nurses,* ed 3, Philadelphia, 1993, FA Davis.

Drago S: Banking on your own blood, *Am J Nurs* 92(3):61-64, 1992.

Fischbach F: *A manual of laboratory diagnostic tests,* ed 4, Philadelphia, 1992, JB Lippincott.

Flyge H: Meeting the challenge of neutropenia, *Nursing* 23:60-64, 1993.

Hammond L, Machemer S: Myths and facts about blood and its components, *Nursing* 23(9):29, 1993.

Harous J, Antony H: Your guide to trouble-free transfusions, *RN* 56(11):26-35, 1993.

Lederer JR and others: *Care planning pocket guide: a nursing diagnosis approach,* ed 5, Redwood City, Calif, 1993, Addison-Wesley.

Luckmann J, Sorenson K: *Medical surgical nursing: a psychophysiological approach,* ed 4, Philadelphia, 1993, WB Saunders.

MacDermott B, Deglin J: *Understanding basic pharmacology: practical approaches for effective application,* Philadelphia, 1994, FA Davis.

Mantik S, Collier I: *Medical-surgical nursing. Assessment and management of clinical problems,* ed 3, St Louis, 1992, Mosby.

McConnell E: Clinical do's and dont's. Administering blood therapy safely, *Nursing 92,* 22(8):91, 1992.

McConnell E: What's wrong with this patient? *Nursing* 23(7):70-71, 1993.

Mills D: When blood won't clot, *RN* 55(11):28-33, 1992.

Monahan F, Drake T, Neighbors M: *Nursing care of adults,* Philadelphia, 1994, WB Saunders.

National Blood Resource Education Program's Nursing Education Working Group: Transfusion nursing: trends and practices for choosing blood components and equipment, *Am J Nurs* 91(6):42-56, 1991.

Pagana K, Pagana T: *Mosby's diagnostic and laboratory test reference,* St Louis, 1992, Mosby.

Panlilo A, Parrish C: Blood contacts during surgical procedures, *JAMA* 265(12):1533-1537, 1991.

Phipps WJ, Long B: *Medical surgical nursing: a nursing process approach,* ed 5, St Louis, 1995, Mosby.

Pollin S, DeLuca E: How to use the new weapon against anemia, *RN* 55(1):36-38, 1992.

Pugliese G: Universal precautions: now they're the law, *RN* 55(9):63-69, 1992.

Querin J, Stahl L: 12 simple sensible steps for successful blood transfusions, *Nursing* 20(10):68-81, 1990.

Rivers R, Williamson N: Sickle cell anemia: complex disease, nursing challenge, *RN* 53(6):24-29, 1990.

Rhodes A: A minor's refusal of treatment, *MCN Am J Matern Child Nurs* 15(4):261, 1990.

Spratto G, Woods A: *RN magazine's nurse's drug reference,* Albany, NY, 1994, Delmar.

Sympson G: CATR: a new generation of autologous blood transfusion, *Crit Care Nurse* 11(4):60-64, 1991.

Thibodeau GA, Patton KT: *Anatomy and physiology,* ed 2, St Louis, 1993, Mosby.

Thompson J, Mc Farland G, Hirsch J, Tucker S: *Mosby's clinical nursing,* ed 3, St Louis, 1993, Mosby.

US Department of Health and Human Services: *National blood resource education program's transfusion therapy guidelines for nurses,* 1-24, Washington, DC, 1990.

Vallerand HA, Deglin JH: *Davis' guide to IV medications,* ed 2, Philadelphia, 1994, FA Davis.

CHAPTER 23

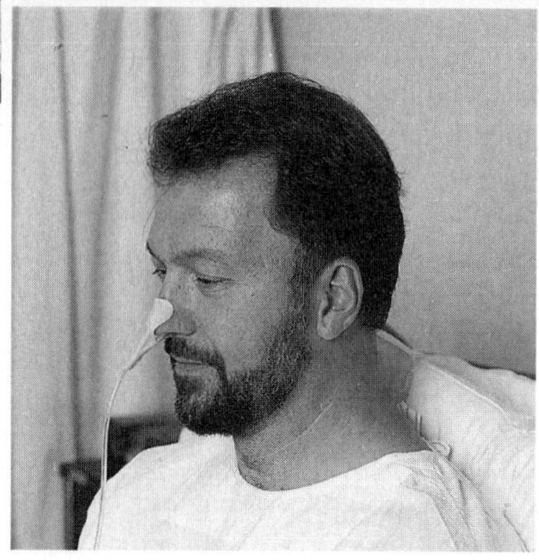

Gastrointestinal Function

CHAPTER OBJECTIVES

1. Describe the pathway of food through the gastrointestinal tract.
2. Explain the following diagnostic tests, including purpose, procedure, and preparation of the patient: endoscopy, gastrointestinal series, liver function tests, cholecystography, and cholangiography.
3. Discuss the nursing care of the patient with the following gastrointestinal disorders: diverticulitis; inflammatory bowel disease; intestinal obstruction; peptic ulcer; cirrhosis of the liver.
4. Discuss the care of the ostomy patient, including skin care, application of appliances, psychologic aspects, and nutritional management.
5. Describe the nursing care of the patient with a gastric decompression and enteral feeding, including routine care measures, problem solving, and prevention of complications.
6. Discuss the purpose of total parenteral nutrition and the potential side effects of administering it too rapidly.
7. Describe the modes of transmission of the various strains of viral hepatitis and nursing measures to control transmission.
8. Discuss the nursing care of the patient with cirrhosis of the liver and hepatic coma.
9. Identify nursing interventions to prevent complications following cholecystectomy.

KEY WORDS

anastomosis
cholangiography
cholecystectomy
cholecystography
cirrhosis
colostomy
diverticulitis
dysphagia
enteric fistula
esophageal varices
esophagogastroduodenoscopy
hepatitis
hernia
hiatus hernia
ileostomy
pancreatitis
paralytic ileus
peptic ulcer
peristalsis
total parenteral nutrition

STRUCTURE AND FUNCTION OF THE GASTROINTESTINAL SYSTEM

The gastrointestinal (GI) system, or alimentary tract, is also called the digestive system because its function is the digestion and absorption of food. The system begins in the mouth and terminates at the anus (Figure 23-1). The mouth is also called the *buccal* or *oral cavity.* Three sets of salivary glands secrete through ducts that open into the mouth. The teeth and tongue are considered accessory organs of digestion. The esophagus, which is approximately 10 inches long, leads from the mouth to the stomach. It descends through the thoracic cavity behind the trachea and the heart. A muscle, the **gastroesophageal sphincter,** controls the opening between the esophagus and the stomach. The muscle relaxes to permit the passage of food or fluids, after which it contracts to prevent backward flow. The stomach is a pouchlike structure located in the right upper quadrant of the abdominal cavity under the liver and the diaphragm. It is divided into three parts: the fundus, the upper part nearest the esophagus; the middle section, or body; and the pylorus, which is the lower part. Located between the stomach and the small intestine is the *pyloric sphincter,* which relaxes to permit passage from the stomach into the small intestine and contracts to prevent the contents of the intestine from returning to the stomach.

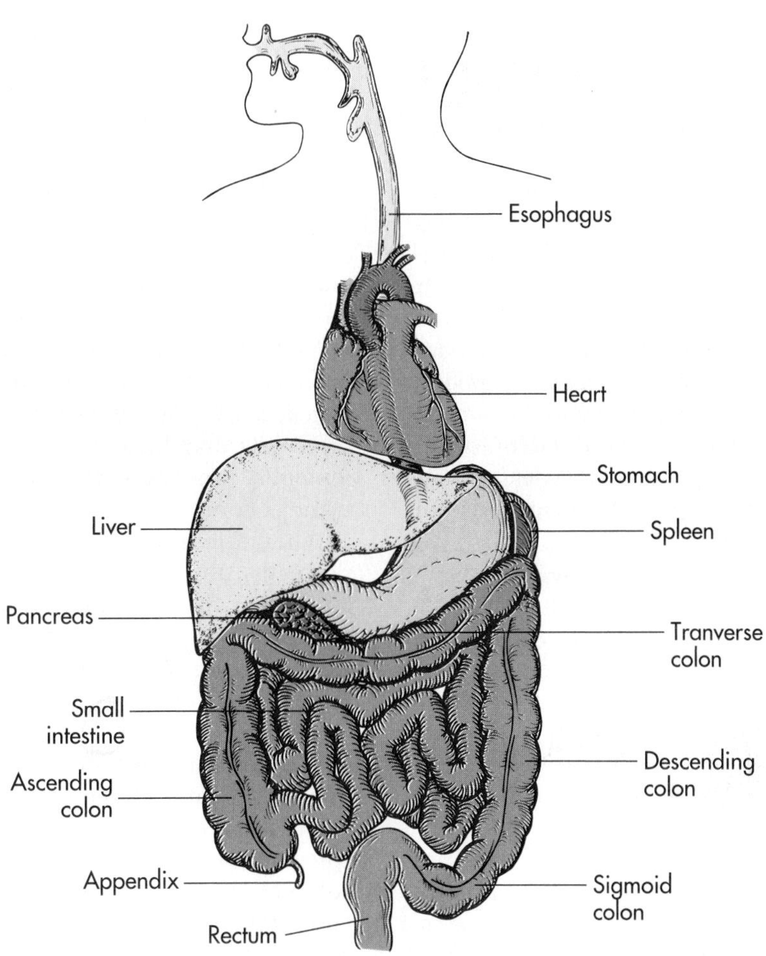

Figure 23-1 Anatomy of the gastrointestinal system. (From Potter PA, Perry AG: *Basic nursing,* ed 3, St Louis, 1995, Mosby.)

The small intestine, which is approximately 20 feet long, is divided into three segments: the *duodenum,* the *jejunum,* and the *ileum.* Most of the digestion and absorption of food takes place in the small intestine.

The large intestine or colon extends from the ileocecal valve to the anus. It is divided into seven segments: the *cecum,* the *ascending colon,* the *transverse colon,* the *descending colon,* the *sigmoid colon,* the *rectum,* and the *anus.* The large intestine is responsible for the absorption of water and electrolytes and the transport and elimination of waste matter. The ileocecal valve is located at the junction between the last section of small intestine (the ileum) and the first section of the large intestine (the cecum). The valve regulates the forward passage of intestinal contents from the ileum into the cecum and prevents the reflux of contents backward into the small intestine. The vermiform appendix, a small, wormlike appendage, is located at the lower end of the cecum. Two sets of sphincter muscles, the internal and external sphincters, are located within the anal canal and control defecation. The alimentary tract is lined with muscles that contract involuntarily to produce the wavelike contractions called **peristalsis** (McCance and Huether, 1994).

The liver, gallbladder, and pancreas are accessory organs of digestion. They assist the process of digestion by contributing specific secretions and enzymes essential for normal digestion and use. The liver, located in the right upper quadrant of the abdomen, under the diaphragm, is the largest of the organs. It has many digestive and metabolic functions. The gallbladder is shaped like a pear and lies under the liver. It stores and concentrates bile and releases it into the duodenum during the process of digestion. The pancreas is a slender organ, fishlike in shape, which is located at the back of the stomach with a portion extending into a C-shaped curve of the duodenum. Located within the pancreas are small masses of cells called *islands of Langerhans,* which secrete insulin (McCance and Huether, 1994).

Because much of the care of the patient depends on the specific parts of the gastrointestinal system affected, the nurse is encouraged to review in greater detail the structure and function of the system.

DIGESTION AND ABSORPTION

Digestion is the process by which food is prepared so that it may be absorbed and used by the body. Absorption is the process by which nutrients pass into the circulation so that they may be carried to the body tissues. Digestion is accomplished by two processes: (1) mechanical digestion and (2) chemical digestion.

During mechanical digestion, which begins in the mouth, food is cut and ground into small pieces (mastication). Its passage from the mouth to the stomach is facilitated by lubricating mucus from the salivary glands and the mucus-secreting glands along the esophagus. Food entering the stomach from the esophagus passes through the gastroesophageal sphincter. The muscle relaxes to allow food to enter the stomach, then contracts to prevent its backward flow. When the semiliquid contents of the stomach *(chyme)* enter the small intestine (duodenum), their passage is controlled by the pyloric sphincter, which relaxes and contracts in much the same way as the gastroesophageal sphincter. Food is moved along the entire route by wavelike muscular contractions (peristalsis). Mechanical digestion may be best described as a cutting, grinding, and churning process. As this action goes on, numerous enzymes are secreted that chemically act on the various food constituents.

Chemical digestion is the action of enzymes on proteins, carbohydrates, and fats, breaking them into simple compounds in preparation for absorption. Ptyalin is secreted in the mouth and acts on starches; however, this action is limited and largely destroyed by the hydrochloric acid in the stomach. Several hormones are secreted into the blood and transported to the stomach and small intestine to assist with the process of digestion. The major hormones affecting digestion are secretin, gastrin, and cholecystokinin. The breakdown of proteins begins in the stomach. Hydrochloric acid is secreted in the stomach, and the acidity must remain at about pH 2 for enzyme action. There is little action on fats in the stomach. The major part of chemical digestion occurs in the small intestine, where all of the food constituents undergo enzymatic action. An enzyme from the pancreas aids the digestion of fats. Bile produced in the liver and stored in the gallbladder is released into the duodenum and is required to dissolve fats and fat-soluble vitamins. Other vitamins, minerals, and water that are present require no enzyme action.

When chemical action is complete, through several processes, absorption begins. Carbohydrates and proteins enter the circulation through the portal system, whereas fats enter the lymph vessels and eventually reach the portal system near the thoracic duct. The large intestine (colon) has several functions before the cycle is complete. There are no enzymes in the large intestine. After the residue from the small intestine passes through the ileocecal valve and enters the colon, water and some electrolytes such as sodium and chloride are absorbed into the blood. Bacteria in the colon putrefy undigested foods, synthesize vitamin K and vitamins B_{12}, B_2, and B_1, and produce gas that assists in propelling the feces toward the anus. The urge to defecate is a reflex stimulated by distention of the rectum. Voluntary relaxation of the rectal sphincter assists defecation. It takes 24 to 40 hours for feces to pass through the large intestine.

The liver plays an important role in the metabolism of carbohydrates, fats, and proteins. It assists in the regulation of blood glucose by converting carbohydrates to glycogen, storing glycogen, and then converting it to glucose as needed. When glycogen stores are low, the liver deaminates (removes the ammonia) from amino acids to make glucose and glycogen or ketones for energy. It synthesizes and catabolizes fatty acids and neutral fats to form ketone bodies and active acetate (sources of cell energy). Its role in protein metabolism includes synthesis of amino acids and supply of plasma proteins for tissue repair. It synthesizes the proteins, prothrombin, and fibrinogen necessary for blood coagulation. The liver stores vitamins, including vitamin K and the other oil-soluble vitamins, and is the primary site of vitamin B_{12} storage.

There are many factors that affect the process of digestion and absorption. Elderly persons who have lost their teeth and have no dentures or poorly fitting ones will have problems with mastication. Thus the mechanical process of cutting and grinding will be compromised. The patient who must remain in a recumbent position may have difficulty in swallowing because food does not pass down the esophagus as easily as in a sitting position. Emotions affect the secretion of enzymes or may cause severe and painful contractions of the sphincter muscles. Pathologic disease may affect any part of the system; some may be treated medically, whereas others may require surgery. The lack of specific nutrients or sufficient calories may result in malnutrition or starvation.

ASSESSMENT OF THE GASTROINTESTINAL SYSTEM

Many conditions can disrupt the normal functioning of the gastrointestinal system. Specific pathologic conditions, traumatic injury, metabolic abnormalities, immunologic alterations, as well as normal age-related changes can interrupt normal function. Medications and other treatment measures often have an effect on the gastrointestinal system as well. For example, some chemotherapy drugs and antibiotics are known to cause nausea, vomiting, and diarrhea. Similar symptoms may occur in several different diseases, and the nurse assists the physician by making careful observation of the patient's complaints and assessment findings and reporting and recording them. The nurse performs a systematic assessment to ensure a thorough examination of the patient. The nurse determines from the patient or the family the normal pattern for the patient and any significant changes noted in weight, diet and appetite, and bowel elimination. Additionally, the nurse asks the patient about the use of laxatives or enemas and of alcohol. The nurse asks about any problems or concerns that the patient has. The nurse also observes the patient's mental state for signs of depression, anxiety, apprehension, and restlessness. The nurse obtains specific information about the onset, duration, and severity of any GI symptoms or complaints. Specific symptoms the nurse should ask the patient about include pain, distention, dyspepsia (indigestion), dysphagia (difficulty swallowing), nausea, vomiting, diarrhea, constipation, fecal incontinence, and bloody vomitus or stool. Because a serious imbalance of electrolytes can occur with many GI problems, it is essential for the nurse to assess for any signs and symptoms of electrolyte loss (see Chapter 8). Tissue turgor and the condition of mucous membranes should be assessed to determine the state of hydration.

Physical examination of the abdomen by inspection, auscultation, percussion, and palpation contributes essential information about GI status. When assessing and reporting information about the patient, the nurse should use and make reference to specific anatomic locations on the abdomen (Figure 23-2). The nurse records and reports all abnormal findings to the physician.

When assessing abdominal pain, the nurse asks the patient to describe the location and characteristics of the pain. Abdominal pain is usually described as throbbing, aching, stabbing, dull, intermittent, or constant. The nurse observes the abdomen for distention and notes whether the distention is localized to one or more areas of the abdomen or is generalized across the entire abdomen. If the patient complains of nausea, the nurse determines whether the nausea is constant or intermittent and whether the nausea is followed with vomiting. If the nausea is intermittent, does anything precipitate the nausea, like medications, hunger, or eating? If the patient is vomiting, the amount and characteristics of the vomitus are determined. Stools are observed for frequency, color, consistency, presence of mucus, bright red blood, coffee-ground appearance (indicating old blood), odor, and macroscopic parasites (worms).

DIAGNOSTIC PROCEDURES

Several diagnostic tests and procedures are performed to evaluate GI and biliary function. Some are performed to aid the physician in establishing a diagnosis when symptoms of a disease are present. Tests may be done to rule out the existence of a specific disease, and some may be done as a preventive measure to discover a disease before symptoms occur, when treatment may be most advantageous (Wallach, 1992).

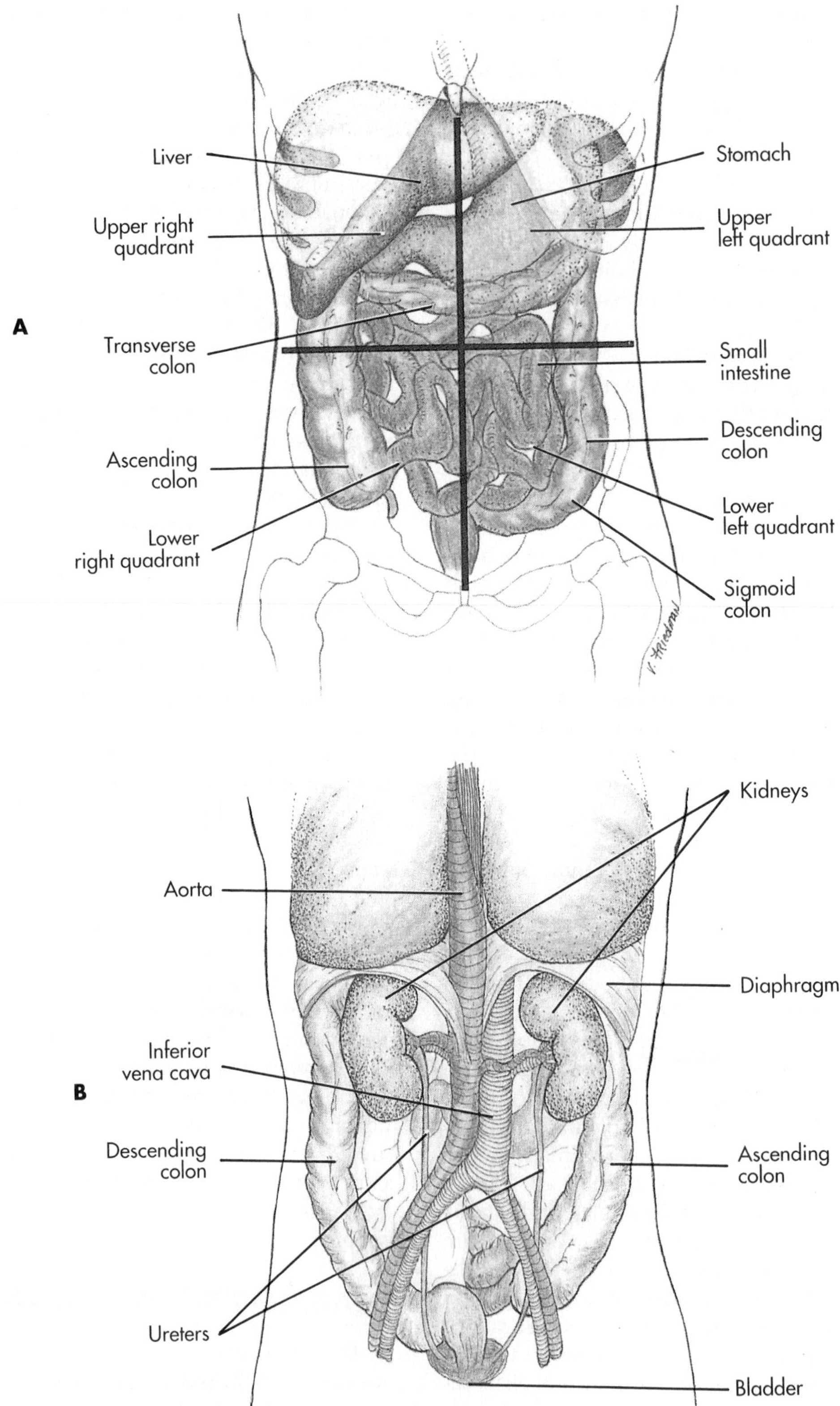

Figure 23-2 **A,** Anatomic areas of the abdomen described in *quadrants*—right and left upper quadrants; right and left lower quadrants. **B,** Posterior view. (From Potter PA, Perry AG: *Basic nursing,* ed 3, St Louis, 1995, Mosby.)

There may be some variation in procedures among physicians and hospitals. The nurse should understand the physician's orders and laboratory or x-ray protocols (Doughty, 1993).

Abdominal X-ray Examination

The abdominal x-ray examination is noninvasive and is used to assess the size and position of organs, to determine the presence of any masses, and to determine the distribution of intestinal gas, fluids, or calcifications. No patient preparation is needed. Several different x-ray films may be taken to examine the abdomen from various directions. Because of this, the patient may need to assume various positions during the examination.

Endoscopy

The upper gastrointestinal tract may be examined by endoscopy. This procedure (**esophagogastroduodenoscopy,** or EGD) allows direct visualization of the mucosal surface and luminal structures of the esophagus (esophagoscopy), the stomach (gastroscopy), or the duodenum (duodenoscopy). Another form of endoscopy (lower endoscopy) allows visualization of the large intestine (colonoscopy), or just the lower portions of the large intestine (proctoscopy, sigmoidoscopy).

The endoscope is an instrument containing a cluster of glass fibers that transmit light and return an image to a scope at the head of the instrument (fiberoptics). Pictures can be taken of suggestive lesions by attaching a camera to the head of the scope; a biopsy can be performed through the scope when desired. In addition to its use in diagnosing inflammatory, ulcerative, infectious, and neoplastic diseases of the gastrointestinal tract, it can be used for the removal of a foreign body.

For a complete EGD or any portion of this examination, the patient is usually kept NPO (nothing by mouth) for 6 to 12 hours before the procedure. An intravenous line is started or a heparin lock is inserted for intravenous administration of fluids, if needed, and medications. A surgical consent form must be signed before the patient is medicated; the patient should be instructed on the purpose and procedure. The patient is medicated with a sedative such as diazepam (Valium) or midazolam (Versed) before the procedure. Atropine may be given to reduce secretions and to act as a vagolytic to protect the patient from profound bradycardia during the insertion and manipulation of the endoscope. Vital signs should be taken before any medication is given and again before the patient is transferred to the examination room.

Before insertion of the flexible tube of the endoscope, the vital signs are taken once more, and the blood pressure cuff is left in place to monitor the patient's blood pressure during the procedure. The patient's throat is sprayed with an anesthetic, and a mouth guard is inserted to protect the teeth and keep the mouth immobile. The nurse maintains the patient on a cardiac monitor throughout the procedure because of the potential for cardiac arrhythmias. Additionally, a finger or ear pulse oximeter is used to monitor the patient for respiratory compromise, especially during an upper endoscopy.

The patient is positioned on the left side with the head of the bed elevated. The tube is inserted through the mouth and into the esophagus with the head bent forward. The physician may instruct the patient to change the position of the head and chin as the tube is passed through the various parts of the gastrointestinal tract. Additional medication for relaxation is given intravenously if needed. Air is sometimes instilled to flatten tissue folds; water or normal saline may be instilled to rinse materials from the lens or from a lesion. Suction may be applied to remove fluid and secretions. The patient will experience feelings of pressure as air is inserted. The tube is withdrawn when the physician has completed visualization or biopsy of the organ in question (Doughty, 1993).

After the test is completed, the patient's vital signs are taken before transfer. If the patient is an outpatient, further observation is performed in the recovery area. The hospitalized patient can be returned to his or her room. Until the patient is fully awake and stable, vital signs are taken often, and the patient is observed closely for respiratory problems. Food and fluid are withheld until the gag reflex returns. The nurse tests for the presence of the gag reflex by touching the back of the throat with a tongue blade. In the recovery period, the patient will experience a sore throat and some belching from the instillation of air. More severe pain in the throat, neck, stomach, back, or shoulder is not expected and could indicate perforation; the physician should be notified immediately and the patient's vital signs should be monitored. Elevation of temperature is another indication of perforation. Patients should be instructed to observe their vomitus or stool for blood and report it immediately.

Colonoscopy

The colonoscope is inserted via the rectum. The large intestine must be thoroughly cleansed to be clearly visible. The patient remains on a clear liquid diet for 24 hours before the examination. In addition, a thorough bowel cleansing with a laxative such as Golytely or Colyte is given the evening before the examination. Tap water or saline enemas are administered until clear returns are noted 3 to 4 hours before the examination. Soapsuds enemas are not given because they irritate the mucosa and stimulate mucous secretions that may hinder the examination. A sedative may be given intramuscularly or intravenously to help the patient relax. Vital signs, cardiac rhythm, and oxygen saturation are monitored as outlined for the patient undergoing EGD.

The patient is positioned on the left side, and the colonoscope is generously lubricated and inserted into the rectum. The patient will experience pressure and an urge to defecate. The nurse instructs the patient to breathe deeply and slowly through the mouth to relax the abdominal muscles. Air may be introduced to distend the intestinal wall. Flatus will escape around the instrument when air is instilled, and the patient is instructed not to try to control it. Suction can be used to remove blood or liquid feces. When the instrument is advanced to the descending sigmoid junction, the patient is assisted to the supine position, if necessary, to facilitate advancement of the instrument. This procedure is contraindicated in patients who are pregnant or have diseases of the bowel that would predispose them to perforation, such as ischemic bowel disease, acute diverticulitis, peritonitis, and active colitis. Following the examination, the patient's vital signs are monitored per the routine postoperative procedure, and the patient is observed for side effects of the sedatives and for perforation. Malaise, rectal bleeding, abdominal pain and distention, fever, and mucopurulent discharge should be reported to the physician immediately. The patient will pass large amounts of flatus and may be embarrassed unless privacy is provided. A normal diet can be resumed after recovery from sedation. Some blood may be present in the stool if a polyp is removed.

Proctoscopy and Sigmoidoscopy

Proctoscopy and sigmoidoscopy are examinations that enable the physician to visualize the lower portion of the gastrointestinal tract. The proctoscope is used to examine the rectum, whereas the sigmoidoscope can be inserted further to visualize the lower 10 inches of the gastrointestinal tract. The use of the flexible fiberoptic instrument allows further examination of the colon beyond the range of the rigid sigmoidoscope and is less uncomfortable for the patient.

Preparation for both procedures includes the administration of an enema before the examination. Diet and fasting orders will vary with the physician; they should be checked and followed closely.

The procedure is performed with the patient in the knee-chest or lateral position. The patient usually assumes a kneeling position on a special proctoscopy table that "breaks" in the middle so that he or she can bend at the waist. The patient is secured to the table while it is rotated so that the head is lowered and the buttocks are elevated. This position facilitates insertion of the instrument and allows the physician to assume a comfortable position during the procedure. The patient will feel pressure during insertion and advancement of the instrument and when air is instilled to distend the bowel lining. The position and procedure may be embarrassing to the patient. After the examination the patient is observed for signs of perforation as in the postoperative interventions for other endoscopic procedures.

Ultrasonography

Ultrasound examination may be ordered for examination of the gallbladder and biliary system, the liver, spleen, and pancreas to determine the presence of abscesses or to evaluate the stage of rectal cancer. High frequency sound waves are channeled into the region to be examined, and the echoes that result are converted to electric impulses, which are displayed as a pattern of spikes or dots on an oscilloscope screen. The pattern of the dots varies with tissue density and reflects the size, shape, and position of the organ being examined. There is no exposure to radiation. The ultrasound picture resembles an x-ray picture, but closer examination will reveal the series of dots or spikes that create the image. When a good view is obtained, photographs are taken for later study (Doughty, 1993).

The patient is instructed to fast for 8 to 12 hours before the examination to reduce the amount of gas in the bowel, which hinders transmission of ultrasound. When the gallbladder is to be examined, the patient is given a fat-free meal the evening before to promote accumulation of bile in the gallbladder. During the procedure the room may be darkened slightly to improve visualization on the oscilloscope. The test will take 15 to 30 minutes for each organ being examined. A water-soluble lubricant is applied to the face of the transducer, and then transverse scans are taken at frequent intervals and at angles appropriate for the organ being examined. After the procedure, the lubricant is washed from the abdomen and the patient may resume his or her usual diet. No other follow-up care is necessary. The presence of barium within the GI tract will interfere with ultrasound, so the ultrasound should be performed before any barium studies or delayed for at least 48 hours after any barium studies.

Computerized Tomography

Computerized tomography (CT) involves the passage of multiple x-ray beams through the upper abdomen while detectors record the strength of the x-ray beam as it is deflected off various tissues (tissue attenuation). This information is reconstructed by a computer as a three-dimensional image on an oscilloscope screen. Because attenuation varies with tissue density, CT can distinguish various tissues. The patient is kept NPO for at least 8 hours before the procedure. Oral contrast medium is administered approximately 4 hours before the procedure to accentuate different densities. Defects in the tissue are seen as different in density from normal tissue. Intravenous contrast may be given before to the procedure as well.

The patient is positioned supine on a radiographic table in the center of the scanner. Transverse x-ray films are taken and recorded on magnetic tape. This information is fed into the computer, and selected images are photographed. **The patient must be observed for an allergic reaction (iodine sensitivity) to the contrast medium.** CT may be ordered for examination of the biliary tract, liver, and pancreas or to diagnose tumors. Barium interferes with visualization of tissues during CT scanning; therefore, CT scan should be performed prior to barium studies or delayed for at least 4 days after barium studies.

Magnetic Resonance Imaging (Abdominal)

Magnetic resonance imaging (MRI) uses radiofrequency and a strong magnetic field to produce images of tissue. Different tissues produce different signals, and these variations are interpreted by the MRI computer to produce the images of various structures. Tissues with large amounts of water, such as blood vessels, produce stronger signals; whereas very dense structures, such as bone, produce weak signals. For this reason, MRI is most useful in evaluating soft tissue and blood vessels. Abdominal MRI is used to assist in evaluating abscesses, fistulas, and sources of GI bleeding. Patients are usually kept NPO for 6 to 8 hours before an abdominal MRI. Because of the strong magnetic field used in the MRI process, it is essential to determine whether the patient has any metallic devices or implants, such as earrings, rings, braces, pacemakers, or shrapnel. Some of these metal devices or implants may be contraindications to the use of MRI. The patient is instructed to remove any metal-containing devices that can be removed. The nurse must report any metal-containing implants or devices that are not easily removed, such as braces or pacemakers, to the MRI department before beginning the procedure. No post-examination follow-up is required.

Gastrointestinal Series

The gastrointestinal series (upper or lower) uses a radiopaque contrast material to provide an outline of the GI tract. These tests aid in the identification and diagnosis of abnormal conditions of the GI tract, tumors, ulcerative lesions, and problems with motility.

Upper GI series

An upper GI series provides visualization of contrast material (usually barium) as it passes through the esophagus and into the stomach and small intestine, if needed. The actual passage of the contrast material can be visualized with a fluoroscope as it moves down the esophagus. X-ray films are taken over time as the stomach and small intestine fill with the contrast material. It may take up to several hours for the contrast material to pass through the small intestines. The patient is kept NPO for 6 to 8 hours before the examination. After the examination, the nurse monitors the color and consistency of stool to ensure that the barium contrast material is completely passed. If the barium is not completely expelled within 2 to 3 days, a stimulant laxative (milk of magnesia, citrate of magnesia) is usually administered. If barium is not cleared from the GI tract, it can form a hard mass and lead to an impaction or an intestinal obstruction.

Lower GI series (barium enema)

If the physician needs to visualize the lower intestinal tract above the sigmoid, an enema containing barium is administered. The radiologist observes the filling of the colon with the fluoroscope, after which x-ray films are taken (Figure 23-3). If both upper and lower GI series are to be done, the patient should have the lower GI series first because it will take several days to completely eliminate the barium from the upper series.

A thorough bowel cleansing is necessary for a quality study of the lower GI tract. The patient is usually given a clear liquid diet for 24 hours before the lower GI series. Laxatives and enemas are administered to clear the colon of stool. After the examination, the nurse monitors for evacuation of the barium contrast and administers laxatives as needed as with the upper GI series.

In some clinical situations, it may be necessary to perform the study of the lower GI tract with a water-soluble contrast material (Gastrografin). For example, the use of barium contrast for a patient with suspected

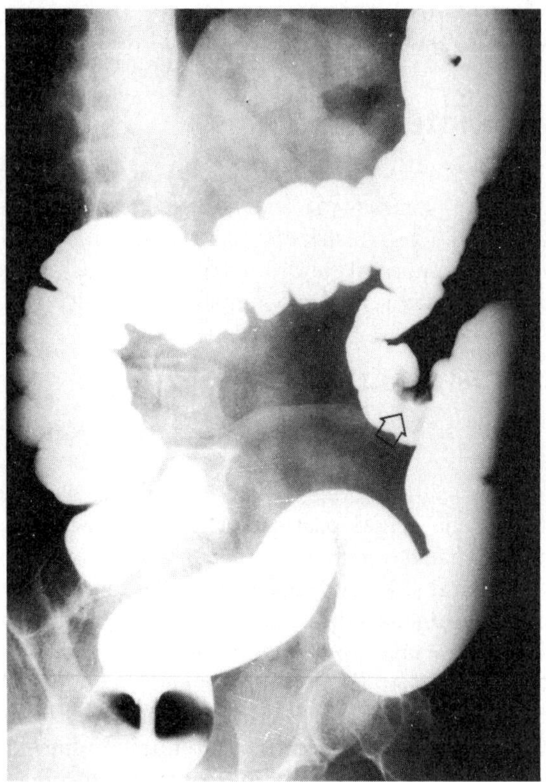

Figure 23-3 Barium enema. (From Pagana KD, Pagana TJ: *Pocket guide to laboratory and diagnostic tests,* St Louis, 1986, Mosby.)

GI perforation is contraindicated because of the risk of peritoneal contamination. The procedure is the same as the barium enema but with a different contrast medium. Patient preparation is similar to that of barium studies, except that bowel cleansing will depend on the patient's diagnosis. Laxatives and enemas are usually eliminated in the patient with a suspected bowel perforation. Gastrografin is iodinated, so the nurse determines if the patient has any known allergies or sensitivity to iodine or other contrast materials. Postprocedure enemas or laxatives are not needed because the medium is not constipating and is easily eliminated.

Gastric Analysis and Histamine Test

The test for gastric analysis is performed to examine the acidity of the stomach contents. Cells of the stomach secrete hydrochloric acid, which aids digestion. The value of acid measured in the stomach is useful in the diagnosis of diseases of the upper GI tract, such as peptic ulcers, carcinoma, and Zollinger-Ellison syndrome. The patient receives nothing by mouth after supper the evening before the test, and in the morning a tube is passed through the nose into the stomach. A large syringe is attached to the tube, and the contents of the stomach are aspirated. Usually several specimens are secured at intervals according to the physician's direction. Each specimen must be carefully labeled with the time it was taken, as well as its numerical order. A clamp is placed on the tube between specimens, and the tube is taped to the patient's face. The physician may wish to stimulate the flow of gastric secretions and will order a subcutaneous injection of histamine or betazole (Histalog). This is known as the histamine test. The gastric secretions are then aspirated at 15-minute intervals for 1 hour or longer. Because some patients are sensitive to histamine and may have a reaction, a tray with a syringe containing a 1:1000 solution of epinephrine should be ready for emergency use.

The procedure is explained to the patient, and the patient is assured that although the procedure may be uncomfortable, it is not painful. An emesis basin is given to the patient because gagging may produce vomiting during the procedure. The test may be performed in the physician's office or in an outpatient clinic. The procedure may be carried out by the nurse under the physician's direction, or it may be done by a laboratory technician.

Stool Analysis

Stools may be examined for bacteria, parasites, or blood, or a chemical analysis may be made. The process of digestion changes blood that might be coming from the stomach or the intestine so that it will not be observed in the stool on inspection. Chemical examination is then necessary to detect *occult* (hidden) *blood.* In some instances the patient may be given a meat-free diet for 3 days before the test because these substances may cause a false positive reaction, whereas in other situations any random stool may be sent to the laboratory. Stools may also be examined for other substances that may indicate disorders of the biliary tract, pancreas, or some problem of digestion of food.

Stool specimens may be examined for various types of parasitic infections. The specimen is obtained and kept in various ways, depending on the type of parasite sought. Most stool specimens must be taken to the laboratory as soon as they are obtained and must be kept warm.

Cholecystography (Oral)

Through the use of a radiopaque dye, it is possible to visualize the gallbladder and the extrahepatic biliary system with **cholecystography.** This assists the physician in detecting calculi (stones), inflammatory conditions, or tumors of the gallbladder. After a low-fat evening meal, the patient is given a synthetic radiopaque drug, usually iopanoic acid (Telepaque) orally. The number of tablets ordered is based on the weight of the patient. The tablets should not be crushed and should be taken one at a time, at 5-minute intervals, with one or two sips of water. Thereafter, nothing is permitted by mouth. If the tablets are vomited, or if the patient shows any other signs of intolerance to the dye (itching, cramps, diarrhea, flushing), the physician should be notified. In the morning a cleansing enema may be ordered so that the presence of stool in the intestine does not obstruct visualization of the gallbladder. After the x-ray films are taken, a high-fat diet may be given to stimulate the gallbladder to contract, expelling the dye into the bile ducts. X-ray films are again taken to visualize the biliary system. The nurse should be sure that the examination has been completed before permitting the patient to have food. The patient is observed for any toxic symptoms resulting from the radiopaque drug.

Cholangiography

Cholangiography allows for visualization of the biliary ducts. It may be used when a patient cannot tolerate or is unable to absorb the oral agents. The contrast medium may be injected into the blood (intravenous cholangiography), into a *T tube* inserted after a cholecystectomy (T-tube cholangiography), or through the skin directly into the ductal system (percutaneous cholangiography). The patient is informed that the procedure may involve being placed on a tilting x-ray examination table that rotates into vertical and horizontal positions and that injection of the contrast medium may cause nausea, vomiting, hypotension, flushing, and urticaria. A severe reaction may produce anaphylactic shock. Before the examination, a consent form is signed and a patient history is taken to determine hypersensitivity to iodine, seafood, or contrast media used in other diagnostic tests. During the procedure, the patient is monitored for any response to the contrast. Vital signs are checked often during and after the procedure until they are stable.

Nursing Responsibilities for Tests and Diagnostic Procedures

When the physician writes the order for examinations and tests, the forms must be properly completed and the laboratory or x-ray departments notified without delay. Several tests and procedures require special patient preparation before the procedure, such as diet modification, NPO status, or bowel cleansing. The nurse determines what specific preparation is necessary and initiates patient preparation.

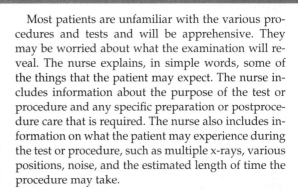

PATIENT/FAMILY TEACHING

Most patients are unfamiliar with the various procedures and tests and will be apprehensive. They may be worried about what the examination will reveal. The nurse explains, in simple words, some of the things that the patient may expect. The nurse includes information about the purpose of the test or procedure and any specific preparation or postprocedure care that is required. The nurse also includes information on what the patient may experience during the test or procedure, such as multiple x-rays, various positions, noise, and the estimated length of time the procedure may take.

Specimens to be collected by the nurse are obtained promptly, labeled properly, and sent to the laboratory. The patient is prepared and transported to the x-ray department or laboratory at the scheduled hour. If for any reason an appointment cannot be kept at the specified time, the department should be notified as early as possible. Medications ordered before and in preparation for tests and studies are administered promptly and recorded. Any patient receiving intravenous dye is carefully assessed for allergies before the examination and for reactions after the procedure.

Many patients, especially the elderly, are at risk for fluid and electrolyte problems related to special preparations for these tests and procedures. Restricted dietary and fluid intake, as well as repeated bowel cleansing procedures, could result in severe dehydration and electrolyte depletion. The nurse must evaluate the patient for potential problems and discuss with the physician the need for intravenous fluid and electrolyte replacement in high-risk patients.

LABORATORY STUDIES

Laboratory studies of blood, urine, and stool provide information about gastrointestinal, hepatic, and biliary function. Serum electrolytes, hematocrit and hemoglobin, white blood cell count, and serum osmolarity and bicarbonate contribute valuable but nonspecific information about pathologic conditions. Some tests, however, provide more specific information about GI, hepatic, pancreatic, and biliary function, as well as about nutritional status (Table 23-1) (Doughty, 1994; Wallach, 1992).

Carcinoembryonic Antigen

Carcinoembryonic antigen (CEA) is a protein seen on the membrane of many tissues. CEA is also seen on

TABLE 23-1

Laboratory Tests of GI, Hepatic, and Biliary Function

Test	Normal Value
Carcinoembryonic antigen (CEA)	< 5.0 ng/ml
Bilirubin	
Indirect	0.2-0.8 mg/dl
Direct	0.1-0.3 mg/dl
Total	< 1.0 mg/dl
Liver enzymes	
Alkaline phosphatase	30-85 ImU/ml or 42-128 U/L (SI units)
Aspartate aminotransferase (AST) (Formerly SGOT)	8-20 U/L or 5-40 IU/L
Alanine aminotransferase (ALT) (Formerly SGPT)	5-35 IU/L or 8-20 U/L (SI units)
γ-Glutamyl transpeptidase (GGTP)	8-38 U/L men and women ↑ 45 years; 5-27 U/L women ↓ 45 years
Lactic dehydrogenase (LDH)	45-90 U/L or 115-225 IU/L
Ammonia	15-110 μg/dl or 47-67 umol/L (SI units)
Serum proteins	
Albumin	3.5-5.0 g/dl
Globulin	2.0-3.5 g/dl
Total	6.4-8.3 g/dl
Clotting factors	
PT	11.5-14 sec
PTT	25-40 sec
Nutritional factors	
Albumin	3.5-5.0 g/dl
Prealbumin	15-32 mg/dl
Transferrin	250-300 mg/dl
Urine urea nitrogen (UUN)	Positive balance

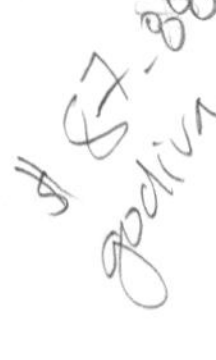

some cancerous tissues of the GI system. However, elevated levels of CEA are not diagnostic of GI cancer because the level may be elevated with other cancers as well as noncancerous diseases. For this reason, CEA levels are not a good tool for identifying GI cancers. CEA levels are a valuable monitoring tool for evaluating a patient's response to treatment or for monitoring the patient for recurrence of disease.

Liver and Biliary Function

Bilirubin tests

Bilirubin tests may be performed on blood, urine, or feces. Bilirubin, a pigment resulting from a breakdown of hemoglobin, is excreted with bile into the small intestine, where it is converted to urobilinogen. Some of the urobilinogen is excreted, and some is returned to the liver, where it is reconverted into bilirubin. Normally, little bilirubin appears in the blood, but when obstruction of the bile ducts or liver cell damage occurs, bilirubin is picked up by the blood, resulting in jaundice. Thus in jaundice there is an increase of bilirubin in the blood. Bilirubin is normally excreted in feces and urine in the form of urobilinogen. Elevated levels of serum bilirubin are associated with hemolysis of RBCs (indirect), liver cell damage, or biliary obstruction (direct and total).

Liver enzymes

Alkaline phosphatase. Alkaline phosphatase is synthesized primarily in the liver and in bone. Elevated levels of alkaline phosphatase are seen in many various disease processes, such as bone fractures and bone metastases, and are not specific to the GI system. Test results are evaluated in light of the patient's history, signs and symptoms, and physical assessment.

Aspartate aminotransferase. Aspartate aminotransferase (AST) is an enzyme found in cardiac, liver, skeletal muscle, kidney, and cerebral tissue. It functions in the synthesis of amino acids. When cell damage occurs, AST is released and serum levels rise.

Alanine aminotransferase. Alanine aminotransferase (ALT) is found in high concentrations in liver tissue. Lower concentrations are seen in cardiac and other tissue. Like AST, ALT is an enzyme that also functions in normal protein metabolism. Elevated levels of ALT are indicative of liver cell damage.

Gamma-glutamyl transpeptidase. Gamma-glutamyl transpeptidase (GGTP) is an enzyme found primarily in the kidneys but also in the liver, pancreas, and prostate. Elevated levels are seen in biliary disease, chronic alcoholism, acute pancreatitis, gallbladder disease, liver cancer, and cirrhosis.

Lactic dehydrogenase. Lactic dehydrogenase (LDH) is an enzyme found in almost all cells. It is found in the liver, heart, kidney, skeletal muscle, brain, and red blood cells. It is released when cells are damaged. Elevated levels of LDH indicate cell injury, but the elevation is not specific to what tissue is injured. There are five different *isoenzymes* that are specific to certain tissue types. LDH_4 and LDH_5 are most specific to liver and skeletal muscle tissue damage.

Ammonia

Ammonia is the end product of protein metabolism. Normally ammonia is absorbed into the blood from the intestine and transported to the liver via the portal vein. In the liver, ammonia is converted to urea for excretion by the kidneys. When liver cells are damaged and cannot convert ammonia to urea, or when portal blood is shunted away from the liver via collateral circulation, serum ammonia levels rise.

Serum Proteins

Serum proteins (albumin, globulin, transferrin) are synthesized in the liver. Therefore reduced levels of these proteins may be indicative of reduced liver function.

Blood Clotting Factors

The liver plays a major role in coagulation by synthesizing coagulation factors. Additionally, bile salts in the GI tract are required for the absorption of vitamin K in the ileum. Vitamin K is necessary for the liver to synthesize prothrombin. Abnormalities in liver or intestinal function may alter the synthesis of coagulation factors. *Prothrombin time (PT)* and *partial thromboplastin time (PTT)* are used to evaluate coagulation status.

Nutritional Status

Dietary intake and GI function affect nutritional status. Selected laboratory tests are used to evaluate nutritional status. Blood levels of *albumin, prealbumin,* and *transferrin* depend on protein intake and the liver's ability to synthesize the specific proteins and are therefore markers of nutritional status. Decreased values reflect either inadequate protein intake or inability of the liver to synthesize proteins. Urine urea nitrogen (UUN) is also used to assess protein balance. The value is determined by subtracting the amount of protein excreted in the urine from the amount of dietary protein. Normal UUN is a positive number, indicating that more protein was ingested than excreted.

THERAPEUTIC TECHNIQUES OF THE GASTROINTESTINAL TRACT

Gastric Lavage

Gastric lavage refers to the washing out of the stomach. Gastric lavage is used to remove large amounts of blood accumulated from upper GI bleeding, to remove ingested poisons, or to neutralize any ingested caustic agents. A large-bore tube is passed through the mouth into the stomach. Approximately 4000 ml of solution (which may be tap water, physiologic saline, 5% solution of sodium bicarbonate, or in case of poison, the specific antidote or activated charcoal) is used. Not more than 500 ml of solution is instilled into the stomach at one time. It is then siphoned back and the procedure is repeated. In the case of poison, usually the siphoned solution may need to be saved for laboratory analysis. Emotional and physical support of the patient is very important during this procedure.

Gastrointestinal (Gastric) Decompression

Gastric decompression is used to remove air (gas) and fluids from the upper gastrointestinal tract. A nasogastric tube (Levin tube or Salem sump) is most commonly used for this purpose. The tube is generously lubricated with a water-soluble jelly and passed through a nostril, down the esophagus, and into the stomach. After the tube is inserted, placement in the stomach must be checked. There is no foolproof method other than a chest x-ray examination of verifying correct tube placement. Common bedside methods used to check for correct tube placement include aspiration of gastric contents, pH testing of contents, and air instillation. To check for tube placement by aspiration, the nurse should attach an irrigating syringe to the drainage port of the tube and attempt to aspirate stomach contents. The aspiration of stomach contents into the syringe suggests correct tube placement. The normal pH of stomach contents is low because of the presence of hydrochloric acid, so if pH testing of the contents aspirated from the tube is acidotic (between a pH of 2 and 4), correct placement of the tube in the stomach is assumed. If the nurse is unable to aspirate stomach contents, a small amount of air (10 to 30 ml) can be injected through the tube while auscultating the gastric bulb (upper middle abdomen) for the "rush" of air. After correct placement is confirmed, the tube is taped in place to secure its position. The tube should be taped in such a fashion as to prevent pressure injury to the nostril (Figure 23-4; Box 23-1). The tube is then attached to either continuous or intermittent low suction (60 to 80 mmHg) (Figure 23-5).

Gastric decompression is commonly used to prevent or treat a postoperative ileus and to reduce pressure from accumulated fluid on anastomotic suture lines in the patient with upper GI surgery. Gastric decompression is also used for patients who have an intestinal obstruction with a large accumulation of secretion.

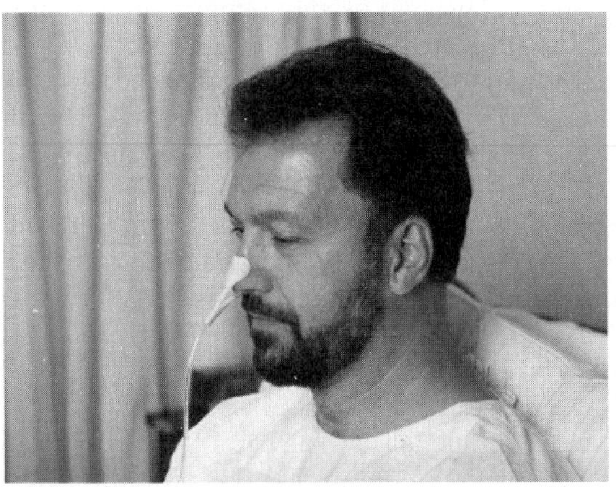

Figure 23-4 Secure nasogastric tube with tape to maintain correct placement and to prevent damage to the nasal tissues.

The length of time the tube is left in place depends on the patient's condition. It is dependent on the return of peristalsis (bowel sounds) and the amount and characteristics of the drainage. As long as the patient has a gastric decompression tube in place, the nurse is responsible for maintaining tube patency, recording the amount and characteristics (color, odor, pH, and heme) of the drainage, and assessing for the presence of bowel sounds.

Intestinal Decompression

Intestinal decompression may be necessary when an obstruction along the intestinal route is suspected or in the case of paralytic ileus. Several types of long tubes may be used for this purpose, including the Harris tube, Miller-Abbott tube, or Cantor tube (Figure 23-6). These are long, soft rubber tubes with a balloon at or near the end and eyes through which secretions may be drained. The Miller-Abbott tube has two lumens; one opens into the balloon, into which mercury is placed; the other is attached to suction. The tube is inserted through the nostril and is advanced along the intestine by peristaltic action or by the weight of the mercury. Secretions along the route are removed by low suction. The tube usually remains in the intestinal tract for several days and then is removed gradually (Figure 23-7).

All decompression tubes are generally attached to some type of suction apparatus, and it is important that the equipment used be in working order. The tubing for *gastric* suction is pinned or clipped to the patient's

BOX 23-1

Guidelines of Care for the Patient with Gastrointestinal (Gastric) Decompression

1. Maintain patency of decompression tube.
2. Irrigate tube as necessary with 30 ml normal saline. Check with physician before irrigating tube in patients with esophageal or gastric surgery.
3. Tape nasogastric tube to nose or cheek; *do not* tape intestinal decompression tubes; ensure that no pressure is placed on nostril.
4. Administer nothing by mouth unless ordered; physician may permit sips of water, ice chips, or hard candy.
5. Cleanse nostril through which tube is passed at least once every 8 hours; lubricate with water-soluble jelly.
6. Administer mouth care every 2 hours; rinse mouth with water or nonalcohol mouthwash; lubricate lips and oral mucosa with water-soluble jelly or solution.
7. Pin nasogastric tube to gown to prevent displacement with turning; loop intestinal decompression tube on bed to prevent displacement.
8. Attach tube to low suction unless otherwise ordered.
9. Empty and measure drainage bottle every 8 hours and record.
10. Observe and record color, appearance, odor, pH, and presence of blood, bile, or mucus.
11. Notify physician if tube is not draining despite irrigation.
12. Assess for signs of fluid and electrolyte deficit; evaluate fluid balance: total fluid in minus total fluid out.

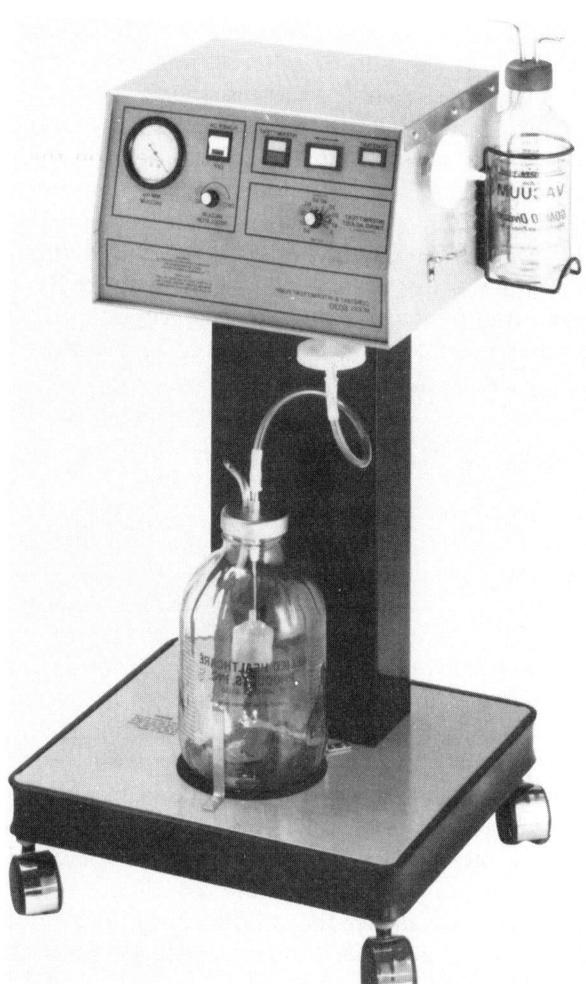

Figure 23-5 Gomco thermotic pump. (Courtesy Allied Healthcare Products, St Louis, Mo.)

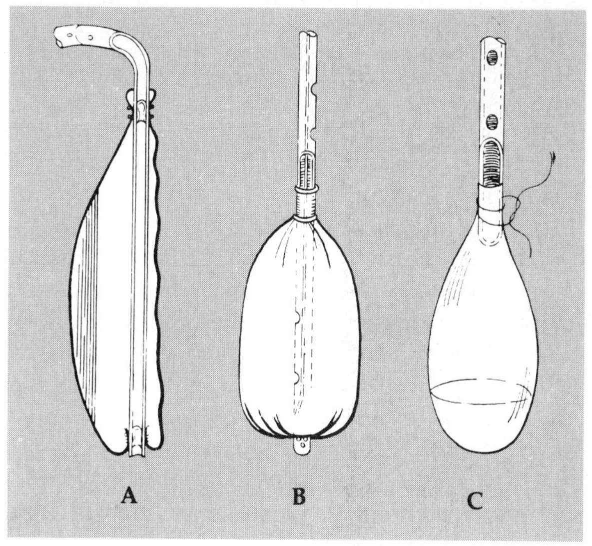

Figure 23-6 Decompression tubes. **A,** Harris tube. **B,** Miller-Abbott tube. **C,** Cantor tube.

gown, allowing sufficient slack to permit the patient to turn without displacement of the tube. Care should be taken to prevent the tubing from becoming kinked or obstructed by the patient lying on it. Patients usually complain of considerable discomfort from the nasogastric tube. The nostrils become dry and crusted from increased mucous secretions. The throat is irritated, and the mouth and lips are dry from mouth breathing. The patient often receives nothing by mouth but should be allowed to rinse the mouth often with water or a mouthwash that does not contain alcohol. Water-soluble moisturizers, such as K-Y jelly or Mouth Moisturizer, are recommended for use on lips and within the mouth to promote moisture. Lemon and glycerine swabs should be avoided. The acid in the lemon can cause tissue irritation as well as decalcification of teeth; glycerine absorbs water, leading to drying and irritation of the mucous membranes. The nares around the tube are cleansed with applicators and warm tap water or a water-soluble jelly. Some physicians may allow the

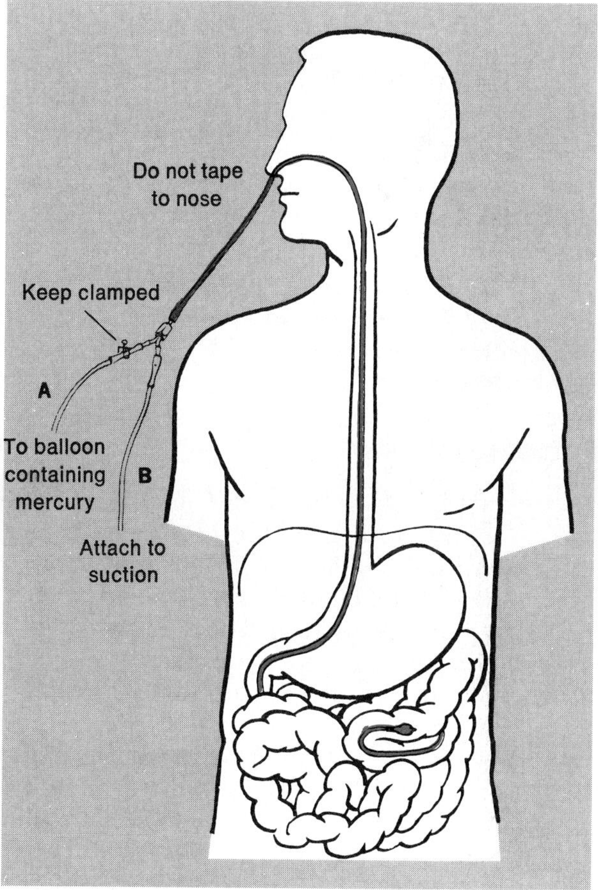

Figure 23-7 Intestinal decompression tube in place. Note that tube is not taped to nose. **A,** Arm of Y tube leading to balloon containing mercury or air must be kept clamped. **B,** Other arm of Y tube is attached to rubber tubing leading to suction.

patient to have occasional chipped ice, sips of water, or hard fruit candy to relieve throat discomfort. Chewing gum results in some swallowing of air; therefore some physicians disapprove of it.

Drainage tubes may become blocked with blood or mucus, which obstruct the flow. The physician often orders irrigation of the tube with sterile physiologic saline solution every 2 hours or as necessary to keep it patent and draining. Not more than 30 ml of solution should be injected (gently) through the tube at one time. Careful aspiration of the solution may be necessary to ensure patency of the tube, but any vigorous effort to aspirate the tube should be avoided. Irrigating solution is *not to be aspirated from long intestinal decompression tubes.* If the suction apparatus is working properly and the tube is patent, the solution will return. Accurate records of irrigation solution used must be maintained, and the amount must be deducted from the total gastric drainage. The secretions in the drainage bottle are measured at least every 8 hours and recorded. The appearance, odor, and presence of blood, bile, or mucus is noted. If the nurse observes that the tube is failing to drain despite efforts to irrigate it, the physician is immediately notified.

When intestinal decompression tubes are used, they should *not* be taped to the nose, because they are designed to move through the intestine by gravity and peristaltic action. Caution must be used in irrigating these tubes to ensure that the solution is injected into the opening that is attached to suction. The other opening leads into the balloon containing air or mercury and it is kept clamped shut. To avoid error, both outlets should be labeled. Measurement and observation of drainage are the same as those done with the gastric tube.

Enteral Feeding

Enteral feeding is used to provide nourishment to patients who are unable to meet their nutritional needs with an oral diet. *Enteral* refers to any location within the GI tract, usually via the stomach, the duodenum, or the jejunum. Enteral feeding is the preferred alternative to normal eating for providing nutrition when the GI tract is able to tolerate and absorb an adequate amount of nutrients. *If the gut works . . . use it.* Enteral feeding may be administered as the sole source of nutrition or as a supplement to oral or intravenous nutrition. A tube for feeding may be inserted into the stomach or duodenum either through the nose (nasogastric, nasoduodenal) or directly into the stomach or duodenum (gastrostomy, duodenostomy). If the patient is to be fed into the jejunum, the tube is placed during surgery. Jejunostomy tube feeding is usually reserved for patients who have had extensive surgical resection of the upper GI tract, such as total gastrectomy or Whipple procedure. It allows the patient to receive nutrition via the GI tract while bypassing the area just operated on.

A small-bore, flexible tube is preferred for nasoenteral feeding to minimize the discomfort and complications associated with the larger bore, hard tubes used for gastric drainage. The tube is introduced through the nose into the stomach in the same manner as a Levin tube or Salem sump. If the tube is to be placed into the duodenum, a slightly longer and weighted tube is used to help the tube move forward past the pylorus and into the duodenum. Placement of feeding tubes is confirmed by x-ray examination before administering feedings or medications. Tubes are flushed with 20 to 30 ml of water intermittently and after administering any medications, to prevent clogging of the tube.

Enteral feeding may also be administered via a gastrostomy tube—a tube placed directly into the stomach with an exit site on the surface of the abdomen. *Percutaneous endoscopic gastrostomy* (PEG) is a method of placing a gastrostomy tube through the skin (percutaneous) with internal placement guided and visualized through an endoscope. PEG tubes are usually placed when long-term gastrostomy feeding is anticipated. Displacement of the tube, perforation of the mucosa, and gastric reflux are potential complications of the PEG. Displacement of the PEG tube, either inward or outward, is a complication that the nurse assesses. The nurse measures the length of the tube from the skin to the feeding adaptor and compares the length with prior measurements. If the PEG tube migrates forward, it may obstruct the pyloric outlet, causing nausea and vomiting. Perforation of the gastric mucosa by the tube causes gastric contents to leak into the peritoneal cavity, causing peritonitis, with signs of temperature, abdominal pain, and rigidity. Reflux of gastric contents and enteral feedings causes chemical irritation to the skin. The nurse keeps the PEG site clean and dry. The site is cleansed with mild soap and water, and initially a dry dressing is applied. After complete healing, a cover dressing is no longer necessary. If gastric reflux occurs, the nurse applies a protective barrier wafer to protect the skin around the insertion site.

Liquid feedings or medications are introduced through the tube and may flow by gravity or be controlled by pump. Feedings may be administered continuously at a set rate or intermittently at a prescribed volume. Fewer complications are associated with continuous tube feeding. The patient should be positioned with the head of the bed elevated at least 30 degrees if not contraindicated, or in the side-lying position to prevent aspiration. Signs of pain, gastric or abdominal distention, or vomiting are reported to the physician. Routine assessment of appropriate tube placement is completed by the nurse. For intermittent feedings, placement is checked by aspiration or air instillation before each feeding. With continuous feedings, the nurse checks for correct tube placement at least once each shift. The nurse observes the patient for any changes in respiratory rate, breathing pattern, or breath sounds to assess for aspiration of the feedings into the lungs. Diarrhea is a common complication associated with enteral feeding. It may occur from changes in the absorptive function of the GI tract as a result of prolonged periods of no GI feeding, or it may result from the high osmotic nature of tube feeding formulas. Decreasing the rate and volume and diluting the tube-feeding concentration with water are measures that may reduce the diarrhea.

Total Parenteral Nutrition

Total parenteral nutrition (TPN) or *hyperalimentation* is an intravenous technique used to provide for the nutritional needs of the patient who cannot or should not digest or absorb nutrients via the GI tract. The patient's nutritional deficits are carefully determined, and an appropriate formula is prepared for nutritional support. Patients selected for this procedure are generally poorly nourished as a result of surgery, trauma, or disease and are unable to adequately meet their own nutritional needs. Patients with gastrointestinal disorders often fall into this category because of an interruption of the normal digestion and absorption processes of the system.

TPN is administered as a concentrated solution of at least 10% dextrose in water, proteins, and electrolytes and trace elements. Emulsified fats may also be added to the formula. Because these solutions are so concentrated, a large vessel must be used so that the amount of plasma in the vessel can sufficiently dilute the solution to prevent complications. The infusion rate is kept constant for proper dilution to occur, as well as for the prevention of complications that could arise from sporadic infusion of such a concentrated solution so high in glucose. Nausea and headache are often early signs of too rapid administration. Later symptoms may include severe dehydration and convulsions (Box 23-2).

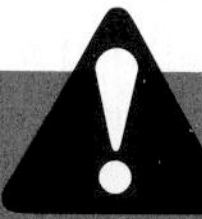

NURSE ALERT

TPN should be administered using an intravenous pump to keep the rate of administration constant. Do not speed up the rate to "catch up" if the infusion falls behind schedule. Speeding up the rate may cause a dangerous increase in blood glucose.

BOX 23-2 **Nursing Process**

TOTAL PARENTERAL NUTRITION (TPN)

ASSESSMENT

Weight loss
Fluid and/or electrolyte deficit (symptoms specific to deficit)
Inadequate food intake

NURSING DIAGNOSIS

Altered nutrition: less than body requirements related to inability to ingest/digest food or to absorb nutrients

NURSING INTERVENTIONS

Monitor intake and output.
Monitor vital signs.
Measure blood glucose (fingerstick) every 6 hours.
Maintain constant intravenous flow rate.
Monitor insertion site and report any evidence of redness, swelling, oozing, or tenderness.
Be familiar with additives to TPN (especially insulin).
Use sterile technique when caring for central line and TPN supplies.
Maintain sterile occlusive TPN dressing.
Change intravenous tubing at least every 24 hours.
Change intravenous dressing at least every 72 hours.
If infusion is interrupted, infuse 10% dextrose in water until TPN is restarted.
When discontinuing TPN therapy, taper rate over 2-4 hours.
Keep TPN solution refrigerated until needed.
Never use TPN line for medications, blood draw, or CVP readings.
Use filter and infusion device per hospital policy.
Weigh patient daily.
Monitor serum electrolytes, albumin.

EVALUATION OF EXPECTED OUTCOMES

Cessation of weight loss or gain
Maintenance of fluid and electrolyte balance
Normal blood glucose levels
Absence of infection through the intravenous line or at venipuncture site

SURGERY OF THE GI TRACT AND ACCESSORY ORGANS

Surgical procedures of the GI tract and accessory organs usually involve an incision into the thoracic or abdominal cavity and sometimes into both. An incision into the thoracic cavity is called a *thoracotomy;* an incision into the abdomen cavity is called a *laparotomy.* The thoracic cavity may be entered for surgical procedures involving the esophagus and sometimes the stomach. The abdominal cavity is opened for most other surgical procedures involving the GI tract and accessory organs. Surgical procedures within the abdominal cavity may include surgery on the stomach, the small intestine, the large intestine, and the accessory organs of digestion. Additionally, the upper part of the uterus, fallopian tubes, and ovaries are within the abdominal cavity. Therefore for many gynecologic surgical procedures, the abdomen may be opened for the surgical removal of any or all of the pelvic organs. Abdominal surgery may also involve certain other structures within the abdominal cavity such as lymph nodes and blood vessels, or it may provide for drainage of blood or pus. An *exploratory* laparotomy may be performed when it is not possible to make an accurate diagnosis before surgery.

Preoperative Nursing Care

The preoperative nursing care of all patients who undergo surgery of the GI tract and accessory organs is essentially the same, with slight variations based on the specific surgical procedure (see Chapter 18). Most patients are admitted to the hospital on the day of surgery or may even have their procedures performed in an outpatient surgical center. Only patients who require more extensive preoperative assessments or procedures are admitted to the hospital before the day of surgery. Therefore it is most common for patients to have their preoperative assessments, testing, and preparations completed outside the hospital setting. Coordination and communication of nursing assessments and interventions among nurses who work with the patient from preadmission through the surgical procedure are essential to ensuring thorough patient preparation and lack of duplication.

The nurse evaluates the patient's understanding of the surgery and identifies areas in which further clarification is needed. The patient's feelings and fears about the surgery are determined beforehand so that problems that may be encountered during the postoperative period are identified. During this time, the nurse offers encouragement, relieves anxiety, and reassures the patient that efforts will be made to meet his or her individual needs.

Cleansing enemas are often completed before abdominal surgery, unless an inflammatory condition contraindicates this procedure. If the large bowel is to be entered during surgery, a laxative, such as Golytely or Colyte, may be administered, and a series of cleansing enemas and oral antibiotics is given to "sterilize" (a term commonly used for the process of reducing bacterial count in the lower gastrointestinal tract) the bowel and reduce risks of peritonitis postoperatively. The nurse ensures that the patient understands the rationale and procedures for these preoperative procedures, especially if they will be completed before admission to the hospital. The nurse may wish to call the patient at home before the day of surgery to verify that the procedures are completed.

Required laboratory studies, chest x-ray examinations, ECGs, and any other diagnostic tests to be completed preoperatively are based on the patient's diagnosis and surgical procedure, age, and medical history. Laboratory studies commonly performed before major surgery on the GI tract or accessory organs include complete blood count, serum electrolytes, hematocrit, hemoglobin, blood glucose, prothrombin time, partial thromboplastin time, liver function tests, blood urea nitrogen, serum creatinine, and urinalysis. If the patient is at high risk for nutritional deficits (malnutrition, obesity, eating disorder, malabsorption), serum proteins and prealbumin are usually obtained.

The most important aspect of preoperative nursing care is patient teaching. The patient must know what to expect in preparation for surgery and the expected postoperative course and understand the method and importance of turning, coughing, and deep breathing; care of the wound and dressings; antiembolism exercises; pain control; and ambulation. The nurse evaluates the patient's understanding of the preoperative instructions by observing behavior that indicates that the patient has in fact learned. For example, a patient who has learned about coughing and deep breathing would be expected to demonstrate the technique and explain the importance of performing it regularly. All preoperative teaching and evaluation of patient learning is documented in the patient record.

Postoperative Nursing Care

Postoperatively, the nurse observes the patient's vital signs (heart rate, respiratory rate, temperature, and blood pressure); observes for abdominal distention, nausea, and vomiting; and notes the passing of stool or flatus. Peristalsis is usually interrupted after abdominal surgery, producing a period of adynamic or paralytic ileus for 12 to 36 hours. Normal intestinal function usually resumes without treatment. Food and fluids are usually withheld until the patient has passed flatus. A nasogastric tube may be inserted to drain intestinal contents until peristalsis returns. Intravenous infusions are given to provide necessary fluids, electrolytes, and nutrients until oral feedings can be resumed. If a patient begins to vomit after surgery, oral intake is usually withheld, and any emesis and distention is reported to the physician.

Distention can be detected by observing and palpating the abdomen. The degree of distention can be determined by measuring the abdomen at the largest portion with a tape measure and marking the area with a pen so that a comparison of later measurements will be accurate. Measurements are made once each shift and by the same person every day if possible, and they are evaluated to determine whether the distention is increasing or decreasing. The characteristics of bowel sounds assist with diagnosing the cause of distention. For example, high-pitched bowel sounds are heard in the area proximal to an obstruction. To listen for bowel sounds, the diaphragm of the stethoscope is placed over all four quadrants, and sounds are listened to for 3 to 5 minutes. Normal bowel sounds are gurgling, swishing, or tinkling noises.

Paralytic ileus, or the inability of the intestinal tract to move its contents because of an absence of peristalsis, is a complication associated with abdominal surgery and inflammation or infection within the abdominal cavity. Bowel function is also affected by pH and electrolyte imbalance, anesthetics, narcotics and other drugs, the extent of the tissue trauma, and the concentration of albumin in the plasma. When normal intestinal function is slowed or stopped, gas, fluid, and waste products collect in the intestines. This results in a rapid increase of pressure within the intestine, distention, and pressure on surrounding areas such as the diaphragm. Decompression is vital at this time to prevent atelectasis and life-threatening complications such as intestinal perforation (see Box 23-1).

Patients who have surgery of the GI tract or accessory organs are at high risk for fluid and electrolyte imbalance in the early postoperative period as a result of fluid losses from tubes and drains, bleeding, or leakage of fluid from the intravascular space to the interstitial space (third space fluid shift). The nurse maintains accurate records of fluid losses from all sources (urine, nasogastric and other drainage tubes, dressings, etc.) and all fluids administered (intravenous lines, blood, medications, etc.). The nurse also assesses other parameters of fluid status such as thirst, mucous membranes, skin turgor, serum osmolarity, and heart rate.

COLOSTOMY AND ILEOSTOMY NURSING CARE

Both **colostomy** and **ileostomy** provide an artificial opening through which fecal matter may be eliminated. A colostomy may be temporary or permanent. Until recently, an ileostomy was almost always permanent, but new surgical techniques may be used to create an *ileoanal reservoir* (a pouch that connects the ileum to the anus) that allows stool to be evacuated through the anus. Often a temporary ileostomy is the first stage of this reconstructive procedure.

The most common reasons patients require a fecal ostomy (either ileostomy or colostomy) are cancer, inflammatory bowel disease (Crohn's disease or ulcerative colitis), trauma, perforated diverticulitis, **enteric fistula** (an abnormal connection between sections of the intestine, between the intestine and peritoneal cavity, or between the intestine and the skin), or intestinal obstruction. Part or all of the diseased or injured colon is removed, and a stoma is created for elimination of stool.

Most ileostomies are created at the distal end of the ileum. Colostomies can be constructed at any point in the large intestine but are most commonly constructed in the cecum (cecostomy), or the transverse, descending, or sigmoid sections of the colon. The location of the stoma usually depends on the part of the intestine that is being exteriorized. For example, an ileostomy or cecostomy stoma is usually located in the right lower quadrant of the abdomen; the descending and sigmoid colostomy stoma is usually located in the left lower quadrant; the transverse colostomy stoma may be located in the right or left upper quadrant and occasionally in the midline position.

There are three types of stomas: an **end stoma,** a **double-barreled stoma,** and a **loop stoma** (Figure 23-8). An end stoma is created by cutting the bowel and bringing the proximal (functioning) end out to the skin as a single stoma. The distal end of the bowel may be removed or left in the abdomen. If the distal end of the bowel is left in the abdomen, it is sutured closed and left in place (Hartmann's pouch), or it may be sutured closed and affixed to the peritoneum near the end stoma. If the distal end of the bowel is surgically removed, the ostomy is likely to be permanent. However, some patients with ulcerative colitis may have the distal bowel removed and the rectal stump left in place for reconstructive surgery in the future (see the section on ileoanal reservoir). If the distal bowel is left in the abdomen, it is possible to reconnect the bowel and close the stoma (ostomy "takedown") (Hampton and others, 1992).

A double-barreled stoma is created when both the proximal and distal ends of the cut bowel are brought to the surface of the skin as two separate stomas. The proximal end is the functioning portion of the bowel; the distal end is called a *mucous fistula.*

With a loop stoma, a loop of bowel is brought up through the skin and an opening is made into the anterior wall of this bowel loop to provide for fecal drainage. The posterior wall of the loop stoma remains

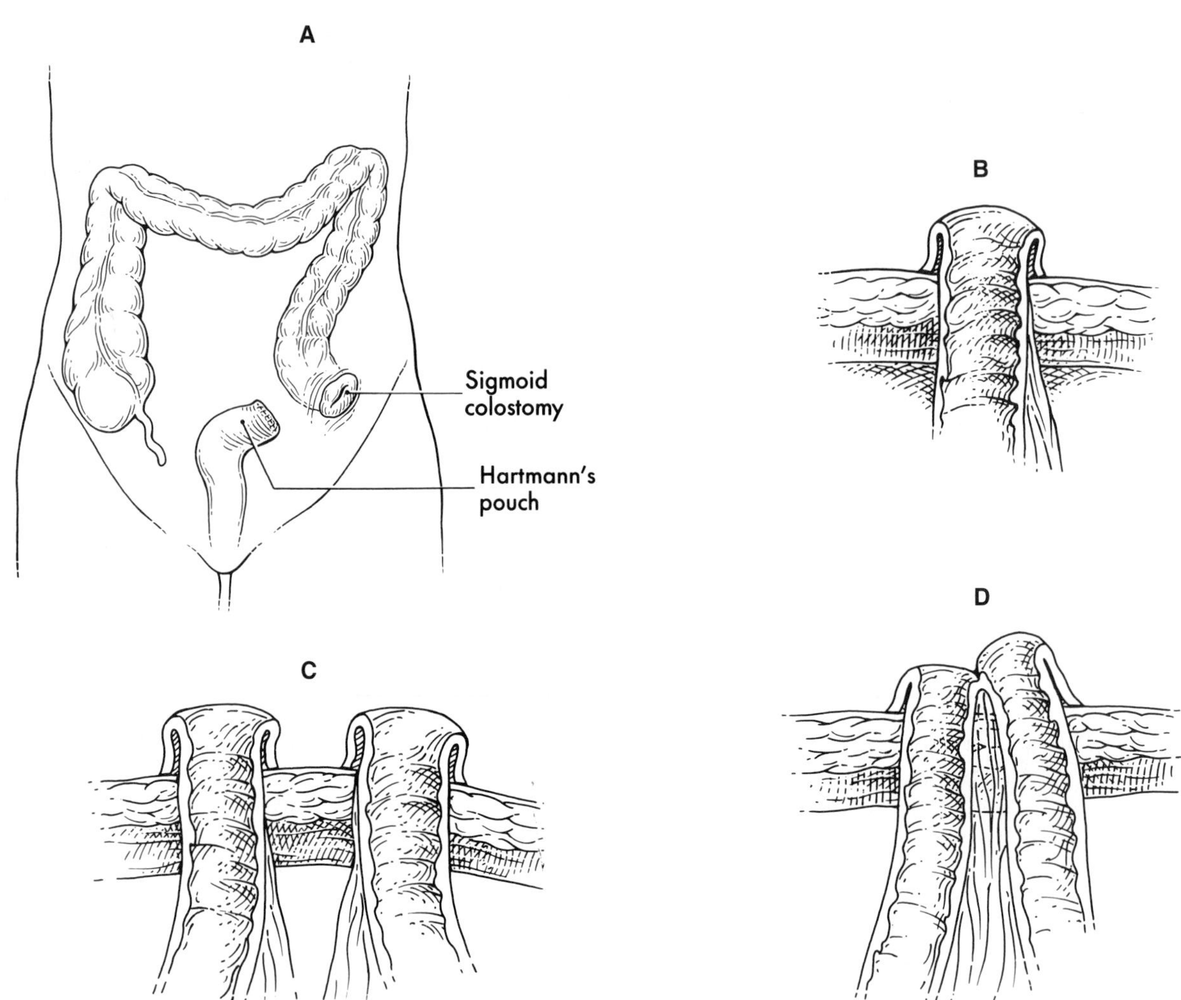

Figure 23-8 Types of stomas. **A,** End stoma of sigmoid colostomy, anterior view. **B,** Cross-section view of end stoma. **C,** Cross section of double-barreled stoma. **D,** Cross section of loop stoma. (From Hampton BG, Bryant RA: *Osteotomies and continent diversion,* St Louis, 1992, Mosby.)

intact, so a single stoma has both a proximal and distal os. Usually a plastic rod or bridge is positioned beneath the loop of bowel to secure its position on the surface of the skin and to prevent it from retracting back into the abdomen. The ostomy pouch should be labeled "bridge underneath" so that the pouch is removed gently from the skin and the bridge is not accidently displaced during pouch removal. The bridge is usually removed 7 to 10 days after surgery by the physician. A loop stoma is usually much larger than other stomas and is usually temporary.

The nursing care of the ostomy patient both preoperatively and postoperatively is generally the same as for all patients with GI surgery (see Chapter 18). Stoma assessment, GI function, and patient teaching are additional nursing considerations for the ostomy patient in the postoperative period. In the first few postoperative days, the nurse assesses the appearance of the stoma with each set of vital signs. A normal, healthy stoma is red and moist. Changes in color of the stoma could indicate ischemia and potential necrosis. If the stoma appears blue or black, or if it is not visible (retracted), the nurse should notify the physician immediately. The stoma and mucous fistula, if present, are pouched immediately after surgery or on the first postoperative day to protect the skin from drainage and to prevent contamination of the surgical wound. When applying the pouch, the skin is cleansed with plain water. If petroleum jelly–gauze was applied in the operating room, it must be removed and the skin cleansed with water and defatted for the ostomy pouch to adhere. A drainable pouch instead of a closed-end pouch is used so that it can be emptied without being removed. The amount, color, and consistency of the drainage and the presence of flatus is measured, assessed, and recorded.

Evacuation of stool from a descending or sigmoid colostomy may be regulated by using routine irrigation. After a period of daily irrigations, the patient may become regulated enough to wear a small, closed pouch or gauze dressing; most prefer the security of the small pouch. Irrigations should not begin until approximately 6 weeks after surgery. Patients who have chemotherapy or radiation should not be irrigated. An enterostomal therapy (ET) nurse should evaluate the patient for the safety of routine irrigations.

GI function normally returns within a few days after surgery. A small amount of serosanguinous drainage may flow from the stoma site immediately after surgery, but this drainage does not signal the return of GI function. Usually, the patient first begins to pass flatus, followed by the passage of stool. An ileostomy usually begins to function within 2 to 3 days after surgery. Stool draining from an ileostomy is initially watery and may amount to 1800 to 2000 ml each day. But after a period of time (a few days to a couple of weeks), it is expected that the drainage will decrease in volume to approximately 500 to 1000 ml each day and change in consistency to a loose, pastelike quality similar to that of toothpaste. The nurse must closely monitor the ileostomy patient for signs of dehydration and electrolyte imbalance in the early postoperative period.

When a new colostomy begins to function is dependent on the location of the stoma within the colon; more proximal stomas regain function before the more distal stomas. Cecostomy function is likely to return within 2 to 3 days, as in an ileostomy, whereas it may take 5 to 7 days for a descending or sigmoid colostomy to begin to function. The amount and characteristics of stool from a colostomy depend on the location of the colostomy along the length of the large intestine. The large intestine normally absorbs approximately 900 to 1000 ml of the fluid that comes from the ileum. As stool passes along the length of the large intestine, more fluid is absorbed, and the stool volume decreases and becomes more formed. The cecum is adjacent to the ileum of the small intestine, so the amount and characteristics of the stool will be similar to those of ileostomy drainage. Stool from a transverse colostomy is usually "mushy" or partially formed because it has less water content than an ileostomy or cecostomy. Water content of stool from the descending or sigmoid colostomy is more similar to normal stool and may be partially or fully formed.

Patient Education

Patient education begins as early in the preoperative period as possible and continues until the patient is secure and confident in the management of the stoma, diet, and lifestyle changes (Hampton, Bryant, 1992; Wilson, 1993).

Psychosocial

The nurse helps the patient to recognize and acknowledge the changes in body image that the new stoma presents. The nurse recognizes that the patient may need to grieve the loss of "normal" body image and function and the loss of a body part. By talking with the patient and listening to the patient express fears and concerns about body and lifestyle changes, the nurse can help the patient to progress through periods of anger and denial and toward acceptance. The nurse asks the patient about previous experiences with other people who have ostomies. Previous positive or negative experiences will often affect the way the patient views this change. The nurse also allows family members or significant others to discuss their reactions to the ostomy. The nurse provides information about ostomy support groups to both patient and family (Box 23-3).

Care of stoma and management of fecal drainage

The nurse instructs the patient on how to assess and care for the stoma and surrounding skin. The nurse emphasizes the appearance of a normal stoma and the surrounding skin and instructs the patient to call the physician or the ET nurse with any changes from nor-

BOX 23-3

SUPPORT SERVICES FOR OSTOMY PATIENTS

UNITED OSTOMY ASSOCIATION

The United Ostomy Association helps ostomy patients return to normal life through mutual aid and moral support. It publishes *Ostomy Quarterly* and other educational materials. Contact the American Cancer Society for more information.

OSTOMY VISITOR PROGRAM

The Ostomy Visitor Program is a service of the American Cancer Society provided to ostomy patients. A trained volunteer who has an ostomy will visit the patient to provide support and assistance to the patient with an ostomy. Contact the American Cancer Society for more information.

ENTEROSTOMAL THERAPY NURSES

An enterostomal therapy nurse has specialized training in the care of patient with ostomies. This nurse provides assistance to patients and family members through preoperative and postoperative teaching and counseling, ostomy supplies, and skin and stoma problem management. Contact Wound, Ostomy, Continence Nurses Society (714)476-0268 for more information.

BOX 23-4 Guidelines for Colostomy Irrigation

1. Provide for patient privacy.
2. Remove ostomy pouch.
3. Apply irrigation sleeve; direct drainage into toilet or close bottom of sleeve to collect irrigation returns.
4. Use lukewarm solution for irrigation; use 500 to 1000 ml; fill and prime irrigation bag; attach cone tip adaptor.
5. Lubricate cone tip adaptor; gently insert cone tip into stoma; hold cone tip in place to prevent back flow.
6. Instill irrigating solution over 5 to 10 minutes; remove cone tip adaptor.
7. Expect returns within 30 to 45 minutes.
8. Remove irrigation sleeve; reapply ostomy pouch.

Modified from Hampton BC, Bryant RA: *Ostomies and continent diversions,* St Louis, 1992, Mosby.

mal. The pouch is emptied when it is one-third to one-half full to prevent it from pulling off from the weight of the drainage. Initially, the pouch is changed every 3 to 4 days or whenever it leaks. The size of the stoma normally decreases in the first 6 to 8 weeks after surgery, so the patient is instructed to change the size of the pouch opening as the stoma changes in size. After the stoma shrinks to its permanent size, the pouch can be changed every 5 to 7 days, or as needed. The patient may bathe or shower with the pouch on or off. Skin problems should be prevented, but when they arise, the ET nurse should be consulted. Barrier wafers or topical medications are often helpful in treating ostomy skin problems; sometimes specialized pouching equipment may be needed for difficult to manage stomas. There is no odor from a well-pouched stoma. If odor occurs, it is likely due to leakage of drainage from around the pouching equipment. Patients should be informed that the only time they will have odor is when they open the pouch to remove flatus or to drain the contents (Box 23-4).

Diet

Most ostomy patients require little or no modification in diet after their surgery. The nurse emphasizes the importance of eating a balanced diet. The patient is instructed about which foods may cause problems with odor, gas, diarrhea, or obstruction. Each person reacts differently to foods; therefore new foods should be added gradually to the diet to identify any that stimulate bowel activity and gas formation. Fresh vegetables and fruits, nuts, whole grains, bran, and other high-fiber foods increase stool volume and gas; however, some people find that a steady high-fiber diet eventually decreases gas and fecal odor. Yogurt and buttermilk may reduce odor, probably because of the bacteria normally present in these foods, as will green leafy vegetables like parsley and spinach that contain chlorophyll.

Ileostomy patients are at high risk for fluid and electrolyte imbalances because the fluid reabsorption function of the colon no longer exists. Symptoms of electrolyte imbalance include headache, fatigue, drowsiness, nausea, and anorexia. Some patients complain of muscle cramps, but they are more likely to complain of flaccid muscles, weakness, and fatigue resulting from a deficiency of potassium. These patients are encouraged to drink at least 6 to 8 glasses of water a day to prevent dehydration. Patients are instructed to notify the doctor if there is a significant increase in drainage from the stoma.

Sexual dysfunction

Sexual dysfunction may result from various surgical procedures involving the creation of an ostomy. Male patients may be incapable of achieving an erection, and female patients may experience changes in vaginal lubrication and expansion when the surgical procedure involves the nerves and blood supply of the pelvis or resection of parts of the vagina. Surgical procedures that commonly affect sexual function include abdominal perineal resection and total proctocolectomy. The nurse discusses the changes in sexual function as a result of surgery with both the patient and the partner. More importantly, the nurse discusses with the patients alternative methods of achieving sexual pleasure with their partners. Ostomy support groups and sexual counseling may be particularly helpful for these patients.

Enterostomal Therapy Nurse

The ET nurse is specialized in the care of patients with wounds, ostomies, and incontinence. The ET nurse is a resource for ostomy patients, their families, and other nurses involved in the care of the ostomy patient in both the hospitalized and the community settings. All ostomy patients should be referred to an ET nurse as early in their surgical course as possible. Before surgery, the ET nurse marks the site on the abdomen where the stoma should be placed. The ET nurse tries to select a site that avoids skin folds and

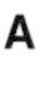

A

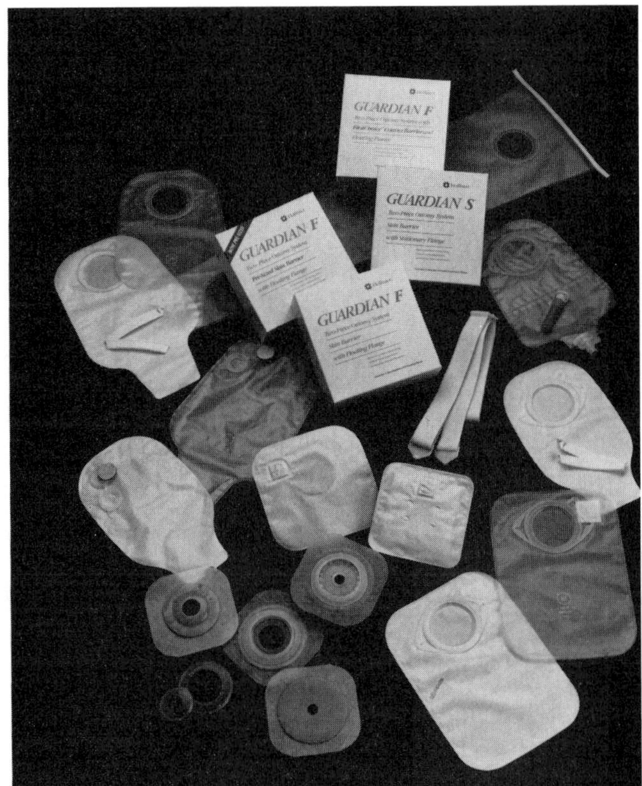

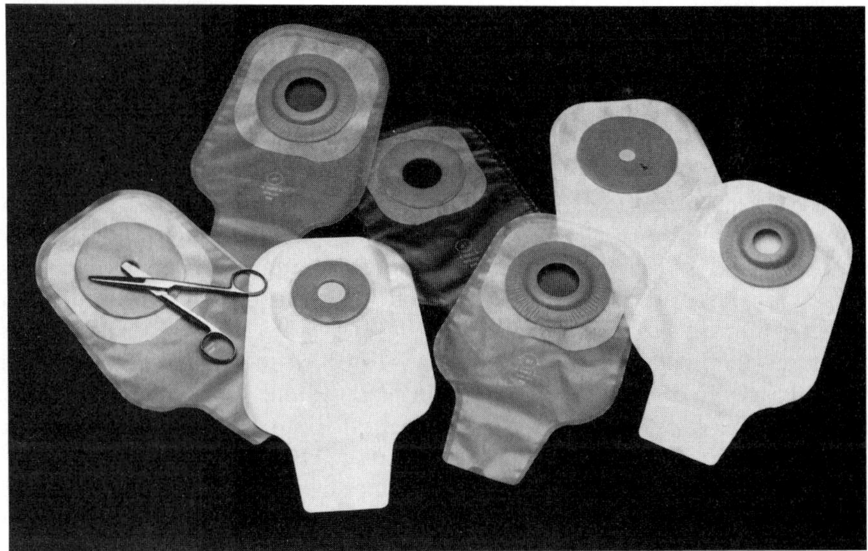

B

Figure 23-9 Ostomy equipment. **A,** The Guardian two-piece ostomy system by Hollister provides a complete selection of skin barrier styles (cut-to-fit, presized, convex, nonconvex, floating flange, and stationary flange), pouch styles (drainable, closed, and urostomy), irrigator drains, and stoma caps. Drainable and closed pouches are available with transparent or opaque pouch film in small or full sizes. Guardian pouches securely attach to Guardian skin barriers and are used by people with colostomies, ileostomies, and urostomies. **B,** The FirstChoice one-piece drainable ostomy pouches by Hollister provide a complete selection of preattached skin barrier styles (cut-to-fit, presized, convex, and nonconvex) with either transparent or opaque pouch film. FirstChoice drainable ostomy pouches are used by people with colostomies and ileostomies. (Courtesy of Hollister, Inc.)

scars that could interfere with good pouch adherence and makes it easier for the patient to perform stoma care and pouching.

The ET nurse plays a major role in preoperative and postoperative patient/family education and counseling. The ET nurse will provide information about the disease process necessitating the ostomy procedure and will discuss the surgical options, the effects of the surgical procedure, and postoperative care and management. The ET nurse also provides psychosocial support to patients and families throughout the preoperative and postoperative period.

The ET nurse is an expert in ostomy supplies and ostomy management and is a resource for the selection of pouching equipment and supplies that will maximize the patient's quality of life and facilitate self-care (Figure 23-9). If the patient develops problems with skin irritation or inadequate appliance adherence, the

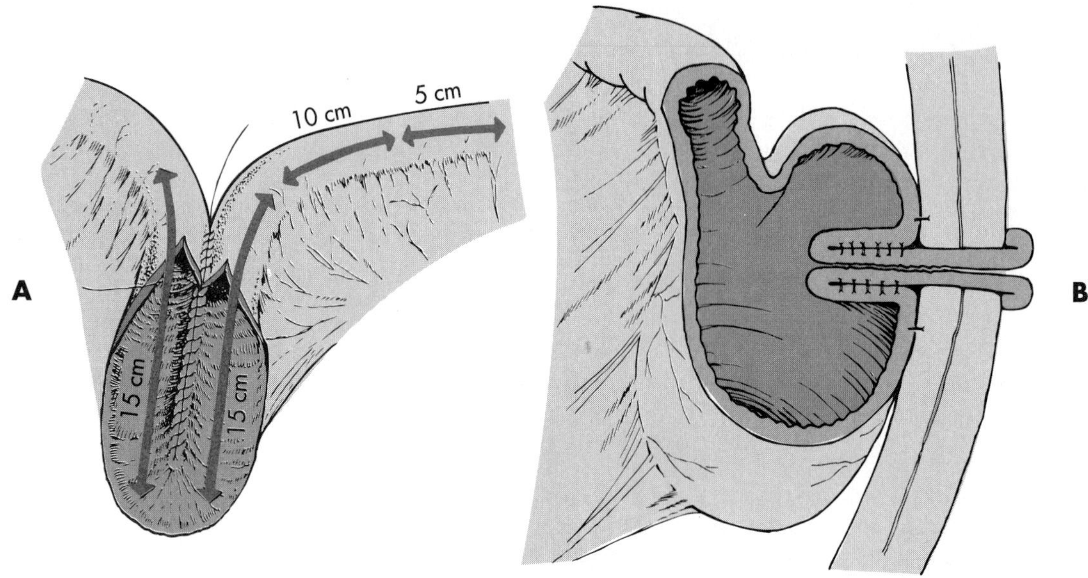

Figure 23-10 Kock's pouch for continent ileostomy. **A,** Pouch created from ileum. **B,** Nipple valve to control release of contents and provide for drainage by inserting tubing. (From Hampton BG, Bryant RA: *Ostomies and continent diversions,* St Louis, 1992, Mosby.)

ET nurse can suggest appropriate additions or changes in stoma care to manage these difficulties.

CONTINENT POUCH ILEOSTOMY AND ILEOANAL RESERVOIR

The continent pouch ileostomy and the ileoanal reservoir are two procedures developed to provide surgical alternatives that maintain fecal continence, thus eliminating constant stool drainage from the ileostomy. These procedures are being done on an increasing number of patients with chronic ulcerative colitis and familial adenomatous polyposis (FAP) who formerly required a permanent ileostomy (Hampton, Bryant, 1992; Wilson, 1993).

With the continent or pouch ileostomy (Kock's pouch), the patient has a stoma but does not need to wear a stoma pouch because a reservoir to collect and hold the stool is surgically created using a section of the terminal ileum (Figure 23-10). The last few inches of ileum are used to create a *nipple valve,* which controls the release of stool from the stoma in much the same way as the anal sphincter controls the collection of stool in the normal bowel. A catheter is usually placed through the stoma into the pouch to allow for continuous drainage of stool from the ileum until the newly created pouch is fully healed (3 to 4 weeks). During this time the catheter may be irrigated to remove mucus from the pouch. Once the new pouch is healed and the catheter is removed, a tube is inserted into the pouch at gradually lengthening intervals to evacuate drainage from the pouch (every 2 hours, then every 3 hours, then every 4 hours). This process allows the pouch to gradually increase in capacity; eventually the pouch is able to hold 500 to 1000 ml and requires draining only two or three times a day. A small, absorbent dressing is taped over the stoma, and the patient will be drainage free for another 5 or 6 hours. Ultimately, the drainage procedure takes no more than 5 or 10 minutes. Patients may choose to have either the continent ileostomy or the ileoanal reservoir procedure if they feel their quality of life would be better than if they had an ileostomy that necessitated wearing a pouch. They will require support in the transition from the "sick role" to health and in adjusting to the stoma and self-care procedures (Box 23-5).

Ileoanal reservoir (IAR) is a collective term for a number of surgical procedures that can be used to retain "normal" evacuation of stool via the anus by means of constructing an anal reservoir or pouch to provide for the collection of stool between evacuations. Ileoanal reservoir procedures are usually performed in stages and, if performed in stages, require a temporary ileostomy to allow the reservoir to heal before making the final surgical connection.

If the IAR is constructed in stages, the first stage involves removal of the entire colon, construction of the reservoir pouch from the ileum, connecting the reservoir pouch to the anus, and constructing a temporary ileostomy. Postoperative care is generally simi-

BOX 23-5 Guidelines of Care for Drainage of Continent Ileostomy Pouch

1 Sit or stand at toilet.
2 Lubricate the catheter (usually 28 F Silastic) generously with water-soluble jelly.
3 Slowly and gently insert catheter through stoma and valve into the pouch to premarked site on the catheter; if catheter is difficult to pass, relax, take deep breaths, and gently advance catheter during exhalation or instill small amount of water or air into the catheter to relax pouch valve.
4 May instill 20 to 25 ml lukewarm water into pouch to dilute thicker stool.
5 Remove catheter when drainage is complete; usually takes 5 to 10 minutes.
6 Clean catheter thoroughly with mild soap and water, allow to dry; strong detergents may erode catheter.
7 Store supplies in plastic bag or kit for easy transport.

lar to that of patient with abdominal surgery and a new ileostomy. Because the ileostomy is created in a more proximal section of the ileum, the nurse should expect up to 1500 to 2400 ml/day. The patient may have the urge to defecate and may pass mucus from the rectum. Fecal incontinence, usually mucoid in nature, may occur through the first few weeks postoperatively. The physician may order irrigations of the ileoanal reservoir to remove foul-smelling mucous secretions. When the ileoanal reservoir is completely healed, usually 8 to 10 weeks after the initial surgery, the temporary ileostomy is closed. Fecal output via the anus usually begins within 2 to 3 days. Fecal drainage is in fact ileostomy drainage via the rectum, so perianal skin irritation is a common complication of this procedure. Skin sealants and moisture barrier products must be used to prevent breakdown. Toilet paper and soap should not be used to cleanse the perianal area. Baby "wipes" provide a convenient, soothing method for cleansing. Soft tissues moistened with water can also be used to dab clean the perianal area. Initially the patient will have frequent bowel movements (10 to 12/day), but the frequency should decrease over time.

Pouchitis (inflammation of the pouch) can occur in patients with either a continent pouch ileostomy or an ileoanal reservoir. Symptoms associated with pouchitis are new onset of frequent bowel movements, pain, fecal urgency, and bleeding. It is usually treated with antibiotics.

GASTROINTESTINAL MANIFESTATIONS OF ILLNESS

Anorexia

Anorexia, lack of appetite, is a nonspecific symptom that is associated with a variety of illnesses and diseases. Anorexia may appear in conjunction with other nonspecific GI symptoms such as nausea, diarrhea, or pain, or it may be an isolated presenting symptom. A multiplicity of factors may cause anorexia. Emotional stress and psychologic disorders are often associated with lack of appetite. Anorexia may be a symptom of some specific GI problems, such as intestinal obstruction, and may also be associated with problems related to other illnesses and disease, such as chronic renal disease and heart disease. Prolonged anorexia can lead to severe nutritional deficits unless treatment is instituted.

Nausea and Vomiting

Nausea is a subjective feeling of the need to vomit. Like anorexia, nausea may appear with other GI symptoms and may be caused by a variety of factors. Nausea may be a symptom associated with GI problems or may be associated with other systemic problems. The association of nausea with other symptoms, like vomiting, pain, anorexia, and abdominal distention may be helpful in diagnosing the specific problem.

Vomiting is the forceful expulsion of gastric or duodenal contents through the mouth. Vomiting is a reflex that can be stimulated in a variety of ways. The vomiting center lies in the cerebral medulla; stimulation of this center induces the vomiting reflex. Vomiting may be induced by direct stimulation of the cerebral vomiting center; by increased stimulation of the semicircular canals, as in motion sickness; or by stimulation of certain nerve fibers located in the pharynx, the stomach, the intestine, the kidneys, the heart, or the uterus. Vomiting is usually preceded by a wave of nausea. *Projectile vomiting* is spontaneous vomiting that is not preceded by nausea. Projectile vomiting is associated with cerebral tumors and aneurysms and with increased intracranial pressure.

Assessment

The nurse assesses the patient for potential causes of nausea or vomiting, including stress, foods, and medications. The nurse also looks for associated symptoms such as pain, abdominal distention, constipation, or diarrhea. The nurse measures the amount of vomitus and carefully inspects the contents. Specifically, the nurse examines the vomitus for the presence or absence of undigested food particles, bile, and blood. The presence of blood in the vomitus is an indication that the patient is bleeding from some source in the upper GI tract. The blood may be bright red, which is usually indicative of recent or rapid bleeding, or it may appear as "coffee-ground" emesis with a dark red or black appearance, which is indicative of blood mixing with gastric secretions.

Any specific odor of the vomitus is also noted; fecal odor of the vomitus is associated with intestinal obstruction, peritonitis, or enteric fistulas. Prolonged vomiting predisposes the patient to dehydration, electrolyte and acid-base imbalances, weakness, and nutritional deficiency, so the nurse must monitor the patient closely for these complications.

Intervention

Nursing interventions are aimed at preventing aspiration, maintaining fluid and electrolyte balance, and providing symptomatic relief. If the patient is able, the nurse places the patient in a sitting or in a side-lying position with the head slightly flexed forward to prevent aspiration during vomiting. Deep breathing and swallowing often suppress the urge to vomit. Warm fluids such as weak tea or carbonated beverages may be given in sips if tolerated by the patient. Dry crackers or toast may be added if liquids are tolerated. Fried or spicy foods are to be avoided until all symptoms have resolved. If oral intake of bland fluids continues to produce vomiting, intake is withheld for a period of time and then reintroduced slowly. Intravenous fluid replacement may be necessary to maintain adequate fluid and electrolyte balance during prolonged vomiting. In some cases the patient is given nothing by mouth, and a nasogastric tube is placed to remove gastric contents to prevent further vomiting.

Antiemetic agents are used to relieve the symptoms of prolonged and severe nausea and vomiting (Table 23-2). Antiemetics may be administered orally, intramuscularly, intravenously, or rectally. The nurse monitors the patient for the effectiveness of the antiemetic agent. If the agent does not relieve the symptoms, the nurse notifies the doctor.

Additional nursing measures in caring for the patient with nausea and vomiting include keeping an emesis basin within easy reach and emptying the basin quickly after patient use. If clothing or linens are soiled by vomitus, clean replacements are provided immediately. Providing mouth care after vomiting and applying a cool cloth to the forehead or back of the neck may increase patient comfort.

Diarrhea

Diarrhea is the passage of stool that is characterized by increased frequency and increased water content. The causes of diarrhea vary but are usually classified by how excessive water content gets into the GI tract: *secretory, osmotic,* or *mixed* (McCance, Huether, 1994). Water is either "pushed" into the lumen of the GI tract by secretion or it is "pulled" into the lumen by osmosis; diarrhea often occurs as a result of a combination of secretory and osmotic factors. *Secretory diarrhea* occurs as a result of an abnormal increase in the production ("push") of intestinal secretions (water and electrolytes) and usually occurs as a result of GI mucosal inflammation or infections with toxin-producing organisms. Secretory diarrhea is usually high in volume (greater than 1 L/day) and high in sodium content.

Osmotic diarrhea is characterized by poor water reabsorption from the GI tract and occurs as a result of an increased amount of water being "pulled" into the GI lumen by hyperosmolar contents. This type of diarrhea may be caused by certain drugs, such as cathartics, sorbitol, lactulose, antacids, and some antibiotics, as well as certain surgical procedures or disease processes that increase the speed at which contents pass through the GI tract, reducing the time for reabsorption. Osmotic diarrhea contains high levels of potassium.

Mixed diarrhea is associated with increased intestinal motility, as well as a combination of secretory and osmotic factors. Increased motility decreases the time allowed for adequate water and electrolyte reabsorption by the intestine. It is believed that this increased motility stimulates factors that increase secretion and malabsorption of intestinal fluids.

The consequences of diarrhea depend on both the cause and the severity. Severe dehydration and electrolyte imbalance can result from prolonged loss of GI secretions through diarrhea. Major patient care considerations include fluid and electrolyte imbalance and perianal skin irritation.

Assessment

The nurse monitors the color, odor, volume, and consistency of diarrhea stool and inspects the stool for the presence of blood, mucus, or undigested food. Additionally, the nurse assesses for any associative factors that relate to the diarrhea. How often are the diarrhea stools occurring? How long has the diarrhea persisted? Are the episodes of diarrhea related to eating? What specific foods? Has the patient recently traveled

TABLE 23-2

Pharmacology of Drugs Used in Gastrointestinal Function

Drug (Generic and Trade Name); Route and Dosage	Action/Indication	Common Side Effects and Nursing Considerations
ALUMINUM HYDROXIDE (Amphojel) **ROUTE:** PO, liquid **DOSAGE:** 5 to 30 ml 3 to 6 times daily	Used in treatment of peptic, duodenal, and gastric ulcers	Constipation; contraindicated for unknown severe abdominal pain; use cautiously in hypercalcemia and hypophosphatemia
ALUMINUM HYDROXIDE AND MAGNESIUM HYDROXIDE (Maalox) **ROUTE:** PO, liquid **DOSAGE:** 5 to 30 ml or 1 to 2 tabs 1 and 3 hr after meals and at bedtime	Used in treatment of peptic ulcer pain and to promote healing of duodenal and gastric ulcers; used in a variety of GI complaints, including hyperacidity, indigestion, and reflux esophagitis	Constipation and diarrhea; contraindicate for unknown severe abdominal pain; use with caution in renal insufficiency
ALUMINUM HYDROXIDE, MAGNESIUM HYDROXIDE, AND SIMETHICONE (Mylanta) **ROUTE:** PO, liquid **DOSAGE:** 5 to 30 ml 1 to 3 hr after meals and at bedtime	Antacid and antiulcer; same as above	Same as above
AMOXICILLIN OR TETRACYCLINE (Pepto-Bismol and Flagyl) **ROUTE:** PO; Flagyl can also be given IV **DOSAGE:** Amoxicillin or tetracycline 500 mg tid × 2-4 weeks; Pepto-Bismol 2 tabs qid × 2-4 weeks; Flagyl 500 mg tid last 7 to 10 days of treatment regimen	Treatment for gastric and peptic ulcers caused by *Helicobacter pylori.*	Rashes and diarrhea with amoxicillin; contraindicated if hypersensitive to penicillin; nausea, vomiting, and diarrhea with tetracyclines; headache, dizziness, nausea, vomiting, abdominal pain, anorexia, diarrhea in flagyl
CIMETIDINE (Tagamet) **ROUTE:** PO, IV, IM (rarely) **DOSAGE:** PO 300 mg 4 times daily; IV 900 mg infused over 24 hours	Prophylactic and active treatment of duodenal ulcers	Confusion; use with caution in renal disease
CISAPRIDE (Propulsid) **ROUTE:** PO **DOSAGE:** 10 to 20 mg 4 times daily 15 minutes before meals and at bedtime	Used in management of heartburn associated with esophageal reflux disease (GERD)	No common side effects
DIPHENOXYLATE, ATROPINE (Lomotil) **ROUTE:** PO **DOSAGE:** 2.5 to 5 mg 3 to 4 times daily (not to exceed 20 mg/day)	Used in treatment of diarrhea	Dizziness, lightheadedness, drowsiness, constipation, and dry mouth; use with caution if opioid addicted, in inflammatory bowel disease, and with children sensitive to atropine
DOCUSATE SODIUM (Colace) **ROUTE:** PO and rectal **DOSAGE:** 50 to 500 mg once daily	Stool softener used in prevention of constipation	Excessive use may lead to dependence; should not be used if prompt results are desired

continued

TABLE 23-2

Pharmacology of Drugs Used in Gastrointestinal Function—cont'd

Drug (Generic and Trade Name); Route and Dosage	Action/Indication	Common Side Effects and Nursing Considerations
BISACODYL (Dulcolax, Fleet laxative) **ROUTE:** PO and rectal **DOSAGE:** 5 to 15 mg (up to 30 mg); rectal 10 mg suppository	Used in treatment of constipation, particularly that associated with prolonged bedrest and constipating drugs	Nausea and abdominal cramps
FAMOTIDINE (Pepcid) **ROUTE:** PO and IV **DOSAGE:** PO 20 mg daily at bedtime; IV 20 mg q 12 hr and higher doses may be used	Used in short-term and maintenance treatment of active duodenal ulcers	Dizziness, headache, and constipation; use with caution in renal disease
LOPERAMIDE (Imodium-A-D, Pepto Diarrhea Control) **ROUTE:** PO **DOSAGE:** 4 mg initially, then 2 mg after each loose stool; 4 to 8 mg/day in divided doses (not to exceed 16 mg/day)	Used for acute diarrhea and chronic diarrhea associated with inflammatory bowel disease	Drowsiness and constipation; contraindicated in patients who must avoid constipation; use with caution in liver disease
MAGNESIUM CITRATE **ROUTE:** PO **DOSAGE:** 100 to 300 ml	Used as a laxative to evacuate the bowel in preparation for surgical or radiographic procedures	Diarrhea; contraindicated in hypermagnesemia, hypocalcemia, anuria, heart block, and any degree of renal insufficiency
MINERAL OIL (Fleet mineral oil) **ROUTE:** PO and rectal **DOSAGE:** 5 to 45 ml as a single or divided dose; rectal 60 to 150 ml as a single or divided dose	Used to soften impacted feces in the management of constipation	Use cautiously in elderly or debilitated
NIZATIDINE (Axid) **ROUTE:** PO **DOSAGE:** 150 mg bid or 300 mg at bedtime	Used in short-term treatment and maintenance preventive treatment of active duodenal ulcers	Use with caution in liver and renal impairment; concurrent antacid administration may interfere with absorption
PSYLLIUM (Metamucil) **ROUTE:** PO **DOSAGE:** 1 to 2 tsp packets in a full glass of liquid 2 to 3 times daily	Used in management of simple or chronic constipation particularly, that associated with a low fiber diet; also used for chronic watery diarrhea	No common side effects
RANITIDINE (Zantac) **ROUTE:** PO or IV **DOSAGE:** 150 mg bid or 300 mg at bedtime; IV 50 mg q 6 to 8 hr	Used in management of short-term and long-term active duodenal ulcers	Headache and malaise; use with caution in elderly, and in renal and liver impairment; antacids may decrease absorption
SUCRALFATE (Carafate) **ROUTE:** PO and liquid **DOSAGE:** 1 gram qid 1 hr before meals and at bedtime	Used in short-term management of duodenal ulcers	Constipation; antacids may decrease absorption

outside the country? What medications, especially new medications, is the patient taking? Are any other symptoms associated with the diarrhea? Pain? Abdominal cramps? Nausea? Vomiting? Abdominal distention?

Stool samples may be obtained and sent for analysis to assist with determining the nature and cause of the diarrhea. Laboratory analysis of stool samples can determine the presences of bacterial toxins, ova and parasites, blood, fat, electrolytes and osmolarity, and WBCs. Upper and lower endoscopy or a barium enema may also be used to assist with the diagnosis.

General physical assessment parameters, including blood pressure, heart rate, and temperature, as well as assessment of hydration status and intake and output should be monitored. Serum WBC count may also be evaluated to assess for infectious causes; serum electrolytes are evaluated to assess the need for replacement therapy.

Intervention

Care of the patient with diarrhea is directed at eliminating or controlling the cause, controlling symptoms, preventing complications, and providing for patient comfort. Specific foods or medications that are poorly absorbed or precipitate inflammation are discontinued if possible. Antibiotics are administered for infectious causes of diarrhea. Antiinflammatory agents are used in the treatment of diarrhea caused by inflammatory bowel disease. Antidiarrheal agents are used to control the frequency of diarrhea episodes by decreasing peristalsis; bulk-forming agents are used to reduce the water content of the diarrhea stool. Fluid and electrolyte maintenance or replacement therapy is administered as needed.

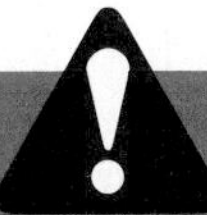

NURSE ALERT

Agents that control diarrhea by effecting peristalsis, such as codeine, diphenoxylate, or loperamide should not be given to patients who have diarrhea from any type of infectious agent, ulcerative colitis, or pseudomembranous colitis because of the risks of toxic complications. Additionally, always check with the physician before administering antidiarrheal agents to patients with acute abdominal pain, GI bleeding, intestinal obstruction, or abdominal inflammation.

Careful cleansing and protection of the perianal skin area is essential to prevent skin breakdown caused by frequent soiling and the caustic nature of the diarrhea stool. Gentle washing with tap water, mineral oil, or special products available for perineal skin cleansing are used to remove stool from the skin surface. Topical application of skin sealants or moisture barriers can provide further protection from breakdown. Agents with vitamin A, D, or E can also be applied to prevent or treat perianal skin breakdown. If severe diarrhea persists, the nurse may choose to apply a fecal incontinence collector. The use of rectal tubes to collect fecal drainage is discouraged because of the potential for injury to the rectal mucosa and anal sphincter.

To provide patient-comfort measures, the nurse ensures easy access to the bathroom or places a bedpan within easy reach. Room deodorizers are used to control foul odors. Soiled linen and clothing are changed immediately.

EATING DISORDERS

Eating disorders are abnormal eating behaviors that result in physical and psychologic illness or injury. Primary eating disorders are *anorexia nervosa* and *bulimia*. Eating disorders are primarily psychologic disorders that are associated with physical manifestations and physical complications. Psychologic disturbances associated with eating disorders are depression and obsessive-compulsive behavior.

Anorexia Nervosa

Anorexia nervosa is characterized by an abnormal preoccupation with food and the fear of becoming fat. Patients with anorexia nervosa perceive themselves as overweight and react by severely restricting their food intake and induce starvation to achieve a desired body image. Excessive exercising used to achieve weight loss may also be evidence of anorexia nervosa. The major symptom of anorexia nervosa is marked cachectia; other symptoms include amenorrhea, sleep disturbances, intolerance to the cold, and skin changes. Patients may try to cover up their weight loss by wearing long sleeves, long pants, or long skirts despite the weather. The major complications are those related to prolonged starvation and severe fluid and electrolyte imbalances and can be associated with major damage to the heart and liver (Sleisenger, Fordtram, 1993).

Bulimia

Bulimia is also characterized by an abnormal preoccupation with food and eating. But unlike anorexia nervosa, bulimia is characterized not by starvation but by alternating episodes of eating abnormally large quantities of food and calories (*binging*) with induced intestinal *purging* by means of vomiting or laxatives or both. Patients with bulimia are not usually cachectic like those with anorexia nervosa. Generally symptoms and complications related to bulimia are associated with the metabolic alterations caused by binging and purging. Gum disease and dental caries are commonly seen and are caused by injury from acidic vomitus.

Interventions

Treatment of patients with eating disorders include nutritional management and psychologic intervention. Psychotherapy is instituted as a prime focus of the treatment plan.

Nutritional management is guided by the findings of a thorough nutritional and metabolic assessment. Mild to moderate malnutrition may be managed outside the hospital, but severe malnutrition will require hospitalization. Oral nutrition is preferred, but if adequate nutrition cannot be provided by the oral route, enteral feeding will be initiated. Occasionally TPN is required as a primary or supplementary source for nutritional replacement.

SPECIFIC DISEASES AND DISORDERS OF THE GASTROINTESTINAL SYSTEM

Inflammatory Diseases

Stomatitis

Inflammation of the mouth results from several causes and may affect the entire mouth or only a small part of the mucous membrane. Among the causes of stomatitis are vitamin deficiency, infection by specific organisms such as fungi or bacteria, certain drugs including chemotherapy, and some viral diseases. Symptoms may include a burning sensation; pain; formation of ulcers; the presence of membranes as in diphtheria; tender, bleeding gums; a disagreeable odor; and sometimes fever. Treatment depends on identifying and treating the cause. Vincent's stomatitis, commonly called *trench mouth,* often occurs in epidemics and is fairly common. The condition responds readily to penicillin and good oral hygiene.

Thrush (candidiasis) is caused by a fungal organism, *Candida albicans.* The disease appears as small, white patches on the mucous membrane of the mouth and tongue. The same organism is responsible for monilial vaginitis in the adult, and newborn infants may become infected as they pass through the birth canal. The infection may be spread in the nursery by the carelessness of nursing personnel. Handwashing, care of feeding equipment, and cleanliness of the mother's nipples are important to preventing spread. There are several methods of treatment, including 1 to 4 ml of nystatin (Mycostatin) dropped into the infant's mouth several times a day. Thrush may also occur in adults who are receiving broad-spectrum antibiotics, particularly chlortetracycline or tetracycline, or immunosuppression therapy. Treatment for the adult is the same as for the infant.

The possibility of transmission of some inflammatory diseases of the mouth has been questioned. However, when bacterial disease is known to exist, nurses should use every precaution to protect themselves and all other patients. Nursing care consists of cleansing the mouth and teeth of any foreign material, rinsing the mouth, and lubricating the lips. The mouth is inspected using a flashlight and tongue blade. The frequency of oral care depends on the patient's condition, and whatever procedure is used should meet the needs of the patient and should be consistent and effective. The nurse identifies patients who are in need of special mouth care and should encourage good oral hygiene in all patients.

Gastritis

Gastritis is an inflammatory disorder affecting the mucosal surface of the stomach. The disease may be acute or chronic. Acute gastritis is usually caused by injury to the mucosal surface. This injury may be caused by irritating drugs or agents, such as aspirin, alcohol, or nonsteroidal antiinflammatory agents. Acute gastritis is also associated with uremia and liver disease. Clinical manifestations of acute gastritis include anorexia, vague abdominal distress, epigastric pain, and potential bleeding. Treatment consists of discontinuing the irritating drugs or substances and the use of antacids and acid-inhibiting drugs such as Cimetidine, Tagamet, or Pepcid. If bleeding is present, Sulcrafate may be used to promote healing. Healing should occur within a week.

Chronic gastritis is a progressive disease and often occurs in the elderly. Chronic gastritis causes the stomach mucosa to thin and atrophy. The most common type of chronic gastritis is called antral gastritis and exhibits the inflammatory changes associated with the bacteria *Helicobacter pylori.* Another type of chronic gastritis, called atrophic gastritis, is characterized by atrophy of the gastric mucosa and a decrease in acid secretion. The patient with chronic gastritis may report vague signs and symptoms, such as poor appetite, nausea, and epigastric pain. Bleeding may be the only symptom the patient reports. Treatment consists of avoiding irritating agents such as aspirin or alcohol; eating small, frequent meals; and adhering to a bland diet. Vitamin B_{12} may be given if the patient has associated pernicious anemia.

Enteritis

Inflammation of the intestine accompanying gastritis is called *gastroenteritis*. Enteritis occurs in conjunction with some infectious diseases, such as typhoid fever, dysentery, tuberculosis involving the intestines, and most cases of food infection. The severity of the condition depends on the virulence of the organism causing the condition. The primary symptoms are diarrhea and abdominal cramping. When the infection is from food, the symptoms occur within a few hours after the contaminated food has been eaten. Fever may or may not occur, but dehydration and weakness are usually present. Diarrhea is present in many types of infections and may be the forerunner of serious infections, especially in children.

Treatment is based on identifying the cause by using stool examination or cultures from suspected food. Precautions should always be taken until the cause of the diarrhea has been established. Bedrest is indicated, and only liquids are given by mouth. When vomiting is present, oral fluids may be withheld, and the appropriate electrolyte solutions are administered parenterally to replace those lost through diarrhea and vomiting. Antibiotic or sulfonamide drugs may be ordered by the physician in treating some types of enteritis.

Inflammatory bowel disease

Inflammatory bowel disease (IBD) is an umbrella term used in referring to diseases of the large and small intestines. IBD is characterized by inflammation with tissue changes that are caused by this chronic inflammation. Most commonly, IBD refers to Crohn's disease and ulcerative colitis. It is estimated that as many as 2 million people in the United States suffer from IBD. Recent research points to a complex interplay between genetic and environmental factors as the cause of IBD. These factors join to produce an exaggerated, inappropriate, or prolonged inflammatory response. Genetic markers for Crohn's disease and ulcerative colitis have been discovered. Environmental factors under suspiciion include infectious agents, food additives, and birth control pills. Once the defective genes can be identified, medications can be developed to correct or neutralize the genes. Although the exact cause is unknown, it is known that IBD is not caused by emotional stress. Psychologic stress may cause exacerbation of the symptoms of IBD or may alter the course of the disease, but it does not initiate the disease process (Doughty, 1994; Hampton, Bryant, 1992) (Box 23-6).

PATIENT/FAMILY TEACHING

Inflammatory bowel disease

The nurse should instruct the patient and family in the following:

- Disease process and precipitating factors
- Medication action, dosage, and side effects
- Long-term steroid therapy and importance of compliance
- Skin care
- Dietary guidelines
- Stress management
- Medical follow-up
- Community resources (e.g., dietician, support groups, social service)

Crohn's disease. Crohn's disease, also referred to as *regional enteritis*, is a chronic, progressive inflammatory disease that can affect any part of the GI tract from mouth to anus but most commonly involves the small and large intestine. The mortality rate is not high, but the disease often results in a significant alteration in lifestyle and requires chronic medical therapy and often surgery. All layers of the bowel wall are affected by this disease. Inflammatory lesions tend to appear in patches, with normal segments interspersed between diseased segments. It has been suggested that Crohn's disease is a disorder of the lymphoid tissue. This would explain the frequent involvement of the terminal ileum and anus, both of which have a rich lymph supply.

Extension of the ulcerative lesions through all layers of the bowel predisposes the patient to abscess and fistula formation. Fistulas often involve other loops of the small intestine, the colon, the bladder, the vagina, or even the abdominal wall. Anal fissures, perianal abscesses, and partial bowel obstruction are other complications associated with Crohn's disease. Fever, abdominal pain, and diarrhea are symptoms commonly seen with Crohn's disease. Patients with Crohn's disease may also exhibit anorexia, weight loss, and malnutrition.

This disease occurs most often in young adults, and there seems to be a higher incidence among Jewish persons. The disease often results in disability and incapacity and requires long medical or surgical treatment.

BOX 23-6 **Nursing Process**

INFLAMMATORY BOWEL DISEASE

ASSESSMENT

Vital signs
Abdomen for pain, bowel sounds, contour, firmness
Fluid volume status
Weight
Nutritional status
Stool frequency and appearance
Rectal bleeding
Laboratory studies (electrolytes, B, folic acid, hemoglobin, hematocrit, WBC)
Coping mechanisms

NURSING DIAGNOSES

Pain related to bowel inflammation, frequent diarrhea, perirectal excoriation
Altered nutrition: less than body requirements related to malabsorption, diarrhea, anorexia
Risk for fluid volume deficit related to excessive diarrhea, blood loss, or poor oral intake
Risk for infection related to poor nutritional status and immunocompromised state
Diarrhea related to inflammation of bowels
Anxiety related to change in health status
Ineffective individual coping related to stress, disease process, pain, lack of rest, or lack of support
Knowledge deficit related to chronic disease, change in treatment, new information

NURSING INTERVENTIONS

Administer medications as prescribed and evaluate effectiveness.
Provide heating pad to abdomen if indicated.
After defecation, cleanse anal area and apply topical soothing ointment if indicated.
Keep room as free from odor as possible.
Administer TPN/IV fluids as prescribed.
Provide diet high in protein, calories, vitamins, and minerals.
Provide small, frequent meals.
Avoid food high in fat, fiber, spicy foods, milk products, raw vegetables, fruits, nuts, or whole grains.
Encourage optimal nutrition.
Test stool for occult blood.
Maintain handwashing before providing nursing care.
Provide/instruct on perianal hygiene.
Promote skin and mouth care.
Provide opportunity to discuss feelings, concerns, frustrations.
Encourage diversional activities.

EVALUATION OF EXPECTED OUTCOMES

Acceptable pain level
Stable weight
Controlled diarrhea
No evidence of dehydration
No evidence of infection
Patient/family understand disease and management
Able to verbalize anxiety and coping measures

Assessment. The symptoms are mild and intermittent at first. Exacerbations often follow dietary indiscretions (milk, milk products, fatty foods), emotional upsets, or illness. Abdominal pain, cramping, tenderness, flatulence, nausea, fever, and diarrhea will occur in an acute attack. The more typical picture is the chronic type with diarrhea accompanied by mild pain. It may be aggravated by illness or emotional upsets but is usually less severe than diarrhea associated with ulcerative colitis. The stool is usually soft or semiliquid and may be quite foul smelling and fatty. Urgency to expel stools may awaken the patient at night. A large amount of flatus is also likely to be present. The passing of gross blood is rare and would indicate extensive ulceration.

Diagnosis is made by a series of x-ray examinations, including an upper gastrointestinal tract series (barium swallow) and a barium enema. Proctosigmoidoscopy may be beneficial to rule out other diseases such as ulcerative colitis or diverticulitis or to obtain a rectal biopsy.

Intervention. Treatment of Crohn's disease is not specific or curative but is supportive, palliative, and aimed at attaining remission of the disease. Goals of treatment are aimed at reducing inflammation and controlling symptoms. Medical treatment initially attempts to reduce active inflammation and is more likely to be successful early in the course of the disease before permanent structural changes have developed. Loperamide hydrochloride (Immodium) is used to treat cramping. Antiinflammatory (Prednisone) and immunosuppressive (azathioprine) agents, as with ulcerative colitis, are used in the treatment plan. Although the exact mechanism of action in Crohn's disease is unknown, metronidazole (Flagyl) may also be used; it is suspected that the drug acts as an immunosuppressant. Following recent clinical trials, mesalamine (Pentasa) is used to reduce inflammation. Its antiprostaglandin activity is thought to be the effective action. Methotrexate, a drug used to treat arthritis, is being used experimentally as a safer alternative to prednisone (Hanauer, 1995). Nutritional support and dietary modifications are part of the treatment plan in Crohn's disease. A diet with reduced roughage and low residue will reduce the diarrhea associated with the inflammatory process.

Surgical intervention as a treatment for Crohn's disease is delayed until symptoms can no longer be controlled or significant complications have developed. Surgical treatment is aimed at correcting complications or removal of the affected portion of the intestinal tract or both. Strictures may require surgical treatment with stricturoplasty to increase the diameter of the bowel or resection to remove the stricture. An ostomy is performed only when the rectum and anus must be bypassed temporarily or removed (Doughty, 1994).

Nursing care is centered around rest, relief of pain and diarrhea, and psychologic support.

Ulcerative colitis. Ulcerative colitis is one of the most serious diseases of the gastrointestinal tract. Although the disease has been reported since 1875, the specific cause is still unknown. There appears to be little evidence that the disease is caused by pathologic organisms. Possible causes include food allergies, immunologic reaction, infections, destructive enzymes, and autoimmune reactions. Once the disease becomes established, it often becomes chronic. The disease may be acute, progressing rapidly to a fatal outcome, or it may remain low grade. The disease usually attacks young adults and may be found in children and adolescents; it almost always occurs before 30 years of age.

Ulcerative colitis affects the mucosal surface of the colon and rectum. It begins in the rectum and spreads upward through the colon, eventually involving the entire colon. It is characterized by chronic, persistent inflammation, and fibrosis and narrowing of the bowel lumen occurs. Because of the associated frequent diarrhea and poor absorption of nutrients, the disease can lead to chronic nutritional deficiency, anemia, and electrolyte imbalances. Cancer of the colon is a known complication of long-term chronic ulcerative colitis. The disease may be controlled medically but is cured only by surgical intervention and removal of the diseased colon.

Assessment. Ulcerative colitis is characterized by frequent loose, bloody, mucoid stool. Although pain is not the hallmark symptom associated with ulcerative colitis, patients often complain of a mild, cramping-type pain occurring in the left lower quadrant. This pain is often associated with the urge to defecate and is relieved with defecation.

Symptoms begin rather insidiously, with increasing distress and frequency of stools until the individual may have as many as 20 to 30 stools a day. The presence of ulcers on the lining of the intestine results in blood loss and anemia and possibly in severe hemorrhage. The patient becomes debilitated, pale, weak, and thin, and electrolytes are constantly being depleted from the severe diarrhea. Because of the nutritional deficiency, symptoms of vitamin deficiency may occur. Diagnosis is made on the basis of the history and physical examination, including sigmoidoscopy, x-ray examination, and stool specimens.

Intervention. Treatment includes physical and psychologic rest; nutrition, fluid, and electrolyte management; control of inflammation; and prevention of infection. Symptoms are managed with antiinflammatory agents such as Sulfasalazine, aspirin, or a sulfapyridine-aspirin drug combination. Steroids (Prednisone) are used during severe episodes of the disease to reduce inflammation. Immunosuppressive agents such as azathioprine (Imuran) or 6-mercaptopurine may also be used (Doughty, 1993; Shannon and others, 1992). These agents target the local and systemic immunologic response.

Anticholinergics and antidiarrheal agents are used to control GI spasm and frequency of stool. Azulfidine is also used to help control the frequency of stool. In this instance it is not used for its antibiotic effect but because it decreases diarrhea and associated symptoms. It also reduces the incidence of relapse when used on a long-term basis. Its specific action is unknown, but it is retained by the connective tissue of the intestinal mucosa and submucosa. Remission and improvement occur in 70% of the patients. A hot water bottle or electric heating pad to the abdomen and hot sitz baths may provide some relief for abdominal cramps.

A diet high in proteins, calories, and vitamins and minerals is encouraged. Foods that are high in fat, fiber, and residue are avoided. Because the appetite is poor, the patient will need much encouragement to eat, and consideration should be given to the patient's food desires because he or she will often know which foods cause him or her the most discomfort. Food intake should be carefully noted because diet is important in treating patients with ulcerative colitis. Because of nutritional and fluid deficiencies, the skin is dry; superfatted soap should be used, followed by lanolin. Special mouth care must be given several times a day, with the application of appropriate moisturizers to the mouth and lips.

During the acute stage of the disease, the patient may be receiving intravenous infusions and blood transfusions. Perforation of intestinal ulcers may occur, resulting in hemorrhage and peritonitis. Any drop in blood pressure, increase in pulse rate, or abdominal pain should be reported. The patient is usually given a mild sedative drug to promote psychologic rest and decrease anxiety.

The psychologic care of the patient with ulcerative colitis requires the empathic understanding of everyone concerned with his or her care. The patient is often insecure, sensitive, and apprehensive. A carefully prepared nursing care plan contributes to the continuity of care, which is important in meeting the patient's needs for a feeling of security. Because the patient's behavior may be characterized by periods of depression and changes in mood, the nurse must be prepared to accept such changes and continue to provide intelligent, personalized nursing care. The nurse should refer the patient to support groups for patients with IBD.

Patients with ulcerative colitis should have a quiet, pleasant environment and should be protected from chilling and secondary infection. Because diarrhea constitutes one of the major problems, bathroom facilities should be readily available; a bedside commode or, if the patient is not ambulatory, a padded bedpan should be within reach of the patient. After defecation the anal area should be carefully cleansed and a soothing ointment applied. The frequency, amount, and character of stools should be observed and recorded. Enemas are avoided because of the risk of bowel perforation. Room deodorizers are used to eliminate unpleasant room odors, and plans should be made for airing the room daily.

If medical management is unsuccessful, surgery is indicated to remove the diseased colon. Surgical alternatives for the patient with ulcerative colitis include colectomy with the creation of a permanent ileostomy, colectomy with the creation of an ileoanal reservoir, or colectomy with an ileoanal anastomosis. The decision to treat the patient medically or surgically is dependent on the severity of the disease, the patient's age, and the patient's preference.

Patient and family teaching. Because of the chronicity of IBD, patient teaching is integral to successful disease management. The patient is instructed on how to control diet and stress to reduce acute exacerbations of the disease. The nurse and dietician work with the patient to make a list of do's and don't's for eating: Do eat small frequent meals; eat food high in carbohydrates, proteins, and minerals. Don't eat foods high in fat, fried foods, spicy foods, milk and milk products; don't eat raw vegetables, fruits, nuts, whole grains. A complete and balanced dietary plan can be developed that incorporates the patient's food preferences.

The patient is taught the expected actions of medications in controlling symptoms of the disease, as well as how to monitor response to the medical treatment. Instructing the patient in stress management techniques is a valuable adjunct to the medical and surgical management of IBD.

Appendicitis

One of the most common causes of an acute abdominal condition is *appendicitis.* The risk of fatal complications is increased when treatment is delayed. Factors that have helped reduce deaths from appendicitis during past years include early recognition of the disease, improvement in surgical techniques and anesthesia, the use of antibiotics, and intensive nursing care.

Pathophysiology. Appendicitis is an inflammation of the vermiform appendix, a projection of bowel tissue located at the apex of the cecum where the small and large intestine meet. The lumen of the proximal end of the appendix is shared with that of the cecum, whereas the distal end is closed. The walls of the appendix contain lymphoid cells, and although the appendix has been generally considered to have no specific function, it is now believed to share with other lymphoid tissues of the body the function of preventing infection. The appendix fills and empties regularly in the same way as the cecum. However, the lumen is narrow and is easily obstructed. It is most commonly believed that appendicitis develops as a result of an obstruction of the lumen of the appendix and subsequent bacterial overgrowth. When the lumen becomes obstructed, the blood supply is disrupted, the appendix becomes distended and hypoxic, and inflammation occurs. Pathogenic bacteria present in the intestinal tract, often *Escherichia coli,* begin to multiply in the appendix, and infection develops with the formation of pus. If distention and infection are severe enough, the appendix may perforate, with spillage of intestinal contents and bacteria into the peritoneum. If this occurs, the infectious material may be walled off and the infection localized with an appendiceal abscess. If it is not localized, the infectious material spreads to the abdominal cavity and generalized peritonitis occurs. Perforation with subsequent peritonitis and abscess formation is the most serious consequence of acute appendicitis.

Assessment. Diagnosis of acute appendicitis is made based on the presence of a typical pattern of signs and symptoms. The symptoms most characteristic of acute appendicitis are pain, fever, elevated WBC, anorexia, and nausea and vomiting. Pain may be felt in the lower right quadrant of the abdomen, halfway between the umbilicus and the crest of the ileum (*McBurney's point*), or experienced near the umbilicus. *Rebound tenderness* in the right lower quadrant may be present (Figure 23-11).

NURSE ALERT

To test for the presence of rebound tenderness, place the patient in a supine position. Extend fingertips at a 90 degree angle directly over the abdomen in an area away from the suspected area of tenderness. Gently press fingers deep into the abdomen and remove them quickly. Quick removal of the fingers causes the abdominal organs to "rebound" to their normal position. If the patient has "rebound tenderness," a sharp pain will be felt in the area of peritoneal irritation.

Interventions. Surgical removal of the appendix (appendectomy) is the definitive treatment for acute appendicitis; often the procedure is performed as an emergency operation. When appendicitis is suspected, surgery is usually done as soon as the diagnosis has been completed to avoid rupture and complications.

In a clean appendectomy (without rupture), recovery is usually rapid. The patient is discharged from the hospital quickly, often within 24 hours, and may resume most normal activities within 5 to 7 days. If the appendix has ruptured before surgical intervention, intraoperative irrigations with balanced electrolyte and antibiotic solutions are used to cleanse the peritoneal cavity of intestinal spillage. Drains are often placed in the wound, and the wound is left open to heal by secondary intention to prevent abscess formation.

The nurse closely monitors the patient for signs and symptoms of local and systemic infection following surgery for a ruptured appendix. Specific attention is given to monitoring temperature, heart rate, WBC count, pain, the appearance of the surgical wound, and the presence and characteristics of any wound drainage (Box 23-7).

The postoperative care is directed toward preventing wound infection and pulmonary complications.

PATIENT/FAMILY TEACHING

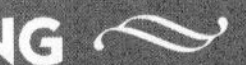

Appendicitis/appendectomy

The nurse should instruct the patient and family on the following:

- Activity restrictions (no heavy lifting after surgery)
- Progressive activity as tolerated
- Wound care
- Signs and symptoms of infection
- Dietary guidelines
- Follow-up medical care
- Medication action, dosage, and side effects

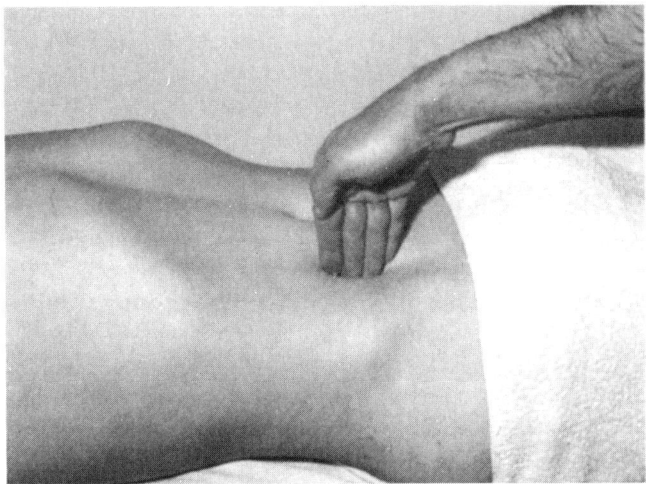

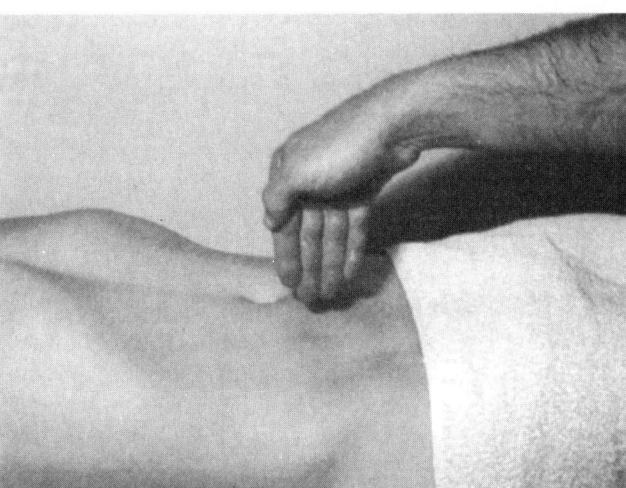

Figure 23-11 Testing for rebound tenderness. (From Seidel HM and others: *Mosby's guide to physical examination*, ed 3, St Louis, 1995, Mosby.)

BOX 23-7 **Nursing Process**

APPENDICITIS/APPENDECTOMY

ASSESSMENT

Preoperative
Abdominal pain
Abdomen for bowel sounds, contour, firmness, rebound tenderness
Vital signs
For anorexia, nausea, or vomiting
CBC
Postoperative
Vital signs
Comfort level
Fluid volume status
Respiratory status
Abdomen for bowel sounds, contour, firmness
Surgical incision and drains, if present

NURSING DIAGNOSES

Pain related to inflammation or surgery
Risk for infection related to perforation of appendix
Risk for fluid volume deficit related to preoperative vomiting, surgery, or third spacing
Ineffective breathing pattern related to pain and analgesic effect
Knowledge deficit related to new diagnosis, home care needs

NURSING INTERVENTIONS

Administer analgesics as ordered.
Provide comfort measures.
Administer antibiotics if ordered.
Provide aseptic wound care.
Administer IV fluids as prescribed.
Provide clear liquids in small amounts when po intake instituted.
Maintain accurate I&O.
Encourage coughing, deep breathing, and ambulation.
Instruct on splinting of incision with movement and cough.
Help patient turn every 2 hours while in bed.
Refer to visting nurse for assist with dressing changes if indicated.

EVALUATION OF EXPECTED OUTCOMES

Meets discharge criteria for postsurgical patient (p. 487)
Evidence of wound healing without purulent drainage and erythema
Temperature within normal limits
No evidence of respiratory distress
Lungs clear
Tolerating diet without distress
Tolerating diet without nausea
Acceptable pain level
Return to preoperative self-care level

Ambulation usually begins the day of surgery. When drainage is necessary because of an abscess, dressings must be changed as necessary and disposed of carefully.

Patient and family teaching. Before being discharged from the hospital, the patient is taught how to assess the wound for signs and symptoms of infection, including redness, tenderness, and drainage, and to report these findings to the physician. Patients may require specific wound care instructions if the surgical wound is not closed before discharge. Any limitation on physical activity, especially lifting, is carefully explained.

Diverticular disease: diverticulosis and diverticulitis

Diverticula are pouches of mucosa and submucosa that protrude or herniate through the circular muscles of the intestinal wall (Figure 23-12). Diverticula can occur anywhere in the large bowel but are most commonly found in the sigmoid colon. They are rarely found in persons under age 40, but it is estimated that one of every three persons over age 60 has some diverticula. There is increasing evidence that a low-fiber diet may contribute to the development of diverticula. When diverticula are present, the individual is said to have *diverticulosis.* **Diverticulitis** occurs when fecal matter penetrates the thin-walled diverticula, resulting in inflammation and abscess formation outside the bowel.

Pathophysiology. The exact cause of diverticular disease is unknown, but there seems to be a strong correlation with factors that contribute to increased colonic pressure and weakened points in the muscle wall of the colon in the development of the disease. The role of diet in the development and progression of the disease is also a factor.

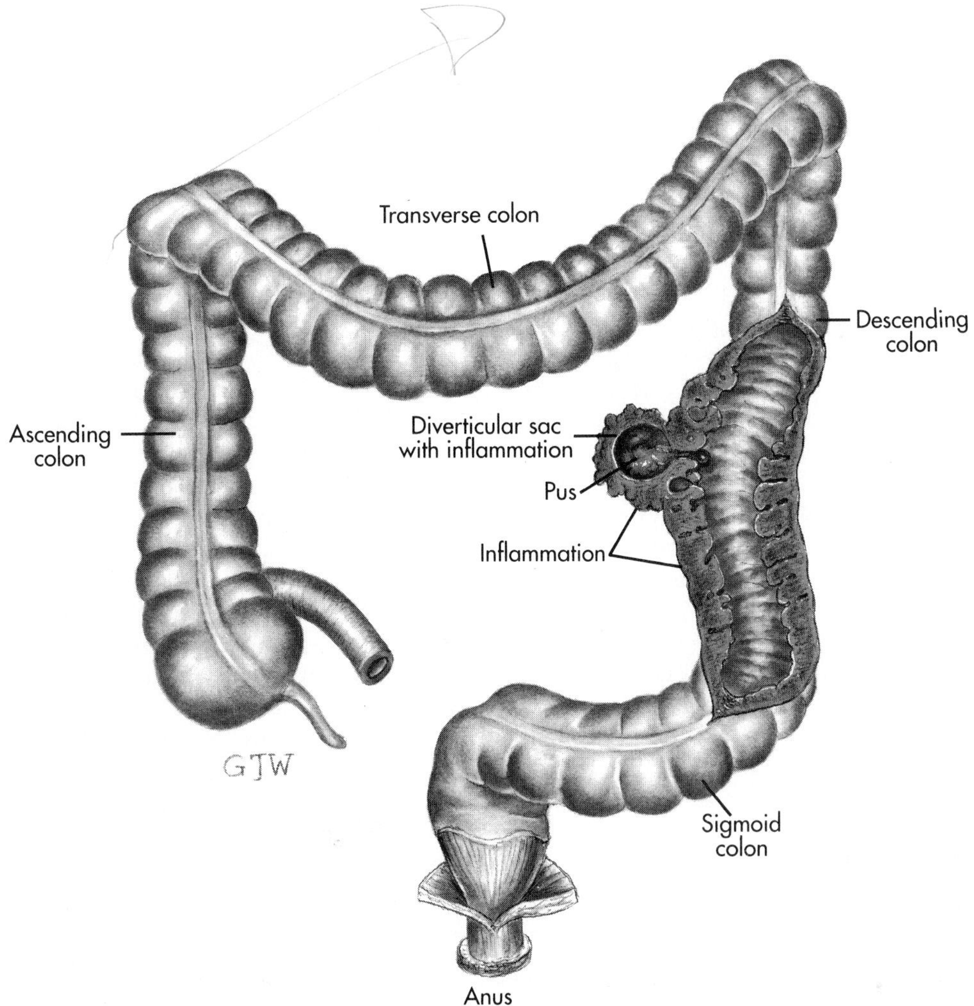

Figure 23-12 Diverticula located in descending colon. (From Doughty DB, Jackson DB: *Gastrointestinal disorders,* St Louis, 1993, Mosby.)

Diverticula develop when the muscles of the colon hypertrophy or become thickened. Both the circular and longitudinal muscles and the muscular fibers (teniae coli) are involved. Little sacs develop between these circular fibers. Increased pressure in the colon results in the protrusion of mucosa through the weakened muscle in the little sacs, resulting in diverticula and diverticulosis (Marchiondo, 1994; McCance, Huether, 1994).

Once diverticula develop, there is the possibility that the protrusion will continue and inflammation and perforation of the sac will occur, resulting in diverticulitis. This complication can be in the form of microperforations into the fat layer around the bowel or larger macroperforations opening into the peritoneal space. Microperforations result in the formation of abscesses and localized peritonitis. Macroperforations produce severe, generalized peritonitis. The body responds as it does to any inflammatory process (pain, fever, elevated WBC). Complications of diverticulitis include fistulas, septicemia, obstruction, and hemorrhage.

Those who theorize that diet plays a role in diverticular disease believe that a diet low in fiber causes muscle thickening that predisposes the individual to formation of diverticula. Reduced fiber in the diet results in less bulk in the stool. The lumen of the bowel is not forced to widen, and the pressure within that lumen is therefore increased (intracolonic pressure). The sigmoid is normally the narrowest segment of the bowel; interestingly, it is the most common site of diverticula. Fiber also affects stool transit time—the time it takes for stool to move through the bowel. Stool that moves faster will have less water absorbed and will thus be softer and easier to eliminate. Increased intracolonic pressure is believed to be the cause of the muscle hypertrophy, which leads to the formation of diverticula.

Assessment. The patient with diverticulosis may not display any problematic symptoms. Diarrhea, constipation, distention, or flatulence, along with mild to moderate complaints of cramping pain over the lower abdomen, are associated with diverticulosis. When diverticula perforate and diverticulitis develops, the patient will complain of mild to severe pain in the lower left quadrant of the abdomen and will have fever and an elevated white blood cell count and sedimentation rate. If the condition goes untreated, septicemia and septicemic shock can develop. The septic patient will be hypotensive, have a rapid pulse rate, and may have a change in mental status. Obstruction can occur, and the patient will experience abdominal distention, nausea, and vomiting. Hemorrhage occurs in approximately 10% to 20% of patients; it may be mild and go unnoticed for some time or be severe and result in shock.

Interventions. Management for diverticulosis is based on a high-fiber diet, including vegetables, fruits, and whole grains, fiber supplements (if needed), and a bulk-forming laxative.

If inflammation develops, the treatment plan will change to a low-fiber diet, intravenous fluid replacements and gastric decompression as necessary, and antibiotics. Microperforation resulting in localized abscess is treated with a combination of antimicrobials effective against gram-negative, gram-positive, and anaerobic organisms. Fluids and electrolytes must be administered intravenously, and a nasogastric tube is inserted and attached to suction. Analgesics, usually morphine sulfate or Meperidine, are given to manage pain. Surgical intervention may be indicated for repeated bouts of diverticulitis, especially if they result in a partial bowel obstruction.

Macroperforations always require surgical intervention. A temporary or permanent colostomy or bowel resection with a reanastamosis may be performed depending on the severity of the disease and the extent of complications.

Nursing intervention is aimed at monitoring vital signs and fluid balance, providing relief of pain, and assessing the response to treatment. The patient is observed closely for signs of septicemia and shock. The schedule for antibiotic therapy must be strictly followed. When surgery is necessary, nursing interventions follow the recommendations for the specific procedure performed (Box 23-8).

Patient and family teaching. Patients are taught the importance of dietary control of diverticular disease. Working with the patient, the nurse and the dieti-

BOX 23-8 **Nursing Process**

DIVERTICULOSIS/DIVERTICULITIS

ASSESSMENT

Vital signs
Abdomen for pain, bowel sounds, contour, firmness
Dietary history
Patterns of elimination
Laboratory studies (WBC, sedimentation rate)

NURSING DIAGNOSES

Pain related to bowel inflamation or microperforation
Risk for infection related to bowel microperforation
Risk for injury: peritonitis related to bowel perforation
Constipation related to inadequate diet or fluid intake
Anxiety related to lifestyle modification
Knowledge deficit related to causative factors of disease and dietary modifications

NURSING INTERVENTIONS

Provide comfort measures.
Medicate as needed with analgesics.
Promote relaxation and diversional activities.
Administer IV fluid as ordered.
Administer antibiotics as ordered.
Provide dietary modification depending on acuity of illness (acute diverticulitis, NPO to clear liquids to low fiber diet; diverticulitis, high fiber diet).
Refer to dietician if indicated.
Encourage liberal fluid intake if not contraindicated.
Spend time providing emotional support.
Encourage ventilation of feelings, fears, concerns.

EVALUATION OF EXPECTED OUTCOMES

Absence of abdominal pain
No evidence of infectious process
Soft, formed bowel movements
Identifies symptoms that indicated need for medical treatment
States necessary dietary modifications

PATIENT/FAMILY TEACHING

Diverticulosis/Diverticulitis

The nurse should educate the patient and family about the following aspects of these conditions:

- Disease process
- Dietary modifications—high fiber diet inclusive of vegetables, fruits, whole grains, and bulk-forming laxatives.
- Importance of avoiding corn, nuts, and seeds
- Liberal fluid intake
- Avoidance of increasing intraabdominal pressure (e.g., constipation, improper lifting, and restrictive clothing)

cian develop a dietary plan based on the stage of the disease. Diverticulosis is managed with a diet rich in fiber and whole grains. During episodes of acute inflammation, however, modifications in diet are needed; low fiber is used during these episodes to decrease irritation and minimize inflammation.

Peritonitis

Peritonitis is an inflammation of the peritoneum and the abdominal cavity and is often a complication of a bacterial infection. Infection may develop from a perforated peptic ulcer or ruptured appendix. It may be caused by infection from the internal female organs. Although infrequent, it may occur from trauma to abdominal organs or be carried by infection in the bloodstream. Peritonitis may also occur as a complication of peritoneal dialysis. Every patient who has had surgery of the GI tract is at risk for the development of peritonitis. The inflammatory process may be localized, with abscess formation, or it may be generalized, with bacteria spreading throughout the entire abdominal cavity. Sometimes peritonitis occurs without any known cause.

Assessment. Generalized peritonitis is an extremely serious condition characterized mainly by severe abdominal pain. The patient usually lies on her back or side with the knees flexed to relax the abdominal muscles; any movement is painful. Nausea and vomiting occur. Constipation or diarrhea may occur early, but as the condition progresses, peristalsis ceases and paralytic ileus develops. The abdomen becomes distended, tense, rigid, and very tender. The pulse is weak and rapid, and blood pressure falls. Leukocytosis and marked dehydration occur. Without quick and appropriate intervention, the patient may die.

Intervention. Interventions for peritonitis include antibiotics to treat infection, fluid and electrolyte replacement, pain management, and relief of paralytic ileus. The patient is placed in a semi-Fowler's position for comfort. Pain medication, preferably morphine, is administered to relieve pain. The patient is maintained NPO. A nasogastric tube is inserted and connected to suction to keep the stomach empty and to help relieve the ileus. Intravenous fluids are administered to prevent dehydration and to maintain electrolyte balance. Antibiotic therapy is started; usually a broad-spectrum antibiotic is used until the exact infectious agent is identified through cultures. Further care or indications for surgery depend on the cause of the peritonitis and the patient's condition.

The nurse monitors all vital signs, including blood pressure, heart rate, and temperature, and examines the abdomen for distention, pain, and the presence of bowel sounds. Additionally, the nurse carefully monitors and records all intake and output, including intravenous fluids, vomitus or NG drainage, and urine. The patient is observed for pain, and the type of pain and its location are described, recorded, and reported. The patient often realizes the seriousness of his or her condition, and the nurse should facilitate expression of fears and provide emotional support.

Intestinal Obstruction

An obstruction of the small or large intestine may occur when any condition exists that prevents the free passage of bowel contents through the intestine. The obstruction may be partial or complete, but it is always considered serious. Some intestinal obstructions resolve or correct with only conservative medical treatment, but most obstructions require surgical intervention.

Pathophysiology

An intestinal obstruction has many causes, some of which include a strangulated hernia, twisting of the bowel (volvulus), cancer, postoperative adhesions, paralytic ileus, and stricture. The most common causes are postoperative adhesions and hernia. Obstruction may occur in the small or the large intestine. Obstruction in the large intestine is less dramatic than when it occurs in the small intestine. When an obstruction cuts off the blood supply, as in a strangulated hernia, part of the intestine becomes necrotic, and gangrene develops. Most obstructions occur in the small intestine and affect the normal homeostasis of the body. The continuous vomiting causes loss of electrolytes and loss of hydrochloric acid from the stomach, leading to alkalosis. The loss of water and sodium from the body may cause acidosis and severe dehydration.

Assessment

The symptoms of obstruction vary according to location and extent of the obstruction. When the obstruction is high in the small intestine, symptoms appear earlier and are more acute than when the large intestine is obstructed. The early symptoms are abdominal pain, abdominal distention, vomiting, and constipation. The pain is often wavelike, and vomiting may be projectile. The gastric contents are first vomited, but as peristalsis is reversed, bile and fecal matter from above the obstruction are vomited. When the obstruction is in the colon, vomiting may not occur. The patient may eliminate blood or pus via the rectum, but no fecal matter or flatus passes. Extreme thirst occurs; the tongue and mucous membranes of the mouth and lips become parched. Abdominal distention develops and is greater when the obstruction is in the colon. Signs of shock may appear, and without treatment, the patient may die within a few hours.

Intervention

A nasogastric tube is inserted and attached to low suction to remove intestinal secretions and gas that have accumulated proximal to the obstruction. Some physicians may insert a long intestinal decompression tube, such as the Miller-Abbott, instead of the nasogastric tube. The patency of the tube is checked often and is maintained by irrigating the tube every 1 to 2 hours with 30 ml of normal saline. The volume, characteristics, and consistency of the drainage are observed and recorded. Drainage is tested for the presence of blood (refer to the section on gastric decompression). A long intestinal decompression tube is intended to travel down the intestinal tract and should never be taped.

The patient is given nothing by mouth. Intravenous fluids are administered to correct the dehydration and replace the electrolytes lost through vomiting or intestinal drainage. All vomitus or drainage is accurately described, and any fecal matter should be saved to be examined for occult blood.

Temperature, heart rate, blood pressure, and respiratory rate are taken at least every 4 hours; more frequent assessments are made if the patient exhibits signs of hypovolemic shock. The nurse may elevate the head of the bed 30 to 40 degrees to prevent respiratory difficulty that might occur as a result of abdominal distention, to help prevent aspiration, and to encourage passage of small intestine contents into the colon. Careful records of urinary output are maintained, and if retention occurs, the patient should be catheterized. The patient is assisted with frequent cleansing of the mouth and changes in position. The environment is kept well ventilated and free of odors by prompt care of vomitus and the use of a deodorizer if necessary.

Surgery for intestinal obstruction depends partly on the cause of the obstruction, its location, and the condition of the patient. In some cases surgery may be relatively simple, whereas in other situations the cause may complicate the surgical procedure. In obstructions resulting from a strangulated hernia, cutting off the blood supply may have caused the bowel to become gangrenous, and resection of the affected bowel may be necessary. Before surgery, the patient may be given a small enema under low pressure. Intravenous fluids are administered to replace electrolytes lost through vomiting, and TPN may be initiated to provide nutritional elements. After surgery, if the bowel has been resected, oral feeding is withheld to give the anastomosis time to heal. A nasogastric tube attached to suction aids in keeping the stomach empty. Accurate intake and output records are maintained. Other postoperative care is the same as that for any abdominal surgery.

Tumors

Oral cancer

Tumors of the lips, tongue, and mouth may be benign or malignant; cancer of the tongue is the most common type of tumor of the mouth. Although the cause of mouth cancer is unknown, it is believed that irritation resulting from smoking, alcohol consumption, dental appliances, and rough, jagged teeth are predisposing factors. Malignant tumors of the mouth metastasize early to adjacent structures such as the lymph nodes in the neck and muscle tissue. Cancer of the mouth is often associated with leukoplakia, a condition characterized by the formation of white patches on the mucous membrane of the tongue or cheek. Cancer of the mouth is more common in men than in women and is responsible for 3% to 6% of deaths from cancer. When the disease is discovered early, the prognosis is good.

Malignant lesions may involve the lips, tongue, or mucous membrane lining the mouth, and surgery or radiation or both may be used in the treatment. Any surgery of the mouth interferes with the normal functions of respiration, speech, and eating and will involve certain nursing problems. The mouth cannot be rendered completely free of pathogenic organisms but should be kept as clean as possible to prevent infection.

Preoperative care of the mouth for patients with malignant tumors requires meticulous attention. The teeth should be brushed before and after meals, and dental floss should be used to remove any particles between the teeth. Dentures and bridges are cared for in the same manner. Warm mouthwashes or irrigations with an antiseptic solution may be ordered by the physician. If necrotic tissue is present, various preparations may be used to loosen the tissue and deodorize the mouth. A solution of 1 teaspoon of salt and 1 teaspoon of baking soda in 1 quart of warm water may be used for frequent mouthwashes. In addition, 1.5% hydrogen peroxide may be used as a mouthwash with moderate pressure irrigation. Depending on the site and the extent of the lesion, eating may be difficult. The diet should contain soft food and be free of acids and citrus foods, which may cause pain; frequent small feedings may be more desirable than large meals three times a day. The emotional factors involved in this type of surgery require that the nurse have an understanding of the patient's feelings. The patient may fear permanent disability or disfigurement and should be given as much information before surgery as is necessary to help relieve his or her anxiety. If the malignancy involves the lymph nodes in the neck, a radical neck dissection may be done in an attempt to remove all affected tissue.

After surgery, the patient's speech will be affected, and a pad and pencil should be at the bedside. The patient may have a tracheotomy or a tracheostomy, and nursing care is the same as that outlined in Chapter 20. A nasogastric tube may be inserted through the nostril and connected to suction. The physician will order the position in which the patient should be placed. Depending on the suture line and the extent of surgery, suction of secretions and mucus may be gently done, or a wick of gauze may be placed in the mouth and allowed to drain into an emesis basin. The physician may order mouth irrigations to be performed, using a prescribed solution and sterile equipment. Intravenous infusions may be given. If a radical neck dissection has been done, blood transfusions may be needed, and a large pressure dressing may be applied to help prevent edema and splint the affected body part. Some patients may have a wound drain (Hemovac, Jackson-Pratt) placed to remove blood and serous drainage from the wound bed.

The method of feeding will depend on the site and the extent of the surgery. Enteral feeding is often required in the early postoperative period. When a portion of the tongue has been removed, a thread is often passed through the remaining portion of the tongue and fastened to the outside of the cheek with adhesive tape to keep it from obstructing the airway. The patient is watched carefully for hemorrhage and respiratory difficulty because edema may occur and obstruct the airway. A tracheostomy tray, suction and suction catheters, and oxygen should always be available for emergency use.

Cancer of the mouth may be treated by external radiation or by implanting radium needles or radon seeds (see Chapter 10). When radium needles are used, they are attached to threads fastened to the outside of the cheek with adhesive tape, and the patient must be cautioned against pulling on the threads. The threads must be checked and counted several times a day and recorded on the patient's chart. A pad and pencil or slate should be provided for the patient because talking will be difficult. Mouth hygiene is important, and a spray may be ordered and used while the needles are in place. Any equipment used must be carefully inspected for radium that may have become dislodged. The physician will give directions concerning food and fluids. The patient should always be watched carefully for hemorrhage, edema, or choking.

Esophageal cancer

Cancer of the esophagus occurs mostly in men and accounts for over 6000 deaths each year in the United States. Despite all therapy, the 5-year survival rate for esophageal cancer is poor—at only about 4%. In the majority of cases only palliation is possible.

Dysphagia (difficulty in swallowing) with the ingestion of solid foods is the prime symptom in 90% of cases; weight loss may also occur. Because pain does not occur until the disease is well advanced, and swallowing difficulty may be intermittent in the beginning, there is usually a delay in reporting symptoms to a physician. This is unfortunate because metastasis does not occur until after extensive local infiltration. Hence, the slightest dysphagia should be investigated promptly and thoroughly with *esophagoscopy*, esophagrams, and cytologic examinations of esophageal washings. The tumor metastasizes to the lymph nodes in the neck and chest and eventually to the liver and the bones. The patient becomes thinner and more malnourished as the disease progresses. Radiation may be used for palliation when metastasis has occurred. The only hope for cure is early diagnosis and surgical removal of the lesion. The tumor and lymph nodes may be removed and the esophagus anastomosed to the stomach (esophagogastrostomy), or a portion of the intestine may be anastomosed between the esophagus and the stomach after the tumor is removed. If the patient is not a candidate for major surgery or if the tumor is inoperable, a gastrostomy may be performed for feeding purposes.

Gastrostomy care. The patient with a gastrostomy has an opening into the stomach through which a tube has been inserted for the purpose of feeding (Figure 23-13). The stomach may be sutured to the abdom-

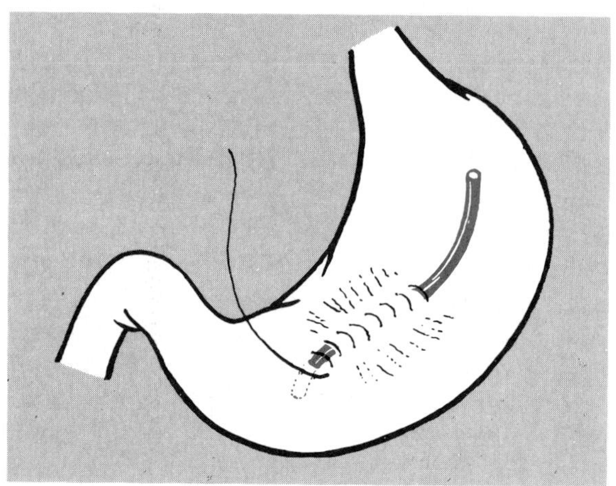

Figure 23-13 Gastrostomy tube is inserted into stomach and secured with sutures. End of tube or catheter is brought out through opening in abdomen so that feedings may be given.

inal wall to prevent stomach contents from entering the abdominal cavity, and the catheter is secured into a small incision. Routine care of the gastrostomy site includes cleansing of the skin around the tube with soap and water or an antibacterial agent. A dressing is usually placed around the tube insertion site. The tube is secured in place to prevent accidental dislodgement. The nurse should refer to specific hospital protocols for tube care. If the gastrostomy tube inadvertently becomes dislodged or is removed, the nurse should notify the physician.

Nursing management of the patient with a gastrostomy tube includes caring for the skin, maintaining patency of the tube, good oral care, and administering the prescribed feeding as ordered by the physician. Often there is a slight seepage of secretions around the tube, which will cause excoriation of the skin. Careful washing with mild soap and water, thorough drying, and the application of a bland ointment will usually keep the skin in a healthy condition. If the tube becomes blocked, it may be gently irrigated with a bulb syringe and physiologic saline solution. Force should not be used to irrigate the tube, and if the tube is not easily unplugged, the physician should be notified.

Most institutions use commercially prepared solutions. The specific formula, volume, rate, and concentration of the enteral feeding is prescribed by the physician. Formulas should be at room temperature, not cold when administered. Cold feedings may cause cramping and diarrhea. The patient is placed with the head of the bed elevated or in a side-lying position to prevent aspiration during feeding. The amount of feeding taken should be recorded so that the physician may determine if the amount of food that the patient is receiving provides sufficient calories (refer to the section on enteral feeding).

The patient with a gastrostomy feeding tube has an emotional adjustment to make that may be difficult. The realization that he or she will not be able to eat normally may be traumatic, and the patient will need a great deal of support and encouragement. As the patient begins to accept this method of feeding, he or she should be encouraged to participate in administering the feeding and caring for the skin. If this method of feeding will be long term or permanent, it is important for a member of the family to be taught the preparation of the diet, as well as the gastrostomy care and feeding of the patient. After the patient leaves the hospital, the home health nurse may visit the patient to supervise, instruct, and provide encouragement.

Stomach cancer

The incidence of cancer of the stomach in the United States has declined by more than 35% during the past 3 decades and continues its downward trend annually. However, higher incidence of cancer of the stomach is found in other nations of the world. Men are more likely to develop cancer of the stomach than women; incidence is most likely between the fifth and sixth decades of life.

Pathophysiology. The cause of cancer of the stomach is unknown, but environment, genetics, and the presence of the bacteria *Helicobacter pylori* are factors implicated in the disease. Diet is probably the most significant environmental factor associated with the development of cancer of the stomach. The incidence is high in parts of the world where there is heavy consumption of smoked fish and smoked meat, such as Japan, Iceland, Chile, and Hawaii. Diets rich in starch, pickled vegetables, salted meats and fish, as well as nitrates and nitrites correlate with an increased risk for cancer of the stomach. *H. pylori* is a known cause of gastritis and atrophic changes associated with gastritis, and has been implicated as a possible factor predisposing patients to gastric cancer. Additionally, an increased incidence of cancer of the stomach is noted in patients with Type A blood and in families in which a member has gastric cancer.

Cancerous lesions of the stomach cause obstruction, either into or out of the stomach; bleeding; or metastasis to adjacent or vital organs.

Assessment. The early symptoms are so poorly defined that most individuals delay medical treatment until the malignancy is well established. Often symptoms related to the metastasis rather than the cancer itself prompt the patient to consult the physician. Symptoms include dysphagia, loss of appetite, a feeling of fullness after meals, epigastric distress, nausea, vomiting, weight loss, anemia, vomiting blood that has a coffee-grounds appearance, blood in the stools that appears dark and tarry, and pain. A palpable mass may be felt through the abdominal wall, but this often indicates that the condition is inoperable. Early diagnosis is most important.

Diagnostic tests include upper GI endoscopy and upper GI barium studies. Gastric analysis is performed; cytologic examination using Papanicolaou's technique to determine the presence of cancer cells may be done following lavage. Emesis may be saved for examination, and stool specimens are examined for the presence of occult blood.

Intervention. The only surgical treatment is a subtotal or total gastrectomy. The malignant growth often causes a severe malnutrition, and several days of preoperative nutritional support may be required before surgery. Chemotherapy and radiation therapy are part of the postoperative treatment plan.

Interventions for the patient after a total gastrectomy are slightly different from those after a subtotal gastrectomy because the chest cavity must be entered to remove the entire stomach. There will be little nasogastric drainage because secretions are normally formed in the stomach, which has been removed. Small frequent feedings, beginning with tap water and slowly progressing to bland foods, are given. Often a period of enteral tube feedings is required to provide or supplement oral nutrition. The patient should be given easily digested foods, eat slowly, and chew the food thoroughly. Because the intrinsic factor normally produced by the stomach is now missing, vitamin B_{12} cannot be absorbed, and a regular injection of vitamin B_{12} is necessary to prevent pernicious anemia. The patient may undergo chemotherapy. A combination of chemotherapeutic agents (5-fluorouracil, doxorubicin, and mitomycin C) has been found to be more effective than single-drug therapy. Radiation may be used with chemotherapy, but radiation alone has not proven effective against gastric cancer.

Cancer of the small intestine

Malignant lesions develop less often in the small intestine than in other segments of the gastrointestinal tract. Symptoms, which include intestinal obstruction, bleeding, and upper abdominal pain, do not appear early. Treatment is surgical removal of the tumor. The prognosis is poor because these tumors tend to metastasize early into the liver and local lymph nodes. A considerable portion of the bowel wall becomes involved before symptoms appear, making early diagnosis almost impossible.

Colorectal cancer

Cancers of the colon and rectum are the most prevalent internal cancers in the United States, occurring equally in men and women. Early detection and treatment lead to a good prognosis, but most patients are still diagnosed and operated on late in the course of the disease. Etiologic factors are not definite, but certain conditions appear to be more prone to malignant changes, including ulcerative colitis and diverticulosis. Evidence suggests that a low-fiber diet is related to colorectal cancer. Evidence also suggests that a diet rich in beef and saturated fats leads to an increased incidence of colorectal cancer. It is theorized that carcinogens are formed from degraded bile salts and that stool, which remains in the large bowel for a longer period as a result of too little fiber to stimulate its passage, may overexpose the bowel to these carcinogens. Another theory relates diverticulosis to low-fiber diets, proposing that the lack of fiber necessitates stronger muscle contractions to excrete hard stools, increasing pressure on the colon wall, which leads to outpouching, or diverticula. Thus the reduced weight of stool and the increased time it takes for stool to pass (transit time), which results from a low-fiber diet, have been related to both diverticulosis and cancer of the colon. As stated earlier, the individual with diverticulosis is already considered more prone to malignant changes.

Assessment. Symptoms may partly depend on the portion involved. Rectal bleeding is still the most common symptom. Alternating constipation and diarrhea is common, along with excessive flatus, cramplike pains in the lower abdomen, and abdominal distention. Obstruction is most likely to occur if the tumor is on the right side or in the transverse colon, in which fecal contents are still fluid. The individual may complain of weakness, loss of appetite, and loss of weight, and anemia may be present. Hemorrhoids and cancer often coexist. Rectal bleeding can never be assumed to be the result of hemorrhoids alone without an examination that rules out cancer. The diagnosis is made on the basis of abdominal and rectal examinations, which include a barium enema and a gastrointestinal series, proctoscopic and sigmoidoscopic examination, and examination of the stools for occult blood. Three fourths of all colon and rectum cancers can be detected with the aid of the sigmoidoscope, and it is important to include this examination in the routine physical examination for all adults over 40 years of age. Any change in normal bowel habits should be reported to the physician.

Intervention. Treatment is always surgical, but preoperative radiation therapy may also be used, along with chemotherapy. The type of surgery depends on the anatomic position of the carcinoma. Whenever possible, the tumor is removed and an end-to-end anastomosis (bringing together the healthy sections of the colon after the tumor has been removed) is performed. If the tumor has obstructed the bowel, a temporary colostomy may be done to divert bowel contents, and resection is done after the obstruction has been decompressed. If the tumor is in the sigmoid or rectum, an abdominoperineal resection is performed, removing the rectum and constructing a colostomy on the abdominal wall. Patients who have inoperable disease may be treated with radiation therapy or chemotherapy. A colostomy may be performed to divert the bowel contents if an inoperable tumor is causing obstruction.

Preoperative. The psychologic preparation of the patient is extremely important. If the physician anticipates that a colostomy will be necessary, the patient should be prepared for it. The patient needs to understand that he or she may expect to lead a normal life (refer to the section on surgery of the GI tract and accessory organs).

Postoperative. Postoperative care includes the care of all tubes, such as a nasogastric tube, a urinary drainage catheter, or drains placed in the perineal wound. The character and appearance of all drainage is observed and recorded. Considerable bloody and serosanguinous drainage is expected to occur from the perineal wound for the first 24 hours. Dressings are changed or reinforced often, and the patient is observed closely for signs and symptoms of hemorrhage or severe volume depletion. Antibiotics are usually administered after surgery to prevent or control infection for the first 24 to 48 hours. The patient receives nothing by mouth, but intravenous fluids are given to maintain hydration and replace electrolytes. If an abdominoperineal resection was done, the perineal wound may have been packed, and the packing is removed gradually by the physician within the first few days after surgery. When all packing has been removed, irrigation of the wound may be ordered for once or twice a day. The physician orders specific directions regarding how the wound is to be irrigated and the solution to be used. Irrigation is a mechanical method of removing tissue and debris. Routine care is given for the colostomy.

Patients who have had an abdominal perineal resection usually have more difficulty with ambulation as a result of the perineal wound, and the nursing procedures of encouraging deep breathing and coughing, turning the patient, and giving leg exercises are of special importance. Postoperative pain control measures are essential to providing for early ambulation and good pulmonary hygiene.

Benign tumors

Benign tumors may occur anywhere in the gastrointestinal tract and usually take the form of polyps, which occur most often in the stomach and the large intestine. Symptoms may resemble those of malignant growths, but surgical procedures are less radical. The diagnosis is made by proctoscopic and x-ray examination.

Peptic Ulcer

A **peptic ulcer** is an erosion of the mucosal and submucosal surface of the lining of the upper GI tract. Erosions may be confined to the mucosal or submucosal layers, or they may go as deep as the muscle layer and may penetrate the serosa into the abdominal cavity (perforated ulcer). Peptic ulcers are most often found in the upper duodenum just below the pylorus (duodenal ulcers) but are also found in the stomach (gastric ulcers) and in the lower esophagus—in other words, all the places bathed by the gastric juices.

The exact cause of peptic ulcers is unknown, but there is evidence of hereditary predisposition. *H. pylori* has recently been associated with the incidence and development of peptic ulcers. The incidence in relatives of an ulcer patient is three times higher than in persons unrelated to someone with an ulcer. Men are afflicted more often than women, and ulcers are often more common in people with type O blood (Sleisenger, Fordtran, 1993). Emotional stress, hurried and irregular eating, and excessive smoking are considered predisposing factors. Ulcers seem to develop in people who are emotionally tense, but a definite link has not been established.

Ulcers can be caused by pancreatic tumors, which secrete excessive amounts of the hormone gastrin (Zollinger-Ellison syndrome). For reasons that are unknown, the incidence of both gastric and duodenal ulcers has declined over the last two decades. It has been estimated that about 10% of adults in the United States will have a peptic ulcer at some time in their lives.

Pathophysiology

Peptic ulcers occur when the lining of the lower esophagus, stomach, and duodenum are "digested" by the digestive juices, gastric acid, and pepsin. The lining is usually protected from its own juices by a barrier of mucus and epithelium. Erosion occurs when there is an increase in the concentration or activity of gastric acid or pepsin or when there is a decrease in the normal resistance of the protective barrier.

Gastric juices are released in three phases. The first is the cephalic, or psychic, phase, a reflex action in response to parasympathetic fibers in the vagus nerve. This reflex action takes place when food is seen, smelled, or even imagined. Second, in the gastric phase, juices are secreted in response to a hormone, gastrin, which is formed by cells in the antrum of the stomach. Gastrin is released when partly digested proteins are present. The third is the intestinal phase. When hydrochloric acid enters the duodenum, it stimulates the secretion of the hormone secretin. Secretin stimulates bicarbonate secretion by the pancreas, and these alkaline secretions enter the duodenum and neutralize the acid. Secretin also inhibits the production of gastric juices during the gastric phase.

The glands in the mucosa lining of the stomach secrete the substance that provides the protective barrier. These mucous secretions are a mixture of mucopolysaccharides and mucoproteins. This mucus absorbs pepsin and protects the stomach by allowing hydrochloric acid to pass through to the surface of the gastric mucosa very slowly. This gastric mucosal barrier prevents the mucosa from being digested by its own secretions. The ability of the mucosa to resist digestive action is also influenced by blood supply, acid-base balance, the condition of the mucosal cells, and the ability of the epithelium to regenerate.

It was once thought that people with peptic ulcers simply secreted more acid than others. This has been found to be true for those with duodenal ulcers and gastric ulcers near the duodenum, but people with gastric ulcers seem to secrete subnormal amounts of acid.

In times of stress, the sympathetic nervous system takes over and prepares the body for "fight or flight" by inhibiting the blood flow to the digestive organs and decreasing the production of juices. In some people chronic stress seems to enhance the action of the parasympathetic system on the abdominal organs, thus stimulating gastric juice production and the entire digestive process. These persons will develop a peptic ulcer in response to chronic stress.

Severe injury or illness, burns, head injury or intracranial disease, and ingestion of alcohol or drugs that act on the gastric mucosa often result in gastric erosions called "stress ulcers." The exact mechanism is unknown, but it is thought to be caused by a decrease in blood supply, which in turn causes a decrease in energy metabolism within the gastric mucosa. The gastric mucosal barrier is then disrupted, and its protective ability decreases. Gastric juices are then allowed to act on the mucosa, and multiple lesions develop very rapidly.

The major consequences of peptic ulcers are obstruction, bleeding, and perforation.

Assessment

Symptoms may vary with the location and severity of the ulcer (Table 23-3). If the ulcer erodes through a blood vessel, bleeding or severe hemorrhage may result. In the case of hemorrhage, the vomited blood has a bright red or coffee-grounds appearance. If slow bleeding occurs, the blood generally passes through the intestinal tract, and stools are dark and tarry in appearance.

Pain is a characteristic symptom and is described by the patient as dull, burning, gnawing, or boring; it is located in the midline of the epigastric region. With a gas-

TABLE 23-3

Comparison of Gastric and Duodenal Ulcers

	Gastric Ulcer	Duodenal Ulcer
Location	In antrum of stomach	In first 1-2 cm of duodenum
Incidence	Usually between 40 and 70 years Common in elderly women Higher mortality rate then duodenal ulcers	Usually between 40 and 60 years More common in men than women Occurs more often than gastric ulcers
Risk Factors	Stress, ulcerogenic drugs (ASA, NSAIDS), alcohol, smoking, gastritis	COPD, cirrhosis, pancreatitis, alcohol, smoking, chronc renal failure, stress
Pain characteristics	Occurs 1-2 hours after eating Described as heartburn or indigestion May be relieved by food May cause weight loss	Occurs 2-4 hours after eating Episodic (pain/eat/relief cycle) Described as heartburn or back pain Relieved by food or antacid May cause weight gain
Effects	High recurrence; fewer remissions May develop into gastric cancer More likely to be associated with hemorrhage than duodenal ulcers	Occurs seasonally (spring and fall) Remission and recurrence pattern Seldom malignant Likely to perforate

BOX 23-9 **Nursing Process**

PEPTIC ULCER DISEASE

ASSESSMENT

Vital signs
Level of comfort (abdominal or epigastric pain, pain associated with meals, nausea)
Stool and emesis for blood
Abdomen for bowel sounds, contour, firmness
Overall skin color
Fluid volume status
Laboratory studies (hemoglobin, hemocrit, coagulation profile)
Stress management

NURSING DIAGNOSES

Pain related to action of gastric secretions on inflamed mucosa
Knowledge deficit related to medications and diet prescribed to promote healing and over-the-counter drugs that must be avoided
Altered nutrition: more than body requirements related to frequent ingestion of food to prevent ulcer pain
Sleep pattern disturbance related to pain at night
Anxiety related to inability to manage stress
Risk for fluid volume deficit related to sudden hemorrhage at ulcer site
Risk for injury: peritonitis related to possible perforation

NURSING INTERVENTIONS

Offer and administer analgesics as needed.
Administer medications as ordered (antacids, anticholinergics, histamine blockers)
Provide oral hygiene as indicated.
Provide quiet environment.
Plan treatments to provide rest periods.
Spend 15 minutes each shift when patient is awake, listening to concerns and encouraging expression of feelings.
Provide diversional activities as needed.
Explain all procedures and anticipate needs.
Maintain IV fluids as ordered.
Reinforce dietary instructions and restrictions.
If patient smokes, facilitate efforts to avoid smoking.

EVALUATION OF EXPECTED OUTCOMES

Absence of pain
Absence of blood in stool
Vital signs stable and within normal limits
Ability to select and eat foods for well-balanced diet that complies with dietary modifications
Understands medications
Verbalizes fears and concerns

tric ulcer, the pain occurs 60 to 90 minutes after eating; with a duodenal ulcer, 2 to 4 hours after eating. The pain of a duodenal ulcer is relieved by eating or antacids, and patients usually have pain during the night that awakens them. They are usually free of pain when they wake in the morning because the flow of gastric secretions is lowest at this time. The pain is caused by the irritation of the ulcer by the gastric acid; exposed sensory nerve endings at the edges and base of the ulcer or increased motility and spasm of the muscle at the ulcer site are thought to produce the pain. Although pain is the typical symptom, many variations are found in its presence or absence, its character, and its duration.

Nausea and vomiting may or may not be present and, when present, are often the result of pyloric obstruction, which may result from ulcerous inflammation or scarring. Many patients are anemic because of loss of blood but are usually well nourished because they eat to relieve the pain. The diagnosis is established through a gastrointestinal series, endoscopic examinations, and examination of stool specimens for occult blood. The histamine test and cytologic examination of gastric washings may be done to rule out malignancy. If the patient with a suspected gastric ulcer fails to secrete hydrochloric acid after an injection of histamine, it is likely that he or she has a malignancy in the stomach.

Intervention

The goals of therapy are to relieve pain, heal the ulcer, prevent complications, and prevent recurrence (Box 23-9). Symptoms may be relieved before the ulcer heals, which may take 4 to 8 weeks. The patient should understand that he or she must continue treatment even though the symptoms disappear. Treatment includes rest, diet, medication (antacids, anticholiner-

PATIENT/FAMILY TEACHING

Peptic ulcer disease

The patient and family should understand the following when dealing with peptic ulcer disease:

- Dangers of aspirin and over-the-counter drugs containing aspirin
- Dietary restrictions of caffeine and alcohol
- Medication action, dosage, and side effects
- Importance of long-term maintenance
- Stress management

gics, histamine blockers), and in some cases, surgery. Increasing evidence that the bacteria *H. pylori* is involved in the cause has led to the use of antibiotic therapy.

Rest. The patient must have physical rest and relief of tension. Diversional activities such as reading, watching television, or making crafts are encouraged. Stress should be reduced for the patient whenever possible. Everything that is done, as well as the goals of treatment, are carefully explained; being informed reduces the patient's anxiety. The patient must identify those factors that aggravate the condition, and a good listener is necessary for the patient to vent his or her feelings and examine his or her lifestyle. Listening alone may help, and nurses may discover problems that are appropriate to refer to the physician, social worker, or other qualified professionals.

Diet. The traditional milk and cream (sippy) diet is no longer used, although patients will still ask about it. It has been found that although milk products do buffer gastric acid, the high protein and fat in milk stimulates further acid production. Some authorities recommend a diet that eliminates only those foods that stimulate secretion, highly seasoned foods, highly fibrous foods, and those that cause pain to the patient. An even more liberal approach eliminates only those foods that cause pain. When milk is prescribed, skim milk is used. In the early stages of healing, the patient will need to be more cautious and may be given small, frequent feedings. Foods that stimulate gastric acid secretion and motility, such as extremely hot or cold foods, coffee, alcohol, and seasonings, are avoided at first and then used with moderation to test tolerance. Because gastric contractility is increased when the stomach is empty or overly full, small, frequent feedings are indicated.

Drug therapy. Antacids are used to bring relief of symptoms, but there is no conclusive evidence that they promote healing. Antacids may be ordered every hour at first, and the frequency is then gradually reduced. Some antacids, such as sodium bicarbonate, are absorbed systemically and may cause alkalosis. An antacid made of calcium carbonate (Dicarbosil, Tums) is not desirable because it produces rebound gastric secretion. The calcium carbonate also is absorbed into the bloodstream, producing hypercalcemia and possible renal damage with long-term treatment. Magnesium and aluminum hydroxide mixture (Maalox) may cause loose stools, whereas magnesium trisilicate and aluminum hydroxide (Gelusil) and aluminum hydroxide gel (Amphojel) may be constipating. Some patients alternate these two drugs to prevent problems in elimination. Camalox is a mixture of the two but also contains small amounts of calcium carbonate, which stimulates acid secretion. Antacids can affect the absorption of some drugs; therefore they should be given 1 to 2 hours before or after other drugs. In the event of constipation or diarrhea, the patient should consult his or her physician. No cathartics should be taken unless prescribed by the physician because they increase peristaltic activity.

Anticholinergics, such as methantheline (Banthine) and propantheline (Pro-Banthine), may be prescribed with antacids because they block stimulation from the vagus nerve, which causes the secretion of hydrochloric acid. They also decrease gastric motor activity and permit antacids to remain in the stomach longer. Anticholinergics should be used with caution, however, because they can cause gastric obstruction.

The introduction of cimetidine (Tagamet) in the late 1970s brought about dramatic results in treating ulcers. Cimetidine, ranitidine (Zantac), and famotidine (Pepcid) are classified as histamine blockers; they act by blocking the action of the histamine H_2 receptors, thereby inhibiting the secretion of hydrochloric acid. These drugs relieve the pain and promote healing of the ulcer. Their effectiveness in treating ulcers has greatly reduced the need for surgical intervention. Because antacids can decrease the absorption of cimetidine, they should not be given concurrently (Shannon and others, 1992).

Other agents used in the treatment of peptic ulcer disease include sucralfate, omeprazole, and misoprostol. Sucralfate is a cytoprotective agent used to promote ulcer healing. The drug coats the surface of the ulcer and protects it from gastric secretions. Omeprazole (Prilosec) is an antisecretory agent that suppresses gastric acid production. Misoprostol (Cytotec) is a synthetic prostaglandin that serves to inhibit gastric acid secretion and provides mucosal protection (Shannon and others, 1992).

It is generally agreed that smoking, caffeine, and alcohol should be eliminated by the patient with an ulcer. Smoking reduces the bicarbonate content of pancreatic juice, which is the neutralizer of gastric acid in the duodenum. An extremely tense patient may be better off smoking than trying to quit, but there are few who fall into this category. Both regular coffee and decaffeinated coffee stimulate acid output. Tea, cocoa, cola, and chocolate also contain caffeine and should be avoided. Alcohol reduces the ability of the mucosa to resist the effects of gastric secretions. It should be avoided while the ulcer is healing and taken only occasionally after the ulcer has healed. An ounce of liquid antacid taken half an hour before a drink limits the alcohol's effect on the mucosa.

Mucosal resistance is also reduced by many medications, including acetylsalicylic acid (aspirin), steroids, phenylbutazone, reserpine, indomethacin, and many over-the-counter drugs containing aspirin. Aspirin may also act as an anticoagulant and precipitate hemorrhage at the ulcer site. The patient must be alert to avoid medications that contain aspirin and should be taught to read labels thoroughly for ingredients.

Complications

The major complications occurring in peptic ulcer are hemorrhage, perforation, and obstruction. When a large hemorrhage occurs, measures are taken to control the bleeding and to restore the volume of circulating fluid. The patient is transfused with red blood cells or plasma expanders, such as hetastarch (Hespan), and intravenous fluids are administered to maintain urinary output and electrolyte balance.

A nasogastric tube is inserted to remove acid and the protein load from the stomach, prevent nausea and vomiting, and monitor blood loss. While the tube is in place, the patient needs frequent mouth care and cleansing and lubrication of the nostril through which the tube is passed. The tube is checked often to see that it is patent and draining. All intake and output are recorded, with a description of the color and consistency of the gastric drainage. Nothing is given by mouth to promote physiologic rest for the stomach and avoid further irritation. Fluids and electrolytes are given by intravenous infusion. Because gastric drainage removes fluids and electrolytes from the body, the nurse monitors the patient for signs of fluid and electrolyte imbalance. Dry skin, oliguria (urine output of less than 30 ml/hr), increased heart rate, and hypotension indicate a deficit in fluid volume (hypovolemia). Shallow respiration could indicate metabolic alkalosis, and muscle weakness may be a sign of potassium and sodium deficiencies.

Perforation occurs when an ulcer erodes through the wall of the stomach or the duodenum and the intestinal contents are released into the peritoneal cavity. The result is peritonitis. Emergency surgery is required to close the perforation. The gastric contents that have escaped into the peritoneal cavity are aspirated by suction during the operation. A solution containing antibiotics may be placed in the abdominal cavity before the abdomen is closed.

Surgical procedures include gastrectomy (gastric resection), vagotomy (resection of the vagus nerve to decrease secretion of gastric acids), and antrectomy (removal of a large amount of the acid-secreting mucosa of the stomach) or vagotomy and pyloroplasty (enlarging of the pyloric sphincter to allow reflux from the duodenum).

Another complication of peptic ulcer disease is obstruction of the pyloric sphincter, which results from scarring and fibrosis caused by the healing or breakdown of an ulcer. The muscle becomes spastic, edematous, and stenosed, gradually obstructing the passage from the stomach to the pylorus. Surgery is usually required to relieve the condition, and vagotomy with pyloroplasty is the procedure most often used.

Gastric resection (gastrectomy)

Peptic ulcers that do not respond well to medical management and chronic peptic ulcers may be treated surgically by performing a gastric resection or *gastrectomy*. A total or subtotal gastrectomy may be done, and several different types of surgical procedures may be used. Usually the ulcer and a large amount of acid-secreting mucosa of the stomach are removed (antrectomy), and the remaining portion of the stomach is anastomosed to the small intestine (gastroenterotomy). The remaining portion of the stomach may be joined to the duodenum (Billroth I) or jejunum (Billroth II) (Figure 23-14). A patient whose duodenum is deformed as a result of a duodenal ulcer requires the remainder of the stomach to be joined to the jejunum, whereas a patient whose duodenum is normal may have the remainder of the stomach joined to the duodenum.

A vagotomy may be done at the same time. This procedure includes resection of the vagus nerve to decrease secretion of hydrochloric acid and gastric motility. A vagotomy with a pyloroplasty or segmental resections are used because of the lower incidence of side effects and a low ulcer recurrence rate.

The patient who is about to have a gastrectomy has probably been ill for a long time and feels discouraged and worried, often fearing that the condition may be cancer. During this time an explanation of the various treatments and procedures and the reasons for them will help relieve tension and apprehension. During the preoperative period the patient is encouraged not to smoke and is given an explanation of what to expect after surgery.

A

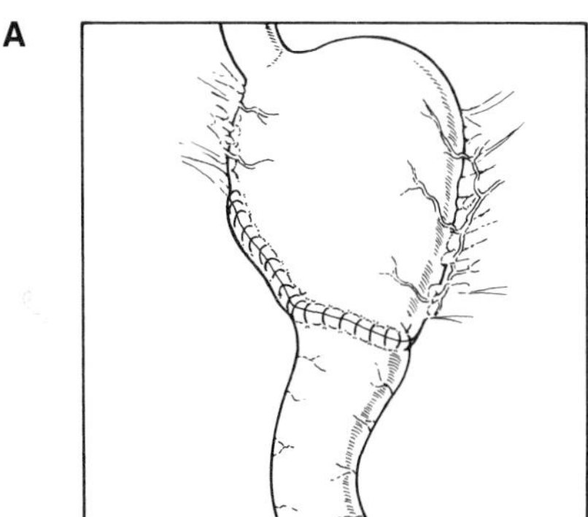

B

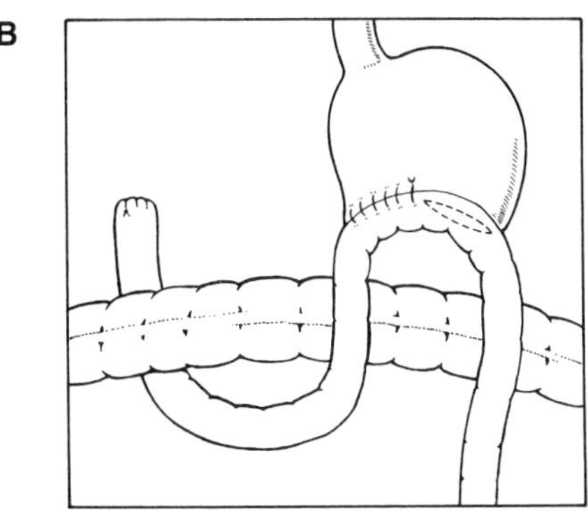

Figure 23-14 **A,** Bilroth I operation: completed anastomosis. **B,** Bilroth II operation. (From Doughty DB, Jackson DB: *Gastrointestinal disorders,* St Louis, 1993, Mosby.)

After surgery, the patient has a nasogastric tube connected to suction and is given nothing by mouth for 24 to 48 hours. Drainage from the gastric tube is watched carefully. Initially, the drainage may be bright red, but this changes to dark brown or dark red within 6 to 12 hours after surgery. Within 24 to 36 hours the drainage becomes greenish-yellow, indicating normal secretions containing bile. If large amounts of bright red blood continue, the physician should be notified. Dressings are observed for any evidence of bleeding, which should be reported promptly. The nurse monitors the nasogastric suction often to ensure that it is working properly. Distention of the stomach will strain the suture line.

NURSE ALERT

When a patient has had esophageal or gastric surgery, the nurse should *never* try to reposition the tube if the tube is not draining well. *The physician should be notified immediately.* Manipulation of the NG tube may cause injury to the anastomosis and may lead to perforation.

PATIENT/FAMILY TEACHING

Gastrectomy

The nurse should ensure that the patient and family understand the following:

- Surgical procedure
- Wound care
- Signs and symptoms of infection and other reportable complications
- Dietary modification (e.g., low-carbohydrate, low-fat, and high-protein diet)
- Importance of small, frequent meals
- Avoidance of spicy foods
- Dumping syndrome
- Avoidance of aspirin containing products, caffeine, alcohol, and tobacco
- Smoking cessation, if indicated
- Stress management
- Medication action, dosage, and side effects
- Medical follow-up care

Vomiting usually indicates obstruction or kinking of the drainage tube in the stomach; the surgeon is notified immediately. There may be an order to irrigate the tube with 30 ml of normal saline to keep the tube open. No irrigation should be done unless ordered. Intravenous fluids are given to maintain fluid balance in the body. All intake, including fluids, and all output, including gastric drainage, are measured and recorded. The mouth and the area of the nares near the tube must have frequent care.

The nasogastric tube is removed when peristalsis returns and sutures begin to heal. The nurse assists the physician in determining the return of peristalsis by listening for bowel sounds with a stethoscope and by questioning the patient about passing flatus. Oral fluids, beginning with water, may be started before the tube is removed; if so, the tube is clamped during and shortly after oral intake. Diet is gradually resumed on the physician's order, usually beginning with small, frequent feedings, and increased as tolerated by the patient. Any feeling of fullness, nausea, or vomiting are reported (Box 23-10).

When a total gastrectomy is performed, the entire stomach is removed and the small intestine (jejunum) is anastomosed to the esophagus. Patients having this procedure must be given injections of vitamin B_{12} for the rest of their life. The stomach mucosa secretes the intrinsic factor that is essential for the absorption of this vitamin from the intestinal tract; without it, no vitamin B_{12} will be absorbed. In addition, the patient must eat small, frequent meals. A complication that oc-

BOX 23-10 **Nursing Process**

GASTRECTOMY

ASSESSMENT

Vital signs
Level of comfort
Abdomen for bowel sounds, contour, firmness, passage of flatus
Surgical incision and/or dressing
Surgical drains
Fluid volume status
Character and amount of nasogastric drainage
Respiratory status
Patterns of elimination
Laboratory studies (electrolytes, hemoglobin, hematocrit, WBC)

NURSING DIAGNOSES

Altered nutrition: less than body requirements related to change in absorption of nutrients and passage of food/fluids
Pain related to surgical incision, abdominal distention, presence of NG tube
Risk for fluid volume deficit related to excessive losses
Risk for infection related to invasive procedure, nutritional deficit
Risk for altered breathing pattern related to pain, high abdominal incision, sedation from analgesics and immobility
Anxiety related to surgery and lifestyle changes
Knowledge deficit related to dietary and lifestyle modifications

NURSING INTERVENTIONS

Explain all treatments and procedures.
Maintain suction of NG tube.
Irrigate NG tube only if ordered.
Do not reposition NG tube under any circumstances.
Provide oral hygiene.
Administer IV fluids as prescribed.
Progress diet as tolerated, as ordered, advancing from clear liquids to bland diet with frequent, small feedings.
Administer analgesics as needed.
Provide comfort measures (massage, relaxation, diversion).
Ambulate as soon as possible.
Encourage coughing and deep breathing every 2 hours.
Encourage to splint incision with turning or coughing.
Provide aseptic wound care.
Encourage expression of feelings and concerns.

EVALUATION OF EXPECTED OUTCOMES

Meets discharge criteria for postsurgical patient (p. 487)
Maintains stable weight
Pattern of elimination established
Tolerating diet without nausea and vomiting
No evidence of dehydration
Wound healing without evidence of infection
No respiratory distress
Acceptable pain control
Verbalizes understanding of diet and lifestyle modifications

casionally occurs with some extensive gastric surgeries is the *dumping syndrome,* which is characterized by a sensation of nausea, weakness, and faintness after meals, commonly accompanied by profuse perspiration and palpitations and a sense of fullness in the epigastric area. It is believed that these symptoms may be caused by the rapid emptying of large amounts of food and fluid through the gastroenterostomy into the jejunum, rather than passing through the entire stomach and the duodenum before entering the jejunum. The intestinal contents are more hypertonic than they would be if they had passed through the entire stomach and the duodenum, and they attempt dilution by drawing fluid from the circulating blood volume into the intestine, consequently reducing the blood volume and producing a syncopelike syndrome. This may occur after many of the surgical procedures used to treat gastric ulcer, and approximately 20% of patients experience this reaction after gastric surgery. Dumping generally subsides within 6 months to 1 year and may be avoided by eating frequent, small meals; avoiding chilled foods and fluids; lying down after meals; reducing carbohydrates in the diet; and taking fluids between meals rather than with meals. The physician may prescribe sedatives and antispasmodics to delay gastric emptying.

Patient and family teaching

After discharge from the hospital, the patient is given instructions concerning diet and the importance of eliminating irritants such as coffee, alcohol, tobacco, and aspirin. Foods that contain many spices are usually prohibited. The patient needs to follow a regimen that is relatively free from tension. Specific teaching related to medications to be taken after discharge is be included. If the patient has had surgery as part of the treatment of ulcer disease, specific postoperative instructions pertinent to the specific surgery are given to the patient. Diet, activity, wound care, and symptoms that should be reported to the physician are included in discharge teaching.

Hernia

A **hernia** is the projection of a loop of an organ, tissue, or structure through a congenital or acquired defect. Most hernias have their origin in the abdomen.

One type of hernia is the *umbilical hernia,* which is often seen in infants as the result of a congenital weakness of the abdominal wall. A *femoral hernia,* more common in women, occurs at the point where the femoral artery passes into the femoral canal. An *inguinal hernia,* seen more commonly in men, occurs when part of the intestine projects through the inguinal canal. Hernias may also develop at the site of an incision *(incisional hernia);* they develop because of impaired wound healing. If the protruding structure can be returned by manipulation to its own cavity, it is called a reducible hernia. If it cannot, it is called an irreducible or *incarcerated* hernia. The size of the defect through which the organ passes largely determines whether the hernia can be reduced. When the blood supply to the structure within the hernia becomes occluded, the hernia is said to be *strangulated* and gangrene may result, requiring immediate surgery.

Assessment

There may be no symptoms associated with a hernia other than swelling or protrusion on the abdomen or groin when the patient coughs, stands, lifts heavy objects, or strains in any other way. The nurse looks for maneuvers that contribute to the protrusion, the degree (size) of the protrusion, and any pain noted with the hernia. Pain is an ominous sign with hernias and usually signals the need for surgical intervention.

Intervention

The treatment of choice for all hernias is surgery. However, sometimes surgery is inadvisable because of the patient's condition or some other reason. For such persons a mechanical appliance called a *truss* may provide some relief and prevent the hernia from enlarging.

The surgical procedure for repair of a hernia is called *herniorrhaphy.* To prevent recurrence of the hernia and facilitate closure of the defect, a *hernioplasty* may be performed, using fascia, filigree wire, mesh, or a variety of plastic materials to strengthen the muscle wall.

The preoperative care for the repair of a hernia is the same as that for any uncomplicated abdominal surgery. Postoperative care includes prevention of wound infection and avoidance of any strain on the wound for approximately 2 weeks. Early ambulation is encouraged to prevent abdominal distention. After repair of an inguinal hernia, tenderness and swelling of the scrotum may be reduced by applying ice packs. If scrotal edema does occur, the use of a suspensory may provide some relief. The urinary output is watched because retention sometimes occurs and catheterization may be necessary. Food and fluids are usually permitted as soon as nausea ceases. Any evidence of abdominal distention or coughing after hernia repair is reported to the physician immediately. Hernia repair is generally performed in an ambulatory surgical center. The repair is completed in the morning, and the patient rests at home in the evening.

Patient and family teaching

The patient is instructed to avoid any strenuous activity, including lifting, to prevent recurrence of the hernia. The physician will advise the patient when normal activity can be resumed. Discharge instruction must also include a plan for avoiding constipation (straining). Increased fluids (6 to 8 glasses of water a day) and a balanced diet rich in bulk and fiber will help prevent constipation. Stool softeners or bulk-forming agents may be needed.

Hiatus (hiatal) hernia

The **hiatus hernia** (*hiatus* meaning opening), or *diaphragmatic hernia,* is a common pathologic disorder of the upper gastrointestinal tract. It is the protrusion of part of the stomach through the diaphragm and into the esophagus. It is caused by a weakness in the area where the esophagus passes through the diaphragm. Hiatus hernia occurs with conditions that cause increased intraabdominal pressure, such as obesity or pregnancy, or with conditions that cause decreased diaphragm muscle strength, such as aging.

Diagnosis is made by esophagoscopy and barium and x-ray examination. Cytologic studies are usually made to eliminate a diagnosis of cancer.

Pathophysiology

Before entering the stomach, the esophagus passes through a small opening in the diaphragm. Under normal conditions the opening in the diaphragm encircles the esophagus securely. Thus the esophagus is held within the thoracic cavity, whereas the stomach remains in the abdominal cavity. For some reason, often congenital, the esophageal sphincter fails to remain tight, permitting the opening to become enlarged and relaxed. When this occurs, the upper portion of the stomach may protrude upward through the relaxed muscle into the thoracic cavity. Often this type of hernia may occur when the individual is in a prone position, and it will return to its normal position when the individual is in an upright position.

Assessment

When symptomatic, a hiatus hernia may cause the person considerable distress. The primary symptom is *heartburn* caused by the gastric contents of the stomach being regurgitated into the esophagus. There may be substernal or epigastric pain, most notably after eating, that may radiate, simulating angina pectoris. Vomiting and abdominal distention may occur.

Intervention

Treatment includes dietary measures with small meals consisting of bland foods. Antacids may be given if symptoms are not relieved. The patient is advised not to smoke and to avoid wearing a girdle or tight-fitting belts or clothes. Sleeping with several pillows at night may provide comfort. Straining for bowel elimination, coughing, and bending are discouraged. If the condition does not respond to conservative treatment, surgery may be performed. The surgical approach may be thoracic, and the patient will have a thoracotomy and chest drainage. The surgery may also be abdominal, in which case the nursing care is the same as that for other types of abdominal surgery.

Hemorrhoids

Hemorrhoids (piles) are dilated veins similar to varicose veins. They may occur outside the anal sphincter as external hemorrhoids or inside the sphincter as internal hemorrhoids. The small, bluish lumps characteristic of external hemorrhoids may disappear spontaneously, leaving a small skin tag. Occasionally the hemorrhoid will become thrombosed, and a blood clot will develop within the vein. In addition to hemorrhoids, anal fissures (cracks in the mucous membrane) and an anal fistula (a duct extending from one tissue surface to another) may be present. Hemorrhoids result from numerous factors, including prolonged constipation, heavy lifting, straining in an effort to defecate, and pregnancy or large pelvic tumors. Certain forms of liver disease and high blood pressure may also contribute to the disorder.

Assessment

Symptoms may include an awareness of a mass in the rectum near the anus. Constipation is almost always present. Bleeding may occur and will appear as bright red blood that is not mixed with feces. The dilated veins may become thrombosed, causing severe pain. Although hemorrhoids rarely become malignant, bleeding and constipation are symptoms of cancer of the rectum. For this reason, all patients with these symptoms should have a thorough examination to rule out cancer, including a sigmoidoscopy and barium enema.

Hemorrhoids do not cure themselves, and medical or surgical care is necessary. Individuals have been reluctant to talk about the problem and even to seek medical care. When bleeding occurs, severe anemia may result unless medical care is obtained.

Intervention

When the patient comes in for an examination, the nurse should be aware that this has been a difficult decision and should assure the patient of absolute privacy and should protect his or her self-respect. Medical treatment of the patient with hemorrhoids consists of warm compresses to stimulate circulation and healing and analgesic ointments such as dibucaine (Nupercaine). Sitz baths help to reduce pain and edema, and bulk stool softeners such as Metamucil or Fibercon, bran, and other natural food fibers are recommended to assist in the passage of fecal material. Steroid suppositories may be given to relieve inflammation. External hemorrhoids may be excised in the physician's office. Internal hemorrhoids occasionally are treated with injection of a solution that will cause sclerosing or hardening of the dilated vein. This causes the vein to shrink and adhere to underlying muscles as it heals with fibrous tissue. Internal hemorrhoids may also be treated by ligating them with rubber bands. Tight bands are applied with a special instrument in the physician's office, causing constriction, necrosis, sloughing, and scarring. Fixation to underlying muscle is also accomplished with infrared photocoagulation, in which the tissue is destroyed by creating a small burn to cause inflammation. Scarring cryotherapy destroys the tissues by freezing. The Nd-YAG laser is also used for fixation and excision of hemorrhoids.

Hemorrhoidectomy

Standard treatment involves surgical excision of the hemorrhoid (hemorrhoidectomy), leaving the wounds open or closed. A laxative may be given before surgery. After surgery the patient is often positioned on the stomach, but he or she may lie on his or her back with a support under the buttocks. Although this surgery is not considered a major procedure, pain may be acute, and narcotics may be given and analgesic ointments applied. Sitz baths are given to relieve pain and promote healing. If a spontaneous bowel elimination does not occur within 3 days, an oil retention enema may be given, followed by a cleansing enema. Dressings may or may not be used. Difficulty in voiding may occur. A soft diet is permitted on the evening of the surgery; a full diet is given on the first postoperative day. The patient is advised to include fiber and plenty of fluids and to exercise moderately to promote regular bowel function.

Functional Disorders

Functional disorders can occur without a demonstrable pathologic disease. However, most functional conditions may also occur when there is a pathologic condition. Therefore they should not be considered lightly, and every effort should be made to determine the presence or absence of disease. These complaints can be psychosomatic, and these patients may benefit from counseling and psychotherapy.

Indigestion

Indigestion may be the result of disease somewhere in the body, but as a functional disorder, it does not have a pathologic basis. Some hypersensitive persons who are tense and anxious may become aware of normal sensations present in the stomach, usually related to the digestive process. These individuals may interpret such sensations as pain. They complain of pain in the upper abdomen, usually related to the eating of food. They may describe the pain in a variety of ways and often attribute their discomfort to specific foods. Often these people resort to the habitual use of sodium bicarbonate or some popularly advertised antacid, which may provide temporary relief. Treatment is based on examination to rule out the existence of disease and the encouragement of improved mental health.

Constipation

Constipation is the most common disorder of the gastrointestinal tract and is as old as the human race. Many people still believe that failure to have a daily bowel movement results in absorption of poisons, and they attribute several complaints to this "absorption of poison." There is no single cause for constipation; it may be the result of several factors, including nervous tension, poor diet, inadequate fluid intake, lack of sufficient exercise, and inadequate toilet facilities. It must be kept in mind that constipation is a symptom of many organic diseases. During an acute illness constipation may occur because of reduced food intake and reduced intestinal motility. This type of constipation is usually relieved as soon as health returns. The patient in the hospital may repress the need to defecate because he or she does not want to ask for the bedpan or because of lack of privacy.

Constipation may occur during the latter part of pregnancy as a result of pressure on the lower bowel, or it may be a complication after delivery in the postpartum period. The patient may be able to relieve the disorder during the antepartum period by drinking more water and eating fresh fruit and vegetables and food containing roughage. Laxatives should be taken only on the physician's order.

Elderly people often suffer from constipation as a result of the slowing down of the digestive process and inadequate diet. Often they have a cabinet full of laxatives and fall prey to popular advertisements in an effort to have a daily bowel movement.

Treatment must be based on the type of constipation and the patient's individual needs, and the presence of possible organic disease must be ruled out. Diet modifications are the easiest way to relieve constipation. Fresh fruits and vegetables, whole grains, and bran increase the fiber content of the diet and promote fecal evacuation. Adequate hydration is also important in preventing constipation; 6 to 8 glasses of water a day is appropriate for the people with no fluid restrictions. Several laxatives and stool softeners are on the market under the trade names of Peri-Colace, Dialose, Sof-Cil, and Milkinol. Laxatives should not be used regularly without consulting a physician and should be discontinued as soon as possible. Bulk-forming agents are also useful in relieving symptoms of constipation.

Cardiospasm and pylorospasm

Sphincter muscles are located between the esophagus and the stomach (gastroesophageal sphincter) and between the stomach and its outlet into the duodenum (pyloric valve). Normally, these muscles contract to prevent the backward flow of food material and gastric secretions and relax to allow food to enter the stomach from the esophagus and to permit the passage of food from the stomach into the duodenum. Under certain conditions these muscles fail to relax at the proper time and may contract vigorously. These severe contractions are called *spasms*. They give rise to symptoms of inability to swallow, regurgitation of food, epigastric pain, and vomiting. Spasms of the pyloric sphincter may be associated with peptic ulcer, but emotional factors are believed to be the primary cause of *cardiospasm* and *pylorospasm*. Treatment may include regulation of the diet, administration of antispasmodic and sedative drugs, and psychologic support. If cardiospasm is severe, dilation of the constricted esophagus may be necessary.

Anal sphincter spasm

Sphincter muscles surrounding the anus and rectum relax to permit defecation. When the individual has severe hemorrhoids or fissures (cracks) in the anus or mucous membrane of the rectum, spasms of the sphincter muscles may occur. Difficult and painful defecation may then result. The treatment is correction of the cause or dilation of the sphincter muscles.

Hyperacidity

Hyperacidity, commonly called *heartburn*, may occur as the result of a pylorospasm that contributes to reverse peristalsis. The gastric juice in the stomach is forced up through the cardiac valve into the esophagus, which creates the characteristic burning sensation.

Psychic vomiting

Psychic vomiting occurs in persons with emotional and psychologic problems. It may occur after every meal or infrequently, particularly when the individual is faced with a tense situation. Often the amount of food vomited is small and is regurgitated rather than vomited; thus it does not interfere with normal nutrition. However, if large quantities of food are regurgitated at frequent intervals, the individual may become malnourished. Psychic vomiting is not uncommon in children and frequently occurs after breakfast. If the child expects to face an unpleasant situation at school, it may provide a means of escape.

Air swallowing

Air swallowing is a functional condition in which the person swallows air and then belches it up with a loud noise. Persons often master the technique so well that it is impossible for others to detect the individual swallowing the air.

DISEASES AND DISORDERS OF THE ACCESSORY ORGANS OF DIGESTION

Diseases and Disorders of the Liver

Viral hepatitis

Viral **hepatitis** is an infectious disease that attacks the liver. A variety of similar but distinct viruses cause hepatitis. The mode or transmission and incubation periods differ among the various forms of the virus. The most common strains of the hepatitis virus are types A, B, and C. Hepatitis types D and E, although less common, cause injury to the liver and are associated with severe liver damage and liver failure (Doughty, Jackson, 1993; Kucharski, 1993) (Box 23-11).

The source of the virus causing type A hepatitis is primarily human feces. It is spread by the oral intake of food, milk, or water contaminated with the virus. There is some evidence that the virus can also be transmitted by the parenteral introduction of the hepatitis virus through blood, blood products, or the equipment

BOX 23-11

TYPES OF VIRAL HEPATITIS

Hepatitis A Transmitted by the fecal-oral route; incubation period about 4 weeks (2 to 7 weeks range); rarely causes chronic liver disease

Hepatitis B Transmitted by the parenteral route and exposure to infected body fluids (e.g., urine, saliva, feces, semen, breast milk); incubation period about 2 to 3 months (1 to 6 months range); may progress to chronic liver disease

Hepatitis C *(previously called non-A non-B)* Transmitted primarily by the parenteral route; may be transmitted by sexual or maternal-fetal contact; incubation period approximately 4 to 6 weeks (2 to 25 weeks range); often progresses to chronic liver disease

Hepatitis D Found only in patients with hepatitis B; transmitted by the parenteral route; increases the severity of the hepatitis B infection; contributes to progression to chronic liver diseases with hepatitis B infection

Hepatitis E Transmitted by the fecal–oral route; causes endemic form of hepatitis C; causes serious infections and commonly progresses to liver failure

used for venipuncture or other procedures that require penetrating the skin. The virus is excreted in the feces long before clinical symptoms appear. The carrier is thought to be most infectious just before the onset of symptoms. An individual may have and carry the disease but not be diagnosed because it can occur in a mild form that is not severe enough to produce jaundice.

The source of the virus that causes hepatitis B is the blood of persons who have the infection or who are carriers of the virus. The virus is present in semen, saliva, and blood and is transmitted by sexual contact or blood products, usually through accidental needle sticks or the sharing of needles by intravenous drug users.

Hepatitis C is also transmitted in the blood and is the major cause of transfusion-related viral hepatitis. It is often seen in parenteral drug abusers and is common among personnel working in renal transplantation units.

Pathophysiology. A diffuse inflammatory reaction occurs, and liver cells begin to degenerate and die. As the liver cells degenerate, the normal functions of the liver are affected. Degeneration, regeneration, and inflammation may occur simultaneously and may distort the normal lobular pattern of the liver and create pressure within and around the portal vein areas. These changes may be associated with elevated aminotransferase (AST, ALT) levels, a prolonged prothrombin time (PT), and a slightly elevated serum alkaline phosphatase level.

In most instances of nonfatal viral hepatitis, regeneration begins almost with the onset of the disease. The damaged cells and their contents eventually are removed by phagocytosis and enzymatic reaction, and the level returns to normal. The outcome of viral hepatitis is affected by such factors as the virulence of the virus, the preexisting condition of the liver, and the supportive care provided when symptoms appear.

Assessment. Symptoms may be mild or severe and include loss of appetite, fatigue, nausea and vomiting, chills, headache, and a temperature that may range from 100° F to 104° F (38° C to 40° C). Jaundice usually appears in 4 to 7 days but may not occur before 30 days and may be absent altogether in some patients. Temperature usually returns to normal when jaundice appears, but anorexia and nausea persist. Children usually have a milder form of infectious hepatitis, with no jaundice and with symptoms predominantly appearing as those of an intestinal or respiratory illness.

Jaundice is caused by the inability of the liver to satisfactorily remove the waste products of red blood cell destruction (bilirubin) from the bloodstream. Bilirubin is a pigment that gives bile and stools their normal color. When obstruction to the elimination of bilirubin occurs, the pigment accumulates in the bloodstream and is ultimately deposited in the body tissues. It can first be detected in the sclera. The urine becomes dark as the kidney attempts to remove the excess pigment from the bloodstream. Pruritus, abdominal pain with tenderness over the liver, and photophobia occur. A diagnosis of hepatitis is based on symptoms, liver function tests, and a liver biopsy, with prothrombin and clotting time tests preceding the biopsy.

Intervention. There is no specific treatment for hepatitis. Therapy is planned to strengthen the patient's resistance to the infection, and rest and nutrition are primary considerations. Antibiotics may be administered to prevent secondary infection, and antihistamines may be given to relieve the itching associated with jaundice. Fluid intake is encouraged during the acute stage, and if a sufficient amount is not taken, intravenous infusions may be given.

Diet is of major importance and should provide all the necessary nutrients. Because the appetite is poor, the patient will need considerable encouragement to eat, and records of food intake and calorie count are maintained. If eating does not provide sufficient calories and nutrients, enteral feedings or parenteral nutrition is used to supplement or replace oral intake.

Prevention is the most important goal in controlling hepatitis. Patients, their families, and healthcare providers must be knowledgeable about how the virus is transmitted and take the steps needed to prevent its spread. Handwashing is the mainstay for prevention of all disease transmission. Patients and family members must be instructed on proper handwashing technique. Using standard precautions will control exposure to potentially contaminated blood and body fluids and excrement (CDC, 1994). In the case of diapered infants and children or other incontinent patients with hepatitis, contact precautions are implemented to prevent the spread of infection (CDC, 1994).

PATIENT/FAMILY TEACHING

Hepatitis

The patient with hepatitis and his or her family should understand the following:

- Disease process and transmission
- Long-term treatment regimen
- Possible complications
- Energy conservation techniques
- Importance of compliance with therapy
- Avoidance of blood donation

The patient's environment is made as pleasant as possible. Tepid baths, rubs, and oral care are important, and a soothing lotion is used to provide relief from skin pruritus associated with jaundice. The patient may have concerns about problems created by a long illness and the resulting financial difficulties. The nurse makes appropriate referral to social services to explore financial options for the patient. The nurse encourages the patient and provides diversional activities to relieve the monotony of convalescence. With children the problems of a long convalescence may be greater, and it will require the help of everyone involved to keep them occupied and contented. Physical and emotional support is essential to recovery during this long convalescence (Box 23-12).

A more severe course will be seen in the patient with a fulminating viral hepatitis that involves a sudden and severe degeneration and atrophy of the liver that may lead to hepatic failure and death. Fulminating viral hepatitis causes acute massive necrosis, finally destroying enough of the liver to cause death.

Cirrhosis

Cirrhosis is a chronic liver disease in which diffuse destruction and regeneration of liver cells occur and in which there is an accumulation of fibrous connective tissue. This accumulated fibrous tissue distorts the normal lobular structure of the liver and obstructs the normal biliary and vascular channels in the liver. The

BOX 23-12 **Nursing Process**

HEPATITIS

ASSESSMENT

Energy level
Activity tolerance
Vital signs before and after activity
Weight
Fluid volume status
Skin
Pruritus, anorexia, fatigue, jaundice
Laboratory studies (liver enzymes, albumin)

NURSING DIAGNOSES

Activity intolerance related to viral infection, fatigue, weakness
Altered nutrition: less than body requirements related to anorexia, fatigue, nausea, decreased metabolism of nutrients by liver
Risk for fluid volume deficit related to vomiting, diarrhea, decreased intake
Risk for infection related to malnutrition and inadequate secondary defenses
Risk for impaired skin integrity related to accumulation of bile salts onto skin
Risk for diversional activity deficit related to lack of energy, isolation, lengthy course of disease
Situational low self-esteem related to isolation, length of illness, jaundice
Knowledge deficit related to new condition and unfamiliarity of disease

NURSING INTERVENTIONS

Prevent spread of disease by handwashing and proper handling of blood, body fluids, and feces.
Use disposable dishes and utensils (HepA).
Provide quiet environment.
Promote rest.
Coordinate nursing activity in blocks of time.
Increase activity as tolerated.
Provide diversional activities when energy levels adequate.
Determine food preferences.
Provide diet high in calories and carbohydrates and limited in fat.
Provide small, frequent meals.
Monitor I&O.
Weigh every day before breakfast.
Encourage fluids.
Provide comfort measures to skin (tepid bath, lotion).
Avoid soap on skin.
Encourage discussion of feelings.
Discuss prolonged recovery.

EVALUATION OF EXPECTED OUTCOMES

Verbalizes understanding of disease process, transmission, and treatment
Reports an increase in activity tolerance
Able to perform self-care activities
Stable weight
No evidence of dehydration
Skin intact
Absence or decrease in pruritus
Verbalizes self-acceptance

basic cause is not clearly understood but appears to be repeated injury to the liver cells. Although the liver cells have a great potential for regeneration, repeated scarring decreases their ability to be replaced. Cirrhosis is more common in men who are middle aged or older, but it may occur in younger persons. In the United States cirrhosis as a cause of death is outranked only by heart disease, cancer, and cerebral hemorrhage in the 45- to 61-year-old age group.

There are three primary types of cirrhosis: alcoholic (Laennec's), biliary, and postnecrotic (named because of the initiating cause of the disease). However, despite the initiating cause, the final result is essentially the same for each type. The most common form of the disease in the United States is Laennec's cirrhosis, which is caused by the effects of alcohol on liver tissue.

Pathophysiology. Cirrhosis is a disease that develops slowly and usually progresses gradually over a period of years. There is a slow destruction of the functional cells of the liver (hepatocytes). As the cells degenerate, they become infiltrated with fat and the organ increases in size (fatty cirrhosis). The regenerated nodules are separated by bands of fibrous scar tissue. This scarring process restricts the flow of blood within the organ, which contributes to its further destruction (Doughty, 1993; McCance, Huether, 1994). As the blood supply continues to be diminished and the scar tissue increases, the organ becomes atrophied. The damaged liver cannot metabolize protein normally; therefore protein intake may result in an elevation of blood ammonia levels.

Liver cell damage reduces the liver's ability to synthesize albumin. The progressive liver damage also obstructs the flow of blood through the liver. This obstruction of the circulation results in *portal hypertension,* or increased pressure in the veins that drain the gastrointestinal tract. This increased pressure forces fluid and albumin into the peritoneal cavity, which is called *ascites.* Reduced synthesis of protein and the leaking of existing protein result in hypoalbuminemia (reduced protein or albumin level in the blood), which reduces oncotic pressure of the blood, leading to leakage of serum out of the blood vessels into the interstitial tissue. Protein must be present in adequate amounts to create colloidal osmotic pressure and "pull" the fluid back into the blood vessels after it escapes from the capillaries. As fluid leaves the blood and the circulating volume decreases, the receptors in the brain signal the adrenal cortex to increase secretion of aldosterone to stimulate the kidneys to retain sodium and water. The normal liver inactivates the hormone aldosterone, but the damaged liver allows its effects to continue (hyperaldosteronism). Retention of fluid and sodium then results in increased pressure in the blood vessels and lymphatic channels, adding to the problem of portal hypertension. Ascites is therefore a result of portal hypertension, hypoalbuminemia, and hyperaldosteronism.

Because of the obstruction to blood flow through the liver, collateral vessels develop as a mechanism to divert the blood from the portal vein back to the inferior vena cava and the heart. These collateral vessels develop primarily in the esophagus *(esophageal varices),* the rectum *(hemorrhoids),* and on the surface of the abdomen *(caput medusae).* These vessels dilate and distend as a result of increased portal pressure and increased volume in the blood vessels. All of the collateral vessels, but primarily the esophageal varices, may rupture, causing severe hemorrhage.

Skin lesions appear on various parts of the body (spider angiomas), which appear as small, dilated blood vessels. Pressure on the center of the lesion causes its temporary disappearance.

Assessment. Early symptoms of cirrhosis include loss of appetite, nausea and vomiting, fever, and jaundice. When enough cells of the liver become involved to interfere with its function and obstruct blood flow through the liver, the gastrointestinal organs and the spleen become congested and cannot function properly. The patient loses weight and may experience diarrhea and constipation. Anemia occurs because of nutritional deficiency. Epistaxis, purpura, hematuria, spider hemangioma, and bleeding gums may also occur. The patient becomes weak and depressed.

Late symptoms include ascites, hematologic disorders, splenic enlargement, and hemorrhage from esophageal varices or other distended gastrointestinal veins. The patient may lapse into a coma, and death may occur.

Intervention. Interventions used to manage the patient with cirrhosis vary with the symptoms and their severity, but there is no cure for the disease (Box 23-13). Diet is the one important factor; when the patient has no appetite, it may take more than encouragement to persuade him to eat. Food is best served when the patient feels like eating. Small, frequent meals may be better tolerated by the patient.

A high-protein diet is used to maintain body needs and to provide for tissue repair. But a protein-limited diet will be needed if serum ammonia levels become elevated. Salt (sodium) is restricted to reduce edema and ascites, and potassium supplements may be necessary to replace potassium lost in gastric drainage and as a result of diuretic therapy. Careful records of food intake and calorie counts are maintained. Strict fluid intake and output records are maintained, and the patient is weighed daily.

Special attention is given to the skin because of poor nutritional status, and tissue edema may contribute to the development of decubiti. Oral care is given often and regularly. A mouthwash before meals may make

BOX 23-13 **Nursing Process**

CIRRHOSIS

ASSESSMENT

Vital signs, including temperature, pulse, blood pressure, respirations
Neurologic status, including state of arousal, mood alterations, confusion, neuromuscular activity
Ascites
Peripheral edema
Fluid balance
Laboratory values, including electrolytes, AST, ALT, bilirubin, ammonia, PT, PTT, platelets, hematocrit, WBC, BUN, and creatinine
Active or occult bleeding
Pain level on 0 to 10 scale
Breath sounds and oxygenation
Nutritional status
Jaundice
Compliance with therapeutic plan

NURSING DIAGNOSES

Risk for altered tissue perfusion related to ascites, fluid and electrolyte losses, or bleeding
Fluid volume excess related to increased intraabdominal pressure and decreased osmotic gradient
Pain related to ascites, liver inflammation
Ineffective breathing pattern related to ascites, altered level of consciousness
Risk for infection related to diminished immunologic response
Altered thought process related to encephalopathy
Risk for injury related to neurologic changes
Altered nutrition: less than body requirements related to anorexia and fatigue
Noncompliance with diet modification and alcohol restriction
Risk for impaired skin integrity related to decreased activity, ascites, peripheral edema, elevated bilirubin level

NURSING INTERVENTIONS

Check vital signs at least every 4 hours and more often if evidence of bleeding is noted.
Observe mental status and neuromuscular activity; note and report any changes.
Observe for edema by checking dependent areas for pitting (indentation) with pressure.
Observe for ascites by measuring abdominal girth at least daily.
Monitor laboratory values and note changes from baseline.
Weigh daily.
Check all gastrointestinal drainage for blood.
Position patient in low or semi-Fowler's position to facilitate breathing.
Administer oxygen, if ordered.
Help patient to take deep breaths.
Turn patient or help patient with turning every 2 hours while in bed.
Maintain IV fluid therapy as ordered.
Maintain accurate I&O records.
Assist with paracentesis if performed by physician.
Medicate patient for pain, as ordered.
Assist with activities of daily living as needed to conserve energy.
Provide adequate rest.
Provide oral hygiene before meals.
Give frequent, small feedings individualized to patient's preference and dietary restriction; provide nutritional supplements as needed.
Cleanse skin with tepid water (avoid soap) and apply moisturizing lotions to relieve pruritus.
Protect patient from harm.
Orient to time, place, or person as indicated.
Make referral for alcohol abuse treatment, if appropriate.

EVALUATION OF EXPECTED OUTCOMES

Maximum gas exchange maintained as evidenced by acceptable SaO_2 and clear breath sounds
Adequate tissue perfusion and absence of elevated temperature
Acceptable pain level
Skin integrity maintained
Adequate nutritional status maintained with stable weight and implementation of dietary modifications
Demonstrates self-monitoring activities: weight, edema, jaundice, abdominal girth, bleeding, temperature
Identifies signs and symptoms to be reported to physician immediately, including weight gain, increased abdominal girth, elevated temperature, bleeding or tarry stools, changes in memory or behavior
Demonstrates knowledge and correct use of prescribed medications and reasons to avoid nonprescription medications
Demonstrates knowledge of the dangers of alcohol use
Alert and oriented

food a little more appetizing. The patient's environment should be quiet and conducive to rest, and precautions should be taken to prevent exposure to secondary infections.

Diuretic therapy is used to decreased peripheral edema and ascites. Hydrochlorothiazide (Hydrodiuril) and spironolactone (Aldactone) are the most common agents used. The diuretic action reduces fluid and sodium; spironolactone minimizes potassium loss associated with diuresis.

When ascites is present, the patient may be more comfortable if placed in a supine position with the head of the bed elevated to reduce pressure on the diaphragm and to ease the work of breathing. When ascites is present and interferes with the respiratory status, an abdominal paracentesis may be done.

When diet and medication fail to control ascites, a peritoneovenous shunt, also called the LeVeen shunt, may be performed. It is a surgical procedure in which a specially designed tube containing a one-way pressure valve is placed so that one end is in the peritoneum. The other end is threaded through the subcutaneous tissue of the chest wall and placed in the jugular vein or superior vena cava (Figure 23-15). The segment of tubing that lies in the peritoneum is perforated to allow passage of peritoneal fluid into the tubing. When the pressure valve is open, fluid enters the tubing, flows upward, and empties into the superior cava, where it is then recirculated with the blood. The valve is triggered by the patient's breathing. When the patient inhales, the diaphragm descends and causes an increase in pressure in the fluid in the peritoneum (intraperitoneal fluid pressure) and a decrease in the pressure in the superior vena cava (intrathoracic superior vena cava pressure). This change in pressure causes a pressure difference between the two locations, causing the valve to open and forcing the fluid to flow from the peritoneum, into and up the tube.

Although this procedure controls ascites, there are additional risks involved. The tube can become occluded, ascitic fluid can leak from the incision site, and the blood can become too diluted. As with any surgical procedure, there is a risk of wound infection, and the candidate for a LeVeen shunt is predisposed to infection because of general debilitation and a poor nutritional state.

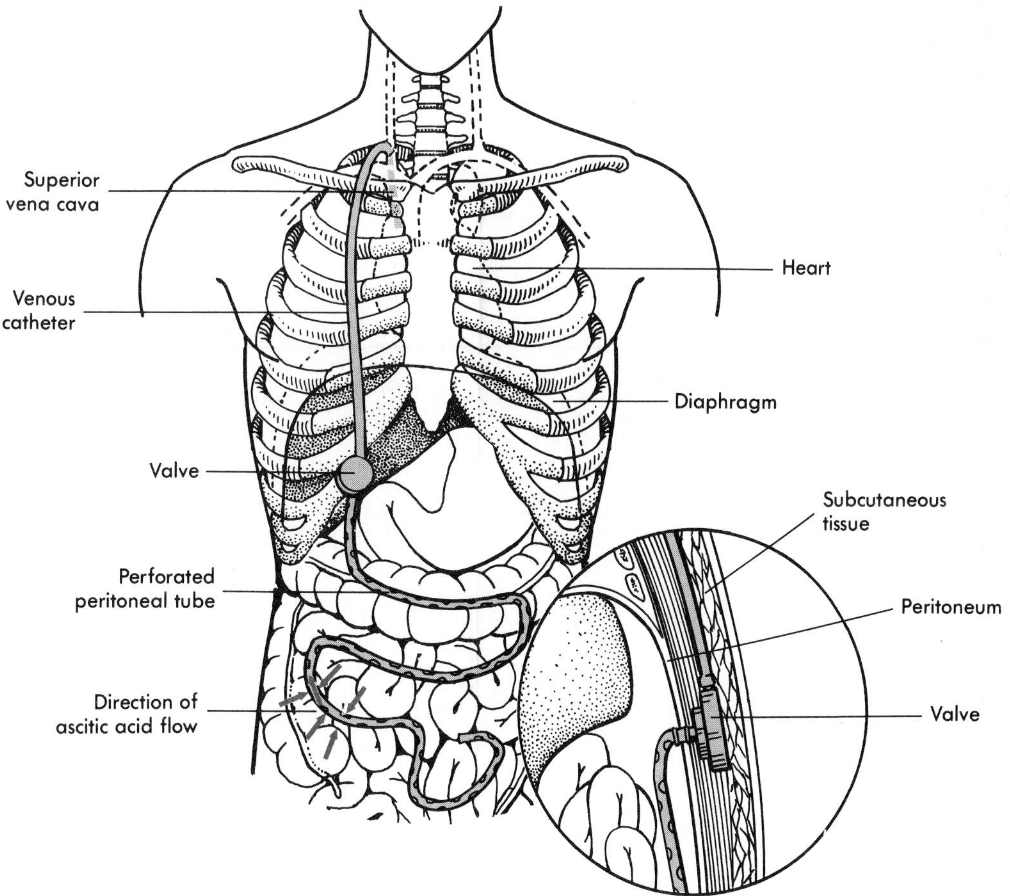

Figure 23-15 LeVeen shunt showing placement of catheter. (From Phipps WJ and others: *Medical-surgical nursing: concepts and clinical practice,* ed 5, St Louis, 1995, Mosby.)

Gastrointestinal bleeding occurs in 40% to 60% of cirrhosis patients. Bleeding may occur secondary to erosive gastritis, peptic ulcer, or esophageal varices. An endoscopy is performed to determine the exact cause of bleeding. Blood transfusions are given to replace blood loss and treat anemia. Severe hemorrhage may be treated by intravenous infusion of vasopressin (Pitressin) or somatostatin. If medication does not stop or control bleeding, an esophageal tamponade tube (Sengstaken-Blakemore or Minnesota) may be inserted. A tamponade tube has two balloons that can be inflated to put pressure on the bleeding vessels in an attempt to stop the bleeding (Figure 23-16).

The tube is usually inserted through the mouth, down the esophagus, and into the stomach. When correct placement is ensured, the balloon in either the stomach alone or the balloons in both the stomach and esophagus are inflated to press against the bleeding vessels and control the hemorrhage. The gastric drainage port is attached to low intermittent suction to remove secretions and blood from the stomach. When the gastric balloon alone or both the gastric and esophageal balloons are inflated, secretions above the balloon must also be removed to prevent aspiration. If a Sengstaken-Blakemore tube is used, a Salem sump tube is passed into the esophagus through the mouth or nose and attached to low suction to drain the secretions; the Minnesota tube has its own esophageal drainage port, and this port is attached to suction to drain the secretions. Tamponade therapy should not continue for more than 24 to 48 hours in order to prevent ischemia and necrosis to the mucosal surface of the stomach or esophagus.

Other interventions. Surgical and radiologic procedures may be performed to lower portal venous pressure or to treat ascites. The increased portal pressure found with liver disease can be reduced by shunting some of the portal blood directly into the inferior vena cava (Figure 23-17). This reduces the flow of

PATIENT/FAMILY TEACHING

Cirrhosis

The nurse should provide the patient and family with the following information:

- Diet instructions, with attention to special restrictions
- Medication instructions, including actions, dosage, side effects and over-the-counter medications to avoid unless prescribed
- How to self-monitor weight, edema, jaundice, abdominal girth, bleeding, temperature

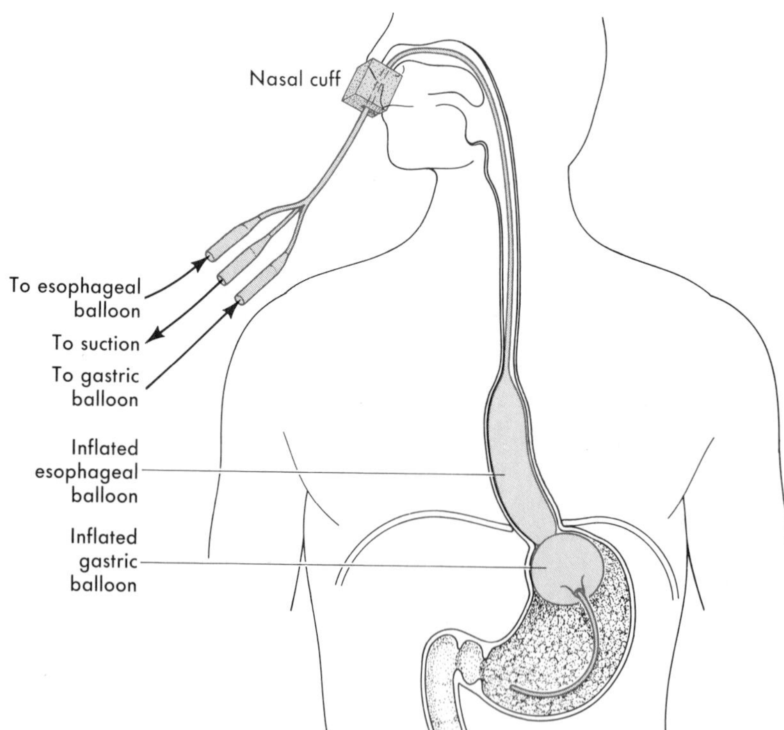

Figure 23-16 Sengstaken-Blakemore tube. (From Beare DB, Myers JL: *Adult health nursing,* ed 2, St Louis, 1994, Mosby.)

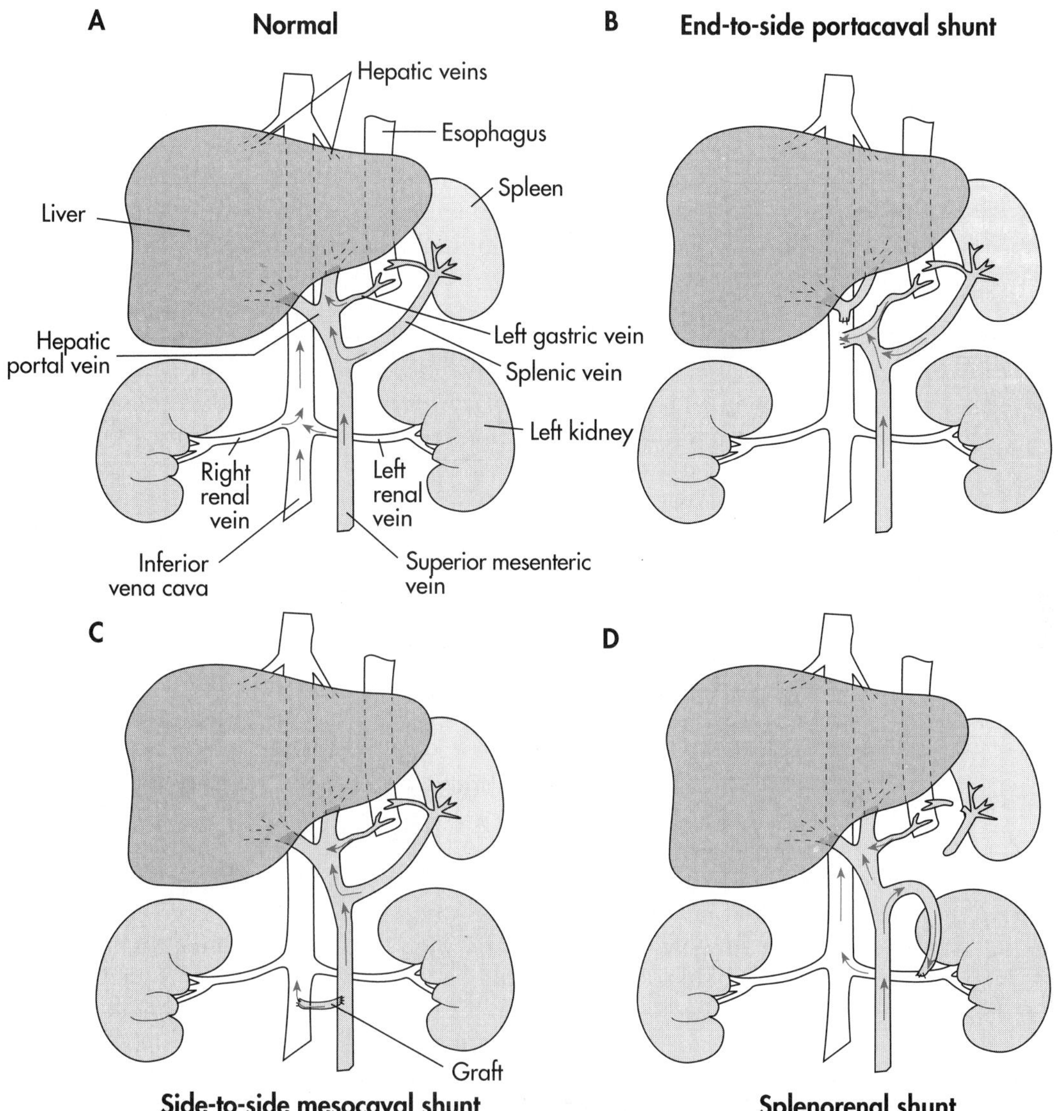

Figure 23-17 Portosystemic shunts. **A,** Normal portal circulation. **B,** End-to-side portacaval shunt. Large amount of blood is diverted from its usual route to the liver and flows directly into the inferior vena cava. The portal vein and vena cava are anastomosed just outside the liver. Encephalopathy is a danger because ammonia and other toxins enter the systemic circulation directly instead of going to the liver for detoxification. **C,** Side-to side mesocaval shunt. In this more conservative procedure, a graft is added between the superior mesenteric vein and the inferior vena cava to reduce blood flow to the liver and to reduce pressure. **D,** Distal splenorenal shunt. In this selective shunt the splenic vein is connected to the renal vein to reduce the pressure in the varices without drastically decreasing liver perfusion via the portal vein. Often the spleen is removed with this procedure.

blood through the portal vein. With a *portacaval shunt,* the portal vein is anastomosed directly to the inferior vena cava so that the liver is bypassed. With the *splenorenal shunt,* the splenic vein is anastomosed to the left renal vein, and the spleen is removed. A more conservative procedure relieves portal pressure by adding a graft *(mesocaval shunt)* between the superior mesenteric vein and the inferior vena cava. This is elective surgery that may be only palliative in nature.

An alternative procedure used to reduce portal venous pressure, the *transiugular intrahepatic portosystemic shunt* (TIPS), is performed in the radiology department and does not require taking the patient to surgery. During the TIPS procedure, a catheter is inserted into the jugular vein and passed through the hepatic vein and the liver and into the portal vein. A stent is then positioned in the liver tissue itself to provide an unobstructed passage of blood from the portal vein through the liver into the hepatic vein and back to the inferior vena cava, thus reducing portal venous pressure (Adams, Soulen, 1993).

Liver transplantation

Liver transplantation is considered in the treatment of various forms of liver disease. However, to be considered for transplantation, the patient must have irreversible, end-stage liver disease that cannot be managed by other forms of medical or surgical care. Advanced cirrhosis from biliary or alcoholic disease and from hepatitis is the most common indication for liver transplantation in adults.

Before transplantation is performed, a complete assessment of the patient is completed that includes physiologic and psychologic factors. The scarcity of donor organs limits the number of patients who can receive this treatment.

Hepatic coma

Hepatic coma is a degenerative condition of the brain that follows liver failure. It is thought to be the result of increasing levels of ammonia in the bloodstream, which results in hepatic encephalopathy. Symptoms progress from inappropriate behavior, confusion, flapping tremors, and twitching of the extremities to stupor and coma.

Interventions. The underlying cause must be treated and the patient given supportive care that will prevent further damage to the liver. The patient is given the supportive care necessary for any patient who has liver disease and who is unconscious. However, special measures such as central venous pressure monitoring and tracheostomy care may be necessary. The urinary output is monitored carefully because renal failure may occur. Intravenous infusions and intermittent positive-pressure breathing therapy may also be needed. Drugs that are normally detoxified by the liver are avoided if possible. Hepatic coma is usually associated with elevated serum ammonia levels, so interventions are initiated to correct this problem. Dietary protein is restricted to minimize the accumulation of serum ammonia. Neomycin is a nonabsorbable antibiotic that is administered into the GI tract and removes normal GI bacteria that function in the digestion and absorption of protein, the major source of serum ammonia. Lactulose is administered singly, or in combination with neomycin, to promote the evacuation of protein from the GI tract through diarrhea. Hemodialysis may also be used to remove ammonia from the blood.

ETHICAL DILEMMA

Mr. Hyatt is a 56-year-old man with a 30-year history of alcohol abuse and severe alcoholic cirrhosis. He has had multiple hospital admissions for problems related to his liver disease, including major bleeding from esophageal varices and endoscopic sclerotherapy. He is admitted to the hospital now with severe ascites and encephalopathy. Mr. Hyatt is in a coma with no hope of recovery without liver transplantation. His family wishes that "everything be done" for him.

Should this patient be considered for a liver transplant? How would you analyze the ethics issues in this case?

Diseases and Disorders of the Biliary System

The *biliary system* consists of the gallbladder and the ducts leading from the liver to the gallbladder and then to the duodenum. About 1 liter of bile per day is formed in the liver and excreted into the left or right hepatic ducts, which merge to become the common hepatic duct (Figure 23-18). Bile passes through the hepatic duct to the cystic duct that leads to the gallbladder, where it is stored and concentrated. When needed for digestion, bile is released from the gallbladder into the cystic duct, flows through the common bile duct, and empties into the duodenum. Bile salts are the metabolically active components of bile. In the intestine, they act on fat to make it more soluble and to break it up into tiny particles that can pass through the intestinal wall. Cholesterol and lecithin in bile keep bile salts in suspension. Bile facilitates the absorption of fat-soluble vitamins, iron, and calcium and activates the release of pancreatic and intestinal enzymes (McCance, Huether, 1994; Sleisenger, Fordtran, 1993).

Disorders of the biliary system are common in the United States and are responsible for the hospitalization of more than one-half million people per year. Disorders include tumors (which are rare); infections; congenital malformations; and the two most common conditions, *cholecystitis* (inflammation) and *cholelithiasis* (stone formation).

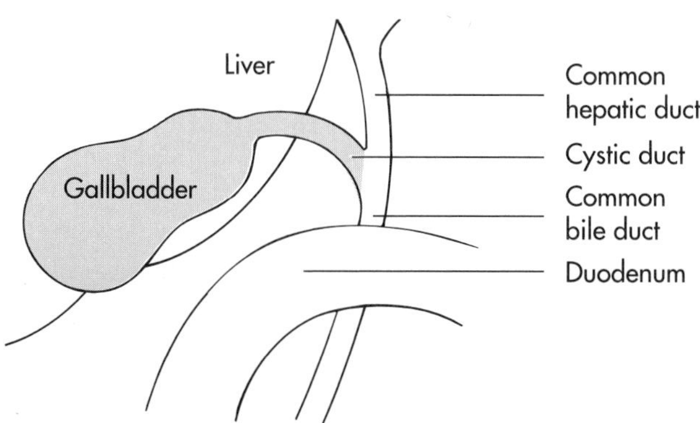

Figure 23-18 Biliary system. Gallbladder and ducts.

Cholecystitis

Cholecystitis, an inflammation of the gallbladder, is more common in women than men, and sedentary, obese persons are more likely to be affected. The incidence increases with age, becoming highest in persons in their 50s and 60s.

Pathophysiology. Cholecystitis can be caused by an obstruction, a gallstone (cholelithiasis), or a tumor. A large variety of organisms may contribute to acute inflammation of the gallbladder. Because the bile cannot leave the gallbladder, more water is absorbed, and the bile becomes more concentrated and irritates the walls of the gallbladder. A typical inflammatory response occurs, and the gallbladder becomes enlarged and edematous. Chronic inflammation results in thickening of the walls, which become fibrous, replacing normal muscle and mucosal tissues. This can further affect the ability of the gallbladder to empty and concentrate bile. As the tissues of the gallbladder become damaged, bacteria or other irritants can become trapped and contribute to a chronic inflammatory process. There is danger of rupture of the gallbladder and spread of infection to the hepatic duct and liver. When the disease is severe enough to interfere with the blood supply, the gallbladder wall may become gangrenous.

Assessment. Cholecystitis may be an acute or chronic problem. With an acute attack, there is a sudden onset of nausea and vomiting and severe pain in the right upper quadrant of the abdomen; chronic cholecystitis is evidenced by several milder attacks of pain and a history of fat intolerance. The attacks may be so mild that the patient avoids medical attention until he or she develops jaundice or severe pain from obstruction in the biliary ducts. During an acute attack, the patient is usually febrile, with temperatures often as high as 40° C.

Intervention. Treatment usually requires surgical removal of the gallbladder **(cholecystectomy),** but some physicians prefer to wait until the acute infection subsides. Others prefer to operate immediately to avoid the risk of rupture and subsequent peritonitis. If treated medically, the patient is maintained at NPO; a nasogastric tube is passed and attached to low suction if nausea or vomiting is present; intravenous fluids are used to maintain adequate hydration and electrolyte replacement; and antibiotics are administered to prevent or treat infection. Pain management is a key medical and nursing issue. Patients with cholecystitis and cholelithiasis often experience intense pain located in the right upper quadrant of the abdomen that may radiate to the back and shoulders. Meperidine (Demerol) is the "traditional" agent of choice for pain management in patients with gallbladder disease because it does not cause spasm of the sphincter of Oddi. However, morphine sulfate, because of its superiority in pain control, is more often being used as long as spasms do not increase. When the inflammation subsides, a diet low in fat is resumed. Nursing intervention includes monitoring fluid and electrolyte balance and vital signs, observing for symptoms, and relieving pain. If surgery is planned, routine preoperative nursing care for abdominal surgery is implemented.

Cholelithiasis

Cholelithiasis is the presence of stones in the gallbladder or in the bile ducts. Approximately 10% of the people in the United States have stones in the gallbladder, and approximately 6000 people die each year as a result of this disorder. Before the age of 50 years, cholelithiasis is more common in women; the incidence is equal in men and women after age 50 years. It is more common in diabetic persons, women who have been pregnant, and obese people.

Pathophysiology. Stones are composed primarily of cholesterol, bilirubin, and calcium. They may be large, measuring inches across, or very small stones, referred to as gravel. The cause of gallstone formation is not fully understood, and there are numerous theories. Evidence suggests that gallstones form when the bile excreted by the liver is abnormally high in cholesterol and lacks the proper concentration and proportion of bile salts. Individuals with an increased cholesterol level may be predisposed to the formation of gallstones.

When the balance of cholesterol, lecithin, and bile salts is disturbed, precipitation of bile salts may cause the formation of gallstones. Stasis of bile from delayed emptying may result in excess saturation of bile with cholesterol and promote the precipitation of bile salts. Infection can create an area of irritation that may become a site for stone formation. Inflammation may cause gallstones, and stones may also cause inflammation.

Assessment. Symptoms result from the inflammation in the gallbladder and the presence of stones or from obstruction to bile flow from the liver or gallbladder. Pain occurs under the right rib cage in the upper right quadrant of the abdomen and may radiate to the back and shoulders. Decreased flow of bile produces fat intolerance with symptoms of abdominal distention, nausea and vomiting, and flatulence. Symptoms may first appear after ingestion of a meal high in fat content. With severe disease, pain and tenderness are increased, with elevation of temperature, increased pulse and respiratory rates, and an increase in the WBC count. Serum cholesterol level is elevated. Pain is more severe when the bile passages are obstructed by a stone. The pain may be referred to the back and shoulders and may last for several hours; it is usually accompanied by nausea and vomiting and profuse perspiration. The obstruction to bile flow may cause jaundice. Cholecystography, cholangiography, ultrasound, or CT scan is usually performed to assess for the presence and location of stones.

Intervention. Some mild attacks of cholelithiasis may be treated medically. Antispasmodic drugs are used to decrease spasms of the sphincter of Oddi, a nasogastric tube is inserted and attached to suction for the patient with nausea and vomiting, and intravenous fluids are administered to maintain hydration. Pain is managed pharmacologically with meperidine or morphine. Positioning the patient supine with the head of the bed elevated 45 to 60 degrees and the knees flexed, or side lying in a knee-chest position, supplements drug therapy in the management of pain. After the acute phase a low-fat, low-cholesterol diet may be recommended to prevent future attacks.

Traditionally cholelithiasis has been treated by surgical removal of the gallbladder (cholecystectomy). Alternative treatment methods are available for some patients. Extracorporeal shockwave lithotripsy (ESWL) and oral dissolution of gallstones with bile acids are being used with increased frequency.

ESWL is the application of shockwaves to bombard and disintegrate the gallstone. With the use of ESWL, recovery time and patient discomfort are significantly reduced. A major drawback of ESWL is the likelihood of recurrence of the gallstones. Because the procedure is new, further studies are needed to validate this. Following ESWL, oral dissolution therapy is prescribed for many patients to dissolve the remaining fragments.

Oral bile acids, chenodeoxycholic acid, and ursodeoxycholic acid (UDCA) are currently used to dissolve small cholesterol gallstones. Taken in pill form, this treatment option is used alone or in conjunction with ESWL. It is very expensive, ranging from $1300 to $1600 per year, and it may need to be continued for up to 2 years. There is a high (up to 40%) incidence of recurrence of the stones over a 5-year period.

Cholecystectomy

Surgical removal of the gallbladder (cholecystectomy) is indicated when the patient has chronic or acute cholecystitis or cholelithiasis. Careful evaluation and examination of the patient's general condition are made before the surgery (see Chapter 18). If jaundice is present, tests of liver function and prothrombin time are usually included in the preoperative evaluation.

In cholecystectomy an incision is made just under the ribs in the right upper quadrant of the abdomen (right subcostal incision). The gallbladder is excised from the posterior liver wall. The physician can also explore the common bile duct (choledochostomy). After common duct exploration a T tube is inserted to allow adequate bile drainage during healing of the duct (Figure 23-19). The T tube also provides a route for post-operative cholangiography if desired (T-tube cholangiogram). The T tube is placed in the common bile duct with one arm directed toward the hepatic duct and the other toward the duodenum. A Jackson-Pratt or Penrose drain is often inserted and brought out through a stab wound to provide an escape route for drainage caused by inflammation of tissues in the operative area. The drain is removed when drainage stops.

More commonly, the cholecystectomy is performed using a laser and a laparoscope. *Laser laparoscopic cholecystectomy* can reduce a patient's hospital stay to 24 hours or less and recovery time to a few days. The large abdominal incision is avoided because the gallbladder is visualized through a laparoscope inserted through a small incision in the navel. The scope acts like a television camera, projecting a magnified view of the abdominal organs on a color video screen. The laser and other instruments are introduced into the abdomen through three tiny openings. The gallbladder is grasped with a forceps, the bile is aspirated with a needle, and the organ collapses. It is detached with the laser and removed through the laparoscope. If stones are present, they are removed before the gallbladder is detached. The laser seals the operative area and adhesive strips close the tiny opening. The incision in the navel is closed with a single suture. Eliminating the large incision results in less pain, less blood loss, rapid return of bowel function, and prompt return to normal food intake. It is considered an option for patients with chronic pain but not for those with acute cholecystitis.

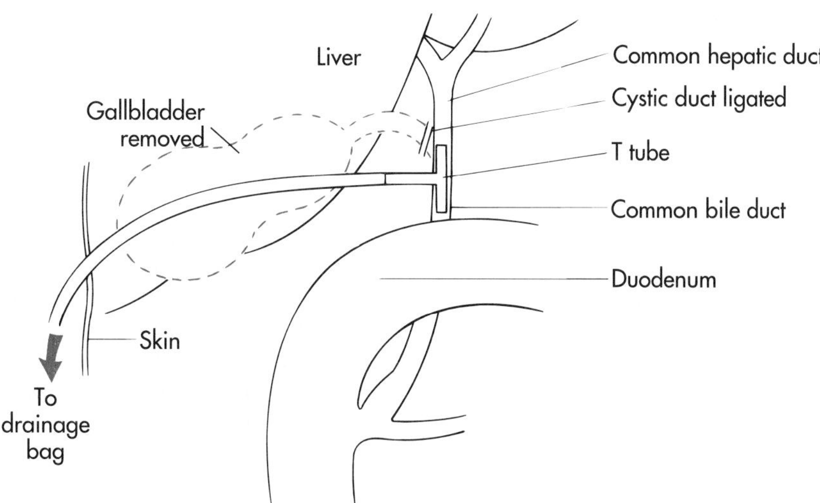

Figure 23-19 T tube in common duct.

Postoperative interventions. Vital signs are monitored and dressings are observed carefully and often for drainage or hemorrhage. Wet dressings at the incision site and around drain sites are changed to prevent skin maceration and infections. (The nurse should consult hospital protocols to determine if this is a nursing or physician role.) The patient is placed in the Fowler's position to facilitate both surgical site and T-tube drainage. The patient is encouraged and assisted as necessary to turn often while in bed, to ambulate at least four times a day, and to perform leg exercises to prevent embolism. Deep breathing exercises are extremely important in the patient with surgery in the upper quadrants of the abdomen. The patient needs considerable encouragement because of the location of the incision. Upper abdominal incisions are more painful and are more likely to interfere with deep breathing maneuvers. The patient will tend to avoid taking deep breaths because expansion of the rib cage and chest wall is painful. The nurse can assist by splinting the incision with a towel or small pillow. Respiratory therapy or the use of an inspiration spirometer are ordered to ensure adequate lung ventilation and expansion. Pain medication must be administered often in the early postoperative period to facilitate movement and deep breathing. Early ambulation is pivotal in preventing postoperative complications. When the patient is fully awake and vital signs are stable, he or she is usually dangled and assisted out of bed on the night of surgery or early on the first postoperative day.

Fluid balance is maintained with intravenous therapy; potassium is usually added to compensate for loss from surgery. A nasogastric tube may be inserted and connected to suction to prevent nausea, vomiting, and abdominal distention. The nurse ensures that the tube is draining properly, and if it becomes obstructed, it is irrigated with physiologic saline solution. The patient is given nothing by mouth while the nasogastric tube is in place, although sips of water or ice chips may be allowed to keep the mouth moist (refer to the section on gastric decompression).

Dressings may have to be changed often to keep the patient comfortable and prevent excoriation of the skin. Montgomery straps may be used to prevent skin irritation from frequent removal of adhesive tape. A small drainage pouch may be applied to the drain site to collect drainage and protect the skin.

If a T tube has been inserted in the common bile duct, the long segment of the tube is brought out to the skin through a small stab wound and sutured to the skin (see Figure 23-19). The site of the T tube is assessed carefully for signs of inflammation and infection and leakage of bilious drainage. A large amount of bile staining the dressing could indicate leakage around the T tube and/or blockage of the tube. The T tube is attached to a drainage bag. Bile will flow into the bag instead of down the common bile duct if the bile duct is edematous. Positioning the drainage bag at the abdominal level rather than at a lower point will create more resistance for the flow of bile into the bag. Bile will only flow into the bag if the resistance in the common duct is greater. The greater the edema, the greater the resistance in the common duct. If positioned at the abdominal level, it is secured by pinning it to tape applied to the skin. Otherwise, the weight of the bag would pull on the long tube and cause tension on the insertion site in the common duct. The bag must be positioned so that the tube is not kinked, otherwise bile will not be able to drain from the liver. The position of the bag and tube and the color and amount of drainage

PATIENT/FAMILY TEACHING

Cholecystectomy, cholecystostomy, choledochostomy

The nurse should ensure that the patient and family are taught routine preoperative procedures, including deep breathing exercises, use of incentive spirometry, splinting of incision when coughing, and leg exercises for deep vein thrombosis prophylaxis.

are assessed, measured, and recorded at frequent intervals during the first 24 hours. The T tube is emptied as often as necessary to keep it no more than half full. The T tube is expected to drain 300 to 500 ml in the first 24 hours after surgery. This amount will decrease as edema decreases because the bile will then flow to the duodenum; it should be less than 200 ml a day by the fourth day. After oral intake is resumed, the physician may order the tube clamped for approximately 1 hour during meals to aid in the digestion of fat.

The T tube may be left in place for up to 10 days, and some patients are discharged from the hospital with the tube still in place. The physician will remove the tube when the common bile duct is patent for drainage of bile. The patient must be observed for jaundice, as evidenced by yellowing of the skin, sclera, and mucous membranes. Dark-colored urine and lack of color in the stool (clay-colored) indicate an obstruction in the biliary ducts. These symptoms should be reported to the physician immediately. If the patient was jaundiced before surgery, there should be a clearing of the skin, sclera, and mucous membranes, and the stool and urine should return to normal color.

Bowel sounds are checked at least daily to determine the return of peristalsis. A clear liquid diet is usually ordered 24 to 48 hours after surgery and increased as tolerated. Some physicians wait for the return of bowel sounds to begin the patient on a clear liquid diet, whereas others believe the clear liquid diet will encourage the return of peristalsis, which is also facilitated by ambulation.

When a solid food diet is started, it will usually be low in fat. Many patients who were troubled with flatulence or nausea after eating certain foods will continue to experience these problems after a cholecystectomy. The patient should be instructed to experiment with different foods, trying small amounts of those that previously caused discomfort and gradually eliminating those that continue to do so.

Throughout the postoperative period, the patient must be observed for complications. Jaundice will appear if the common duct is occluded by stones or there is stricture of a duct. A decrease in blood pressure and a rise in the pulse rate are signs of bleeding. Dressings must be observed for hemorrhage and leakage of bile. An elevated temperature could indicate peritonitis or wound infection. Pancreatitis may occur following cholecystectomy. There is also the discouraging possibility that the symptoms experienced before surgery will return. This may be caused by another stone in the ducts, but sometimes the cause cannot be identified.

At the time of discharge, the patient is instructed on any restriction in activity or diet. The diet is usually low in fat. The patient should be able to describe the restrictions and identify the signs of complications that should be reported to the physician (Box 23-14).

Cholecystostomy

A cholecystostomy is an opening into the gallbladder. It is usually considered a temporary measure and may be performed if the patient cannot tolerate a cholecystectomy. An incision is made in the fundus (the top, rounded section) of the gallbladder. The gallbladder is then emptied of stones, and a tube with a large lumen is sutured into the gallbladder for drainage during the postoperative period (see Box 23-14).

Choledochostomy

A choledochostomy is the opening and exploration of the common bile duct, usually performed to remove stones. A T tube is inserted for drainage, as already described for cholecystectomy. The procedure is usually performed in conjunction with a cholecystectomy (see Box 23-14).

Pancreatitis

Pancreatitis is an inflammation of the pancreas and is caused by premature activation of pancreatic enzymes that results in autodigestion of pancreatic tissue and altered organ function. Pancreatitis is known to occur most commonly in patients with biliary tract disease and in patients with a history of excessive alcohol intake. However, the exact cause is unknown. Acute pancreatitis is characterized by intense pain in the epigastric region, nausea and vomiting, elevation of temperature, and increased leukocyte count (WBC). Decreased serum calcium and jaundice are associated with more severe cases of inflammation. Fluid and electrolyte depletion, respiratory complications, and infection are seen. In patients with the most severe form of

BOX 23-14 **Nursing Process**

CHOLECYSTECTOMY, CHOLECYSTOSTOMY, OR CHOLEDOCHOSTOMY—POSTOPERATIVE CARE

ASSESSMENT

Vital signs, including temperature, pulse, blood pressure, respirations
Pain level on 0 to 10 scale
Breath sounds and oxygenation
Abdominal distention
Surgical wound area and surgical dressing
Surgical tubes and drains, including nasograstric tube, T tube, penrose, or self-suction drain (Jackson Pratt)
Learning needs related to self-care and diet changes

NURSING DIAGNOSES

Risk for altered tissue perfusion related to fluid and electrolyte losses or bleeding
Pain related to abdominal incision
Ineffective breathing pattern related to pain and splinting of abdominal incision
Risk for injury related to accidental obstruction of biliary drainage
Risk for impaired skin integrity related to wound drainage
Knowledge deficit related to diet modifications, activity restrictions, and signs of biliary obstruction after discharge

NURSING INTERVENTIONS

Check vital signs every 15 minutes until stable, then at least every 4 hours.
Assist patient with taking deep breaths; help to splint incision with coughing.
Medicate patient for pain as ordered.
Assist patient with turning, or turn patient every 2 hours while in bed.
Assist patient with ambulation as early as permissible.
Maintain intravenous fluid therapy as ordered.
Maintain accurate I&O records.
Maintain patency of nasograstric tube, if in place.
Observe for nausea, vomiting, and abdominal distention.
Observe color of skin and sclera for jaundice, indicating obstruction of bile flow.
Note color and consistency of stool.
Observe surgical dressing for drainage; reinforce or change per hospital standards; avoid use of tape by using Montgomery straps if frequent dressing changes are needed.
If T tube is in place:
Maintain patency of T tube and prevent tension of tube.
Place patient in low to semi-Fowler's position to promote drainage from T tube.
Observe, describe, and record amount and characteristic of drainage at least every 8 hours.
Empty bag when half full.
Clamp tube in intervals prescribed by physician.

EVALUATION OF EXPECTED OUTCOMES

Meets discharge criteria for postsurgical patient
Understands activity restrictions, such as driving and lifting limitations; signs and symptoms of wound infection; diet modifications (low fat)
Maximum gas exchange maintained as evidenced by no respiratory distress, acceptable Sa_{O_2}, and clear breath sounds
Adequate tissue perfusion and absence of elevated temperature
Acceptable pain level
Absence of bile duct injury
Skin integrity maintained
Evidence of wound healing
Adequate nutritional status maintained and implementation of dietary modifications
Return to preoperative self-care level

the disease, hemorrhage into the pancreatic tissue and the abdominal cavity occur as the pancreas is destroyed by its own enzymes, and the patient becomes critically ill (Brodrick, 1991).

Chronic bouts of pancreatitis may occur, leading to the formation of scar tissue within the pancreas, which often interferes with normal pancreatic function.

In treating patients with mild forms of pancreatitis, food and fluids are withheld to avoid stimulating pancreatic activity, and intravenous fluids are administered. The most common complaint is severe, constant pain radiating to the back and both sides. The pain is treated with morphine sulfate or meperidine. Mild to severe pain continues; weakness, jaundice, and diarrhea may occur; and the patient becomes weak and debilitated. These patients need good nursing care and emotional support.

Respiratory complications, such as pneumonia and pleural effusion, are commonly seen in patients with acute pancreatitis. Additionally, patients may develop pseudocysts (sacs filled with fluid and debris from the injured tissue) within the pancreas, harboring purulent material that may lead to overwhelming infection. Large pseudocysts often put pressure on adjacent organs, such as the stomach or duodenum, and cause symptoms. Pseudocysts often require surgical drainage or excision. Occasionally part of the pancreas is resected to remove a portion of the organ that is diseased and causing additional problems by the obstruction of biliary ducts.

Treatment for pancreatitis is essentially supportive. Patients with more severe symptoms are kept strictly NPO; a nasogastric tube is placed to remove gastric secretions that stimulate pancreatic secretion and to relieve nausea and vomiting. Fluid and electrolyte replacement is the mainstay of care. The patient often requires several liters of fluid per day to maintain adequate hydration and replacement of losses. Antibiotics are administered to treat any infections. Preventive measures are instituted to support respiratory function, such as turning and deep breathing exercises. However, many patients require the administration of supplemental oxygen, or even mechanical ventilation, to maintain good gas exchange. Insulin therapy may be needed to treat elevated blood sugars that occur as a result of decreased insulin secretion by the diseased pancreas.

Tumors

Malignant or benign tumors may occur in any of the accessory organs of digestion and are usually associated with some symptoms related to organ function. Patients with cancer of the accessory organs of digestion experience loss of appetite, loss of weight, general weakness, secondary anemia, and a general feeling of discomfort. Tumors of the pancreas are usually malignant and are often not diagnosed until the tumor is significantly advanced. Tumors may appear in the head, body, or tail of the organ. Nonspecific symptoms of pain, jaundice, anorexia, nausea, vomiting, and weight loss are seen. Often symptoms are mistaken for symptoms of biliary tract disease. A *Whipple procedure* may be performed to remove tumors located at the head of the pancreas. The procedure involves the removal of part of the stomach, duodenum, and the head of the pancreas; biliary and pancreatic ducts are anastomosed to the jejunum (Figure 23-20).

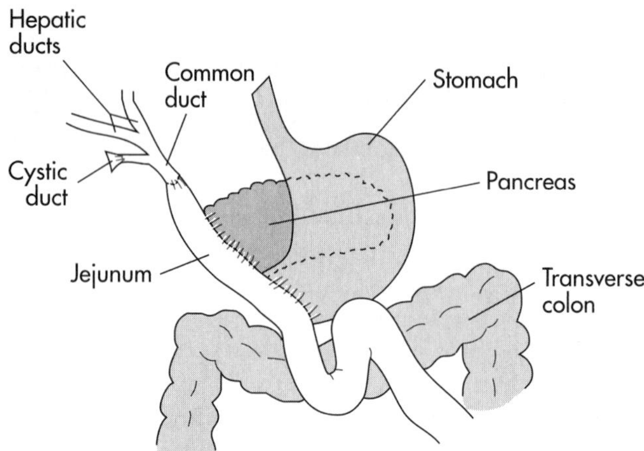

Figure 23-20 Whipple procedure includes resection of distal portion of the stomach, the duodenum, and part of the pancreas. The gallbladder is removed and the biliary ducts are connected to the jejunum. The remaining stomach and pancreas are anastomosed to the jejunum.

Removal of the entire pancreas, *total pancreatectomy*, is another alternative for treatment or cure of tumors located at the head of the pancreas. Unfortunately the prognosis for cancer of the pancreas is poor despite surgical intervention and chemotherapy.

Sources of tumors of the liver may be primary (hepatoma) or metastatic. Most metastatic liver tumors originate from tumors in the breast or GI tract. Chemotherapy is used in the treatment of both primary and metastatic tumors of the liver. Surgical treatment for liver tumors involves removing the affected lobe or lobes (lobectomy).

Liver transplantation is rarely (although sometimes) considered as a treatment option for malignant tumors of the liver because of the risk of recurrent disease. If the patient has a resection of diseased lobes of the liver, careful preoperative preparation and expert postoperative nursing care are necessary. After surgery, the patient is observed for hemorrhage, which is always a possibility. All vital signs are checked at frequent intervals. The patient may have chest tubes connected to closed chest drainage and will have a nasogastric tube connected to suction. Food and fluids are withheld for several days, and mouth care is important. Ambulation is usually delayed for several days.

Cancer of the gallbladder and bile ducts is rare. When it occurs, it generally begins in the biliary ducts and metastasizes to the liver.

Nursing Care Plan

PATIENT WITH CIRRHOSIS

Mr. Barton is a 45-year-old male who enters the emergency department of the veteran's hospital complaining of fever, burning on urination, constipation, general malaise, and anorexia. He states he began feeling poorly 3 nights ago and noticed that his "eyeballs were turning yellow just like last time." He states he gave up drinking 4 years ago. He has no known food or drug allergies.

Past Medical History

History of chronic alcoholism since age 30

Appendectomy at age 15, no other surgeries

Pneumonia at age 40; has smoked 1 to 2 packs of cigarettes per day since age 12

Multiple VA admissions for chronic nutritional anemia related to alcoholism

Patient is poor historian; old records not available

Both parents are deceased, causes unknown

Psychosocial Data

Has 2 siblings, sister (with whom he lives), and younger brother who lives out of state; states he has no contact with brother

Sister works as receptionist for lawyer and has 2 adult children living in the home

Family relations described as "strained"

Lives with sister since second divorce 2 years ago; previous divorce 6 years earlier. First marriage lasted 12 years; states he supports and visits 3 daughters from first marriage (ages 13, 15, and 17); conflicting stories of involvement with them

Works as a carpenter at a local insurance company; states he enjoys work and rarely misses going to work; considers himself as a "master cabinet maker" and works with woods as a hobby

States he has few close friends

Attends AA meetings "when he thinks of it"

Served in the Army during Vietnam as a clerk/cook

Denies use of drugs and/or alcohol for 4 years

Assessment Data

General: Thin male who appears malnourished; pale skin color

Height: 5 ft 10 in; weight 140 lbs, 20% below ideal body weight (IBW)

Oriented × 3 (time, place, and person)

Skin: Intact, olive coloring with some scaly patches on anterior chest (2 to 3 cm); patient states some pruritis.

Eyes: Obvious yellow sclerae; EOM intact

Respiratory: Nonproductive cough, especially in the morning; rales heard in bilateral bases; regular rate and rhythm, 22-24

Cardiovascular: Apical rate 78; regular; point of maximal impulse at apex; no bruits, all pulses intact

Abdominal: Soft, slight distention; bowel sounds hypoactive (14-16), heard in all four quadrants; liver palpable at right costal margin with firm, sharp edges and small nodules

Genitourinary: Complaining of burning on urination; urine dark amber, cloudy

Vital signs: T 100, P 68-72, R 20, BP 110/64

Laboratory Data

Hgb 9.4, Hct 29, BUN 45, AST 96

ALT 52, Total bilirubin 7.2

Alk Phosp 20, Serum amylase 24 IU/L

WBC 4500, Platelets 200,000

Electrolytes within normal limits

Urine pH 5.1, specific gravity 1.028

4 + albumin, many RBC, casts

Urine culture—*E. coli* present

Medications

Folic acid 1 mg po daily

Feosol 120 mg bid

Prednisone 20 mg daily

Multivitamin tab 1 daily

Nembutal 100 mg po hs

Ascorbic acid tab 1 daily

Tylenol 325 to 650 mg po prn fever/discomfort

continued

NURSING DIAGNOSIS

Altered urinary elimination pattern related to infection as evidenced by cloudy urine, burning sensation, and culture of *E. coli*

NURSING INTERVENTIONS

Observe voiding patterns.

Document urine color, characteristics, and I & O, as well as patient's daily weight.

Identify patient's fluid choices (ginger ale, water, and orange juice).

Force fluids up to 800 to 1000 ml per shift.

Instruct patient regarding need for personal cleaning of perineal area to avoid stool contamination of urethra.

Provide supportive measures as indicated (Tylenol ordered).

Assist with general hygiene.

Encourage patient to express feelings regarding discomfort.

EVALUATION OF EXPECTED OUTCOMES

Fluid intake equals output

Expresses feelings of comfort

Discusses need for attention to personal hygiene and identifies daily practices of self-care

Does not show evidence of skin breakdown, infection, or other complications

Maintains urinary continence

NURSING DIAGNOSIS

Denial related to alcoholism as evidenced by statements of abstinence for 4 years

NURSING INTERVENTIONS

Provide for specific amount of uninterrupted non-care-related time daily.

Encourage patient to express feelings related to present problem, its severity, and potential impact on life pattern.

Encourage patient to cite significant losses in his relationships and to identify any insight into his own role in these losses.

Listen to patient with nonjudgmental acceptance. Correct any gross misperceptions.

Discuss "enabling" behaviors and their role in fostering his alcoholism.

Discuss his relationship with his sister and each daughter. Encourage honesty in his descriptions.

Discuss the philosophy of AA and explore his member contacts. Identify the need for regular attendance at meetings.

EVALUATION OF EXPECTED OUTCOMES

Discusses present health problems and their relationship to alcohol abuse

Describes ADLs and reports any stressors that contribute to the need for a drink

Identifies need to maintain consistent contact with AA members and to attend meetings on a regular basis

Identifies an increasing awareness of reality either verbally or behaviorally

NURSING DIAGNOSIS

Altered nutrition: less than body requirements related to poor eating habits and anorexia

NURSING INTERVENTIONS	EVALUATION OF EXPECTED OUTCOMES
Obtain and record patient's weight daily. Determine food preferences and provide them within the limits of planned caloric needs (high carbohydrate, high calorie, and high protein). Prefers pasta, some lean meats, salads, and fruits. Dislikes many vegetables and fiber foods (states his best meal is breakfast). Give small, frequent feeds. Elevate head of bed during meals. Check tolerance for foods after each meal. Perform a daily calorie count. Refer to dietician or nutritional support team for dietary management. Monitor bowel sounds once per shift. Teach principles of basic four food groups. Involve sister in instruction. Discuss foods high in fiber. Try to identify one that patient approves. Provide oral hygiene before meals. Discuss role of alcohol as appetite suppressant, and physiologic damage of taking drink with no food in stomach.	Maintains present weight of 140 lbs and shows a gradual increase of 1 to 2 lbs by the end of the week Takes in between 1800 to 2200 calories per day Patient (and his sister) discuss the basic four food groups, list sample foods in each group, and plan a sample diet menu for 1 week post-discharge based on proper food nutrient exchanges Continues to eat quality breakfasts and identifies foods that can be eaten for snacks

NURSING DIAGNOSIS

Social isolation related to inadequate personal resources as evidenced by statements of "few friends," history of two divorces, and estranged relationships with brother and daughters

NURSING INTERVENTIONS	EVALUATION OF EXPECTED OUTCOMES
Assign the same caretaker to build a trusting relationship. Plan a 15-minute period every shift to sit with patient; if he does not talk, allow silence. Involve patient in planning his own care. Maintain on bed rest while acutely ill, but monitor for quality interactions. Discuss patient's living accommodations and lifestyle outside of hospital. Refer to social services for follow-up if necessary. Praise sister for visiting. Inquire into past friendships that hold potential for renewal.	Interacts in a positive manner (eye contact, pleasant voice) Expresses feelings toward significant persons in his life Identifies need to be involved with support groups Uses available resources States a plan to participate in social activities

KEY CONCEPTS

- A thorough bowel cleansing is necessary for study of the lower GI tract: clear liquid diet for 24 hours, laxatives, and enemas. Laxatives and liquids are necessary following barium studies to clear barium.
- Gastric decompression removes air and fluids from the upper gastrointestinal tract. The tube is secured to the nose to maintain position in the stomach.
- Intestinal decompression requires a tube that is not taped so it is free to descend into the lower gastrointestinal tract.
- Total parenteral nutrition is administered in a large vessel, and the rate of infusion must be kept constant because the solution is so high in glucose.
- When surgery involves the large bowel, antibiotics are given preoperatively to reduce the bacterial count and the risk of peritonitis postoperatively. This is commonly referred to as "sterilizing" the bowel, even though the bowel is not actually sterile as a result.
- After gastrointestinal surgery, the patient must be observed for resumption of normal function: return of bowel sounds, passing flatus, absence of distention, and nausea and vomiting.
- A normal, healthy stoma is red and moist and is visible above the surface of the skin. If it retracts below the skin or if changes in color occur, indicating ischemia and potential necrosis, notify the physician.
- A continent pouch ileostomy (Kock's pouch) does not require wearing a stoma pouch to collect stool because a reservoir has been created. It is drained continually until it heals, and eventually will need to be emptied only two or three times a day by inserting a tube.
- Severe dehydration and electrolyte imbalance can result from prolonged loss of GI secretions through diarrhea.
- The patient with anorexia nervosa or bulimia will require nutritional management and psychologic intervention.
- Crohn's disease (regional enteritis) involves sections of inflamed tissue anywhere in the GI tract, causing pain and diarrhea. It is possibly a disorder of lymphoid tissue. The patient is predisposed to abscess and fistula formation and bowel obstruction.
- Ulcerative colitis involves the colon and rectum, and the inflammation results in fibrosis and narrowing of the bowel lumen. Cancer of the colon is a complication in the long term. The patient has frequent, loose, bloody, mucoid stools with some mild cramping pain in the left lower quadrant.
- Patients with inflammatory bowel disease need support in dealing with complications and in handling the difficulties associated with frequent, loose, foul-smelling stools.
- Signs and symptoms of appendicitis typically include fever, elevated WBC, anorexia, nausea and vomiting, and pain in the lower right quadrant of the abdomen, halfway between the umbilicus and the crest of the ileum (McBurney's point) or near the umbilicus. Rebound tenderness may be present in the right lower quadrant.
- Diverticula are pouches of mucosa and submucosa that protrude or herniate through the circular muscles of the intestinal wall. A low-fiber diet may contribute to the development of diverticula.
- Diverticulitis occurs when fecal matter penetrates the thin-walled diverticula, resulting in inflammation and abscess formation outside the bowel. The patient will have mild to severe abdominal pain in the LLQ, fever, and elevated WBC and sedimentation rate. Septicemia and septicemic shock can develop if untreated.
- Symptoms of bowel obstruction include abdominal pain, distention, vomiting, and constipation. Shock may develop. A nasogastric tube may be inserted to remove gas and secretions. Surgery may be necessary.
- Cancer of the tongue is the most common type of tumor of the mouth, believed to be predisposed by irritation resulting from smoking; consumption of alcohol; dental appliances; and rough, jagged teeth. Leukoplakia (white patches) may be seen on the mucous membrane of the tongue or cheek.
- Dysphagia (difficulty in swallowing) is the prime symptom of cancer of the esophagus.
- Nursing management of the patient with a gastrostomy tube includes caring for the skin, maintaining patency of the tube, good oral care, and administering the prescribed feeding. Force should not be used to irrigate the tube if it becomes blocked.
- The bacteria *Helicobacter pylori,* which is associated with chronic gastritis and peptic ulcer, is also a factor in developing cancer of the stomach. Diet is probably the most significant environmental factor.
- Evidence suggests that a low-fiber diet, rich in beef and saturated fats, leads to an increased incidence of colorectal cancer. Rectal bleeding is the most common symptom.
- Peptic ulcers are found in the stomach (gastric ulcers) and in the duodenum. Pain is a characteristic symptom, described as dull, burning, gnawing, or boring. It is located in the midline of the epigastric region. Gastric ulcer pain occurs 60 to 90 minutes after eating. Pain with duodenal ulcer occurs 2 to 4 hours after eating and is relieved by eating or antacids. There will be bright red bleeding or coffee-grounds emesis with hemorrhage and dark, tarry stools with slow bleeding.
- Pain with hernia signals the need for surgical intervention.

presence of stones, tumors, or any other pathologic condition is detected. Patient care is similar to cystoscopic examination and retrograde urography (Richard, 1986).

Urodynamic studies

Various tests exist that evaluate bladder function and all phases of voiding; for example, a cystometrography measures bladder pressure during bladder filling and voiding. The nurse should refer to Gray (1992) for a thorough explanation of these tests and patient care.

Radioisotope Studies

Renography

A small amount of radioactive material is administered intravenously; it circulates through the kidney and is excreted in the urine. This test measures renal function. A graphic record (renogram) is made that traces the radioisotope through the kidney and assesses renal blood flow, glomerular filtration, and tubular secretion. Patient preparation includes an explanation of the test and an assessment of the patient's ability to sit or lie quietly for 30 to 60 minutes. There is no special postexamination patient care.

Renoscan

The renoscan is a procedure that outlines the kidney by external scanning. After intravenous injection of a radioactive isotope, a scanning device, such as a scintillator, is passed over the patient's back directly above each kidney and counts the activity of the isotope. In the presence of tumors or nonfunctioning areas, the radioactive material will not be detected by the scan. Patient care is the same as for renography.

Ultrasonography

Ultrasound is a noninvasive procedure that provides almost immediate information. High-frequency sound waves are reflected over the desired body areas, transmitted to an oscilloscope, and recorded. There is no discomfort associated with ultrasound, but it is important to realize that the patient must be able to tolerate a prone position for approximately 30 minutes.

Computerized Tomography

Computerized tomography (CT) combines the basic principles of radiography with computer technology. Instead of broad x-ray beams passing through the patient to be captured on x-ray film, CT scanning uses a thin x-ray beam that is visualized on a computer screen. While the patient rests in a recumbent position, the thin x-ray beams are transmitted rapidly through the patient and assembled and integrated by digital computers. This information is developed into a cross-sectional image shown on the screen that gives a remarkable definition of body anatomy (Walsh, 1992).

Magnetic Resonance Imaging

Magnetic resonance imaging (MRI) is an imaging method that provides superior visual information about soft tissue. Short pulses of low-energy radio waves are introduced into the hydrogen nuclei of the tissue cells to create a magnetic field, and the resulting complex series of events is assembled as a tomogram that is far superior to the image provided by a CT scan (Richard, 1995a). It does not differentiate benign from malignant tumors. The patient must assume a recumbent position throughout the test.

Renal Biopsy

Tissue obtained from a renal biopsy is examined microscopically, which helps to determine the nature and extent of renal disease. Biopsy of renal tissue may be accomplished by the open or closed method. Both are invasive procedures that require sterile technique. An *open renal biopsy* requires an operation with general anesthesia. An incision is made, the kidney is exposed, the biopsy needle is inserted into the kidney, a piece of tissue is extracted, and the area is closed and sutured.

The procedure for a *closed renal biopsy* (also called a percutaneous renal biopsy) is as follows. A local anesthetic is given, and the patient is placed in a prone position with a pillow under the abdomen. A patient who has undergone a kidney transplant is positioned to maximize access to the transplanted kidney, which is usually in the groin area. The patient is instructed to hold his or her breath while the biopsy needle is inserted through the skin and into the kidney. Confirmation that the needle is in the kidney is provided when the needle moves when the patient breathes, because the kidneys are in contact with the diaphragm and move with ventilation. A small fragment of tissue is obtained and the needle is withdrawn. After a specimen is obtained, pressure must be applied to the site along with a pressure dressing.

With either method of renal biopsy, hemorrhage is the most common complication. The patient must maintain bedrest for 24 hours in a supine position with a pressure dressing. The patient is assessed for pain and given analgesics as needed. Vital signs are evaluated often, as is the biopsy site and the dressing. The patient is encouraged to drink fluids to keep the urine diluted and prevent clot formation in the kidney, which could obstruct urine flow. Urine is evaluated for hematuria. The patient is also observed for signs and symptoms of urinary tract infection (Richard, 1995a). The patient may be fearful of the possible diagnosis, and waiting for the biopsy results may be stressful. Hence the nurse provides emotional support during this time.

THERAPEUTIC PROCEDURES AND NURSING IMPLICATIONS

Diuretics

Diuretics are substances and/or drugs that increase the urinary output. The excretion of large amounts of urine is **polyuria,** and polyuria after the administration of a diuretic is called **diuresis.** Diuretics have different physiologic actions in the kidney and are classified according to their actions, whether the action occurs in the nephron, and if the diuretics are potassium-sparing or potassium-depleting. The more thoroughly renal physiology is understood, the easier it is to understand the action and side effects of diuretics and to take care of patients receiving them.

Table 24-2 lists several diuretics. Alcohol and caffeine suppress the release of antidiuretic hormone (ADH) from the pituitary gland. When ADH is not present in the collecting duct, a copious dilute urine is secreted. Spironolactone (Aldactone) inhibits aldosterone from causing sodium reabsorption and potassium secretion in the distal tubule. Because sodium attracts water, excess water is excreted with the sodium. Potassium is reabsorbed and not excreted in excess in the urine. Ethacrynic acid (Edecrin) and furosemide (Lasix) inhibit the reabsorption of sodium, primarily in the ascending loop of Henle, and increase potassium excretion. An elevated concentration of electrolytes in the nephron attracts water, which increases the fluid volume and flow rate and decreases potassium reabsorption in the distal tubule (Shannon, Wilson, 1992).

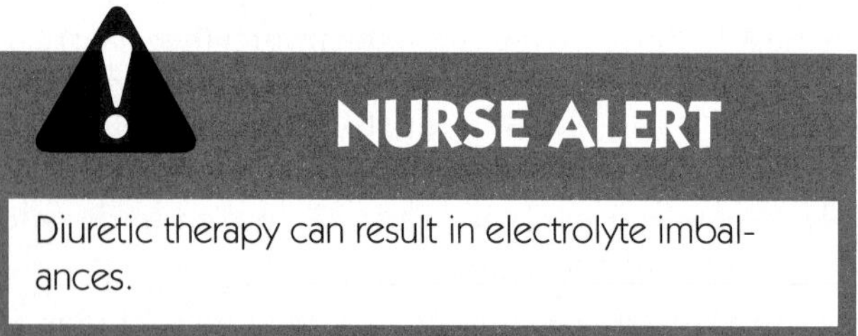

Diuretic therapy can result in electrolyte imbalances.

Major side effects of diuretics are an exaggeration of their physiologic actions. For instance, all diuretics cause **polyuria,** and with prolonged polyuria there is water loss that can result in a fluid volume deficit. Dehydration, therefore, is an important side effect that nurses and patients need to watch for. Signs and symptoms of fluid volume deficit are decrease in weight, concentrated urine, hard stool, sunken eyeballs, dry mouth, poor skin turgor, dizziness, orthostatic hypotension, increased hematocrit, and increased plasma osmolality. If a fluid volume deficit becomes severe enough, blood flow to the kidney can be so reduced that renal failure results (Kellick, 1992; Richard, 1995b).

The most reliable method for assessing body fluid changes is by weight. The patient should be weighed daily and, if possible, fluid intake and output should be recorded. The patient should be weighed at the *same* time each day with the *same* amount of clothing and on the *same* scale. A good time to weigh is usually before breakfast, after the bladder has been emptied. The nurse should balance the scale before each weighing and should use a metric scale, if possible, because it is easier to calculate fluid changes on a metric scale. Fluid intake and output changes should correlate with daily weight changes. For example, if the weight change from one day to the next is a loss of 1 kg, then the fluid change should also be a loss of 1 L (1 kg = 1 L = 2.2 lbs).

Patients should be taught how to weigh themselves and how to record fluid intake and output. Patients should also be taught about the action, onset, and duration of diuretics so they will not be alarmed at the increased voiding and will know when to expect it and how long it will last. Diuretics are administered at certain times so that the patient's sleep is not disturbed.

Most diuretics cause potassium depletion by interfering with its reabsorption. Some diuretics directly affect the potassium reabsorbing mechanisms. Other diuretics, especially those that act proximal to the distal tubule, increase the volume of fluid in the nephron. An expanded fluid volume increases the fluid flow rate, which sweeps potassium and other substances along so fast that they do not have time to be reabsorbed.

The nurse is alert to signs and symptoms of hypokalemia, such as undue fatigue, weakness, loss of appetite, loss of muscle tone, muscle cramping in the legs, arrhythmias, constipation, and abdominal distention. Blood levels of potassium are evaluated often. Dietary and/or drug potassium supplements are given as needed (Guzzetta, Dossey, 1992; Lancaster, 1995; Shannon, Wilson, 1992).

Provision for Urinary Drainage

There are several types of urinary drainage procedures. The most common method is to allow the urine to flow by gravity. It is recommended that a closed drainage system be used for all patients needing urinary drainage. Closed systems have the drainage tube sealed to the container, whereas open systems are not sealed and allow air and microorganisms to enter the system freely.

TABLE 24-2

Pharmacology of Drugs Used for Urinary Disorders

Drug (Generic and Trade Name); Route and Dosage	Action/Indication	Common Side Effects and Nursing Considerations
ACETAZOLAMIDE (Diamox) **ROUTE:** PO, IV, IM **DOSAGE:** PO, glaucoma, 250-1000 mg/day in 1-4 divided doses or 500 mg/kg/day in 1-4 divided doses; IM, IV, 250-500 mg, may repeat in 2-4 hr	A carbonic anhydrase inhibitor used primarily as a diuretic to lower intraocular pressure in cerebral edema; also used as adjunct therapy in seizure disorders	Tiredness, weakness, metallic taste, anorexia, weight loss, and paresthesias; use with caution in diabetes and hepatic disease
BELLADONNA AND EXTRACT OF OPIUM (B & O Supprettes) **ROUTE:** Rectal **DOSAGE:** 1 q 3-4 hr/prn bladder spasms	Drug used in the treatment and management of bladder spasm pain	Use with caution in the addicted patient
BETHANECHOL (Urecholine) **ROUTE:** PO, SC **DOSAGE:** PO, 10-50 mg bid to qid; SC, 2.5 mg tid to qid	Drug used for urinary retention in postpartum and postoperative urinary retention resulting from neurogenic bladder	Heart block, abdominal discomfort, diarrhea, vomiting, salivation, urgency, flushing, and sweating; contraindicated in obstruction of the GI or GU tract; use with caution in asthma, ulcers, epilepsy, and hyperthyroidism
BUMETANIDE (Bumex) **ROUTE:** PO, IV **DOSAGE:** PO, 0.5-2 mg/day (up to 10 mg/day; larger doses may be required in renal insufficiency); IV, 0.5-1.0 mg, may give 1-2 more doses q 2-3 hr (not to exceed 10 mg/24 hr)	Drug used as a diuretic in edema secondary to congestive heart failure or hepatic or renal disease	Hypotension, hearing loss, metabolic alkalosis, hypovolemia, dehydration, hyponatremia, hypokalemia, hypochloremia, and hypomagnesemia; much more potent than lasix; use with caution in severe liver disease
CYCLOSPORINE (Sandimmune) **ROUTE:** PO, IV **DOSAGE:** PO, 15 mg/kg/day (first dose before transplant) for 1-2 weeks, taper by 5% weekly to maintenance dose of 5-10 mg/kg/day; IV, 5-6 mg/kg/day (⅓ PO dose) initially, change to PO as soon as possible	Drug used in the prevention and treatment of rejection in renal, cardiac, and hepatic transplantation (with glucocorticoids)	Tremor, hypertension, hirsutism, gingival hyperplasia, nausea, vomiting, diarrhea, nephrotoxicity, hepatotoxicity, infections, and hypersensitivity reactions; use with caution in severe hepatic impairment, renal impairment, and any active infection; in children, larger and more frequent doses may be required
EPOETIN ALFA (Epogen) **ROUTE:** IV, SC **DOSAGE:** SC, IV, 100 U/kg 3 times weekly initially, then adjust dosage by changes of 25 U/kg/dose to maintain target range of HCT; usual maintenance dose is 25 U/kg 3 times weekly	Drug used for the treatment of anemia associated with chronic renal failure; also used for the management of anemia secondary to AZT therapy in HIV-infected patients	Hypertension; contraindicated in uncontrolled hypertension; use with caution in history of seizures

continued

TABLE 24-2

Pharmacology of Drugs Used for Urinary Disorders—cont'd

Drug (Generic and Trade Name); Route and Dosage	Action/Indication	Common Side Effects and Nursing Considerations
FUROSEMIDE (Lasix) **ROUTE:** PO, IV **DOSAGE:** PO, IV, 20-80 mg/day initially (up to 600 mg may be necessary; doses up to 1 g/day have been used in CHF and renal failure); when maintenance dose is determined, dose may be given every other day 2-3 times weekly	Diuretic drug used in the management of edema secondary to congestive heart failure, hepatic, or renal disease; also used alone or in combination with antihypertensives in the treatment of hypertension	Metabolic acidosis, hypovolemia, dehydration, hyponatremia, hypokalemia, hypochloremia, and hypomagnesemia; use with caution in severe liver disease, electrolyte depletion, diabetes mellitus, and anuria or increasing azotemia
HYDROCHLOROTHIAZIDE (Hydro-chlor, Hypodiuril, Thiuretic Esidrex) **ROUTE:** PO **DOSAGE:** 25-100 mg/day in 1-2 doses (up to 200 mg/day); as a diuretic may be given every other day or 3-5 days/week	Diuretic drug used alone or in combination with other agents in the management of mild to moderate hypertension; also used alone or in combination in the treatment of edema associated with CHF, renal dysfunction, cirrhosis, and glucocorticoid and estrogen therapy	Hypokalemia and hyperuricemia; contraindicated in anuria; use with caution in renal or severe hepatic impairment
MANNITOL (Osmitrol) **ROUTE:** IV **DOSAGE:** 50-100 g as a 5%-25% solution; may precede with a test dose of 0.2 g/kg over 3-5 min	Diuretic drug used as an adjunct in the treatment of acute oliguric renal failure; also used as an adjunct in the treatment of edema and in the reduction of intraocular pressure	Transient volume expansion, hyponatremia, hypernatremia, hypokalemia, hyperkalemia, and dehydration; contraindicated in anuria, dehydration, and active intracranial bleeding
NEOSTIGMINE (Prostigmin) **ROUTE:** SC, IM **DOSAGE:** SC, IM, 250 μg-500 μg q 4-6 hr for 2-3 days for prevention and treatment of bladder atony and abdominal distention	Used in the prevention and treatment of postoperative bladder distention and urinary retention or ileus; also used to increase muscle strength in myasthenia gravis	Excess secretions, bronchospasm, bradycardia, abdominal cramps, nausea, vomiting, diarrhea, excess salivation, and sweating; contraindicated in mechanical obstruction of the GI or GU tract; use with caution in asthma, ulcers, cardiac disease, epilepsy, hyperthyroidism, and pregnancy
PHENAZOPYRIDINE (Pyridium) **ROUTE:** PO **DOSAGE:** 200 mg tid for 2 days	Drug used to provide relief from urinary tract symptoms that may occur in association with infection or following urologic procedures; symptoms include pain, itching, burning, urgency, and frequency	Bright-orange urine; contraindicated in glomerulonephritis, severe hepatitis, uremia, or renal insufficiency or failure
SPIRONOLACTONE (Aldactone) **ROUTE:** PO **DOSAGE:** 25-400 mg/day in 2-4 divided doses	Diuretic drug most commonly used to counteract potassium loss induced by other diuretics in the management of edema or hypertension	Nausea, vomiting, diarrhea, and hyperkalemia; contraindicated in hyperkalemia, renal insufficiency, menstrual abnormalities, or breast enlargement; use with caution in hepatic dysfunction and in the elderly or debilitated

Collection sets in widespread use contain sterile drainage tubing that is permanently connected to plastic containers. Most containers are flexible bags that have drains at the bottom of the bags to allow the urine to be emptied frequently. The end of the drain is protected by a cap, and the tube is fastened to the container when it is not being used. Most containers have valves at the top where the drainage tubing enters, to prevent bacteria from invading the drainage tubing and traveling upward toward the urethra and bladder. Filter air vents are also located on the top of the containers and allow air to enter the system but prevent bacteria in the air from contaminating the urine. All collection containers have bed hangers, which keep the containers in an upright position and off the floor (Figure 24-5).

NURSE ALERT

Urinary drainage catheters should remain patent and allow free flow of urine.

Inserting a bladder catheter

The nurse should use standard (universal) precautions throughout the procedure. The nurse should explain the procedure to the patient, including the fact that catheterization usually does not hurt. Pain could be associated with a lower urinary tract obstruction and must be reported to a physician. Occasionally during catheter insertion men will tighten their muscles, and resistance will be felt as the catheter is advanced. Men say this is uncomfortable and even painful. Deep slow breathing helps people relax.

Although most bladder catheter insertion sets contain the equipment necessary, the nurse should read the list of what is in the set before beginning the procedure. A good light source is essential. The perineal area is washed with soap and water and dried. The patient is positioned as comfortably as possible, with the head of the bed as flat as possible. The legs and abdomen are draped with a sheet, and only the perineal area is exposed. The nurse should bring the bed up to the center of gravity, about waist level, so that good body mechanics can be used to reach the area.

Sterile technique should be used to insert the catheter. The nurse should open the insertion set following the manufacturer's directions. The nurse should put on a mask, if necessary, don gloves, and assess all the equipment in the set (e.g., fill the balloon with the sterile solution to make sure it does not leak and then deflate the balloon). The nurse should position all the cleaning items, lubricating jelly, catheter, and other equipment so that they can easily be reached with one hand. The nurse should tell the patient what is being done throughout the procedure. With a female, the labia should be separated with one hand, and the urinary meatus area should be cleansed with single strokes that go from anterior to posterior. The goal is to get the urinary meatus as clean as possible. The area should be cleansed 3 to 5 times. With a male, the penis should be held slightly upward and the foreskin retracted if present. The urinary meatus should be cleansed 3 to 5 times.

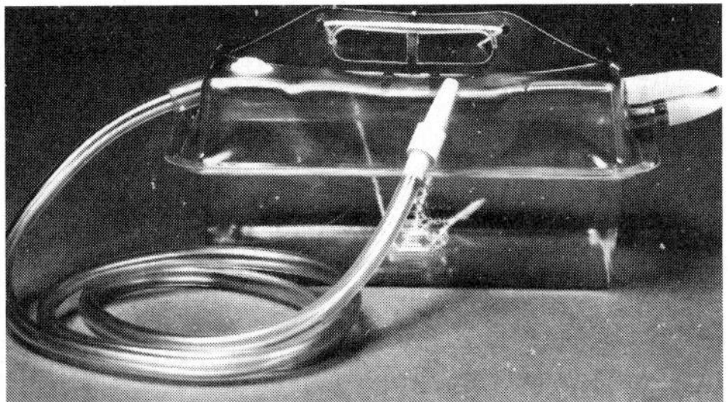

Figure 24-5 Urinary collection set. Drain box container. (Courtesy Abbott Laboratories, North Chicago, Ill.)

Once the urinary meatus is cleansed, the nurse should lubricate the bladder catheter, insert it into the meatus, and gently push it through the urethra until urine appears in the drainage tubing. The nurse should push the catheter a little further and hold it there until the balloon has inflated. The drainage tubing should be secured to the thigh, and the rest of the tubing should be positioned so that it is without kinks and lower than the bladder. The drainage bag should be positioned so that it is lower than the tubing and off the floor. The nurse should lower the bed into its lowest position and make the patient safe and comfortable. The nurse should observe and record the urine characteristics and the patient's response to the procedure.

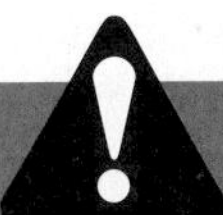

NURSE ALERT

Bladder catheterization is done using only sterile technique and only when absolutely necessary.

Catheter care

Most bladder catheters are made of rubber, whereas drainage tubing is clear plastic. Determination of urine clarity or color should be made by observing the urine in the tubing; the urine collected in the drainage bag does not give an accurate assessment. Specimens must only be taken from the port with a sterile syringe.

Patients whose condition necessitates the presence of indwelling catheters over extended periods are very susceptible to infection. This is especially true of chronically ill patients. A point to remember to help prevent infection is that the catheter should provide free flow of urinary drainage and should be comfortable for the patient. It should be secured to the inner upper thigh in females to eliminate tension on the bladder, and laterally to the thigh or lower abdomen in males to avoid pressure on the urethra at the penoscrotal junction, which can cause the formation of a fistula. The drainage tubing may be placed over the thigh, downward between the legs, or under the patient's leg near the popliteal space. Excess tubing should be coiled on the bed and not allowed to loop below the collection container. Many collection sets provide an apparatus so that the tubing may be attached to the sheets in a proper manner. Care must be taken that the tubing does not become kinked or obstructed. If the urine flow is blocked, stasis occurs and provides a good medium for bacteria to grow. The entire system should remain sterile and should not be disconnected. The collection set and tubing should not be lifted or elevated because drainage may flow back into the bladder.

Using a catheter of the proper size is also important. If the catheter is too small, leakage may occur around it; if it is too large, it may be uncomfortable for the patient. Retention catheters are available in various sizes, with balloons of 30- and 5-ml capacity. For most patients a size 16 or 18 French catheter with a 5-ml balloon is satisfactory and will be both comfortable and adequate for free drainage. Often when a 30-ml balloon is used, the tip of the catheter may bend on the balloon and obstruct the flow of urine.

Free urinary drainage is facilitated when the patient receives adequate amounts of fluid. Adequate fluid intake helps prevent accumulation of mucus, minerals, and exudate, which may adhere to the catheter and cause obstructions. Adequate fluids also eliminate the necessity for irrigation. Crusts and secretions around the vulva or penis and around the catheter should be removed, and the general area should be cleansed as needed. There are differing opinions about cleansing methods, but washing the area gently with soap and water is now thought to be adequate. Trauma to the meatus should be avoided.

When it is necessary for patients to have retention catheters indefinitely, the catheter and its tubing should be changed every 7 to 10 days or more often if it becomes encrusted with organic deposits.

Pyelostomy, nephrostomy, ureteral, and cystostomy catheters

Several surgical procedures are performed on the urinary system in which the patient will return from the operating room with a catheter placed in the *kidney pelvis (pyelostomy)* or in the kidney **(nephrostomy).** The nephrostomy catheter or tube is brought out through an incision in the flank and sutured to the skin (Figure 24-6). *Ureteral catheters* are passed through the urethra and bladder and to the ureters and the kidney pelvis.

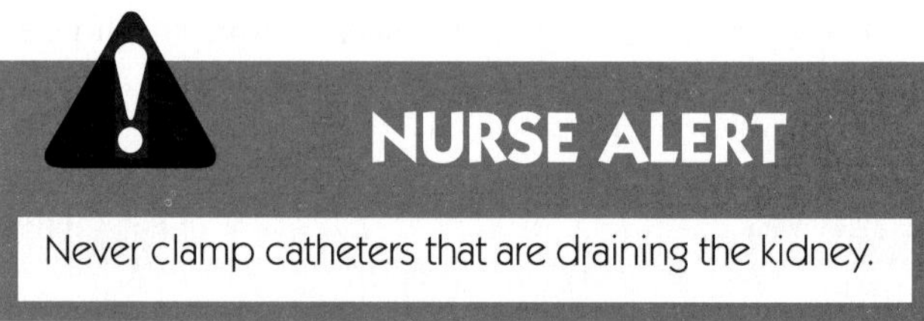

NURSE ALERT
Never clamp catheters that are draining the kidney.

These catheters are attached to free drainage. Any catheter placed in the kidney pelvis is never clamped because obstructing the flow of urine causes increased pressure in the kidney pelvis, resulting in hydronephrosis and subsequent damage to the kidney. Care must be taken to prevent any displacement of these catheters because reinsertion may not be possible. The nurse should observe the catheters often to be sure they are opening and draining, and any evidence of failure to drain must be reported to the physician immediately. All drainage is measured and recorded.

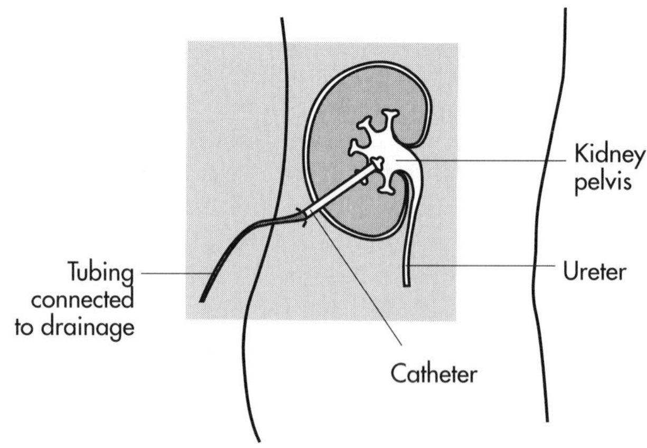

Figure 24-6 A nephrostomy catheter in the kidney pelvis. The catheter is brought out through a skin incision in the flank, sutured to the skin, and connected to tubing and gravity drainage.

Sometimes a catheter is placed in the bladder through an abdominal incision (**cystostomy** or *suprapubic tube*) and is attached to drainage at the bedside. All the equipment that is used for pyelostomy, nephrostomy, and ureteral and cystostomy drainage must be kept sterile (Table 24-3).

Catheter irrigation

A physician's order is needed for catheter irrigation. If the fluid intake is adequate and no blood clots occur, it should not be necessary to irrigate the urethral catheter unless the procedure is specifically ordered. Thirty milliliters of physiologic saline solution, 0.9% NaCl, is usually sufficient to determine the patency of the catheter. After irrigation, the solution should return by gravity. If the irrigating fluid flows in well but does not return, a clot is usually present at the end of the catheter. The nurse should remember that catheter irrigation is done to keep the catheter open and draining and not to irrigate the bladder.

If the patient has a bilateral pyelostomy and irrigations are ordered, separate equipment must be maintained for each catheter. The irrigating equipment and solution must be sterile; only 2 to 3 ml is used for the irrigation, depending on the physician's order. The solution must be injected with extreme care and gentleness, and its return by gravity should be observed. Failure of the solution to return must be reported, and additional solution should not be injected.

If a urethral catheter needs frequent irrigation, it may be practical to set up closed intermittent irrigation using a Y connector (Figure 24-7). A bottle of sterile irrigating solution is elevated on a stand, and sterile tubing leads from the irrigating solution to the Y connector, which is attached to the catheter. The third arm of the Y connector is attached to the drainage tubing. By releasing a clamp on the tubing to the irrigating solution, the nurse allows the desired amount of solution to flow into the patient's bladder. A clamp on the drainage tubing prevents the solution from immediately draining into the collection set. When the desired solution has entered the bladder, that clamp is turned off, and the clamp on the drainage tubing is released, allowing the solution to drain from the bladder under force of gravity. The drainage tubing is left unclamped until the next irrigation. The physician will order the kind of solution, the amount, and the interval for irrigation.

If continuous irrigation is necessary, the patient must have a triple-lumen Foley catheter (or a cystostomy tube and a urethral catheter) in the bladder to provide for continuous flow into and out of the bladder. The irrigation equipment is the same except that a drip-o-meter may be attached to the irrigating solution to regulate the rate of flow; the drainage tubing is left unclamped. In both intermittent and continuous closed bladder irrigation, it is important to keep an accurate record of the amount of irrigating solution used and to subtract this amount from the measurement of total drainage.

Catheter removal

Removal of the indwelling bladder catheter is preceded by explaining the procedure to the client and collecting all equipment: gloves, absorbent pad (e.g., chux, blue pad, or several paper towels), syringe, and bedside commode, urinal, and/or bedpan if the person is unable to get to a toilet. The syringe should be the same size or larger than the balloon on the catheter. Usually the volume of the balloon is printed on the port that leads to the balloon.

The nurse should use standard (universal) precautions during the entire procedure. The nurse should wash hands, provide privacy, and place the commode, urinal, and/or bedpan within close reach. The nurse should don gloves and place the absorbent pad under the catheter and drainage tube and between the client's legs. The nurse should deflate the balloon by attaching the syringe to the balloon port and aspirating the fluid from the balloon. The nurse should ensure that the balloon is entirely deflated by pulling strongly on the plunger of the syringe. A partially inflated balloon can injure the urinary tract as the catheter is removed. The nurse should gently untape the catheter from the skin, place one hand under the absorbent pad, and hold the catheter with the other hand. The patient should be informed that the catheter is about to be removed. The nurse should ask the patient to take a long, deep breath through the nose and to slowly exhale through the mouth while the nurse gently pulls out the catheter. The purpose of the breathing exercise is to relax the patient. The absorbent pad is wrapped around the catheter, the amount of urine in the collection bag is measured and recorded. The catheter is inspected, and the physician is notified if it is not intact.

After the catheter is removed, the client is instructed about and observed for urinary incontinence and retention. With prolonged bladder catheterization, the bladder is continually emptied and hence does not have an opportunity to function as a muscle, loses tone, and needs time to recover. Additionally, the urethral muscular sphincters, forced open by the presence of the catheter, lose tone and need time to recover. The loss of bladder and sphincter tone can result in a variety of situations. Flaccid bladder and sphincters result

TABLE 24-3

Urinary Drainage Systems

Catheter and Origin	Irrigation	Clamp
Indwelling bladder catheter	Only if needed to assess or maintain patency; use sterile equipment with each irrigation; approximately 30 ml of sterile normal saline or an amount as ordered; gently instill saline and let it gravity drain.	To obtain specimen or as ordered, for example, with bladder retraining
Cystostomy catheter (suprapubic tube)	If necessary to disconnect system, close three-way stopcock before disconnecting to maintain column of urine in catheter and to maintain siphon action.	On physician's order the suprapubic tube may be clamped 4 hours, then drained 30 minutes so bladder fills, and patient attempts to void through urethra while the tube is clamped
Ureteral catheters (through bladder and ureters to kidney pelvis)	Irrigate according to physician's order; irrigate with 2 or 3 ml of sterile solution	Never
Pyelostomy (kidney pelvis)	Only with physician's order; use 2 or 3 ml of sterile solution as ordered; irrigate gently with gravity return; separate sterile equipment for each catheter	Never
Nephrostomy (kidney)	Only with physician's order and sterile equipment	Never

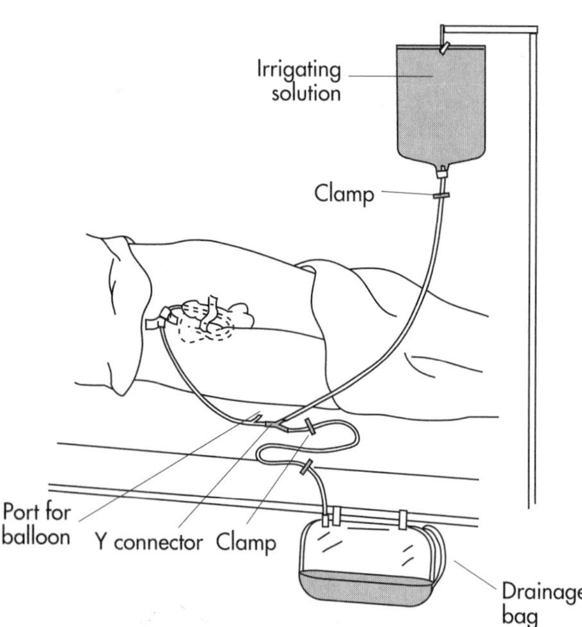

Figure 24-7 Retention catheter inserted for urinary drainage and a closed system with Y connector for intermittent irrigation. Continuous irrigation requires a triple lumen catheter. One lumen is for irrigating solution instillation, another lumen is for urine and irrigation solution drainage, and a third lumen is for instilling fluid to inflate the balloon.

in incomplete bladder emptying and dribbling of urine. Sphincters that contract produce urinary retention. A contracted bladder with decreased capacity can result in frequent urination.

The nurse should encourage the patients to assist in keeping a record/diary of the amount and appearance of urine and the time voided. Patients should be taught about the micturition process and that it is important to maintain their hydration status by drinking a glass of water every 1 to 2 hours. Patients should be encouraged to void every 1 to 2 hours, and to do Kegel exercises four times a day to strengthen the muscles used in urination. A Kegel exercise is done correctly when one can stop and start the flow of urine. These exercises, however, must be done when the patient is not urinating.

Sometimes the patient is unable to void normally, and catheterization and/or replacement of the retention catheter may be necessary. The patient may void only small amounts because the bladder cannot empty completely. The bladder capacity is temporarily decreased and the patient complains of abdominal discomfort shortly after the catheter is removed because he or she is unable to void and the bladder is full.

Bladder muscle retraining may be helpful before removing a retention catheter. The catheter is clamped

Measuring Output	Drainage Tubing	Care of Site
Empty drainage bag every 8 hours or more often if filled to capacity.	Place over thigh and secure to avoid trauma to urethra; maintain closed system with drainage bag attached to beds.	Cleanse entire perineal area with soap and water as needed.
Empty drainage bag every 8 hours or more often if filled; measure and record voided urine on separate record if catheter is clamped and patient voids.	Secure to lower abdomen; attach catheter to closed drainage system.	Apply sterile dry dressing to site; dressing may become saturated from leaking urine.
Measure and record separately for each kidney; observe output hourly.	Tape to thigh; maintain closed system and patency.	Care as for bladder catheter if it enters meatus; apply sterile dry dressing if brought out on flank or abdomen.
Measure drainage from each kidney and record separately.	Secure to flank; maintain patency and closed system.	Apply sterile dry dressing; change often to keep dry.
Measure drainage and record separately.	Secure to flank; maintain patency and closed system.	Apply sterile dry dressing; change often to keep dry.

and unclamped on a schedule for 12 to 48 hours. For instance, the catheter is clamped for 1 hour and then unclamped for 5 to 15 minutes for 4 to 6 hours. The catheter is clamped for two hours and then unclamped for 5 to 15 minutes for 6 to 8 hours, and so on (Mondoux, 1994).

If blood appears in the urine (hematuria) after a bladder catheter is removed, the physician is notified. It is often necessary to maintain fluid intake and output records for several days, especially if the client has had urinary tract surgery.

Patient and family teaching

Many patients are dismissed from the hospital to their homes with indwelling catheters, draining wounds, and permanent appliances. There should be a planned program that teaches the patient self-care insofar as he or she is competent. This includes three steps: (1) observation, (2) participation, and (3) practice under supervision. The patient will observe the nurse in the various procedures; at the same time the nurse explains, step by step, what is being done and the reason for it.

As the patient is able, he or she begins to assist the nurse or participate in the procedures, gradually assuming more and more of the care. Finally the nurse allows the patient to give all the care while observing to correct any mistakes and provide positive feedback.

When the patient leaves the hospital, he or she should feel secure about knowing what to do and how to do it. There may be catheters or dressings that the patient cannot reach, and a member of the family or another person should be instructed in the care. In addition, hospitals should provide written instructions with a list of the home equipment needed for the patient or the family. In planning care for patients with urologic conditions, it has been found that each patient has her or his own special needs.

There should be a referral system between the hospital and the home health agency, and when it can be arranged, the home health nurse should visit the patient in the hospital before discharge. Information should be available to the home health nurse concerning the care needed and the instructions given the patient. The home health nurse will supervise or assist with the necessary care after discharge. The continuity of care between the hospital and the home provides a feeling of security for the patient and facilitates the process of rehabilitation.

URINARY INCONTINENCY

Urinary incontinency is the inability to retain urine and is a symptom and not a disease. Urinary incontinency can be temporary or permanent. There are many causes for incontinence, including side effects from drugs. Physiologic reasons could include injury or disease to some part of the urinary pathway such as the bladder, sphincters, spinal cord, and cortex. There could be psychologic or emotional reasons such as fear, stress, a feeling of loss of control of one's life, sorrow, and excitement. Table 24-4 summarizes the different types and causes of urinary incontinencies.

It is important to assess carefully for the cause of urinary incontinency and not just assume that it is some incurable physical problem. It may require multiple conversations with the person to determine the cause. Some people are uncomfortable and even ashamed to discuss their elimination problems because they think that urine is a socially unacceptable topic related to sex. The urinary tract is part of the male reproductive tract and very close to the female reproductive tract. Many people are uncomfortable discussing anything that remotely relates to sex. People believe myths, such as the belief that with aging one will automatically become incontinent of urine. People are humiliated and devastated by incontinency because they feel like an infant who cannot control urination. They feel that adults are supposed to void in appropriate places at appropriate times.

Urinary incontinency is a sensitive emotional and physical problem that must be approached with compassion and solved professionally. The nurse should sit down, provide privacy, express concern about their incontinency, and encourage them to vent their feelings. The nurse should demonstrate listening by repeating back to them what they have said using their words. The nurse should ask clients the following questions: When did the incontinency start? What does the incontinency mean to you? Is it a problem for you? How has it altered your life? How do you think it can be changed? Do you want help with the incontinency? The nurse should encourage the person to keep a diary of when the incontinency occurs and the feelings associated with it. The information can help to identify the cause. Patients may need to undergo an examination and physical tests of the urinary tract to assess for a cause of incontinency.

Some general goals or outcomes of care for the person with urinary incontinency are to maintain self-esteem, self-worth, skin integrity, and fluid balance or hydration, as well as to increase knowledge of micturition and incontinency. When incontinency occurs, the

TABLE 24-4

Classification of Urinary Incontinency

Type	Cause	Description
Functional incontinency	Impaired mobility, musculoskeletal function, cognitive function, and physical and environmental barriers to toilet facilities	Urinary tract is intact and functional; unable to reach toilet facilities in time to void
Stress incontinency	Urinary sphincter dysfunction and/or weak pelvic floor muscles associated with obesity, multiple pregnancies, and prostatectomy surgery	Involuntary loss of urine with increased intraabdominal pressure such as coughing, sneezing, laughing, and straining with a bowel movement and with physical exertion such as lifting and jumping;
Urge incontinency	Involuntary bladder contractions associated with neurologic disorders (CVA and Parkinson's disease), bladder irritation (infection and tumors), and large intake of alcohol and caffeine	Feels the urge to void, and shortly afterward has an involuntary loss of urine; incontinence can occur as often as every 2 hours
Reflex incontinency	Disease and/or trauma to the spinal cord above the sacral micturition center at S2-S4 associated with spinal cord disease (tumor and injury) and multiple sclerosis	Constant loss of urine without the sensation to void
Overflow incontinency	Bladder is overdistended and has not emptied completely because of an obstruction in the lower urinary tract associated with an enlarged prostate gland or constricted urethra	Continual and/or persistent loss of urine; also referred to as dribbling

nurse should treat the person with respect. The skin should be cleaned with soap and water and patted dry. Cornstarch can be applied to decrease skin irritation. The nurse should change clothes and bed linens immediately and wash them or send them to the laundry. Urine containers should be emptied immediately and the room should be kept well ventilated. These interventions will help keep the environment clean. The nurse should offer to take the patient to the toilet or offer the bedpan or urinal to prevent incontinency. The nurse should encourage hourly fluids, except for the 2 hours before sleep, which helps maintain fluid balance, keeps the urine dilute, decreases fabric staining, odors, and skin irritation (Gray, 1992; Mondoux, 1994).

The nurse should set goals with the patient and create an individualized program based on what is most important to the patient. Many people socially isolate themselves, change their lifestyle drastically, decrease their fluid intake to dangerously low levels so that they will urinate less, and worry about incontinency all the time. Instead of worrying and imagining themselves being incontinent, patients can visualize and imagine their urinary tracts being healthy and being continent.

If hospitalized, patients may feel that they are a nuisance and are sometimes treated as such by the staff; they are put in diapers and further humiliated. The diapers cause skin breakdown, which is very painful to the patient and increases hospital stay and staff work. Some people are immediately catheterized and then are at risk for urinary tract infection, which is dangerous, costly, and enhances urinary incontinency. Only as a last intervention should an absorbent pad be used with incontinency. The pad should be small, covering the perineal area only, and be changed whenever wet or every 2 hours to preserve skin integrity.

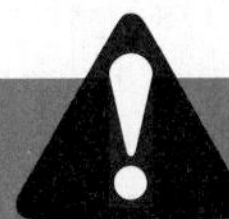

NURSE ALERT

Urinary incontinency, an inability to retain urine, is a symptom requiring investigation and is not a disease.

DISEASES AND DISORDERS OF THE URINARY SYSTEM

Pathogenic organisms may gain entrance to the urinary tract by the blood stream or from infections elsewhere in the body. The result may be an inflammatory process or an infection that may spread from the urethra upward to other parts of the system. Obstructions may occur along the tract from stones, strictures, tumors, or a kinked ureter. Tumors, either benign or malignant, may result in serious injury to the bladder, urethra, or kidneys. Injuries elsewhere in the body may also affect the kidney. Some diseases of the kidney may be the result of allergic factors, and others may be the result of degenerative changes.

Noninfectious Diseases

Glomerulonephritis is a term that encompasses several conditions affecting the glomerular capillaries of the kidney. Early classifications were based on the clinical picture of the disease. Since the advent of percutaneous renal biopsy and sophisticated techniques of electron microscopy, the newer classifications of the glomerulopathies are based on histologic and immunologic findings.

Acute poststreptococcal glomerulonephritis

Pathophysiology. Acute poststreptococcal glomerulonephritis (APSGN) is usually preceded by a recent infection of the pharynx or the skin (impetigo) caused by beta-hemolytic streptococcus. Antibodies develop and combine with an unknown antigen, possibly a protein (M) of the streptococcus, and form an *immune complex*. These immune complexes become trapped in the glomerular basement membrane (GBM) and cause inflammation. The inflammatory response in the glomeruli results in the passage of red blood cells and protein into the urine.

It is not yet known why some people develop the immune complex and APSGN after a streptococcal infection and others do not. The disease is most common in children, appears suddenly, and usually clears up with no residual damage. It may progress to a chronic form of the disease, however, when the patient is an adult.

Assessment. Urine output is reduced (oliguria) and will be rusty colored from the presence of red blood cells. Edema results from increased capillary permeability and is seen in the face, eyelids, and hands in the morning and in the legs at night. A significant number of patients have circulatory congestion from fluid and sodium retention, resulting in dyspnea, cough, and pulmonary edema. Protein is found in urine, but blood levels of protein remain normal. The BUN and serum creatinine levels will be increased. Most patients will have mild to moderate hypertension at the onset that diminishes as the body eliminates the excess fluid.

Some cases will be more severe, resulting in **anuria** (absence of production of urine) and subsequent uremia. The prognosis is favorable if there is no preexisting renal disease or if proteinuria is not heavy or persistent. Patients may have some urinary abnormalities for several years after recovery. Follow-up studies are now revealing residual pathologic conditions, but evidence is not conclusive. Adults who develop the disease are more likely to develop chronic renal disease as a complication, resulting in end-stage renal failure (Beare, Myers, 1994).

Intervention. Treatment of acute glomerulonephritis is aimed at relieving the symptoms of hypertension, circulatory congestion, and edema. The patient will probably be allowed as much activity as can be tolerated. Bedrest is indicated in the acute stage until hematuria and proteinuria subside.

Fluids and sodium are restricted if there is circulatory congestion or hypertension. Diuretics can be used, but vigorous diuresis and dehydration should be avoided. Antihypertensives are used to reduce the elevated blood pressure. Treatment of hypertension prevents additional damage to the renal microvasculature. Protein intake must be restricted if nitrogenous protein waste levels in the blood become increased (azotemia), but vigorous protein restriction is avoided.

Steroids and cytotoxic agents may help control the deposition of immune complexes (Lancaster, 1995). Antibiotics do not help the patient but may be given to the family to prevent them from having the antibody reaction to the antigen associated with the preceding infection.

An increase in urine output and a corresponding weight loss signal improvement. The urine begins to clear itself of albumin and red blood cells, the blood pressure decreases, and the patient feels better. This usually begins about 3 weeks after the onset of the edema. When the weight and blood pressure are stable, edema and hematuria are gone, and the BUN level is decreased, dietary and activity restrictions may be lifted (Box 24-1).

Nephrotic syndrome (nephrosis)

Pathophysiology. The increased permeability of the glomeruli allows protein to leave the blood and enter the urine, producing proteinuria. The reduced serum protein level causes a decrease in plasma oncotic pressure. The inadequate plasma oncotic pressure reduces the natural force that draws fluid back into the capillary from the interstitial spaces. The excess fluid remaining in the interstitial space results in edema (see Chapter 8). An unknown factor stimulates hepatic lipoprotein synthesis, which results in hyperlipidemia. Cholesterol and low-density lipoproteins are the first to elevate, followed by triglyceride levels. Fatty casts are found in the urine.

Assessment. The term *nephrotic syndrome* is used to describe the patient with massive proteinuria, hyperlipidemia, hypoalbuminemia, and edema. The edema accompanying the nephrotic syndrome causes a puffy face, distended eyelids, a bloated abdomen (ascites), and swelling in the lower extremities. The skin may have a waxy pallor because of the edema.

The syndrome has multiple causes and is characterized by increased glomerular permeability, which results in protein and fat found in the urine. Nephrotic syndrome is not a disease but is a group of symptoms found in many diseases affecting the glomeruli. It occurs with some infectious diseases, poisoning from chemical substances, toxemia of pregnancy, shock resulting from external burns, and coronary occlusion and may follow a transfusion with incompatible blood. It is seen in membranous, proliferative glomerulonephritis and poststreptococcal glomerulonephritis. It is also found in diabetic glomerulosclerosis, systemic lupus erythematosus, renal vein thrombosis, syphilis, and some neoplastic conditions (Beare, Myers, 1994; McCance, Huether, 1994).

Intervention. Treatment usually consists of administration of diuretics to decrease the edema. Dietary restraints depend on the severity of the symptoms, but the diet should include high-protein foods and restrictions on sodium. Corticosteroids and cyclophosphamide (Cytoxan) are used in severe cases. Intravenous albumin is not usually administered because it is rapidly lost from the permeable glomeruli, but it may be used if edema is severe and generalized *(anasarca)*. The individual is encouraged to continue normal activity unless the edema is severe.

Prevention and control of infection are important because the patient is highly susceptible, and infection is one of the chief causes of death. Nursing care requires the monitoring of diuretic therapy; it includes weighing the patient daily as well as measuring the girth of the abdomen and extremities, intake and output, and the protein and sodium intake. The patient may be anorectic, and small frequent feedings may be necessary to ensure an adequate protein intake. The disorder may be acute or chronic, and the primary causative disease must be cured or controlled to relieve the condition.

Infectious Diseases

An infection can originate anywhere along the urinary tract and can spread from one area to any or all areas of the tract (Figure 24-8). Urinary tract infection (UTI) is a broad term that includes a variety of clinical diseases. Cystitis and pyelonephritis are discussed in the following sections.

The urinary tract has several defenses against infection. The major defense is micturition. Approximately 99% of all microbes are washed out with voiding, which is why it is so important for a person with a UTI to drink lots of fluids. Additionally, a large fluid intake can help to prevent a UTI. Other defenses are the acid-

BOX 24-1 **Nursing Process**

ACUTE POSTSTREPTOCOCCAL GLOMERULONEPHRITIS

ASSESSMENT

Recent sore throat or skin infection
Changes in urine volume and color
Signs and symptoms of edema
Elevated blood pressure, pulse, and respirations

NURSING DIAGNOSES

Activity intolerance related to fatigue and weakness secondary to renal dysfunction
Anxiety related to unknown prognosis
Impaired physical mobility related to inactivity secondary to prolonged bedrest
Fluid volume excess, edema related to decreased renal excretion
Knowledge deficit: signs and symptoms of fluid and electrolyte imbalance and side effects of corticosteroids and cytotoxic agents
Risk for infection related to increased susceptibility secondary to corticosteroid therapy, immobility, invasive procedures
Risk for impaired skin integrity related to edema, bedrest
Altered nutrition: less than body requirements, related to anorexia and restrictions of protein and sodium
Altered urinary elimination related to decreased renal excretion of potassium.

NURSING INTERVENTIONS

Maintain activity as tolerated.
Measure and record intake and output—report reduced output.
Measure urine output hourly if indwelling catheter present.
Observe urine for color and sediment and record.
Test urine for protein (albumin).
Restrict fluids as ordered, based on urinary output and body weight.
Restrict protein intake as ordered, based on blood levels of nitrogenous wastes and urine output.
Give high carbohydrate diet.
Check temperature, pulse, and respirations every 4 hours; report elevated temperature, galloping or irregular pulse, dyspnea, and coughing.
Check blood pressure every 4 hours—notify physician if systolic pressure is over 160 mm Hg or diastolic pressure is over 110 mm Hg.
Weigh patient daily.
Observe for edema and note location.
Measure abdomen daily to evaluate ascites.
Observe signs of hyperkalemia; administer ion resin exchanges for hyperkalemia.
Observe mental status at least once each shift and report changes, including confusion, headache, sleepiness, or tremors.
Institute seizure precautions if mental changes observed.
Teach patient about disease process and treatment.

EVALUATION OF EXPECTED OUTCOMES

Weight stable at level maintained before edema
Blood pressure stable
Urine negative for albumin and red blood cells
Absence of edema
Urine output appropriate for intake

ity and high osmolality of urine, which decreases bacterial growth; the bladder mucosa, which is somewhat resistant to bacterial attachment; prostate fluid, which contains an antibacterial substance; and the male urethra, which is longer than the female urethra.

NURSE ALERT

Urinary tract infections can best be prevented by drinking a lot of water and avoiding invasive urinary tract procedures.

Cystitis

Pathophysiology. **Cystitis** is an inflammation of the lining of the bladder. It may be acute or chronic and is more common in females than males. The female urethra is shorter and straighter than the male urethra and therefore is more easily contaminated. In addition, the prostatic secretions in the male have antibacterial properties. Cystitis may be caused by bacteria that enter through the urinary meatus, or it may occur through catheterization, during which organisms in the urethra are carried into the bladder. Cystitis in women can occur after sexual intercourse for unknown reasons. Infections may also be carried from the upper urinary tract, beginning with the kidney and involving the ureters and the bladder. In this instance

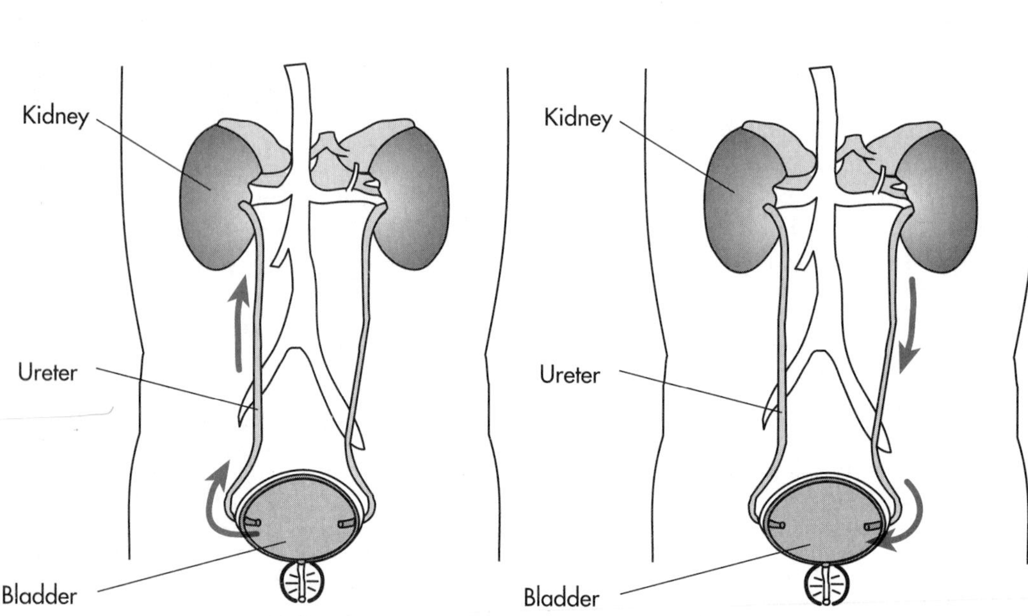

Figure 24-8 Urinary tract infection. **A,** Bacteria enter the bladder, ascend the ureter, and invade the kidney. **B,** Bacteria originate in the kidney and with micturition descend through the ureter and into the bladder. Arrows indicate the direction that bacteria can move. (From Richard CJ: *Comprehensive nephrology nursing,* Boston, 1986, Little, Brown.)

the infectious organism gains entrance to the kidney by way of the bloodstream. Cystitis may result from nonbacterial factors such as injury to the lining of the bladder caused by instruments or a catheter.

Assessment. Symptoms are frequent urination, including nocturia, severe pain and burning in the urethra with urination, and a sensation of bearing down or pressure in the bladder and suprapublic area. Examination of the urine may show the presence of pus and may reveal blood. Specific pathogenic organisms are often not found. (Phipps and others, 1995).

Intervention. The first criterion of treatment is to establish the cause of the problem. Antispasmodic drugs, sulfonamide or antibiotic drugs, and preparations to acidify the urine may be ordered. Nitrofurantoin (Macrodantin) inhibits bacterial enzymes, is effective against *Escherichia coli, Staphylococcus aureus,* and *Streptococcus faecalis* but can change urine to a brown color. (Shannon, Wilson, 1992). The patient is encouraged to drink water freely. Hot sitz baths and the application of heat to the abdomen may relieve pain. Phenazopyridine (Pyridium), a urinary antiseptic, may be given to relieve discomfort, but it can change the urine to orange and stain clothing.

Nursing interventions should include teaching the patient to prevent recurrence of cystitis. The patient should be instructed to have regular follow-up examinations to rule out the presence of asymptomatic infections and to take medications as prescribed with a full glass of water. The patient should be advised to continue taking medication for the full time prescribed, even though symptoms may be relieved or disappear. Women who experience frequent urinary tract infections should be instructed to do the following:

1. Cleanse the perineal area from front to back after each voiding and bowel movement.
2. Increase fluid intake and void every 2 to 3 hours during the day to empty the bladder and reduce growth of bacteria.
3. Void before and after sexual intercourse.
4. Wear absorbent cotton panties or those lined with cotton in the crotch.

Pyelonephritis

Pyelonephritis is an acute pyogenic infection involving the parenchyma in one or both kidneys. Although *pyelitis* (infection of the kidney pelvis) may occur alone, it is considered rare.

Pathophysiology. Pyelonephritis is caused by bacteria: the *Proteus* group, *E. coli,* and *Pseudomonas;* less common causes are the streptococcus and the staphylococcus bacteria. The infection may be brought to the kidney by the bloodstream or the lymphatic system

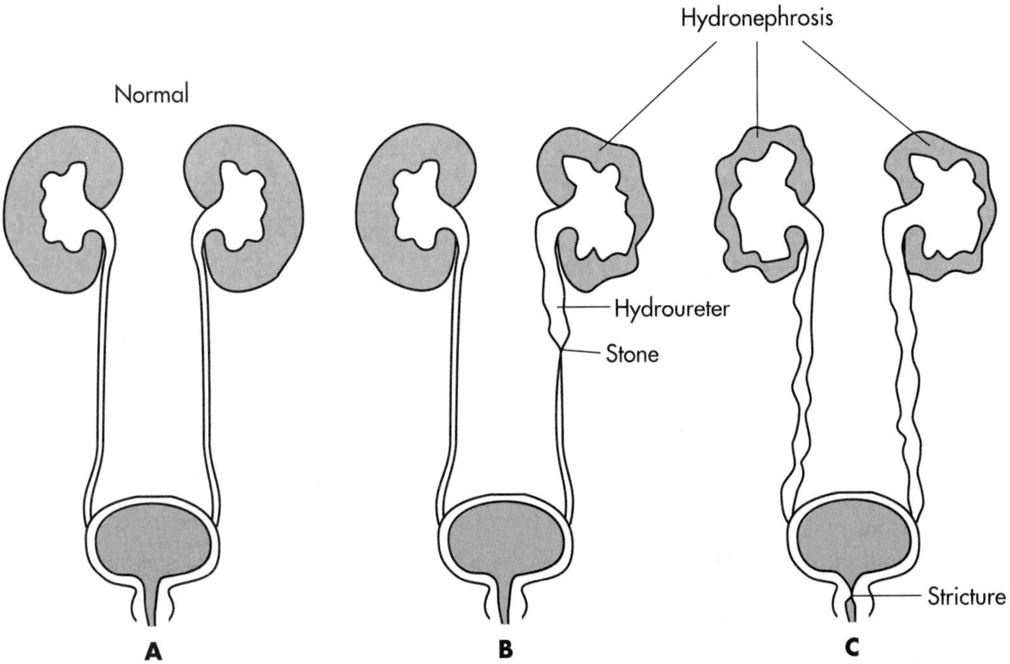

Figure 24-9 Obstructions of the urinary tract. Dilation occurs above the point of obstruction. **A,** Normal urinary tract. **B,** Unilateral urinary tract obstruction from a stone in the left ureter resulting in hydroureter and hydronephrosis. The right kidney and ureter are normal. **C,** Bilateral urinary tract obstruction from a urethral stricture as a result of an enlarged prostate gland; results in bilateral hydroureters and hydronephrosis. (From Phipps WJ and others: *Medical-surgical nursing,* ed 5, St Louis, 1995, Mosby.)

from infection elsewhere in the body. It may also spread upward from the bladder. Factors that contribute to the disorder include obstructions that restrict urinary flow and examinations, such as cystoscopy and catheterization. Pyelonephritis may occur in persons with some neurologic diseases or with conditions that require long periods of immobilization during which urinary calculi may develop.

Assessment. The kidney becomes edematous and inflamed, and the blood vessels are congested. The urine may be cloudy and contain pus, mucus, and blood. Small abscesses may form in the kidney. The diagnosis is made by microscopic examination of the urine and urine cultures; an intravenous urography may be done. The symptoms may occur abruptly with fever, chills, severe malaise, an elevated leukocyte count, aching, pyuria, and white blood cell cysts. There may or may not be pain in the back (Richard, 1995a).

Intervention. The treatment of the patient depends on locating and eliminating the cause. Sensitivity tests are done, and the appropriate antibiotic is administered. Bedrest is required during the acute period. Vital signs are recorded twice a day, and the patient is weighed daily. Fluid intake is encouraged, and all intake and output should be recorded. The patient should be observed for any difficulty in voiding, such as pain and burning. Urine should be observed for color. The patient should be kept warm and protected from drafts or chilling and respiratory tract infections.

With proper intervention, the patient with pyelonephritis has a normal temperature, urinalysis without abnormalities, no back or flank pain, and no fatigue.

Obstructions of the Urinary System

Obstructions of the urinary system may be caused by stones, tumors, kinking of a ureter, a congenital anomaly, or an enlarged prostate gland in a male (see Chapter 26) and be located anywhere from the kidney to the urinary meatus. Any prolonged obstruction will lead to serious anatomic and physiologic pathology.

With an obstruction, pressure develops in the urinary tract as urine backs up. The obstruction may be high enough to cause damage to the kidney, resulting in a decreased glomerular filtration rate; a decreased excretion of creatinine, urea, and other substances; and dilation of the kidney and/or ureter (Figure 24-9). Dilation of the kidney is called *hydronephrosis,* and dilation of the ureter is called *hydroureter*. Once hydronephrosis begins, it cannot be reversed. It can, however, be stopped by relieving the obstruction, which allows urine to flow freely. Hydroureter does not result in loss of function. Hydronephrosis, however, can result in renal failure as more and more kidney tissue is damaged (Figure 24-10) (Richard, 1995a).

Renal calculi

Pathophysiology. A stone is called a **calculus,** the formation of stones is called **lithiasis,** and the presence of stones in the kidney is called *nephrolithiasis.* When stones occur in any other part of the urinary system, the location determines the term used, as in ureteral calculi. The exact cause of the formation of renal calculi is unknown, but some factors that contribute to their formation are known. Paraplegic patients and patients who are required to remain on a regimen of bedrest for long periods are likely to develop calculi because of stasis of urine and the release of increased amounts of calcium from bone. Some common organisms that cause infection of the bladder and kidney cause the urine to become alkaline. Calcium phosphate, a compound readily excreted by the kidneys, cannot dissolve in the alkaline urine and will form crystals around a shred of tissue or other substance in the kidney, resulting in stone formation. Patients requiring continuous urinary drainage often will develop kidney or bladder stones as a complication. Pathologic disorders such as senile osteoporosis, gout, infection, hyperparathyroidism, and disorders affecting the pH and concentration of the urine are believed to be contributing factors.

Assessment. Stones may be like tiny gravel, and the patient may be asymptomatic. Large stones with irregular branches may be present in the kidney pelvis; they are known as *staghorn calculi* and require surgical intervention (Figure 24-11). When stones occur in the kidney, pain may be present on the involved

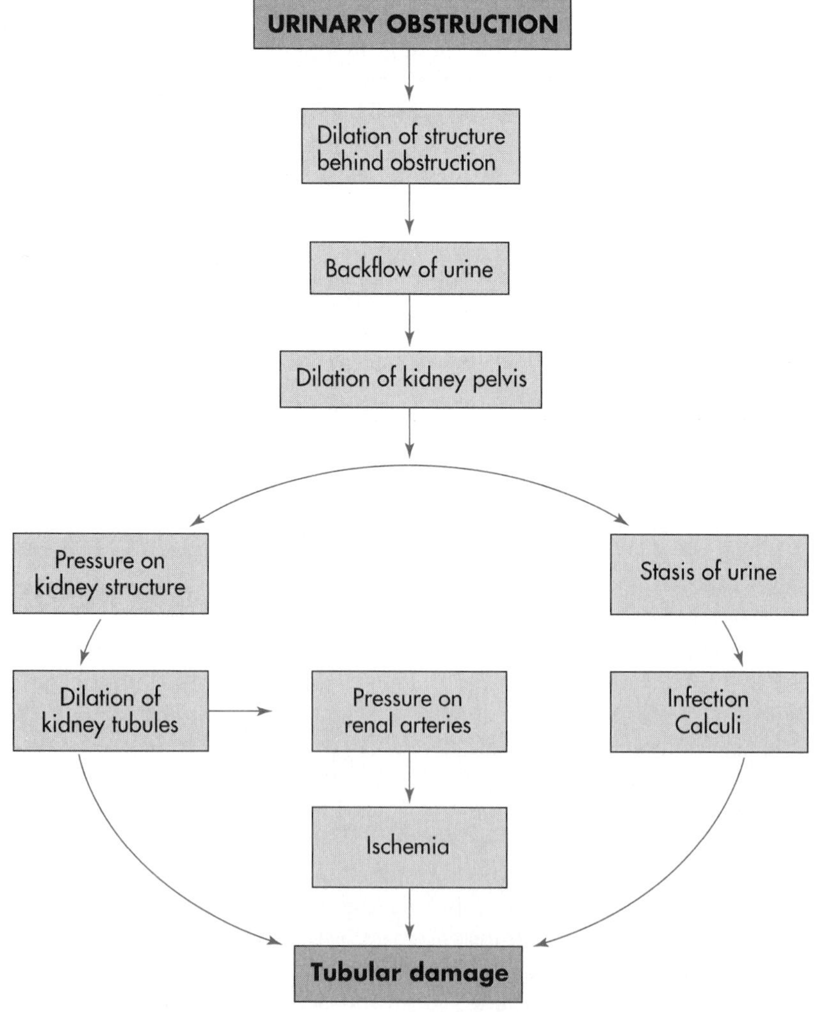

Figure 24-10 Pathophysiology of uncorrected urinary obstruction. (From Phipps WJ and others: *Medical-surgical nursing,* ed 5, St Louis, 1995, Mosby.)

side and usually radiates from the flank to the crest of the ileum. Pus may be present in the urine, resulting from infection at the back of the stone. Hematuria, usually microscopic, results from injury to the mucous membrane from the rough, jagged edges of the stone (McCance, Huether, 1994; Richard, 1986).

Ureteral colic is caused by a stone passing down or becoming lodged in the ureter. The pain is excruciating and radiates down the ureter and may extend to the thigh and the urethra. Nausea, vomiting, and sweating occur, and the patient feels weak and may faint.

Intervention. All urine from patients with renal calculi is voided, poured through a straining device, and carefully inspected for stones. The patient is encouraged to drink at least 3000 ml of fluid in 24 hours because increasing urinary output will facilitate passage of the stone. If infection is present, the appropriate antibiotic may be ordered. The patient is encouraged to remain active because stones are more likely to be passed if the patient is ambulatory.

Narcotics are required to relieve the pain, and an antispasmodic drug such as methantheline bromide (Banthine) or propantheline bromide (Pro-Banthine) may be ordered to relieve spasm (Box 24-2).

Prevention is also important. Patients confined to bed should be turned regularly every 2 hours. Long periods of immobilization result in a loss of calcium from

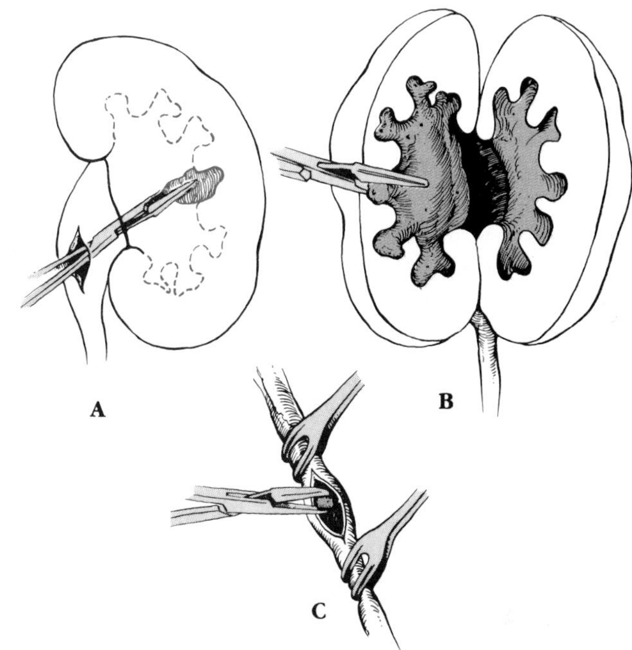

Figure 24-11 Removal of renal calculi from the upper urinary tract. **A,** Pyelolithotomy. The stone is removed through the renal pelvis. **B,** Nephrolithotomy. A staghorn calculus is removed through a lateral bisection of the kidney. **C,** Ureterolithotomy. The stone is removed from the ureter. (From Phipps WJ and others: *Medical-surgical nursing,* ed 5, St Louis, 1995, Mosby.)

BOX 24-2 **Nursing Process**

RENAL CALCULI

ASSESSMENT

Stone fragments when straining urine
Decreased urine output
Pain in the abdominal region, lower back, and/or upper thighs

NURSING DIAGNOSES

Anxiety related to fear of disease process, invasive medical procedure
Pain related to passage of calculi, invasive procedure
Knowledge deficit related to limited understanding of disease process, prescribed treatment
Altered urinary elimination related to obstructing calculi

NURSING INTERVENTIONS

Teach patient about disease process and treatments.
Encourage activity and ambulation.
Encourage patient to verbalize fears and concerns.
Explain all diagnostic tests, nursing measures, and physiology of ureteral colic and bladder spasm.
Give analgesics as often as ordered to relieve pain.
Encourage fluids to produce high urinary output of dilute urine—offer 200 ml every 2 hours while awake and 400 ml during night.
Strain all urine and observe for sediment, crystals, and stones; report findings; save any solids and send to laboratory for analysis; instruct patient to do the same.
Instruct patient and supervise dietary restrictions indicated by nature of stone as analyzed by laboratory.

EVALUATION OF EXPECTED OUTCOMES

Absence of pain
Urine output of 1400 to 1600 ml every 8 hours
Absence of calculi
Can verbalize diet restrictions and be able to select appropriate foods for restricted diet

the bones and an increase of calcium in the bloodstream. High levels of calcium in the blood contribute to the formation of kidney stones. Adequate hydration will dilute the urine so that stones are less likely to form (Phipps and others, 1995). Isometric exercise and weight-bearing exercise will reduce calcium lost from the bone. The use of the tilt table, the circle bed, rocking bed, and overhead trapeze provides exercise for the patient and helps in the prevention of stone formation.

Patients who require intervention for removal of large stones have several options. In place of conventional open surgical techniques, percutaneous stone removal and extracorporeal shock-wave lithotripsy are used successfully for stone removal or dissolution. Percutaneous stone removal is achieved through a nephroscope under fluoroscopy after the patient has received a local anesthetic. This method has the greatest success rate with renal pelvic and caliceal stones (Walsh and others, 1992). The nephrostomy tube is left in situ for several days.

Extracorporeal shock-wave lithotripsy is a noninvasive procedure that uses high-energy shock waves to pulverize renal stones into tiny fragments that are excreted in the urine (Lancaster, 1995). This procedure can be done with the patient in a tank of water or lying on a table similar to an x-ray table. Before the treatment begins, the procedure is explained and all questions are answered. Patients usually receive a sedative, maybe an epidural or general anesthetic, cardiac monitoring, and maybe oxygen, and have an IV placed. Patients must lie still while the high-energy waves are directed toward the stone through electrodes. Patients experience different degrees of discomfort during the procedure and appropriate analgesics are administered. X-ray examinations are performed throughout the procedure to evaluate the effectiveness of the treatment and assess for position of the stone.

Patient and family teaching. The shock waves pulverize the stone into dust and/or small gravel. To facilitate passage of these particles through the urinary tract, the client is instructed to drink 3 to 4 L of water every day for at least a week. It is critical that patients understand the importance of drinking the fluid to pass the pulverized stone because without copious urine, the stone fragments can cause an urinary tract obstruction. Patients have discomfort, hematuria, and bruising at the electrode sites and are tired after treatment. Analgesics are prescribed for the pain. Although lithotripsy is done in outpatient settings, it can also be done in the hospital. Usually patients are advised to rest for several days before returning to work and daily routines.

Tumors of the Urinary Tract

Kidney

Tumors of the kidneys are generally malignant and usually result from metastasis from the lung. The malignancy is often spread to the lungs and bones by the bloodstream. The primary symptom is blood in the urine; other symptoms are weight loss and fatigue. The treatment is a nephrectomy and may be only palliative because metastasis may have occurred.

Bladder

Tumors of the bladder may be benign or malignant. A complete urologic examination, including cystoscopy and a biopsy, is done to diagnose the problem. Cancer of the bladder is more common in men over age 50. Smoking and exposure to dyes, chemicals, and ionizing radiation increase the risk of developing cancer of the bladder. The bladder is also a site of metastasis of cancer originating in the male prostate or female lower reproductive tract. The most common symptom is gross, painless hematuria. Urinary tract infection often develops as a complication of malignancy and produces symptoms of frequency, urgency, and dysuria. A distant metastasis may produce pelvic or back pain.

For malignancy, a partial or complete cystectomy may be performed. A complete cystectomy necessitates urinary diversion. Radiation therapy or chemotherapy may be initiated. Chemotherapy may be given systemically or locally by instilling a solution into the bladder. Immunotherapy is in the experimental stage but offers hope for the future. BCG (Bacille Calmette-Guérin) has been instilled into the bladder and allowed to remain a given time before withdrawal. This treatment offers the advantage of actual contact with the tumor.

Traumatic Injuries

Injuries to the urinary system often occur in connection with injuries to other parts of the body. Injuries may be caused by gunshot wounds, penetrating wounds from sharp objects, and crushing injuries with fracture of the pelvis, which may cause rupture of the bladder or the urethra. Injuries resulting from external violence such as falls or blows may result in simple injury to the kidney or may completely shatter the kidney. All trauma victims should be observed for blood in the urine. The patient in shock will have a reduced blood supply to the kidney, and the urine output will be reduced. Initial interventions are aimed at stabilizing vital signs and maintaining circulation and oxy-

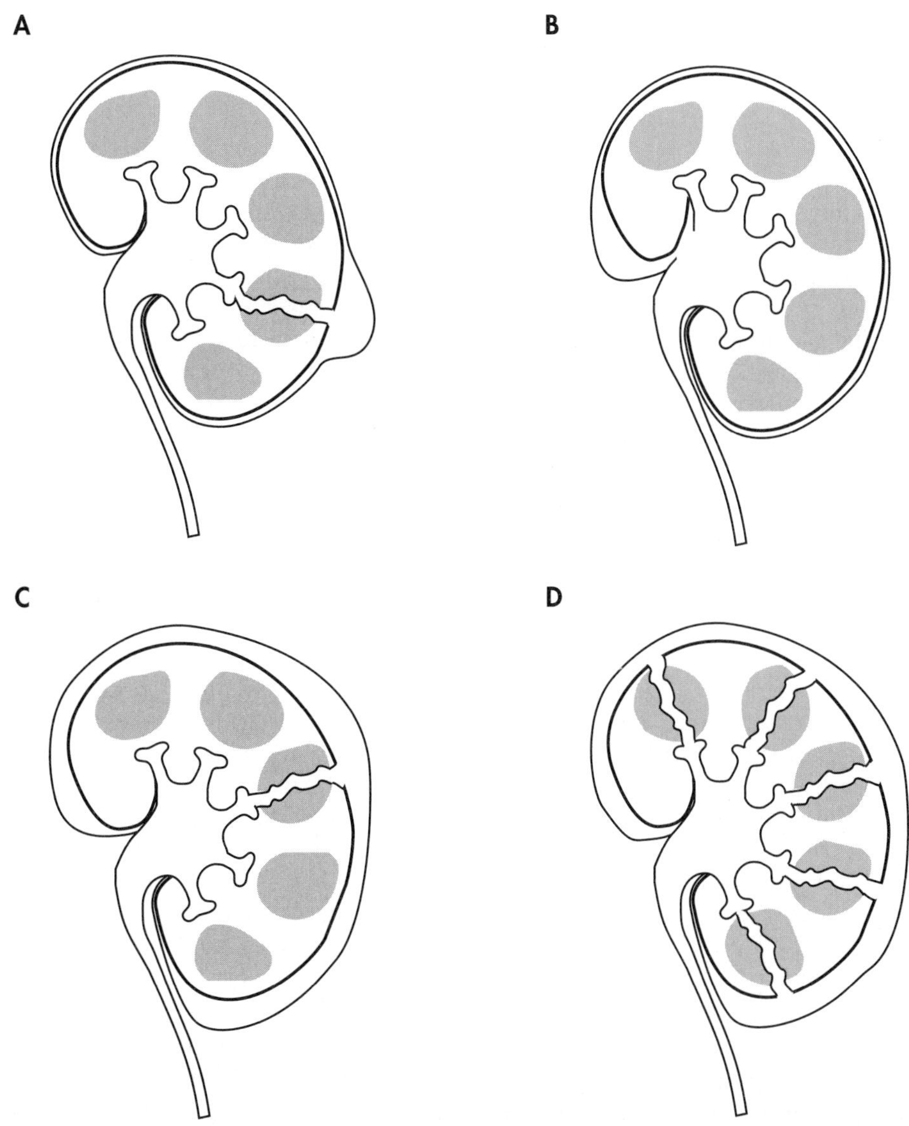

Figure 24-12 Four degrees of renal trauma. **A,** Urine is extravasating from split in renal parenchyma but confined under renal capsule. **B,** Urine is extravasating through tear in renal pelvis. **C,** Urine is extravasating through rent in kidney and capsule and surrounds kidney and renal pelvis. **D,** Kidney is shattered, and urine is extravasating in all areas.

genation of tissues. Assessment of the extent of injury determines the method of treatment, which may be conservative or may require surgical intervention (Figure 24-12) (Richard, 1986).

Renal Failure

Renal failure is a broad term for kidneys that are unable to meet the demands of the body. It is described as acute or chronic, according to the time required for the development of the condition and whether it is short-lived or prolonged.

Acute renal failure

Acute renal failure may develop insidiously or suddenly, but the kidneys suddenly stop functioning. Acute renal failure proceeds through several well-defined stages.

Pathophysiology. The causes of acute renal failure are numerous, but decreased renal blood flow and nephrotoxins are the most common causes. Postoperative shock produces hypotension that prevents the kidney from filtering the blood adequately. This decreased flow and lack of oxygen to the kidney may cause acute renal failure. Other causes include burns, blood transfusion reactions, infections, antigen-antibody reactions (acute glomerulonephritis), and obstructions.

Changes that occur in the kidney include necrosis and a sloughing of the lining of the renal tubules. Areas of the nephron rupture, resulting in the formation of scar tissue. Blood chemistries show an increase in the BUN, plasma creatinine, and potassium and a decrease in pH (acidosis) and bicarbonate. Generalized edema, pruritus, headache, disturbance of vision, hypertension, and vomiting occur, and there is an odor of urine on the breath. The patient appears acutely ill.

Assessment. The first stage is the *onset stage,* the time from the precipitating event to the onset of oliguria or anuria, usually a short period. Next is the *oliguric-anuric stage,* in which output is less than 400 ml in 24 hours. This may last only for a day or two, or it may last as long as 2 weeks. Then the kidney starts to recover and enters the *diuretic stage,* when urinary output increases and the BUN level stops rising and eventually falls to normal range. The *convalescent stage* begins when the BUN level is stable and ends when the patient returns to normal activity and urine output is normal. This may take several months, and some patients may develop chronic renal failure.

Intervention. Treatment begins with determining the cause and correcting it if possible. Management focuses on fluid balance, electrolyte balance, nutrition, preventing infection, and educating the patient. The patient is kept alive while the kidney heals itself. The mortality rate is approximately 50%, and the leading cause of death is infection (Richard, 1986).

There is a tendency for nurses to become preoccupied with the patient's urine volume and blood chemistries and to forget that they are dealing with a very frightened human being. Nurses should be alert for and respond to the patient's behavior and provide the support and understanding needed in this difficult time.

Because daily weights and fluid output guide fluid replacement, careful recording is done. The diet is high in carbohydrates to prevent the breakdown of fats, which produces ketosis, and low in protein and potassium to reduce BUN and hyperkalemia. Fluids are restricted. Protein is increased as the nephron units begin functioning and BUN decreases. If the level of serum potassium continues to increase and becomes dangerously high, an exchange resin is administered to release the excess potassium. Medications should be evaluated to determine potential buildup. Conservative treatment is continued, and dialysis is indicated when the clinical condition or biochemical state is deteriorating. Peritoneal dialysis may be used unless very rapid dialysis is required or repeated dialysis is anticipated; in such cases hemodialysis is used (Box 24-3) (Gutch and others, 1993).

Chronic renal failure

Chronic changes in renal failure may be considered on a continuum that ranges from impairment to insufficiency to failure. *Renal impairment* is detected by changes in concentration and dilution of the urine. *Renal insufficiency* becomes apparent when the kidney cannot meet the demands of dietary or metabolic stress. *Renal failure* appears when the normal demands of the body cannot be met. As many as 80% of the nephrons may be lost before renal functional losses are detected. Hypertrophy and hyperplasia of the remaining nephrons permit an increase in their workload and in their ability to maintain function (McCance, Huether, 1994). **Uremia** is a term that has been used for years to describe terminal renal failure and literally means urine in the blood. Although it is less popular now, the term is still used.

Pathophysiology. As renal function diminishes, the kidney loses its ability to adapt to varying intakes of foods and fluids. Polyuria and an inability to concentrate the urine are early signs of chronic renal failure. Oliguria and anuria occur later. An output of less than 400 ml of urine per day indicates failure.

The kidneys may be small and contracted or large and irregular in shape. The nature and extent of the underlying disease affect the rate of progression and the complicating factors. The most common causes are pyelonephritis, chronic glomerulonephritis, glomerulosclerosis, chronic urinary obstruction, severe hypertension, diabetes, gout, and polycystic kidney disease (McCance, Huether, 1994; Richard, 1995a).

Assessment. Patients with **chronic renal failure** have a characteristic dusky, yellow-tan, or gray color from retained urochrome pigments. The pallor of anemia is obvious. Pruritus and crawling or tickling sensations cause the patient to scratch the skin, producing excoriations that become infected. Abnormalities in clotting and capillary fragility permit large bruises and purpura to develop. The skin is dry and scaly because of a decrease in oil gland activity and in subcutaneous tissue. Uremic frost appears as white or yellowish crystals on the skin and is a late sign of chronic renal failure that is rarely seen if dialysis is implemented.

The patient will develop a nonbacterial stomatitis caused by the action of the urea-splitting flora of the oral cavity on the increased urea in the tissues. This gives rise to a metallic taste in the patient's mouth. Anorexia, nausea, and vomiting are common. Metabolism of urea in the intestinal tract forms ammonia, which causes formation of ulcers that may then hemorrhage, causing melena. High levels of urea in the blood produce a general feeling of lethargy advancing to drowsiness, confusion, and eventual coma.

Elevation of the serum potassium level accompanies the loss of sodium and the elimination of hydrogen

BOX 24-3 **Nursing Process**

ACUTE RENAL FAILURE

ASSESSMENT

Recent history of severe fluid depletion, exposure to nephrotoxins, and obstruction in the urinary tract
Volume of urine
Rise in plasma creatine and BUN
Feelings of malaise

NURSING DIAGNOSES

Anxiety related to prognosis
Decreased cardiac output related to arrhythmias, drug intolerance, stress on heart function
Pain related to infection, muscle cramps
Ineffective individual coping related to anger, anxiety, denial, dependent behavior, depression
Altered family processes related to complex therapies, hospitalization, illness of family member
Fear related to disease process, hospitalization, invasive medical procedure, powerlessness, real or imagined threat to well-being
Fluid volume excess related to decreased output
Grieving related to actual or perceived loss
Knowledge deficit related to limited understanding of disease process or prescribed treatment
Altered nutrition: less than body requirements related to dietary restrictions, loss of appetite, nausea and vomiting
Powerlessness related to disease process, hospitalization
Ineffective breathing pattern (impaired gas exchange) related to fluid overload
Personal identity disturbance related to body image, personal identity, role performance, self-esteem
Altered thought processes related to impaired perception of reality
Altered urinary elimination related to decreased kidney function, decreased urine output

NURSING INTERVENTIONS

Teach patient about disease process and treatment.
Measure and record urine output hourly; report if less than 30 ml/hr.
Report any reduction in urine output.
Restrict and regulate fluid intake as ordered and as permitted by output and weight gain.
Weigh patient daily.
Observe signs of fluid excess—dyspnea, tachycardia, pulmonary edema, distended neck veins, peripheral edema.
Observe signs of elevated serum potassium (hyperkalemia) and administer ion exchange resins as ordered.
Turn patient every 2 hours.
Have patient cough and deep breathe every 2 hours.
Provide emotional support, anticipating needs.
Limit dietary protein as necessary during oliguric phase.
Restrict sodium intake as ordered.
Anticipate treatment with dialysis.

EVALUATION OF EXPECTED OUTCOMES

Blood chemistries to level before illness
Urine output greater than 30 ml/hr
Weight decreased to level maintained before illness
Absence of edema and respiratory distress
Lungs clear
No signs/symptoms of infection
Patient and family verbalize fears and concerns

ions from the kidneys (the body's attempt to reduce acidosis). The high potassium level may cause arrhythmias. For some reason calcium is not absorbed in the gastrointestinal tract, and low levels of calcium may produce muscle irritability followed by tetany or convulsions if not corrected. Acidosis progresses, depleting bicarbonates and stimulating the respiratory center to increase respirations. Thus a deep sighing form of breathing is a symptom of renal insufficiency, whereas in the late stages of uremia, hyperventilation is amplified to rid the body of carbonic acid along with water in the form of carbon dioxide.

Anemia accompanies chronic renal failure because the kidney is unable to produce erythropoietin. This causes air hunger and a mild dyspnea. Belching and hiccups are also common.

Hypertension will develop to compensate for the decreased oxygen-carrying capacity of the blood in anemia, and retinopathy may then occur.

Intervention. Ongoing teaching is the most important nursing intervention implemented for the patient with renal failure (Brundage, Swearingen, 1994). Chronic renal failure is treated by restriction of nutrients and fluids to levels that the kidneys are able to manage effectively, and by dialysis or renal transplantation. If dietary management is initiated early, the buildup of toxins can be prevented or minimized and the impaired functional abilities of the kidneys can be more effective for a longer time. Transplantation and dialysis are discussed later in this chapter.

Usually the diet is complex and is managed by a renal dietician (Lewandoski, 1994). The diet contains enough protein to prevent tissue wasting but not so much as to contribute to the overload of its metabolic end products (urea). When even a minimum amount of protein cannot be handled by the kidneys, dialysis is required. The diet is high in calories from carbohydrates and fats, consisting of at least 2500 to 3000 calories daily. Without sufficient calories from carbohydrates and fats, the liver will form glycogen from amino acids (glyconeogenesis) and increase the metabolic end products of protein in the blood. Other dietary restrictions are related to the patient's degree of acidosis. Potassium is retained; therefore foods high in potassium could be restricted. Sodium is controlled at a level sufficient to replace sodium loss without causing fluid retention. Table salt is almost always eliminated, and commercially prepared low-salt foods are used. Boiling and processing fruits and vegetables removes potassium.

Fluid balance is of prime importance. The patient may have fluids equal to the amount excreted in the urine plus 300 to 500 ml to compensate for insensible fluid loss (e.g., through the lungs, perspiration). Fluids in excess of the amount that can be eliminated are retained in the body, and the patient gains weight. Accurate records of all intake and output, as well as daily weights, are essential to the calculation of fluid replacement. Weighing the patient at the same time each day on the same scale with same amount of clothes is important.

The patient often complains of thirst, but the thirst associated with renal failure cannot be relieved by ordinary means. Factors that the nurse must consider in relation to the patient's thirst include the total amount of fluid allowed, condition of the patient's mouth, fluid output, diet, physical activity, and the patient's mental state. There are ways in which the nurse can space the fluid without giving more fluid than the amount permitted.

When fluids are restricted, the following methods of administering medications should be considered: (1) giving several medications at mealtime, (2) giving small pills and capsules rather than large ones that may require larger amounts of water to swallow, (3) using solid forms of medications rather than liquid forms, (4) using small glasses rather than large glasses (a small glass full of water has a better psychologic effect than a large glass with a small amount of water), and (5) realizing that a small amount of cold water will be more satisfying than warm water.

Dietary and fluid restrictions may be eased once the patient begins dialysis, but some treatment plans continue rigid control on the premise that this will prevent complications and improve the prognosis.

Thorough and frequent oral hygiene is necessary to relieve the effects of stomatitis and the metallic taste in the mouth. Vinegar (0.25% acetic acid) used as a mouthwash helps to neutralize ammonium. Hard candy, gum, and cold liquids help improve the taste in the mouth. The more critical the patient's condition, the more mouth care will be required, and in some cases it may have to be given hourly. Whatever method is used must meet the needs of the patient. The mouth may be dry because of dyspnea or because of the effects of receiving oxygen. Humidification of the air will provide moisture and relieve dryness.

Patients who are given a regimen of bedrest may develop decubiti or pulmonary complications and should be turned regularly and encouraged to breathe deeply. The use of an alternating air pressure pad may provide comfort for some patients. Skin care is extremely important in the care of patients with chronic renal failure. Mild soap such as Basis, a baking soda solution, or bath oil may be used to cleanse the skin. Lanolin or other ointments may be ordered to relieve itching. Nails should be kept short so that the patient will not scratch and traumatize the skin. Edematous areas should be supported with pillows and circulation stimulated through active or passive exercises. Edematous extremities should be elevated above the level of the heart.

If the patient's vision is failing, care should be taken to prevent injury. Padded side rails should be used for patients who are confused or disoriented. The nurse should be sure that an oral airway is kept at the bedside or nearby in case convulsions should occur.

The administration of Epoetin alfa, a form of recombinant human erythropoietin, has improved the signs and symptoms of anemia in many patients with chronic renal failure (Kammerer, 1994; York, 1994).

Blood transfusions may be necessary, and only washed donor cells may be used, especially if the patient is awaiting transplant. Antigens should not be introduced into the body unnecessarily because the formation of antigen-antibody complexes may limit the patient's ability to accept a donor kidney. Blood transfusions, together with hyperkalemia, fluid retention, and hypertension, may result in congestive heart failure. In treating congestive heart failure, it must be remembered that drugs normally excreted by the kidney, such as digoxin, will require reduced dosages and that diuretics that depend on glomerular filtration will not be effective.

Patients with chronic renal failure should be encouraged to participate in self-care activities and to remain active if their condition permits (Brundage, 1994).

DIALYSIS

Hemodialysis

Hemodialysis is an extracorporeal mechanical method of removing waste products and establishing equilibrium of electrolytes and water when the kidneys are unable to perform their functions. Hemodialysis is accomplished by the use of the artificial kidney called a *dialyzer* and may be used in (1) chronic renal failure, (2) acute renal failure, and (3) drug poisoning. Hemodialysis will not cure the damage caused by renal disease but will remove waste products from the body and prevent damage to other organs until further treatment can be instituted and healing of the kidney takes place.

The process of hemodialysis is as follows: blood leaves the body and flows through sterile tubing, a sterile *dialyzer* (also called an artificial kidney), more sterile tubing, and back to the body (Figure 24-13). The dialyzer is composed of two compartments that are separated by a semipermeable membrane, which is similar to cellophane. In one compartment is the patient's blood, and in the other compartment is the dialyzing solution that is chemically similar to blood. As the blood and the dialyzing solutions circulate on the two sides of the semipermeable membrane, waste products leave the bloodstream, cross the membrane, and enter the dialyzing solution, which is changed periodically. Therefore the dialysis process occurs across the semipermeable membrane inside the dialyzer. The dialyzer is attached to a hemodialysis machine that has different pumps and safety devices.

There are three basic circulatory accesses to remove and return the blood. The *external arteriovenous shunt* requires the insertion of cannulas in an artery and a vein, usually on the forearm (Figure 24-14). Cannulas are attached to the dialysis tubing during hemodialysis treatment, but otherwise they are attached to each other by a connector. This shunt is intended for short-term use.

An alternative to the arteriovenous shunt is the insertion of a specially designed, double-lumen *catheter* through the subclavian or jugular vein. The catheter is designed so that blood is removed from a point proximal to the insertion site, routed through the dialyzer,

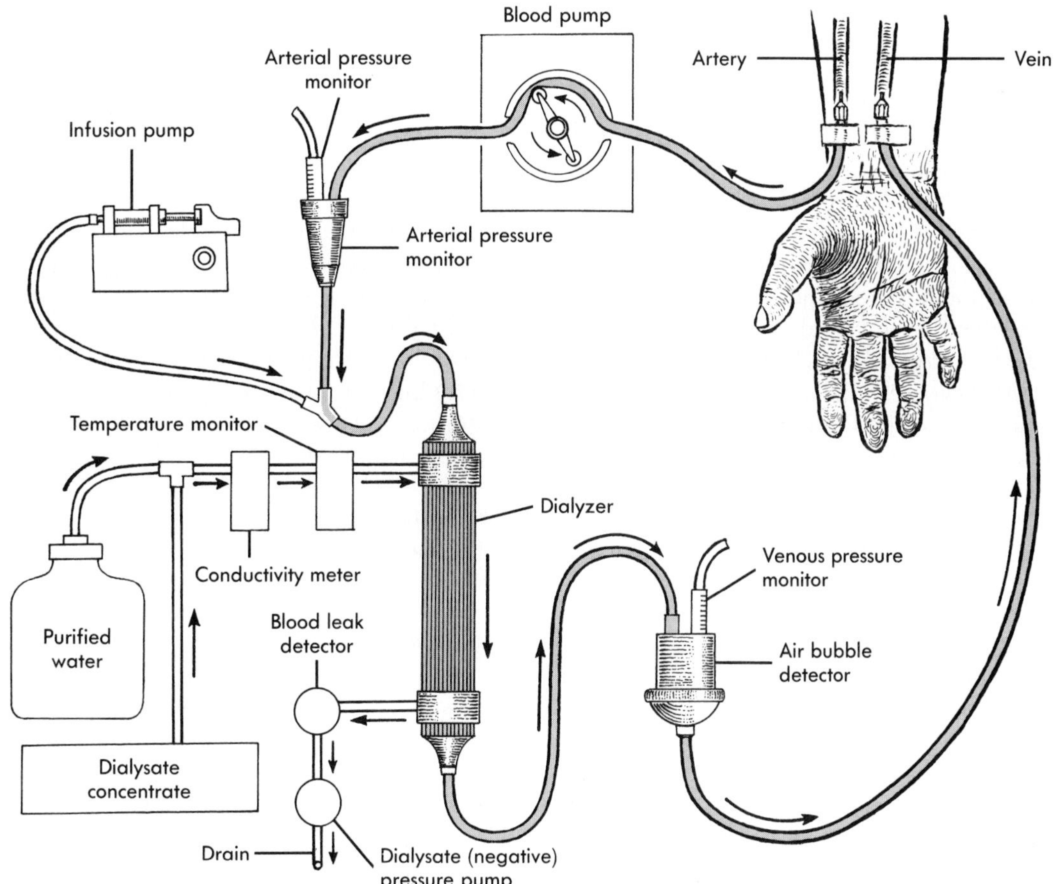

Figure 24-13 Components of a hemodialysis system. (From Thelan and others: *Critical care nursing,* ed 2, St Louis, 1994, Mosby.)

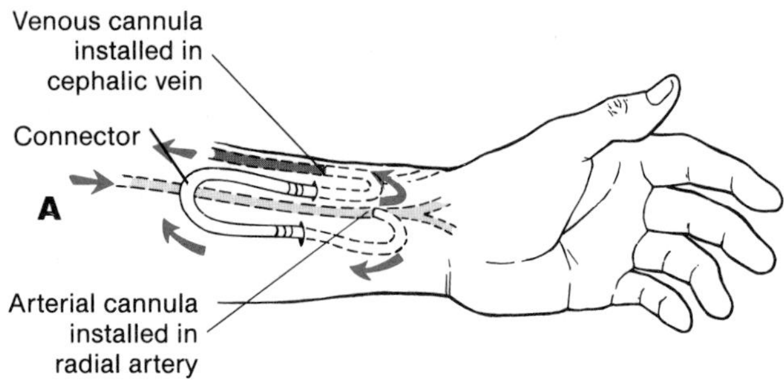

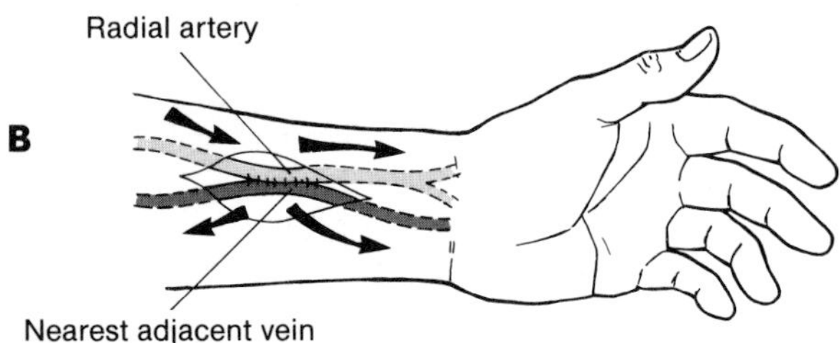

Figure 24-14 Hemodialysis circulatory accesses. **A,** External arteriovenous shunt. A cannula is inserted into a vein, and another cannula is inserted into an artery. The two cannulas are joined by a connector. Arrows indicate the direction of blood flow. **B,** Arteriovenous fistula. An artery and vein are surgically anastomosed. Blood flows through the artery into the vein and arterilizes the vein. Arrows indicate the direction of blood flow.

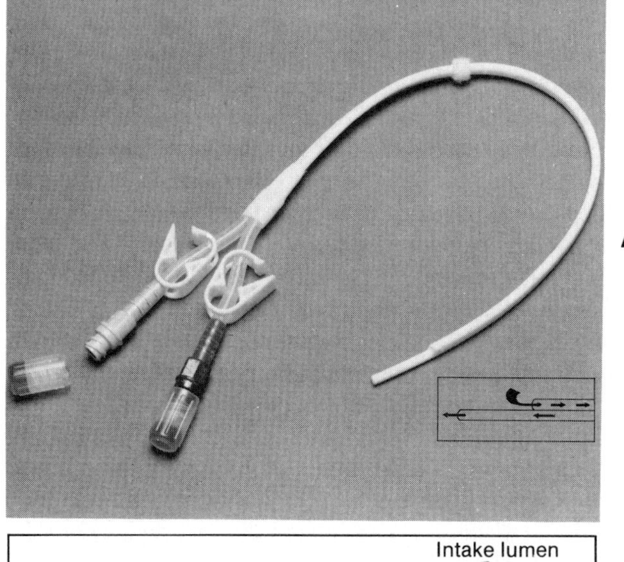

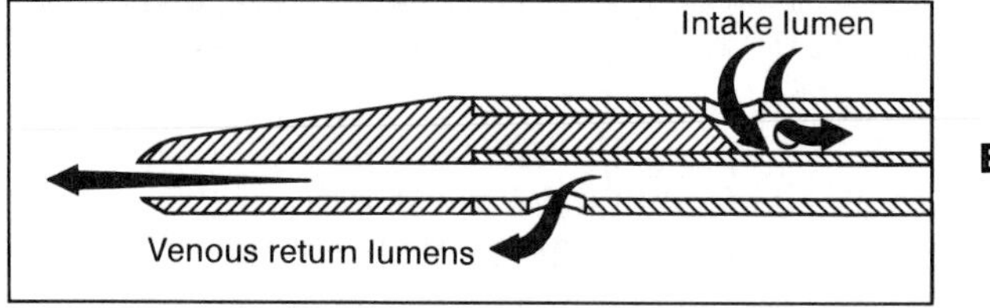

Figure 24-15 **A,** This double lumen hemodialysis catheter is available for subclavian and femoral insertion. **B,** (Enlargement of small insert in **A.**) The distance between the venous return lumen and the return intake lumen ensures minimal recirculation. (Photos courtesy of Quintron Instrument Company, Seattle, Wash.)

and returned through a distal hole in the catheter (Figure 24-15). The subclavian or jugular site is easier to protect and maintain than the shunt site in the forearm. It can be used for a number of weeks. The site must be cleansed and redressed regularly, as for any long-term infusion catheter. The other method used to conduct dialysis involves an *arteriovenous fistula,* in which a vein is surgically anastomosed to an artery. The vein then becomes distended, and the vessel wall thickens and can be palpated easily so that needles can be inserted for dialysis hook-up (see Figure 24-15).

Patients can be maintained on dialysis therapy and their lives prolonged pending the possibility of a kidney transplant. When long-term dialysis is necessary for end-stage renal disease, the patient may go to a dialysis center, usually two or three times weekly, and remain approximately 4 to 6 hours for the treatment. Some patients receive their treatment at night and go about their normal activities during the day. Smaller, portable units have been developed that allow the patient to be dialyzed anywhere. Many patients, with the help of an assistant, dialyze themselves at home.

Patients receiving dialysis therapy need a great deal of psychologic support and encouragement (Korniewicz, O'Brien, 1994). Most patients realize the seriousness of their condition. They may become depressed and question why they are being kept alive. The patient's family plays a most important role.

Personnel who work with hemodialysis patients must be specially educated in anatomy, physiology, pathology of the kidney, and pharmacology. Usually each dialysis center has its own education program, lasting 6 to 12 weeks. (Gutch and others, 1993; Lancaster, 1995; Richard, 1986).

Peritoneal dialysis. Peritoneal dialysis was the original substitute for a nonfunctioning kidney. It can be performed in any hospital with minimum equipment, as well as when the patient is ambulatory. In all types of peritoneal dialysis, a fluid is instilled into the peritoneal space by gravity, allowed to remain there long enough to collect waste products and excess electrolytes that have been left in the blood by the nonfunctioning kidney, then drained from the space and discarded (Figure 24-16). While in the peritoneal space, the fluid, called *dialysate,* bathes the peritoneal membrane. The waste products and electrolytes pass through the capillaries in the membrane, by the processes of osmosis and diffusion, into the dialysate.

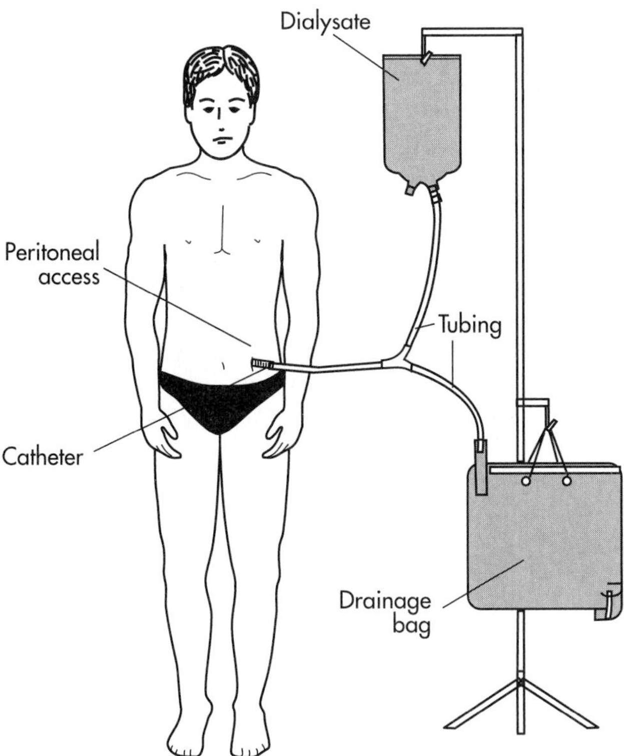

Figure 24-16 Peritoneal dialysis system.

The chemical composition of the dialysate is designed to promote removal of products from the blood in the same way it functions in hemodialysis.

The catheter is inserted into the peritoneal cavity using a technique that is similar to abdominal paracentesis. A trocar, a large needle with a large bore, is inserted through a tiny incision made in the skin of the abdomen. During insertion, a stylet is in place in the bore of the trocar; after insertion, the stylet is removed, and a catheter with tiny holes running the length of all sides is inserted through the trocar. The trocar is then withdrawn, and the catheter remains in the peritoneal cavity.

Next, 2000 ml of dialyzing solution is allowed to run into the peritoneal cavity and remain for 30 to 60 minutes. The solution is warmed before it is instilled to improve its effectiveness and to prevent chilling of the patient. The fluid is then drained by gravity. When 100 to 200 ml of solution remains in the cavity, another bottle of solution is connected, and the process is repeated. Sterile technique is observed when inserting the catheter and caring for the site. All connections to the tubing and the addition of bottles of solution must be done in a manner that prevents contamination of the inside of the tubing, the site, and the solution.

During the procedure the patient should be observed for signs of abdominal or respiratory distress, changes in vital signs, and bleeding. The amount of fluid instilled and drained should be carefully recorded. The patient should be weighed before and after the procedure. The catheter is removed when the process is completed. If the procedure is to be repeated in a day or two, the pathway to the peritoneal cavity may be kept open with a sterile plastic tube specially designed for this purpose. A sterile dressing is applied to the site; the incision is small and does not require repair with sutures.

Considering the time required for this procedure to remove the waste products, it is easy to see how hemodialysis came to be the preferred method for the patient with chronic renal failure. It is not practical to spend 24 hours every other day confined to bed or a hospital unit while receiving a peritoneal dialysis treatment. Although hemodialysis does restrict the patient, it is at least less time consuming.

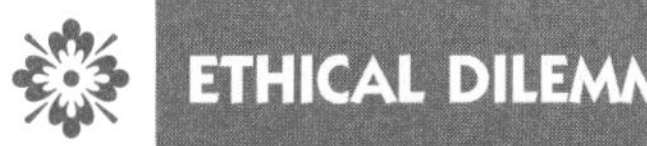

ETHICAL DILEMMA

Mr. Williams, a 68-year-old man, has been receiving hemodialysis treatments for 9 years in the dialysis center where you work. Recently his overall health has been deteriorating significantly. His cognitive abilities are also markedly decreased. He has a power of attorney for healthcare on his chart, which gives his healthcare agent the authority to discontinue dialysis when it no longer contributes to his general health.

The daughter who is his healthcare agent understands his wishes but says she doesn't know if she can carry them out because her out-of-town sister says it would be wrong to stop dialysis.

How would you analyze this case?

Continuous Ambulatory Peritoneal Dialysis

Continuous ambulatory peritoneal dialysis (CAPD) removes some of the restrictions from the patient with end-stage renal disease. It allows the patient to receive dialysis during the night while asleep at home or while ambulatory at home, work, or play. A catheter is inserted surgically and is left in place and covered by a sterile dressing. The catheter is placed in the peritoneal space through an incision, and the distal end is tunneled through a 3- or 4-inch section of subcutaneous tissue on the abdomen, then brought out to the surface of the abdomen. This tunnel creates a barrier to prevent infection of the peritoneal cavity if the catheter site should become infected. The patient is taught to meticulously care for the catheter and site, using a sterile technique. Before and after connecting the dialysate tubing, the connection is disinfected with a povidone-iodine (Betadine) soak for about 20 minutes.

For nighttime dialysis, the dialysate instillation is regulated by a machine that automatically starts the flow of solution, times the period it remains in the cavity, and then allows the fluid to drain by gravity. Safety mechanisms are built into the machine to prevent fluid from being instilled if the previous instillation has not drained adequately. Multiple bottles of dialysate are hooked up to the machine, and it automatically instills each bottle in sequence. Used dialysate is likewise collected in multiple bottles that are weighed by the machine to verify complete elimination before the next bottle is instilled. An alarm sounds to waken the patient if any problem is sensed by the machine.

For daytime dialysis with continuous ambulatory peritoneal dialysis, the patient attaches a small bag of dialysate to the catheter, instills it, then rolls it up and tucks it in an inconspicuous place while the dialysate is instilled. Later the dialysate is drained into the same bag and discarded. The procedure is repeated as necessary to maintain the waste products in the blood at a safe level, usually four times each day. Research and development of new products and techniques continue to make life more livable for the patient dependent on dialysis.

RENAL TRANSPLANTATION

A renal transplantation is the procedure of placing a normal kidney from a donor into a person with nonfunctioning kidneys. The most successful transplants are those done with a sibling or family member with the same blood and tissue typing. By carefully matching the donor kidney with the recipient, kidneys from unrelated people and from cadavers are transplanted with fair success (Budinger, Donnelly, 1994; Lancaster, 1995).

The patient may undergo a bilateral nephrectomy in preparation for the transplant if the kidneys are severely infected or if the patient has severe diastolic hypertension. This patient will experience a sense of loss, even though the absent kidneys were not functioning. The kidneys may both be left in place for transplant surgery because the donor kidney is placed in the iliac fossa and receives its blood supply from the iliac arteries (Figure 24-17). Dialysis is necessary until the transplantation can be accomplished.

Postoperative care is centered around careful observation of hourly urine output and maintaining patency of the indwelling catheter along with the maintenance of intravenous fluid and electrolyte therapy.

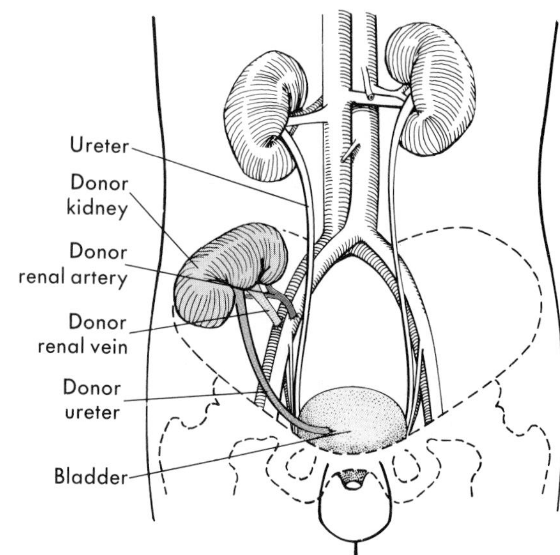

Figure 24-17 Location of a transplanted kidney showing the anastomosis of the renal artery, renal vein, and ureter. (From Phipps WJ and others: *Medical-surgical nursing,* ed 5, St Louis, 1995, Mosby.)

Massive diuresis or oliguria may be possible. Additional nursing measures are similar to those of any major surgical procedure. A central venous pressure line may be in place to monitor fluid needs. The patient is weighed daily to monitor fluid retention. The patient must be observed carefully for signs of *rejection* of the donor kidney, which include decreased urine output, increased blood pressure, fever, and swelling and tenderness at the site of the implanted kidney.

The major problem in transplantation is that of rejection. Before surgery the patient's immunologic responses are suppressed, and immunosuppressive therapy is continued long after discharge. Cyclosporine (Sandimmune), a drug obtained from soil fungus, has revolutionized the success of organ transplantation, including kidney transplants (Trusler, 1990). Cyclosporine may be used as a single immunosuppressant agent or in conjunction with steroids. Cyclosporine may be administered intravenously or orally. Because cyclosporine is prepared in an oil base, patients may find it unpalatable. Administering it with food or diluting it in chocolate milk may help the patient ingest the drug. Therapeutic levels of cyclosporine are carefully monitored with a radioimmunoassay because ironically, elevated levels of cyclosporine are nephrotoxic.

Other drugs that may be used are azathioprine (Imuran), prednisone, and methylprednisolone (Solu-Medrol). The visible side effects of steroid therapy, namely moon face and weight gain, may be the greatest problem for the patient during recovery. As immunosuppressive therapy is withdrawn, the physical appearance returns to normal.

The patient will also be given furosemide (Lasix) to control fluid retention, aluminum phosphate gel (Phosphaljel) to protect the stomach during steroid therapy, hydralazine (Apresoline) and methyldopa (Aldomet) for the control of blood pressure, and sulfisoxazole (Gantrisin) and nystatin (Mycostatin) to prevent infections.

Rejection of the transplanted kidney may occur soon after surgery, or it may be delayed for months or even years after transplantation. The possibility of rejection is a very important factor to the patient. The patient must be encouraged and facilitated in expressing concerns about rejection and the long-term prognosis. The patient must be prepared for discharge and convalescence by being taught the importance of taking medications, keeping appointments with the physician or clinic, and keeping track of how he or she feels. Psychologically, the patient must adopt the new kidney.

OPERATIVE CONDITIONS OF THE URINARY SYSTEM

Many conditions affecting the urinary system require both medical and surgical treatment, and operative procedures are seldom done until a thorough urologic examination has been completed. The preoperative care of patients does not differ greatly from that of other surgical patients. When surgery involves the kidney, the patient's blood is typed and cross-matched in case transfusion should be necessary. The postoperative care differs from other kinds of surgery in that drains, tubes, or catheters are placed to remove urine.

Many patients will have draining wounds after surgery on the urinary system. Although patients may have understood this before surgery, when they are faced with the discomfort of wet dressings, the odor of urine, and the resulting skin irritation, they may become irritable and depressed and feel that adjustment is impossible. It may challenge the nurse to find ways to overcome these problems.

Because dressings need to be changed often, Montgomery straps or laced dressings could be used to avoid skin irritation from adhesive tape. Small dressings changed often will keep the patient more comfortable than large bulky ones that become saturated, heavy, and foul smelling. A ureterostomy cup may be applied and attached to free drainage, or the disposable plastic urostomy bags may be used for some patients. Wound drainage bags are available that may be effective in some drainage problems. Any device used is only an adjunct to good nursing care, which includes cleansing the skin and protecting wounds from infection.

Cystectomy

A **cystectomy** is the surgical removal of the bladder and may be partial or complete. The surgery may be necessary because of malignant tumors involving the bladder and adjacent structures. When the bladder is removed, the ureters are transplanted by one of the methods discussed in the following section to provide for urinary drainage. The nursing care is the same as that for patients having abdominal surgery. The prostate gland may have been removed through a perineal wound, and such wounds must be observed for evidence of hemorrhage. The patient will have a nasogastric tube connected to suction siphonage and will be given nothing by mouth for several days. During this time the patient should receive special mouth care at frequent intervals.

If a partial resection of the bladder has been done, a catheter will be inserted into the remaining bladder, and precautions must be taken to prevent any pulling on the catheter. The tubing should be pinned to the sheet and sufficient slack allowed to permit the patient to turn.

Urinary Diversion: Ureteral Transplants

Several types of procedures are used to divert the flow of urine when required for treatment of bladder cancer, invasive cancer of the cervix, neurogenic bladder, and congenital anomalies. The *ureterosigmoidostomy* involves implanting the ureters into the large bowel, which is left intact so that both urine and feces are eliminated rectally. This technique is rarely used today because of the undesirable effects on the perianal skin resulting from chronically liquid stool. A variation of this procedure is the formation of an isolated rectal pouch into which the ureters are implanted while the remainder of the bowel is diverted to form a sigmoid colostomy.

A second procedure, *cutaneous ureterostomy,* involves direct implantation of the terminal ends of the ureters onto the skin (Figure 24-18). The ureters may be joined so that there is only one stoma, or each ureter may be brought to the skin separately, forming two stomas. A third procedure, the *ileal conduit,* is a common method of urinary diversion at present (Figure 24-19). In this procedure a section of the ileum is resected from the small bowel, and its blood supply is preserved. The remaining small bowel is then anastomosed so that

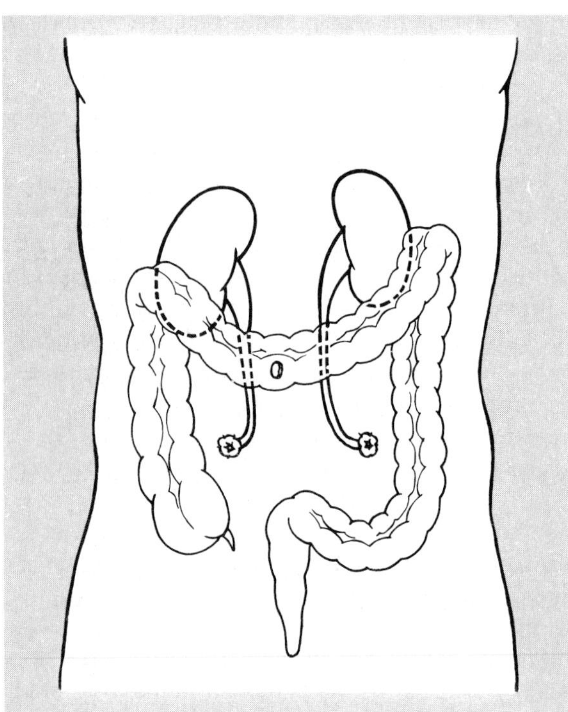

Figure 24-18 Cutaneous ureterostomy in which ureters are brought through the skin onto the abdomen.

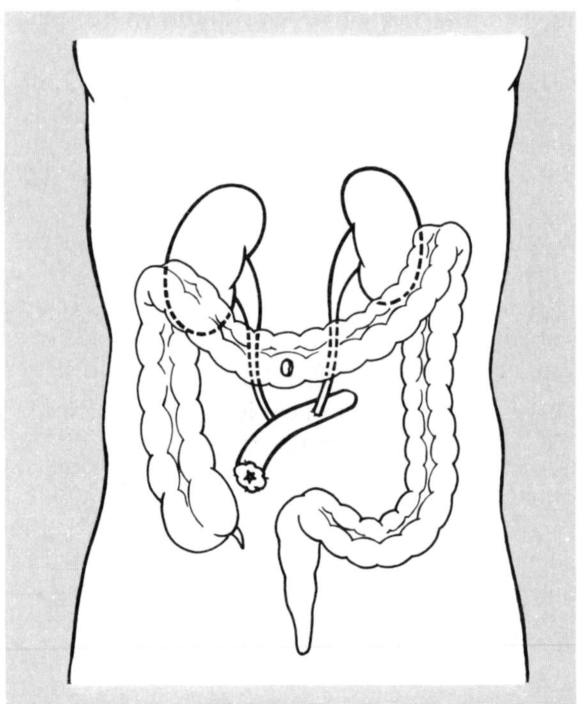

Figure 24-19 Ileal conduit. A small section of the ileum is resected from the small intestine. One end of the resected portion is sutured closed, and the other end is brought to the skin surface. The ureters are transplanted into the resected ileum.

normal bowel function will be maintained. The resected segment of ileum is sutured closed at one end, forming a pouch, and the other end is sutured to the skin, forming a stoma. The ureters are transplanted into this segment of ileum, which forms a conduit that serves as a passageway for urine to flow from the body. It does not serve as a reservoir for urine.

A variation of the ileal conduit is the *continent urostomy* (or *Koch's pouch*), in which the pouch is formed from the ileum. In this instance the reservoir can hold up to 800 ml of urine. A large segment of the ileum is structured into an internal pouch with two nipple valves. The ureters are implanted into the reservoir, and a portion of the ileal reservoir is brought out transcutaneously and fashioned into a stoma. Patients are taught to catheterize this pouch approximately four times a day, and they do not need to wear an external urinary appliance. A small bandage over the stoma is sufficient (Beare, Myers, 1994).

Cutaneous ureterostomy

When the ureters have been transplanted to the abdominal wall skin, the patient may have soft rubber catheters in place for about 1 week if the ureters are small. It is important that the catheters drain adequately so that hydronephrosis does not develop.

If cutaneous ureterostomies heal properly, the patient can use ostomy bags instead of catheters for drainage. The bags may be applied to the skin with adhesive disks and may require changing only every 2 or 3 days. The technique for applying the bag is not difficult, but it does take practice. When the bag is first applied, the nurse must make sure that there is adequate drainage from the kidney. If the patient complains of any back pain, the appliance should be removed at once and reapplied. Sometimes obstruction to drainage is caused by angulation of the ureter or by temporary ureteral edema.

If the ureter is angulated or if there is stomal stenosis, the kidney will need to be drained permanently with a catheter. If the patient must wear ureteral catheters, he or she is taught to irrigate these each day. Patients must return to the physician every 2 to 4 weeks to have the catheters changed, or they are taught to change their own catheters. The catheters are anchored to the skin with adhesive tape, or a catheter disk with a belt is used. The catheters are attached by tubing to a drainage receptacle. This procedure is not commonly used, since infections occur often, causing a series of complications.

Ileal conduit (ileobladder)

The **ileal conduit** is a method of urinary diversion that results in fewer fluid and electrolyte problems and provides an added barrier to infection (the conduit). Preoperatively, the patient will have little or no special preparation of the bowel because the ileum is considered sterile. Careful preoperative measurement and inspection of the abdomen for optimum placement of the stoma will facilitate movement and application of an appliance for urinary drainage postoperatively.

Postoperative complications related to abdominal surgery must be prevented. The abdomen should be observed for any changes that might indicate inflammation. Paralytic ileus can occur as a result of manipulation of the bowel. There is a possibility of urine leakage at the suture lines, which allows urine to enter the peritoneal cavity; the resultant inflammation causes pain, fever, nausea, and vomiting. The patient's abdomen will feel rigid and will be sensitive to the touch. A nasogastric tube is usually inserted to decompress the bowel until peristalsis returns. Oral intake is restricted or prohibited while the nasogastric tube is in place.

The patient returns from surgery with a catheter in place or with a temporary transparent appliance attached to the skin to collect urine. If the catheter is used, it is attached to a sterile gravity drainage system. The appliance is also attached to a drainage system to provide for the flow of urine, which will be continuous. Urinary flow must be maintained; if it is allowed to distend the conduit, it will cause back pressure on the kidneys, damaging them, or it will rupture the suture lines. The nurse must watch closely for low abdominal pain and decreased urinary output. Urine output may be measured hourly in the early postoperative period.

When the stoma has healed, a permanent (reusable) appliance is fitted to the patient. Disposable appliances are available (Figure 24-20) but expensive; therefore patients may choose a reusable appliance. Proper application of the appliance will prevent leaking and irritation of the skin. The stoma is covered with gauze or a tampon to absorb urine while the area around the stoma is cleaned. A skin barrier such as Stomahesive may be applied directly to the skin before the appliance is applied, or the skin may be prepared in some other manner. It is essential to keep the skin dry before applying the appliance, or it will not adhere. Permanent appliances have a faceplate that is attached to the skin with cement or a double-faced adhesive. The collection pouch is attached to the faceplate. A permanent appliance can be worn for 3 to 7 days if applied properly. It is recommended that the patient purchase a second appliance so that one may be cleaned and aired while the other is worn.

The psychologic problems that result from urinary diversion are similar to those occurring from diversion of the intestinal tract. The surgery is a traumatic experience, and the patient must adapt to an altered body image. The patient must be supported and reassured when learning to care for the urostomy and encouraged to continue everyday activities once recuperation from surgery has occurred. It may be beneficial to consult an ostomy nurse specialist (Box 24-4).

Cystotomy

A cystotomy is a surgical incision into the bladder and may be performed for various reasons, including the correction of prostatic hypertrophy in connection with suprapubic prostatectomy. It may be performed to remove tumors or stones from the bladder.

The preoperative care of the patient is the same as that for other abdominal surgery. When the patient returns from surgery, a drainage tube will have been inserted into the bladder, which may be connected to a drainage bag. The dressings will have to be changed often to keep the patient dry and comfortable. The skin must be kept clean, and a protective ointment may be used to prevent irritation. Blood pressure and pulse must be checked often during the immediate postoperative period, and the patient must be turned from side to side to prevent pulmonary complications.

Ureterotomy and Lithotomy

Surgery on the ureter is generally performed to remove a stone, to repair a severed ureter, or to do plastic repair of a stricture. If the stone is in the ureter, a *ureterolithotomy* is performed. Removal of the stone from the kidney is a *nephrolithotomy,* and removal of the stone from the kidney pelvis is a *pyelolithotomy* (see Figure 24-11). Patients having a stone removed from the lower third of the ureter will have an abdominal incision, and care is similar to that for any patient with abdominal surgery. However, the incision will drain urine for several days after surgery because the ureter cannot be closed with watertight sutures or strictures will form. Stones removed from the upper two thirds of the ureter and the kidney will necessitate a flank or kidney incision.

The postoperative care of the patient is directed toward the care of tubes and maintaining drainage. Occasionally a catheter is inserted into the ureter, which serves as a splint while healing occurs. It is important that the catheter be kept in place at all times. When

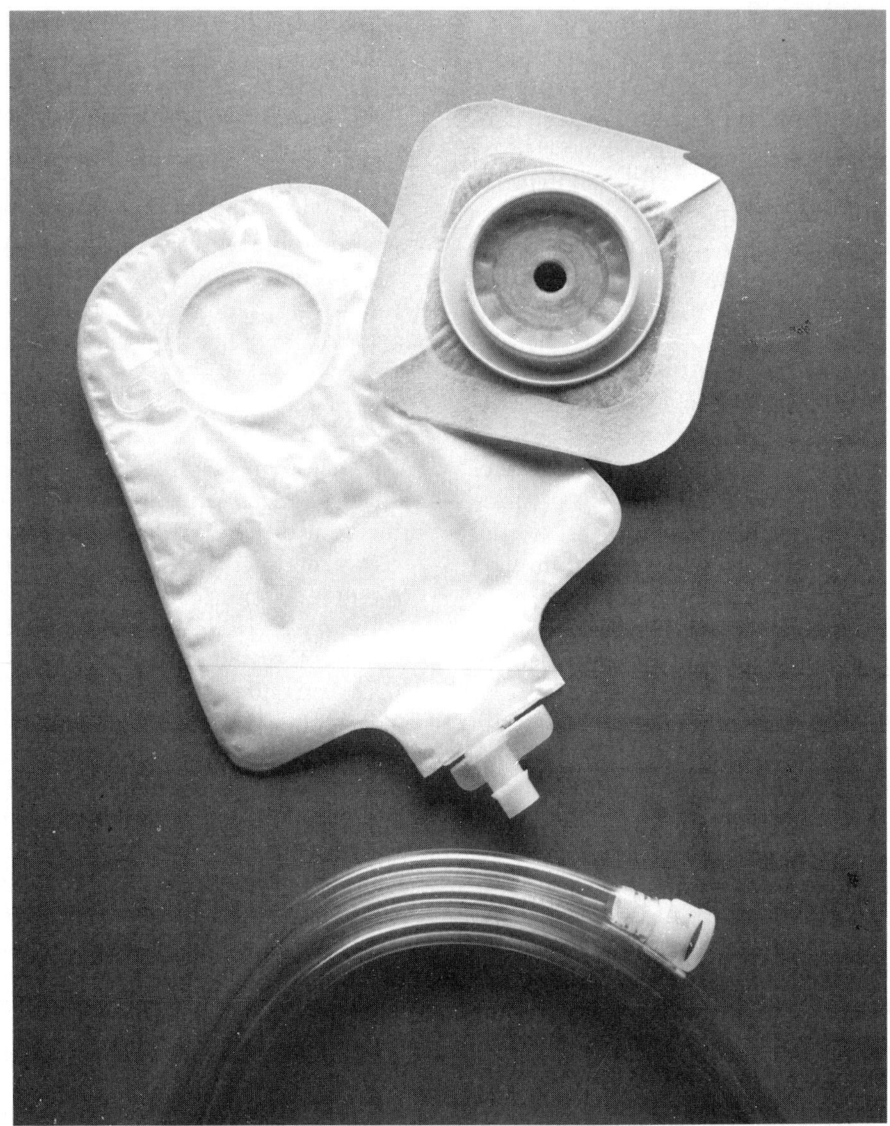

Figure 24-20 Disposal appliances for ileal conduit or other urinary diversion (e.g., urostomy). Faceplate *(upper right)* attaches to skin as barrier, and drainable bag attaches to flange on skin barrier. Drainage tube can be attached for nighttime use. (Courtesy of Hollister, Inc.)

there is urinary drainage onto the skin, there must be frequent change of dressings and cleansing of the skin to prevent irritation and maceration. All urinary drainage should be measured and recorded (Box 24-5) (Beare, Myers, 1994; Richard, 1995b).

Nephrectomy and Nephrostomy

A **nephrectomy** is the surgical removal of the kidney and may be done because of tumors or chronic infection, or to provide a kidney for transplantation. No matter what the reason for the nephrectomy, the patient needs emotional support and an opportunity to express and discuss feelings about the loss of a body part.

A small drain may be placed in the wound for incisional drainage. When the patient has had a nephrectomy, there may be a minimal amount of drainage from the wound for the first 24 to 48 hours, which gradually diminishes.

Dressings should be checked often for evidence of fresh bleeding because hemorrhage is always a possibility. Vital signs are watched, and any significant change in the pulse rate with restlessness should be reported to the physician. Gastrointestinal complications with nausea, vomiting, and abdominal distention may occur. Fluids by mouth may be restricted and a nasogastric tube inserted, which should be connected to suction drainage.

The most important postoperative concern is that

BOX 24-4

Nursing Process

URINARY DIVERSION—POSTOPERATIVE PHASE

ASSESSMENT

Signs and symptoms of urinary tract infection and systemic infection
Decrease in urine volume and cloudiness
Urinary tract pain
Daily bowel movement

NURSING DIAGNOSES

Activity intolerance related to anxiety, pain, weakness, fatigue
Anxiety related to fear, prognosis
Constipation related to decreased activity, painful defecation
Pain related to surgical procedure
Ineffective individual coping related to anxiety, depression
Fear related to disease process, hospitalization, powerlessness, real or imagined threat to well-being, surgical procedure
Fluid volume deficit related to abnormal fluid loss, decreased fluid intake
Impaired home maintenance management related to home environment obstacles, inadequate support system
Knowledge deficit related to limited understanding of disease process, prescribed treatment
Personal identity disturbance related to body image, role performance, self-esteem
Sexual dysfunction related to altered bladder control, body image, depression, impotence, physiologic limitations
Altered urinary elimination related to diversion

NURSING INTERVENTIONS

Administer standard immediate postoperative care, such as frequent vital signs.
Measure and record intake and output.
Report absence of urinary drainage immediately.
Maintain intravenous fluid and electrolyte infusions.
Provide mouth care every 4 hours while patient is awake.
Maintain patency of nasogastric tube, and cleanse and lubricate nostril through which tube passes.
Monitor return of peristalsis by observing for flatus, listening for bowel sounds once every 8 hours.
Administer nothing by mouth until ordered, based on return of bowel function.
Administer analgesics as ordered to relieve pain and facilitate movement.
Turn patient every 2 hours and encourage coughing, deep breathing, and leg exercises.
Ambulate as early as orders permit.
Maintain patency of drainage tubes.
Facilitate expression of feelings about altered body image.
Assess integrity and color of the stoma every shift.
Teach about disease process and treatment.

Cutaneous ureterostomy

Maintain patency of ureteral catheters.
Put ureterostomy cups or urostomy bags in place after catheters removed.
Dilate ureters with sterile catheters as ordered to ensure patency and prevent ureteral stricture.

Ileal conduit

Maintain drainage bag over stoma or catheter in stoma to collect urine; attach catheter to gravity drainage.
Empty drainage bag every 2 hours; attach to gravity drainage bag at night.
Control odor of urine and in appliance:
- Avoid odor-producing foods.
- Give cranberry juice.
- Add commercial deodorizers to bag.
- Wash permanent appliance with detergent and water and rinse in vinegar water; air dry overnight; patient uses two permanent appliances (alternating one each day) or uses disposable appliances.

Change appliance and cleanse skin as follows:
- Remove appliance.
- Bend over to drain conduit before cleansing skin.
- Clean cement from skin with adhesive solvent.
- Wash skin with soap and water.
- Apply stomahesive skin barrier or powder for skin irritation.
- Apply cement or liquid adhesive or double-faced adhesive disks and appliance.

Instruct patient and gradually involve the patient in care until self-care possible.

EVALUATION OF EXPECTED OUTCOMES

Adequate urinary drainage maintained
Discomfort relieved
No signs or symptoms of infection
Actively participates in care
Adequate nutritional and fluid states maintained
Describes disease process, surgical intervention, and responsibility for care
Relates less anxiety from fear of unknown, loss of control, or misinformation
Shares feelings about control of elimination and bodily changes
Patient and family verbalize fears and concerns
Skin integrity maintained

BOX 24-5 **Nursing Process**

LITHOTOMY—POSTOPERATIVE PHASE (URETEROLITHOTOMY, PYELOLITHOTOMY, NEPHROLITHOTOMY)

ASSESSMENT

Decrease in urine volume
Passing of stone fragments in the urine
Healing of skin and operative site
Signs and symptoms of urinary tract infection
Pain
Daily bowel movement

NURSING DIAGNOSES

Activity intolerance related to anxiety, pain, weakness, fatigue
Constipation related to decreased activity, painful defecation
Pain related to surgical procedure
Ineffective individual coping related to anxiety, depression
Fear related to disease process, hospitalization, powerlessness, real or imagined threat to well-being, surgical procedure
Fluid volume deficit related to abnormal fluid loss, decreased fluid intake
Knowledge deficit related to limited understanding of disease process, prescribed treatment

NURSING INTERVENTIONS

Weigh daily.
Use standard immediate postoperative care.
Anticipate drainage from wound; secure dressing with Montgomery straps.
Change sterile dressing as often as necessary to keep dry; use caution to prevent displacement of penrose drain in wound.
Maintain patency of bladder catheter.
Measure and record intake and output.
Observe color of urine.
Relieve pain with analgesics as ordered.
Splint incision during movement and coughing.
Assist males to stand when voiding.
Instruct on disease process and treatment.

EVALUATION OF EXPECTED OUTCOMES

Maintains adequate urinary drainage
Discomfort relieved
Actively participates in care
Relates less anxiety from fear of unknown or misinformation
Describes disease process, surgical intervention, and care
Adequate nutritional fluid status maintained
No signs or symptoms of infection

good urinary drainage be established from the remaining kidney. The patient may have a retention catheter in place, which is connected to gravity drainage; if the patient does not void, catheterization may be ordered. All intake and output must be carefully measured and recorded.

The patient will find it difficult to breathe deeply because of the location of the incision. In some cases the thoracic cavity may have been opened, and the patient will have chest tubes connected to underwater drainage. Medication for pain should be given, after which the incision may be splinted and the patient ecouraged to breathe deeply. The patient will be positioned according to the approach used for surgery. The patient is usually out of bed on the first postoperative day and ambulatory soon after. Most patients are able to tolerate a regular diet by the fourth postoperative day, with a fluid intake of approximately 3000 ml.

When the patient leaves the hospital, he or she is advised to avoid heavy lifting and straining for 6 weeks, to maintain fluid intake, and to avoid alcohol. The patient should be advised to avoid respiratory tract infections and activities that might result in injury to the other kidney.

A *nephrostomy* is an incision into the kidney pelvis for the purpose of drainage. The postoperative care of the patient with a nephrostomy or pyelostomy is the same as that for nephrectomy except for the presence of catheters, which are attached to drainage (see Figure 24-7). The nurse should watch carefully to be sure that the catheters do not become plugged with a blood clot. The physician's orders concerning turning the patient onto the affected side should be clearly understood. Drainage must be accurately measured and recorded, and dressings about the tubes or wound may need to be changed often. The skin may be kept clean by washing with mild soap and water and dried to prevent irritation. If tubes have been placed in both kidneys, both tubes should be placed on one side of the bed.

Nursing Care Plan

PATIENT WITH CHRONIC RENAL FAILURE

Ms. Barton is a 39-year-old female who comes into the outpatient dialysis unit for hemodialysis treatments three times per week because of chronic renal failure secondary to diabetic nephropathy. An internal arteriovenous fistula in her left arm is used as an access for dialysis. Physically, she has been tolerating the dialysis treatments well, with only mild dizziness at the end of each session.

The dialysis nurses have noted, however, that Ms. Barton gets irritated approximately 1 hour into the treatment. She calls to the nurses to check the machine, solutions, or her blood pressure, all of which are normal.

Ms. Barton has been on dialysis treatments on a regular basis for 6 months. She is on the transplant list, awaiting a matched donor.

Past Medical History

- Diagnosed as having juvenile diabetes (insulin dependent) at age 8
- Good control until adolescence; multiple hospitalizations from age 12 to 19; periods of noncompliance, denial of the diabetes, and growth spurts
- Appendectomy at age 16
- First pregnancy at age 21; baby a fetal demise at 39 weeks
- Second pregnancy at age 22; complicated by preeclampsia; C-sectioned at 36 weeks, viable male infant weighing 10 lbs
- Third pregnancy at age 26; mild toxemia, repeat C-section at 36 weeks, viable female infant weighing 9 lbs 15 oz
- Abdominal hysterectomy (uterus only) at age 29
- Hospitalized at ages 30 and 37 for severe episodes of vomiting leading to ketoacidosis
- Major illness at age 38, characterized by intractable vomiting, diarrhea, ketoacidosis, and coma; diabetic nephropathy and retinopathy identified at that admission; being followed closely by specialists for both conditions

Psychosocial Data

- Incomplete as to biologic family; adopted as an infant; is in the process of petitioning the courts to obtain birth records to identify genetic relatives in the hopes of locating a matched donor
- Currently a housewife; not employed outside of the home
- Has completed 2 years of junior college; now attending a 4-year program, wants to obtain a degree as a counselor
- Divorced for 10 years; states she has a "friendly" relationship with her ex-husband due to the children
- Has 2 children: 17-year-old Dan Jr., a high school sophmore, and 13-year-old Lisa, who is in the 8th grade
- Is living with her boyfriend David, who is supportive and caring
- Current living situation for 6 years; both children spend every other weekend with their father and stepmother
- Receives disability through Social Security, also on Medicaid (title 19)
- Ex-husband is a lawyer, contributes child support payments on a regular basis
- Owns own home—multi-level split style, but master bedroom on first floor
- Quality relationships with adoptive parents, siblings and ex-in-laws
- *Religion:* Lutheran, active in church, sings in the choir
- *Hobbies:* Likes to read, garden, knit, and draw; is an avid hockey fan, has season tickets to local professional team

Assessment Data

- Height 5 ft 4 in, weight 118 lbs
- Oriented × 3 (time, place, and person)
- *Skin:* Dry and scaly; dusky color at times; usually pale but has been noted to be gray; signs of irritation from scratching evident on chest and arms; no signs of infection; small areas of broken skin on right chest wall; A-V fistula in left forearm (is right handed)
- *EENT:* Full extraocular movements (EOMs); wears glasses for nearsightedness; last ocular visit 3 months ago; teeth in good repair; visits dentist regularly
- *Respiratory:* Regular rate and rhythm (18-20); all lung fields clear to percussion and ascultation
- *Breasts:* Firm; no nipple discharge; no masses or tenderness on palpation; practices breast self-examination monthly; had mammogram 6 months ago, negative findings
- *Abdominal:* Soft, nontender, nondistended; midline scar noted
- *Cardiovascular:* Apical rate 68; best heard at apex; S1, S2 heard; all peripheral pulses felt
- *Musculoskeletal:* Full range of motion; joints not inflamed or painful; steady gait

Laboratory data

- Blood sugar (fasting) = 128; does own blood sugar daily
- Hgb 9.4, Hct 27, WBC 8500, Platelets 300,000
- Electrolytes within normal limits now; before dialysis, potassium was high
- Screened on a weekly basis
- BUN 38; had been as high as 76

continued

Nursing Care Plan

PATIENT WITH CHRONIC RENAL FAILURE—cont'd

Past Medical History	Psychosocial Data	Assessment Data
Immunizations up-to-date; last tetanus booster 3 years ago No known food or drug allergies Has never smoked	Does not feel well enough to drive after dialysis treatments, so David brings her to the dialysis center during his lunch hour at noon and returns to pick her up at 6 PM (treatment time is from 1 to 6 PM, Monday, Wednesday, and Friday)	Creatinine clearance varies depending on when tested in relation to dialysis; felt to have some residual nephron function *Medications* NPH insulin 46 units daily Regular insulin 8 to 10 units on a sliding scale Colace 100 mg po prn Centrum vitamin tab 1 po daily

NURSING DIAGNOSIS

Diversional activity deficit related to long hours of treatment and relative immobility during treatment, as evidenced by statements of boredom and frequent turning of the channel selector of the television set

NURSING INTERVENTIONS	EVALUATION OF EXPECTED OUTCOMES
Encourage patient to discuss drawing and sketching in detail. Ask her what parts of these activities are most meaningful. Initiate a discussion of past artwork and have her describe specific details that give her pleasure. Focus on what patient *can* do with one hand and her other senses while sitting for 5 hours, rather than on what she *cannot* do. Encourage patient to use her analysis of the meaningful aspects of gardening to find something related to these activities. If necessary, prompt patient with ideas related to her analysis, such as listening to tapes on gardening, drawing plans for use of oils or colored pencils, writing stories about painting, or planning hockey moves. Let patient know that the environment can be adapted for her use (such as moving a larger table near by, allowing her time to set up before hooking up the dialysis machine). Have patient identify what she needs for her chosen daily activities and plan together how to obtain the materials. Observe for periods of frustration and assist. Let patient know that changes in her plans are possible (e.g., adding new activities).	Feels free to discuss the prolonged immobility and her negative feelings toward it Identifies the personal meaning of her usual diversional hobbies and incorporates these into her treatment times Identifies those diversional activities that appeal to her while immobilized Selects certain activities to engage her time and mind while immobilized Plans a range of diversional activities and feels comfortable in asking for assistance in setting them up Chooses a desired activity that she can engage in Satisfactorily engages in her chosen diversional activity during periods of immobility

NURSING DIAGNOSIS

Fluid volume excess related to compromised regulatory mechanisms, as evidenced by changes in neurologic, cardiovascular, respiratory, and renal status

NURSING INTERVENTIONS

Assess for and report signs and symptoms of fluid volume excess: significant weight gain (greater than 0.5 kg/day), elevated BP and pulse, (BP may not be elevated if fluid has shifted out of vascular space), development of an S3 or S4 gallop rhythm, change in mental status, crackles and diminished or absent breath sounds, dyspnea, orthopnea, peripheral edema, distended neck veins, or elevated central venous pressure.
If respiratory difficulty, help patient into a semi-Fowler's position to facilitate breathing.
Administer oxygen as needed.
Remind patient of the necessity of restricting fluids to 500 ml plus amount of urine output daily.
Discuss the importance of weighing herself daily and comparing and contrasting findings.
Remind her to phone the dialysis center if her weight gain is over 4 lb per day.
Reinforce teachings regarding measuring specific gravity testings.
Discuss a sodium and potassium-restricted diet.
List foods that are to be avoided. Refer her to a dietician to incorporate food restrictions into the ADA diet exchanges.
Teach patient to test all stools for occult blood. Have her give a return demonstration.
Provide a diet high in calories from carbohydrates and fats.
Reinforce with patient the importance of monitoring I&O. Remind patient of the need for frequent oral hygiene.
Discuss the use of hard sugarless candy, gum, and cold liquids to help improve the taste in her mouth.

EVALUATION OF EXPECTED OUTCOMES

At home, or in the dialysis center, does not experience symptoms of fluid volume excess
Can cite the importance of self-monitoring and self-regulating all necessary parameters (e.g., weight, fluid intake and output)
Identifies what symptoms to report to her physician and the dialysis center
States the importance of immediately reporting any changes to either her physician or the dialysis center
Does not experience fluid volume excess as evidenced by stable weight, stable BP and pulse, absence of gallop rhythm, usual mental status, normal breath sounds, absence of dyspnea, peripheral edema, distended neck veins, and central venous pressure within the normal range
Avoids any complications of excess fluid volume
Has normal skin turgor
Electrolytes within the normal range
States her ability to breathe comfortably
Takes the responsibility of teaching her children/significant other these untoward changes
Keeps her fluid intake at 500 ml plus the amount of urine output daily
Baseline weight of 118 to 120 lbs maintained
Urine specific gravity remains within 1.005 to 1.020

NURSING DIAGNOSIS

Powerlessness related to chronic illness, as evidenced by statements of ambivalent feelings about dependence on others

NURSING INTERVENTIONS

Encourage patient to express her feelings.
Set aside time for meaningful discussions regarding daily happenings.

EVALUATION OF EXPECTED OUTCOMES

Describes strategies for decreasing anxiety
Demonstrates increased control by participation in decision making related to healthcare

continued

NURSING INTERVENTIONS—cont'd	EVALUATION OF EXPECTED OUTCOMES—cont'd
Accept her feelings of powerlessness as normal. Plan to be present (if possible) during situations where feelings of powerlessness are likely to be greatest, and offer therapeutic use of self. Identify and develop patient's coping strategies, strengths (sense of humor), and resources (extended family) for support. Discuss situations that provoke feelings of anger, anxiety, and powerlessness to search for areas that she can control. Encourage participation in self-care; provide positive reinforcement for her attempts; make her feel like a member of the health team by asking her opinion. Provide opportunities for her to make decisions relating to care, treatment, positioning, and ambulation. Encourage family and significant other to support her without taking control. Explain rules, policies, procedures, and schedules to decrease areas of potential conflict. Modify the environment when possible to promote a sense of control.	Actively participates in planning and carrying out some aspects of care and treatment; communicates a renewed sense of power and control over the current situation Acknowledges her fears, feelings, and concerns about the current situation Participates in self-care activities such as personal hygiene Decreases her level of anxiety by citing stressors and identifying ways to change responses (control for her) Expresses feelings of regained control Accepts and adapts to lifestyle changes Projects and daydreams about the time when her kidney transplant will alter her illness and treatment needs

NURSING DIAGNOSIS

Altered sexuality patterns related to illness and medical treatment as evidenced by statements of concern about sexuality

NURSING INTERVENTIONS	EVALUATION OF EXPECTED OUTCOMES
Initiate a trusting therapeutic relationship with patient. Provide time for privacy. Encourage her to express her feelings openly in a nonthreatening, nonjudgmental atmosphere. Discuss with patient and significant other expressions of affection to enhance their relationship, as well as past supportive roles, especially in times of crisis. Offer a referral to counselors or support persons/groups (e.g., I Can Cope).	Describes crying episodes, the treatment plan, and all the effects on her sexual desire Identifies at least three activities to enhance pleasure and communication with significant other Indicates a willingness to follow through with a referral if the sexuality problem remains unresolved Voices her feelings about potential or actual changes in sexual activity/desire Identifies ways to enhance pleasure and improve interpersonal communication with significant other Regains a sexual desire after recovery from depression

KEY CONCEPTS

- The nephron is the structural-functional unit of the kidney.
- The nephron forms urine by filtering the blood and altering the filtrate to return necessary substances to the blood and excreting unnecessary substances in the urine.
- The kidney produces four hormones: erythropoietin, which stimulates the formation of erythocytes; vitamin D, which increases calcium and phosphate absorption from the intestine, bone, and kidney; kinin, which causes vasodilation; and prostaglandin, which causes vasodilation and vasoconstriction.
- Micturition is the process of releasing urine from the body and is controlled by voluntary and involuntary influences.
- Urinalysis provides important information about kidney function.
- A sterile urine specimen is collected by catheterization and clean-catch, and routine specimens are collected during voiding.
- Diagnostic tests such as x-ray, pyelography, ultrasonography, computerized tomography, and magnetic resonance imaging provide information more about structure than function.
- Renal biopsy is an invasive test that obtains kidney tissue for microscopic examination and that provides information about renal structure and function.
- An important nursing responsibility associated with all diagnostic tests is to educate the patient about pretest procedures, what will occur during the test, and posttest care.
- Major side effects of diuretic therapy are fluid loss and electrolyte imbalances.
- Bladder catheterization is done using only sterile technique and when absolutely necessary because of the risk of urinary tract infection.
- Urinary incontinency is the inability to retain urine, is a symptom and not a disease, and needs to be investigated for the cause.
- Acute poststreptococcal glomerulonephritis is a disease that affects the glomerular capillaries and usually follows a recent sore throat.
- A urinary tract infection can best be prevented by drinking large quantities of water and by avoiding invasive procedures into the urinary tract.
- Cystitis is an infection of the bladder, and pyelonephritis is an infection in the kidney.
- Obstructions of the urinary tract can be caused by stones, tumors, kinking of a ureter, a congenital anomaly, or an enlarged prostate gland and be located anywhere in the urinary tract.
- Acute renal failure is the sudden loss of renal function, and the focus of patient care is to keep the patient alive until the kidney heals, especially by preventing infection.
- Chronic renal failure is when renal function is lost over a period of time, and the focus of patient care is implementing treatments that substitute for the lost kidneys.
- Dialysis is a treatment that cleans the blood of waste products and excess water. Peritoneal dialysis is done within the body, and hemodialysis is done outside the body.
- Renal transplantation is the procedure of placing a normal kidney from a donor into a person with nonfunctioning kidneys.
- After surgery on the urinary tract, it is highly possible that drains, tubes, and/or catheters will be placed to drain urine. A major nursing responsibility associated with these devices is that they remain patient and allow the free flow of urine.
- People relate to their urinary tract in a variety of ways because of its association with the reproductive system and because it produces urine, a socially unacceptable topic to some people.
- It is important that nurses assess each patient's psychologic and emotional responses to a urinary tract problem.

CRITICAL THINKING EXERCISES

1 What is the difference between voluntary control and the spinal cord reflex of urination?

2 Why is urinary incontinency a symptom and not a disease?

3 How does the urinary tract change with the normal aging process?

4 Why is it important for people who have had an excretory urography and/or lithotripsy to drink a lot of water?

REFERENCES AND ADDITIONAL READINGS

Beare PG, Myers JL: *Principles and practice of adult health nursing,* ed 2, St Louis, 1994, Mosby.

Brundage DJ: *Renal disorders,* St Louis, 1992, Mosby.

Brundage DJ, Swearingen PA: Chronic renal failure: evaluation and teaching tool, *ANNA J* 21(5):265-270, 1994.

Brunner LS, Suddarth DS: *Textbook of medical-surgical nursing,* ed 7, Philadelphia, 1993, Lippincott.

Budinger JM, Donnelly SS: Nursing care protocols for the kidney/islet cell transplant recipient, *ANNA J* 21(2):123-128, 1994.

Corbett JV: *Laboratory tests and diagnostic procedures with nursing diagnosis,* ed 3, Norwalk, Conn, 1992, Appleton & Lange.

Droller M: Immunotherapy and genitourinary neoplasia, part III, *Infect Control Urol Care* 16(4):12, 1992.

Dworkin LD: Why kidneys fail, *Mt Sinai J Med* 59(1):13-22, 1992.

Gray M: *Genitourinary disorders,* St Louis, 1992, Mosby.

Gutch CF, Stoner MH, Corea AL: *Review of hemodialysis for nurses and dialysis personnel,* ed 5, St Louis, 1993, Mosby.

Guzzetta CE, Dossey BM: *Cardiovascular nursing holistic practice,* St Louis, 1992, Mosby.

Kammerer JK: Case study of the anemic patient: epoetin alfafocus on CQI and patient management, *ANNA J* 21(5): 282-285, 1994.

Kellen M and others: Predictive and diagnostic tests of renal failure: a review, *Anesth Analg* 78(1):134-142, 1994.

Kellick KA: Diuretics, *AACN Clinical Issues* 3(2):472-482, 1992.

Korniewicz DM, O'Brien ME: Evaluation of a hemodialysis patient education and support program, *ANNA J* 21(1):33-40, 1994.

Lancaster LE: Renal response to shock, *Crit Care Nurs Clin North Am* 2(2):221, 1990.

Lancaster LE, editor: *Core curriculum for nephrology nursing,* ed 3, Pitman, NJ, 1995, American Nephrology Nurses Association.

Lewandoski J: Issues in renal nutrition, *Nephrol Nurs Today* 3(4):1-8, 1994.

Malasanos L and others: *Health assessment,* ed 4, St Louis, 1989, Mosby.

McCance KL, Huether SE: *Pathophysiology the biologic basis for disease in adults and children,* ed 2, St Louis, 1994, Mosby.

Mondoux LC: Patients won't ask, *RN* 15(2):35-40, 1994.

Phipps WJ, Long BC, Woods NF, Cassmeyer UL: *Medical surgical nursing concepts and clinical practice,* ed 5, St Louis, 1995, Mosby.

Porush JG, Faubert PF: *Renal disease in the aged,* Boston, 1991, Little, Brown.

Radke KJ: The aging kidney: structure, function, and nursing practice implications, *ANNA J* 21(4):181-190, 1994.

Richard CJ: *Comprehensive nephrology nursing,* Boston, 1986, Little, Brown.

Richard CJ: Assessment of renal structure and function and causes of renal failure. In Lancaster LE, editor: *Core curriculum for nephrology nursing,* ed 3, Pitman, NJ, 1995(a), American Nephrology Nurses Association.

Richard CJ: *Renal function.* In Copstead LE, editor: *Pathophysiology,* Philadelphia, 1995(b), WB Saunders.

Shannon MT, Wilson BA: *Govoni and Hayes drugs and nursing implications,* ed 7, Norwalk, Conn, 1992, Appleton & Lange.

Trusler LA: OKT 3: nursing considerations for use in acute renal failure transplant rejection, *ANNA J* 17(4):299-303, 1990.

Walsh PC, et al.: *Campbell's urology,* ed 6, Philadelphia, 1992, WB Saunders.

York A: Current perspectives: iron management during therapy with recombinant human erythropoietin, *ANNA J* 20(6):645-652, 1994.

CHAPTER 25

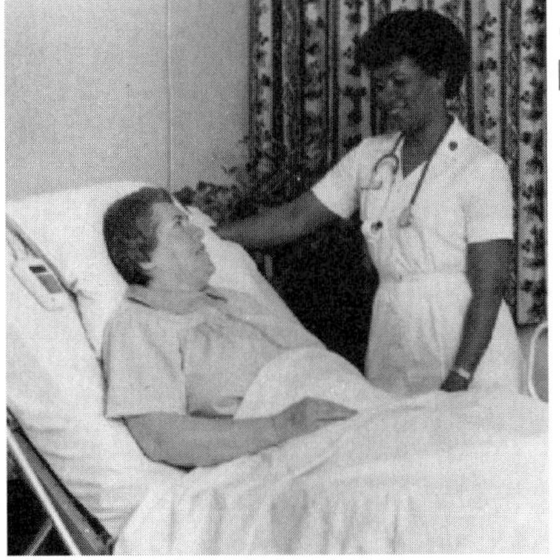

Women's Reproductive Health

CHAPTER OBJECTIVES

1 Discuss the physiology of menstruation and menopause.
2 Identify the physiologic changes of puberty and discuss the teaching role of the nurse in the care of the teenage girl.
3 Contrast the efficacy, risks, and benefits of the various contraceptive options.
4 Identify patients at high risk for osteoporosis and discuss the risks and benefits of hormonal replacement.
5 Discuss the use of open-ended questions in assessing sexuality.
6 Identify the purpose and nursing responsibilities for the following diagnostic tests: Papanicolaou smear, breast examination, and pelvic ultrasound.
7 Contrast the treatment of vaginitis caused by the *Trichomonas* organism with that caused by *Candida albicans*.
8 Describe the symptoms and treatment of vaginal fistulas.
9 Identify the primary goal of nursing care following colporrhaphy.
10 Describe the cause and treatment of endometriosis.
11 Discuss the risk factors for cervical cancer and the recommended screening interval for Papanicolaou smears.
12 Identify the early symptoms of ovarian cancer.
13 Discuss the assessment and relationship of pelvic inflammatory disease (PID) and ectopic pregnancy.
14 Discuss medical indications for vulvectomy and hysterectomy. Discuss their effects on female sexuality.
15 Describe the goals of care for the patient following hysterectomy.
16 Contrast possible treatments for breast cancer and discuss methods of breast reconstruction following a mastectomy.
17 Discuss the need for abortion counseling and the use of active listening to support the patient's decision-making process.
18 Contrast a normal postabortion recovery with a complicated recovery.

KEY WORDS

abortion
amenorrhea
bartholinitis
climacteric
colporrhaphy
colposcopy
culdoscopy
curettage
dilation and curettage (D & C)
dysmenorrhea
endometriosis
fimbriated
hysterectomy
laparoscopy
mammography
mastectomy
mastitis
menarche
menopause
menorrhagia
metrorrhagia
ovulation
Papanicolaou (Pap) smear test
pelvic exenteration
pessary
puberty
vaginitis

STRUCTURE AND FUNCTION OF THE REPRODUCTIVE SYSTEM

The reproductive system includes the external genitalia of the female, as well as the internal organs associated with reproduction. The female breasts also play a role in sexual function and dysfunction. Sexual and reproductive development are influenced by the endocrine system, and the nervous system is involved in human sexual response.

The Female Reproductive System

The region encompassing the female external genitalia is usually referred to as the *vulva* (Figure 25-1). The vulva includes the mons pubis, a pad of fatty tissue that protects the pubis. During puberty the mons becomes covered by hair, and its sebaceous glands become more active. The labia majora are two elongated folds of skin extending from the mons to the perineum (Figure 25-1). At puberty, hair begins to grow along the outside surfaces of the labia, while the inside surfaces start to secrete lubricants from their sebaceous glands. Lying within the labia majora are two thinner, hairless folds of skin known as the labia minora. The labia minora are richly supplied with sebaceous glands, nerves, and blood vessels. During sexual excitement, they become engorged with blood and lubricated by secretions. The upper folds of the labia minora meet to form the clitoral hood or prepuce, which shields the clitoris beneath. The clitoris consists of spongy erectile tissue that becomes swollen with blood during sexual arousal. The clitoris is exquisitely sensitive because of a rich network of nerves, but only a small part of the clitoris is visible, as the deeper shaft lies beneath the skin. The labia minora protect an area called the

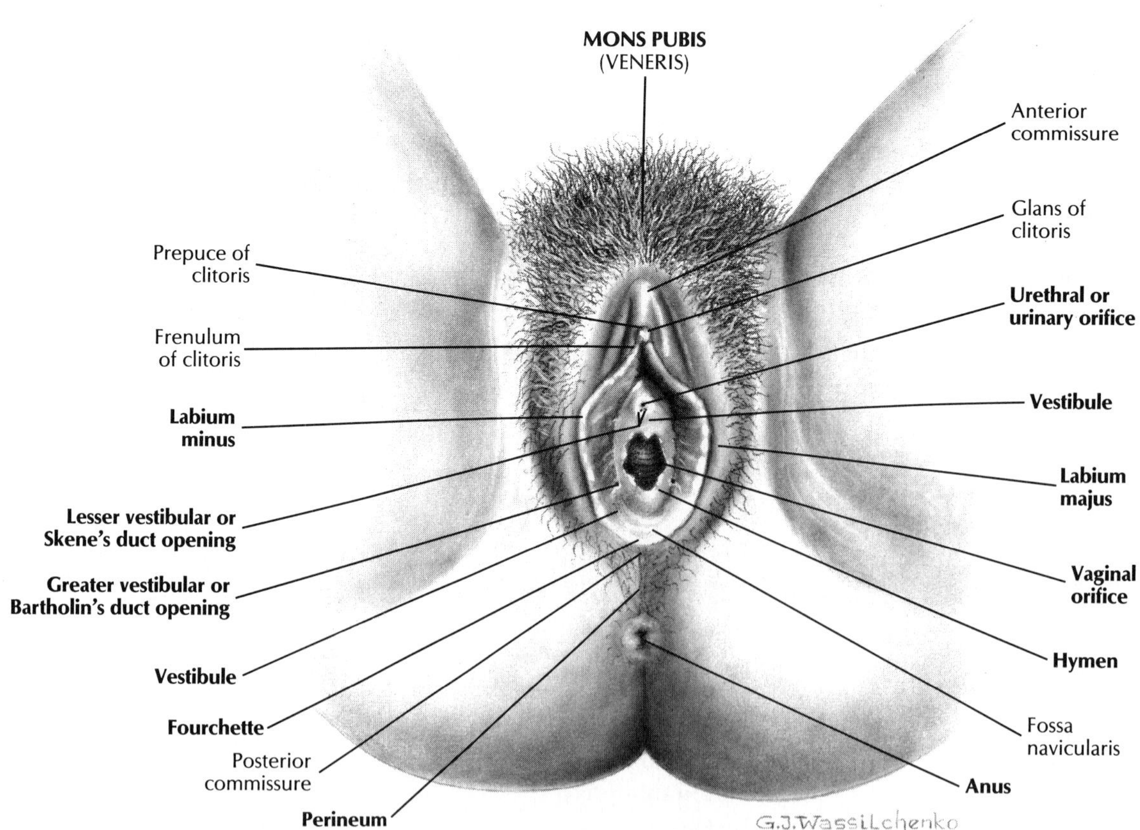

Figure 25-1 External female genitalia. (From Bobak IM, Jensen MD: *Maternity and gynecologic care,* ed 5, St Louis, 1993, Mosby.)

vestibule, within which lies the urinary meatus (urinary opening) and below it the introitus (vaginal opening). The hymen is a fragile band of tissue that encircles or covers the introitus. Even in virgin girls the hymen allows the passage of menstrual blood and will usually accommodate a tampon without tearing. However the hymen can be torn accidentally during exercise, trauma, and digital examination as well as during intercourse, and thus it is an unreliable indicator of virginity. The *perineum* is a muscular area that lies between the anus and the vaginal outlet. The area of the perineum where the labia minora join posteriorly is called the *fourchette.* The vagina is an elastic, muscular canal that extends from the introitus to the cervix. The space surrounding the cervix is called the vaginal fornix. During the childbearing years the epithelium that lines the vagina is arranged in transverse folds called *rugae.* These folds allow the mucosal layer to stretch during coitus and childbirth. The vagina is lubricated by secretions from two sets of glands, *Bartholin's glands* and *Skene's glands,* located near the introitus. During sexual stimulation the vagina becomes engorged with blood, and this pushes some fluid to the surface of the epithelium, serving as additional lubrication. Before puberty the vaginal pH is nearly neutral (7.0), but after puberty and until menopause the vaginal pH is more acidic (4.5). This acidity helps to protect women from infection during their most sexually vulnerable years. After menopause the vaginal pH becomes more alkaline and the epithelium thinner and less protective. The vagina acts as an outlet for menstrual flow, serves as the birth canal during childbirth, and functions as an organ of sexual pleasure. Although the vaginal walls are only sparsely supplied with nerves, the introitus is sensitive and can be highly excitable.

The *uterus* is a pear-shaped, hollow, muscular organ composed of three layers: the inner, *endometrial* layer, which is shed during menstruation; the muscular middle layer, or *myometrium,* which contracts during childbirth; and the outer layer, or *perimetrium.* The bulging, upper part of the uterus is called the *fundus* (Figure 25-2). The lowest portion extends downward into the vagina and forms the cervix. The cervix has a narrow canal that has openings at the entrance and exit, called the *internal os* and *external os.* This passageway is called the *endocervical canal.* Usually the endocervical canal is less than an inch in circumference, but during childbirth the canal widens to ten centimeters to permit passage of the fetal head. The endocervical canal is

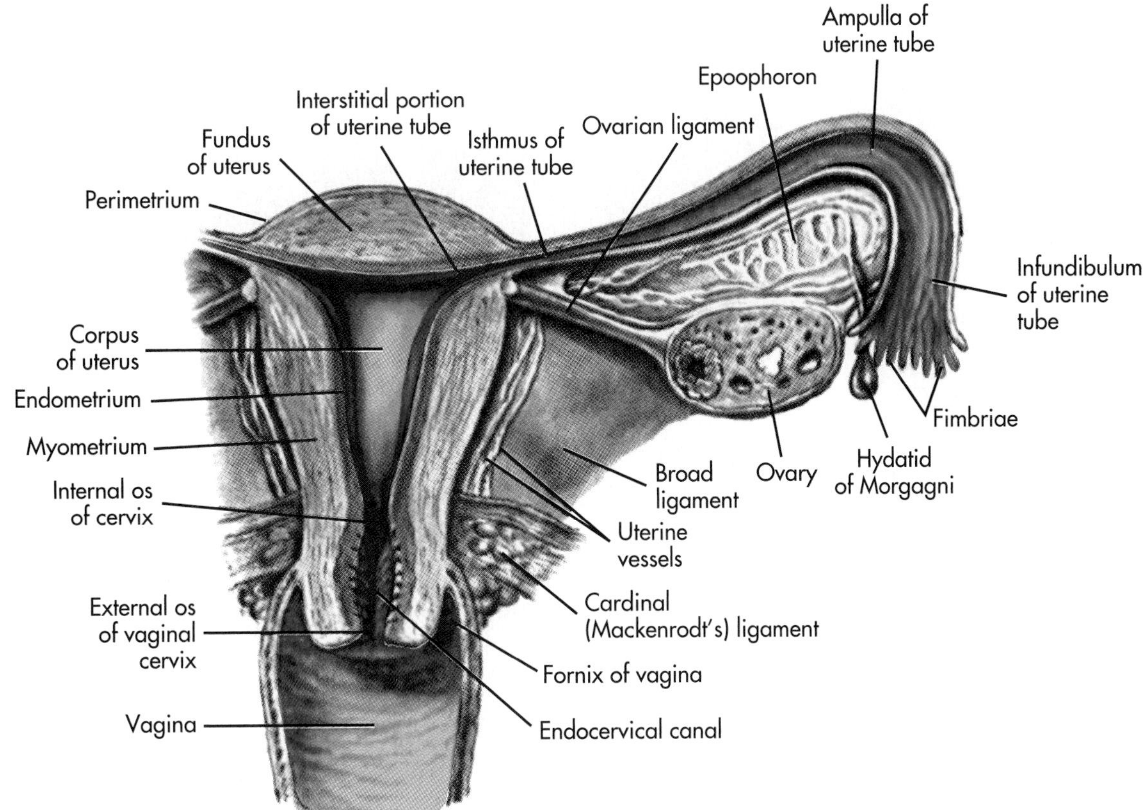

Figure 25-2 Cross sections of uterus, fallopian tube, and ovary. (From Bobak IM, Jensen MD: *Maternity and gynecologic care,* ed 5, St Louis, 1993, Mosby.)

lined with columnar epithelial cells. These cells are taller and plusher than the squamous epithelial cells that line the vagina and outer cervix. The junction of these cells, called the *transformation zone,* is usually located within the endocervical canal and thus is not visible during the pelvic examination. The squamocolumnar junction (transformation zone) is the area where most cervical cancer begins. In young girls or women on birth control pills, the transformation zone may extend from the endocervical canal and may be visible during the pelvic examination as a red, plush, circular area on the cervix. This is considered a normal finding. The endocervical canal also contains a thick plug of cervical mucus that acts as a barrier to infection. The uterus is not a fixed organ but lies suspended in the pelvic cavity by the round, broad, and uterosacral ligaments. Typically the uterus is anteverted (tilted forward) (Figure 25-3), but it may also be found midline or retroverted (tilted backward). The two fallopian tubes are attached to and open into the upper part or fundus of the uterus. The distal end of the tubes flares out and is known as the *infundibulum.* It has a **fimbriated** or fringed end and opens into the abdominal cavity; the ovaries are located near the distal end of each tube. At ovulation the fringed ends of the fallopian tubes move, producing a current that helps draw the ovum into the tubes. Fertilization usually occurs in the distal third of the fallopian tubes. Cilia and muscular contractions of the tubes keep the fertilized ovum moving toward the uterus for implantation. If fertilization does not occur, the ovum disintegrates and is shed during menstruation.

The white, almond-shaped ovaries are attached to the uterus by a ligament. In a woman of reproductive years, each ovary is approximately 1 to 1½ inches long, 1 inch wide, and 1 inch thick. After menopause the ovary becomes smaller and is not typically palpable during the pelvic examination. Each ovary consists of a cortex and a medulla; the ovarian follicles form within the cortex. During the menstrual cycle, one follicle matures more quickly than the others and releases an ovum that is transported down the fallopian tube toward the uterus. The follicle then becomes a structure known as the *corpus luteum,* the function of which is to secrete hormones that maintain pregnancy should the ovum be fertilized. If the ovum is not fertilized, the corpus luteum disintegrates after a few days, and menstruation occurs shortly afterward.

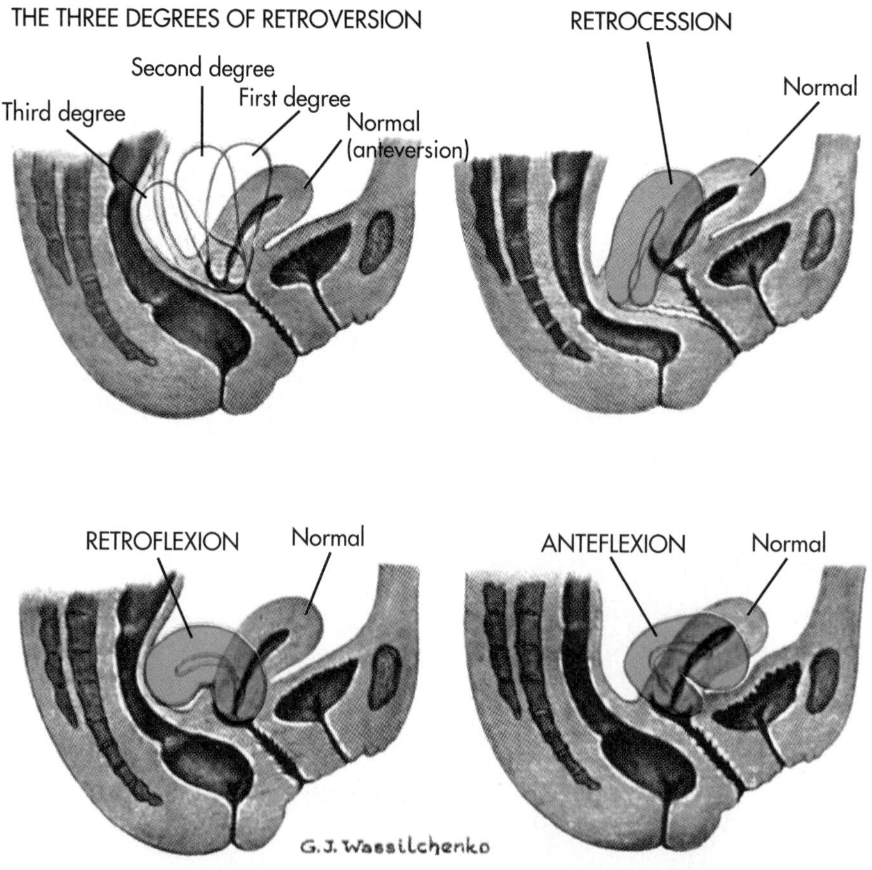

Figure 25-3 Uterine positions. (From Bobak IM, Jensen MD: *Maternity and gynecologic care,* ed 5, St Louis, 1993, Mosby.)

The female breast is composed of milk-producing glands called *acini;* the lactiferous ducts, which collect and deliver milk during lactation; and the nipple. The nipple is surrounded by a darkened area called the *areola.* The pigment of the areola deepens during pregnancy and with the use of oral contraceptives. The nipple is composed of erectile tissue and responds to tactile stimulation and cold temperatures by becoming erect. Nipples are usually everted but occasionally can be inverted (pushed inward). Nipple inversion usually has no effect on breast-feeding because the nipple becomes everted by the infant's sucking. *Montgomery's glands* are small elevations on the areola surrounding the nipple, and they secrete a lubricating and protective substance during lactation. The form of the breast is provided by subcutaneous and fatty tissue supported by the pectoralis major and pectoralis minor muscles. A girl's breasts may develop unevenly during puberty, although both breasts usually become approximately equal in size. In some normal women a noticeable disparity in breast size persists. As women age, the breasts tend to stretch and become less firm. The female breast has a rich lymphatic system that drains from the breast to various nodes in the axilla.

The Menstrual Cycle

Menstruation is a cyclic process in females, occurring at fairly regular intervals between puberty and menopause and spanning a period of approximately 30 to 35 years. The onset of menstruation, or **menarche,** is a normal physiologic process and does not indicate a state of illness or disability. The average age of menarche in the United States is 12.8 years, with the normal range of onset occurring between 10.5 and 15.5 years (Lappe, 1994).

A wide variation exists in the cycle and duration of the menstrual flow. A cycle of every 28 days may be normal for some women, but for others it may be shorter or longer. Menstrual cycles ranging between 21 and 35 days are normal for most women. The usual amount of blood loss is 1 to 6 ounces. Ovulation is the discharge of an ovum from a follicle in the ovaries. It occurs approximately 2 weeks before the onset of menstruation, regardless of the duration of the menstrual cycle. Ovulation begins some time after menarche, and a girl may not ovulate for up to 2 years after her first period. Ovulation ceases at some time during menopause.

The first day of bleeding is considered the first day of the menstrual cycle (Figure 25-4). As levels of estrogen and progesterone decline from the preceding cycle, the lining of the uterus (endometrium) is shed during menstruation. Usually this is accomplished in 2 to 7 days. Simultaneously several follicles begin to develop in the ovary during these first few days of the cycle. As the hypothalamus of the brain senses the low estrogen and progesterone levels from the preceding cycle, it responds by secreting gonadotropin-releasing hormone (GnRH), which acts on the anterior pituitary and causes it to release follicle-stimulating hormone (FSH). This hormone helps the follicles to mature. In the group of developing follicles, one will become dominant because of its greater receptivity to FSH. All the developing follicles produce estrogen, which acts on the anterior pituitary to decrease FSH. As the level of FSH declines, only the dominant follicle with its larger number of FSH receptors can continue to thrive. This follicle then continues to produce increasing amounts of estrogen, and the other follicles atrophy. From this follicle will come the mature ovum (egg) for the cycle.

Meanwhile the endometrium of the uterus becomes thicker in response to increased estrogen production in the ovary. Increasing estrogen also changes the character of the cervical mucus to a copious, stretchy, clear secretion that aids sperm transport. When the mucus may be stretched into a strand several inches long, it is known as *spinnbarkheit mucus.* This period in the menstrual cycle is known as the *follicular phase* with reference to the follicular development occurring in the ovary, and as the *proliferative phase* with reference to events occurring in the uterus.

As the ovum and follicle near maturity, the rising levels of estrogen trigger the release of luteinizing hormone (LH) by the pituitary gland. This hormone in turn stimulates the ovary to produce progesterone and androgen a few days before ovulation begins. When the increasing level of estrogen produced by the follicle reaches a critical threshold, it causes a surge in LH production. This surge assists the final maturation of the egg and allows for rupture of the follicle so that the ovum may enter the fimbriated end of the fallopian tube. This phase of the menstrual cycle is known as ovulation.

After the ovum is released, the ruptured follicle is transformed into a small body filled with yellow fluid called the *corpus luteum.* If the ovum is fertilized by a spermatozoon in the fallopian tube, it descends the tube to implant in the thick, vessel-rich lining of the uterus. If fertilization does not occur, the ovum leaves the body through the vagina. Whether or not the ovum is fertilized, the endometrium prepares for a possible pregnancy. After the follicle ruptures and becomes the corpus luteum, it produces the hormone progesterone, which makes the endometrium more vascular and glandular, enabling it to secrete glucose to an embryo. The production of FSH is now inhibited. This period is known as the *luteal phase* in reference to ovarian events, and as the *secretory phase* in reference to endometrial changes. If the ovum is fertilized, the developing embryo produces the hormone human chori-

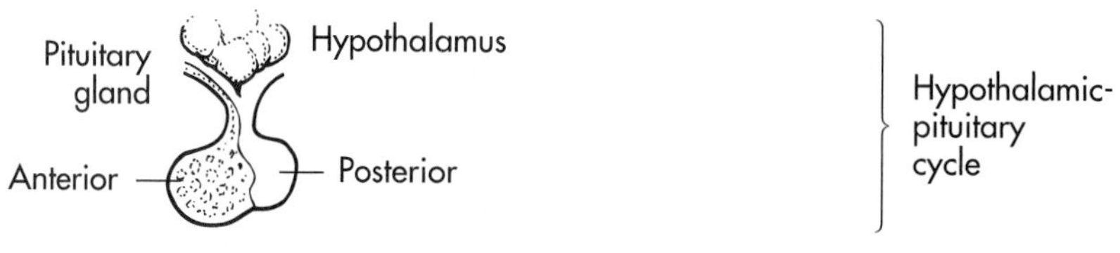

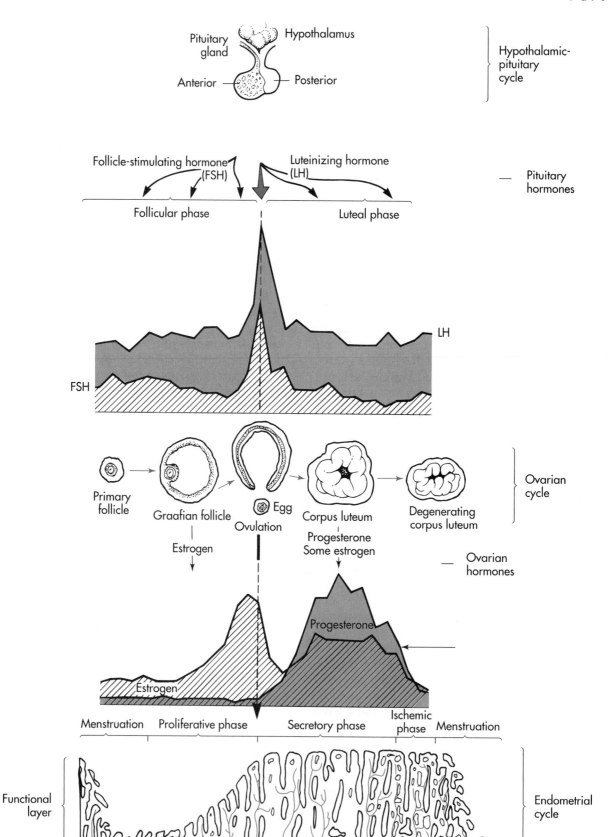

Figure 25-4 Menstrual cycle: hypothalamic-pituitary, ovarian, and endometrial. (From Bobak IM, Jensen MD: *Maternity and gynecologic care,* ed 5, St Louis, 1993, Mosby.)

onic gonadotropin (HCG), which sustains the corpus luteum and allows it to continue producing estrogen and progesterone until the placenta can assume these functions. The corpus luteum must remain functional for the first 7 to 9 weeks of the pregnancy before the placenta can assume production of sufficient estrogen and progesterone. If the ovum is not fertilized, the prepared endometrium degenerates, and menstrual flow begins approximately 2 weeks after ovulation. After menstruation, the cycle begins again.

Disturbances of Menstrual Function

Dysmenorrhea

Painful menstruation **(dysmenorrhea)** is the most common complaint associated with the menstrual process; at least one half of all women experience some degree of physical discomfort. The discomfort may occur with or without the presence of a pathologic condition. When pain and discomfort are severe enough to incapacitate the individual, a medical examination should be performed to rule out disease. Sometimes pain may result from fibroid tumors of the uterus, ovarian cysts, chronic inflammation of the fallopian tubes, pelvic inflammatory disease, displacement of the uterus, endometriosis, or narrowing of the cervical canal.

Hypercontractility of the uterus resulting from higher than normal levels of prostaglandins may be the cause of dysmenorrhea. Prostaglandins stimulate smooth muscle contraction, and the uterus is composed of smooth muscle.

The discomfort of cramps, backache, and leg pain can often be relieved by rest, a heating pad or hot-water bottle applied to the abdomen, and a few simple exercises (Figure 25-5). Heat is an especially effective treatment because it reduces muscle tone and increases circulation, thereby increasing oxygen to the muscle and relieving the ischemia.

Recent studies have shown that drugs inhibiting the production of prostaglandin (antiprostaglandins) have been effective in reducing or eliminating pain or other undesirable symptoms that sometimes accompany menstruation. Several over-the-counter (OTC) preparations are available for the treatment of dysmenorrhea. Aspirin, a drug commonly recommended to relieve dysmenorrhea, has been identified as having antiprostaglandin activity, which explains its effectiveness. Other drugs known to have antiprostaglandin action include ibuprofen (Motrin) and naproxen (Anaprox). They are thought to be more effective than aspirin in reducing the production of prostaglandins (Table 25-1). These drugs were previously used primarily for their antiinflammatory action in diseases such as arthritis. In addition to reducing uterine cramping, antiprostaglandin drugs are thought to reduce the gastrointestinal symptoms of indigestion, nausea, vomiting, and diarrhea that accompany menstruation in some women. Prostaglandin activity is thought to also increase contractility in the gastrointestinal tract, which also causes these symptoms.

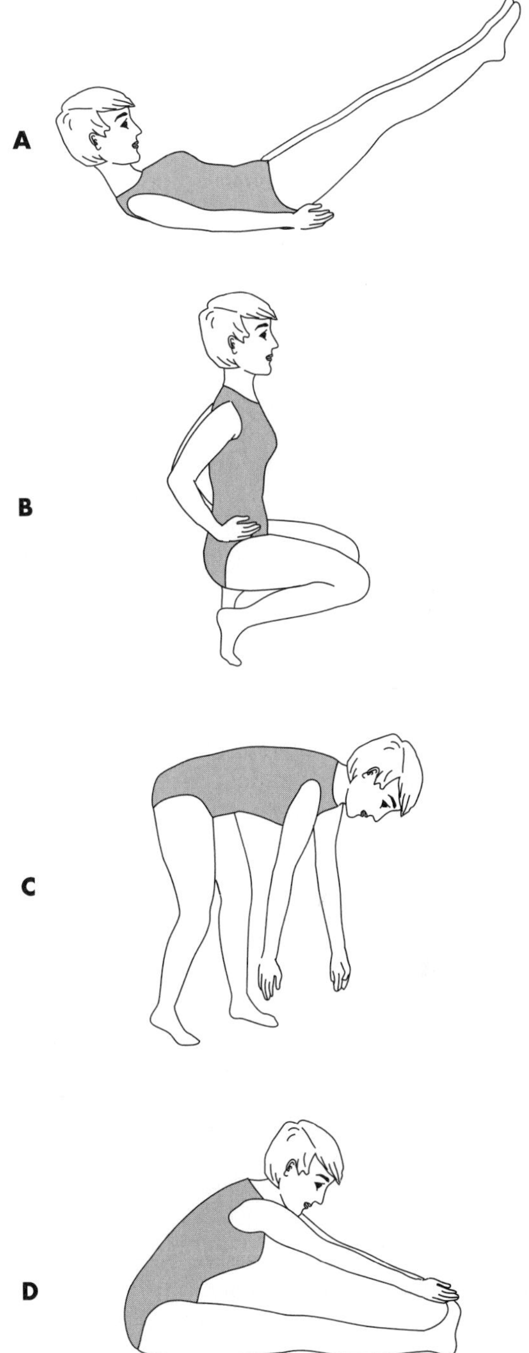

Figure 25-5 Sitting-up exercises for dysmenorrhea. **A,** Supine position with head and legs raised simultaneously; arms should be kept at side and legs straight. **B,** Deep knee bends; back should be kept straight. **C,** Monkey walk; keep hands flat on floor and walk about on hands and feet. **D,** Toe touching; keeping back straight and the legs straight, bend and touch toes with hands.

It is recommended that these drugs be taken with the onset of menstruation and only for the second, third, or fourth days of the menstrual cycle in which the indi-

TABLE 25-1
Nonsteroidal Antiinflammatory Agents for Dysmenorrhea

Antiinflammatory Agent	Dosage
ibuprofen (Motrin and others)	400 mg every 4 hours
ketoprofen (Orudis)	25-50 mg every 6-8 hours
mefenamic acid (Ponstel)	500 mg initially, followed by 250 mg every 6-8 hours
naproxen (Naprosyn)	500 mg initially, followed by 250 mg every 6-8 hours
naproxen sodium (Anaprox)	550 mg initially, followed by 275 mg every 6-8 hours

vidual normally experiences discomfort. These drugs should only be taken to control symptoms. If taken in a limited dose, the chance of side effects is reduced.

There has been very little research in the area of dysmenorrhea despite its incidence to some degree in many women and its regularly incapacitating effect on many others.

Amenorrhea

Amenorrhea is the absence of menstruation, which is normal during prepuberty, after menopause, and during pregnancy and lactation. Amenorrhea may occur with some diseases, such as tuberculosis, nephritis, anorexia nervosa, and certain endocrine disturbances. It may also occur as a result of change of climate, emotional factors, or strenuous exercise. Nurses must be aware that nongynecologic surgery may cause amenorrhea for a period of time. A woman of the appropriate age who has never menstruated is said to have primary amenorrhea, whereas suppression of menstruation once it has become established is called secondary amenorrhea. The treatment is based on the underlying cause and must be determined on an individual basis.

Menorrhagia

Menorrhagia refers to excessive menstrual flow, either in amount or duration. The condition can be associated with some pelvic pathologic conditions such as uterine fibroids or an endocrine disturbance. It may also be associated with sexually transmitted diseases, spontaneous abortion, IUD use, or anovulatory cycles. Medical examination is always indicated, and if bleeding is severe, the individual may need endometrial biopsy or dilation and curettage (D & C) of the endometrium.

Metrorrhagia

Metrorrhagia is bleeding that occurs between regular menstrual periods and usually indicates the presence of some abnormal pathologic condition. It may be associated with a malignant condition of the reproductive system or may result from benign lesions of the cervix or the uterus. It may also result from trauma, ectopic pregnancy, cervicitis, oral contraceptive use, vaginal infections, or IUD use. Postcoital spotting is often associated with benign or malignant lesions of the cervix and infections.

Oligomenorrhea

Oligomenorrhea is infrequent menses (i.e., menses occurring less often than every 40 days). Oligomenorrhea may occur normally with anovulatory cycles, as in the young girl just beginning menstruation. It can also occur at times of stress or change, such as leaving home for college and during the perimenopausal period. Marathon runners, athletes, and women with anorexia nervosa may experience oligomenorrhea secondary to changes in muscle and fat distribution. A woman whose menses are more than 90 days apart may need to have menstruation regulated to prevent buildup of the endometrial lining, which can predispose her to endometrial cancer. Oral contraceptive pills and Provera are sometimes used to regulate menses.

Toxic shock syndrome

Although not related to menstrual function, *toxic shock syndrome* (TSS) may affect healthy young women during their menstrual periods. This illness was first reported to the Centers for Disease Control in 1980. TSS also occurs in nonmenstruating women and in men, but data suggest it is especially associated with the use of high-absorbency tampons by women who have *Staphylococcus aureus* colonized in the vagina. Nonetheless, approximately 45% of TSS cases are not related to menstruation. It is estimated that between 1 and 17 women per 100,000 menstruating women annually will develop TSS (Colbry, 1992). TSS is characterized by the sudden onset of fever of 102° F (39° C) or higher, an erythematous macular rash (usually on the palms and soles) that desquamates in 7 to 24 days, systolic blood pressure below 90 mm Hg (in an adult), and involvement in three or more other organ systems. The systems most commonly involved are the gastrointestinal, muscular, mucous membrane, renal, hematologic, hepatic, central nervous, and cardiopulmonary. Nausea, vomiting, and diarrhea are common.

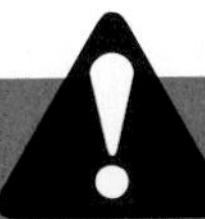

NURSE ALERT

The danger signs of toxic shock syndrome are a sudden onset of fever (102° F [39° C] or higher); hypotension (systolic pressure below 90 mm Hg); and a diffuse, erythematous, macular rash.

Danger signs of TSS may be accompanied by a sore throat, headache, decreased urine output, and confusion. Laboratory studies reveal elevated levels of blood urea nitrogen (BUN), serum creatinine, creatine phosphokinase (CPK), serum glutamic-oxaloacetic transaminase (SGOT), bilirubin, and leukocytes in the blood (leukocytosis).

Treatment involves antibiotic therapy with beta-lactam antistaphylococcal antibiotics such as nafcillin, oxacillin, or cephalosporin and fluid and electrolyte replacement. Careful monitoring of fluid intake, urinary output, and vital signs is necessary. Early detection and treatment improves the prognosis. Women who recover from TSS should be instructed to avoid tampon use altogether or until eradication of *S. aureus* in the vaginal flora can be documented. The risk of previously unaffected women developing TSS can be reduced if they wear tampons during only part of the day or night and during only part of their menstrual cycle. All women should be warned about the danger of high-absorbency tampons (Box 25-1).

BOX 25-1

PATIENT TEACHING

Guidelines for Tampon Use

Use tampons during time of moderate to heavy flow; change every 1 to 3 hours.
Avoid tampon use during times of light flow when vaginal walls are drier (usually at the beginning and end of the menstrual period).
Avoid tampon use at night. Use sanitary pads.
Avoid using superabsorbent tampons.
If high fever, vomiting, and diarrhea occur while using a tampon, see a healthcare professional at once.
If skin rash, sore throat, weakness, and flulike muscle aches occur while using a tampon, see a healthcare professional at once.
Stop using a tampon immediately if any of the above symptoms develop while wearing a tampon.
Avoid using tampons if you have a history of TSS, or stop using them for 3 to 4 months after the acute infection until cultures are negative for *S. aureus*.

Premenstrual syndrome

The condition known as *premenstrual syndrome (PMS)*, also called premenstrual tension, has been the subject of many current research studies. However, as yet there is no known cause of PMS nor any universally accepted treatment. PMS is a set of both physical and emotional symptoms that begin approximately 7 to 10 days before the beginning of the menstrual period. Symptoms commonly associated with PMS include irritability, depression, insomnia, fatigue, weight gain, edema, mastalgia, abdominal distention, headache, and backache. These symptoms usually disappear with the onset of the menstrual period. PMS symptoms may occur as a woman gets older and may worsen over time.

Because PMS is highly individualized, a nurse should help a woman to identify her symptoms. The nurse should advise her to keep a log of her symptoms and note their severity on her calendar over several months. The nurse might inquire whether certain events in her life trigger symptoms and counsel her accordingly. The patient can be encouraged to anticipate days that may be especially difficult and plan low-stress activities at these times. Women may also find that open communication with their families on this subject helps to increase understanding.

Because the exact cause of PMS is not known, a great variety of methods is used to treat the condition. Nutritional supplements such as calcium; magnesium; vitamins A, B_6, and E; and even primrose oil have all been suggested for relief of PMS (Lichtman, Papera, 1990). The nurse could suggest that the woman eat a diet low in sodium and high in complex carbohydrates 7 to 10 days before the beginning of the menstrual cycle and avoid caffeine and alcohol. Improved nutrition and exercise have been suggested as a means to control symptoms. Joining a self-help group may be useful to women who have low self-esteem from lack of understanding of PMS. Medication may be prescribed for the relief of the more severe symptoms. A diuretic such as chlorothiazide (Diuril) may be prescribed to relieve the edema resulting from water and sodium retention. Other medications that have been tried include progesterone, oral contraceptives, bromocriptine, and aldosterone (Lichtman, Papera, 1990).

PHASES OF REPRODUCTIVE FUNCTION THROUGHOUT THE LIFE CYCLE

Puberty

Puberty is the period during which the body prepares for reproductive ability. It begins in females at about age 10. Secondary sex characteristics begin to make their appearance. The size of the external reproductive organs increases, axillary and pubic hair grows, and the breasts become larger. In the female the first menstrual period is termed *menarche.* There is some variation in age at onset of puberty and menarche. The first menstrual period usually occurs between the ages of 12 and 13; however, it may occur anytime from age 10 to 15 years. Menarche usually occurs after the peak of the growth spurt. The average girl will continue to grow 2.5 inches in height after menarche (Lichtman, Papera, 1990). The first menstrual cycles are usually anovulatory, and so they are likely to be irregular for the first 1 to 2 years after onset of menstruation. Menstrual cramps are also uncommon during these first cycles. If menses has not begun by age 15 or 16 years, a gynecologist should be consulted to rule out endocrine imbalance, an imperforate hymen, or congenital anomalies. The hymen normally has an opening that allows menstrual flow to occur, but if it is imperforate, there is no opening and the flow is held back.

The sequence of physical changes in girls during puberty varies by individual. Typically the first sign of puberty is the appearance of the breast bud (Figure 25-6). The development of pubic hair usually follows, with axillary hair appearing approximately 2 years after pubic hair (Figure 25-7). There are increases in height and weight as well as changes in body contour and genital development. Puberty is considered precocious if menarche begins before age 10 or secondary development occurs before age 8 (Lichtman, Papera, 1990). This may be a result of early physiologic maturation, but it could also result from an ovarian or adrenal tumor. Reassurance can be offered once pathologic causes of precocious puberty have been explored.

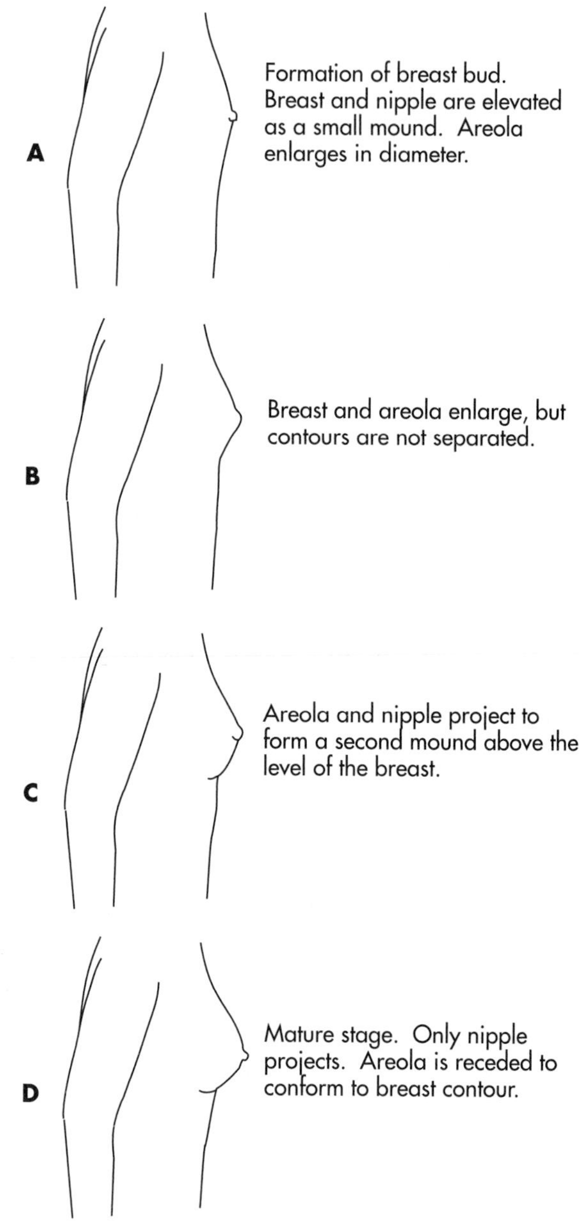

A
Formation of breast bud. Breast and nipple are elevated as a small mound. Areola enlarges in diameter.
B
Breast and areola enlarge, but contours are not separated.
C
Areola and nipple project to form a second mound above the level of the breast.
D
Mature stage. Only nipple projects. Areola is receded to conform to breast contour.

Figure 25-6 Development of breasts in girls.

Menstruation and hygiene

The nurse may be involved in counseling and teaching girls about menstruation. This process must always begin with an assessment of the individual's knowledge and feelings about menstruation. The nurse can then proceed to clarify any misconceptions and provide additional knowledge appropriate to the age and developmental level of the girl. Using terms such as *the curse* or *sick time* connotes a negative attitude and makes menstruation seem like an abnormal process. A more positive attitude about the normalcy of menstruation is fostered by the use of proper terminology, such as *menstruating* or *having my period.* In addition to basic information regarding the process of menstruation, instruction should include hygiene measures and methods of sanitary protection. Either tampons or sanitary pads can be safely used by girls of any age. However, the possibility of toxic shock syndrome (TSS) related to

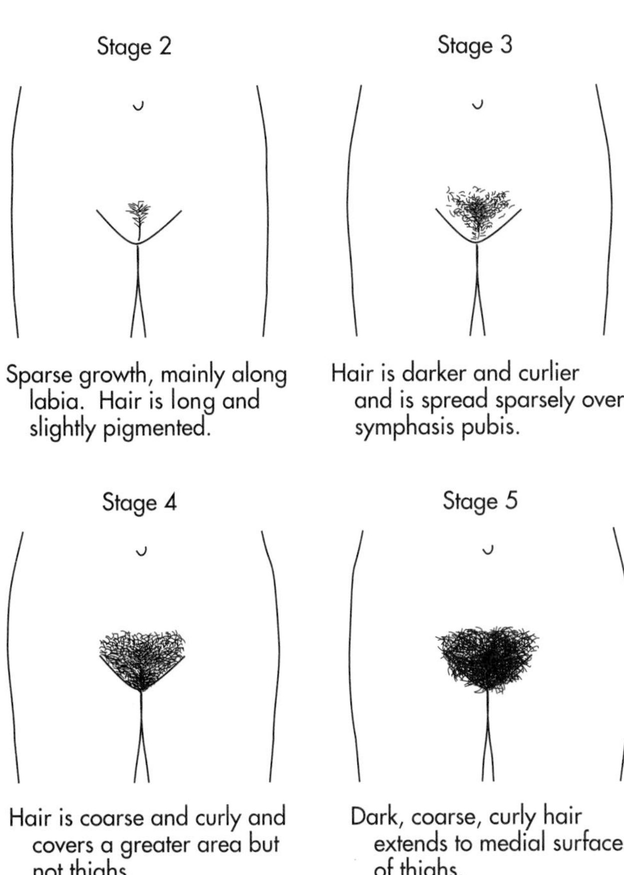
Stage 1: Hair in pubic area similiar to that on abdomen
Stage 2
Stage 3
Sparse growth, mainly along labia. Hair is long and slightly pigmented.
Hair is darker and curlier and is spread sparsely over symphasis pubis.
Stage 4
Stage 5
Hair is coarse and curly and covers a greater area but not thighs.
Dark, coarse, curly hair extends to medial surfaces of thighs.

Figure 25-7 Development of pubic hair in girls.

tampon use has resulted in some specific guidelines regarding their use (see discussion on toxic shock syndrome earlier in this chapter). A young girl may need to lubricate the tampon before it can be comfortably inserted. Even if not completely saturated, sanitary pads and tampons should be changed about every 3 to 4 hours to prevent irritation and odor. But if tampons are changed too frequently, removing the dry tampon can irritate vaginal walls and increase the risk of TSS. The nurse should encourage handwashing before and after changing a tampon or pad to prevent infection.

The nurse has numerous opportunities to instruct patients in personal hygiene measures. Cultural differences influence the habits and opinions of an individual; some cultures place great importance on cleanliness, others do not. The practice of douching was once considered by some to be essential to feminine hygiene. Routine douching is now discouraged because it is known to irritate the vaginal mucosa and upset the normal protective flora of the vagina to resist infection. Genital odor rarely comes from the vagina but instead stems from the interaction of bacteria with oils secreted by the skin of the vulva. Old menstrual blood and seminal fluid remaining after coitus sometimes produce odor. A simple and effective douching solution can be prepared using 30 ml of white vinegar in a quart of warm water. The solution is placed in a douche bag and instilled into the vagina under gentle pressure. Commercial preparations *are not* more effective and may contain perfumes that are irritating to the vaginal mucosa. Significant odor or discharge may indicate a retained tampon, foreign body, or infection and should be further assessed. Soap and water cleansing of the perineal area is all that is normally necessary for feminine hygiene.

All females should be encouraged to lead a normal life during menstruation. A program of personal hygiene, as well as sleep, rest, proper diet, and exercise should be continued. Exercise, with a few exceptions, is considered helpful in relieving minor discomfort. Although many taboos previously existed concerning swimming or bathing, there is no valid evidence of harm resulting from these activities. A daily warm bath or shower is important because there is often increased activity of the sweat glands during this time. Coitus may be objectionable to women during their periods, and they may choose to avoid it for aesthetic reasons. Women may also be at higher risk for infections during menses because the cervical os is dilated slightly to allow the passage of blood.

Recent research has linked the discomfort associated with menstruation to the activity of prostaglandins, and treatment with antiprostaglandin drugs has been successful (see the discussion on dysmenorrhea earlier in this chapter).

Psychosocial development in adolescence

Adolescence is a period of rapid physical growth, bodily change, and psychosocial development. Teenagers feel a need to assert their independence from family and experiment with new behaviors. Peer relationships assume increasing importance, and adolescents are preoccupied with issues of body image, peer groups, and self-esteem. Elkind has termed the adolescent's belief in their own invulnerability, "the personal fable of omnipotence" (Lichtman, Papera, 1990). This personal fable allows adolescents to assume physical and emotional risks because they believe they are unique and immune from harm. Girls, for instance, may engage in unprotected sex and become pregnant. In addition they may believe that it is wrong to use birth control because to do so would indicate that they are planning to engage in sexual activity. They may also become pregnant to fill a sense of personal emptiness, resolve a dependency conflict with a parent, to find an excuse to leave the parental household, or to achieve self-individuation (Trad, 1994). Sexual risk-taking and exploration is common among adolescents, and teenage pregnancy is a significant problem in the United States. Adolescent girls are also more susceptible to sexually transmitted disease because of the cellular structure of vaginal and cervical tissue in adolescence. Nurses may play an important role in assessing emerging sexuality and risk-taking behaviors. Appropriate preventive measures such as birth control and condoms may need to be offered as well as education regarding physical and emotional changes.

Gender development

In each stage of physical and emotional growth there are tasks related to the development of behaviors associated with the particular sexual role. Any condition or situation that interferes with the completion of these tasks may affect the development of sexual role behavior, but the process continues and evolves throughout the lifetime of an individual.

Sexual role or gender role is the public expression of behavior that implies masculinity or femininity. Gender identity is defined as the private or personal experience of one's maleness or femaleness. It is usually, but not always, congruent with the individual's gender or biologic sex. The development of gender identity and sexual role behavior is a complex process influenced by biologic, psychologic, and social factors.

Gender identity begins with the biologic event of conception, when the X or Y chromosome of the male combines with the X chromosome of the female. An XY pair influences the undifferentiated gonad of the embryo to become a testis at a gestational age of about 6 weeks; an XX pair differentiates the gonad as an ovary at about 12 weeks.

The appearance of the external genitalia is the next factor in the development of sexual role behavior. The parents tailor child-rearing practices in accordance with their perception of their child's gender. The child eventually becomes aware of his or her body, including the genitalia. The child's body and the responses of others to it influence juvenile gender identity.

At puberty the production of hormones affects sexual desire and further development of the genitals. These changes at puberty, combined with social influences, determine adult gender identity (Box 25-2).

BOX 25-2

PATIENT TEACHING ACROSS THE REPRODUCTIVE LIFESPAN

PATIENT TEACHING AT ADOLESCENCE

Explain the menstrual cycle
Discuss menstrual hygiene
Reassure about normal development
Assess birth control needs
Discuss peer pressure
Teach assertiveness and self-protection
Encourage healthful diet and adequate calcium intake

PATIENT TEACHING IN THE REPRODUCTIVE YEARS

Assess birth control needs and discuss options
Discuss sexuality
Encourage regular screening for cervical cancer
Teach monthly breast self-examination
Encourage low-fat diet, adequate calcium intake, smoking cessation, moderate alcohol intake
Advise on precautions in pregnancy (no drugs, tobacco, or alcohol)
Assess for family violence and role stress

PATIENT TEACHING IN THE PERIMENOPAUSAL YEARS

Assess sexual comfort; teach use of lubricants, if needed
Assess risk of osteoporosis
Discuss risks and benefits of hormonal replacement therapy
Encourage low-fat diet with adequate calcium
Assess for role stress and adaptation to change
Teach need for cancer screening (breast, cervical, colon)
Encourage breast self-examination, mammography, and regular checkups

The Reproductive Years

Patterns of childbearing are different for women of different cultural and economic circumstances. Some women bear children in their early teens, and others postpone motherhood until their late 30s or early 40s. Still others decide not to bear children at all, and some women who wish to have children may eventually prove to be infertile. "Women of reproductive years" is thus a wide category, ranging from early teens to menopause. During this period, women are concerned with establishing and maintaining intimate relationships, and most women also have concerns about contraception. Decisions about birth control are needed to space childbearing or prevent it altogether. Homosexual women do not share these concerns about birth control but may have different issues centering on becoming pregnant by the use of donor semen.

For a majority of women in their reproductive years, contraception is a significant concern. The well-informed nurse is able to provide much of the education and counseling that women need to make these contraceptive decisions. A complete discussion of obstetrics is outside the scope of this book, and the nurse is advised to consult a comprehensive obstetric text (see the abortion and ectopic pregnancy discussions later in this chapter).

Birth control (contraception)

Birth control, or contraception, is the voluntary prevention of pregnancy. The selected method of birth control depends on individual preferences, religious beliefs, and cultural considerations. A complete history, physical examination, and laboratory tests may precede the prescription of some forms of contraception. Methods of birth control include hormonal methods such as oral contraceptives, Norplant, and Depro-Provera; intrauterine devices (IUDs); diaphragms; cervical caps; condoms; foams; suppositories; jellies; and natural family planning (Table 25-2).

Combined oral contraceptives. Combined oral contraceptive pills (OCP) were approved by the Federal Drug Administration (FDA) in 1960. Since then they have been extensively studied and found to be safe and effective. Although brands differ, all combined oral OCPs contain some form of estrogen and progestin. Since the early research on the pill in the 1960s, the dose has been considerably lowered, and most women choosing this method today are started on a low-dose birth control pill. Although the serious side effects are theoretically possible at low doses, the likelihood of their occurrence is extremely low. Nonetheless, according to a 1980 Gallop poll, approximately 75% of women who are 35 years or younger consider the use of oral contraceptives to be very risky (Table 25-3) (Kaunitz, 1992). Most women named cancer as their chief concern. In fact, oral contraceptives have been shown to markedly *decrease* a woman's risk of developing ovarian and endometrial cancer. Oral contraceptives used for 1 year reduce a woman's risk of ovarian cancer by 40%, and OCPs used for 10 years reduce the risk of ovarian cancer by 80%. Further this protection appears to last for more than a decade after discontinuation of use (Kaunitz, 1992). Endometrial cancer risk is reduced by 50% after 12 months of OCP use, and this protective effect persists for more than 15 years after discontinuing use. At present there is no clear evidence of increased risk of breast cancer with use of the birth control pill. Thus the nurse can perform an important role in dispelling the myths that women may have about the risks of cancer with use of the birth control pill.

Mechanism of action and effectiveness. The combined birth control pill prevents pregnancy primarily by suppressing ovulation. In addition, progestin in the pill thickens cervical mucus, making it less possible for sperm to ascend the endocervical canal. The birth control pill is 97% to 99.9% effective. No differences in effectiveness among brands have been described. A higher potency pill is sometimes recommended for women who are taking medications for seizure disorder because these medications decrease the effectiveness of the pill (Table 25-4).

Risks, benefits, and side effects

Cardiovascular complications such as stroke, heart attack, blood clots, and hypertension are extremely rare, as are hepatic adenomas. The risk of cardiovascular complications increases in women over age 35 who smoke. Smokers over the age of 35 should be encouraged to consider other birth control methods.

Side effects are usually minimal but may occur in certain women, especially in the first few months of OCP use. These include nausea, headache, dizziness, spotting, weight gain, breast tenderness, and cholasma (increased pigmentation of the face). Taking OCP at bedtime or with food should minimize nausea. Taking pills at the same time each day may help to prevent breakthrough bleeding. Occasionally OCPs need to be changed to find the right match for the individual woman. Many brands are available, so this can be easily accomplished. The nurse should take side effects seriously, because patients may discontinue OCP use if they experience troublesome side effects. The noncontraceptive benefits in terms of cancer protection have been described above. In addition, birth control pills protect the patient from uterine fibroids, benign breast masses, pelvic inflammatory disease (PID), and ovarian cysts. The pill also decreases menstrual blood loss and lessens menstrual cramps. OCPs may be protective of fertility by preventing PID and ectopic pregnancy. No delay in return to fertility is to be expected when a woman discontinues OCP use.

Patient use. Birth control pills are prescribed in 21- or 28-day cycles. In the 28-day pack, the last week of pills are inactive and may contain small amounts of iron. These inactive pills allow the women to stay in the habit of taking a daily pill. A woman may be instructed to start her first pack on the first day of menses or on the first Sunday after the onset of menses. If she is prescribed a 21-day pack, she takes 3 weeks of pills and waits 1 week to begin the next pack. She can expect her period in the week she is not taking pills. Alternatively if she is prescribed a 28-day pack, she begins a new pack immediately upon finishing all the pills in the previous pack. She can also expect her menses in the week prior to starting a new pack of OCP. Women should be encouraged to take OCP at approximately the same time each day to increase the effectiveness of the birth control pill and decrease the likelihood of breakthrough bleeding. If a woman misses a pill, she should take it as soon as she remembers or take it with the next scheduled pill. If she misses two pills, she may take two pills together for 2 days until she is caught up, but she should also be advised to use a backup method of

TABLE 25-2

Pharmacology of Drugs Used for Women's Reproductive Health

Drug (Generic and Trade Name); Route and Dosage	Action/Indication	Common Side Effects and Nursing Considerations
CLOMIPHENE (Clomid) **ROUTE:** PO **DOSAGE:** PO 50-100 mg q × 5 days or 50-100 mg q beginning on day 5 of the cycle; may be repeated until conception occurs or 3 cycles of therapy have been completed	Ovulation stimulant used in female infertility	Headache; depression; nausea; vomiting; constipation; rash; and dermatitis; contraindicated in hepatic disease or undiagnosed vaginal bleeding; use with caution in hypertension, depression, convulsions, or diabetes
CLONIDINE (Catapres) **ROUTE:** PO, transdermal patch **DOSAGE:** PO, 0.1 mg bid, then increase by 0.1 mg/day or 0.2 mg/day until desired response; range 0.2-0.8 mg/day in divided doses; transdermal patch available in 2.5, 5.0, 7.5 mg patches delivering 0.1, 0.2, 0.3 mg/24 hr respectively	Primarily used as an antihypertensive, but also used for treatment of dysmenorrhea and menopausal syndrome	Drowsiness; dry mouth; and withdrawal phenomenon; use with caution in serious cardiac, cerebrovascular, and renal disease, pregnancy, and elderly; do not discontinue abruptly
DANAZOL (Danocrine) **ROUTE:** PO **DOSAGE:** Endometriosis, initial dose 500 mg bid, then decrease to 400 mg bid × 3-9 mo; fibrocystic breast disease, 100-400 mg q in 2 divided doses × 2-6 mo	Androgen used in the treatment of endometriosis, prevention of hereditary angiodema, and fibrocystic breast disease	Cholestatic jaundice; contraindicated in severe renal, cardiac, or hepatic disease; use with caution in seizures or migraine headaches; may increase effects of anticoagulants
ESTRADIOL, ESTRADIOL CYPIONATE, ESTRADIOL VALERATE **ROUTE:** PO, IM, topical **DOSAGE:** Menopause, ovarian failure, PO 1-2 mg q × 3 wk on, 1 wk off or 5 days on, 2 days off; or IM 0.2-1.0 mg q wk; breast cancer, PO 10 mg tid × 3 mo or longer; atrophic vaginitis, vaginal cream 2-4 g qd × 1-2 wk, then 1 g 1-3 times a week; kraurosis vulvae, IM, 1-1.5 mg 1-2 wk	Nonsteroidal synthetic estrogen used for menopause, breast cancer, prostatic cancer, atrophic vaginitis, kraurosis vulvae, hypogonadism, castration, primary ovarian failure, and prevention of osteoporosis	Gynecomastia, testicular atrophy, impotence, thromboembolism, stroke, pulmonary embolism, myocardial infarction, and cholestatic jaundice; contraindicated in breast cancer, thromboembolic disorders, and reproductive cancer; use with caution in hypertension, asthma, blood dyscrasias, gallbladder disease, congestive heart failure, diabetes, bone disease, depression, migraine headaches, convulsant disorders, hepatic and renal disease, and family history of cancer of the breast or reproductive tract
LEUPROLIDE (Lupron) **ROUTE:** SC **DOSAGE:** 1 mg/day	Antineoplastic gonadotrophin-releasing hormone used in the management of endometriosis	Edema, hot flashes, impotence, decreased libido, amenorrhea, vaginal dryness, gynecomastia; contraindicated in thromboembolic disorders, pregnancy, and undiagnosed vaginal bleeding; use with caution in edema, hepatic, cerebrovascular accident, myocardial infarction, seizures, hypertension, or diabetes; monitor liver function tests.

TABLE 25-2

Pharmacology of Drugs Used for Women's Reproductive Health—cont'd

Drug (Generic and Trade Name); Route and Dosage	Action/Indication	Common Side Effects and Nursing Considerations
LEVONORGESTREL IMPLANT (Norplant System) **ROUTE:** Subdermal caps implanted in the upper arm **DOSAGE:** Implanted during first 7 days after onset of menses; may remain × 5 yr	Synthetic progestin contraceptive used in the prevention of pregnancy over a 5-yr period	Possibly a change in appetite or weight gain; no common side effects; contraindicated in thrombophlebitis, undiagnosed genital bleeding, liver tumors, breast carcinoma, and liver disease; use with caution in depression, psychosis, lactation, fluid retention, and contact lens wearers
MEDROXYPROGESTERONE ACETATE (Depo-Provera) **ROUTE:** PO, IM **DOSAGE:** Secondary amenorrhea, PO 5-10 mg q × 5-10 days; endometrial/renal cancer, IM 400-1000 mg/wk; uterine bleeding, PO 5-10 mg q × 5-10 days starting on 16th day of menstrual cycle	Progesterone derivative used for uterine bleeding, secondary amenorrhea, endometrial and renal cancer, and as a contraceptive	Depression, nausea, gynecomastia, testicular atrophy, impotence, spontaneous abortion, thromboembolism, stroke, pulmonary embolism, myocardial infarction, or cholestatic jaundice; contraindicated in breast cancer, thromboembolic disorders, reproductive cancer, or genital bleeding; use with caution in lactation, hypertension, asthma, blood dyscrasias, gallbladder disease, congestive heart failure, diabetes, bone disease, depression, migraine headache, convulsive disorders, hepatic or renal disease, and family history of cancer of the breast or reproductive tract
MIFEPRISTONE (RU-486) **ROUTE:** PO **DOSAGE:** 1 tablet; may be used as an immediate contraceptive if given within 24 hr after intercourse	This drug is a progestin antagonist and when given to females early in pregnancy, in most cases (85%) results in abortion of fetus; it can also be used as a contraceptive, which is given once a month during the midluteal phase of the cycle when progesterone is normally high	Significant uterine bleeding and the possibility of incomplete abortion
NORETHINDRONE **ROUTE:** PO **DOSAGE:** 5-20 mg q days 5-25 of menstrual cycle; endometriosis, 10 mg q × 2 wk, then increased by 5 mg q × 2 wk, up to 30 mg/day	Progesterone derivative used to control abnormal uterine bleeding, amenorrhea, and endometriosis	Nausea, thromboembolism, stroke, pulmonary embolism, myocardial infarction, cholestatic jaundice, and spontaneous abortion; contraindicated in breast cancer, thromboembolic disorders, reproductive cancer, and genital bleeding; use with caution in lactation, hypertension, asthma, blood dyscrasias, gallbladder disease, congestive heart failure, diabetes, bone disease, depression, migraine headache, convulsive disorders, hepatic or renal disease, and family history of breast or reproductive tract cancer

continued

TABLE 25-2

Pharmacology of Drugs Used for Women's Reproductive Health—cont'd

Drug (Generic and Trade Name); Route and Dosage	Action/Indication	Common Side Effects and Nursing Considerations
NORGESTREL **ROUTE:** PO **DOSAGE:** 1 tablet q day	Progesterone derivative used as a contraceptive	Nausea, gynecomastia, testicular atrophy, impotence, thromboembolism, stroke, pulmonary embolism, myocardial infarction, cholestatic jaundice, and spontaneous abortion; contraindications and precautions same as above
TAMOXIFEN CITRATE (Nolvadex) **ROUTE:** PO **DOSAGE:** 10-20 mg bid	Antineoplastic, antiestrogen hormone used in advanced breast carcinoma that has not responded to other therapy in estrogen-receptor-positive patients (usually postmenopausal)	Nausea, vomiting, rash, hot flashes, headache, and lightheadedness; use with caution in leukopenia, thrombocytopenia, lactation, and cataracts; withhold drug if WBC is < 3500 or platelet count is < 100,000
Common drugs for vaginitis		
CLOTRIMAZOLE (Lotrimin) **ROUTE:** Topical, intravaginal **DOSAGE:** Topical, rub into affected area bid × 1-8 wk; intravaginal 1 applicator × 1-2 wk hs	Local antifungal, antiinfective used for infections of the vagina and vulva	Infrequent burning, itching, stinging, redness, and local hypersensitivity reactions
METRONIDAZOLE (Flagyl) **ROUTE:** PO, IV, topical **DOSAGE:** Anaerobic infections, PO, 7.5 mg/kg q 6 hr (not to exceed 4 g/day), IV, initial dose 15 mg/kg, then 7.5 mg/kg q 6 hr (not to exceed 4 g/day); trichomoniasis, PO, 250 mg q 8 hr for 7 days (single 2 g dose or 1 g bid for 1 day may be used); bacterial vaginosis, topical, 5 g bid for 5 days	Antiinfective used for treatment of anaerobic infections, including such gynecologic infections as trichomoniasis, and bacterial vaginosis	Headache, dizziness, nausea, vomiting, abdominal pain, anorexia, and diarrhea; contraindicated in first trimester of pregnancy; use with caution in blood dyscrasias, history of seizures or neurologic problems, and severe hepatic impairment; PO administrations should be administered with food
MICONAZOLE, MICONAZOLE NITRATE (Monistat, Monistat 3) **ROUTE:** IV, bladder irrigation, topical, intravaginal **DOSAGE:** IV, 200-3600 mg/day in divided doses q 8 hr; bladder instillation, 200 mg q 6-12 hr by continuous infusion; topical, apply to affected area bid; intravaginal, 1 suppository inserted vaginally once daily at bedtime × 3 consecutive days	Antifungal used in the treatment of fungal infections, including vulvovaginal candiasis	Headache, phlebitis, and pruritis at IV site; patients with recurrent vulvovaginal yeast infections may represent chronic illness requiring other interventions
NYSTATIN (Mycostatin) **ROUTE:** Intravaginal, topical **DOSAGE:** Intravaginal, one tablet (100,000 units nystatin) daily for 2 wk; topical, cream and ointment applied liberally to affected areas bid or as indicated until healing complete	Antifungal used in the treatment of vaginal *Candida* infections	Nystatin is well tolerated by all age groups; insert vaginal tablets high into the vagina with applicator

TABLE 25-2

Pharmacology of Drugs Used for Women's Reproductive Health—cont'd

Drug (Generic and Trade Name); Route and Dosage	Action/Indication	Common Side Effects and Nursing Considerations
TERCONAZOLE (Terazol 3, Terazol 7) **ROUTE:** Intravaginal, topical **DOSAGE:** Intravaginal, 1 suppository (80 mg) administered at bedtime × 3 consecutive days; topical, 0.4% or 0.8% vaginal cream is administered with applicator intravaginally at bedtime × 3 consecutive days	Antifungal, antiinfective used for vaginal and vulvovaginal candidiasis	Headache; patients with recurrent vulvovaginal infections may indicate a chronic illness requiring other interventions

TABLE 25-3

Voluntary Risks in Perspective

Activity	Chance of Death in a Year
Risks for men and women of all ages who participate in	
Motorcycling	1 in 1,000
Automobile driving	1 in 6,000
Power boating	1 in 6,000
Rock climbing	1 in 7,500
Playing football	1 in 25,000
Canoeing	1 in 100,000
Risks for women age 15-44 years	
Using tampons	1 in 350,000
Having sexual intercourse (PID)	1 in 50,000
Preventing pregnancy	
Using birth control pills	
Nonsmoker	1 in 63,000
Smoker	1 in 16,000
Using IUDs	1 in 100,000
Using diaphragm, condom, or spermicide	None
Using fertility awareness methods	None
Undergoing sterilization	
Laparoscopic tubal ligation	1 in 67,000
Hysterectomy	1 in 1,600
Vasectomy	1 in 300,000
Continuing pregnancy	1 in 11,000
Terminating pregnancy	
Legal abortion	
Before 9 weeks	1 in 260,000
Between 9 and 12 weeks	1 in 100,000
Between 13 and 15 weeks	1 in 34,000
After 15 weeks	1 in 10,200

From Hatcher RA and others: *Contraceptive technology,* ed 16, New York, 1994, Irvington Publishers. Used with permission.

birth control (such as condoms and foam) for 1 week (Box 25-3). Because some antibiotics may decrease the effectiveness of the birth control pill, a woman should be advised to use a backup method of contraception should she be placed on antibiotics. Birth control pills become effective as contraception after 1 week. Therefore a backup method of contraception should be used during the first week of use, if she begins on the Sunday after her menses. If she begins on the first day of menses, a backup method of contraception is not considered necessary.

Progestin-only pills (Mini pills). Progestin-only pills are not as effective as combined OCP and tend to cause irregular menstruation. However, they can be used by lactating women without disruption of milk production, and they may be an appropriate alterna-

TABLE 25-4

Percentage of Women Experiencing a Contraceptive Failure During the First Year of Typical Use and the First Year of Perfect Use and the Percentage Continuing Use at the End of the First Year, United States.

	% of Women Experiencing an Accidental Pregnancy Within the First Year of Use		% of Women Continuing Use at One Year
Method (1)	Typical Use (2)	Perfect Use (3)	(4)
Chance	85	85	
Spermicides	21	6	43
Periodic abstinence	20		67
Calendar		9	
Ovulation method		3	
Symptothermal		2	
Postovulation		1	
Withdrawal	19	4	
Cap			
Parous women	36	26	45
Nulliparous women	18	9	58
Sponge			
Parous women	36	20	45
Nulliparous women	18	9	58
Diaphragm	18	6	58
Condom			
Female (Reality)	21	5	56
Male	12	3	63
Pill	3		72
Progestin only		0.5	
Combined		0.1	
IUD			
Progesterone T	2.0	1.5	81
Copper T 380A	0.8	0.6	78
LNg 20	0.1	0.1	81
Depo-Provera	0.3	0.3	70
Norplant (6 capsules)	0.09	0.09	85
Female sterilization	0.4	0.4	100
Male sterilization	0.15	0.10	100

From Hatcher RA and others: *Contraceptive technology,* ed 16 revised, New York, 1994, Irvington Publishers. Used with permission.
Emergency Contraceptive Pills: Treatment initiated within 72 hours after unprotected intercourse reduces the risk of pregnancy by at least 75%.
Lactational Amenorrhea Method: LAM is a highly effective, *temporary* method of contraception.

tive for women who should not take combined contraceptive pills. Thus women at risk for the estrogen-related side effects of the combined pill may be advised to use a progestin-only pill. In the older woman (ages 35 to 50) whose fertility is diminished, the lessened efficacy may not be as great an issue as for the younger woman. Mini pills are immediately reversible and have no effect on long-term fertility.

Mechanism of action and effectiveness. Progestin-only pills thicken cervical mucus, making it more difficult for sperm to penetrate the endocervical canal and ascend into the uterus. The progestin-only pill does not inhibit ovulation as reliably as combined OCPs. It does, however, promote a thin, atrophic endometrium that is inhospitable to the fertilized ovum. In the first year of typical use, the proportion of women becoming pregnant on the progestin-only pill ranges from 1.19% to 13.29% (Hatcher and others, 1994). Taking pills even a few hours late markedly reduces efficacy, as does use of anticonvulsants. Because lactation tends to inhibit ovulation, the progestin-only pill is almost 100% effective for lactating women.

BOX 25-3

PATIENT TEACHING

Missed Oral Contraceptives

One pill missed

Take the missed pill as soon as remembered and the next pill at the usual time.

Two pills missed in a row (in the first 2 weeks of cycle)

Take two pills for 2 days and use a backup method of birth control for the next 7 days.

Two pills missed (in the third week of cycle) or three or more pills missed in a row any time

Sunday start: Continue taking pills once a day until the next Sunday. Start a new pack that Sunday. Use a backup method of birth control from the time of the missed pills until 1 week into the new pack of pills.

Non-Sunday start: Throw out the remainder of the pill pack. Start a new pill pack that day. Use a backup method of birth control for the next 7 days.

Risks, benefits, and side effects. Because mini pills contain no estrogen, they do not cause the complications related to estrogen that may occur with the combined pill. They are more likely to cause menstrual disturbance, which may include frequent bleeding or amenorrhea. Although not well studied at present, mini pills may also decrease bone density, adding to a woman's risk of osteoporosis later in life. Mini pills may cause lighter bleeding patterns or amenorrhea, which lessens a woman's risk for anemia. They may also lessen the cramping associated with endometriosis. Thickening of cervical mucus helps protect a woman from PID. Mini pills are also thought to protect women from developing endometrial and ovarian cancer, as do combined OCPs.

Patient use. Women who have contraindications to estrogen (Box 25-4) or who have developed severe headaches or hypertension while on estrogen may consider use of progestin-only pills as well as other progestin-only methods (see Norplant and Depro-Provera discussions later in this chapter). For lactating women the progestin-only pill is an excellent choice. The nurse should counsel women to take progestin-only pills at exactly the same time each day to promote their effectiveness. If a woman tends to be forgetful about taking pills, the progestin-only pill may not be an effective method of contraception for her.

Emergency contraception: postcoital pill. Emergency contraception is safe and effective. It has been available for two decades but remains an underused form of birth control. Some clinicians are disinclined to use it because the FDA has not approved birth control pills for this use and because they feel women will come to rely on it for contraception. These assumptions need to be challenged. "As long as condoms break, inclination and opportunity unexpectedly converge, men rape women, diaphragms and cervical caps are dislodged, people are so ambivalent about sex that they need to be swept away, IUDs are expelled, and pills are lost or forgotten, we will need emergency postcoital contraception" (Hatcher and others, 1994). The contraceptive method most often used in an emergency involves commonly available but specifically formulated birth control pills given in two doses 12 hours apart (Table 25-5). Other birth control pills have not been used for this purpose. Postcoital insertion of an IUD can also be used as an emergency contraceptive, and high-dose progestin-only pills are available outside the United States for emergency contraception. Ideally treatment should be initiated as early as possible; 12 to 24 hours after unprotected intercourse is ideal, but it may be given up to 72 hours after intercourse.

BOX 25-4

CONTRAINDICATIONS TO ESTROGEN

CVA
Ischemic heart disease
Uncontrolled hypertension
Deep-vein thrombosis
Insulin-dependent diabetes with vascular disease
Classic migraine with neurologic impairment
Active liver disease
Pregnancy

Mechanism of action and effectiveness. Hormonal methods interrupt ovarian hormone production and interfere with the preparation of the endometrium for implantation. These methods may also have an effect on transportation of the egg in the fallopian tube and thus inhibit fertilization (Hatcher and others, 1994). Effectiveness for an individual may be difficult to estimate because the risk of pregnancy varies depending on the timing of intercourse with relation to the menstrual cycle. At midcycle, the risk of pregnancy is the highest. One act of intercourse at ovulation has been estimated to carry a 15% to 26% risk of pregnancy (Hatcher and others, 1994). Use of emergency contraception pill treatment reduces the risk of pregnancy by approximately 75% (Hatcher and others, 1994).

Risks, benefits, and side effects. Women who cannot take birth control pills should also not take hor-

TABLE 25-5

Emergency Contraceptive Pill Options

Brand Name	Number of Tablets for Each Dose (Two Doses, 12 Hours Apart)
Ovral	4
Lo/Ovral, Nordette, or Levlen; Triphasil or Tri-Levlen (yellow pills only)	4

From Hatcher RA and others: *Contraceptive technology,* ed 16, New York, 1994, Irvington Publishers. Used with permission.

monal emergency contraception. The most common side effects of this method are nausea and vomiting. Dizziness, headache, and abdominal pain occur less often. Menses usually occurs within 1 week of a woman's regular, expected period.

Patient use. The largest barrier to use of this method is making women aware of its availability. The nurse should counsel all patients about the availability of emergency contraception. In particular, women using barrier methods should be informed that this method is available should they experience a failure of that method. Women should be advised to return for a pregnancy test if menses does not begin within 3 weeks of treatment. Women should also be advised that they may experience nausea and vomiting. Some clinicians advise that an extra dose be taken if the patient vomits within 1 hour of a dose. Women need careful instruction and preparation about what to expect in order to use this method comfortably.

Norplant. The Norplant system is a long-acting, reversible method of birth control. Research and development for Norplant began in 1966, and the first clinical trials began in Chile in 1974. By the end of 1989, more than 55,000 women in 44 countries had used Norplant for contraception in clinical trials (Wyeth-Ayerst Laboratories, 1991). Norplant was approved for use by the FDA in the United States in 1989 and first marketed in 1990 by Wyeth-Ayerst Laboratories. By the end of 1990, an additional 550,000 women had used Norplant worldwide (Wyeth-Ayerst Laboratories, 1991).

The Norplant System provides effective and continuous contraception for up to 5 years. Six thin, flexible capsules made of silastic tubing are filled with levonorgestrel (Figure 25-8). These capsules are inserted in a fan-shaped pattern just under the skin on the inside of a woman's upper arm. Small amounts of levonorgestrel then continuously diffuse through the capsule walls to maintain an effective blood level of the hormone. Although they may be palpable, the capsules are usually invisible under the skin. Norplant may be a good choice of contraception for women who cannot remember to take birth control pills and who wish a contraceptive method that does not depend on special action at the time of intercourse (see Table 25-5).

Mechanism of action and effectiveness. Norplant maintains a constant low level of hormone in the body. It prevents pregnancy by inhibiting ovulation, thickening cervical mucus, and decreasing the receptivity of the endometrium toward implantation. With an annual failure rate of 0.09% in the first year of use, Norplant is one of the most effective contraception methods available (Hatcher and others, 1994). The chance of accidental pregnancy rises only slightly with subsequent years of use. Because of the low blood levels of Norplant, women who are on antiseizure medication should be advised to consider alternative contraception because most antiseizure medications induce hepatic enzymes that break down levonorgestrel, the hormone contained in Norplant.

Risks, benefits, and side effects. The most commonly reported side effect is a change in the menstrual bleeding pattern. Some women have prolonged bleeding, others may have erratic spotting, and still others amenorrhea. The type of bleeding pattern a woman will experience on Norplant cannot be predicted. Usually the monthly blood loss does not exceed that of normal menses. Some women also complain of headaches on Norplant and, more rarely, women have complained of nervousness, nausea, dizziness, acne, weight change, mastalgia, hirsuitism, and hair loss. The average weight gain on Norplant over 5 years is under 5 pounds, which is a typical pattern for women irrespective of contraceptive choice. There is a small risk of infection at the insertion site. A patient may also have a ¼ inch scar at the site of insertion; no sutures are required.

Noncontraceptive benefits. The noncontraceptive benefits of Norplant use are similar to those of the progestin-only pill.

Patient use. Norplant is inserted under local anesthetic during minor, in-office surgery. Usually insertion can be accomplished within 15 minutes, although removal may be more difficult and time consuming.

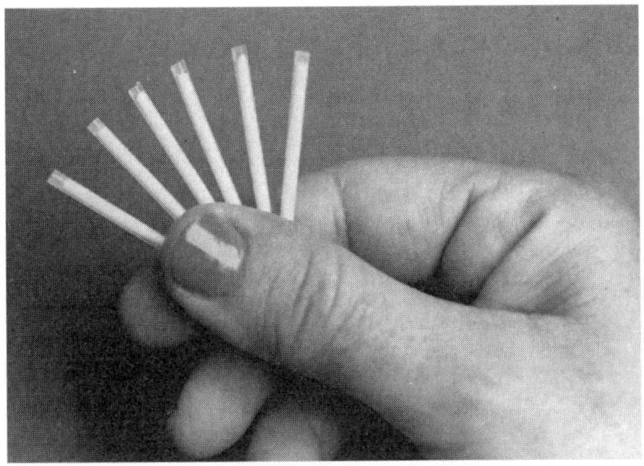

Figure 25-8 Norplant System implants. (Courtesy of Wyeth-Ayerst Laboratories, Philadelphia.)

An incision of about ¼ inch is made in the skin and the capsules are inserted by use of a trocar. A steri-strip is applied to close the incision, and a dry sterile dressing with a gauze bandage is applied over the incision. Patients should be advised to leave the dressing in place in order to protect the arm for 3 to 5 days. A woman may notice substantial bruising after the dressing is removed. She should be advised to return if she notices pus or bleeding at the insertion site.

Before having the Norplant inserted, the patient should have been advised of the likelihood of a change in menstrual periods and the possibility of other side effects (see the previously discussed risks, benefits, and side effects). Women with Norplant insertions should be advised to call back in the event of frequent bleeding, because a cycle of low-dose oral contraceptive pills or conjugated estrogens can be prescribed temporarily to control bleeding. Norplant will become effective as contraception within 24 hours. Normally it is inserted during menses in order to ensure that a woman is not already pregnant at the time of insertion. If it is inserted at another time, a pregnancy test is done before insertion, and an alternate method of contraception should be used for the remainder of that cycle.

Depro-Provera. Depro-Provera (DMPA) is a long-acting, injectable contraceptive that acts to prevent pregnancy for 3 months per injection. DMPA was used by 8 to 9 million women worldwide before it was approved in the United States (Hatcher and others, 1994). Depro-Provera is available as a 150 mg dose of medroxyprogesterone acetate suspension suitable for intramuscular injection in the deltoid or gluteus maximus muscles. In the United States it is typically provided in single dose vials of 150 mg of DMPA in 1 ml of fluid.

Mechanism of action and effectiveness. DMPA is given by intramuscular injection every 12 weeks. It inhibits ovulation by suppressing FSH and LH levels and, like other progestin-only contraceptives, it promotes a thick cervical mucus that functions as a barrier to sperm and an atrophic endometrium that resists implantation of a fertilized ovum. DMPA has a first-year failure rate of 0.3%. Its efficacy continues beyond the 12-week dosing regimen, and women may be given a subsequent injection up to 14 weeks after the prior dose.

Risks, benefits, and side effects. Because DMPA contains no estrogen, it may be suitable for women who have contraindications to oral contraceptive pills. Its side-effect profile is similar to Norplant and the progestin-only pill. The most prominent side effect is menstrual-cycle disturbance. During the first year of use, women may be more likely to experience frequent bleeding or spotting. However, the longer a woman continues on DMPA, the more likely it is that she will experience amenorrhea. Weight gain is more likely than with other progestin-only contraceptives. A weight gain of 2 to 5 pounds is possible in the first year of use. DMPA provides a higher dose of hormone than Norplant and so is less likely to be deleteriously impacted by antiseizure medication. In addition it may actually improve seizure control. Some concern exists about the effect DMPA may have on bone density over time. More research is needed to clarify this effect. The noncontraceptive benefits of DMPA use are similar to those of the progestin-only pill.

Patient use. Injections should be scheduled every 3 months. If the first injection is given within 5 days of the onset of menses, no backup method of contraception is necessary because DMPA becomes effective within 24 hours. If it is given at another point in the cycle, backup contraception must be used for 2 weeks. Although DMPA is reversible, patients should be advised that there may be a 6-month delay in return to fertility. Injection should be given intramuscularly in the deltoid or gluteus maximus muscles. The nurse should *not* massage the area of injection since this may decrease the effectiveness of DMPA (Hatcher and others, 1994).

Women should be prepared to expect menstrual changes on DMPA. Patients can be told that troublesome spotting or break-through bleeding can usually be managed by a cycle or more of combined OCP. Pa-

ETHICAL DILEMMA

In the family planning clinic where you are employed, you overhear a discussion between two other nurses about a decision to prescribe Norplant for a 17-year-old unwed mother of two. She admits to being sexually active and admits that she often forgets to take her contraceptive pills.

What are the ethical issues in the use of Norplant?

tients should also be told that amenorrhea is likely to increase the longer they remain on DMPA, but that this is not harmful.

Intrauterine device. The intrauterine device (IUD) was developed in the 1930s, but its use first became widespread in the 1960s. At present there are only two kinds of IUDs available in the United States. Lawsuits by women who developed PID and became infertile caused other IUDs to be withdrawn from the market. In particular, an IUD known as the Dalkon Shield was associated with a greater chance of infection and subsequent infertility. Despite its current low popularity in the United States, the IUD remains popular worldwide and is an important option for well-selected women.

The CuT 380A (ParaGard) intrauterine copper contraceptive is approved for 10 years of use. It is manufactured in a polyethylene T-shape with barium sulfate added to create x-ray visibility. Thin copper wire is wound around the vertical arm of the T, and a single filament string is looped through the bottom of the T (Figure 25-9A). In contrast, the progesterone T (Progestasert System), which releases small amounts of progesterone, is approved for only 1 year of use. Because it must be replaced annually, it offers no advantages to the copper T but is an option for women allergic to copper (Figure 25-9B).

A new IUD called the Levonorgestrel IUD is available in Europe and is likely to be approved for use in the United States soon. It releases 20 μg of levonorgestrel into the uterus daily and is designed for 5 years of use.

Mechanism of action and effectiveness. The manner in which the IUD works is unclear, although it appears to immobilize sperm, speed transport of the egg through the fallopian tube, and effect changes in the endometrium that make implantation unlikely. Its efficacy depends on many factors, including age and parity of the user, as well as clinical experience in inserting the IUD. The first year failure rates for typical IUD users are 0.8% for the ParaGard and 2% for the Progestasert System (Hatcher and others, 1994). The new levonorgestrel IUD has a better efficacy rate and may also reduce the incidence of PID and lessen menstrual bleeding.

Risks, benefits, and side effects. Women with IUDs are at increased risk for PID. Because there is a slight increased risk just after the time of insertion, the long-acting copper T rather than the Progestasert System, which needs annual replacement, is preferable. Women who are not in mutually monogamous relationships have a higher risk of PID and subsequent infertility. It is unknown whether the IUD puts a woman at greater risk for contracting HIV. A small risk of uterine perforation at the time of insertion is directly related to clinician experience. Approximately 2% to

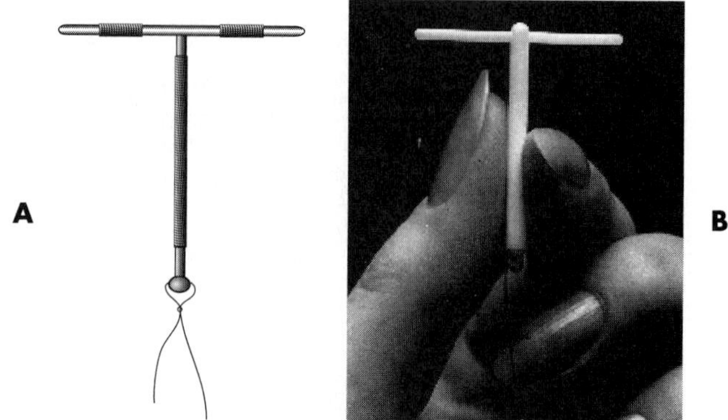

Figure 25-9 Intrauterine devices. **A,** ParaGard T380A. Intrauterine copper contraceptive. **B,** Progestasert Intrauterine Progesterone Contraceptive Systems provides contraceptive effect for 1 year. (Courtesy of ALZA Corp, Palo Alto, Calif.)

10% of first-time IUD users spontaneously expel their IUDs (Hatcher and others, 1994). If expulsion is undetected, pregnancy can result. Pregnancy with the IUD in place results in spontaneous abortion half the time, but if the IUD is removed in early pregnancy, this rate of abortion can be halved. The IUD should not be left in place during pregnancy because severe pelvic infections with a high mortality rate can result. Most IUD users notice that menses are heavier, and between 10% to 15% of women will choose to have their IUDs removed because of heavy bleeding or cramping during their periods (Hatcher and others, 1994).

Patient use. The IUD is usually inserted during the menses after a bimanual examination to rule out pregnancy and determine the position of the uterus. An analgesic before the procedure is helpful, and sometimes a local anesthetic is used. Because the material of the IUD has shape memory, it can be inserted by means of a narrow, plastic inserter high up into the fundus of the uterus where it resumes its original shape when released. The IUD is usually easily removed by steady traction on the string extending through the cervical canal. The nurse should counsel women to check for the IUD strings often during the first few months after insertion. Thereafter a woman should check the IUD string after each menses or with any unusual cramping. Patients should be advised to return for care if the IUD string feels longer or the plastic tip of the IUD is felt. Women should be advised that pelvic pain and fever could indicate a serious infection and that they should seek treatment immediately. Likewise they should seek attention if they learn that they have been exposed to a sexually transmitted disease. The IUD appears to be best tolerated in women who have borne children and who are in mutually monogamous relationships.

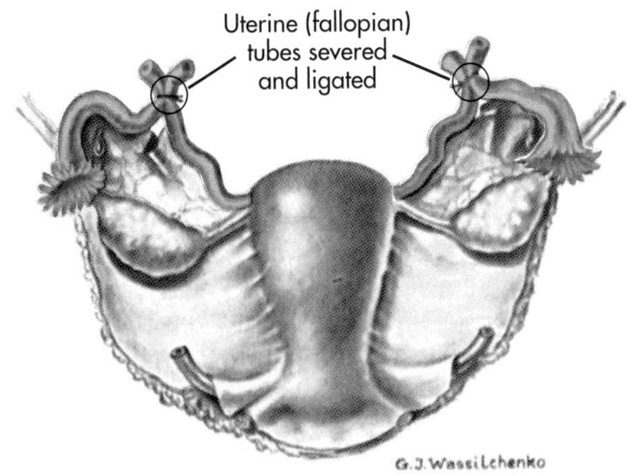

Figure 25-10 Tubal sterilization (tubal ligation). (From Bobak IM, Jensen MD: *Maternity and gynecologic care*, ed 5, St Louis, 1993, Mosby.)

Surgical contraception. In the past 20 years improved surgical techniques and the use of a local anesthetic with light sedation have contributed to the safety of female sterilization. Approximately 1 million women now choose this method of contraception annually in the United States (Hatcher and others, 1994). The couple should consider both vasectomy (see Chapter 26) and female sterilization. Vasectomy is a safer and simpler procedure that can be performed during an office visit. Sterilization for both men and women should be considered permanent because current techniques to reverse the procedures are not dependable.

Mechanism of action and effectiveness. Sterilization involves tying or blocking the fallopian tubes to prevent sperm from reaching and fertilizing the ovum (Figure 25-10). Efficacy is quite high but varies slightly depending on the surgical procedure used and the skill of the surgeon. The failure rate for all techniques is 0.49% of women becoming pregnant in the first year of use (Hatcher and others, 1994). Different surgical techniques and incision sites may be used in the postpartum period.

Risks, benefits, and side effects. Sterilization for women is a safe procedure. Fatality rates in the United States are approximately 3 deaths per 100,000 women, which compares favorably with maternal mortality rates of 7.9 deaths per 100,000 women (Hatcher and others, 1994). Local anesthesia with light sedation can be used for both minilaparotomy and laparoscopic procedures. Local anesthesia has fewer complications than general anesthesia. Possible complications to surgery include infection, uterine perforation, and injury to bladder or intestine. However, complications to surgery occur in less than 1% of all sterilizations (Hatcher and others, 1994). New evidence suggests that tubal sterilization reduces a woman's risk of contracting ovarian cancer by 70% (Edwards, 1994). Even when researchers adjusted for influences that reduce a woman's risk of ovarian cancer, such as parity, use of the birth control pill, and age, the results were upheld. A biologic explanation for this effect has not yet been proposed, nor has a comparison of the effects by different tubal ligation techniques.

Patient use. Women should be advised that sterilization should be considered a permanent contraceptive method because procedures to reverse it are difficult and often unsuccessful. Patients should discuss how their plans might change were they to divorce or lose their present children to death or illness.

Patients should not eat 8 to 12 hours before the surgery and should be instructed to bathe or shower just before arrival for surgery. Because 1-day surgery will be performed, a patient arriving for surgery should have someone with her to drive her home. In addition she should arrange for an adult to accompany her at home for at least 24 hours after surgery in case complications develop. Women with small children will need assistance caring for their children on the day of surgery and a day or two immediately following. Women should be advised that the pain following surgery is usually managed with oral analgesics. After surgery, women should be advised to rest for at least 24 hours and to gradually resume normal activities over the next week. They should be counseled to avoid heavy lifting and sexual intercourse for 1 week after surgery. Typically the sutures dissolve, and women are allowed to bathe 2 days after surgery. Warm baths may relieve the gaseous distention that can occur with laparoscopy. A follow-up visit is usually scheduled for 1 week after surgery. Patients should be counseled to report signs of an infection such as fever, syncope, or increasing abdominal pain. Abnormal bleeding or pus or other fluid from the incision site should also be reported. Women should be advised that they should seek medical attention immediately if they believe they have become pregnant, because a high rate of ectopic pregnancies is associated with failure of the procedure.

Barrier methods of contraception. Barrier methods of contraception include the diaphragm, cervical cap, female condom, male condom, spermicides, foam, and vaginal contraceptive film (VCF). Except for the cervical cap and diaphragm, which must be fitted by a clinician, all these methods are available without prescription. This may enhance their use by teenagers or women without access to medical care. Without exception, these methods are use-dependent, that is, a woman or man must choose to use them at the time of intercourse. Use-dependence often affects compliance.

Mechanism of action and effectiveness. Most barrier methods rely on a mechanical barrier together with

BOX 25-5

PATIENT TEACHING

Diaphragm Use

Check for holes or rips before each use. Place one tablespoon of contraceptive cream or jelly into the cup of the diaphragm and around the rim.

Fold the diaphragm in half and gently push it into the vagina as far as it will go. You may be lying down, squatting, or standing with one knee raised when you do this.

Check the diaphragm's location by feeling for your cervix with one finger. The cervix should be covered by the latex dome of the diaphragm, and the rim of the diaphragm should be tucked comfortably behind the public bone.

If you have intercourse more than once, you should insert more contraceptive cream or jelly with an applicator before each act of intercourse.

Remove the diaphragm 6 to 8 hours after the last act of intercourse. Hook your index finger under the rim and pull down to remove.

Wash the diaphragm with mild soap and warm water. Dry carefully. If desired, the diaphragm can be dusted with cornstarch, but *never* dust with talcum powder.

a spermicide to prevent migration of sperm through the endocervical canal. Some methods, such as condoms, rely principally on a mechanical barrier, while others, such as foam and VCF, rely on a spermicide for their effectiveness. Efficacy rates vary depending on use. Typical failure rates for barrier methods range more widely from the perfect-use failure rate than with contraceptives such as Norplant, Depro-Provera, or the IUD. (see Table 25-2). It should be noted that of the vaginal barrier methods, the diaphragm may offer greater efficacy for parous women than the cervical cap (Trussell, 1993).

Risks, benefits, and side effects. Aside from a generally higher risk of pregnancy, barrier methods are quite safe, with few if any side effects. Some couples may be allergic or irritated by the latex in condoms or the nonoxynol-9 in spermicidal products, but these problems are uncommon. TSS is a rare possibility with use of vaginal barrier methods. The syndrome is caused by the toxins released by a strain of staphylococcus bacteria and is more often associated with tampon use during menses (see TSS discussion earlier in this chapter). Two or three cases of TSS per 100,000 women annually may be attributed to using vaginal barrier methods (Hatcher and others, 1994).

Of all the contraceptive methods available, the male and female condoms afford the greatest protection from sexually transmitted disease. All women at risk should be encouraged to use condoms, regardless of other contraceptive methods employed, to protect themselves from infection. Although spermicides have a bactericidal action, which offers some protection against sexually transmitted infections such as gonorrhea and syphilis, they do not offer the protection afforded by barrier methods such as condoms. Nor is there general agreement on whether spermicides decrease the transmission of HIV because of their spermicidal activity or possibly increase it because of the irritant effect of spermicides on vaginal and cervical mucosa that would facilitate entry of HIV.

Patient use.

Diaphragm. The diaphragm has been in use for more than 60 years in the United States. The diaphragm is a dome-shaped rubber cup with a compressible rim that must be sized to the individual woman. The woman should be instructed in its use and allowed the opportunity to practice inserting it before the office visit is concluded (Box 25-5). Before insertion the woman should apply about a tablespoon of contraceptive jelly or cream into the cup of the diaphragm and spread it around the rim and interior surface of the dome. Then she should fold the diaphragm in half and push it gently into the vagina. The anterior rim should be tucked up behind the pubic bone and the posterior rim behind the cervix, thus covering the cervix (Figure 25-11). This can be checked by having the patient palpate for the cervix, which will feel somewhat firm and rubbery behind the dome. The diaphragm should be left in place for 6 to 8 hours after intercourse. If intercourse is desired again before the diaphragm should be removed, a second application of contraceptive cream should be inserted with an applicator and the diaphragm left in place for an additional 6 to 8 hours. The woman should check the diaphragm for tears or holes before each use and clean it with mild soap and warm water after use. When fit correctly, the diaphragm should be completely comfortable for the woman, and her partner is usually unable to feel the device during coitus. The nurse should follow recommended cleaning and disinfecting practices for all fitting rings (diaphragms) used to size women during the fitting procedure.

Cervical cap. The Prentif cervical cap is the only cap approved for use in the United States (Figure 25-12). It is devised to fit snugly over the cervix. Before insertion, the dome is filled with approximately 1 tablespoon of contraceptive jelly or cream. It can be more difficult to fit a cervical cap than a diaphragm. Insertion and removal may be slightly more difficult for the woman as well. Some women are unable to be fitted for a cap because of their cervical anatomy. The

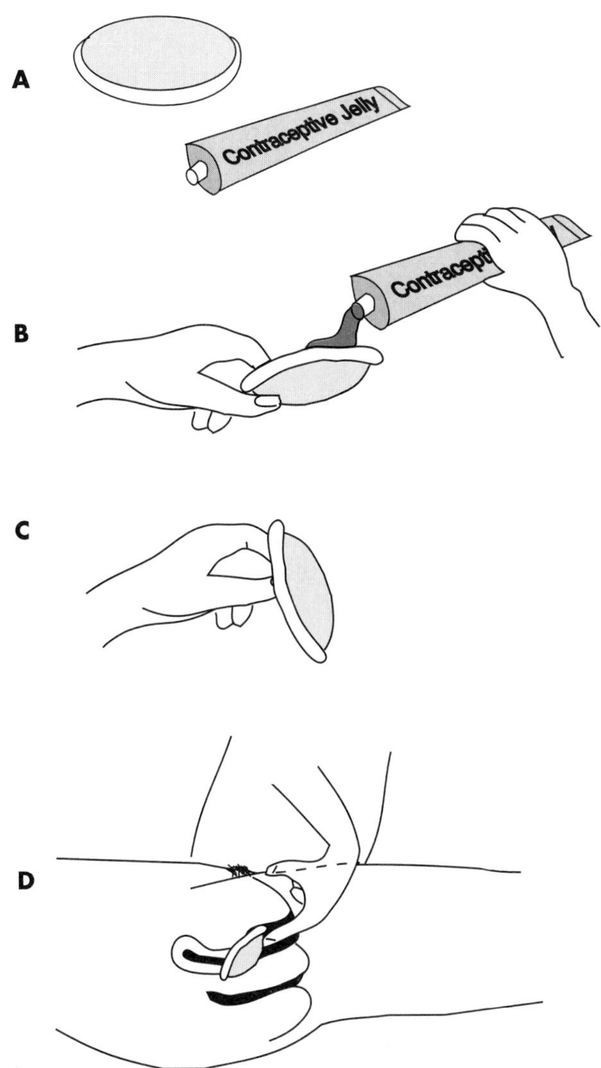

Figure 25-11 Diaphram insertion technique.

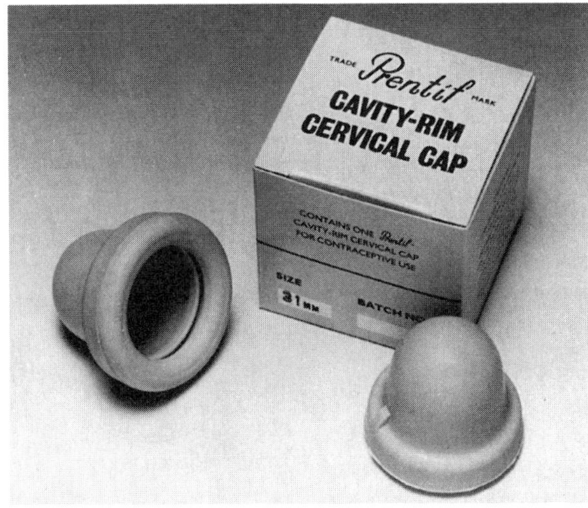

Figure 25-12 Cervical cap. (Courtesy of Cervical Cap Ltd, Los Gatos, Calif.)

cervical cap may be left in place up to 48 hours, and repeated applications of spermicides are not necessary with subsequent acts of intercourse. It must be left in place for at least 6 hours after the last act of intercourse. Care of the cervical cap is similar to the diaphragm, and the same precautions should be followed by the nurse for disinfection of caps used for fitting and sizing.

Female condom. The Reality female condom is a thin polyurethane sheath with a flexible ring at either end. The open ring is intended to lie outside the vagina, and a ring at the end of the pouch serves to anchor the device deep inside the vagina (Figure 25-13). The female condom is less likely to tear than the male condom, but like the male condom, it may become dislodged during intercourse.

Male condom. Most condoms are manufactured from latex, but natural "skin" condoms are available and are made from the intestinal membranes of lambs. Natural or "skin" condoms do not offer the same protection from STDs because they allow passage of some smaller viruses through the membrane. In laboratory tests hepatitis B, herpes simplex, and HIV have been shown to pass through the "skin" condoms. For men and women with latex sensitivity, the female condom, which is made of polyurethane, may be suggested as an alternative. Two new kinds of condom made of polyurethane and natural rubber are also expected to be available in the near future. Alternatively a latex condom could be worn under or over a natural skin condom so that the partner with sensitivity to latex is shielded from direct contact. Condoms should be unrolled carefully over the erect penis before any contact between penis and vagina occurs. It is recommended that ½ inch of empty space be left at the end of the condom to reduce breakage. Some condoms are designed with a "reservoir tip" for this purpose. The condom should be unrolled so that the rolled rim is on the outside of the condom. If a condom is unrolled incorrectly, it is better to use a new condom rather than attempt to reverse the first one, because potentially infectious body fluids could otherwise be transmitted.

Natural family planning

Natural family planning includes the basal body temperature, rhythm, and cervical mucus methods. They consist of abstaining from intercourse during carefully calculated times and require planning and dedication to be effective.

Infertility

Infertility is usually defined as the inability of a couple to conceive after 1 year of sexual relations without contraceptive measures. Approximately 40% of all in-

Open end

A

OPEN END
Covers the area around the opening of the vagina.

CLOSED END
Used for insertion and helps hold the pouch in place.

Closed end

Index finger

B

HOW TO HOLD THE POUCH
Hold closed end between thumb and middle finger. Put index finger on pouch between other two fingers

Closed end

Open end

C

TO INSERT,
Squeeze the inner ring. Insert the pouch as far as possible into the vagina. Make sure closed end is past the pubic bone.

D

MAKE SURE PLACEMENT IS CORRECT
Pouch should not be twisted. Open end should be outside the vagina.

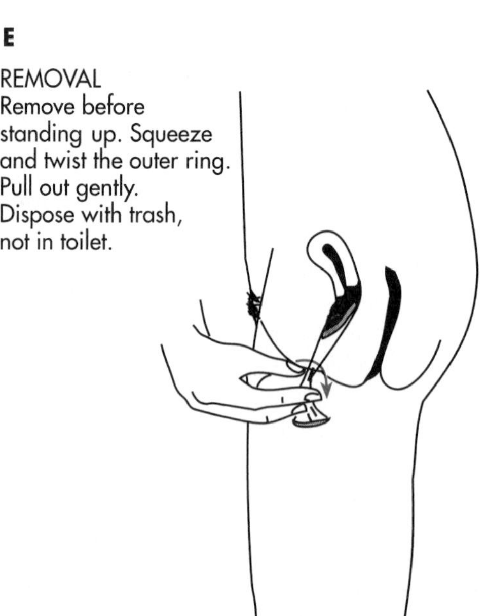

E
REMOVAL
Remove before standing up. Squeeze and twist the outer ring. Pull out gently. Dispose with trash, not in toilet.

Figure 25-13 Female condom.

fertility problems are a result of male factors, and approximately 40% are a result of female factors. Combined male and female factors account for 10% of problems, and 10% are unexplained. Aging has only a moderate effect on female fertility, and this effect is demonstrated only for women in their late 30s and older (Hatcher and others, 1994). The probability of conception remains roughly the same over time for an individual couple as long as health and sexual behavior remain constant. Because fecundity peaks in a given population at the age most women choose to bear children, statistics on fecundity do not give an accurate indication of the possibilities for pregnancy in an individual woman. Also, statistics for pregnancy in couples older than the norm are affected by including in this group women who have attempted pregnancy for many years and have been unable to conceive.

The causes of diminished fertility in women are numerous and range from simple lack of coital frequency and poor timing to anatomic and hormonal problems. Timing of intercourse is important because there may be only a few hours each cycle when a ripe ovum is ready for fertilization. Sperm, on the other hand, survive more than 72 hours in the female genital tract (Hatcher and others, 1994). Optimal timing of intercourse around the expected time of ovulation can be assisted by monitoring the basal body temperature (BBT) of the woman. In order to do this, a woman must take her temperature at approximately the same time each morning before arising from bed. She should use a special BBT thermometer calibrated in tenths of a degree from 97° F to 99° F. With such a thermometer, she can record fine distinctions in temperature on a menstrual cycle chart, which can then be used as an aid to predict ovulation. For most women a slight dip in temperature occurs just before ovulation, followed by a sustained and sharp rise in temperature after ovulation. BBT monitoring is useful for timing intercourse and for coordinating tests that a woman may need to further evaluate infertility.

PID may cause infertility when the infection is severe enough to cause scarring and blockage of the uterus or fallopian tubes. The risk of developing PID is increased by untreated sexually transmitted disease, postpartum and postabortion infections, and use of the IUD. Infections of human papillomavirus (HPV) may cause chronic cervicitus, cervical dysplasia, or cervical cancer, and treatment of any of these conditions may damage the mucus-producing cells of the cervix, affecting sperm transport or causing cervical incompetence. Cervical incompetence could result in pregnancy loss or preterm delivery. Of course infertility also results from surgery (necessitated by cancer of the cervix, endometrium, or ovaries) that removes the organs of reproduction.

Structural causes of infertility can be found in women with an absent or bicornate uterus. Endometriosis results in implantation of endometrial tissue from the uterus in ectopic locations, which then swell and bleed at menses. This may result in adhesions and tubal blockage significant enough to prevent conception in some women. Abdominal or pelvic surgery may also cause adhesions and contribute to infertility. Fibroid tumors may also cause difficulties in implantation and subsequent pregnancies.

Endocrine imbalances in the thyroid, pituitary, and ovaries can all contribute to infertility. Thus hypothyroidism, prolactinoma, polycystic ovarian disease, and premature ovarian failure can all affect fertility. Some women do not ovulate with each cycle (anovulatory cycles), which decreases their chances of becoming pregnant. Both women and men can develop antibodies that immobilize sperm and cause them to clump rather than ascend the uterus. Other causes of infertility are malnutrition, extreme weight gain or loss, excessive exercise, exposure to toxic agents or radiation, and the use of certain drugs.

Infertility of whatever cause can be an emotionally devastating diagnosis for a couple. A woman may feel acutely the potential loss of her role as a mother. The diagnosis may even affect her sense of femininity and sexual identity. It can cause feelings of grief, shame, and anger. Certainly the evaluation and treatment of infertility invades the private domain of a couple's sexual life. A detailed sexual history must be taken, and the couple is advised to time intercourse to coincide with ovulation, which may markedly decrease their sense of pleasure and spontaneity. Also the repeated inability to conceive in cycle after cycle adds to the couple's growing sense of futility and failure, which may affect their desire for coitus. Clinical tests that the couple may find invasive or embarrassing may cause further stress.

Infertility can rightly be called a life crisis. Women may resent other women who have children and feel isolated from others who, they believe, cannot understand their feelings. Family members and friends can ask intrusive questions or make insensitive comments that cause further anguish. Sometimes women feel their lives are on hold while they are trying so hard to become pregnant. They may not feel as though they can make other long-range plans or commitments. One partner may also blame the other for being the "cause" of infertility, or one partner may care more about resolving the problem, increasing the stress in the relationship. It is important for the nurse to explore the emotional feelings of both partners and to help them understand their responses to this crisis. Self-help groups can also be of great benefit. When infertility is untreatable, couples may need assistance with adoption or reconceptualizing their lives without children.

The assessment of infertility should proceed from basic concerns such as frequency and timing of intercourse to a physiologic assessment of both partners.

Thus both partners should have focused physical examinations that look for contributing causes of infertility at the same time that the woman begins to keep BBT records. Assessment of the male is done first because it is noninvasive. Semen is usually analyzed twice for live-sperm count as well as for morphology and motility. If the semen is normal and the couple have still not conceived after 2 to 3 months of BBT monitoring, then a postcoital test is done to assess adequacy of the semen when exposed to vaginal secretions. The couple is instructed to have intercourse the evening before or the morning of the examination. The examination is scheduled for 1 to 2 days before ovulation according to BBT records. A specimen is obtained from the cervix and examined microscopically for particular characteristics conducive to sperm transport. Motility and the number of sperm are also assessed. If a cause is not found, subsequent visits may assess the woman's hormonal status, adequacy of the endometrium, and patency of the fallopian tubes. Blood tests, endometrial biopsy, and hysterosalpingogram are commonly used in this further assessment. Counseling and encouragement should occur on each visit, and the work up should proceed in a logical fashion from least invasive to more invasive examinations.

Female infertility is treated with a range of approaches, according to the cause. Cervical mucus disorder can be treated by placing sperm directly into the uterus. Hormonal imbalances are alleviated by treating the underlying cause. Ovulation can also be induced by drugs, if necessary. Uterine and tubal abnormalities or obstructions may be treated by surgical intervention. In other cases procedures such as GIFT or IVF can offer success when more conventional methods fail (Box 25-6).

BOX 25-6

ALTERNATE PROCEDURES FOR TREATING INFERTILITY

GIFT

Gamete Intrafallopian Tube Transfer

Sperm and oocytes are placed into the fallopian tube during laparoscopy. A pregnancy rate of 29% per treatment cycle results (Hatcher and others, 1994).

IVF

In-vitro Fertilization

Mature ova and sperm are incubated in a special medium, and fertilized ova are placed in the uterus. A pregnancy rate of 19% per treatment cycle results (Hatcher and others, 1994).

Menopause (Climacteric)

Menopause is defined as the cessation of menses associated with reduced ovarian function. It is diagnosed when a year has passed since the last menstrual period. The climacteric refers to the transition period during which reproductive function gradually diminishes and is eventually lost. Menopause is often referred to as "the change of life"; however for many women there is no appreciable change in the normal pattern of living. Menopause is a normal, physiologic process and simply means that the period of female reproductivity has come to an end.

In the majority of women, menopause occurs between 45 and 55 years of age, but it may occur earlier or later. Artificial menopause may be induced by the surgical removal of the ovaries or by deep internal radiation and radium placed in the vaginal canal. Although some women may stop menstruating abruptly, the usual pattern is a gradual tapering off. The flow may gradually decrease, with some irregularity of periods. When the production of the ovarian hormone (estrogen) falls below the level necessary to stimulate the endometrium, menstruation ceases. The uterus, vagina, and ovaries decrease in size.

Several changes in the epithelial cells occur in the postmenopausal woman that affect the vagina and urinary tract. Vaginal dryness, urinary frequency, and dysuria may result. Urinary tract infections may also occur more often in the menopausal woman because of thinning of the epithelial layer. At menopause the vaginal epithelium becomes pale and fragile and more susceptible to infection or trauma. There is a gradual loss of rugae and elasticity of the vagina, which together with decreased lubrication may lead to complaints of dysparunia. Because of atrophied tissue of the external genitalia, vulvar puritus may also be experienced. These changes are caused by the loss of estrogen and will resolve with replacement estrogen. Loss of tone in the supporting ligaments may promote uterine prolapse or bulging of the uterus through the vaginal wall (rectocele, cystocele). Atrophic changes in breast glandular tissue results in alteration of breast shape as well as diminished size.

A lack of estrogen also contributes to the development of osteoporosis and a rise in heart disease risk. By age 65, women experience the same risk for heart disease as do 55-year-old men (Maddox, 1990). Estrogen may reduce the risk of heart disease and osteoporosis. Alternatively, osteoporosis may be treated by increased calcium intake, vitamin D supplements, and weight-bearing exercises, which prevent some loss of bone density after menopause. Most postmenopausal women are calcium deficient. The recommended intake of calcium for postmenopausal women not on hormone replacement therapy (HRT) is 1500 mg daily, which is equivalent to five 8-ounce glasses of skim milk. For a woman on HRT, 1000 mg of calcium daily should be adequate.

With the cessation of menses, many women do not experience any symptoms severe enough to require medical care. Hot flashes, which are warm feelings about the face and neck accompanied by sweating, are experienced by 75% to 85% of postmenopausal women. These often occur at night, and for some women may significantly interrupt sleep (Maddox, 1990). Some women may also complain of headaches, nervousness, palpitation, dizziness, insomnia, and irritability. When the symptoms are severe enough to require medical care, some form of estrogen therapy is often advised.

There is a great deal of discussion and some disagreement concerning the use of supplementary estrogens in menopausal women for the prevention of osteoporosis and heart disease. There is no single correct answer, and treatment must be individualized. Risk of osteoporosis and coronary disease, together with menopausal symptoms and medical history, must be evaluated by the medical provider and woman to arrive at the most appropriate plan. *Estrogen therapy* is most effective in relieving hot flashes and night sweats. A patient with a history of uterine or breast cancer is not usually treated with estrogen, although this point of view is now being challenged. Patients receiving estrogen should have a regular examination for cancer of the uterus and breast. A woman with an intact uterus should not take unopposed estrogen, because this significantly increases the risk of endometrial cancer. For most women estrogen is usually prescribed with progesterone to eliminate this risk. If prescribed, estrogens may be administered orally, vaginally, or by transdermal patch. One form in common use is a naturally occurring estrogen (Premarin) derived from the urine of pregnant mares. When administered in combination with Provera, a progesterone preparation, the excess risk of uterine cancer is eliminated. However, a woman may continue to have menses while on this combined therapy, and some women find this an unappealing side effect. Mild sedatives, tranquilizers, or mood-elevating drugs may be prescribed to alleviate psychologic symptoms. Emphasis should be placed on the normalcy of menopause, and women should be encouraged to pursue interests, hobbies, activities, and careers.

NURSING ASSESSMENT OF THE PATIENT WITH PROBLEMS OF THE REPRODUCTIVE SYSTEM

The nursing assessment of female patients should include information on the onset of menses and menopause, a record of all pregnancies and their outcomes, the type of birth control (if used), and the date of the last Papanicolaou (Pap) smear test. If the woman is still menstruating, the date of the first day of her last menstrual period should be recorded, as well as the length in days and the frequency and character of flow of each period or any bleeding between periods. The nurse should also note if the woman is experiencing any of the symptoms related to premenstrual syndrome (PMS). These symptoms include weight gain, abdominal bloating, pelvic fullness, and a variety of emotional responses. (PMS is discussed in more detail earlier in this chapter.) The type and character of any pain or discomfort accompanying menstruation should also be reported. In the menopausal female, symptoms of hot flashes, headache, nervousness, palpitation, dizziness, insomnia, and irritability should be identified, if present. Urinary symptoms such as stress, incontinence, urgency, or frequency are indicative of gynecologic problems.

Nursing is concerned with total patient care. Illness or disease can adversely affect an individual's interest in sex or ability to function sexually. If a patient's condition or treatment raises sexual concerns or limits sexual ability, the nurse should provide an opportunity to discuss the situation with the patient. An attitude of nonjudgmental concern and caring on the part of the nurse helps provide an atmosphere conducive to discussion. It is also important to provide privacy when discussing sexual concerns so that the patient knows confidentiality will be maintained. When privacy is provided and there are no distractions, the patient is better able to focus on sexual questions.

The nursing assessment of the patient with problems of the reproductive system is used to help the patient talk about sexual concerns and to help the nurse plan care, give information, or make referrals on the basis of the patient's problems. The assessment is best accomplished late in the interview when a nurse-patient relationship has been established. The assessment does not need to be long and detailed. Its primary focus is to help the patient identify sexual concerns.

When assessing sexual functioning in the female, the nurse should know that chronic illnesses such as hypertension, arthritis, and diabetes, as well as medications can decrease sexual desire and sexual response. Many individuals who take antihypertensives such as propranolol (Inderal) and methyldopa (Aldomet) may find that they have a diminished libido. This effect of medication on libido has been better studied among men than women, but problems of sexual function affect both partners. A woman may have suffered sexual abuse or rape at some time in her life and have subsequent difficulty enjoying sexual intimacy. Women may experience depression, anxiety, and sexual dysfunction for months to years after a sex-

BOX 25-7

QUESTIONS USED IN A SEXUAL ASSESSMENT

TEENAGER

You are starting to develop sexually. Has anyone talked to you about what that means?

Some girls your age have questions about the ways their bodies are developing. Do you have any?

What is the sexual climate at your school like? Are lots of kids sexually active?

Do you feel pressured by your friends to be sexually intimate?

Do you need a birth control method now?

Do you have any questions about birth control methods that I might answer?

ADULT WOMAN

Are you satisfied with your sexual life?

Do you think your partner is satisfied with your sexual life?

Do you experience pain or discomfort during intercourse?

Have you felt forced or pressured by your partner to have sex?

Have you ever or are you now being sexually abused?

OLDER WOMAN

In addition to the questions for the adult woman above:

What are your expectations for sex now that you are past menopause? Are things different than you expected?

Are there any illnesses that affect your sexuality?

Has your partner had any illnesses or surgeries that have affected your sex life?

ually traumatic event. Referral for group or individual therapy or to a rape crisis center may be helpful.

Women may be troubled by sexual dysfunction but find it difficult to approach the topic with a healthcare provider. Nurses can introduce the subject by simply inquiring whether a patient is satisified with her sexual life. Keeping questions open-ended and allowing the patient to take the lead in the discussion promotes privacy and a sense of concern for the individual (Box 25-7). The nurse should remember that words, tone of voice, and the phrasing of questions are important when assessing sexual function. It is important that the nurse not reveal personal sexual value systems when asking questions or making comments. The nurse should ask for clarification or additional information when an answer is unclear or incomplete. Words that the patient understands should be used. In some cases, this may mean using slang or "street words." The patient and the nurse should both be comfortable with word choices so that they both understand what the other is saying. Patients differ greatly in the degree of openness with which they will discuss symptoms related to reproductive and sexual function. Learning to talk about sexual concerns and feelings is often difficult for both the nurse and the patient. For the nurse it is a skill that will develop with careful practice.

Women often do have problems that they wish to discuss. The most common problem presented to the nurse is discomfort during intercourse. If pain at the beginning of coitus is predominant, lack of lubrication may be a cause, and the nurse can suggest that the couple engage in a longer period of foreplay until the woman is aroused or use a water-based lubricant such as K-Y jelly to lubricate the introitus. A physical examination should rule out other causes such as herpes simplex, fissures, or other genital lesions. Pain during the thrusting phase of intercourse may be caused by the penis striking against the cervix or uterus. Some women have relatively short vaginal vaults, or the position of their uteruses may cause this type of discomfort. Changing position so the woman has more control over the angle of coitus can help this problem. Of course, infections, PID, and uterine fibroids should be excluded. Other problems that women may report are anorgasmia (inability to have an orgasm) and decreased libido. Assessment of these problems can be complicated and needs to consider both physical and psychologic causes, including issues within the relationship.

NURSING RESPONSIBILITIES FOR DIAGNOSTIC PROCEDURES

Physical Examination

Examination of the patient begins with a complete history, which includes the menstrual history, history of any pregnancies or past illnesses, and history of the present illness. The physical examination of the patient includes palpation of the breasts for evidence of cysts or tumors and examination of the pelvis. Nurses are employed in many physician's offices, and it is important for them to be familiar with the procedure for pelvic examination and their responsibilities in assisting the physician.

Pelvic examination

The nurse must understand that this examination may not be easy for the patient and may have been long delayed. The nurse should try to relieve the patient's anxiety, fears, and embarrassment by maintaining a caring attitude and explaining the procedure to her.

Often children have gynecologic problems and are

brought to the physician by the parent. Young children are likely to have a profound sense of modesty, and they may resist exposure for examination. Efforts should be made to secure the child's confidence and cooperation. The child should not be restrained, because this may cause traumatic results that can affect future behavior.

In preparation for the examination the patient should be instructed to void and evacuate the bowel, if necessary. Clothing below the waist should be removed to allow visualization of the genitalia and palpation of the abdomen. The breast examination is usually performed at the same time. Therefore all clothing should be removed, and the patient should be dressed in an examination gown.

Positioning the patient

The patient is usually placed in the lithotomy position with both legs elevated in stirrups and the lower third of the table pushed back and out of the way. The patient is then asked to slide her buttocks down so they extend just over the edge of the table. If an examination table is not available or if the patient cannot be moved to one, the examination can be performed in bed with the buttocks elevated on a firm surface such as a wrapped bedpan. The patient should be carefully draped, and unnecessary exposure should be avoided. A sheet or bath blanket positioned diagonally should cover the chest, abdomen, and both legs; the lowest corner can be lifted to visualize the genitalia.

Examination procedure

The procedure begins with a visual inspection of the external genitalia. Then a speculum examination is performed to visualize the cervix and obtain the Pap smear. A sample of cells is obtained and placed on a slide that is immediately sprayed with a fixative. The Pap smear is sprayed with a fixative or immersed in alcohol to fix the cells to the slide. Other cultures or a wet prep may also be obtained at this time, depending on the patient's symptoms and risk factors. Then a bimanual examination of the uterus is performed. The clinician inserts two fingers of a gloved hand into the vagina up to the cervix, while using the other hand to place gentle pressure on the lower abdomen over the uterus. Pressure on the abdomen applies pressure to the fundus. The position of the uterus and the condition of the ovaries are checked at this time. Cervical motion tenderness might indicate a pelvic infection. Finally a bimanual rectovaginal examination is performed by inserting the second finger into the vagina and the third finger into the rectum. The other hand is placed on the abdomen to palpate rectal and pelvic abnormalities. A clean glove should be used because infections from the vagina, such as gonorrhea, can be inadvertently transmitted to the rectum by the clinician. The nurse stays during the procedure to provide support to the patient, assist the examiner, focus the light, and provide instruments or equipment as needed. When the examination is complete, the patient should be cleansed of any lubricating jelly or offered tissues. The patient can then be assisted to a sitting position on the table and should be encouraged to stay sitting until she is sure she is not dizzy. The clinician may wish to speak to the patient at this time or may return later after the patient has dressed to discuss further treatment.

Handling and cleaning of examination equipment, cultures, wet preps, or Pap smears should be performed with caution and while wearing latex gloves because many pelvic diseases are infectious. Many clinicians do not always follow clean technique and subsequently contaminate objects in the room with their gloved hands. The light, fixative spray, and tube of lubricating jelly are most likely to be contaminated. The nurse should discuss with the clinician how to prevent this from occurring so that objects do not need to be discarded because of contamination. Care should be taken with a reusable tube of lubricating jelly that the clinician's gloved hand does not touch the dispensing end of the tube.

Types of Diagnostic Procedures

Laboratory tests

The laboratory tests conducted along with a pelvic examination include urinalysis; the *Papanicolaou cytologic test* (Pap smear) for cancer; and smears and cultures from the vagina, cervix, and urethra, which may be examined for both infectious and noninfectious organisms. A complete blood count and a serologic test for syphilis also are usually done.

Pap smears are used to detect early cases of cervical cancer. For women of average risk, routine smears are recommended once yearly for 3 years, then, after three negative tests, once every 2 or 3 years. The patient's or her family's history may reveal high risk and indicate more frequent testing. Patients with more than three lifetime sexual partners, onset of first intercourse before age 20, and patients who smoke or have a history of human papiloma virus (HPV) are at higher risk for cervical cancer and should be screened yearly. Many physicians recommend that their patients have a Pap smear and vaginal examination every year. A woman should begin routine testing at age 20 or before if sexually active. After an abnormal test, annual Pap smears are recommended thereafter. The woman must understand the purpose of the test and the interpretation of results. Douching 24 hours before the test is contraindicated because cellular discharges to be ex-

TABLE 25-6

A Comparison of Pap Smear Cytologic Classifications

Dysplasia	Bethesda System	Papanicolau System
Normal	Within normal limits	Class I
Condyloma (HPV)	Low-grade squamous intraepithelial lesion (SIL)	Class II
Mild dysplasia	Low-grade SIL	Class II or III
Moderate dysplasia	High-grade SIL	Class III
Severe dysplasia	High-grade SIL	Class IV
Carcinoma in situ	High-grade SIL	Class IV
Invasive cancer	Squamous cancer	Class V

amined may be washed away and negate the test. Sexual intercourse should also be avoided, and the Pap smear should not be collected at the menses. The patient should void, be placed in the dorsal lithotomy position, and then draped. The nurse may be asked to assemble the proper equipment for the physician, including a glass slide, vaginal speculum, wooden swab or spatula, a fixing solution of alcohol or formalin, and a cytology laboratory requisition. In some situations nurses obtain the sample for the smear, and often the nurse applies the sample to the glass slide after it is collected by the physician. Many Pap smear classification systems are in use, but currently the Bethesda System is the predominant one (Table 25-6). Sometimes minor infections may affect the Pap smear. Atypical Pap smears usually are repeated at 3, 6, and 12 months after the first atypical result. If the Pap smear is more seriously abnormal, colposcopy can be performed. Minor abnormalities often resolve without treatment.

Colposcopy

Colposcopy involves the examination of the cervix and vagina with an instrument called a colposcope, which contains a magnifying lens and light. The test is used after an abnormal Pap smear or to further examine suggestive lesions seen during a vaginal examination. A biopsy may be performed, and photographs may be taken of suggestive lesions with the colposcope and its attachments. Patients whose mothers received DES (diethylstilbestrol) during pregnancy are monitored regularly with the colposcope. The patient is positioned in a lithotomy position, and the colposcope is used to inspect the vagina. If a biopsy has been performed, the patient must be instructed to abstain from sexual intercourse and to avoid inserting anything into the vagina except a tampon until healing of the biopsy site is confirmed.

Cervical biopsy

A cervical biopsy is the surgical excision of tissue from the cervix for the purpose of histologic examination. Samples are taken from three or more sites around the cervix. The sites are determined by direct visualization with colposcopy or by iodine staining (Schiller's test). It is indicated in women with suggestive cervical lesions and should be performed when the cervix is least vascular, usually 1 week after menses. If findings indicate advanced dysplasia or carcinoma in situ, a cone biopsy may be performed with the patient under general anesthesia to obtain a larger tissue specimen and allow a more accurate evaluation of the extent of dysplasia. Before this, a consent form must be signed, and the patient should void before the biopsy. The patient is instructed to avoid strenuous exercise for 8 to 24 hours after the biopsy. The patient should be allowed to rest briefly before going home. A tampon may be inserted by the physician after biopsy to help stop bleeding. The patient should be instructed to leave it in place for the time ordered by the physician, usually 8 to 24 hours. Some bleeding is expected, but bleeding heavier than menstrual flow should be reported to the physician. Douching and intercourse should be avoided for about 2 to 6 weeks, as instructed. A foul-smelling, grayish-green vaginal discharge will appear in a few days and remain for as long as 3 weeks. This discharge is caused by the healing of the cervical tissue, and the patient should be told to expect this.

Culdoscopy

A culdoscope is a long, metal, lighted instrument that can be inserted into the vagina and through Douglas' cul-de-sac, a pouch that lies between the uterus and the rectum. The test is usually performed in the operating room with the patient in the knee-chest position. An incision is made in the posterior fornix of the vagina, and the culdoscope is introduced through this incision to provide visualization of the pelvic organs. Preparation is routine for minor vaginal surgery, and postoperative care includes checking vital signs and observing for hemorrhage and infection. The incision usually heals rapidly, and douching and sexual activity are to be avoided for about 1 week or until permitted by the physician. Air embolism is a rare complication of this procedure.

Laparoscopy

A laparoscope is a small, fiberoptic instrument that is inserted through a small incision in the anterior abdominal wall. The procedure is used to detect abnormalities as well as to perform minor surgical procedures, such as lysis of adhesions, ovarian biopsy, tubal sterilization, removal of foreign bodies, and treatment of sites of endometriosis. Because laparoscopy is performed under anesthetic, the patient must fast for at least 8 hours before surgery. There is a danger of hemorrhage following the test and the possibility of peritonitis following the spilling of intestinal contents if a visceral organ is accidentally punctured. The patient will experience pain at the puncture site following the test. There also will be pain in the shoulder resulting from the air that was introduced into the peritoneal cavity to allow better visualization of the organs. Following the test, vital signs should be monitored according to routine postoperative instructions, urinary output should be checked, and the patient should be ambulated. A normal diet may be resumed gradually, and activity will be restricted for 4 to 7 days as ordered by the physician. The pain in the abdomen and shoulder should disappear within 24 to 36 hours and will be relieved by aspirin or acetaminophen as ordered.

Hysterosalpingography

A hysterosalpingogram is an x-ray examination used to visualize the uterine cavity, the fallopian tubes, and the area around the tubes. To determine tubal and uterine abnormalities, fistulas, and adhesions, a radiopaque substance is injected into the uterus and up into the fallopian tubes as fluoroscopic x-ray films are taken. The structure and patency of the tubes may be examined. The presence of foreign bodies can also be detected; however, pelvic ultrasound is more commonly used for this purpose. Following the test, the patient may experience cramps and a vagal reaction resulting in a slow pulse rate, nausea, and dizziness. These symptoms should subside quickly. The patient must be watched for signs of infection, such as fever, pain, increased pulse rate, malaise, and muscle ache.

Pelvic ultrasonography

In this test high frequency sound waves are passed into the area to be examined and are reflected to a transducer. The transducer then converts the sound energy into electric energy and forms images on an oscilloscope screen, which is similar to x-ray film. Pelvic ultrasonography is used to detect foreign bodies; to distinguish between cysts and tumors; to measure organ size; to detect multiple pregnancies or fetal abnormalities; to evaluate the size, gestational age, growth rate, position, and viability of the fetus; and to determine the location of the placenta and the fetus during amniocentesis. The patient must have a full bladder during the examination to improve the image produced by the sound waves and to provide a landmark to define pelvic organs. The patient is asked to drink liquids, approximately 6 to 8 glasses of water, before the test and is instructed not to void. Immediately following the test, the patient should be allowed to empty her bladder. Alternatively a transvaginal ultrasound can be used, which is performed with the bladder empty. A narrow probe is inserted into the vagina, and the sound waves emit directly into the pelvis. There is some question about the effects of ultrasound. There has been no evidence of harm to the fetus or the mother during the 20 years it has been in use. However a hypothetical risk exists that cannot be ignored. The patient must be fully informed regarding the benefits and potential risks of ultrasonography.

Breast examination

The clinician palpates the breasts during the examination. In recent years emphasis has been placed on teaching women to palpate their own breasts monthly. Early cancer of the breast is curable, and if every woman would take time to carefully examine her own breasts at regular intervals, many benign and malignant tumors would be discovered early. Nurses should become familiar with the procedure of breast self-examination (BSE) so that they may teach patients, friends, or members of their families (Figure 25-14).

Mammography

Mammography is a radiographic (x-ray) technique used to detect breast cysts or tumors, especially those not palpable on physical examination. The test uses relatively low radiation levels but is contraindicated during pregnancy. The patient stands and is asked to place one of her breasts on a table above an x-ray cassette. A compressor is placed on the breast, and the patient is instructed to hold her breath while a picture is taken from above. The machine is rotated, the patient

How to do BSE

1. Lie down and put a pillow under your right shoulder. Place your right arm behind your head.
2. Use the finger pads of the three middle fingers on your left hand to feel for lumps or thickening. Your finger pads are the top third of each finger.

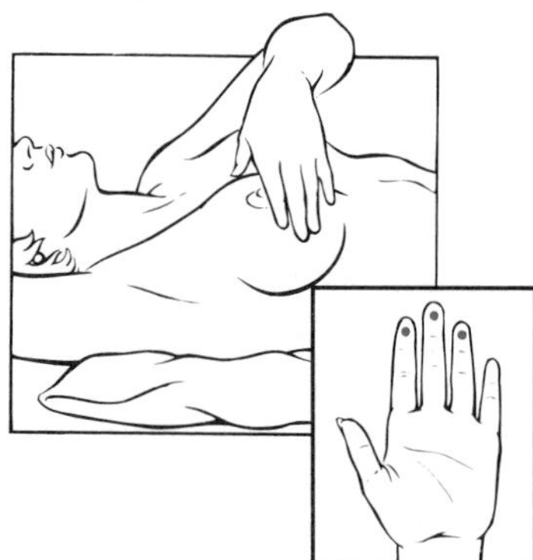

3. Press hard enough to know how your breast feels. If you're not sure how hard to press, ask your health care provider. Or try to copy the way your health care provider uses the finger pads during a breast exam. Learn what your breast feels like most of the time. A firm ridge in the lower curve of each breast is normal.

4. Move around the breast in a set way. You can choose either the circle (A), the up and down line (B), or the wedge (C). Do it the same way every time. It will help you to make sure that you've gone over the entire breast area and to remember how your breast feels each month.

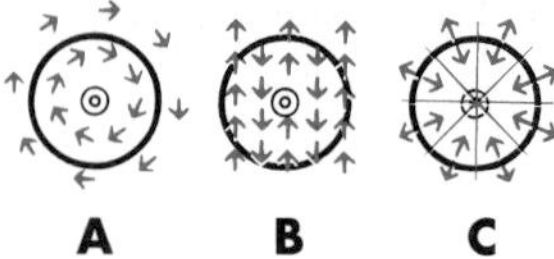

5. Now examine your left breast using right hand finger pads.

You might want to check your breasts while standing in front of a mirror right after you do your BSE each month. You might also want to do an extra BSE while you're in the shower. Your soapy hands will glide over the wet skin making it easy to check how your breasts feel.

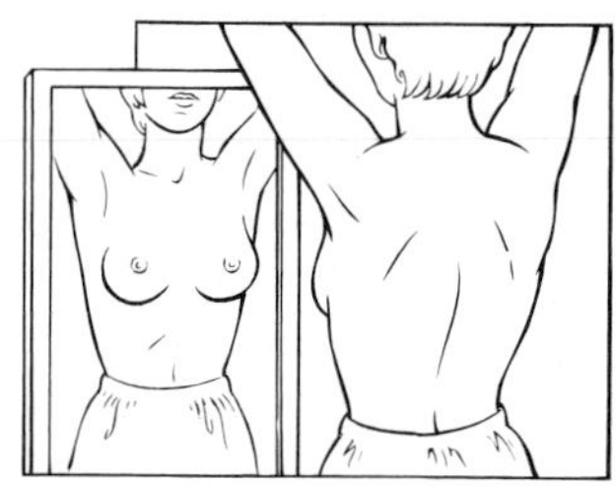

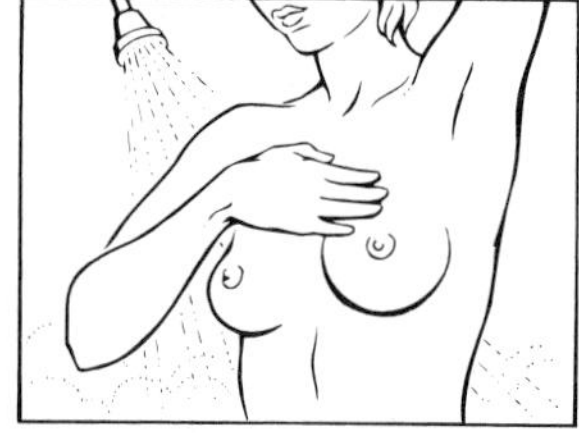

Figure 25-14 Breast self-examination. (Courtesy of American Cancer Society.)

is repositioned, and a lateral view is taken. The procedure is then repeated on the other breast. Abnormal tissues is evident on the developed films. The current recommendations of the American Cancer Society are as follows:

- Women 40 to 49 years of age should have a mammogram every 1 to 2 years.
- Women 50 years of age and older should have an annual mammogram (American Cancer Society, 1994; Mettlin, Smart, 1994).
- Women who have a family history of breast cancer in a first degree relative or who have other risk factors should have an annual mammogram (Table 25-7).

Needle localization biopsy

Needle localization biopsy uses the skills of both a radiologist and a surgeon. The radiologist places a needle in a solid breast mass with the use of x-rays to aid in placement. The needle is left in place, and the patient is transported to 1-day surgery, where a surgeon performs an open biopsy. This technique is useful for small, nonpalpable breast masses discovered by mammogram.

Stereotactic biopsy

Stereotactic biopsy is needle-directed and performed by a radiologist. A core of tissue is removed by a hollow needle guided to the location of a solid mass with the help of x-rays. It is currently available only at large teaching hospitals because it requires specialized x-ray equipment. It is useful in the evaluation of breast mass and is less invasive than open biopsy.

Rubin's test (tubal insufflation)

Rubin's test is done when sterility is suspected to determine if the fallopian tubes are open. The test consists of injecting carbon dioxide gas into the uterine

TABLE 25-7

American Cancer Society Recommendations for Breast Cancer Screening in Asymptomatic Women

Age	Examination	Frequency
20-40	Breast self-examination	Monthly
	Clinical examination	Every 3 years
40-49	Breast self-examination	Monthly
	Clinical examination	Annually
	Mammography	Every 1-2 years
50 and over	Breast self-examination	Monthly
	Clinical examination	Annually
	Mammography	Annually

cavity under controlled pressure. If the tubes are open, the gas escapes through the tube into the peritoneal cavity, where it is absorbed. The test is usually done 2 to 6 days after the end of the menstrual period. The test is contraindicated if pregnancy is suspected, if any infection is present, or if the patient has recently had a dilation and curettage procedure. When the examination is finished and the patient sits up, she will experience discomfort in the right shoulder and neck. This pain is referred to the shoulder and neck from irritation of nerves under the diaphragm where the gas collects. The patient should be assured that the discomfort will last only a few minutes because the gas is absorbed quickly. An absence of pain or discomfort indicates that the tubes are not open.

Pregnancy tests

The most common tests for pregnancy are based on finding *human chorionic gonadotropin (HCG)* in serum or urine. The urine tests are widely available in kit form and are fairly accurate, simple, and inexpensive. The manufacturers of these kits claim that HCG can be detected in urine 42 days after the last menstrual period. Improper collection of the specimen, proteinuria, hormone-producing tumors, and other factors can produce false-positive or false-negative readings.

Dilation and curettage

Dilation and curettage (D & C) is a procedure in which the cervical os is dilated, and the inside of the uterus is scraped with a curette. There are three basic reasons for this procedure: 1) to secure tissue from the lining of the uterus (endometrium) for examination, 2) to control uterine bleeding, and 3) to clear the uterine cavity of any residue left after an incomplete abortion. D & C is a surgical procedure requiring an anesthetic. Preoperative preparation of the patient is the same as that for most other surgical patients. Postoperative care includes observation of the patient for excessive vaginal bleeding and urinary retention. The surgery is usually scheduled on an outpatient basis, and the patient is discharged the same day that surgery is performed.

THE PATIENT WITH DISEASES AND DISORDERS OF THE REPRODUCTIVE SYSTEM

Conditions Affecting the Female External Genitalia and Vagina

Vulvitis

Vulvitis may be either an acute or chronic inflammatory condition of the vulva. There are many causes, including an irritating vaginal discharge, infectious diseases, untreated diabetes, contraceptive pills, and trauma caused by scratching. There usually is severe itching and burning with redness and, in some patients, ulceration. Treatment consists of identifying and treating or removing the cause. Clothing that rubs or irritates the condition should be eliminated. Patients should be questioned about overzealous hygiene because excessive washing may be a cause of vulvitis.

Vaginitis

Vaginitis is one of the most common disorders affecting the female. This condition affects females of any age group, from infants to the elderly.

Pathophysiology. Vaginitis is an inflammation of the vagina. Many factors are associated with its occurrence. *Trichomonas vaginalis* is a flagellated protozoan and is a common cause of vaginitis. It is considered to be sexually transmitted in most cases. Vaginitis may also be caused by *Candida albicans*, a yeastlike fungus. This form is commonly found in women with diabetes and during antibiotic or steroid therapy. Atrophic vaginitis occurs after menopause and is caused by low levels of estrogen, resulting in a thinning of the vaginal lining. Bacterial vaginosis is caused by a proliferation of one or more bacterial anaerobes in the vaginal flora. Vaginitis may be caused by faulty hygiene, tight clothing, illness, or emotional stress.

Assessment. The patient with vaginitis complains of burning and itching of the vulva and vaginal discharge and may report that she has pain on urination or with intercourse. Examination of the vaginal walls often shows a profuse foamy (bubbly) exudate if the cause of the vaginitis is *T. vaginalis*. If *C. albicans* is the causative agent, a thick cheeselike discharge is more typical. Bacterial vaginosis produces a milklike discharge with a foul or fishy odor.

Intervention. Most patients with vaginitis caused by *Trichomonas* organisms are treated with metronidazole (Flagyl), in a 2 g single dose (see Table 25-2). Both partners should be treated at the same time to avoid reinfection. Douches using 1 tablespoon of vinegar to 1 pint of warm water may be ordered to help remove excessive discharge and provide local comfort. Many treatments for vaginitis caused by *C. albicans* can be purchased over the counter. The vaginal cream is inserted at bedtime with a specially designed applicator. Terazol vaginal cream may be prescribed for 7 days or terazol double-strength suppositories for 3 days. Bacterial vaginosis is treated with a 2 g single dose of metronidazole (Flagyl) or with 500 mg given twice a day for 7 days. Patients should be advised to avoid alcohol while on this medication. Flagyl should be avoided during pregnancy. Atrophic vaginitis in women past menopause is treated with estrogen vaginal creams. Pain during intercourse can be relieved with the use of vaginal lubricants. In all cases of vaginitis, patients should be instructed to maintain adequate cleanliness, especially after elimination; to ingest or apply medications as ordered; and to restrict sexual activity to allow the vagina to heal.

Bartholinitis

Bartholinitis is inflammation of the Bartholin's glands, which are located on either side of the vaginal opening. The condition may result from any of several pathogenic bacteria and can be seen in untreated gonorrhea. The ducts from the glands may become occluded by the inflammatory condition, and abscess formation occurs. The abscess may rupture spontaneously, or an incision and drainage may be necessary. Treatment includes administration of the appropriate antibiotic and hot sitz baths. The patient is usually treated in the physician's office or in an outpatient clinic. On the other hand, Bartholin cysts may not be painful and often remain untreated. If they become markedly enlarged, minor surgery can be performed to remove the cyst.

Vesicovaginal and rectovaginal fistula

A vesicovaginal fistula is an abnormal opening from the bladder to the vagina. Rectovaginal fistula is an abnormal opening between the rectum and the vagina. A fistula can occur congenitally or be caused by injury during childbirth or vaginal surgery or result from tissue damage as a result of Crohn's disease or invasive carcinoma. Surgical repair is indicated if the fistula does not heal. Healing is promoted by an increase in dietary vitamin C and protein, cleansing of the area with douches and enemas, rest, and oral antibiotics. A temporary colostomy may be necessary to keep the site clean. Soiling from leakage of urine or stool into the vagina is disturbing for the patient. Sitz baths, deodorizing douches, perineal pads, and protective pants are necessary preoperatively. For those with an irreparable fistula, hygiene and comfort are ongoing concerns. Daily sitz baths and use of "baby wipes" to cleanse the perineum after elimination reduce irritation. If the fistula is repaired surgically, a Foley catheter may be inserted postoperatively to prevent strain on the suture line caused by a full bladder.

Relaxation of the pelvic musculature: rectocele, cystocele, and uterine prolapse

Pathophysiology. The uterus is normally supported by pelvic muscles. These muscles can atrophy with age or weaken with childbearing, thus allowing the uterus to descend, impinge on other structures of the bladder and/or rectum, and protrude through the vaginal wall. A rectocele is the bulging of the rectum against the vaginal wall; a cystocele is the bulging of the bladder against the vaginal wall; and uterine prolapse is the collapse of the uterus into the vagina. In severe cases of uterine prolapse, the cervix may protrude through the external vaginal opening.

Assessment. These conditions cause a feeling of downward pressure, especially when the patient stands or walks. Stress incontinence and urinary frequency and urgency accompany cystocele. Rectal pressure, constipation, heaviness, and hemorrhoids are associated with rectocele. Uterine prolapse produces more severe urinary symptoms such as incontinence and retention. Constipation, backache, and vaginal discharge result from the increased pressure exerted by the prolapsed uterus. Some degree of prolapse occurs in many women, but treatment is not usually initiated unless symptoms are problematic.

Intervention. Uterine prolapse can be treated by inserting a **pessary** to support the uterus, by transvaginal surgical correction, or by removing the uterus (hys-

BOX 25-8 **Nursing Process**

COLPORRHAPHY (REPAIR OF RELAXED PERINEAL MUSCLES)

ASSESSMENT

Vital signs (often)
Dressing/vaginal drainage (often)
Intake and output
Elimination patterns
Lung and bowel sounds
Level of comfort
Self-esteem and self-concept

NURSING DIAGNOSES

Pain related to inflammation at surgical site
Risk for injury (strain on sutures at site of surgical repair) related to full bladder, straining during defecation
Risk for infection related to contamination by fecal material and obstruction of vaginal drainage
Urinary retention related to inflammation of bladder and neck and urethra
Altered sexuality patterns related to postoperative restrictions on sexual intercourse for 6 weeks
Knowledge deficit related to restrictions on physical activity
Alteration in self-concept related to hospitalization
Altered role performance related to surgery and restricted activity level
Risk for impaired skin integrity related to decreased activity level
Risk for respiratory infection related to anesthesia and decreased activity level

NURSING INTERVENTIONS

Monitor routine vital signs until stable.
Maintain patency of indwelling urinary catheter.
Have patient void every 4 hours after catheter is removed to prevent strain on sutures from full bladder.
Give and instruct patient on low-residue diet to promote soft stool.
Avoid cleansing enemas.
Apply ice pack to perineum first 24 hours postoperatively; heat lamp to perineum 20 minutes tid beginning second postoperative day if prescribed.
Administer perineal care with sterile solution qid and after each voiding or defecation.
Apply anesthetic and antiseptic sprays to perineum as prescribed.
Maintain low Fowler's position.
Encourage deep breathing exercises every 2 hours; however, discourage coughing.
Encourage ventilation of feelings and concerns.
Inform patient that loss of vaginal sensation is usually temporary.

EVALUATION OF EXPECTED OUTCOMES

Meets discharge criteria for the postsurgical patient (p. 487)
Has soft, formed stool
Voids in adequate amounts without difficulty
Verbalizes ways to decrease the risk of reherniation of the bladder
Selects foods from a menu that complies with restrictions of a low-residue diet and promotes bowel function
Correctly performs perineal care
Identifies restrictions on activity and coitus during recovery

terectomy). Surgery is the preferred treatment, but a pessary is used if the woman plans further pregnancies or is unable to withstand surgery. A pessary is a small appliance placed in the vagina to reposition the uterus. A sterile lubricant is applied for insertion, and the pessary is removed and cleaned about every 2 months by the physician to prevent infection. The pessary may cause vaginal irritation or erosion. Therefore frequent and regular examinations by the physician are important. The patient must immediately report any unusual vaginal discharge or changes in voiding.

Pelvic floor exercises (Kegel exercises) are prescribed for women who experience prolapse after childbirth. The women alternately contracts and relaxes both the gluteal and perineal floor muscles to strengthen muscle tone. Hysterectomy may be necessary in severe cases of uterine prolapse. (See the section on care of the patient with vaginal or abdominal hysterectomy later in this chapter.)

Surgical repair of a cystocele involves shortening the muscles that support the bladder through a procedure called anterior **colporrhaphy;** repair of a rectocele is called posterior colporrhaphy (Box 25-8). Both repairs may be done at the same time and are then referred to as an anteroposterocolporrhaphy or anteroposterior repair.

Preoperative intervention: colporrhaphy. Preoperative care for colporrhaphy is especially important in ensuring as clean an operative area as possible. Patients may be admitted to the hospital before surgery and given a cathartic, followed by enemas to be sure the bowel is completely empty. A liquid diet for 24 hours before surgery helps to keep the bowel empty. The surgeon may order a cleansing vaginal douche on the evening before and the morning of surgery. The entire vaginal area is shaved, including the pubis and rectal area.

Postoperative intervention: colporrhaphy. The postoperative care of the patient having colporrhaphy includes checking vital signs and observing often for hemorrhage. A retention catheter is usually inserted into the urinary bladder to keep it empty and to prevent pressure on sutures. It is important to keep the fecal residue as soft as possible. Some physicians order a liquid diet for several days, or they may order stool softeners to be given every night. An oil retention enema may be ordered, but cleansing enemas should not be given. A small, soft, rubber tube should be used for the oil retention enema, and the patient must be instructed not to strain when defecating. External sutures may or may not be present, depending on whether perineal repair has been done. The nurse should understand the physician's orders concerning perineal care because some physicians want the area to be kept completely dry. The heat lamp may be used two or three times a day for 20 to 30 minutes. If a solution rather than plain water is to be used in giving perineal care, the physician will order it. All equipment and supplies must be sterile to prevent infection.

The patient is usually kept in a low Fowler's position to prevent pressure or strain on the sutures. When ambulation is allowed, the patient should be taught to roll out of bed. After discharge from the hospital, the patient should be advised against standing for long periods or lifting heavy objects for several weeks. Coitus must be avoided until healing is complete, which is approximately 6 weeks.

Malignant lesions of the vulva

Malignant lesions of the vulva are relatively rare. They account for 3% to 4% of all gynecologic malignancies and occur most often in women after menopause (Lichtman, Papera, 1990). Although these lesions are easily visible, many women wait years before seeking medical attention. Cancer of the vulva is also being diagnosed in women between 20 to 40 years of age. There may be a correlation between onset of this disease and a history of infection with herpes simplex virus and papilloma viruses. These cancers grow slowly and metastasize late. Chronic vulvar dystrophies such as leukoplakia are considered premalignant. Malignant lesions can be of the in situ variety, involving just the tissues at the site of origin, or the invasive type. If lesions are invasive, extensive local spread occurs, particularly into the lymphatic channels.

Assessment. The most common complaint of patients with early vulvar cancer is pruritus (itching). The precancerous lesions of leukoplakia may be present and are seen as thickened white patches on the mucous membranes of the vulva. The patient often gives a history of having used various salves, ointments, and lotions for symptoms of mild soreness before finally seeking medical care. Cardiovascular and degenerative diseases are often present because of the typical older age of these patients. Later symptoms include edema of the vulva and pelvic lymphadenopathy.

Intervention. Radiation therapy may be used if the disease has progressed beyond the operable stage. If the malignancy can be surgically removed, a vulvectomy is indicated.

A vulvectomy includes the removal of the external female genitals. It may be a partial procedure for biopsy purposes, a simple procedure for removal of a benign or an in situ type lesion, or a radical procedure for invasive malignant lesions. A simple vulvectomy is the removal of the vulva along with a margin of skin adjacent to the vulva. A radical vulvectomy includes the excision of skin from the symphysis pubis to the anus and may include removal of the inguinal lymph nodes in the groin on both sides. The excised areas are covered with a skin flap.

Preoperative care includes the same care as reviewed in Chapter 18. Wide areas of skin preparation should include the inguinal regions, vulva, and pubic and perineal areas. The emotional preparation of the patient is important, and the nurse should listen to any apprehension or fears that the patient expresses. Fear of disfigurement and loss of a body part are common. Both before and after surgery the patient may show signs of a grief reaction, such as depression, anger, denial, or withdrawal.

When the patient returns from surgery, a Foley catheter will be in the urinary bladder to prevent constriction of the urethra. Dressings may need to be changed often for several days because of the serous drainage from the wounds. A T binder may be used to hold dressings in place. The patient is placed in a low Fowler's position to prevent strain on the sutures. The patient should be turned every 2 hours, and when on her side, a pillow should be placed lengthwise between her legs to support the upper leg and prevent strain. The wound is cleansed according to the physician's orders. Solutions often used for cleansing include hydrogen peroxide and warm physiologic saline solution. The surgeon may prefer that wounds be exposed and that a heat lamp be used because it stimulates circulation and promotes healing. Some physicians may order sitz baths, whereas others may believe that such baths increase the danger of wound infection. The patient is usually given a low-residue diet. Analgesics are required for several days, and recovery is generally slow. The patient may be ambulatory by the third day, but the nurse should remember that ambulation must be gradual for the older person. Leg edema is common after surgery, and some patients may develop chronic leg edema. Elastic stockings, elevation of the legs, and avoidance of long periods of sitting or standing help to provide better venous return. An important nursing function is the prevention of wound infection. Care should be taken to provide privacy when caring for the wound and to avoid any unnecessary exposure of the patient.

Acceptance of and adjustment to her change in appearance may be difficult, and the patient may need support in helping her partner accept the change in her appearance. The patient may experience difficulty in coitus because of loss of tissue in the supporting structures of the labia and vagina and possible constriction of the vaginal orifice. Constriction may require dilation or surgical revision.

Expected outcomes. With proper intervention the patient with a vulvectomy does the following:

- Has her self-esteem intact as indicated by attention to personal hygiene and appearance
- Verbalizes concerns about the change in appearance of her vulvar region and shares concerns with her husband or significant other
- Has wound approximated and healing with no signs of infection
- Voids regularly in amounts greater than 150 ml
- States plans for restricting activity postoperatively that will strain operative area
- States plans for restriction of sexual activity until permitted by physician
- Verbalizes understanding that constriction of vaginal orifice may occur postoperatively and may require reconstructive surgery
- States plans for follow-up visit to physician

Vaginal cancer

Cancer of the vagina, particularly in young women, is also rare, but the incidence is higher in women who were prenatally exposed to the hormone DES.

Early detection makes it possible to completely remove the malignant area in the vagina. The vagina can then be reconstructed using a split-thickness graft from the buttocks applied to a Silastic mold, which is sutured to the labia. The mold is removed a few days postoperatively, after the graft shows evidence of taking.

A lighter, more comfortable mold is created with a condom filled with tampons that is inserted until healing is complete.

DES syndrome

DES (diethylstilbestrol) is a synthetic form of estrogen that was prescribed for approximately 5 to 6 million women in the United States between 1941 and 1971. It was commonly used to treat women who were pregnant and who had the following: 1) one prior miscarriage; 2) diabetes; 3) toxemia; or 4) slight bleeding during pregnancy. A prescription audit showed that the drug was still being prescribed during pregnancy as late as 1974, despite the FDA announcing in 1971 that the drug was contraindicated in pregnancy. This FDA restriction followed the discovery that several young women developed adenocarcinoma of the vagina and that each of them was the daughter of a woman who had ingested DES during pregnancy. Studies were then conducted on other young women who had been exposed to DES in utero, and characteristic benign genital tract abnormalities were found in the majority. Follow-up studies continue to determine the risk of these women for developing malignancies. Daughters of women who took DES are encouraged to have a yearly gynecologic examination and frequent colposcopy to screen for cervical and vaginal cancer.

Conditions Affecting the Cervix and Uterus

Cervicitis

Cervicitis may be the result of an acute inflammatory condition of the vagina, or it may be a chronic condition resulting from lacerations occurring at the time of delivery, erosion, cysts, or a specific infection such as gonorrhea. The cause of erosion is not always known. Cervicitis may occur in any woman, often producing no symptoms, and is detected only on a routine pelvic examination. Most physicians believe that untreated chronic cervicitis predisposes women to cancer of the cervix. Treatment includes examination and studies to exclude cervical cancer. Cervical erosions may be cauterized or treated with cryotherapy (freezing). If the condition does not respond to conservative treatment, the patient may be admitted to the hospital and placed under general anesthesia to have the cone-shaped portion of the cervix removed (conization).

Endometriosis

Endometriosis is the growth of endometrial tissue in abnormal sites, usually in the peritoneal cavity. The ovaries and the peritoneum are the most common sites. The uterus is an organ that sheds cells periodically. These are endometrial cells, and occasionally they become seeded throughout the pelvis and other organs. The exact cause is unknown. Although these endometrial cells are not in the uterus, they are stimulated by the ovarian hormones and bleed into the nearby tissue, resulting in an inflammatory process. Adhesions, strictures, cysts, and infertility can result.

The patient is usually asymptomatic until she is between 25 and 40 years of age. Symptoms that gradually begin to occur are pain during menstruation that becomes progressively worse, fatigue, pressure in the pelvic organs, and general discomfort. Treatment with drugs that suppress ovulation for a time delays the stimulation of the cells and increases the chance of fertility when administration of the drug is stopped. When endometriosis is severe, removal of the uterus, fallopian tubes, and ovaries may be necessary.

Tumors

Fibroid. A fibroid, or myomatous tumor, is a benign growth of muscle tissue of the uterus. It occurs in 20% to 30% of all women and develops slowly between the ages of 25 and 40. Menorrhagia, abnormally long or heavy bleeding with menstrual periods, is the characteristic symptom. If the fibroid tumor becomes large enough to cause pressure on other structures there may be backache, constipation, and urinary symptoms. Treatment is surgical removal. If the fibroid tumor is small, a myomectomy is performed to remove just the tumor. If the tumor is large or produces excessive bleeding, a hysterectomy is performed, preserving the ovaries if possible.

Cervical and uterine cancer. Cervical cancer is the second most common form of malignancy affecting the female reproductive organs. Postcoital spotting is the predominant symptom, but this is common with any kind of cervical lesion or inflammation and is not restricted to cervical carcinoma. Unfortunately cancer of the cervix may not cause any symptoms during the early stages, and the condition can be far advanced before any signs appear. Although cervical cancer may occur in young adults, the incidence increases with age, with the greatest incidence occurring in patients between ages 30 and 50. Only 30% of high-grade SIL (squamous intraepithelial lesions) indicated on Pap smears will ever progress to carcinoma in situ (CIS). There is an increased incidence of cervical carcinoma in young women whose mothers took DES during pregnancy as treatment to prevent spontaneous abortion. The Pap smear test is widely used and has had a primary effect on the decreasing mortality associated with cervical cancer. CIS is a preinvasive, asymptomatic carcinoma that can only be diagnosed by microscopic examination. Once it is diagnosed, it can be treated early without radical surgery, and a cure results. CIS of the cervix is essentially 100% curable. All women over 20 years of age or who are sexually active should have a pelvic examination and Pap smear every 3 years after three negative examinations 1 year apart. High-risk women should be examined more often, and many gynecologists prefer to see their patients yearly. Risk factors for cervical cancer include first sex partner at an early age, multiple sex partners, smoking, history of HPV infection, and history of radiation to the pelvis.

Uterine cancer occurs somewhat later in life, usually affecting postmenopausal women. The most common symptom is vaginal bleeding. There is no relationship between the amount of bleeding and the existence of cancer. Sometimes only slight spotting occurs.

Treatment of cervical and uterine cancer varies with the extent of the cancer and age of the patient. For cervical CIS a conization or laser surgery may be performed, which removes a portion of the cervix. Other patients may have a simple hysterectomy. Radical surgery and radiation therapy are used for more advanced cancer (see Chapter 10).

Conditions Affecting the Ovaries and Fallopian Tubes

Cysts and tumors

Many different types of ovarian tumors and cysts are benign. However, others may be malignant. Ovarian cysts may cause no symptoms or may result in a disturbance of menstruation, a feeling of heaviness, and slight bleeding. If a pedicle (a stemlike structure) is present, the cyst may become twisted on the pedicle, cutting off the blood supply. If this occurs, immediate surgery is required.

Cancer of the ovary represents 26% of all female genital cancer and 4% of all cancer seen in women (Lichtman, Papera, 1990). The risk of ovarian cancer increases with age, with the highest rates occurring in women age 65 to 84. It has been called the silent disease because early warning signs that prompt medical attention rarely occur. As a result, ovarian cancer causes more deaths than cancer of the uterus. Vague lower abdominal discomfort and mild digestive complaints are early symptoms for some women. Later symptoms include pelvic pain, anemia, and ascites. The ovary may be the primary site of the cancer, or the cancer may occur as a result of metastasis from the gastrointestinal tract, breast, pancreas, or kidneys. Treatment for cancer of the ovary depends on the severity of the malignancy. Surgical removal of the tumor is the preferred treatment. This may include radical excision of the uterus, ovaries, tubes, and omentum. Chemotherapy follows surgery.

Pelvic inflammatory disease

Pelvic inflammatory disease (PID), also termed pelvic infection, is an inflammatory condition of the pelvic cavity that may involve the fallopian tubes (salpingitis), ovaries (oophoritis), pelvic peritoneum, or pelvic vascular system. The disease can be acute or chronic and can be caused by gram-negative bacteria, staphylococcus, streptococcus, or sexually transmitted organisms such as gonorrhea or chlamydia. It can be confined to one structure or be widespread in the pelvic cavity (See Chapter 11). Pathogens invade the pelvic organs during sexual intercourse, childbirth, the postpartum period, or abortion, or they may spill into the cavity following rupture of an infected organ such as the appendix. PID is more common in women using IUDs.

Pathophysiology. Pathogenic organisms are usually introduced from the outside and enter the cervix from the vagina, move up through the uterus to the fallopian tubes, exit from the tubes, and enter the pelvic cavity. They may also enter the pelvis through thrombosed uterine veins or through the lymphatics of the uterus. When the pathogens lodge in the fallopian tubes, the inflammatory process results in purulent material and subsequent adhesions, strictures, and obstruction. Infertility results when the tubes become occluded. Partial tubal obstruction predisposes the woman to ectopic pregnancy. Whereas the sperm may be small enough to pass through the stricture or obstructed area, the fertilized ovum is too large to make the return trip to the uterus and remains in the tube, where it begins to develop. Adhesions may produce symptoms severe enough to require removal of the uterus, fallopian tubes, and ovaries.

Assessment. Acute PID is characterized by severe abdominal pain, pelvic pain, malaise, nausea, vomiting, and fever with leukocytosis. A foul-smelling, purulent vaginal discharge may be present. The symptoms may be so mild that the woman ignores them. They may subside before the patient seeks medical care, and the disease then goes untreated. Lack of treatment or inadequately treated acute PID results in the chronic form. The patient then complains of a chronic dull pain in the lower abdomen, backache, constipation, malaise, low-grade fever, and menstrual disturbances. Acute symptoms can also appear during periods of exacerbation. The patient's complaints are often vague and nonspecific. Examination reveals pain and tenderness in the lower abdomen, which increases with a vaginal examination. Masses are felt if the fallopian tubes or ovaries are enlarged or if an abscess is present. Abscess formation is common in Douglas' cul-de-sac. If adhesions are present, the pelvic organs will be less movable. Smears and cultures are taken from the vagina, cervix, or Douglas' cul-de-sac to identify the causative organism and determine the most effective antibiotic. Laparoscopy may be performed to diagnose the disease. In this way the physician is able to visualize the reproductive organs and surrounding tissues.

Intervention. Hospitalization may be required so that the patient can receive intensive antibiotic therapy. Activity is restricted to bedrest, and the patient is placed in a mid-Fowler's position to prevent upward flow of drainage and the formation of abscesses high in the abdomen. Intravenous fluids may be necessary if the patient's condition requires restricted intake. The antibiotics are given intravenously at first to ensure that blood levels of the drug are adequate to be effective against the causative organism. Heat to the abdomen or hot sitz baths may be ordered to improve circulation and provide comfort. Analgesics are necessary for pain. Blood pressure, temperature, pulse, and respirations should be taken every 4 hours until the fever subsides. The patient should be observed for any increase or decrease in pain and any change in amount, color, odor, or consistency of vaginal drainage. Surgical removal of involved organs may be necessary.

Expected outcomes. After proper intervention the patient with PID:

- Is afebrile.
- Has absence or reduction of pain and vaginal drainage.
- Identifies the point of entry and route of travel of organisms causing PID.
- Identifies signs and symptoms of recurrence.
- Lists all medications to be taken after discharge, including time and frequency of each dose.
- Demonstrates compliance with restrictions on activity, medication regimen, and recommendations for follow-up care.

Surgical Intervention for Conditions Affecting the Cervix, Uterus, Ovaries, and Fallopian Tubes

Hysterectomy

Hysterectomy is the surgical removal of the uterus. A hysterectomy may be performed through an incision into the abdominal cavity (abdominal hysterectomy), or the uterus may be removed through the vagina (vaginal hysterectomy). In premenopausal women, the ovaries are usually not removed unless some abnormal condition exists. Depending on the existing condition, the physician may remove one or both ovaries or one or both fallopian tubes. Removal of both ovaries is called *bilateral oophorectomy,* and removal of both fallopian tubes is called *bilateral salpingectomy.* When the entire uterus, tubes, and ovaries are removed, the operation is called *panhysterosalpingo-oophorectomy,* or *panhysterectomy.* It may also be referred to as a *total abdominalhysterectomy with bilateral salpingo-oophorectomy* (TAH BSO). Removal of the body of the uterus, leaving the cervix in place, is termed a *subtotal hysterectomy.* In a total hysterectomy the entire uterus is removed, but the tubes and ovaries are left in place. The patient should understand that a hysterectomy does not necessarily mean that any organs will be removed other than the uterus. However, if there is evidence of disease affecting other organs, those organs are removed at the same time as the uterus.

Surgery involving the female reproductive tract is upsetting to most women. Often the patient perceives the procedure as a threat to her femininity. If the patient is of childbearing age, she may be disappointed because she can no longer have children. Patients often worry about the process of healing and the resumption of sexual activity. If cancer is suspected or found, she may have a fear of death. The more thoroughly the patient is prepared for the surgery, the more satisfactorily she will recover, both physically and emotionally (Box 25-9).

Abdominal hysterectomy.

Preoperative intervention. Preoperative care for the abdominal hysterectomy patient is the same as that for patients having other types of abdominal surgery. The surgical preparation of the skin includes the abdomen, pubis, and perineum. The physician may order an antiseptic vaginal douche, and a Foley catheter may be inserted to keep the bladder from

BOX 25-9 **Nursing Process**

HYSTERECTOMY

ASSESSMENT

Vital signs (often)
Dressing/vaginal drainage (often)
Intake and output
Elimination patterns
Lung and bowel sounds
Level of comfort
Signs and symptoms of menopause

NURSING DIAGNOSES

Pain related to surgical incision and abdominal distention
Altered sexuality patterns related to restrictions on sexual intercourse
Ineffective individual coping related to loss of reproductive function
Dysfunctional grieving related to loss of reproductive organ
Knowledge deficit related to onset of menopause and postoperative limitations
Risk for infection related to interruption in integrity of skin and/or vaginal mucosa
Disturbance in self-concept (body image, self-esteem, and/or role performance) related to loss of reproductive organ and function
Urinary retention related to pelvic edema and discomfort
Altered peripheral tissue perfusion related to venous congestion in pelvis

NURSING INTERVENTIONS

Administer routine nursing care immediately after anesthesia.
Check abdominal or perineal dressing for hemorrhage; change as needed according to hospital policy.
Maintain intravenous infusion, as ordered.
Administer nothing by mouth until peristalsis returns.
Maintain patency of indwelling catheter or check for bladder distention every 8 hours; straight catheterization, as necessary.
Catheterize for residual urine after voiding, if ordered.
Apply heat to abdomen for gas pains, if ordered.
Encourage deep breathing and coughing every 2 hours.
Apply plastic or pneumatic stockings, if ordered.
Avoid sharp flexion of knees or thighs.
Do not place pillows under the knees.
Dangle the patient the evening of surgery.
Encourage leg exercises until ambulating.
Provide emotional support.
Encourage ventilation of fears and concerns related to loss of reproductive capacity.

EVALUATION OF EXPECTED OUTCOMES

Meets discharge criteria for the postsurgical patient (p. 487)
Voids regularly, with amounts greater than 150 ml and residual amounts less than 60 ml
Tolerates regular diet without nausea or distention
Has no signs and symptoms of complications
Demonstrates self-esteem evidenced by attention to personal hygiene and appearance
Expresses fears and concerns regarding loss of reproductive capacity and sexual identity
Identifies restrictions on activity and coitus during recovery
Verbalizes an understanding of surgical menopause

filling during surgery and causing strain postoperatively.

Postoperative intervention. Postoperative nursing care is concerned with the prevention of urinary retention, intestinal distention, and venous thrombosis. If a retention catheter was inserted, it should be kept patent and attached to closed drainage. If it is not, the patient must be checked often for bladder distention. The incidence of urinary retention is greater after a hysterectomy than after other types of surgery, because some trauma to the bladder unavoidably occurs. Urinary retention leads to discomfort from distention and increases the danger of urinary tract infection. Before administering drugs for pain, the nurse should be sure that the discomfort is not from an overdistended bladder. Most patients are given intravenous fluids for 1 or 2 days, and the additional fluid may contribute to bladder distention. Every method should be used to assist the patient to void before catheterization. Efforts should be instituted early, not delayed until the patient is miserable because of an overdistended bladder. If the patient does not have an indwelling catheter and is unable to void, catheterization every 8 hours may be necessary.

Intestinal distention is common following a hysterectomy. A nasogastric tube may be inserted. A small tapwater enema or a Harris flush may be ordered to help relieve distention. Early ambulation helps to return the bowel to normal function. As soon as bowel sounds have returned and flatus is being expelled, the patient is allowed liquids by mouth with a gradual return to solid food.

Patients undergoing pelvic surgery are more susceptible to venous stasis and phlebitis because of trauma to blood vessels. Patients who have varicose veins in the extremities must be carefully observed. The nurse should *not* raise the knee gatch, place pillows under the knees, or place the patient in a high Fowler's position. Active exercise should be started as soon as the patient is fully conscious because early ambulation helps prevent venous stasis. Some surgeons order elastic antiembolism stockings to prevent stasis and to support venous flow.

Sedation such as meperidine (Demerol) may be ordered for relief of pain. Slight vaginal drainage may occur for a day or two, but any unusual bleeding should be reported to the physician. The nurse should routinely check vital signs and observe the abdominal dressing for evidence of bleeding. Most patients without complications are released from the hospital in approximately 5 days (see Box 25-9).

Vaginal hysterectomy.

Preoperative intervention. Skin preparation involves shaving the pubis and perineum. Some physicians order prophylactic antibiotics and some an antiseptic vaginal douche. A primary source of postoperative infection is the vaginal vault. A Foley catheter is inserted to drain the bladder during surgery, and an enema is given.

Postoperative intervention. If a repair has been done along with the hysterectomy, the Foley catheter remains in place for 4 or 5 days to prevent pressure on the sutures. Otherwise it is removed postoperatively, and the patient must be observed for bladder distention and assisted to void. Other postoperative nursing care is essentially the same as that for repair of relaxed muscles.

Discharge teaching: hysterectomy. Before the patient is discharged, she should know what changes to expect. She will no longer menstruate, and she should not have coitus until her physician permits it, usually after the first checkup in 4 to 6 weeks. She may have worries concerning her ability to continue to share sexual pleasure. When a hysterectomy is performed, the vaginal floor is reconstructed with ligaments, and most women should have the same capacity for sexual stimulation after surgery as before. Pain experienced during intercourse (dyspareunia) should be reported to the physician. Normal physical activity and light work may be done when the woman returns home. However, lifting heavy objects and more difficult activity must be avoided for a few weeks. Most women may return to work within 6 weeks.

Pelvic exenteration

Complete or total pelvic exenteration consists of the removal of the rectum, distal sigmoid colon, urinary bladder and distal ureters, internal iliac vessels and their lateral branches, all pelvic reproductive organs, and lymph nodes. In women, in addition, the entire pelvic floor and peritoneum, levator muscles, and perineum are excised. Urinary and fecal diversions are done. *Pelvic evisceration* and *pelvic sweep* are terms used interchangeably with pelvic exenteration.

The procedure is sometimes modified. An anterior pelvic exenteration removes the bladder and distal portion of the ureters while the proximal portions are implanted in an ileal conduit. In women the vagina, adnexa, pelvic lymph nodes, and pelvic peritoneum are removed as well. The normal bowel structure is preserved. In posterior pelvic exenteration the colon and rectum are removed, and in women the uterus, vagina, and adnexa are also removed. Pelvic exenteration is indicated for carcinomas that are locally destructive and capable of growing to great size but that do not tend to metastasize and for tumors that are radioresistant or incurable by less radical surgery. The tumor must be confined to the pelvis without metastatic spread to distant sites and must be operable within the pelvis. The patient should be of an age and general physical and mental condition that make rehabilitation a reasonable goal. Exenteration is an alternative to lethal disease, but the patient and spouse or supportive person must have a stronger than usual desire to live in order to cope with altered methods of fecal and urinary elimination and sexual intercourse. Their psychologic and sociologic status must be carefully evaluated preoperatively.

Preoperative care must focus on the patient's psychologic needs, as well as physical preparation of the bowel with a low-residue diet, laxatives, a saline enema, and antibiotic therapy. A sulfonamide drug regimen for bowel cleansing may be used, but there is some controversy regarding the use of antibiotics for bowel cleansing. Antiembolism stockings are applied, and a nasogastric tube may be inserted the morning of surgery. Before surgery, the woman douches daily with an antiseptic solution. Vitamin K therapy to promote blood coagulability may begin 2 to 3 days before surgery. The patient must be prepared to remain in bed for up to 1 week postoperatively as healing begins.

After surgery, the vital signs and blood pressure are taken every hour for approximately 48 hours. Then they are assessed every 4 hours for 7 days or as long as necessary. Rectal temperatures are contraindicated. Intravenous therapy is maintained up to 4000 ml daily. All intake and output are measured. The operative site, the dressings, and all drainage tubes are also assessed hourly for the first 48 hours. Dressings should be reinforced and changed as ordered. Specific nursing care is indicated by the extent of the procedure, the status of the wounds and/or ostomies that were created, and the patient's response to the surgery.

Self-worth. Exenterative surgery has a drastic effect on body image. Loss of the reproductive organs and the ability to have sexual intercourse may be a major handicap to the patient's rehabilitation. Society's emphasis on physical attractiveness makes it even more difficult for the patient to maintain a positive self-concept and strong sexual role identity after the loss of the ability to function in a reproductive capacity. Sexual readjustment may be a problem of great magnitude for the patient and his or her sexual partner. Vaginal reconstruction is possible, but it is usually done as a follow-up procedure. Segments of colon or ileum or skin grafts over a stent can be used. It is important for the nurse to facilitate the patient's expression of fears and concerns and to communicate the patient's needs to other members of the healthcare team and community resources. Ostomy clubs can be of help to patients in their efforts to regain social mobility and maintain a realistic yet hopeful outlook on life.

Conditions Affecting the Breast

Acute mastitis

Mastitis is an inflammation of the mammary gland (breast) that often occurs during lactation but may occur anytime. It is usually the result of the entrance of bacteria through a crack or fissure in the nipple. The infection may block one or more of the milk ducts, causing the milk to stagnate in the lobule. The infection may spread throughout the breast tissue and cause abscess formation. The infection usually causes an elevation of temperature, with pain and tenderness of the breast. The treatment consists of administration of antibiotic drugs, application of heat or cold, and support of the breast. Incision and drainage of an abscess may be necessary. Because the invading organism in mastitis is often the staphylococcus, isolation and care as outlined in Chapter 11 should be followed.

Physiologic nodularity (fibrocystic breast disease)

Physiologic nodularity is a common occurence in premenopausal women. It is characterized by the formation of a nodular type of benign cyst in the breast. The exact cause is unknown. Many women go through life unaware of the condition or neglect diagnosis and treatment. The condition is benign and does not produce an inflammatory condition. Although it generally involves both breasts, it may be accentuated in one breast. The cysts may occur singly or may be numerous and vary in size and tenderness over the menstrual cycle. Pain may be present and may become worse during the menstrual period. Treatment is usually conservative after cancer has been ruled out. However, the patient should examine her own breasts monthly and remain under medical supervision. In most instances there is no increased risk of breast cancer.

Tumors

Tumors of the breast can be benign or malignant. Benign tumors are not tender and are freely movable. An exact diagnosis can be made only by careful microscopic examination of the cells. Benign tumors should be surgically removed.

Breast cancer

Breast cancer is the most common cancer in women, but it is now second to lung cancer in the number of deaths from cancer in women. It is estimated that 1 out of every 9 women in the United States will develop cancer of the breast in her lifetime. One of every 100 cases is seen in males (Ellorhorst-Ryan, Goeldner, 1992). Women who do not bear children or who bear children after the age of 35 have a slight increase in risk for breast cancer. There appears to be a lower incidence of breast cancer among women who breast-feed their infants for at least 3 months. However, some authorities question this factor. A small proportion of breast cancers appear to run in families. The most significant risk factor is age; risk increases with each decade. The cause of breast cancer is poorly understood despite extensive research (Box 25-10).

BOX 25-10

RISK FACTORS FOR BREAST CANCER

Family history: mother/sister
Nulliparous
First pregnancy after age 35
Menarche before age 11
Menopause after age 50
History of cancer in one breast
Diet high in fat and protein
Obesity

Time is an important factor in the diagnosis and treatment of breast cancer. If discovered in the early stages, the possibility of cure is high. When the disease is localized in the breast, 85% of patients will survive 5 years or longer. The 5-year survival rate is decreased to less than 50% when axillary nodes are involved.

Assessment. The American Cancer Society has outlined a program for breast self-examination and has sought to encourage women to examine their breasts monthly to detect abnormalities (see Figure 25-14). Women are advised to begin monthly self-examinations of their breasts at age 20. Annual examinations by a clinician are recommended for women over age 50. Women between age 20 and 40 should be examined every 3 years. The American Cancer Society recommends mammograms every 1 to 2 years between ages 40 and 49. It is strongly recommended that women over the age of 50 have mammograms annually (American Cancer Society, 1994; Baird, 1991; Ellorhorst-Ryan, Goeldner, 1992). However, mammography screening is not 100% effective: 10% to 14% of breast cancers found by physical examination are missed by mammography (Baird, 1992). Nurses should therefore continue to teach and encourage breast self-examination.

The development of breast cancer is insidious, and pain is usually absent in the early stages. The only sign that may be present is a small, firm lump in the breast, not well defined or movable, which may be discovered only by careful examination. As the tumor increases in size, it attaches itself to the chest wall or to the skin above. A dimpling of the skin may be present, the nipple may be retracted or inverted, and a discharge from the nipple may be present. In some cases reddening of the skin may develop and, if the tumor is large, a change in the contour of the breast may be present. Without treatment the axillary lymph nodes become involved, ulceration may occur, and metastasis to the lungs, bones, liver, and brain may occur. A gradual state of ill health occurs, with weight loss and poor appetite later in the illness.

Carcinoma of the breast usually occurs in a single area in one breast. Almost half of these tumors occur in the upper outer quadrant and another fourth in the central or inner half of the breast. Tumors in the upper outer quadrant tend to metastasize first to the axillary lymph nodes, whereas those from the central portion metastasize to the internal mammary chain lymph nodes (Figure 25-15).

Assessment should include exploration of the patient's feelings about treatment choices, which may include breast conservation surgery, modified mastectomy, and reconstructive surgery. Reconstruction can be more successful when tissue is conserved at the time of surgery. Methods of and indications for breast reconstruction are covered later in this chapter.

Breast conservation surgery (lumpectomy). Early-stage breast carcinoma can be treated by breast conservation surgery (lumpectomy) combined with partial axillary node dissection and radiation or a modified mastectomy and lymph node dissection. When the malignancy is less than 1½ inches, it is common for the physician to offer breast conservation surgery as an alternative to mastectomy. Informed patients who refuse a mastectomy are seen as a major force in advancing research on conservative management of breast cancer. Several studies performed over the last 20 years have shown that rates of survival, distant metastasis, and local recurrence are similar in patients treated with lumpectomy plus radiation and mastectomy plus radiation (Knobf, 1994). If the likelihood of "cure" is considered equal, one can consider the cosmetic advantage of removing only the malignant tumor and a small amount (¼ to ½ inch) of surrounding breast tissue.

In breast conservation surgery, the surgeon removes a minimum amount of skin, and the breast tissues are approximated to preserve the appearance of the breast where the tumor has been removed. The incision is made to follow the contour of the breast. A separate incision is made in the axilla to dissect the axillary nodes for biopsy. At least five nodes lying lateral to (level I) and under (level II) the pectoralis minor muscles should be removed for review. If the nodes are removed from the lower two thirds of the axilla, the patient has better function and tolerance and less postoperative edema. If the nodes are negative, the axilla need not receive radiation therapy. Radiation treatments are given to the tumor site and the whole breast up to five times weekly for 6 to 7 weeks.

Mastectomy. The surgical removal of the breast for treatment of malignancy can be simple, modified radical, or radical. In a *simple mastectomy* the skin and tissue of the breast are removed, the edges of the remaining skin are sutured together, and the lymph nodes are left in place. Some surgeons think that preserving the lymph nodes is important in controlling the spread of malignant cells.

A *modified radical mastectomy* involves removal of all breast tissue and an axillary node dissection, but the pectoralis major and minor muscles are left in place.

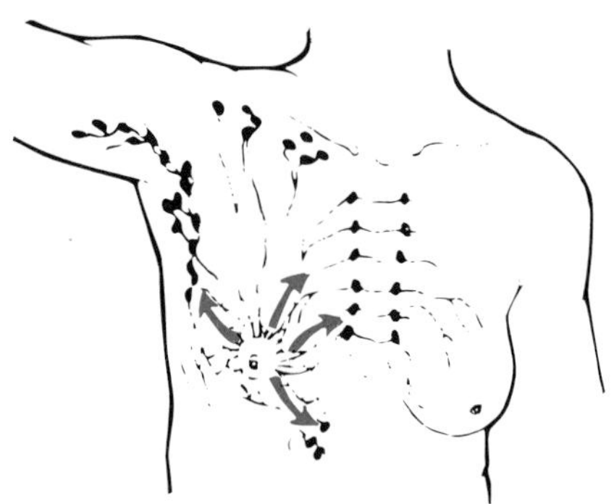

Figure 25-15 Mode of dissemination of breast cancer. (From Bouchard R, Owens NF: *Nursing care of the patient,* ed 4, St Louis, 1981, Mosby.)

Preserving these muscles prevents the formation of a hollow depression below the clavicle, thus reducing disfigurement. Hand and arm swelling are uncommon, and arm and shoulder motion are rarely affected. For more advanced cancer, irradiation may precede or follow a surgical procedure, but sufficient time must be allowed before or after surgery to avoid interference with healing.

A radical mastectomy involves removal of the breast and the underlying tissues, including the muscles, axillary lymph nodes, vessels, and perhaps the entire mammary lymph node chain and supraclavicular nodes. The extent of surgery depends on the spread of the neoplasm. However, a radical mastectomy is rarely performed today. When the malignant tumor is localized and examination of the lymph nodes is negative, most surgeons believe that a modified radical mastectomy should be done.

Breast reconstruction after mastectomy. Although a mastectomy is a curative treatment, the amputation of a breast is usually viewed as a tragic event, accompanied by loss of body image. Advances in the techniques of reconstructive mammoplasty hold the promise of restoring the contour and consistency of breast tissue to many mastectomy patients. Early detection and treatment make the patient a good candidate for less extensive surgery. Most women experience some dissatisfaction with any type of external prosthesis, whether it be difficulty in wearing clothing or lack of normalcy in sexual relationships. It is becoming more common to replace the missing breast with an internal prosthesis or an implant of the patient's own tissues. Consultation with a plastic surgeon before mastectomy provides the opportunity to explore the possibilities for reconstruction and to perform the surgical procedure in a manner that is more likely to result in success.

The patient considering reconstruction can choose between an artificial implant or a procedure that utilizes her own tissues (autogenous implant). The artificial implant usually involves insertion of a temporary expander that is gradually filled with saline to stretch the breast tissue before insertion of the permanent implant. Some patients can receive the implant immediately without stretching the skin. The autogenous implant uses tissue and muscle from the back or the abdomen to create a new breast. Either procedure can be performed immediately after mastectomy or can be elected at a later date. The options for breast reconstruction must be considered carefully, and some patients are not ready to make the decision at the time of mastectomy.

Skin expansion with implant. A saline implant is inserted immediately or sometime after the breast tissue is removed in a modified radical mastectomy (Figure 25-16). Saline is added gradually to inflate the implant and stretch the breast tissue. The tissue does stretch, just as abdominal tissue stretches during pregnancy. The permanent implant is then inserted in a second surgical procedure. After the incision has healed, the nipple and areola are reconstructed during an outpatient procedure. The nipple is created from a flap of skin, and the areola can be created either by injecting dark color, as done with a tattoo, or by using darker tissue from the inner thigh. The permanent implant is filled with saline and has a textured surface intended to reduce the amount of scar tissue that forms around it. If scar tissue does form, it may create a firm capsule that needs to be broken up manually or surgically. Silicone gel implants used previously are not often used because of continued controversy. There is conflicting evidence of the dangers of silicone leaking into the system. While there is any question, surgeons and patients are hesitant to use silicone implants.

Flap reconstruction. An autogenous implant involves the use of the patient's own tissue taken from another part of her body (Figure 25-17). Use of the latissimus dorsi from the back was the first donor site. Now the tissue of the abdomen over the rectus muscle is more commonly used. The flap of skin and muscle may remain attached to the blood supply and be tunneled under the skin to the breast site, or it may be completely dissected and the blood supply reestablished through microsurgery (Figure 25-18). The abdominal area is reconstructed to restore abdominal strength and prevent hernia. The nipple and areola are reconstructed in the same manner as with a saline implant. The reconstructed breast can be very close in form and appearance to a natural breast. However, normal sensation cannot be restored with breast reconstruction.

Preoperative intervention The emotional preparation of the patient may be more important than the physical preparation. When a biopsy is positive, the patient and the physician together decide on the best course of action. The possibility of reconstructive

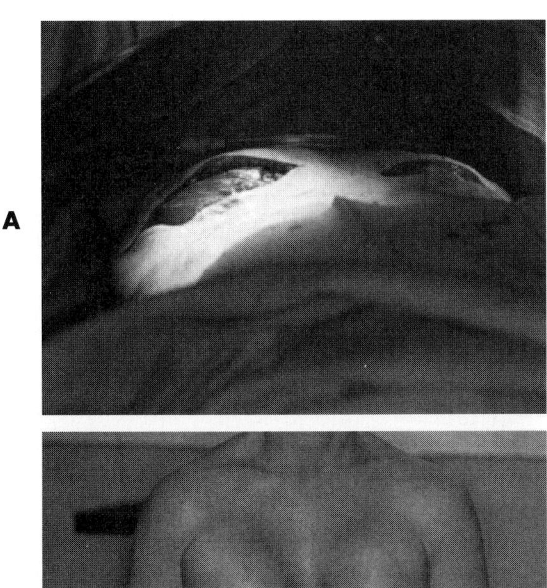

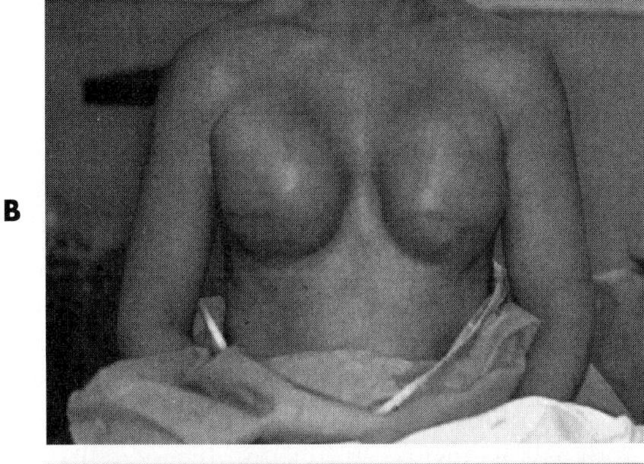

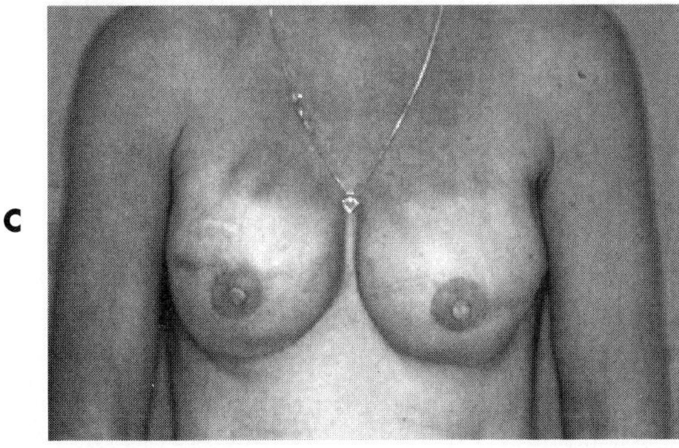

Figure 25-16 Breast reconstruction. Immediate reconstruction via tissue expansion, eventual insertion of saline-filled breast implants, and nipple and areola reconstructions. **A,** Removal of bilateral breasts. **B,** Hyperexpansion phase using temporary, saline-filled implants; **C,** Final results after insertion of permanent implants and nipple and areola reconstruction. (Courtesy Michael A Epstein, MD, Elk Grove Village, Illinois)

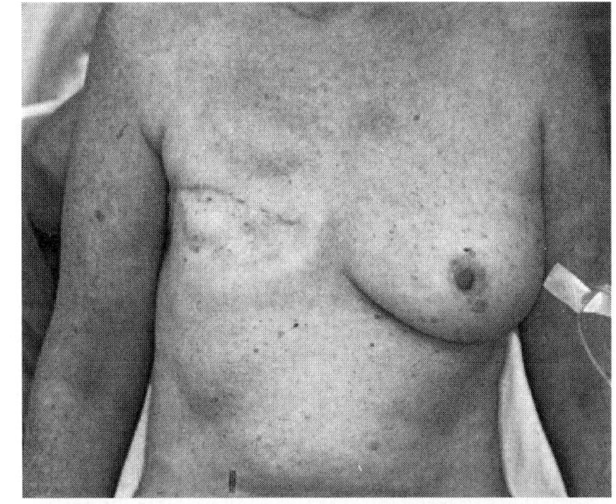

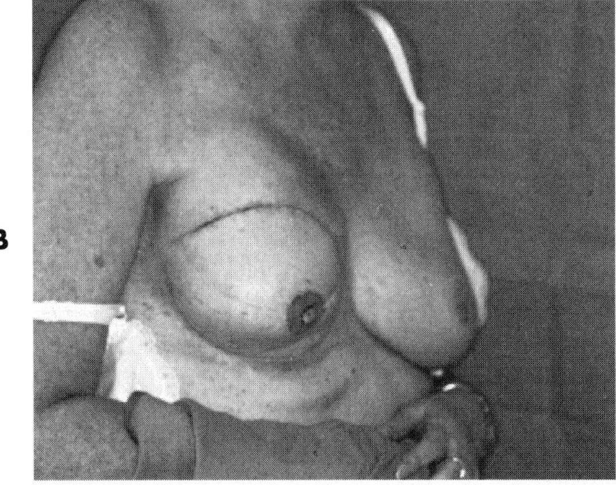

Figure 25-17 Reconstruction 2 years postmastectomy using TRAM procedure. **A,** Two years postmastectomy. **B,** After reconstruction with autogenous implant (TRAM) and nipple and areola reconstruction. (Courtesy Michael A Epstein, MD, Elk Grove Village, Illinois)

surgery can be discussed at this time (Table 25-8). Although this improves the patient's ability to accept the diagnosis and loss, it remains an enormous psychologic trauma. The patient's partner may be unable to provide the understanding that she needs and should be given the opportunity to express feelings and concerns. It is important to discuss the patient's fears openly, and this is best done by a nurse who has established a therapeutic relationship with the patient and family. The relationship must begin on the day of admission. The nurse should demonstrate an awareness of the patient's concerns and help her to express them. Identifying and labeling fears makes them more manageable. The nurse should respond to all questions in a way that keeps the patient talking. The "Reach to Recovery" program, sponsored by local chapters of the American Cancer Society, sends volunteers who have had breast surgery and reconstructive surgery to speak to patients at their request. Providing an opportunity to discuss the effects of a mastectomy with someone who has had one often gives needed reassurance to the patient facing or recuperating from such surgery. Unfortunately these services are not available in all communities.

The physical preparation of the patient requires that a wide area of skin be shaved, including the axilla. If the patient's condition permits, a pint of blood is taken preoperatively for administration at the time of surgery, if needed, to avoid a chance of reaction to donated blood. Other preparation is the same as that for other types of major surgery.

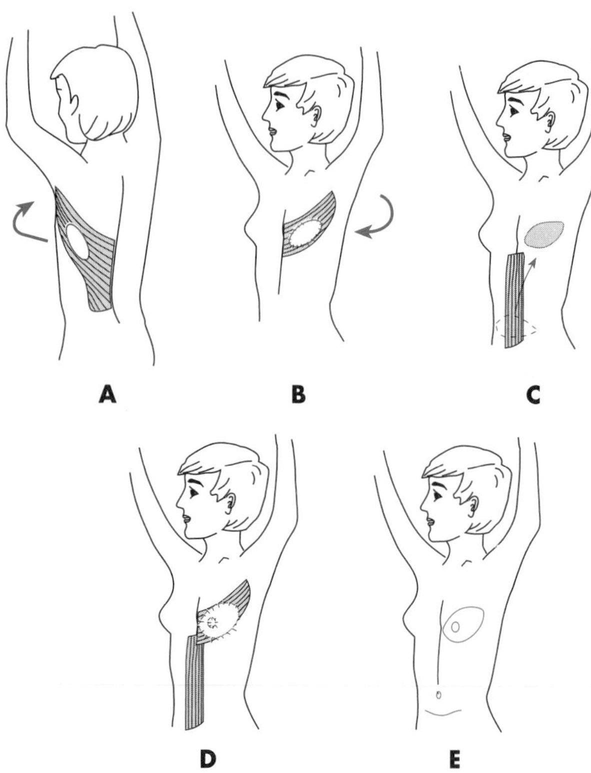

Figure 25-18 Flap surgery, breast reconstruction.

Postoperative intervention. Postoperative nursing care should include checking vital signs and observing for symptoms of shock or hemorrhage, because many large blood vessels are involved in the procedure. Jackson-Pratt (JP) drains, attached to low suction, may be placed in the axilla to facilitate drainage. Dressings are usually applied rather tightly and may cause some pain and discomfort. When the vital signs are stable, the patient is placed in a 45-degree Fowler's position to promote drainage. The position should be changed often, and deep-breathing exercises should be encouraged. The patient may have some pain and should be given pain-relieving medication. The arm is elevated on a pillow with the hand and wrist higher than the elbow and the elbow higher than the shoulder joint. This facilitates the flow of fluids by the lymph and venous routes and prevents lymphedema. The arm should be observed for signs of circulatory disturbance such as coldness, lack of radial pulse, cyanosis, or blanching. The arm should also be observed for edema, numbness, or inability to move the fingers, which should be reported immediately. Fluids are permitted as soon as nausea ceases, and diet is usually ordered as tolerated. The patient may need help in cutting meat and in arranging food conveniently because use of the arm on the affected side may be difficult. When drawing blood, administering intravenous fluids, or taking blood pressure, the nurse should use the unaffected arm. The patient is discharged 2 to 3 days postoperatively (Box 25-11).

NURSE ALERT

Swelling and discomfort in the arm may result after mastectomy. The nurse should check for coolness, cyanosis, and lack of a radial pulse. The arm can be elevated with pillows to aid drainage.

Rehabilitation. One of the primary aims of rehabilitation is to restore the use of the affected arm as soon as possible to prevent contracture. The physician determines the time at which exercises may be started. Some exercises that help the patient regain use of the arm are shown in Figure 25-19. A small handbook entitled "Help Yourself to Recovery" is available from the American Cancer Society for use by the nurse in teaching patients. If a "Reach to Recovery" visitor is requested, she brings a kit containing this manual along with a small pillow to aid in positioning, a length of rope and ball to use in exercising, and a temporary prosthesis made of washable cotton. The kit also contains information about permanent prostheses. The visitor demonstrates and helps the patient with the exercises if indicated by the physician. Conversation centers on clothing, prostheses, and returning to day-to-day routines. When the patient is discharged, the home health nurse may visit the patient to encourage and reassure her and to supervise exercises.

Another important area for patient teaching is monthly self-examination of the chest wall and remaining breast if she has had a mastectomy, or both breasts if she has had breast conservation surgery. Evaluation of the patient's ability to perform breast self-examination and her understanding of its importance is essential. A discussion of nursing diagnoses and intervention for the patient following breast cancer surgery appears earlier in this chapter.

Choosing a prosthesis. The patient should not be fitted for a prosthesis for at least 6 weeks after surgery to allow for adequate healing. A list of recommended fitters in the patient's geographic area assists the patient in her selection. Information about types of prostheses available is also helpful. The "Reach to Recovery" visitor usually has this information. The public health nurse may be of help to the patient in following up suggestions concerning a prosthesis.

Breast prostheses are available in a variety of types, sizes, weights, and prices. They may be filled with rubber, air, fluid, or a gelatinlike substance. The ideal

TABLE 25-8

Breast Cancer Treatment Options, Side Effects, Complications, and Patient Issues

Procedure	Description Procedure	Hospitalization	Side Effects	Potential Complications Short-term	Potential Complications Long-term	Patient Issues
Modified radical mastectomy	Removal of breast; preservation of pectoralis muscle; axillary dissection	Hospital stay 1-4 days	Chest wall tightness; phantom breast sensations; arm swelling; sensory changes	Skin flap necrosis; seroma; hematoma; infection	Muscle atrophy; muscle weakness; lymphedema	Loss of breast; incision; body image; need for prothesis; impaired arm mobility
Breast conservation surgery with radiation therapy	Wide excision of tumor; axillary dissection; radiation therapy	Hospital stay 1-3 days; radiation 6-7 weeks	Breast soreness; breast edema; skin reactions; arm swelling; sensory changes (surgery-arm); sensory changes (breast-XRT); fatigue	Moist desquamation; hematoma; seroma; infection	Fibrosis; rib fractures; lymphedema; myositis; pneumonitis	Prolonged treatment; impaired arm mobility; change in texture and sensitivity of breast
Immediate reconstruction-implant	Implantation of prosthesis under musculofascial layer of chest wall	Hospital stay 1-4 days	Discomfort (greater than mastectomy alone due to elevation and stretching of muscles)	Skin flap necrosis; wound separation; seroma, hematoma; infection; delayed wound healing; cellulitis	Capsular contractions; loss of implant; questionable risks of silicone implants	Body image; prolonged physician visits (expander implants); opposite breast (desire for additional procedures); prolonged postoperative recovery
Immediate reconstruction-flap procedures	A musculocutaneous flap (muscle, skin, blood supply) transposed to chest wall area	Hospital stay 5-7 days	Pain related to two surgical sites and extensiveness of the surgery			

From Knobf MT: Treatment options for early stage breast cancer, *Med Surg Nurs* 3(4):249, 1994.

BOX 25-11

Nursing Process

MASTECTOMY

ASSESSMENT

Vital signs (often)
Dressings and drain (often)
Lymphedema of the affected arm
Intake and output
Elimination patterns
Lung and bowel sounds
Level of comfort
Self-esteem/self-concept

NURSING DIAGNOSES

Anxiety related to uncertainty of prognosis or decisions about treatment
Pain related to incision in skin and muscles of chest wall
Ineffective breathing pattern related to incision in chest wall
Risk for injury to lymphatic system related to obstruction of lymph drainage
Risk for infection related to interrupted skin integrity and presence of drainage
Ineffective individual or family coping related to loss of breast and perceived loss of attractiveness
Disturbance in self-concept (body image and/or self-esteem) related to loss of breast
Knowledge deficit related to prosthesis or reconstruction, activity restrictions, rehabilitation exercises, and support groups

NURSING INTERVENTIONS

Maintain in bed in semi-Fowler's position to promote drainage.
Elevate affected arm with pillows above level of heart.
Use *unaffected* arm only for blood pressures, venipunctures, and injections.
Encourage early movement of affected arm, and exercise as soon as medically permitted.
Check dressings for signs of hemorrhage; reinforce as necessary.
Maintain patency and suction of drain, if present.
Maintain intravenous fluids as ordered; do not infuse in arm on affected side.
Encourage deep breathing, coughing, and turning every 2 hours.
Encourage active range of motion exercises of the legs.
Encourage expression of grief related to loss of breast and possible change in self-image.
Discuss sexuality if indicated.
Discuss the "Reach to Recovery" program and encourage participation.
Encourage early use of temporary breast forms and well-fitting brassiere as soon as permitted by physician.
Provide information on available community resources (Visiting Nurse Association, American Cancer Society, prosthetic suppliers).

EVALUATION OF EXPECTED OUTCOMES

Meets discharge criteria for the postsurgical patient (p. 487)
No edema in arm of affected side
Demonstrates exercises as ordered by physician
Verbalizes fears, concerns, and feelings related to loss of breast and change in body image
Donor site of graft (if present) is dry and healing, with granulation tissue present
States plans for use of appropriate temporary prosthesis and identifies need to postpone fitting of permanent prosthesis until physician permits
Demonstrates procedure for breast self-examination and verbalizes understanding of need to perform it monthly on remaining breast or breast tissue
Maintains self-esteem, evidenced by attention to personal hygiene and appearance
Discusses fears and concerns with significant other

weight of the prosthesis to provide proper balance and the type of brassiere to offer comfortable support must be considered. A properly fitting prosthesis is essential to allow for normal posture and to provide a natural appearance under clothing. A natural appearance is important because it can help the patient regain a positive self-image.

Inoperable conditions. When patients have delayed medical care and surgery so that the cancer has become invasive and therefore inoperable, radiation, chemotherapy, or both may be used to retard the damaging effects of the malignant growth. The goal is to improve the quality of the patient's life while increasing the duration of survival with the least number of untoward effects for the patient. The patient cannot be cured, but if she responds to treatment, she can live a longer and less painful life than if not treated. Radiation, chemotherapy, and hormonal therapy can be used. Treatment decisions need to be considered individually and center on the woman's age, health status,

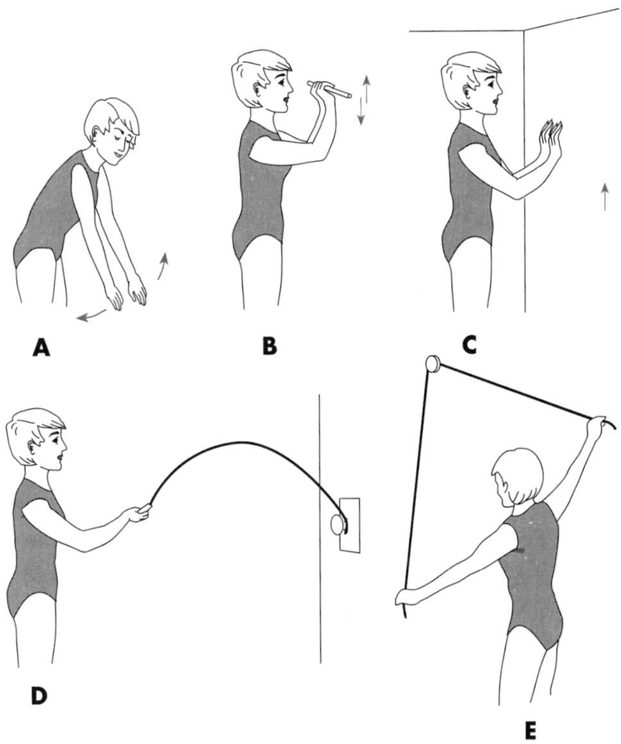

Figure 25-19 Arm exercises after mastectomy. **A,** Pendulum swinging with arms relaxed and swinging free. **B,** Arm raising over head. **C,** Wall climbing by standing with face to wall and climbing wall with hands, with fingers reaching as far as possible. **D,** Rope swinging with length of rope tied to doorknob and swinging with shoulder motion. **E,** Rope sliding by placing length of rope over pulley and sliding rope up and down.

tumor staging and type, axillary node status, and hormone receptor status of the tumor. A woman needs assistance from her healthcare team in choosing treatment options (see Table 25-8).

CONDITIONS OF PREGNANCY

Abortion

The term **abortion** means the termination of pregnancy at any time before the fetus has attained the stage of viability, which is approximately 20 to 24 weeks. There are two main types of abortion: *spontaneous* and *induced* (Box 25-12). The layperson uses the word "miscarriage" to denote a spontaneous abortion. It is estimated that 15% of all pregnancies end in spontaneous abortion. At least half of these are the result of a defective fetoplacental unit, genetic defects, or implantation abnormalities.

The exact causes of spontaneous abortions are unknown, but evidence indicates that some abortions are the result of defective germ plasm. Falls are not believed to be a significant cause.

BOX 25-12

CLASSIFICATION OF ABORTION

- Spontaneous abortion
  - Habitual
  - Threatened
  - Inevitable
  - Incomplete
  - Complete
  - Missed or retained
  - Septic
- Induced abortion
  - Therapeutic
  - Legal
  - Criminal or illegal

It is customary to use the weight of the fetus as a criterion for defining abortion. Many authorities maintain that the fetus must weigh less than 500 g and have a crown-rump length of less than 16.5 cm. In many states a birth certificate is prepared for any pregnancy terminating after the twentieth week of gestation, or when the fetus weighs 500 g or more.

Types of abortions

Habitual abortion. A woman is said to undergo habitual abortion when three or more successive pregnancies are spontaneously interrupted. The situation commonly creates a severe emotional problem when a woman wants to have children.

Threatened abortion. Threatened abortion is indicated when vaginal bleeding or spotting occurs during the first 20 weeks of gestation. The cervix is not dilated, and with conservative treatment the pregnancy may continue uninterrupted. Treatment of threatened abortion includes limiting activity, and bedrest may be prescribed for 24 to 48 hours. If the bleeding stops, it usually does so within 48 hours. The woman should be encouraged to avoid stress and fatigue and may be instructed to avoid intercourse until the pregnancy seems stable.

Inevitable abortion. In inevitable abortion, the vaginal bleeding may be only spotting, or hemorrhage may occur with passing of clots. The cervix is dilated, and mild pelvic cramping gradually increases until all or part of the uterine contents are expelled. There is no chance of saving the pregnancy.

Incomplete abortion. In incomplete abortion, only a portion of the products of conception has been expelled; bleeding continues and may cause severe hemorrhage. The part retained is usually fragments of the placenta. It is necessary to hospitalize the patient and prescribe a regimen of bedrest. Sedative drugs are administered, and blood transfusions are given if the hemorrhage has been severe. Oxytocin may be administered to stimulate contractions of the uterus. If the residue is not expelled and bleeding continues, the patient is prepared for surgery, taken to the operating room, and given a light anesthetic. Then a D & C is performed.

Complete abortion. In complete abortion, all products of conception are expelled. Many complete abortions occur without any major difficulty, but a physician should be seen to determine whether any of the products of conception remain and to administer Rho(D) immune globulin, if necessary.

Missed abortion. In a missed abortion, the fetus dies and is retained for 8 weeks or more before the 20th week of gestation. Weekly examinations of the fibrinogen level in the blood are done. No attempt is made to empty the uterus unless the level of fibrinogen begins to fall. Oxytocin may be administered to stimulate contractions and cause the fetus to be expelled.

Septic abortion. Evidence of septic abortion includes an elevation of temperature to 104° F (40° C) or more, with threatened or incomplete loss of the products of conception. The presence or absence of any other focus of infection is ruled out before establishing a diagnosis of septic abortion. The sepsis may be caused by any of several pathogenic organisms. If caused by *Clostridium perfringens,* a spore-forming organism, a powerful exotoxin is liberated. The patient is critically ill with an elevated temperature; the pulse is rapid; and headache, malaise, abdominal tenderness, and indications of pelvic peritonitis occur. The patient is isolated, and medical aseptic technique is carried out. Cultures from the cervix and the uterus are taken, and the appropriate antibiotics are administered. Intravenous fluids and blood transfusions may be given, and hydrocortisone and oxytocin (Pitocin) may be ordered. Septic abortion often results in serious complications, including acute renal failure, congestive heart failure, hemorrhage, and severe shock. The patient's condition is considered in the physician's decision to do a D & C. However, opinions differ concerning the time when a D & C should be done. In some cases a hysterectomy may be performed.

NURSE ALERT

Fever, severe abdominal pain, and bleeding heavier than a normal menses after an abortion may indicate a complication.

Therapeutic abortion. Therapeutic abortion is the termination of pregnancy by a physician during the first trimester of pregnancy. Therapeutic abortion is usually indicated when the life or health of the mother must be protected. It is considered when there is hazard to the fetus, such as rubella in the mother. Reputable physicians secure medical consultation or approval by an established committee before performing a therapeutic abortion.

Legal abortion. Legal abortion, the termination of a pregnancy at the request of the woman, is now available in all states as the result of a Supreme Court ruling. On January 22, 1973, the U.S. Supreme Court ruled that all antiabortion laws were unconstitutional in the United States. In general the court made the following ruling concerning abortion:

1. During the first 12 weeks, the state could not bar a woman from obtaining an abortion by a licensed physician.
2. Between 12 and 24 weeks the state could regulate the performance of an abortion in ways reasonable to the woman's health.
3. During the third trimester the state could regulate and prohibit abortion except those deemed necessary to protect the woman's health or life (Hatcher and others, 1994).

In 1976 the U.S. Congress passed the Hyde amendment, which forbids the use of federal funds for abortions except for situations in which the woman's life is threatened. As a result women with personal funds or private insurance are able to have abortions, whereas poor women who use federal funds for healthcare are denied the same opportunity. Legal abortion has nonetheless become the most commonly performed surgical procedure in the United States, with 1.4 million abortions performed annually (Hatcher and others, 1994). On June 29, 1992, the Supreme Court ruled that states might impose restrictions such as waiting periods, parental notification, hospitalization requirements, and specific informed-consent requirements. Thus the provision of abortion may vary considerably from state to state.

Intervention

Interventions are planned according to the type of abortion, prognosis, and nursing diagnosis. All pregnant women should be taught to report any signs of vaginal bleeding or spotting to their healthcare provider. Women experiencing bleeding or spotting must be observed for hemorrhage. An exact pad count must be kept, and the pads may be weighed to determine the amount of blood loss. All clots and tissue must be saved for inspection and possible laboratory testing. The nurse must be aware of hospital policy concerning the disposal of the products of conception. The nurse should also understand and encourage the woman's religious beliefs and practices that might be appropriate at this time.

In preparing the woman for a D & C, the nurse uses the same procedures as those for the nonpregnant woman. Administration of medication, intravenous fluids, or blood transfusions is carried out according to physician's orders. An informed consent must be obtained.

Postoperatively vital signs should be monitored routinely. The woman must be observed for vaginal bleeding and any signs of infection. She should be taught good hygiene practices and good nutrition. Because there has been blood loss, she should be instructed to eat foods high in iron, folic acid, vitamin C, and protein. The nurse should listen to her speak about the meaning of the loss of the pregnancy. The nurse should recognize that abortion may precipitate grief and that the grieving process takes time before it is resolved. The woman may need advice about birth control before discharge. A method of birth control may need to be prescribed by the physician, so the patient should be encouraged to consult with her physician before discharge.

Abortion counseling

Most women approach the decision to terminate a pregnancy with some ambivalence, fear, and doubt. They worry about making the right decision for themselves, their families, and the unborn child. Sometimes the pregnancy is desired, but the woman may choose to abort after learning of fetal abnormalities in the second trimester. Under these circumstances the decision to abort may be particularly difficult and accompanied by regret and grief. More often the pregnancy is unplanned and not desired. On learning that she is pregnant, a woman may experience feelings of shock, disbelief, and anger. Before she can make a decision, she must cope with feelings generated by the confirmation of her pregnancy. The nurse must allow her time to process her feelings. All options for continuing the pregnancy as well as support systems for the pregnancy should be addressed. If she is considering abortion, she will need information about the procedure, its safety, and its cost in order to make her decision. She may feel overwhelmed by such a decision and may need help assessing both her feelings about the pregnancy and her life plans. The nurse should try to remain empathetic and objective. Active listening on the part of the nurse, such as paraphrasing and clarifying what the patient tries to communicate, may help the woman to identify concerns and conflicts. A woman's decision may be complicated by an abusive partner, lack of financial resources, fear of parental involvement, and unfamiliarity with making important life decisions. Whether she maintains or terminates the pregnancy, the decision is ultimately hers to make.

Whatever the feelings of the individual nurse, the patient who enters the hospital seeking an abortion should never face hostility or discrimination. The decision to seek an abortion may be a difficult one, and these patients have problems and worries similar to those of any other hospitalized patient. Nurses who believe that they cannot morally assist with an abortion should not work in a setting in which they are performed.

Types of legal abortions

First trimester legal abortion. Five out of every six abortions are performed before the 13th week of pregnancy (Hatcher and others, 1994). The most common method used in the first trimester is vacuum aspiration. The procedure is relatively simple and safe. Local anesthesia in the form of a paracervical block is typically used. Although general anesthesia may be used, doing so adds to the risk of the procedure and to the cost. To perform suction **curettage,** the physician completes a bimanual examination to determine gestational size and uterine position. An injection of a local anesthetic such as lidocaine may be used before the cervix is dilated. Alternatively laminaria (dried seaweed) may be used to gently dilate the cervix up to 1 day before the procedure. After the cervix is dilated, the vacuum cannula is introduced into the uterus and negative pressure is applied, which evacuates the contents of the uterus. Curettage is performed to complete evacuation of the uterus. The products of conception are examined briefly, weighed to confirm complete evacuation, and then sent for closer scrutiny to a pathologist. The vacuum aspiration procedure may be done on an outpatient basis up to the 14th week of gestation. The nurse may be responsible for sterilization of equipment and assisting the physician during the procedure. The nurse may also play a central role in preparing the patient and offering emotional support during the surgery. The patient remains in recovery under the observation of a nurse for 1 to 3 hours after the procedure. The nurse checks vital signs and provides emotional support. The patient should be instructed to check and report the amount of vaginal bleeding to the nurse before leaving the recovery area. At discharge, the patient should be instructed to immediately report bleeding heavier than normal menses, severe or increasing abdominal pain, or fever greater than 100° F (37.8° C) (Table 25-9). If future contraception needs have not been addressed previously, they should be discussed at this point. Birth control pills or DMPA may be started on the day of the procedure. Rho(D) immune globulin should be given to women with Rh negative blood to avoid the risk of

TABLE 25-9

Patient Teaching—What to Expect After an Abortion

	Expected Effect	Warning Signs
Vaginal bleeding	Bleeding lasting up to 2 weeks Spotting up to 4 weeks No bleeding	Bleeding heavier than menses Bleeding more than 2 weeks Foul odor
Cramps	Menstruallike Mild to moderate, relieved by mild analgesia	Severe, persistent, uncramplike abdominal pain
Temperature (oral)	Less than 100° F	100° F or higher
Menses	Resume within 4 weeks or after first package of oral contraceptives completed	No menses within 8 weeks Continued symptoms of pregnancy
Other	Fatigue	Appearance of rash or hives if antibiotics were given

From Lichtman R, Papera S: *Gynecology well-woman care,* Norwalk, Conn, 1990, Appleton & Lange.

sensitization and problems in future pregnancies. Some physicians prescribe a short course of antibiotics or oxytocic drugs, such as Methergine, to contract the uterus. The woman should be instructed not to put anything into her vagina for 2 weeks after the abortion. That is, she should not douche, use tampons, or engage in sexual intercourse. Bleeding and cramping may vary, but discomfort is usually relieved with mild analgesics. She should return for a checkup 2 weeks after the procedure. She can expect her next period 4 to 6 weeks after the procedure. She should contact her healthcare provider if she does not get her period as expected, because this could indicate a continued pregnancy or adhesions of the uterus (Asherman's syndrome).

Medical abortion. Mifepristone (RU-486) is a synthetic steroid that can be used together with prostaglandins in the first trimester to induce abortion without the need for surgery. Combining RU-486 with an oral prostagalndin such as Cytotec has been shown to have a 98.7% success rate as an abortifacient in the first trimester of pregnancy (Dipierri, 1994). RU-486 has only recently been available in the United States. If it is approved for use in the United States after clinical trials, the privacy of an abortion decision will be increased because the administration of RU-486 is a medical treatment rather than a surgical procedure. Women would no longer need the services of abortion clinics to terminate early pregnancies.

Second trimester abortion. Second trimester abortions account for less than 10% of all abortions performed in the United States (Hatcher and others, 1994). The most common surgical procedure used is dilation and evacuation, which may be used up to 20 weeks but is typically performed between 13 to 16 weeks gestation. An ultrasound is usually obtained to confirm gestational age. Because the products of conception are greater in amount in the second trimester, the cervix requires greater dilation and osmotic agents such as lamineria are often used to achieve this. The uterine contents are evacuated by vacuum cannula as with first trimester abortion. Less frequently, agents such as hypertonic saline, hypertonic urea, and prostaglandin E2 are used to induce abortion late in the second trimester. In these instances the usual procedure involves removing amniotic fluid by amniocentesis and instilling one of the above agents in its place. A local anesthetic is used, and most clinicians use lamineria to dilate the cervix. Oxytocin accelerates the uterine contractions and hastens expulsion of the fetus.

Ectopic Pregnancy

Ectopic pregnancy is gestation anywhere outside the uterus. An ectopic pregnancy rarely occurs in the abdomen or the ovary. The most common site for an ectopic pregnancy is in the fallopian tube. When the ovum becomes implanted in the fallopian tube, it is referred to as *tubal pregnancy.* Infrequently a tubal pregnancy may be palpated during bimanual examination in the area near the uterus, but the first indication of tubal pregnancy often occurs when the tube ruptures. The incidence of ectopic pregnancies increased threefold between 1970 and 1983 to a rate of 14 per 1000 pregnancies (Catlin and Wetzel, 1991). Tubal pregnancy results from some condition within the tube that slows or prevents passage of the ovum through the tube to the endometrium of the uterus. Conditions such as inflammation from disease, narrowing of the tube, and an elongated or immature tube create a situation conducive to tubal pregnancy. Thus

BOX 25-13 **Nursing Process**

ABORTION OR ECTOPIC PREGNANCY

ASSESSMENT

Vital signs (often)
Vaginal bleeding (often)
Intake and output
Lung and bowel sounds
Level of comfort
Coping mechanisms

NURSING DIAGNOSES

Fluid volume deficit related to blood loss
Risk for infection related to retained products of conception
Pain related to uterine cramping
Spiritual distress related to loss and grief
Ineffective individual coping related to death of fetus

NURSING INTERVENTIONS

Save all peripads, blood-soaked linens, clots, and tissue.
Monitor intravenous infusions.
Observe for bladder distention; catheterize as ordered.
Encourage verbalization of concerns and feelings related to loss.
Provide spiritual support and refer for religious practices if requested.

EVALUATION OF EXPECTED OUTCOMES

Meets discharge criteria for the postsurgical patient (p. 487)
Vaginal drainage reduced and free of unusual odor
Voids without difficulty
Verbalizes concerns and feelings

a medical history of PID, tubal ligation, or previous ectopic pregnancy increases a woman's risk for this problem.

As the embryo increases in size, the tube stretches until it can no longer remain intact. The tube may rupture, releasing the entire products of conception into the abdominal cavity *(ectopic abortion)*. The rupture may be small, with the embryo remaining within the tube, but severe bleeding may occur as a result of damage to the blood vessels. The length of time the tube remains intact with the developing varies but averages 7 to 8 weeks from the last menstrual period (Catlin and Wetzel, 1991).

Assessment

With an ectopic pregnancy, often the patient has missed one period and has noted slight spotting, but she may not know that she is pregnant. In the majority of patients rupture results in sudden acute abdominal pain. The pain may extend to the shoulder and the rectal area. The patient becomes faint and pale, and she may be in shock. Hemorrhage may be severe, and acute secondary anemia results. In other cases the clinician may consider the diagnosis based on nonspecific symptoms such as bleeding and a uterine size that does not correlate with the last menstrual period. In a nonemergency situation, a patient may be evaluated by serial HCG levels and pelvic ultrasound. Ultrasound should be able to detect an interuterine gestational sac by 5 to 6 weeks gestation.

Intervention

A ruptured tubal pregnancy is always an emergency and requires immediate surgery. There may be little time for preoperative preparation. The patient is treated immediately for shock by blood transfusions or intravenous infusion of lactated Ringer's solution. When an ectopic pregnancy is not yet ruptured, there are more choices available for treatment. These include laparoscopic surgery and treatment with methotrexate or etoposide, which induces dissolution of the fetal tissue coupled with close observation when the pregnancy is small and HCG low and declining (Hatcher and others, 1994). In cases of this last sort, spontaneous abortion and reabsorption of tissue may occur without surgical intervention.

NURSE ALERT

Abdominal pain, nausea, and referred pain to the shoulder in early pregnancy may indicate an ectopic pregnancy.

Postoperative care of the patient is the same as that for other abdominal surgery. Transfusions with whole blood may be necessary to combat anemia. Uterine bleeding occurs for several days, and the patient must be observed for any unusual bleeding from the abdominal incision or from the vagina (Box 25-13).

KEY CONCEPTS

- Teaching a patient about menstruation must begin with an assessment of her knowledge and feelings about menstruation, then proceed to clarify misconceptions and provide additional knowledge appropriate for her age and developmental level, using positive terms.
- Contraceptive methods vary in effectiveness, and the patient must be guided and assisted in reviewing choices and selecting the most appropriate method.
- Infertility can be a life crisis and emotionally devastating for a couple. Causes are multiple, and systematic evaluation is required.
- Supplementary estrogen therapy in menopausal women is most effective in relieving hot flashes and night sweats and is generally accepted as important in preventing osteoporosis and heart disease. Treatment must be individualized.
- If a patient's condition or treatment raises concerns about limitations of sexual ability, the nurse should provide an opportunity for discussion. This is best done after the nurse-patient relationship is established. It also requires privacy and an attitude of nonjudgmental concern and caring.
- Vesicovaginal and rectovaginal fistulas require increased vitamin C and protein intake and careful hygiene to promote healing and comfort. Sitz baths, deodorizing douches, perineal pads, and "baby wipes" should be used to cleanse the perineum after elimination.
- Colporrhaphy is the surgical procedure used to repair cystocele (bulging of the bladder against the vaginal wall) and rectocele (bulging of the rectum against the vaginal wall). The primary goal of postoperative care is prevention of strain on the suture lines.
- Endometriosis is an inflammatory condition of endometrial cells located outside the uterus. The inflammation causes pain during menstruation, fatigue, pressure in the pelvic organs, and general discomfort.
- Vague lower abdominal discomfort and mild digestive complaints are early symptoms of ovarian cancer in some women.
- Pelvic inflammatory disease (PID) may demonstrate symptoms so mild that they are ignored and untreated. Chronic PID then results. PID can result in infertility and predispose a woman to ectopic pregnancy.
- Postoperative care of the patient with a hysterectomy is concerned with prevention of urinary retention, intestinal distention, and venous thrombosis. The surgery should not usually affect capacity for sexual stimulation.
- The American Cancer Society recommends that women 40 to 49 years of age should have a mammogram every 1 or 2 years, and those 50 and over and those with a family history in first degree relatives should be scheduled annually.
- With 10% to 14% of breast cancers found during physical examinations and missed by mammography, breast self-examinations should be taught and encouraged.
- The patient must understand treatment choices available for breast cancer: breast conservation surgery (lumpectomy), modified mastectomy, and reconstructive surgery.
- The emotional preparation of the patient for breast surgery is as important as the physical preparation. The patient's selection of course of action must be facilitated, and the patient must be able to openly express fears, feelings, and concerns.
- Legal abortion has become the most commonly performed surgical procedure in the United States, with 1.4 million performed annually. Federal funds may not be used for abortion except for situations in which the woman's life is threatened.
- Women considering a termination of pregnancy should have counseling to cope with and process feelings and to explore options; support systems for continuing the pregnancy; and information about abortion procedures, safety, and cost. Active listening is essential.
- Abdominal pain, nausea, and referred pain to the shoulder in early pregnancy may indicate an ectopic pregnancy.

CRITICAL THINKING EXERCISES

1. Consider your approaches in taking sexual histories from an adolescent and a postmenopausal woman.
2. Contrast oral contraceptive pills and Norplant with regard to risks and benefits.
3. What are the risks and benefits of hormonal replacement therapy for postmenopausal women?
4. Contrast the pros and cons of lumpectomy and modified radical mastectomy as treatments for breast cancer.
5. Explain a colposcopy to your 45-year-old patient.

REFERENCES AND ADDITIONAL READINGS

American Cancer Society: *Cancer facts and figures—1994,* Atlanta, 1994, American Cancer Society.

Baird SB, editor: *A cancer source book for nurses,* Atlanta, 1991, American Cancer Society Professional Education Publication.

Bates B: *A guide to physical examination and history taking,* Philadelphia, 1991, JB Lippincott.

Bostwick J: Breast reconstruction following mastectomy, *Ca Cancer J Clin* 45(5):289-304, 1995.

Brucks JA: Ovarian cancer, *Nurs Clin North Am* 27(4):835-845, 1992.

Catlin AJ, Wetzel WS: Ectopic pregnancy: clinical evaluation, diagnostic measures and prevention, *Nurs Pract* 16(1):38-46, 1991.

Clark-Coller T: Dysfunctional uterine bleeding and amenorrhea, *J Nurse-Midwifery* 36(1):49-62, 1991.

Colbry SL: A review of toxic shock syndrome: the need for education still exists, *Nurs Pract* 17(9):39-43, 1992.

Dest VM, Fisher SM: Breast cancer: dreaded diagnosis, complicated care, *RN,* 57(6):49-54, 1994.

Dipierri D: RU 486, mifepristone: a review of a controversial drug, *Nurs Pract* 19(6):59-61, 1994.

Edwards S: Women who have undergone a tubal sterilization have a reduced risk of contracting ovarian cancer, *Family Planning Perspectives* 26(2):90-91, 1994.

Ellorhorst-Ryan JM, Goeldner J: Breast cancer, *Nurs Clin North Am* 27(4):821-833, 1992.

Gorsky RD and others: Relative risks and benefits of long-term estrogen replacement therapy: a decision analysis, *Ob & Gyn* 83(2):161-165, 1994.

Hatcher RA and others: *Contraceptive technology,* ed 16, New York, 1994, Irvington.

Hinkle LT: Education and counseling for Norplant users, *JOGNN* 23(5):387-391, 1994.

Holm K, Penckofer S, Chandler P: Deciding on hormone replacement therapy, *Am J Nurs* 95(8):57-60, 1995.

Ivey CL, Gordon SI: Breast reconstruction: new image, new hope, *RN,* 57(7):49-53, 1994.

Jones KD, Lehr ST: Vulvodynia: diagnostic techniques and treatment modalities, *Nurse Pract* 19(4):34-46, 1994.

Johnson JR: Caring for the woman who's had a mastectomy, *Am J Nurs* 94(5):25-31, 1994.

Kahane DH: The management of the psychosocial impact of breast cancer, *Nurse Pract Forum* 4(2):105-109, 1993.

Kaunitz AM: Oral contraceptives and gynecologic cancer: an update for the 1990s, *Am J Obstet Gyncol* 167(4, pt2):1171-1176, 1992.

Knobf, MT: Treatment options for early stage breast cancer, *Med Surg Nurs* 3(4):249-259, August 1994.

Lappe JM: Bone fragility: assessment of risk and strategies for prevention, *JOGNN* 23(3):260-268, 1994.

Lichtman R, Papera S: *Gynecology well-woman care,* Norwalk, Conn. 1990, Appleton & Lange.

Maddox MA: Women at midlife: hormone replacement therapy, *Nurs Clin North Am* 27(4):959-969, 1992.

McCance KL, Huether SE: *Pathophysiology: the biologic basis for disease in adults and children,* St Louis, 1990, Mosby.

McMullin M: Holistic care of the patient with cervical cancer, *Nurs Clin North Am* 27(4):847-857, 1992.

Mettlin C, Smart CR: Breast cancer detection guidelines for women aged 40 to 49 years: rationale for the American Cancer Society reaffirmation of recommendations *CA: Cancer J for Clinicians* 44(4):248-255, 1994.

Phippen ML, Wells MP: *Perioperative nursing handbook,* Philadelphia, 1995, WB Saunders.

Sarazin SK, Seymour SF: Causes and treatment options for women with dyspareunia, *Nurse Pract* 16(10):30-41, 1991.

Stevens-Simon C: Clinical applications of adolescent female sexual development, *Nurse Pract* 18(12):18-29, 1993.

Tierney LM, McPhee SJ, Papadakis MA: *Current medical diagnosis and treatment,* Norwalk, Conn., 1994, Appleton & Lange.

Trad PV: Teenage pregnancy: seeking patterns that promote family harmony, *Am J Family Therapy* 22(1):42-55, 1994.

Trussell, J: Contraceptive efficacy of the diaphragm, the sponge and the cervical cap, *Family Planning Perspectives* 25(3):100-135, 1993.

Wood NJ: The use of vaginal pessaries for uterine prolapse, *Nurse Pract* 17(7):31-38, 1992.

Woodward JA: The triple C approach to the detection of cervical cancer, *Nurse Pract Forum* 1(1):31-39, 1990.

Wyeth-Ayerst Laboratories: *Norplant system levonorgestrel implants product monograph,* 1991.

CHAPTER 26

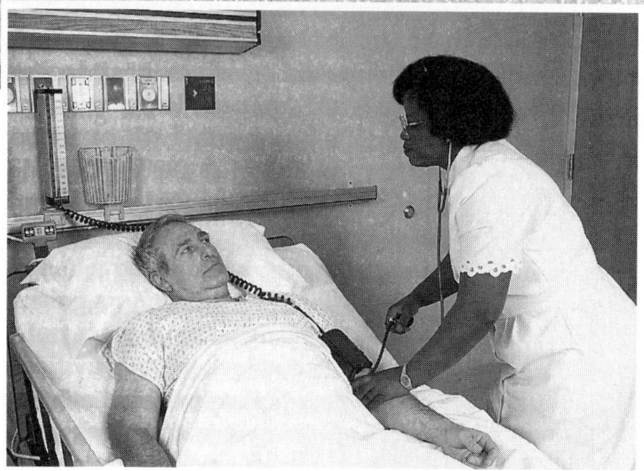

Men's Reproductive Health

CHAPTER OBJECTIVES

1 Discuss methods and techniques involved in the assessment of sexual function in the male patient.
2 Outline the assessment and treatment of conditions commonly affecting the male reproductive tract.
3 Describe the method of testicular self-examination (TSE) and discuss the importance of teaching TSE to male patients.
4 Describe the operative procedure and discuss the perioperative interventions for the following types of prostatectomy: transurethral, suprapubic, perineal, and retropubic.
5 Discuss the preoperative and postoperative interventions for the following methods of prostatectomy: transurethral, suprapubic, perineal, and retropubic.
6 Identify those procedures for prostatectomy that may result in incontinence, impotence, or sterility.
7 Discuss the methods for correcting erectile dysfunction.

KEY WORDS

androgens
benign prostatic hypertrophy
circumcision
Cowper's glands
dilation
epididymis
epididymitis
genitalia
glans penis
gonads
hydrocele
pelvic exenteration
phimosis
prostate gland
prostatitis
prepuce
puberty
scrotum
semen
seminal vesicles
spermatozoa
testes
testosterone
varicocele

STRUCTURE AND FUNCTION OF THE REPRODUCTIVE SYSTEM

The major function of the reproductive system is to create new life. The reproductive system includes the external **genitalia** and the internal organs associated with reproduction. Sexual and reproductive development are influenced by the endocrine system, and the nervous system is involved in human sexual response.

The male reproductive organs include the penis, **testes,** vas deferens, **seminal vesicles,** and the accessory glands. The penis and the **scrotum** are the external genital organs of the male. The internal structures or organs include the testes **(gonads)** and seminiferous tubules, **epididymis,** ductus deferens (vas deferens), seminal vesicles and ejaculatory ducts, urethra, **prostate gland,** and bulbourethral glands **(Cowper's glands).** The penis is composed mostly of erectile tissue that is divided into three sections: two *corpora cavernosa* and one *corpus spongiosum.* The penis is the primary organ of sexual pleasure in the male. It also contains the urethra (Figure 26-1). The urethra is a long channel that runs from the floor of the bladder through the corpus spongiosum to the external opening, called the *urinary meatus.* The meatus is normally found at the end of the penis in the center of the **glans penis,** which is a bulging structure covered by a loose, retractable skin called the **prepuce,** or foreskin. The upper section of the urethra passes through the center of the prostate gland. The prostate secretes an alkaline fluid that is transported by ejaculatory ducts that pass through it.

The testes are enclosed in and supported by the scrotum. Their location outside of the body allows them to maintain the sperm at a temperature lower than the rest of the body, which is essential for fertility. The testes produce sperm and **testosterone.** As sperm are produced, they collect in the epididymis, which is located along the upper side of the testes. The sperm are transported through the vas deferens to the ejaculatory ducts, where they are mixed with fluids from the seminal vesicles and the prostate gland.

Penile erection is controlled by the central, autonomic, and somatic nervous systems working together. The erection is caused by engorgement of the erectile tissue with blood. During coitus the seminal fluid and sperm are ejaculated into the upper urethra near the prostate and travel through the penis and into the vagina.

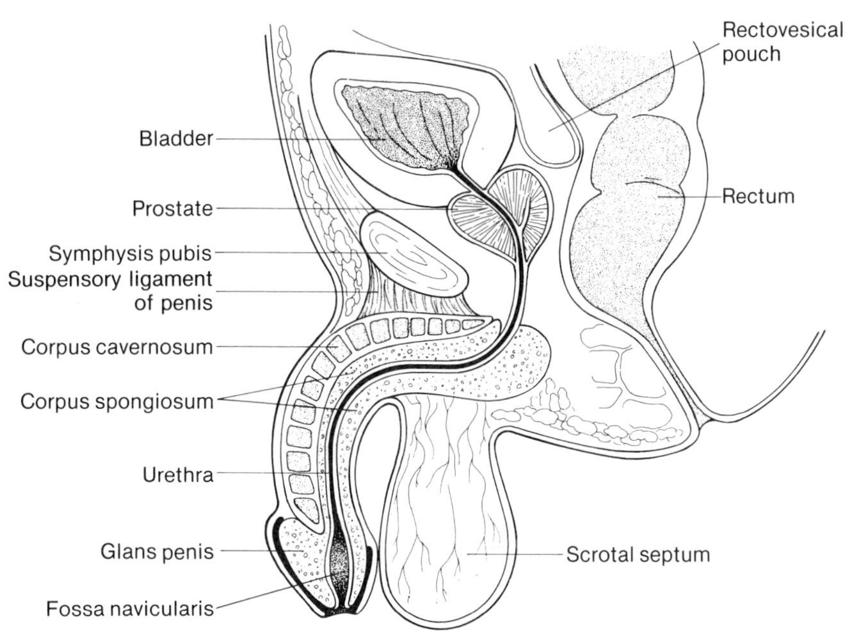

Figure 26-1 Male reproductive organs.

The breasts of the male do not contain the milk-producing glands or the subcutaneous and fatty tissue found in the female breast.

NURSING ASSESSMENT OF MEN WITH PROBLEMS OF THE REPRODUCTIVE SYSTEM

The history is a particularly important part of the assessment of the reproductive system. The nurse must be aware that the patient and his partner may be reluctant to discuss sexual habits with a nurse. This is particularly true of older couples and people who live in conservative parts of the country. If the patient's reading and writing levels are adequate, a form is often provided to the patient, and he writes out his own history. In other cases the nurse must be able to get the history verbally from the patient. In all cases, the nurse's questions must be tactful and clear so that a complete history can be obtained (Box 26-1). Male patients must be assessed for signs and symptoms of prostate enlargement. They include (1) difficulty in voiding, (2) reduced urine stream pressure, (3) difficulty in starting or stopping the urine stream, (4) a feeling of bladder fullness after voiding, or (5) dribbling of urine. The nurse should also determine whether there has been any change in the size of the testes and whether there is any pain during voiding.

When assessing sexual functioning, the nurse should know that chronic illnesses such as hypertension, arthritis, and diabetes, as well as medication therapy can decrease sexual desire and sexual ability. Many individuals who take antihypertensives such as propranolol (Inderal) and methyldopa (Aldomet) may find that they have a diminished libido. Men may have difficulty establishing an erection. The nurse should inform these individuals that their illness or medication may affect sexual desire and performance and that they should notify the physician if problems occur. Many times a solution to the problem can be found, such as changing or lowering the dose of the medication.

The nurse should ask about the presence of any unusual discharge from the penis and any itching or lesions on the genitalia. Changes in the breast also should be documented. The male breast may enlarge in response to hormonal changes during puberty or in certain disease states. Medications such as digoxin also may cause breast enlargement. This abnormal enlargement is referred to as *gynecomastia.* Pain during intercourse (dyspareunia) or sexual dysfunction also should be investigated.

Because reproductive health and sexual function or dysfunction are topics not easily approached without establishment of rapport, the nurse may use the patient's self-history to facilitate discussion and gathering of pertinent information. The self-history may be one that the patient has already filled out, or it may be a self-history form that the nurse helps the patient to fill out. In either case, the indication of sexual problems in a self-history allows the patient to take the initiative and gives the nurse the opportunity to verbalize and assess these areas. Patients differ greatly in the degree of openness with which they will discuss symptoms related to reproductive and sexual function. This methods gives the patient the opportunity to set the pace.

BOX 26-1

QUESTIONS ONE MIGHT USE IN A SEXUAL ASSESSMENT

You are starting to develop sexually. Has anyone talked to you about what that means?

What things in your past have affected the way you feel about your sexuality today? Religion? Parents? Friends?

Most of us have heard some sexual myths while growing up. Are there any that come to mind?

Are there things in your present health status, lifestyle, or living situation that affect or influence your sexuality?

How has your illness (or surgery) affected your sex life?

What are your expectations for sex now that you have had a prostatectomy?

PHASES OF REPRODUCTIVE FUNCTION THROUGHOUT THE LIFE CYCLE

Puberty

Puberty is the period during which the body prepares for reproductive ability. In males puberty begins about age 12, and secondary sex characteristics begin to make their appearance then. The size of the external reproductive organs increases, axillary and pubic hair grow, and the male voice deepens.

With the increase in size of the sexual organs in the male at puberty, continuous production of sperm begins in the testes in response to the *follicle-stimulating hormone (FSH)* secreted by the anterior pituitary. When the reproductive system begins to function, the male will experience nocturnal seminal emissions ("wet dreams"), usually around age 14. Nocturnal seminal emissions (NSE) are a physiologic benchmark of puberty in males, and they are characterized by a release, or ejaculation, of semen during sleep. The muscles of the body become larger and give the male a more mature appearance.

All children need preparation for puberty through sex education. From the moment of birth, infants begin to respond to and reflect the attitudes of others who care for them. Parents are usually the most influential caretakers during the developing years, so they have a great impact on their children's attitudes toward sexuality. Young children are curious and need direct, truthful answers to their questions. Although sex education in schools still arouses controversy, it is generally being accepted and incorporated into elementary and junior high school curricula. Often it is the school nurse or health teacher who is requested to teach basic sex education, usually to small groups of children.

Sexual Role Behavior

At each stage of physical and emotional growth, there are learned skills that are related to behavior patterns associated with the particular sexual role. Any condition or situation that interferes with the mastery of these skills may affect the development of sexual role behavior, but the process continues and evolves throughout the lifetime of an individual.

Sexual role or *gender role* is the public expression of behavior that implies masculinity or femininity. *Gender identity* is defined as the private or personal experience of one's maleness or femaleness. It is usually, but not always, congruent with the individual's *gender* or *biologic sex*. The development of gender identity and sexual role behavior is a complex process influenced by biologic, psychologic, and social factors.

Gender identity begins with the biologic event of conception, when the X or Y chromosome from the male parent combines with an X chromosome from the female parent. An XY pair of chromosomes influences the undifferentiated gonad of the embryo to become a male at a gestational age of approximately 6 weeks, whereas an XX pair of chromosomes differentiates the gonad as a female at approximately 12 weeks of gestation. If the fetus develops testes, two hormonal secretions of the testes initiate the masculinization of the external genitalia. The first hormone, müllerian-duct inhibiting factor, suppresses development of the uterus, fallopian tubes, and upper vagina. The second hormone, testosterone, promotes the growth of the wolffian ducts, from which develop the internal male reproductive structures and external genitalia. The appearance of the external genitalia is the next factor in the development of sexual role behavior. The parents tailor child-rearing practices in accordance with their perception of a daughter or son. The child eventually becomes aware of his or her body, including genitalia. The child's body and the responses of others to it influence juvenile gender identity.

At puberty the production of hormones affects sexual desire and further development of the genitals. These changes at puberty, combined with social influences, determine adult gender identity. Gender identity and sexual identity are sometimes the same, but sexual identity is also used to indicate sexual orientation (e.g., heterosexual, homosexual, bisexual).

Male Climacteric

Climacteric occurs in males but is usually less pronounced than in women, and many men will exhibit no symptoms. The male climacteric refers to the midlife changes that take place in the body both physiologically and psychologically. It is the normal pattern of reproductive aging or changes in men, which is quite different from that in women. It begins about age 45 and continues until the man is 80 to 90 years of age. Some men may associate their approaching retirement with a loss of sexual power. Although sperm production may diminish, it does not stop completely. Some men do experience flushing and chills and may exhibit psychologic symptoms.

EXAMINATION OF THE MALE PATIENT

Physical Examination

The reproductive system of the male patient is intricately related to the urinary system. Therefore patients with disease or dysfunction of the reproductive system are usually cared for by a physician who specializes in urology (urologist). Most men prefer to be examined by a male without a female present. Examination includes inspection and palpation of the external genitalia for abnormalities of structure, for signs of infection such as discharge and swelling, and for skin lesions. The penis is inspected for the presence and position of the urinary meatus. In the uncircumcised male the prepuce, or foreskin, must be retracted and the glans examined. If the foreskin does not retract easily, the patient may have **phimosis** (a tight prepuce that cannot be retracted).

The scrotum should be examined for size, symmetry, and the presence and size of both testes. The testes are also examined for masses, swelling, and movability. Examination often finds that the left testis is lower than the right, and this is normal. The scrotum contracts and becomes smaller when cold, so it is easier to examine the testes when the scrotum is relaxed. For this reason, men are advised to examine the testes monthly, while in a warm tub or shower. Routine self-examination is of great value in early detection of testicular cancer and is recommended as a monthly procedure for all men age 15 and over.

The prostate gland is examined through the rectum by a procedure known as the digital rectal examination (DGE). A gloved and lubricated finger is inserted into the rectum to palpate the prostate and determine its size, shape, and consistency.

Male breasts are examined for enlargement, lesions, discharge, and masses. The incidence of breast cancer in males is less than 1%, but men should be instructed to observe and report any discharge, masses, or changes in size, shape, and color of the breast.

If sterility is suspected, several examinations may be performed. Among the first are an examination of **semen** to determine the presence and characteristics of **spermatozoa** and a physical examination to locate obstructions along the tubal route. A voided urine specimen may be collected after massage of the prostate gland for examination for cancer cells or tubercle bacilli. A biopsy of the prostate gland or the testes may also be done.

Laboratory Tests

The laboratory tests include urinalysis, a complete blood count, and usually a serologic test for syphilis. Smears and cultures from the urethra are examined for both infectious and noninfectious organisms. Prostatic smears also may be obtained through massage of the prostate gland by a gloved finger placed in the rectum, after which a urine specimen is collected for laboratory examination.

Semen analysis is a relatively simple and inexpensive procedure for evaluating fertility in the male. It is also used to detect semen in a rape victim, to identify the blood type of an alleged rapist, or to prove sterility in a paternity suit. After a vasectomy, semen is analyzed to determine whether the surgical procedure was effective.

Semen may be collected after masturbation, after coitus, or by interrupting coitus. If the man prefers to collect the sample at home, the specimen must be protected from direct sunlight and extremes in temperature to avoid killing the sperm. When evaluating fertility, the physician may recommend refraining from intercourse from 2 to 5 days before collecting the specimen. The specimen must be brought in for examination within 3 hours after collection. The male is instructed either to masturbate and ejaculate into a clean container; to interrupt coitus just before ejaculating, withdraw the penis, and deposit the ejaculate in a container; or to collect during coitus by using a condom that has been washed with soapy water and dried to remove any spermicide. The entire specimen must be collected. The specimen is analyzed for volume of seminal fluid and for microscopically determined sperm count, sperm motility, and shape *(morphology)* of the sperm. When collecting semen from a female after rape or for evaluation of fertility, the physician uses a vaginal speculum and aspirates the specimen by using a small syringe without a cannula or needle.

CONDITIONS AFFECTING THE MALE GENITALIA

Congenital Malformation

Congenital malformations in the male involve the bladder, the urethra, and the penis. *Exstrophy of the bladder* is a major defect in which the abdominal wall has failed to close and the anterior bladder is open onto the abdomen. A direct passage of urine to the outside occurs, and it is difficult to keep the patient dry. *Epispadias* is a condition in which the male urethra is open somewhere along the upper surface (dorsal) of the penis, whereas in *hypospadias* the urethra is open at some point along the undersurface (ventral) of the penis. Most cases of hypospadias are minor and require no corrective surgery. Severe urethral defects require extensive urethroplasty and plastic surgery. If surgery is required, no circumcision is done because the foreskin will be used in the procedure (Cumes, 1993). When surgery for exstrophy of the bladder is done, a long hospitalization is usually necessary. The surgery is not always successful and is associated with some risk.

Conditions Affecting the Testes and Adjacent Structures

Epididymitis

The epididymis is a coiled tube approximately 20 feet long that lies on top of the testes in the scrotum and collects the spermatozoa. Any of several bacteria may cause an infection, including the streptococcus, staphylococcus, and colon bacilli. Infection of the epididymis **(epididymitis)** may occur after prostatitis or an infection of the urinary tract, and it often occurs as a complication of gonorrhea. The patient may be ill with fever, chills, headache, nausea, and vomiting. Painful swelling of the scrotum occurs, and it may be unilateral or bilateral. Treatment is to place the patient on a regimen of bedrest and support the scrotum. Heat or cold may be applied, and the appropriate antibiotic is given. If abscesses form, incision and drainage may be required.

Orchitis

Orchitis, an infection of the testicles, may result from injury or from any one of several infectious diseases such as influenza, pneumonia, or gonorrhea. It may also occur as a complication of mumps. Symptoms include fever, nausea, and painful swelling of the testicles. The treatment is the same as that for epididymitis.

Hydrocele and varicocele

A **hydrocele** is a collection of fluid between the testes and their outermost covering, the tunica vaginalis testis. The condition is often associated with some other disease or injury. Several methods of treatment are used, including aspiration of the fluid; injection of a sclerosing solution, which causes the walls of the sac containing the fluid to adhere; and surgical removal of the sac, which is often the treatment method most likely to ensure cure. The scrotum should be supported with bandages or a commercial suspensory. A **varicocele** is a form of varicosity that involves the veins of the spermatic cord. It is usually a painless and harmless condition, but if it causes pain, the scrotum should be supported. If support fails to relieve the discomfort, ligation of the veins may be done.

Tumors

Tumors of the male reproductive tract are usually malignant. They commonly occur in the testes, the prostate, and on the penis. *Penile* tumors account for a small percentage of cancer in men. They are usually the result of poor hygiene practices and are rarely seen in men who were circumcised as infants. Treatment involves removal of the cancerous tumor, and partial or total removal of the penis may be necessary.

Testicular tumors are the second most common malignancy in men between the ages of 25 and 35, and they account for 1% to 2% of all tumors in men of this age group. The incidence of testicular cancer is higher in men with cryptorchidism (undescended testes). However, the disease does occur in the general population of men in most age groups, so all men should be aware of the symptoms (Box 26-2). Regular testicular self-examination (TSE) is currently recommended as an effective method for detecting cancer in its early stages (Figure 26-2). All males age 15 and older should perform TSE once a month, during a warm bath or shower.

BOX 26-2

WARNING SIGNS OF TESTICULAR CANCER

A lump in either testicle
Any enlargement of a testicle
A feeling of heaviness in the scrotum
A dull ache in the lower abdomen or the groin
A sudden collection of fluid in the scrotum
Pain or discomfort in a testicle or in the scrotum
Enlargement or tenderness of the breasts

Testicular carcinoma has a highly metastatic character (Beare, 1994). Treatment includes surgical removal of the testes and radiation. Chemotherapy is used in metastatic disease. A primary role for the nurse in caring for these patients is to provide emotional support. These men may express fear and anxiety about their sexual functioning and about the outcome of cancer treatment. They may also experience alterations in role performance and may grieve over the cancer diagnosis and the upcoming treatments.

Postoperative care includes assessing the dressing over the scrotal wound, maintaining patency of the catheter if present, providing scrotal support, and maintaining the patient in a comfortable position. Men who have been treated for cancer in one testicle have approximately a 1% chance of developing cancer in the other testicle. They should be checked yearly by their doctors and should be encouraged to do testicular self-examination monthly.

Phimosis

Phimosis is a condition in which the orifice of the prepuce is too small to allow retraction over the glans penis. The condition is often congenital but may result from local inflammation or disease. The condition is rarely severe enough to obstruct the flow of urine, but it may contribute to local infection because it does not permit adequate cleansing. The male may experience dyspareunia (painful intercourse) because of phimosis, urinary tract infection, or insufficient lubrication. A surgical procedure **(circumcision)** may be performed in which part of the foreskin is removed, leaving the glans penis uncovered. This reduces infections, allows for repair and healing of damaged tissue, and allows for additional lubrication during intercourse. To prevent phimosis resulting from inflammation, circumcision is often performed on newborn infants before they leave the hospital. The procedure is also performed in a ritual ceremony, known as a bris, in the Jewish religion.

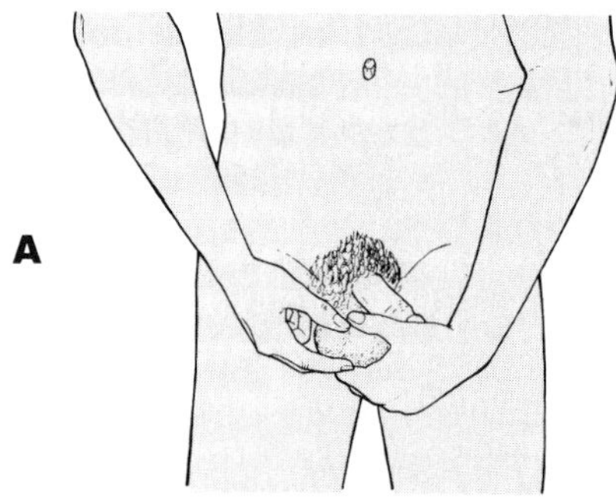

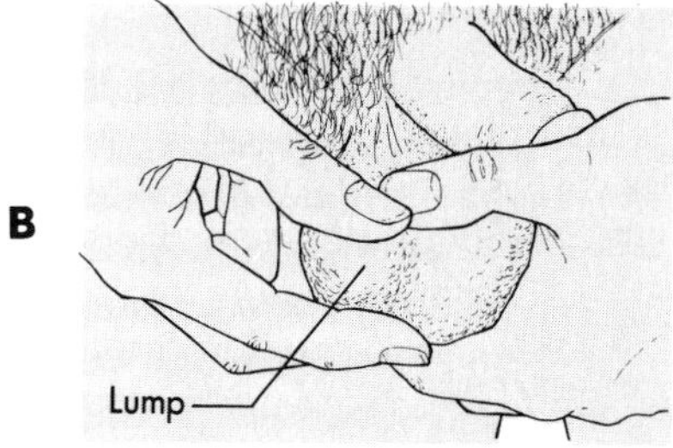

Figure 26-2 Testicular self-examination (TSE). **A,** Hold testis with both hands; palpate gently between thumb and forefingers. **B,** Abnormal lumps or irregularities should be reported to physician. Monthly TSE is recommended for all men age 15 and older and is most effective when performed during a warm bath or shower. (Modified from Phipps WJ and others: *Medical-surgical nursing,* ed 5, St Louis, 1995, Mosby.)

Cryptorchidism (undescended testicle)

During embryonic life, the testes are in the abdomen, and during the last 2 months before birth they descend into the scrotum. In some instances they remain in the abdomen or the inguinal canal. One or both testicles may be involved. They sometimes descend during the first few weeks of life. By 1 year of age the incidence of undescended testes is less than 25%. If the testes fail to descend, treatment with certain hormones is usually initiated. If results are not secured, surgery may be done, but it is not always successful. Although the condition is fairly common in newborn infants, only a small number of adults are seen with an undescended testicle, which indicates that the condition is generally self-correcting.

Ectopic testes

Ectopic testes means that undescended testes are outside the normal path for descent. Because their location may subject them to greater risk of injury, intervention to place them into the scrotum is done early. Hormone treatment has no effect on ectopic testes.

Torsion of the spermatic cord

A kinking and twisting of one of the spermatic cords also twists the enclosed artery and interrupts the blood flow to the testicle being supplied. This sequence of events can lead to ischemia and severe pain, and the pain may be aggravated by scrotal elevation. The patient with torsion of a spermatic cord is prepared for surgery, and the testicle is surgically fixed to the scrotal wall. If gangrene is present, the testicle is removed. The opposite testis (testicle) is usually anchored to its adjacent wall at the same time to prevent torsion of the spermatic cord on that side. Postoperative care includes application of ice to relieve swelling and discomfort. Care should be taken to place the ice cap under the scrotum, and the nurse should see that it is removed for short intervals every hour to prevent ice burn. The scrotum can also be elevated by using a folded towel (Long, Phipps, 1993).

Penile ulceration

Ulceration on the penis may result from many conditions, including syphilis, herpes virus, chancroid, and tuberculosis. Examination should be made as soon as possible so that proper diagnosis and treatment may be started immediately (see Chapter 11).

Conditions Affecting the Prostate Gland

The prostate is a firm, partially glandular, partially muscular body that surrounds the urethra at the bladder neck. It has five lobes. Conditions affecting the prostate include prostatitis, cancer, and benign prostatic hypertrophy.

Prostatitis

Prostatitis is an infection of the prostate gland by bacteria or a virus. It can occur in an acute or a chronic form. Symptoms of acute prostatitis include fever, chills, lower back pain, perineal discomfort, dysuria, and urinary urgency and frequency. After the diagnosis is confirmed by culture of the urine and prostatic secretions, the patient is treated with antibiotics, rest, increased fluid intake, and analgesics.

Chronic prostatitis may affect as many as 80% of all men between the ages of 30 and 50. It may go undiagnosed for years until the patient seeks medical treatment at the onset of symptoms such as pain in the perineum, lower back pain, or persistent urinary tract infections. Treatment includes antibiotic therapy and periodic digital massages of the prostate to increase the flow of infected prostatic secretions. The chronic inflammation may cause an increase in prostate size, which may result in obstruction of urinary flow and require surgical correction.

Another form of prostatitis does not involve bacterial infection. It is a chronic prostatitis also called *prostatosis.* It may be caused by excessive consumption of alcohol or caffeine and may also be a psychologic problem in a man with sexual dysfunction. There is congestion in the prostate gland, which is found on physical examination to be nontender and of normal consistency. The patient experiences mild urinary frequency and urgency; lower back pain; and discomfort in the rectum, urethra, and perineal area. The patient also may experience a moderate loss of libido. The symptoms are usually self-limiting, and treatment involves removing the cause of the problem.

OLDER ADULT CONSIDERATIONS

Certain problems of the urinary tract/reproductive system are commonly found in the elderly male population. Many of the urinary problems are directly related to an enlarged prostate. Overflow incontinence, urinary tract infection, and urinary retention are three of the most common ones. Impotence can be related to medications that the elderly male may be taking for health problems such as cardiac ailments or hypertension. A careful voiding history and medication record is important when assessing urinary/reproductive problems in the elderly male. Fluid intake and output estimates are important to obtain because the patient who is dribbling urine may have limited his fluid intake in an attempt to control the problem on his own. This self-imposed fluid limitation may cause dehydration in the elderly.

Cancer of the prostate gland

The prostate gland is the second most common site of cancer among men 55 to 74 years of age in the United States. It is the third leading cause of death from cancer in men of that age group. Prostate cancer is the most common type of cancer found in African-American men. It is catching up with lung cancer as the leading cause of cancer-related deaths in men of African descent. Prostate cancer tends to occur at an earlier age in African-American men, and by the time it is diagnosed, almost 50% of the patients in this group already have advanced disease. As a result of this delayed diagnosis, the survival rate among African-American prostate cancer patients is lower than in the overall group of men with prostate cancer (American Cancer Society, 1994).

Early detection, surgery, radiation therapy, hormone therapy, and chemotherapy drugs have improved the prognosis for prostate cancer during the last 15 years. Ninety-two percent of those with localized disease and 78% of those with metastatic disease survive 5 years or more (American Cancer Society, 1994).

Early detection of prostate cancer by routine rectal examination of prostate nodules can lead to early treatment. For this reason, all men over age 40 should have annual routine rectal examinations done by their physicians. The American Cancer Society recommends that men age 50 and over have an annual prostate-specific antigen (PSA) blood test in addition to the rectal examination. If the PSA blood level is elevated, it is considered an indicator of possible prostate cancer.

Detection of firm nodules on the posterior lobe of the prostate indicates malignancy. The lesion may be the size of a marble before it can be palpated. Newer diagnostic techniques that use ultrasound can detect lesions as small as 2 mm. Early symptoms are rarely present, but the patient may complain of dysuria and frequent urination. Later the patient will experience a sciatic type of pain, urinary retention, and hematuria. The disease is usually far advanced by the time these symptoms appear (Gray, 1992). Laboratory findings in the advanced stages include an elevated serum acid phosphatase (Smeltzer, Bare, 1992). Acid phosphatase is an enzyme that is normally present in large concentrations in the prostate gland. If metastatic carcinoma of the prostate gland ruptures the capsule surrounding the gland, the enzyme is released into the bloodstream. An elevated alkaline phosphatase indicates bony metastases.

If the diagnosis is made while the malignancy is still a small nodule within the gland and no metastasis has occurred, a radical resection of the prostate gland is usually curative (Gray, 1992). However, when cancer of the prostate gland is extensive, treatment may be only palliative. The goal of treatment at this stage is to slow the growth rate of malignant cells and to provide relief from pain. Several procedures may be used, including *cryosurgery* (freezing prostatic tissues) and radiation therapy. Surgical removal of the testes *(orchiectomy)* eliminates the male sex hormones that contribute to growth of prostate cancer cells. Giving estrogen (stilbestrol) in small doses also helps to slow the growth of malignant cells (Groenwald and others, 1993). A combination of the hormone estradiol and the cytotoxic agent estramustine phosphate (Emcyt), also known as nitrogen mustard, has also been shown to be effective in halting progression of the disease. The hormone is believed to act as a carrier of the nitrogen mustard to the hormonally receptive cancerous tissue. The drug is taken by mouth, produces few side effects, and in some patients rapidly relieves pain. It has proved effective in more than one third of patients who did not respond to hormone therapy alone (Cumes, 1993).

Benign prostatic hypertrophy

Benign prostatic hypertrophy (BPH) is a common and treatable disease found in more than half of all men over the age of 50. It is simple nonmalignant enlargement of the prostate gland. As the gland enlarges, it presses the urethra and causes urinary symptoms to develop. The urinary stream begins to slow, and urination becomes frequent and painful, eventually progressing to complete urinary retention. Most men have some symptoms by age 55, and many will eventually require surgery (transurethral resection of the prostate) to remove blockage of the urethra.

Prostatectomy

There are several methods by which the prostate gland may be removed, and the physician determines which method is best suited for the particular patient and his diagnosis. Nursing care is determined by the type of surgery (Box 26-3).

BOX 26-3

FOUR METHODS OF PROSTATECTOMY

1. Suprapubic prostatectomy is accomplished by an incision through the abdomen; the bladder is opened, and the prostate gland is removed with the finger from above.
2. Transurethral prostatectomy is done by approaching the prostate gland through the penis and bladder using a resectoscope, a surgical instrument with an electric cutting wire for resection and cautery, to cut the lobes away from the capsule.
3. Perineal prostatectomy requires an incision through the perineum between the scrotum and the rectum.
4. Retropubic prostatectomy is the method in which an incision is made into the abdomen above the bladder, but the bladder is not opened. The prostate gland is removed by making an incision into the capsule that encases the gland.

Each situation will present certain special problems of nursing care. Additional problems may occur because most patients are men who are well past age 50 and who may have other diseases from degenerative changes.

Preoperative intervention. The patient is usually admitted to the hospital before surgery. Because of the urinary frequency, the patient should be shown the location of the bathroom and given a urinal immediately on admission to the clinical unit.

Numerous laboratory tests are completed. Among the first are urinalysis and urine culture. These tests often indicate infection because one third of the patients with prostatic hypertrophy have infected urine because of urinary retention. BUN and serum creatinine tests are done to determine renal function. Hemoglobin and coagulation time are done to evaluate the ability to withstand blood loss and control bleeding. Acid phosphatase and alkaline phosphatase are done to determine metastases if malignancy is suspected. An intravenous pyelogram is done to rule out renal mass or other abnormalities. An electrocardiogram, as well as a cystoscopic examination with biopsy, may also precede a prostatectomy. Because the prostate gland is very vascular, blood loss during surgery may be extensive. Blood typing and cross matching are usually ordered in case transfusion therapy is necessary. The nurse should be sure that the physician's orders for the various examinations are understood and that the request forms are properly completed and routed to the appropriate departments.

Catheter drainage may or may not be ordered before surgery, but accurate records of urinary output must be maintained and should include the interval and the amount of urine voided. Many patients if properly instructed can help with maintaining the record. An enema will be given the night before the surgery to reduce the risk of straining during defecation, which could cause bleeding after surgery. Antiembolism stockings will be applied the morning of surgery. Nurses should be familiar with nursing diagnoses and interventions commonly seen in patients after prostatectomy (Box 26-4).

Postoperative intervention: transurethral resection of the prostate (TURP). A transurethral prostatectomy has three major advantages: the patient is ambulatory soon after the surgery, recovery is generally rapid, and a shorter hospitalization is required. Postoperatively, the patient will have a Foley catheter connected to continuous closed-bladder irrigation (CCB or CBI) to reduce clot formation (Figure 26-3). Gentle traction may be applied to the catheter by taping it against the thigh. This action pulls the catheter balloon down against the bladder and helps to control bleeding

BOX 26-4

Nursing Process

PROSTATECTOMY

ASSESSMENT

Vital signs as indicated
Incision and surgical dressing, if present
Surgical drains and tubes
Level of comfort
Breath sounds and oxygenation
Extremities for adequate tissue perfusion
Fluid volume status
Patency of urinary catheter
Bleeding/clots from urinary catheter, hourly
Mental status for confusion or disorientation
Understanding of possible impact of surgery on sexual functioning
Laboratory studies: hemoglobin; hematocrit; electrolytes, especially Na

NURSING DIAGNOSES

Anxiety related to uncertain outcome of surgery
Pain related to bladder spasms or surgical incision
Risk for altered tissue perfusion related to hemorrhage or deep vein thrombosis
Risk for injury related to straining during defecation
Risk for infection related to indwelling urinary catheter
Risk for urinary retention related to edema of urethra after catheter removal
Risk for fluid volume excess related to excessive absorption of irrigating solution
Risk for body image disturbance related to surgery involving reproductive organs
Sexual dysfunction: impotence related to actual or perceived effects of prostatectomy on sexual functioning
Sexual dysfunction: retrograde ejaculation and altered fertility related to surgical procedure

NURSING INTERVENTIONS

Maintain NPO until a diet is ordered.
Maintain intravenous fluids as ordered.
Measure and record intake and output.
Maintain patency of indwelling catheter.
Instruct patient not to void around catheter.
Maintain gentle traction for 24 hours if ordered.
Administer continuous or intermittent catheter irrigation as ordered.
After the catheter is removed, instruct the patient to perform perineal exercises: press buttocks together, hold as long as possible, relax and repeat 10 to 20 times per hour.
Encourage the patient to void whenever he feels the urge.
Inform the patient to expect dribbling of urine.
Observe for urinary retention or incontinence.
Maintain fluid intake of 2000 ml/day if not contraindicated.
If dressings are present, change prn to keep dry.
Ambulate as ordered; avoid sitting.
Administer antispasmodics and analgesics as ordered.
Provide a low-residue diet during the healing period following perineal prostatectomy; provide a regular diet 24 to 48 hours postoperatively after other procedures as ordered.
Administer a stool softener and mild laxatives as ordered.
Avoid rectal temperatures and enemas.
Apply antiembolism stockings while the patient is in bed.
Allow the patient time to express his feelings and fears.
Discuss the potential effects of surgery on sexual functioning.
Refer the patient for sexual counseling as indicated.

EVALUATION OF EXPECTED OUTCOMES

Meets discharge criteria for the postsurgical patient (p. 487)
Hematocrit and hemoglobin stable
Urinary drainage reddish-pink to light pink 24 hours postoperatively with continuous irrigation; cherry red and clear with intermittent irrigation; urine clear in 7 to 10 days
Free of bladder spasms
Absence of pain and pallor in lower extremities
Absence of symptoms of fluid and/or electrolyte imbalance
Maintains self-esteem as evidenced by attention to personal hygiene and appearance
Verbalizes fears, concerns, and feelings

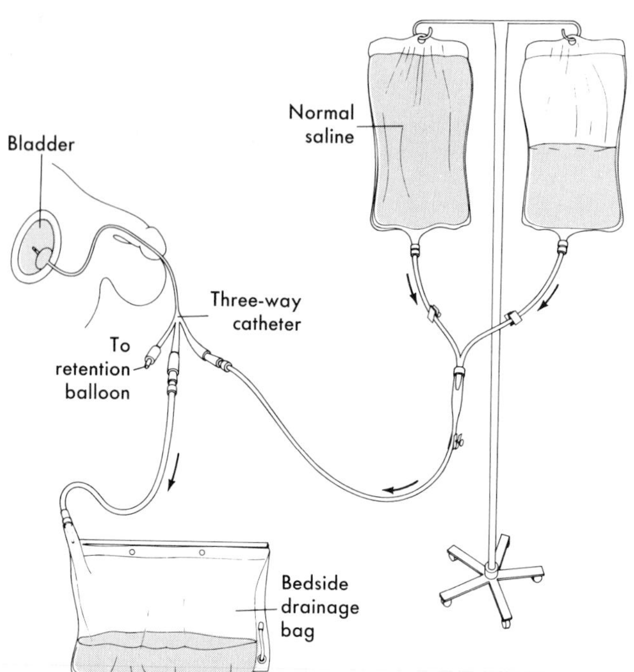

Figure 26-3 Continuous irrigation of the bladder requires a three-way Foley catheter that allows simultaneous infusion and drainage of irrigating solution (normal saline) through the bladder. The solution, infused rapidly into the bladder and drained into a bedside drainage bag, is assessed for evidence of excessive bleeding. The drainage bag should be emptied every 1 to 2 hours. (From Beare PG, Myers JL: *Adult health nursing,* ed 2, St Louis, 1994, Mosby.)

(Figure 26-4). The irrigation system should be assessed every hour to be sure that patency is maintained and obstruction prevented. Closed drainage with intermittent irrigation by 20 to 30 ml normal saline is sometimes used, but clots are more likely to form and obstruct the catheter and/or cause painful bladder spasms. The patient should be advised not to try to void around the blocked catheter because doing so will contribute to bladder spasm. The patient must be observed closely for hemorrhage, which is always a possible complication. Careful monitoring of the catheter drainage will alert the nurse if hemorrhage should occur.

When continuous closed-bladder irrigation is used to clean the bladder, the drainage is expected to be reddish-pink to light pink within 24 hours after surgery. Without continuous irrigation, the urine will be cherry red but clear. A deeper color indicates hemorrhage. Bright red drainage with numerous clots and viscous consistency accompanied by a falling blood pressure indicates arterial bleeding and usually requires that the patient return to the operating room for further cautery.

Venous bleeding is more common and is darker and less viscous than arterial bleeding. It can usually be controlled by applying traction to the catheter so that the ballooned end inside the bladder applies pressure to the prostatic fossa (Figure 26-4). This technique should be done by the physician but may be done by an experienced nurse who has been trained in the procedure. Traction is rarely maintained longer than 24 hours, and this limitation avoids trauma to the external urinary sphincter.

If continuous irrigation is not ordered or maintained, a blocked catheter can result and can cause bladder distention and spasms. If drainage stops, the catheter is usually irrigated with a catheter tip (Toomey) syringe and sterile normal saline. If gentle suction dislodges clots or tissue remnants, irrigation should be repeated after the initial sterile saline instillation has drained. Irrigation should be repeated at least every 4 hours until the drainage is entirely free of clots. If the catheter will not clear, the urologist will need to remove it and insert another.

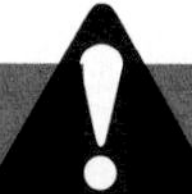

NURSE ALERT

Patients undergoing continuous bladder irrigation after prostate surgery are at high risk for fluid and electrolyte imbalances because of absorption of the irrigation fluid. They should be monitored closely for signs and symptoms of bradycardia, hypertension, tachypnea, confusion, agitation, vomiting, headache, and tremor (Beare, Myers, 1994). Any of these changes should be reported promptly.

As the urinary drainage clears, continuous irrigation is discontinued and straight drainage is maintained. The drainage may become deeper pink because there is no irrigation solution to dilute the color. With increased fluid intake, the color lightens and eventually returns to normal in 7 to 10 days.

Stool softeners and mild laxatives will be ordered to prevent constipation. Straining must be avoided for 6 weeks after discharge to prevent pressure of the rectum against the prostatic fossa, which delays healing.

Most complications are likely to occur in the first 24 hours postoperatively. Blood pressure should be taken every 2 hours. Temperature should be taken every 4 hours; a temperature above 101° F (38.3° C) by mouth indicates infection. A pulse rate below 60 beats/minute should be reported because bradycardia can result if spinal anesthesia was used for a

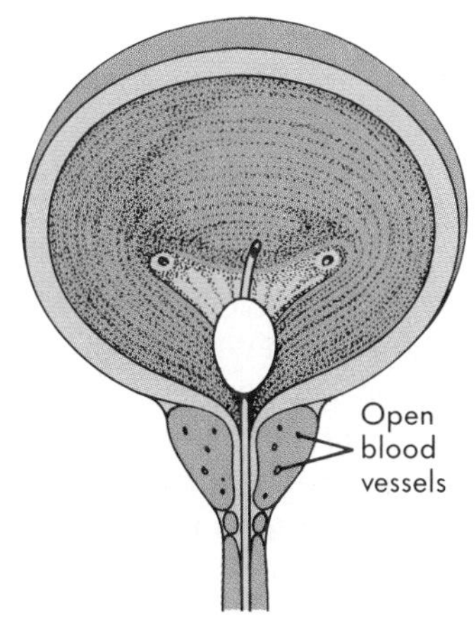

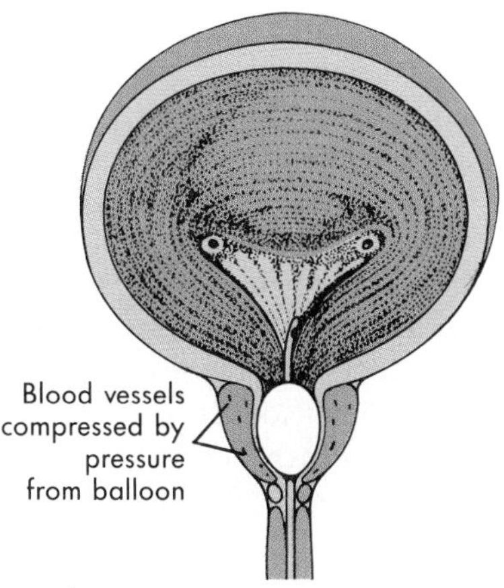

Figure 26-4 Gentle traction is maintained against the prostatic vascular bed to prevent excessive bleeding following transurethral resection. (From Beare PG, Myers JL: *Adult health nursing,* ed 2, St Louis, 1994, Mosby.)

prolonged time. An elevation in pulse accompanied by a drop in blood pressure indicates hemorrhage and shock.

The patient is ambulated on the first postoperative day. He should avoid sitting because it increases intraabdominal pressure and promotes bleeding. Ambulation should be increased to frequent short walks, and the patient should wear antiembolism stockings while in bed. He should be helped to turn and deep breathe at frequent intervals. When the catheter is removed, the patient will normally void small amounts (approximately 15 to 30 ml), and the amount of each voiding will remain small until the bladder is stretched to normal capacity.

Patient/family teaching. Because the bladder capacity is small, the patient should void whenever he has the urge for at least 2 months. This will prevent pressure of a full bladder on the surgical site before it is fully healed. The patient may experience dysuria, which may be helped by warm tub baths. Some patients have difficulty voiding, and others are incontinent after the catheter is removed. Incontinence usually is caused by bladder irritation and weakened sphincter muscles. Perineal exercises performed by tightening and releasing the gluteal muscles should improve control. Voiding problems usually disappear with time.

After discharge, the patient should void whenever he has the urge, avoid straining during defecation, and avoid constipation by taking prescribed stool softeners and laxatives and by eating adequate fiber and fluids. Spicy foods should be avoided. Sexual activity can be resumed in 6 to 8 weeks. Erectile function should not be permanently affected but may be temporarily altered.

Suprapubic prostatectomy. When a suprapubic prostatectomy has been done, the surgeon may place some agent such as gauze packing or a hemostatic bag in the depressed area where the gland was located to prevent hemorrhage. In addition, there will be some provision for urinary drainage through the abdominal incision. Drains or tubes such as a cystostomy tube may be used. Not all urologists use this method. If only small drains are used, a ureterostomy cup may be used to collect urine and to keep the patient dry. In other cases large abdominal dressings may be used. The abdominal dressings may need to be changed often to keep the patient dry, and enclosing them in some type of impervious material may help. In any procedure used, the patient must be watched closely for hemorrhage. The patient also will need medication for pain because bladder spasms may be severe and painful. The nurse should help and encourage the patient to turn often, and deep breathing exercises are especially important to prevent pulmonary complications. Ambulation for these patients is delayed. The catheter must be kept open and draining.

Retropubic prostatectomy. The patient recovering from a retropubic prostatectomy has less discomfort than do patients who have had prostatectomies by other methods. The patient has a retention catheter and should be observed for hemorrhage. There are few or no bladder spasms, and there is no urinary drainage on the abdominal dressing. If urinary drainage is noted on the abdominal dressing, or if purulent drainage, fever, or increased pain with ambulation occurs, the physician should be notified. These symptoms may indicate deep wound infection or pelvic abscess (Long, Phipps, 1993).

Perineal prostatectomy. Perineal prostatectomy involves removal of part or all of the prostate gland through a perineal incision. It may be performed because of benign prostatic hypertrophy or for cancer of the prostate gland. When the surgery is for cancer, radical prostatectomy may be performed, removing the entire prostate gland, including the capsule, seminal vesicles, and the adjacent tissue. The remaining urethra is anastomosed to the bladder neck. Because the internal and external sphincters of the bladder lie close to the prostate, the patient is likely to experience some degree of urinary incontinence. He will also be impotent and sterile. Both the patient and his sexual partner must be made aware of the consequences of radical prostate surgery (Patrick and others, 1991).

A modified radical approach may also be performed for cancer of the prostate gland. In this procedure the nerves controlling erection are saved. Erectile function may be disturbed for 6 to 12 months, but most patients will eventually regain erection capabilities. This greatly improves the patient's outlook on the effects of the procedure. It is recommended only for well-localized prostatic lesions.

The preoperative preparation of the patient for perineal prostatectomy is essentially the same regardless of whether the underlying disease is benign or malignant. The bowel is prepared by giving a laxative and enemas. An antibiotic or sulfonamide drug is often given preoperatively, and only clear liquids are allowed on the day before surgery.

When the patient returns from surgery, he will have a retention catheter, which should be connected to sterile closed drainage. Extreme care should be taken to ensure that the catheter does not become blocked or displaced. There is less possibility of hemorrhage and bladder spasms in the perineal approach to the prostate gland. Urinary drainage that may appears on the perineal dressings will gradually decrease over a period of a few hours. In a perineal prostatectomy, temporary fecal incontinence may occur. The patient should be taught perineal exercises, and beginning them early will strengthen the rectal and urethral sphincter muscles. Patients who have had simple perineal prostatectomy for benign prostatic hypertrophy have no problem with urinary control.

For some patients the catheter is removed in approximately 1 week, whereas for others it may not be removed for several weeks. The patient should be instructed to perform perineal exercises and to void whenever he feels the urge. All patients should receive at least 3000 ml of fluid daily. After the first 24 to 48 hours, most patients are allowed solid food, except for those recovering from a perineal prostatectomy. During the immediate postoperative period, the patient receives nothing by mouth. Liquids or a low-residue diet may be given later and should continue until there has been time for healing.

Cryosurgical ablation for prostate cancer

A new surgical procedure known as cryosurgical ablation has been performed since 1993 as an investigational procedure in cases of prostate cancer. It involves freezing the entire prostate gland and the portions of the seminal vesicles closest to the prostate. The prostate is turned into an iceball, while the prostatic urethra is maintained above core body temperature by irrigation with water heated to 110° F (44° C). The areas to be treated are located by the physician with transrectal ultrasound. Cryosurgical ablation is used as an alternative to radiation therapy for patients with localized tumors and for patients whose medical condition contraindicates radical prostatectomy. If it is proven successful, this procedure could be used instead of the radical prostatectomy, which would leave the patient with fewer complications.

Cryosurgical ablation of the prostate is believed to cause the death of prostate cells by dehydration. Freezing the cells causes hypovolemia, and the reduced fluid in the cells results in concentrations of electrolytes in the cells high enough to reach toxic levels. As the freezing continues, the cell membranes rupture. Thermal shock causes cell protein to change in structure. Blood flow to the area ceases, and the result is vascular necrosis.

After cryosurgery, the bladder needs to be retrained. Urine drains through a suprapubic tube, which is inserted during surgery. On the first postoperative day the tube is clamped and the patient attempts to void when he feels the need. After voiding, he unclamps and drains the tube and measures any urine remaining in the bladder. Any urine obtained after voiding is called postvoiding residual (PVR) urine. Eventually, the amount of PVR will be minimal. The patient must be taught to care for the suprapubic catheter and site, to empty and measure PVR, to drink plenty of fluids, and to take stool softeners to avoid straining at stool. The patient can expect to be discharged on the second postoperative day, and he goes home with the suprapubic tube in place (Brenner, Krenzer, 1995).

ETHICAL DILEMMA

Mr. O'Leary has been diagnosed with prostate cancer. His doctor knows that Mr. O'Leary's wife died 9 months ago and that he is eagerly looking forward to a long vacation with a son and his family. He decides not to tell Mr. O'Leary about the cancer so it won't ruin his trip.

How would you analyze this case?

Conditions Affecting Erectile Function

Any condition affecting erectile function causes the male a period of impotence. *Erectile dysfunction* is the failure to achieve penile erection in a manner sufficient for successful intercourse. This condition has many causes, and the incidence tends to increase with age. *Hormonal disorders* that disturb the hypothalamic-pituitary-gonadal circuit often cause erectile dysfunction (Cumes, 1993). *Vascular disorders* have a major effect on penile erection because it is a vascular event. Both arterial and venous disorders can be responsible for erectile dysfunction. *Neurologic disorders* of erectile function are caused by conditions that affect the brain, spinal cord, or peripheral nervous system (Aikey, 1992). Other causes include advanced syphilis, amyotrophic lateral sclerosis, and diabetes. *Surgical procedures* can compromise peripheral neural tissue or vascular erectile tissue in the penis. Radical prostatectomy is an example of a surgical procedure that may cause impotence. Trauma to the lower urinary tract and pelvis also can cause erectile dysfunction.

Treatment is based on the cause of the impotence and is planned after a complete history and physical examination are done. The nurse should remember that sexual dysfunction might be a result of physiologic, psychologic, and sociocultural factors. Restoration of the erectile function does not remove underlying psycologic causes of impotence, nor does it have any effect on the man's ability to achieve orgasm or ejaculation. The female nurse must realize that the male patient may be embarrassed and hesitant to speak to or be examined by a female nurse.

Erectile dysfunction caused by hormonal abnormalities can be treated by medications. Exogenous **androgens** can be given orally or parenterally to correct this disorder. If infertility is also involved, a combination of drugs is used to treat both (Table 26-1).

When erectile dysfunction is caused by vascular disorders, surgery can sometimes be done to correct or increase the blood supply to the penis. Some patients respond well to vasodilation medications, and they are taught to inject a vasodilator, usually papaverine, into the corporal bodies of the penis (Beare, Myers, 1994). Side effects of injected vasodilators include sustained painful erection (priapism) and fibrous plaque development at the injection sites.

Other methods of treating erectile dysfunction make use of mechanical devices. One type is the vacuum pump device (Figure 26-5) that uses suction to pull blood into the cavernous bodies. To keep the blood in the penis and maintain the erection, a restrictive device is then placed at the base of the penis. Prosthetic devices (Figure 26-6) can be surgically implanted in the corporal bodies on either side of the penis. They are easy to use, but some devices are difficult to conceal in clothing. The main complications with these devices are infection and erosion of the device through the skin. Postoperative care includes assessing the penile or scrotal incision for infection and noting the amount and type of drainage during dressing changes. Penile and scrotal swelling usually lasts 3 to 5 days.

The patient who has had a penile implant should be advised that healing will proceed faster if he avoids strenuous exercise and sexual contact for at least 3 weeks. The patient should operate the device under

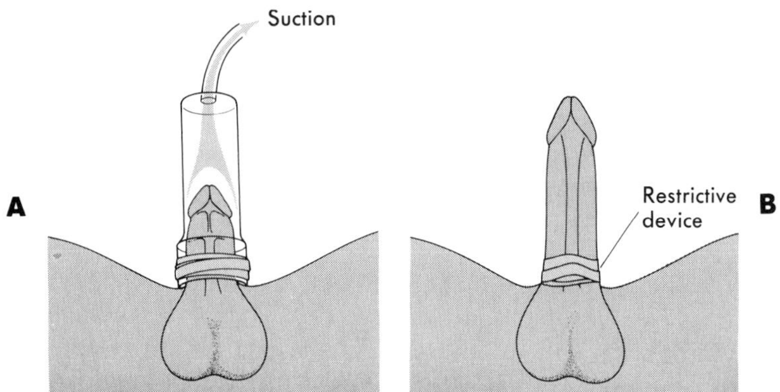

Figure 26-5 **A,** Mechanical devices create a vacuum to shunt blood into the penis. **B,** A restrictive device or tourniquet for maintaining penile engorgement must be used for successful intercourse. (From Beare PG, Myers JL: *Adult health nursing,* ed 2, St Louis, 1994, Mosby.)

TABLE 26-1

Pharmacology of Drugs in Men's Reproductive Health

Drug (Generic and Trade Name); Route and Dosage	Action/Indication	Common Side Effects and Nursing Considerations
DIETHYLSTIBESTROL (DES) **ROUTE:** PO, IV **DOSAGE:** PO, 1-3 mg/day; IV, 500 mg-1 g/day initially until response is obtained (5 or more days), then 250-500 mg 1-2 times weekly	Hormone and antineoplastic agent used palliatively in advanced, inoperable metastatic prostate and breast carcinoma	Headache, edema, hypertension, intolerance to contact lenses, nausea, weight changes, breakthrough bleeding in females, dysmenorrhea, amenorrhea, testicular atrophy, impotence, acne, oily skin, gynecomastia, and breast tenderness; contraindicated in thromboembolic disease and undiagnosed vaginal bleeding; use with caution in renal, cardiac, and hepatic disease; may increase risk of endometrial carcinoma
FINASTERIDE (Proscar) **ROUTE:** PO **DOSAGE:** 5 mg once daily	Used in treatment of benign prostatic hyperplasia	Use with caution in hepatic impairment or obstructive uropathy; can cause impotence or decreased libido
PAPAVERINE (Cerespan, Pavabid) **ROUTE:** PO, IM, IV **DOSAGE:** PO, 100-300 mg 3-5 times daily; IM, IV, 30 mg initially, then 30-120 mg q 3 hr if necessary	Adjunct treatment with alpha-adrenergic blockers in the management of male impotence due to organic causes	Contraindicated if history of heart block; use with caution in glaucoma and in sickle cell, liver, and coagulation-defect diseases
PRAZOSIN (Minipress) **ROUTE:** PO **DOSAGE:** 1 mg 2-3 times daily initially (give first dose at bedtime); increase gradually to maintenance dose of 6-15 mg/day in 2-3 divided doses (not to exceed 20-40 mg/day)	Treatment for mild to moderate hypertension; also used in the management of urinary outflow obstruction in patients with BPH	Dizziness, drowsiness, headache, weakness, first-dose orthostatic hypotension, palpitations, and nausea; use with caution in renal impairment, angina, and with diuretics
TERAZOSIN (Hytrin) **ROUTE:** PO **DOSAGE:** 1 mg at bedtime, may be increased gradually to 5-10 mg/day	Antihypertensive used in the treatment of mild to moderate hypertension and in the management of outflow obstruction in patients with prostatic hypertrophy	Dizziness, weakness, headache, nasal congestion, and nausea
TESTOSTERONE **ROUTE:** IM **DOSAGE:** 25-50 mg 2-3 times/wk	Used for treatment of hypogonadism in androgen-deficient males; also used for erectile dysfunction and as palliative treatment of androgen-responsive breast cancer	Edema, clitoral enlargement, change in libido, decreased breast size, acne, priaprism, facial hair, oligospermia, impotence, and gynecomastia; contraindicated in males with breast or prostate cancer, hypercalcemia, or severe liver, renal, or cardiac disease

direct supervision of his doctor to be sure that he is able to do it properly, and he should be instructed to promptly report any dysfunction in the device or any signs of infection.

Pelvic Exenteration

Pelvic exenteration is a surgical procedure indicated for carcinomas that are locally destructive and capable of growing to great size but do not tend to metastasize. It is also indicated for tumors that are radioresistant or incurable by less radical surgery. The tumor must be confined to the pelvis without metastatic spread to distant sites and must be operable within the pelvis. The patient should be of an age and general physical and mental condition that make rehabilitation a reasonable goal. Exenteration is an alternative to lethal disease, but the patient and the spouse or supportive person must have a stronger than usual desire to live in order to cope with altered methods of fecal and urinary elimination and sexual intercourse. Their psychologic and sociologic status must be carefully evaluated well before the surgery.

Pelvic exenteration is done for both sexes and for adults in all age ranges. Complete or total pelvic exenteration consists of the removal of the rectum, distal sigmoid colon, urinary bladder and distal ureters, internal iliac vessels and their lateral branches, all pelvic reproductive organs, and lymph nodes. Urinary and fecal diversions are done. *Pelvic evisceration* and *pelvic sweep* are terms used interchangeably with pelvic exenteration.

The procedure is sometimes modified. An anterior pelvic exenteration removes the bladder and distal portion of the ureters, while the proximal portions are implanted in an ileal conduit. The normal bowel structure is preserved. In posterior pelvic exenteration, the colon and rectum are removed.

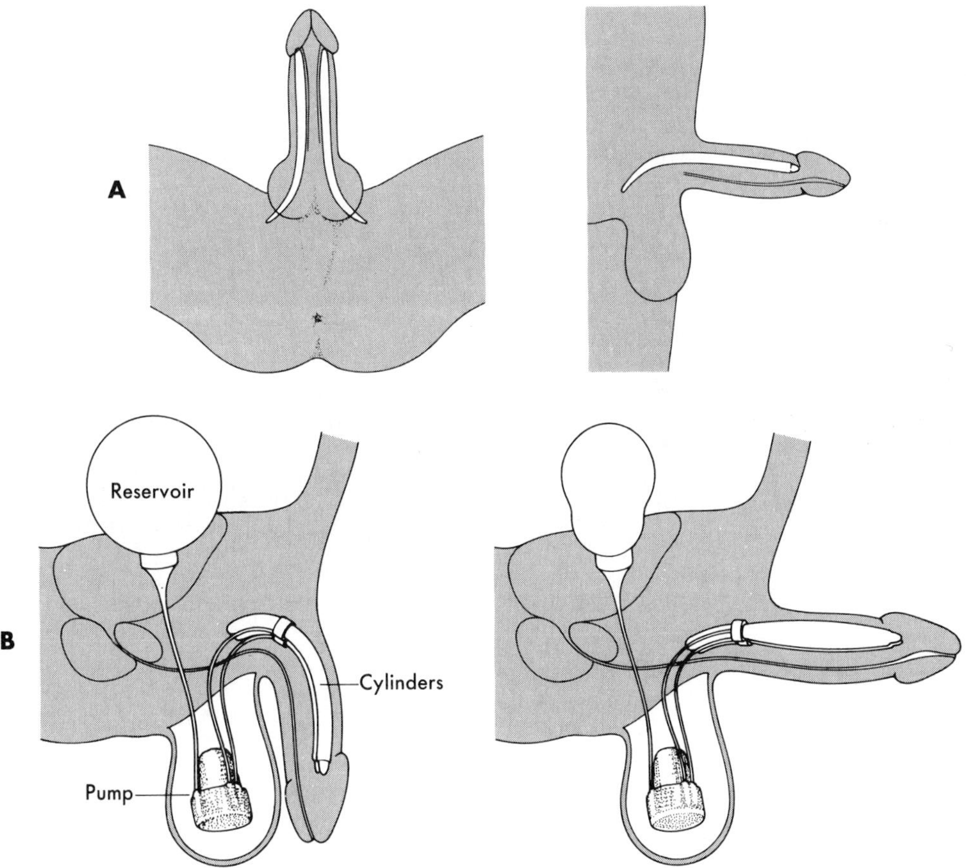

Figure 26-6 **A,** A semirigid prosthesis is implanted in the corpora cavernosa and remains in an erect position that may be difficult to hide in clothing. **B,** The Scott Inflatable Prosthesis has both erect and flaccid positions designed to mimic normal erectile function. (From Beare PG, Myers JL: *Adult health nursing,* ed 2, St Louis, 1994, Mosby.)

The patient is admitted 5 or 6 days before surgery, and preoperative care must focus on the patient's psychologic needs as well as on physical preparation of the bowel. Bowel preparation is accomplished with a low-residue diet, laxatives, a saline enema, and antibiotic therapy. Despite the controversy regarding the use of antibiotics for bowel cleansing, a sulfonamide drug regimen for bowel cleansing may be used. Antiembolism stockings are applied, and a nasogastric tube may be inserted the morning of surgery. Vitamin K therapy to promote blood coagulability may begin 2 or 3 days before surgery. The patient must be prepared to remain in bed for up to 1 week after surgery as healing begins.

Postoperatively, the vital signs and blood pressure are taken hourly for approximately 48 hours. They are assessed every 4 hours for 7 days, or as long as necessary. Rectal temperatures are contraindicated. Intravenous therapy is maintained up to 4000 ml daily, and all intake and output are measured. The operative site, the dressings, and all drainage tubes are also assessed hourly for the first 48 hours. Dressings should be reinforced and changed as ordered. Specific nursing care is indicated by the extent of the procedure, the status of the wounds and ostomies that were created, and by the patient's response to the surgery.

Exenterative surgery has a drastic effect on body image. Loss of the reproductive organs, loss of the ability to have sexual intercourse, and loss of the structures necessary for normal elimination all may be major handicaps to the patient's rehabilitation. Society's emphasis on physical attractiveness will make it even more difficult for the patient to maintain a positive self-concept and strong sex/gender role identity. Sexual readjustment may be a problem of great magnitude for the patient and the sexual partner. It is important for the nurse to encourage the patient to express his fears and concerns and to communicate the patient's needs to other members of the health team and to community resources. Ostomy clubs can be of help to patients in their efforts to regain social mobility and maintain a realistic yet hopeful outlook on life.

Nursing Care Plan

PATIENT HAVING SURGERY FOR IMPLANTATION OF PENILE PROSTHESIS

Mr. Bartlett is a 58-year-old male with a history of insulin-dependent diabetes for the last 20 years. He is entering the hospital for implantation of a penile prosthesis after a history of impotence for the last 2 years. His wife of 32 years accompanies him to the hospital. Additional medical data reveal that he has a history of hypertension controlled by medication. He does not drink alcohol and stopped smoking 15 years ago.

Past Medical History	Psychosocial Data	Assessment Data
Transurethral resection of prostate for benign prostatic hypertrophy 1 year ago; no complications postoperatively Follows ADA diet with good control Takes 25 units of regular insulin with 15 units of NPH insulin q am Takes methyldopa (Aldomet) 25 mg/day for his blood pressure No known allergies to food or drugs	Lives locally with wife, in a two-story house with a small yard Has 4 adult children; two live locally; the other two are no more than 4 hours away High school graduate and is retired from a local textile factory; wife works part-time at the library Plays golf, fishes, and takes walks for recreation	Patient is alert and oriented × 3 Afebrile *Respiratory:* Lungs clear, able to demonstrate effective cough, rate 18-20, regular depth and rhythm *Abdominal:* Soft, nontender, nondistended, bowel sounds present in all four quadrants. Skin clear with no lesions present *Cardiovascular:* Apical pulse 72-80, rate regular, pedal pulses palpable bilaterally ***Laboratory data*** Hgb 14, Hct 42, electrolytes within normal limits, serum glucose 156, Urinalysis and other laboratory data within normal limits Chest x-ray and ECG within normal limits

NURSING DIAGNOSIS

Pain related to penile incision, postoperative edema, and indwelling urinary catheter

NURSING INTERVENTIONS	EVALUATION OF EXPECTED OUTCOMES
Assess the patient's pain. Have patient describe pain on a scale of 1 to 10. Provide comfort measures as needed: repositioning, ice packs, analgesics. Anticipate need for analgesics, administer as per orders. Use bed cradle to keep bed linens off the operative site. Tape catheter to abdomen to keep penis perpendicular to body.	Describes pain on scale of 1 to 10 Verbalizes need for comfort measures Able to provide self-care measures such as positioning Verbalizes decrease or pain after comfort measures

NURSING DIAGNOSIS

Risk for infection related to surgical incision and indwelling urinary catheter

NURSING INTERVENTIONS	EVALUATION OF EXPECTED OUTCOMES
Assess dressing for drainage and odor. Change dressing as needed, using sterile technique. Monitor vital signs for elevations/changes. Provide catheter care at least bid. Monitor urinary drainage for changes in color and clarity. Encourage fluid intake of at least 2000 ml/day. Administer antibiotics as per orders.	No infection at surgical site No urinary tract infection Able to demonstrate incision care and dressing change before discharge Able to verbalize signs and symptoms of infections at surgical site before discharge Able to verbalize signs and symptoms of urinary tract infection before discharge

NURSING DIAGNOSIS

Body image disturbance related to need for penile prosthesis and need for exposure of genitalia to healthcare professionals

NURSING INTERVENTIONS	EVALUATION OF EXPECTED OUTCOMES
Assess patient's verbalization about the prosthesis, the level of participation in his own care, and embarrassment. Assess whether patient's expectations of surgery have been met or unmet. When inspecting the surgical site, maintain a professional demeanor to decrease embarrassment. Allow patient time for expressions of feelings.	Patient and wife discuss feelings about prosthesis and altered body image Discusses and participates in self-care Verbalizes both negative and positive feelings about implant

continued

NURSING DIAGNOSIS

Altered sexuality patterns related to preoperative impotence, placement of prosthesis, expectations of self and partner after surgery

NURSING INTERVENTIONS	EVALUATION OF EXPECTED OUTCOMES
Assess patient's and wife's behavior when discussing expectations after surgery.	Patient and wife openly discuss expectations of surgery on their sexual relationship
Assess patient's and wife's knowledge and expectations for their sexual relationship after surgery.	Patient and wife verbalize concerns and feelings about surgery
Allow time for patient/wife to verbalize concerns and feelings about surgery.	Patient and wife have clear understanding of differences among erection, ejaculation, fertility, and orgasm

KEY CONCEPTS

- The major function of the reproductive system is the creation of new life.
- The reproductive organs of the male include the penis, testes, vas deferens, seminal vesicles, and the assessory glands.
- Penile erection is controlled by the central, autonomic, and somatic nervous systems working together.
- The patient history is particularly important when assessing problems with the reproductive systems. A patient's culture and religious background may make it difficult for him to talk to the nurse about his problems.
- Chronic illnesses and their medications can affect sexual functioning.
- Puberty is the period of growth and development when secondary sex characteristics begin to appear.
- Nocturnal seminal emissions are a physiologic sign of puberty in males.
- Sexual role or gender role is the public expression of behavior that implies masculinity or femininity.
- Gender identity is the private or personal experience of one's maleness or femaleness. It is not always congruent with the individual's gender role.
- Male climacteric refers to the midlife physical and psychologic changes that take place in males.
- Physical examination of the male patient includes inspection and palpation of the external genitalia for abnormalities of structure and signs of infection such as discharge, swelling, and skin lesions.
- Congenital malformations of the male involve the bladder, the urethra, and the penis.
- Tumors of the male reproductive tract are usually malignant.
- Testicular tumors are the second most common malignancy in men between the ages of 25 and 35.
- Regular testicular self-examination (TSE) is recommended as an effective method for detecting cancer in its early stages.
- A primary role for the nurse when dealing with patients with testicular cancer is to provide emotional support.
- Conditions affecting the prostate gland include prostatitis, cancer, and benign prostatic hypertrophy.
- Many urinary problems of the elderly are signs of prostate enlargement.
- Cancer of the prostate gland is the second most common site for cancer among men between the ages of 55 and 74.
- Prostate cancer is the most common type of cancer found in African-American men.
- Benign prostatic hypertrophy is simple, nonmalignant enlargement of the prostate gland.
- Erectile dysfunction is the failure to achieve penile erection in a manner sufficient for successful intercourse.
- Erectile dysfunction can be caused by hormonal, vascular, or neurologic disorders, or by surgical procedures, trauma, and psychologic problems.
- Correction of the erectile dysfunction does not have an effect on the ability to achieve orgasm or ejaculation, nor does it remove underlying psychologic problems.
- Pelvic exenteration is indicated for carcinomas that are locally destructive and can grow to great size without metastasis.
- Total pelvic exenteration consists of the removal of the rectum, distal sigmoid colon, urinary bladder, distal ureters, all pelvic reproductive organs, and lymph nodes.

CRITICAL THINKING EXERCISES

1 Develop a teaching plan for a patient undergoing a transurethral prostatectomy.
2 Identify at least three nursing diagnoses appropriate for the patient undergoing suprapubic prostatectomy and list at least two interventions for each diagnosis.
3 Prepare a teaching plan to help a patient decrease his chances of developing a urinary tract infection after prostate surgery.
4 Identify at least three psychosocial nursing diagnoses for the patient undergoing a penile prothesis implantation and list at least two interventions for each diagnosis.
5 Discuss possible complications of continuous bladder irrigations; what are the signs and symptoms to monitor for?
6 Discuss at least three reasons why someone might have difficulty talking with the nurse about his expectations of sexual outcomes after penile implantation.

REFERENCES AND ADDITIONAL READINGS

Acute Pain Management Guideline Panel: *Acute pain management: operative or medical procedures and trauma. Clinical practice guideline,* Rockville, Md, February 1992. Agency for Health Care Policy and Research, Public Health Service, US Department of Health and Human Services, AHCPR Publication No 92-0032.

Aikey, C: Erectile dysfunction, *Urolog Nurs* 12(3):96-100, 1992.

American Cancer Society: *Cancer facts and figures,* New York, 1994, The Society.

Beare P, Myers P: *Principles and practices of adult health nursing,* ed 3, St Louis, 1994, Mosby.

Brenner ZR, Krenzer ME: Update on cryosurgical ablation for prostate cancer, *Am J Nurs* 95(4):44-49, 1995.

Bucket-Piccolino A, Costa FJ: No-scalpel vasectomy (NSV) procedure and nursing care, *J Urolog Nurs* 11(2):83-92.

Cant S: Infertility: causes and treatment, *Nurs Stand* 7(13-14):28-30, 1992.

Cumes DM: Transurethral prostate resection: a frustration free surgical method, *AORN J* 58(2):302; 304-308; 311; 1993.

Gray ML: *Genitourinary disorders,* St Louis, 1992, Mosby.

Greifzu S, Tiedemann D: Prostate cancer: the pros and cons of treatment, *RN* 58(6):22-27, 1995.

Groenwald SL and others: *Cancer nursing: principles and practice,* ed 3, Boston, 1993, Jones and Bartlett.

Groenwald SL: *Psychosocial dimensions of cancer,* Boston, 1991, Jones and Bartlett.

Lewis JH: Treatment options for men with sexual dysfunction, *J ET Nurs* 19(4):131-42, 1992.

Long B, Phipps WJ: *Medical surgical nursing,* ed 3, St Louis, 1993, Mosby.

Moore S and others: Nerve-sparing prostatectomy, *Am J Nurs* 92(4):59-64, 1992.

Patrick M and others: *Medical-surgical nursing: pathophysiologic concepts,* ed 2, Philadelphia, 1991, JB Lippincott.

Scherer JC: *Introductory medical-surgical nursing,* ed 5, Philadelphia, 1991, JB Lippincott.

Smeltzer SC, Bare BG: *Brunner and Suddarth's textbook of medical-surgical nursing,* ed 7, Philadelphia, 1992, JB Lippincott.

Smith DB, Babaian RJ: The effects of treatment for cancer on male fertility and sexuality, *Cancer Nurs* 15(4):271-275, 1992.

Spencer RT and others: *Clinical pharmacology and nursing management,* ed 4, Philadelphia, 1993, JB Lippincott.

Suddarth DS, Brunner LS: *The Lippincott manual of nursing practice,* ed 5, Philadelphia, 1991, JB Lippincott.

Thibodeau GA: *Textbook of anatomy and physiology,* ed 2, St Louis, 1993, Mosby.

Thompson JJ and others: *Clinical nursing,* ed 4, St Louis, 1993, Mosby.

Travis M, Gwozdz DT: Nursing case management for patients with TURP, *Urolog Nurs* 13(2):48-54, 1993.

Waxman ES: Sexual dysfunction following treatment for prostate cancer: nursing assessment and interventions, *Oncol Nurs Forum* 20(10):1567-1571, 1993.

Willis D: Taming the overgrown prostate, *Am J Nurs* 92(2):34-42, 1992.

CHAPTER 27

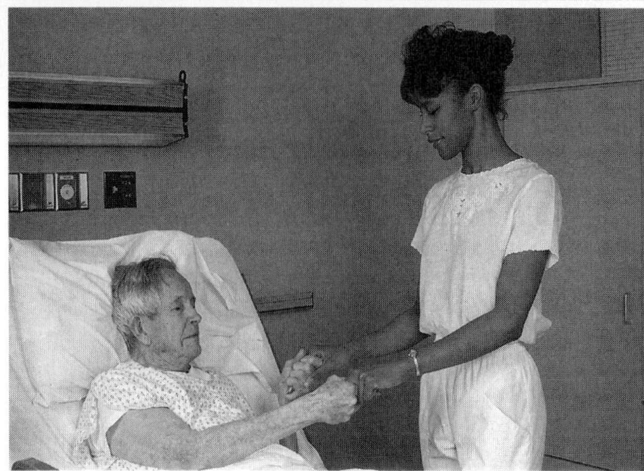

Endocrine Function

CHAPTER OBJECTIVES

1 Discuss the nursing responsibilities to identify potential problems of the endocrine system.
2 Describe nursing interventions to manage patient responses to hypersecretion or hyposecretion of specific endocrine glands.
3 Describe the pathophysiology, course, prognosis, and treatment of diabetes mellitus.
4 Compare and contrast the risk factors, onset, and course of the acute complications of diabetes mellitus.
5 Outline the actions that patients and providers take to prevent, detect, and treat diabetic complications.
6 Discuss the palliative treatment goal of diabetes to reduce symptoms, control hyperglycemia, and prevent complications.
7 Describe some examples of patients' responses to diabetes mellitus that indicate the uniqueness of this disease.
8 Describe nursing interventions that foster self-care of diabetes activities of daily living.
9 Describe some special educational needs of the elderly patient with diabetes.

KEY WORDS

acetone
aldosterone
atrophy
calibrated
catecholamines
cretinism
diabetic
endogenous
endogenous glucagon
exogenous
exogenous glucagon
glucagon
glycohemoglobin
goiter
hirsutism
homeostasis
hormone
hyperglycemia
hyperglycemic, hyperosmolar, nonketotic coma
hypoglycemia
insulin reaction
ketoacidosis
ketonuria
ketosis
lipodystrophy
metabolism
myxedema
renal threshold
tetany
type I diabetes
type II diabetes
ultrasonogram

ENDOCRINE GLANDS AND THEIR FUNCTION

The endocrine glands, or ductless glands, are sometimes called glands of internal secretion because they do not have ducts to carry their secretions to the outside, as do the exocrine glands. Instead the secretions pass directly into the tissue fluid, from which they are picked up by the blood. The secretions of the endocrine glands are chemical substances called hormones, and they act as chemical messengers, ultimately altering the activity of various body organs. Some of these hormones have been reproduced synthetically in the laboratory, whereas others are natural and are extracted from the glands of animals. The nurse who administers medications gives many of these commercially prepared hormone products, which are marketed under various trade names. Both the overproduction or underproduction of certain hormones may result in serious disease. In some cases the very life of the individual may depend on an adequate supply of a particular hormone. When for some reason the gland fails to supply the normal requirement, a commercial preparation must be given to compensate for the deficiency. The most significant example of this situation is the use of insulin in treating diabetes mellitus.

Endocrine glands have many functions, and they are so interrelated and interdependent that to separate their activities and their importance would be extremely difficult. They regulate the metabolic processes that control energy production, fluid and electrolyte balance, growth, development, reproduction, and lactation. Hormones from endocrine glands help to maintain **homeostasis** and regulate blood pressure and neuromuscular contraction. They assist in maintaining fluid and electrolyte and acid-base balance. Secretions from some glands stimulate other glands to activity. A description of the endocrine glands (Figure 27-1) and their chief hormones follows.

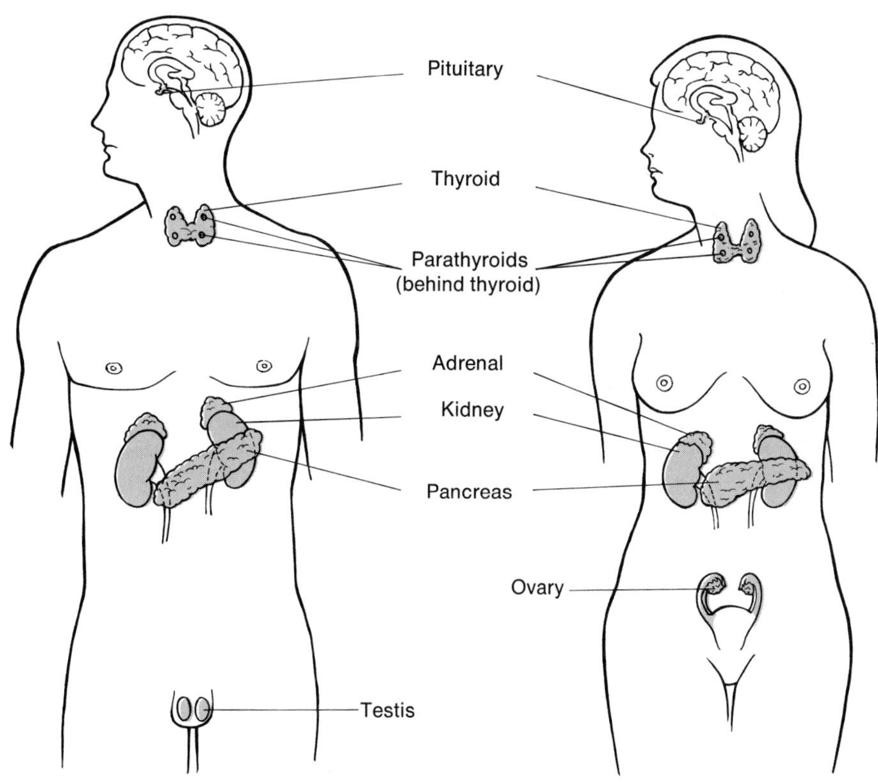

Figure 27-1 Location of the endocrine glands.

The *thyroid* gland is the largest of the endocrine glands. It consists of two lobes and is located in the neck below the pharynx and anterior to the trachea; one lobe is on each side of the trachea. The two lobes are connected with a strip of thyroid tissue called the *isthmus.* The thyroid gland stores iodine and secretes three hormones: thyroxine (T_4), triiodothyronine (T_3), and thyrocalcitonin (calcitonin). The primary function of the thyroid gland is regulation of **metabolism,** the rate at which nutrients are oxidized to provide energy for the body. Both T_4 and T_3 produce similar effects; T_4, however, acts more slowly and is longer lasting than T_3. Any disturbance in the secretion of T_4 may result in hyperthyroidism or hypothyroidism. A congenital absence of the thyroid gland causes **cretinism** in the infant, a deficiency of secretion may result in *myxedema* in the adult, and increased secretion may result in Graves' disease. Calcitonin is a hormone secreted by the thyroid gland that acts to decrease the level of calcium in the blood by increasing the movement of calcium from the blood into the bones.

The *parathyroids* are usually four small glands, but there may be more or fewer. They are arranged in pairs and embedded in the posterior lateral lobe of the thyroid gland. The parathyroids release parathormone, which helps to maintain the homeostasis or relative consistency of the calcium levels in the blood and body fluids. The presence of this hormone tends to increase calcium in the blood and to increase the excretion of phosphates.

The *adrenal* (suprarenal) *glands* are small bodies located above each kidney. Each gland is divided into two parts, the medulla and the cortex, and each part secretes different hormones. One hormone secreted by the medulla is epinephrine, prepared commercially as Adrenalin. Epinephrine has many uses, such as elevating the blood pressure, acting as a vasoconstrictor, and relaxing the bronchioles as in asthma. Because epinephrine is naturally released in stress situations and in anger, it is sometimes called the fight hormone.

The other hormone secreted by the medulla is norepinephrine, which functions as a pressor hormone to maintain blood pressure. The adrenal cortex secretes hydrocortisone (cortisol), corticosterone, aldosterone, and small amounts of sex hormones. Hydrocortisone and corticosterone have many functions in the body, but they primarily promote normal metabolism and resist stressful situations. **Aldosterone** regulates the level of sodium in the blood and body fluids. When a deficiency of cortisone and hydrocortisone occurs, Addison's disease results. Hypersecretion of ACTH (adrenocorticotropic hormone) resulting in excess cortisol causes Cushing's syndrome (Scherer, 1991).

BOX 27-1

HORMONES SECRETED BY THE ANTERIOR LOBE OF THE PITUITARY GLAND

growth hormone (somatotropin) Stimulates growth of bone and soft tissues

prolactin (lactogenic hormone) Initiates milk secretion

thyrotropin Promotes and maintains the development of the thyroid gland

adrenocorticotropic hormone (ACTH) Promotes and maintains the development of the adrenal cortex

follicle-stimulating hormone (FSH) Stimulates the development of reproductive organs

luteinizing hormone (LH) Stimulates the development of reproductive organs and secretion of progesterone and estrogens in the female and testosterone in the male

melanocyte-stimulating hormone (MSH) Stimulates pigmentation of the skin

The *pituitary body* (hypophysis) is often referred to as the master gland because it is important in regulating many of the functions of the other glands. The pituitary gland is located in the sphenoid bone in the skull and secretes several hormones. It consists of two lobes, the anterior lobe and the posterior lobe.

The release of seven hormones is controlled by the anterior lobe of the pituitary gland, the adenohypophysis (Box 27-1). The hypothalamus releases hormones that either stimulate or inhibit the release of hormones by the anterior lobe of the pituitary gland. The target organs of these hormones are illustrated in Figure 27-2.

The posterior lobe of the pituitary gland secretes two hormones, vasopressin (antidiuretic hormone, or ADH) and oxytocin. ADH affects the amount of urine excreted because it causes a faster reabsorption of water from the kidney into the blood. When extremely large amounts of urine are excreted, this indicates an inadequate amount of ADH, a disorder known as diabetes insipidus. Oxytocin affects uterine contractions and lactation and is used in obstetrics to promote uterine contraction after delivery, thus preventing excessive bleeding.

In the female the *gonads,* or sex glands, include

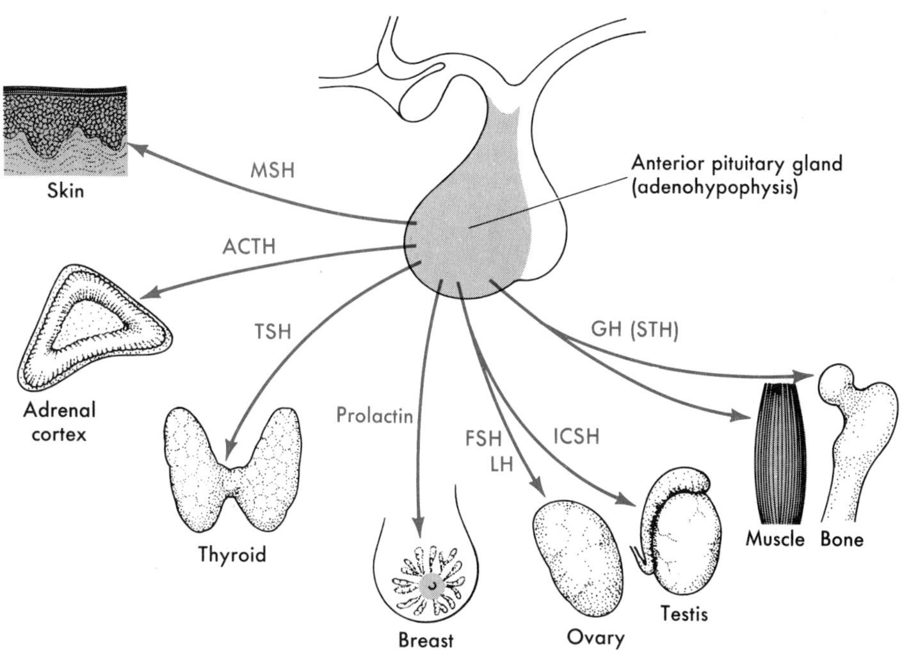

Figure 27-2 Target organs of hormones released by the anterior lobe of the pituitary gland. (From Beare P, Myers J: *Adult health nursing,* ed 2, St Louis, 1994, Mosby.)

the ovaries, which secrete estrogen, progesterone, and small amounts of androgens. Male sex glands are the testes, which secrete testosterone and androsterone. These hormones are important in the development of sex characteristics and in the reproductive process.

The *pancreas* has both exocrine and endocrine functions. Pancreatic acinar cells have an exocrine function, whereas cells known as the islets of Langerhans have an endocrine function. There are two types of islet cells: *alpha cells,* which secrete **glucagon,** a hormone that elevates the blood sugar; and *beta cells,* which secrete insulin. Insulin is necessary for the use of sugar by the body.

NURSING ASSESSMENT OF THE PATIENT WITH ENDOCRINE PROBLEMS

Endocrine problems are often difficult to assess because each hormone secreted by endocrine glands has different effects. Therefore the approach to assessment of the patient with an endocrine problem is to start with the health history. It should be determined if the patient has any cardiovascular, pulmonary, renal, neurologic, or other hormonal problems. Hypertension should be noted, along with any previous endocrine disorders.

Signs and symptoms of endocrine disorders are varied as a result of the multiple systems that may be affected. Symptoms that should be assessed include changes in smell, taste, speech, skin, personality, and energy level. Potential problems such as visual disturbances, headaches, muscle weakness, excessive hunger, thirst, and urinary frequency should be assessed.

A history of medications taken by the patient is also important. Many medications have effects on the endocrine glands and could possibly contribute to the symptoms displayed by the patient.

Physical assessment of the endocrine system is difficult because the thyroid gland is the only endocrine gland that is palpable. The primary assessment tool used for the endocrine system is inspection. Data should be collected on the individual's general appearance, apparent age, facial expression, and stature. Facial features and hair distribution should be assessed. The thyroid gland should be palpated to determine if it is enlarged or if any nodules are present (Ober, 1993).

NURSING RESPONSIBILITIES FOR DIAGNOSTIC TESTS AND PROCEDURES

Many of the tests used to initially diagnose a possible endocrine disorder, to follow its course, and to evaluate the results of therapy are performed on blood and urine. The amount and type of specific hormones can be estimated through chemical analysis of the blood and urine. When an excess or deficiency is suggested, further tests and procedures may be done to determine the effect on the whole body. Many of these tests require nursing interventions to ensure that specimens are collected properly. Some procedures require withholding food and fluids and collecting urine specimens. To ensure that the test results provide reliable information about endocrine status, procedures must be followed accurately.

NURSE ALERT

A patient's history of allergy should be determined and clearly noted before any tests.

Procedures

Blood chemistry

Analysis of endocrine gland functions is often done by hormone assay. Serum levels of hormones such as T_3 or T_4 indicate if appropriate amounts of hormones are being secreted. However, not all hormone levels can be easily determined by blood level. Insulin secretion can best be estimated by measurement of blood glucose levels. High blood glucose levels indicate that insulin secretion is insufficient for the body's metabolic needs.

Urinalysis

A 24-hour urine collection may be necessary for hormone analysis. The collection may start at any hour. The nurse should secure a clean container sufficient to hold all urine voided for the 24-hour period. The procedure should be explained to the patient to avoid error, and the hour at which the collection was started should be carefully noted. Because the test measures substances *produced* within a 24-hour time frame, the bladder must be empty at the start of the test. The patient is asked to void and the specimen is discarded, but all other urine voided after that hour is saved. The collection is completed at exactly the same hour the next day, at which time the patient voids, and that urine becomes the last part of the specimen. It is the responsibility of the nurse to see that the patient voids the last specimen exactly 24 hours from the time the collection started. For ease of collection, 24-hour urine tests are usually collected from 7:00 AM one morning until 7:00 AM the next morning.

Several precautions need to be taken in conducting urinalysis. First, the bottle should be clearly labeled with the patient's name, room number, and the date and time the collection began. Second, all urine must be collected and saved. Finally, the container holding the urine must be maintained as specified for the diagnostic test. A preservative or refrigeration may be required. Patients should be taught to collect their urine and pour it into bottles containing preservatives and to never void directly into a bottle containing a chemical. If the preservative used is an acid, the patient should be instructed to notify the nurse when he or she voids, and the nurse should pour the urine into the bottle to ensure patient safety.

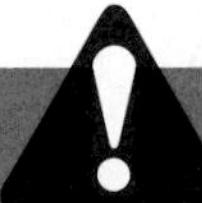

NURSE ALERT

Universal precautions must be followed when collecting all urine and blood samples. The nurse should wear gloves while obtaining specimens and wash hands after completing the collection.

Radioactive iodine uptake

The test for radioactive iodine uptake measures the ability of the thyroid gland to concentrate ingested iodine. A small amount of radioactive iodine is administered orally to the patient, either in capsule form or in a colorless, odorless drink. The amount is called a *tracer dose*. After 24 hours the amount of radioactive iodine stored in the thyroid gland is measured by a Geiger counter—a type instrument called a *scintillator*, which is held near the thyroid gland. Persons with overactive glands are found to store a high percentage of the iodine, whereas those with underactive glands take up a small amount of the iodine.

Thyroid ultrasonogram

The patient is brought to the x-ray area, and a radiologic technique visualizes the tissue structure. In an

ultrasonogram, ultrasonic waves reflect the organ, and a picture of the findings appears on an oscilloscope and paper printout.

Thyroid scan

The patient is given radioactive iodine-131 (^{131}I), and the uptake is quantitatively measured by the external passing of the scintillator over the throat. The scintillator is connected to a recording device that provides a record of the activity. The scan is used in connection with other tests and is used to differentiate between a nonmalignant condition and a possible malignancy of the thyroid gland.

Triiodothyronine (T_3) resin uptake test

In the T_3 resin uptake test, a blood specimen is secured from the patient, and ^{131}I is added to the blood in the laboratory. Normally the red blood cells take up 11% to 19% of the iodine. In hypofunction of the gland, less is taken up, whereas in hyperfunction more is taken up by the red blood cells. The advantage of the test is that the patient does not have to be given the ^{131}I.

Nursing Responsibilities

Several thyroid function tests use ^{131}I. The nurse may not be directly concerned with the test but may have important responsibilities related to the various tests. These responsibilities include reassuring the patient and encouraging cooperation. Patients should realize that they will not become radioactive as a result of the test. Care must be taken to ensure that the patient does not receive iodine before the test. Drugs that contain various iodine preparations, contrast mediums used in x-ray examinations, iodine used as a skin antiseptic, (Betadine), and iodized salt are all forms of iodine that should be avoided. The nurse should question the patient about any hypersensitivity to iodine before any testing with this drug is done.

Other diagnostic tests to detect or monitor the course of endocrine disturbances require some patient education. There are two noninvasive tests. For computed tomography (CT scan), patients should be told that a picture of their gland will be taken by a machine that moves around them. *Magnetic resonance imaging* (MRI) is a noninvasive test that uses a magnet, radiowaves, and computers to take an image of the entire body. It is a painless scanning and requires no special preparation. The presence of any metal within the patient's body, such as pacemakers, heart valves, or clips, must be known before the test.

For invasive tests such as arteriography a contrast medium is injected into a vein and travels to the organ to be examined. X-ray pictures of the gland are taken once it is visualized on the screen. When the medium is injected, some people may feel a warm sensation, which is normal.

NURSING RESPONSIBILITIES FOR THERAPEUTIC PROCEDURES

The treatment for endocrine disorders varies greatly, depending on the type of disorder. There are, however, some nursing responsibilities that are the same regardless of the problem. First and foremost is maintenance of the patient's airway. The airway should be patent, and the patient should be ventilating. Fluid and electrolyte balance should be monitored as necessary by recording fluid intake and urinary output and daily weights. Vital signs should be assessed, and the neurologic status of the patient should be monitored when indicated.

Endocrine disorders are often traumatic, both physically and emotionally, and support should be given to the patient and family. Many endocrine disorders such as diabetes and Addison's disease require lifelong treatment that may be costly and inconvenient to the patient. Feelings of frustration are commonly experienced, and the nurse should help the patient and family deal with these feelings by encouraging them to talk openly about the disorder and about the changes that need to occur in their lifestyles.

Patient education is an essential component of the treatment of endocrine disorders and is the responsibility of both the nurse and the physician. Both patient and family must understand the disorder and be prepared to deal with the lifestyle changes it may necessitate. Patients who understand the need for the diabetic meal plan will be more likely to comply with the diet than those who do not understand it. Medications to be taken by the patient should be explained. Patients, significant others, and families should know the expected results, possible side effects, and methods to minimize side effects when possible (Table 27-1). The nurse should also educate the patient regarding possible complications of the disorder. For example, patients with diabetes should know the difference between **ketoacidosis** and **insulin reaction** and the emergency treatment for both. Patient education is often the difference between compliance and noncompliance, and compliance is necessary for successful treatment of a disorder.

Support groups are available for patients to assist them in dealing with chronic endocrine problems, es-

TABLE 27-1

Pharmacology of Drugs Used for Endocrine Disorders

Drug (Generic and Trade Name); Route and Dosage	Action/Indication	Common Side Effects and Nursing Considerations
CHLORPROPAMIDE (Diabinese) **ROUTE:** PO **DOSAGE;** 100-250 mg every day initially, then 100-500 mg maintenance dose according to response; not to exceed 750 mg/day	Antidiabetic oral hypoglycemic agent used for noninsulin dependent diabetics	Headache, weakness, dizziness, and drowsiness; contraindicated in juvenile or brittle diabetes; use with caution in elderly and cardiac, thyroid, renal, or hepatic disease
FLUDROCORTISONE ACETATE (Florinef) **ROUTE:** PO **DOSAGE:** 0.1-0.2 mg every day	Drug used to promote increased reabsorption of sodium and loss of potassium from the renal tubules; used in adrenal insufficiency	Flushing, sweating, and hypertension; contraindicated in acute glomerulonephritis; use with caution in CHF and osteoporosis
GLIPIZIDE (Glucotrol) **ROUTE:** PO **DOSAGE:** 5 mg initially, then increase to desired response; do not exceed 15 mg once a day dose or 40 mg/day in divided doses	Antidiabetic second generation sulfonylurea used for stable noninsulin dependent diabetes	Headaches, weakness, dizziness, and drowsiness; contraindicated in juvenile or brittle diabetes; use with caution in the elderly and with cardiac, severe renal, severe hepatic, and thyroid disease
LEVOTHYROXINE (Synthroid, Levothroid, T4) **ROUTE:** PO, IV **DOSAGE:** PO, 12.5-50 μg as a single daily dose initially, and may be increased every 2-4 weeks; usual maintenance dose is 75-125 μg/day	Drug used for replacement or substitution therapy in diminished or absent thyroid function of many causes	Irritability, insomnia, nervousness, tachycardia, arrhythmias, and weight loss; contraindicated in recent MI or thyroidtoxicosis; use with caution in cardiac disease, severe renal insufficiency, uncorrected adrenocortical disorders, and in the elderly; can be safely used in pregnancy
PREDNISONE **ROUTE:** PO **DOSAGE:** 5-60 mg/day single dose or divided doses; maintenance dose may be given daily or every other day	Drug used systematically and locally in a wide variety of chronic diseases, including inflammations, allergic, hematologic, neoplastic, and autoimmune conditions; also used for replacement therapy in adrenal insufficiency	Depression, euphoria, hypertension, nausea, anorexia, decreased wound healing, petechiae, ecchymoses, fragility, hirsutism, acne, adrenal suppression, muscle wasting, osteoporosis, increased susceptibility to infection, and a moon face or buffalo hump appearance; chronic treatment leads to adrenal suppression; never abruptly discontinue drug; use of the drug may mask presence of infections, and it should be administered at the lowest possible dose for the shortest time period

TABLE 27-1

Pharmacology of Drugs Used for Endocrine Disorders—cont'd

Drug (Generic and Trade Name); Route and Dosage	Action/Indication	Common Side Effects and Nursing Considerations
STRONG IODINE SOLUTION, LUGOL'S SOLUTION **ROUTE:** PO **DOSAGE:** Strong iodine solution 0.1-0.3 ml (3-5 drops) tid	Drug used as an adjunct with other antithyroid drugs in preparation for thyroidectomy	Hypothyroidism, diarrhea, and hypersensitivity; use with caution in tuberculosis, bronchitis, hyperkalemia, and impaired renal function
TOLAZAMIDE (Tolinase) **ROUTE:** PO **DOSAGE:** 100 mg/day for fasting blood sugar < 200 mg/dl or 250 mg/day for FBS > 200 mg/dl; dose should be titrated to patient response (1 g or less/day)	Antidiabetic first generation sulfonylurea used in noninsulin-dependent diabetes	Headache, dizziness, hypotension, and bradycardia; contraindicated in juvenile and brittle diabetes; use with caution in the elderly and with cardiac, thyroid, renal, and hepatic disease
TOLBUTAMIDE (Orinase) **ROUTE:** PO **DOSAGE:** 1-2 g/day in divided doses, titrated to patient response	Antidiabetic first generation sulfonylurea used for noninsulin-dependent diabetes	Headache and weakness; contraindicated in juvenile or brittle diabetes; use with caution in the elderly and with cardiac, thyroid, renal, and hepatic disease
VASOPRESSIN (Pitressin) **ROUTE:** IM, SC, nasal spray **DOSAGE:** Diabetes insipidus, IM, SC 5-10 units bid to qid as needed; abdominal distention, IM 5 units, then every 3-4 hr increasing to 10 units if needed; nasal spray as ordered	Antidiuretic hormone used for diabetes insipidus, abdominal distention postoperatively, and bleeding esophageal varices	Contraindicated in chronic nephritis

pecially diabetes. Most states have local chapters of the American Diabetes Association and the Juvenile Diabetes Association, and these associations will provide lists of support groups, diabetes camps, and special education classes.

THE PATIENT WITH DISEASES AND DISORDERS OF THE ENDOCRINE SYSTEM

Disorders of the Thyroid Gland

Simple (endemic) goiter

Any enlargement of the thyroid gland is called a **goiter.** *Endemic,* or *simple,* goiter results when dietary iodine is insufficient for synthesis of thyroxine. To compensate for the insufficiency, the pituitary secretes excessive amounts of thyroid-stimulating hormone (TSH), causing the gland to hypertrophy. Iodine deficiencies in food and water exist in certain areas of the United States, and it is in those areas that the occurrence of endemic goiter has been greatest. The marketing and use of iodized salt has reduced the incidence of this type of goiter.

Increased physiologic demands such as pregnancy, lactation, puberty, infections, and other body changes can also result in an inadequate iodine supply to meet the demands. For instance, endemic goiter is more common in girls and usually occurs just before puberty, after which it may completely disappear. Usually these types of goiter produce no symptoms unless they grow large and exert pressure on adjacent structures such as the trachea. When this occurs, patients may experience mild neck discomfort, a chronic cough, difficulty in swallowing, and respiratory difficulty (Lammon, Hart, 1993).

The best treatment for goiters is prevention with adequate amounts of dietary iodine. However, once goiters have developed, treatment is aimed at decreasing the size of the gland with iodine and thyroid preparations. Large goiters may be surgically removed to relieve pressure or to improve appearance. Usually a subtotal thyroidectomy is performed. Persons living in areas where there is a known deficiency of iodine in the water and soil should be encouraged to use iodized salt and eat foods rich in natural iodine, such as leafy vegetables and seafood.

Hyperthyroidism (Graves' disease)

Hyperthyroidism is caused by an overactive thyroid gland that produces an excess of thyroid hormone. The condition may be idiopathic, or it may result from hypertrophy, neoplasms, inflammatory processes, or autoimmune disorders. Often the condition follows infections or emotional stress. The disease is known by several names, including toxic goiter, thyrotoxicosis, exophthalmic goiter, and Graves' disease. The increase in hormone production increases all metabolic processes of the body and gives rise to a characteristic set of symptoms.

Assessment. The appetite is increased, but there is weight loss, and the individual is thin. There is an increase in systolic blood pressure, and the pulse rate is greatly increased, even while the individual is at rest. There may be enlargement of the thyroid gland. The skin is warm, and the patient perspires freely and is sensitive to heat. Palpitation, tachycardia, and atrial fibrillation may occur. When the fingers are extended, a fine tremor may be observed. Fatigue, weakness, a disturbance in menstruation, a disturbance in sleep, and constipation or diarrhea may exist. Profound personality changes may be present, with irritability, excitability, and crying episodes, which may occur spontaneously. Such personality changes are often difficult for friends and family members to understand. It is therefore important that nurses provide emotional support for the family and for the patient, to help them understand that a person's emotional state is related to hormonal changes and should subside as the hormone levels decrease. There may be a bulging of the eyeballs, known as *exophthalmos,* which gives the patient a startled expression. This is a result of retraction of the upper eyelid resulting from fluid retention in extraocular muscles. Excessive tearing, blurred vision, and a feeling of pressure behind the eyes may occur. Treatment may or may not relieve symptoms. (Figure 27-3)

The symptoms of hyperthyroidism are a result of an accelerated metabolic rate and the resulting increase in all physiologic processes. It should be noted that women over the age of 50 often do not present the standard symptoms of hyperthyroidism but instead show the cardiovascular symptoms, which could include shortness of breath, palpitations, or chest pain (Scherer, 1991).

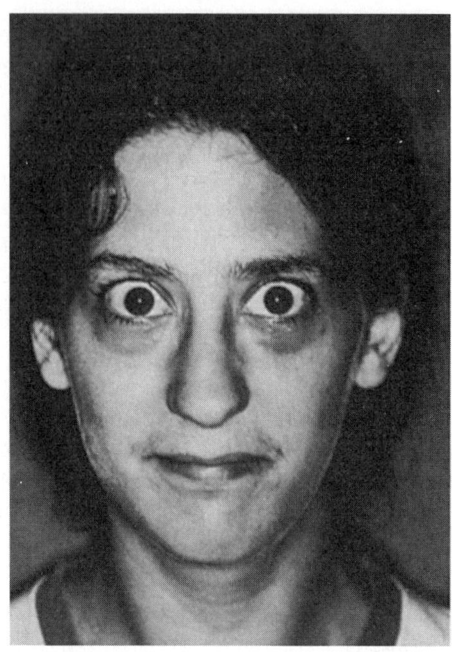

Figure 27-3 Exopthalmos occurring in hyperthyroidism. Note severe upper- and lower-lid retraction. (From Rose L, Kaye D: *Fundamentals of internal medicine,* St Louis, 1983, Mosby. In Phipps WJ and others, *Medical surgical nursing,* ed 5, St Louis, 1995, Mosby.)

Diagnostic tests show an above-normal increase in metabolic rate. A rapid and increased iodine uptake is indicated in the radioactive iodine uptake test.

Intervention. The treatment of patients with hyperthyroidism is directed toward reducing the activity of the thyroid gland and the excessive production of thyroxine (Box 27-2). The disease may be treated with antithyroid drugs, the surgical removal of the gland, or therapeutic doses of radioactive iodine.

Iodine preparations, propylthiouracil, and saturated solutions of potassium iodide (SSKI) may be given to reduce the symptoms of hyperthyroidism. They prevent the release of thyroxine but are effective only for temporary periods. Liquids are usually diluted with fruit juice, water, or milk and are administered through a straw to prevent staining of the teeth. Side effects include a metallic taste, epigastric discomfort, nausea, and vomiting. Iodine preparations are most useful before thyroid surgery or in emergency situations but are rarely used for long-term therapy.

Propranolol (Inderal) relieves many of the symptoms of hyperthyroidism, tachycardia, and hyperten-

BOX 27-2 **Nursing Process**

HYPERTHYROIDISM

ASSESSMENT

Mental status: decreased attention span, emotional lability
Cardiovascular: increased systolic blood pressure; decreased diastolic blood pressure; tachycardia at rest; arrhythmia; complaints of palpitation, chest discomfort, and dyspnea
Skin: flushed, warm
Hair: fine, thinning
Eye: lid retraction, decreased visual acuity, complaints of eyes tiring easily
Metabolic changes: decreased weight; increased food intake; decreased serum cholesterol and triglycerides; complaints of intolerance of heat, fatigue, sleep disturbance, and change in libido
Musculoskeletal: muscle weakness, decreased muscle tone, tremors

NURSING DIAGNOSES

Altered nutrition: less than body requirements related to increased metabolism
Altered thought processes related to personality changes
Sleep pattern disturbance related to increased metabolism
Ineffective thermoregulation associated with increased metabolism
Knowledge deficit related to altered metabolism
Anxiety related to inability to control illness
Ineffective individual and family coping related to personality changes

NURSING INTERVENTIONS

Keep environment quiet and calm.
Limit visitors.
Monitor vital signs and temperature.
Promote diet high in protein, vitamins, calories, and fluids.
Discourage intake of caffeinated foods (coffee, cocoa, chocolate, cola, tea).
Monitor for potential adverse effects of medications (rash, fever, conjunctivitis, generalized discomfort).
Protect eyes from trauma, especially if exophthalmos exists.
Weigh patient daily.
Observe for respiratory problems, tetany, or voice changes after thyroidectomy.
Observe for signs of complications of hyperthyroidism (thyrotoxicosis, thyroid crisis, or thyroid storm), including elevated temperature, rapid pulse and respirations, pain, dyspnea, confusion, restlessness, and alteration in level of consciousness.
Provide emotional support to patient, significant others, and family.
Educate patient, significant others, and family to watch for adverse effects of medications and for signs of thyroid crisis.

EVALUATION OF EXPECTED OUTCOMES

Verbalizes the rationale for reducing environmental stimuli
Follows a diet high in protein, vitamins, calories, and fluids
Avoids intake of caffeine
Describes the medication regimen and potential side effects of medications
Discusses the need for protection of eyes from trauma
Weighs self daily
Recognizes signs of complications of hyperthyroidism

sion. The β-andrenergic blockers help prevent critical complications from thyroid hormone excess. Because of its effectiveness, it is often used in conjunction with antithyroid drugs.

Radioactive iodine may also be given for hyperthyroidism. The drug acts the same as nonradioactive iodine, and after an oral dose it enters the bloodstream and becomes concentrated in the thyroid gland, where it destroys the cells. This treatment is inexpensive and is easily administered. Persons involved with patient care should wear gloves when giving radioactive iodine and when disposing of the patient's excreta. The major side effect is hypothyroidism.

Each patient must be considered as an individual, and patience and tact may be required in meeting nursing needs. If exophthalmos is present, the eyes need to be protected from irritation. The environment should provide rest and quiet and be free from annoying distractions. Because the patient is sensitive to warmth, the room should be private, well ventilated, and cool. Visitors should be limited to family and significant others, and efforts should be made to interpret the patient's erratic behavior as a part of the disease. The patient needs emotional as well as physical quiet and should be protected from situations that increase emotional tension and anxiety. Psychotherapy may be beneficial.

The diet should be high in calories and vitamins, with carbohydrate supplements. Extra servings should be available, and between-meal feedings may be given if sufficient calories are not taken with the regular meals. Patients should be permitted to choose food, especially if the appetite is poor, and a visit from the dietician may be helpful in ascertaining the patient's likes and dislikes. If the patient is to be cared for at home, the visiting nurse may visit the home and help plan the patient's care.

Thyroidectomy

The surgical removal of part or all of the thyroid gland may be done because of malignancy, exophthalmic goiter, or any other severe condition affecting the gland and adjacent structures. A thyroidectomy is not an emergency procedure, and the patient must have a normal thyroid functioning before surgery is done. This may require 2 to 3 months of drug therapy. Surgery is usually done only in cases of a carcinoma or large goiter. Nursing care after thyroid surgery requires more than routine postoperative care because of the location of the incision. Swelling around the incision can cause airway obstruction, and a tracheotomy tray should be available for emergency intervention. The patient should be observed for **tetany** as a result of problems with calcium metabolism related to injury to the parathyroid gland and also for voice changes as a result of injury of the vocal cords.

Thyroid crisis (storm) is a rare complication that can occur before surgery or during the initial postoperative period. It may also occur following severe physical or emotional stress. Increased amounts of thyroid hormones are released into the bloodstream, resulting in a sudden increase of metabolism. The heart rate, pulse rate, and temperature are elevated, and the patient is apprehensive, restless, and may finally become comatose and die. The patient is given oxygen, intravenous fluids, and sedatives and is placed on a hypothermia blanket to control temperature. The administration of cardiac drugs may be indicated if heart failure is imminent. This serious complication is the reason why the patient must be stabilized with antithyroid drugs preoperatively.

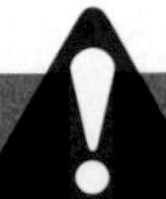

NURSE ALERT

Marked tachycardia, fever greater than 100° F (37.8° C), flushing, sweating, agitation, and restlessness are symptoms of a thyroid storm (thyrotoxic crisis). Delirium and coma can occur within 24 hours.

Hypothyroidism

Hypothyroidism is the result of an undersecretion of thyroxine by the thyroid gland or in some cases a complete lack of secretion. It may occur after surgical removal of the gland if too much thyroid tissue is removed. When the production of thyroid hormones is decreased, the symptoms are almost the reverse of those characterizing hyperthyroidism. Three conditions are recognized as resulting from hypothyroidism: myxedema, juvenile myxedema, and cretinism, all of which are actually forms of the same deficiency occurring at different ages.

Myxedema is the term applied to hypothyroidism in adults. The symptoms usually occur gradually and include sensitivity to cold, dryness of the skin and hair, weight gain despite a loss of appetite, and a gradually appearing dull facial expression with thickening of the lips and puffiness around the lips and eyes (Figure 27-4). The individual becomes lethargic and may fall asleep at intervals; the speech is slurred, and response

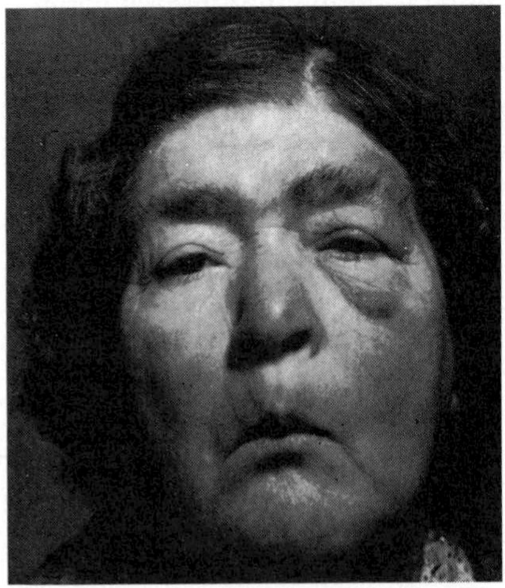

Figure 27-4 Adult with severe hypothyroidism showing typical puffiness around eyes. (From Schottelius and others: *Textbook of physiology,* ed 18, St Louis, 1978, Mosby. In Phipps WJ and others: *Medical surgical nursing,* ed 5, St Louis, 1995, Mosby.)

is slow. Impaired memory, personality changes, and depression may also occur. The pulse is slow, and the patient complains of severe fatigue.

The treatment is to replace the deficient hormone by administering synthetic triiodothyronine (T_3), levothyroxine, or desiccated thyroid. Replacement therapy is done gradually, and it may require 2 weeks or more for effects to be noticeable. A complete subsiding of symptoms may require up to 2 months or more of therapy, and once therapy is begun, it must be continued for life. Because thyroid hormone increases the metabolism, the patient's cardiovascular status must be monitored, especially during the initial weeks of therapy.

Juvenile myxedema is similar to adult myxedema and varies in degree of severity. When the disease is moderately severe, both physical and mental growth is delayed. Puberty is also delayed, and the child tends to be lethargic. The treatment is administration of levothyroxine or desiccated thyroid, which is well tolerated by the child. The dose administered is sufficient to relieve the symptoms but not large enough to result in hyperthyroidism. The dosage needs to be readjusted periodically with increasing metabolic needs. Children are usually treated in ambulatory care facilities.

Emotional support is particularly important for these children. In addition to the normal changes of

BOX 27-3

Nursing Process

HYPOTHYROIDISM

ASSESSMENT

Mental status: slowing of intellectual functions, altered memory, somnolence, lethargy or confusion
Cardiovascular: peripheral edema, bradycardia, observe for cardiorespiratory complications
Skin: cool, pale, may become dry and thickened
Hair: thin
Metabolic: weight gain, decreased appetite, tiredness, weakness, intolerance to cold, constipation, increased serum triglycerides and cholesterol
Neurologic: slowed speech, deepened voice, lethargy progressing to coma, slow reflexes, paresthesia
Reproductive: decreased libido, change in menses

NURSING DIAGNOSES

Altered nutrition: more than body requirements related to decreased metabolism
Altered thought processes related to personality changes
Ineffective thermoregulation related to decreased metabolism
Chronic low self-esteem related to depression
Knowledge deficit related to altered metabolism
Ineffective individual and family coping related to personality changes

NURSING INTERVENTIONS

Keep environment warm.
Promote care of skin with lotions.
Monitor effects of medications, especially those depressing central nervous system; drugs may be potentiated because of decreased metabolism.
Assess for signs of infection carefully because resistance to infection may be decreased.
Prevent constipation by encouraging good bowel habits: exercise and eat diet high in fiber, fruits, and fluids.
Prevent hypoxia by encouraging deep breathing and moving.
Promote good nutritional status by decreasing caloric intake if necessary to promote weight loss.
Support patient and family emotionally during treatment, which usually leads to dramatic reversal of symptoms.
Educate patient and family to watch for side effects of therapy, such as tachycardia, sleeplessness, palpitations, and anxiety.

EVALUATION OF EXPECTED OUTCOMES

Verbalizes principles of good skin care and demonstrates an ability to perform this care
Describes the medication regimen and potential side effects of medications (tachycardia, sleeplessness, palpitations, anxiety)
Discusses signs of infection (redness, warmth, fever)
Practices good bowel habits by exercising and eating a diet high in fruits, fiber, and fluids
Follows a well-balanced diet and monitors weight
Performs deep-breathing and moving exercises every 1 to 2 hours

adolescence, they must also deal with the changes caused by hypothyroidism and its treatment. Adolescence is often associated with feelings of rebellion; therefore teaching the importance of management of hypothyroidism and compliance with therapy is essential.

Cretinism is the result of a complete absence of thyroid secretion from birth, which may be caused by absence of the gland or its failure to secrete thyroxin. Intrauterine development is usually normal, but the characteristics of the condition may begin in the first few weeks after birth. The first symptoms are difficulty in breast-feeding, failure to thrive, protrusion of the tongue, dry skin, constipation, and a hoarse cry. If the condition is not recognized early, irreversible damage may occur in physical and mental development. Because the effects of cretinism are easily prevented with an early diagnosis, many states have mandated testing of thyroxine (T_4) levels after birth. Box 27-3 summarizes interventions for the patient with hypothyroidism.

Tumors of the thyroid gland

Tumors occurring in the thyroid gland may be benign or malignant and may be associated with hyperthyroidism. Enlargement of the thyroid from benign tumors is referred to as *nodular goiter,* and the tumors may be single or multiple. Some of the tumors secrete thyroxine because they consist of the same type of cells as those found in normal thyroid tissue. If they secrete appreciable amounts of the hormone, hyperthyroidism develops, and the symptoms are the same as those generally associated with hyperthyroidism. Surgical removal is generally indicated for the nodular type of tumors.

Carcinoma of the thyroid may be any of several types. Some types grow slowly and metastasize first to the lymph nodes, then to the lungs and bones. Other types progress rapidly, and some may be fatal within a few weeks. Surgery has proven to be the most satisfactory method of treatment, although radioactive iodine and x-ray therapy may be used in conjunction with surgery for some types. The nurse may care for patients for whom treatment is only palliative. The same physical care and emotional support are necessary as for all patients with terminal cancer.

Disorders of the Parathyroid Glands

Hyperparathyroidism is one of the most common endocrine disorders. Excessive secretion of parathormone (hyperparathyroidism) may be caused by a benign tumor of one of the glands. The purpose of the hormone is to maintain a constant calcium balance in the blood. Too much parathyroid hormone causes a calcium imbalance by allowing the calcium in the bones to be removed and migrate into the bloodstream. The bones become weak, tender, and painful, and spontaneous fractures may occur. The appetite may become poor, constipation may be present, and there may be fatigue, depression, weight loss, and loss of muscle tone, which makes walking difficult for the patient. An increase in the blood calcium level occurs, and renal calculi composed chiefly of calcium salts may form in the kidney. Small tumors, which are detected by x-ray examination, may form in the bones. The treatment is surgical removal of the tumor or removal of the overactive gland. Following surgery, all symptoms should disappear, and the bones gradually strengthen.

When too little parathormone is secreted (hypoparathyroidism), the level of blood calcium decreases and phosphorus increases in the blood. The deficiency of the hormone may result from injury to the glands or the removal of too much parathyroid tissue during a thyroidectomy. The primary symptom is tetany resulting from the decreased level of blood calcium. There is lack of muscular coordination, resulting in tremor and muscular spasm. Laryngeal spasm and generalized convulsions may occur. The treatment is to elevate the blood calcium level by the administration of calcium salts, parathormone extract, and vitamin D. Depending on the severity of the condition, calcium gluconate in physiologic saline solution, parathormone solution, and vitamin D may be administered intravenously.

Disorders of the Adrenal (Suprarenal) Glands

The body has two adrenal glands located immediately above the kidneys. Each adrenal gland consists of two parts, which function as separate glands. The outer part, the adrenal cortex, produces several different hormones that are essential to life. These include the glucocorticoids, the mineralocorticoids, and sex hormones. The glucocorticoids *cortisone* and *hydrocortisone* regulate much of the cell activity of the body and maintain an optimum internal environment for the body cells. They also regulate the body's ability to adapt to constant changes in the external environment. The mineralocorticoids help regulate electrolyte metabolism. **Aldosterone** is the most important mineralocorticoid, and its primary function is to maintain homeostasis of sodium concentration in the blood. Small amounts of the male hormone androgen and female hormone estrogen are also secreted by the adrenal cortex. The adrenal medulla secretes the **catecholamines** epinephrine and norepinephrine, two hormones that tend to increase and prolong the effects of the sympathetic nervous system. Epinephrine and norepinephrine primarily affect smooth muscle, cardiac muscle, and glandular activity and are responsible for the "fight or flight" response to stress situations.

Addison's disease

Hypofunction of the adrenal cortex resulting in insufficient secretion of hormones causes Addison's disease. The specific cause for the **atrophy,** or wasting away, of the gland is unknown, but it often is diagnosed after the patient has undergone stressful situations such as injury, infection, or surgery. Autoantibodies that react against adrenal tissues have been discovered in a significant number of patients. This finding suggests that Addison's disease may be an autoimmune process.

Symptoms result from inadequate amounts of adrenocortical hormones in the blood and body fluids. Common gastrointestinal symptoms are nausea, vomiting, anorexia, diarrhea, and abdominal pain. The patient may fatigue easily and show signs of hypoglycemia such as nervousness, increased perspiration (diaphoresis), headache, and trembling. These symptoms result from inadequate amounts of circulating cortisone and hydrocortisone. The normal fluid and electrolyte balance is interrupted, and the patient has a deficiency of sodium and chloride and an excess of potassium because of insufficient aldosterone. Often the skin develops a bronze color, and the patient appears tanned (Peterson, 1992).

Addison's disease is treated by reestablishing a state of normal hydration and then replacing hydrocortisone and fludrocortisone (Florinef) (see Table 27-1). Both of these medications should be given after meals because they may cause gastrointestinal upset. Once therapy is begun, it is essential that the patient understand that Addison's disease is a lifelong disorder and that medications should not be adjusted or stopped except under the guidance of a healthcare professional. Patients should avoid undue stress, both mental and physical, and should carry a Medic Alert tag or card identifying them as having Addison's disease and listing emergency measures to be taken. An addisonian crisis is a serious exacerbation of the disease and may produce a severe drop in blood pressure, leading to shock, coma, and death. When this occurs, fluids are replaced with normal saline solution, and hydrocortisone may be given intravenously.

Education is extremely important for patients with Addison's disease and their families because mild physical or emotional stress, as well as minor infection, can bring on an addisonian crisis. Patients and families must have knowledge of the signs and symptoms of inadequate or excessive steroid levels and understand the need to report symptoms promptly.

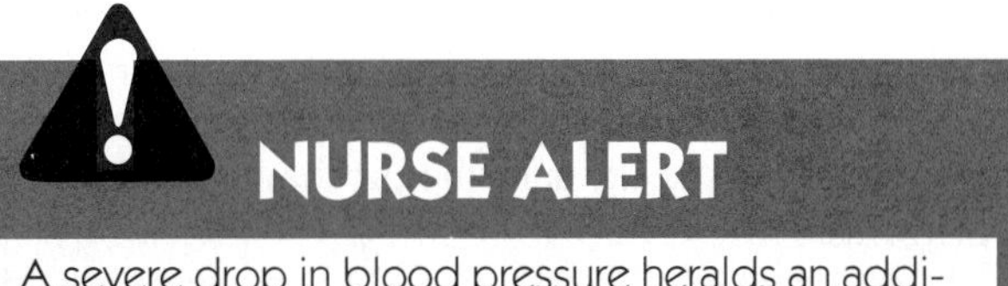

A severe drop in blood pressure heralds an addisonian crisis.

Secondary hypoadrenalism

Steroid (hydrocortisone) therapy is commonly used in the treatment of asthma and ulcerative colitis. Long-term treatment with steroids leads to atrophy of the adrenal glands. If steroid therapy is withdrawn too suddenly, symptoms similar to those of Addison's disease occur. The patient feels lethargic and weak and may become hypotensive. The response to stress such as surgery may be severe depression; therefore it is important to know if a patient going into surgery has been receiving steroid therapy. Withdrawal from steroid therapy must be done very slowly to allow the adrenal glands to recover.

Cushing's syndrome

Hyperfunction of the adrenal cortex produces an excessive secretion of hormones from the gland and results in Cushing's syndrome. The cause is usually a tumor in the anterior pituitary gland or a tumor of the adrenal cortex.

Characteristic symptoms of Cushing's syndrome reflect exaggeration of the normal functions of adrenal hormones. These include weakness with muscle wasting; fat accumulation in the face, neck, and trunk creating a "humpback" appearance; hemorrhagic tendencies; changes in secondary sex characteristics including **hirsutism;** hypertension; obesity; menstrual irregularities; hyperglycemia; irritability; and symptoms of fluid and electrolyte imbalance. The patient's appearance may be upsetting, especially to the woman

OLDER ADULT CONSIDERATIONS

Elderly patients with acute symptoms, including weakness and confusion, need careful assessment for adrenal insufficiency.

Determine whether elderly patients have been taking corticosteroids for a chronic disease.

affected by Cushing's syndrome, and the patient may withdraw from others.

Nursing care should convey acceptance and reassurance. Treatment usually involves surgical removal of the tumor, if possible. However, if the pituitary gland is involved, a hypophysectomy (removal of the gland) or irradiation of the pituitary gland may be performed.

A variety of chronic diseases are treated with adrenal steroids, although no adrenal disease is present. Examples of such diseases are rheumatoid arthritis, leukemia, emphysema, and ulcerative colitis. Drugs such as prednisone have potent antiinflammatory effects, which can be of great therapeutic value. However, most patients treated with adrenal steroids develop Cushing's syndrome to a variable degree, and serious complications and side effects can occur. Careful observation, notation, and reporting by the nurse is a requirement. Some side effects of prednisone may be decreased if the desired therapeutic result can be obtained when the drug is given on alternate days.

Patient and family teaching. Side effects of prednisone may be minimized through patient education. For those individuals who are susceptible to weight gain, caloric control should be initiated at the beginning of steroid therapy. Females who develop a moon face should be instructed in makeup techniques and clothing to minimize the appearance of that side effect (e.g., avoid wearing turtlenecks). Families should be instructed to expect mood swings in individuals who are taking steroids.

Pheochromocytoma

Pheochromocytoma is a catecholamine-producing tumor of the adrenal medulla. These tumors are generally small and benign, with only a tiny number being malignant. Pheochromocytoma is believed to be associated with neurofibromatosis and tumors of the thyroid gland and may be hereditary.

Symptoms result from the hypersecretion of epinephrine and norepinephrine. The characteristic symptom is hypertension. However, the hypertension may be variable, being persistent and chronic or occurring in intermittent attacks. Because of the elevated blood pressure, pheochromocytoma is often confused with essential hypertension. Other symptoms may include severe headache, excessive sweating, nausea, vomiting, palpitation, and nervousness with acute anxiety. During an acute attack, tachycardia, hyperglycemia, and polyuria may occur.

The diagnosis of pheochromocytoma may be made by testing the urine for elevated levels of metanephrine (a by-product of epinephrine metabolism), using a 24-hour urine collection. When collecting the specimen, the urine should be kept on ice in a dark container with a preservative (hydrochloric acid). Pheochromocytoma may also be diagnosed by urine levels of vanillylmandelic acid (VMA), by intravenous pyelography, or by aortography. A CT scan, MRI, or ultrasound may also be useful for diagnosis. The treatment is removal of the tumor.

Adrenalectomy

Adrenalectomy is the surgical removal of the adrenal gland, usually because of a pathologic disorder such as a tumor. The preoperative preparation of the patient is the same as that for other abdominal surgery. The postoperative care may require the administration of hydrocortisone if the adrenal cortex has been removed. When surgery has been done because of pheochromocytoma, the patient's condition may be critical for the first 48 hours. Shock may occur because of the abrupt fall in blood pressure. Blood pressure must be monitored continuously and the patient observed for hemorrhage, which may be external or internal. Urinary output must be observed for signs of oliguria. Vasopressor drugs are administered intravenously. Caution should be used when administering narcotic drugs for pain because some have a tendency to cause hypotension. After the critical period the recovery progresses normally. If both adrenal glands are removed, the patient needs hormone replacement therapy for the rest of his or her life.

Disorders of the Pituitary Gland

The *hypophysis,* or pituitary gland, has been called the *master gland* because it exerts some control over the other endocrine glands. The anterior lobe secretes several hormones, including growth hormone, and the posterior lobe secretes two hormones, including the antidiuretic hormone (ADH).

A hypersecretion of the anterior lobe of the pituitary gland may result from a tumor affecting certain cells. The condition causes *acromegaly* in the adult and is characterized by the following symptoms: the features become coarse, the bones become large and heavy, the hands and feet become broad and massive, the chin protrudes, and the tongue enlarges. These effects are primarily caused by the effects of increased amounts of growth hormone circulating throughout the body. Surgical removal of the tumor may be extremely difficult, and radiation therapy may be used in treatment of the condition. A congenital deficiency of the growth hormone results in *dwarfism* (midget), whereas a tumor affecting the growth hormone in childhood or

PATIENT/FAMILY TEACHING

Disorders of the pituitary gland

Give the patient written instructions at discharge on the following:

- Importance of taking all medication
- Signs and symptoms of dehydration
- Need to monitor weight
- What to do if nasal congestion is present and one of the medications is taken by inhalation

(DeWit, 1992)

adolescence causes the individual to grow extremely tall, resulting in *gigantism.*

Diabetes insipidus is a disease caused by failure of the posterior lobe of the pituitary gland to secrete sufficient amounts of ADH. ADH functions to increase the amount of water reabsorbed from the kidney tubules, and in its absence large amounts of urine are excreted, as much as 10 L daily. Excessive fluid and electrolyte losses occur, producing symptoms such as dehydration, insatiable thirst, weakness, weight loss, and anorexia. Treatment includes parenteral fluids and ADH replacement therapy either parenterally or through nasal spray. Daily accurate intake and output is especially important to ensure that the patient is receiving the therapeutic dose of medication (Scherer, 1991).

Because the pituitary gland regulates many functions of the body and controls other functions through its influence on the other glands, many disorders may result from an oversecretion or undersecretion of its various hormones. Because many of these conditions occur only rarely, a discussion of them is not included here.

Disorders of the Pancreas

Diabetes mellitus

Diabetes mellitus is the most common endocrine disorder in the United States. The American Diabetes Association estimates that there are 13 million people in the United States with type II diabetes. More than 6 million are over age 65. Approximately 1 in every 20 Americans is or will be affected by this metabolic problem. Diabetes mellitus is a chronic, currently incurable health problem that results from defects in insulin action or secretion. It is a heterogeneous group of anatomic and chemical problems characterized by high blood-glucose levels. In addition to the initially observed problem with carbohydrate metabolism, individuals who have diabetes mellitus also have a deficit in their conversion of proteins and fats.

Although the etiology of diabetes mellitus is currently unknown, there are probably diverse causes. Known risk factors for developing diabetes mellitus are heredity, environment, and lifestyle. Blood relatives of people who have diabetes, especially type II, are more likely to develop diabetes than are individuals not related to anyone with the disease. Overweight individuals and those who lead a sedentary lifestyle are more prone to develop type II diabetes mellitus. Certain viruses and autoimmune factors have been associated with the development of the disease and are thought to play a role in its etiology. Chickenpox-type viruses have been associated with the development of type I diabetes mellitus. The present thinking is that diabetes develops as a result of a combination of risk factors.

Diabetes is the leading cause of blindness, heart attack, stroke, and gangrene. Improvements in therapeutic techniques have increased the average life span of the individual who has diabetes, but prevention through health education of the complications of the disease are appropriate.

Pathophysiology. The symptoms of diabetes mellitus result from insulin deficiency. Insulin is secreted by the beta cells in the islets of Langerhans in the pancreas. The deficiency may result because of diminished or absolute lack of insulin or as a result of resistance to insulin action at the cell level. Lack of enough usable insulin causes **hyperglycemia,** a high blood-glucose level.

An adequate supply of insulin in the body is necessary for the body cells to combine oxygen and glucose to produce the energy necessary for body functions. In the absence of insulin several metabolic changes occur. Glucose accumulates in the blood and is excreted in the urine. The body is then required to use proteins and fat for energy, which under certain conditions will lead to metabolic acidosis.

Diabetes mellitus is classified as either insulin dependent (IDDM), **type I;** or as noninsulin dependent (NIDDM), **type II** (Table 27-2). Formerly IDDM individuals were classified as having juvenile-onset, or brittle diabetes. NIDDM individuals previously were described as having stable, or adult-onset, diabetes. Clinically many patients lie between the two extremes, and nursing interventions are directed toward individual responses to diabetes and its treatment, regardless of classification. But because the pathogenesis, treatment, and possible complications of the types differ, the two classes are discussed separately.

Assessment. The two classifications differ in respect to insulin dependency, onset and symptoms, and intensity of treatment. Type I diabetes commonly has a

TABLE 27-2

Comparison of Type I and Type II Diabetes Mellitus

Type I (IDDM)	Type II (NIDDM)
Less than 10% of known cases of diabetes mellitus	90% of all known cases of diabetes mellitus
Any age, peaks at 5 and 11	Over age 30
Usually thin	Obese
Abrupt symptoms	Few symptoms
Ketosis prone	Nonketosis prone
Severe insulinopenia	Insulin levels normal, depressed, or elevated
Dependent on insulin for life	Not dependent on insulin for life
Autoimmune disease	Autosomal dominant inheritance
At risk for complications of retinopathy, neuropathy, and nephropathy	At risk for microvascular and macrovascular complications

sudden onset marked by an excessive concentration of glucose in the blood and the presence of the three *poly*'s associated with diabetes: polyuria, polydipsia, and polyphagia accompanied by weight loss. Type II diabetes is characterized by a slow insidious onset and may go undetected for years.

Lack of insulin or a problem with its use at the cellular level initiates a chain of events that accounts for the initial symptoms of type I diabetes. With an insulin deficiency, glucose cannot enter the cell and accumulates in the bloodstream. This is evidenced by hyperglycemia. Because the body cannot use this glucose for food or energy, it keeps piling up until the kidneys excrete it. Glucose is dissolved in fluid in the bloodstream, so when it is excreted by the kidneys (glycosuria), not only is it wasted, but so is the water in which it is dissolved. This accounts for the *polyuria*, or excessive urination. The increase in the amount of fluid lost makes the individual very thirsty, *polydipsia*, so the patient drinks extra liquids to maintain fluid balance. Instead of being absorbed into the cell, glucose is lost in urine. Because those calories were not used, the appetite mechanism is stimulated and the individual becomes very hungry and eats an excessive amount of food, which is known as *polyphagia*. There is no weight gain because calories are wasted when the glucose is excreted into the urine.

Diabetes is a complex phenomenon. The analogy of insulin helping to unlock the cell wall so that circulating glucose can enter into the cell has been used as a learning device for patients. The absorption of glucose into the cell, the resultant circulating glucose level, and its potential spill into urine are different, depending on the presence or absence of available insulin.

Individuals who develop type I diabetes are usually young, of normal weight or have recently experienced weight loss, and often show signs of polyuria, polydipsia, polyphagia, and **ketosis** (an accumulation of ketone bodies in the blood and tissues). When left untreated, other symptoms that result include dry skin and mucous membranes, constipation, and signs of fluid and electrolyte losses. These undiagnosed individuals may develop diabetic ketoacidosis and die unless this process is stopped by **exogenous** insulin (insulin that is produced outside the body). Most people who have type I diabetes eventually require insulin to manage their diabetes.

Type II diabetes symptoms are usually so mild that the condition may exist undetected and untreated for a considerable period. Often individuals are middle-aged and overweight. They have some **endogenous** (produced within the body) insulin, but its secretion may be slow or subnormal. When this diabetes exists for a long time and is untreated, symptoms of varied severity may occur. These symptoms include skin infections such as boils and carbuncles and arteriosclerotic conditions, particularly of the eyes, kidneys, lower extremities, and coronary and cerebral blood vessels. Some people who have type II diabetes are able to control the disease with diet and exercise alone, others require the addition of an oral hypoglycemic agent, and a third group requires insulin.

Treatment goal. The therapeutic goal of diabetes management is to maintain a blood glucose level that is as close to normal as possible while allowing the patient to maintain a normal lifestyle. Diabetes cannot be cured, but its symptoms can be controlled and its pathologic course may be kept in check. The therapeutic management of diabetes mellitus is palliative. The goals of hyperglycemia reduction, prevention of acute complications (insulin reaction; diabetic ketoacidosis; and **hyperglycemic, hyperosmolar, nonketotic coma**), and forestalling chronic complications (microvascular and macrovascular angiopathies) guide clinicians as they plan the diabetic regimen with the individual.

Priorities of nursing care are first concerned with immediate patient needs and then with long-range needs because diabetes at the present time is a lifetime disease. Patients must assume a great deal of responsibility for their self-care management and become partners with clinicians who provide needed healthcare. Because individuals who have diabetes become managers of their chronic illness on a day-to-day basis, they are not always in a patient role. Therefore instead of always labeling people who have diabetes as patients, the should be referred to as persons or individuals. The word **diabetic** should only be used as an adjective to describe a component of the regimen, such as diabetic meal plan. The label *diabetic* should never be used to refer to a person.

Diagnostic tests. The range of clinical symptoms of new-onset diabetes mellitus is from none to coma, depending on the type of diabetes and the length of time it is undetected. The sooner individuals who have diabetes mellitus are diagnosed and begin to control their disease, the more the chronic problems associated with the disorder can be prevented. Because type II diabetes first appears with such mild symptoms, it may go undetected for years. Screening programs are effective in early diagnosis. In contrast, individuals who have type I diabetes mellitus often have the recognizable classic symptoms of diabetes or progress to a state of acidosis that prompts them to seek healthcare. The initial diagnosis of diabetes mellitus is accomplished by analyzing the patient's blood or urine for the presence and amount of glucose.

Neither glucose nor acetone are normally present in urine. Their presence indicates the possibility of diabetes mellitus and the need for additional diagnostic tests. Glucose in urine means that the blood-glucose level has exceeded the **renal threshold,** which is the blood-glucose level for an individual that must be reached before circulating glucose is removed from the blood by the kidneys. The presence of **acetone,** one of the ketone bodies produced in abnormally large amounts in uncontrolled diabetes mellitus, in the urine means the body has rapidly broken down fats to use as energy and that some of the breakdown product has been removed from the bloodstream and is present in the urine. Severe dieting or a high-fat diet can also cause **ketonuria,** an excess of ketone bodies in the urine.

Glucose is always present in the blood. The amount varies according to a number of factors. Whether the blood sample is venous, capillary, or arterial affects glucose levels. The type of blood specimen, such as whole, plasma, or serum, also influences the value of the glucose detected. Fluctuations in amount of glucose occur secondarily to the type of foods the individual has eaten. How recently and how much food has been consumed is also a factor. Laboratory analyses can differ, so the upper and lower range of normal for a specific setting must be determined. All these factors must be known before a decision regarding the presence or absence of diabetes can be made on the basis of blood glucose level. The amount of glucose is reported in the number of milligrams (mg) present in 100 milliliters (100 ml) of fluid. One deciliter (1 dl) equals 100 ml and is the standard way the value is reported. A value of 100 mg/dl means that 100 mg of glucose are present in 100 ml of plasma.

Consistency in the diagnosis of diabetes is being achieved by the use of criteria recommended by the National Diabetes Data Group of the National Institutes of Health (Sperling, 1988). The diagnosis of diabetes can be made for nonpregnant adults when one of the following signs is present: (1) classic symptoms of diabetes and hyperglycemia with a random plasma glucose level of 200 mg/dl or greater; (2) a fasting venous plasma glucose level at least equal to 140 mg/dl on two occasions; or (3) an elevated venous plasma glucose level once after drinking glucose and before the 2-hour point *and* at the 2-hour point in an oral glucose tolerance test. A fasting plasma glucose level over 130 mg/dl should be an indication for further testing in children. Diabetic ketoacidosis can occur rapidly in young children, so early diagnosis and treatment is especially important.

An oral glucose-tolerance test is done after an individual has eaten a high carbohydrate diet for 3 days. The person fasts from the evening before the test until the last specimen has been obtained. The day of the test, an initial fasting blood sample is drawn and sent to the laboratory. The patient is given a pure glucose drink. Consuming the very sweet-tasting drink on an empty stomach may make the person feel a little nauseous. Because the test is terminated if vomiting occurs, the nurse should instruct the patient to assume a comfortable position during the test. Blood samples are collected at various specified intervals until the test is complete. An elevated glucose level at the 2-hour point usually indicates some disorder of carbohydrate metabolism.

Another common test is a 2-hour postprandial blood sugar test that is drawn exactly 2 hours after the patient finishes the specified meal. Individuals who do not have diabetes mellitus would have a 2-hour postprandial blood-glucose level that had returned to the normal fasting range.

NURSE ALERT

The patient who has blood-glucose tests in the morning should be told that breakfast will not be served until after the blood specimen has been taken.

Immediately after the diagnosis is made, healthcare providers monitor the status of the individual's diabetes and responses to treatment. Patients are taught to self-monitor their own condition as soon as possible. Patients learn the rationale for and techniques to correctly obtain the desired specimen and test it for the presence and amount of glucose or acetone.

Urine testing provides an approximation of the individual's blood-glucose level. An individual's renal threshold determines when blood glucose spills over into urine. For adults with no renal problems, this threshold is approximately 170 to 200 mg, which means the blood glucose level must be least 170 mg before any glucose could be wasted into the urine. Individuals determine their own renal threshold by recording their blood-glucose values and comparing them with their urine glucose values. The lowest blood glucose value at which glucose spills into the urine is an estimate of the renal threshold.

When insulin is being used, the timing of specimen collection varies. Urine specimens are collected approximately 30 minutes before mealtime and at bedtime. Patients should be instructed to test a second voided specimen to avoid testing urine that has been allowed to pool in the bladder since a previous meal. Individuals who control their disease by diet alone or with an oral hypoglycemic agent may test their urine after meals. Clinitest, Tes-Tape, or strips may be used to test urine. The product used should reflect the patient's choice and abilities. Because urine testing for glucose is a retrospective test and shows what blood-glucose levels were 1 to 2 hours earlier, clinicians encourage blood glucose testing as a more accurate measurement.

Urine testing is the only method patients can use to test for ketones. The patient should be instructed to test urine for ketones if there is a large amount of glycosuria, if there is a blood-glucose level over 240 mg/dl, or if there are symptoms of illness. When acetone is present in the urine, the body has metabolized fatty acids. This can occur during a usual overnight fast, and a trace amount may be expected every morning. Conversely, larger amounts of ketone bodies can be a sign that the person requires more insulin.

Because it is desirable to keep the blood glucose in a range close to normal, a more accurate appraisal of blood glucose can be achieved by testing blood glucose levels. Morning blood glucose determinations should be done on specimens collected in a fasting state. Insulin or oral agents should be held until after the specimen has been obtained. The patient having blood-glucose tests in the morning should be told that breakfast will not be served until after the blood specimen has been taken.

Self-monitoring of blood-glucose levels may be done with the use of commercial products such as visual strips or meters. A finger stick is done, and capillary blood is placed on the test strip. After a certain amount of time, the reagent strip turns to a color indicating the amount of glucose in the blood. A color comparison of the strip to the chart indicates the amount of glucose present. Meters can automate the calculation and give a readout of the glucose level. Home measurement of blood glucose is recommended for all individuals on insulin therapy.

In 1994 the American Diabetes Association issued a policy statement strongly recommending that certain classes of patients self-monitor their blood-glucose levels (American Diabetes Association, 1994a). Some patients require frequent insulin dose adjustments on the basis of blood-glucose levels. These patients include those who are (1) receiving intensive insulin therapy by insulin pump or multiple daily injections, (2) pregnant or plan to be, or (3) prone to hypoglycemia but who may not experience warning signs of hypoglycemia. In another policy statement, the American Diabetes Association stressed the importance of blood-glucose self-monitoring to meet treatment goals. They stated that patients must be taught blood-glucose self-monitoring if their treatment goals included maintenance of specific blood sugar levels, prevention of severe hyperglycemia, prevention of frequent hypoglycemia, and insulin adjustment to meet lifestyle changes (American Diabetes Association, 1994b).

Individuals who are taught to monitor their diabetes at home need to follow the same precautions that nurses in healthcare facilities take with similar diagnostic products. The most important precaution is the most basic: Read and carefully follow the manufacturer's directions! The individual should wait the exact number of seconds required before examining the strip or solution for color change. He or she should be sure to use the specific color chart or automatic device designed for the test. The individual should observe the reagents and color strips to be sure they have not discolored or gone bad, which would make them inaccurate. The individual should test the calibration of instruments used to ensure their accuracy and should clean them regularly according to package directions. He or she should store all testing materials in a place safe for both the product and the people who live in the same environment. There are many glucose meters on the market today. Most are extremely easy to use, and the nurse can assist the patient by following package or video instructions. Patient technique should be observed before discharge to ensure proper home use. All blood-glucose monitoring requires patients to puncture the skin to obtain blood samples. Companies are working on noninvasive blood-glucose testing using near-infrared light that can see through the skin. Although the new technology could be expensive, it would reduce many problems with technique and compliance (National Diabetes Information Clearinghouse, 1993).

Glycohemoglobin levels are another diagnostic test used in diabetes. Glycosylated hemoglobin forms when glucose in the blood attaches to the hemoglobin in the red blood cells. The higher the blood-glucose level, the more glucose is attached and the higher the result. Because urine and blood-glucose levels reflect the present, they are easily influenced by recent events and are useful in determining daily insulin or dietary requirements. The glycohemoglobin level represents the degree of glucose control achieved during the previous several weeks and is a general indicator of long-term metabolic control. Glycohemoglobin production increases in the presence of hyperglycemia. An elevated glycohemoglobin level means that the patient's blood-glucose levels were consistently high for 6 to 8 weeks previously. Because the palliative goal of diabetes therapy is to achieve good metabolic control without complications, glycohemoglobin levels are assessed periodically.

Providers and patients must exercise some general precautions regarding the use and interpretations of diabetic diagnostic tests. The specific test and range of normal may differ from setting to setting. The important consideration is not to memorize lists of laboratory values but to know what the normal ranges of values are in the setting in which the specimen was analyzed.

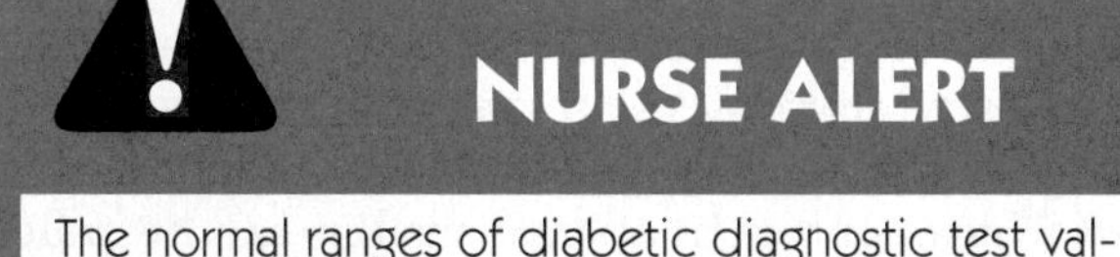

NURSE ALERT

The normal ranges of diabetic diagnostic test values vary according to the setting.

Meal plan. There is no standard "diabetic diet." Meal plans are developed for the individual patient on the basis of caloric needs, nutritional requirements, and usual eating habits. Many patients with type II, mild diabetes are maintained on only their food intake and exercise. Some meal plans control calories and are commonly prescribed for older, obese patients who do not require insulin therapy. The metabolic picture of obese patients with type II diabetes often improves after they reduce their weight.

For patients who have unstable type I diabetes, the meal plan is first calculated and then the amount of insulin necessary to metabolize it is established. A meal plan controls the amount of protein, fat, cholesterol, carbohydrate, fiber, and calories. The amount of food is divided into specific amounts to be eaten at meals and for snacks at predetermined times.

Usually the food-exchange lists prepared jointly by the American Diabetes Association, the American Dietetic Association, and the United States Public Health Service are used in planning the patient's therapeutic meal plan. Seven lists of exchangeable foods have been defined: (1) foods with a minimum caloric content that are allowed as desired; (2) vegetables; (3) fruits; (4) bread; (5) meat; (6) fats; and (7) milk. Each item on a specific list is equal in nutritional value, and similar amounts are interchangeable with one another (Figure 27-5). A specified number of exchanges is allowed for each meal and snack according to the caloric needs of the patient and the prescribed plan (Table 27-3).

The individual's usual lifestyle, preferences, and cultural differences are considered when the meal plan is established. Because the discipline of dietary restrictions and the need to eat at prescribed time intervals are so demanding, it is crucial that the meal plan be accommodated into the patient's routine as much as possible. Creativity of healthcare providers exercised within therapeutic guidelines can help minimize the tedium of following the same plan day after day. Individuals can be taught how to eat at fast-food chains and to correctly "augment" their diet. For instance, a person who craves a large glass of orange juice in the morning but is allowed only 4 ounces can be taught to add 4 ounces of sugar-free orange tonic to their juice. Eight ounces of frosty, cold, orange-juice–tasting liquid can be had for one fruit exchange.

In 1994 the American Diabetes Association released new dietary guidelines for people with diabetes. Sugars and starches are now one food category and can be exchanged. However, food containing carbohydrates must still be measured. If a high-sugar food is selected, one gets a smaller amount than with a low-sugar counterpart. For example, ⅓ cup of frosted flakes would be equal to ¾ cup of corn flakes. Many high-sugar foods contain fat and should be avoided (American Diabetes Association, 1994b).

Diet therapy for people who have type I diabetes follows a specific time frame. When the action of insulin is at its peak, patients must have enough circulating glucose in their bloodstream to move into the cells. A specific amount of carbohydrate, protein, and fat in the form of food exchanges is calculated. The time frame for eating the exchanges is specified. Thus a package of peanut butter crackers eaten 3 hours after lunch, instead of being a casual snack, is an important component of an individual's diabetes therapy. A bedtime snack also prevents reactions during the night. Patients can be taught to exchange meals and snacks to accommodate special events in their lives.

Insulin. Many individuals who have diabetes require insulin. In the United States, insulin is commer-

Food Guide Pyramid
A Guide to Daily Food Choices

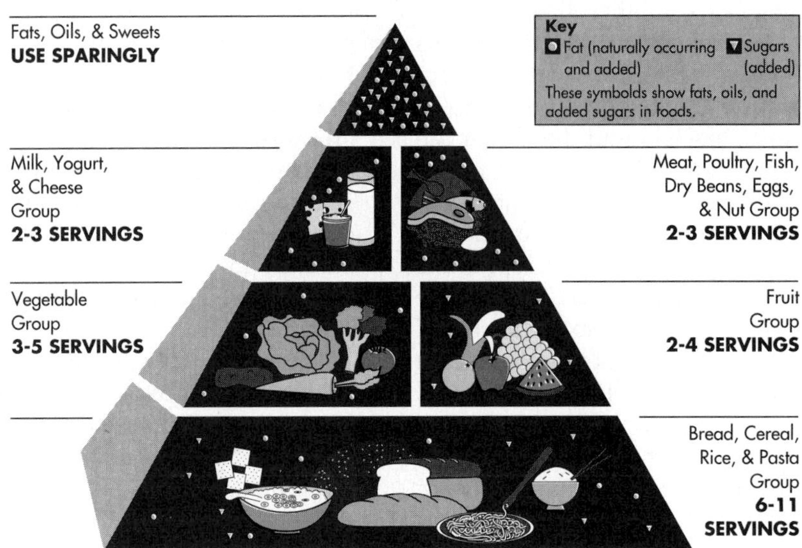

Figure 27-5 The food guide pyramid, a guide to daily food choices. Each food group provides some, but not all, required nutrients. (From US Department of Agriculture, Human Nutrition Information Service, 1992.)

cially derived from the pancreas of a pig or cow, or synthesized in a laboratory. The new synthetic human insulins (Humulin, Novolin) are the purest forms of insulin. Patients should not switch to synthetic insulin without close monitoring of dosage by the healthcare provider. The amount of insulin needed depends on the individual and varies at different times for the same person. The type of insulin needed also varies. The purpose of administering insulin is to replace a deficiency. Its action is to enable the body to metabolize food, absorb glucose into the cell, and thus lower the blood glucose level. Many types of insulin are in current use. Each insulin has three expected time frames: (1) *onset* is the time between the injection of insulin and when it starts to be effective in the body, (2) *peak* is the time when the insulin action is at its highest, and (3) *duration* is the length of time the insulin effect is expected to last in the body. Insulins are classified according to their time frame of action and duration of effect as one of three types: (1) fast acting or short duration, (2) intermediate acting or medium duration, and (3) slow acting or long lasting (Table 27-4).

Product information circulars or current drug books provide precise data about the composition of specific insulins and their action. For patients, however, a range of possible times is not as helpful as learning when *their* insulin starts to work, peaks, and disappears. Healthcare professionals examine patient records of blood and urine glucose and acetone levels and relate those values to food eaten, exercise, and symptoms of possible insulin reactions. They learn the approximate times after an injection that the insulin has its onset, peak, and duration for that individual. Adjustments in dose are then made until the best dose and type of insulin is found to achieve the individual's goal of blood-glucose levels. Insulin used on a daily basis may be stored at room temperature for 1 month, as long as it is not exposed to direct sunlight or kept near a heat source. Unopened insulin can be stored safely in the refrigerator until the expiration date on the bottle.

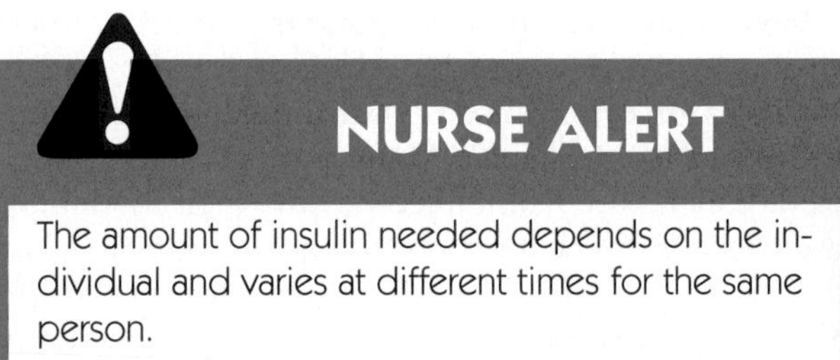

Insulin is administered in units that have been standardized so that it is the same no matter where it is purchased or from which pharmaceutical manufacturer it comes. Insulin is available in concentration of 100 units/ml centimeter (U-100) and in a 10 ml vial in the United States. Insulin syringes are **calibrated** in units of 100 to correspond to that concentration of insulin (100 units/ml). Small gauge (28-29), short

TABLE 27-3

1200 Calorie Meal Plan

	Breakfast	Lunch	Afternoon Snack	Dinner	Evening Snack
Time	7 AM	12 PM		6 PM	
No. of choices					
Lowfat milk	½ cup	½ cup			½ cup
Vegetable		1		2	
Fruit	1	1		1	
Bread	1	1	1	1	1
Meat		1	1	2	
Fat	1	1		1	

Cholesterol 153 g, Protein 61 g, Fat 41 g

TABLE 27-4

Types of Insulin Available in the United States

Type	Action	Duration (hours)	Peak of Action (hours)
Regular (beef/pork or pure pork)	Fast acting	5-6	2-4
Novolin, regular	Fast acting	5-8	2-5
Humulin, regular	Fast acting	6-8	2-4
Velosulin	Fast acting	5-8	2-5
Lente (beef/pork or pure pork)	Intermediate acting	18-24	6-16
NPH (beef/pork or pure pork)	Intermediate acting	18-24	6-12
Novolin lente	Intermediate acting	18-24	7-15
Humulin NPH	Intermediate acting	14-24	6-12
Humulin ultralente	Long lasting	24-28	8-20
Humulin 70-30	Insulin mixture	12-24	4-8
Mixtard 70-30	Insulin mixture	12-24	4-8
Novolin 70-30	Insulin mixture	12-24	4-8

Modified from Sperling MA: *Physicians' guide to insulin dependent (type I) diabetes,* Alexandria, Va, 1988, American Diabetes Association.

(½ inch) needles are used. One-milliliter (U-100) syringes are suitable for patients with higher dosages. Low-dose syringes that hold 50 units of U-100 concentrated insulin are available for those who require minimum amounts of insulin. U-30 and U-25 insulin syringes are available especially for use by children or those with impaired vision. The most important consideration is that the patient understand that each line on the U-100 syringe equals 2 units, whereas on all other syringes each line equals 1 unit.

The skills required to inject insulin are less complex than the skills of drawing insulin into a syringe. The patient may be fearful of the first self-administered injection. Routine planned time by the healthcare professional with the patient is vital, and the teaching can commence as soon as possible.

Before teaching the mechanical skills for drawing insulin, the patient should be assessed for ability to see the syringe markings and manual dexterity to handle the equipment. The patient should be taught to always check the label on the bottle. The insulin bottle should be gently rolled to ensure that all sediment is mixed into the liquid (Figure 27-6). The insulin vial should be placed on a firm surface, and its top should be cleaned with alcohol. The syringe should be handled carefully so as not to stress the small needle, and sterile technique should be used. The patient should then remove the needle cover and draw in the amount of air equal to the amount of insulin to be removed from the vial. The air is injected into the vial, and the vial is inverted in the patient's hand so that the tip of the needle is covered by insulin and the bottle is not resting on the needle. The plunger is pulled halfway down the syringe, and air bubbles are eliminated. Then the correct amount of insulin is withdrawn from the vial.

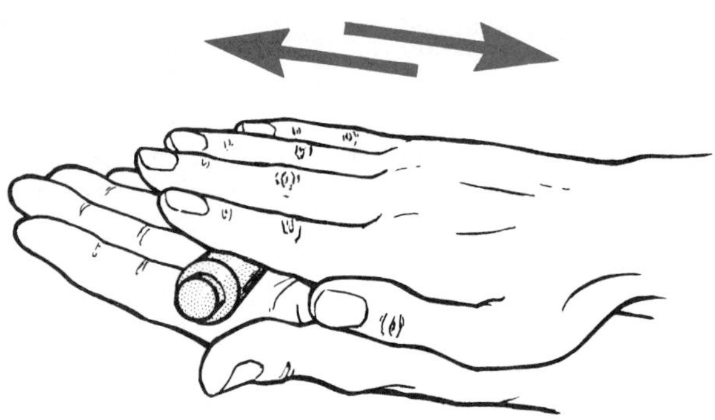

Figure 27-6 Method for mixing insulin. Vial is rolled between the palms.

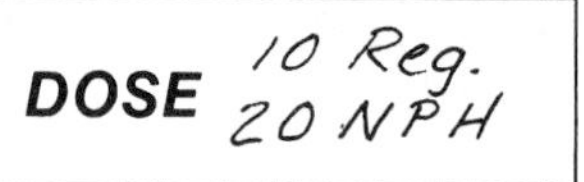

INSTRUCTIONS FOR MEASURING INSULIN

Mixed Dose

1. Turn cloudy bottle upside down and roll between hands.
2. Wipe off tops of bottles with cotton and alcohol.
3. Pull plunger to ..20.. . Put needle through top of cloudy bottle and push plunger down, putting air into bottle. Take needle out empty.
4. Pull plunger to ..10.... . Put needle through top of clear bottle and push plunger down. Leave needle in bottle.
5. Turn bottle upside down and pull plunger halfway down syringe. Push all insulin back in bottle;
6. Pull plunger halfway down syringe and check for bubbles.* If no bubbles present, push plunger to ..10.. units of regular insulin and take out needle.

   *If bubbles present, repeat step 5 before completing step 6.
7. Turn cloudy bottle upside down and stick needle through rubber top.
8. Pull plunger slowly to ..30... units. (..10.. + 20..). Take out needle.
9. Wipe skin with alcohol and cotton and pinch.
10. Pick up syringe like a pencil and push needle straight into skin. Push plunger down.
11. Release pinch, press alcohol next to needle and pull out.

Figure 27-7 Instructions for measuring a mixed dose of insulin.

If the patient is receiving two insulins that can be mixed in the same syringe, some modifications are made to the procedure. Additionally careful reading of each bottle label is imperative. To ensure patient consistency and avoid contamination, the shorter-acting insulin should be drawn first. Both insulin vials are cleansed and placed on a firm surface. The amount of air to be injected into the longer-acting insulin is drawn and injected into the vial, and the needle is removed. Then the correct amount of air for the shorter-acting insulin is injected into that bottle, the vial is inverted, the bubbles are removed, and the insulin is removed. Without letting any of the shorter-acting insulin leave the syringe, the longer-acting bottle is entered, the needle tip is covered, and the correct amount of insulin is withdrawn.

Patients are given careful instructions so that dose errors are avoided. If the patient's dose is 10 units of Regular insulin and 20 units of NPH insulin, the following instructions would be given so that the patient would correctly draw up a total dose of 30 units:

1 Draw up 20 units of air, inject it into NPH vial, and remove the syringe.
2 Draw up 10 units of air, inject it into the Regular vial, invert the bottle, cover the needle with insulin, fill the syringe halfway, remove the air bubbles, push-pull the plunger until there are exactly 10 units of insulin and no air in the syringe, and remove the syringe from the vial.
3 Without losing any of the Regular insulin in the syringe, inject the needle into the NPH vial, cover the tip of the needle with NPH insulin, and slowly pull the plunger back until it reaches 30 on the syringe.
4 Remove the needle from the NPH bottle and proceed with the injection (Finding, 1992).

A total dose of 30 units (10 Regular, 20 NPH) was drawn into the same syringe. If too much insulin is pulled from the NPH bottle, it may not be pushed back into either bottle. The syringe is discarded, and the patient must begin the process again. Because mixing insulin may be a problem for some patients, taking two separate injections may be one safe solution. Premixed insulins may be purchased (Novolin or Humulin 70/30) when the required dose is 30% Regular insulin and 70% NPH insulin (see Table 27-3). Sample instructions for measuring insulin are found in Figure 27-7.

The method currently used for injecting insulin is to place the insulin in the space between the subcutaneous tissue and the muscle. Once the correct dose is prepared, the patient is taught to clean the skin and to pinch up a large fold of skin and fat. Holding the syringe like a pencil, the needle is injected into the skin at a 90-degree angle all the way to the hub. The insulin should be injected through the subcutaneous tissue into the loose space made by the pinch. Once all the insulin has been injected, the pinch of skin is released before the needle is withdrawn to avoid loss of insulin. The first time the patient self-injects insulin, the nurse should select a site that is easily reached, such as the thigh or abdomen. The patient should be guided through the procedure and assisted as needed.

The sites for injection should be rotated with each injection to prevent **lipodystrophy,** which may interfere with absorption and lead to the formation of scar tissue. Possible injection sites should be chosen on the basis of the condition of the skin, patient preferences, manual dexterity, and the sensitivity of the individual to site changes. Preferred sites are the lateral surface of the upper arms, the abdominal tissue just below the rib cage, the anterolateral surfaces of the thigh, and the upper buttock (Figure 27-8). Any atrophied or hypertrophied area should be avoided, including scar tissue, nevi, or moles. If insulin is given in the same site for a time, scar tissue may form, which leads to erratic absorption of the insulin. The site chosen for the insulin injections affects the rate of absorption. The most rapid absorption is from the abdomen, and the arm site is second. Patients should be instructed to use these sites if blood glucose levels are elevated.

Once the prescribed dose of insulin has been injected, the patient should record the amount and site in a record book. The used syringe and needle should be placed in a covered container (e.g., coffee can) before disposal.

A family member or significant other should be taught the insulin administration technique for when assistance is needed. For patients who have problems meeting acceptable skill levels in any components of the insulin administration process, problem-solving should be done so that individuals are as independent as possible. For instance, if a patient cannot see well enough in the morning to accurately draw up insulin, but can manipulate injecting insulin, there are several alternatives. A visiting nurse can draw up a weeks' supply and leave them, a neighbor could be asked for daily assistance, or a magnifier or close gauge could be used on the syringe. If the person can see better at the end of the day, which is not uncommon, the insulin for the next day can be drawn up the night before and stored in the refrigerator.

There are also several devices on the market to aid patients with injections. Some patients with unstable diabetes and changing lifestyles may be candidates for intensive treatment. The first is multiple injections of insulin, and the second is the use of the insulin pump. Both of these treatments require motivation and special education but do allow for greater flexibility in meal scheduling and exercise programs.

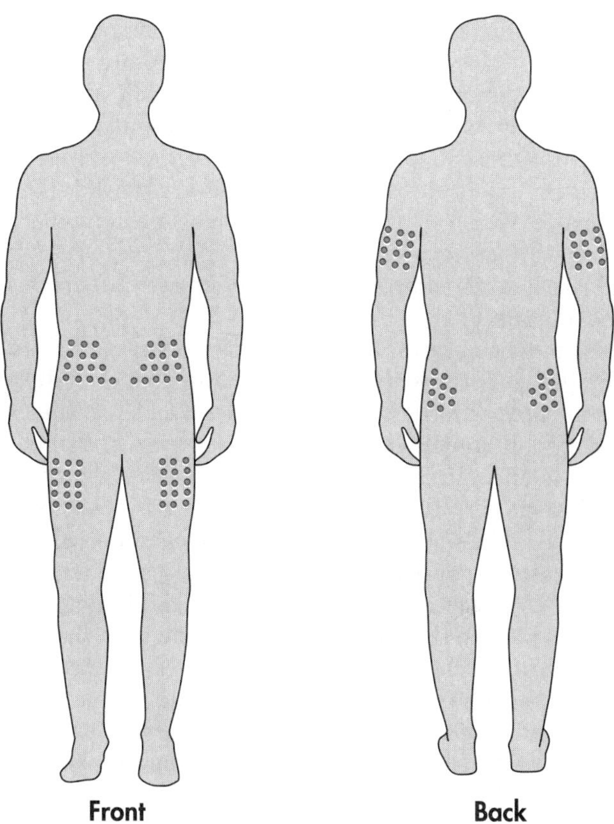

Figure 27-8 Rotation sites for insulin injections. (From Potter PA, Perry AG: *Basic nursing: theory and practice,* ed 3, St Louis, 1995, Mosby.)

Oral agents. Several oral hypoglycemic drugs stimulate the islet cells of the pancreas to secrete more insulin. For these agents to be effective, the individual must secrete endogenous insulin but requires additional insulin to maintain metabolic control. Oral hypoglycemic agents (OHAs) are suited for people who have type II diabetes. These patients cannot achieve control with diet therapy alone and do not require exogenous insulin to provide acceptable metabolic control. There are some possible complications from each of the drugs, the most common being **hypoglycemia.** Because sulfonylureas are detoxified in the liver, individuals who have liver problems must be monitored closely. The action of the drugs may be more intense in this group because the potential delay in their breakdown may cause an accumulation of the drug and increase the risk of hypoglycemia.

OHAs are not oral insulins. This is an important concept for the patient and family to understand. OHAs are currently sulfonylurea drugs. They are taken once or several times daily, depending on their duration of action (see Table 27-1). Like insulin, OHAs are classified on the basis of how long they act. Tolbutamide (Orinase) is a short-acting OHA (6 to 12 hours) and is taken several times daily. Acetohexamide (Dymelor) and tolazamide (Tolinase) are intermediate acting (12 to 24 hours), so they are taken once or twice daily depending on their duration of the effect for specific individuals. Chlorpropamide (Diabinese) has a long duration (up to 60 hours), so it is taken daily. There are oral agents on the market, glipizide (Glucotrol) and glyburide (DiaBeta or Micronase), that are known as second-generation sulfonylurea drugs. These require much lower dosages to be effective and therefore lower incidence of side effects.

There has been some controversy regarding the use of OHAs. Because insulin therapy imposes such discipline on individuals' daily activities, OHAs are suited for certain people. If a patient has the type of diabetes that is uncontrolled by diet and more endogenous insulin stimulated by OHAs maintains their metabolic control, then one of those drugs may be indicated.

Hygiene. People who have diabetes are believed to have a lowered resistance to infection, and their abrasions or wounds may heal more slowly than those of individuals who do not have diabetes. These observed phenomena may be secondary to an etiologic factor of immunologic suppression or may exist because of the effect of high blood-glucose levels when diabetes is uncontrolled. The nursing implication from these observations is that hygiene for people who have diabetes must be a component of their therapeutic regimen. General skin care to prevent the accumulation of pathogenic organisms and prevent drying should be carried out daily.

Because many patients are at risk for foot problems because of potential vascular complications from their diabetes, the most important aspect of hygiene is proper care of the feet. Feet should be washed daily with warm water (avoid hot water) and mild soap and dried well. The area between the toes should be especially dry, and no lotion or lanolin should be applied. Nails should be filed slightly longer than the shape of the toe. Corns and calluses should be smoothed with a pumice stone or emery board. Patients should be told to avoid bathroom surgery and to consult a podiatrist for very tough toenails or corns that require cutting. Feet should be examined daily, and any problem should be reported to the healthcare provider.

Even a trivial injury should be reported early, because care for a minor problem can prevent its escalation into a major one. Other aspects of foot care include wearing properly fitting shoes, not going barefoot, and avoiding anything constricting (e.g., round garters or tightly fitting knee-high hose) that could decrease circulation to the feet. Shoes should be broken in gradually. Heating devices for the feet (e.g., hot water bottles) should never be used, and feet should never be soaked.

Exercise. One of the American pioneers in diabetes treatment, Dr. Elliot Joslin, viewed diet, exercise, and insulin as three "frisky ponies" that together control diabetes. After insulin became readily available as a therapy, the Joslin Clinic noted that patients who returned to farm work or other active jobs were in better metabolic control than their patients who had a more sedentary lifestyle. Exercise is believed to exert its physiologic benefit by changing the cell wall permeability so that movement of glucose into the cell is increased, by directly lowering blood-glucose levels because glucose is used for energy, and by increasing the uptake of free fatty acids. Exercise also increases the level of high-density lipoproteins and lowers cholesterol and triglyceride levels. This is very important because individuals who have diabetes are at a greater risk for cardiovascular diseases.

Just as diet and insulin therapies are individualized, so too are exercise regimens. Healthcare professionals are aware of potential complications from exercise and characteristics of those individuals for whom exercise would be considered dangerous. Therefore the specific exercise plan should be mutually decided by the patient (to fit into daily activities) and provider (to prescribe the proper amount and adjust the diet and insulin as necessary). Exercise may be contraindicated for some individuals. Others may need cardiovascular screening before an exercise prescription is given.

Weight control, lower insulin requirements, and a sense of well-being are positive outcomes of an ongoing exercise program. Integrating regular exercise into a daily routine can be difficult. For those who integrate the activities required of diabetes management into their routine, the addition of an exercise plan may be especially difficult. This underscores the importance of the patient and provider collaborating in the development of diabetes ADLs that are acceptable to the individual who has the diabetes. No matter how ideal a plan may appear, it will not be effective if it is not determined by the patient.

Insulin reaction. The goal of diabetes therapy is to prevent or delay the onset of chronic complications without precipitating acute complications. Achieving a near-normal blood-glucose level at all times is ideal but very hard to achieve in actuality. Shifts in blood-glucose levels are inevitable, and these may result in one of the acute complications of diabetes. An insulin reaction, or hypoglycemic (low blood glucose) reaction, is the most common acute complication of diabetes, especially in patients who use insulin. Individuals who use insulin should be taught to expect some insulin reactions, to learn when they are most likely to have a hypoglycemic event, and to recognize their own early warning signs. Both patients and providers must incorporate prevention, detection, and management of reactions into the overall treatment plan.

An insulin reaction results from either a drop in blood-glucose level to an amount not tolerated by the individual (usually under 60 ml/dl of blood) or from a

TABLE 27-5

Characteristics of Hyperglycemia and Hypoglycemia (Insulin Reaction)

	Hyperglycemia	Hypoglycemia (Insulin Reaction)
Cause	Dietary excesses	Dietary deficit, (too little food or delayed meals)
	Too little insulin	Too much insulin
	Infection	
	Decreased exercise with same dietary intake	Increased exercise without dietary supplement or insulin reduction
	Another disease or condition that taxes available insulin	
	Emotional stress	
Symptoms	Early	Early
	Gradual loss of appetite	Lassitude
	Increased thirst	Lethargy
	Nausea and vomiting	Inability to concentrate
	Dry skin, flushed face	Hunger
	Headache	
	Weakness	
	Late	Late
	Diabetic acidosis	Trembling sensation
	Kussmaul's respirations	Profuse perspiration
	Sweet, fruity odor to breath	Irritability
	Decreased blood pressure	Generalized muscle weakness
	Increased pulse	Blurred or double vision
		Headache
		Tingling sensation of lips or tongue
Blood glucose	Greater than 240 mg/dl	Less than 60 mg/dl
Urinary glucose	Positive	Negative
Progression	Gradual	Rapid
Intervention	Regular insulin	Simple carbohydrates by mouth (orange juice, sugar)
	Fluid and electrolyte replacement	20-30 ml of 50% glucose intravenously
	Mannitol if cerebral edema is present	1-2 mg of glucagon subcutaneously or intramuscularly

very rapid drop in blood-glucose level. In the second case, a blood test would reveal a "normal" blood-glucose level, but the individual would still experience and exhibit the symptoms of a reaction. Once individuals recognize their reaction patterns, their opinion of whether or not they are in reaction is what determines if treatment is required. When in doubt, treat!

Hypoglycemic reactions are caused by too little circulating glucose. The reaction may be caused by too much insulin or exercise and not enough food. An increased amount of insulin, not enough food at the time insulin is peaking, alcohol consumption, or strenuous exercise without an insulin decrease or food increase may precipitate a reaction. Reactions come on very rapidly. They can be very mild or extremely severe. The most common symptoms are a trembling sensation, profuse perspiration, irritability, and dizziness. Additional signs may be generalized muscle weakness, headache, tingling sensations of the lips or tongue, blurred or double vision, an unsteady gait, palpitations, pallor, and hunger (Table 27-5). Without immediate treatment, the patient may become confused, lose consciousness, and develop seizure activity.

The immediate treatment is to raise the blood-glucose level. Unless a patient is hospitalized and hypoglycemia can be evaluated (blood tests are usually required before glucose is given), a simple carbohydrate should be ingested. Some patients monitor their blood-glucose level before treating to make an appraisal of how much carbohydrate they need. Such monitoring allows patients to gain a closer approximation of what symptoms they experience at various levels. Under no circumstances should treatment be delayed, because symptoms rapidly progress. If a suspected reaction is treated with 4 ounces of ginger ale and later on it is discovered that the patient was in error when the diagnosis was made, there is no harm done. Extra calories from the ginger ale are better than the risk of not treating or waiting too long.

Patients should be taught to carry a simple carbohydrate with them at all times so they can immediately treat suspected reactions and prevent serious ones. In a hospital setting, a conscious patient who experiences an insulin reaction is treated with fruit juice, regular soda, honey, jelly, or milk. If a patient is unconscious, nothing is given by mouth. One of two methods is used to quickly raise the blood-glucose level. The length of time the patient has been unconscious and the setting in which the patient was found determine which to use. If the patient is unconscious at home or if it is known that the patient just became unconscious, then glucagon would be the first treatment to use. **Endogenous glucagon** is a hormone secreted by the alpha cells of the islets of Langerhans. In the presence of low blood-glucose levels, glucagon is secreted and stimulates the liver to break down glycogen, which in turn releases glucose into the bloodstream and raises the blood-glucose level. An **exogenous glucagon** preparation would be given subcutaneously or intramuscularly to stimulate a glucose release from stored glycogen.

Once conscious, the patient should ingest some easily absorbed carbohydrate and then some more complex food. Family members are taught to administer glucagon by using one of the patient's insulin syringes and a glucagon kit. A side effect of glucagon is nausea, so the patient and families should be told of this during the teaching session. After the initial treatment of an unconscious reaction, the patient and family should be instructed to investigate the cause of the low blood sugar. Repeated unconscious reactions should be avoided.

If the patient does not immediately respond to the glucagon or if the patient has been unconscious for awhile, intravenous glucose is required. Approximately 20 to 30 ml of a very concentrated glucose solution (50%) is given, and patients usually respond rapidly. Additional complex carbohydrates, protein, and fat are provided as soon as the patient can tolerate them because the intravenous glucose rapidly passes from the bloodstream into the cells. Insulin reactions should not be overtreated. The day after a reaction, the patient may normally experience "rebound hyperglycemia." The ideal treatment for an insulin reaction is to give enough but not too much extra carbohydrate. One suggestion is to wait 10 minutes after giving carbohydrates; if the symptoms have not disappeared in that time, the carbohydrate should be repeated.

When patients begin taking insulin, they may experience a reaction while their dose is being adjusted. Experiencing a reaction at this time may help them recognize what a reaction feels like and give them confidence in treating future reactions. As individuals gain more experience with their illness, they should be able to detect initial warning signs and learn their particular signs of impending reaction. For example, a growling stomach may indicate an impending insulin reaction.

Patients need to be taught when to expect reactions and how to prevent them. Once they learn when their insulin peaks, they should be instructed to eat an appropriate snack a little in advance to prevent hypoglycemia. If strenuous weekend-only exercise is planned, then depending on body size and whether one wishes to gain or lose weight, either less insulin is used that day or more food is taken. Regularity in times of insulin administration, eating, and exercise is the best way to prevent insulin reactions. Personal identification (e.g., Medic Alert) should be worn. These alerts indicate the disease and the possibility of a hypoglycemia reaction.

NURSE ALERT

Increased exercise in people with poorly controlled diabetes may result in ketoacidosis.

Diabetic acidosis (ketoacidosis). If the question, "Why treat diabetes?" is posed, the first response would be "to prevent diabetic acidosis." This serious acute complication of diabetes leads to death if untreated and is always considered an emergency. Ketoacidosis may occur in an undiagnosed individual, and it may be the first indication of the disease. Ketoacidosis is more prevalent in individuals who have type I diabetes. Although it is unusual, it may occur in individuals who do not require insulin to manage their diabetes.

The immediate cause of diabetic ketoacidosis (DKA) is always lack of insulin and the subsequent accumulation of glucose and waste products from increased fat and protein metabolism. The onset is gradual and can be caused by any events that result in decreased available insulin or increased insulin requirements. Too little insulin, the flu, infection, or stress are some possible causes of DKA. Because the pathophysiology of DKA is similar to untreated type I, uncontrolled diabetes, early DKA symptoms are similar to the classic signs of new-onset, type I diabetes. Initial symptoms are polyuria, polydipsia, and polyphagia, which may go unnoticed until some other symptoms such as nausea, vomiting, appetite loss, weakness, headache, dry skin, and flushed face occur (Table 27-4). Often patients think they have these symptoms because they have a virus. This is why all sick days are treated as if they might mean an impending DKA.

Unchecked DKA can lead to complex metabolic processes that result in fluid and electrolyte loss, dehydration, starvation, and reduction in the acid-base buffering system. Late symptoms of DKA are related to these metabolic sequelae and include sweet, fruity breath; decreased blood pressure; increased pulse; and *Kussmaul's respirations.* Kussmaul's respirations, characteristic of late DKA, are a rhythmic cycle that includes a pattern of loud, deep, and rapid respirations followed by apnea. Body chemistries reflect this picture of metabolic acidosis. Patients exhibit high blood-glucose levels, low pH and carbon dioxide, and altered electrolytes and have fatty acid breakdown products (ketones) in the urine. A blood-glucose level may be well over 1000 mg/dl. This complication is the exact opposite of an insulin reaction. Usually the classic signs and symptoms of DKA allow the diagnosis to be made quickly. If symptoms are unusual and there may be doubt as to which acute complication has occurred, the patient should be treated for an insulin reaction. If the patient has DKA that is incorrectly diagnosed as an insulin reaction and glucose is given, the only harm done is the waiting for a few minutes to see if the glucose is effective.

Patients with DKA look and feel seriously ill. They may become comatose if treatment is delayed. Emergency treatment is necessary to reverse the hyperglycemia, dehydration, acidosis, and electrolyte imbalance. Quick-acting insulin is given intravenously and is followed by subcutaneous or intravenous infusion of insulin. Rapid infusion of intravenous fluids is used to reverse the dehydration. Electrolytes are closely monitored, and supplements are given as required. These seriously ill patients require intensive nursing care, most prominently, observation and management of symptoms. The treatment goal for DKA is to reverse the metabolic imbalance without causing fluid overload or hypoglycemia.

Once the patient's condition has been stabilized, the cause of the DKA must be discovered. Alterations in diabetes management and education of the patient and others should be tailored to prevent future occurrences.

Hyperglycemic, hyperosmolar, nonketotic coma. A severe, but less commonly seen acute complication of diabetes is hyperglycemic, hyperosmolar, nonketotic coma (HHNC). Individuals who do not require insulin to manage their diabetes are susceptible to this problem. It is more common among elderly patients and may occasionally be the first indication that the individual has type II diabetes. The syndrome was named from its observed clinical signs and symptoms. There is no ketoacidosis, but the other defining characteristics of the problem, hyperglycemia and hyperosmolality, are very intense. Extreme dehydration is treated with massive amounts of fluid replacement, and very small amounts of insulin are used to reverse the hyperglycemia. These patients are critically ill and require intense monitoring as their metabolic problems are reversed.

Once the critical phase has passed, the cause of the HHNC must be discovered. Often it is secondary to an infection or another illness. This explains a general rule of thumb in diabetes management. No matter what other disease process may be present, metabolic control of diabetes must be concurrent with other disease management.

Chronic complications. The second answer to the question, "Why treat diabetes?" is to prevent, minimize, or delay the onset of chronic complications. Macrovascular and microvascular changes, functional disturbances in the nervous system, and infection are the major categories of impairment of long-term or uncontrolled diabetes mellitus. A syndrome called diabetic *triopathy* results when severe pathologic changes have occurred in the peripheral nerves (neuropathy), eyes (retinopathy), and kidneys (nephropathy). The primary focus of the treatment of the complications of diabetes is early detection and initiation of treatment to delay or minimize progression.

According to the American Diabetes Association, diabetes and its complications are the fourth leading cause of death by disease in the United States. Diabetes is a major health problem because approximately 2.3 million hospital days are attributed to it. A clinical study was started in 1985 to examine the relationship between efforts to lower blood glucose and the long-term complications of diabetes. This clinical research was conducted in 29 centers across the United States, and the results were released by the Diabetes Association in 1993. The results of the Diabetes Control and Complication Study showed that improved blood-glucose control reduced the risk of clinically meaningful retinopathy by 76%, nephropathy by 54%, and neuropathy by 60%. This study clearly demonstrates that near-normal glucose levels are the best means of preventing diabetic complications (McCarren, 1993).

Individuals who have diabetes often develop macrovascular changes caused by atherosclerosis. These changes usually occur earlier and are more severe than in individuals without diabetes. Some specialists estimate the anatomic changes of a patient's cardiovascular system to be consistent with that expected according to their chronologic age plus the number of years they have had diabetes. These patients are in high-risk groups for problems with their peripheral vascular system, such as intermittent claudication or gangrene. Stroke and coronary artery disease also result from macrovascular changes.

Microvascular problems are caused by changes in the capillary basement membrane. High levels of circulating glucose in uncontrolled diabetes are believed to cause thickening and damage to these small vessels. Capillaries in the eye and kidney can be affected and cause retinal problems, leading to blindness. Other vision changes may occur from cataracts secondary to prolonged hyperglycemia. Also, glomerulosclerosis may cause renal failure.

High blood-glucose levels probably account for the increased susceptibility that individuals with diabetes have for infections. Metabolic imbalances also contribute to problems that are evidenced in the central or peripheral nervous systems. Sensory and motor fibers can be affected and contribute to the "at-risk" foot. The ease with which individuals who have diabetes can acquire infection; poor circulation, which impedes healing; and diminished sensation to lower extremities guide patient teaching regarding foot care. Patients are taught to observe their feet daily because an abrasion or infection may be present but not felt.

Other complications. Surgery for any reason causes physiologic stress regardless of whether one has diabetes or not. The individual who has mild type II diabetes that is under metabolic control by diet alone may require insulin for several days when hospitalized for major surgery. Patients who previously required insulin have increased insulin requirements. One half of the anticipated insulin dose is usually given preoperatively and the remainder in the recovery room. An intravenous glucose solution runs during the perioperative period. Blood-glucose levels are monitored closely, and supplemental insulin or glucose is administered as required.

Routine tests that require nothing by mouth can complicate the hospitalization of individuals who have diabetes. The length of the procedure and sensitivity of the patient to periods of fasting or withholding insulin determine what is ordered for each individual. Some patients may tolerate half of their usual insulin dose (including rapidly acting insulin), whereas others may need to receive an intravenous glucose infusion.

Patients should learn how to adjust their diet when they go out to dinner and how to eat from a restaurant menu. When excessive "sick days" are taken, more tailoring of the therapeutic plan may need to be made. Sick days should be treated as days of impending DKA or HHNC. Blood-glucose levels and urine ketones need to be monitored every 4 hours, and patients must be in contact with their healthcare provider during the duration of the illness. Extra insulin may be needed even if only fluids such as ginger ale instead of a full diet are all that can be tolerated. Patients should be reminded that they must always take their insulin dose even if they are unable to eat because of nausea and vomiting.

OLDER ADULT CONSIDERATIONS

Noninsulin-dependent diabetes mellitus is common in elderly people.

Symptoms related to diabetes mellitus are often masked by other illnesses and may be atypical in the elderly.

Cognitive impairment may lead to inconsistent medication administration or erratic eating problems in older adults.

Visual or sensory defects and functional limitations should be assessed when planning care for the older adult with diabetes mellitus.

Patient and family teaching. The American Association of Diabetes Educators has issued a position statement that recommends a careful adjustment of diet, exercise, and medications and suggests that individualized education be based on the person's intellect, motivation, physical ability, and social and personal resources. Individual cultures must be acknowledged and incorporated into the development of the entire plan of care.

One patient may be taught how to eat at a fast-food restaurant chain by following a specific list of what to order. Another individual may have the ability to exchange foods quite accurately and by following a few suggestions could eat within the diet at almost any restaurant. This same patient might be taught a sophisticated algorithm to increase the usual insulin dose by 20% during a sick day. Conversely another individual might be told, "Call your provider to find out what to do whenever you have the flu."

The most important feature of patient teaching is that its success depends on both the ability and willingness of individuals to incorporate their therapeutic plan into their daily routine. In collaboration with their healthcare provider, individuals' plans of care must be stylized to their beliefs, values, and attitudes. If a plan does not work, a new one must be developed jointly. A patient should not be labeled "noncompliant," but rather an effort must be made to establish a joint alliance of patient and provider.

Nursing interventions for people who have diabetes are directed toward the diagnosis and treatment of

	DAY OF ADMISSION	DAY 1	DAY 2	DAY 3
Tests:	Admission labs Blood glucose ECG (if indicated)	Blood glucose level 4-6 times daily	Blood glucose level 4-6 times daily CXR (if indicated) Dx test as indicated	Blood glucose level 4-6 times daily
Consults:	Order consults as needed	Call in consults: eye, exercise, pods/vasc. surg., etc.	Consult done	—
Activity:	Out of bed Tour	Out of bed	Out of bed	Out of bed
Diet:	Dietary history (24 hr. recall)	RD assessment Meal plan Goals	Individual follow-up as needed	D/C diet reviewed
Education:	Pretest Start education	DNE assessment Education goals Classes	Individual follow-up of survival skills	D/C instructions: survival skills reviewed; post-test; behav. obj.
Nurse and/or physician:	History; physical Treatment plan Patient goals established, including discharge plan	Instruct drawing up insulin; patient to inject Instruct visual blood testing technique	Demo/return demo: insulin/BG skills by patient and/or family Team conference	Demo/return demo: insulin/BG skills by patient and/or family
Medications:	Insulin Other orders	Insulin adjusted	Insulin adjusted	Insulin: D/C dose
Treatments:	Weight Vital Signs	—	—	—
Discharge planning:	Social service consult	Discharge planning started	Patient notified of D/C date Family involved or VNA consult prn	D/C plan entered into computer

Figure 27-9 Critical pathway for patients new to insulin.

their actual and potential responses. A critical pathway for a stable, newly diagnosed hospitalized patient who needs insulin therapy is included in Figure 27-9. The steps of the nursing process are the organizing framework to summarize general nursing interventions for people with diabetes, regardless of setting (Box 27-4).

The type of diabetes, general health status, personal ability, regimen complexity, and individual differences are some of the factors that determine expected outcomes for specific patients. Outcome criteria determine when patients are prepared to be the self-care manager of their disease, require additional assistance, or require a change in their therapeutic plan.

Patients need to have adequate knowledge about their diabetes. They should have an understanding of the rationale that determines their individual care plan and should possess the requisite skills to manage their therapeutic regimen. An integration of patients' cognitive and behavioral skills should be demonstrated as they monitor, make decisions, and carry out their diabetes activities of daily living. Good metabolic control without acute complications is the expected therapeutic outcome.

Patients should understand the rationale for their treatment on the basis of the pathophysiologic condition that exists. This includes specific components of their therapy, such as monitoring glucose level, giving medications, acting on the basis of blood and urine testing, and eating the correct foods. Blood and urine chemistry levels should be as close to normal range as possible. Normal ranges include a fasting venous plasma glucose level of 100 to 150 mg/dl, no sugar or acetone in preprandial urine specimens, a glycohemoglobin level less than 1.5 times normal (acceptable range for an individual with diabetes would be approximately 4.5% to 9%), and a 2-hour postprandial blood glucose level close to fasting range. Nurses are responsible for ensuring that patients demonstrate knowledge of the prevention, detection, and treatment of complications such as hypoglycemia and hyperglycemia (see Box 27-4).

Because there is no known cure for or prevention of diabetes mellitus, early detection and careful treat-

BOX 27-4

Nursing Process

DIABETES MELLITUS

ASSESSMENT

Mental status: anxiety, fear
Cardiovascular: dizziness, palpitations, changes in blood pressure and pulse
Respiratory: changes in respiratory rate and depth, breath odor
Skin: changes in skin turgor, temperature, and color
Gastrointestinal: polyphagia, nausea, vomiting, polydipsia (excessive thirst), abdominal pain or bloating
Metabolic: changes in blood glucose levels
Urinary: glycosuria, polyuria
Neuromuscular: tiredness; lethargy; weakness; tremors; headache; visual changes; changes in level of consciousness; change in reflexes, muscle mass, and strength
Fluid status: intake and output, tongue appearance, moisture of mucous membranes, firmness of eyeballs

NURSING DIAGNOSES

Altered nutrition: less than body requirements related to insulin deficiency
Anxiety related to inability to control illness
Risk for fluid volume deficit related to polyuria
Chronic low self-esteem related to chronicity of illness
Knowledge deficit related to complex management of illness
Ineffective individual and family coping related to chronicity of illness
Risk for infection related to metabolic changes
Impaired tissue integrity related to metabolic change

NURSING INTERVENTIONS

Monitor blood glucose levels (normal fasting level: 100-150 mg/dl).
Promote nutritional status by planned meal plan.
Monitor vital signs.
Weigh patient daily.
Encourage moderate levels of activity, which lower blood sugar levels.
Test urine for ketones if blood glucose is more than 240 mg/dl.
If patient is taking oral hypoglycemic agents, observe for adverse effects such as nausea, vomiting, rash, photosensitivity, and alcohol intolerance.
Monitor for signs of insulin reaction, such as diaphoresis (excessive perspiration), shaking, tachycardia, and anxiety.
Observe for signs of diabetic ketoacidosis, such as nausea, vomiting, facial flushing, weight loss, polydipsia, and positive urine tests for ketone.
Provide emotional support for patient and family.
Educate patient and family regarding basic pathophysiology and management of diabetes.
Foster independence in self-care management.
Assess patient's health status, psychosocial functioning, and social support.
Assess patient's and significant others' ability to comprehend and integrate their diabetes ADLs into their usual lifestyle pattern.
Observe condition of feet and skin.
Collaborate with patient, family, and diabetes clinicians to identify a therapeutic plan that provides the best metabolic control possible within the limitations of patient ability and acceptability.
Decide how best to implement the plan so that patient becomes independent in self-management techniques as soon as possible without becoming overwhelmed.
Incorporate the therapeutic plan of the patient care setting into the patient's individualized care plan. For example, use laboratory results of blood glucose values so patient can relate how he or she feels in relation to varying blood glucose levels; if the patient takes urine tests, he or she can learn renal threshold.
Promote patient confidence and independence in carrying out diabetes ADLs. For example, under decreasing supervision, patient should draw up and inject own insulin, perform urine or blood test, and select foods for meals and snacks.
Evaluate patient's skill level and coping ability so refinements can be made in care plan.
Collaboratively determine patient outcome expectations regarding the degree of metabolic control to be achieved, specific patient and significant other responsibilities in the home setting, and mechanisms to evaluate diabetes control, regimen ease/difficulty, and adherence to the therapeutic plan.

EVALUATION OF EXPECTED OUTCOMES

Blood and urine chemistries close to normal range
Basic pathology of diabetes explained
Rationale for treatment regimen explained
Prevents, detects, and treats hypoglycemia and hyperglycemia
Foods exchanged properly
Manages self-care on a sick day
Healthcare provider called appropriately
Complications prevented

ment are the current therapeutic interventions. Individuals who develop diabetes become managers of their chronic illness and become partners with healthcare providers who prescribe therapy. Interventions must be guided to assist patients to successfully live with this disorder so that its catastrophic complications are prevented. Nurses with creativity and ingenuity can make the difference between a regimen that is impossible for the patient to accept and one that accommodates culture and lifestyle. The pharmaceutical companies that make insulin and the companies that manufacture diabetes equipment (meter syringes) are wonderful resources for educational materials. These materials are available free of charge and can be obtained in several languages to meet the needs of a culturally diverse population.

Hypoglycemia

An abnormally low level of blood glucose may also occur in the absence of diabetes. It may be caused by disease of the liver or pancreas or disease of the pituitary or adrenal glands. The symptoms include hunger, weakness, anxiety, pallor, headache, sweating, and rapid pulse. One type known as functional hypoglycemia has an unknown cause. The symptoms are variable and often occur several hours after meals or exercise. The attacks may last from minutes to days. Treatment is based on relieving the immediate attack, followed by removing the cause when it is known. In mild attacks orange juice or hard candy may relieve the symptoms, whereas for patients with severe cases glucose may be administered intravenously. Patients may be given low-carbohydrate, high-protein intake with restriction of simple sugars; frequent small meals are usually prescribed. This type of meal plan should help prevent hypoglycemic episodes.

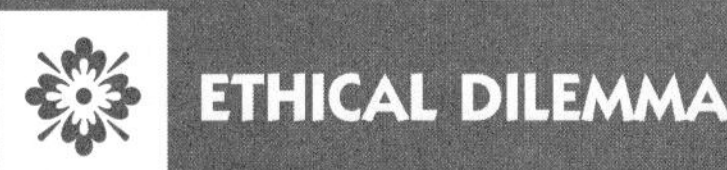

ETHICAL DILEMMA

Ms. White is a 32-year-old with brittle diabetes. She is often admitted to your unit because of the severity of her disease. She is, in the words of one of your colleagues, "a crabby, unlikable patient."

How would you analyze this case?

Nursing Care Plan

PATIENT WITH HYPERTHYROIDISM

Mrs. Reynolds is a 34-year-old female who is admitted to the medical unit for a diagnostic work-up after having palpitations, tachycardia, and an enlarged thyroid gland that was identified on a routine health visit to her private medical doctor (PMD).

Significant in her history is the fact that she has lost 20 pounds within the last 2 months without exercising or dieting. Her menstrual cycle has been erratic for the last 6 months, with no menses for the last 3 months. She denies being pregnant. She states she is currently stressed over her husband's projected employment transfer to the west coast and away from her extended family. She complains of heat intolerance and frequent episodes of "sweating." She states she is easily fatigued and has had periods of insomnia and constipation. She describes herself as feeling irritable and having crying outbursts without warning.

Past Medical History	Psychosocial Data	Assessment Data
Tonsillectomy and adenoidectomy, age 10 years Appendectomy at 14 years old; no other surgeries Hospitalized × 3 for childbirth; all routine vaginal deliveries without complications [Im]munizations up to date No known food or drug allergies; has received antiobiotics in past without problems	Married 12 years; quality relationship with husband; dated 6 years while in college and after; only stressor due to husband's frequent traveling with his work (consultancy business and sales) Own home; has cleaning lady once per week	Thin, frail-appearing woman with obvious exophthalmos; height 5 ft 8 in; weight 118 lbs *Skin:* Warm with evidence of recent diaphoresis; no rashes, lesions, or bruises *Musculoskeletal:* Steady gait; full range of motion all joints Fine tremors noted when fingers extended *Neck:* Diffuse swelling anterior portion neck; isthmus of gland palpable; no specific nodules palpable

continued

Nursing Care Plan

PATIENT WITH HYPERTHYROIDISM—cont'd

Past Medical History	Psychosocial Data	Assessment Data
Both parents alive and in good health; both employed full time and supportive to their children Two brothers in good health; both lawyers Identical twin sister recently diagnosed with Grave's disease Family history of hypertension in maternal grandmother, age 79 Adult onset diabetes in paternal uncle, age 70; good management Cancer of the breast in maternal aunt, deceased age 52 Excellent health behaviors: yearly physical, Pap smear, mammogram Has never smoked; denies use of alcohol and/or drugs; some use of over-the-counter (OTC) cold remedies/analgesics (aspirin, Tylenol)	Works part-time as librarian in media center at grammar school Has three children: Steve, age 9; Melissa, age 6; and Adam, age 5; all in excellent health Jewish faith; children attend Hebrew school Has private health insurance *Hobbies:* Avid reader, gardening, some traveling; is a gourmet cook	*Respiratory:* Lungs clear to percussion and auscultation; RR 24-26; regular rate and rhythm *Cardiovascular:* BP 146/84. (normal baseline = 118/72); apical pulse 96-100; no bruits; all peripheral pulses symmetrical; atrial flutter documented on ECG *Abdominal:* Bowel sounds heard all four quadrants; slight distension ***Laboratory data*** Hgb 12.1, Hct 37.8, WBC 8000, platelets 320,000, BUN 16, electrolytes WNL Thyroid ultrasonogram reveals marked diffuse swelling bilaterally Thyroid scan reveals a nonmalignancy condition T_3 triiodothyronine (T_3) resin uptake test = 24% of iodine uptake. ***Medications*** SSKI 300 mg po every 4 hours; dilute in 4 oz orange juice Inderal 20 mg po QID Colace 100 mg po daily Multivitamins tab 1 po daily Tylenol 300 mg po prn headache

NURSING DIAGNOSIS

Altered nutrition: less than body requirements related to increased metabolism, as evidenced by rapid weight loss and chronic fatigue

NURSING INTERVENTIONS	EVALUATION OF EXPECTED OUTCOMES
Weigh patient daily (same time, same scale) and record results. Monitor fluid I & O (likes milkshakes as between-meal snacks). Provide high-calorie, high-carbohydrate diet. Assist her with menu choices and discuss rationale for choices. She likes pasta, some creamed soups, and fresh fruits. Patient hates broccoli. Refer to dietician for teachings related to incorporating special dietary needs into gourmet cooking. Monitor bowel sounds once per shift. Check for episodes of constipation. Hold colace if loose stools. Teach same to patient. Provide oral hygiene at least twice per day. Remind patient to try to eat at least 90% of each meal tray. Record results on calorie count sheet.	Remains at or above specified weight (125 lb) and shows a steady increase of 2 lb bimonthly Consumes at least 90% of meals served and all of in-between snacks Plans appropriate diet for discharge for 1 week postdischarge; can explain the rationale for her choices

NURSING DIAGNOSIS

Body image disturbance related to exopthalmic appearance as evidenced by statements of anxiety and wearing dark glasses

NURSING INTERVENTIONS	EVALUATION OF EXPECTED OUTCOMES
Assess patient's usual coping patterns. Encourage discussion of feelings by initiating comments related to self-esteem and self-worth. Cite behaviors of progress. Introduce patient to available personnel (by mutual consent) who have had similar condition (not rare condition). Praise efforts to participate in self-care. Discuss hairstyle changes that might enhance self-image. Actively listen for expressions of anxiety. Guide thinking along positive channels. Protect eyes from trauma. Monitor for complete closure while asleep to prevent corneal drying.	Discusses the change in her body image Takes an active role in planning hygiene and self-care Expresses at least two positive feelings about herself daily Identifies coping strategies that aid situations

NURSING DIAGNOSIS

Sleep pattern disturbance related to increased metabolism

NURSING INTERVENTIONS	EVALUATION OF EXPECTED OUTCOMES
Ask patient what factors are conducive to sleep. Discourage intake of caffeinated foods such as coffee, cocoa, tea, chocolate, and cola drinks. Keep environmental restful and calm. Plan to provide period for uninterrupted sleep. Provide patient with normal sleep aids such as back rubs, pillow, food, drinks, and personal hygiene measures. Ask patient to discuss sleep pattern from previous night. Teach patient relaxation techniques such as meditation, guided imagery, and muscle relaxation exercises. Plan medication schedule to allow for maximum rest. Limit visitors to those persons specified by patient. Reduce environmental stimuli at bedtime (dim lights, soft music, closed doors).	Sleeps at least 6 hours without interruption and expresses a feeling of being well rested Does not exhibit signs and symptoms of sleep deprivation Discusses lifestyle changes to induce sleep after discharge to home Performs relaxation techniques at bedtime

continued

NURSING DIAGNOSIS

Knowledge deficit related to physical status as evidenced by statements of "immediate recovery"

NURSING INTERVENTIONS	EVALUATION OF EXPECTED OUTCOMES
Ascertain what patient already knows about Graves' disease. Urge her to ask questions. Suggest she write down major concerns. Determine if she enjoys learning through media (is a librarian) such as videotapes, audiotapes, or books. Begin negotiating learning objectives with her. Plan mutual establishment of goals. Set times for discussion and include her husband if needed. Discuss possible adverse side effects of medications. Answer any questions pertaining to the possibility of surgery.	Discusses newly acquired knowledge Develops realistic learning goals Identifies specific changes in her lifestyle needed to promote optimal health Discusses a reasonable time frame for condition to subside Feels free to question the possibility of surgery if necessary

KEY CONCEPTS

- Endocrine glands secrete hormones that act as chemical messengers, ultimately altering the activity of a variety of body organs.
- Endocrine glands include the thyroid gland, the parathyroid glands, the adrenal glands, the pituitary body, the gonads, and the pancreas.
- All patients requiring therapeutic procedures for endocrine disorders require maintenance of a patent airway, monitoring of fluid and electrolyte balance, assessment of vital signs and neurologic status, emotional support, and education about their condition.
- A simple goiter is an enlargement of the thyroid gland that occurs when dietary iodine is insufficient for synthesis of thyroxine. Iodized salt has reduced the incidence of this condition.
- Hyperthyroidism, or Graves' disease, is caused by an overactive thyroid gland that produces an excess of thyroid hormone.
- The symptoms of hyperthyroidism are a result of an accelerated metabolic rate and resulting increase in all physiologic processes. Common symptoms include increased appetite, weight loss, increased systolic blood pressure and pulse rate, sensitivity to heat, arrhythmias, palpitation, tremors, weakness, and bulging of the eyeballs as a result of lid retraction.
- Treatment of patients with hyperthyroidism is directed toward reducing the activity of the gland by antithyroid drugs, surgical removal of the gland, or therapeutic doses of radioactive iodine.
- Hypothyroidism is the result of an undersecretion of thyroxine by the thyroid gland. Myxedema, juvenile myxedema, and cretinism are alternate forms of this deficiency that occur at different ages.
- In adults, symptoms of hypothyroidism occur gradually, including sensitivity to cold, dryness of the skin and hair, weight gain, and a dull facial expression with puffiness around the lips and eyes.
- Treatment of hypothyroidism replaces the deficient hormone.
- Disorders of the parathyroid glands interfere with the calcium balance in the blood.
- Tetany results from a decreased level of blood calcium.
- Surgery for hyperthyroidism or replacement of deficient parathormone extract, calcium salts, and vitamin D for hypothyroidism will control the conditions.
- The adrenal cortex produces several different hormones that are essential to life. Cortisone and hydrocortisone regulate cell activity and the internal environment of the body. Aldosterone is a mineralocorticoid that maintains homeostasis of sodium

KEY CONCEPTS—cont'd

concentration in the blood. The catecholamines, epinephrine and norepinephrine, increase and prolong the effects of the sympathetic nervous system.

- Addison's disease is hypofunction of the adrenal cortex. It is a lifelong disease requiring consistent hormone replacement. Addisonian crisis is a serious exacerbation of the disease.
- Hyperfunction of the adrenal cortex results in Cushing's syndrome. Fat accumulation in the face, neck, and trunk; weakness; muscle wasting; fluid and electrolyte imbalance; irritability; and other symptoms are common. Adrenalectomy may be performed.
- Disorders of the pituitary gland are not common. However, hypersecretion of the anterior lobe of the pituitary gland can result in conditions such as acromegaly in the adult, as well as diabetes insipidus.
- The most common endocrine disorder is diabetes mellitus, a disorder resulting from insulin deficiency. Diabetes mellitus is classified as either insulin dependent type I or as noninsulin-dependent type II.
- Insulin is necessary for the body cells to combine oxygen and glucose to produce the energy necessary for body functions.
- The therapeutic goal for diabetes management is to maintain as close to normal a blood glucose level as possible while allowing the patient to maintain a normal lifestyle. This is done through administration of insulin or oral hypoglycemic agents, control of diet, and prevention of complications.
- Hyperglycemia and hypoglycemia are serious complications and should be avoided. Over time, diabetes mellitus can result in changes throughout the body.

CRITICAL THINKING EXERCISES

1. Compare the pathophysiology and resulting signs and symptoms for hypothyroidism and hyperthyroidism.
2. Explain ketosis and compare in type I and type II diabetes.
3. Design a patient teaching plan for a patient with diabetes insipidus.
4. Discuss four special teaching strategies in teaching the elderly patient with diabetes.

REFERENCES AND ADDITIONAL READINGS

Anderson RM, Fitzgerald JT, Oh MS: The relationship between diabetes related attitudes and patients' self-reported adherence, *Diabetes Educ* 19(4):287-292, 1993.

American Diabetes Association: Census statement: self-monitoring of blood glucose, *Diabetes Care* 18(1): 81-85, 1994a.

American Diabetes Association: Position statement: implications of the diabetes control and complications trial, *Diabetes Care* 11:1517-1520, 1993.

American Diabetes Association: Position statement: nutrition recommendations and principles for people with diabetes mellitus, *Diabetes Care* 17(5):519-522, 1994b.

Burch WM: *Endocrinology for the house officer,* ed 2, Baltimore, 1990, Williams & Wilkins.

Christensen MH and others: How to care for the diabetic foot, *Am J Nurs* 91(3):50-58, 1991.

Collier JH, Brodbeck CA: Assessing the diabetic foot: plantar callus and pressure sensation, *Diabetes Educ* 19(6): 503-508, 1993.

Deakens DA: Teaching elderly patients about diabetes, *Am J Nurs* 94(4):38-42, 1994.

DeWit SC: *Kean's essentials of medical surgical nursing,* ed 3, Philadelphia, 1992, WB Saunders.

Epstein CD: Fluid volume deficit for the adrenal crisis patient, *DCCN* 10(4): 210-217, 1991.

Finding JW: Cushing's syndrome an etiologic workup, *Hosp Pract* 27(10):107-112, 114-118, 121-122, 1992.

Franz MJ and others: Nutrition principles for the management of diabetes and related complications, *Diabetes Care* 17(5):490-500, 1994.

Harris MI, Cowie CC, Howie LJ: Self-monitoring of blood glucose by adults with diabetes in the United States population, *Diabetes Care* 16(8): 1116-1122, 1993.

Herman W, editor: *The prevention and treatment of complications of diabetes,* ed 2, Atlanta, 1991, National Center for Chronic Disease Prevention and Health Promotion.

Hershamn JM and others: A savvy approach to thyroid testing, *Patient Care,* 26(3): 134-137, 140-142, 144-145, 1992.

Keegan A, editor: 1994 Buyer's guide to diabetes supplies, *Diabetes Forecast* 46(10): 49-78, 1993.

Kistel F: Using blood glucose meters—part I, *Nursing 93* 23(3): 34-42, 1993.

Kistel F: Using blood glucose meters—part II, *Nursing 93* 23(4): 50-53, 1993.

Kistel F: Using blood glucose meters—part III, *Nursing 93* 23(5): 51-54, 1993.

Lammon C, Hart G: Recognizing thyroid crisis, *Nursing 93* 23(4): 33, 1993.

Lebovitz HE, editor: *Therapy for diabetes mellitus and related disorders,* Alexandria, Va, 1991, American Diabetes Association.

Lundman B, Norberg S: Coping strategies in people with insulin-dependent diabetes mellitus, *Diabetes Educ* 19(3): 198-204, 1993.

McCarren M: DCCT—the results, *Diabetes Forecast* 46(9):48-51, 1993.

Mundy GR: Evaluation and treatment of hypercalemia, *Hosp Pract* 29(6): 79-84, 1994.

National Diabetes Information Clearinghouse: Noninvasive blood glucose monitoring, *Diabetes Dateline* Spring 1993, Clearing House.

Ober PR, editor: Endocrine crisis, *Endocrinology Metab Clin North Am* 22(2):181-453, 1993.

Peterson A, and others: How to keep adrenal insufficiency in check, *Am J Nurs* 93(10): 316-320, 1992.

Policoff SP: Diseases your doctor may miss, *Ladies Home J* 107(6): 104, 106-109, 1990.

Sperling MA, editor: *Physicians guide to insulin dependent (type I) diabetes,* Alexandria, Va, 1988, American Diabetes Association.

Scherer JC: *Introductory medical surgical nursing,* ed 5, Philadelphia, 1991, JB Lippincott.

Schmidt LE and others: The relationship between eating patterns and metabolic control in patients with noninsulin dependent diabetes mellitus, *Diabetes Educ* 20(4): 317-321, 1994.

Steuer R: The light at the end of the meter, *Diabetes Self-Manage* 10(3): 42-44, 1993.

Tucker SM: *Patient care standards,* ed 5, St Louis, 1992, Mosby.

Yucka C, Blakeman N: Pheochromcyloma—the great mimic, *Cancer Nurs* 14(3): 136-140, 1991.

Zehrer CL, Gross CR: Patient perceptions of benefits and concerns following pancreas transplantation, *Diabetes Educ* 20(3):217-219, 1994.

CHAPTER 28

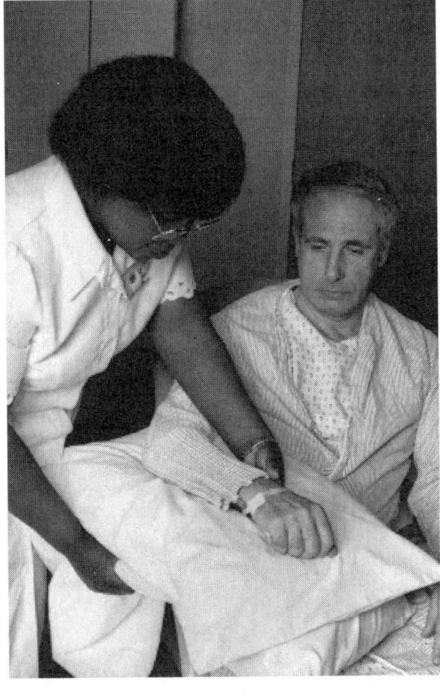

Neurologic Function

CHAPTER OBJECTIVES

1 Define the basic structure and function of the nervous system.
2 Discuss the purposes of the various neurodiagnostic procedures.
3 Interpret the signs and symptoms of neurologic disturbances.
4 Recognize the significance of alterations in the patient's neurologic status.
5 List the characteristics of major neurologic conditions.
6 Identify the reasons underlying medical interventions for neurologic conditions.
7 Describe nursing interventions for patients with neurologic dysfunction.

KEY WORDS

aphasia
ataxia
aura
autonomic hyperreflexia
automatism
cerebrospinal fluid (CSF)
cholinergic crisis
coma
concussion
confusion
consciousness
craniotomy
dysphagia
flaccid
hemianopia
hemiplegia
hemorrhagic
herniation
hyperreflexia
intracranial pressure
ischemic stroke
laminectomy and diskectomy
lethargic
meninges
Monro-Kellie hypothesis
muscle spasms
myasthenic crisis
neglect
nuccal rigidity
obtunded
paraplegia
quadriplegia
reflex
rigidity
seizure
spinal shock
stupor
tremor

STRUCTURE AND FUNCTION OF THE NERVOUS SYSTEM

The nervous system is the body's most highly organized and complex system. It controls the motor, sensory, and autonomic function of the body. The nervous system receives sensory information from the body's internal and external environment, interprets sensory input into the brain, and determines the body's responses to these sensory messages. In this way the nervous system controls and coordinates all the body's systems so they function as an integrated whole.

The nervous system is divided into the central nervous system and the peripheral nervous system. The *central nervous system* is composed of the brain and the spinal cord. The *peripheral nervous system* is made up of 12 pairs of cranial nerves that arise from the brain stem, 31 pairs of spinal nerves that arise from the spinal cord, and the autonomic system. Information to and from the brain and spinal cord is carried by the cranial and spinal nerves respectively.

The *autonomic nervous system,* a division of the peripheral nervous system, carries information to smooth muscle (heart, lungs, intestines, bladder) and glands (salivary, adrenal, pancreas). The autonomic nervous system acts automatically; its functions are carried out without the individual's awareness. The autonomic nervous system is divided further into the sympathetic and parasympathetic nervous system. The *sympathetic nervous system* produces generalized physiologic responses to prepare the individual for "fight or flight." Increased heart rate and blood pressure; an increased blood supply to the brain, skeletal muscles, and heart; and vasoconstriction of the blood vessels of the skin are examples of these responses. The *parasympathetic nervous system* produces more localized effects in particular organs, such as slowing the heart rate and increasing peristalsis. The parasympathetic nervous system balances the effects of the sympathetic nervous system, maintaining the body in a state of equilibrium.

The brain is divided into three major areas: the cerebrum, the brain stem, and the cerebellum (Figure 28-1). The *cerebrum* is divided further into two cerebral hemispheres. The left hemisphere controls the right side of the body, and the right hemisphere, the left.

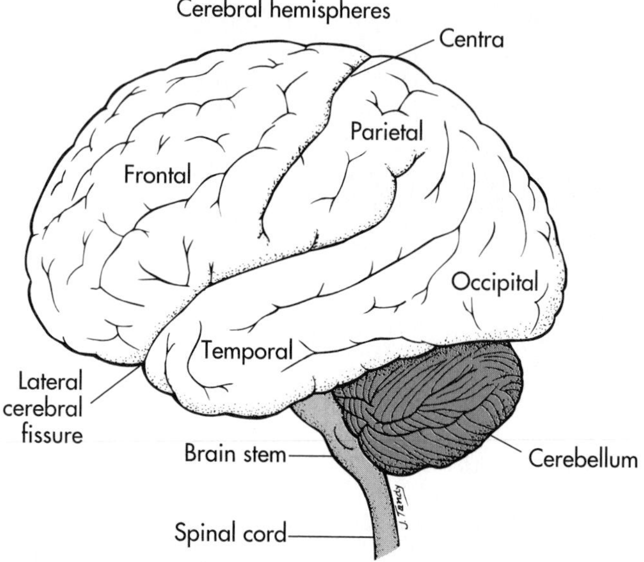

Figure 28-1 Major parts of the brain.

The hemispheres are composed of pairs of frontal, parietal, temporal, and occipital lobes. The cerebrum receives, analyzes, and stores information for future use and controls conscious voluntary movements. The *cerebellum,* attached to the brain stem, assists in the coordination of voluntary movement and maintenance of muscle tone. The *brain stem* is the pathway for impulses between the brain and spinal cord. The vital centers for control of respiration, cardiac function, and vasoconstriction of blood vessels are located here. All the sensory and motor pathways must pass through the brain stem on their way to the brain. Many of these pathways cross over in the brain stem, which explains why injury to one side of the brain may result in loss of function on the opposite side of the body.

The *spinal cord* is a slender cylinder of nerve tissue extending from the brain stem to the level of the first lumbar vertebrae (Figure 28-2). The spinal nerves that innervate the legs extend beyond the end of the spinal cord to approximately the level of the hip. The function of the spinal cord is to transmit sensory information from the periphery to the brain and motor responses from the brain to nerves supplying muscles and glands. The spinal cord also

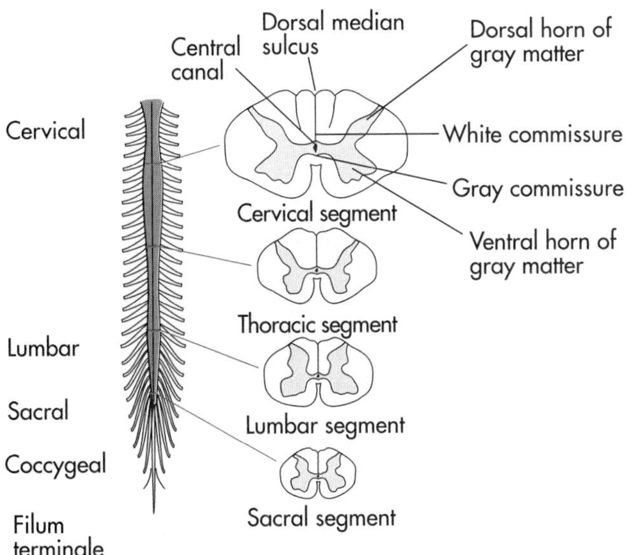

Figure 28-2 Spinal cord showing cross-sections.

serves as the connection for the reflex pathway (as illustrated by eliciting the deep-tendon reflexes) that bypasses the brain.

The brain and spinal cord are protected from injury by a bony covering, by the meninges, and by the cerebrospinal fluid. The skull or cranium is the bony covering of the brain; the spinal cord is encased within the *vertebral column*. The **meninges** are connective-tissue coverings that completely enclose the brain and spinal cord. In addition to providing protection, the meninges contain the blood vessels that supply the brain and spinal cord. The brain and spinal cord are suspended in **cerebrospinal fluid** (CSF), a clear, watery liquid that fills the ventricles of the brain and extends down into the spinal canal around the spinal cord. It provides moisture and lubrication and cushions the brain and spinal cord from injury.

ASSESSMENT OF THE PATIENT WITH NEUROLOGIC DYSFUNCTION

The Neurologic Examination

The neurologic examination is usually carried out by the physician to determine the presence or absence of neurologic dysfunction, to diagnose diseases of the nervous system, and to localize disease within the nervous system. An advanced practice nurse may also conduct a neurologic examination. The nurse's ability to interpret this data is helpful in identifying specific areas of concern and focus when planning the overall care of the patient. For example, a patient with a middle cerebral artery distribution stroke is likely to have hemiparesis, or weakness involving one side of the body. It would be important for the nurse to make that assessment and apply this information when planning the patient's daily care. The patient might, for example, need assistance with activities of daily living and with mobilizing.

The purpose of the basic neurologic examination is to localize the site of a pathologic condition. The nurse provides support to the patient and observes the patient's responses to the examination. These data help the nurse to establish a baseline of neurologic function that is used as a point of comparison for ongoing assessments.

The examination includes the systematic evaluation of the patient's mental status; cranial nerve function, including those of the senses (vision, hearing, taste, smell); motor function (e.g., muscle strength and tone); sensory function (e.g., perception of light touch, pain, temperature, and position sense); cerebellar function (e.g., gait and coordination); and deep-tendon reflexes (e.g., knee jerk, ankle jerk).

The mental status portion of the examination consists of observations regarding the patient's behavior, emotional status, affect, and mood. In addition, formal testing of level of orientation, memory, and higher level cognitive function is carried out. The cranial nerve examination provides information regarding the functioning of the 12 pairs of cranial nerves (Table 28-1) as well as some information about the function of their point of origin, the brain stem.

Evaluation of the pupils is an important part of the cranial nerve examination. It provides vital information about central nervous system function. When assessing pupils, it is important to note their size, shape, and reaction to light. Normally the pupils are equal in size, are round, and constrict when light is shone into the eye. Deviation from these norms may indicate an increase in intracranial pressure and should be reported immediately.

Motor system examination is conducted systematically, beginning with the upper limbs and the trunk and proceeding to the lower extremities. Consideration is given to muscle size, tone, and strength and to the presence of involuntary movements. Conducted in the same systematic manner, the sensory examination evaluates the patient's ability to perceive various types of sensation with the eyes closed. Perception of pain, temperature, light touch, and position sense (proprioception) are common modalities included in the test.

TABLE 28-1

Cranial Nerves and Their Functions

Nerve	Function
I Olfactory	Sense of smell
II Optic	Visual acuity
III Oculomotor	Movement of eye muscles Upper lid opening Pupillary reflexes
IV Trochlear	Movement: superior oblique eye muscles
V Trigeminal	Sensory of face Motor to muscles of chewing
VI Abducens	Movement of lateral rectus eye muscle
VII Facial	Motor to muscles of facial expression Sensory: taste, anterior two-thirds of tongue
VIII Acoustic	Auditory acuity Position in space: balance
IX Glossopharyngeal	Sensory position in space Motor to uvula Soft tissue of palate Sensory: taste in posterior one third of tongue
X Vagus	Motor to muscles of pharynx and larynx
XI Hypoglossal	Motor to tongue
XII Spinal accessory	Motor to sternocleidomastoid muscles and trapezius muscles

From Malasanos L, Barkauskas V, Stoltenberg-Allen K: *Health assessment,* ed 5, St Louis, 1994, Mosby.

OLDER ADULT CONSIDERATIONS

- Peripheral nerve cells, fibers, and brain cells decrease in number with aging, becoming more pronounced after age 70. This decrease is not necessarily associated with decreased cognitive ability.
- Slowing of nerve impulse transmission may result in a longer reaction time and diminished reflexes in the elderly. Tremors are common.
- The sense of pain is diminished in the elderly, and they may be free of pain in such acute disorders as myocardial infarction or pneumonia.
- Recovery from stress is slower and incomplete with increased age.
- There are fewer periods of deep sleep and frequent periods of wakefulness in the elderly, although the total sleep time is approximately the same as that in younger people.
- Confusion is not normal behavior for the elderly. Reversible confusion can be a result of such conditions as anemia, electrolyte imbalances, hypoxia, drug therapy, pain, and sensory deficit or overstimulation.
- Thickening of vessel walls and atherosclerosis and arteriosclerosis may increase the incidence of TIAs. A complete assessment should follow a TIA.
- Cerebrovascular accidents increase after the age of 55.

The assessment of cerebellar function includes the observation of gait and the patient's ability to perform coordinated tasks with the upper and lower extremities. The reflex examination provides important information about the status of the central nervous system. The **reflex** response is elicited when the tendon is suddenly stretched as by the tap of a reflex hammer. Reflexes commonly assessed include the biceps, triceps, and brachioradialis in the upper extremities and the patellar and achilles reflexes in the lower extremities. The plantar response (Babinski reflex) is a superficial reflex that is included in this portion of the examination. The presence of a Babinski reflex indicates damage at a higher level in the central nervous system.

The findings of the neurologic examination may indicate the need for further assessment with the help of diagnostic tests.

Lumbar Puncture

A lumbar puncture consists of withdrawing a small amount of fluid (usually 8 to 10 ml) from the lumbar subarachnoid space via a hollow needle with a stylet. The procedure, done for diagnostic purposes, is usually performed in the patient's room or in an outpatient clinic.

Before the examination, the nurse should explain the procedure to the patient, emphasizing the need to remain completely still. During the procedure, the patient is placed in the side-lying position near the edge of the bed with the knees pulled up, the back bowed, and the chin and knees together (Figure 28-3). A local anesthetic is used to minimize discomfort, but the patient may experience slight pressure at the insertion site or feel pain that extends down the legs. Using strict aseptic technique, the needle is placed between L3 and L4 or L4 and L5 (level with the top of the hip bones), which is below the level of where the spinal cord ends at L1. CSF pressure is then measured with a

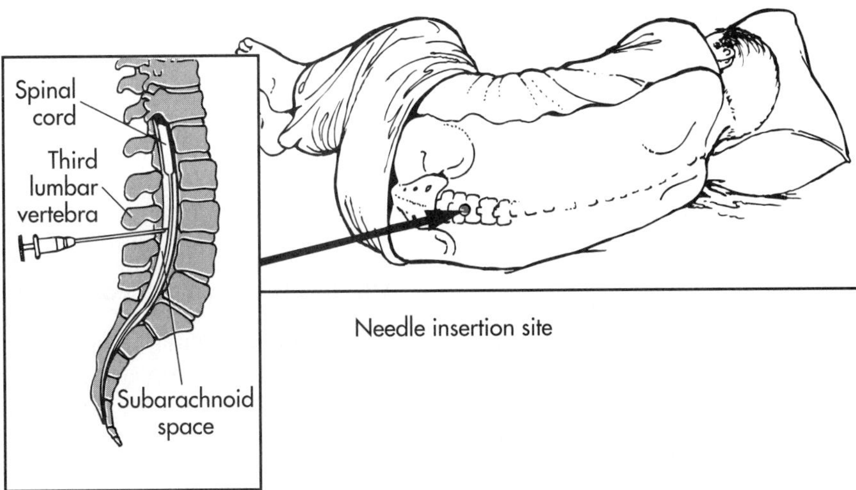

Figure 28-3 Patient position for lumbar puncture. An imaginary line can be drawn from the iliac crests, above L4 and L5. (From Beare PB, Myers JL: *Adult health nursing,* ed 2, St Louis, 1994, Mosby.)

manometer. Specimens of spinal fluid are collected in test tubes. Typical laboratory tests done on the fluid include the measurement of glucose, cell count, and protein, as well as a gram stain and culture and sensitivity tests.

Throughout the procedure, the nurse should provide emotional support and encourage the patient to relax and lie quietly. The nurse should observe and record any significant reactions to the procedure, noting any changes in pulse, respiratory rate, or skin color.

Following a lumbar puncture, the patient should be advised to maintain flat bedrest for between 6 to 12 hours. Fluids are forced and vital signs and neurologic signs are monitored often. The loss of cerebrospinal fluid or leakage of fluid at the puncture site may cause a mild to severe headache. A mild analgesic is generally administered (e.g., acetaminophen, codeine). Because the headache is often aggravated by an upright position, flat bedrest is advised.

Neuroradiologic Studies

Cerebral angiography and myelography are contrast studies that allow for detection of pathologic disorders of the brain and spinal cord. The procedures are done in the diagnostic radiology department and usually require only a local anesthetic or mild sedation. The nurse is responsible for providing care to the patient before and after the procedure.

Cerebral angiography

A cerebral angiogram consists of injecting a radiopaque contrast medium into an artery for visualization of the cerebral arterial system. As the contrast medium circulates in the arterial system, intracranial lesions (tumors) or cerebrovascular abnormalities (aneurysms) can be seen. The puncture site (generally the femoral or brachial artery) is cleaned aseptically and local anesthetic is injected. The injection of contrast medium follows. Patients with a sensitivity to the contrast media may experience nausea and vomiting at this time. Following the procedure, pressure must be applied to the puncture site for 5 to 10 minutes. Vital signs and neurologic status are monitored often. The nurse should also carefully inspect the site to ensure that bleeding has not occurred or that a hematoma has not developed. The patient must remain on bedrest with the punctured extremity immobilized for 8 hours. Pulses distal to the puncture site should also be monitored. Normal activities can usually be resumed following the period of bedrest.

Myelography

A myelogram is an x-ray examination of the spinal cord and vertebral canal following injection of a contrast medium (dye) through a lumbar puncture. The purpose of the procedure is to identify partial or complete obstructions that interfere with the flow of the contrast medium (e.g., spinal cord tumors or ruptured intervertebral disks).

A water-soluble contrast medium (metrizamide [Amipaque]) has replaced the oil-based medium that was commonly used in the past because it is self-absorbing and nonirritative and causes fewer side effects. The frequency of myelography as a diagnostic tool has decreased since the advent and accessibility of CT and MRI scans.

Following the procedure, vital signs and neurologic status should be monitored as ordered. Fluids are usually encouraged to aid in eliminating the contrast medium. It is generally advisable to keep the head of the patient's bed elevated 30 to 45 degrees for 12 to 24 hours to prevent the contrast material from entering the intracranial vault, because this has the potential to cause seizures.

Computed tomography

Computed tomography (CT scan) is a diagnostic technique used to study the structure of the brain. It is noninvasive, involves low exposure to x-rays, and is low risk to the patient. It has virtually revolutionized the diagnosis of neurologic disorders. Its three-dimensional views of the brain contents allow for differentiation among intracranial tumors, cysts, edema, and hemorrhage. Narrow X-ray beams pass through the head and are either absorbed or transmitted, depending on the density of tissue. Through interpreting changes in density from that of normal tissue, a diagnosis can be made. To intensify imaging, a contrast medium may be used. This is particularly helpful if a tumor or abscess is suspected.

The nurse should explain the procedure to the patient, indicating that the patient will remain flat with the head immobilized throughout the scan. The patient may resume normal activities once the procedure is completed.

Magnetic resonance imaging

Magnetic resonance imaging (MRI) is now available in most medical centers. MRI scans are similar to CT scans except that radiofrequency waves rather than x-rays are used. The images obtained are unmatched for sharpness and detail and provide information about the anatomy of the brain as well as the chemistry and the physiology of the tissue. It is useful in diagnosing tumors, hemorrhage, vascular malformations, and neurodegenerative disorders in addition to other pathologic conditions. Little preparation of the patient is required before an MRI scan. The nurse should explain the scan to the patient, including the possibility of claustrophobia during the procedure. A mild sedative (e.g., diazepam [Valium], lorazepam [Ativan]) might be helpful if this is a problem. All external metals such as jewelry must be removed before the scan. Patients with metallic implants cannot be exposed to MRI. After the procedure, the patient can resume normal activity.

Positron emission tomography

Positron emission tomography (PET) scanning is a noninvasive technique that provides information about biochemical and physiologic functioning. It is helpful in diagnosing diseases that alter the metabolism and cerebral blood flow within areas of the brain (e.g., Alzheimer's disease, cerebrovascular disease, mental illness). Its major advantage is the increased clarity of images provided over conventional radionuclide scans. The necessary equipment for generation of these images, however, is available in only selected, major research centers.

Electroencephalography

Electroencephalography (EEG) is a graphic recording of the brain's electric activity and can be performed on patients of any age. The EEG is not considered conclusive but may be helpful in locating the site of a lesion or in determining the presence of epilepsy. The test is performed by placing small electrodes at specified locations on each side of the patient's scalp. The electrodes are connected by wires to a recording machine, which transcribes the electric activity on graph paper. The EEG is performed in a darkened room and takes 1 to 2 hours to complete. Before the test, the patient is instructed to avoid stimulants or depressants of any type (e.g., coffee, tea, colas, alcoholic beverages, or sedatives). The scalp should be clean, but no other preparation is necessary. No specific follow-up nursing care is required.

Electromyography

Electromyography (EMG) is a diagnostic test that measures and records the electric activity of muscles. The EMG is useful in detecting dysfunction of the motor neuron, the neuromuscular junction, or muscle fibers. Either surface electrodes are applied to the patient's skin, or needle electrodes are inserted into the muscle. Patients should be assured that they are in no danger of being electrocuted. However, some discomfort may be felt when the muscles are stimulated.

The procedures previously outlined are among the most commonly performed for the diagnosis of disorders of the nervous system. Nursing care before and after the procedures may differ depending on the specifics of the patient's situation, hospital protocol, or physician's preference. Some of these procedures require signed consent from the patient.

Patients and families also need accurate information and the opportunity to ask questions and express concerns. The patient undergoing these procedures is likely to be stressed as a result of the factors that brought him or her to seek treatment and may be anxious about what the findings will mean.

GENERAL CONSIDERATIONS IN NEUROLOGIC NURSING

Altered States of Cerebral Functioning

Consciousness can be thought of as being on a continuum from a state of complete wakefulness to that of sleep or coma. The reticular formation, a portion of the brain stem, is responsible for maintaining wakefulness. Unconsciousness, or a state in which the patient is unresponsive to sensory stimuli and lacks awareness of self, is a symptom of many conditions, some of which involve the central nervous system directly and others that do not. For a patient to be in a **coma,** the cerebral hemispheres, the brain stem, or both must be damaged.

The cerebral cortex, responsible for higher level mental function, is also the portion of the brain involved with thought, association, discrimination, judgment, and memory. These functions may be disrupted or disturbed following a head injury or in certain diseases.

The nurse, who often has the most frequent contact with the patient, may be the first to note changes in levels of consciousness. It is the nurse's responsibility to assess and record accurately any changes in the patient's neurologic status. Even subtle changes in behavior may be important in the diagnosis and treatment of the patient's condition. Therefore any changes should be documented carefully and reported at once.

One tool available to the nurse for accurate reporting of level of consciousness is the Glasgow Coma Scale (GCS). Originally developed for use with patients with closed head injuries, it has become widely used in the United States for all patients with altered levels of consciousness. The GCS evaluates three aspects of behavioral responses that reflect cerebral functioning: eye opening, best verbal response, and best motor response. Each area is scored by the degree of responsiveness (Box 28-1).

BOX 28-1

GLASGOW COMA SCALE SCORING

EYES OPEN
4 Spontaneously
3 On request
2 To pain stimuli (supraorbital or digital)
1 No opening

BEST VERBAL RESPONSE
5 Oriented to time, place, person
4 Engages in conversation, confused in content
3 Words spoken but conversation not sustained
2 Groans evoked by pain
1 No response

BEST MOTOR RESPONSE
5 Obeys a command ("Hold out three fingers.")
4 Localizes a painful stimulus
3 Flexes either arm
2 Extends arm to painful stimulus
1 No response

Phipps WJ and others: *Medical-surgical nursing: concepts and clinical practice,* St Louis, 1995, Mosby.

Scores assigned to each section are based on the patient's best response in that area. The individual subcategory scores are totaled to determine the overall level of consciousness score, which can range from 3 to 15. The less responsive the patient, the lower the score. The tool has been used with some success in predicting morbidity and mortality following head injury. Patients with GCS scores of 3 to 4 within the first 24 hours of coma have been found to have only a 7% chance of achieving independence as compared with those who have scores of 11 or more, of whom 82% regain independence (Jennett, Teasdale, 1977).

There are many terms used to describe various states of consciousness, but there is no agreement on the specific manifestations of each state. Because no precise terminology exists for conveying information regarding level of consciousness from one clinician to another, confusion often exists regarding the accuracy of assessing these patients. When used appropriately, the GCS decreases the subjectivity and confusion associated with assessment of level of consciousness.

Despite the confusion of terminology, there are several terms used commonly in clinical discussions to describe altered states of consciousness. These include confusion, lethargy, obtundation, stupor, and coma.

Confusion refers to some level of disorientation, either to time, place, or person. The confused patient has some difficulty in following commands and may be agitated, restless, or irritable. The **lethargic** patient is generally oriented to time, place, and person but exhibits a slowing of mental processes, speech, and motor activities. The patient who is **obtunded** often sleeps when not stimulated but can follow simple commands and is appropriately conversant when aroused. **Stupor** refers to the patient who is generally unarousable even to vigorous stimulus. The patient's verbal output may consist only of incomprehensible sounds, but he or she responds appropriately to painful stimuli. The patient in a **coma** appears to be in a sleeplike state with eyes closed and does not respond appropriately to external stimuli (Box 28-2).

Increased Intracranial Pressure

An understanding of the concept of increased intracranial pressure is fundamental when caring for the patient with neurologic problems. Uncontrolled and untreated intracranial hypertension can lead to irre-

BOX 28-2 **Nursing Process**

THE UNCONSCIOUS PATIENT

ASSESSMENT

LOC
Neurologic status
Vital signs
Respiratory status
Laboratory studies: ABGs, pulse oximetry, electrolytes
Fluid volume status
Nutritional status

NURSING DIAGNOSES

Ineffective airway clearance related to neurologic deficit
Total incontinence related to unconsciousness
Ineffective breathing pattern related to unconsciousness
Risk for impaired gas exchange related to unconsciousness
Impaired swallowing related to unconsciousness
Risk for injury related to unconsciousness
Impaired physical mobility related to unconsciousness
Altered nutrition: less than body requirements related to altered intake pattern
Altered oral mucous membranes related to unconsciousness
Self-care deficit related to unconsciousness
Risk for impaired skin integrity related to decreased mobility

NURSING INTERVENTIONS

Ensure an open airway; insertion of an oral airway or tracheostomy may be necessary.
Position patient in lateral or semiprone position to facilitate drainage of oral secretions.
Aspirate tracheal and oral secretions by suctioning patient as necessary.
Check vital signs, neurologic signs (pupillary reaction, reflexes), and levels of consciousness every 15 minutes for first several hours and then every hour for 24 hours.
Turn patient every 2 hours.
Maintain proper body alignment by positioning patient to prevent foot drop, wrist drop, and joint contracture.
Carry out passive range-of-motion exercises on all joints at least four times a day.
Use sheepskin pads, water mattresses, or alternating air flotation systems to prevent pressure sores.
Protect eyes from irritation and corneal ulceration—use eye shields, eye irrigations with physiologic saline, or eye lubricants and ointments as ordered by physician.
Monitor intravenous fluids or tube feedings closely; do not give unconscious patients oral fluids.
Carry out frequent oral hygiene.
Monitor patient's urinary output closely; if indwelling catheter is in place, tape to abdomen for male patient.
Administer suppositories or enemas or both as necessary to maintain bowel elimination.
Provide emotional support and reassurance to family; allow family members to assist in care when feasible.

EVALUATION OF EXPECTED OUTCOMES

Maximum pulmonary function maintained
Aspiration prevented
Skin integrity maintained
Adequate nutrition status maintained

versible neurologic pathology and possible cardiopulmonary arrest.

Intracranial pressure (ICP) is the pressure exerted by the cerebrospinal fluid within the ventricles of the brain. Although ICP fluctuates in response to multiple factors, it is normally less than 10 mm Hg when measured at the level of the ventricles in the brain. The **Monro-Kellie hypothesis** provides the basis to the understanding of pathophysiologic changes related to increased intracranial pressure. The hypothesis states that the skull is a rigid compartment that is filled to capacity with three components: blood, brain, and cerebrospinal fluid. If any one component increases in volume, another component must decrease for the overall volume to maintain constant, or a rise in ICP will occur. Increased intracranial pressure, or intracranial hypertension, is defined as a elevation of ICP of 15 mm Hg or higher.

A variety of conditions, which will be discussed throughout this chapter, can cause increased ICP. These include the following:

- **Conditions that increase brain volume** (e.g., abscesses, tumors, hematomas, aneurysms)
- **Conditions that increase blood volume** (e.g., obstruction of venous outflow)
- **Conditions that increase CSF volume** (e.g., hydrocephalus, tumors that produce CSF [choroid plexus papilloma])

One of the principal goals of neurologic assessment is the early detection of signs and symptoms of increased ICP (Box 28-3). It is imperative that the nurse establish a neurologic baseline for all patients at risk for the development of increased ICP and perform ongoing assessments of the individual as often as the situation dictates. Any changes in the baseline neurologic examination should be reported immediately so that treatment for increased ICP can be initiated. Increased ICP should be considered a neurologic emergency.

Early signs and symptoms of increased ICP may include a deterioration in the level of consciousness (e.g., confusion or drowsiness), changes in pupillary response to light, motor weakness on one side of the

BOX 28-3

EARLY AND LATE SIGNS AND SYMPTOMS OF INCREASED INTRACRANIAL PRESSURE

Early Signs and Symptoms	Late Signs and Symptoms
Changes in LOC: Restlessness, irritability, personality changes, mild confusion, agitation, lower Glasgow Coma Score (GCS)	LOC: Difficult to arouse, require more stimulus, any decrease in Glasgow Coma Score (GCS), coma
Pupils: Ptosis, ovoid pupil, delayed or sluggish reactivity, unilateral change in pupil size	Pupils: Unilateral enlarging pupil, progressing to fixed, dilated "blown pupil"; papilledema; later bilateral fixed, dilated
Vision: Blurred, diplopia, decreased visual acuity	Motor: Dense weakness, decorticate or decerebrate posturing, flaccid muscles
Motor: Pronator drift, decreased grasp, paresis	Sensory: May only posture to painful stimulus
Sensory: Decreased response to touch or pinprick	Headache: Worsening with projectile vomiting
Headache: Early morning headache with nausea/vomiting	Speech: May only groan/moan to painful stimuli
Speech: Slow or slurred	Respiratory: Irregular respirations, Cheyne-Stokes progressing to central neurogenic hyperventilation, ataxia, and respiratory arrest
Memory: Slightly impaired	Vital signs: Rising systolic BP with widening pulse pressure, bradycardia followed by tachycardia, temperature changes as hypothalamus is compressed, Cushing's response
Appearance of cranial incision: Postoperative bulging or swelling	Cardiac: Q-waves with ST depression, elevated T waves, supraventricular tachycardia, sinus bradycardia, A-V block, PVCs, and an agonal rhythm leading to cardiac arrest
Vital signs: No change	Cranial nerves: Related to supratentorial or infratentorial lesion and edema with brain stem reflexes (corneal, gag)
Cranial nerves: May or may not show changes initially	Abnormal reflexes: Babinski sign
Seizure activity: May or may not occur depending on cause	

From Barker E: *Neuroscience Nursing,* St Louis, 1994, Mosby.

body, headache, possible seizures, and vomiting. If increased ICP is left untreated, the patient's level of consciousness may continue to deteriorate, pupillary dilation may occur on one side, and changes in vital signs may occur. Vital-sign changes include slowing of the pulse, widening of the pulse pressure, and respiratory rate irregularities. These changes, however, are late and are often indicative of impending herniation. **Herniation** is defined as the abnormal protrusion of a portion of the brain through one of the defects or natural openings in the skull. If increased ICP remains untreated, herniation of a portion of the cerebrum can occur, resulting in pressure on the brain stem. Death can follow as a result of pressure on the vital structures of the medulla.

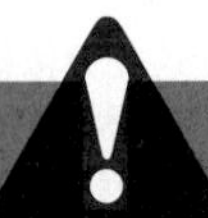

NURSE ALERT

Deterioration in a patient's level of consciousness accompanied by changes in pupillary response, motor weakness, headache, seizures, or vomiting may indicate that intracranial pressure is increasing.

Medical treatment of patients with increased ICP focuses on the rapid diagnosis of the condition, the support of body systems, and the control of intracranial hypertension. Medications such as osmotic diuretics (Mannitol) and corticosteriods (Decadron) are often used. Mannitol's osmotic effect causes water to be drawn from the edematous brain, reducing brain volume and decreasing ICP. The use of Decadron is somewhat controversial, and its action is not completely clear. It is thought, however, to be effective in reducing cerebral edema.

Control of temperature, blood pressure, and respiratory rate (by mechanical hyperventilation) are all important in the management of increased ICP. Drainage of CSF through an intraventricular catheter allows not only for control of ICP but also for constant monitoring of the ICP. Other methods of ICP monitoring include the use of a subarachnoid screw or bolt or the use of a fiberoptic transducer-tipped catheter. Surgical intervention aimed at removal of tumor, hematoma, or abscess or decompression by debulking of infarcted or necrotic cerebral tissue also helps to reduce intracranial hypertension.

Nursing intervention with this population is aimed primarily at early detection of signs of increased pressure and control of any factors that may increase cerebral pressure further (Box 28-4).

CARE OF THE PATIENT WITH TRAUMA TO THE NERVOUS SYSTEM

Trauma is the leading cause of death in persons between the ages of 1 and 44 years of age (Ross, Pitts, Kobayashi, 1992). Central nervous system trauma, including injury to the brain and spinal cord, contributes significantly to death in more than half of these trauma victims. Those that survive are often left with permanent disability, including paralysis, memory loss, personality changes, and speech disturbance. The incidence of traumatic injuries of this type are two to three times higher in males than in females, and over half are associated with alcohol and drug use. Nearly one half of all head injuries are caused by motor vehicle accidents. Public education in the prevention of accidents and the use of safety measures such as seat belts, air bags, and helmets is essential to lower the incidence of devastating injury from trauma.

Head Injuries

The term *head injury* refers to any injury involving the scalp, the skull, or the brain. Head injuries are classified as *closed* if the skull covering the brain remains intact and *open* when injury penetrates the skull. Injuries to the scalp include abrasions, contusions, and lacerations. These injuries are debrided and surgically closed as necessary.

Skull fractures are classified in several ways. A fracture may be (1) linear (simple), in which the fracture resembles a line or single crack in the skull; (2) comminuted, in which the bone is fragmented into many pieces; or (3) depressed, where there is inward depression of bone fragments. Basal skull fractures involve fractures of the bones of the base of the skull. The consequences of these fractures are more serious than those of the cranial vault because they are often associated with dural tears and result in leakage of CSF. The nurse should carefully observe any patient with brain injury for serous or bloody drainage from the ears or nose. This drainage may indicate leakage of CSF. Such an opening may allow infection to be introduced into the cranial cavity from the nose or ears, causing meningitis. Nasal procedures (such as insertion of nasogastric tubes or nasal suctioning) should be avoided in such patients. If frank drainage is observed, a sample of the fluid should be checked for glucose, which is an indication of the presence of CSF.

Injuries to the brain can be classified as diffuse or focal. A **concussion** is considered a diffuse injury and is defined as a transient, temporary, neurogenic dysfunction caused by mechanical force to the brain (Hickey, 1992). The degree of severity of a concussion is deter-

BOX 28-4 **Nursing Process**

INCREASED INTRACRANIAL PRESSURE

ASSESSMENT

Neurologic status
Vital signs for changes in status
Fluid volume status
ICP
Respiratory status
Nutrition status
Laboratory studies (e.g., CBC, electrolytes, ABGs)

NURSING DIAGNOSES

Sensory/perceptual alterations related to neurologic deficit and decreased consciousness
Self-care deficit related to neurologic deficit and decreased consciousness
Impaired physical mobility related to neurologic deficit and decreased consciousness
Ineffective airway clearance related to neurologic deficit and decreased consciousness
Risk for ineffective breathing pattern related to neurologic deficit and decreased consciousness
Altered nutrition: less than body requirements related to neurologic deficit and decreased consciousness
Risk for injury related to neurologic deficit and decreased consciousness
Impaired swallowing related to neurologic deficit and decreased consciousness
Total incontinence related to neurologic deficit and decreased consciousness
Altered thought processes related to neurologic deficit and decreased consciousness

NURSING INTERVENTIONS

Elevate head approximately 30 degrees to improve cerebral drainage.
Check vital signs, blood pressure, neurologic signs, and level of consciousness every hour for first 24 hours.
Minimize situations that cause an increase in intracranial pressure—for example, vomiting, coughing, straining during bowel movements, or changing position.
Maintain an open airway and use oxygen therapy as ordered to prevent decreased oxygenation of brain tissue.
Monitor intravenous fluids closely; do not overhydrate by infusing intravenous solutions or blood transfusions rapidly.
Accurately measure intake and output.
Know the differences between symptoms of increased intracranial pressure and shock.
Check with physician about hyperventilating patient to keep $Paco_2$ at 25 to 30 mm Hg.
Report immediately to physician any changes in patient's condition.

EVALUATION OF EXPECTED OUTCOMES

Injuries prevented
Maximum pulmonary function maintained
Aspiration prevented
Skin integrity maintained
Adequate nutrition status and fluid intake maintained
Participates in self-care as appropriate
Relates rationale for interventions

mined by the length of loss of consciousness and the persistence of memory deficits that are often associated with the injury. Other symptoms include headache, drowsiness, confusion, dizziness, and irritability.

A cerebral contusion is a bruising of the surface of the brain resulting in areas of hemorrhage. The signs and symptoms of a contusion are related to the anatomic structures involved. They may be relatively minor if the contusion is small, whereas larger contusions often produce significant deficits and problems with increased ICP. Treatment depends on the degree of injury.

Traumatic intracranial hemorrhage is a common complication of head injury (Figure 28-4). An *epidural hematoma* refers to hemorrhage into the potential space between the inner table of the skull and the dura. Hematomas often form under the site of a skull fracture when laceration of an artery has occurred. Treatment is always surgical, and early diagnosis is imperative. Because bleeding is often arterial, death can result if left untreated.

A *subdural hematoma* results from bleeding into the subdural space between the dura and the arachnoid layers. Bleeding is generally caused by rupture of the small vessels that bridge the subdural space. Small subdural hematomas may be treated medically because they are often absorbed. Larger hematomas require surgical evacuation.

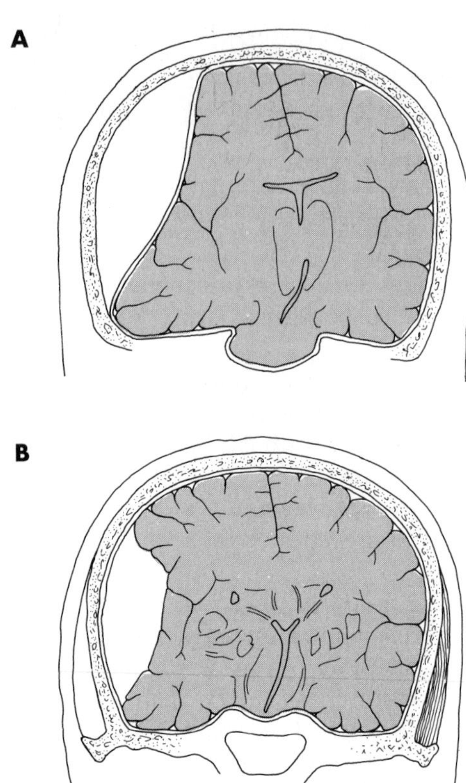

Figure 28-4 **A,** Epidural hematoma in the temporal fossa, usually a result of laceration of the middle meningeal artery. **B,** Subdural hematoma, usually a result of laceration of the subdural veins. (From Price S, Wilson L, editors: *Pathophysiology: clinical concepts of disease processes,* ed 4, St Louis, 1991, Mosby.)

Bleeding may also occur within the brain itself, resulting in *intracranial hemorrhage* or *hematoma* formation. They are often associated with serious brain injuries such as contusions, lacerations, and other types of hematomas. Signs and symptoms include headache, deterioration in level of consciousness, hemiplegia on the contralateral side, and dilation of the pupil on the side of the clot. Craniotomy is beneficial when there is a distinct clot that can be evacuated. Most of these patients are at risk for problems related to increased ICP.

On arrival at the emergency department, the priorities of management include maintenance of airway, breathing, and circulation. A careful history and physical examination are carried out, and a CT scan is done once the patient is hemodynamically stable. Frequent neurologic assessments should be done because the level of consciousness is an important indicator of neurologic function. The patient should also be examined carefully for additional injuries to the cervical spine, abdomen, chest, and extremities. The treatment of head injury is primarily aimed at reducing and controlling cerebral edema and preventing compression of intracranial contents from depressed skull fractures, hemorrhage, or hematoma.

Increased ICP following acute head injury is most often caused by cerebral edema. Osmotic diuretics such as mannitol reduce cerebral edema. Limiting fluid intake to 1200 ml per 24-hour period also reduces brain swelling. Fluid and electrolyte balance should be monitored closely because sodium and water retention often occur as a result of increased secretion of antidiuretic hormone (ADH).

Seizure activity caused by cerebral irritation can occur and must be prevented and controlled with anticonvulsants such as phenytoin (Dilantin) and phenobarbital. Hyperthermia can occur as a result of injury to the hypothalamus. As cerebral metabolism increases when the patient is hyperthermic, it is important to monitor the temperature closely and treat fevers promptly with antipyretics.

The importance of maintaining a clear and patent airway to ensure effective respirations cannot be over-emphasized. Impaired respiratory function can result in decreased oxygen supply to brain tissue and contribute to cerebral edema. The nurse should observe the patient closely for any changes in respiratory function, hyperventilation, hypoventilation, or irregular respiratory rates. Any sign of respiratory dysfunction should be reported immediately so treatment can be initiated.

The nutrition needs of the patient should be addressed early because the metabolic rate following head injury increases markedly. Patients may require long-term nutrition management via a gastrostomy tube. Stress ulceration of the stomach and duodenum are also a concern in this population. These ulcers are thought to result from disturbances in the autonomic nervous system as a response to injury. Treatment and prevention are similar to that for any patient with an ulcer.

The aftermath of brain injury depends on the severity of damage to the brain tissue. The majority of patients with minor injuries recover without any residual effects. Some patients may suffer from headaches, dizziness, and mental changes for several months after injury. Seizures as a result of scar tissue may occur in some patients. Patients with moderate to severe injury require rehabilitation in an inpatient setting. The patient and family need guidance and support throughout the acute period and during rehabilitation to adjust to any residual deficits (Box 28-5).

Spinal Cord Injuries

Injuries to the spinal cord resulting in loss of motor and sensory function are by far one of the most devastating traumatic injuries that healthcare providers encounter. Recent studies indicate that traumatic spinal cord injuries occur most often between ages 16 and 30. Eighty-two percent of all victims are male (Cochran,

BOX 28-5 **Nursing Process**

ACUTE HEAD INJURY

ASSESSMENT

Neurologic status (loss of consciousness, orientation, motor function, pupil size and reaction to light, EOMs, speech, thought processes)
Vital signs
ICP, if indicated
Cranial nerve function
Respiratory status
Oxygen saturation
Fluid balance status
Daily weight
Swallowing ability, gag reflex, ability to cough
Seizure activity
CSF leak (nasal, ear, or head wound drainage)
Pain/headache
Attention span, memory, concentration, if applicable
Nutrition status
Individual/family coping and knowledge of status
Laboratory studies: ABGs, electrolytes, BUN, CBC, serum osmolarity, albumin

NURSING DIAGNOSES

Altered cerebral tissue perfusion related to edema, increased ICP, hemorrhage, vascular spasm
Risk for fluid volume deficit related to vomiting, diaphoresis, fever
Fluid volume excess related to SIADH
Ineffective airway clearance related to decreased loss of consciousness
Risk for injury (seizures, falls) related to intracranial bleed, electrolyte disturbance, motor impairment
Altered nutrition: less than body requirements related to decreased LOC, restriction of intake, impaired gag reflex, dysphagia
Pain related to trauma
Impaired physical mobility related to cerebral injury, activity restrictions
Altered thought processes related to cerebral injury
Ineffective individual/family coping related to change in health status and lengthy hospitalization
Knowledge deficit related to new injury and long-term care

NURSING INTERVENTIONS

Record regular and frequent neurologic status to determine any change in condition.
Report elevated ICP (> 15 mm Hg), increased or decreased urine output (< 30 ml/hr or > 200 ml/hr).
Defer nursing care as appropriate if elevated ICP.
Elevate head of bed 30 degrees.
Maintain head in midline position.
Administer medications as prescribed (hyperosmotic agents, anticonvulsants, calcium-channel blockers, analgesics).
Administer central nervous system depressants with caution.
Protect from injury with seizure precautions, side rails up and bed in low position.
Reorient as indicated.
Explain all procedures and treatments.
Restrain only if absolutely necessary.
Restrict fluid and free water if indicated.
Encourage deep breathing if capable.
Administer oxygen as prescribed.
Suction secretions prn only as necessary (hyperoxygenate and hyperventilate before event).
Prepare for or provide care related to mechanical ventilation if indicated.
Turn or reposition q 2 h.
Administer tube feedings or TPN as prescribed.
Avoid insertion of nasogastric tube until basal skull fracture ruled out.
Minimize environmental stimuli.
Avoid startling patient.
Provide active/passive ROM tid.
Increase activity as tolerated when stable.
Do not converse about patient at bedside.
Encourage family to bring in pictures, favorite music, etc.
Place familiar items within view.
Encourage family involvement in care and provide support.
Refer family to social service if indicated.

EVALUATION OF EXPECTED OUTCOMES

Absence of new neurologic deficit
Overall improvement in neurologic status
No evidence of fluid volume deficit/excess
Urine specific gravity between 1.005 to 1.0025
No evidence of respiratory distress
Clear breath sounds
Normal ABGs for patient
No secondary injury or trauma
Free from seizures
Stable weight
Family able to describe treatment/nursing care

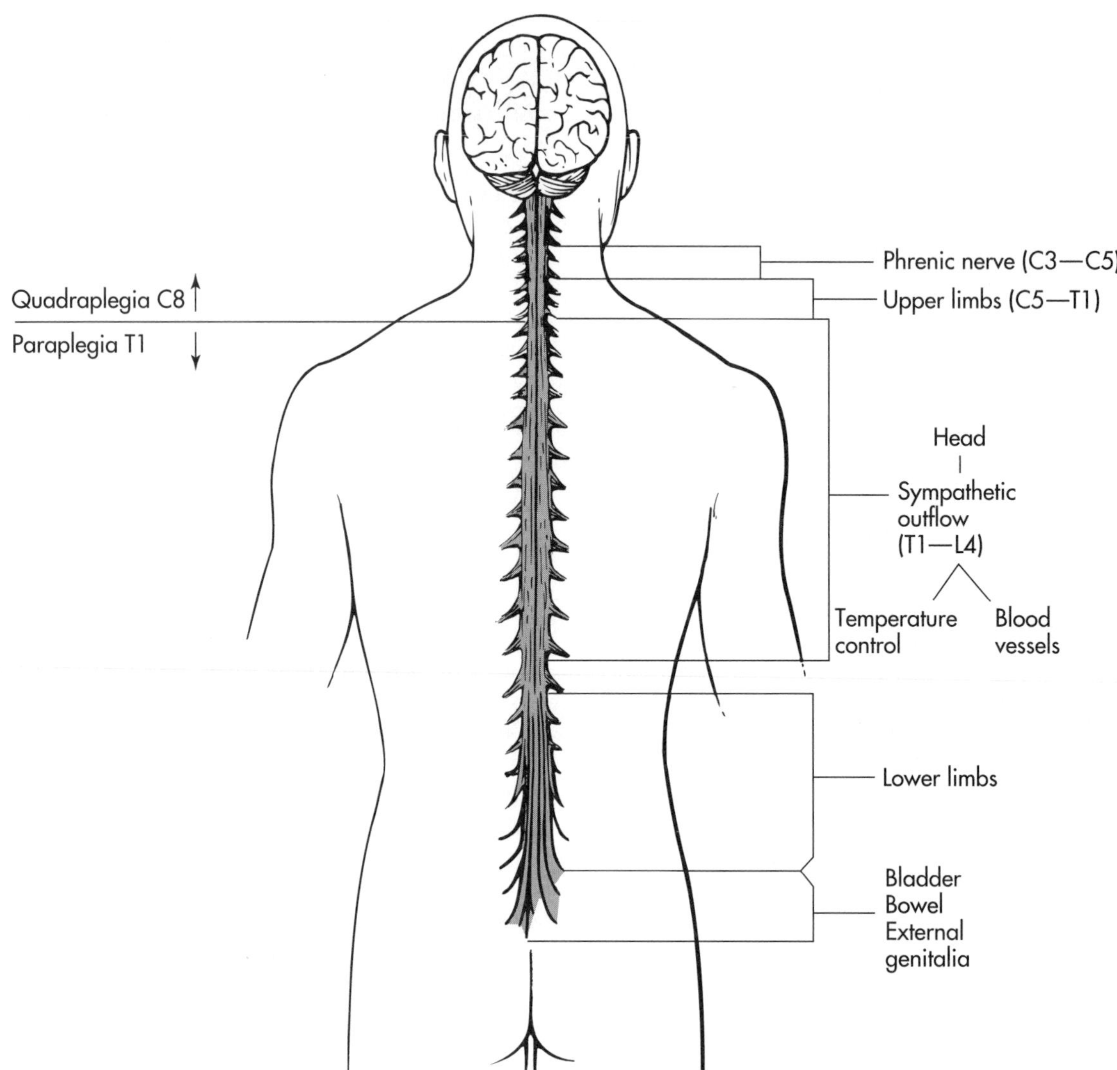

Figure 28-5 Symptoms, degree of paralysis, and potential for rehabilitation depend on the level of the lesion. (From Lewis SM, Collier IC: *Medical-surgical nursing: assessment and management of clinical problems,* ed 3, St Louis, 1992, Mosby.)

Kessler, Wittenborn, 1994). Motor vehicle accidents account for the majority of injuries, whereas falls and acts of violence are ranked second and third. Injuries resulting in complete transection of the spinal cord are more devastating and result in complete loss of motor and sensory function below the level of the injury (Figure 28-5). An injury in the cervical or high-thoracic region may result in **quadriplegia,** whereas an injury in the thoracic or lumbar region results in **paraplegia** (Figure 28-6).

Emergency intervention

Any person with a suspected spinal cord injury should be handled with extreme caution to prevent further damage to the cord. Until proven otherwise, every trauma patient should be treated as if he or she has a spinal cord injury. Spinal cord injury should be highly suspected in any person who cannot move the arms or legs, complains of tingling or lack of feeling in any extremity, or complains of neck or back pain. The person should not be moved until properly trained emergency personnel are available to immobilize and stabilize the head, neck, and back with a cervical collar and a back board.

Early intervention

Early interventions for a patient with spinal cord injury is aimed at reducing the effects of the injury, maintaining alignment of the spine, and stabilizing the spine to prevent further damage. Treatment of this population of patients is best carried out at designated trauma centers. During the initial period, the patient should be monitored closely for signs of shock and circulatory collapse. In patients with cervical cord injury,

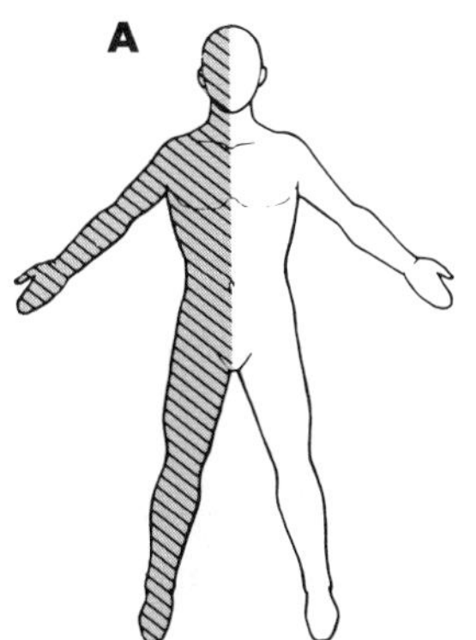

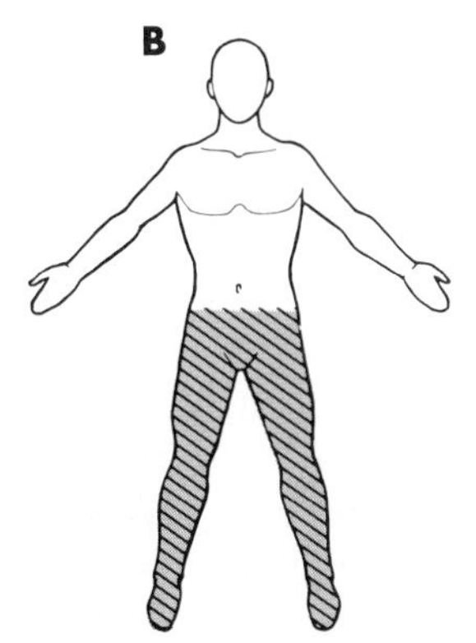

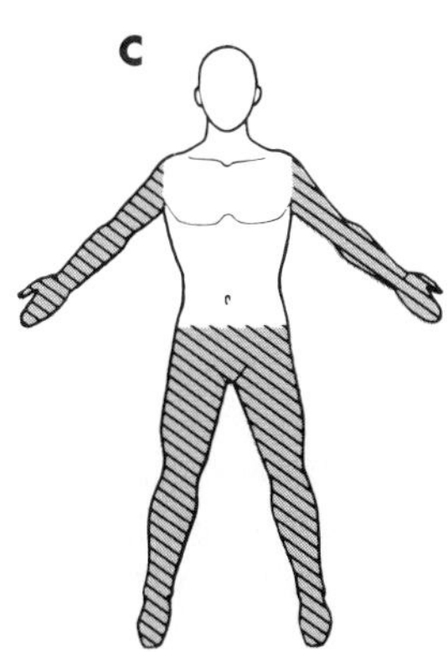

Figure 28-6 Damage to central nervous system may result in paralysis of some or all extremities. **A,** Hemiplegia. **B,** Paraplegia. **C,** Quadriplegia.

the muscles of respiration may be affected, and mechanical ventilation is often necessary (Box 28-6).

High-dose intravenous steroids should be administered over the first 24 hours because these have been shown to improve the overall outcome of the patient's neurologic function. Restoration of alignment and stability of the cervical spine is accomplished with cervical tongs and the halo device. The halo (metal ring) is attached to the skull using four pins. Once in place, the ring can be attached to traction or to a body jacket that allows for increased mobility (Figure 28-7; Box 28-7). Some institutions also use the Roto Rest Kinetic Treatment Table to care for patients who require a great degree of immobilization. If the spinal cord is being compressed by bony fragments, surgical intervention is often the treatment of choice.

NURSE ALERT

People with suspected spinal cord injuries should not be moved until trained emergency personnel can immobilize and stabilize the head, neck, and back with a cervical collar and back board.

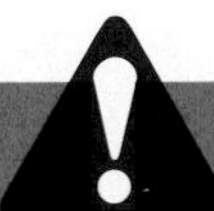

NURSE ALERT

A decreasing heart rate of 40 to 50 beats/minute, decreasing blood pressure, and loss of reflexes below the level of the lesion can be life-threatening, early complications of spinal cord injury (neurogenic shock).

Spinal shock

Immediately after a spinal cord injury, a period of complete inactivity of the nervous system occurs below the level of the injury. This period of **spinal shock** may last from 1 week to several months and is characterized by **flaccid** paralysis; loss of sensation, reflex activity, and autonomic function below the level of the injury; and bowel and bladder dysfunction. Because of the loss of muscle tone, the patient is extremely susceptible to many of the complications of immobility, particularly pressure ulcers, thrombophlebitis, and renal calculi. Conscientious and expert nursing care during this acute period can help prevent many of these complications.

Daily care

After the injury, a disturbance of the heat-regulating mechanism occurs, and the patient does not perspire below the level of the injury. The loss of temperature regulation results in a phenomenon referred to as *poikilothermy*—the tendency of the body to take on the temperature of the surrounding environment. If the environment is hot, the patient's temperature rises; if the environment is cold, the patient's temperature falls. The patient should be instructed to avoid extremes in temperature to prevent the undesirable effects of hyperthermia or hypothermia. In addition, the skin must receive meticulous care. Powder should be avoided because it holds moisture and contributes to maceration of the skin. Wrinkles in sheets and clothing must be removed to ensure that pressure ulcers do not develop.

The patient with quadriplegia cannot use a traditional push-button bell signal to summon help. Special devices such as a bladder-type call bell should be obtained to allow the patient the maximum amount of independence possible.

BOX 28-6

Nursing Process

SPINAL CORD INJURY

ASSESSMENT

Acute phase

Respiratory status
Ability to cough
Oxygen saturation
Vital signs
Neurologic status (muscle movement of upper and lower extremities, sensation, proprioception, deep-tendon reflexes, sphincter contraction, and perianal sensation)
Peripheral pulses, capillary refill
Laboratory studies: ABGs, electrolytes, CBC

Ongoing

Respiratory status
Vital signs
Neurologic status for change
Ability to perform self-care activities
Baseline ROM
Skin integrity
For signs/symptoms of dysreflexia
For complaints of excessive warmth or coolness below level of injury
Coping skills
Perception of illness on self and lifestyle
Level of anxiety

NURSING DIAGNOSES

Inability to sustain spontaneous ventilation related to high-cervical injury
Altered systemic tissue perfusion related to spinal shock
Ineffective breathing pattern related to loss of abdominal and intercostal muscle function, immobility
Impaired physical mobility related to paralysis, paresis
Risk for impaired skin integrity related to immobility
Ineffective thermoregulation related to loss of compensatory feedback to temperature change
Altered urinary elimination related to injury effect on nerve innovation to bladder
Constipation related to decreased mobility, decreased sensation, decreased control of defecation
Risk for injury: dysreflexia related to loss of sympathetic nervous response below level of injury
Anxiety related to sudden change in health status
Body image disturbance related to paralysis, change in lifestyle
Powerlessness related to dependence on others
Knowledge deficit related to change in health status

NURSING INTERVENTIONS

Acute phase

Administer oxygen as prescribed.
Assist with intubation as indicated.
Provide care related to mechanical ventilation as indicated.
Suction prn.
Maintain stability of neck with any movement.
Administer IV fluids as prescribed.
Avoid elevation of head of bed.
Apply MAST suit as prescribed.
Assist with application of spinal immobilizing device.
Administer medications as prescribed (anticholinergics, sympathomimetics, corticosteroids).
Provide information/reassurance as indicated.

Ongoing

Logroll every 2 hours.
Provide ROM tid.
Apply antiembolic stockings, remove for 30 to 60 minutes bid.
Apply abdominal binder when out of bed if indicated.
Provide support to prevent foot drop.
Consult with PT and OT.
Keep skin clean and dry.
When up in wheelchair, shift weight every 30 minutes.
Provide appropriate pressure reducing/relieving devices.
Encourage deep breathing and coughing.
Use assisted cough as indicated.
Maintain room temperature at 70° F if indicated.
Provide/remove blankets and clothing as indicated.
Initiate bladder and bowel programs (intermittent catheterization, Crede or trigger techniques, rectal suppository).
Encourage ventilation of feelings.
Provide accurate information regarding status.
Provide support as indicated.
Include patient in decision making.
Encourage independence.
Encourage high fiber and 2500 ml intake.
Provide pin care if indicated.
Prevent stimulation of sympathetic nervous system below level of injury (full bladder, pressure, trauma).
Monitor BP for complaint of headache, flushing, diaphoresis, or blurred vision.

BOX 28-6 **Nursing Process**

SPINAL CORD INJURY—cont'd

EVALUATION OF EXPECTED OUTCOMES

Respiratory status stable
ABGs within normal limits for patient
Neurologic status stable
Vital signs within normal limits for patient
Palpable peripheral pulses
Maintenance of full range of motion
No evidence of foot drop
Skin intact
Urinary/bowel program established
Effective management of dysreflexia if it occurs
Discusses feelings and coping methods
Participates in self-care activities
Verbalizes beginning adjustment to injury and change in lifestyle
Verbalizes understanding of rehabilitation

Respiratory care. Depending on the degree of injury, the patient develops varying degrees of respiratory difficulty. Paralysis of the diaphragm occurs with injuries at the level of C4 or above. The patient with low-cervical or high-thoracic lesions must also be monitored carefully, and vigorous pulmonary toilet must be part of the daily plan of care. It is important to remember that during the acute phase, ascending edema can rapidly cause respiratory difficulties. The patient who is not on ventilatory support needs particularly close monitoring during this early phase.

Cardiovascular system. Because of the loss of input from higher centers in the brain, vasodilation of the blood vessels occurs below the level of the injury. Blood pools in the lower extremities, causing problems with vasodilation, hypotension, vascular stasis, and edema. The use of thigh-high elastic stockings and abdominal binders can help control the pooling of blood in the abdomen and lower extremities. Elevation of the legs also helps control edema. The prophylactic use of subcutaneous heparin (if not contraindicated) is also helpful in the prevention of disseminated vascular thrombosis.

Musculoskeletal system. Prolonged immobility has many negative effects on the bones, joints, and muscles. Keeping the body in functional alignment is essential to prevent contractures. The use of soft foot supports, trochanter rolls, and hand splints or rolls can help maintain normal functional position of joints. Passive range of motion to all joints and a regular turning schedule are imperative in the prevention of contractures and pressure ulcers. Involvement of rehabilitation services (physical and occupational therapists) is imperative during this phase.

Gastrointestinal system. Peristalsis is lost during the immediate postinjury phase, and paralytic ileus often develops. Abdominal distention can interfere with respiratory function; therefore decompression with a nasogastric tube is sometimes necessary. When the patient begins to eat, a high-protein, high-calorie diet is preferable. Fluid intake should be at least 3 L per day to aid in the prevention of urinary tract infections and renal calculi formation. H_2 blockers (Ranitidine, Cimetidine) and antacids are also used in the prevention of stress ulcers and upper gastrointestinal hemorrhage.

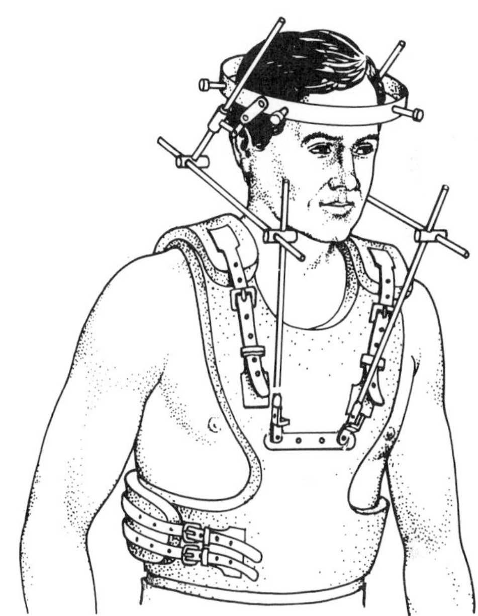

Figure 28-7 Halo vest. (From Beare PB, Myers JL: *Adult health nursing,* ed 2, St Louis, 1994, Mosby.)

Because bowel function is affected, fecal incontinence and impaction should be guarded against. A bowel retraining program should be initiated soon after bowel sounds return. (For more information about bowel retraining see Chapter 15.) Stool softeners (Colace, PeriColace) should be used on a routine basis. Bisacodyl (Dulcolax) or glycerin suppositories should be administered every 1 to 2 days until bowel retraining is complete. Because the goal of the retraining program is to establish a predictable pattern of elimination for the patient, suppositories should be administered at the same time every day. Digital stimulation

BOX 28-7 Guidelines of Care for Patient in Halo Brace

Nursing Interventions	Rationale
1 Explain routine care and procedure to patient.	Provides basis for patient cooperation and education regarding care while in halo
2 Using proper body mechanics, position patient to perform care. Patient is flat on back to gain access to anterior aspect and side lying for posterior aspect.	Decreases risk of injury to patient is repositioned by grasping shoulders, lower extremities, and posterior portions of vest; patient is *never* lifted, turned, or pulled by strut bars
3 Open one side of vest to visualize desired area.	Maintains vest stability
4 Cleanse skin with soap and water.	
5 Perform visual assessment, noting any reddened or open area.	Identifies any high risk or broken areas of skin
6 Chest physiotherapy may be performed while patient is on side and vest is open.	Allows greater access to thorax, especially at lower lobes
7 Auscultate breath sounds while vest is open.	Allows for identification of adventitious breath sounds over a greater area
8 Rebuckle vest and reposition patient.	Maintains vest stability
9 Open alternate side of vest and repeat hygiene and assessment measures.	
10 Perform pin care every 8 hours.	To prevent crust formation and decrease risk of pin infection
a Mix 1 oz each of hydrogen peroxide and sterile saline in sterile container.	Half-strength solution used for pin care; solution expires within 24 hours of mixing
b Dip sterile cotton swab in solution and cleanse around pin. Repeat if necessary to remove old blood, crusts, or exudate.	Sterile technique used for pin care while patient is hospitalized; use clean swab for each pin site cleansed
c Rinse with sterile cotton swab soaked in saline only.	Not necessary to apply povidone-iodine (Betadine) or antibacterial ointments at pin sites
d Note pin integrity to insertion area.	Pin should be set tightly at insertion site; disengaged pin or tenting of skin beneath pin suggests patient is no longer in effective traction and should be reported immediately to the physician
e Identify any signs and symptoms of localized infection.	Redness, swelling, pain, and exudate are symptoms to be reported to physician

Modified from Beare PG, Myers JL: *Adult health nursing,* ed 2, St Louis, 1994, Mosby.

may be required, particularly during the early stages of the bowel program. Enemas should be avoided and should be used only when all other methods fail.

Genitourinary system. In the patient with severe spinal cord injury, urinary retention often occurs. An indwelling catheter usually is inserted while the patient is in the emergency department. For the female quadriplegic patient, an indwelling catheter may be necessary if she is unable to manage self-catheterization. For the male quadriplegic and for the paraplegic patient, intermittent catheterization is the method of choice because it is less likely to result in chronic urinary tract infection.

Patients are catheterized intermittently to maintain urine volumes less than 500 ml for each void. Consistent volumes greater than this can result in overstretching of the bladder and can increase the potential for the development of **autonomic hyperreflexia,** which is an emergency condition occurring in the patient with cervical or high-thoracic injury. It occurs as a result of an exaggerated and uncontrolled response of the sympathetic nervous system to external stimulation. Some of the common causes are bladder or bowel distention, enemas, digital rectal stimulation, bladder irrigation, infection, or skin ulcers. The condition is characterized by pounding headache, markedly elevated blood pressure (sometimes as high as 300 mm Hg systolic), flushed face, "goose flesh," and a period of tachycardia followed by bradycardia. Once the cause of the attack has been identified and corrected, the symptoms usually subside without further treatment. When the symptoms of hyperreflexia occur, the nurse should immediately check for bladder distention, obstruction of the Foley catheter, or other causes so the problem can be corrected. If the bladder is distended, the patient should be catheterized immediately. In cases of fecal impaction, a local anesthetic ointment should be inserted into the rectum before any attempt is made to remove the impaction. The preceding emergency nursing measures should be attempted immediately. The physician should be notified that the patient has had an episode of autonomic hyperreflexia or if these measures are ineffective. If the above interventions fail, rapid-acting antihypertensive medications such as metoprolol (Lopressor) are required. The patient and family should have a complete understanding of this problem and how to correct it before the patient is discharged.

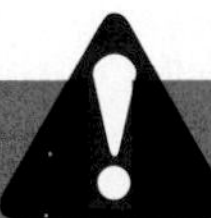

NURSE ALERT

Pounding headache, markedly elevated blood pressure, flushed face, "goose flesh," and a period of tachycardia followed by bradycardia may herald autonomic hyperreflexia. This is an emergency condition occurring in patients with cervical or high-thoracic injuries. Check immediately for bladder distention, obstruction of the Foley catheter, impaction, or other stressful conditions. Antihypertensive medications may be necessary.

Rehabilitation

The process of rehabilitation begins immediately, and the primary objective of care is to assist the patient in achieving an optimum level of physical and mental function within the limits of the disability. The extent of functional return for patients with spinal cord injury depends on the type and extent of the spinal cord damage. The higher the level of injury, the more muscles involved and the greater the degree of disability. With long-term physical and occupational therapy, the patient can learn to use remaining functional muscles and adaptive devices to achieve independence in daily activities. Ambulation with or without bracing may be attempted in select patients with lumbar or sacral injuries. The nurse plays an important role during this period in teaching the patient and family aspects of self-care so that many of the potential complications of chronic disability can be prevented.

Bladder and bowel reconditioning are considered major goals during rehabilitation (see Chapter 15). If the patient can regain continence of bladder or bowel function, the patient's self-confidence and potential for successful rehabilitation improves. Once spinal shock has passed, bladder and bowel reconditioning should be initiated. A rigid program of regulated fluid intake and attempts to void is begun. Many patients are able to empty their bladders through stimulation of the voiding reflex by tapping over the bladder area, stroking the inner thighs, or pulling pubic hairs. Catheterization for residual urine is done routinely to prevent distention and to determine the effectiveness of bladder emptying. The goal of bowel reconditioning is to achieve a regular schedule of emptying the bowel by methods previously cited. The time selected should be convenient for the patient after discharge. As soon as the patient can maintain an upright position, he or she should be assisted to the toilet to facilitate evacuation.

Sexual counseling has been an area commonly neglected in the past. Many patients with spinal cord injuries have concerns regarding their potential for normal sexual activity. The nurse should be aware that some patients may be embarrassed or reluctant to ask questions related to sexual functioning. If the nurse does not feel comfortable with or capable of answering questions, a referral to the appropriate resource person should be made.

Adjustments to disability are difficult, with extreme changes in body image being required. The grief process, including such emotions as anger, depression, denial, and withdrawal, can be anticipated. Often the patient does well when interacting with others who have similar problems.

Intervertebral Disk Trauma

The intervertebral disks are fibrocartilaginous disks located between the vertebral bodies. Disks allow for limited flexibility of the spine and act as shock absorbers to protect the vertebrae from jars and jolts. Sometimes these disks rupture, and the soft, gelatinous substance in the center (nucleus pulposus) escapes (Figure 28-8). The disk material may compress the spinal cord or exert pressure on the nerve root, causing neurologic symptoms. The disks in the lumbar region are most commonly affected, although cervical disk herniations are not infrequent.

Lower back pain is generally the initial symptom. The pain eventually radiates over the buttock and down the leg to the ankle or foot. The patient may experience tingling or numbness in the foot and **muscle spasms** in the leg. Motor weakness may also occur.

Heavy lifting or twisting of the back usually precipitates the onset of pain. In cases of herniation of cervical disks, hyperextension of the neck (whiplash) may be the precipitating factor. Rupture of the interverte-

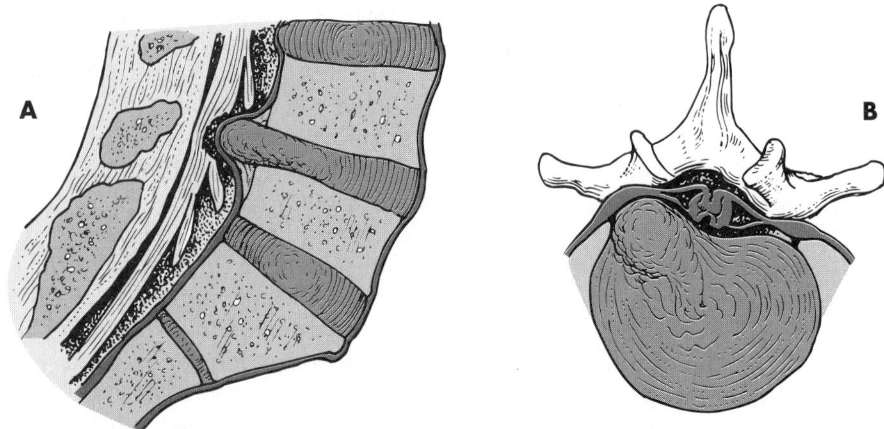

Figure 28-8 Ruptured intervertebral disc. Diagram shows herniation of the nucleus pulposus. **A,** Herniation presses on the structures of the spinal cord. **B,** Herniation may press on the exit of the spinal nerve and produce pain and other symptoms. (From Barker E: *Neuroscience nursing,* St Louis, 1994, Mosby.)

bral disk is now considered to be one of the major causes of severe, recurrent lower back pain.

Nursing intervention

Conservative methods of treating ruptured intervertebral disks are tried initially unless symptoms of cord compression are present. A short period of bedrest followed by limitations in activity are necessary. Pain is often treated with nonsteroidal antiinflammatory medications (NSAIDS) if the patient has no sensitivities or contraindication to the use of this class of drugs. In severe cases, stronger analgesics such as codeine may be required. Muscle relaxants such as cyclobenzaprine (Flexeril) and diazepam (Valium) often are helpful. Lying on the side with knees and hips flexed helps relieve the tension on the lumbar and sacral nerves. Another position of comfort for the patient with lower back pain is on the back with the head of the bed elevated and the knees elevated. This helps to lengthen the muscles of the back and legs to prevent muscle spasms. A small pillow placed under the lumbar region of the back also helps relieve the tension. Physical therapy, applying moist heat or ice to the lumbar area, or light massage often is helpful in reducing symptoms. With cervical disk problems, a cervical collar usually is worn to keep the neck in a neutral or slightly flexed position. If conservative treatment is ineffective or neurologic symptoms increase, surgical intervention may be necessary.

The nurse can be helpful in teaching the patient correct body mechanics when bending, lifting, or turning in bed. The patient should be advised not to twist or strain the back during movement. General care of the patient is similar to that of any patient who is immobilized for a period of time. Attention should be given to maintaining adequate fluid intake and elimination. Mild laxatives may be necessary.

Surgical intervention

A **laminectomy and diskectomy** is a surgical procedure that is performed to remove bone, cartilage, or herniated intervertebral disk material. The posterior arch of the vertebra is removed so that the spinal cord or nerve root is exposed, and the disk is removed. A spinal fusion also may be done during the operation. Spinal fusion consists of the placement of a piece of bone (either from another area of the body, such as the hip, or from cadaveric bone graft) onto the vertebrae for grafting purposes. This provides a firm, bony union in a weakened area of the vertebral column. Metal wires or rods also may be attached to the vertebrae to provide additional support to the area. A laminectomy may involve the cervical, thoracic, or lumbar vertebrae. However, the thoracic vertebrae are less often involved. A partial laminectomy, or hemilaminectomy, can be performed to remove a herniated disk. In this case, spinal fusion is not necessary because the defect that results is negligible.

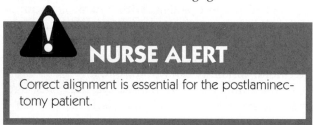

NURSE ALERT

Correct alignment is essential for the postlaminectomy patient.

BOX 28-8 **Nursing Process**

POSTOPERATIVE CARE—LAMINECTOMY PATIENT

ASSESSMENT

Neurovascular status to lower extremities
Vital signs
Respiratory status
Bladder/bowel functioning
Pain level
Ability to perform self-care activities

NURSING DIAGNOSES

Pain related to surgical procedure
Impaired physical mobility related to surgical procedure
Self-care deficit related to impaired mobility
Risk for ineffective breathing pattern related to discomfort
Sensory/perceptual alterations related to surgical procedure
Risk for infection related to surgical intervention and immobility
Risk for altered urinary elimination related to surgical procedure

NURSING INTERVENTIONS

Check postoperative orders carefully.
Place patient on firm mattress.
Keep head of bed flat until ordered otherwise.
Check patient's vital signs and monitor motor and sensory function in all extremities—report any muscle weakness and numbness or tingling to the surgeon.
Observe dressing for signs of hemorrhage or cerebrospinal fluid leakage.
If cervical laminectomy was performed, closely observe quality and rate of respirations.
Maintain correct body alignment at all times.
Turn patient in logroll fashion with a turning sheet every 2 hours; caution patient not to attempt to turn self.
Check for urinary retention; catheterize patient as necessary.
Assist patient to ambulate when ordered; encourage patient to walk erect and not to bend forward.
Avoid having patient sit in chair for long periods—use only straight-back chair.

EVALUATION OF EXPECTED OUTCOMES

Maximum pulmonary function maintained
Aspiration prevented
Infections prevented
Participates in self-care as appropriate
Demonstrates understanding of rationale for interventions
Reports increased comfort following pain relief measures
Maintains continency, voids voluntarily

Preoperative. Preoperative care of the patient is essentially the same as that for most surgical patients (see Chapter 18). The patient is often apprehensive and needs reassurance. An explanation of what to expect postoperatively helps relieve anxiety.

Postoperative. General postoperative care is also similar to that of other types of surgical procedures. After a laminectomy, the patient's spine must be kept in a position of correct alignment. Turning and activity orders vary according to the surgeon. The patient is often allowed out of bed on the evening of surgery. Activity progresses slowly over several days, and the patient is often discharged on the third postoperative day.

When a spinal fusion is performed, recovery is slower. Ambulation occurs gradually, and the patient should be taught to bend from the hips, keeping the back straight. Sitting is likely to be the least comfortable position, but when sitting, a straight-back chair is preferable (Box 28-8).

CARE OF THE PATIENT WITH A TUMOR OF THE BRAIN AND SPINAL CORD

All tumors of the brain, whether benign or malignant, are potentially fatal unless treated. Death from untreated tumors results from the compressive effects of a space-occupying lesion or from progressively increasing ICP. Tumors can originate within the brain tissue (gliomas) or from the meningeal coverings of the brain (meningiomas). Malignant tumors may result from metastasis from lesions elsewhere in the body, but primary tumors of the brain rarely metastasize outside the brain. Brain tumors tend to occur in young adult life or middle age.

Symptoms of intracranial tumors are caused by localized destruction or compression of brain tissue and vary according to the location and size of the lesion. Initially tumors may exist with very few noticeable symptoms. Often a slight slowing of mental functioning or change in personality is the only abnormal behavior. Occasionally seizure activity, particularly when onset occurs in middle age, is a dramatic early sign.

The specific symptoms presented provide clues to the location of the tumor. The nurse can help localize the site of the tumor by observing and recording focal symptoms such as motor weakness, hearing or vision disturbances, dizziness, or speech or sensory deficits.

The generalized classic symptoms of brain tumors are those of gradually increasing ICP. Headaches tend to occur at night or on awakening in the morning. The location and nature of the headache varies considerably but increases in intensity as the tumor grows. Coughing, straining, or stooping often aggravates the headache. Nausea and vomiting appear in approximately one third of patients and may accompany the headache. Some patients may vomit unexpectedly and forcibly (projectile vomiting) without any preceding nausea. Other late symptoms include papilledema, dizziness, and changes in level of consciousness.

Before planning surgery, the exact location of the tumor must be determined. In addition to a complete history and neurologic examination, CT scan, MRI, and angiogram are often helpful in diagnosis.

When possible, brain tumors are treated by surgical excision. For tumors that are malignant and infiltrative, complete excision is impossible. If complete removal of the tumor is not accomplished, surgery is often followed by radiation therapy or chemotherapy. Radiation therapy is the treatment of choice for inoperable or incompletely resectable tumors. Many chemotherapeutic agents are not effective for brain tumors because they do not cross the blood-brain barrier.

Craniotomy

A **craniotomy** is a surgical opening through the cranium for the purpose of removing a tumor, evacuating hematomas, or relieving ICP. The preoperative preparation of the patient and family includes a thorough explanation of the intended procedure and possible outcomes. The nurse can be most helpful in providing emotional support and accurate information during this stressful period. Corticosteroids such as dexamethasone (Decadron) are usually administered preoperatively to reduce cerebral edema.

Careful monitoring of neurologic status is important in the postoperative period. The patient is at risk for problems related to increased ICP, particularly on the third postoperative day, when swelling peaks. Principles of care are similar for all patients with intracranial surgery (Box 28-9).

During convalescence, the patient may continue to have the neurologic deficits that existed before surgery. The physical therapist is helpful in the evaluation of the need for posthospital rehabilitation, as well as for assistance with ambulation and motor strengthening. The patient needs constant encouragement and reassurance and should be urged to be active within the limits of his or her abilities.

Spinal Cord Tumors

Spinal cord tumors occur approximately one tenth as often as brain tumors, and the majority are benign. They affect males and females equally and are generally seen in the 20- to 60-year age range. Approximately 50% of spinal cord tumors occur in the thoracic region, 30% in the cervical region, and 20% in the lumbar region. Spinal cord tumors may originate from spinal cord tissue (intramedullary) or from the surrounding tissue (extramedullary). Metastatic lesions to the vertebral column from various primary sites can cause pressure on the cord or may involve the cord itself.

Symptoms of spinal cord tumors depend on the anatomic location of the tumor, the tumor type, and the spinal nerves involved. Some general symptoms include pain, motor and/or sensory deficits, and bowel/bladder dysfunction. The diagnosis is made by MRI, CT scan, or myelogram. Treatment is often surgical removal of the tumor by laminectomy, radiation therapy, or both. Prognosis depends on the type of tumor and the degree of compression and resulting spinal cord ischemia. If the cord is not permanently damaged, the symptoms of neurologic deficit may be reversible.

CARE OF THE PATIENT WITH CEREBROVASCULAR DISEASE

Cerebrovascular disease continues to be the third most common cause of death in the United States and the most common cause of permanent neurologic disability in the adult population. However, the death rate has declined since the 1970s, largely as a result of improved health habits (e.g., a decrease in cigarette smoking, improved exercise habits) and improved medical management of diseases such as hypertension and hypercholesterolemia (Whitney, 1994). Present mortality data show a greater frequency of stroke among men than among women and a greater frequency in the nonwhite than the white population. The incidence of hypertension and atherosclerosis bears a direct relationship to the incidence of cerebrovascular disease.

Pathophysiology

Strokes can be classified into two major categories, **ischemic** and **hemmorrhagic** (Figure 28-9). An ischemic stroke has either a thrombotic or embolic

BOX 28-9

Nursing Process

POSTOPERATIVE CARE—CRANIOTOMY PATIENT

ASSESSMENT

Neurologic status (loss of consciousness, pupil size, reaction of pupils to light, motor movement and strength)
Vital signs
Any change in status
Head dressing
ICP
Laboratory studies (CBC, electrolytes, ABGs)
Fluid volume status
Respiratory status
Seizure activity
Pain level

NURSING DIAGNOSES

Pain related to surgical intervention
Risk for impaired physical mobility related to surgical intervention
Self-care deficit related to neurologic deficit
Risk for ineffective breathing pattern related to neurologic deficit
Risk for sensory perceptual alterations related to altered consciousness
Risk for impaired verbal communication related to neurologic deficit
Risk for infection related to surgical intervention
Risk for altered nutrition: less than body requirements related to altered level of consciousness

NURSING INTERVENTIONS

Position patient according to site of surgery—do not place on operative side if large tumor or bone was removed; elevate head of bed.
Check vital and neurologic signs at frequent intervals.
Observe patient for signs of increased intracranial pressure and seizure activity.
Observe dressings for signs of bleeding and leakage of cerebrospinal fluid.
Maintain asepsis in handling all dressings.
Observe for signs of neurologic deficits (paralysis, sensory loss, difficulty in swallowing or speaking).
Maintain activity or position restrictions as ordered.
Do not place patient in Trendelenburg's position without physician's order.
Do not suction patient through nose.
Ice bags may be used to relieve headache and facial edema; analgesics may be necessary.
Prevent straining by patient; avoid use of restraints, enemas; avoid coughing or vomiting.
Provide calm, quiet environment.

EVALUATION OF EXPECTED OUTCOMES

Maximum pulmonary function maintained
Aspiration prevented
Infections prevented
Adequate nutrition status maintained
Communicates effectively
Participates in self-care as appropriate
Demonstrates understanding of rationale for interventions
Reports increased comfort following pain relief measures

During convalescence the patient may continue to have the neurologic deficits that existed before surgery. The physical therapist is helpful in the evaluation of the need for posthospital rehabilitation, as well as for assistance with ambulation and motor strengthening. The patient needs constant encouragement and reassurance and should be urged to be active within the limits of his or her abilities.

mechanism. A thrombotic stroke results from the narrowing and ultimate occlusion of a blood vessel by an atherosclerotic plaque. Before an actual thrombotic stroke occurs, many patients experience *transient ischemic attacks (TIAs)*. A TIA is characterized by the sudden onset of a neurologic deficit that lasts less than 24 hours and leaves the patient at his or her neurologic baseline. It is a warning sign of a stroke, and if intervention is taken, the patient is often spared a significant neurologic event.

An embolic stroke is the second type of ischemic event. It involves the blockage of a cerebral blood vessel by a small clot and is most often caused by tiny emboli that are carried to the brain as a result of atrial fibrillation. The onset and progression of symptoms are usually rapid as a result of the sudden ischemia in the brain.

Hemorrhagic stroke occurs either as an intracerebral or subarachnoid hemorrhage. Intracerebral hemorrhage involves bleeding into the brain tissue as a result of rupture of a small blood vessel, often as a result of hypertension. The site of hemorrhage is usually deep within the brain tissue. A major hemorrhage can cause herniation and death. Subarachnoid hemorrhage oc-

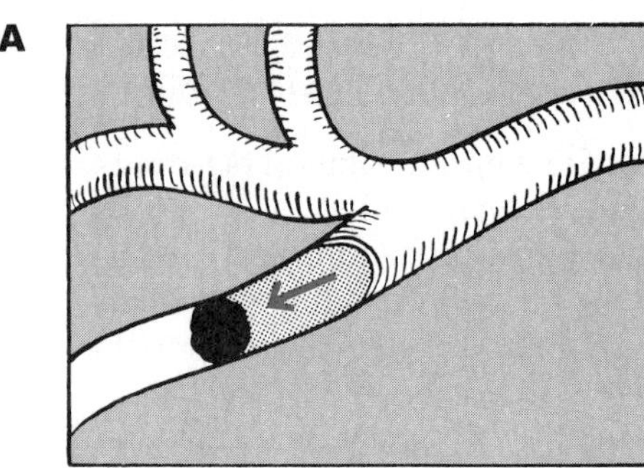

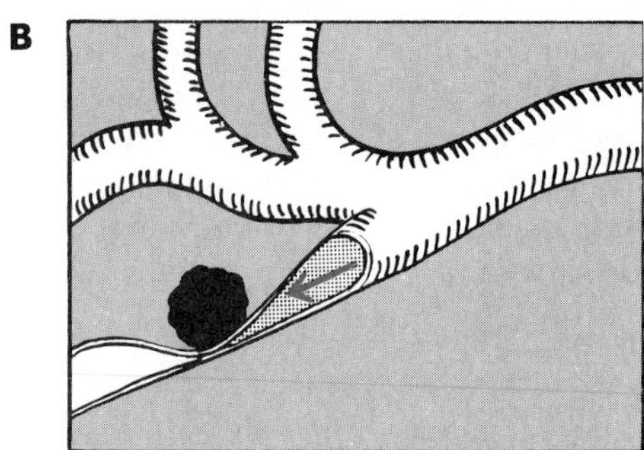

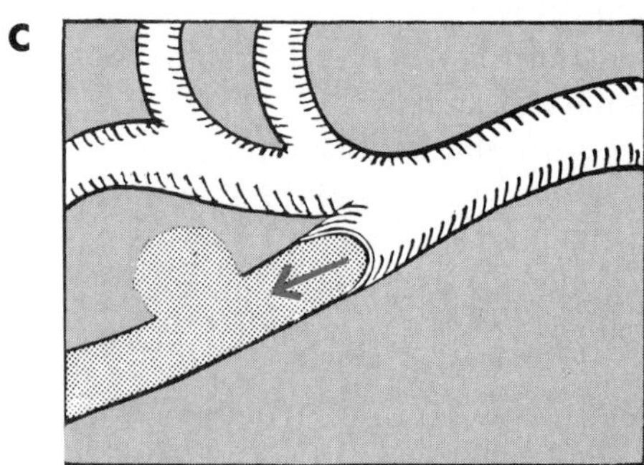

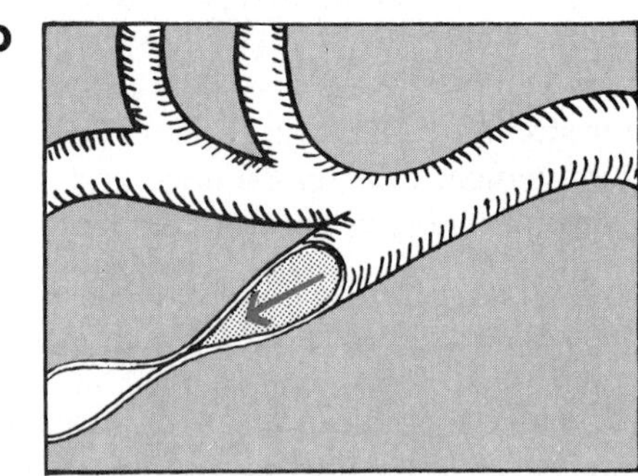

Figure 28-9 Causes of cerebrovascular accident. **A,** Formation of blood clot in blood vessel, resulting in occlusion and ischemia. **B,** Pressure on blood vessel from a blood clot, tumor, or anything that compresses the blood vessel, resulting in ischemia. **C,** Rupture of blood vessel with hemorrhage into adjacent tissue. **D,** Closing of blood vessel from spasm or contraction, causing blockage of blood flow and ischemia.

curs as a result of bleeding into the subarachnoid space and is often a result of a ruptured aneurysm or arteriovenous malformation (AVM).

Assessment

The early signs and symptoms of stroke depend on the cause, location, and extent of the insult. TIAs precede many thrombotic events. Symptoms may include slurring of speech, visual changes, dizziness, headache, confusion, or motor weakness. These symptoms may progress to involve more permanent deficits if left untreated. Hemorrhagic events occur more suddenly and without warning. Headache, seizures, and rapid deterioration in level of consciousness may occur.

NURSE ALERT

A transient ischemic attack (TIA) is a warning sign of a stroke. Common symptoms include slurring of speech, visual changes, dizziness, headache, confusion, or motor weakness that last 24 hours or less.

The patient with a stroke involving the right side of the brain has hemiplegia (paralysis) involving the left side of the body, because the motor nerve pathways cross from one side of the brain to the other in the brainstem (see Figure 28-5). If the left side of the brain is involved, the patient has hemiplegia on the right side. Because the speech center (Wernicke's and Broca's area) is located in the left hemisphere, the patient may also have difficulty speaking or understanding the spoken word (**aphasia**). The patient with involvement of the right hemisphere tends to have perceptual problems. He or she may not recognize the hemiplegic side as being a part of himself or herself and may ignore it altogether (**neglect**). In addition, the patient may be impulsive and often presents as a safety risk. Other problems include difficulty swallowing (**dysphagia**), bladder and bowel incontinence, and loss of vision toward the hemiplegic side (**hemianopia**) (Figure 28-10).

Intervention

During the acute phase, medical management and nursing care are directed toward maintaining cerebral circulation to prevent ischemia of cerebral tissue. With thrombotic events, anticoagulant therapy may be

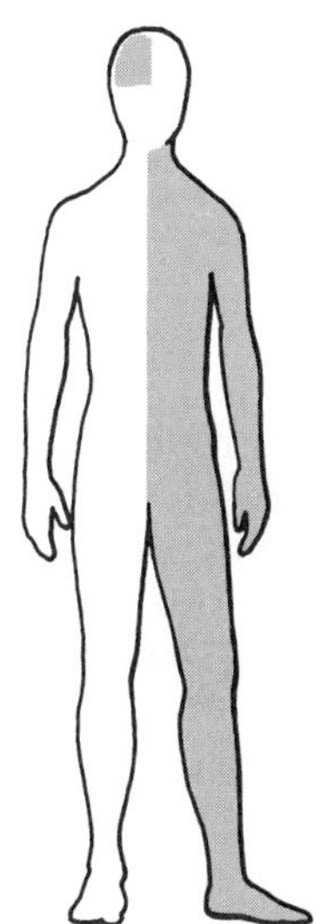

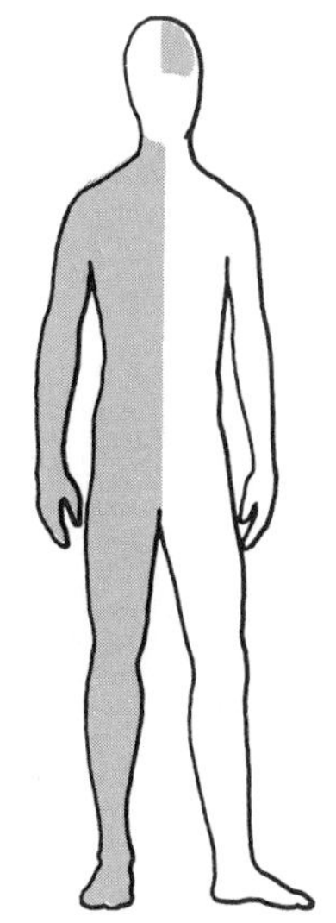

Left brain damage:
• Paralyzed right side
• Speech-language deficits (if left brain dominant)
• Behavioral style: slow, cautious
• Memory deficits: language
• Distress and depression in relation to the disability

Figure 28-10 Manifestation of right-sided and left-sided stroke. (From Lewis SM, Collier IC: *Medical-surgical nursing,* ed 3, St Louis, 1992, Mosby.)

started to prevent further thrombotic events. If cerebral hemorrhage is suspected, anticoagulation is contraindicated. Careful monitoring of vital and neurologic signs is imperative during this phase. Any signs of increased ICP should be reported. If the patient survives the acute insult, the prognosis for life is good. With active rehabilitation, the patient may return to his or her previous level of functional independence. The intense, interdisciplinary approach of a stroke management team provides the patient with the best opportunity to regain lost function. The patient and family are an integral part of the therapy program and should be included in developing the plan of care if possible.

The process of rehabilitation following a stroke begins at admission, and care must be taken to implement principles of rehabilitation during the acute phase. The patient who is hemiplegic or hemiparetic and relatively immobile is at risk for contractures, pressure ulcers, thrombosis, and edema. Proper positioning and frequent turning is imperative to prevent these complications. During position changes, the joints should be put through a full range of motion. The patient should be taught to use the unaffected arm to exercise the hemiplegic extremities as soon as possible (Box 28-10).

Complications of Stroke

Aphasia

If the stroke has affected the left hemisphere of the brain (right hemiplegia), damage to the speech center may occur, resulting in aphasia. Aphasia is described as *receptive* or *expressive.* With receptive aphasia, the patient has difficulty understanding the written or spoken word, whereas with expressive aphasia, the patient has difficulty speaking and writing. Sometimes the patient is able to sing simple songs, count, or recite the alphabet and make statements such as "Good morning" or "How are you?" but is unable to communicate effectively. This phenomenon is called *automatic* or *primitive* speech. Several guidelines are useful when talking with the patient with aphasia (see Box 28-10). When the patient is stable, a referral to a speech therapist is made. Not being able to speak can be extremely frustrating to the patient, and encouragement and emotional support are essential during this period.

Dysphagia

Difficulty in chewing and swallowing (dysphagia) may occur as a result of damage to the ninth and tenth cranial nerves, which control the gag and swallow reflexes. Before oral food and fluids are given to the stroke patient, the swallow and gag reflexes should be checked by the nurse. This is done by stroking each side of the oropharynx with a tongue blade and assessing the response. If the reflexes are impaired, a feeding tube might be necessary to ensure adequate nutrition intake. If the patient is able to eat, frequent oral hygiene, particularly after each meal, is necessary because the patient may tend to accumulate food on the affected side of the mouth. Measures to facilitate chewing and swallowing are often helpful (see Box 28-10).

Nursing Process

ROBLEMS ASSOCIATED WITH CEREBROVASCULAR ACCIDENT (CVA)

ASSESSMENT

Neurologic status
Speech and language ability
Tactile sensation and joint position
Evidence of body neglect
Ability to perform ADLs
Respiratory status
Presence of gag reflex
Vital signs
Motor function of upper and lower extremities

NURSING DIAGNOSES

Impaired verbal communication related to aphasia and hemiplegia
Impaired swallowing related to hemiphagia and cranial nerve damage
Sensory/perceptual alterations related to aphasia, hemianopia, and cerebral hemisphere damage
Impaired physical mobility related to hemiplegia
Self-care deficit related to hemiplegia
Risk for injury related to visual and perceptual problems and hemiplegia
Risk for incontinence related to hemiplegia
Risk for ineffective airway clearance related to hemiplegia
Altered nutrition: less than body requirements related to impaired swallowing, hemiphasia, and cranial nerve damage.
Risk for altered oral mucous membranes related to neurologic deficits
Risk for anxiety related to hemiplegia, aphasia, dysphagia, hemianopsia, and perceptual problems
Body image disturbance related to aphasia, hemiphasia, and cerebral hemisphere damage

NURSING INTERVENTIONS

Aphasia
Talk slowly in normal tone of voice.
Use simple words, phrases, and short sentences.
Allow patient sufficient time to answer.
Eliminate distracting noises or stimuli.
State question that can be answered by "yes" or "no" or nod of head—determine reliability of patient's answers.
Listen carefully to patient's attempts to speak.
Do not force patient to talk if unable.

Dysphagia
Place patient in upright position with head slightly flexed.
Determine presence of gag and swallow reflexes before attempting any oral fluids or foods.
Place food in mouth on nonparalyzed side.
Encourage patient to eat slowly and to concentrate on coordinating chewing, breathing, and swallowing.
Ice tongue before feeding to increase muscle tone—may use popsicles or iced utensils.
Avoid giving patient milk and milk products, which cause thick, stringy secretions.
Give foods that are stimulating to taste and form a ball (e.g., chilled pureed fruit).

Hemianopsia
Place patient so activity is toward nonparalyzed side.
Approach patient from nonparalyzed side.
Place personal objects within patient's vision.
As patient recovers, encourage to turn head toward paralyzed side to increase viewing area.

Perceptual problems
Provide sensory stimulation to affected side.
Have patient touch and handle affected extremities.
Use mirrors to improve sitting and standing balance.
Teach patient to check position of affected extremities visually.
Label clothes right, left, top, and bottom to reduce confusion in dressing.

EVALUATION OF EXPECTED OUTCOMES

Injuries prevented
Maximum pulmonary function maintained
Aspiration prevented
Skin integrity maintained
Adequate nutrition status maintained
Demonstrates improved ability to express self
Expresses decreased frustration with communication
Participates in self-care as appropriate
Reports satisfaction in self-care despite limitations
Demonstrates understanding of rationale for interventions
Describes own anxiety and coping patterns; uses coping mechanisms effectively
Demonstrates ability to understand and express self
Achieves or maintains control of own body
Shares feelings of changes in perception of self

Hemianopia

Hemianopia is the loss of one half of the normal field of vision. The loss of vision occurs as a result of damage to the visual pathways as they travel from the eye to the visual center in the occipital lobe of the cerebral cortex. The vision loss occurs on the same side as the hemiplegia. The patient may often seem unresponsive to stimuli when in actuality the lack of response is a result of vision loss (Figure 28-11).

Hemianopia can be diagnosed by having the patient name or point to all objects seen without moving the head. The nurse should then compare what is named to its location around the patient. Modification of the patient's care plan may decrease stress and anxiety over the vision loss. As cerebral edema subsides, the vision loss may lessen or disappear.

Bowel and bladder incontinence

Damage to the centers in the brain that control bladder and bowel function (located in the frontal lobes) can result in decreased awareness of bladder fullness and the need to defecate. The problem may be one of urgency, frequency, or incontinence. When incontinence persists, a program of retraining is necessary. The patient should be taken to the toilet or commode every 2 hours. Intake and output, as well as voiding patterns, should be carefully documented. Such data may be helpful in planning a voiding schedule for the patient. Constipation may become a problem because of decreased mobility. Stool softeners and the addition of fiber to the diet may be helpful. A consistent morning or evening bowel program helps to establish a routine evacuation pattern.

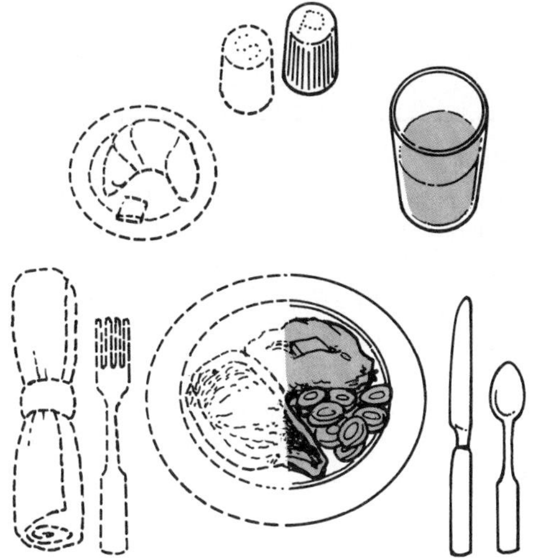

Figure 28-11 Spatial/perceptual deficits in stroke. Perception of a patient with homonymous hemianopsia shows that food on the left side is not seen and thus is ignored. (From Lewis SM, Collier IC: *Medical-surgical nursing,* ed 3, St Louis, 1992, Mosby.)

Perceptual problems

If the patient's stroke involves the parietal lobe of the right cerebral hemisphere, perceptual ability may be impaired. Some common disorders of perception include disturbances of body image and difficulty with recognizing objects through the senses (vision, hearing, or touch). Measures to provide increased sensory input can help overcome some of these problems.

CEREBRAL ARTERY ANEURYSM

A cerebral aneurysm is a distention of the arterial wall that develops because of a weakness in the vessel wall. It is the most common cause of subarachnoid hemorrhage. Most patients are adults between the ages of 35 and 60 (MacDonald, 1989). Although the cause of cerebral aneurysm is unclear, it is thought to occur as a result of a congenital defect in the arterial wall lining or as a result of a degenerative process that affects the wall. At the time of rupture, blood is forced into the subarachnoid space under high pressure, causing an increase in ICP.

Before bleeding, most patients are asymptomatic. At the time of rupture, the patient usually experiences an explosive headache, often described as "the worst headache of my life." In addition there may be vomiting, motor weakness, seizure activity, and decreased level of consciousness. These symptoms are related to the increased ICP that results from the addition of blood into a contained space.

Following the initial rupture, the patient is at risk for rebleeding. With rebleeding, the survival rate decreases. Rebleeding usually occurs around the 7th day following the initial hemorrhage. *Cerebral vasospasm* (narrowing or constriction of the vessel) is another complication of subarachnoid hemorrhage. It can result in ischemia to the brain and infarction if tissue death is severe. The clinical signs of vasospasm vary depending on the arterial distribution that is affected but often include decreased level of consciousness and motor weakness.

Surgery is usually indicated for treatment of cerebral aneurysm. The timing of surgical intervention is crucial in obtaining the best outcome. If the patient is relatively stable neurologically, early surgery within the first 1 to 3 days posthemorrhage is advisable. If significant neurologic deficits are present initially, it may be advisable to wait until the patient is more stable before proceeding with surgery. Obliteration of the aneurysm from circulation during a special vascular neuroradiologic procedure may also be an option. Medical management aimed at controlling hypertension, fever, and seizures is a priority. The calcium channel blocker nimodipine is administered to reduce the risk of vasospasm.

BOX 28-11 **Nursing Process**

CEREBRAL ANEURYSM

ASSESSMENT

Neurologic status
Vital signs
Seizure activity or evidence of meningeal irritation
Changes in status
Evidence of intracranial bleed (e.g., change in WC, vital signs, hemodynamic pressures)
Fluid volume status
Muscle strength and coordination
Laboratory studies: CBC, electrolytes, BUN, creatinine, serum osmolarity, coagulation studies

NURSING DIAGNOSES

Risk for altered body temperature (hyperthermia) related to neurologic deficits
Constipation related to decreased mobility
Pain related to headache
Impaired verbal communication related to pain
Fear related to surgery and prognosis
Risk for injury related to ischemia or seizure activity
Knowledge deficit related to aneurysm and care
Impaired physical mobility related to headache, neurologic deficit
Risk for impaired gas exchange related to neurologic deficit
Self-care deficit related to decreased mobility
Body image disturbance related to impaired mobility and neurologic deficit
Altered thought processes related to pain, neurologic deficit
Altered tissue perfusion of brain cells related to altered cerebral blood supply

NURSING INTERVENTIONS

Monitor neurologic and vital signs every 15 minutes initially and every hour thereafter.
Notify the physician of any changes in vital signs or neurologic status.
Assess and document location and severity of headache.
Administer and evaluate effectiveness of prescribed medications.
Reposition patient at least every 2 hours.
Maintain seizure precautions.
Provide support to patient and family.

EVALUATION OF EXPECTED OUTCOMES

Injuries prevented
Maximum pulmonary function maintained
Aspiration prevented
Adequate nutritional status maintained
Skin integrity maintained
Demonstrates improved ability to express self
Normal body temperature maintained
Participates in self-care as appropriate
Demonstrates understanding of rationale for interventions
Indicates increased comfort following pain relief measures
Shares feelings of changes in perception of self

Nursing interventions are directed toward monitoring neurologic status and vital signs, preventing additional injury from ischemia or seizure activity, and providing support to the patient and family (Box 28-11).

CARE OF THE PATIENT WITH A SEIZURE DISORDER

A **seizure** is a sudden, excessive, disorderly discharge of electric impulses from nerve cells in the cerebral cortex (Hartshorn, Byers, 1992). Seizures may occur at any age and are associated with a variety of diseases and disorders. They may also occur following a traumatic injury to the brain. Children are especially prone to seizures with temperature elevation. Seizures do not always follow any single pattern or form; their characteristics depend on the area of the brain from which they originate.

Seizure disorder and *epilepsy* are two terms used to identify recurrent episodes of disturbances in cerebral functioning resulting in convulsive movements, loss of consciousness, and abnormal sensory or behavioral manifestations. Approximately ½% to 2% of the U.S. population has some form of this disorder (Hickey, 1992). Eighty percent of this group has the first seizure before the age of 20. Epilepsy has been one of the least understood conditions since ancient times, often clouded in superstition. Today the cause of seizures is better understood. In some cases the cause may not be specifically identified (idiopathic epilepsy). An inherited tendency is thought to play a role with some individuals. Other causes include metabolic disturbances, congenital malformations in the brain, trauma, and neurologic conditions of the cerebral cortex. Although several types of seizures exist, this discussion will be limited to the most commonly observed in the major categories of *partial* and *generalized* seizures.

Partial Seizures

Partial seizures are seizures that begin with a localized focus. *Simple partial seizures* are characterized by convulsive twitching in one part of the body. The patient is generally awake and alert throughout the episode. *Complex partial seizures,* also called temporal lobe seizures, involve a loss of contact, although consciousness usually remains undisturbed. The patient is able to interact with the environment, but these interactions are not appropriate. He or she may also exhibit **automatisms** or automatic movements such as lip-smacking or picking at clothing.

Generalized Seizures

Tonic-clonic seizures are characterized by generalized convulsions and loss of consciousness. The patient may have some warning or sign of the approaching attack, which is called an **aura,** but almost immediately becomes unconscious, often falling. The attack may be immediately preceded by a cry, which occurs as the thoracic and abdominal muscles go into spasm, forcing air out of the lungs. The body becomes rigid, the legs extend straight, the jaws clench tightly, and the hands grip tightly (clonic phase). A temporary cessation of respiration with cyanosis may occur at this time. The eyes are often wide open, and the pupils dilate. In a few seconds the clonic phase begins, with all the muscles beginning to jerk and twitch violently. Bowel and bladder incontinence and profuse salivation occur. The clonic phase is of short duration, but the patient may remain unconscious or drowsy. A deep sleep lasting from several minutes to several hours may follow. On awakening, the patient often does not remember having the seizure but may complain of fatigue or generalized muscle aches.

Absence seizures are a mild form of generalized seizures in which an aura is not present and only momentary loss of consciousness occurs. Tonic-clonic convulsions do not occur, and only a slight twitching of the face or a nod of the head may be observed. A patient with absence seizures may have several attacks per day. These seizures are common in children under the age of 10 and often are outgrown at puberty. Because of the frequency of these attacks, children may have problems in school.

Status epilepticus is a condition in which seizures recur without recovery between them. Respirations are disturbed, blood pressure is often elevated, and sweating and fever occur. If left untreated, the condition may continue for hours or days. Status epilepticus is a medical emergency and should be treated without delay to avoid permanent neurologic deficit.

Intervention

The treatment of seizure disorders is aimed at eliminating factors that precipitate seizures and controlling seizures through the regular administration of antiepileptic medications. A program that includes regulation of diet, rest, stress, and medications should be followed. Medication is prescribed for the purpose of preventing seizures, and any attempt on the part of the patient to reduce, skip, or otherwise alter the schedule of dosage may cause the return of seizures. Drugs used in the treatment of seizures include phenytoin (Dilantin), phenobarbital, primidone (Mysoline), carbamazepine (Tegretol) and ethosuximide (Zarontin) (Table 28-2). Drugs may be used singly or in combination to enhance their action and decrease toxic side effects. All medication is administered in divided doses, and the patient should be observed for toxic effects such as skin rash, nervousness, drowsiness, fatigue, **ataxia,** and nystagmus. Because of the possible toxic effects from these medications, drug levels should be monitored by medical personnel on a regular basis. White blood cell count should also be monitored periodically because some medications cause depression of bone marrow. Surgical intervention may be useful in treating a small number of patients with well-defined and localized seizures that do not respond to antiepileptic medications.

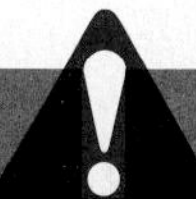

NURSE ALERT

When caring for the patient with a seizure disorder:

- Do not leave the patient unattended during a seizure.
- Prevent injury from falling.
- Place the patient's head in a lateral position.
- Place patient on the floor or bed.
- A plastic airway or padded tongue blade should be inserted between the patient's back teeth *only* if the patient's jaw is relaxed.
- Observe and record all aspects of the seizure.

The nurse should be aware of all patients who are admitted to the hospital with a history of seizures. Necessary precautions for the care of the patient with seizures should be taken. In addition, the nurse should

TABLE 28-2

Pharmacology of Drugs for Neurologic Disorders

Drug (Generic and Trade Name); Route and Dosage	Action/Indication	Common Side Effects and Nursing Considerations
AMANTADINE (Symmetrel) **ROUTE:** PO **DOSAGE:** 100 mg 1-2 times daily	Drug used in the initial and adjunct treatment of Parkinson's disease	Dizziness, ataxia, insomnia, hypotension, and mottling; use with caution in seizure disorders, liver, cardiac and renal disease, and elderly
BENZTROPINE (Cogentin) **ROUTE:** PO, IM, IV **DOSAGE:** PO, 0.5-6 mg/day in 1-2 divided doses; IV and IM doses for acute dystonic reactions 1-2 mg initially, then 1-2 mg PO bid	Drug used for adjunctive treatment of all forms of Parkinson's disease, including drug induced extrapyramidal effects and acute dystonic reactions	Dry eyes, blurred vision, constipation, and dry mouth; contraindicated in tardive dyskinesia and glaucoma; use with caution in elderly
CARBAMAZEPINE (Tegretol) **ROUTE:** PO **DOSAGE:** Start with 200 mg bid and increase by 200 mg/day until therapeutic range is achieved; range is usually 800-1200 mg/day in divided doses every 6-8 hours	Anticonvulsant drug used for prophylaxis of tonic-clonic, mixed, and complex-partial seizures	Drowsiness and ataxia; contraindicated in bone marrow suppression; use with caution in cardiac and hepatic disease and in elderly men with benign prostatic hypertrophy
CARBIDOPA (Sinemet) **ROUTE:** PO **DOSAGE:** 75/300-150/1500 mg/day in 3-4 divided doses, can increase up to 200/2000 mg/day	Drug used in the treatment of Parkinson's disease and other forms of parkinsonism	Involuntary movements, nausea, and vomiting; contraindicated in glaucoma, patients receiving MAO inhibitors, malignant melanoma, and undiagnosed skin lesions; use with caution with history of psychiatric, cardiac, or ulcer disease
ETHOSUXIMIDE (Zarontin) **ROUTE:** PO **DOSAGE:** 250 mg bid initially, may increase by 250 mg/day every 4-7 days up to 1.5 g/day given in divided doses bid; usual maintenance dose is 20 mg/kg/day	Anticonvulsant drug used in the management of absence seizures (petit mal)	Anorexia, gastric upset, nausea, vomiting, cramping, weight loss, and diarrhea; do not discontinue abruptly; use with caution in hepatic or renal disease
LEVODOPA (Dopar, Larodopa) **ROUTE:** PO **DOSAGE:** 500-1000 mg/day given in divided doses every 6-12 hr initially; increase by 100-750 mg/day every 3-7 days until response occurs or 8000 mg/day is reached; usual maintenance dose is 2000-8000 mg/day	Drug used in the treatment of parkinsonian syndrome	Involuntary movements, nausea, and vomiting; contraindicated in glaucoma, patients receiving MAO inhibitors, malignant melanoma, undiagnosed skin lesions; use with caution in cardiac, psychiatric, or ulcer disease
NEOSTIGMINE (Prostigmin) **ROUTE:** PO, SC, IM **DOSAGE:** PO, 15 mg every 3-4 hr initially, increase at daily intervals until optimal response achieved; usual maintenance dose is 150 mg/day to 375 mg/day, SC, IM, 0.5 mg	Drug used to increase muscle strength in symptomatic treatment of myasthenia gravis	Excess secretions, bronchospasm, bradycardia, abdominal cramps, nausea, vomiting, diarrhea, excess salivation, and sweating; contraindicated in mechanical obstruction of the GI or GU tract; use with caution in asthma, ulcers, cardiac disease, epilepsy, hyperthyroidism, and pregnancy

TABLE 28-2

Pharmacology of Drugs for Neurologic Disorders—cont'd

Drug (Generic and Trade Name); Route and Dosage	Action/Indication	Common Side Effects and Nursing Considerations
PHENOBARBITAL **ROUTE:** PO, IV **DOSAGE:** PO, 60-250 mg/day, single dose or 2-3 divided; IV, 100-320 mg as needed initially (total of 600 mg/24-hr period); 10-20 mg/kg has been used for status epilepticus	Drug used as an anticonvulsant in tonic-clonic (grand mal), partial, and febrile seizures; can also be used as a preoperative sedative and hypnotic	Hangover, laryngospasm (IV only), and angiodema; contraindicated in CNS depression, uncontrolled severe pain, and known alcohol intolerance; use with caution in hepatic, renal, cardiac, elderly, and drug addicted; chronic use as a hypnotic may lead to dependence
PHENYTOIN (Dilantin) **ROUTE:** PO, IV **DOSAGE:** Anticonvulsant, PO, loading dose of 1 g or 20/mg/kg as extended release capsules in 3 divided doses at 2-hr intervals; maintenance dose 300-400 mg/day; usual maximum dose is 600 mg/day; status epilepticus, IV, 15-20 mg/kg; rate not to exceed 25-50 mg/min, followed by 100 mg every 6-8 hr	Anticonvulsant drug used in the treatment and prevention of tonic-clonic seizures and complex partial seizures; also can be used an an antiarrhythmic	Nystagmus, ataxia, diplopia, gingival hyperplasia, hypotension (IV only), nausea, and rashes; contraindicated in sinus bradycardia and heart block (antiarrhythmic use); use with caution in severe liver disease and elderly; drug dosage may need to be increased in obese patients
TRIHEXYPHENIDYL (Artane) **ROUTE:** PO **DOSAGE:** 1-2 mg/day initially, increase by 2 mg every 3-5 days; usual maintenance dose is 5-15 mg/day in 3-4 divided doses	Drug used in the adjunct management of parkinsonian syndrome due to many causes, including drug-induced parkinsonism	Sedation, extrapyramidal reactions, constipation, and photosensitivity; contraindicated in glaucoma, bone marrow depression, and severe liver or cardiac disease; use with caution in elderly, debilitated, diabetes, respiratory disease, and epilepsy

be aware of all antiepileptic medications that the patient is taking, because many of these drugs interact with other medications.

Once a seizure has begun, the main responsibilities of the nurse are to protect the patient from injury and to accurately observe and record the patient's behavior before, during, and after the event (Box 28-12). A careful and accurate recording from the initial onset of the seizure until its completion can assist in locating the site of the origin of the seizure as well as in planning further care and treatment. Observation of the patient's seizure should include the following:

- Exact time of onset, duration, and ending of seizure
- Presence or absence of aura
- Level of consciousness before, during, and after event
- Progression and type of muscular activity, parts of body involved
- Presence of cyanosis or respiratory difficulty
- Presence or absence of urinary or fecal incontinence
- Movement of tongue or eyes
- Postseizure behavior
- Any injury that may have occurred during the seizure

Patient and Family Teaching

One of the most important responsibilities of the nurse in caring for the patient with a seizure disorder is patient and family education. The patient should understand the nature of the seizure activity, the medication program, the potential side effects of drugs, and the danger of not taking medications exactly as prescribed. The nurse should also emphasize the importance of adequate rest, a well-balanced diet, and avoidance of situations that may precipitate a seizure, such as extreme physical exertion, infection, and emotional stress. The patient should be advised not to par-

BOX 28-12 **Nursing Process**

SEIZURES

ASSESSMENT

Frequency, duration, and type of seizure activity
Aura prior to seizure
Respiratory status during and after seizure activity
Loss of consciousness, orientation, memory, speech, and pupillary response postseizure
Knowledge regarding safety and treatment

NURSING DIAGNOSES

Risk for injury related to uncontrolled movement
Ineffective airway clearance related to muscle spasm
Ineffective breathing pattern related to muscle spasm
Risk for total incontinence related to change in consciousness
Impaired swallowing related to muscle spasm
Impaired physical mobility related to muscle spasm
Self-care deficit related to change in consciousness
Impaired verbal communication related to change in consciousness
Knowledge deficit related to condition and prognosis

NURSING INTERVENTIONS

Do not leave patient unattended; do not attempt to move patient.
Insert plastic airway or padded tongue blade between patient's back teeth *only* if patient's jaw is relaxed; do not attempt to forcibly open patient's jaw if teeth are clenched.
Keep padded side rails up at all times; may be lowered during seizure.
Maintain patent airway and adequate ventilation; suctioning and oxygen may be necessary.
If patient is standing, lower carefully to floor and place pad under head.
Accompany patient with frequent seizures when ambulating.
Administer anticonvulsive medications as ordered; notify physician if patient is unable to take medication for any reason.
Accurately record all aspects of the seizure.
Respect dignity of patient—provide privacy if possible.

EVALUATION OF EXPECTED OUTCOMES

Injuries prevented
Maximum pulmonary function maintained
Aspiration prevented
Participates in self-care as appropriate
Relates rationale for interventions
Demonstrates ability to understand and to express self
Demonstrates understanding of interventions

ticipate in activities such as working near dangerous machinery, climbing ladders, or swimming alone. Driving an automobile is permitted if seizures have been under complete control for an extended period of time. State laws differ regarding this point. The Epilepsy Foundation of America can provide information and support to the patient and family regarding the many issues of living with a seizure disorder.

CARE OF THE PATIENT WITH CENTRAL NERVOUS SYSTEM INFECTION

Meningitis

Meningitis is an inflammation of the meninges covering the brain and spinal cord. Common bacterial causes of the disease are meningococcal, pneumococcal, streptococcal, and *Haemophilus influenzae* infections. Any number of viruses can also cause viral meningitis. The causative organism may reach the meninges through the bloodstream after a systemic infection. Meningitis also may develop by direct extension from an adjacent infected area, such as in otitis media or mastoiditis. The disease often occurs in sporadic epidemics and is a threat where crowded conditions exist. Children are more commonly affected than adults because of their tendency to develop ear infections.

Assessment

The onset of symptoms varies according to the causative organism. Clinical symptoms usually develop within 48 hours, but meningococcal meningitis has a more rapid onset of 8 to 12 hours. The diagnosis is made through analysis of CSF, including a culture to determine the causative organism. Symptoms of meningitis include a headache, a severely rigid and stiff neck or **nuccal rigidity,** fever, lethargy, and confusion. As the disease progresses, nausea, vomiting, photophobia (intolerance to light), and seizures may occur.

Intervention

Treatment for meningitis includes prompt administration of appropriate antibacterial therapy. Intravenous fluids usually are given during the acute phase, although fluid restriction may be advised to prevent cerebral edema. Analgesics (codeine) may be used to relieve the headache. The patient should be placed in a quiet, slightly darkened room because of the photophobia and headache. Seizure precautions should be instituted. Isolation precautions are necessary for patients with meningococcal infections and may be required in some areas for all types of meningitis until the causative organism has been identified. Extreme caution should be used to avoid transmission of the disease by contamination with respiratory secretions.

General supportive measures necessary for any acutely ill patient are necessary, including regular turning intervals, maintenance of good body alignment, and accurate monitoring of fluid intake and urinary output. Measures to control fever and seizures may be necessary. The patient should be observed for evidence of increased ICP. The outcome cannot always be predicted. Some sequelae that occur after meningitis include visual impairment, deafness, cognitive deficits, and personality changes.

Encephalitis

Encephalitis is an acute febrile illness with evidence of involvement of brain tissue. It may be caused by viruses, bacteria, fungi, chemical substances, toxins, or injury. It also may occur with or following one of the acute infectious diseases of childhood (measles or rubella) or may be a complication of measles, chickenpox, or rabies vaccination (postviral encephalitis). Residual neurologic deficits may follow encephalitis, including a slowly developing parkinsonian syndrome. The disease occurs sporadically and in epidemics. The greatest incidence is during the late summer or fall months.

Viral encephalitis is caused by several viruses, including the herpes simplex virus. Among the viral infections most commonly encountered are those caused by mosquitoes (arthropod-borne encephalitis). The virus is transmitted to humans by the bite of an infected mosquito. It cannot be transmitted from person to person. Evidence indicates that the virus is harbored by several species of wild birds or horses. The mosquito becomes infected through biting these infected birds or animals. These forms of arthropod-borne encephalitis have been classified as St. Louis encephalitis, eastern equine encephalitis, western equine encephalitis, and Japanese B encephalitis. St. Louis encephalitis is the most common type, and epidemics may have a mortality rate as high as 60% to 70%. Very young and elderly persons are most commonly affected, although persons of all ages may contract the disease. Each of the viral types is caused by a different virus, although they may be related.

Assessment

The symptoms are fairly uniform for all types of encephalitis. The onset is sudden, with an elevation of temperature to 104° F to 105° F, increased pulse rate, and severe headache unrelieved by analgesics. Symptoms include nausea; vomiting; **tremor** of the hands, tongue, and lips; stiffness of the neck; speech difficulty, and drowsiness. In severe cases seizures, coma, and death may occur suddenly.

Intervention

For patients with viral encephalitis no specific treatment is indicated. Isolation is not required because encephalitis is not transmitted from person to person. Nursing care requires careful observation of the patient, because progress of the disease may be rapid. The patient is critically ill, and nursing care is based on symptoms. Variations in level of consciousness and mental status should be considered in planning care for the patient. If respiratory difficulties occur, mechanical ventilation may be necessary. Seizures are not uncommon, and necessary precautions should be taken. Fluids may be given intravenously, and a diet high in calories and proteins should be given either by mouth or via a nasogastric tube. Residual deficits may result, requiring prolonged periods of rehabilitation.

Acquired Immunodeficiency Syndrome (AIDS)

Neurologic involvement is often seen in adults and children with HIV infection. It is thought that approximately 40% of patients with AIDS have documented neurologic complications (Ake and Perlstein, 1987). Involvement of the central nervous system may be seen through opportunistic infections (toxoplasmosis and cryptococcus), tumors (CNS lymphoma), and AIDS dementia complex. The patient is admitted for episodic treatment of these problems, but the majority of care is often managed through an outpatient healthcare provider. Beyond the specifics of management for each of the above noted problems, the nurse's role involves providing support, patient education, and community-based referrals for long-term management (see Chapter 13).

NURSING CARE OF THE PATIENT WITH DEGENERATIVE DISEASES INVOLVING THE CENTRAL NERVOUS SYSTEM

Degenerative diseases of the central nervous system refer to conditions in which premature degeneration of nerve cells and pathways occurs with no identifiable cause. Familial factors, toxic agents, metabolic defects, and viral and immunologic mechanisms all have been suspected as possible etiologies. These conditions may develop over a period of years and result in some degree of chronic disability. Nursing care is concerned primarily with the care given to any patient with a chronic illness. Other concerns are to provide encouragement and emotional support for the patient and family and to help the patient be independent and self-sufficient as long as possible. The major degenerative conditions that will be reviewed here are multiple sclerosis, amyotrophic lateral sclerosis, Parkinson's disease, Alzheimer's disease, and Guillain-Barre syndrome. Myasthenia gravis, although not a degenerative disease, is discussed because of its similarities with the other conditions.

Multiple Sclerosis

Multiple sclerosis (MS) is a chronic disease of the central nervous system and is characterized by remissions and exacerbations. The disease affects the myelin sheaths (segmented coverings around nerve fibers), resulting in numerous areas of demyelinization of nerve fibers of the spinal cord and brain. Later, patches of sclerotic nerve fibers (plaques) develop at these sites. The symptoms and severity of the disease are quite variable depending on the location and extent of the lesions. Remissions of symptoms occur when partial healing in the area of demyelination occurs. The disease is chronically progressive because residual disability usually increases after each exacerbation.

The first symptoms of the disease begin between the ages of 20 and 40 in nearly two thirds of all cases, with the peak incidence occurring between ages 30 and 35. An estimated 250,000 people in the United States currently have MS (Hainsworth, 1994).

Assessment

The onset of the disease may be acute or may develop slowly over months or years. Diagnosis of the disease in its early stages is difficult because MS symptoms are varied and often vague. Among the earliest symptoms are double vision (diplopia), spots before the eyes (scotoma), blindness, tremor, weakness or numbness of a part of the body, and fatigue. As the disease progresses, nystagmus, paralysis, disorders of speech, urinary frequency and urgency, and muscle uncoordination occur. Severe spasticity of muscles resulting in contractures is a late manifestation. Approximately one third of all patients with MS develop changes in mental status. Symptoms and their severity reflect the area of the brain that is involved.

Intervention

MS is treated symptomatically and supportively. During acute exacerbations, the patient may be given corticosteroids, but this is controversial. A concentrated program of physical and occupational therapy is important to maintain functional independence as long as possible. Precipitating factors that cause exacerbations, including fatigue, cold, hot baths, and infections, should be avoided. Because of sensory loss and motor weakness, safety measures must be instituted to prevent injury. Heating pads should be avoided, and patients should be instructed to check water temperature with uninvolved body parts. They should be cautioned about scatter rugs and polished floors, which may cause falls. They also should receive nutrition counseling to ensure a well-balanced diet high in vitamins.

An important responsibility of the nurse during hospitalization is patient and family education concerning all aspects of the disease process, methods of preventing complications of pressure ulcers and contractures, and ways to conserve energy to avoid fatigue. Work and social activities should be continued as long as possible, although alteration of the the work schedule may be necessary to avoid fatigue. Self-help devices are available to patients with considerable disability. The National Multiple Sclerosis Society is an excellent source of information for patients and families.

Amyotrophic Lateral Sclerosis

Amyotrophic lateral sclerosis (ALS) is a progressive degenerative disorder of the motor neurons of the spinal cord, brain stem, and motor cortex and results in muscular weakness and atrophy. Approximately 30,000 persons in the United States are affected, with 5000 new cases per year (Hickey, 1992). The disease affects men more than women, and the age of onset is often between 40 and 70 years. Its cause is unknown, but a slow-acting virus is suspected.

Symptoms of ALS include progressive muscle weakness. Muscle twitchings are an early sign. As the disease progresses, brain stem involvement causes difficulty in speech, chewing, and swallowing. No known treatment of the disease exists. In the terminal stage, the patient is often completely functionally dependent. Death occurs as a result of respiratory failure. Nursing care is aimed at supportive and symptomatic measures to improve the patient's well-being. The ALS Foundation is available to provide assistance to families and patients following diagnosis and throughout the course of the disease.

Parkinson's Disease

Parkinson's disease is a chronic, progressive disease affecting the basal ganglia, a group of nerve cell bodies (nuclei) located deep within the cerebral hemispheres. It is considered to be one of the most common neurologic disorders of the aged, with the first symptoms becoming apparent between ages 50 and 60. Parkinson's disease often begins with only unilateral involvement and progresses to severe disability with confinement to bed or wheelchair.

Research has shown that patients with Parkinson's disease have a deficiency of dopamine, a compound found normally in large amounts in the basal ganglia. Dopamine is necessary for the normal transmission of nerve impulses in the basal ganglia. Deficiencies of dopamine result in involuntary movements and disturbances of muscle tone and posture. The exact cause of the disease is unknown, but a number of factors associated with deficiency of dopamine include encephalitis, arteriosclerosis, toxic substances (carbon monoxide and mercury), and certain tranquilizer drugs.

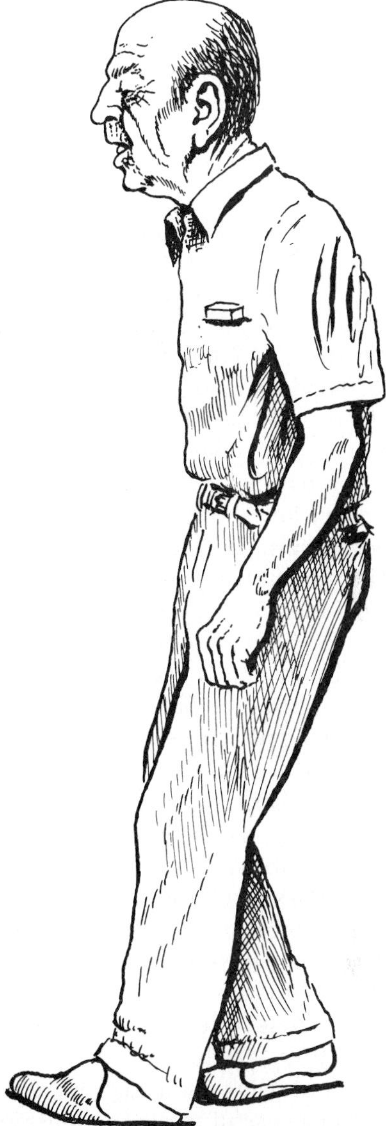

Figure 28-12 This patient displays several outward characteristics of Parkinson's disease. (From Rudy E: *Advanced neurological and neurosurgical nursing,* St Louis, 1984, Mosby.)

Assessment

Parkinson's disease is characterized by tremors, imbalance (postural instability), muscle rigidity, and slow movement (bradykinesia). The tremor, often the first sign reported, can best be described as a pill-rolling motion of the fingers. The tremor is rhythmic and rapid and may be limited to the fingers and hand or may involve the entire body. Typically the tremor is more noticeable with the hand at rest and may disappear with voluntary movement of the hand. It is aggravated by stress and anxiety and usually disappears with sleep. **Rigidity** of the muscles results in jerky, uncoordinated "cogwheel" movements. All complicated movements are slow and difficult to perform. The patient's gait is typically a shuffle, with the patient taking very small steps. Some patients begin to take smaller and faster steps (propulsive gait), resulting in a danger of falling, and associated movements such as arm swing may be lost. Postural disturbances also result from rigidity. A stooped posture with the head and body flexed forward often results, and the extremities remain flexed continuously (Figure 28-12). Other symptoms include a masklike facies; slow, monotonous speech; and drooling. Depression often results because these patients have difficulty talking and tend to withdraw from people because of their physical appearance. Cognitive changes do occur in early Parkinson's disease and sometimes indicate the onset of a more global pathologic process.

Intervention

Treatment of Parkinson's disease is symptomatic, supportive, and palliative and includes drug therapy, a physical therapy regimen, and psychotherapy if necessary. Although there is no cure for the disease, the symptoms can be well controlled with an appropriate medical regimen.

Levodopa (L-Dopa), the immediate precursor of dopamine, is effective for long-term management of the disease. L-Dopa has proven to be particularly effective in alleviating the symptoms of tremor and rigidity. The drug is converted to dopamine after passing the blood-brain barrier into the brain. The dosage of the drug is increased gradually until maximum benefit is gained with the fewest side effects. Many patients are troubled with nausea and vomiting, postural hypotension, and cardiac arrhythmias. Probably the most disturbing side effect to the patient is the abnormal involuntary movements (choreiform movements) of the tongue, jaw, and neck, resulting in lip smacking and protrusion of the tongue. Agitation, delusions, and insomnia may occur. Carbidopa (Sinemet) is a preparation that enhances the therapeutic response to L-Dopa but reduces the side effects. It is effective because it decreases the peripheral metabolism of L-Dopa, making more L-Dopa available for use in the brain. Carbidopa reduces the amount of L-Dopa required by 75%. Giving small, divided dosages also tends to reduce the side effects of L-Dopa. Ingestion of large amounts of protein and pyridoxine (vitamin B_6) reduces the therapeutic effect of L-Dopa. Pyridoxine has no effect on carbidopa.

Several other drugs have been used for their symptom-relieving effects, including the anticholinergics trihexyphenidyl (Artane) and benztropine (Cogentin). Other drugs found useful include antihistamines and amantadine (Symmetrel). These drugs may be given in combination with L-Dopa for their synergistic effect.

In select patients, any of several surgical procedures may be performed. Stereotactic surgery (destruction of areas controlling specific functions) may be done in cases in which drug therapy has been unsuccessful. In this procedure, destruction of a well-defined area of the basal ganglia is accomplished with alcohol or liquid nitrogen after burr holes have been made in the skull and a cannula inserted.

Nursing care of the patient with Parkinson's disease is aimed at maintaining independence. The nurse can contribute significantly to the patient's successful adaptation in the home through a program of patient and family teaching that emphasizes drug therapy, diet, elimination, and daily exercise. The patient should be encouraged to work and participate in social functions as long as possible. Family members may need support and education to understand the disease and anticipate necessary adjustments in the home (Box 28-13).

Alzheimer's Disease

Alzheimer's disease is a chronic degenerative disease that causes gradual, progressive loss of cognitive function. Women are affected more often than men, and the disease usually involves people over 45 years of age. It is the major cause of dementia in the elderly (see Chapter 14). The cause of Alzheimer's disease is unknown, although atherosclerosis, heredity, and autoimmune response are suggested as possible contributors (Burns, Buckwalter, 1988).

Alzheimer's disease has been characterized as progressing in three stages. The first stage is characterized by forgetfulness, a decline in interest in people and environment, and problems with work performance. In the second stage, memory loss, irritability, and wandering behavior are exhibited. The final stage is characterized by weight loss, inability to communicate, incontinence, and loss of motor skills (e.g., standing and walking). Death is often caused by infection (e.g., aspiration pneumonia). The progression is usually gradual and develops over an average period of 7 years. Nursing care of the patient varies depending on symptoms. Supervision, protection from injury, encouragement in the participation in activities of daily living, and nutrition support are key principles of management during the last two stages. At present, no known treatment exists. Support for the patient and family is essential, with the involvement of social service and community resources.

Guillain-Barre Syndrome

Guillain-Barre syndrome is an acute inflammatory polyneuropathy believed to be an autoimmune response to a viral infection. It is one of the most common disorders of the peripheral nervous system. Sensory symptoms may occur in the absence of any motor symptoms, but if motor involvement occurs, sensory symptoms always are evident. Motor symptoms may begin with weakness, disturbance of gait, and paralysis. The motor weakness is ascending; it begins in the ankles and wrists and gradually extends up the extremity until complete paralysis results. Pain may also be experienced by some patients.

Guillain-Barre syndrome is divided into three stages: acute onset, which begins with development of symptoms and ends when no additional symptoms or deterioration is observed (usually 1 to 3 weeks); plateau, which lasts from 1 to 3 weeks; and recovery, which may

BOX 28-13 **Nursing Process**

PARKINSON'S DISEASE

ASSESSMENT

Motor system, functional ability, activities of daily living, mental status, and emotional state
Rigidity and slowness of body movement
Patterns of mobility
Communication patterns
Medication information
Nutrition status and swallowing ability
Home environment

NURSING DIAGNOSES

Impaired physical mobility related to coordinated movements
Self-care deficit related to altered movement patterns
Anxiety related to inability to control illness
Risk for injury related to altered movement patterns
Constipation related to altered movement pattern
Ineffective individual and family coping related to chronicity of illness
Hopelessness
Knowledge deficit related to drug therapy regimen
Body image disturbance related to change in body movement

NURSING INTERVENTIONS

Observe for L-Dopa side effects—check pulse rate and rhythm four times a day; take blood pressure in lying and standing position.
Administer L-Dopa with meals to decrease nausea.
Reduce stress- and anxiety-producing situations—allow patient plenty of time to perform such activities as eating and dressing.
Encourage patient to exercise and use all muscles and joints—range-of-motion exercises should be done several times a day.
Carry out regular daily exercise program to maintain function.
Practice writing and singing aloud.
Use march music and lines placed at intervals on the floor to encourage larger steps.
Encourage exercises to improve balance.
Use stool softeners and suppositories as necessary to prevent constipation.
Involve family and patient in all aspects of planning and giving care.
Provide emotional support to patient and family—be calm and reassuring.

EVALUATION OF EXPECTED OUTCOMES

Takes appropriate precautions to prevent injury
Sets realistic goals
Participates in self-care as appropriate
Reports satisfaction with self-care despite limitations
Relates rationale for interventions
Describes own anxiety and coping patterns; uses coping mechanisms effectively
Demonstrates ability to understand and express self
Demonstrates initiative and autonomy in making decisions
Describes methods to prevent constipation

last for up to 2 years depending on the extent of involvement and loss of function. Permanent disability may be an outcome, although most patients experience gradual recovery over a 1- to 2-year period (Griswold, Guanci, Ropper, 1984).

Acute Guillain-Barre syndrome is managed medically with steroids, plasmapheresis, and respiratory support if needed. Nursing interventions focus on assessment of baseline neurologic and respiratory function and careful monitoring for changes from this baseline. Respiratory insufficiency is a primary concern, and the patient may need mechanical ventilatory support during the acute phase. Nursing care is crucial in the prevention of the complications of immobility. Deep vein thrombosis and pulmonary embolism are of major concern, as are gastrointestinal complications of the ileus and impaction. Most patients have difficulty with communication and are understandably anxious and fearful. Constant support and reassurance of a positive outcome is a primary role of the nurse during the acute phase.

Myasthenia Gravis

Myasthenia gravis is a chronic, progressive disease characterized by muscle weakness. It is caused by a deficiency in neuromuscular transmission at the point where the motor nerve joins a skeletal muscle (myoneural junction). Although the exact cause of the problem is unclear, the etiology is believed to be related to an autoimmune process.

Normally nerve endings produce a substance called acetylcholine, which carries the nerve impulse from the nerve fiber to the muscle and causes it to contract. The muscle produces an enzyme, cholinesterase, which inactivates the acetylcholine. The patient with myasthenia gravis produces either too little acetylcholine or too much cholinesterase. The result is insufficient muscle contraction or weakness.

Myasthenia gravis occurs most often between 20 and 30 years of age. Women are affected two times as frequently as men up to the age of 40. After 40, men are equally affected (Marshall, 1990). Drug treatment is the major approach to management of the disease. The prognosis is poor without treatment.

Assessment

The primary symptom is muscle weakness, which affects almost every muscle in the body except those of the heart, intestines, and bladder. Muscle strength is characteristically stronger in the morning and becomes progressively weaker with continued use. The weakness may range from a slight reduction of strength after repeated use of a particular muscle to complete paralysis. Symptoms are aggravated by emotional upset, alcoholic intake, lack of rest, and respiratory tract infections. As a result of the muscle weakness, ptosis of the eyelids and weakness of the muscles of swallowing, chewing, and speaking are common. Shortness of breath may develop with walking.

The diagnosis of myasthenia gravis is made on the basis of history, physical examination, and electromyography. Administration of a test dose of neostigmine or edrophonium (Tensilon) produces dramatic improvement in muscle strength and is usually diagnostic for the disease.

Intervention

Treatment of patients with myasthenia gravis depends on the severity of the disease. Maintenance doses of anticholinesterase drugs have been found effective in controlling symptoms. These include neostigmine (Prostigmin) and pyridostigmine (Mestinon). These drugs prevent the breakdown of acetylcholine by cholinesterase. The optimum dose for the patient is the smallest possible dose that produces the greatest muscle strength. Overdosage can produce generalized weakness (cholinergic crisis). Dysphagia and respiratory weakness during a cholinergic crisis may be so severe that mechanical ventilatory assistance is necessary. Corticosteroids may be used for patients who do not respond to these drugs. The purpose of the corticosteroids is to mediate the body's autoimmune response.

Because thymic tumors have been associated with myasthenia gravis, surgical excision of the thymus gland is performed in certain cases. The remission rate is approximately 40% to 50% if the procedure is done in the early stages. Plasmapheresis, the process of washing acetylcholine receptor antibodies from the plasma, is also a helpful treatment for severe myasthenia gravis. An improvement in muscle strength is generally noted 24 to 48 hours after the first exchange.

Nursing care of the patient with myasthenia gravis should emphasize careful monitoring and follow-up. The patient's status may change, requiring an adjustment in medication dosage. A **myasthenic crisis,** often difficult to distinguish from a cholinergic crisis, may occur. In an exacerbation of the disease, a decreased response to anticholinesterase medication develops. Emergency measures are usually necessary at this time.

Myasthenia gravis is a chronic disease that affects every aspect of the patient's life. It afflicts young people in the prime of life and can be a terrifying, life-threatening condition. Apprehension and fear may be great because the patient never knows when he or she may lose the ability to swallow, breathe, or move. The patient needs consistent reassurance and support around the uncertainty of the illness. Measures to conserve energy and muscle strength should be emphasized in preparing the patient for discharge. The patient should carry a Medic Alert identification card or wear a Medic Alert bracelet to ensure proper treatment during emergency situations. Helpful information can be obtained from the Myasthenia Gravis Foundation, Inc.

REHABILITATION FOR NEUROLOGIC DISORDERS

Rehabilitation of the patient with a neurologic disorder begins on admission. Although it may be simpler and faster for the nurse to perform various tasks for the patient, the patient should be encouraged to perform activities that do not cause undue frustration. The patient should not be rushed during these activities. A sense of accomplishment is important. New learning experiences should be attempted only when the patient is well rested.

Independence in mobility, either walking or by using a wheelchair, helps to reduce the patient's feelings of helplessness. The nurse is involved in teaching the patient to transfer from bed to wheelchair and wheelchair to toilet by leading with the nonparalyzed side of the body. In assisting the patient to walk, the nurse should support the patient's weak side. A belt placed around the patient's waist and held in back by the nurse helps to maintain balance. A sling may be used to support the affected arm when the patient is walking to prevent separation of the shoulder joint (subluxation).

The patient who has suffered a neurologic insult has experienced a sudden, drastic change in body function that may be overwhelming. Although intellect may remain intact, the patient's body no longer reacts according to wishes. The patient may not be able to speak intelligibly, move at will, or control the most basic body functions. The patient's perception of himself or herself has been altered suddenly, and emotional reactions are to be expected. The patient may succumb to outbursts of anger, tears, or extreme withdrawal as a means of expressing fear, anxiety, and frustration. Nurses must provide opportunities for the patient to communicate in whatever way possible. Being calm and reassuring, recognizing small gains, and giving constant encouragement stimulates the patient to continuous progress.

The nurse shares with other team members the responsibility of preparing the patient for discharge. Team members may include a physical therapist, occupational therapist, speech therapist, neuropsychologist, dietician, and social worker. Both the patient and family should be involved in planning for care after discharge. The patient's home situation should be assessed, and necessary physical changes should be made before discharge. The family should be encouraged to maintain as normal a home environment as possible, considering the patient's capabilities. Constant and consistent patient and family education is important to ensure adequate care with the least amount of stress on family members. If the family understands what to anticipate, a smoother adjustment to the home situation is made by both the patient and family.

ETHICAL DILEMMA

Cognitive impairment disorder is a group of disorders that is growing because of the aging of the population. What ethical issues, questions, and dilemmas can you identify and analyze that may occur in a patient with one of these diagnoses (e.g., Alzheimer's disease)?

Nursing Care Plan

PATIENT WHO IS CONFUSED

Mr. Wilson is a 19-year-old male who was brought into the trauma center by the police after having been found wandering aimlessly along a dirt road by a passing motorist. Details of the patient's accident are still not complete, but the police found an overturned smashed motorcycle approximately 500 feet from where the patient was discovered. On arrival, it was noted that the patient was not wearing a helmet and had a strong odor of alcohol on his breath. A blood-alcohol level was drawn as well as other drug toxicology studies, but the results are being kept confidential on the advice of his lawyer. Identification was made via a wallet found near the cycle. His vital signs have been stable but difficult to obtain because he has been combative since his arrival. Physical examination has also been hard to accomplish because of his altering states of cooperation.

He has a large facial laceration extending from just above the right eyebrow to the center midhair line (approximately 8 cm). Frontal swelling is noted along his forehead. Skull x-ray examinations are negative for a fracture, and he has had a cranial CT scan. The laceration was sutured with 6-0 nylon sutures and xylocaine.

He is moving all extremities without evidence of pain or tenderness. Abdominal trauma is being questioned because he has guarding and wincing on palpation of the left upper quadrant. Serial hematocrits have been stable, ruling out a ruptured spleen. Vital signs are stable, and his pupils are equal and reactive to light. He has been uncooperative in testing his hand grasp. His condition is felt to be stable, but he is being admitted for observation because of the ingestion of unknown substance(s) and possible loss of consciousness at the scene of the accident. His score on the Glasgow Coma Scale is 12, with orientation only to self.

continued

Nursing Care Plan

PATIENT WHO IS CONFUSED

Past Medical History

- Provided by anxious parents, who were notified once identification had been established
- Generally good health; recently passed Army physical examination and was awaiting orders to attend basic training; had plans to join the Reserves to obtain its college assistance program
- Immunizations up-to-date; last tetanus booster 2 years ago because of a foot laceration with sutures
- No known food or drug allergies
- No history of hospitalization/surgeries

Psychosocial Data

- Lives with parents and three younger brothers
- Second year of college; business major
- Reported to be in scholastic jeopardy due to low grades
- Active in sports, likes basketball best
- Has part-time job at local McDonald's
- Has had driver's license since age 16
- One conviction of driving while intoxicated (DWI), age 18
- Has attended mandatory DWI classes; license just renewed
- Covered by parents' health insurance
- Protestant religion; no active church involvement
- Said to have many girlfriends, recently depressed over loss of special girlfriend

Assessment Data

- Well-developed, well-nourished male who is oriented to self only; cannot state orientation to time, place, or persons
- Does not appear to recognize parents
- Vital signs stable: T99, P 84, R 22, BP 126/78
- *Skin:* Color good; multiple abrasions on right forehead; sutures dry and intact; no evidence of infection
- Abrasions also on right chest wall; no drainage
- No rashes, no edema
- *Head:* Patent nares; no discharge
- Cut on upper lip; central upper incisor loose
- *EENT:* Full extra ocular movements (EOMs); pupils round, equal, and react to light accomodation; visual acuity intact
- No complaints of dizziness or diplopia
- *Respiratory:* Regular rate and rhythm; no use of accessory muscles
- Chest movements symmetrical; clear to percussion and ascultation; no rales, rhonchi, or rubs
- *Abdominal:* Soft; slight tenderness in upper left quadrant, with some guarding on palpation; nondistended; bowel sounds present all quadrants
- *Musculoskeletal:* Moving all extremities well; full range of motion
- Equal grasps and sensations; DTRs intact, 2+ and symmetrical
- Babinski sign negative; unable to test for Romberg's sign
- Is right-handed
- *Neuro:* Follows commands inconsistently; speech rambling; some echolalia
- No memory of events before accident
- Cannot name president of United States or identify basic colors
- Will count to 10 only; no ability to add or subtract
- Periods of increased agitation and crying
- Unable to test all cranial nerves due to lack of cooperation
- Will shrug shoulders, blink, raise eyebrows, smile, frown, and yawn
- *Cardiovascular:* Apical pulse 82 and regular; no diaphoresis

Laboratory data

- Hct stable at 34-36; checked every 3 hours for first 24 hours
- Hgb 12.2; oxygen saturations stable at 96-98
- Platelets, electrolytes, liver function tests (LFTs), BUN, FBS all within normal limits

Nursing Care Plan

PATIENT WHO IS CONFUSED—cont'd

Past Medical History	Psychosocial Data	Assessment Data
		Urinalysis WNL; no gross or microscopic hematuria Chest x-ray and flat plate of abdomen all negative *Medications* No medications IV 1000 ml D5W in Ringer's Lactate at 80 ml per hour IV removed by patient; decision to restart pending tolerance of po fluids Clear liquid diet; advance as tolerated; nursing judgment

NURSING DIAGNOSIS

Sensory/perceptual alterations related to head trauma and question of drug ingestion as evidenced by confusion, anxiety, and apprehension

NURSING INTERVENTIONS

Assess patient for signs and symptoms of decreased cerebral tissue perfusion: dizziness, syncope, blurred or dimmed vision, diplopia, or any change in his visual field.
Monitor for a decreased level of consciousness, seizures, paresthesis, motor weakness, paralysis, and unequal pupils, (late sign) or an absent pupillary reaction to light.
Monitor vital signs every 2 hours until stable. Report any deviations from the baseline.
Orient patient to reality: call him by name. Tell him your name and why you are with him.
Give background information (time, place, and date) often throughout the day.
Orient him to his environment, including sights and sounds. (Example: "This is a hospital. I am a nurse caring for you. You are hearing the food cart go down the hall.")
Have parents bring in photos and personal articles from home.
Talk to patient while providing care. Encourage the family to discuss past and present events with him.
Arrange to be with him at predetermined times to avoid feelings of isolation.
Turn on the TV and radio for short periods of time, based on his interests to help him orient to reality.
Hold his hand while talking to soothe him.
Monitor his response.
Continually monitor neurologic signs and report changes immediately.

EVALUATION OF EXPECTED OUTCOMES

Does not show signs of altered tissue perfusion related to an interruption in cerebral blood flow
Level of consciousness does not deteriorate
Communicates in a lucid manner
Reestablishes a sleep-wake cycle
Shows an interest in external environment
Demonstrates an increased ability to react to reality
At discharge, oriented to self, person, place, and time
Periods of agitation, anxiety, and confusion diminished or absent

continued

NURSING INTERVENTIONS—cont'd	EVALUATION OF EXPECTED OUTCOMES—cont'd
Always approach in a calm, gentle manner to avoid startling him. Encourage regular sleep patterns and routines. Encourage the family to visit often. Provide reassurances and explanations to aid their understanding of his condition. Suggest that friends send cards rather than visit or call during the acute stage.	

NURSING DIAGNOSIS

Risk for injury related to the question of drug ingestion and cerebral trauma

NURSING INTERVENTIONS	EVALUATION OF EXPECTED OUTCOMES
While orienting patient to the environment, state his boundaries. Assess his ability to use the call bell. Keep the side rails up at all times, with the bed in the low position and the wheels locked. Keep a light on at night to prevent falls. Conduct a close watch on him, especially when agitated. Teach the family about the need for safe illumination, especially if he has distorted images. Monitor his gait when he ambulates. Have two people if he is unsteady. Have a system in place to call for assistance if he is extremely agitated. Assist patient when eating. Monitor for safe use of utensils. Have him do as much self-care as possible (e.g., brushing teeth). Praise him for any attempts. Discuss the need for nonskid slippers or sneakers when ambulating. Assess his visual acuity before ambulation. Discuss safety after returning home with his parents. Inquire into their ability to remain home with him until he feels safe. Discuss the impact of patient's confusion on his younger siblings.	Remains safe and free of injury while in a confused state Identifies factors that could increase potential for injury Cooperates in keeping himself free from harm Parents incorporate safety teachings into discharge plans Cooperates in applying safety measures to prevent injury Family develops strategies to maintain safety upon discharge to home Optimizes ADLs within sensiomotor limitations

NURSING DIAGNOSIS

Impaired verbal communication related to the questionable history of drug ingestion and the cerebral trauma, as evidenced by periods of crying, echolalia, and garbled speech

NURSING INTERVENTIONS	EVALUATION OF EXPECTED OUTCOMES
Speak slowly and distinctly when addressing patient. Stand where he can see and hear you.	Needs are met consistently Patient and family communicate at a satisfactory level

NURSING INTERVENTIONS—cont'd

Reorient him to reality. Use a large calendar and reality orientation boards.
Use short simple phrases and yes and no questions, especially when his frustration level is high.
Be prepared to repeat the words or directions.
Monitor for signs of understanding (nodding his head, frowning).
Encourage his attempts at communication.
Listen carefully for identifiable words. Provide reinforcement when he is lucid.
Allow ample time for a response.
Do not answer questions for him. Teach his family the same.
Do not pretend to understand if you do not. This only adds to his confusion.
Remove distractions from environment during his attempts to communicate (e.g., lower the sound on the TV).
Adjust his care plan as progress develops.

EVALUATION OF EXPECTED OUTCOMES—cont'd

Correctly answers two direct questions
By the time of discharge, echolalia is gone and speech is no longer garbled
Communicates basic needs (e.g., use of the urinal, need for privacy) to staff and his family via gestures and sign language before regaining oral ability

NURSING DIAGNOSIS

Pain: headache related to cerebral trauma as evidenced by crying and wincing with head movement and swelling in the frontal area of his head

NURSING INTERVENTIONS

Determine how patient usually responds to pain.
Assess for nonverbal signs of headache (wrinkled brow, clenched fists, squinting, rubbing head, avoidance of bright lights and noises).
Assess for any verbal attempts at communication of pain.
Assess for factors that seem to aggravate head pain.
Implement measures to relieve the pain (quiet environment, dim lights, avoidance of any sudden movements).
Provide nonpharmacologic measures for headache relief (e.g., cool cloth to forehead, back rub, distraction).
Involve family to assist in soothing pain by gentle touch.
Administer nonnarcotic analgesics if ordered.
Monitor results. Consult physician if above action fails to relieve headache.

EVALUATION OF EXPECTED OUTCOMES

By body language, indicates that aggravating factors have been decreased or eliminated
Cooperates more fully in his neurologic assessments and participates in nursing care activities
Obtains relief from headache as evidenced by verbalization of headache relief, relaxed facial expression, and body posturing
Shows increased participation in activities

KEY CONCEPTS

- The purpose of the neurologic examination is to determine the presence or absence of neurologic dysfunction and to localize the site of a pathologic condition.
- Common diagnostic testing procedures include lumbar puncture and neuroradiologic studies such as cerebral angiography, myelography, computed tomography, magnetic resonance imaging, positron emission tomography, electroencephalography, and electromyography.
- Care of patients with altered states of cerebral functioning is a primary function of the neurologic nurse. Any changes in a patient's neurologic status should be assessed, documented, and reported immediately.
- The Glasgow Coma Scale is a tool available to nurses for accurate reporting of a patient's level of consciousness.
- Deterioration in the level of consciousness, changes in pupillary response to light, motor weakness, headache, seizures, and vomiting may indicate increased intracranial pressure requiring immediate treatment.
- Acute head injury often results in fracture of the skull, hemorrhage into cerebral tissue, and cerebral edema. Emergency management includes maintenance of the airway, breathing, and circulation.
- Cerebral edema results in increased intracranial pressure that must be controlled.
- Injuries to the spinal cord result in loss of motor and sensory function. Early intervention is aimed at reducing the effects of the injury, maintaining alignment of the spine, and providing stabilization to prevent further damage.
- Autonomic hyperreflexia is an emergency condition occurring in patients with cervical or high-thoracic injuries. Acute hypertension and tachycardia followed by bradycardia occur. Nurses should check immediately for stressful conditions such as bladder distention or catheter obstruction. Antihypertensive medications may be necessary.
- Rehabilitation of the patient with spinal cord injury begins immediately. Major goals are bladder and bowel reconditioning, sexual counseling, and psychologic support.
- Intervertebral disk trauma may compress the spinal cord or exert pressure on the nerve root, causing severe back pain. A laminectomy may be performed to remove bone, cartilage, or herniated intervertebral disk material. Correct alignment is crucial during the postoperative period.
- Careful observation and assessment can help localize the site of brain and spinal cord tumors. Careful monitoring of neurologic status is important in the postoperative craniotomy or laminectomy period.
- Transient ischemic attacks (TIAs) are characterized by the sudden onset of a neurologic deficit that lasts less than 24 hours with no residual effects. It is a warning sign of stroke (cardiovascular accident).
- Acute care of the stroke patient includes maintenance of cerebral circulation to prevent ischemia of cerebral tissue. Aphasia, dysphagia, hemianopia, bladder and bowel incontinence, and perceptual problems present challenges for care and rehabilitation.
- Aneurysms of the cerebral arteries are treated surgically. Nursing interventions are directed toward monitoring neurologic status, preventing injury from seizures or ischemia, and providing support to the patient and family.
- Nursing responsibilities while the patient is experiencing a seizure are to protect from injury and accurately observe and record behavior before, during, and after the event.
- Prompt administration of appropriate antibacterial therapy, supportive measures, and rehabilitation are interventions for infections of the nervous system.
- Degenerative diseases involving the central nervous system develop over a period of years and result in some degree of chronic disability. Nursing care is supportive and is based on actual or potential problems.

CRITICAL THINKING EXERCISES

1 What are important nursing considerations in caring for a patient during a seizure? What behaviors should you observe and record during the seizure?
2 Discuss some ways that the patient with multiple sclerosis might conserve energy and avoid becoming overly fatigued.
3 What is the difference between a cholinergic and a myasthenic crisis? Discuss some important nursing considerations to prevent these situations from occurring.
4 What are the important factors in the care of a patient in Halo traction? Why?

REFERENCES AND ADDITIONAL READINGS

Ackerman LL: Alteration in level of responsiveness: a proposed nursing diagnosis, *Nurs Clin North Am* 28(4): 729-45, 1993.

Ake JM, Perlstein LM: AIDS: Impact on neuroscience nursing practice, *J Neurosci Nurs* 19(6):300-304, 1987.

Alter M, Henry GL, Kramer DA: Altered mental status, *Patient Care* 25(13):64-68, 70, 73, 1991.

Barker E: *Neuroscience nursing*, St Louis, 1994, Mosby.

Beck C, Heacock P: Nursing interventions for patients with Alzheimer's disease, *Nurs Clin North Am* 23:95-124, 1988.

Booth B: The knowledge nurses need to educate patients about stroke, *Nurs Times* 90(15):32-34, 1994.

Boyer CL: Three cancer complications that can't wait, *Nurs* 23(10):34-42, 1993.

Burns EM, Buckwalter KC: Pathophysiology and etiology of Alzheimer's disease, *Nurs Clin North Am* 23:11-29, 1988.

Chase JA: Spinal stenosis: when arthritis is more than arthritis! *Nurs Clin North Am* 26(1):53-64, 1991.

Cochran JW, Kessler ES, Wittenborn, R Jr: Neurologic disease: 5 scenarios to manage, *Patient Care* 28(10):32-36, 38, 41, 1994.

DeYoung S, Grass RB: Coma recovery program, *Rehab Nurs* 12:121-124, 1987.

Dodson WE, Leppik IE, Pedley TA: Are you up-to-date on seizures? *Patient Care* 25(11):162-166, 168, 173-174, 1991.

Eisenhart K: New perspectives in the management of adults with severe head injury, *Crit Care Nurs Q* 17(2):1-12, 1994.

Faye EE, Materson RS, Zazove P: Help people with disabilities to help themselves, *Patient Care* 28(2):65-68, 71-72, 74-76, 1994.

Feingold, DJ, Peck, SA, Reinsma, EJ, and Ruda, SC: Complications of lumbar spine surgery, *Orthop Nurs* 10(4) 39-58, 1991.

Griswold K, Guanci MM, Ropper AH: An approach to the care of patients with Guillain-Barre syndrome, *Heart Lung* 13(1):66-72, 1984.

Hainsworth M: Living with multiple sclerosis: the experience of chronic sorrow, *J Neurosci Nurs* 26(4):237-240, 1994.

Hall M, Yetman L, Brandys C: Multidisciplinary approaches to management of acute head injury, *J Neurosci Nurs* 24(4): 199-204, 1992.

Hartshorn J, Byers V: Impact of epilepsy on quality of life, *J Neurosci Nurs* 24(1):24-29, 1992.

Hickey JV: *The clinical practice of neurological and neurosurgical nursing*, ed 3, Philadelphia, 1992, JB Lippincott.

Kurz JM: Predicting alcohol-withdrawal seizures, *Am J Nurs* 94(11):56, 1994.

Langford R: Keeping control...incontinence—the bane of many MS sufferers' lives—is treatable, *Nurs Times* 90(27): 58, 60, 1994.

Lugger KE: Dysphagia in the elderly stroke patient, *J Neuro Nurs* 26(2):78-84, 1994.

MacDonald E: Aneurysmal subarachnoid hemorrhage, *J Neurosci Nurs* 21(5):313-321, 1989.

Malasanos L, Barkauskas V, Stoltenberg-Allen K: *Health assessment*, ed 4, St Louis, 1990, Mosby.

Marshall SB and others: *Neuroscience critical care: pathophysiology and patient management*, Philadelphia, 1990, WB Saunders.

Meissner JE: Caring for patients with multiple sclerosis, *Nurs* 24(8):60-61, 1994.

Nayduch D, Lee A, Butler D: High-dose methylprednisolone after acute spinal cord injury, *Crit Care Nurs* 14(4):69-72, 77-78, 1994.

Newton C, Mateo MA: Uncertainty: strategies for patients with brain tumor and their family, *Canc Nurs* 17(2):137-140, 1994.

Ottewell C: From the patient's point of view ... a survivor of a major traumatic closed head injury, *J Cog Rehabil* 12(3):8-10, 1994.

Peterson R: A nursing intervention for early detection of spinal cord compressions in patients with cancer, *Canc Nurs* 16(2):113-116, 1993.

Ross A, Pitts L, Kobayashi S: Prognosticators of outcome after major head injury in the elderly, *J Neurosci Nurs* 24(2): 88-93, 1992.

Simmons B: What do you think? What are some strategies for managing the "difficult patient" on a spinal cord injury unit?, *Sci Nurs* 11(2):62-3, 1994.

Smith DC: The terminally ill patient's right to be in denial, *Omega* 27(2):115-21, 1993.

Whitney, F: Drug therapy for acute stroke, *J Neurosci Nurs* 26(2):111-117, 1994.

CHAPTER 29

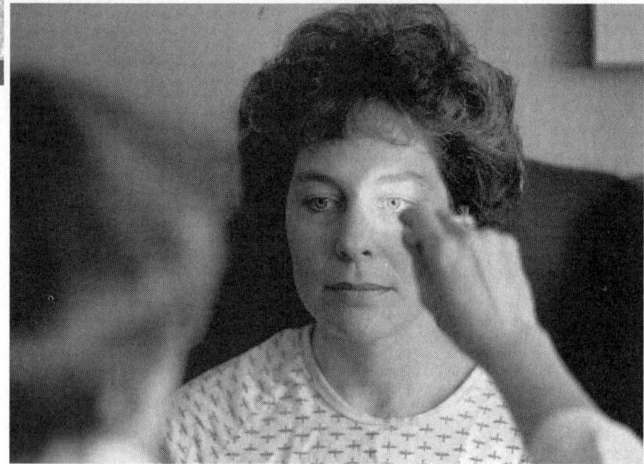

Vision

CHAPTER OBJECTIVES

1. Correlate each anatomic part of the eye and its associated structures with its function in achieving sight.
2. Identify the purpose and procedure for common diagnostic tests involving the eye.
3. Describe the normal versus the abnormal refraction of the eye.
4. Explain the importance of screening for amblyopia in children.
5. Explain why and how to detect and remove contact lenses from an injured or unconscious patient.
6. Discuss the methods of interacting with visually impaired people.
7. Describe the method of punctal occlusion in the administration of ophthalmic medications.
8. Differentiate the signs and symptoms of conjunctivitis and acute glaucoma.
9. Discuss the relationship between injury to the cornea and corneal ulcers.
10. Describe the medical and surgical treatment for glaucoma.
11. Identify the symptoms of cataracts and describe the nursing considerations that follow cataract surgery.
12. Identify the signs and symptoms of retinal detachment.
13. List the conditions that are considered true ocular emergencies.
14. Describe potential hazards in the environment that may result in eye injuries and list ways to prevent them.
15. Identify normal eye changes in the aging process.

KEY WORDS

amblyopia
astigmatism
cataract
conjunctivitis
diplopia
emmetropia
epiphora
glaucoma
hyperopia
keratoplasty
myopia
ophthalmologist
optometrist
opticians
phacoemulsification
photophobia
pseudophakia
refraction
tonometry
trabeculoplasty
vitrectomy

STRUCTURE AND FUNCTION OF THE EYE

The eye is a highly specialized sense organ, a large portion of which lies protected within a bony cavity, with only the anterior portion exposed (Figure 29-1). The eye has three coats. The external, or fibrous, coat comprises the white, opaque *sclera,* covering four fifths of the eye, and the *cornea,* a transparent, avascular, curved layer covering the anterior one fifth of the eye. The cornea bends light rays entering the eye and focuses the resulting images slightly behind the retina. The sclera, the protective outer layer of the eye, has an opening at the back of the globe, through which the optic nerve and blood vessels pass. The anterior surface of the sclera and the posterior surface of the eyelids are covered by the *conjunctiva,* a transparent mucous membrane that aids in tear-film dispersion.

The middle, or vascular, coat is also known as the *uveal tract* and consists of the choroid, iris, and ciliary body. The *choroid* lies between the sclera and retina and is firmly attached on its inner surface to the retina. The blood supply of the choroid nourishes the retina, and the choroid's dark pigmentation prevents internal reflection of light. The *iris* is the colored part of the eye that can be seen through the cornea. It is composed of muscle fibers that regulate the amount of light entering the eye by changing the size of the *pupil,* the circular opening in its center. Behind the iris lies the crystalline

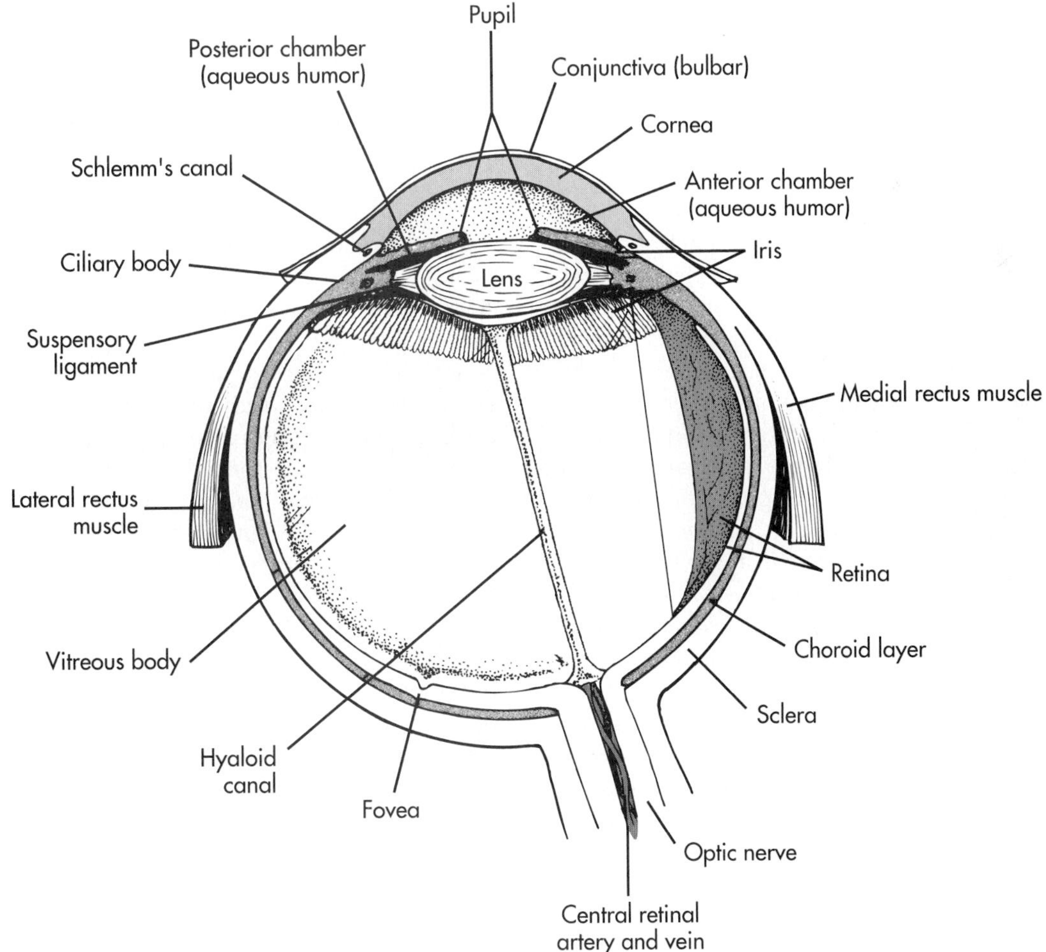

Figure 29-1 Cross section of the eye. (From Phipps WJ and others: *Medical-surgical nursing: concepts and clinical practice,* ed 5, St Louis, 1995, Mosby.)

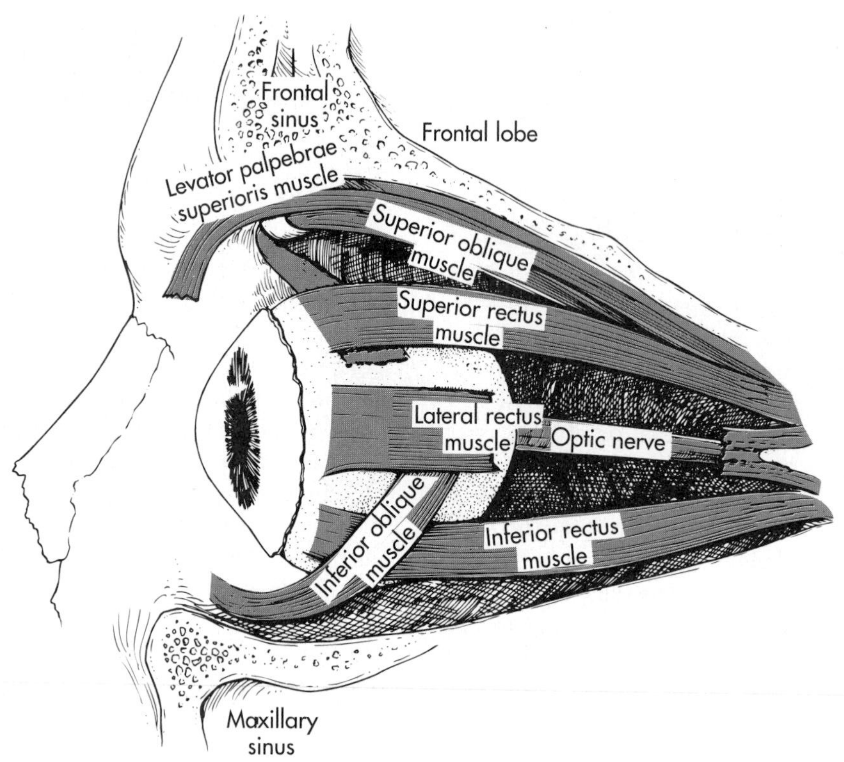

Figure 29-2 Extraocular muscles of the eye. Both oblique muscles insert behind the equator of the globe. The inferior oblique muscle passes inferior to the body of the inferior rectus muscle but beneath the lateral rectus muscle. (From Newell FW: *Ophthalmology: principles and concepts,* ed 7, St Louis, 1992, Mosby.)

lens, a biconvex, transparent structure enclosed in a capsule of transparent elastic membrane that changes shape to focus light rays precisely on the retina. The shape of the lens is controlled by the ciliary muscle contained in the external aspect of the *ciliary body.* The internal surfaces of the ciliary body secrete *aqueous humor,* the watery fluid that fills the anterior and posterior chambers of the eye—the spaces in front of and behind the iris. The fluid passes from the posterior chamber, through the pupil, to the anterior chamber, and then is drained off through spaces at the angle formed by the iris and cornea, through the *trabecular meshwork,* and into a complex circular venous channel called *Schlemm's canal.* The ciliary body connects the choroid with the periphery of the iris.

The third and inner coat is the *retina,* a delicate membrane in which the fibers of the optic nerve are spread out in a complicated network of nerve cells, rods, and cones lined with pigment epithelium. The rods are responsible for peripheral and night vision, whereas the cones are for central vision and color vision. The posterior portion of the retina is called the *optic fundus.* Near its center lies a circular, depressed, white to pink area where the optic nerve enters the eyeball, this is the *optic disc.* It contains no photoreceptor cells; thus it is insensitive to light and is known as the blind spot. Just lateral to the optic disc is a small, oval, yellowish area called the *macula lutea* or macula. At the center of the macula is a depression known as the *fovea centralis,* the area of most acute vision. Blood is supplied to the retina by its central artery, which enters the eyeball with the optic nerve. Drainage is accomplished through a corresponding system of retinal veins that join to form the central vein of the retina, which exits along the path of the optic nerve. The space between the lens and the retina is the *vitreous chamber,* which composes four fifths of the volume of the eye. It contains a colorless, transparent gel called the *vitreous gel,* or *vitreous humor.*

Vitreous humor maintains the shape of the eye and provides structural support for the retina. If the vitreous were to be lost and not replaced, such as by a penetrating injury, the eye would collapse.

The eye rests on a cushion of fat within its bony orbit. Six voluntary *(extrinsic)* muscles attached to the outside of the sclera control the movements of the eyes. The action of these extraocular muscles is coordinated to allow binocular vision, the concerted use of both eyes working together. Branches of several cranial nerves control these muscles. Involuntary *(intrinsic)* muscles within the eye control the shape of the lens and the size of the pupil (Figure 29-2).

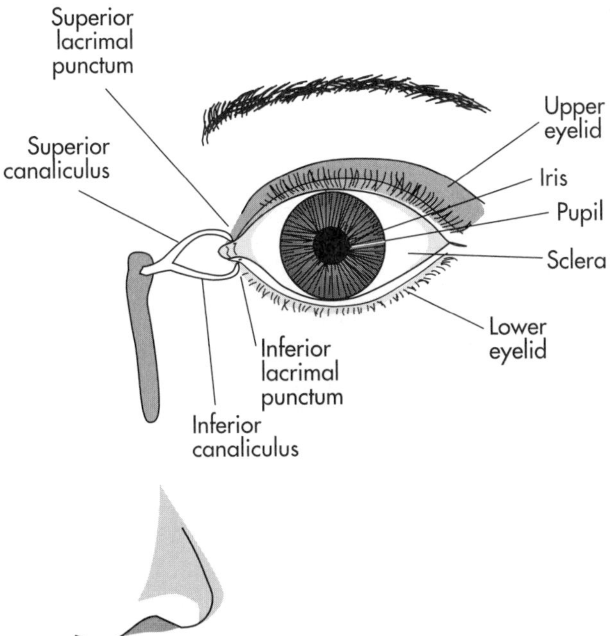

Figure 29-3 External landmarks.

The accessory organs of the eye include the eyebrows, eyelids and their muscles, eyelashes, bulbar and palpebral conjunctiva, lacrimal glands and tear ducts, and sebaceous glands.

The eyebrows and eyelids protect the eyeball and help spread the tear film over the eye. Muscles within the lid help close the lid. The lacrimal glands secrete tears, which flow across the eye into the lacrimal sac. The fluid passes openings in the nasal aspect of the upper and lower lids, called puncta. From this point, tears flow through the nasolacrimal duct into the back of the nose (Figure 29-3) (Smith, Nachazel, 1980).

Vision is the result of light rays passing through the eye and focusing on the retina. The cornea is responsible for two thirds of this bending, or **refraction,** of light. The lens is responsible for the other third. When an image is produced on the retina, visual receptors are stimulated and cause a nerve impulse to be transmitted via the optic nerve to the visual center in the brain, the occipital lobes. (Vaughan, Asbury, Riordan-Eva, 1992).

NURSING ASSESSMENT OF THE PATIENT WITH EYE PROBLEMS

The assessment for conditions and diseases of the eye begins with a thorough nursing history that includes general medical health, family history, and allergies. Previous surgery, current medications, visual aids or glasses/contact lenses, and visual symptoms should be noted. The chief complaint, such as change in vision, floaters, or discharge, as well as the duration of the problem are documented. Clinical observations of the eye include (1) general condition of the lids and lashes; (2) eye movement; (3) color of the sclera; (4) tear function; (5) pupil size, color, and shape; (6) position of the eye within the orbit; (7) systemic complaints of nausea and vomiting; and (8) level of cognizance (Boyd-Monk, Steinmetz, 1987; Hunt, 1992).

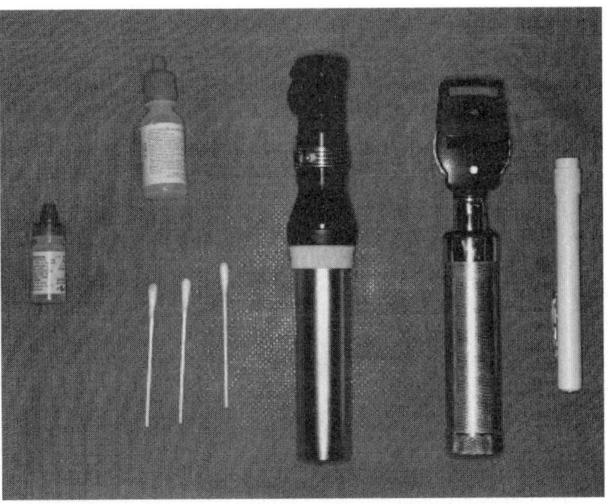

Figure 29-4 Examination instruments and supplies.

Physical Examination

A complete physical examination is important in the treatment of many diseases of the eye (Figure 29-4). Often systemic diseases can be diagnosed by their ocular manifestations. When the underlying cause is diabetes, hypertension, rheumatoid arthritis, thyroid dysfunction, or leukemia, treatment of the underlying condition must accompany any treatment of the eye. The ophthalmologist may consult an internist or may order x-ray examinations, blood studies, or neurologic examinations to aid in diagnosis and subsequent treatment of systemic disease (Boyd-Monk, Steinmetz, 1987).

Eye Examination

Several eye tests are used to evaluate visual acuity or to detect eye diseases and disorders. A variety of professionals provide these comprehensive services. Included are ophthalmologists, optometrists, opticians, nurses, orthoptists, technicians, and photographers. **Ophthalmologists** are medical doctors who have completed 4 years of residency and, in some instances, one to 3 years of additional training in a subspecialty. They diagnose and treat patients with eye disease and vision problems by performing surgery or by prescribing medications, glasses, or contact lenses (American Academy of Ophthalmology, 1992; Vaughan, Asbury,

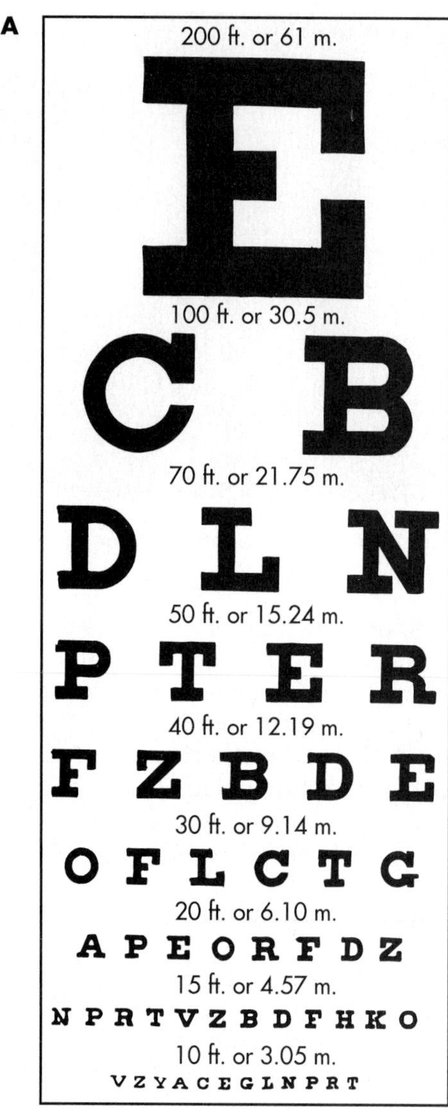

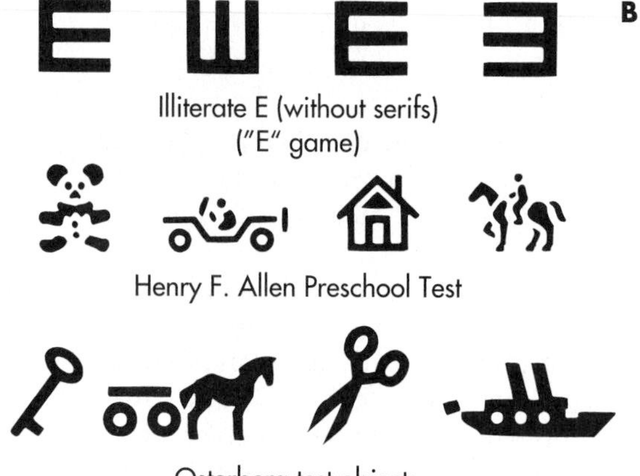

Figure 29-5 **A,** Snellen chart used in testing vision. **B,** Symbols used in testing distance vision in children and illiterate adults. (Modified from Newell FW: *Ophthalmology: principles and concepts,* ed 7, St Louis, 1992, Mosby.)

Riordan-Eva, 1992). **Optometrists** have a degree in optometry after attending optometry school for 4 years after obtaining a baccalaureate degree. They examine eyes, prescribe glasses and contact lenses, check intraocular pressure, and prescribe exercises for various eye-muscle problems. They provide low-vision examinations, visual devices, and adaptive training for patients with limited vision (American Academy of Ophthalmology, 1992; Vaughan, Asbury, Riordan-Eva, 1992). **Opticians** are technicians who make and fit eyeglasses, contact lenses, and vision aids as prescribed. Some states require formal licensing to practice as an optician.

The eye examination begins with an evaluation of the general health and appearance of the external structures of the eye. Obvious defects of the orbit, eyelids, eyelashes, and lacrimal system should be noted (Hunt, 1992). Visual assessment follows the general examination.

Visual acuity

Visual acuity is the measurement of the smallest object a person can identify at a given distance from the eye. The most common method for determining acuity of distance vision is testing with a *Snellen's eye chart,* a method used in schools, industry, physicians' offices, and screenings (Figure 29-5). The chart consists of rows of letters arranged in various sizes that a person views from a measured distance to the chart—usually 20 feet. By use of a mirror projection system, the actual distance can be less. If individuals are able to read the letters marked 20 at a distance of 20 feet, they have 20/20 vision which is "normal vision."

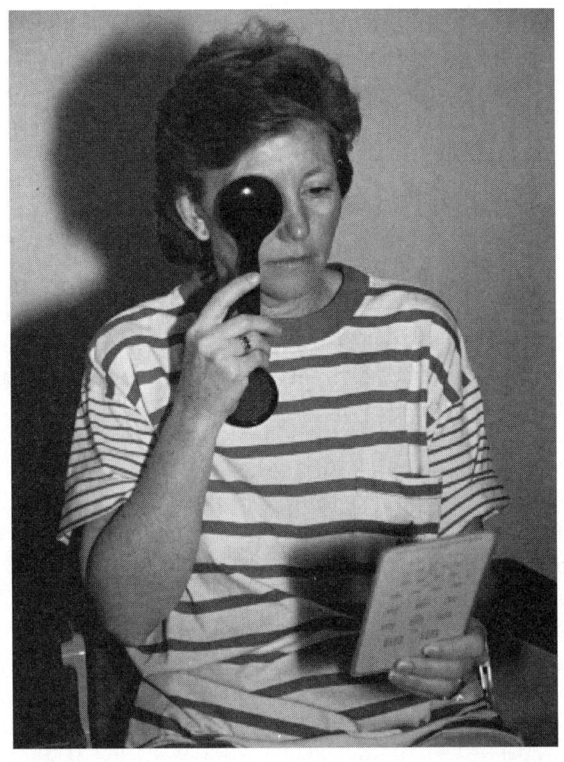

Figure 29-6 Assessing near vision with Jaeger chart.

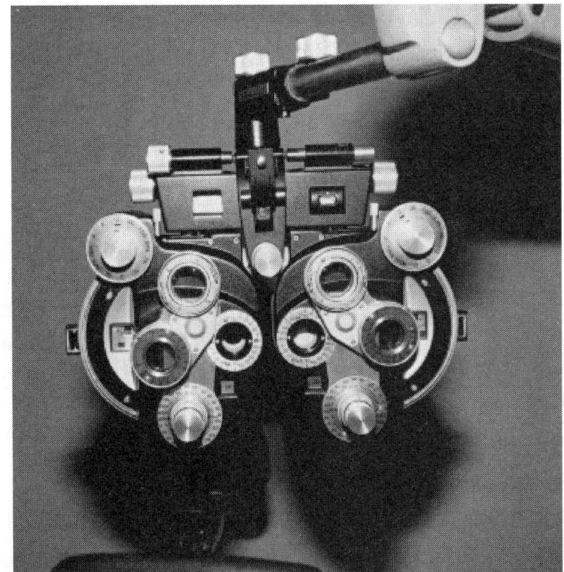

Figure 29-7 Phoropter stores lenses used in determining the refraction error of the eye.

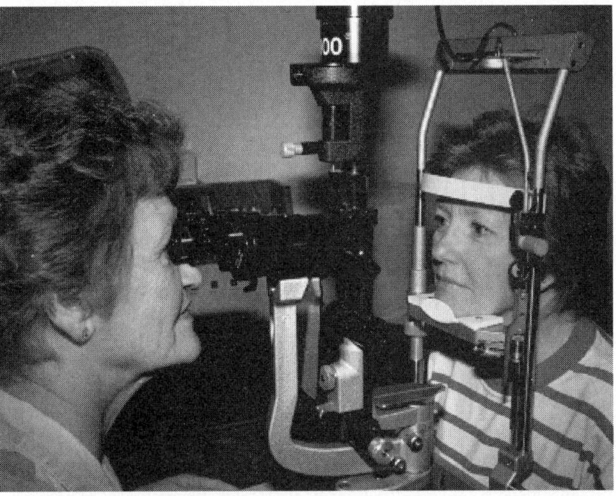

Figure 29-8 Examination of the eye with slit lamp.

However, if only rows marked at 30, 40, or 200 are read correctly the person is said to have 20/30, 20/40, or 20/200 vision. If lenses are used to correct the vision to 20/20, the person has no vision loss. If visual acuity can be corrected to no better than 20/50, the person has a vision deficit. It is not unusual for each eye to have a slightly different acuity. If a person normally wears glasses or contact lenses, the test is performed both with and without the corrective lenses.

In younger children, illiterate adults, or those with language problems, a chart with the letter E can be used. With this E chart, the person points in the direction faced by the open side of the E, which may be rotated to be open at the top, bottom, right, or left. Various other object charts have been designed for use with children. Near-distance visual acuity is tested with *Jaeger's eye chart* (Vaughan, Asbury, Riordan-Eva, 1992). The procedure is similar to that of Snellen's chart but uses smaller graduated letter sizes on a handheld card. The distance is measured at 14 inches (Figure 29-6).

Refractometry

The *phoropter* is a machine that houses various combinations of prescriptive lenses in an apparatus. The patient looks through the phoropter so that the amount of refraction (bending of light) needed to focus images on the retina to achieve normal or 20/20 vision can be determined (Figure 29-7). The patient's response to changes in lens power is used subjectively to determine the best achievable vision.

Retinoscopy

The instrument for objectively measuring the refraction of the eye is a retinoscope. A streak of light is passed across the eye, and the reflex of the pupil is noted. Because it is an objective measurement, it is most useful for small children and for adults with disease conditions of the eye (Vaughan, Asbury, Riordan-Eva, 1992).

Slit-lamp examination

The slit lamp is a lighted binocular microscope (Figure 29-8). The light beam can be projected onto the eye in various widths and intensities. It is used to assess all the structures within the eye, as well as the lids, lashes, and conjunctiva. The light beam provides a three-dimensional view of the eye and helps determine abnormalities in any of the structures, including the aqueous fluid, lens, and vitreous. With additional lenses, cameras, or laser attachments, other examinations and treatments are possible. Dilating drops are used when pupil dilation is needed in the examination. Fluorescein stain is used to diagnose corneal abrasions and ulcers (Vaughan, Asbury, Riordan-Eva, 1992).

Tonometry

Tonometry is the measurement of intraocular pressure (IOP), which normally ranges between 12 and 21 mm Hg (Berson, 1987). This pressure is the result of the balance between aqueous production and absorption from the eye. In glaucoma, there is an imbalance resulting from a defect in one or the other of these mechanisms. Tonometry can be a contact or noncontact method. Contact method includes the *Schiötz tonometer* or *applanation tonometer* (Figure 29-9). Although the Schiötz method is an older technique, it is still used as a portable, handheld method in the operating room and sometimes at the bedside. Because the applanation tonometer provides the most accurate measurement of IOP, it is used most often. Anesthetic drops (0.5% proparacaine) and fluorescein dye are placed in the eye, and the tonometer, which can be an attachment to the slit lamp, is placed on the cornea for the numerical reading. The Tono-pen is a handheld, battery-powered applanation tonometer. It is more expensive than the Schiotz and needs daily calibration. The *noncontact tonometer,* or "air-puff" method, is less precise but does not require anesthetic drops. Pressure from air on the cornea is calibrated by the machine. It can be used by a variety of trained ophthalmic personnel (Vaughan, Asbury, Riordan-Eva, 1992).

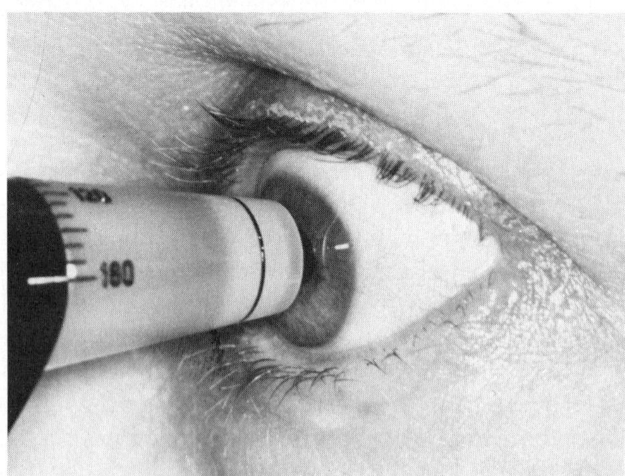

Figure 29-9 Applanation tonometer provides a more precise measurement of intraocular pressure. (From Saunders WH and others: *Nursing care in eye, ear, nose, and throat disorders,* ed 4, St Louis, 1979, Mosby.)

Fundus photography

Special cameras are used to provide documentation of the retina and fundus of the eye. This is particularly important in following the progression of optic nerve damage associated with **glaucoma.**

Perimetry

This test is used to assess central and peripheral visual fields. It is used to measure the progression of glaucoma, to help determine the location of a brain lesion, or to establish a loss of vision as a result of a cerebral vascular accident. Three methods are used: *tangent screen, Goldmann perimetry,* and *computerized automated perimetry.* The tangent screen is the fastest and simplest method for determining the loss of central field vision (central 30 degrees). An examiner uses a test object brought in from the periphery, and the patient signals when the object is seen. The Goldmann perimeter, a more accurate test, evaluates all of the peripheral vision (Figure 29-10). The patient faces a hol-

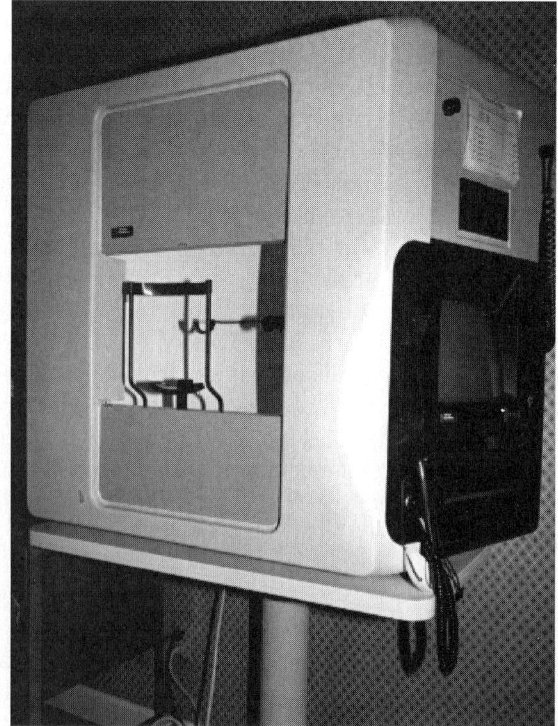

Figure 29-10 Perimeter used to evaluate the visual fields of patients with glaucoma and tumors.

low, white, spherical bowl. Lights of variable size and intensity are presented by the examiner, and the patient indicates when they are seen. The computerized automated perimeter uses the same method as Goldmann perimetry but with a computer program, which eliminates examiner bias. This sophisticated equipment is the most sensitive of all the perimetry methods and has the advantage of comparing recent results with previous testing of the patient (Vaughan, Asbury, Riordan-Eva, 1992).

Ophthalmoscopy

The ophthalmoscope is used to visually examine the vascular and nerve tissue in the fundus of the eye, including the retina, retinal vessels, optic disc, and macula (Figure 29-11). With the handheld or *direct ophthalmoscope,* no dilating drops may be necessary if room lighting can be reduced enough for pupillary dilation. Mydriatic drops may be instilled if pupil dilation is necessary for appropriate visualization. The direct ophthalmoscope provides a highly magnified view (×15) of the entire fundus. It also is used to check the red reflex of the eye, and if a slit lamp is unavailable it can be used to view the conjunctiva, cornea, and iris. The *indirect ophthalmoscope* provides a less magnified, wider view of the fundus. The examiner uses a hand-held lens and head-mounted ophthalmoscope. Because the examiner uses both eyes for the test, a three-dimensional view can be accomplished, which is helpful in diagnosing elevations or tumors in the back of the eye. The indirect ophthalmoscope is used preoperatively or intraoperatively for retinal-detachment repair. The intensity of the light source often is not well tolerated by the patient.

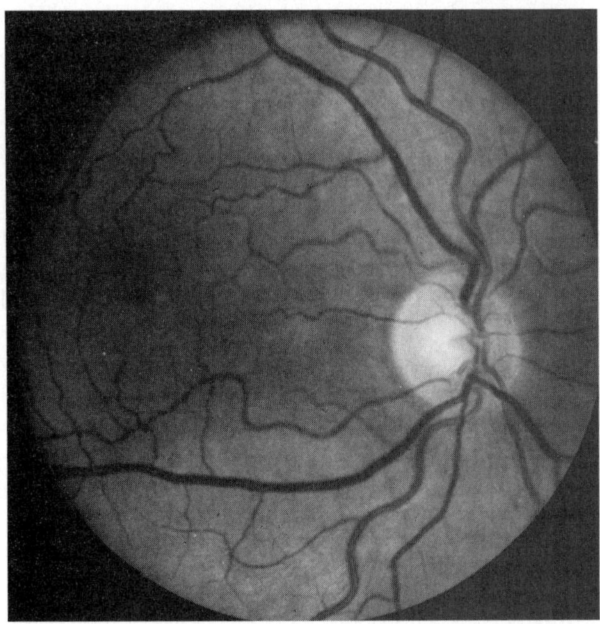

Figure 29-11 Normal fundus photograph. Optic nerve and retinal blood vessels as seen with ophthalmoscope. (From Saunders WH and others: *Nursing care in eye, ear, nose, and throat disorders,* ed 4, St Louis, 1979, Mosby.)

Keratoscopy

To determine the surface condition of the cornea, a keratoscope is used. Concentric circles are projected onto the cornea, and if the distance between the circles is uniform, the cornea is considered normal. Distortion of the circles indicates corneal abnormalities. Keratoscopy is used for penetrating keratoplasties and refractive surgeries.

Pachymetry

The central thickness of the cornea is measured by pachymetry. Patients with corneal edema are monitored to evaluate changes in corneal thickness that can be caused by endothelial cell loss.

Keratometry

The keratometer measures the curve of the cornea in two 90 degree meridians to determine the spherical shape of the cornea. An uneven corneal curvature is called **astigmatism.** Contact lens fitting and intraocular lens power calculations require keratometer measurements (Boyd-Monk, Steinmetz, 1987).

Specular microscopy

Corneal endothelial cell counts are determined by specular microscopy. Corneal decompensation can occur when there is a low cell count. Patients with corneal decompensation are at a higher risk for corneal edema after intraocular surgery or inflammation (Cataract Management Guideline Panel, 1993).

Glare testing

Glare testing is done to determine the disturbance in vision that light can cause when striking opacities in the ocular media. Patients with complaints of glare in daylight or while gazing at oncoming traffic may have normal vision in a darkened room. Glare symptoms are found in patients with cataracts and corneal abnormalities (Cataract Management Guideline Panel, 1993; Vaughan, Asbury, Riordan-Eva, 1992).

Contrast sensitivity testing

Contrast sensitivity testing determines the ability of the patient to detect subtle shading differences between lines and their background. The ability to determine contrast differences can be affected before visual acuity changes can be determined by Snellen's chart. Cataracts, retinal lesions, and optic nerve disease can be the causes. The government's Cataract Management Guideline Panel (1993) has suggested that research be done in older adults to determine the usefulness of this technique for diagnosing functional impairment in a cataract patient.

Fluorescein angiography

The technique for visually examining retinal circulation is fluorescein angiography. Fluorescein dye is injected through a vein in the arm. Fundus photos are then taken in rapid sequence to document the flow of blood through the vessels of the retina. These black-and-white photos are essential for diagnosis and treatment of retinal conditions, especially diabetic retinopathy. Patient preparation for the test includes an assessment for allergies to the dye. Fluids or a light meal are allowed. The pupils are dilated with mydriatic drops. Normally, blood vessels of the retina fill with dye in 12 to 15 seconds after injection. However, delayed photographs may be taken 20 minutes after the initial dye injection to diagnose leakage from the vessels. A small percentage of patients may be nauseated and vomit. For 24 hours the urine will be yellow-orange. An increase in oral fluids will hasten excretion of the dye. Dark glasses will lessen sensitivity to light caused by pupil dilation (Boyd-Monk, Steinmetz, 1987; Smith, Folk, Losch, 1992).

Ocular ultrasonography

Ocular ultrasonography involves transmitting high frequency sound waves through the eye and the measurement of their reflection from ocular structures. A-scan is used to measure the axial length (cornea-to-retina measurement) of the eye—a measurement needed for calculating the intraocular lens power for cataract surgery. It is also used to determine tumor growth. B-scan provides a view of ocular structures when opacities in the cornea, lens, or vitreous make a view of the fundus difficult. Lesions within the eye and retinal detachments can be diagnosed with this technique.

Amsler's grid test

The Amsler grid is composed of horizontal and vertical lines that form 5-mm squares. It is used to detect scotomas, or blind spots, in the central 20 degrees of visual field and to evaluate the presence, stability, or progression of macular degeneration (Figure 29-12). Covering one eye and wearing any corrective lenses usually worn, the patient is instructed to stare at a dot centrally located on the grid. The patient should be able to see the dot, and the lines on the grid should appear straight. All four sides of the grid should be visible. The patient is asked to describe and outline any area where the grid is distorted or absent. A pathologic condition of the macula is suggested if the patient describes a gray area or an area where lines are missing or distorted *(metamorphopsia).* This test is for initial screening only and must be followed by ophthalmoscopy, visual field testing, and fluorescein angiography to further evaluate the presence of disease.

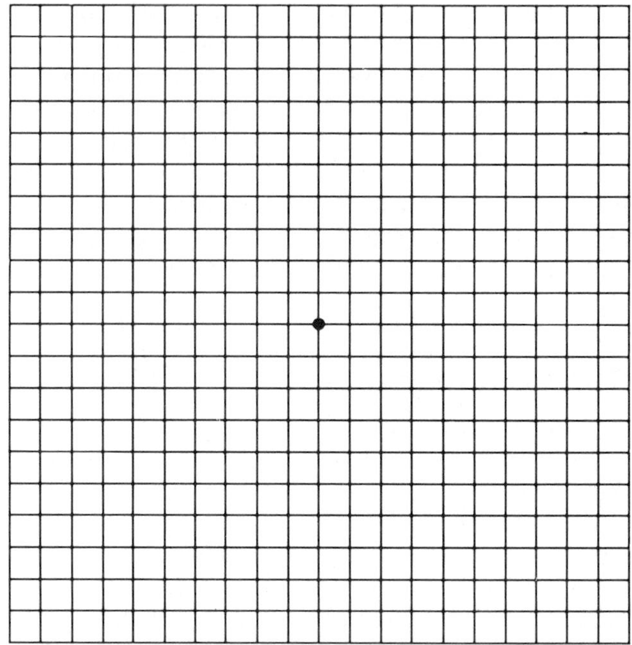

Figure 29-12 The Amsler grid. (From Phipps WJ and others: *Medical-surgical nursing: concepts and clinical practice,* ed 5, St Louis, 1995, Mosby.)

Schirmer's tearing test

The function of the major lacrimal glands responsible for tearing can be tested by inserting a strip of filter paper into the lower conjunctival sac. The amount of moisture absorbed by the paper is timed, measured, and compared to the normal level. The accessory lacrimal glands of Krause and Wolfring, responsible for maintenance of adequate corneal moisture, can be tested by instilling a topical anesthetic before inserting the paper. The anesthetic inhibits the reflex tearing by the major lacrimal glands that is caused by the filter paper so that only the basic tear film produced by the accessory glands is measured.

Exophthalmometry

Exophthalmometry uses an instrument called an exophthalmometer to measure the forward protrusion of the eye and to evaluate an increase or decrease in the

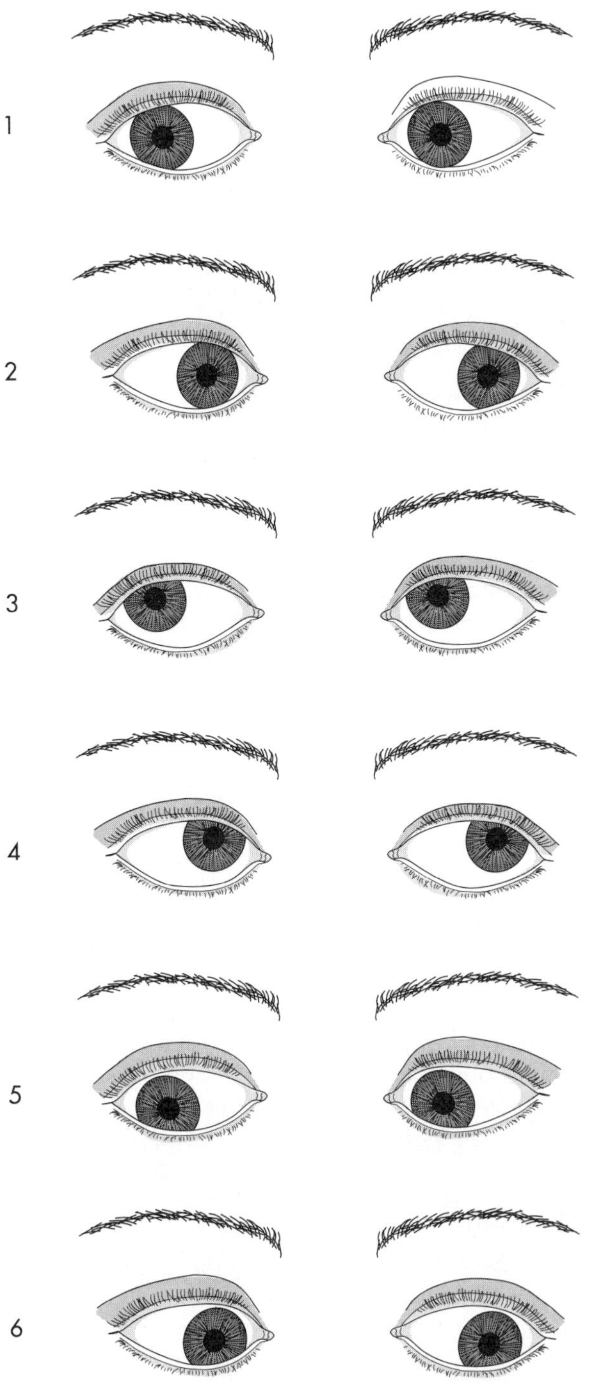

Figure 29-13 Six cardinal positions of gaze and eye positions contracting to produce that eye rotation.

condition known as exopthalmos, the abnormal forward protrusion of the eye. This condition is seen in thyroid diseases and other conditions that displace the eye in the orbit.

Tensilon test

To evaluate ptosis (drooping) of the eyelids that is caused by myasthenia gravis, an edrophonium

TABLE 29-1

Six Cardinal Positions of Gaze

Direction of Gaze	Muscles Involved
Right	Right lateral rectus-left medial rectus
Left	Left lateral rectus-right medial rectus
Up and right	Right superior rectus-left inferior oblique
Up and left	Left superior rectus-right inferior oblique
Down and right	Right inferior rectus-left superior oblique
Down and left	Left inferior rectus-right superior oblique

(Tensilon) test is done. A positive response (eliminating the lid droop) after injection of the edrophonium confirms the diagnosis of myasthenia gravis (Boyd-Monk, Steinmetz, 1987).

Cardinal fields of gaze

To evaluate the extraocular muscles of the eye for possible abnormalities, the patient is asked to look in each of six directions known as the cardinal fields, or positions, of gaze (Figure 29-13; Table 29-1).

Cover/uncover test

The cover/uncover test for evaluating strabismus requires a cooperative patient able to fixate on an object. When the "fixing" eye is covered, the fellow eye is checked for movement, either inward or outward. A deviation is present if the uncovered eye moves. Each eye is checked individually.

THE PATIENT WITH VISION PROBLEMS

Refractive Errors of the Eye

Normal vision

Light rays enter the eye through the cornea, which is responsible for two thirds of the refractive or light-bending power of the eye. Light passes through the anterior chamber; the pupil; the lens, which is responsible for the remaining one third of the eye's refractive power; and the vitreous cavity. The light rays must focus directly on the retina for normal vision, also known as 20/20 or **emmetropia** (Figure 29-14). If this does not happen, the defect is known as a *refractive er-*

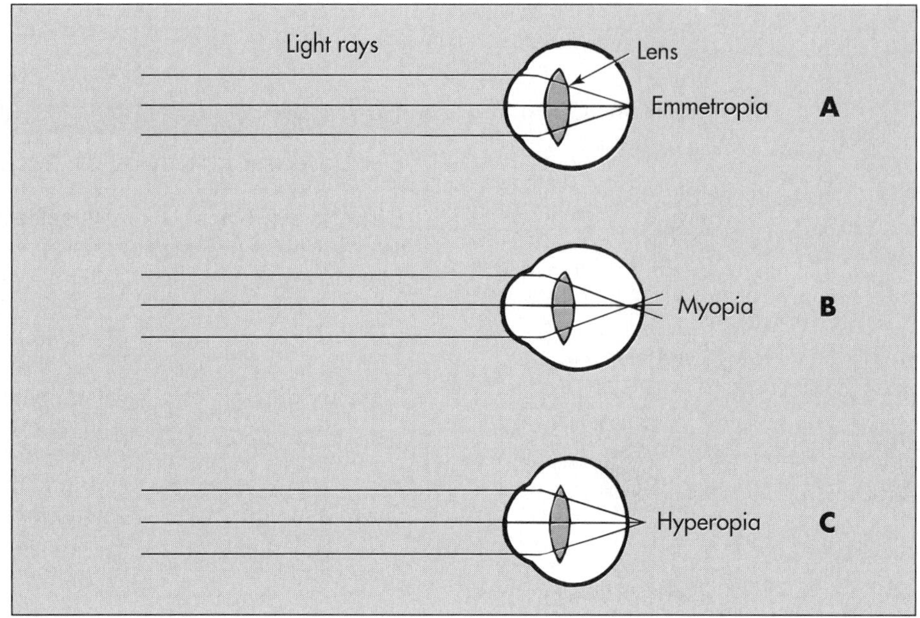

Figure 29-14 Refractive conditions of eye. **A,** Light rays entering eye are brought to focus directly on retina, resulting in normal vision emmetropia. **B,** Light rays focus in front of retina, resulting in nearsightedness myopia. **C,** Light rays focus at back of retina, resulting in farsightedness hyperopia.

ror. The patient may complain of eyestrain, headache, and blurring of distance or near vision. To correct a refractive error, a person should have a thorough eye examination and be fitted with appropriate lenses. This examination, called a **refraction,** can be done by an ophthalmologist or optometrist.

Myopia (nearsightedness)

Persons with **myopia** usually have a longer eyeball than normal. Incoming light from distant objects focuses in front of the retina. Near vision is fine, but distance vision is poor. A concave lens corrects the focus. Myopia may continue to progress in young persons, and frequent increases in lens strength may be required until the condition stabilizes. A technique called radial keratotomy has been developed to correct this defect (see p. 987).

Hyperopia (farsightedness)

Hyperopia is less common than myopia. The eyeball is often shorter than normal, which causes the light rays to focus on a spot behind the retina. Distance vision is clear, but near objects are blurred. A convex lens corrects the focus. A Snellen's chart examination may not show this condition, so a Jaeger's chart should be used for testing a near-vision defect.

Presbyopia

The ability to focus on near objects (accommodation) diminishes with age. This inability, called presbyopia, is caused by a loss of elasticity of the lens and ciliary body muscles. Consequently, most people over age 40 require magnifying glasses or bifocals for reading and closeup work. Bifocal glass styles are designed to individualize patient needs. The flat-top design is used for closeup work. For tasks that require not only close work but also a wide field of vision, "Franklin bifocals," which extend the magnifying portion of the lens all the way across the bottom of the lens, are better suited. Progressive lenses provide a gradual lens-power change from top to bottom, with no visible line. They give a distance, mid-range, and close vision range. However, they are harder to adjust to for some people and are more costly.

Astigmatism

Astigmatism is an irregularity or defect on the corneal surface or lens of the eyeball that blurs vision. Slight defects occur in most people, but they are not significant enough to cause any vision problem. However, when the irregularity is pronounced, light rays do not bend equally, and the patient experiences eyestrain and blurred vision. These patients tend to see better if glasses are worn at all times.

Strabismus

Strabismus is a misalignment of one or both eyes. Children are the age group primarily affected, but adults may also have the condition. The deviation or turning can be inward (esotropia), outward (exotropia), upward (hypertropia), downward (hypotropia), or in a rotary direction. If the deviation is present under binocular viewing conditions (using both eyes at once), it is called a *tropia*. If the deviation is present only after binocular vision is interrupted by covering one eye, it is called a *phoria*. Strabismus affects 2% to 3% of the population. It should be noted that to avoid the double vision caused by the deviation, a child will suppress the vision of the weaker eye (lazy eye). Treatment for strabismus includes patching of the eye, pharmacologic drugs, and motility exercises or glasses to stimulate vision. Surgical procedures for correction are designed to strengthen or weaken the muscles (Boyd-Monk, Steinmetz, 1987).

Amblyopia

If a child does not receive treatment for strabismus before the age of seven, a permanent vision defect (**amblyopia**) develops in the weaker eye, and it is not treatable with glasses or contact lenses. Amblyopia can be caused by strabismus, cataracts, or refractive errors in children. The child should have visual rehabilitation started without delay so that binocular vision can be preserved. Initially newborns need to have each eye evaluated for corneal light reflex, pupillary response, and presence of a red reflex. Uncoordinated eye movements may be present until an infant is 3 to 4 months of age (Berson, 1987). Persistent deviations should be evaluated by a physician. The primary care physician can check the infant's vision during routine checkups. The eyes should be able to follow and fixate on an object. From 2 to 4 years of age, or during the prereading age, picture cards or the single E chart can be used to check visual acuity. Each eye is checked individually. If both eyes have equal vision of 20/40 or better, no referral to a specialist is necessary. However, an ophthalmologist should evaluate vision if there are abnormalities or if there is a family history of strabismus or other eye disease (Berson, 1987).

Contact Lenses

Contact lenses are an alternative to wearing glasses. Cosmetically, people prefer them. They are designed to move with the eye and to provide better peripheral vision, depth perception, and visual acuity than glasses. The contact lens is a small, thin, polished plastic/silicone/cellulose disc whose outer surface is shaped or ground to correct the vision abnormality. It rests on the tear film over the corneal surface and is held in place by capillary traction and the upper lid. A variety of contact lens styles are available today. The original hard lenses are worn by relatively few users today. Soft and gas-permeable lenses are most common. Hard lenses, designed to be removed daily, are easy to care for and are less expensive, but they do not allow oxygen to reach the cornea. Soft and gas-permeable lenses do allow oxygen to reach the cornea. Soft lenses offer little correction for astigmatism and require greater care than gas-permeable and hard lenses. Wearing time for soft lenses is longer, and the cost is higher.

Contact lenses have been associated with corneal abrasions and infections. Among the risk factors for these injuries are prolonged wearing time, improper fit of the lens, scratched or torn lenses, hyposecretion of tears, improper hygiene, and decreased oxygen to the corneal surface. "Bandage," or therapeutic, soft lenses are used to treat lid disorders, corneal epithelial defects, corneal erosions or ulcers, wound leaks, and small corneal perforations. A contact lens may be prescribed to correct the vision of a patient who has had cataract surgery on one eye but did not receive an intraocular lens implant (Vaughan, Asbury, Riordan-Eva, 1992).

Contact lenses should be removed in an injured or comatose patient to prevent damage (abrasions) to the corneal epithelium (Figure 29-15; Box 29-1). If the eyes are not fully closed, the contact lenses may begin to adhere to the corneal surface. This happens because the tear film is not spread over the eye with normal lid blinking. Prolonged lens wear with decreased oxygen to the cornea can lead to keratitis and scarring.

Vision Loss

Blindness is legally defined by the Internal Revenue Service as a visual acuity that is not correctable to at least 20/200 in the better eye or a visual field no greater than 20 degrees at its widest diameter. The area of vision lost can be the central field, the peripheral field, or a portion of the peripheral field in one or both eyes. Generally, vision loss can be thought of as a decrease in vision significant enough to prevent a person from performing activities of daily living without dependence upon others or upon visual aids. Vision loss may be congenital or acquired, and it may occur suddenly or gradually over time. Macular degeneration, glaucoma, diabetic retinopathy, cataract, and optic atrophy are major causes of blindness in the United States. Worldwide, blindness is attributed to cataract, trachoma, glaucoma, onchocerciasis (river blindness), xerophthalmia (nutritional blindness due to vitamin A deficiency), and trauma (Grimes, Scardino, Martino, 1992; Vader, 1992).

Color Blindness

The inability to distinguish colors may be congenital or acquired, and it may be partial or com-

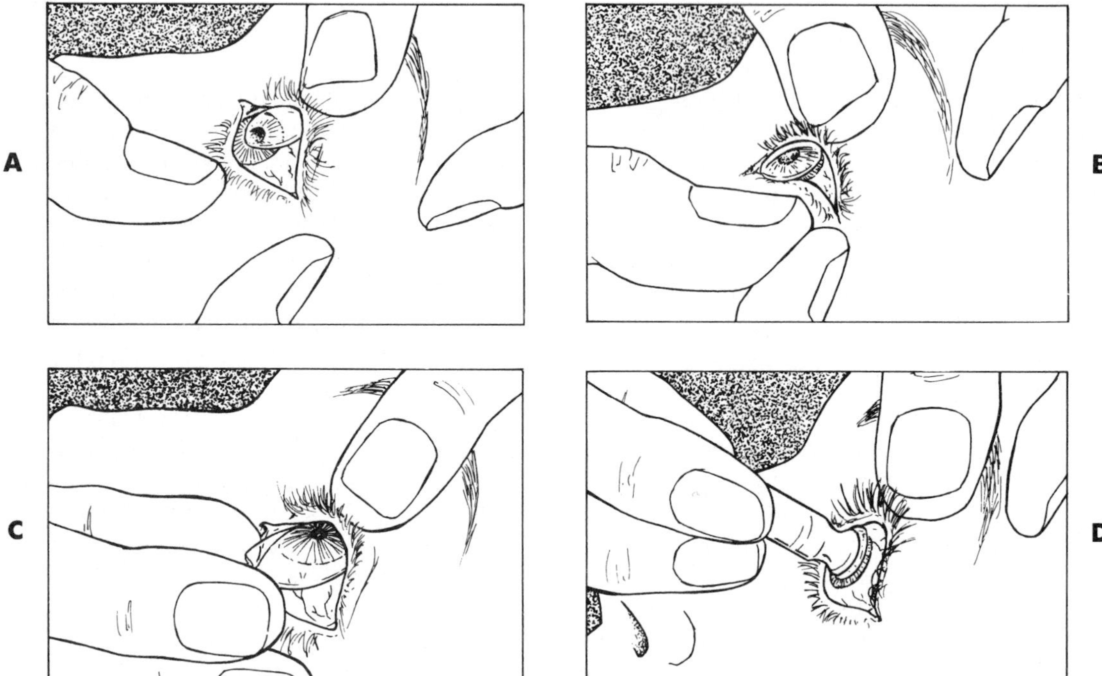

Figure 29-15 **A,** To remove hard lens, place thumb or finger directly on margin of lid at base of eyelashes and raise lid. Use same procedure with other hand to lower bottom lid. Recenter lens before removing. **B,** Slowly bring lids together, trapping contact lens between lid margins. Eyelid will break tear-layer adhesion of contact lens, which will be ejected as lid forces it outward. **C,** Soft lens will move as lids are manipulated. If it does not seem slippery, it must be moistened with saline solution before attempting to remove it to avoid peeling epithelial tissues from corneal surface. To remove soft lens, raise upper lid with one hand and pinch lens with fingers of other hand. It will be removed easily if it is moist and may be removed even it it is off center in eye. **D,** Kits that contain contact lens suction cup are available in many emergency rooms. Suction cup is effective for removing hard and scleral lenses but cannot be used with soft lenses.

BOX 29-1

SUGGESTED EMERGENCY CARE FOR PATIENTS WEARING CONTACT LENSES

DETERMINE IF PATIENT IS WEARING CONTACT LENSES:
- Ask
- Check I.D. Card
- Check Medic Alert Medallion
- Look for contact lenses

IF YOU SUSPECT THE LENSES ARE STILL ON THE EYE:
- Apply adhesive tape strip to patient's forehead or adjacent area and label "Contact Lenses"
- Consult emergency aid file when time permits

IF THE LENSES ARE FOUND:
- Place in a case or bottle and label with patient's name (Mark "right" or "left," if known)
- Record on emergency tag

Provided as a public service by the
AMERICAN OPTOMETRIC ASSOCIATION

Reprinted with permission of the American Optometric Association, St Louis, Mo.

plete. Red-blue–sensitive and green-sensitive pigments in the retina are responsible for normal color vision. Defects in one or more of these pigments are responsible for color blindness. Congenital defects are sex linked and occur mostly in males. Retinal or optic nerve disease can also cause color vision abnormalities. The most common type of color blindness is red-green blindness, in which persons see these colors as yellow or blue. One or both eyes can be involved. Awareness of this defect is important to drivers, who must use some feature other than color to distinguish the difference in traffic lights. Some states require color vision testing when applying for a driver's license. Color vision testing can be accomplished with the Ishihara test (polychromatic plates). A person with normal color vision can identify all patterns or symbols on the test field, whereas a patient with a deficiency cannot. This problem affects approximately 8% of males and less than 1% of females. True color blindness, called achromatopsia (the inability to see any colors), is rare (Vaughan, Asbury, Riordan-Eva, 1992).

NURSING INTERVENTIONS FOR EYE DISORDERS

Several specific procedures are necessary for the patient with eye problems. The nurse should be familiar with these procedures and understand the basis for using each one on a selected patient. Handwashing and clean equipment are essential. In some instances, sterile supplies and equipment may be required.

Normal pupillary response is the response of the pupil to light (PERRLA, = pupils equal, round, react to light, and accommodation). The pupil of one eye should constrict simultaneously when the opposite pupil is exposed to light, even when the unexposed eye is blind. To check the pupils, the nurse should dim the lights and use a penlight. The nurse should stand in front of the patient and have the patient look straight ahead at an object. The nurse should direct the flashlight beam onto one pupil from the side and then repeat for the other eye. Head trauma, eye medications, and other drugs—therapeutic or recreational—can affect pupil size and response (Hunt, 1992).

Other procedures include routine or compression eye dressings, medication application, lid hygiene and irrigation, everting the lids, and warm and cold compresses (Figure 29-16; Boxes 29-2 to 29-6).

Overview of Ophthalmic Medications

Medications for ophthalmic diagnosis and treatment are used in many forms (Table 29-2). Topically, they are applied as drops or ointment. Ointments tend to cloud the vision, so they are better used at night or when the eye is closed. They do provide better lubrication than drops. Drops should be instilled before an ointment if both are ordered. Some drops may produce local irritation, causing redness, blurred vision, stinging, foreign body sensation, or tearing. Discolored solutions should be discarded. Special storage such as refrigeration or storing away from light is required for some eye medications. Combinations of antibiotics with antiinflammatory medications are prescribed for external diseases such as blepharitis and bacterial corneal ulcers. Separate bottles or tubes of medication should be used for each eye if both are infected, and each bottle should be labeled properly (Boyd-Monk, Steinmetz, 1987; McCoy, 1992).

Parenteral or oral medications are used for systemic effect in various conditions. Injections are given subconjunctivally or intraocularly into the anterior chamber or the vitreous cavity. Doses for these injections are calculated and given with great care. The incorrect dosage could be toxic, and corneal decompensation or retinal tissue destruction is possible.

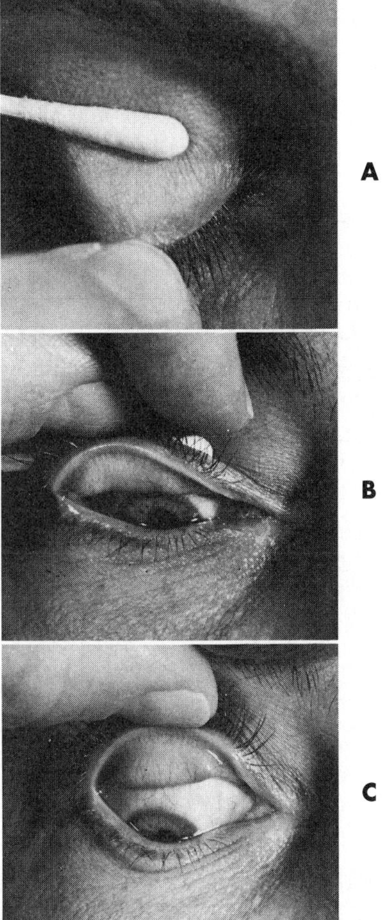

Figure 29-16 Eversion of upper eyelid. Patient is instructed to look downward, and lashes of upper eyelid are grasped between thumb and index finger. **A,** Cotton-tipped applicator is placed at level of tarsal fold. **B,** Eyelid is folded back on applicator while patient continues to look downward. **C,** Applicator is removed. (From Newell FW: *Ophthalmology: principles and concepts,* ed 7, St Louis, 1992, Mosby.)

As with all treatments, meticulous handwashing before and after applying medications is a must. Universal precautions should be followed with all patients, according to OSHA guidelines.

The following drugs that are used for treatment of systemic disease can be toxic to the eye and cause irreversible damage:

1 Corticosteroids cause cataract formation. Children are more susceptible than adults.
2 Isotretinoin (Accutane), a vitamin A analog used for treating acne, can cause increased intracranial pressure and damage the optic nerve. A vision check needs to be done within 6 weeks of initial therapy.

BOX 29-2

EYE DRESSINGS

ROUTINE DRESSING

Close the affected eye and place a patch over the globe.

Tape diagonally from the middle of the forehead to the cheek.

Apply a shield, if required, over the patch and tape in a similar method.

PRESSURE DRESSING

For a pressure patch, use two patches and tape as for a routine dressing (Figure 29-16).

BOX 29-3

INSTILLATION OF EYE DROPS

1 Wash your hands before and after doing any procedure on the eye.
2 With one hand, put a finger on the patient's cheek just below the eye on the bony socket. Gently pull down until a small pocket is formed between the eyeball and lower lid.
3 Have the patient tilt his or her head back and look up. Put a drop into the pocket that you have formed (conjunctival sac).
4 Have the patient gently close both eyes for a minute to let the drop absorb.
5 If another drop is to be instilled, wait 3 to 5 minutes before the next one is put in.
6 The same procedure is followed for putting in ointments. A strip of ointment approximately ½ inch long is squeezed into the conjunctival sac from the inner to outer side of the eye. If drops and ointment are given at the same time, the ointment goes in last.
7 Avoid touching any part of the eye with the medication container.
8 To prevent systemic absorption of drugs, the puncta (small openings to the nasolacrimal ducts located on the medial aspect of the upper and lower lids) should be occluded. After instilling the drop, press the index finger over the inner canthus until you can feel the bone beneath the skin. Release after 30 seconds.
9 Store medications properly.

NOTE: Some medications need to be refrigerated or stored away from light.

3 Hydroxychloroquine (Plaquenil), an arthritis and lupus drug, is toxic to the rods and cones in the retina. A baseline examination should be followed by checks every 3 to 6 months while medication is being taken.
4 A tuberculosis drug, ethambutol (Isoniazid) can cause optic neuropathy.

The nurse should monitor the vision closely in any patient taking any of these medications.

Conjunctivitis

Conjunctivitis is an inflammation of the conjunctiva of the eye. Symptoms include a burning or scratching sensation, foreign-body sensation, tearing, swelling, drainage, and increased blood in the vessels (hyperemia). It may be a result of an allergy or a viral or bacterial infection. *Allergic conjunctivitis* usually subsides when the allergen is removed, but the itching and redness can be treated with vasoconstrictive drops and cold compresses. Severe cases may require systemic antihistamines or steroids. *Viral conjunctivitis* is caused by herpes simplex, herpes zoster, adenovirus, and other viruses. After the causative organism is identified, topical antiviral drugs are used. It should be noted that although steroids can be used in allergic conjunctivitis, they are contraindicated in viral conjunctivitis.

The most common type of conjunctivitis is often referred to as *pink eye.* In temperate climates, it is often caused by the pneumococcus organism. In tropical climates, the Koch-Weeks bacillus is the most common cause. It is often encountered as an epidemic among school children and is spread through droplet infection. There is redness, burning, and mucopurulent discharge. The infection starts in one eye and rapidly spreads to the other (Vaughan, Asbury, Riordan-Eva, 1992). The eyelids are usually stuck together in the morning, and warm moist compresses may be applied to separate the lids. Eye irrigations using physiologic saline may be ordered, and once the specific organism is identified, the disease is treated with a sulfonamide or other antibiotic drug (see Box 29-5). Steroid therapy is contraindicated before the infection is identified. Drops are used during the day, and an ointment is used at night. Lid hygiene should be performed before medication is applied (see Box 29-4). Persons with the infection should use their own towels and washcloths and avoid public pools. Children should not attend school until the infection has cleared (approximately 1 week). Meticulous handwashing is necessary to prevent the spread of infection. *Bacterial conjunctivitis* is caused by staphylococcus, streptococcus, diplococcus, *Escherichia coli,* and other bacteria. Universal precautions, including use of gloves for patient care during irrigations, lid hygiene, and medication application, are required.

BOX 29-4

LID HYGIENE FOR POSTOPERATIVE CARE

1 Wash hands before and after the cleansing.
2 Assemble the solution (normal saline or tap water), cotton balls, gauze or a clean washcloth.
3 Position the patient sitting comfortably, possibly near the sink if tap water is used.
4 Wipe the eye with a moistened cotton ball or gauze from the nasal to the temporal side of the eye. Avoid getting solution into the unaffected eye.
5 Each time the procedure is done, use fresh, clean supplies.

BOX 29-5

EYE IRRIGATION/CLEANSING

1 Wash hands before and after the procedure. Use gloves.
2 Assemble necessary equipment, including cotton balls, normal saline or other solution, kidney basin or towel to absorb the solution.
3 Position the patient comfortably with the head turned to the affected side.
4 Direct the irrigating solution over the eye from the nasal to the temporal side of the eye. Avoid getting solution into the unaffected eye.
5 Use a separate set of supplies for each eye if both eyes are involved.
6 Do not instill the solution forcefully. The eyelid can be gently held open for a thorough cleansing.

Ophthalmia neonatorum refers to any purulent conjunctivitis of the newborn acquired from an infected birth canal. State laws require that erythromycin 0.5% or tetracycline 1% ophthalmic ointment or drops be instilled in the eyes of all newborn infants to prevent the disease. Prophylactic drugs are given no later than 1 hour after birth. Although ophthalmia neonatorum can occur as a result of maternal gonorrhea, it is now most commonly caused by chlamydia. Silver nitrate does not prevent chlamydial infections. If mothers have a known disease, infants may require systemic therapy as well as prophylaxis.

Untreated chlamydia causes *trachoma,* identified by the World Health Organization as the leading cause of blindness in the world (Vaughan, Asbury, Riordan-Eva, 1992). Initially, this infection leads to scarring of

BOX 29-6

EVERTING THE LIDS

This procedure is done to inspect the eye for a foreign body or to irrigate the lid margins.

1 Assemble equipment, including cotton-tipped applicators, irrigation solution, fluorescein strips, and a light source (a slit lamp if available).
2 Gently pull down the lower lid on the orbital rim to expose the conjunctival sac of the lower lid.
3 For the upper lid, use a cotton-tipped applicator. Grasp the lashes with the finger and thumb and gently fold the lid back over the applicator.
4 Once the lid is folded, remove the applicator so the lid can rest against the conjunctiva for inspection.
5 To close the eyelid, the patient need only blink or close eyelids slowly and reopen again (see Figure 29-16).

the conjunctiva and interferes with tear film. This leads to corneal infections, scarring, and eventual blindness. Treatment is with sulfonamides, tetracycline, or erythromycin administered orally for 3 to 5 weeks. All members of the family must be treated if they are infected. Proper hygiene practices and improved sanitation can eliminate trachoma. Evaluation of a "red eye" as a result of conjunctivitis should not be confused with angle-closure glaucoma (Table 29-3).

Corneal Disorders

The cornea, or clear window at the front of the eye, has five layers. One or more of these layers can be involved in a disease process or injury that will necessitate replacing the defective cornea with a human donor cornea. Because the cornea has no blood supply or lymphatics, tissue typing is normally not required.

Corneal abrasions and *ulcers* destroy the normal barrier of corneal epithelium and expose the other layers to infection from a variety of organisms. Included are yeasts, viruses, fungi, protozoa, and gram-positive or gram-negative organisms. Pseudomonas, a gram-negative organism, is one of the most common contaminants in used bottles of eye drops and used tubes of mascara. Invasion by the herpes simplex virus is easily identified, with the aid of fluorescein stain, by its characteristic appearance resembling a linear branch with feathered edges (Ostler, 1993; Vaughan, Asbury, Riordan-Eva, 1992).

Symptoms of abrasions and ulcers include pain, **photophobia** (light sensitivity), and **epiphora** (tearing). Symptomatic diagnosis is confirmed by slit-lamp

Text continued on p. 986.

TABLE 29-2

Pharmacology of Drugs Used for Vision

Drug (Generic and Trade Name); Route and Dosage	Action/Indication	Common Side Effects and Nursing Considerations
Antibiotics		
BACITRACIN OINTMENT (Ak-tracin) **ROUTE:** Ocular **DOSAGE:** ½-inch strip of 500 units/g ointment 2-4 times daily	Antibacterial used for minor gram-positive infections	Do not use with silver nitrate; can delay wound healing
CIPROFLOXACIN (Ciloxan) **ROUTE:** Ocular **DOSAGE:** 1-2 drops 15-30 min until infection is controlled, then 1-2 drops 4-6 times daily	Quinolone antibacterial used for corneal ulcers and bacterial conjuncitivits	Watch for local irritation; not to be used for pseudomonas
ERYTHROMYCIN OPTHALMIC (Ilotycin) **ROUTE:** Ocular **DOSAGE:** 0.5% ointment to conjunctiva 1 or more times daily	Used for treatment of superficial ocular infections and for prophylaxis in opthalmia neonatorum; useful when penicillin-based opthalmic drug cannot be used because of hypersensitivity	Staph resistance may develop
GENTAMICIN (Garamycin, Genoptic) **ROUTE:** Ocular **DOSAGE:** 1-2 drops of solution q 2-4 hr, or ointment 2-3 times daily	Bactericidal used for pseudomonas, gram-negative infections, and other localized infections	Incompatible with erythromycin, chloramphenicol, and not effective against streptococci; use with caution in renal patients
POLYMYXIN B SULFATE (Aerosporin) **ROUTE:** Ocular **DOSAGE:** 1-3 drops q 1 hr; dosage interval may be increased as response occurs	Bactericidal used for pseudomonas and gram-negative infections	Not effective for gram-positive infections; may be toxic to renal patients
TETRACYCLINE (Achromycin) **ROUTE:** Ocular **DOSAGE:** Thin strip of ointment q 2-4 hr, or 1 drop of suspension q 6-12 hr (may be used more often); single dose for opthalmia neonatorum	Bacteriostatic used against gram-positive and gram-negative infections and for prophylaxis in opthalmia neonatorum	Use with caution in hepatic or renal failure
TOBRAMYCIN (Tobrex) **ROUTE:** Ocular **DOSAGE:** 1 cm of ointment 2-3 times daily (q 3-4 hr for severe infections), or 1-2 drops of solution q 4 hr (q 30-60 min for severe infections)	Bacteriocidal used for pseudomonas, staphylococcus, and gram-negative infections	Prolonged use may result in overgrowth of nonsusceptible organisms
Antifungals		
AMPHOTERICIN B (Fungizone) **ROUTE:** Ocular **DOSAGE:** 3% ointment 1-2 drops daily or as ordered	Used against *Candida,* histoplasmosis, and blastomycosis	Use with caution in renal or electrolyte abnormalities; watch closely for adverse reactions; give test dose before maintenance dose

TABLE 29-2

Pharmacology of Drugs Used for Vision—cont'd

Drug (Generic and Trade Name); Route and Dosage	Action/Indication	Common Side Effects and Nursing Considerations
NATAMYCIN (Natacyn) **ROUTE:** Ocular **DOSAGE:** 1-2 drops q 4-6 hr	Used for treatment of fungal keratitis, blepharitis, or fungal conjuctivitis	
Antivirals		
IDOXURIDINE (Herplex, Stoxil) **ROUTE:** Ocular **DOSAGE:** 0.5% ointment; 0.1% solution, 1 drop q hr when awake, and q 2 hr at night	Used for herpes simplex keratitis	Refrigerate solution and keep from light; should not be mixed with other eye solutions; watch for signs of hypersensitivity
TRIFLURIDINE (Viroptic ophthalmic solution 1%) **ROUTE:** Ocular **DOSAGE:** 1-2 drops q 2-3 hr initially, then q 4 hr when awake	Used against primary keratoconjuctivitis and recurrent epithelial keratitis caused by herpes simplex virus, types I and II	Stinging upon instillation; use with caution in pregnancy
VIDARABINE (Vira-A Opthalmic) **ROUTE:** Ocular **DOSAGE:** ½-inch strip of ointment into lower conjunctival sac 5 times daily at 3-hr intervals	Used against herpes simplex keratitis and herpes zoster keratitis	Use cautiously with steroids; not for long-term use
Glaucoma		
ACETAZOLAMIDE (AKZol, Diamox) **ROUTE:** PO, IV **DOSAGE:** PO 250-500 mg 1-2 times daily; IV 250-500 mg daily	Carbonic anhydrase inhibitor used in treatment of narrow-angle glaucoma	Nausea, vomiting, diarrhea, anorexia, headache, skin rash, confusion, and paresthesia; do not give to sulfa-sensitive patients; contraindicated in kidney or liver dysfunction
BETAXOLOL (Betoptic) **ROUTE:** Ocular **DOSAGE:** Instill 1 drop of 0.5% solution or 1-2 drops of 0.25% suspension bid	Beta blocker, decreases aqueous formation	Local irritation and insomnia; contraindicated in pulmonary, renal, or cardiac disease, including congestive heart failure
GLYCERIN (Osmoglyn) **ROUTE:** PO, ocular **DOSAGE:** PO, 1-1.5 g/kg as a single dose, may be followed by 500 mg/kg q 6 hr; ocular, 1-2 drops q 3-4 hr	Alcohol used for management of edema of the superficial layers of the cornea and reduction of intraocular pressure	Use with caution in diabetics; onset is 10 min and duration 45 min; serve over ice with lemon
LEVOBUNOLOL (Betagan) **ROUTE:** Ocular **DOSAGE:** 1-2 drops daily or bid	Beta-adrenergic-blocking agent used for short-term reduction of IOP due to glaucoma	Decreases heart rate; may cause headaches, nausea, dizziness, and depression; contraindicated in asthma, emphysema, diabetes, and bradycardia

continued

TABLE 29-2

Pharmacology of Drugs Used for Vision—cont'd

Drug (Generic and Trade Name); Route and Dosage	Action/Indication	Common Side Effects and Nursing Considerations
MANNITOL (Osmitrol) **ROUTE:** IV **DOSAGE:** 5%-10% solution continuously up to 200 g IV, while maintaining 100-500 ml urine output/hr and a positive fluid balance	Osmotic agent used for angle-closure glaucoma and preoperative or postoperative control of IOP	Nausea, vomiting, urine retention; contraindicated in pulmonary edema, congestive heart failure, and renal disease
TIMOLOL MALEATE (Timoptic) **ROUTE:** Ocular **DOSAGE:** Initially 1 drop 0.25% solution bid; reduce maintenance dose to 1 drop daily	Beta-adrenergic-blocking agent used for chronic open-angle glaucoma, secondary glaucoma, aphakic glaucoma, and optic hypertension	Nausea, vomiting, urine retention; not for use in pulmonary edema, congestive heart failure, or renal disease; does not affect pupil size or visual acuity; can cause apnea in infants
Nonsteroidal antiinflammatory		
DICLOFENAC (Voltaren) **ROUTE:** Ocular **DOSAGE:** 1 drop of 0.1% solution 4 times/day × 2 weeks, beginning 24 hr after procedure	For management of inflammation after cataract extraction	May enhance digoxin, methotrexate, cyclosporin, and lithium
FLURBIPROFEN (Ocufen) **ROUTE:** Ocular **DOSAGE:** Instill 1 drop into eye undergoing surgery approximately q ½ hr, beginning 2 hr before surgery; give total of 4 drops	Given preoperatively to inhibit miosis during intraocular surgery	May increase incidence of bleeding postoperatively; do not use with anticoagulants such as Coumadin
Miotics		
CARBACHOL INTRAOCULAR (Miostat) **ROUTE:** Ocular **DOSAGE:** Physician instills 0.5 ml into the anterior chamber, before or after securing sutures	Used to produce pupilary miosis during ocular surgery and for open-angle glaucoma	Prolonged constriction contraindicated in acute iritis and corneal abrasion
ECHOTHIOPHATE IODIDE (Phospholine Iodide) **ROUTE:** Ocular **DOSAGE:** Instill 1 drop of 0.03%-0.125% solution into conjunctival sac daily	Used in treatment of primary open-angle glaucoma and conditions obstructing aqueous flow	Discontinue several weeks preoperatively; causes respiratory depression with succinylcholine
Mydriatics and cycloplegics		
ATROPINE (Atropisol, Isopto Atropine) **ROUTE:** Ocular **DOSAGE:** 1 drop 2-4 times/day	Anticholinergic agent used for treatment of uveitis, amblyopia, iritis, posterior-segment surgery, and some anterior-segment surgery	Systemic reactions (tachycardia, increased blood pressure); side effects may last up to 2 weeks; antidote is physostigmine
CYCLOPENTOLATE HYDROCHLORIDE (Cyclogyl, AK-Pentolate) **ROUTE:** Ocular **DOSAGE:** 1-2 drops, up to 3 doses	Used for diagnostic procedures requiring mydriasis and cycloplegia	Photophobia and local irritation; onset 15-30 min, with up to 24-hr duration; use with caution if patient hypertensive

TABLE 29-2

Pharmacology of Drugs Used for Vision—cont'd

Drug (Generic and Trade Name); Route and Dosage	Action/Indication	Common Side Effects and Nursing Considerations
EPINEPHRINE **ROUTE:** Ocular **DOSAGE:** 1:1000 to 1:40,000; used in irrigation solution for intraocular injection	Adrenergic agent dilates pupil intraoperatively	Use with caution in cardiac, diabetic, and hypertensive patients
PHENYLEPHRINE (AK-Dilate, Mydfrin, Neo-Synephrine 2.5% or 10% drops) **ROUTE:** Ocular **DOSAGE:** 1-3 drops, up to 3 doses, for refraction; 1 drop qid for uveitis	Adrenergic agent used for diagnostic tests, preoperatively, and for uveitis	Onset 5-10 min, with duration 3-5 hr; can cause systemic hypertension; monitor BP and pulse; use with caution with MAO inhibitors
SCOPOLAMINE (Isopto-Hyoscine 3% drops) **ROUTE:** Ocular **DOSAGE:** 1-2 drops tid	Used for diagnosis, to induce refraction, and for iridocyclitis	Onset in 40 min, with duration 3-5 days
TROPICAMIDE (Mydriacyl, Tropicacyl 1% drops) **ROUTE:** Ocular **DOSAGE:** Instill 1 drop of 1% solution; may repeat in 5 min; additional drop in 20-30 min if necessary	Used for diagnosis, to induce refraction, and for fundus photography	Onset in 20-30 min, with duration 4-6 hr; local irritation and blurred vision
Steroidal antiinflammatory		
DEXAMETHASONE (Decadron, Hexadrol, Maxidex) **ROUTE:** Ocular, IV **DOSAGE:** Ocular, 1-2 drops 4-6 times daily, or hourly as prescribed; IV, 2-mg doses up to 12 mg daily	Used for ocular inflammation in intraocular surgery	Contraindicated for viral or fungal infections; can increase IOP or cause cataracts
HYDROCORTISONE (cortisol) **ROUTE:** Ocular **DOSAGE:** 1-2 drops 4-6 times daily, or hourly as prescribed	Antiinflammatory and immunosuppressant used for treatment of sympathetic opthalmia, chemical burns, corneal graft rejection, intraocular lens surgery, and conjunctivitis	Retards corneal regeneration; contraindicated for fungal and viral conditions and glaucoma; increased susceptibility to fungal and viral infections with long-term use. To discontinue drug, it must be tapered slowly
PREDNISONE (Deltasone, Meticorten) **ROUTE:** Ocular **DOSAGE:** 1-2 drops 4 to 6 times daily and then taper properly to discontinue; may be ordered every hour	Same as for hydrocortisone (above)	Same as for hydrocortisone (above)
PREDNISOLONE (Pred-Mild, Inflamase, AK-Pred) **ROUTE:** Ocular **DOSAGE:** Same as for prednisone (above)	Same as for hydrocortisone (above)	Same as for hydrocortisone (above)

TABLE 29-3

Evaluating a Red Eye

	Acute Glaucoma	Bacterial Conjunctivitis	Viral Conjunctivitis	Allergic Conjunctivitis
Corneal opacity	Yes	No	0 to +	0
Hyperemia (increased blood in vessels)	++	+++	++	+
Pupil	mid-dilated; nonreactive	normal	normal	normal
Anterior chamber depth	shallow	normal	normal	normal
Intraocular pressure	high	normal	normal	normal
Discharge	none	++ to +++	++	+
Preauricular nodes	none	none	+	none
Signs and symptoms	no exudates—itching, blurred vision, pain, photophobia, colored halos, nausea and vomiting—affects one eye	large amount of discharge—mucopurulent, yellowish exudate—affects one or both eyes	moderate exudate—watery or yellow tinged—affects one or both eyes	small amount of exudate—white, stringy—affects one or both eyes

examination with fluorescein staining. Correctly identifying the source of the infection is most important. A variety of medications is available for use, and the choice of drug depends on the causative organism. Initial treatment for an abrasion includes antibiotic drops or ointment, cool packs, and dark glasses to decrease the photophobia. With a larger abrasion or severe pain, a pressure dressing is applied for comfort and to limit eye movement. This patch also prevents the lid from opening and closing and rubbing over the abraded area. Pain medication may be prescribed. Serious abrasions and ulcers are treated more aggressively with topical and periocular antiinfective agents. Occasionally, systemic drugs are given. Most superficial ulcers heal without complication when treated. Deep ulcers may perforate and tend to scar.

Strict adherence to the regimen of drop administration for corneal ulcers is vital to preserve the cornea and prevent scarring. Initially, "fortified" eye drops (individualized to the patient's ulcer) are prepared by the pharmacist or the physician and are given every 5 minutes for 30 minutes, then every hour around the clock until the cornea improves. Nighttime drops may be given every 2 hours. After 72 to 96 hours, a commercial drop is substituted. Patient compliance with this regimen is difficult because the frequency of drops conflicts with normal activities and sleep. Usually hospitalization is required to achieve this type of therapy. Patients need to understand how important the schedule is in preserving vision.

Other treatments for persistent defects that fail to heal are *bandage contact lenses* or adhesives (Vaughan, Asbury, Riordan-Eva, 1992). Lateral tarsorrhaphy or suturing the eyelids closed can be a temporary or permanent procedure used to treat corneal complications as a result of trauma, coma, dry-eye syndrome, neurologic lid diseases, or strokes.

Dystrophies and Degenerative Corneal Diseases

Other abnormalities of the cornea can be congenital or acquired. In all conditions, an opacity is found in one or more of the layers. This clouding interferes with vision. *Keratoconus*, or coning of the cornea, is a degenerative disease of unknown cause. The onset is in the teenage years. Xerophthalmia, a condition caused

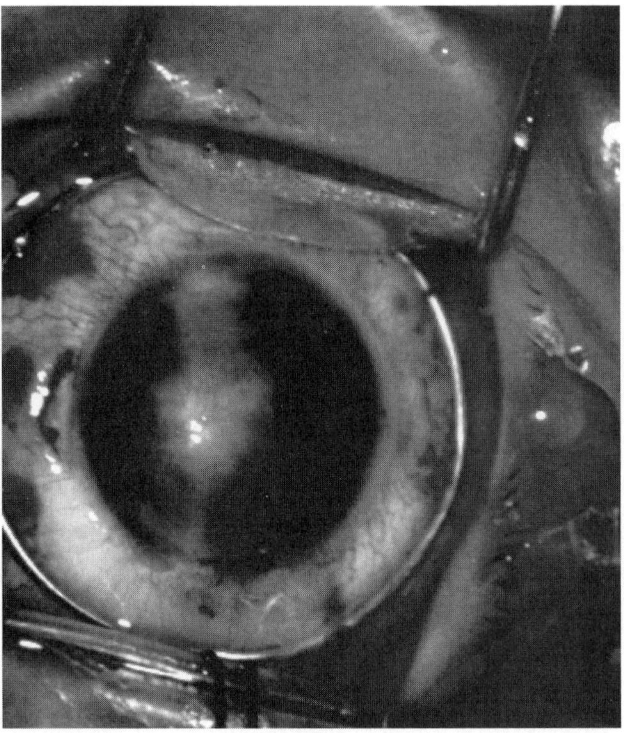

Figure 29-17 Preoperative view of corneal scar across the visual axis. (Photo courtesy of Dr. J. B. Rubenstein, Chicago, Ill.)

by vitamin A deficiency, is found primarily in Africa and Latin America. Symptoms can progress from night blindness to actual decompensation of the cornea. Corneal dystrophies are bilateral hereditary conditions of the cornea that appear later in life, after the second decade. They may progress slowly or be stationary for long periods and not require treatment. However, corneal decompensation accompanied by a decrease in visual acuity may require a full-thickness graft (penetrating keratoplasty [PKP]) (Ostler, 1993). *Pseudophakic bullous keratopathy,* or edema of the cornea as a result of an intraocular lens implant, accounts for approximately 40,000 PKP procedures a year in the United States. Acquired conditions that require surgery include trauma and lacerations that leave a scar across the visual axis (pupil) of the cornea (Figure 29-17).

Corneal Transplantation

Corneal transplantation **(keratoplasty)** is the surgical technique of replacing the patient's cornea with a human donor cornea (Box 29-7). A full-thickness graft is called a *penetrating keratoplasty* (PKP). A partial-thickness graft, lamellar keratoplasty, is a technique seldom used today. Donor tissue is stored in a preservative medium that extends tissue viability to 10 days after expiration of the donor (Box 29-8) (Ostler, 1993). This extension of viable storage has significantly decreased the number of patients on waiting lists. Scheduling for surgery procedures can be done on an urgent basis rather than on an emergent one. The patient can follow a normal routine without staying by a phone for news about the availability of tissue. Depending on the individual city or state, donor tissue may be in a limited supply.

A network of eye banks is set up by cities, states, and regions across the United States. This efficient and cost-effective linking of patient and tissue information ensures that the cornea is where it is needed when it is needed.

Preoperative evaluation of the patient includes a complete eye examination with keratometry readings, pachymetry, specular microscopy, and assessment of tear function if indicated. Routinely, surgery is performed under local anesthesia, with sedation and monitoring. Occasionally, general anesthesia may be indicated for reasons similar to those requiring general anesthesia for cataract extraction surgery. During the operative procedure the diseased central portion of the patient's cornea is removed and replaced with the donor tissue. The graft is sewn in place with a 10-0 or 11-0 suture in a running (continuous) or interrupted (individually tied) suture technique (Figure 29-18). When the procedure is completed, antibiotic and steroid injections are given subconjunctivally to prevent infection and inflammation. A patch and shield are routinely placed over the eye, and regular eye glasses may be worn during the day to protect the eye.

Depending on the reason for the procedure, the patient can be an outpatient, 23-hour observation patient, or hospital inpatient. Uncomplicated cases are done on an outpatient basis similar to that for cataract surgery. Patients need to have a thorough understanding of postoperative medication orders and drop administration. They also need to know that compliance with this regimen and daily vision checks are equally important. Signs of rejection are redness, sudden loss of vision, or pain (RSVP), and any one of these must be reported to the ophthalmologist immediately. Follow-up visits are weekly for 2 to 3 weeks, every other week for 2 months, and then monthly until 6 months after surgery. Because the cornea is avascular, it heals slowly and sutures remain in place for up to 1 year. For this reason, seat belts are recommended every time the patient is in a car, and contact sports should be avoided (see Box 29-7).

Other surgical procedures on the cornea are designed to correct refractive errors of the eye. They include astigmatic keratectomy and radial keratotomy. *Radial keratotomy,* or RK, consists of 4 to 16 pie-shaped cuts into the cornea, from a clear optical zone in the center to the outer portion of the cornea, but not as far

BOX 29-7 **Nursing Process**

INTRAOCULAR SURGERY (CATARACT EXTRACTION, PENETRATING KERATOPLASTY, TRABECULECTOMY, VITRECTOMY)

ASSESSMENT

Vital signs per routine
Eye dressing
Level of comfort
Ability to care for self
For signs of disorientation

NURSING DIAGNOSES

Anxiety related to fear of loss of sight or to symptoms of disease and prospective treatment
Pain related to surgical inflamation or increased IOP
Self-care deficit related to decreased visual acuity or physical limitations
Noncompliance to surgical protocol related to memory impairment, anxiety, or instructions not heard or seen well
Knowledge deficit related to condition, treatment, medication administration, or activity restriction
Risk for infection related to invasive surgery
Sensory/perceptual alterations: visual related to disease and to surgical dressing postoperatively (especially important if both eyes are involved or if patient is monocular)
Diversional activity deficit related to decreased vision

NURSING INTERVENTIONS

Preoperative
Review previous teaching done by the physician and staff, including written postoperative instructions for outpatients.
Orient the patient to the surroundings, admission routine, and surgical environment.
Facilitate the patient's expression of fear about the possibility of decreased vision.
Ensure that the patient has followed restrictions to take nothing by mouth.
Inform patient that a patch and shield will be worn immediately after surgery and that glasses may be substituted during waking hours.
Review administration of drops or ointment as ordered.
Inquire who will take the patient home.

Postoperative
Orient the patient to the surroundings.
Position the patient for comfort in bed or a recliner: supine with the head of the bed elevated 30 degrees or more.
Ensure that the patient complies with activity restrictions on the basis of procedure or the physician's order.
Allow the patient to watch television but prohibit reading.
Provide a light diet the first day.
Announce your presence when entering the room.
Approach from the unoperated side.
Place a call bell or signal within easy reach of the patient.
Raise side rails as needed to protect the patient from injury.
Administer medications as prescribed.
Keep the eye patch or shield in place as ordered.
Help the patient with meals, ambulation, and personal hygiene as needed.
Report severe pain to the physician immediately.
Question whether the home environment will be manageable and whether help will be needed.

EVALUATION OF EXPECTED OUTCOMES

Meets discharge criteria for the the postsurgical patient (p. 487)
Expresses fears and concerns
Vision improved or maintained (not applicable for enucleation patients)
Able to ambulate with help
Uses other senses to avoid bumping eye when patched
Verbalizes understanding of instructions
Demonstrates ability to administer own medications
Able to return to normal activity, or has assistance until normal activity resumes
Knowledgeable about modifications at home to enhance safety

as the corneoscleral junction (limbus) (Figure 29-19). The amount of correction desired determines the number and depth of incisions. This reshaping or flattening of the cornea is done with a calibrated diamond knife. Lasers are also being used in clinical trials for myopia and central superficial corneal opacities. Controversy still surrounds this procedure as an option to eliminate the need for glasses or contact lenses. (The goal of these surgeries is to have the patient be less dependent on eyeglassess.) After the procedure the patient may have pain or discomfort, photophobia, or foreign-body sensation. Complications include corneal perforation, fluctuation in vision, persistent glare, regression of the correction, hyperopia, astigmatism, infection, and the need to continue wearing glasses or contact lenses. Long-term follow-up will determine risk and benefit factors more clearly. Most insurance companies consider radial keratotomy a cosmetic procedure, so the expenses incurred are the patient's responsibility.

NURSE ALERT

Cornea safety. Ultraviolet radiation can cause acute inflammation of the cornea (keratitis). Wearing goggles with UV filters protects people who are exposed to the sun (skiers, sunbathers, outdoor workers), as well as people who are employed as arc welders.

BOX 29-8

CORNEAL DONOR CRITERIA

- Age between 1 and 75 years
- Negative medical history for the following:
  - AIDS or risk for HIV infection
  - Active hepatitis
  - Sepsis
  - Lymphoma or active leukemia (other cancer types are okay)
- Ventilator support not required before tissue retrieval
- Routine testing of donors for the following
  - AIDS
  - Hepatitis B and C
  - Serology
- Donation within 6 to 12 hours after cardiopulmonary death (dependent on circumstances); keep lightweight eye packs over upper orbit
- Verbal consent by next of kin, followed by signed consent

Uveitis

The uveal tract includes the ciliary body, iris, and choroid. Anterior uveitis refers to inflammation of the iris and ciliary body. Posterior uveitis refers to inflammation of the choroid. Uveitis usually affects one eye, and it is more common in younger people. Symptoms are dependent on the structure involved. They include photophobia, blurred vision, irregular pupil, and deposits on the posterior corneal surface. Uveitis is

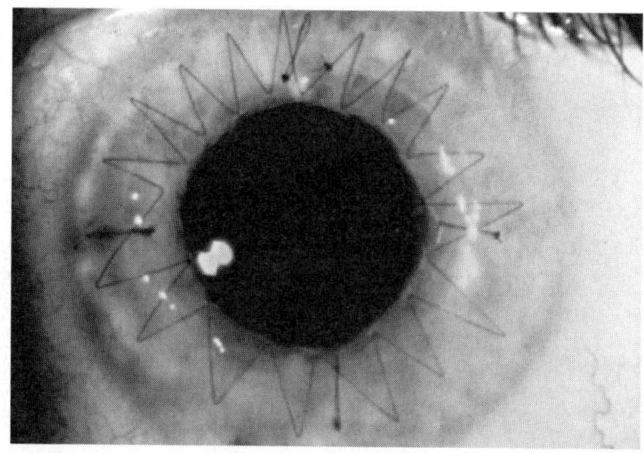

Figure 29-18 Sutures placed in corneal transplant. (Photo courtesy of Dr. R. J. Epstein, Chicago, Ill.)

A

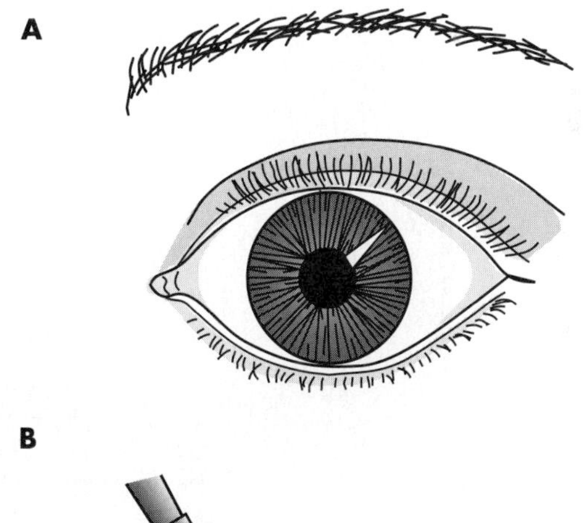

B

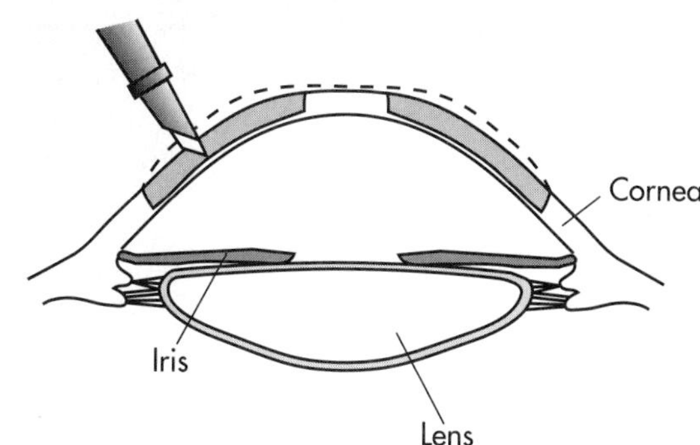

Figure 29-19 Radial keratotomy for myopia. Nearly full-thickness incisions of the cornea are made with a calibrated diamond blade in a radial fashion with sparing of the central cornea. **A,** Frontal view. **B,** Axial view.

found in patients with toxoplasmosis, tuberculosis, sarcoidosis, and syphilis. Treatment is with appropriate antiinfective drugs, steroids, and dilating drops. Atropine or cyclopentolate prevent the formation of synechiae (adhesions). Children are sensitive to atropine, and toxicity may occur unless precautions are taken. Medications should be kept out of reach, and parents who will be giving atropine should be instructed on the toxic effects of an overdose and on the use of punctal occlusion to prevent systemic absorption of topical eye medications (Boyd-Monk, Steinmetz, 1987).

Sympathetic Ophthalmia

Sympathetic ophthalmia is a rare bilateral condition occurring after a penetrating injury to the eye. The exact cause of the uveitis is not known but is thought to be an autoimmune response to the injury. It can occur 10 days to several years after the initial trauma (Vaughan, Asbury, Riordan-Eva, 1992). In rare instances it has occurred after intraocular surgery for cataract and glaucoma. The patient complains of photophobia, redness, and blurred vision. Local and systemic steroids and atropine can be given as initial treatment. However, enucleation is recommended for severely injured, sightless eyes to prevent inflammation in the "sympathizing" eye. The patient needs a thorough explanation of the treatment and risks involved. Complete bilateral blindness can develop over time without treatment (Boyd-Monk, Steinmetz, 1987; Vaughan, Asbury, Riordan-Eva, 1992).

Glaucoma

Glaucoma is a disease that is characterized by a gradual, painless loss of peripheral vision that results in a tunnel-vision effect (Figure 29-20). It affects

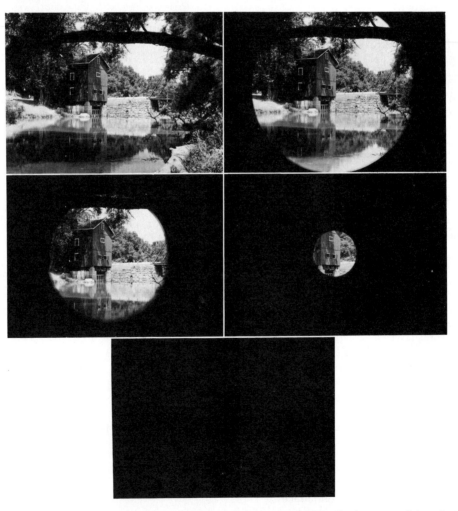

Figure 29-20 Gradual loss of sight from glaucoma so insidiously destroys vision that the person is unaware of impending blindness until extensive and irreversible damage is present. Note loss of peripheral vision. (From Saunders WH and others: *Nursing care in eye, ear, nose, and throat disorders,* ed 4, St Louis, 1979, Mosby.)

0.4% to 0.7% of those over age 40 in the United States and 2% to 3% of those over age 70 (Vaughan, Asbury, Riordan-Eva, 1992). Vision loss is caused by an increase in IOP, which damages the optic nerve. This damage is referred to as "cupping" of the disc. In a normal fundus examination, the ratio of cup size to optic disc diameter is less than 1:3. The optic disc has a depression (cup) that relates to the size of the optic nerve sheath fibers. In glaucoma, the optic disc increases in depth and diameter. The blood vessels are also displaced.

Because peripheral vision is lost slowly, the patient is not aware of any changes until much vision is lost. This is why glaucoma is commonly referred to as the "sneak thief" of sight. Testing for glaucoma is done with a tonometer (see Figure 29-8), which measures IOP. Persons age 40 and older should have their IOP measured every 2 or 3 years during their regular eye examination. More frequent testing is recommended when there is a family history of glaucoma. The local Society for the Prevention of Blindness regularly provides information about the disease and about free testing in the community.

The two main types of glaucoma are angle-closure glaucoma, or narrow-angle glaucoma, and open-angle glaucoma, or chronic open-angle glaucoma (Figure 29-21). In angle-closure glaucoma, the iris pushes up against the cornea and blocks the flow of aqueous, which is an ocular emergency.

In chronic open-angle glaucoma, the blockage is located near the trabecular meshwork and Schlemm's canal. Symptoms are apparent only after vision is lost and may include frequent mild headaches, halos around lights, intermittent blurred vision, difficulty with night vision or adaption to dark rooms and movie theaters, loss of peripheral vision, and frequent change of glasses. Diagnosis of the disease is made by assessing intraocular pressure (normal range is 12 to 20 mm Hg), optic disc abnormalities, and visual field loss. Treatment is designed to decrease the IOP medically by decreasing the pupil size (miotic drops) or by decreasing aqueous production (carbonic anhydrase inhibitors) or both (Table 29-2). When maximum medical therapy fails, laser treatments or operative procedures are needed to preserve the remaining vision.

Argon laser iridectomy is a noninvasive procedure used to treat angle-closure glaucoma. For this procedure to be done easily, the cornea must be clear. It is considered a preventive procedure when used to treat narrow-angle glaucoma before an actual attack. Surgical iridectomies are rarely done today. The argon laser can also be used for a noninvasive procedure called a laser **trabeculoplasty.** Initially, an area covering approximately 180 degrees of the trabecular meshwork is treated. If pressure remains elevated, the remaining 180 degrees can be treated in a similar fashion. Frequently, the IOP increases after both types of laser surgery. The pressure is checked before the patient is released, approximately 1 to 2 hours after the procedure (Nowell, 1990).

Surgical *trabeculectomy* or filtration surgery may be required if other methods fail to control IOP. A portion of the trabecular meshwork is surgically incised to create an alternate drainage channel for the aqueous (Spires, 1991). This fistula then allows aqueous to be absorbed underneath the conjunctiva. Nursing interven-

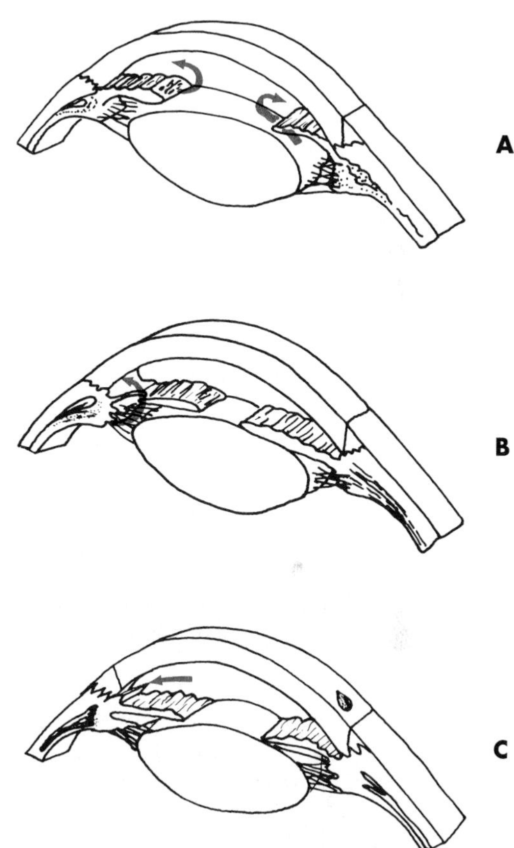

Figure 29-21 **A,** In the normal eye, aqueous produced by ciliary body flows through trabecular meshwork into Schlemm's canal to return to general circulation. **B,** In acute congestive, or narrow-angle, glaucoma, angle of anterior chamber is too narrow and aqueous cannot enter canal. Treatment includes use of miotics to constrict pupil and widen angle, as well as laser trabeculoplasty and peripheral iridectomy to provide supplementary channel. **C,** In chronic wide-angle glaucoma, the problem is in overproduction or decreased absorption of aqueous by the trabecular structures. When maximum medical therapy is no longer effective or tolerated or if there is a compliance problem, laser trabeculoplasty or filtration surgery may be indicated to improve aqueous outflow. (Modified from Kornzweig AL: Visual loss in the elderly, *Hosp Prac* 12(7) and from Reichel W, editor: *The geriatric patient,* New York, 1978, HP Publishing. Reprinted with permission.)

tions are those stated for intraocular surgery in Box 29-3, with an additional consideration: strict aseptic administration of eye drops is essential. The intraocular contents are now separated from external contamination by one layer, the conjunctiva, and bacteria have easier access to the inner eye. Complications of the procedure include a flat anterior chamber, soft eye, failure to filter, hyphema, endophthalmitis, cataract formation, and corneal decompensation. Failure to filter (drain) after the surgery has been attributable to scar tissue forming and blocking the site. Two antimetabolite drugs, mitomycin and 5-fluorouracil (5-FU), have been used to decrease the scarring, but dosage levels and administration technique have not yet been established. Glaucoma implants to shunt aqueous from the anterior chamber to a disc sewn to the sclera are in the developing stages and are being used on some patients.

As a last resort for uncontrolled glaucoma, *cyclocryopexy* or cryosurgery is done. A freezing probe is used to destroy a portion of the ciliary body that produces the aqueous. Because of the tissue destruction, patients undergoing this procedure experience much pain. Treatment includes pain medication, steroids, and atropine.

Compliance with prescribed regimens is important to glaucoma patients, but it is difficult for many reasons: (1) daily drops do not improve existing vision; a patient who also has a cataract may experience decreased vision because of pupil constriction; (2) systemic medications have bothersome or toxic side effects; (3) drops may be difficult to administer because of physical limitations such as arthritis; and (4) treatment is a lifelong concern (Box 29-9).

Cataract

A cataract is an opacity in the lens of the eye that may cause a loss of visual acuity and loss of the ability to function autonomously (Figure 29-22). The Agency for Health Care Policy and Research (AHCPR) describes functional impairment as a result of a cataract in the adult as the decreased ability to (1) perform everyday activities such as driving, using the phone, taking medicine; (2) engage in hobbies and leisure activities such as reading and viewing television; and (3) work at one's occupation (Cataract Management Guideline Panel, 1993).

Because the lens focuses light rays on the retina, a clouding of this structure causes a painless loss of vision that can progress over time. Cataracts associated

BOX 29-9 **Nursing Process**

GLAUCOMA

ASSESSMENT

Visual loss
Loss of peripheral vision
Level of comfort
Ability to care for self

NURSING DIAGNOSES

Sensory/perceptual alterations: visual related to disease process
Anxiety related to possible loss of vision
Self-care deficit related to decreased visual acuity
Pain related to sudden increased IOP
Diversional activity deficit related to decreased vision
Risk for injury (trauma) related to decreased vision
Knowledge deficit related to new condition, treatment, and medications

NURSING INTERVENTIONS

Listen actively to patient concerns.
Help patient manage visual limitations.
Assist with personal hygiene as indicated.
Reduce clutter in the immediate environment.
Administer medications as ordered.
Provide analgesics as needed for acute glaucoma.
Prepare patient for surgical intervention as indicated.
Recommend that family members be examined regularly.

EVALUATION OF EXPECTED OUTCOMES

Maintains current vision without further loss
Expresses concerns and anxiety
Verbalizes understanding of condition and treatment
Demonstrates correct instillation of eye medications
Able to care for self with assistance if necessary
Exhibits safety measures in home environment
Maintains acceptable level of comfort

with the aging process are called senile cataracts. Other causes are congenital defects, intraocular infections, and trauma—surgical, blunt, or radiation. Factors that may influence formation of cataracts are diabetes, drugs, ultraviolet (UV) radiation, and nutritional deficiencies. Most cataracts are not visible to the naked eye until they become very dense, but an ophthalmoscopic examination or slit lamp examination can detect the opacities at earlier stages (Ruehl, Schremp, 1992).

Symptoms of cataract formation include difficulty in reading, driving at night, seeing well in bright light, increased sensitivity to glare, decreasing color vision, and double vision.

Diagnosis of cataract begins with a thorough patient history, including medical, surgical, and family history, as well as medications taken. The nurse should document allergies and when visual changes were first noted. The eye examination includes visual acuity tests for distance vision and near vision. Contrast sensitivity and glare disability may be assessed. However, the judgment of the AHCPR panel is that more research is necessary to corroborate the need for these tests (Cataract Management Guideline Panel, 1993).

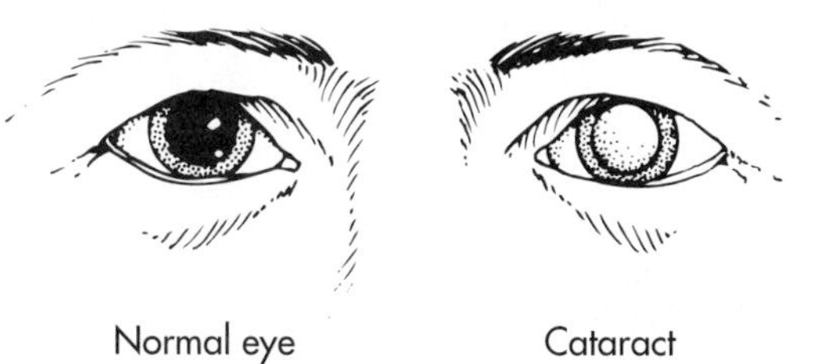

Figure 29-22 Cataract, visible in left eye as white opacity of lens, is seen through pupil. (From Phipps WJ and others: *Medical-surgical nursing: concepts and clinical practice,* ed 5, St Louis, 1995, Mosby.)

The direct ophthalmoscope and slit lamp are used to examine the lens and other structures in the eye so that the general health of the eye can be evaluated. If an intraocular lens implant is to be used to replace the natural lens, A-scan and keratometry are performed to determine the correct lens implant strength.

The cure for a cataract is surgical removal. Cataract extraction is not considered an emergency for the most part, and nonsurgical treatments can be tried. This may include stronger eye glasses, magnification devices, and better illumination. The best judge for surgery is the patient, as well as quality-of-life issues as they relate to his or her visual and functional needs.

Cataract surgery is usually performed on an outpatient basis except in cases where there is a preexisting medical condition. Conditions requiring inpatient care include (1) surgery on the only eye, (2) mental disturbances, (3) physical disability preventing immediate postoperative care, and (4) a medical condition needing observation by a nurse or skilled professional. Most cataract surgery is performed under local anesthesia. However, general anesthesia is indicated in cases of extreme anxiety, a known allergy to local anesthetics, skeletal or other disorders preventing lying still, a language barrier, or inability to cooperate for other reasons (Cataract Management Guideline Panel, 1993).

There are two surgical types of cataract extraction: intracapsular extraction and extracapsular extraction (Figure 29-23). In intracapsular cataract extraction, the lens and surrounding capsular layer are removed intact. Approximately 98% of all cataract surgery is done by extracapsular extraction, and this procedure can be performed by either of two techniques: planned extracapsular cataract extraction or **phacoemulsification** (Ruehl, Schremp, 1992). In planned extracapsular extraction, the anterior portion of the capsule surround-

A 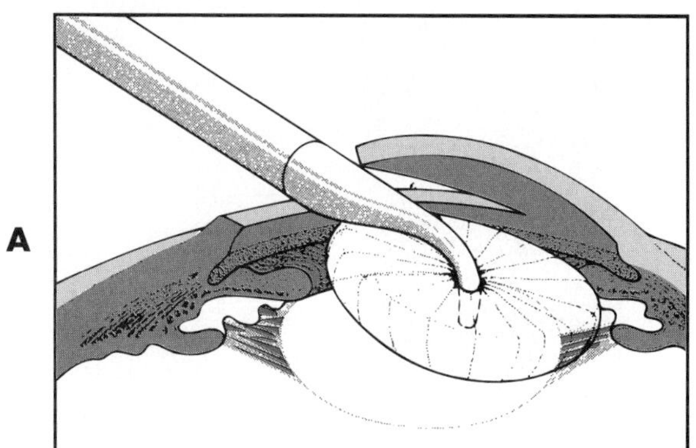

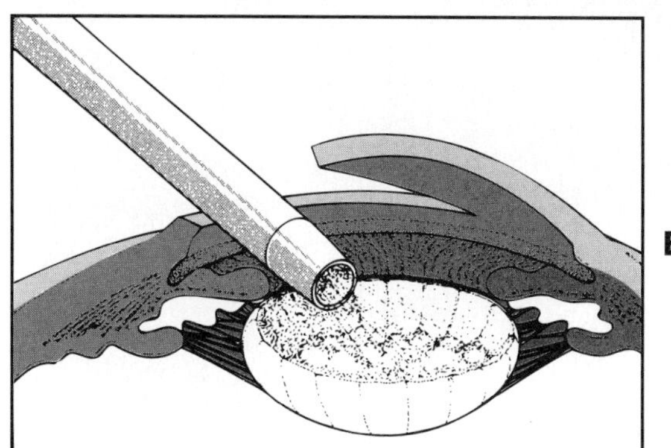 B

Figure 29-23 Cataract extraction. **A,** Intracapsular, when lens and capsule are removed. **B,** Extracapsular, when lens and only the anterior part of the capsule are removed. (From Beare PG, Myers JK: *Principles and practice of adult health nursing,* ed 2, St Louis, 1994, Mosby.)

ing the lens is removed before the lens nucleus is extracted. The cortex of the lens is then removed, leaving behind the posterior portion of the capsule. In phacoemulsification, the surgical incision is smaller because the lens nucleus is fragmented ultrasonically and irrigated and aspirated from the eye. The cortex is removed in a manner similar to extracapsular technique. The lens implant is placed in the posterior remnant of the capsule with either technique (Figures 29-24, 29-25, and 29-26).

The normal eye is described as being phakic because it has a lens. When the lens is removed, the eye becomes *aphakic* (absence of lens) and cannot accommodate or refract light properly. Therefore a replacement lens is needed. Glasses or a contact lens can be used after cataract surgery, but the usual lens choice is the intraocular lens implant (IOL). With the IOL the eye is considered **pseudophakic** (having an artificial lens). Lens implants are manufactured from polymethylmethacrylate (PMMA), silicone, or hydrogel. They are designed in various sizes and shapes with structures to hold them in a stable position within the eye (Ruehl, Schremp, 1992). The artificial lens is not able to accommodate (change focus) so glasses may still be needed by the patient to achieve the best near or distance vision. Most lens implants are placed in the posterior capsule today. However, anterior chamber lenses, those placed in front of the iris, are used in certain cases where support of the capsule is absent (Ruehl, Schremp, 1992).

Complications of cataract surgery include vitreous loss, inflammation, increased IOP, macular edema, retinal detachment, hyphema, endophthalmitis, and expulsive hemorrhage.

After cataract surgery a patch and shield are placed over the operative eye. Written instructions from the physician should be reviewed with the patient. Because depth perception is compromised, mobility guid-

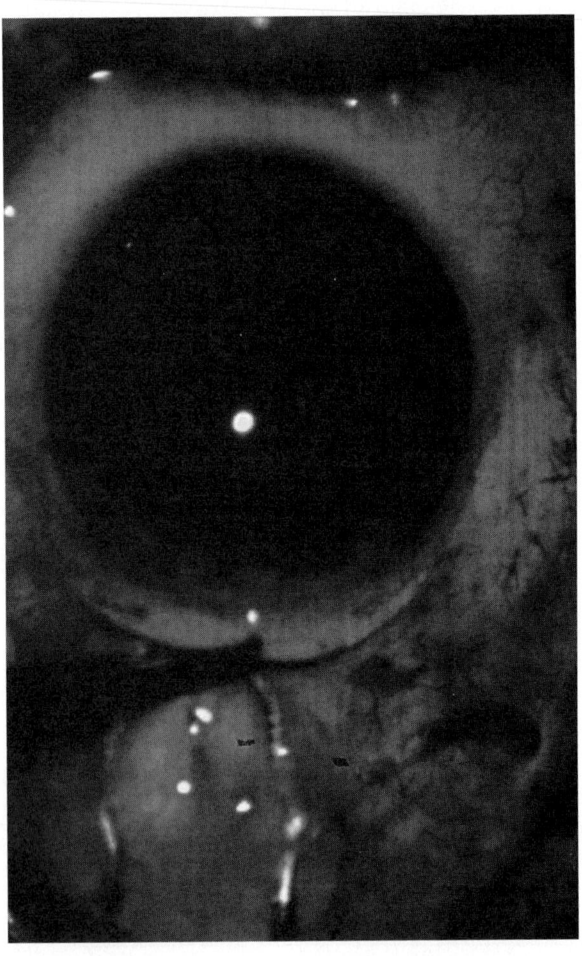

Figure 29-24 Delivery of the lens nucleus as seen in planned extracapsular surgery. (Photo courtesy of Dr. J. B. Rubenstein, Chicago, Ill.)

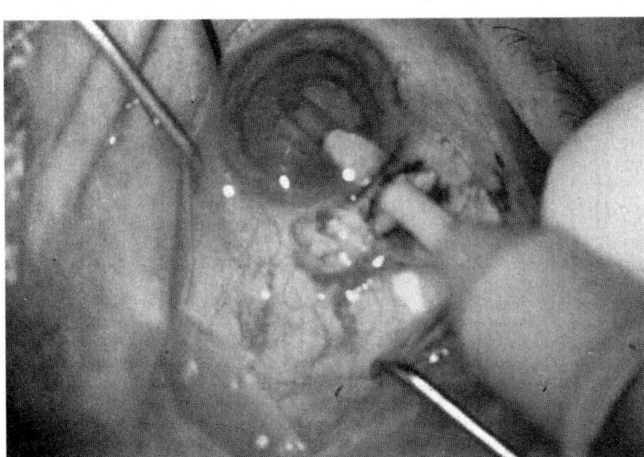

Figure 29-25 Ultrasonic aspiration of lens nucleus with phacoemulsification instrument. (Photo courtesy of Dr. J. B. Rubenstein, Chicago, Ill.)

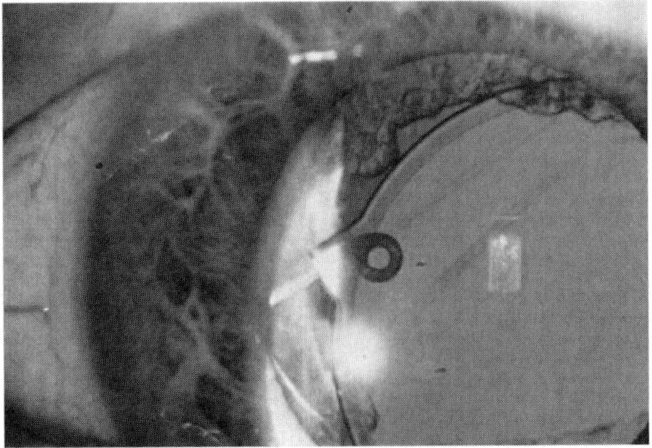

Figure 29-26 Intraocular lens implant following cataract extraction. (Photo courtesy of Dr. R. J. Epstein, Chicago, Ill.)

ance is needed. Discharge instructions include leaving the dressing in place with a protective shield, avoiding strenuous activity and reading, eating moderately, and notifying the physician of severe pain. Heavy lifting, straining at elimination, and bending the head lower than the waist are examples of activities to avoid. Lid hygiene should be done daily. Common sense instructions are to wash hands before and after drop/ointment instillation, avoid falling or bumping the eye, and wear sunglasses for glare or photophobia. The ophthalmologist examines the patient the first postoperative day, at 1 week, 3 weeks, and 6 weeks after surgery unless there are complications. Total visual rehabilitation takes from 6 to 12 weeks.

Vitreous Pathology

Normal vitreous can be observed by means of a slit-lamp examination. This transparent, colorless gel can become clouded with cell debris or membranes from acquired systemic diseases such as diabetes and hypertension. "Floaters" or "flashing lights" are often symptoms that a patient describes to the physician. This light flash is caused by cells floating across the pupillary space and casting a shadow on the retina. This can occur normally with age as the vitreous gel liquifies or as blood cells or pigments float into the gel. However, persistent floaters or showers of neon-type lights need to be evaluated for possible treatment (Vaughan, Asbury, Riordan-Eva, 1992). An immediate decrease in vision could be a symptom of vitreous hemorrhage, especially in patients with diabetic retinopathy. Inflammation or infection also can cause the vitreous to cloud.

Endophthalmitis, an extensive intraocular infection, may occur after penetrating injuries to the globe or as a postoperative complication of intraocular surgery. To properly diagnose and treat endophthalmitis, a vitreous tap is done to identify the cause of the infection. Current treatment for endophthalmitis includes antibiotic therapy (systemic, intraocular, intravitreal, and topical), with or without **vitrectomy** (removal of diseased vitreous). Symptoms include pain and decreased vision, although pain is not always present. Signs are corneal haze, periorbital bruising, haze or cells in the anterior chamber, hypopyon (pus or cells in the anterior chamber), and decreased red reflex.

Vitrectomy

Conditions for which vitrectomy may be necessary include endophthalmitis, vitreous hemorrhage, retinal membranes, cytomegalovirus (CMV) retinitis, and traction retinal detachment. It is also done in conjunction with scleral buckling for retinal detachment repair. In cases with dense vitreous opacities, B-scan ultrasonography can be used to locate membranes and intraocular foreign bodies, as well as normal vitreous and retinal structures.

Pars plana vitrectomy is a microscopic technique in which three incisions are made in the globe. One provides infusion to maintain the pressure within the eye, and the other two are for an illumination probe and the vitreous cutting instrumentation (Figure 29-27). Laser or cautery may also be used through one of these incisions. Contact lenses are used on the cornea during the surgery to provide a better view of the inside of the eye. Air, surgical gases, or silicone oil can be instilled through the infusion port to provide pressure to the retina. Unlike air, some of these gases expand after a few days. Therefore, IOP is carefully monitored during this time. Slowly the gases are resorbed and replaced by intraocular fluids. Changes in air pressure may influence the gas bubble, so flying in airplanes is to be avoided.

Vitrectomy usually requires a 23-hour observation status, and the preoperative patient may be admitted to the hospital the day of surgery. Other patients may be hospitalized for 2 or 3 days. They often have systemic disease problems that must be evaluated by the physicians (ophthalmologist, internist, anesthesiologist) before surgery is performed. Instructions to the patient for activity, postoperative positioning, comfort expectations relating to pain or nausea, and eye medication procedures should be provided before surgery. It is important to give emotional support and allow the patient to express fears concerning visual prognosis.

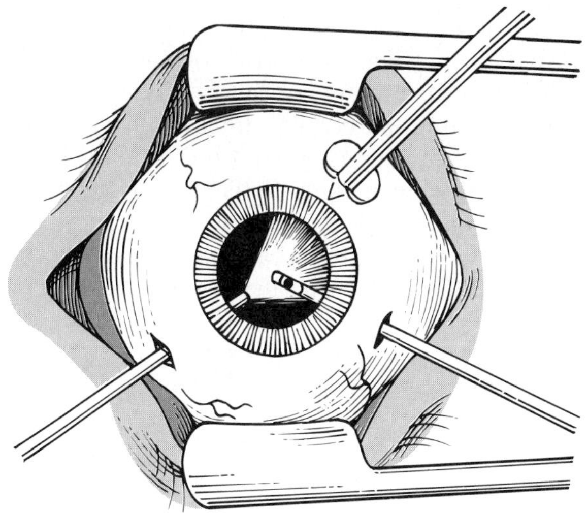

Figure 29-27 The vitrectomy instrument and fiberoptic illuminator are positioned in the anterior vitreous cavity and visualized through the pupil.

Vitrectomy is an intraocular procedure (see Box 29-7). The eye is kept dilated postoperatively with cyclopentolate (Cyclogyl) and tropicamide (Mydriacyl). Other drops include an antibiotic/antiinflammatory medication. Patients with an air or gas bubble in the eye may need to position the head so that the bubble presses on the area of the retina that needs to be flattened. This may require prone position with the head down or turned to the side. While the patient is awake, the bedside table can be used to help maintain this position. A foam head donut provides additional comfort. Marking the eye shield with an arrow indicating the desired bubble position is also helpful. Ice packs can reduce some of the swelling. Additional considerations for vitreous surgery include medication for nausea and for pain caused by edema and increased pressure on the eye.

Strenuous activity is limited for 2 weeks. Driving a car is not allowed, but riding as a passenger is. A patch may be needed for comfort because of epiphora or photophobia. Dark glasses can be worn during the day to protect the eye, but the shield is preferable at night. Aching or cramp-like pains may be common and can be relieved with a nonaspirin medication. Severe pain or change in vision needs to be reported to the physician. Lid hygiene can be followed (see Box 29-4). Results for visual acuity depend on the reason for surgery. If the macula is involved, central vision is compromised.

Retinal Pathology

The entire retina can be visualized with the direct or indirect ophthalmoscope. Abnormalities of the vessels or retinal tissues can be seen, and systemic diseases often reveal themselves by producing characteristic changes in the retina. Treatment of the eye involves treatment of the underlying causes as well. The most common findings are complications related to diabetes mellitus and hypertension. Sickle cell disease, histoplasmosis, leukemia, lupus erythematosus, human immunodeficiency virus (HIV), and metastatic disease can be diagnosed by fundus examination. Abnormalities of the arteries and veins in the retina are indicators for disease elsewhere. The test for diagnosing retinal circulation abnormalities is called intravenous fluorescein angiography (Boyd-Monk, 1990).

Diabetic retinopathy is a progressive disease affecting the blood vessels in the retina. Initially, the blood vessels become more narrow and at times occlude. The narrowed vessels can develop aneurysms that can leak or rupture. New abnormal vessels grow to supply needed oxygen to the tissue, but these vessels also leak fluid. This continuing process results in decreased vision as a result of scar tissue formation. The amount of visual loss depends on the location of the disease (central vs. peripheral vision) (Smith, 1992).

Patients who have had diabetes for 15 years or more are more likely to develop diabetic retinopathy. Research reported by the American Diabetic Association indicates that diabetics are 25 times as likely to experience vision loss and blindness as the general population. Diabetic retinopathy is classified as *background diabetic retinopathy* (BDR) and *proliferative diabetic retinopathy* (PDR). Microaneurysms, hard exudates, hemorrhages, and cotton-wool spots are signs of background diabetic retinopathy. The vision loss is a result of macular edema from the leaking vessels. In proliferative diabetic retinopathy, new blood vessels grow (neovascularization) to supply oxygen to the tissues. These new vessels grow over the macula and retinal surface. Fibrovascular tissue develops because of the continued leakage of blood from these vessels. These newly formed fibrous membranes are attached to the retina and to the posterior vitreous. The pulling of this scar-like tissue may cause a vitreous hemorrhage or a traction retinal detachment, which are the causes for vision loss in PDR.

Treatment for BDR is laser therapy on the specific leaking vessels to reduce the macular edema. This can be done with topical anesthesia only, and more than one treatment may be necessary. Panretinal photocoagulation (PRP), a therapeutic procedure involving scattered laser spots to the peripheral retina, is used for PDR. Local and topical anesthesia are necessary for this procedure (McEvoy, 1994; Smith, 1992), which helps stabilize vision if the neovascularization regresses. Vitrectomy surgery is recommended for longstanding vitreous hemorrhage, traction retinal detachment, or fibrous membranes pulling on the retina or vitreous. Diabetics who experience vision loss as a result of diabetic retinopathy need a planned educational program to help manage their diabetes. With decreased vision, it is more difficult to monitor blood sugar and identify and administer their insulin. Methods for shopping, preparing meals, and instilling eye drops properly need to be individualized. Patient compliance and improved patient outcomes can be increased by appropriate nursing interventions. Patient understanding and knowledge, personal independence, and patient/family use of community resources are areas in which nurses and diabetes educators can collaborate to ensure the best overall health of the individual. A thorough eye examination by an ophthalmologist is recommended for people with type I or type II diabetes. This baseline evaluation can be used to monitor changes that may occur later. Routine yearly examinations are recommended unless vision changes noticeably (Smith, 1992).

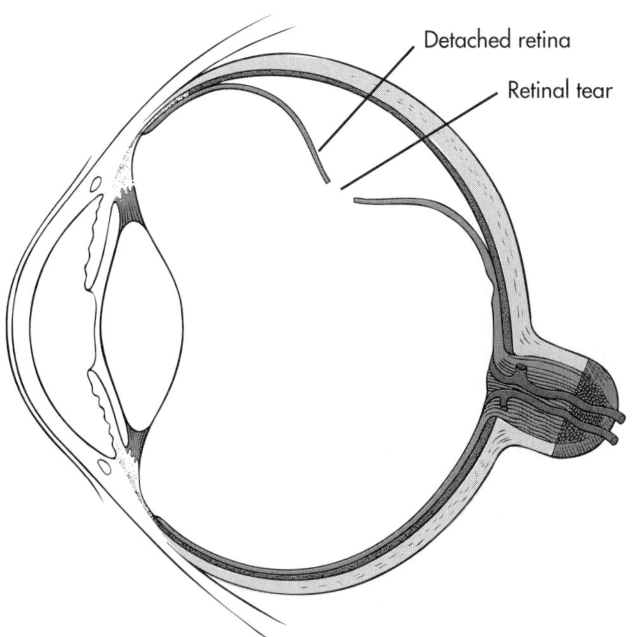

Figure 29-28 Retinal detachment. (From Phipps WJ and others: *Medical-surgical nursing: concepts and clinical practice,* ed 5, St Louis, 1995, Mosby.)

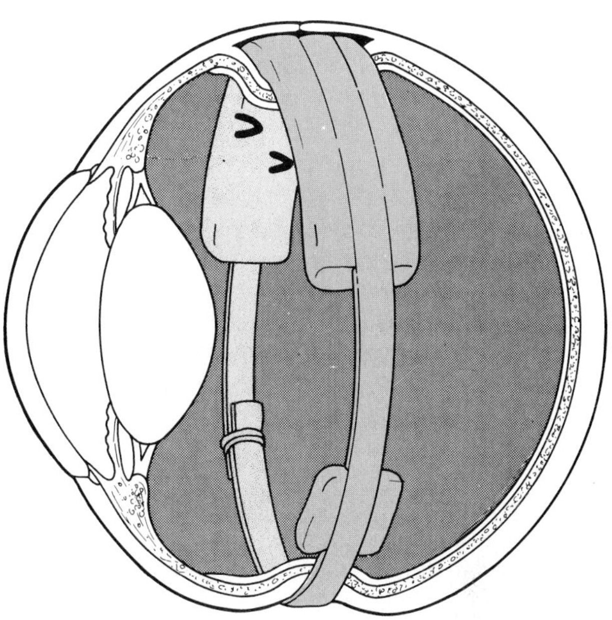

Figure 29-29 Scleral buckle. (From Phipps WJ and others: *Medical-surgical nursing: concepts and clinical practice,* ed 5, St Louis, 1995, Mosby.)

Retinal Detachment

A retinal detachment is a separation of the sensory retina from the pigmented layer with a subsequent subretinal fluid accumulation between the layers (Figure 29-28). Unless the retina is reattached, total blindness will develop. Predisposing factors include lattice degeneration, advanced myopia, cataract surgery, glaucoma, trauma, retinal detachment in the fellow eye, and a family history of retinal detachment.

Symptoms include a "shower" or "flashes" of light, floaters, or visual field defects. Vision is sometimes described as seeing through a veil or cobweb. The vision loss experienced depends upon the location of the detachment. Peripheral vision is affected first, and then the central vision if the macula becomes involved. There can be one or more breaks or holes in the retina, and all breaks need to be found and repaired. Three methods can be used for repair: (1) *scleral buckling* (Figure 29-29), (2) *pneumatic retinopexy* (injecting air into the vitreous space), and (3) *vitrectomy* (Vaughan, Asbury, Riordan-Eva, 1992). Scleral buckling is the traditional technique for a rhegmatogenous (break or hole in the retina) detachment. It is indicated for multiple breaks, lattice degeneration, and vitreous traction. Pneumatic retinopexy is not a procedure that requires hospitalization, but it has drawbacks in that it cannot be used to relieve traction of the vitreous or to repair multiple retinal breaks. However, with either technique—scleral buckling or pneumatic retinopexy—transconjunctival cryotherapy or laser is applied to the break or hole. Patient compliance is required for postoperative positioning of the air. Followup is required at 1, 2, and 4 weeks. Complications include recurrent detachment, increased IOP, more breaks, and endophthalmitis. Vitrectomy is used for complicated detachments, giant retinal tears, detachment as a result of macular holes, and vitreous traction with membranes. Other conditions that may require vitrectomy are recurrent detachments after scleral buckling and opacities in the vitreous.

Scleral buckling procedures can be done with local or general anesthesia. The physician locates the breaks in the retina by using the indirect ophthalmoscope, and cryotherapy is applied to the breaks and other areas of weakness. Various silicone implants are used to reattach the retina. These can be encircling bands to "belt buckle" the globe or radial components sewn to the sclera. Subretinal fluid that has collected may then be drained through a small incision under the "buckle." Complications include redetachment, increased IOP, central retinal artery occlusion, deep sutures, choroidal detachment, infection, extrusion of the implant, and eye muscle disturbance. Prognosis for visual outcome is decreased if the macula is involved. When a patient has a retinal detachment and the macula is still attached, surgery is urgent if central vision is to be preserved. Followup examinations are scheduled for 1 week, 3 weeks, and 6 weeks postoperatively (Box 29-10).

BOX 29-10 **Nursing Process**

EXTRAOCULAR SURGERY (EYE MUSCLES, EYELIDS, ORBIT, LACRIMAL-DUCT PROBING, SCLERAL BUCKLING, ENUCLEATION)

ASSESSMENT

Vital signs per routine
Eye dressing
Level of comfort
Ability to care for self for signs of disorientation

NURSING DIAGNOSES

Anxiety related to decreased vision, cosmesis, or surgical outcome
Impaired physical mobility related to vision or postoperative positioning
Risk for injury related to visual deficit and to decreased depth perception
Knowledge deficit related to surgical repair and to activity restrictions
Sensory/perceptual alterations: visual related to patching and ointment in the eye
Risk for infection related to surgical procedure
Pain related to light sensitivity and to the surgical procedure

NURSING INTERVENTIONS

Listen actively to the patient's concerns.
Provide information and reassurance.
Position the patient according to physician's order.
Ambulate patient with assistance.
Speak slowly and clearly, and repeat if necessary.
Protect the eye with a patch, if needed, to reduce lid edema, to contain drainage, or to shield the eye from light.
Administer medications as ordered.
Provide ice packs to reduce edema.
Provide comfort measures.
Dim the room lights if dilating drops are used.
Provide light meals the first day.

EVALUATION OF EXPECTED OUTCOMES

Meets discharge criteria for the postsurgical patient (p. 487)
Expresses fears and concerns
Vision improved or maintained (not applicable for enucleation patients)
Able to ambulate with help
Uses other senses to avoid bumping eye when patched
Verbalizes understanding of instructions
Demonstrates ability to administer own medications
Able to return to normal activity, or has assistance until normal activity resumes
Knowledgeable about modifications at home to enhance safety

Macular Degeneration

Age-related macular degeneration (ARMD) is a disease associated with central vision loss and affects people age 50 and over (Figure 29-30). The two types of ARMD are "dry" (atrophic) and "exudative" (neovascular). Atrophic macular degeneration accounts for 70% to 90% of the cases (Vaughan, Asbury, Riordan-Eva, 1992). It is caused by a weakening and deterioration of the retinal cells and is seen as visible changes in the retina. Visual changes are variable and may be minimal. These changes may progress or stabilize. No treatment is available. Because the exudative stage can develop later, patients are advised to have their vision monitored with an Amsler grid (Boyd-Monk, 1990). Exudative macular degeneration accounts for 10% of the cases of ARMD but is responsible for 90% of all legal blindness as a result of ARMD. In exudative ARMD, abnormal blood vessels in the retina leak fluid, which results in scar tissue formation. This is followed by a proliferation of more abnormal new vessels (neovascularization). Early symptoms include difficulty with reading, blurred vision, and distortion of straight objects and straight lines. Eventually the entire central vision may be affected in one or both eyes. Peripheral vision, however, is not affected (Vader, 1992). Laser treatment of subretinal neovascularization in selected patients where the fovea is not involved has been done (Olk, 1992). Because this laser treatment itself destroys part of the retinal tissue, some central vision will be affected. Even after successful therapy, recurrent neovascularization may develop within 2 years. Eventually many patients with exudative ARMD become "legally blind" and will need to alter their patterns and habits of daily living. Assessment of the patient's understanding and desire for help is essential for individualized care.

Low-vision referral and evaluation can help the patient use the remaining peripheral vision to the maximum. Recognizing that grieving over vision loss is a natural process, the nurse should encourage the patient to participate in support groups that include other members of the family, who also need help in coping with the loss (Woods, 1992). Low-vision care is available and needs to be a part of ophthalmic health-

A 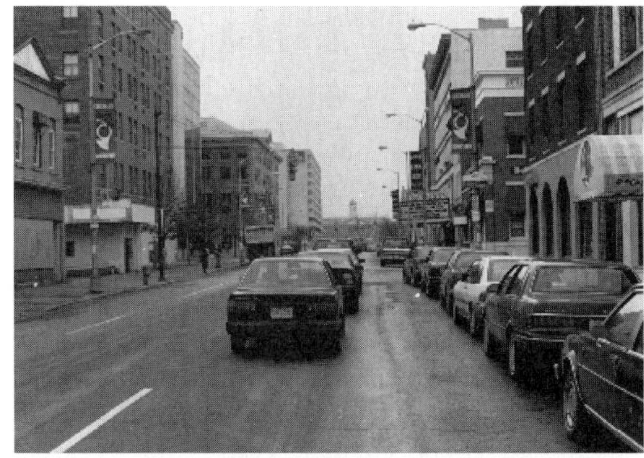 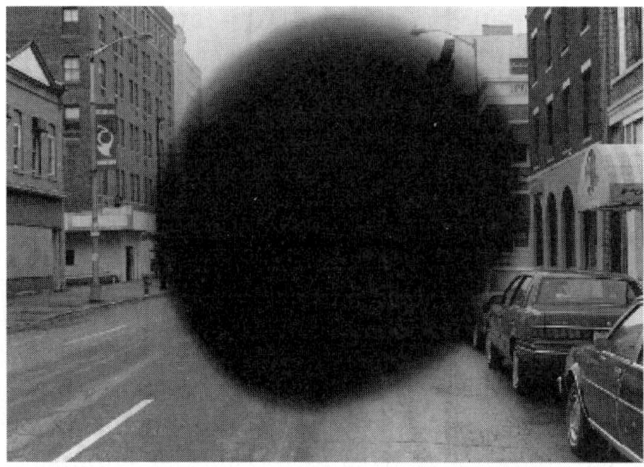 B

Figure 29-30 **A,** The road as it appears to a person with normal central and peripheral fields of vision. **B,** Loss of central field as seen in macular degeneration. The central field of vision is indistinct, whereas the peripheral field of vision remains clear.

BOX 29-11

GUIDELINES FOR INTERACTING WITH THE VISUALLY IMPAIRED

- When approaching, announce yourself each time and call the person by name. State the time of day if appropriate.
- Explain procedures before you begin. Do not touch the person before you speak.
- Let the person know when you are leaving so that the embarrassment of speaking when no one is present can be avoided.
- Remember that hearing is not impaired. Speak in a normal tone.
- When walking, the person grasps your arm and walks a half step behind you.
- Note obstacles on either side when walking.
- Before seating the person, place his or her hand on the back or arm of a chair. Stay nearby while the person sits down.
- At mealtime explain the menu. Arrange the food at clock hours. Explain the hot foods and place them where they will not be spilled.
- In the hospital, orient the patient thoroughly to the environment. Note placement of furniture, phone, and call light.
- Place a sign on the door or over the bed indicating the person's visual status so that all personnel can approach correctly.

BOX 29-12

HOME HELPS FOR THE VISUALLY IMPAIRED

- Encourage family and friends to keep furniture and objects in the same place.
- Place food, cooking utensils, and supplies in specific locations in the refrigerator and cupboards.
- Place clothing in specific locations in the closets and drawers, or label with identifying or distinguishing marks.
- Arrange money in wallet compartments according to denomination or fold different denominations in different ways.
- Investigate low-vision aids that may be of help, including magnifiers, large-print books and magazines, colored lenses, high-contrast paint, voice-activated phones, calculators, tapes, clocks, and watches. Also investigate special radio receivers that provide programming on a full range of subject matter such as employment, news, business, and sports.

care (Boxes 29-11 and 29-12). Centers designed for rehabilitation teach the patient how to maintain his or her independence and function in activities of daily living. Special services are individualized to each patient. Optical and nonoptical aids are available. Mobility training, educational assessment, job rehabilitation, and counseling help the patient and the family to adjust to the vision loss. National, state, and local agencies provide special services. Catalogs and literature are available from the U. S. Department of Health and Human Services. Among the other agencies that provide resources are the American Foundation for the Blind, American Printing House for the Blind, Guide Dogs for the Blind, and National Society for the Prevention of Blindness.

Retinopathy of Prematurity

Retinopathy of prematurity (ROP), previously called retrolental fibroplasia (RLF), is a bilateral retinal disease that has been increasing. This is attributed to the increased survival rate of low-birth-weight (<1000 g) infants and the possibility that premature birth may trigger the onset of ROP (American Academy of Ophthalmology, 1994-95). Other factors may include high oxygen concentration and increased partial pressure of carbon dioxide (Pco_2) (Spires, 1991). Retinal vessels begin to develop at 16 weeks of gestation and are complete at 40 weeks. In a premature infant, an attempt to complete this vascularization process results in development of abnormal vessels. These vessels may then bleed and form scars, which may result in retinal detachment.

Careful screening for ROP in all premature infants should begin in the neonatal intensive care unit at 4 to 6 weeks after birth. Follow-up examinations are done every 2 weeks thereafter until the retina is fully vascularized. Most early stages of ROP resolve spontaneously. Cryotherapy is used to help regress the proliferation of abnormal vessels that cause retinal detachment, and some of the newer treatments for ROP show some promise. A study is being done to evaluate the effectiveness of indirect laser photocoagulation as a treatment alternative to cryotherapy. Repair of total retinal detachment through a vitrectomy approach is becoming more successful, and studies show that early cryotherapy reduces the rate of retinal detachment. Parent education while the infant is hospitalized is most important. ROP can lead to blindness, and there is high risk for myopia, amblyopia, strabismus, glaucoma, and cosmetic defects. Parents need to know early in the premature infant's life that appropriate follow-up by an ophthalmologist gives the infant the best chance for visual rehabilitation.

Ocular Malignancies

Although it is rare and affects relatively few people, *choroidal melanoma* is the most common adult primary intraocular tumor. It is found mostly in patients between ages 53 and 60 but has been documented in teens and older adults (Servodidio, Abramson, 1992). Symptoms include blurring of vision, defects in the visual field, "floaters," pain, or "flashing" of light. Decrease in visual acuity and defects in the visual field are the most common presenting signs. The size of the tumor is determined by A-scan ultrasonography and fundus examination. After the diagnosis has been made, a metastatic workup that includes a liver scan is done to determine whether the disease has spread into the orbit or through the sclera into the blood. Treatment options include enucleation, radiation, or radioactive plaque therapy. Follow-up is required every 6 to 12 months for life (Servodidio, 1991). Teaching aids to demonstrate the location of the tumor inside the eye can also be used to explain the plaque placement if that is the treatment used. Ocular prostheses should be available to show the patients if they so desire. Written postoperative instructions that can be individualized need to be used in conjunction with the verbal teaching plan.

Retinoblastoma

The most common childhood intraocular tumor is retinoblastoma (1 per 17,000 live births). Most cases appear by the age of 3, and the tumor can affect one or both eyes. A parent who has the disease has a 50% chance of having an affected child. The most obvious sign is the characteristic "cat's eye reflex," a bright reflection from the pupil. Other signs are strabismus, tearing, inflammation, pain, and poor vision. A metastatic workup should follow a positive diagnosis. Treatment includes enucleation, external beam radiation, or irradiation plaque therapy. Vision prognosis in the fellow eye is excellent. Discharge planning involves teaching the parent how to care for the enucleation site by maintaining lid hygiene and instilling ointment or drops. Follow-up appointments are essential for evaluating a recurrence. Support groups and counseling help the parents to deal with guilt feelings associated with the disease, and genetic counseling can be suggested (Servodidio, 1993). Changes in the visual fields of successfully treated retinoblastoma patients can challenge the child's ability to keep up in school. With limited peripheral vision, reading can be a problem. Maximizing available vision helps the child cope with daily activities, school, and sports in ways that maintain safety.

Human Immunodeficiency Virus

Ocular conditions, infectious or noninfectious, develop in 75% of persons with HIV (Plona, Schremp, 1992). Kaposi's sarcoma, which produces lesions on the eyelids and conjunctiva, is not infectious. Non-Hodgkin's lymphoma and HIV retinopathy also are considered noninfectious. Keratitis, particularly that caused by herpes simplex or herpes zoster, is one of the opportunistic infections that develop because AIDS patients are immunosuppressed.

Cytomegalovirus (CMV) retinitis is a sight-threatening infectious disease involving the retina. It usually begins in one eye but progresses to the other. Characteristic granular spots are evident in the retina. These spots enlarge, denoting retinal necrosis and vision loss. Current treatments for CMV retinitis are ganciclovir and trisodiumphosphonoformate, both of which must be monitored for bone marrow toxicity. Vitrectomy with silicone oil injection to treat retinal detachment caused by this virus is being evaluated.

Treatment for Kaposi's sarcoma may be indicated for cosmesis or to allow better closing of the eyelids.

Other treatment includes radiation or injection of chemotherapeutic drugs into the lesion.

Knowledge of ocular manifestations of AIDS and the treatment protocols will help in the total care of the AIDS patient. Nurses also should encourage patients to maintain their independence for as long as possible by making use of the resources available for educating low-vision persons and their families (Plona, Schremp, 1992).

Enucleation

Indications for surgical removal of the eyeball (enucleation) include severe trauma; malignant tumors; a painful, blind eye; and cosmesis. The surgery may involve the entire eye and related structures or only the contents of the eyeball (evisceration). Before the surgery takes place, the patient's knowledge of the diagnosis and treatment needs to be confirmed. Discussion of the permanence of the procedure should be accompanied by an explanation of the postoperative appearance, orbital implant, prosthesis, and the fitting procedure. A sympathetic, understanding approach is essential. The nurse should encourage questions. Self-concept will be changed by loss of the eye, so the grieving process is normal in these individuals. However, in cases in which the eye has caused severe pain, the patient may look forward to the relief provided by this surgery.

Immediate postoperative care includes a pressure dressing for 24 hours. The patient should be assessed for pain or hemorrhage, and if anticoagulants are part of the patient's preoperative routine, they are withheld during the immediate postoperative period. Excessive coughing and sneezing should be avoided. Ice packs may be applied to reduce swelling and pain.

When the eye socket has healed (2 to 6 weeks), the patient is fitted with a prosthesis. The prosthesis is made to fit over the ball implant that was surgically placed under the conjunctiva and Tenon's layer of the orbit. The prosthetic eye is made of plastic and is fitted and crafted by an oculist to match the iris, sclera, and veins of the other eye. Plastic is preferred to glass because it is more durable and lasts longer. Care, cleaning, insertion, and removal instructions need to be given to the patient. If the prosthesis needs to be stored, it should be stored in water or contact lens solution. Occasionally, people with artificial eyes will complain of a dry eye, which can be treated with artificial tears or lubricant. Points to reinforce with the patient are (1) when wiping the eye, wipe toward the nose with the eyes closed; this procedure prevents the prosthesis from dislodging; (2) alcohol, ether, chloroform, and other abrasive agents can damage the eye; (3) when participating in water sports, the eyes should be protected with goggles, or the prosthesis should be removed; (4) the remaining seeing eye should be protected with safety devices such as safety glasses, even if no eyeglass correction is needed; and (5) at yearly visits to the oculist, the cells and protein buildup on the artificial eye can be cleaned. Vision loss is more than just loss of sight. Learning to live with the loss requires adjusting and adapting. Body image, loss of a familiar lifestyle, occupational considerations, and financial concerns need to be addressed.

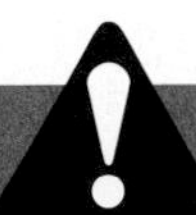

NURSE ALERT

Injuries to the retina caused by viewing a solar eclipse without proper filters or by observing the sun directly can result in eclipse retinopathy (solar retinitis). The edema may clear with no visual loss, or a permanent blind spot in the macula may result.

Lid Disorders and Defects

Marginal blepharitis is a chronic inflammatory process involving the margin of both eyelids and may be caused by bacteria, allergy, or degenerative diseases. The most common type of blepharitis is seborrheic. The patient often has a history of a similar scalp condition commonly known as dandruff, and the skin and scalp are often excessively oily. The first symptoms of the eyelids may be itching and burning. The lids are red and inflamed, with fine crust-like scales at the base of the eyelashes. Ulceration of the lids may develop. Treatment consists of application of warm, moist compresses and lid scrubs to remove the crusts. Medications such as sulfacetamide ointment may be prescribed for bedtime application in patients prone to the disease. Cleanliness of the hair, skin, and scalp is important in controlling the disease. Severe lid infections, or cellulitis, require systemic antibiotics to prevent spread of the infection into the orbit and then to the brain.

A *sty* (external hordeolum) is an infection of Zeis' or Moll's glands in the eyelid. An internal hordeolum is an infection of a meibomian gland. Sties are characterized by a small, inflamed swelling at the edge of the eyelid. As the swelling increases, the sty may rupture spontaneously and drain, after which healing occurs. Staphylococcus is often the causative organism, and systemic antibiotic therapy may be necessary. The condition can become chronic, and some cases require incision and drainage.

Chalazion is a sterile, granulomatous inflammation of a meibomian gland. It is found in the upper and lower eyelids and begins with an inflammation and tenderness. It does not have the acute signs of inflammation seen in a sty. The most common symptom is a painless swelling that develops over several weeks. In the early stages, warm, moist compresses may help reduce the inflammation. Antibiotics or steroids also may be injected into the lesion. Chalazions may need to be removed surgically, and any recurrences need to have biopsies performed to rule out malignancy.

Anatomical lid defects interfere with vision. Turning in of the lid, *entropion*, can be the result of aging, scar formation, or a congenital defect. Surgery is needed to prevent corneal irritation and damage caused by the lashes rubbing over the corneal surface. *Ectropion*, turning out or sagging of the lid, is also common in older people and is corrected by shortening the lower lid. Patients with this defect experience symptoms of exposure keratitis, tearing, and irritation. *Ptosis*, or drooping of the upper eyelid, can be congenital or acquired. To rule out myasthenia gravis as the cause, an edrophonium (Tensilon) test is performed. Surgery can be done to correct either congenital or acquired ptosis. Postoperative care includes ice compresses to decrease swelling and antibiotic ointment to prevent infection and to keep the cornea moist.

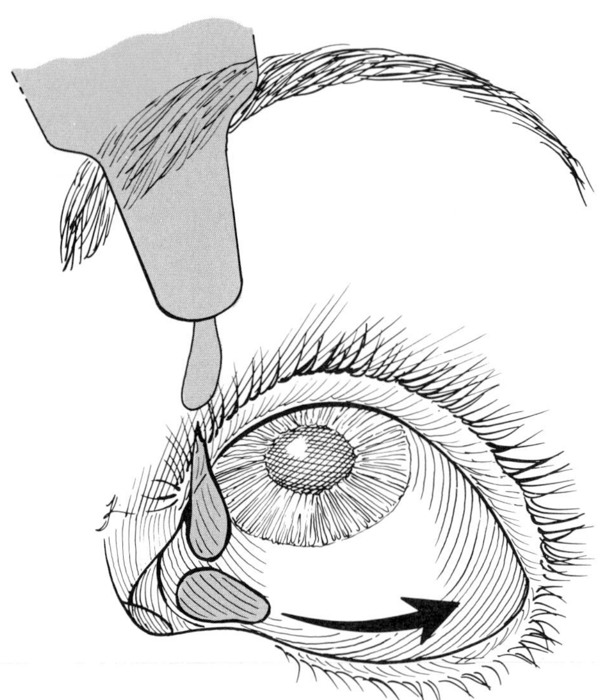

Figure 29-31 Irrigating the eye. Fluid is directed along conjunctiva and over eyeball from inner to outer canthus. (From Long BL, Phipps WJ: *Medical-surgical nursing: a nursing process approach*, ed 3, St Louis, 1993, Mosby.)

Lacrimal System Disorders

Dry-eye syndrome or *keratoconjunctivitis sicca* is the result of abnormalities of the tear film, eyelid surface, or corneal surface. Patients complain of a foreign-body sensation, itching, unusual mucous secretion, and burning. The condition is often associated with rheumatoid arthritis and autoimmune diseases. A Schirmer's test is done to assess tear production. Punctal occlusion, temporary or permanent, may be done to keep tears in the conjunctival sac. *Punctal obstruction* can be a congenital defect or the result of scarring as a result of infections, topical medications, or systemic chemotherapy. Blockage of the tear ducts causes a slight discharge and irritation of the eye. Patency needs to be established for normal tear flow. *Dacryocystitis* is an infection of the lacrimal sac. It can be the result of chronic infection, trauma, or a stone in the duct. Symptoms are purulent discharge and tearing (epiphora). Acute cases are treated with systemic antibiotics. Chronic cases may require surgery in which an opening is made between the lacrimal sac and the nose (Boyd-Monk, Steinmetz, 1987; Vaughan, Asbury, Riordan-Eva, 1992).

EYE EMERGENCIES AND TRAUMA

It is important to know which eye emergencies and trauma need immediate or urgent treatment and which ones can be referred. Treatment for chemical burns and sudden painless loss of vision should be done within minutes to preserve sight. *Chemical burns* should be irrigated immediately with copious amounts of water or noncaustic liquids such as milk. To prevent injury to the other eye, the head should be turned toward the affected eye for irrigation (Figure 29-31; Box 29-13). After 15 to 20 minutes of irrigation, the patient can be transported to a physician's office or emergency room. Here the injury and visual acuity are assessed, and testing for the type of chemical is done with litmus paper. Treatment includes cycloplegic medication, steroids, and antibiotics. To prevent *sudden vision loss* as a result of an occlusion of the central retinal artery, attempts to vasodilate the patient's retinal circulation should be made. Vasodilation can be accomplished by rebreathing into a paper bag, the idea being that the carbon dioxide buildup may help dilate the vessels. Intermittent pressure on the globe for several seconds with sudden releasing of the fingers may alter the IOP enough to dislodge the embolus. The chance of restoring sight is negligible after 30 minutes. For other eye emergencies treated in the office or emergency room, the first step is to assess the visual acuity of the injured eye. Although the patient may not want to cooperate, it is essential for medical and legal reasons. The actual ability to see may allay the anxiety related to the injury. The nurse should test both eyes and document visual acuity before the accident.

BOX 29-13

EYE IRRIGATION FOR CHEMICAL INJURIES (TRAUMA)

1 Assemble equipment necessary, including 1000 ml IV irrigating solution (normal saline, lactated Ringer's, or balanced salt), IV tubing, lid retractors, cotton applicators, and topical anesthesia per physician or ER standing protocol.
NOTE: Water is the most available fluid and should be used initially if other solutions are not readily available.
2 Position patient in a reclining position with head turned toward affected side.
3 Place a towel or kidney basin near the lateral canthus.
4 Hold the eye open if necessary. NOTE: Often the patient cannot hold the eye open because of severe pain.
5 Direct the flow of irrigating solution from nasal to temporal side of eye (inner to outer canthus).
6 If both eyes are affected, irrigate them alternately. Have a second liter of fluid available. Use 1000 ml of solution for each eye.
7 Have patient evaluated by an ophthalmologist.

Sudden vision loss as a result of *angle-closure glaucoma* or *temporal arteritis* needs to be treated within hours. In addition to decreased vision, the patient with angle-closure glaucoma will have pain, headache, and vomiting as a result of increased IOP.

Lacerations and *rupture of the globe* need to be evaluated by the ophthalmologist. The nurse should not attempt to remove a protruding foreign object from the globe and should not apply pressure to the globe. A protective shield made from a cup or box can be used to protect the eye from further injury. The fellow eye can be patched to decrease movement of both eyes. The nurse should not let the patient eat or drink anything until he or she is seen by the physician because surgery may be necessary. The incidence of infection is high, and extensive trauma may require enucleation.

Blunt trauma to the eye is evaluated by x-ray or other radiographic tests to rule out orbital fractures. The shock wave created by the trauma can also be responsible for internal damage, including hyphema, vitreous hemorrhage, and retinal detachment (Vaughan, Asbury, Riordan-Eva, 1992).

Corneal abrasions and *foreign bodies* cause significant discomfort to the patient in the form of pain, photophobia, epiphora, and conjunctival redness. Fluorescein dye is used to evaluate abrasions. Because this dye can stain contact lenses, they should be removed before the dye is used. Foreign bodies often can be removed with a small needle or instrument after the cornea is anesthetized. The eyelids should be everted before inspection and removal of foreign objects, if indicated (see Box 29-8). Treatment includes antibiotic drops, a pressure patch, and often a cycloplegic agent. The unconscious patient is at greater risk for corneal damage if the eyelids do not close. Within hours the patient can develop necrosis and permanent scarring. Closing the lids and applying lubricants decrease this danger.

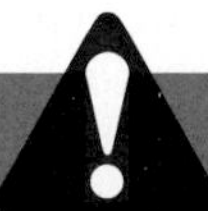

NURSE ALERT

WHEN TO SEEK TREATMENT FOR "BLOOD IN THE EYE."

Subconjunctival hemorrhage—Patch of blood between the transparent conjunctiva/layer and white sclera of the eye; caused by rupture of a small vessel; spontaneous, sudden occurrence, sometimes following an episode of violent coughing, sneezing, or vomiting; painless with no visual symptoms; no treatment needed; reabsorbs in 2 to 3 weeks.

Hyphema—Collection of blood within the eye in the space between the cornea and iris that is normally filled with clear aqueous humor; most often caused by blunt trauma (a blow to the eye); usual treatment is bedrest with bilateral eye patches; IOP monitored because blood cells block the trabecular meshwork; resolves spontaneously; anterior-chamber lavage may be required.

Lid lacerations need to be treated in the same way as lacerations elsewhere. The lids are vascular and bleed freely. Foreign material in the wound needs to be debrided before repair is done. If the lid injury is on the nasal side, injury of the tear duct system should be evaluated. Other structures that may be injured are the lacrimal gland and levator muscle of the lid. Realignment of tissues in lid margin lacerations prevents a "notched" appearance of the lid. Postoperative treatment includes antibiotic ointment, patching, and ice to decrease swelling. If indicated, a tetanus injection may be given.

Swollen lids can be an indication of orbital cellulitis, or inflammation of the fatty tissue of the orbit. The patient may have a history of blunt trauma, dental infection, or sinusitis. Hospitalization and intravenous therapy with a broad-spectrum antibiotic are required to prevent the infection from traveling through the orbit into the brain, where it can cause meningitis or a brain abscess.

EYE SAFETY

Eye safety needs to be everyone's concern. Nurses can provide vital information for prevention of eye injuries. Figures reported by the National Society to Prevent Blindness (NSPB) indicate that 2 to 3 million people every year have an eye injury. It is estimated that 90% of these are preventable and that 45% occur around the home (Berleu, 1991). Prevention is the most effective way to save sight, and identifying potential hazards in the environment is the first requirement. Children—more boys than girls—sustain more injuries than adults, and toys are a frequent cause of their injuries. Sharp, pointed toys or those with projectiles are the most dangerous to the child and other playmates. BB guns and pellet rifles cause irreparable damage (Hunt, 1993). Sports-related injuries can be reduced by use of protective goggles or sunglasses. Children engaged in contact sports should wear helmets and face protection. Monocular or one-eyed patients need high-impact–resistant prescription or nonprescription eyewear.

Chemicals in the home are dangerous for children and adults. Dangerous substances should be kept out of the reach of children. Protective glasses should be worn when using chemicals, painting, or plastering. Contact lenses can trap chemicals under them, and mixing cleaning products can produce toxic gases. Steam from cooking can burn the cornea as well as the face. Bags of microwave popcorn have been reported as causes of injury. Aerosols contain chemicals that are harmful to the eyes. Power tools, "weed whackers," and lawnmowers can project rocks and other debris into the eyes. Ultraviolet light from the sun, sun lamps, or arc welding can cause symptoms similar to corneal abrasions. UV exposure also has been associated with cataract formation (Hunt, 1993; Vaughan, Asbury, Riordan-Eva, 1992).

In the workplace and schools, safety eyewear should be worn if there is a possibility of flying debris, chemical injury, or radiation exposure. Healthcare personnel need to shield their eyes from biohazards when giving patient care. Contact lenses should be avoided in areas of intense heat, flying debris, chemical fumes, and molten metal. Special eyewash stations need to be accessable to all patients in hazardous environments. To avoid injury from sparks or battery acid explosions,

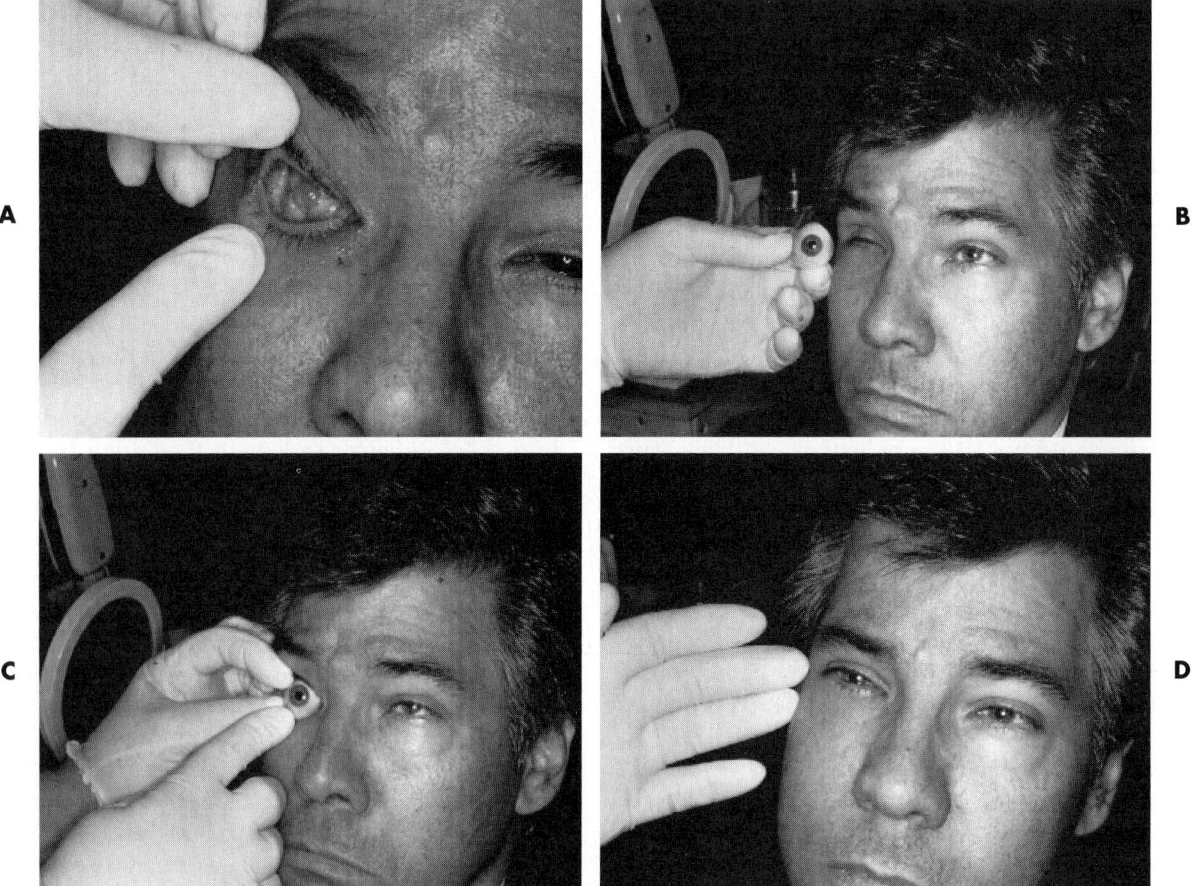

Figure 29-32 Artificial eye placement.

protective goggles should be worn when repairing cars. Fireworks should be avoided. Over 15,000 eye injuries per year are caused by fireworks, and 60% of these injuries affect children. NSPB figures indicate that 40% of the injuries result in permanent damage to the eye (Berlew, 1991). Seventy-five percent of all fireworks injuries are caused by bottle rockets (Hunt, 1993a). If an injured eye must be removed, an artificial eye is placed in the socket (Figure 29-32).

NORMAL AGING AND THE EYE

Because Americans are living longer, healthcare providers can expect to see more of of the normal vision changes associated with advanced age, as well as pathological changes. Loss of vision in the elderly can be caused by cataracts, glaucoma, macular degeneration, or diabetic retinopathy, but poor vision should not be equated with the aging process (Hunt, 1993b). A normal decrease in visual acuity is attributed to diminished elasticity of the lens and the muscles in the ciliary body, both of which affect accommodation. This change occurs at varying rates and times for different people, but it usually becomes noticeable in people who are in their 40s and tends to increase in those who are 50 to 59 years of age before it stabilizes (Vaughan, Asbury, Riordan-Eva, 1992). Other causes for decreased vision are a reduction in the function of the rods and cones, cataract formation, or a miotic pupil. To help improve vision, bifocal glasses, magnifiers, large print books, and easily brightened lighting sources (three-way) can be used. Visual-field loss can be caused by a miotic pupil, lid relaxation, or a decrease in the amount of orbital fat. People who notice this problem should exercise greater caution while driving and crossing streets. Turning the head instead of just moving the eyes will help, as will using the senses of touch and hearing to compensate for the reduced peripheral vision.

Yellowing of the lens and cornea and a decrease in cone function make colors seem less bright and affect depth perception. To offset this deficit, warmer colors can be used. Reds and yellows are seen better. The first and last stair can be painted a lighter color for better visibility, and all stairways should have handrails. Night-vision impairment, dark-adaptation time, and glare problems increase with age because a slowing retinal metabolism and miotic pupil provide less light to the retina. Flat paint on surfaces decreases glare. Sunglasses should be used during the day, and looking directly into car headlights at night should be avoided. Sources of indirect lighting in the home should be positioned appropriately (Woods, 1992).

Vitreous "floaters" or "spots" occur more often in myopic people. As the vitreous liquifies with age, the frequency can increase. A retinal evaluation is advised if the amount and frequency increase noticeably. Tear quality and quantity decrease, and this causes problems associated with dry eyes (Gilchrist, Hunt, 1993). Artificial tears and lubricants to ease this problem are available commercially. The skin of the eyelid thins and loses elasticity, which may cause the eyelid to droop. No treatment is indicated unless symptoms interfere with vision or the person desires cosmetic surgery.

The American Academy of Ophthalmology recommends that adults 65 years and older have an eye examination every 2 years, or sooner with certain risk factors. Reasonably good vision can be expected as people age, and nurses can educate older people to seek early diagnosis and treatment so that their quality of life as it relates to vision can be preserved.

ETHICAL DILEMMA

Bernice Jones is an 89-year-old resident in a nursing home. Previously she had lived with her son and daughter-in-law until problems required nursing assistance 1 year ago. Mrs. Jones has chronic obstructive pulmonary disease (COPD) and aortic stenosis. She has left-sided paralysis as a result of a stroke and uses a wheelchair.

Her son, Bill, and his wife, Carole, have been discussing her complaints about the effects of sunlight on her vision. When checked, her vision was 20/400 in the right eye and 20/30 in the left eye, which had undergone cataract surgery 2 years ago.

Mrs. Jones enjoys the company of her roommate and other residents. She watches TV in her room or in the game room. Her family visits twice a week and talks with her daily.

Bill and Carole want the best care money can buy and are requesting surgery on Mrs. Jones's right eye. They ask your opinion on the second cataract surgery. The doctor feels that she is doing well with her current vision and that her other health problems pose a risk for the procedure.

How would you respond? How would you analyze the ethical issues?

Nursing Care Plan

PATIENT WITH A DETACHED RETINA

The patient is a 26-year-old male who was brought to the emergency department by one of his caretakers after complaining of "blurred vision," and "seeing out of only one half of his right eye."

The patient is a moderately retarded young man who requires assistance in his activities of daily living (ADLs). He can feed and dress himself and is responsible for toileting and hygiene, but he needs assistance with time management and decisionmaking. He is considered trainable and can function semiindependently in many self-care skills.

An opthalmic examination revealed that the patient has a right detached retina, and he was admitted for surgery on the following day. His overall health status is good. He has known allergies to ragweed (hay fever every summer) codeine, xylocaine, and strawberries.

Past Medical History

- Some information from old records
- Premature birth at 32 weeks, unknown cause; required oxygen for first 3 weeks of life; periods of apnea and bradycardia during first month of life
- Bilateral inguinal hernia repair at 3 months
- Grand mal seizures started at age 6, currently under control with carbamazepine (Tegetrol); last seizure 1 year ago
- Mild cerebral palsy—wears short leg braces
- Moderate level mental retardation
- Has never smoked; negative alcohol use
- Has chronic constipation

Psychosocial Data

- Mother age 52, alcoholism × 30 years
- Father age 60, no available data
- Brother age 20 years, history of mental illness and autism
- Lived with biologic family until 7 years old
- Seizures plus social conditions within family prompted Children's Protective Services to intervene
- History of foster families, unknown period of time
- Lived in residential state school from age 14 to 19
- Special education classes until age 21; can write own name, count to 30, and read on a primary level; has very short attention span
- Has lived in current group home for 7 years
- Considers other residents his family; particularly attached to "Joe," his primary caretaker
- Biologic family no longer in area, minimal visits or contacts
- Has Medicaid, Title 19, and Social Security disability income
- Works in local grocery store as bagger; excellent work record and attendance.
- Occasional temper tantrums at home, usually over TV or household chores
- Information provided by Joe, who will remain in continuous attendance daily while patient is hospitalized

Assessment Data

- Height 5 ft 6 in, weight 146 lbs
- Pleasant young man with dull facies
- Oriented × 3 (time, place, and person); dependent on caretaker to respond to some questions, otherwise cooperative
- *Skin:* Intact—no signs rashes or bruises
- *Respiratory:* Regular rate and rhythm (16-18); no use accessory muscles; lungs clear to percussion and ascultation
- *Cardiovascular:* Slight pectus excavatum. apical rate heard best to right of midclavicular line; regular rate and rhythm (68-70); no bruits, all pulses intact
- *Abdominal:* Slight distention—bowel sounds heard in all four quadrants
- *Musculoskeletal:* Full range of motion for all joints; Said to have "unsteady gait" without braces

Laboratory data

- ECG and chest x-ray normal
- Hgb 14.1, Hct 42, WBC 9,000, platelets 325,000
- BUN 14, electrolytes within normal limits
- *Urinalysis:* no abnormalities

Medications

- carbamazepine (Tegretrol) 200 mg bid
- docusate sodium (Colace) 100 mg bid
- Cyclogyl eye drops 1 in right eye q 4 hr
- Predulose opthalmic eye drops 2 OD q 6 hr
- Sodium Sulamyd 30% opthalmic solution 2 drops qid and hs
- prochlorperazine (Compazine) 10 mg IM prn nausea
- diezepam (Valium) 5 mg PO qid
- secobarbital (Seconal) 100 mg PO hs

NURSING DIAGNOSIS

Anxiety related to visual disturbance and being in unfamiliar environment, as evidenced by shaky voice and hesitant responses

NURSING INTERVENTIONS	EVALUATION OF EXPECTED OUTCOMES
Determine patient's level of knowledge. Orient him to his surroundings. Encourage him to "touch" all equipment (BP cuff, stethoscope). Use simple terms in explaining what is expected of him. Encourage any questions. Speak gently when entering room (both eyes patched). Tell him when you are leaving. Remind him that his caretaker is always present. Have patient introduce his attendant caretaker from the group home. Reorient patient as often as necessary as to where he is and why the bed is different from his at home. Provide ample time for patient to respond to care measures. Prepare patient for any changes (eye drops); give short simple explanations geared to his level of understanding. At the first signs of anxiety, hold his hand and reassure him.	Patient demonstrates reduced preoccupation with fears and gives evidence of a level of trust in his caretakers and nurses States (in basic terms) what his visual condition is and that the eye patches are temporary Cooperates with treatment regimen

NURSING DIAGNOSIS

Risk for injury or infection related to eyes patched and sensation of "itchiness" with healing

NURSING INTERVENTIONS	EVALUATION OF EXPECTED OUTCOMES
Keep bed at lowest level to floor. Orient patient to use of and need for side rails; remind patient often to remain on bedrest. Assess his ability to use the call bell; keep it near at all times. Immediately postoperative, take vital signs every 15 minutes until stable and then once per shift for 24 hours. Give tranquilizer medication as ordered to promote cooperation. Keep radio or TV on softly to his favorite stations or programs. Encourage his attendant-caretaker to read to him when awake. Encourage deep breathing exercises when ascultating lungs; remind patient not to cough. Monitor for signs of nausea and medicate with perchlorperazine (Compazine) to prevent vomiting.	Patient's eye incision site remains free of erythema, edema, purulent drainage, and other signs and symptoms of infection Vital signs and laboratory values remain within patient's baseline data Discusses the need for safety measures such as side rails Remains in the designated postoperative position and does not attempt to get out of bed Cooperates in some self-care activities within the sensori-motor limitations posed by his eye patches and enforced bedrest

continued

NURSING INTERVENTIONS—cont'd	EVALUATION OF EXPECTED OUTCOMES—cont'd
Encourage movement of all extremities every shift; keep head positioned as ordered. Advance diet slowly as tolerated (clear liquids first). Teach patient the importance of not rubbing eyes or bandages. Have patient perform handwashing 4 times a day, especially at bedtime or after using the bedpan or urinal. Perform basic infection prevention teachings with attendant-caretaker every shift.	

NURSING DIAGNOSIS

Knowledge deficit related to activity restrictions

NURSING INTERVENTIONS	EVALUATION OF EXPECTED OUTCOMES
Advise patient of need to keep the head still when moving in bed. Maintain bedrest with affected eye patched for 48 hours after surgery. Position patient in the prone position with his head downward and turned slightly (may use small pillow). Instruct patient not to forcefully cough. Remind him of the need to deep breathe every 2 hours when awake. Discuss importance of quiet activities after discharge and the need to avoid crowds or any situation where he might have rapid or jolting movements. Teach patient of need to eat lightly to avoid vomiting. Have him cite his favorite foods. Provide written discharge instructions to his caretakers outlining the specific activity restrictions. Provide caretaker with instruction on daily vision checks. Question whether other residents pose a physical threat to patient. Have patient list his favorite "quiet" activities. Praise his efforts at cooperation. Discuss schedule of follow-up appointments.	Patient and his caretakers discuss effects of visual loss on his lifestyle Can list what he is to avoid and how he is allowed to ambulate (slowly and steadily with no rapid movements) Does not lose any of the previously attained self-care skills because of his hospitalization or surgery Caretakers cite ways to assist patient to attain his maximum level of functioning Caretakers plan quiet activities such as television viewing to avoid situations that provoke temper tantrums

KEY CONCEPTS

- The eye is a highly specialized sense organ that functions much like a camera, focusing light images that fall on the retina into electrical impulses that travel through the optic nerve to the brain, where the image is developed.
- The ophthalmoscope enhances visual examination of the fundus of the retina, including blood vessels, optic disc, and macula. The slit lamp provides a three-dimensional view of all internal structures of the eye. It is also used to view the lids, lashes, and conjunctiva.
- Ocular manifestations of systemic disease can be found during a fundus examination. The blood vessels and retinal pathology reveal the state of vessels elsewhere in the body.
- Visual acuity is measured for distance vision and near vision by use of various charts that are placed at a measured distance from the viewer. The viewer reads the graduated lines of letters or symbols on the charts, and his or her vision is stated in terms of its relation to normal, or 20/20.
- When light rays enter the eye and focus at a point in front of the retina, it is called myopia or nearsightedness. If the light is focused at a point behind the retina, it is hyperopia or farsightedness. Corrective lenses are prescribed to refract, or bend, the light rays to focus on the retina to achieve normal vision.
- Extraocular muscle imbalance in children may cause amblyopia or "lazy eye." This condition may not always appear as "crossed eyes," so early vision screening is important. If amblyopia is not treated by the age of 8, useful binocular vision will never develop.
- Contact lenses that are not removed from an unconscious victim can adhere to the corneal surface if the eyes are not fully closed. This may cause severe damage to the corneal surface.
- Vision loss can be central, peripheral, or a combination of the two and may affect one eye or both. Adult vision loss in the United States is attributed to cataracts, diabetic retinopathy, glaucoma, and macular degeneration.
- Resources for persons with functional vision loss, or low vision, are available in all states. Schools and special clinics provide training for home and work settings. Patients who experience vision loss normally go through the grieving process.
- Punctal occlusion, pressing the finger over the inner canthus to obstruct the inner puncta, is used to prevent systemic absorption of topical eye medications.
- Angle-closure glaucoma can be mistaken for conjunctivitis. Both conditions exhibit increased blood in the superficial vessels, but the patient with acute glaucoma will have a shallow anterior chamber, high IOP, a mid-dilated nonreactive pupil, and no discharge.
- Injury to the corneal epithelium or corneal ulcers destroy the barrier that normally protects the other layers from infection. These infections can cause severe scarring that leads to decreased vision or possible blindness.
- Medical therapy for glaucoma includes drugs that decrease aqueous production or increase aqueous outflow. When maximum medical therapy fails or is no longer tolerated, surgical procedures are indicated for open-angle glaucoma. These include laser iridectomy and trabeculoplasty, glaucoma filtering procedures, and glaucoma shunt insertion.
- Ophthalmic surgical procedures can be divided into intraocular and extraocular procedures. Intraocular procedures include cataract extraction, corneal transplantation, glaucoma filtering procedures, and vitrectomy. Extraocular procedures include surgery on the eye muscles, eyelids, lacrimal system, and orbit.
- A painless loss of vision progressing over time can be a sign of cataract formation. Symptoms include difficulty with reading or driving, with seeing well in bright sunlight, or with discriminating colors. The only cure for a cataract is surgical removal of the diseased lens, which is replaced with an artificial lens implant.
- Symptoms of a retinal detachment include seeing a "shower" or "flash" of light. Vision can be described as seeing through a curtain or veil. Complete loss of central vision occurs only when the macula is involved.
- Ocular malignancies are rare. The most common adult primary intraocular tumor is a choroidal melanoma. Retinoblastoma is the most common type in children.
- Most people with HIV develop infectious or noninfectious ocular conditions. Opportunistic infections affect the cornea because immunosupression allows invasion by numerous organisms.
- The retina can be destroyed by cytomegalovirus (CMV) retinitis.
- True ocular emergencies should be treated within minutes to preserve sight. Emergencies include chemical burns and sudden, painless loss of sight. The first step in assessing an injury is determining visual acuity of the eyes.

continued

KEY CONCEPTS

- Preventing eye injuries is the most important step in saving sight. Nearly half of all eye injuries occur around the home. Toys are a common cause of children's injuries, and chemicals or flying debris injure adults as well as children.
- Visual changes commonly associated with aging include diminished ability to focus on near objects, decreased peripheral vision and color vision, an increase in the frequency of "floaters" or "spots" in the vitreous, and dryness as a result of decreased tear formation.
- Eye examinations every 1 to 2 years help diagnose and treat potential problems that may affect sight.

CRITICAL THINKING EXERCISES

1 Describe safety measures to protect the eyes from injury at home and in the workplace.
2 Describe the normal changes in the eye that are associated with aging and explain how they differ from abnormal changes that need to be treated.
3 What support would you give to a patient with glaucoma who has been told that he must continue treatment for the rest of his life?
4 Develop a list of instructions for the patient with glaucoma.

REFERENCES AND ADDITIONAL READINGS

Allen M, Buse E: Stigmatism and blindness, *J Ophthal Nurs Technol* 10(4):147-152, 1991.

American Academy of Ophthalmology: *At first sight—drugs that are toxic to the eye,* San Francisco, 1989, The Academy.

American Academy of Ophthalmology: *Introducing ophthalmology,* San Francisco, 1992, The Academy.

American Academy of Ophthalmology: Basic clinical and science course, Section 6, *Pediatric ophthalmology and strabismus;* and Section 12, *Retina and vitreous,* 1994-95.

American Society of Ophthalmic Registered Nurses: *Ophthalmic procedures: a nursing prospective,* San Francisco, 1994, The Society.

American Society of Ophthalmic Registered Nurses: *Standards of ophthalmic clinical nursing practice,* San Francisco, 1992, The Society.

Arky R, medical consultant: *Physicians' Desk Reference,* ed 48, Montvale, N.J., 1994, Medical Economics Data Production Company.

Bartley GB, Liesegang TJ: *Essentials of ophthalmology,* Philadelphia, 1992, JB Lippincott.

Berlew JA: Preventing eye injuries—the nurse's role, *Insight* 16(6):24-28, 1991.

Berson FG, editor: *Ophthalmology study guide,* ed 5, San Francisco, 1987, American Academy of Ophthalmology.

Boyd-Monk H: Assessing acquired ocular diseases, *Nurs Clin North Am* 25(4):811-822, 1990.

Boyd-Monk H, Steinmetz CG: *Nursing care of the eye,* Norwalk, Conn, 1987, Appleton & Lange.

Bulachek GM, McCloskey JC: *Nursing intervention: essential nursing treatments,* Philadelphia, 1992, WB Saunders.

Bumpus S, Merchant M: Planning for high-risk ophthalmic ambulatory patients, *Insight* 18(2):16-19, 1993.

Burden N: Ambulatory surgical nursing, Philadelphia, 1993, WB Saunders.

Cataract Management Guideline Panel: *Cataract in adults: management of functional impairment, Clinical Practice Guideline 4,* Rockville, Md, 1993. Agency for Health Care Policy and Research, US Department of Health and Human Services, AHCPR Publication 93-0542.

Clinical guidelines: cataract surgery and its alternatives, *Am J Nurs* 93(1):59-61, 1993.

Fairchild SS: *Perioperative nursing principles and practice,* Boston, 1993, Jones & Bartlett.

Gallagher CM: The young adult with recent vision loss: a pilot case study, *Insight* 16(6):8-14, 1991.

Gilchrist V, Hunt L: Assessment and education of the diabetic with vision loss, *Insight* 18(3):9-12, 1993.

Goldblum K: Knowledge deficit in the ophthalmic surgical patients, *Nurs Clin North Am* 27(3)715-725, 1992.

Grimes MR, Scardino MA, Martone JF: Worldwide blindness, *Nurs Clin North Am* 27(3):807-816, 1992.

Hunt L: Caution: systemic adverse reactions from eye drops medications, *Insight* 16(4):5, 1991.

Hunt L: Ophthalmic nursing assessment, *Insight* 18(3):9-11, 1992.

Hunt L: Ocular emergencies, *Insight* 18(2):24-25, 1993a.

Hunt L: Aging and the visual system, *Insight* 18(3):6-7, 18, 1993b.

Langseth F: The use of 5-fluorouracil in glaucoma filtration surgery, *Insight* 18(2):11-13, 1993.

McCoy K: Ophthalmic drug use in the OR, *Insight* 17(4):10-21, 1992.

McEvoy GK: American hospital formulary service, *EyeENT* 52:1766-1867, 1994.

Nowell P: Lasers in ophthalmology, *Nurs Clin North Am* 25(3)635-643, 1990.

Olk RJ: New approaches to vitreoretinal surgery, *Int Ophthal Clinics* 32(2), Boston, 1992, Little, Brown.

Orticio LP, Swan J: Implementation of the post-discharge follow-up call in the patient care units, *Insight* 17(2):15-19, 1992.

Ostler HB: Disease of the external eye and adnexa, Baltimore, 1993, Williams & Wilkins.

Plona RP, Schremp PS: Nursing care of patients with ocular manifestations of human immunodeficiency virus infection, *Nurs Clin North Am* 27(3):793-805, 1992.

Reeves W: Surgical experiences of the ophthalmic patient, *Insight* 18(1):16-22, 1993.

Richard JM: *A manual for the beginning ophthalmology resident: eye emergencies,* ed 3, San Francisco, 1978, American Academy of Ophthalmology.

Ruehl CA, Schremp PS: Nursing care of the cataract patient: today's outpatient approach, *Nurs Clin North Am* 27(3): 727-743, 1992.

Sandler RL: Glaucoma, *Am J Nurs* 95(3):34-35, 1995.

Servodidio CA: Teaching aids for patients diagnosed with choroidal melanoma, *Insight* 16(6):21-23, 1991.

Servodidio CA: Nursing implications of visual fields in successfully treated retinoblastoma patients, *Insight* 18(1):11-16, 1993.

Servodidio CA, Abramson DH: Choroidal melanoma, *Nurs Clin North Am* 27(3):777-791, 1992.

Smith JF, Nachazel DP: *Ophthalmic nursing,* Boston, 1980, Little, Brown.

Smith SC: Diabetic retinopathy, *Nurs Clin North Am* 27(3): 745-759, 1992.

Smith SC, Folk JC, Losch ME: Effects of collaborated education on patient satisfaction and knowledge, *Insight* 17(1): 20-24, 1992.

Spires R: Retinopathy of prematurity, *J Ophthal Nurs Tech* 10(4):166-170, 1991.

Spires R: Glaucoma filtration surgery and the shell tamponade technique, *J Ophthal Nurs Tech* 13(1):17-20, 1994.

Stein HA, Scott BJ, Stein RM: *A primer in ophthalmology,* St Louis, 1992, Mosby.

Vader LA: Vision and vision loss, *Nurs Clin North Am* 27(3): 705-714, 1992.

Vaughan DG, Asbury T, Riordan-Eva P: *General ophthalmology,* ed 13, Norwalk, Conn, 1992, Appleton & Lange.

Weisbacker CA, Naidoff M, Tippermann R: *Physicians' desk reference for ophthalmology,* Montrale, N.J., 1993, Medical Economics Data.

Wong EK, Wang S, Leopold IH: How ophthalmic drugs can fool you, *RN* 43(3):37-44, 1980.

Woods S: Macular degeneration, *Nurs Clin North Am* 27(3): 761-775, 1992.

CHAPTER 30

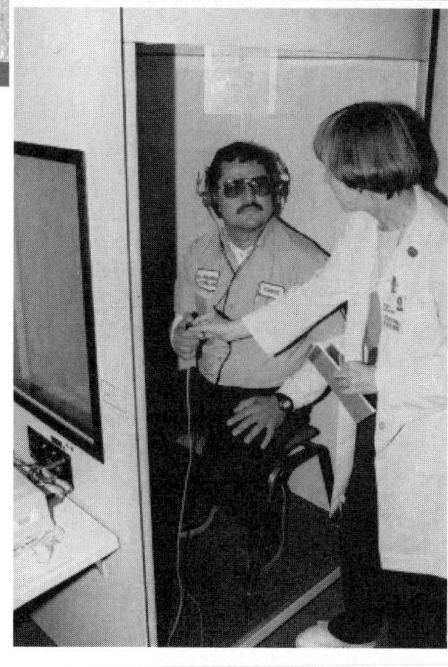

Hearing

CHAPTER OBJECTIVES

1 Associate the anatomic parts of the ear to the functions of hearing and balance.
2 Identify the purpose and procedure for common diagnostic tests involving the ear.
3 List common complaints associated with ear problems.
4 Differentiate between conductive and sensorineural hearing loss.
5 Describe behavioral signs and symptoms of hearing loss in the adult.
6 Describe methods to facilitate communication with the hearing-impaired person.
7 Describe methods that may be used to remove a foreign body from the external ear canal.
8 Discuss nursing care guidelines for the patient with otitis media.
9 Discuss both the preoperative and postoperative nursing care of the patient having ear surgery.
10 Define otosclerosis and describe the surgical procedure (stapedectomy) used to correct the condition.
11 Discuss both preoperative and postoperative care of the patient having a mastoidectomy.
12 Identify activity restrictions for the patient following tympanoplasty.
13 Differentiate between labyrinthitis and Ménière's syndrome.

KEY WORDS

audiologist
audiometry
auditory canal
auricle
cerumen
cochlea
decibel
deafness
endolymph
equilibrium
eustachian tube
incus
labyrinthitis
malleus
mastoiditis
Ménière's syndrome
myringotomy
nystagmus
otitis media
otosclerosis
otoscopy
pinna
perilymph
presbycusis
saccule
semicircular canals
stapedectomy
stapes
tinnitus
tuning fork
tympanic membrane
tympanoplasty
vertigo
vestibule

The ears are a highly specialized, complex set of sense organs and are responsible for both the functions of hearing and balance. The ear consists of three structural parts: external, middle, and inner (Figure 30-1). Each structure has a distinct function that contributes to the processes of hearing and balance.

STRUCTURE AND FUNCTION

External Ear

The external portion of the ear is composed of the visible **auricle** or **pinna** and a passageway called the external **auditory canal** or external acoustic meatus. The auricle acts as a collecting trumpet for sound waves, directing them toward the external auditory canal (external acoustic meatus). Once inside the external auditory canal, the sound waves are further directed toward the tympanic membrane. The external auditory canal is lined with ceruminous (wax-producing) glands and hair follicles. The purpose of the cerumen and hair follicles is to protect both the tympanic membrane and the middle ear. The hair follicles protect the external auditory canal from foreign debris. The ceruminous glands provide lubrication for both the tympanic membrane and middle ear. During the aging process, the hair follicles become coarse, causing a build-up of **cerumen** (wax). Impacted cerumen is a potential source of hearing loss, particularly for the older adult. The external ear is supplied by cranial nerves V (trigeminal) and X (vagus), as well as the cervical nerves.

The **tympanic membrane** (eardrum) covers the end of the external auditory canal, separating the external from the middle ear. The external surface of the tympanic membrane is covered with some of the same ceruminous glands and hair follicles as the external auditory canal. The internal surface of the membrane is covered with a thin, hairless mucous membrane. Normally this membrane appears "pearly" gray and shiny. The tympanic membrane protects the middle ear and vibrates with incoming sound waves to facilitate hearing. It receives its innervation for this vibratory function from a small auricular branch of the vagus nerve, as well as from a portion of the glossopharyngeal and facial nerve fibers.

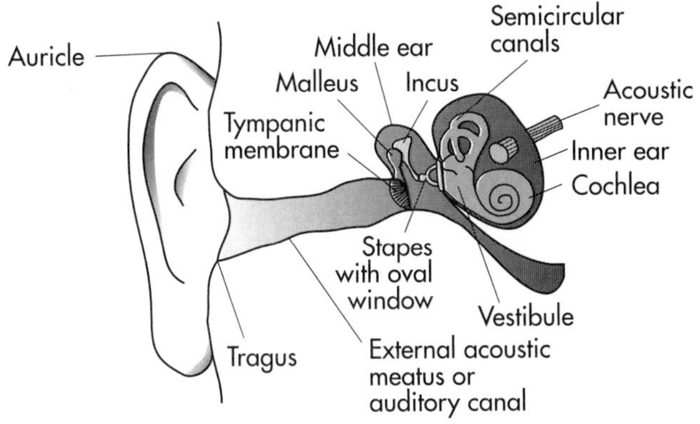

Figure 30-1 Diagram of the ear.

Middle Ear

The middle ear, or tympanic cavity, is a small, air-filled cavity located in the petrous portion of the temporal bone (toward the face). It is separated from the external ear by the tympanic membrane. The middle ear contains the ossicles, oval and round windows, and the eustachian tube. The ossicles (auditory ossicles) are three small bones that traverse the middle ear. Each has been named to describe its shape: the **malleus** (hammer), **incus** (anvil), and **stapes** (stirrup). The malleus is attached to the inner surface of the tympanic membrane, the incus is attached to the malleus, and the stapes is attached to the incus. These bones or ossicles are linked together in a chain, although not rigidly, which allows them to receive sound vibrations from the tympanic membrane and transmit them to the inner ear. The oval and round windows are membrane-covered openings leading from the middle ear to the inner ear. The oval window (fenestra ovalis) is attached to the stapes. The round window (fenestra rotunda) is located below the oval window. These windows provide an exit for sound vibrations from the inner ear, while protecting the middle ear from the inner ear.

The **eustachian tube** connects the middle ear with the nasopharynx. Its function is to equalize the pressure in the middle ear with the atmospheric pressure. The slitlike ending of the eustachian tube is normally closed. During swallowing or yawning, the tube can be opened, allowing air to enter or leave the tympanic cavity in order to balance the pressure on both sides of the tympanic membrane. This allows free movement of the tympanic membrane and prevents it from rupturing. A normally functioning eustachian tube keeps the middle ear free of contaminants from the nasopharynx.

Inner Ear

The inner ear (labyrinth) consists of a system of interrelated cavities. Included in this system is the bony (osseous) labyrinth, membranous labyrinth, **vestibule**, cochlea, and semicircular canals. The membranous labyrinth lies within a portion of the bony labyrinth. The **semicircular canals** contain fluid and hair cells. They are connected to the sensory nerve fibers of the vestibular portion of the eighth cranial nerve. The semicircular canals help to maintain a sense of balance or equilibrium. Two small sacs, the utricle and **saccule**, separate the semicircular canals from the cochlea. These sacs are suspended within the vestibule. They serve as vestibular receptors that respond to the changing positions of the head. The **cochlea** is a snail-shaped tube containing the organ of Corti, the receptor end organ of hearing. There are two fluids found in the inner ear—perilymph and endolymph. **Perilymph** is contained within the space between the bony and membranous labyrinths. It is also found in a portion of the cochlea. **Endolymph** is found within the utricle, saccule, and a portion of the cochlea. These fluids are important in the protection of both the cochlea and semicircular canals. Both organs are suspended in this fluid, which cushions them against abrupt movements of the head.

Process of Hearing

The auditory center for hearing is located in the temporal lobe of the cerebrum. Stimulation of this center results in hearing. Sound waves enter the ear through the auditory canal, causing the tympanic membrane to vibrate. These vibrations are transmitted from the tympanic membrane through the ossicles of the middle ear. One of those ossicles, the stapes, moves against the oval window, causing the vibrations to be transmitted through the fluids in the cochlea to the round window. At the round window these vibrations dissipate. The passing of these vibratory waves from the oval to the round window stimulates the hair cells of the organ of Corti to move, sending a stimulus to the membrane of Corti. These impulses are received by the cochlear branch of the auditory nerve, where they are transmitted to the brain and perceived as sound.

Maintenance of Balance

The vestibular system (saccule, utricle, and semicircular canals) is responsible for the maintenance of **equilibrium** and balance. The semicircular canals contain both endolymph fluid and hair cells. When an individual moves, this endolymph fluid also moves, causing the hair cells to bend. As the hair cells within the semicircular canals bend, they release impulses that stimulate the vestibular branch of the eighth cranial nerve. This allows the brain to reorient the individual and maintain balance. If an individual is stationary, the pressure of gravity on these hair cells maintains balance. Separating the semicircular canals from the cochlea are the utricle and saccule. They also function as vestibular receptors that respond to changes in head position.

NURSING ASSESSMENT OF HEARING LOSS

A nursing assessment should include a thorough patient history of both current and past medical conditions, identification of the patient's chief complaints, a visual examination, and an observation of the patient for signs of hearing loss.

Patient History

A patient history should include information regarding past or current hearing or ear-related problems. For example, symptoms such as **vertigo**, ear pain, discharge, or a recent ear trauma may be important in identifying a structural or hearing problem. The history should include questions regarding hearing acuity and any occupation or hobbies that may involve exposure to excessive noise. A thorough medication history is crucial because many drugs are toxic to the cochlea and vestibule and may cause permanent damage. Others cause dizziness, which could be confused with an ear disorder. The existence of current medical conditions and their medical treatments that are not directly associated with the ear should also be identified. Conditions such as allergies or upper respiratory infections may cause hearing or equilibrium problems.

Visual Examination

The external structure of the ear should be inspected for any signs of injury, redness, swelling, or drainage. The normal external canal is free from lesions and is dry, clean, and not reddened. The presence of any of these symptoms could indicate a possible infectious process, trauma, or the presence of a foreign object and should be reported to the physician for further evaluation. Visual examination also includes **otoscopy**. Otoscopy is the direct visualization of the external auditory canal and the tympanic membrane through an instrument called an otoscope (Figure 30-2; Box 30-1). Otoscopy may reveal signs of common conditions such as a perforated tympanic membrane or acute **otitis media**. Otoscopy is performed before any other auditory or vestibular testing is done.

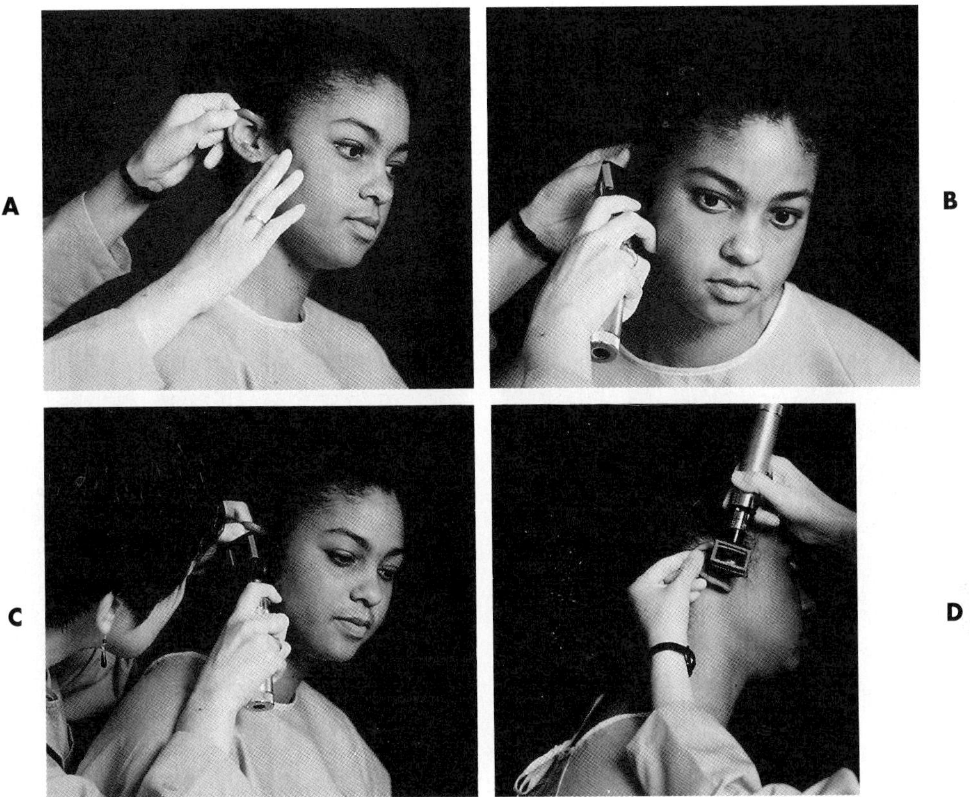

Figure 30-2 Examination of the ear with the otoscope. **A,** Inspection of the meatus. **B,** Patient's head is tipped toward the opposite shoulder. **C** and **D,** Two ways of holding the otoscope. (From Barkauskas VH and others: *Health and physical assessment,* St Louis, 1994, Mosby.)

BOX 30-1

STEPS IN USING AN OTOSCOPE

1. Select the largest speculum that will fit in the ear without causing pain.
2. Tip the patient's head away from you.
3. In adults, straighten the ear canal by pulling the auricle upward and backward. In young children (under the age of 2) and infants, straighten the canal by pulling the auricle downward.
4. Insert the speculum gently to minimize discomfort. The inner two thirds of the external meatus is very sensitive to pressure.
5. Vary the angle at which you insert the speculum into the meatus to obtain the best view of the tympanic membrane.

DIAGNOSTIC TESTING

There are a variety of testing methods used to assess for disorders of the ear. These testing methods are categorized according to their purpose. Auditory testing methods are used to determine hearing acuity. Vestibular testing methods are used to assess for dysfunction of the vestibular system, which affects equilibrium, resulting in dizziness, loss of balance, or **nystagmus** (involuntary rhythmic movement of the eyeball).

Auditory Tests

Voice tests

Voice tests may be done by whispering or speaking in a lower tone of voice. The individual being tested is placed at a distance of 20 feet and turned sideways. The ear to be tested is toward the examiner, the other ear is covered. The individual is asked to repeat each whispered or spoken word. This testing method is of value only as a screening test to identify individuals who require a more thorough examination.

Audiometry

A more accurate examination is done with an audiometer, an instrument that produces tones of varying pitch and intensity. The patient wears earphones that are attached to the audiometer. The individual listens to various tones and is asked to indicate when each sound is heard. **Audiometry** testing provides in-

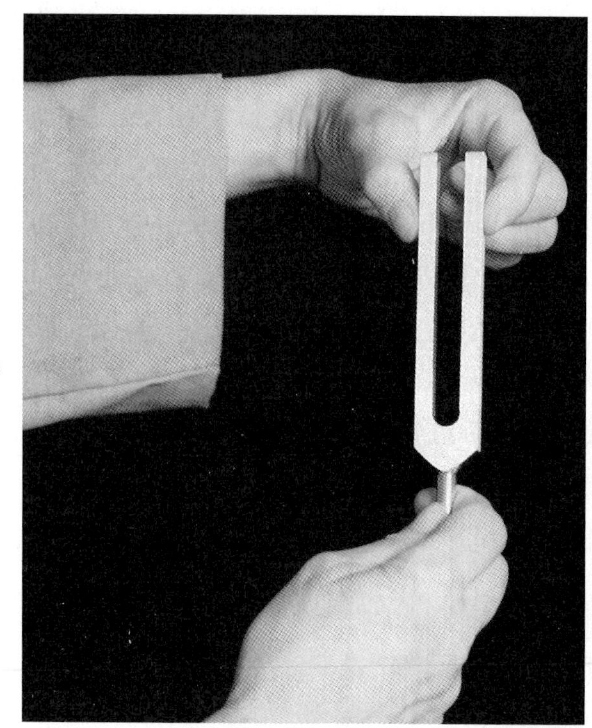

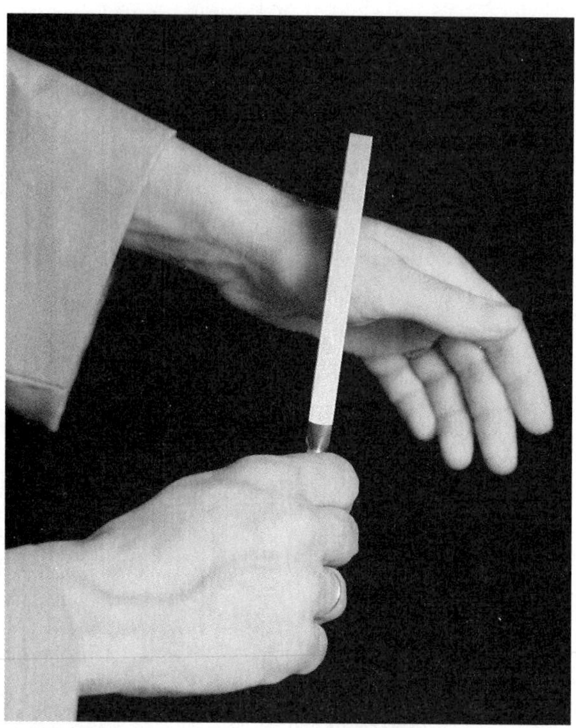

Figure 30-3 Activating tuning fork. **A,** Stroking the fork. **B,** Tapping the fork on the knuckle. (From Barkauskas VH and others: *Health and physical assessment,* St Louis, 1994, Mosby.)

formation concerning both quantitative and qualitative measurements of hearing. It provides the **audiologist** and the otologist (physician who specializes in diseases of the ear) with information that can help determine the type of treatment needed.

Tuning forks

Hearing acuity may also be tested through the use of a **tuning fork** (Figure 30-3). The tuning fork is made to vibrate and is then placed at various locations near the ear. Tuning fork testing is used to differentiate between conductive and sensorineural hearing loss. The Weber test is used to determine hearing loss in one or both ears. It is performed by placing the vibrating tuning fork in the middle of the individual's head at the midline of the forehead (Figure 30-4). The individual will be asked whether the sound is heard equally in both ears or is louder in one ear than the other. The test results are considered normal if the individual hears equally well on both sides. The results are considered to be abnormal if the sound is heard in one ear only. If the individual's hearing loss is of a *conductive* nature, the sound will be louder in the diseased ear. If the hearing loss is of a *sensorineural* nature, the sound will be louder in the normal ear. In the Rinne test, the base of the vibrating tuning fork is shifted between two positions (Figure 30-5). First it is placed on the mastoid process of the temporal bone. While it is still vibrating, the tuning fork is then placed in front of the ear. As the position of the tuning fork is changed, the patient is asked to identify which tone is louder. The patient is also asked to identify when one of the tones is no longer heard. Under normal circumstances the sound will be heard longer in front of the ear. This is consid-

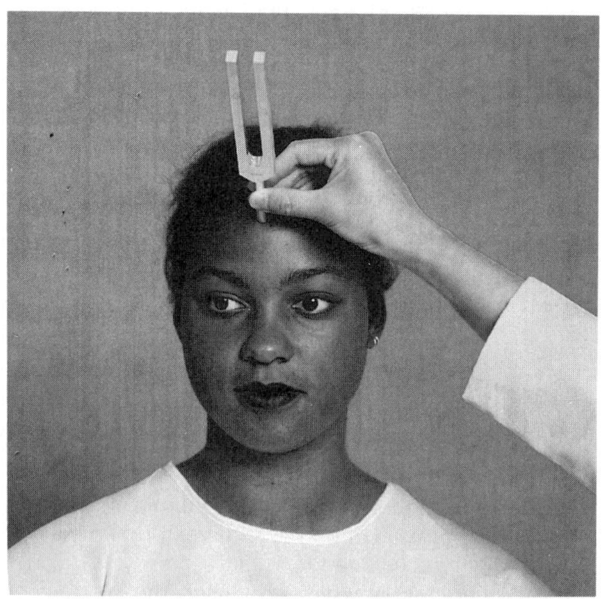

Figure 30-4 Weber test. (From Barkauskas VH and others: *Health and physical assessment,* St Louis, 1994, Mosby.)

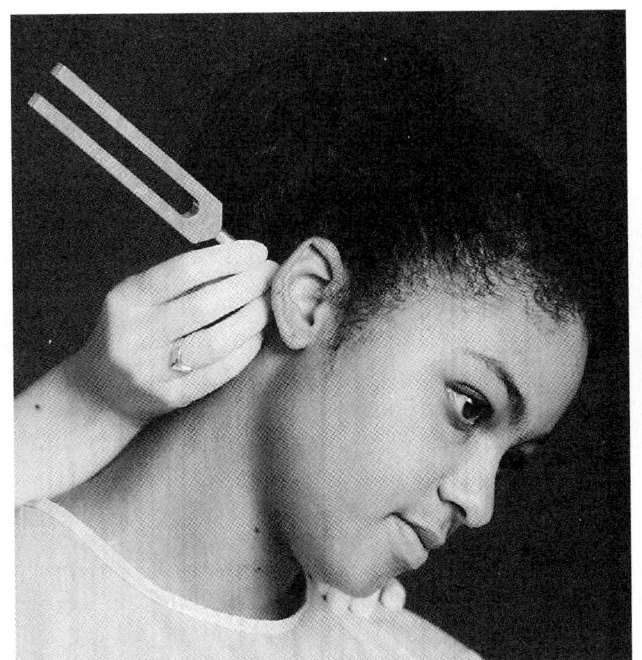

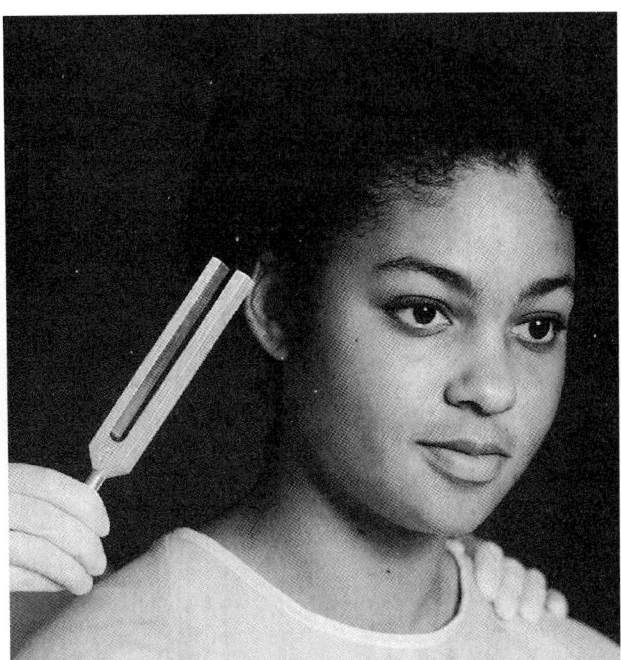

Figure 30-5 Rinne test. **A,** Bone conduction. **B,** Air conduction. (From Barkauskas VH and others: *Health and physical assessment*, St Louis, 1994, Mosby.)

ered to be a normal or positive Rinne tuning fork test result. If the individual is unable to hear the sound through the air in front of the ear, the test is considered to be abnormal or negative. A negative Rinne test result indicates a conductive hearing loss on the side being tested.

Vestibular Tests

Dysfunction in the vestibule or the cerebellum may result in dizziness, loss of equilibrium, or nystagmus. Individuals can be treated for vestibular and cerebellar dysfunction by using either the falling test or past-pointing test. In the *falling test*, the individual is instructed to stand with feet together, stand on one foot, stand heel to toe and then walk forward and backward heel to toe. Each of these exercises is first performed with eyes open and then with eyes closed. Marked swaying or falling indicates dysfunction. In the *past-pointing test* the examiner holds an index finger out at shoulder level. The patient is instructed to reach out and touch the examiner's index finger. The patient is then asked to raise and lower both of his or her arms, attempting to return to the examiner's index finger (point of reference). The patient should be able to return to that point of reference. This would be considered a "normal" test result. Patients with vestibular dysfunction lack a "normal" sense of position. They are unable to return to the point of reference. Instead they deviate to the right or the left of the examiner's index finger.

Electronystagmography

Electronystagmography is a procedure used to evaluate both spontaneous and induced eye movements referred to as nystagmus. The purpose of electronystagmography is to distinguish between normal nystagmus and nystagmus caused by vestibular lesion. Nystagmus following a head turn is normal for a short period of time. Prolonged nystagmus is abnormal. The procedure uses a variety of stimuli, including position changes and hot and cold to elicit nystagmus. The eye movements in response to each stimulus are recorded and evaluated. Electronystagmography is also helpful in diagnosing unilateral hearing loss of unknown origin and identifying the cause of dizziness, vertigo (the sensation of moving in space), or **tinnitus** (ringing in the ears).

HEARING LOSS

Hearing loss or hearing impairment is defined as a "state of diminished auditory acuity that ranges from partial to complete loss of hearing" (Hirsch, Thompson, 1989). Hearing loss can be partial or total. It can also occur in low, medium, or high frequencies, or in combination. Hearing loss can occur in one or both ears, depending on the cause. It may be congenital or it may occur later in life as a result of disease or injury.

Hearing is measured in **decibels** (dB). A decibel is a ratio that compares the relationship between two sound intensities. According to the American Medical Association, a hearing loss of 40 decibels below normal (which is equal to a 22.5% hearing impairment), usually impairs a person's ability to function normally in a social situation and requires intervention, such as a hearing aid or other device that amplifies the sound. True **deafness** is defined as 85 to 90 decibels below normal.

Approximately one out of every 500 adults in the United States is deaf. Deaf persons will have difficulty speaking if their hearing loss is of a congenital nature and they have been without hearing since birth. Those who have lost their hearing after they have learned to speak are usually able to speak quite normally. The inability to speak with normal rhythm and tone because of deafness is not a sign of poor intellectual capacities. Unfortunately there are still people who believe that is the case and use such terms as "deaf mute" or "deaf and dumb." These terms are resented by deaf persons and should not be used. Although there have been many advances made in the treatment of deafness, such as cochlear implants, there is still much to be done to educate people about deafness, particularly regarding their attitude toward it.

Types

Hearing loss may be conductive, affecting only the external or middle ear, or it may be sensorineural (nerve deafness), in which the inner ear is involved. Conductive deafness may be caused by an obstruction of the auditory canal that prevents sound waves from reaching the inner ear. The problem may be an accumulation of cerumen in the auditory canal, or it may be caused by **otosclerosis** in the middle ear that prevents transmission of sound vibrations from reaching the inner ear (Figure 30-6). For these persons, surgery may restore hearing. In some cases there may be a congenital absence of the auditory canal or the tympanic membrane. In conductive deafness only the intensity of sound is affected. Disorders that lead to conductive hearing loss can often be corrected with no damage to hearing or minimal hearing loss.

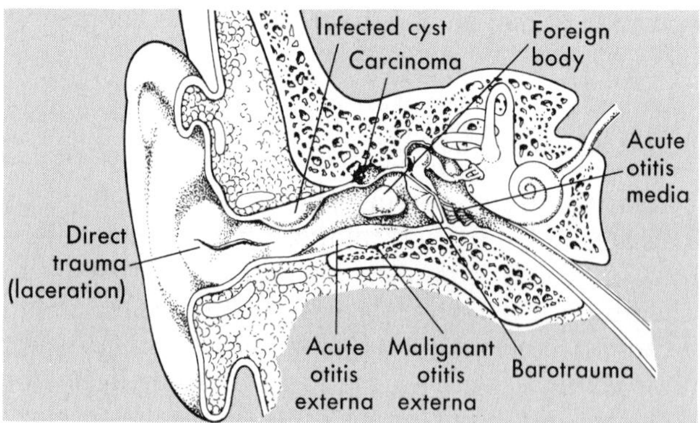

Figure 30-6 Disorders that contribute to conductive hearing loss. (From Beare PG, Myers JL: *Principles and practice of adult health nursing*, ed 2, St Louis, 1994, Mosby.)

In sensorineural deafness, the auditory canal and the middle ear receive the vibrations normally, but the vibrations go no further. This is because of degeneration of the nerve fibers of the auditory nerve or the hearing center in the brain. Damage may result from tumors, head injuries, or other causes such as congenital syphilis that affect cranial nerve VIII. Nerve deafness may occur in babies born to mothers who had rubella during the first trimester of pregnancy. A type of nerve deafness that usually involves high-frequency sounds may occur as part of the aging process (Box 30-2).

Persons with sensorineural deafness experience distortion of sounds along with poor speech discrimination. Often they will speak loudly in an attempt to compensate (Box 30-3). When sensorineural deafness is congenital or acquired during infancy or early childhood, speech is generally affected. Such children usually need training in lip reading and special education. Sensorineural or nerve deafness is permanent and irreversible, but research brings hope for finding a treatment in the future. An electronic cochlea has been devised that is implanted in the inner ear and conducts impulses to the higher centers in the brain. The development of this artificial cochlea has helped and will continue to do so as the implantation technique becomes more refined. However, for the present, most people with nerve deafness must be helped to live without the ability to hear.

BOX 30-2

CHANGES ASSOCIATED WITH AGING

- Pinna becomes elongated because of loss of subcutaneous tissue and decreased tissue elasticity.
- Hair becomes coarse and longer, especially in men.
- Cerumen-producing glands decrease in number; cerumen becomes drier and impacted, causing hearing loss.
- Tympanic membrane loses its elasticity and appears dull and retracted.
- Ossicles decrease movement as a result of calcification.
- Cochlea experiences degenerative changes.
- Vestibular function becomes disturbed, causing vertigo and sensations of being unsteady.
- Hearing acuity diminishes with increased age. Loss of hearing acuity includes loss of ability to hear high-frequency sounds, decreased speech reception (particularly the *f, s,* and *sh* sounds), and increased auditory reaction time.

BOX 30-3

BEHAVIORAL SIGNS/SYMPTOMS OF HEARING LOSS

fatigue Straining to hear conversations is tiresome and often leads to irritability.

speech deterioration "Flat voice," incorrect pronunciation, or omitting words may occur because sounds are produced incorrectly.

indifference Lack of hearing can cause disinterest and depression.

social withdrawal Inattentiveness and withdrawal occur when the person is unable to hear correctly.

insecurity Improper hearing may cause the person to say or respond in the wrong manner, leading to feelings of embarrassment and insecurity.

indecision/procrastination Hearing problems lead to loss of self-confidence, which in turn makes decision making more difficult.

suspiciousness When only parts of conversations are heard, hearing-impaired people suspect that they are being talked about.

false pride Pretending to hear normally to avoid embarrassment often causes others to believe that the person has normal hearing.

loneliness and unhappiness Enforced silence can lead to many frightening experiences, giving the person a sense of not belonging.

dominating conversations By dominating conversations the hearing-impaired person has control of the group, which eliminates embarrassment.

OLDER ADULT CONSIDERATIONS

Presbycusis, impairment of hearing as a result of degenerative changes, is a common cause of sensorineural hearing loss associated with aging. In this case hearing loss is bilateral. Progression of the disease is gradual. Often the older adult will state that hearing is normal but that they cannot understand the words. They can hear the spoken word but it is muffled and often sounds as if the speaker is mumbling. This hearing loss is caused by degeneration or atrophy of several areas of the ear structure, especially the cochlea (Box 30-3).

Management

A common method of improving hearing loss is the use of a hearing aid. The hearing aid is a tiny electronic device designed to amplify sound. Those persons with conduction deafness (in which the problem is intensity of sound) generally benefit from the use of a hearing aid. The hearing aid, however, is of little value to the individual with sensorineural deafness.

The hearing aid consists of three parts: a microphone that picks up sound and converts it into electric signals, an amplifier that intensifies the signal, and a receiver that converts the signal back into an intensified sound. The amplifier can be worn in one or both ears. In the individual with bilateral hearing loss, use of bilateral amplifiers stimulates a stereo effect, which aids in speech discrimination. There are various types of hearing aids, including those that may be used about the head. Hearing aids can be built into glasses, worn behind the ear or worn in the auditory canal (Figure 30-7). Other types may be worn on the torso.

The successful use of a hearing aid depends on the individual's feelings about the disability and the use of the device. Hearing aids amplify all sound, including background noise, which can cause confusion and actually make it more difficult to hear conversation. Not all persons will be able to adjust to this as well as the other aspects of the device. Older adults especially may find it more difficult.

Deafness, whether progressive or sudden in onset, produces anxiety and fear. The possibility of becoming cut off from familiar surroundings, losing friends, losing a job, and becoming isolated often leads to withdrawal. Many individuals deny the disability and refuse assistance. A hearing aid can play an important part in improving residual hearing, thus lessening the emotional impact of hearing loss, but only if it is used.

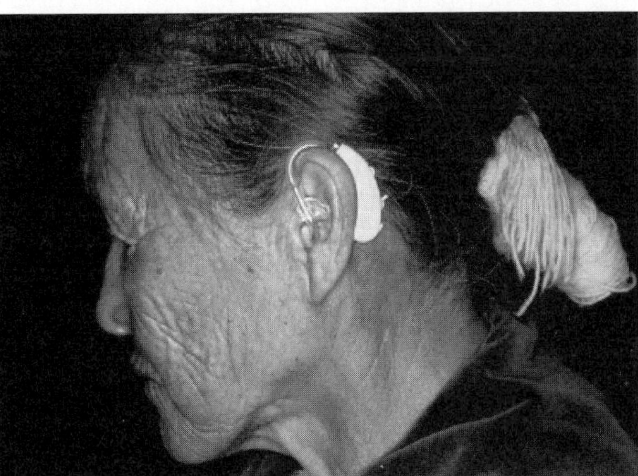

Figure 30-7 One type of hearing aid worn behind the ear.

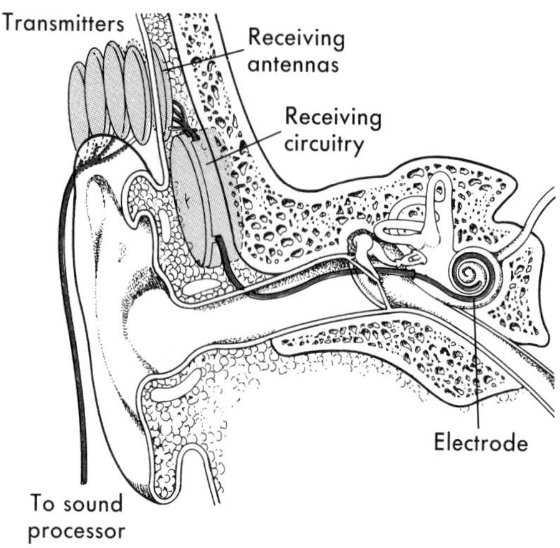

Figure 30-8 Cochlear implant. (From Beare PG, Myers JL: *Principles and practice of adult health nursing*, ed 2, St Louis, 1994, Mosby.)

Proper care of a hearing aid can eliminate problems and increase an individual's confidence in using the device. Individuals should be taught to use the hearing aid only at times and places in which it improves hearing, not at those times when there is a great deal of background noise. Whistling noises can indicate a loose or improperly worn mold. Poor amplification can result from dead batteries, wax build-up, or incorrect volume control. Pain while wearing the mold may indicate an improper fit or a sign of an infection in the ear itself or the surrounding area.

In addition to the hearing aid, there are other devices that are often helpful for individuals with hearing loss. Telephone amplifiers as well as flashing lights are available. A telephone amplifier increases the volume of the sound being carried by the telephone. Flashing lights alert the individual visually rather than through an auditory method. Cochlear implantation has become successful for some individuals with sensorineural hearing loss. The artificial cochlea is a small computer device capable of converting sound waves into electronic impulses, which in turn stimulate the nerve fibers. Although still somewhat experimental, the cochlear implant has improved hearing by 50% in some cases (Figure 30-8). Lip reading and sign language are two additional tools that can enhance communication.

Communication for the individual with a hearing loss can become a hardship. There are several helpful tips that can facilitate communication and assist the individual with the hearing loss:

Always face the individual so that the lips are visible. This is important if the person is relying on lip reading to aid communication.

- Do not raise the voice to any great extent, but do speak more slowly and distinctly than usual.
- Avoid using high tones, because they are more difficult to hear for the deaf person.
- If the individual does not understand what has been said, rephrase the statement using different words to say the same thing.
- Point to the object being talked about whenever possible.
- Some letters and sounds are more difficult to distinguish than others.
- If the individual cannot hear at all and cannot read lips, write out the message.

It is important to communicate in some way with the hearing-impaired person to prevent isolation. Sign language is also a useful tool. The nurse who works often with the hearing impaired should learn how to sign.

DISORDERS OF THE EXTERNAL EAR

Certain disorders of the external ear may affect hearing while causing pain and discomfort (Box 30-4). Common disorders include infection, obstruction, injury, and perforation of the eardrum.

Infections

Boils

Boils are one common type of infection. If large enough, they may obstruct the auditory canal and cause some degree of temporary hearing impairment. The infectious agent that causes the boil to develop is usually a staphylococcal bacteria. The bacteria gains entrance to the subcutaneous tissue through a scratch or injury that occurs while removing ear wax or a foreign body from the external ear canal. Boils can be extremely painful. As the infection develops, swelling in the lining of the auditory canal occurs. This swelling in some cases actually leads to closure of the canal. The severe pain occurs as a result of the swelling because there is no room to accommodate the tissue expansion in the bony canal. Relief may be obtained by the application of nonsterile warm compresses, a hot-water bottle, or an electric heating pad. Treatment may include instillation of drops containing antibiotics or cortisone and a solution of aluminum acetate, known as Burow's solution (Box 30-5; Table 30-1). If the infection extends to the regional lymph nodes, oral or intramuscular administration of antibiotics may be required. Drugs such as acetaminophen or codeine may be needed for pain relief in those patients with a severe infection. Boils have a tendency to recur unless prop-

BOX 30-4

SYMPTOMS OF EAR PROBLEMS

Pain or discomfort in one or both ears
Sudden or gradual hearing loss
Progressive or sudden unilateral hearing loss
Complaints of tinnitus or chronic dizziness
Air-bone conduction gap assessed by special tests
Visible signs of blockage in the ear canal from wax or foreign objects
Congenital or traumatic deformities of the ear

BOX 30-5

EAR INSTILLATIONS

1 Turn the patient's head to the side, with the affected ear upright.
2 In adult patients, the auricle should be pulled upward and backward.
3 In children, the auricle should be pulled downward.
4 Instill the prescribed number of drops (usually 3 or 4) into the ear opening without touching the meatus.
5 Pump the tragus once or twice to remove the air locks and drive the solution forward.
6 To improve contact with the inner ear, have the patient lie on the side, with the affected ear upright, for 5 to 10 minutes before the medication is instilled.

erly treated. Patients should therefore be instructed to complete all antibiotics as prescribed.

External otitis

External otitis is another common infection of the external ear. It can be the result of an infective, inflammatory, or allergic agent that comes in contact with the tissue of the external ear. External otitis is often called "swimmer's ear." Swimming tends to remove cerumen from the ear. Cerumen's primary function is to protect the external ear from bacteria. As the cerumen is removed, bacteria are introduced, causing an infection. Symptoms of external otitis include redness, swelling, and pain of the auditory canal. Treatment consists of a topical antibiotic and steroid, usually in the form of drops. Oral or intravenous antibiotics are administered in severe cases, especially if a cellulitis is present. Acetaminophen can be given and heat may be applied locally to relieve pain.

Other types of infections include those caused by fungi, which are rather uncommon. Various forms of dermatitis may occur, particularly in persons with diabetes. Other generalized infections such as erysipelas or eczema may involve the external ear.

Obstructions

Children often put foreign bodies into their ears, obstructing the auditory canal. Parents and nurses should not attempt to remove foreign bodies because of the danger of pushing them farther into the canal. When the foreign body consists of vegetable matter such as corn, peas, or beans, irrigation should not be done because the fluid will cause the object to enlarge.

Another common cause of obstruction is the accumulation of cerumen, which may plug the canal. Sometimes it pushes against the eardrum and hardens, causing pain and irritation of the eardrum. Cerumen can be softened by placing warmed oil or glycerin in the ear for 2 or 3 days; it is then removed by gentle irrigation with a syringe or a Water Pik on *low* power. Irrigation of the ear is done less often than in the past and should be done under the direction of a physician. Warm water between 105° F and 110° F (40.6° C and 43.3° C) should be used, because water that is too hot or too cold will cause pain or dizziness. Placing the tip of the syringe at the meatus and aiming toward the roof of the ear canal will give the best results. If injury to the tympanic membrane is suspected, irrigation should not be performed.

Insects such as moths can also cause an obstruction, resulting in discomfort and temporary hearing loss. An insect in the auditory canal can generally be killed by instilling a few drops of warm oil into the ear and then irrigating the canal with warm water. If the insect is alive, the physician may gently spray lidocaine in the ear to cause the insect to exit.

Injury

Injury to the external ear may result from a contusion, abrasion, or laceration, or it may be congenital in nature. Occasionally there is loss of the pinna without interference with hearing. However, the congenital absence of the pinna may include absence of the canal and eardrum, resulting in total deafness in the ear.

Perforation

Perforation of the eardrum may occur as a result of a fracture of the skull or a severe blow to the ear. It may also result from a loud noise or from otitis media (infection in the middle ear), in which there is a spontaneous rupture of the eardrum. At the time of the rup-

TABLE 30-1

Pharmacology of Drugs Used in Hearing

Drug (Generic and Trade Name); Route and Dosage	Action/Indication	Common Side Effects and Nursing Considerations
ALUMINUM ACETATE (Burow's Solution, Domeboro) **ROUTE:** Topical solution **DOSAGE:** Topically apply 15-30 minutes as compress or 1-2 drops instilled q 4-8 hr for 3 days or as ordered	Maintains skin acidity, which is protective to skin surface; used for skin irritation, for swimmer's ear to normalize pH, and for infections of external ear canal	Irritation or increasing inflammation; administer a solution warmed to body temperature after ear wax has been removed by irrigation; solutions can be diluted
AMOXICILLIN (Amoxicillin) **ROUTE:** PO **DOSAGE:** 250-300 mg q 8 hr	Used in treatment of otitis media	Rashes and diarrhea; use with caution in severe renal disease; contraindicated in hypersensitivity to penicillins
CARBAMIDE PEROXIDE (Auro Ear Drops, Debrox Drops, Murine Ear Drops) **ROUTE:** Topical **DOSAGE:** Instill several drops in ear canal at bedtime and plug with cotton ball to hold solution in place; remove ear plug in AM; perform bid if wax is thick	Commercial cerumenolytics used to soften ear wax for removal	Common products such as baby oil, mineral oil, and olive oil can also be used
BACITRACIN **ROUTE:** Topical: solution and ointment **DOSAGE:** 1-3 drops or thin layer of ointment 2-3 times daily for 7-10 days	Bacteriostatic, bacteriocidal used against gram-positive and gram-negative bacteria found in cutaneous or ocular infections	Administer and store at room temperature; hypersensitivity reaction rare in local application; usually given in combination with other drugs; parenteral administration highly nephrotoxic
CLOTRIMAZOLE (Lotrimin) **ROUTE:** Topical **DOSAGE:** Apply cream, solution, or lotion twice daily for 1-4 weeks	Topical antifungal used against a variety of cutaneous infections	Local burning, itching, stinging, redness, or local hypersensitivity reactions
DIMENHYDRINATE (Dramamine) **ROUTE:** PO, IM, IV, rectal **DOSAGE:** PO, rectal 50-100 mg q 4-6 hr (not to exceed 400 mg/day); IM, IV 50 mg q 4 hr	Used in the treatment and prevention of nausea, vomiting, dizziness, and vertigo that accompany motion sickness	Drowsiness and anorexia; use with caution in seizure disorder, glaucoma, and benign prostatic hypertrophy
FLUOCINONIDE (Lidex, Topsyn) **ROUTE:** Topical **DOSAGE:** Thin layer 2-4 times daily	Used to decrease swelling and inflammation	Administer and store at room temperature; can cause hypersensitivity reaction; usually given in combination with other products
HYDROGEN PEROXIDE **ROUTE:** Topical **DOSAGE:** 1.5% and 3.0% solutions use as needed; fill ear canal, wait until bubbling stops, and then drain	Destroys bacteria by chemical action	Can be diluted 1:1 with water or saline solution; monitor for irritation, rash, skin breaks, or dryness

TABLE 30-1

Pharmacology of Drugs Used in Hearing—cont'd

Drug (Generic and Trade Name); Route and Dosage	Action/Indication	Common Side Effects and Nursing Considerations
ISOPROPYL ALCOHOL **ROUTE:** Topical **DOSAGE:** 70%-85% solutions, use as needed	Used in dermatitis and eczema to dry ear canal	Toxic reactions are rare
MECLIZINE (Antivert) **ROUTE:** PO **DOSAGE:** 25-50 mg 1 hr before exposure, may repeat in 24 hr	Used in the management and prevention of motion sickness; also used to treat labyrinthitis or Ménière's disease	Use with caution in glaucoma and benign prostatic hypertrophy
NEOMYCIN SULFATE **ROUTE:** Topical **DOSAGE:** Instill 1-3 drops 3-4 times daily for 7-10 days	Antibiotic used to break down protein synthesis, causing bacterial death	Warm to body temperature before administration; doses should be evenly spaced to maintain blood levels
PROCHLORPERAZINE (Compazine) **ROUTE:** PO, IV, IM, rectal **DOSAGE:** PO, 5-10 mg 3-4 times daily; IM, 5-10 mg q 3-4 hr (not to exceed 40 mg/day); IV, 2.5-10 mg, not to exceed 5 mg/min, may be repeated in 30 min; single dose not to exceed 10 mg (not to exceed 40 mg/day); rectal, 25 mg bid	Used in the management of nausea and vomiting and motion sickness	Extrapyramidal reactions, dry eyes, blurred vision, constipation, dry mouth, and photosensitivity; contraindicated in glaucoma and severe cardiac or liver disease
PROMETHAZINE (Phenergan) **ROUTE:** PO, IV, IM, rectal **DOSAGE:** For motion sickness 25 mg 30-60 min before departure, may repeat in 8-12 hr	Treatment and prevention of nausea, vomiting, and motion sickness	Excess sedation, confusion, and disorientation; contraindicated with coma, benign prostatic hypertrophy, and glaucoma; use with caution in sleep apnea, epilepsy, and the elderly
SCOPOLAMINE (Transderm Scōp) **ROUTE:** PO, IM, IV, SQ, ocular, transderm **DOSAGE:** Transderm patch 1.5 mg delivers 0.5 mg over 72 hr and should be applied at least 4 hr before travel; IM, IV, SQ, 0.2-0.65 mg	Prevention of motion sickness; given preoperatively to produce amnesia and decrease salivation	Drowsiness, blurred vision, tachycardia, dry mouth, and urinary hesitancy; contraindicated in glaucoma, and tachycardia; use with caution in elderly and in chronic renal, hepatic, respiratory, or cardiac disease

ture, the individual may experience a sharp pain accompanied by some degree of hearing loss. Generally diagnosis of a perforation is made on the basis of the individual's symptoms as well as an otoscopic examination of the tympanic membrane. Most injuries to the eardrum heal without requiring medical intervention. However, if the perforation is a result of an infection, antibiotic treatment is initiated. Acetaminophen or other analgesics may be given for pain.

DISORDERS OF THE MIDDLE EAR

The middle ear is connected with the posterior part of the nose by the eustachian tube. Equalization of air pressure on both sides of the eardrum is maintained by air entering the middle ear through this tube. Infection from the nose and throat may reach the middle ear through the eustachian tube. Sometimes the tube may become inflamed or plugged with mucus, resulting in diminished hearing. The middle ear contains the or-

BOX 30-6 **Nursing Process**

OTITIS MEDIA

ASSESSMENT

Comfort level
Vital signs
Outer ear for drainage and skin integrity
Patterns of sleep
Hearing
Dizziness

NURSING DIAGNOSES

Pain related to pressure and inflammation in the ear
Risk for injury related to vertigo and diminished hearing
Sensory/perceptual alterations related to disruption in conduction of sound
Sleep pattern disturbance related to ear discomfort
Risk for impaired skin integrity related to ear drainage

NURSING INTERVENTIONS

Provide comfort measures.
Encourage diversional activities.
Provide soothing music at night.
Administer analgesics, antibiotics, and antihistamines as ordered.
Apply localized heat if indicated.
Cleanse outer ear at frequent intervals to keep free of irritating drainage, if indicated.
If ear is draining, place cotton loosely in external ear outside the canal and change often.
Reassure patient that hearing loss is usually temporary.
Speak in a slow, soft voice (loud voices can cause distortion of sound).
Maintain an environment that promotes sleep.
Organize nursing care for minimal interruptions at night.

EVALUATION OF EXPECTED OUTCOMES

Ear pain reduced or eliminated
Outer ear clean and dry
Hearing maintained
Reports restful sleep
No dizziness

gans for transmitting sound to the inner ear, and if they become diseased, deafness may result.

Otitis Media

Infection may enter the middle ear through the eustachian tube as the result of acute upper respiratory tract infections or infectious diseases such as measles or scarlet fever. Children are more susceptible to otitis media because during their early years in life their eustachian tube is more horizontal in its placement than in later years. This favors the transmission of infection from the respiratory passageways into the middle ear. Otitis media is most common in infants because the eustachian tube is shorter, wider, and straighter. In addition, the infant lies flat most of the time, allowing infected materials to move easily from the respiratory tract to the middle ear. Children and adults should be taught to blow their noses with their mouth open to reduce the probability of infection forced from the respiratory tract to the middle ear.

There are several common forms of otitis media: acute, chronic, and serous. Each type affects the structures of the middle ear, varying in cause and incidence. Acute otitis is sudden in onset and usually affects one ear. Chronic otitis follows after repeated acute episodes. It is longer in duration and generally affects both ears. Serous otitis is characterized by persistent fluid behind the tympanic membrane.

Assessment

In all three types of otitis media an infectious agent is introduced into the middle ear, where it causes inflammation of the mucous membranes. This inflammation leads to swelling as well as irritation of the ossicles. In addition, the tympanic membrane becomes red and swollen. The individual with otitis media experiences ear pain, fever, and temporary hearing impairment as a result of the swelling and pressure in the middle ear. A parent should suspect otitis in an infant or young child when crying is accompanied by pulling at the ear, or rolling the head from side to side.

Intervention

Treatment consists of oral antibiotics and acetaminophen for the ear pain. Oral antihistamines will often be prescribed to help decrease the fluid in the middle ear (Box 30-6; see Table 30-1).

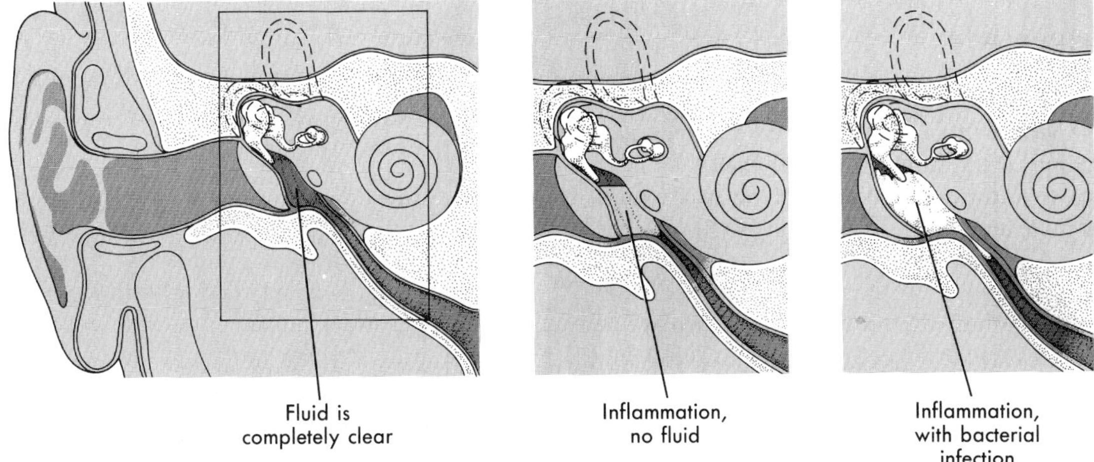

Figure 30-9 Types of middle ear infections: clear fluid, inflammation but no fluid, and purulent otitis media. (From Beare PG, Myers JL: *Principles and practice of adult health nursing*, ed 2, St Louis, 1994, Mosby.)

If the infection is severe, an abscess may form. This condition is called purulent otitis media (Figure 30-9). Purulent otitis media is caused by the streptococcus or staphylococcus organism. Because the mucous membrane lining the middle ear is continuous with parts of the mastoid process, the added danger of extension of the infection into the mastoid cells is always present.

The patient with acute purulent otitis media is usually restricted to bedrest and given amoxicillin for a week. Additional interventions include analgesics to aid in pain relief and antihistamines to decrease the level of fluid in the middle ear.

If the pain continues despite antibiotic therapy and the tympanic membrane continues to bulge because of excess fluid, a myringotomy is usually performed. A **myringotomy** is a surgical incision of a portion of the tympanic membrane. It can be done under a local anesthetic using an ionesthetizer. The ionesthetizer anesthetizes the eardrum through ion transfer with the use of a local anesthetic solution and an electrode in the ear canal. The procedure is usually performed in a physician's office or an outpatient setting.

A myringotomy results in drainage of the middle ear and almost immediate pain relief. Drainage from the ear is generally bloody at first but becomes purulent. Small tissues should be used to remove the drainage, or cotton should be placed loosely at the external opening of the auditory canal so as not to obstruct the flow of drainage. The area around the external ear should be kept clean because the drainage will cause severe irritation if allowed to remain on the skin. Unless proper treatment is given, the condition may become chronic, and the individual may have a draining ear for months or even years. The patient should be protected from chilling and observed for an increase in pain or temperature, which may indicate the need for an additional incision or may be a sign of extension of the infection.

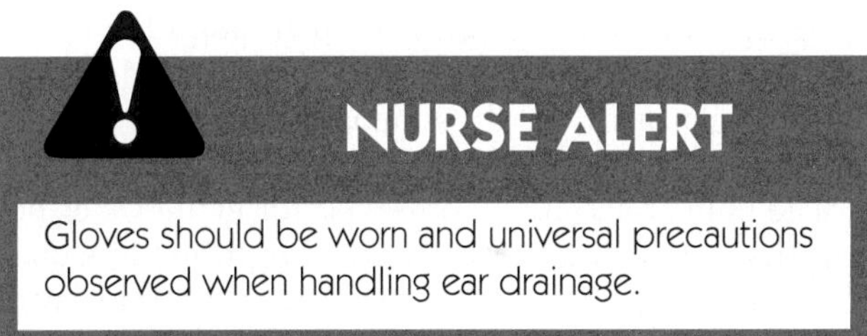

NURSE ALERT

Gloves should be worn and universal precautions observed when handling ear drainage.

Mastoiditis

The mucous membrane lining of the middle ear is continuous with parts of the mastoid process embedded in the temporal lobe. If an infection in the middle ear, such as purulent otitis media, is untreated or inadequately treated, it can continue to the mastoid process and cause **mastoiditis**, inflammation of those cells in the mastoid process. If severe enough, the infection may continue to extend to the brain, causing the formation of a brain abscess or the development of meningitis. In the days before antibiotic therapy, mastoiditis was a leading cause of death in children and of hearing loss in adults. Antibiotic therapy is now aimed at treating otitis media before it progresses to mastoiditis.

Symptoms of mastoiditis include an elevated temperature and pain and tenderness over the mastoid area. There may also be tissue swelling, which tends to push the ear forward. A myringotomy and large doses of oral antibiotics will usually cure mastoiditis. A mastoidectomy, or surgical removal of the infected tissue, is necessary if there is evidence of bone destruction and the infection does not improve with antibiotic therapy.

Mastoidectomy

Preoperative intervention

The preoperative care of the patient undergoing a mastoidectomy is the same as that for the other surgical patients. In addition, particular attention should be focused on hair removal because of the location of the surgery. A careful explanation should be given to all patients concerning removal of hair, and only the necessary amount of hair should be removed. An area of approximately 1½ to 2 inches around the ear is shaved.

Postoperative intervention

When the patient returns from surgery, the ear will be covered with a large pressure dressing that is secured with bandages around the head. The patient should be placed in a semi-Fowler's position. As soon as nausea subsides, oral fluids and a diet as tolerated may be given. Fluids will be administered by the intravenous route if nausea persists. Medication is given to relieve pain as necessary. Temperature, pulse, and respiration rates are measured every 4 hours and recorded. Some drainage may occur through the dressing. If necessary, the nurse may reinforce the dressing, but in most cases, the dressing is changed only by the physician. Antibiotics are usually ordered as indicated.

The patient should be observed for evidence of hemorrhage, which might appear as bright-red blood on the dressing. Stiffness of the neck may occur from positioning during surgery, but stiffness accompanied by headache, visual disturbances, or signs of facial paralysis should be reported to the physician immediately.

Tympanoplasty

Tympanoplasty is the name given to a group of surgical procedures designed to restore hearing loss caused by perforation of the tympanic membrane or necrosis of one of the ossicles of the middle ear, usually following chronic otitis media. The simplest form is a myringoplasty, in which the perforation in the eardrum is closed and reinforced with a tissue graft. Other types of tympanoplasty are more extensive and involve the bones of the middle ear.

Preoperative intervention

There is little preoperative care needed if the patient will be having a simple tympanoplasty such as a myringotomy. The procedure is done under local anesthesia in an outpatient setting. The preoperative care for a patient undergoing a more extensive tympanoplasty will be the same as that for other surgical patients. In either case the patient should be given an explanation of the surgery and should know what to expect postoperatively.

Postoperative intervention

The patient should lie on the unaffected side with the affected ear upward for 12 hours after surgery. The inner dressing in the ear canal is not disturbed, but the outer dressing is changed if it becomes saturated. Because the patient is likely to experience vertigo and nausea after surgery, caution should be taken during ambulation. Antiemetics should be administered as ordered. The patient must keep the ear dry and avoid sneezing and blowing the nose. If it is necessary to blow the nose or if a sneeze occurs, the nurse should instruct the patient to maintain an open mouth to avoid a build-up of pressure in the ear. The patient may not swim or travel by air until healing is complete; however, once the healing is complete, patients will have few restrictions. Antibiotics will be administered for 5 to 7 days postoperatively.

Otosclerosis

The middle ear contains three ossicles, whose function is to transmit sound to the inner ear. Normally the stapes vibrates against the oval window, through which sound reaches the inner ear. In otosclerosis a new growth of bone forms, causing the footplate of the stapes to become fixed in the oval window, preventing it from transmitting sound.

Otosclerosis is the most common cause of conductive deafness. The cause of otosclerosis is unknown, but it is believed that there is a hereditary predisposition to the disorder. Diagnosis is made through evaluation of symptoms as well as an examination of family history. The loss of hearing may first be detected during the adolescent years and may be discovered through audiometer testing. Usually, the loss affects both ears, although one may be more severely involved than the other. The hearing impairment continues to increase slowly until the person reaches 40 years of age or older, by which time the loss may be great. There is currently no medical treatment that cures the disorder or impedes its progress. A surgical procedure called a **stapedectomy** restores hearing in approximately 90% of patients.

Stapedectomy

The stapedectomy is considered the treatment of choice for otosclerosis. In this procedure the stapes is removed and replaced by a small piece of wire or a plastic piston. This is attached to a graft of fat, vein, or Gelfoam, which covers the oval window. Occasionally the footplate of the stapes will be left in place and the

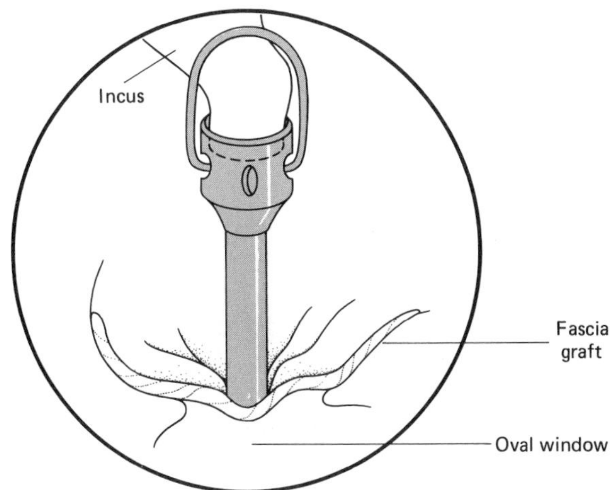

Figure 30-10 One type of stapedectomy. A prosthesis replaces the stapes. The fascia graft over the oval window thins out and becomes contiguous with the adjacent mucoperiosteum. (From Lewis SM, Collier IC: *Medical-surgical nursing: assessment and management of clinical problems*, ed 3, St Louis, 1992, Mosby.)

prosthesis placed through it. Sound travels from the incus to the wire or plastic piece, which vibrates the tissues of the oval window. Liquids of the inner ear then pick up the vibrations, and nerve impulses are initiated (Figure 30-10).

Preoperative intervention

Preoperative preparation of the patient is essentially the same as that for other surgery. A local anesthetic is generally given to avoid the postoperative effects of general anesthesia. The patient should be advised to wash the hair before entering the hospital to avoid the danger of getting water into the ear after surgery. The patient should be given an explanation of the surgery and know what to expect postoperatively.

Postoperative intervention

For the first 24 hours postoperatively, the patient is kept flat in bed and once again instructed not to blow the nose. All head movements should be kept to a minimum. After the initial 24-hour period the patient may be allowed up but should not get up alone. The patient should be helped to get out of bed and walk slowly, keeping head and torso in line and the head level.

There will be packing in the auditory canal and a dressing covering the ear. Slight drainage may appear on the dressing, but any bright red blood should be reported. The patient should be instructed to keep the dressing dry and to avoid getting water in the ear (thus hair washing and swimming are not allowed) and is taught to maintain a sterile technique while changing the dressing. Situations should be avoided in which there are air pressure changes, such as traveling on airplanes with poorly pressurized cabins.

The patient should be carefully observed for signs that might indicate complications such as meningitis or facial paralysis. Facial nerve paralysis may occur immediately postoperatively because of injection of anesthetic near the nerve. Function should return in about 4 hours. Dryness of the mouth or decreased taste sensation may occur from injury to the chorda tympani nerve during surgery. These symptoms will eventually pass but may last for several months. Vertigo may occur from trauma, loss of perilymph, or labyrinthitis.

A sensation of sloshing in the ear may indicate a collection of serous fluid in the middle ear. Otitis media can also occur as a complication of the surgery. Because eating may be painful, administration of an analgesic before meals will increase comfort. A liquid diet is given postoperatively, with a gradual increase to soft foods as tolerated. If nausea and vomiting occur, antiemetics may be ordered.

The patient is generally discharged 3 to 4 days after surgery. It is important that the patient understand that the return of hearing is not immediate but will return gradually over several weeks. Prolonged hospitalization until hearing returns is not indicated.

DISORDERS OF THE INNER EAR

Labyrinthitis

The labyrinth is a system of cavities within the inner ear that communicate with one another. **Labyrinthitis** is an inflammation of these structures and usually results from an extension of infection from the middle ear. The characteristic symptom is severe dizziness (vertigo), causing a disturbance of equilibrium. In patients with severe cases of labyrinthitis, nausea and vomiting may occur. There is generally some hearing impairment as well. Labyrinthitis is usually treated with antibiotics. In addition, the individual is instructed to remain in bed as much as possible and to avoid getting out of bed without assistance because of the danger of falling. If nausea and vomiting are severe, intravenous fluids and antiemetic drugs to control vomiting may be administered.

NURSE ALERT

Care must be taken when ambulating a patient who is experiencing vertigo.

Ménière's Syndrome

Assessment

Ménière's syndrome is characterized by three symptoms occurring together: tinnitus, nausea and vomiting, and vertigo. Unilateral sensorineural hearing loss may be present. The symptoms result from an increase in the endolymph, which causes increased pressure in the inner ear. The cause of the increased endolymph is unknown. However, any factor that increases endolymphatic secretion, such as viral or bacterial infections, allergic reactions, or biochemical disturbances, could potentially be the cause of Ménière's syndrome. Vascular changes in the circulation of the labyrinth as well as psychologic factors have also been suggested as possible causes of the disease.

Intervention

There is currently no specific treatment for Ménière's syndrome. Intervention is aimed at treating the individual symptoms, especially the vertigo, because it is usually severe. Sudden movement may increase the severity of the symptoms. The nurse should provide for patient safety and allow the patient to move in a way that causes the least discomfort. The symptoms of Ménière's syndrome often cause the patient to become anxious or depressed. Good communication and emotional support are necessary when working with these patients.

Often a patient with Ménière's syndrome has a poor appetite. If this is the case, it may be necessary to encourage the patient to eat. In severe prolonged attacks, hyperalimentation supplements or intravenous fluids may be given. The patient is usually prescribed a low-sodium diet to help control edema.

Some patients respond to medical treatment. Vitamins have provided relief to some older patients. Meclizine (Bonine) and nicotinic acid have also been effective in relieving the symptoms of the disease. There is no cure at this time. Drug therapy is aimed at controlling the vertigo and vomiting and restoring normal balance.

Surgery may be performed to relieve severe vertigo. The surgical procedure consists of destruction of the membranous labyrinth. This procedure remains controversial because the remaining hearing in the affected ear is sacrificed during the process. When the loss of hearing is minimal, ultrasonic surgery may relieve symptoms and preserve hearing. Bell's palsy may complicate ultrasonic surgery but will clear in several weeks.

ETHICAL DILEMMA

Mrs. Braun is a 72-year-old woman who has been admitted for surgery. She has a significant hearing loss. You observe the surgeon at her bedside giving her the information she needs to give informed consent for surgery. However, the surgeon is speaking very quickly and very softly. Mrs. Braun is nodding her head as if she understands, but you know she is not hearing a word that the surgeon is saying.

How would you analyze the ethical issues in this case?

KEY CONCEPTS

- Hearing loss can occur as a result of an inflammatory process, an obstruction in the external or middle ear, or damage to the inner ear or auditory nerve.
- Loss of hearing has an impact on both the patient and the family.
- Hearing loss often contributes to feelings of anxiety, loneliness, and isolation. Nursing interventions should be aimed at supporting the patient and assisting him or her to explore the various avenues of communication.
- Older adults are more susceptible to hearing loss as a result of degenerative changes in many of their ear structures.
- The scope and type of testing performed on a patient with an ear disorder depend on the symptoms presented.
- Successful use of a hearing aid depends on the patient's type of hearing loss, desire, and level of understanding of how to properly use the hearing aid.
- Conditions such as an upper respiratory tract infection or allergies can contribute to problems with hearing or equilibrium.
- The pain associated with many of the disorders of the external ear is caused by swelling in the lining of the auditory canal. There is no room to accommodate this tissue expansion in the bony canal.

KEY CONCEPTS

- The location, characteristics, intensity, and duration of ear pain are important nursing assessments.
- Nursing care of the patient with otitis media is aimed at reducing pain and inflammation, keeping the outer ear clean and dry, and maintaining hearing.
- Postoperative care of the patient with ear surgery involves providing a safe environment, pain management, dressing care, positioning, providing hydration and nutrition, psychologic support, and monitoring for infection.
- A patient recovering from ear surgery should be instructed to avoid sneezing and nose blowing or told to maintain an open mouth when sneezing or blowing the nose to avoid middle ear pressure.
- An inner ear disorder is recognized by characteristic symptoms, including vertigo, tinnitus, nystagmus, and hearing loss.
- Potential for injury and sensory/perceptual alterations are two important considerations when caring for a patient with an inner ear disorder.

CRITICAL THINKING EXERCISES

1 Mrs. Johns, who is 78 years of age, fell in her home and suffered an injury to her pelvis. She was admitted to a nursing home and placed on bedrest for 3 months. Mrs. Johns recently developed a severe hearing impairment. Her daughter, who lives in a distant city, came to see her and thought that her mother should have a hearing aid. The daughter contacted a salesman from a manufacturing firm and requested that he see her mother and fit her with a hearing aid. When the prosthesis arrived, a representative of the firm took it to Mrs. Johns and instructed her in its use. Mrs. Johns gave the hearing aid to a visiting neighbor, asking her to take it home and keep it for her.

a What kind of deafness did Mrs. Johns have?
b Had Mrs. Johns been seen by an otologist for diagnosis?
c Did Mrs. Johns think that she needed a hearing aid?
d How long does it take to master the use of a hearing aid?

2 Mrs. Smith, who is 82 years of age, has noticed a progressive loss of hearing. Today she tells you that she has come to see her physician because of her son's insistence. She feels her loss of hearing is just a part of old age and that nothing can be done to correct it.

a What changes in the ear structures associated with aging might Mrs. Smith be experiencing?
b What type of hearing loss might Mrs. Smith be experiencing?
c What testing methods would you expect Mrs. Smith's otologist to perform?
d Why is Mrs. Smith denying her hearing loss?
e What could you say to Mrs. Smith?

REFERENCES AND ADDITIONAL READINGS

Barkauskas VH and others: *Health and physical assessment*, St Louis, 1994, Mosby.

Beare PG, Myers JL: *Principles and practice of adult health nursing*, ed 2, St Louis, 1994, Mosby.

Cremers CW, Beusen JM, Huygen PL: Hearing gain after stapedectomy, partial platinectomy or total stapedectomy for otosclerosis, *Ann Otol Rhinol Laryngol* 100(12):959-961, 1991.

Dennis JM, Neely JG: Basic hearing tests, review, *Otolaryngol Clin North Am* 24(2):253-276, 1991.

Fitzgerald MA, Dietrich TR: *Mastering advanced assessment*, Pennsylvania, 1993, Springhouse.

Fliss DM, Leiberman A, Dagan R: Medical sequelae and complications of acute otitis media, *Pediatr Infect Dis J* 13 (1 suppl 1):534-540, 550-554, 1994.

Giddings NA, House JW: Tympano sclerosis of the stapes: hearing results for various surgical treatments, *Otolaryngol Head Neck Surg* 107(5):644-650, 1992.

Hall JW, Baer JE: Current concepts in hearing assessment of children and adults, *Compr Ther* 19(6):272-280, 1993.

Hirsch JE, Thompson JM: *Clinical nursing*, ed 2, St Louis, 1989, Mosby.

Jacob V and others: Can Rinne's test quantify hearing loss? *Ear Nose Throat J* 72(2):152-153, 1992.

Johnson A: Screening tests for sensorineural deafness, *Nurs Times* 86(44):52-53, 1990.

Johnston DF: A new modification of the Rinne test, *Clin Otolaryngol* 17(4):322-326, 1992.

Lewis SM, Collier IC: *Medical-surgical nursing,* ed 3, St Louis, 1992, Mosby.

Lewis-Cullinan C, Janken JK: Effect of cerumen removal on the hearing ability of geriatric patients, *J Adv Nurs* 15(5): 594-600, 1990.

Lichtenstein MJ: Hearing and visual impairments, *Clin Geriatr Med* 8(1):173-182, 1992.

Mulrow CD: Screening for hearing impairment in the elderly, *Hosp Pract* 26(2A):79, 83-86, 1991.

Munz M and others: Otitis media and CNS complications, *J Otolaryngol* 21(3):224-226, 1992.

Myer CM: The diagnosis and management of mastoiditis in children, *Pediatr Ann* 20(11):633-626, 1991.

Nassif PS, Shelton C, House HP: Otosclerosis, treating progressive hearing loss in young adults, *Postgrad Med* 91(8): 279-282, 287-290, 295, 1992.

Ng M, Jacklev RK: Early history of tuning fork tests, *Am J Otol* 14(1):100-105, 1993.

O'Rourke CM and others: Effectiveness of a hearing screening protocol for the elderly, *Geriatr Nurs* 14(2):66-69, 1993.

Rapin I: Hearing disorders, *Pediatr Rev* 14(2):43-49, 1993.

Roberts A: Systems of life; the ear and hearing, *Nurs Times* 90(2):45-48, 1994.

Seidel HM and others: *Mosby's guide to physical examination,* ed 3, St Louis, 1994, Mosby.

Shea JJ, Domico EH, Lupfer M: Speech perception after multichannel cochlear implantation in the pediatric patient, *Am J Otol* 15(1):66-70, 1994.

Snow JB, Martin JB, Wilson JB: *Principles of internal medicine,* ed 12, New York, 1991, McGraw-Hill.

CHAPTER 31

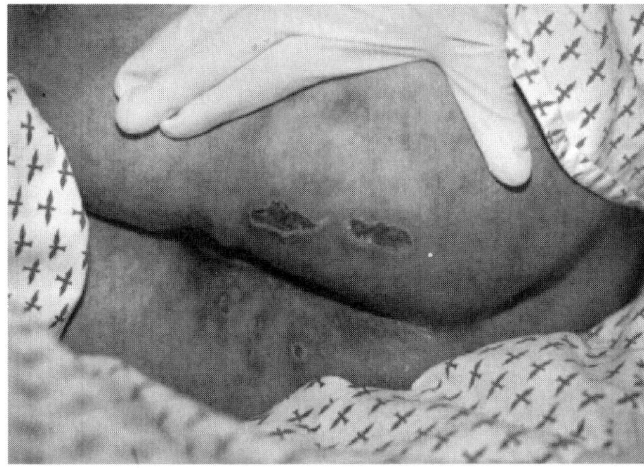

Skin Integrity

CHAPTER OBJECTIVES

1 Identify the functions of the skin.
2 Describe the correct methods for applying open and closed wet dressings and for administering a soak or therapeutic bath.
3 Identify measures to prevent and treat pressure ulcers.
4 Differentiate between the signs and symptoms of folliculitis, furuncles, and carbuncles, and identify the usual causative organism of each.
5 Describe the lesions and transmission of impetigo.
6 Differentiate signs, symptoms, and intervention for the various forms of ringworm (tinea).
7 Differentiate the causes of chafing, prickly heat, plant poisoning, exfoliative dermatitis, and drug dermatitis.
8 Describe lesions and interventions for psoriasis and eczema.
9 Discuss the facts essential to teaching the patient to control systemic lupus erythematosus.
10 Differentiate between herpes simplex types 1 and 2 and herpes zoster.
11 Describe nursing measures to provide relief for the patient with pruritus.
12 Differentiate between the appearance of malignant and benign skin lesions.
13 Describe methods for the prevention and treatment of pediculosis.
14 Identify the causes of the various types of burn injuries.
15 Describe the prevention of airway obstruction and the treatment of burn shock.
16 Evaluate the location, size, depth, and severity of the burn wound.
17 Elicit from the patient or a family member the past medical history of the patient, the age, and allergies to drugs.
18 Describe the three phases of burn care: emergent, acute, and rehabilitative.
19 Describe the following methods of treatment for burns: open (exposure), closed (occlusive) dressings, and topical antimicrobial agents.
20 Discuss the role of the nurse in caring for a patient with skin grafts or artificial grafts.
21 Prepare the burn patient and the family for discharge by teaching the care necessary to support the patient at home and by reviewing the appropriate follow-up care to be provided by the burn team.

KEY WORDS

atopic
atrophy
autograft
bleb
bulla
carbonaceous sputum
circumferential
comedones
crust
debridement
dermis
emergent
epidermis
eschar
escharotomy
fissure
full-thickness skin graft
gumma
heterograft
homograft
hydrotherapy
lichenification
macule
nodule
papule
pressure ulcer
pustule
sebaceous
seborrhea
sebum
shear
shearing force
split-thickness skin graft (STSG)
tangential
telangiectasia
tinea
total body surface area (TBSA)
urticaria
vesicle
wheal

STRUCTURE AND FUNCTION OF THE SKIN

The skin is the largest organ of the body and is often referred to as the integumentary system. It is considered an organ because of its physiologic structure and its many functions (Table 31-1). The functions of the skin are sensory reception, protection, excretion, thermoregulation, communication, vitamin synthesis, maintenance of homeostasis, processing of antigenic substances, and cosmetic adornment. Each function correlates to specific structures and properties in the **epidermis** and **dermis** (Hill, 1994).

The skin is usually thought of as having two distinct layers: the epidermis and the dermis (Figure 31-1); however, a third layer of tissue, the subcutaneous, may be included because of its function in helping to protect other body tissues. The epidermis is the outermost layer, and it actually has four layers or regions, sometimes called strata (stratum basale, stratum spinosum, stratum granulosum, stratum corneum). The three outermost regions consist of dead cells that are constantly being pushed to the surface and shed while new cells are being developed in the innermost region. The principal substance of the outside layer of the epidermis is keratin. Keratin is a protein that provides a waterproof covering that prevents the skin from drying. It has a slightly acidic action, which is the source of the skin's acidity and serves as a barrier to invading pathogens. Hair and nails are a specialized form of keratin that has become dry and firm. The epidermis also contains the pigment melanin, which provides the coloring of the skin and helps prevent skin cancer by shielding the skin from excessive exposure to sunlight. There is an increased synthesis of melanin on exposure to ultraviolet light, and this is the process involved in suntanning. Dark-skinned people have larger melanin pigment granules than light-skinned people. There are no blood vessels in the epidermis, so it receives its nourishment and fluids through seepage of lymph from blood vessels below.

The dermis, or true skin, is closely attached to the epidermis and consists of two layers. The uppermost (superficial) layer contains small elevations that project upward into the epidermis. The reticular or deeper layer contains numerous capillary blood vessels and nerve fibers. This is why bleeding and pain occur when a person pricks a finger. Some of the nerve fibers have receptors for hot and cold, others for touch and pressure, and some are concerned with vasodilation and vasoconstriction. The dermis also contains the sudoriferous (sweat) and sebaceous (oil) glands. All the structures are held together by fibrous and elastic connective tissue. The elasticity of this tissue decreases with the aging process, which causes the skin to take on a wrinkled appearance.

Beneath the dermis is a layer of subcutaneous tissue, also called superficial facia. The subcutaneous

TABLE 31-1

Functions of the Skin

Function	Epidermis	Dermis	Subcutaneous
Protection from dehydration	Keratin renders skin impervious to water, preventing undue water loss	Sebaceous glands render skin impervious to water, preventing undue water loss	
Protection from mechanical injury	Mechanical strength protects underlying structures; layer is thicker where subject to more friction (palms, soles of feet)	Mechanical strength from collagen fibers, elastic fibers, ground substance	Mechanical shock absorber
Protection from infection	Dry external surface inhibits growth of microorganisms Cells reproduce rapidly to repair surface if skin damaged or torn, provided dermis intact	Lymphatic and vascular tissues capable of inflammatory and immune response; first line of defense against microorganisms	
Protection from ultraviolet light	Melanin absorbs UV light and protects subepidermal layers		
Temperature regulation	Sweat glands secrete sweat, taking energy from the skin to reduce skin temperature by evaporating sweat, thus reducing core body temperature	Dilation or constriction of blood vessels will promote or inhibit heat conduction, convection, radiation, and evaporation	
Vitamin synthesis	When exposed to sunlight, synthesizes vitamin D from dehydrocholesterol in malpighian cells; supplements vitamin D taken with food		
Sensory organ	Transmits sensations through neuroreceptor system	Relays sensations to brain	Contains large pressure receptors
Communication	Blushing and facial expressions communicate wide range of emotions		
Preservation of self-image	Epidermal diseases such as psoriasis can alter body image and self-esteem	Dermal diseases such as scleroderma can alter body image and self-esteem	

tissue, closely adherent to the dermis, provides support and, through small arteries and lymphatics, maintains a blood supply to the dermis. Subcutaneous tissue contains large amounts of fat and some sweat glands. The thickness of the skin and the amount of subcutaneous tissue vary on different parts of the body.

The nails, hair, and sebaceous and sudoriferous glands and their ducts are appendages of the skin.

The **sebaceous** glands secrete an oily substance called **sebum,** which keeps the hair from becoming brittle. Sebum also functions to waterproof the hair and skin, promote the absorption of fat-soluble substances into the dermis, and synthesize vitamin D. It may have some antibacterial function (Hill, 1994). The acid coating (pH 4 to 6.8) on the surface of the skin is provided by sebum. The vernix caseosa on the newborn infant is an accumulation of sebum from the sebaceous glands. The sebaceous gland may open into a hair follicle or may open directly onto the skin.

The sweat glands originate as blind coiled tubes with ducts that ultimately open on the surface of the skin as pores. These glands are distributed over the entire body but are more numerous on the forehead, palms of the hands, and soles of the feet. The sweat glands are important because they function in regulating body heat through evaporation of water from the skin surface.

The hair and nails are subordinate to the skin. The appearance of the nails changes during illness, and they may become brittle and easily broken, whereas in old age they may be rough and thickened.

Because of the numerous nerve endings in the skin, its function as a sense organ is of primary importance. Through the sense of touch, the nurse is able to feel the

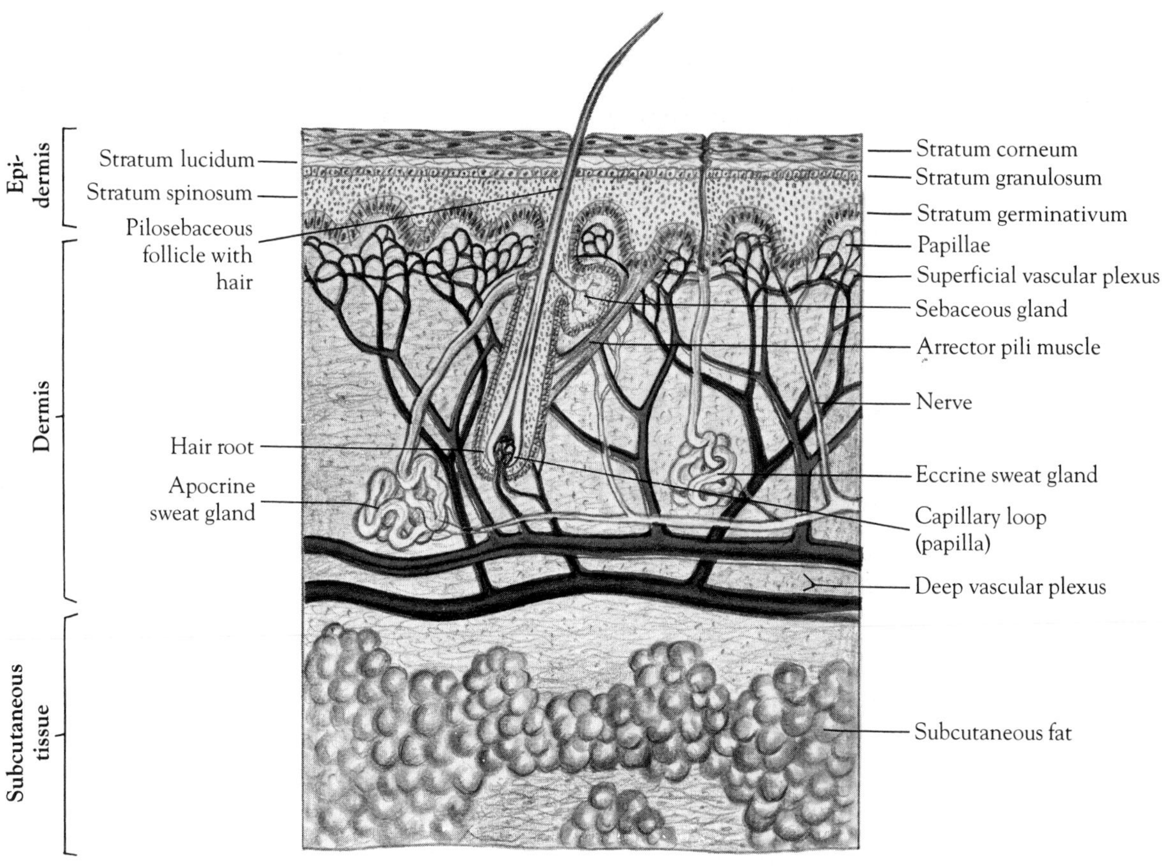

Figure 31-1 Structures of the skin. (From Thompson JM and others: *Mosby's manual of clinical nursing,* ed 3, St Louis, 1993, Mosby.)

patient's pulse or the temperature of the skin. Any disruption of this function can have negative effects. The classic example is the patient with diabetes who develops a foot ulcer because the pain from the incorrectly fitted shoe is not perceived.

The unbroken skin is the first line of defense against pathogenic organisms. The skin protects deeper tissue from injury and loss of body fluids. The excretory function of the skin is limited, but one of its most important functions is to help regulate body temperature. This regulation is accomplished in two ways: (1) evaporation of sweat from the body and (2) dissipation of excess heat into the air when blood vessels dilate, bringing more blood, and thus increased heat, to the skin surface.

NURSING ASSESSMENT OF THE SKIN

In health or disease the normal skin tells many things about an individual, and in many situations it may provide valuable diagnostic clues to disease. Nursing personnel should routinely observe the color of the skin, its texture, presence of rashes or lesions, and characteristics of the hair and nails. Cyanosis, pallor, profuse sweating, and skin rashes are some of the conditions observed that may help to identify disease. In a state of health most persons take their skin for granted and pay too little attention to it, but when disease affects the skin, they become greatly disturbed. Skin that is well cared for and free from disease is a psychologic, social, and economic asset. It contributes to a feeling of well-being, to social acceptance, and to educational and employment opportunities.

ASSESSMENT AND DESCRIPTION OF SKIN LESIONS

Certain types of skin lesions are peculiar to specific disorders and help the dermatologist identify the disease (Figure 31-2). Some diseases are characterized

Lesion

Macule—flat; nonpalpable; circumscribed; less than 1 cm in diameter; brown, red, purple, white, or tan
Examples: Freckles; flat moles; rubella; rubeola; drug eruptions
Note: Classified as patch if greater than 1 cm in diameter

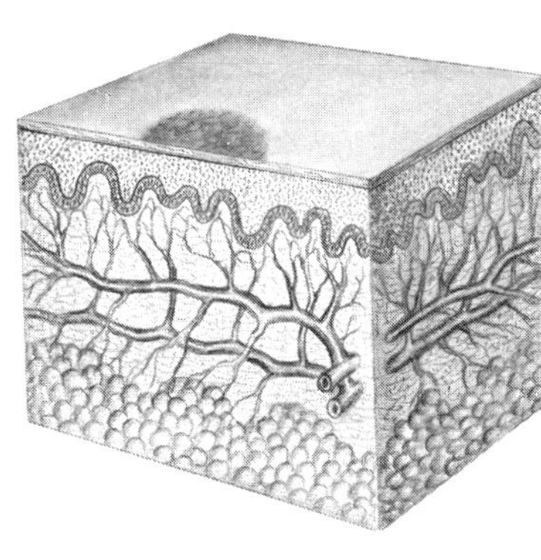

Plaque—elevated; flat topped; firm; rough; superficial papule greater than 1 cm in diameter; may be coalesced papules
Examples: Psoriasis; seborrheic and actinic keratoses; eczema

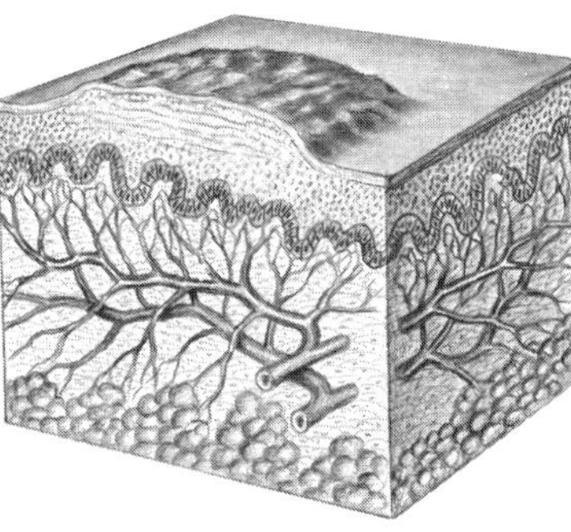

Nodule—elevated; firm; circumscribed; palpable; deeper in dermis than papule; 1 to 2 cm in diameter
Examples: Erythema nodosum; lipomas

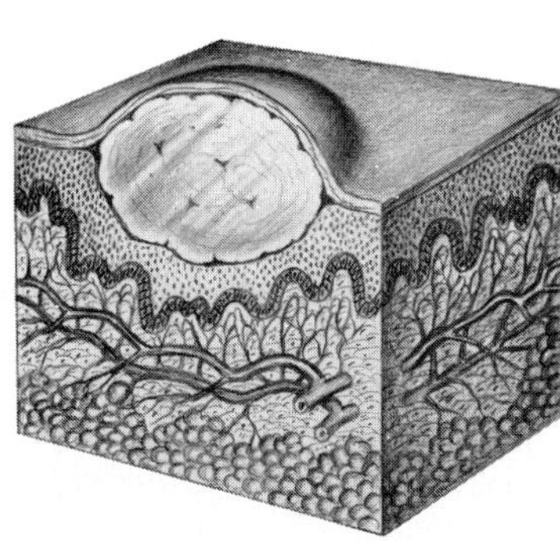

Scale—heaped-up keratinized cells; flaky exfoliation; irregullar; thick or thin; dry or oily; varied size; silver, white, or tan
Examples: Psoriasis; exfoliative dermatitis

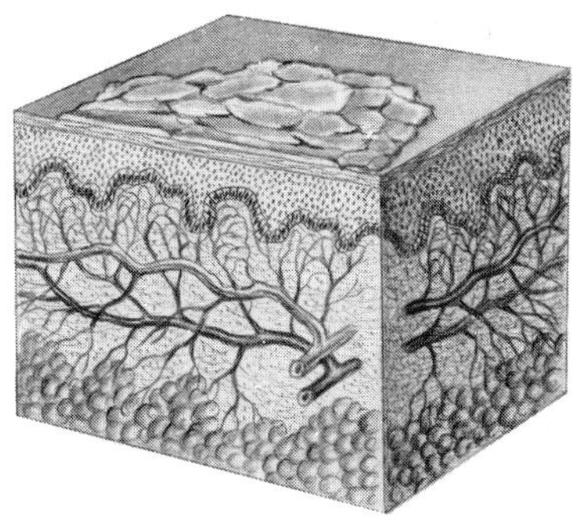

Papule—elevated; palpable; firm; circumscribed; less than 1 cm in diameter; brown, red, pink, tan, or bluish red
Examples: Warts; drug-related eruptions; pigmented nevi; eczema

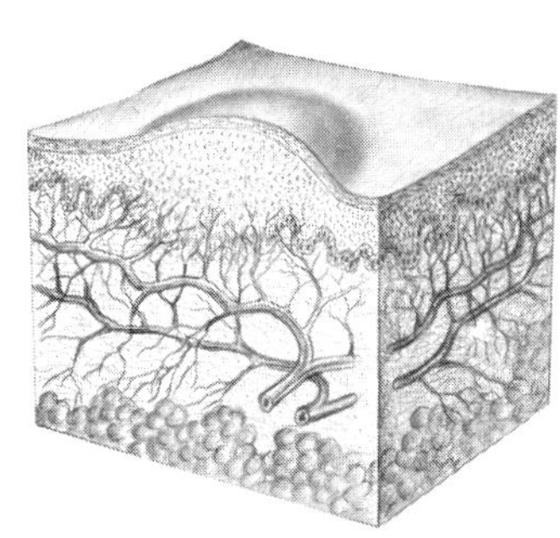

Wheal—elevated, irregular-shaped area of cutaneous edema; solid, transient, changing; variable diameter; pale pink
Examples: Urticaria; insect bites

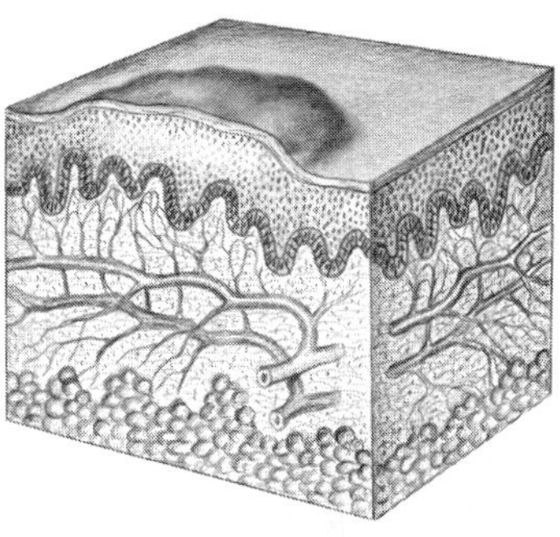

Vesicle—elevated; circumscribed; superficial; filled with serous fluid; less than 1 cm in diameter
Examples: Blister; varicella
Note: Classified as bulla if greater than 1 cm

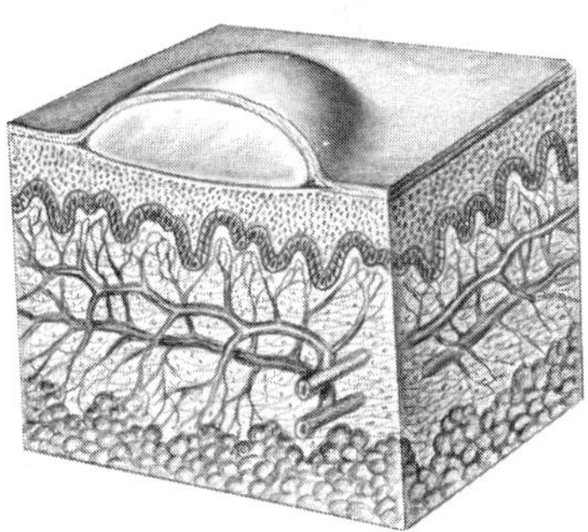

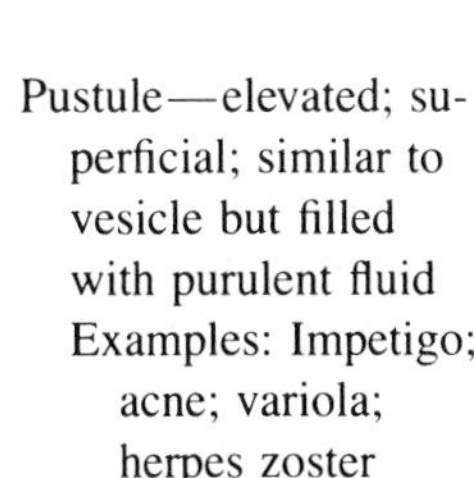

Pustule—elevated; superficial; similar to vesicle but filled with purulent fluid
Examples: Impetigo; acne; variola; herpes zoster

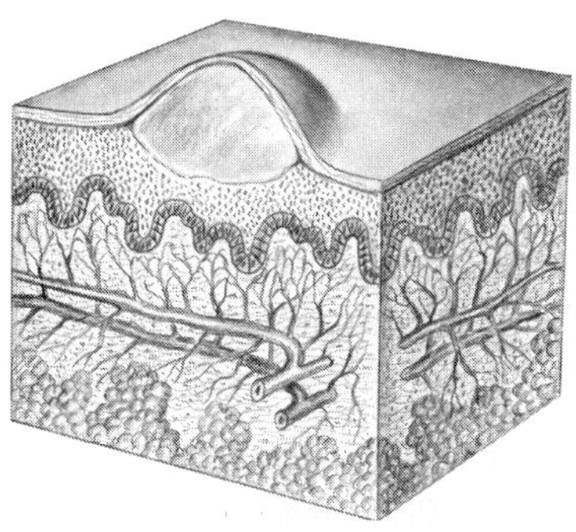

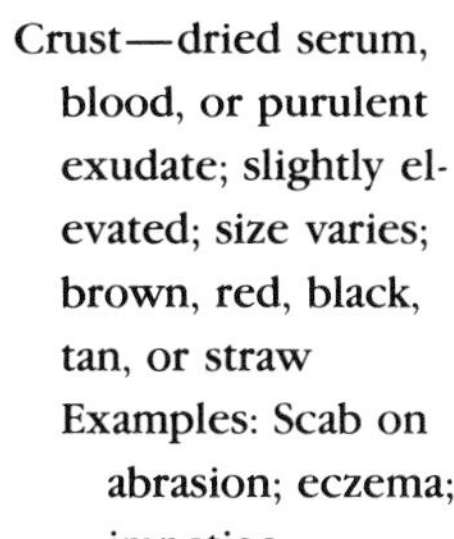

Crust—dried serum, blood, or purulent exudate; slightly elevated; size varies; brown, red, black, tan, or straw
Examples: Scab on abrasion; eczema; impetigo

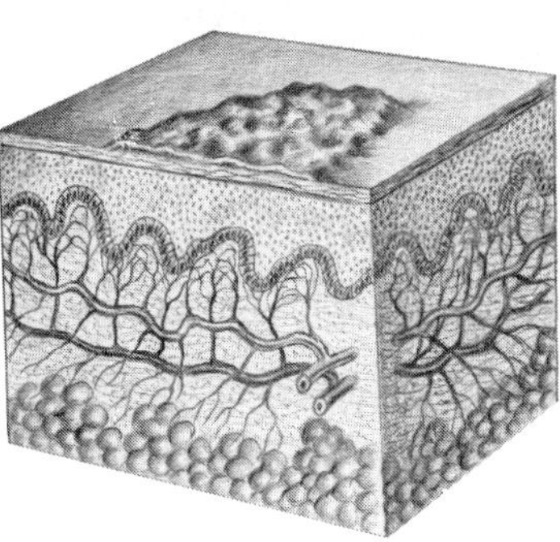

Figure 31-2 Common skin lesions. (From Thompson JM and others: *Mosby's clinical nursing,* ed 3, St Louis, 1993, Mosby.)

BOX 31-1

TYPES OF SKIN LESIONS

atrophy A wasting or thinning of body tissue, typically occurring with the aging process and with some neurologic diseases
bleb An irregular elevation of the epidermis filled with serous or seropurulent fluid; may be large in size and is seen in certain forms of severe dermatitis
bulla A vesicle greater than 1 cm in diameter
crust A dry exudate, commonly called a *scab*, occurring in impetigo, smallpox, chickenpox, and eczema
excoriation An abraded or denuded area of skin; Unless expert care is given to prevent it, may occur where there is drainage, as with a colostomy
fissure A groove, crack, or slit in the skin
gumma A tumorlike lesion similar in appearance to an abscess; characteristic of late syphilis
macule A discolored spot on the skin that may be of various colors and shapes; is neither raised nor depressed
nodule A raised, solid lesion that is deeper in the skin than a papule
papule A small, solid elevation varying from the size of a pinhead to a pea; may be seen in eczema, measles, smallpox, and syphilis
pustule A small elevation filled with pus; characteristic of impetigo and acne vulgaris
scale A small, thin flake of dry epidermis seen in eczema and psoriasis
scar The mark left on the skin after repair of deep tissue loss
ulcer An open lesion on the skin with loss of deep tissue (epidermis and part of dermis), often healing with a scar; classic example is decubitus ulcer
vesicle A blisterlike elevation on the skin containing serous fluid; occurs in herpes simplex, chickenpox, and impetigo
wheal Elevation of varying size and irregular shape; if extensive, may run together; characteristic of various allergic reactions and often referred to as hives

by an orderly sequence of skin lesions. With chickenpox, red macules surmounted by vesicles first appear (lesion is described as a "dew drop on a rose petal"), then umbilication, and finally crusting. Several different types of lesions may be present in an individual at the same time (Boxes 31-1 and 31-2).

BOX 31-2

ASSESSMENT OF SKIN IN DARK-SKINNED INDIVIDUALS

1 Inspection and palpation are equally important in assessing the dark-skinned patient. Skin color changes are best observed in the sclera, conjunctiva, oral mucosa, tongue, lips, nail beds, palms, and soles. Normal variations in pigmentation should be considered when assessing for skin color changes. The oral mucosa may have areas of darker pigmentation in the gums, the cheeks, and borders of the tongue. The lips may have a normal dark blue color. The presence of edema may cause dark skin to appear lighter in color. Changes in skin texture assessed by palpation may be the only indication of the presence of skin rashes.
2 In dark-skinned patients, pallor results in the loss of normal red tones in the skin. The brown-skinned person may have yellow-tinged skin when pallor is present. In the black-skinned patient, pallor produces an "ashen gray" color.
3 Jaundice is best observed in the sclera closest to the center of the eye. The dark-skinned patient may have normal yellow pigmentation present in the sclera. Inspection of the hard palate for a yellow color can confirm the presence of jaundice.
4 Cyanosis may be difficult to detect in the dark-skinned patient. Inspection in areas of lightest pigmentation will often indicate the presence of cyanosis, such as the nail beds, conjunctivae, palms, and soles.
5 Petechiae are best observed in the conjunctiva and oral mucosa. They may also be seen in areas of lighter pigmentation over the abdomen, gluteal folds, or inner aspect of the forearm.
6 Erythema is determined by palpating for increased skin temperature that is usually associated with conditions that produce this skin color change.

From Beare PG, Myers JL: *Adult health nursing,* ed 2, St Louis, 1994, Mosby.

NURSING RESPONSIBILITIES FOR DIAGNOSTIC TESTS AND PROCEDURES

Most skin disorders can be diagnosed from a carefully taken history, the patient's complaints, and observation of the lesion. A personal history should include allergies, sleep habits, occupation, medications, recent travel, contact with others, and level of anxiety.

OLDER ADULT CONSIDERATIONS

Integumentary Assessment

GENERAL APPROACH

Allow more time than for a younger adult.

Articulate clearly; the geriatric patient may be hearing impaired.

Impaired sight, comprehension, or mobility may result in less than optimum cooperation.

Provide clear, concise directions.

HISTORY COLLECTION

Be alert for answers that do not appear appropriate; the patient may not have understood the question correctly because of impaired hearing or comprehension.

Some questions may need to be repeated in a different manner.

PHYSICAL ASSESSMENT

The physical examination itself is not different, but the approach needs to be altered such that the appropriate information is assessed without undue discomfort or embarrassment for the patient.

Maintain an environment with minimal noise, distractions, and interruption.

Decreased elasticity (turgor) is found even in patients with adequate hydration and causes wrinkles.

Dry skin is common secondary to decreased sweat and sebaceous gland production.

Hyperpigmented macules may often be observed and are sometimes referred to as "age" or "liver" spots.

Progressive thinning of all body hair occurs.

Thinning of the epidermis and dermis leads to capillary fragility and therefore easy bruising.

Onychomycosis, a fungal condition of the nails, is a common finding.

From Beare PG, Myers JL: *Adult health nursing,* ed 2, St Louis, 1994, Mosby.

It is also important to find out when and where the lesion first appeared and the direction of its spread, whether it is constant or comes and goes, whether it is wet or dry, and whether pruritus (itching) is present. Four important observations must be made: identification, distribution, shape, and arrangement of the lesion. Careful observation and recording of this information can be of great value to the physician in making the correct diagnosis.

Sometimes the dermatologist may wish to make a bacteriologic study, in which case scraping or swabbing the lesion is necessary. Various types of fungi can be identified by this method. At other times a biopsy may be done for pathologic examination. The nurse's primary responsibility for any diagnostic procedure is to inform the patient of the procedure and answer any questions the patient may have. Skin biopsy is an invasive, though minor, procedure and requires a signed consent. After explaining the procedure to the patient, the nurse should remain with the patient during the procedure to help relieve any anxiety that the patient may have. Postprocedure instructions, which vary according to physician preference, should be carefully explained, and the patient should be told that the nurse is available by phone for assistance if any concerns or questions arise.

NURSING RESPONSIBILITIES FOR THERAPEUTIC PROCEDURES

Nursing care of the patient with skin disorders may involve several nursing procedures, including therapeutic baths, wet dressings, soaks, and the application of various topical medications.

Therapeutic Baths

Therapeutic baths are used for several purposes, including disinfecting and deodorizing, relieving pruritus, achieving a soothing effect, and softening and lubricating the skin. Soap, oils, medications, or a variety of substances such as oatmeal, cornstarch, baking soda, or a combination of these may be used (Table 31-2). One cup of either cornstarch or baking soda may be added to a tub of tepid water to provide a soothing bath for patients suffering from pruritus. For an oatmeal bath, prepare the oatmeal by placing 2 cups of oatmeal and 1 quart of boiling water in a double boiler and cook for approximately 45 minutes. The oatmeal mixture is then put in a gauze bag, and the bag is swished in a tub of water. The cooled oatmeal may be expressed and applied directly to the patient's body, to be washed off before the patient exits the tub. Commercial oatmeal preparations, such as Aveeno, are available and ready to add to the bath water. To prevent the commercial mixtures from lumping, they should be dissolved under running water and then dispersed throughout the bath water.

The temperature of the water for therapeutic baths should be 95° F to 100° F (35° C to 37.8° C), and the tub should be three-fourths full or sufficiently full to cover the involved area. The bath may be given for 10 to 20 minutes several times a day. Warm water should be added to maintain a constant temperature, but the temperature should not exceed 100° F (37.8° C). Very hot water is not good for the skin because of the dry-

TABLE 31-2
Balneotherapy

Type of Bath	Agents	Disease	Purpose
Antibacterial	Potassium permanganate (1:32,000; 1:64,000) Acetic acid Hexachlorophene Povidone-iodine	Infected eczema Dirty ulcerations Furunculosis	Lower skin bacterial load
Colloidal	Starch and baking soda (1 cup each/tub) Aveeno Colloidal Oatmeal (1 cup/tub) Aveeno Oilated Colloidal Oatmeal	Any red, irritated, oozing condition (e.g., atopic eczema)	Relieve itching Soothe
Emollient*	Bath oils: Alpha Keri, Lubath Mineral oil	Any dry skin condition	Cleanse and hydrate the skin Loosen scale
Tar*	Bath oils with tar: Balnetar, Zetar, Polytar Coal tar concentrate (liquor carbonis detergens)	Scaly dermatoses (e.g., psoriasis)	Relieve itching Potentiate UVA/UVB light therapy

From Hill MJ: *Skin disorders: Mosby's clinical nursing series,* St Louis, 1994, Mosby.
*For emollient and tar baths, add 3 to 6 capfuls of therapeutic agent per standard size bathtub.

ing and vasodilation effects, and it is particularly inadvisable for persons with skin diseases.

Because some preparations may cause the tub to be slippery, extreme care should be taken to prevent the patient from slipping in the tub. When the patient is removed from the tub, the skin should be patted dry to avoid irritation or damage, and medication, if ordered, or a bland emollient, should be applied to the moist skin. Measures should be taken to prevent chilling the patient.

Wet Dressings

Wet dressings are used for many types of skin diseases. They may be open or closed and warm or cold depending on the therapeutic effect desired (Table 31-3). Evaporation of the solution in an open dressing initiates vasoconstriction, which provides a cooling effect and relieves the pruritus that accompanies some disease. The moisture will soften crusts and stimulate drainage. Some solutions, such as Dakin's solution, will retard the growth of bacteria on the skin and help prevent infection. Open wet dressings should not be covered with impermeable materials. Because of rapid evaporation, frequent changing or wetting is necessary. Pieces of soft old muslin, fluffs, or abdominal gauze are preferred to cotton, which has a tendency to pack down. Dressings must be clean but not necessarily sterile unless indicated by the overall condition of the patient (e.g., immunocompromised).

Wet dressings under occlusion (closed wet dressings) are used to help hydrate the epidermis to allow more effective absorption of topical medications. The dressings may be used on an isolated area or as total body treatment (mummy wrap) for patients with extensive or generalized involvement. If the area being treated is limited, the nurse should wet the dressing in the prescribed medicated solution and apply it directly to the area. The surrounding skin should be protected from moisture and from the medicated solution by applying petroleum jelly or other suitable protective substances. Wet dressings should be thoroughly saturated but should not drip. Dry towels are wrapped around the closed wet dressing.

A warm, moist dressing is wrapped in thin plastic material and secured. A constant-temperature heating pad may be used to keep the dressing warm, but in that case the dressing should not be wrapped in plastic because of the danger of burning the patient. The nurse should rewet the dressing as needed with an Asepto syringe. However, if drainage is present, it is preferable to remove the entire dressing and reapply a new one. Solutions often used for wet dressings include physiologic saline, magnesium sulfate solution, 0.5% aluminum acetate (Burow's) solution, dilute sodium hypochlorite (Dakin's) solution, and 1:4000 potassium permanganate solution. Boric acid should not be used for widespread, raw areas because of its toxic effects, but it is safe and soothing for small irritated areas. This limited use of boric acid is a major

TABLE 31-3

Solutions for Soaks and Wet Dressings

Solution	Purpose	Dilution
Tap water	To cool and relieve pruritus To loosen eschar and crusts	Tap water at approximately body temperature
Aluminum acetate (Domeborro, Aluwets, Burow's solution)	Same as tap water To promote drying To provide a mild antiseptic effect	 Mix 1 tablet with 1 qt (1L) water (1:40) Mix 1 tablet with 1 pt (500 ml) water (1:20)
Potassium permanganate ($KMnO_4$)	Same as tap water To provide astringent effect To provide antimicrobial effect (especially effective against *Pseudomonas aeruginosa*)	Prepared by pharmacist at dilutions of 0.25% to 0.5%
Normal saline	Same as tap water To provide isotonic solution to skin for cooling and antipruritic effect	0.9% saline solution
Silver nitrate ($AgNO_3$)	Astringent and antibacterial	Prepared by pharmacist at 1:1000 to 1:10,000

From Hill MJ: *Skin disorders: Mosby's clinical nursing series,* St Louis, 1994, Mosby.

disadvantage. Even continuous wet dressings should be removed periodically to allow the skin to dry and to observe the status of the affected area. Cold dressings should be removed every 6 hours for at least 30 minutes. The bed and pillow should be protected when wet dressings are used. Because of the risk of maceration and the decreased frequency of wound observation, continuous wet dressings should be used cautiously and on a limited basis.

When topical medicines such as medicated creams need to be applied, the nurse should wet the dressing material with warm tap water and apply it over the medicine (Tables 31-4 to 31-7). Dry towels (for limited areas) or bath blankets (for mummy wraps) are placed on top of the dressing, which not only keeps the moisture in but also provides warmth for the patient as the dressings begin to cool. These dressings usually are left in place for 20 to 30 minutes, and a lubricating agent is applied over the affected areas to provide occlusion until the next wet dressing is applied. A mummy wrap is the dressing of choice when treating patients with generalized skin disorders that are erythematous, eczematous, or exfoliating (e.g., psoriasis, eczema, mycosis fungoides).

Soaks

Soaks may be ordered to loosen necrotic tissue, promote suppuration, or hydrate the skin to increase the absorption of topical medications. When an extremity is involved, a basin or tub large enough to submerge the part should be secured. The solution, temperature, and frequency and duration of the treatment are prescribed by the physician. Patients with burns may be placed in physiologic saline soaks for the purpose of debridement. Whirlpool treatments can serve the same purposes as soaks.

Paste Boots

Boots are often used for patients with certain types of dermatitis and ulcers on the lower extremities. Several commercial preparations containing water, gelatin, glycerin, and zinc oxide are available. One preparation known as Unna's boot (Dome-paste bandage) is impregnated with the materials, which simplifies its application. The extremity is elevated approximately 30 minutes before applying the boot. An ointment may be applied to the skin lesions and covered with a thin gauze dressing. The paste bandage is then applied from the ankle to the knee, with greater pressure on the ankle and reduced pressure near the knee. This increases venous return and is particularly beneficial in patients with venous stasis ulcers. Two layers of stockinette or an elastic bandage is applied as an outer dressing. The boot is changed every 5 to 8 days.

Emotional Support

Patients with skin disorders may have a long road to travel before recovery is complete. Serious skin problems often become chronic, and the patient must learn to live with this disability. When lesions are on the face

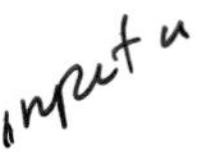

and exposed parts of the body, the fear of disfigurement is always present. The patient is concerned about what others think and that they may fear that the disease is contagious. Real or imagined feelings of being shunned may cause the patient to become isolated and withdrawn. In children and adolescents the impact on personality may be serious. Although few patients with skin disorders may be admitted to the hospital, they are everywhere. Probably few persons escape the experience of some type of skin disorder during their lifetime.

The nurse can be a source of encouragement to patients, whether they are in or out of the hospital. First,

TABLE 31-4

Topical Medications

Class/Content	Purposes	Disadvantages	Inert Examples
Cream			
Oil-in-water emulsion; water content 60% or more	Ease of application Ease of removal Lubrication Delivers medication	Removed by perspiration Low penetration of medication	Dermatology formula Nutraderm
Ointment			
Water-in-oil emulsion; water content 40% or less	Marked lubrication Maintains a layer of medication on skin Delivers medication with enhanced penetration	Greasy sensation May stain clothing May inflame hair follicles	Aquaphor Eucerin Nivea Petrolatum Lanolin
Gel			
Semisolid mixture; between cream and ointment in content; often contains alcohol	Ease of application Greaseless layer of medication	May cause burning on eroded skin	
Powder			
Finely ground solid particles	Absorbs moisture, thereby promoting drying Decreases skin friction Delivers medication best in intertriginous areas	Wears off easily	Talcum Bentonite Cornstarch Zinc oxide
Lotion			
Powder suspended in liquid (water, alcohol, oil)	Cooling effect on evaporation May absorb moisture, promoting dryness Delivers medication as uniform residual film Useful in hairy areas	Wears off easily Can overdry skin	Ken Lubriderm WIBI Cetaphil
Solution			
Powder dissolved in liquid medium	Similar to lotion Useful in hairy areas	Similar to lotion	Vehicle-N C-solve
Aerosol Spray			
Lotion delivered by airborne propellant	Similar to lotion but even more drying Useful in hairy areas	Similar to lotion	
Paste			
Powder mixed in ointment; 50% or more powder content	Leaves a protective coating while delivering medication	Low rate of penetration Messy to use	Zinc oxide paste (Lassar's)

From Hill MJ: *Skin disorders: Mosby's clinical nursing series,* St Louis, 1994, Mosby.

TABLE 31-5
Pharmacology of Drugs Used for Skin Integrity

Drug (Generic and Trade Name); Route and Dosage	Action/Indication	Common Side Effects and Nursing Considerations
ACYCLOVIR, TOPICAL (Zovirax Ointment) **ROUTE:** Topical **DOSAGE:** 5% ointment apply to lesions q 3 hr while awake, 6 times daily × 1 week	Antiviral, interferes with DNA replication; used for simple mucocutaneous herpes simplex and herpes zoster; also used in immunocompromised patients with initial genital herpes	Rash, uticaria, stinging, burning, pruritis, and vulvitis
ALUMINUM ACETATE (Burow's Solution) **ROUTE:** Topical **DOSAGE:** 1:20 or 1:40 solution as wet dressing q 15-30 min for 4-8 hr, or soak for 15-30 min 3 times daily	Used as an astringent for soothing effects of cooling and vasoconstriction; also used for relief from painful inflammation of skin	For external use only; avoid using near eyes
GRISEOFULVIN **ROUTE:** PO **DOSAGE:** Microsize tablets, 250-500 mg q 12 hr or 500 mg once daily; ultramicrosize tablets, 330-375 mg/day in 1 or 2 divided doses	Antifungal antibiotic used for various tinea infections, including ringworm	Headache; contraindicated in severe liver disease; possible cross-sensitivity with penicillin; should not be used for superficial infections that may respond to antifungals
HYDROCORTISONE (Hytone and many others) **ROUTE:** Topical **DOSAGE:** Apply several times a day as ordered	Corticosteroid used as antipruritic and antiinflammatory for psoriasis, eczema, contact dermatitis, and pruritis	Contraindicated in hypersensitivity to corticosteroids; do not use on weeping, denuded, or highly infected areas; avoid sunlight on treated areas
ISOTRETINOIN (Accutane) **ROUTE:** PO **DOSAGE:** 0.5-1.0 mg/kg/day (up to 2 mg/kg/day) in 2 divided doses for 15-20 weeks	Keratolytic agent used for management of cystic acne resistant to more conventional therapy, including topical therapy and systemic antibiotics	Epistaxis, conjunctivitis, cheilitis, dry mouth, nausea, vomiting, pruritis, decreased hemoglobin, decreased hematocrit, hypertriglyceridemia, hypercholesterolemia, decreased high-density lipoproteins, bone pain, and arthralgia; use with caution in diabetes, alcoholism, obesity, and inflammatory bowel disease
KETOCONAZOLE (Nizoral) **ROUTE:** Topical, PO **DOSAGE:** Topical 2% cream, apply 1 or 2 times daily; PO, 200-400 mg/day as single dose	Antifungal used to treat a variety of fungal infections, including dermatologic infections such as tinea corporis; also used for seborrheic dermatitis	Nausea and vomiting; use with caution in severe liver disease and alcoholism
LINDANE, GAMMA BENZENE HEXACHLORIDE **ROUTE:** Topical **DOSAGE:** Apply 1% cream to all infested areas. May repeat in 1 week	Miticide used in the treatment of scabies, head lice, body lice, and crab lice	Contraindicated in history of seizures

continued

TABLE 31-5

Pharmacology of Drugs Used for Skin Integrity—cont'd

Drug (Generic and Trade Name); Route and Dosage	Action/Indication	Common Side Effects and Nursing Considerations
MAFENIDE ACETATE (Sulfamylon) **ROUTE:** Topical **DOSAGE:** Apply topically $\frac{1}{16}$ inch to an affected area 1-2 times daily, and reapply as needed	Sulfonamide, interferes with bacterial wall synthesis; used as an adjunctive treatment in 2nd- and 3rd-degree burns	Bone marrow suppression, fatal hemolytic anemia, and eosinophilia; contraindicated in inhalation injury; use with caution in impaired pulmonary and renal function and in fluid loss and decreased urine output
MINOXIDIL (Rogaine) **ROUTE:** Topical, PO **DOSAGE:** Topically, rub into scalp daily; PO, 5 mg/day not to exceed 100 mg daily; usual range 10-40 mg/day in single dose	Antihypertensive with side effect of stimulating hair growth; used to treat alopecia; also used for severe hypertension not responsive to other therapy	Severe rebound hypertension, drowsiness, dizziness, and sedation; contraindicated in acute myocardial infarction and used with caution in renal disease and congestive heart failure; do not discontinue drug abruptly
MUPIROCIN (Bactroban) **ROUTE:** Topical **DOSAGE:** Apply 2% ointment to affected area tid	Nonpenicillin antibiotic used dermatologically to inhibit bacterial protein synthesis; used against impetigo and other infections	Burning, stinging, and itching
SILVER NITRATE **ROUTE:** Topical **DOSAGE:** Apply as ordered to area affected	Used as antiinfective and astringent and for cauterization of lesions, warts, and burns (low concentration)	Skin discoloration; use a wet dressing for burns; store in cool area; avoid contact with clothing to prevent discoloration
SILVER SULFADIAZINE (Silvadene) **ROUTE:** Topical **DOSAGE:** Apply 1% cream 1 or 2 times daily in layer 1.5 mm thick	Topical antiinfective used in prevention and treatment of infection in 2nd- and 3rd-degree burns.	Use cautiously with sensitivity to sulfonamides and with renal and hepatic disease; may need to premedicate with analgesic before application
TRETINOIN, VITAMIN A ACID, RETINOIC ACID (Retin-A) **ROUTE:** Topical **DOSAGE:** Apply once daily at bedtime	Keratolytic agent used in management of acne vulgaris	Photosensitivity; use cautiously around the mouth, eyes, angles of the nose, or other mucous membranes

TABLE 31-6

Choosing Topical Vehicles

Description of Skin Condition	Example	Topical Vehicle of Choice
Red, hot	Exfoliative erythroderma	Dermatologic wet dressing
Red, irritated, sore, oozing	Contact dermatitis	Lotions or sprays
Acute, red, wet skin; not painful to touch	Atopic eczema	Creams, gels
Chronic, scaly skin with redness	Seborrheic dermatitis	Creams, gels
Thick, hyperkeratotic skin	Psoriasis	Ointments

From Hill MJ: *Skin disorders: Mosby's clinical nursing series,* St Louis, 1994, Mosby.

TABLE 31-7

Potency of Topical Corticosteroids

Potency	Generic Name	Trade Name
Very high	Fluocinonide	Lidex, Topsyn
	Halcinonide	Halog, Halciderm
High	Betamethasone benzoate	Benisone
	Betamethasone dipropionate	Diprosone
	Betamethasone valerate	Valisone
	Diflorasone diacetate	Maxiflor, Florone
Medium	Fluocinolone acetonide 0.025%	Synalar, Synemol
	Triamcinolone 0.1%	Aristocort
	Triamcinolone acetonide 0.1%	Kenalog
	Flurandrenolide	Cordran
Low	Desonide	Tridesilon
	Hydrocortisone valerate	Westcort
Very low	Hydrocortisone	Hytone, Nutracort, Cortril, Synacort

From Hill MJ: *Skin disorders: Mosby's clinical nursing series,* St Louis, 1994, Mosby.

nurses should know that skin disease is rarely fatal and that few skin diseases are contagious. Next, nurses should analyze their own feelings toward the patient. If they find the patient repulsive, they will be unable to give support when it is needed. The nurse must care for the patient with warmth and understanding and convey a feeling of acceptance. Gentleness in removing and applying dressings, keeping wet dressings wet, and carrying out treatments on time will help make the patient feel secure. The nurse should avoid a "hurry-up" attitude and should spend enough time with the patient to reassure him or her of interest and acceptance and encourage expression of his or her feelings about the disease.

PRESSURE ULCERS

Pressure ulcers are defined as local areas of necrosis as a result of vascular insufficiency in an area under pressure (Makelbust, Siegreen, 1991). These ulcers may appear anywhere on the body, but the greatest incidence is over bony prominences (Figure 31-3). Pressure over these areas cuts off the blood supply to the tissue, deprives the cells of nutrition, and prevents elimination of waste from the cells. Anything that hinders the normal cellular functioning will eventually lead to cellular death (necrosis). This results in a pressure ulcer (decubitus ulcer, pressure necrosis). Tissue destruction can occur rapidly. When the skin is broken, there is a rapid destruction of the underlying tissues. The ulcer may become secondarily infected, or the underlying bone may become infected (osteomyelitis). Either of these events complicates the healing process. Pressure ulcers are a cause of considerable morbidity, discomfort, and cost, and they require time-consuming, well-directed nursing interventions.

Sustained pressure is the major cause of pressure necrosis. Both the amount and duration of pressure are important factors. Skin may be able to experience high pressure for a short time without breaking down, whereas low to moderate pressure for an extended period will often result in skin breakdown. For example, the surgical patient may develop a pressure ulcer after a prolonged period on the operating table.

Risk Factors

The most common risk factors for development of a pressure ulcer are existing disease states such as diabetes mellitus, cardiovascular disease, anemias, neuropathies, renal disease, immune deficiencies, and pulmonary disease; immobility; nutritional deficiencies; moisture; friction; shear; and incontinence (Makelbust, Siegreen, 1991).

Preventing the conditions that aggravate pressure ulcers—moisture, friction, and shear—becomes solely the nurse's responsibility in the acute care setting and the caregiver's responsibility in the home. Sustained moisture (incontinence, diaphoresis) overhydrates the skin and results in maceration (softening of the skin as a result of moisture). The protective function of the skin is therefore impaired, which puts the patient at risk for further breakdown and infection. In addition, urinary or fecal incontinence increases the risk of breakdown by chemical irritation.

Friction occurs when a patient is pulled over a surface. This action can strip the epidermis and leave an open erosion. Using lifting devices to move patients rather than pulling them across the sheets greatly decreases this risk factor. The fragile skin of elderly patients is particularly susceptible to friction tears that may lead to infection and further tissue breakdown. **Shear** is another factor related to development of pressure ulcers. Shear occurs when two or more tissue layers slide in opposite, parallel directions and cause subcutaneous blood vessels to become kinked or stretched. This obstructs blood flow to and from the area supplied by those vessels and results in necrosis. Every patient in a hospital bed experiences shear when the head of the bed is elevated 30 degrees or

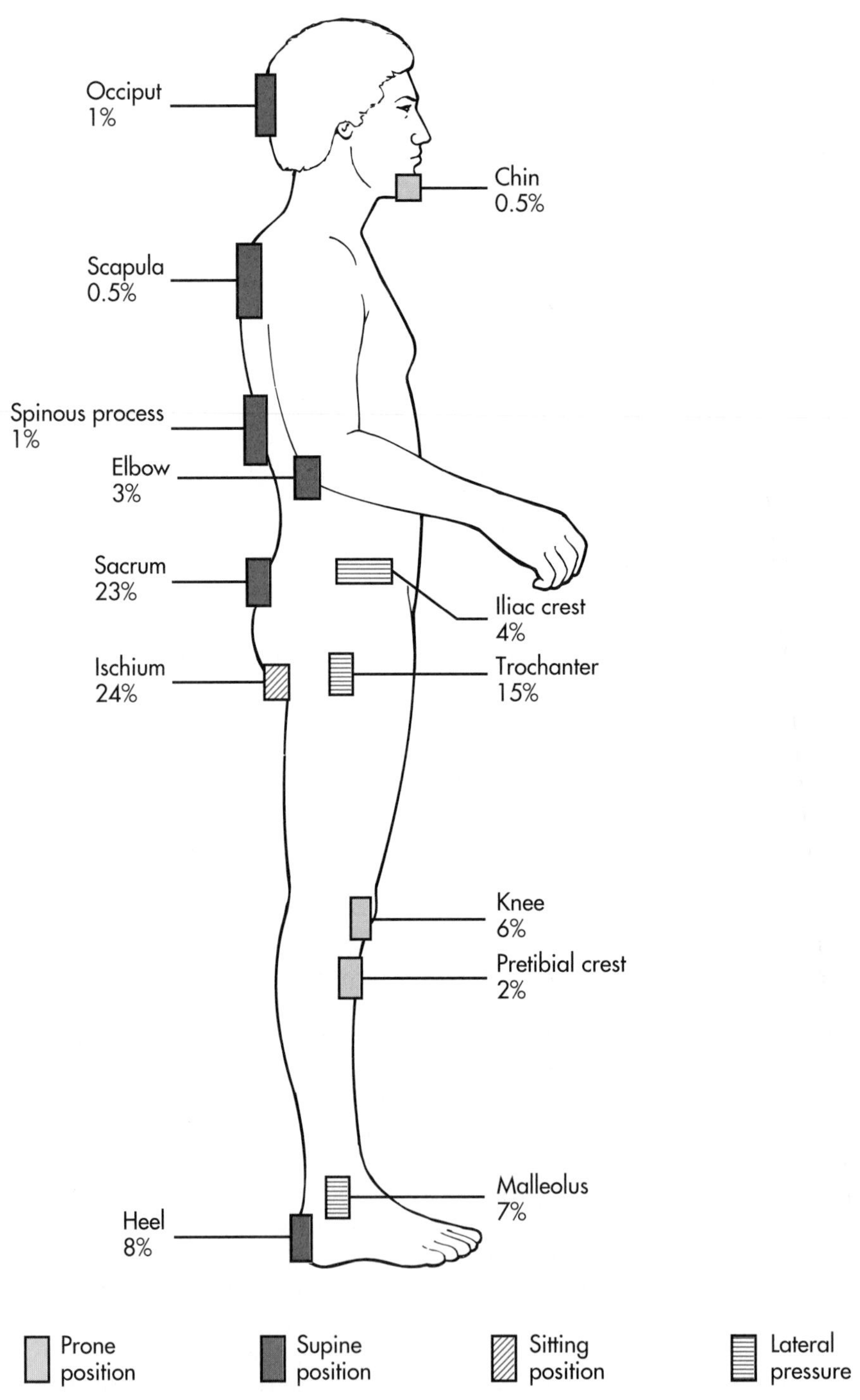

Figure 31-3 Common sites for pressure ulcers and frequency of ulceration per site. (Data from Agris J, Spira M: *Clin Symp* 31(5):2, 1979. In Bryant RA: *Acute and chronic wounds,* St Louis, 1992, Mosby.)

more. As the head of the bed is raised, the patient slides toward the foot of the bed. Those tissues attached to bony structures move with the patient, but the outer skin layers tend to stay in a fixed position, which exerts **shearing force.** The resulting diminished blood flow to the sacral area causes tissue necrosis.

Prevention of Pressure Ulcers

The cost of caring for one patient with a pressure ulcer has been estimated to be $14,000 to $40,000 (Makelbust, Siegreen, 1991). Despite guidelines for preventive measures, pressure ulcers continue to occur. Prevention depends on early recognition of the patient at risk and prompt institution of the appropriate measures necessary to prevent breakdown. Nursing procedures include (1) identifying the patient at risk by use of a risk-assessment scale (e.g., Braden, Gosnell, or Norton); (2) maintaining a dry, unwrinkled bed; (3) using the appropriate pressure-reduction or pressure-relief surface; (4) repositioning the patient at least every 2 hours while in bed and encouraging weight shifts every hour for patients in wheelchairs; (5) constant attention to the overall health status of the patient; and (6) continued observation and reassessment of the skin. A reddened (erythematous) area is the first sign of pressure. In the light-skinned patient a red color change is seen; in the dark-skinned patient the erythematous area may be detected by an increase in skin temperature or by a darkening or lightening of that patient's normal skin color. All patients should be assessed for edema at the suspected pressure site. Edematous skin will feel slick and tight when touched with the back of the finger. Erythema should disappear within a short time after pressure is relieved if no skin damage has been done. If edema occurs and redness remains for 30 minutes after pressure is relieved, pressure ulcer development should be suspected.

Erythematous areas over pressure points should not be massaged because this may cause damage to vasculature. Massaging skin around existing ulcers should be avoided because it may cause unnecessary trauma and spread infection. The use of soap should be limited because the alkali in soap will produce dryness, cracking, and chapping. The old method of using doughnuts and rubber rings is no longer acceptable practice. These devices create rings of pressure that further restrict circulation. Preventing pressure ulcers in long-term and older adult patients requires consistent, diligent nursing care. Ulcers may occur quickly from only slight pressure; this is especially true in the older adult.

The general health and nutritional status of the patient does contribute to the development of pressure ulcers. Protein, vitamin C, and vitamin B are essential for normal cell growth and healing. Inadequate vitamin C contributes to capillary fragility, which makes tissues more susceptible to trauma and interrupted blood flow. Poor nutrition leads to an increased risk of breakdown or impaired healing. Adequate hydration is also necessary to maintain skin turgor and prevent infection.

Devices That Augment Nursing Care

Increased concern for the development of pressure ulcers has resulted in development of products for both the prevention and care of pressure ulcers. To avoid confusion, the products should be looked at generically (e.g., high air loss, low air loss, overlays, beds), which may simplify choices.

Equipment for pressure reduction/relief varies considerably in both effectiveness and cost. Pressure-relieving devices work by redistributing pressure at bony prominences over the larger surface of the entire body. The desired goal is to obtain the largest possible support surface with the lowest possible contact pressure (Makelbust, Siegreen, 1991). The nurse must be able to make a cost-effective choice to deliver the greatest benefit to the patient.

Mattress overlays

The first level of intervention is classified as mattress overlays. These may be convoluted-foam or air products and are either static or dynamic. Overlays provide *pressure reduction* as opposed to *pressure relief.* Convoluted-foam, water-filled, gel, and air-filled overlays are classified as static products. Static products decrease pressure by spreading the weight over a larger area (Bryant, 1992). Convoluted-foam overlays must be at least 4 to 6 inches thick to provide pressure reduction (Figure 31-4). Anything less than 4 inches provides comfort but no significant pressure reduction. Water-filled overlays distribute body weight over the entire support system. Gel flotation pads provide flotation with pressure reduction.

Dynamic products (e.g., alternating air-filled overlays) prevent constant pressure against the skin and enhance blood flow by creating high-pressure and low-pressure areas (Bryant, 1992). These products are indicated for the patient with limited mobility who is at risk for further skin breakdown or who has a stage I, II, or III pressure ulcer. If the patient has documented stage I or stage II pressure ulcers along with excessive moisture (e.g., incontinence, perspiration), an air mattress overlay is indicated (Figure 31-5). Nursing care that includes a turning schedule must be implemented along with the use of any support surface. Patients who have a stage III or IV pressure ulcer or who have multiple

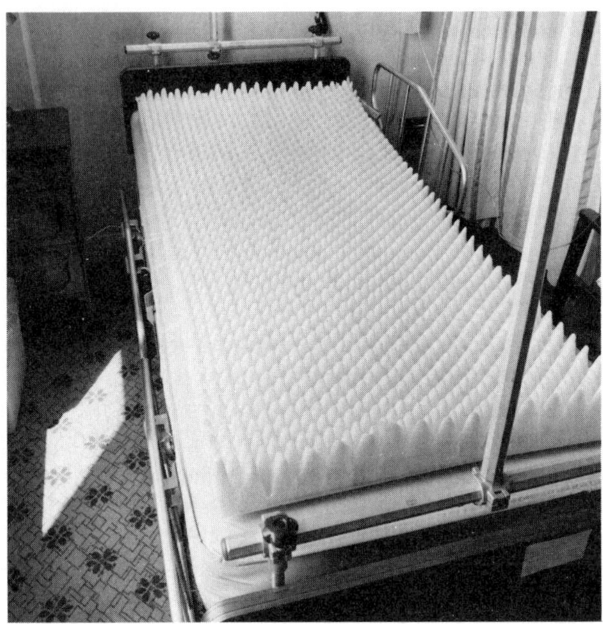

Figure 31-4 Convoluted foam mattress. (From Perry GA, Potter PA: *Clinical nursing skills and techniques,* ed 3, St Louis, 1994, Mosby.)

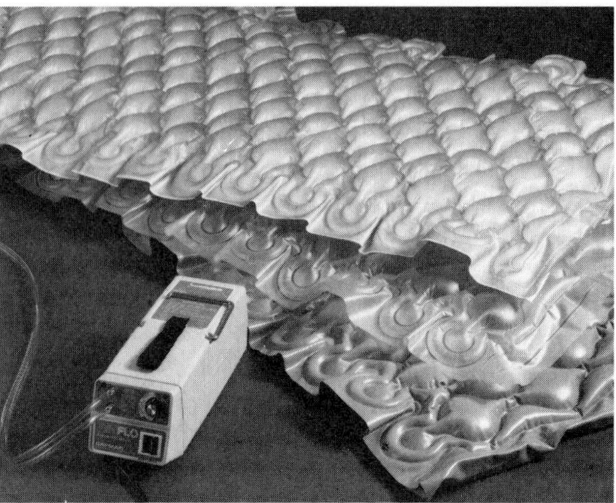

Figure 31-5 Inflated air mattress. (Courtesy Gaymer Industries, Inc, Orchard Park, NY. From Perry AG, Potter PA: *Clinical nursing skills and techniques,* ed 3, St Louis, 1994, Mosby.)

stage II pressure ulcers that involve more than one surface can benefit from a low–air-loss mattress.

Specialty beds

Specialty beds have the technology to allow the bed surface to conform to the body contours, which reduces tissue-interface pressure below capillary closing pressure, thus providing pressure relief. Specialty beds also relieve shear and friction. Specialty beds may be classified as high air-loss, low air-loss, or kinetic.

High–air-loss beds have bactericidal properties because of their temperature, alkalinity (pH 10), and entrapment of the microorganisms by the beads in the bed. High–air-loss beds are recommended for patients with burns or multiple stage III or IV pressure ulcers. They may also be used to rewarm the patient with hypothermia. High–air-loss beds are not recommended for patients with pulmonary disease or unstable spines or for patients who are ambulatory. Low–air-loss beds help reduce moisture and manage pain. They are indicated for patients who need pressure relief and are contraindicated for patients with unstable spines. Patients with stage III or stage IV pressure ulcers, multiple stage II pressure ulcers involving more than one surface, multiple risk factors, end-stage cancer, pulmonary complications, or sepsis, as well as those who need pain management, should be placed on an oscillating low–air-loss bed (kinetic bed). This particular bed provides programmable turning of patients to promote drainage of lung secretions, enhances venous return from lower extremities, and facilitates urine flow. Oscillating support beds provide continuous turning of the patient from side to side to prevent and treat the complications of immobility. This bed may be used with spinal cord injury (Bryant, 1992).

A special function bed has a pressure-relieving surface that provides continuous pulsating air suspension. It has the same indications as the low–air-loss bed, with the addition of pulsation. It is indicated for the patient who needs pain management. Use of this bed is contraindicated for patients in cervical or skeletal traction.

Air-fluidized therapy provides pressure relief on a high–air-loss surface. This specialty bed is indicated for the patient who requires minimal movement to avoid skin damage by shearing forces (posterior grafts, or flaps). Turning schedules are highly recommended. This bed is also contraindicated for patients with unstable spines. The nurse must be aware of fluid intake of patients on air-fluidized therapy. Fluid intake should be sufficient to prevent dehydration.

Treatment of Pressure Ulcers

Many of the wound care products available for treating pressure ulcers must be used in conjunction with the appropriate pressure-reducing or pressure-relieving product. Factors affecting treatment, including the condition of the wound and the general health status of the patient, are continuously changing variables, and treatment choices must be made on the basis of an accurate and ongoing assessment of the wound and patient. Among the products available for treating pressure ulcers are agents for cleansing and debridement, topical medications (antimicrobials, antiseptics, antibiotics), exudate absorbers (beads, pastes), and multiple categories of dressings.

Wound cleansing

The goals of wound cleansing are (1) removal of bacteria and surface contaminants such as slough, foreign bodies, and purulent exudate, and (2) protection of the healing wound (Bryant, 1992). The body's own healing mechanism is very efficient, so any intervention should be aimed at enhancing that mechanism. Effective wound healing can be inhibited by indiscriminate use of some agents. Therefore the choice of cleansing method must be based on the type of wound and the stage of healing.

Hypochlorite solutions, such as Dakin's solution, or chlorpactin, will dissolve necrotic tissue and control odors, but they are toxic to fibroblasts in normal dilutions. Povidone-iodine preparations have broad spectrum effectiveness when used on intact skin or small wounds, but they are toxic to fibroblasts in normal dilutions, have questionable effectiveness in infected wounds, and may cause iodine toxicity when used in large wounds over a prolonged time. Acetic acid is effective against *Pseudomonas aeruginosa* in superficial wounds but is toxic to fibroblasts in standard dilutions and changes the color of exudate, which gives a false assurance of elimination of infection. Lastly, hydrogen peroxide will provide mechanical cleansing and some debridement through effervescent action, but it can cause ulceration of newly formed tissue, is toxic to fibroblasts, and can cause air embolism when used to pack sinus tracts. Moreover, if used for forceful irrigation, hydrogen peroxide can cause subcutaneous emphysema, which mimics gas gangrene (Bryant, 1992). There are several prepared wound cleansers available on the market. Most contain a wetting agent and a blend of moisturizers that help soften **eschar** (scab) and augment debridement. Each product should be used according to the recommendations of the manufacturer. Normal saline is appropriate and safe for all wounds.

Debridement

To enhance the healing process, **debridement** must be done to remove devitalized tissue, particularly in contaminated ulcers. Devitalized, or necrotic, tissue slows the wound-healing process. Debridement can be classified as chemical (topical agents/enzymes), mechanical (surgical, wet-to-dry, hydrotherapy), or autolytic (occlusive dressings).

Chemical debridement is accomplished through the use of enzyme preparations that dissolve necrotic tissue. The enzymes require a moist environment for activation. Enzymatic preparations are made to act on specific necrotic tissue. For example, fibrinolysin-deoxyribonuclease dissolves fibrin clots and hydrolyzes proteinaceous exudate. Sutilains is a proteolytic enzyme, and collagenase digests collagen and denatured protein (Eaglstein and others, 1990). Chemical debridement also may be accomplished by using gauze soaked with Dakin's solution to dissolve necrotic tissue.

Mechanical debridement is accomplished by the use of a scalpel and scissors, irrigation (whirlpool, syringe), or wet-dry dressings. Surgical debridement is aggressive, fast, and selective. Necrotic tissue is removed down to, or just above, viable tissue. Viable tissue is recognized when there is bleeding present. This type of debridement provides a wound bed that stimulates granulation. Carbon dioxide lasers have been used to accomplish this type of debridement. Another form of mechanical debridement is irrigation. Irrigation may be accomplished by putting the patient in a whirlpool tub, by having the patient stand in a shower, or by manual irrigation. Irrigation must be done gently so as not to disturb fragile, healing tissue. Once the wound has begun to granulate, irrigation should be discontinued. Lastly, wet-to-dry dressings are used for mechanical debridement. Wet-to-dry dressings are painful and may cause bleeding; they are also nonselective and may destroy surrounding healthy tissue while trying to remove areas of necrosis or slough.

Autolytic debridement is accomplished with the use of an appropriate occlusive dressing. The dressing uses enzymes normally present in the wound fluid to liquefy the necrotic debris. Dressings that accomplish this goal are occlusive or semiocclusive (hydrocolloidal wafers, paste, or beads).

The choice of the debridement method to be used should be based on the condition of the wound, the amount of exudate present, and the condition of the patient. A patient with a large (stage III or IV) necrotic pressure ulcer who is at very high risk for secondary infection may benefit greatly from aggressive surgical (mechanical) debridement to augment the wound healing process.

Topical medications

Antimicrobials, antiseptics, and antibiotics can be in the form of a cream, ointment, solution, or spray. Topical agents should be chosen for their antibacterial effectiveness and for their ability to enhance, not inhibit, healing. For example, an occlusive ointment may cause maceration or encourage the growth of resistant organisms. Some topical agents interfere with neutrophils, fibroblasts, and endothelial cells in the healing process (Tables 31-4 and 31-5).

Exudate absorbers

Exudate absorbers (absorption dressings) include, but are not limited to, dextranomer beads, hydrophilic powders, pastes, granules, calcium alginates, and other hypertonic dressings. Absorption dressings remove necrotic fluid, obliterate dead space (sinus tracts, undermining), and maintain a moist wound environment. Dead space impairs the wound-healing process and predisposes the patient to abscess formation. All of these dressings expand when they come in contact with the wound fluid, so it is not necessary to pack them tightly into the wound bed. Packing too tightly may impair circulation and damage healthy tissue. Absorptive dressings are suitable for stage III and stage IV pressure ulcers.

Dressing materials

Dressing materials are numerous and varied and should be chosen for their individual actions on the basis of the wound assessment. For simplification they are classified as transparent film dressings, hydrocolloids, foam dressings, hydrogels, and protective barriers. Transparent film dressings are semipermeable adhesive dressings that allow exchange of oxygen and moisture vapor but do not allow passage of fluids or bacteria. They enhance epithelial migration and are indicated for use in superficial (stage I or stage II) dermal ulcers, skin grafts, donor sites, and minor abrasions.

Hydrocolloids are adhesive dressings that absorb small to moderate amounts of exudate while interacting with the wound to form a liquid gelatinous substance that maintains a moist healing environment. They may be used on superficial pressure ulcers and skin tears that produce minimum amounts of exudate. Hydrocolloids may be either occlusive and impermeable to gases or semipermeable. The occlusive hydrocolloids are not suitable for infected wounds, deep wounds with tunnel tracts, or undermining. Semipermeable hydrocolloids are mechanically protective and properly humidify the wound. Hydrocolloids are excellent for autolytic debridement and may be used in stage I, stage II, and some stage III ulcers.

Hydrogels are water-polymer gels that act to provide a moist wound healing environment while absorbing excess exudate. Hydrogels also clean and debride the wound. This type of dressing is appropriate for all stages of wound healing but is most often indicated in stages II and III. Hydrogels may be used in necrotic wounds. They also have the added feature of relieving pain through their cooling properties. They are especially good for burns.

Foam dressings are nonadherent hydrophilic or hydrophobic polyurethane that provide thermal insulation and a moist wound environment. This type of dressing is atraumatic and is indicated for use in stage III and granulating stage IV wounds with a moderate amount of exudate. If the wound has depth or dead space, the foam dressing should be used with packing.

Protective barriers (skin sealants) provide a protective coating, usually in alcohol solution, that is applied to intact skin. This coating forms a second skin and is useful to prep skin before an adhesive is applied. Skin sealants may be applied on stage I wounds because the skin is intact.

Nursing Interventions

A thorough assessment of the patient must be undertaken before any interventions are begun. The individualized plan is then formulated in accordance with the specific needs and condition of the patient. The plan of care must be consistent with goals for patient management, and the goals must be realistic. Several objective factors must be considered when assessing the patient at risk. These factors include general state of the skin, general state of health, mental status, degree of mobility and activity, level of sensory perception, nutritional status, and aggravating factors such as moisture, friction, and shear. Contributing factors must also be taken into consideration when interventions are being developed. These factors include predisposing disease states (diabetes mellitus, cardiovascular disease, anemias, neuropathies, renal disease, pulmonary disease), age, weight, medications, allergies, serial laboratory values (albumin, total protein, hemoglobin, hematocrit, total lymphocyte count), and dietary restrictions. There are several risk-assessment tools in the literature to assist the nurse in this assessment. Some of the tools are the Norton scale, the Gosnell scale, and the Braden scale (Box 31-3).

If a patient is found to be at risk and has no skin breakdown, interventions should be aimed at prevention. Interventions should include placing the patient on a pressure-reducing/relieving surface, inspecting the skin regularly—at least every 8 hours—for redness or evidence of breakdown, instituting measures to reduce shearing forces and friction (keeping head of bed flat or below a 30-degree angle), using a draw sheet to turn the patient, applying cornstarch or powder to surfaces coming in contact with the skin, avoiding direct contact with plastic or vinyl surfaces such as chux or vinyl chairs, and encouraging and assisting ambulation. If the patient is incontinent or diaphoretic, mea-

BOX 31-3

RISK ASSESSMENT SCALES

Pressure Ulcers

NORTON SCALE

- Consists of five parameters: physical condition, mental state, activity, mobility, and incontinence
- Each parameter is rated on a scale of 1 to 4, with one- or two-word descriptions for each parameter
- Scores may range from 5 to 20, with the lower scores indicating increased risk (12 or below)

GOSNELL SCALE

- Consists of five parameters: mental status, continence, mobility, activity, and nutrition
- Each parameter is rated on a scale of 1 to 4 except for mental status, which is rated from 1 to 5, and nutrition, which is rated from 1 to 3, with two- or three-sentence descriptive statements
- Additional variables measured include body temperature, blood pressure, skin tone and sensation, medication, and medical diagnoses (no weight given to these parameters)
- Scores may range from 5 to 20, with the lower scores indicating increased risk (16 or below)

BRADEN SCALE

- Consists of six subscales that reflect (conceptually) degrees of sensory perception, skin moisture, physical activity, nutritional intake, friction and shear, and ability to change and control body position
- Each parameter is rated on a scale of 1 to 4 except for friction and shear subscale, which is rated from 1 to 3; each parameter is accompanied by a brief description of criteria for assigning the rating
- Scores may range from 4 to 23, with the lower scores indicating increased risk (16 or below, or in older population a score of 17 or 18 may be more predictive)

Modified from Bryant RA: *Acute and chronic wounds: nursing management,* St Louis, 1992, Mosby.

sures must be implemented to prevent tissue breakdown caused by moisture. Breathable absorptive pads, fecal incontinence collectors, and external urinary catheters may be used to help manage incontinence. A regular skin cleansing regimen should be instituted and should include use of a skin protectant. Adult absorbent garments are available but should be used judiciously, and the patient should be assessed at least every 2 hours for changing the garment. Poor nutrition and hydration must be addressed if present. Intake and output records should be initiated, fluid intake should be encouraged if not contraindicated, and a dietary consult should be requested for nutritional assessment.

When a pressure ulcer is already present, the previously mentioned interventions and an individualized plan for treatment of the ulcer must be instituted (Box 31-4). Before any plan of care can be initiated, the ulcer must be staged (Figure 31-6). In addition to staging, a new classification system for making decisions regarding wound care has been introduced. It is the red-yellow-black system of wound classification (Cuzzell, 1988). It allows the nurse or physician to look at a wound and quickly assess the interventions needed (debridement, cleansing, dressing type). Red wounds may be acute or chronic. Acute red wounds may be caused by traumatic or surgical injury with frank bleeding or evidence of recent hemostasis. Chronic red wounds have clean pink, bright red, or dark red granulation tissue, which is seen after necrotic tissue is removed. The goal with a red wound is protection, which is accomplished with an atraumatic dressing (hydrogel, hydrocolloid) and/or appropriate topical medication. Cleansing of a red wound is not necessary in most cases.

Yellow wounds have soft necrotic tissue, "slough," or thick, tenacious exudate ranging in color from creamy ivory to yellow green. The goal with a yellow wound is debridement, cleansing, and protection. Debridement by using mechanical or autolytic methods is appropriate.

The black wound is a wound covered by thick necrotic tissue (eschar). The primary goal with this wound is debridement, which may be accomplished mechanically, chemically, or through autolysis. After the eschar is removed, the condition of the wound bed can be accurately assessed for further interventions.

Wounds should be assessed continuously so that treatment procedures can be changed as the wound progresses. For example, a yellow wound will become a red wound when exudate is no longer present and the wound exhibits a red, granulating base. The treatment should then be adjusted to that of a red wound. A wound may possess the characteristics of two different classifications. For example, a wound may have some granulation tissue evident, but slough is also evident. In this case the wound is considered a yellow wound and is treated accordingly. Interventions are always based on the worst scenario, with red being the optimum and black being the worst scenario. The rationale is that the goal of wound care is to have a red wound and that if any part of the wound is not at that stage, interventions must be aimed at advancing the entire wound to the red wound stage.

BOX 31-4 **Nursing Process**

PRESSURE ULCERS

ASSESSMENT

Risk factors (age, mobility, continence, nutrition)
Pressure ulcer for size, depth, drainage, presence of infection, evidence of healing
Bony prominences after each turn
Vital signs (temperature)

NURSING DIAGNOSES

Impaired skin integrity related to shearing force as evidenced by ulcerated area over point of pressure
Risk for injury and infection related to loss of skin barrier
Impaired home maintenance management related to long-term treatment

NURSING INTERVENTIONS

Relieve pressure on the pressure ulcer at all times.
Turn the patient at least every 2 hours.
Apply support surface appropriate to patient's needs.
Keep skin free of excessive moisture, urine, and feces.
Use a draw sheet to lift and turn the patient.
Maintain the head of the bed below a 30-degree angle.
Provide dressings, cleansing, and medication as ordered.
Assist patient and family in setting realistic goals for healing, mobility, and overall recovery.
Refer the patient for in-home nursing care when indicated.

EVALUATION OF EXPECTED OUTCOMES

Ulcer decreased in size
Ulcer free of infection
Pink, healthy granulation tissue apparent, continues to increase
Verbalizes understanding of home care

THE PATIENT WITH DISEASES AND DISORDERS OF THE SKIN

Although most diseases and disorders of the skin are treated by the dermatologist as medical or dermatologic conditions, some require surgical treatment. Both the medical and surgical aspects of the disease are considered in this chapter, and discussion is based on basic pathophysiology.

Disorders of Pigmentation

Lentigo (freckles)

Freckles are collections of skin pigment that result from quantitative changes in melanin. They may occur in certain persons after exposure to the sun in summer and tend to disappear in winter. Persons with severe cases may have the freckles removed by dermal abrasion, but assurance cannot be given that they will not return.

Chloasma (melasma)

Patches of pigmentation that may be yellowish brown, brown, or black occur on various parts of the body. They are more common in women and are often seen during pregnancy, at the time of menopause, or with the use of oral contraceptives.

No treatment is necessary unless the lesions occur on the face and the person is sensitive about them for cosmetic reasons. They may be removed with various bleaching preparations, but the procedure is not recommended.

Disorders of Glands

Seborrhea (oily skin)

Some persons have an excessive secretion of oil from the sebaceous glands that is accentuated on the face, neck, and scalp, where the oil glands are most abundant. It is often associated with other conditions such as acne vulgaris, seborrheic dermatitis, eczema, and seborrheic warts. Although the condition is normal for some persons, particularly women, it not only detracts from personal appearance but also predisposes one to other, more serious skin conditions.

Treatment consists of washing often and thoroughly with soap and water and avoiding the use of greasy creams. Preparations containing salicylic acid or sulfur or both may be rubbed into the affected areas several times a day.

STAGE		APPEARANCE
Stage 1		Redness, no wound. Region of pallor and mottling, followed by erythema. Early lesion: erythema blanches, lesion may be painful. Late lesion: erythema does not blanch, may be soft or indurated; edge is usually irregular.
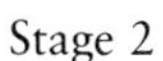 Stage 2	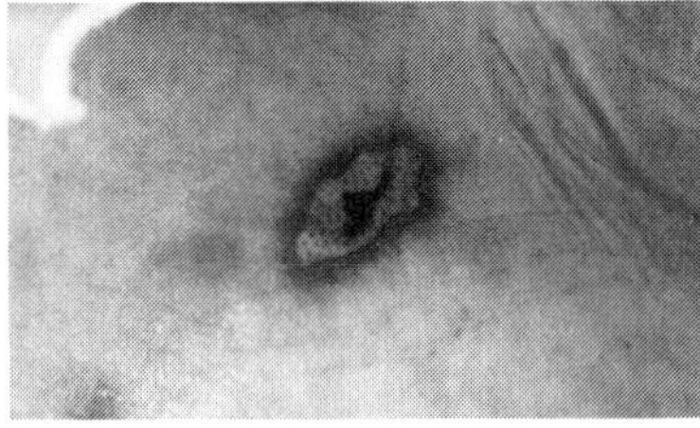	Red wound, clean, healing. Superficial epithelial damage, may range from a heel blister to as much as a 4 mm tissue loss over buttocks. Surrounding area is red and scaly with irregular borders.
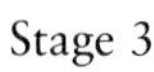 Stage 3	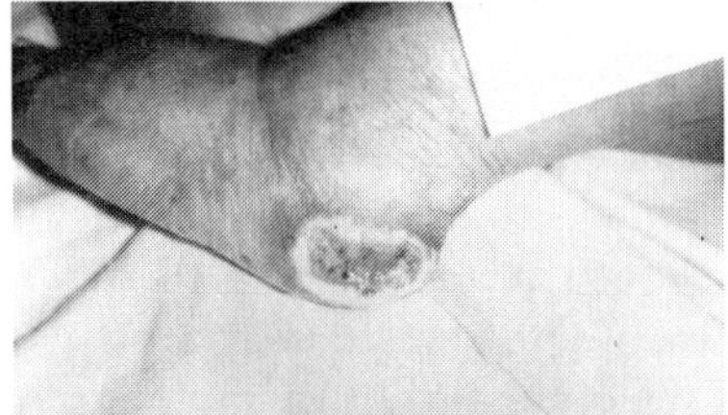	Yellow wound, some exudate. Infection may be present. Destruction of tissue has involved subcutaneous layers. Surface of ulcer will likely be smaller than internal diameters.
Stage 4	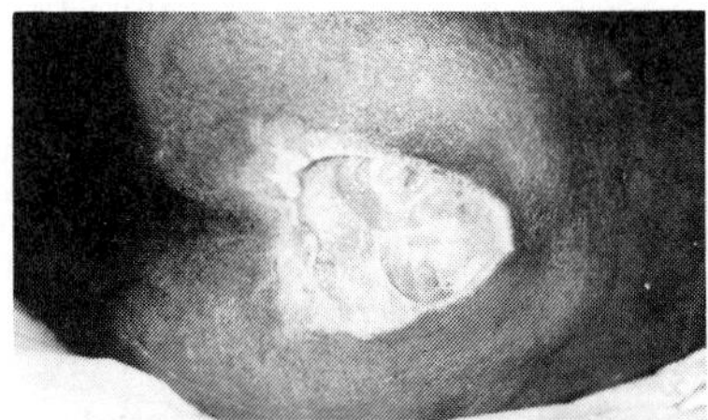	Black wound, necrotic tissue. Tissue destruction extends through subcutaneous layers into muscle and bone. Ulcer edge appears to "roll over" into the defect and is a tough fibrinous ring.
Eschar	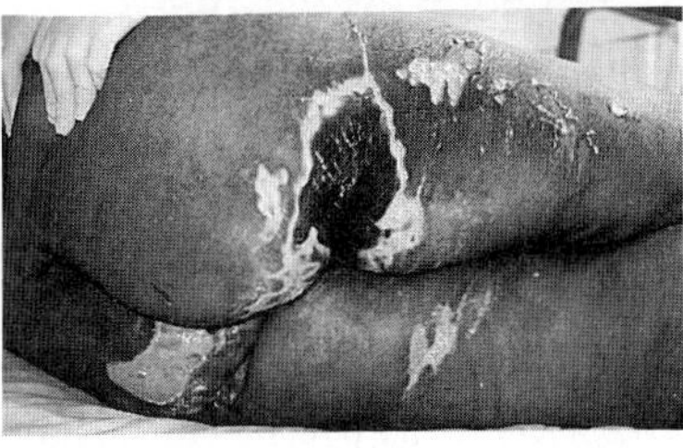	Lesion is covered by a tough membranous layer that may be rigidly adherent to the ulcer base. Stage is difficult to determine until eschar has sloughed or has been surgically removed.

NOTE: Stages describe layers of tissue visually involved. It is important to remember that even at the early stages (1 and 2) what is seen is only a small part of the damaged, swollen tissue underneath.

Figure 31-6 Pressure ulcer stages. (From Perry AG, Potter PA: *Clinical nursing skills and techniques,* ed 3, St Louis, 1994, Mosby.)

Sebaceous cyst (wen)

A sebaceous cyst, commonly called a *wen*, is often seen on the scalp and may become large. It is the result of obstruction of the sebaceous duct in the presence of continued secretions from the gland. These tumors contain an accumulation of sebum, which develops an offensive odor. The treatment is surgical incision, with measures to prevent infection.

Hyperhidrosis (excessive sweating)

Excessive sweating occurs in conjunction with several conditions, including diseases such as tuberculosis and hyperthyroidism, conditions involving severe pain such as that in renal colic, and certain acute heart attacks. It may also occur in some shock states and toxic conditions or after the administration of antipyretic drugs. Under normal conditions excessive sweating usually occurs when a person is exposed to extremes of heat or severe physical exercise. Excessive sweating may predispose the individual to skin disease or irritation.

Treatment is directed toward removing the cause, and nursing care should concern keeping the bed and clothing dry, sponging and drying the skin, and protecting the patient from exposure.

Axillary hyperhidrosis may be controlled by topical application of most of the commercial agents on the market. These preparations act by closing the pores and may occasionally cause a mild irritation. Excessive hyperhidrosis of the feet can be relieved by washing several times daily, drying thoroughly, and dusting with a medicated foot powder.

Anhidrosis (absence of sweating)

Anhidrosis is a normal result of the aging process accompanied by decreased activity of the sebaceous glands, which causes dryness of the skin. It can also be a very serious condition seen in younger individuals in whom the temperature-regulating mechanism (sweating) is disturbed. If temperature regulation is severely affected, the chance of heat prostration increases. This disorder is characteristic of diabetes mellitus, nephritis, hypothyroidism, and several skin diseases and may follow the administration of drugs such as atropine.

There is no specific treatment for the condition except for the use of superfatted soaps and the application of creams or oils. Treatment of the causative factor may provide relief.

Pruritus (Itching)

Pruritus is a symptom that accompanies many disorders, including a variety of skin diseases, systemic diseases, allergic reactions, and anhidrosis in the elderly person. The response of the individual is to scratch, and it is generally useless to tell the person not to scratch because the reply will probably be, "I can't help it." In fact, scratching is almost an automatic, unconscious act.

Whenever possible, treatment is based on removing or treating the cause. In treating small children, splinting of the arms or the use of mitts may be necessary to prevent scratching. Cold wet dressings, emollient baths, and emollient lotion containing phenol or menthol may be used, or the physician may prescribe a lotion containing a steroid drug. Some patients may benefit from antihistaminic drugs.

The nurse should do everything possible to provide comfort for the patient and to relieve the emotional tension often associated with pruritic conditions. Maintaining a cool, even room temperature and providing a quiet environment and some diversional activity will help to relieve itching.

Tumors of the Skin

Tumors of the skin are among the most common of all tumors and generally affect exposed parts of the body such as the face and backs of the hands. Persons whose occupations expose them to wind, sun, and frost are often affected. Most patients with skin tumors are in the older age group. Skin tumors may be benign or malignant, and most malignant tumors can be easily diagnosed and cured. Benign tumors include the keloid, angioma, nevus, wart, and keratoses.

Keloid

The keloid is an overgrowth of fibrous tissue occurring at a scar site. The shape may be irregular and small, or it may increase to the size of the hand. The tumor may develop after inflammation or ulceration from burns or traumatic injuries. It is not known why the condition occurs. It is more common in blacks.

There is no uniform opinion concerning treatment. The lesion may be erythematous, irritated, and painful. Pain may be relieved by injection of a glucocorticoid (Aristocort, Kenacort) diluted 1:5 with lidocaine (Xylocaine). Surgical removal followed by x-ray therapy will be effective in approximately half the cases.

Nevus (mole)

The mole is a nonvascular tumor, many of which are pigmented and may be present at birth. There are many different types of nevi, almost all of which are harmless. However, the raised black mole, although benign, may become malignant if it is located where it is subjected to constant irritation. It is generally advisable for these moles to be excised as a precautionary measure.

Angioma

Angioma is a benign skin tumor that consists of dilated blood vessels. There are several types of angiomas—one is congenital, called a birthmark by many people. The skin may have an area of purplish color known as port-wine stain. The stain is not elevated and may be large. Port-wine stains are commonly found on the face and may cover an entire side of the face. Treatment is usually for cosmetic purposes only and may consist of electrolysis, x-ray therapy, or laser removal.

The spider angioma is an acquired condition and consists of a network of venous capillaries that radiate outward in a spiderlike fashion. It may be related to liver disease and usually fades and disappears as the primary condition improves.

Keratoses

Keratoses are generally considered precancerous lesions, of which there are many types. Some occur in older persons as senile keratoses and are most likely to become malignant. Surgical removal is generally indicated. Some forms of keratoses, such as solar or actinic, appear in persons who have been exposed to the sun and whose skin has been damaged by it. Others are found as seborrheic dermatoses in persons past middle age. These are less likely to become malignant but should be kept under observation.

Malignant tumors

Skin cancer can be prevented, and if diagnosed early, can be cured. The thousands of skin cancer deaths each year can be partially attributed to public ignorance about prevention and to laxity among professionals in assessing skin lesions. Skin cancer may be caused by frequent contact with carcinogenic chemicals such as those found in coal tar, pitch, and pesticides; overexposure or chronic exposure to the sun's ultraviolet rays; repeated scar-producing injuries, especially burns; and radiation treatment. Fair-skinned people are more susceptible to cancer from sun exposure because they have less melanin, which keeps the sun's ultraviolet rays from penetrating the skin. The ultraviolet rays are believed to set off a genetic reaction that results in skin cancer. There are three types of skin cancer: basal cell, squamous cell, and malignant melanoma. The first two types are the most common and are easily cured if detected and treated early. Malignant melanoma is rarer but is the most dangerous to the patient.

Assessment. Assessment begins with a determination of the patient's risk for developing skin cancer. An investigation of lifestyle, occupation, geographic location, and hobbies will reveal factors that predispose the patient to skin cancer. Careful assessment of the skin of the entire body is important, including hidden areas between the toes and fingers and in the folds of the skin.

Basal cell carcinoma is seen most often in fair-skinned people who have had overexposure to the sun. It is usually found on the nose, eyelids, cheeks, rim of the ear, or trunk. There are two forms: nodular and superficial. The nodular form is elevated and firm to palpation and has an ulcerated center, raised margins, and a waxy or pearly border. The superficial type is flat and has a crusted or red center and a raised or pearly border.

Squamous cell carcinoma usually develops on areas exposed to radiation, mainly the head (especially on the lips) and hands. It can be an elevated, nodular mass or a large, fungus-like mass. It spreads more rapidly than basal cell carcinoma.

Malignant melanoma may appear without warning, beginning in or near a mole or other dark spot in the skin. The important warning signs are the ABCDs of melanoma. **A**symmetry: one side does not match the other; **B**order irregularity: the edges are notched, ragged, or blurred; **C**olor: the pigmentation is not uniform; shades of tan, brown, or black appear; dashes of red, white, or blue may be seen in the lesions; and **D**iameter: generally greater than 6 mm (about the size of a pencil eraser). The patient should see a physician if any of the following conditions are observed in a mole: the ABCDs, scaling, oozing, bleeding, spreading of pigmentation, or a change in sensation.

There is an inherited tendency to develop malignant melanoma, and melanoma-prone families can be identified by the presence of numerous large and unusual nevi on the skin. Now known as *dysplastic nevus syndrome (DNS)*, this condition often leads to the development of malignant melanoma and is characterized by many large and unusual moles. The moles often number more than 100 and are usually larger than 5 mm. Their pigmentation is unusual, combining brown, black, red, and pink in a single mole. They are found on the back and chest and may even be found in the scalp and on the breast. Patients with DNS or multiple nevi should be seen regularly by a physician to detect changes warning of malignancy. The patient also must be instructed to regularly and systematically observe the moles so that early detection of change is possible. Any change in size or color of a mole, flaking, ulceration, bleeding, or sudden elevation of a previously flat mole should be reported immediately to the physician. Patients with fewer or no moles must likewise be alert for changes in warts, moles, scars, and birthmarks. Any

BOX 31-5 Guidelines for Protecting the Skin Against Excessive Exposure to the Sun

- Avoid intense sunlight between 10 AM and 3 PM, when ultraviolet rays are the strongest.
- Plan such outdoor activities as walking, gardening, and other hobbies for early morning or late afternoon.
- Wear protective clothing such as hats and long-sleeved shirts.
- Use a sunscreen with a sun protection factor (SPF) of 15 or higher. The sunscreen should be applied 15 to 30 minutes before going out into the sunlight and every 2 to 3 hours during exposure (it may need to be applied more often because of heat, humidity, and sweating). Sunscreen should be applied liberally to the head and neck, with special attention to the nose, rims of the ears, cheeks, and forehead.

From Hill MJ: *Skin disorders: Mosby's clinical nursing series,* St Louis, 1994, Mosby.

unusual finding should be documented completely, including location, size, color, surface characteristics, and appearance of surrounding area. Documentation also should include the patient's observations of the lesion, including time of appearance, recent changes, irritation from clothing, and past treatment.

Intervention. Skin cancer is treated with a number of methods, including excision by standard or laser surgery, radiation, cryosurgery, and electrodesiccation and curettage. More resistant and larger lesions are treated more effectively with a method called Mohs' surgery, named after Frederich Mohs, who developed the technique more than 30 years ago. The technique originally involved the application of a chemical fixative to the visible part of the skin cancer to eliminate blood flow during excision. Modern laboratory procedures and improved surgical techniques have eliminated the need for chemical fixation, and the technique is now performed on fresh tissue. The tissue is examined microscopically as it is removed (by frozen section), and the surgeon continues to remove tissue until microscopic malignancy is excised. The wound can be reconstructed immediately, which was not possible when the chemical fixative was used. It is relatively painless and can be performed on an outpatient basis under local anesthesia. The procedure is now known as microscopically controlled excision or *Mohs' surgery fresh-tissue technique.*

After surgery, instruction in wound care is necessary. If the wound is left open to heal by secondary intention, it will be dressed postoperatively with an appropriate dressing (e.g., hydrocolloid, hydrogel, polyurethane foam, gauze). A topical antibiotic may be applied to the wound before dressing if desired. If the wound is dressed with a hydrocolloid, hydrogel, or a foam, the dressing needs to be changed only every 3 days unless signs of infection or heavy exudate are apparent. If a gauze dressing is used, it should be changed at least once daily. Because the wound is a clean surgical wound, cleansing is not necessary. If cleansing is desired or mandated by protocol, saline is the cleanser of choice. Hydrogen peroxide used to be the cleanser of choice for many years, but because of its cytotoxicity it should be used judiciously, if at all. If a gauze dressing is used, an antibiotic ointment is needed to help maintain a moist wound environment, help provide atraumatic removal of the gauze, and to provide some protection from bacteria. Some antibacterial ointments may cause sensitivity reactions, so the nurse should inform the patient to be aware of any redness, itching, or edema. As is true with any procedure, good handwashing is essential.

The most important intervention in skin cancer is *prevention.* (Box 31-5). Patients should be instructed on the use and importance of sunscreens. The minimum skin protection factor (SPF) that an individual should use is 15. Wearing broad-brimmed hats and limiting sun exposure should be advised. Individuals who are lightskinned and have blue eyes and red or blonde hair are at higher risk for development of skin cancer. Dark-skinned individuals may have a false sense of protection because of their skin color. It should be emphasized that even though their pigmentation offers some protection, they should still use a sunscreen, possibly of a lower SPF, and limit sun exposure. The use of tanning beds is discouraged.

Early detection of a skin cancer is also very important (Boxes 31-6 and 31-7). Patients should be informed of the five signs that should alert them to seek medical intervention. The five signs of skin cancer are (1) a persistent, nonhealing, open sore that bleeds, oozes, or crusts and remains open for 3 weeks or longer; (2) a reddish patch or irritated area, usually on the chest, shoulders, or limbs, that may or may not itch or hurt; (3) a smooth growth with an elevated, rolled border and indented center; (4) a shiny bump or nodule that is pearly or translucent and colored pink, red, white, tan, black, or brown; and (5) a scarlike area that is white, yellow, or waxy and often has poorly defined borders (Hill, 1994).

BOX 31-6

ABCD RULE FOR EARLY DETECTION OF MELANOMA

A = ASYMMETRY
Most true moles tend to be symmetric. Melanomas tend to be asymmetric (one half does not match the other).

B = BORDER
Most true moles have a clear-cut border. Melanomas tend to have a notched, scalloped, or indistinct border.

C = COLOR
True moles may be dark or light, but they usually are uniform in color. Early melanomas have an uneven or variegated color (may range from various hues of tan and brown to black, with red and white intermingled).

D = DIAMETER
Once they have the A, B, and C characteristics, most melanomas are larger than 6 mm in diameter. Moles tend to be smaller. A sudden or progressive increase in the size of a mole should be reported.

From Hill MJ: *Skin disorders: Mosby's clinical nursing series,* St Louis, 1994, Mosby.

Disorders of the Appendages

Alopecia (loss of hair)

Loss of hair may result from several causes, including the normal thinning of hair that is part of the aging process. Hair is sometimes lost after long and debilitating disease or high fever. A characteristic alopecia occurs in early syphilis and is marked by loss of hair in round patches; it may progress until the scalp presents a moth-eaten appearance. Alopecia areata results in patches of baldness that may appear suddenly and tend to spread from the edges. After several round patches of baldness occur, regrowth of hair begins but may not be permanent. Finally, however, the hair is replaced, and spontaneous recovery takes place after several months.

Hypertrichosis and hypotrichosis

Hypertrichosis is an excessive growth of hair in a masculine distribution. It may be congenital, acquired (hormonal dysfunction, porphyria, drugs), or result from a hereditary tendency. In congenital hypertrichosis, hair may cover moles or the skin over a spina bifida. Acquired hypertrichosis that is a result of endocrine disturbance is comonly seen as a growth of hair

BOX 31-7

DANGER SIGNALS SUGGESTING MALIGNANT TRANSFORMATION IN PIGMENTED LESIONS

Change in color
Especially sudden darkening, mottled and variegated shades of tan, brown, and black; red, white, and blue

Change in diameter
Especially a sudden increase

Change in outline
Especially development of irregular margins

Change in surface characteristics
Especially scaliness, erosion, oozing, crusting, bleeding, ulceration, or development of a mushrooming mass on the surface of the lesion

Change in consistency
Especially softening or friability

Change of symptoms
Especially a sense of pruritus

Change in shape
Especially irregular elevation from a previously **flat** condition

Change in the surrounding skin
Especially "leaking" of pigment from the lesion into surrounding skin, or the development of pigmented "satellite" lesions

From Hill MJ: *Skin disorders: Mosby's clinical nursing series,* St Louis, 1994, Mosby.

OLDER ADULT CONSIDERATIONS

Skin Conditions

The aging skin is prone to developing skin cancers. Basal cell carcinoma accounts for 80%.
Changes in the skin occur slowly and gradually.
Carcinomas appear frequently on the nose, eyelid, or cheek from sun exposures.
Seborrheic keratoses are benign epidermal growths frequently seen on face, scalp, trunk, and upper extremities.
Xerosis (dry skin) is the most common skin problem. Emollients such as mineral oil, lanolin, or white petroleum jelly help seal in moisture.

From Beare PG, Myers JL: *Adult health nursing,* ed 2, St Louis, 1994, Mosby.

on the upper lip and on the chin of women. It also may be the result of a hereditary predisposition that is similar in character but not in effect to that which controls male pattern baldness. The most satisfactory method of removing superfluous hair is by electrolysis.

Hypotrichosis is an absence of hair or a deficiency of hair. The condition may be the result of heredity (alopecia universalis), skin disease, drugs, or endocrine factors. When the cause is endocrine disturbance, correction should be made if possible.

Hair transplants

The problem of baldness is more common in men than in women. As an alternative to wearing hairpieces, it is now possible to elect to have a hair transplant for cosmetic purposes. Most balding males retain healthy hair on the back and sides of the head. These hair follicles can be relocated by a transplant procedure in which dozens of small plugs of hair are removed and relocated to the areas where hair is thin or absent. Patterns of grafts are removed from the balding area and replaced by the healthy growing hair grafts from the donor area. Treatment is usually performed in two or three sessions, and each session lasts 1 or 2 hours. Sessions are spaced at least 2 weeks apart to allow adequate healing and to establish circulation through the transplant area. New hair should begin to appear about 12 weeks after the transplant.

Nail disorders

Disorders of the nails may be associated with diseases elsewhere in the body, nutritional status, congenital defects, drugs, or infection. The nails may be soft or brittle. Changes in the shape and contour may occur, and nails may grow into the soft tissues at the sides (ingrown nail). *Paronychia* is an infection in the fold of skin at the margin of the nail. The infection begins on the side of the nail, often from a hangnail or injury, and finally encircles the whole nail. The infection loosens the nail from the matrix and may cause pain. Surgical removal of the affected part of the nail is often necessary. Wet dressings using 1:2000 to 1:10,000 potassium permanganate and the application of neomycin ointment may relieve the condition. Fungal infections of the nails respond poorly to ordinary methods of treatment and may take months to cure.

Infestations

Pediculi (lice)

Three types of pediculi infest human beings: *Pediculus humanus capitis, P. humanus corporis,* and *P. pubis.* Table 31-8 lists the common skin manifestations.

P. humanus capitis is the head louse, which lives on the scalp and attaches its eggs (nits) to the hair. The nits are attached to the hair by an adhesive substance that makes them difficult to remove. The louse bites the scalp to seek nutrition by sucking blood, which causes severe itching and scratching. Severe infestations may result in secondary infections that are associated with enlargement of lymph glands in the neck (Box 31-8). Immediate treatment is required. For many years, the treatment of choice was Kwell shampoo, which contained the active ingredient lindane. Kwell is no longer sold, but generic products containing lindane are available by prescription. Lindane is known to be cerebroneurotoxic, and other preparations such as 1% permethrin (Nix) or pyrethrin (RID) are considered less toxic and have proven as effective as lindane while causing fewer adverse reactions. Nix and RID are available without prescription (University of California at Berkeley, 1995).

P. humanus corporis is a body louse that may be found in the seams of underclothing. Scratch marks

TABLE 31-8

Common Skin Manifestations of Ectoparasites

Ectoparasite	Skin manifestation
Scabies mite	Irregular, linear, gray-brown or pearly burrows less than 1 mm wide, often with a spot at the end; more prominent in the web spaces of the hands, on the flexor surfaces of the wrists, in the axillary folds, and on the buttocks; vesicles and papules may be present; in children, nodular lesions may be present on the upper back, chest, and genitals and in the axillary folds; disseminated papular eruption or crusted exfoliative areas with fissures may be seen in immunocompromised individuals
Lice	Small, erythematous papules and wheals, often with nits attached to hair shaft; cervical adenopathy may indicate severe involvement on the head and often is accompanied by purulent dermatitis, with matting of the hair; louse generally is visible on close observation

From Hill MJ: *Skin disorders, Mosby's clinical nursing series,* 1994, St Louis, Mosby.

may appear on the skin in the area of the involved clothing seams. All personal items such as clothing and bedding must be washed in hot water. With body lice, the extra precaution of ironing the seams of clothing should be recommended. Hats, scarves, hair ornaments, combs, and brushes also must be cleared of lice and their eggs. Although lice can live only approximately 10 days after separation from the host, the eggs may hatch in up to 30 days if kept near body temperature. Body lice are treated with 1% permethrin, pyrethrin, or lindane. Any one of the three pediculicides is applied to the affected skin/scalp after bathing and shampooing, with particular care to avoid the eyes. Lindane is applied to the total body and left on for 2 hours. The treatment may be repeated if necessary. If pyrethrin or permethrin is used, it is left on for 10 minutes, then rinsed thoroughly. This application is repeated daily for 3 consecutive days. As mentioned earlier, pyrethrin (RID) and permethrin (Nix) produce less toxic effects and are available without prescription. A fine-toothed comb should be used to comb nits from hair (scalp and pubic). Patients need to be informed that itching may persist for up to two weeks after treatment.

P. pubis is found primarily in the genital area; however, it may infect the axilla, eyebrows, beard, and eyelashes. The lice may be contracted from toilet seats, bedclothes, clothing, and sexual intercourse. Treatment is the same as for *P. humanis corporis*.

BOX 31-8

COMPLICATIONS OF ECTOPARASITE INFESTATION

- Because of the intense pruritus and scratching associated with scabies, secondary bacterial infections may occur. In immunocompromised individuals, the mite multiplies, unchecked by the cell-mediated response that normally kills a percentage of the mites. As the mites multiply, hyperkeratotic plaques form and fissuring develops. Normal skin flora may be introduced into the blood, resulting in bacteremia, sepsis, and occasionally death.
- Lice infestation may be the source of keratoconjunctivitis, photophobia, and secondary pyoderma, caused by *P. humanus capitis*. Other complications include eczematization, pyodermas, nodular granulomas, urticaria, acarophobia, and delusions of parasitosis. *P. humanus corporis* serves as a vector for epidemic typhus fever *(Rickettsia prowazekii)*, relapsing fever *(Borrelia recurrentis)*, and trench fever *(Rickettsia quintana)* (Hill, 1994).

From Hill MJ: *Skin disorders: Mosby's clinical nursing series*, St Louis, 1994, Mosby.

Scabies (itch mite)

Scabies, an infectious skin disease, is caused by the itch mite, a parasite that burrows under the skin (see Table 31-8). A warm, protected environment fosters the growth of the parasite, and it is spread easily by direct contact with another person who is infested. Even handholding or simply shaking hands can transmit scabies from one individual to another. Contact with infected clothing or linens can spread scabies, but the mite does not jump from one person to the other and does not survive very long in clothing or linens. Outbreaks of scabies were common until World War II and then began a decline, only to make a vigorous comeback in recent years. It is not uncommon to find scabies on patients in nursing homes and hospitals. Scabies may occur as epidemics or endemics. An individual can develop immunity to the disease, but the mechanism of this immunity is not clearly understood.

Assessment. The nurse can prevent the spread of the disease to other patients and also avoid contracting the disease by being alert to the symptoms. A person is more likely to contract scabies from someone whose disease is not diagnosed than from one who has been identified and treated. The disease is recognized by the presence of intense itching and multiform lesions (lesions of many shapes). Papules and vesicles are common, and characteristic S-shaped burrows are often, but not always, present. Secondary bacterial infection and scratching may result in pustules and edema (see Box 31-8). Delay in treatment may lead to an eczematous condition.

The characteristic location of the lesion varies with age. Children have involvement of the palms, soles, head, and neck. Adults rarely have lesions in these areas but do have them on the flexor surfaces of the wrist and elbows, on the waist, buttocks, genitalia in males, and on the breasts in females. Burrows can be found between fingers and around the umbilicus. The characteristic itching intensifies at night. A definite diagnosis may require examination of scrapings taken from lesions on the skin to isolate the mite.

Treatment requires use of an insecticide by the patient and all close contacts. Insecticides may include 5% permethrin cream (Elimite), 1% lindane, or crotamiton (Eurax). The permethrin cream is massaged into the skin from the head to the soles, left on for 8 to 14 hours, and washed off thoroughly. Lindane is applied the same way as permethrin cream, but because of evidence of neurotoxicity with infants and small children, the application time for them is shortened to 2 hours. In addition, if the lindane is applied to the hands of these very young patients, precautions should be taken to keep them from putting their hands in their mouths. Lindane should not be used in pregnant or lactating women. Treatment may be repeated in 7 days if indicated. Crotamiton (Eurax) is applied for 2 to 5 consecutive nights. The patient can bathe 24 hours after the last application. Crotamiton is contraindicated in pregnant or lactating women. Patients should be advised that itching may persist for up to 2 weeks and that they should not use this medication repeatedly to help control the itching because this increases the risk of absorption. Medication may be prescribed specifically to help control the itching (Hill, 1994).

Infections

Bacterial infections

Folliculitis is inflammation of a hair follicle secondary to staphylococcal infection. It commonly occurs on the scalp, the extremities, or the bearded areas of the face. Chronic folliculitis of the beard is called *sycosis barbae.* If hair follicles are permanently damaged, hair will not grow from them.

A *furuncle* (boil) is an acute infection of a hair follicle or sebaceous gland. It usually is caused by a staphylococcus bacterium that produces an abscess of the skin in subcutaneous tissue. The lesion appears with central necrosis and accumulation of pus. Initial lesions are small, indurated, and painful. As the lesions progress, they become elevated, tender, shiny, and bright red, and the patient complains of throbbing pain. Furuncles may resolve spontaneously, but incision and drainage gives almost immediate relief from pain and does hasten healing. Patients may also have fever, malaise, and regional lymphadenopathy. Lesions are most commonly seen on the back of the neck, face, buttocks, thighs, perineum, and breasts, or in the axillae. There may be single or multiple lesions. A carbuncle is similar to a boil, except that the infection infiltrates into the surrounding tissue and results in several boils. Carbuncles are also caused by a staphylococcus bacterium.

A *felon* is an infection of the end of a finger. It may result from a puncture wound such as a pinprick, or it may occur without a known cause. A streptococcus bacterium is a common cause of felons. Clinically, an abscess usually is seen on the distal phalanx of a finger.

Cellulitis is an acute streptococcal or staphylococcal infection of the skin and subcutaneous tissue. The skin becomes erythematous, edematous, hot, and tender to the touch. Lymphatic streaks may develop proximal to the infection (Hill, 1994).

Impetigo is skin infection that is categorized as impetigo contagiosa, caused by group A beta-hemolytic streptococci, or as bullous impetigo, caused by group II *Staphylococcus aureus.* Impetigo contagiosa is found most often in children and may be endemic (Hill, 1994). The initial clinical lesion of impetigo is a vesicular or pustular lesion with a "honey-colored crust" that is considered a definitive sign of impetigo. Lesions of impetigo may be seen on the lower extremities, face, or hands (Figure 31-7). The bacteria are easily spread through direct or indirect contact. It is common for an insect bite to become infected by the staphylococcus or streptococcus organism. Poor health and nutrition, a warm, humid environment, and preexisting pruritic skin eruptions may also predispose a patient to impetigo (Yotter, 1990). Definitive identification of the causative organism may be done by bacterial culture.

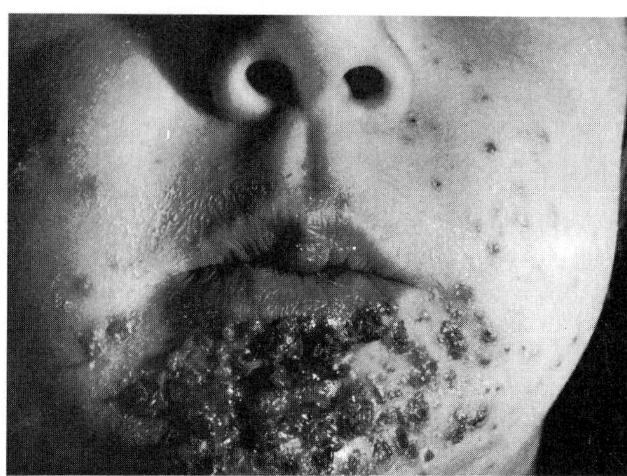

Figure 31-7 Impetigo contagiosa. (From Stewart WD and others: *Dermatology: diagnosis and treatment of cutaneous disorders,* St Louis, 1978, Mosby. In Phipps WJ and others: *Medical-surgical nursing: concepts and clinical practice,* ed 5, St Louis, 1995, Mosby.)

Assessment. Nursing assessment of patients suspected of having a bacterial skin infection includes assessing current health status and performing a physical examination to identify lymphadenopathy and existing skin lesions. Patients with impetigo, cellulitis, furuncles, or carbuncles may appear healthy but complain of fever, chills, headache, and malaise. Lymphadenopathy may be present with any of these infections.

The lesion of folliculitis consists of a pustule surrounded by an area of erythema and appears as a raised dome around the follicle. The pustule weeps, forming a crust, and the hair seems to be growing from the center of the crust. Pain will occur if the infection spreads to the dermis surrounding the follicle.

A furuncle begins as a small, red, edematous, painful area on the skin of the face, neck, axilla, forearm, buttocks, groin, or legs. It may appear as only a tiny pimple and abate spontaneously, or it may continue to in-

BOX 31-9 **Nursing Process**

BACTERIAL INFECTION

ASSESSMENT

Current health status
Skin lesions for characteristics, distribution, and severity
Level of discomfort
Temperature
Lymphadenopathy

NURSING DIAGNOSES

Impaired skin integrity related to inflammatory process
Risk for impaired skin integrity related to exudate
Risk for infection related to inadequate primary or secondary defenses
Body image disturbance related to reaction of others to lesions
Pain related to infectious process

NURSING INTERVENTIONS

Provide local treatment of lesions as ordered.
Use good handwashing technique and instruct the patient in the procedure.
Use antibacterial soap and instruct the patient to use it.
Administer analgesic medication as ordered and evaluate its effect.

EVALUATION OF EXPECTED OUTCOMES

Skin integrity improved
No infection is evident
Pain is relieved

crease in size and exhibit pus formation within a few days. Carbuncles are most commonly found on the back of the neck and upper back. As the infection gradually comes to the surface from the deeper tissue, there will be several openings discharging pus. The site of a felon on a finger is red and edematous, and there is severe, throbbing pain. Both carbuncles and furuncles occur most often in poorly nourished and debilitated individuals and may be a sign of uncontrolled diabetes mellitus.

Cellulitis appears as an erythematous, edematous, hot, and tender area of skin with or without lymphangitic streaks. It may or may not be associated with another skin lesion. Impetigo begins as a vesicopustule on the skin that ruptures and leaves a red, oozing erosion. The erosion becomes covered by a characteristic yellow (honey-colored) crust. The infection may spread from an existing lesion to other parts of the body, so several lesions may be present at the same time.

Interventions. Early treatment of these localized infections prevents complications and systemic spread. General management of these infections includes cleansing of the involved area with an antibacterial soap. The surrounding skin also should be cleansed carefully to prevent spread of the infection.

Warm, moist compresses are used to promote suppuration in folliculitis, furuncles, carbuncles, and felons. If the furuncles or carbuncles do not rupture spontaneously, surgical incision and drainage is necessary. Most patients with folliculitis, furuncles, carbuncles, and felons are cared for in the physician's office.

General management of cellulitis includes immobilization and elevation of the affected limb, hospitalization if necessary, cool compresses for discomfort, or warm compresses to increase circulation. General measures for the management of impetigo includes removal of crusts with soap and water, application of cool compresses, and nutritional interventions as indicated. Patients should be instructed to avoid sharing of clothing, towels, or washcloths.

All skin infections require either topical or systemic antibiotics, depending on the severity. The nurse must educate the patient about any medication, proper use, and possible side effects.

Universal precautions—use of gloves, handwashing, and proper disposal of all contaminated dressings—should be followed at all times when dealing with skin infections. Patients should be instructed to use the same precautions at home to prevent cross contamination while lesions are still draining. Patients should also be instructed not to share clothing and linen while infection is still evident (Box 31-9).

Fungal infections

Fungal infections are superficial infections of the skin and are classified by body region (**tinea** corporis, tinea capitis, tinea cruris, tinea barbae, tenia pedis). Fungi can infect and survive in the dead keratin of the stratum corneum (horny layer) of the epidermis. They also affect the hair and nails. Fungal infection rarely invades deep tissues or involves other organs except in the immunocompromised patient.

Fungal infections must be diagnosed by laboratory examination (KOH wet mount, wood's lamp, or culture). A KOH (potassium hydroxide) wet mount is done by taking a scraping of the suspected lesion, placing it on a microscope slide, adding a drop of KOH, applying a cover slip, heating it slightly, and examining it under the microscope. Hyphae of fungi may be detected under magnification with this technique. A wood's lamp, when shined on suspected lesions, causes the fungus to fluorescence a blue-green. Fungal culture is done by taking scrapings from the suspected lesion and putting them into the appropriate medium. If fungal growth is seen within 1 week, the patient can be told that the culture is positive.

Even though fungal infections are superficial, there are some complications that may occur. These include secondary infections, id reactions, pruritus, and infections that are atypical, generalized, or invasive (usually in immunocompromised patients). An id reaction is a cutaneous response elicited in other areas of the body distant from the primary infection (Hill, 1994).

Tinea capitis. Tinea capitis, better known as ringworm of the scalp, occurs primarily in preadolescent children. The lesion is easily recognized and appears as a scaly bald spot with hairs breaking off at the surface (Figure 31-8A). Occasionally the patient will develop an inflammatory reaction to the fungus and will develop boggy areas with pus called *kerion*. Treatment of ringworm is usually successful with oral griseofulvin. If kerion are present, they should be treated topically with compresses and hydrogen peroxide at the

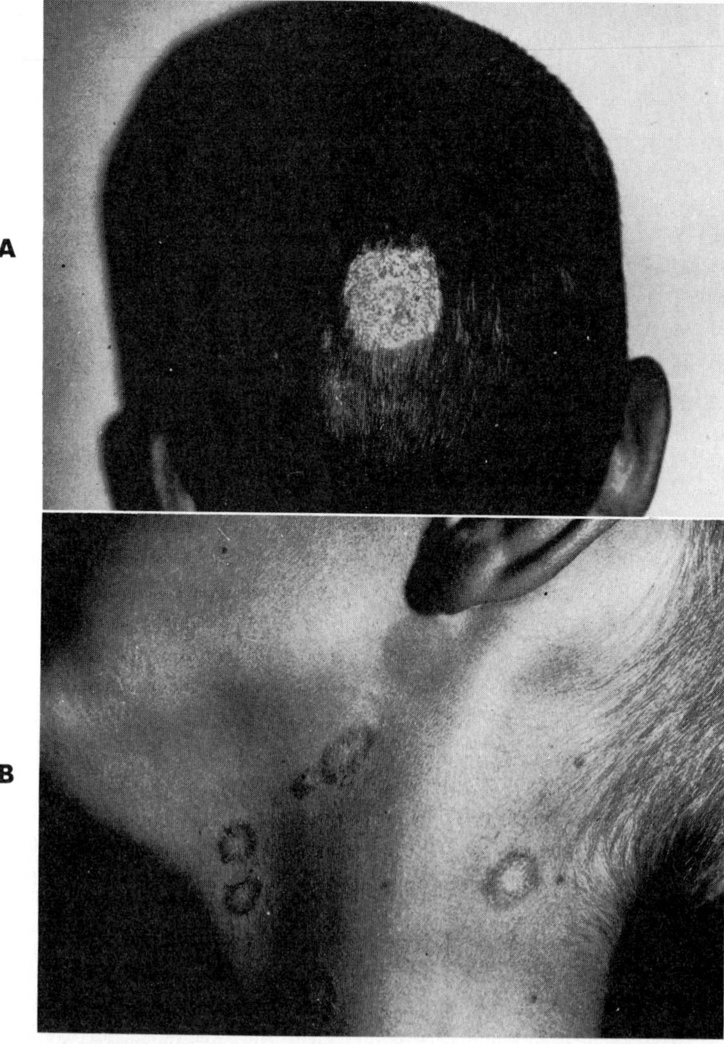

Figure 31-8 **A,** Tinea capitis. **B,** Tinea corporis. (From Stewart WD and others: *Dermatology: diagnosis and treatment of cutaneous disorders,* St Louis, 1978, Mosby. In Phipps WJ and others: *Medical-surgical nursing: concepts and clinical practice,* ed 5, St Louis, 1995, Mosby.)

same time that the oral steroids are given. Patients receiving cortisone should not be given griseofulvin at the same time. When the infection is severe, there may be patches of baldness on the scalp. This loss of hair is usually temporary, and the hair will return when the infection subsides. This infection is contagious, so all members of the family should be examined. The patient's personal toilet articles, such as combs and brushes, should not be used by other members of the family. The individual with tinea capitis is usually treated in the physician's office or in a clinic; however, the patient may have been admitted to the hospital for another condition. If tinea capitis is discovered in a hospital patient, it should be called to the physician's attention, and the nurse should take protective precautions.

Tinea corporis. Tinea corporis is a form of ringworm that occurs on the nonhairy areas of the body, face, neck, and extremities. The characteristic lesion is a papulosquamous annular lesion with raised borders, scaly borders, and central clearing (Figure 31-8B). The lesion increases in size gradually, expanding peripherally. Tinea corporis is more common in hot and humid climates, more common in rural areas, and occurs in both adults and children (Hill, 1994). Treatment with a topical fungicide is satisfactory if only a few lesions are present. For more extensive cases, griseofulvin is used.

Tinea barbae. Tinea barbae, or barber's itch, occurs in the beard and is characterized by a soft nodular type of lesion with accompanying edema of the face. The nodules may break down and become suppurative. The hairs of the beard become loose and slip out, leaving bald areas. Several preparations have been used in the treatment of the condition, including ammoniated mercury ointment, griseofulvin, and copper undecylenate.

Tinea cruris. Tinea cruris is commonly called jock itch and is found in the groin or inner thigh. It is more common in hot weather and is aggravated by friction caused by tight-fitting clothing. The lesion usually affects both sides of the groin equally and may extend to cover the entire groin area, giving a butterfly appearance. The lesions are either hypopigmented or erythematous, and they are well-demarcated, with scaling and central clearing. Pruritus is the main complaint. Maceration of the skin in the skin folds occurs, and secondary bacterial or candidal infection is common. Treatment involves keeping the area cool and dry, wearing loose, absorbent clothing, and applying an antifungal preparation as prescribed.

Tinea pedis. Tinea pedis, or athlete's foot, is a common disorder affecting the feet, although it may be spread to other parts of the body, particularly the hands (tinea manuum). It is rare in children and is not transmitted by simple exposure. It is generally believed that the infection is contracted in showers, around swimming pools, and in similar moist places, but absolute proof of this method of transmission is lacking. Clinical lesions vary and include maceration, scaling, fissuring of interdigital space, erythema of the plantar surfaces, and brittle, discolored nails. Pruritus is a common complaint.

General management of tineas includes keeping intertriginous areas clean and dry and using a medicated powder. With tinea pedis, white cotton socks should be worn. Application of the prescribed topical medication or adherence to the prescribed systemic medication schedule must be emphasized (Table 31-9; Box 31-10).

Viral infections

Viral infections that are contained in or manifested in the skin have distinct symptoms that allow clinical diagnosis without further testing. Rubella, rubeola, human papillomaviruses (warts), herpesviruses (simplex, zoster, and varicella), and human immunodeficiency virus (HIV) are all commonly seen on the skin (Hill, 1994).

Rubella. *Rubella* (German measles, 3 day measles) is a viral infection that appears as erythematous macular/maculopapular lesions that last up to 3 days. Low-grade fever, coryza (rhinitis), malaise, headache, and conjunctivitis may precede the development of a rash by 1 to 5 days. These prodromal symptoms may not appear at all, especially in children. Mode of transmission is airborne, and the virus invades through nasopharyngeal secretions. The incubation period for rubella is 14 to 21 days from infection to presentation of rash. Lymphadenopathy may accompany the presentation of the rash. The rash characteristically begins on the face and spreads from the head toward the hands and feet. Petechial lesions may be seen on the soft palate and uvula. Pharyngitis (inflammation of the pharynx) may also be present (Hill, 1994).

Rubeola. An acute, highly contagious viral disease that is spread by respiratory exposure is *rubeola* (red measles). The prodromes include fever, conjunctivitis, coryza, bronchitis, and Koplik's spots (small, red spots with bluish-white centers) on the buccal mucosa. A red, macular/maculopapular rash appears on the face 3 to 7 days after infection with the virus. The rash will generalize and last from 4 to 7 days. Desquamation is a common occurrence after the rash has resolved (Hill, 1994).

Papillomavirus (warts). Human papillomaviruses cause benign skin growths called *warts.* Warts can be seen in all age groups. They commonly develop at sites of trauma, on the hands, in the periungual region, and on the plantar surfaces, and they usually resolve spontaneously. Individuals with immunosuppression

TABLE 31-9

Summary of Tinea

Type	Distribution	Occurrence	Clinical Features
Tinea corporis	Nonhairy parts of body, face, neck, extremities	More common in hot and humid climates; more common in rural than in urban settings; occurs in both adults and children	Pruritus; papulosquamous annular lesions with raised borders; lesions expand peripherally with central clearing
Tinea cruris	Groin, inner thigh, scrotum or labia not involved	More common in adult men; tends to recur; flare-ups common in summer; aggravated by tight clothes, perspiration, and physical activity	Pruritus; hypopigmented, well-demarcated lesions; dryness and scaling; pustules present at margins; central clearing sometimes present; secondary bacterial or candidal infection and maceration common
Tinea capitis	Scalp	More common in children; contagious	Lesions vary; small, gray scaly patches with short broken hairs; mild, erythematous papules; raised, boggy, inflamed nodules dotted with perifollicular abscesses; thick, yellow, suppurative lesions; lesions may be small and coalesced or may cover entire scalp; hairless patches
Tinea pedis	Feet; begins in third and fourth interdigital spaces and spreads to involve plantar surface; may involve nails	Rare in children; not transmitted by simple exposure	Lesions vary; maceration, scaling, fissuring of interdigital space; vesicular scaling, erythema of plantar surface; chronic, noninflamed, diffuse scaling; nails brittle, discolored; pruritus
Tinea unguium	Toenails and (less commonly) fingernails		Nails thickened, lusterless, and discolored; subungual debris; nail plate crumbling or absent

From Hill MJ: *Skin disorders: Mosby's clinical nursing series,* St Louis, 1994, Mosby.

BOX 31-10

Nursing Process

FUNGAL INFECTION

ASSESSMENT

Skin lesions for characteristics, distribution, and severity
Level of discomfort
Signs of secondary infection

NURSING DIAGNOSES

Impaired skin integrity related to presence of lesions
Risk for infection related to loss of skin's protective barrier
Pain related to skin lesions

NURSING INTERVENTIONS

Cleanse lesions as indicated.
Discourage scratching.
Keep skin surfaces dry.
Administer antihistamines or analgesics as indicated.
Apply topical medications as ordered.
Administer systemic medications as ordered.

EVALUATION OF EXPECTED OUTCOMES

Skin integrity improved
No infection is evident
Pruritis/pain has been relieved

(HIV, drugs), atopic dermatitis, and lymphomas have more severe cases of warts when infected (Hill, 1994). Warts may appear on the genitalia in adults and are transmitted through sexual contact. If genital warts are seen in children, sexual abuse may be the cause.

Herpesviruses. *Herpesviruses* (Herpesvirus hominus) cause opportunistic infections. Opportunistic infections are a consequence of defective functioning of one or more components of the immune system (Beare, Myers, 1994). Herpesvirus hominus is subdivided into *herpes simplex virus type 1* and *herpes simplex virus type 2.*

Herpes simplex. *Herpes simplex 1* (HSV 1) is the most common form of herpes simplex and is found in gingivostomatitis (cold sore, fever blister) (Figure 31-9). *Herpes simplex 2 (HSV 2)* causes genital herpes and is found in lesions of the penis and cervix and in disseminated herpes in the newborn (see Chapter 11).

Each of the two forms of herpes has a primary and a secondary presentation. Primary infections are usually subclinical, but they can become severe and may be life threatening. Secondary presentations, or recurrences, are generally milder and of shorter duration. Subclinical primary infections appear as small vesicles that evolve into ulcerations, then crusts, with healing taking from a few days to 3 weeks. Pain and lymphadenopathy may be associated. Recurrences may have prodromes of tingling or pain in the area of involvement. Recurrent lesions reappear in the same site as the primary lesions (Hill, 1994).

HSV 1 is characterized by the appearance of a group of small vesicles on an erythematous base. It was originally thought that HSV 1 could be found only on the skin and mucous membranes of the lip or nose (see Figure 31-9). This has since been proven incorrect. HSV 1 has been cultured from lesions on the genitalia. The disease often occurs when other acute infections are present but may occur in the absence of any other condition. It was once thought that canker sores (aphthous ulcers) on the mucous membrane of the mouth were also caused by this same virus, but it has now been demonstrated that they are not herpetic lesions. Herpes simplex is usually of short duration, but it is a recurring condition. The virus has the ability to persist in a latent state in certain tissues and to cause repeated infection despite the presence of circulating neutralizing antibodies. The appearance of the lesion, often called a cold sore, is often associated with certain stimuli such as sunlight, menstruation, fatigue, and emotional stress, all of which are thought to trigger viral replication and result in disease.

HSV 2 is found in approximately 20% of the adult population and is more prevalent in lower socioeconomic groups and in sexually active persons. The

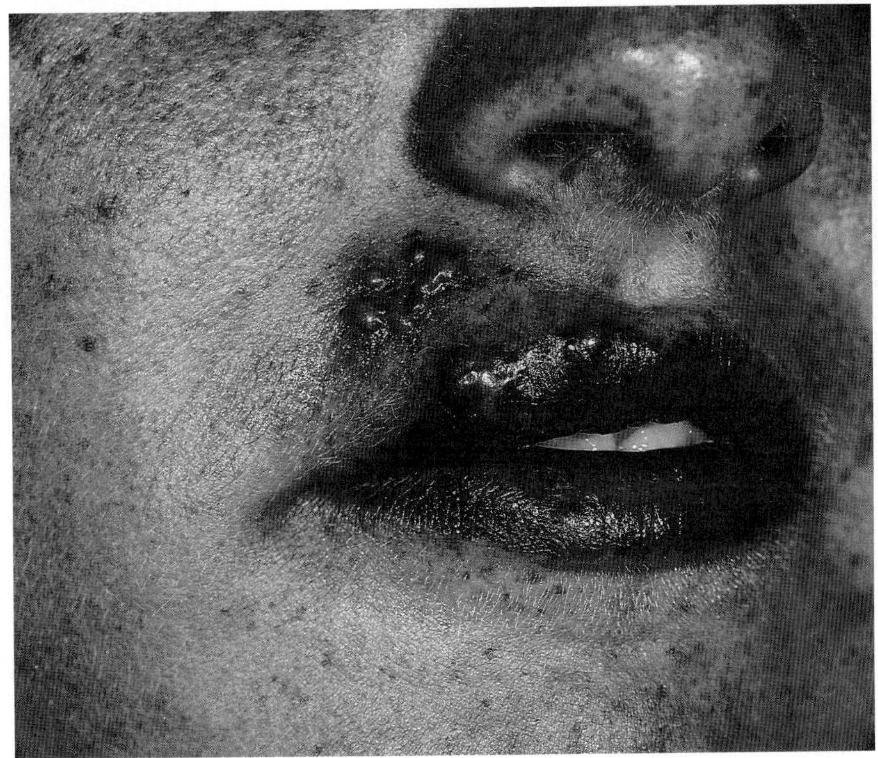

Figure 31-9 Herpes simplex type I. (From McCance KL, Huether SE: *Pathophysiology: adults and children*, ed 2, St Louis, 1994, Mosby.)

virus produces genital herpes and results in ulcerative or necrotizing lesions of the uterine cervix or the vulvar area in women. In men it produces ulcerations on the penis. The ulcerations are painful and tend to recur. It must be remembered that women may have asymptomatic lesions of the cervix that continually shed the virus. It is extremely important to evaluate pregnant women to determine whether vaginal delivery is safe.

Herpes zoster. *Herpes zoster* and *varicella (chickenpox)* are caused by the herpesvirus varicella. A maculopapulovesicular exanthem that has centripetal distribution is the presentation of varicella (chickenpox). Varicella is an acute, highly contagious viral infection. The characteristic lesion is called "dew drop on a rose petal" because of its appearance—a singular vesicle on an erythematous base. Lesions develop in crops, so at any one time there may be primary and secondary (crusted or resolving) lesions present. Varicella is self-limiting, and healing is complete within 2 weeks. In immunocompromised patients, however, varicella is a life-threatening disease. Pruritus is the most disturbing symptom associated with varicella. Treatment is directed at alleviation of symptoms and includes soothing baths (Aveeno, cornstarch), antihistamines, and topical drying agents (calamine, shake lotions).

Herpes zoster (shingles) is often classified as a neurologic disorder because the lesion is located in one or more of the spinal ganglia, with involvement of the skin area supplied by the nerve fibers. The virus can lie dormant in exposed individuals, including those who have developed chickenpox after exposure. Herpes zoster occurs when the dormant virus is activated. Individuals who have not had varicella may develop it after exposure to the vesicular lesions of persons with herpes zoster. Herpes zoster can be a serious condition in any adult and may even lead to death from exhaustion in the older adult and the debilitated. It often occurs in persons with Hodgkin's disease or other cancers because of reduced cell-mediated immunity.

The skin lesions usually follow the dermatomes, which are the segments of the skin surface that are divided according to the nerves that innervate them (Figure 31-10). Because the lesions follow these nerve pathways, they rarely cross the midline of the body and may appear on only one side.

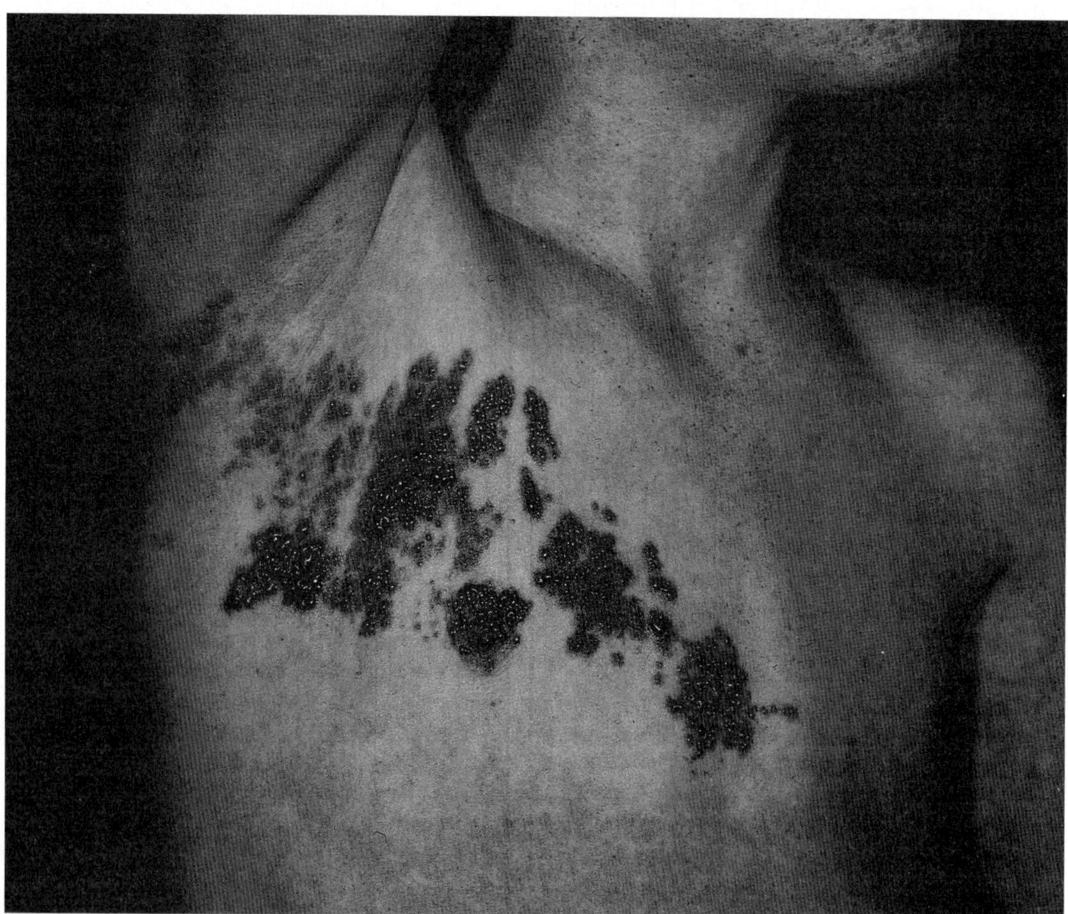

Figure 31-10 Herpes zoster. (From McCance KL, Huether SE: *Pathophysiology: adults and children*, ed 2, St Louis, 1994, Mosby.)

Herpes zoster can be precipitated by trauma, x-rays, or ultraviolet light, or it may be associated with a malignancy. One to 10 days before lesions develop, the patient may experience pain or burning, hyperesthesia (extreme sensitivity to pain or touch), or headache and malaise (uncommon). The patient may also experience a slight fever and loss of appetite before the lesions appear. When the lesions are 1 or 2 days old, an inflamed, edematous area appears where papules are turning into vesicles and are arranged in groups following the sensory nerves from the posterior to the anterior. The most common location of the lesions is the thoracic region, but they may occur on the thighs, lower abdomen, or forehead. Approximately one third of the patients have involvement of cranial nerve V (trigeminal nerve), with lesions on the face, eyes, and scalp. If the lesions do occur along the branch of cranial nerve V, the patient should be observed for facial paralysis and eye or ear disturbances. A neurologic pain occurs in paroxysms and is worse with movement and at night. The pain may persist long after the skin manifestation has subsided; it is then called *postherpetic neuralgia.*

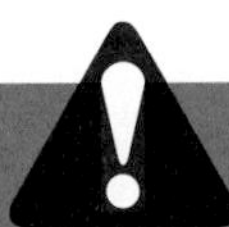

NURSE ALERT

Zoster that crosses the midline, or disseminates, is a sign that the patient may be immunocompromised or may have an internal malignancy.

Herpes zoster is self-limiting, and acyclovir and vidarabine are used in severe cases and in immunocompromised patients. Analgesics are given for pain, and narcotics may be required for severe pain. The injection of a local anesthetic agent into the nerve has been attempted to control pain by blocking its transmission. If begun early enough, this method also seems to provide protection against the development of postherpetic neuralgia. Systemic corticosteroids are used to decrease inflammation and may reduce postherpetic neuralgia. Systemic steroids have no effect on the healing of the skin lesions. Topical shake lotions (calamine, zinc oxide mixture) will help to dry the lesions. If secondary infection is present, antibiotics are given.

Patients with herpes zoster may be hospitalized, and emotional depression often accompanies the disease. The nurse may find the patient irritable and uncooperative. Patience and understanding are needed in caring for these patients.

General management of patients with viral infections are supportive and are directed toward alleviating symptoms (Box 31-11). For pruritus, tepid baths with cornstarch, Aveeno, or baking soda are helpful. Bedrest during febrile periods is suggested. Lesions of herpesvirus should be kept clean and dry, and the patient and family should be educated about the transmission of viral diseases.

Patients with human immunodeficiency virus (HIV) have increased susceptibility to both superficial and disseminated infections (Box 31-12). Superficial infections include scabies, a variety of papillomavirus infections, herpes simplex, and herpes zoster. Chronic

BOX 31-11 **Nursing Process**

VIRAL INFECTIONS

ASSESSMENT

Characteristics, distribution, and severity of lesions/rash
Signs of secondary infection
Lymphadenopathy
Temperature
Nutritional needs

NURSING DIAGNOSES

Impaired skin integrity related to presence of lesions
Risk for infection related to impaired skin integrity
Pain related to skin lesions
Hyperthermia related to disease process
Altered nutrition: less than body requirements related to presence of oral lesions

NURSING INTERVENTIONS

Cleanse the lesions.
Apply topical medications as ordered.
Discourage scratching.
Administer analgesics as needed.
Administer systemic medications as ordered.

EVALUATION OF EXPECTED OUTCOMES

Skin integrity is improved or has been maintained
No evidence of infection
Pain has been relieved
Nutritional status is adequate

BOX 31-12

COMPLICATIONS OF VIRAL INFECTIONS

Rubella
Arthritis/arthralgia
Thrombocytopenic purpura
Myocarditis/pericarditis (rare)
Congenital rubella syndrome (CRS) (frequent)
- Deafness
- Growth retardation
- Cataracts
- Retinitis
- Meningoencephalitis
- Microcephaly
- Mental retardation
- Myocarditis
- Structural defects of the heart
- Death

Rubeola
Photophobia
Clear rhinorrhea
Pharyngitis
Gastrointestinal symptoms (diarrhea)

Warts
Contagious

Herpes simplex
Nutritional problems (gingivostomatitis)
Contagious
Recurrent
Aseptic meningitis (seen in some primary infections of genital herpes)
Possibly fatal in immunocompromised patients

Varicella
Primary varicella pneumonia
Superimposed bacterial infection
Bacterial sepsis/focal abscesses (rare)
Reye's syndrome

Herpes zoster
Scarring
Varicella pneumonitis
Postherpetic neuralgia
Motor weakness (with involvement of cranial nerves)
Bell's palsy
Conjunctivitis
Iritis
Corneal ulcers
Blindness

AIDS
Opportunistic infections
Neoplasia
CNS disease

From Hill MJ: *Skin disorders: Mosby's clinical nursing series,* St Louis, 1994, Mosby.

pruritic eruptions, bacterial infections, and fungal infections are common. Malignant lesions develop at a much higher rate in these patients (Hill, 1994).

Diseases of Epidermal Origin

Diseases of epidermal origin have distinctive characteristics, including erythema and scale. Included in this category are dermatitis (eczema), exfoliative dermatitis (erythroderma), and psoriasis.

Dermatitis (eczema)

The terms dermatitis and *eczema* are used interchangeably, although they do have slightly different meanings. Dermatitis is an inflammatory condition of the skin resulting from a wide variety of causes such as allergy, stress, and unknown factors. In most cases it is characterized by erythema, pruritus, and various types of skin lesions. Eczema is a reactive process rather than a disease. Allergic contact dermatitis is caused by allergy to poison ivy, sumac, oak, or a proven allergen such as nickel. Irritant dermatitis is another cause of eczema. Irritant dermatitis is a result of direct contact with cosmetics, chemicals, dyes, or detergents. Other examples of eczema include nummular eczema (coin-shaped, oozing, crusting patches), seborrheic dermatitis (yellowish-pink scaling of the scalp, face, and trunk), and atopic dermatitis (characteristic distribution of eczema in individuals with a family history of allergic disease) (Hill, 1994).

Eczema/dermatitis exhibits three distinct stages: acute, subacute, and chronic. All three stages may be present at any one time. Acute dermatitis (acute eczema) appears as extensive exudative erosions or as pruritic erythematous papules and vesicles. Subacute dermatitis (subacute eczema) appears as erythematous, excoriated (traumatized by scratching), or scaling papules or plaques (flat or raised patches). Chronic dermatitis (chronic eczema) is characterized by lichenified (thickened, bark-like) skin caused by continuous rubbing or scratching, excoriated papules, nodules, and postinflammatory hyperpigmentation and/or hypopigmentation.

Atopic dermatitis. *Atopic dermatitis* is a chronic eczema marked by remissions and exacerbations.

Atopic refers to the group of allergic diseases involved with this form of eczema, such as asthma, allergic rhinitis (hay fever), and atopic dermatitis. The exact etiology of atopic dermatitis is unknown, although it is known that it occurs in individuals with a family history of allergic diseases (Hill, 1994).

Clinical manifestations of atopic dermatitis include dry, lackluster skin; excoriations; erythema; and **lichenification.** It may appear as early as 2 to 6 months of age and may continue into adulthood. In infants the rash characteristically appears on the face and scalp, and it may develop on the extensor surfaces of the extremities. In older children and adults the rash tends to have a predilection for the large folds of the extremities. Pruritus is the major symptom of the disease. In most cases the pruritus precedes the development of the rash, leading to the statement that atopic dermatitis is "an itch that rashes." Lichenification, excoriation, and secondary infections are the major complications associated with atopic dermatitis.

Exfoliative dermatitis. Another form of dermatitis is *exfoliative dermatitis (erythroderma).* This form of dermatitis involves large areas of skin. It appears as generalized erythema, edema, and desquamation (sloughing of the stratum corneum). Severe exfoliative dermatitis may affect the mucous membranes of the upper respiratory tract and the conjunctivae. Hair loss is not uncommon during the disease process, but hair regrows after the condition is brought under control. Exfoliative dermatitis is seen only in association with other skin diseases such as severe psoriasis, with systemic disease such as malignancy, or as secondary to drug hypersensitivity. With severe erythroderma, the patient experiences fever, chills, malaise, fatigue, skin tightness, and severe pruritus. Because of the generalized vasodilation and shunting of blood to the skin surface, patients must be observed for high cardiac output failure. Water and protein losses caused by the desquamation will lead to dehydration and negative nitrogen balance (Hill, 1994). Exfoliating dermatitis is treated with topical corticosteroids, antihistamines, and bland emollients. Systemic steroids are indicated only in extremely severe cases.

Contact dermatitis. *Contact dermatitis* is usually found on the face, neck, backs of the hands, forearms, male genitalia, and lower legs. The borders of the reaction are commonly well defined, which aids in determining the cause. The lesions may be red, oozing, or scaly. A careful history is essential in determining the cause of contact dermatitis. Removal and avoidance of the offending agent must precede or accompany treatment with antihistamines, bland emollients, cool compresses, and topical steroids. If cutaneous reaction is severe, systemic corticosteroids may be added to the treatment regimen.

Dermatitis venenata. *Dermatitis venenata (plant poisoning)* occurs as the result of contact with certain plants and is referred to as ivy poisoning, sumac poisoning, or poisoning by other specific types of plants. Individual susceptibility is an important factor in this type of dermatitis. Although many different plants and shrubs may cause the condition some of the more common ones are poison ivy, poison sumac, poison oak, and poison elder. Symptoms vary from a mild redness to severe systemic reactions and gangrene. The primary lesions are found on the parts of the body contacted by the irritant, usually the hands, arms, face, and legs. The skin may become erythematous, which may be followed by formation of papules, vesicles, and pustules in a characteristic linear distribution. Facial edema can be seen in patients exposed to airborne allergens (e.g., when the plant is burned). The tissue may be edematous, and severe itching and burning may occur.

When the individual is aware of contact with a poisonous plant, the exposed parts of the body should be washed immediately with soap and water. However, soap and water should not be used once lesions are present. Cool, open wet dressings of 1:20 solution of aluminum acetate (Burow's solution) or physiologic saline solution may be applied 3 times a day for 30 minutes to cool and relieve pruritus. Topical steroid creams and antihistamines may be needed. If lesions and edema are present on the face, systemic steroids may be necessary.

Dermatitis medicamentosa. *Dermatitis medicamentosa (drug dermatitis)* is the term applied to skin eruptions caused by drugs, regardless of the method of administration. Almost any drug may cause a reaction in certain individuals, and with the development of many new drugs and their increased use, the incidence of such reactions can be expected to increase. Drug reactions range from mild erythema to severe, life-threatening conditions. Every type of skin lesion reviewed in this chapter may be seen in various reactions to drugs. Therefore any rash must have drugs considered as a possible cause. A thorough history that includes questions regarding prescribed and over-the-counter drugs must be obtained by any patient showing a rash. The nurse must educate the patient and family about the possible side effects of any drugs that have been prescribed and the importance of reporting any reactions immediately. Dermatitis caused by drugs will usually subside after withdrawal of the medication, but resolution may take up to 2 weeks. Treatment is directed at relief of symptoms.

Psoriasis. *Psoriasis* is a chronic, genetically determined disease of epidermal proliferation. The disease usually begins between the ages of 10 and 35 but may be seen at any age. The exact cause is unknown, but the disease is not contagious. There is no cure, and patients with this disease have episodes of remission and exacerbation. Psoriasis tends to improve during the summer months when the lesions are exposed to ultraviolet rays of the sun. Emotional stress, systemic infections, obesity, excessive alcohol ingestion, injury to the skin, and pregnancy exacerbate the disorder.

Clinically, psoriasis is most commonly seen as well-demarcated erythematous patches or plaques with silver scale, but it may exhibit generalized erythroderma (exfoliative dermatitis) or generalized pustules (Figure 31-11). Removal of scale may result in pinpoint bleeding known as Auspitz sign. Pruritus, if present, is generally severe. There are four basic types of psoriasis: plaque, guttate (drop-like lesions), psoriatic erythroderma, and pustular. Plaque type is the most commonly seen. Guttate psoriasis often occurs after an infection, usually streptococcal, and is commonly seen in school-aged children, so it is often initially misdiagnosed as one of the childhood diseases. Psoriatic erythroderma and pustular psoriasis are the most severe presentations of the disease and may involve the entire body surface. These forms of psoriasis are often resistant to treatment and may last for long periods. Lesions appear symmetrically on the body. Elbows, knees, scalp, genitalia, and the gluteal cleft are the areas most often affected. Lesions may be initiated in areas that have undergone trauma, which is called Koebner's phenomenon. Common complications of psoriasis include psoriatic arthritis and nail dystrophy.

Psoriasis is treated with topical steroids, topical tar preparations, anthralin, salicylic acid preparations, ultraviolet light, bland emollients, and antihistamines. The use of ultraviolet light B (UVB) and tar in combination is known as Goeckerman treatment. Psoralen and ultraviolet light A (PUVA) are also used. Psoralen is a photosensitizing agent that makes the patient sensitive to the ultraviolet-A spectrum of light. Psoralen is given 2 hours before the patient is exposed to UVA. Nausea, sunburn, headache, and photosensitivity may be side effects of the treatment. Patients must be instructed to wear sunglasses that shield against UVA, to wear sunscreens, and, ideally, to avoid sun exposure on the days of treatment. In severe cases antimetabolites (methotrexate) and etretinate may be used. Because of the liver toxicity seen when antimetabolites are given, patients receiving drugs in this category must have a pretherapy liver biopsy and must be monitored during therapy for liver and renal function, white blood cell count, hemoglobin, and hematocrit. Etretinate (synthetic vitamin A or aromatic retinoid) is indicated only for adults and is used with extreme caution in women of childbearing age. Retinoids and vitamin A are not the same compounds, and people should be cautioned not to take large doses of vitamin A in the hope of duplicating the effects of these synthetic drugs.

Systemic steroids are contraindicated as treatment for psoriasis because they produce a "rebound effect," which is a worsening of the psoriasis after withdrawal of the steroids.

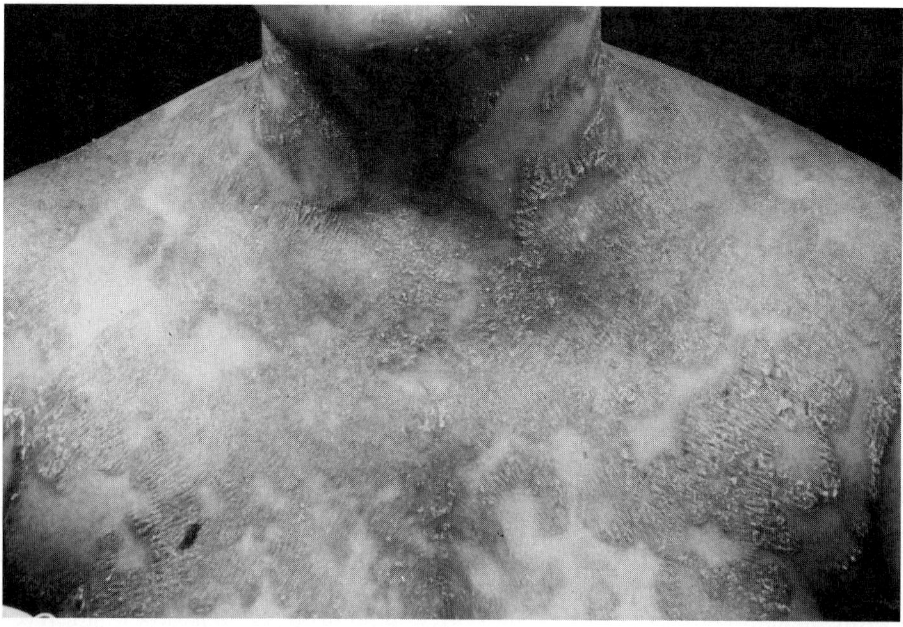

Figure 31-11 Generalized psoriasis. (From Rosai J: *Ackerman's surgical pathology*, ed 6, St Louis, 1981, Mosby. From Phipps WJ and others: *Medical-surgical nursing: concepts and clinical practice*, ed 5, St Louis, 1995, Mosby.)

Most patients with diseases of epidermal origin may be treated as outpatients, but occasionally the severity or extent of involvement warrants confinement for supervised care (Box 31-13). Most often the patients requiring hospitalization are those with erythroderma or pustular psoriasis. The most important part of therapy is the education of the patient regarding the disease process, its symptoms and appearance, and the fact that it is chronic. Patients must feel accepted by the caregiver, and treatment must be individualized.

General management of diseases of epidermal origin include the application of bland emollients to soothe and relieve skin irritability and to provide a temporary barrier, as well as wet wraps or occlusion to help hydrate the skin and to increase absorption of topical medications. In diseases where an allergen or irritant is the cause or suspected cause, the offending agent should be removed or avoided (Box 31-14).

BOX 31-13

COMPLICATIONS OF DISEASES OF EPIDERMAL ORIGIN

Cutaneous dryness (from skin's inability to hold moisture in stratum corneum)
Uncontrolled heat loss (from loss of barrier function)
Pruritus (from dry skin, external irritants, stress)
Infection (from excoriated skin and impaired resistance to cutaneous viral, fungal, and staphylococcal organisms)
Protein and iron loss (with exfoliation)

From Hill MJ: *Skin disorders, Mosby's clinical nursing series,* 1994, St Louis, Mosby.

Acne

Acne is an inflammatory disorder of the pilosebaceous unit of the skin. It appears as eruptions of papules or pustules and is caused when oil delivered to the skin's surface meets with resistance (Hill, 1994). It mainly affects the face, chest, back, and shoulders. Adolescents are most widely affected by the disease, and severe cases may require medical intervention. The disease usually declines in the early twenties, but it can continue into the forties and fifties. It is not uncommon for the first case of acne to occur in the patient's forties, fifties, or even sixties (Laudano, Leach, Armstrong, 1990). Both men and women may be affected, with the higher incidence occurring in males.

The acne begins with the appearance of **comedones** (blackheads) that plug the ducts of the sebaceous glands and are the result of increased secretion of sebum from the glands. The inflammatory process within the duct soon leads to the formation of papules and pustules on the skin.

The papules, pustules, and comedones that characterize acne are found on the face and back. In addition to assessing the location and severity of the lesions, the nurse must assess the patient's reaction to the disorder and understanding of the causes. The psychologic effects are often more serious than the disease. Acne

BOX 31-14 **Nursing Process**

DISEASE OF EPIDERMAL ORIGIN

ASSESSMENT

Lesions for characteristics, distribution, and severity
Signs of secondary infection
Temperature

NURSING DIAGNOSES

Impaired skin integrity related to pathologic process and mechanical factors
Risk for imparied skin integrity related to pruritus
Risk for infection related to skin excoriation and impaired barrier function

NURSING INTERVENTIONS

Apply cool compresses for wet skin or emollients for dry skin.
Apply topical medications as ordered.
Keep room at comfortable temperature to address poor tolerance to temperature changes.
Administer antihistamines as ordered.

EVALUATION OF EXPECTED OUTCOMES

Skin is well hydrated, and inflammation has been reduced
Pruritus has been alleviated
Ability to regulate temperature is restored
No evidence of infection

vulgaris occurs at a time when adolescents are concerned with personal appearance, and the unsightly skin condition may seriously interfere with personality development. It is also important to evaluate the patient's understanding of the treatment prescribed.

Treatment for acne is nonspecific and is directed toward reducing inflammation and infection, reducing blackhead formation, and developing a program of good personal hygiene. The skin should be kept scrupulously clean by washing with soap and water several times a day. A preparation containing hexachlorophene will help to reduce the staphylococcus population on the skin. Keratinous agents that cause drying, such as salicylic acid and resorcinol, may be used to produce a peeling of the skin and the removal of keratinous plugs to prevent the development of comedones and cysts. Cleansing agents are used to remove excess sebum from the skin and thus prevent the development of comedones. Tetracycline, minocycline, or erythromycin may be prescribed by the physician to prevent infection and thus reduce the probability of scarring. Existing comedones can be removed with an extractor by the physician, and pustules can be opened with a blade every week or two. Small doses of estrogens administered to girls just before the menstrual period help relieve the oily condition of the skin and retard the formation of sebum. The patient should be advised against squeezing the lesions, which may worsen the condition and lead to scarring. Emphasis should be placed on developing a program of adequate diet, sleep, and wholesome physical activity. The restriction of certain foods in the diet, such as chocolate or fried foods, does not seem to have any effect on the prevention or treatment of acne. Iodized salt will make acne worse in sensitive people.

The most severe cases of acne, cystic acne, can be treated with isotretinoin (Accutane), a vitamin A derivative called a *retinoid.* This oral medication has potentially serious side effects and must be used with caution. A female who becomes pregnant while taking the drug has a high risk of birth defects in the infant. Other possible side effects include dry skin, hair loss, eye irritation, nosebleeds, and muscle and joint pain. Increased blood levels of cholesterol and triglycerides occur in 25% of patients and increase the risk of heart disease. The cost is approximately $150 per month for the medication alone. After a few months of treatment the condition can be cured.

When scarring is severe, the physician may recommend removal of the scars by chemical face peeling or dermabrasion. Chemical face peeling is also performed in the treatment of fine wrinkles, and both procedures are used to remove abnormal pigmentation, freckles, or scars caused by trauma or other skin diseases as well as by acne. Chemical face peeling involves the application of a phenol-base chemical to the entire face, followed by a mask of waterproof adhesive. The medication causes a burning sensation, and the patient will require medication to control apprehension and relieve pain. After 6 or 8 hours the face becomes edematous. The patient is not allowed to move about for 48 hours, except to go to the bathroom. The dressings are removed after 48 hours, and the appearance of the skin will be similar to that of a second-degree burn. During the next 24 hours a bacteriostatic medication, thymol iodide powder, is applied with a cotton applicator to the entire surface three or four times. After this series of treatments, a lubricating ointment such as A and D ointment is applied to facilitate the separation of the crust that forms on the skin. After an additional 24 hours the face may be washed with plain water. Facial redness will persist for several weeks, and the patient will not feel comfortable being seen by others for as long as 3 or 4 weeks. Cosmetics may be applied at the end of 3 weeks, but exposure to the sun is not permitted for 3 to 6 months because the natural protective mechanism against the sun, melanin, is diminished.

An alternative to chemical face peeling is dermabrasion, or surgical planing. This procedure involves scraping, sandpapering, and brushing the skin to remove the epidermis and some superficial dermis. The remaining dermis produces new cells and forms a new epethelial layer in the dermabraded areas. The procedure can be performed by hand with coarse, abrasive paper or mechanically by using a rapidly rotating wire brush. The patient must be fully informed about the procedure and the appearance of the skin after its completion. After the procedure, pressure dressings may or may not be used, depending on the physician's preference. If dressings are used, they are removed after 48 hours, and the skin has the appearance of a recent sunburn. A crust begins to form, and petroleum jelly or cocoa butter may be used to relieve tightness. The crust separates in about 14 days, and the skin appears red. The patient must avoid direct sunlight for 3 to 4 months and use a sunscreen to protect the skin from exposure to the sun. It should be emphasized to the patient that even with repeat treatment deep scarring may not be completely eliminated, only improved. All patients who are candidates for dermabrasion should be questioned as to their expectations of the outcome of treatment. Some patients set their expectations too high, and these expectations need to be addressed before the procedure is undertaken.

Rosacea

Rosacea (acne rosacea, or adult acne) is a fairly common inflammatory condition that affects the blood vessels in the central part of the face. It may resemble and be associated with acne, appearing as a rosy red pustular eruption without comedones (Hill, 1994). Rosacea primarily affects women over 30 years of age. When it is seen in men, it is more severe. Clinically it appears as erythema and dilated vessels **(telangiectasia)** with a predilection for the center of the face. Patients have a pronounced tendency to flushing or blushing that is generally pronounced with the intake of alcohol, hot drinks, or spicy food, as well as with exposure to external irritants and extremes of hot or cold.

Rhinophyma (pronounced enlargement of the nose) may be seen in men in the later stages of rosacea. Rhinophyma is an overgrowth of sebaceous tissue and can be surgically corrected. Other complications that accompany rosacea include ocular disorders, including blepharitis, conjunctivitis, keratitis, and iritis.

Rosacea may be treated with topical acne medications and systemic antibiotics. A primary component of treatment is the avoidance of aggravating factors.

Cutaneous Disorders

Manifestations of systemic disease

Lupus erythematosus is not strictly a disease of the skin and could be appropriately placed in a number of chapters in this text. It is a chronic inflammatory disease involving the connective tissues of the body. Because these tissues are found in almost all regions and areas of the body, almost any part or organ may be affected. The disease may be confined to the skin, as in discoid lupus erythematosus (DLE), or may become generalized, as seen in systemic lupus erythematosus (SLE).

Discoid lupus erythematosus. Discoid lupus erythematosus (DLE) is a skin ailment characterized by disklike lesions with raised, reddish edges and sunken centers. They are most likely to appear on the arm, neck, face, and scalp and may leave scars when they subside. DLE is rarely fatal, but it is irritating and painful. Few patients with the discoid form go on to develop the systemic form.

Systemic lupus erythematosus. The cause of systemic lupus erythematosus (SLE) is unknown, but theories include autoimmunity, predisposition, and drugs. The autoimmune theory proposes that SLE is an abnormal reaction of the body against its own tissues. The predisposition theory identifies such factors as physical or mental stress, streptococcal or viral infection, exposure to sunlight or ultraviolet light, vaccines, and x-ray treatments as predisposing certain persons to this disease. Because it has been observed in successive generations of some families, genetics may also be a predisposing factor. The drugs suspected of triggering SLE include sulfa forms, penicillin and other antibiotics, certain birth control pills, and individual drugs such as hydralazine and procainamide. Women are 10 times as likely to have SLE as men, and most of these women are of childbearing age. These patients are more susceptible to having miscarriages, premature births, and stillbirths. The fetus who reaches fullterm is not usually affected by the mother's disease. The disease is also more common in blacks than whites, and it is rare in Asia. The incidence has been estimated at somewhere between two and five people per 100,000 persons.

Pathophysiology. SLE can affect the skin, kidneys, central nervous system, heart, lungs, blood vessels, serous membranes, joints, and muscles, either singly or in combination. The inflammation occurs in connective tissue common to all organs, so involvement usually becomes more widespread with time. Because it can affect so many organs, it is difficult to describe a classic group of symptoms and to distinguish it from other diseases. The Diagnostic and Therapeutic Criteria Committee of the American Rheumatism Association has issued a list of 14 preliminary criteria. The presence of four or more of the 14 criteria either serially or simultaneously during any interval of observation constitutes a diagnosis of SLE (Box 31-15).

Pregnant women who demonstrate signs of preeclampsia should be tested for SLE because this may be the early signs of the disease. Approximately 75% of all patients with SLE live 5 years or longer after diagnosis, and this disease is most likely to prove fatal in the patient with kidney or neurologic involvement. Early diagnosis and treatment improve the prognosis, and developments in hemodialysis and renal transplant techniques are improving the outcome for those who experience renal failure. The life expectancy following diagnosis has almost doubled in the last 15 years.

Assessment. Symptoms vary from patient to patient because the same organs may not be involved. The patient who has not been instructed well enough to understand this may become confused and lose confidence in the physician when discussing treatment with other SLE patients. The earliest symptoms often include fatigue, chills, occasional fever, and stiff aching joints on arising, usually followed several months later by a rash on the face and scalp and loss of hair in patches (alopecia). Approximately 70% of patients develop skin eruptions, and approximately 40% develop a characteristic butterfly rash over the bridge of the nose and the cheek. The rash and hair loss become worse on exposure to the sun. The rash sometimes spreads to the arms, trunk, or legs, causing a flushed, sunburned look or a scarred, patchy, coinlike look. Chest, stomach, and muscle pain may occur, or fluid may accumulate in the feet, ankles, or chest. Peri-

BOX 31-15

SYSTEMIC LUPUS ERYTHEMATOSUS

Systemic lupus erythematosus is indicated by the presence of four or more of the following symptoms:

1 Facial erythema (butterfly rash)—diffuse flat or raised rash over the bridge of the nose; may be present on only one side of the face
2 Discoid lupus erythematosus—patches of redness or thickened red, raised, coin-shaped patches covered with scales and involving plugged follicles; may be present anywhere on the body, including the face
3 Raynaud's phenomenon—intermittent attacks in which the hands or some of the fingers of each hand become cold, pale, painful, and then deeply cyanotic; symptoms are relieved by warming the hands
4 Alopecia—rapid loss of large amounts of scalp hair
5 Photosensitivity—an unusual skin reaction from exposure to sunlight
6 Ulcers in the mouth or nose
7 Arthritis without deformity but involving pain on motion, tenderness, swelling in the joints of the feet, ankles, knees, hips, shoulders, elbows, wrists, hands
8 LE cells—an unusual cell can be identified in the blood of patients with systemic lupus erythematosus; if one of these cells is seen in two or more specimens, or two in one specimen, the test is considered positive
9 Chronic false-positive serologic test for syphilis
10 Profuse proteinuria—over 3.5 g of protein excreted in the urine per day
11 Cellular casts—examination of the urine reveals casts that may be red blood cells, hemoglobin, granular, tubular, or mixed in type. When casts are found in the urine, they indicate a pathologic condition in the kidney. They are named to reflect their composition and shape; for example, red blood cell casts are composed of red blood cells, indicating a leakage of red blood cells into the urine. Many contain albumin because albumin often pours out into the urine in diseases involving the kidney. Because systemic lupus erythematosus sometimes causes a type of glomerulonephritis, the presence of casts in the urine can be considered one of the criteria for diagnosis
12 Pleuritis or pericarditis or both—patient experiences pleuritic pain, a pleural rub is heard by the physician, or x-ray examination reveals thickening and fluid in the lungs; pericarditis is detected by electrocardiogram or can be heard by the physician as a rub
13 Psychosis or convulsions or both—uremia and drugs must be ruled out as a cause
14 One or more of the following—hemolytic anemia, leukopenia (white blood count less than 4000/mm^3 on two or more occasions), thrombocytopenia (platelet count less than 100,000/mm^3)

carditis is the most frequent cardiac involvement. Women may experience irregular menstrual periods and may have difficulty in conceiving a child during an exacerbation of the disease. Pregnancy is less safe when there are kidney or neurologic abnormalities, so the pregnant patient with SLE must be watched closely. The blood pressure may become highly elevated. Protein, casts, and red blood cells in the urine indicate renal involvement. The site of the renal involvement usually is the glomeruli, which become inflamed as a result of the deposit of immune complexes in the glomerular basement membrane. Convulsions, cranial nerve involvement, and psychoses may occur with central nervous system involvement. Symptoms tend to come and go, and most can be relieved and even reversed with proper treatment.

Because of the widespread effect of the disease, a number of laboratory tests are performed to aid in diagnosis. In addition to routine blood work, chest x-ray examinations, electrocardiograms, and urinalysis, the urine is examined for creatinine clearance to evaluate kidney function. More specific tests include blood tests for the LE cells, as well as the ANA (antinuclear antibody) and the anti-DNA test, which are positive.

Intervention. Treatment is aimed at reducing the inflammatory process. High doses of aspirin are prescribed, often in combination with magnesium-aluminum hydroxide (Ascriptin) to reduce stomach distress. Indomethacin (Indocin) is also an antiinflammatory and should be taken at bedtime with a snack to prevent stomach distress and provide maximum relief from early morning joint stiffness and pain. Corticosteroids such as prednisone are used for more severe symptoms. The topical steroid flurandrenolide 0.05% is prescribed in ointment form (Cordran ointment) for the facial lesions and as a lotion (Cordran lotion) for the scalp.The patient must use a sunscreen when outdoors. Hydroxychloroquine (Plaquenil), an antimalarial drug whose action in the treatment of SLE is unknown, is prescribed only for severe skin lesions and may cause macular degeneration, which results in permanent blindness. Frequent eye examinations must be made to detect the early signs of this side effect. Immunosuppressive therapy is being used experimentally with patients who do not respond to conservative treatment. Patients must consult their physicians before receiving any immunizations or before taking birth control pills and over-the-counter drugs such as vitamins. The patient who is receiving steroids should be instructed to wear a Medic Alert bracelet. Hot baths or showers are used to relieve joint pain and stiffness, and an exercise program is prescribed to maintain mobility, strength, and endurance.

In addition to providing measures to relieve pain and supervising prescribed exercises, nursing care is concerned with patient education. The patient must understand the disease, its symptoms, and the treatment prescribed in order to control the disease. Return of symptoms or the onset of new symptoms must be reported immediately. The response to drug therapy must be carefully observed and reported to the physician. The patient must make alterations in lifestyle to obtain more rest and avoid exposure to the sun. It may be necessary for the patient to wear clothing that completely covers the body and head, to use a sunscreen on those small areas of exposed skin, and to avoid the sun at midday, when it is strongest. Fluorescent lighting is another source of ultraviolet light that may need to be avoided. The patient's self-concept may be affected by the disease as well as by the restrictions imposed with treatment. It is important to make the patient feel comfortable and free to express concerns and ask questions. The patient's family must also understand the disease and its treatment to be able to provide the support necessary for the patient to live with the disease. It is important to inform the patient of community groups available for supplying information and support. The Lupus Foundation of America and the Arthritis Foundation are two national sources. There may be a local "lupus club," and if so, the patient should be advised of its availability but not pressured to join. With early diagnosis and control of the disease, aided by discoveries resulting from research into its causes and treatment, the patient will be able to make the most of the years ahead.

Erythema intertrigo (chafing)

Chafing occurs when two skin surfaces rub together. It results in redness and may cause maceration of the skin. Common sites are the areas between the thighs, in the axillae, and under the breasts. In infants, chafing may occur in the folds of the skin, particularly around the neck. Obese persons are more likely to be affected. Treatment includes cleansing with mild soap and water, patting the area dry, and powdering with cornstarch. Good personal hygiene and avoidance of strong or irritating soaps are important practices. In extreme cases the application of hydrocortisone cream (Hytone) may be required. Before applying a hydrocortisone cream, the area should have a KOH prep done to rule out fungal infection.

Miliaria (prickly heat)

Miliaria is a condition in which the flow of sweat from the eccrine sweat glands, which are found on all skin surfaces, is hindered. The cause of miliaria includes both environmental and physiologic factors. Persons exposed to extremes of temperature and humidity for long periods, those overprotected by clothing, those with high body temperature, and obese persons are most likely to suffer from attacks of prickly heat. Infants swathed in excessive clothing and blankets are especially susceptible. The condition occurs more commonly during hot weather.

Assessment. Tiny red papules appear on the skin, usually on the trunk but sometimes covering the entire body. The lesions are accompanied by burning, prickling, and itching. An infant with prickly heat will be restless and fretful.

Intervention. Treatment consists of cooling or soothing baths and thorough drying by patting. Emollient baths such as the starch bath may provide relief for persons with severe cases. The application of calamine lotion is generally effective, and cornstarch or other nonirritating powders may be used. The condition is usually of short duration and can be prevented by avoiding extremes of heat and humidity and by wearing absorbent and porous clothing.

Hypersensitivity Reactions

Urticaria

Urticaria is the presence of hives or wheals (Figure 31-12). The condition may be associated with a number of systemic diseases, such as hepatitis, Hodgkin's disease, lupus erythematosus, leukemia, rheumatic fever, dental and sinus infections, and infestations. It may be seen as a cholinergic response to heat, cold, or ultraviolet light, or as a reaction to certain foods. Genetic predisposition and psychogenic factors have also been seen as causative agents. Often the cause is not readily apparent, which is disturbing to patient and healthcare workers alike. Urticaria may be acute, lasting less than 12 hours, or chronic, lasting more than 6 weeks. Select cases of urticaria may be accompanied by respiratory distress, hoarseness, abdominal pain, vomiting, diarrhea, arthralgia, headaches, or central nervous system dysfunction. Angioedema (swelling of

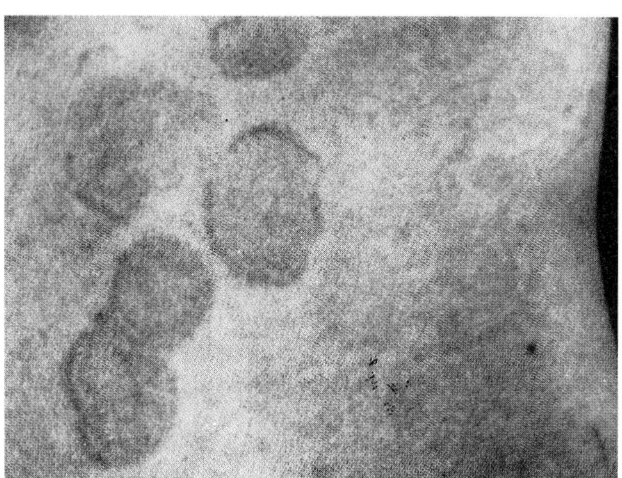

Figure 31-12 Urticaria. (From Stewart WD and others: *Dermatology: diagnosis and treatment of cutaneous disorders,* St Louis, 1978, Mosby. In Phipps WJ and others: *Medical-surgical nursing: concepts and clinical practice,* ed 5, St Louis, 1995, Mosby.)

the face) is the most severe complication seen with urticaria. This is a medical emergency, and the patient should seek treatment immediately. When urticaria appears suddenly, it should be determined whether the patient is taking any new drugs. If so, they should be stopped immediately and the physician notified.

Erythema multiforme

Erythema multiforme is a reactive skin disorder in which the individual lesions have a characteristic target (iris or bullseye) configuration (Figure 31-13). The lesions can be caused by drugs or by viruses such as herpes simplex and vaccinia. They also can be caused by systemic infections such as pneumonia, meningitis, or measles, and in some cases the cause cannot be identified. The lesions may last long enough to cause erosion of the lips, eyelids, and genitalia. Large areas of skin may eventually slough, and the disease can be fatal. Stevens-Johnson syndrome, the most serious form of erythema multiforme, has a mortality rate of 15% to 20%.

Assessment. The lesions are called iris or bullseye lesions because they are depressed in the center and have a raised, reddened border. They are found on the skin and the mucous membranes. Fever, chest pain, and joint pain may precede the eruption.

Intervention. The underlying cause must be discovered and eliminated, if possible. If the patient is taking any drugs, all except those essential to life should be discontinued. Large doses of steroids are given, and the lesions will disappear within 2 weeks if a drug is responsible. Baths, soaks, and dressings are used to reduce the discomfort of the lesions. Adequate fluids and nutrition promote healing. Special mouth care is needed if lesions appear there.

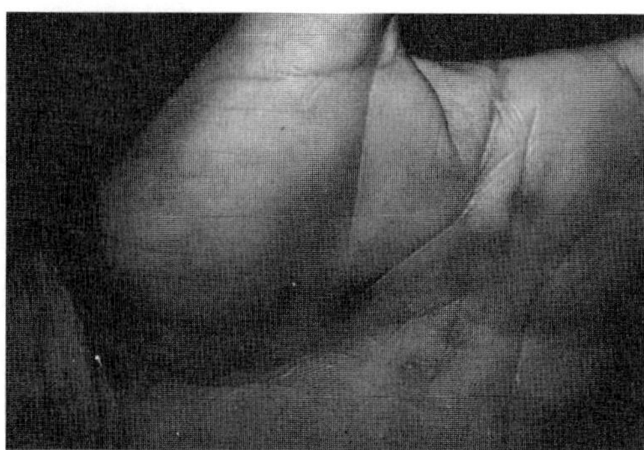

Figure 31-13 Erythema multiforme. (From Thompson JM and others: *Mosby's clinical nursing,* ed 3, St Louis, 1993, Mosby.)

BURNS

Burns are the result of tissue injury to the skin resulting from excessive exposure to thermal, chemical, electrical, or radioactive agents. It is the third leading cause of accidental death in the United States, especially for individuals between the ages of 15 and 45. There are approximately 2 million burn cases each year in the United States, and approximately 7% to 8% of these patients require hospitalization. Approximately one fourth of those hospitalized have major burns or significant associated injuries that require treatment in a specialized burn unit or burn center.

History of Burn Centers

The knowledge that has been gained on the treatment of burn wounds was acquired after World War II and the dropping of the atomic bomb. The U.S. Army Medical Division was sent to Japan to care for the victims after this disastrous event. It was here that doctors and scientists studied fluid shift changes, cosmetic surgery, and radiation therapy. When the division returned, it advised the government that this group of acutely ill patients had special needs. It was then that the U.S. government gave 138 contracts to emergency centers around the nation to establish specific units where all burn victims could be treated. The first of these units or centers was the Brooke Army Medical Center in San Antonio, Texas. The second center was established at the Shriner's Hospital for Children in Boston, Massachusetts. In 1958 the University of Michigan, in Ann Arbor, became the site of the National Institute of Burn Medicine, where the American

TABLE 31-10

Causes and Factors Determining Depth of Burn Injury

Depth	Cause	Appearance	Color	Sensation
Superficial partial-thickness (first-degree)	Flash flame, ultraviolet light (sunburn)	Dry, no blisters Minimal or no edema Blanches with fingertip pressure and refills when pressure is removed	Increased redness	Painful
Deep partial-thickness (second-degree)	Contact with hot liquids or solids Flash flame to clothing Direct flame Chemicals Ultraviolet light	Large, moist blisters that will increase in size Blanches with fingertip pressure and refills when pressure is removed	Mottled with dull, white, tan, pink, or cherry red areas	Very painful
Full-thickness (third-degree)	Contact with hot liquids or solids Flame Chemicals Electrical contact	Dry with leathery eschar Charred vessels visible under eschar Blisters rare, but thin-walled blisters that do not increase in size may be present No blanching with pressure	White, charred dark tan Black Red	Little or no pain Hair easily pulls out

From Phipps WJ and others: *Medical-surgical nursing: concepts and clinical practice,* ed 5, St Louis, 1995, Mosby.

Burn Association is housed. All research is kept on file at this institution and is available to anyone who wishes to study the treatment of burns.

Types of Burns

Burns are usually acquired in two ways: (1) by involvement in an uncontrollable fire or explosion and (2) through contact of some part of the body with a hot object or liquid, acidic, or flaming substances. Thermal burns are usually caused by flammable liquids and clothing, space heaters, gasoline from pilot lights, and scalds from hot coffee or overheated tap water spilled directly on the victim. Electrical burns occur with downed power lines, unprotected wall sockets, lightning, or defective wiring. Radiation burns are caused by exposure to the sun or treatment for cancer. Chemical burns result from contact with mixtures of acid, alkali, and phosphorous.

Classification by Severity

The American Burn Association classifies a burn as minor, moderate, or major, on the basis of the following criteria:

- **Minor burn** Deep partial-thickness burns involving less than 15% **TBSA (total body surface area)** in adults or less than 10% TBSA in children, or a full-thickness burn of less than 2% TBSA that does not involve special care areas (e.g., face, eyes, ears, hands, feet, or perineum); patient has no preexisting disease
- **Moderate burn** Deep partial-thickness burns of 15% to 25% TBSA in adults or 10% to 20% in children, or full-thickness burns of less than 10% TBSA not involving special care areas; patient has no preexisting disease or concurrent injuries
- **Major burn** Deep partial-thickness burns totaling more than 25% TBSA in adults or 20% in children; all full-thickness burns of 10% TBSA or more; other factors such as inhalation or electrical injuries and the age and health status of the individual are considered in classifying a burn as major (Phipps, 1995)

Classification by Burn Depth

Burns are classified as partial-thickness or full-thickness, depending on which layers of the skin have been damaged (Table 31-10 and Figure 31-14). Partial-

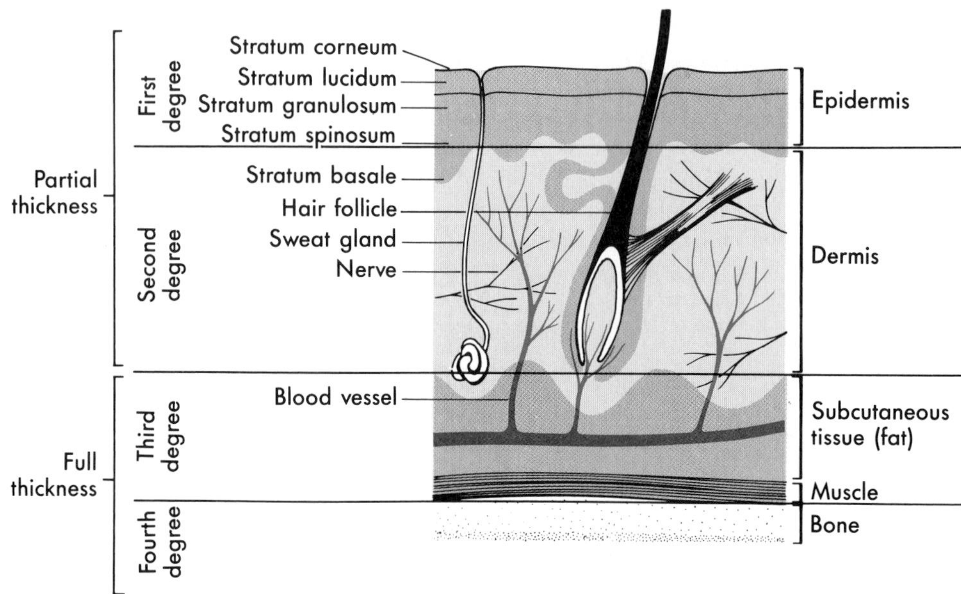

Figure 31-14 Layers of skin involved in burn injury. (From Beare PG, Myers JL: *Adult health nursing,* ed 2, St Louis, 1994, Mosby.)

thickness burns destroy and damage tissue into the dermis. A superficial or shallow partial-thickness burn will be red, warm, and painful. An example of this is a mild sunburn reaction. The epidermis is damaged, but this keratinized layer is rapidly replaced by underlying cells. Because the nerves are intact, there is pain with this type of burn. This was previously classified as a *first-degree burn.*

A deep partial-thickness burn involves the dermis and epidermis and is characterized by redness and blisters that usually increase immediately in size. There are enough epithelial cells remaining around the hair follicles and sweat glands to produce new skin, provided the cells are not destroyed during treatment. The length of time to heal without complications is from 10 days to 2 weeks. This burn can be identified easily if the patient's skin blanches after slight fingertip pressure is applied. This type of burn was previously classified as a *second-degree burn.*

Full-thickness burns destroy all of the layers of the skin, extending into the subcutaneous tissue, and may involve muscles, tendons, and bone. If the patient's hair can be pulled out easily it is considered to be a full-thickness burn. Full-thickness burns appear leathery and may be white, brown, tan, red, or black. Small, thin-walled vesicles may be present. There is no sensation of pain at first because sensory nerve fibers in the dermis have been destroyed. Sensation and pain do return as the tissues recover. Because burns are usually a mixture of full- and partial-thickness injuries, some pain is present. Full-thickness burns must be grafted to heal because there are no skin cells remaining and regeneration is therefore impossible. These burns were previously classified as *third-degree* and *fourth-degree burns.*

Determination of Burn Extent

Various methods are used to estimate the amount of body surface area affected by a burn injury. Regardless of the method used to determine the estimate, the extent of the injured area is expressed as a percentage of the total body surface area (TBSA). This measurement is used to determine fluid and nutritional needs of the burn patient. The "Rule of Nines," the Lund-Browder classification (Figure 31-15), and Berkow's formula are three ways to *estimate* the extent of the burn wound. Different burn centers around the country have their own pictorial representations for estimating the extent of burns. For all methods the person making the estimate colors a chart by using red for areas of full-thickness, or third-degree, burns and blue for deep partial-thickness, or second-degree, burns. With the Rule of Nines one adds the percentages listed for each burned area. For example, burns on the right arm and anterior trunk would total 27% TBSA.

A child who is age 12 or older is considered to be an adult and can be measured by the Rule of Nines to estimate the burned area. However, when a younger child is burned, these measures must be adjusted. The percentage of TBSA represented by an infant's head is twice the percentage represented by the head of an adult, whereas the percentage of a 10-year-old child's

A

The Rule of Nines	
Head and neck	**9%**
Right arm	**9**
Left arm	**9**
Posterior trunk	**18**
Anterior trunk	**18**
Right leg	**18**
Left leg	**18**
Perineum	**1**
	100%

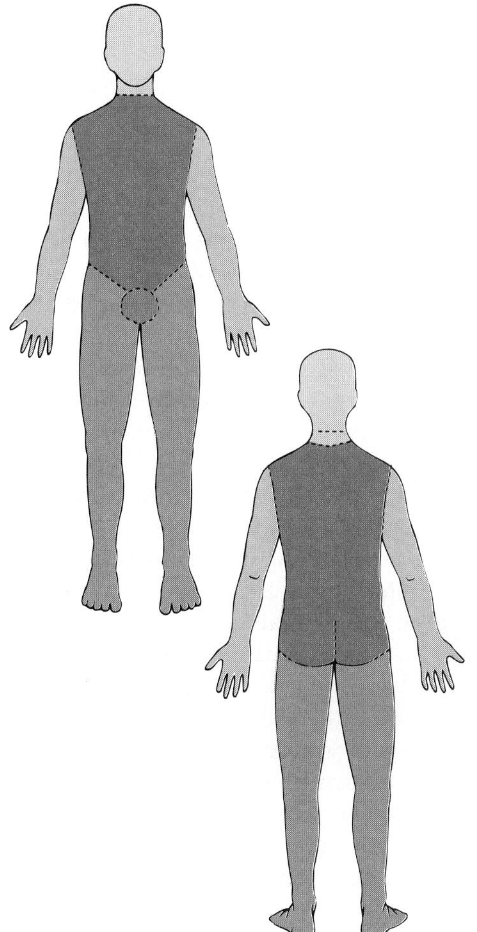

B

Lund and Browder Chart

AREA	AGE-YEARS 0-1	1-4	5-9	10-15	ADULT	% 2°	% 3°	% TOTAL
Head	19	17	13	10	7			
Neck	2	2	2	2	2			
Ant. Trunk	13	17	13	13	13			
Post. Trunk	13	13	13	13	13			
R. Buttock	2½	2½	2½	2½	2½			
L. Buttock	2½	2½	2½	2½	2½			
Genitalia	1	1	1	1	1			
R.U. Arm	4	4	4	4	4			
L.U. Arm	4	4	4	4	4			
R.L. Arm	3	3	3	3	3			
L.L. Arm	3	3	3	3	3			
R. Hand	2½	2½	2½	2½	2½			
L. Hand	2½	2½	2½	2½	2½			
R. Thigh	5½	6½	8½	8½	9½			
L. Thigh	5½	6½	8½	8½	9½			
R. Leg	5	5	5½	6	7			
L. Leg	5	5	5½	6	7			
R. Foot	3½	3½	3½	3½	3½			
L. Foot	3½	3½	3½	3½	3½			
					Total			

Figure 31-15 Estimating burn size. **A,** Rule of Nines. **B,** Lund-Browder classification. (Modified from Lund C, Browder N: The estimation of areas of burns, *Surg Gynecol Obstet* 1944.)

head is about one and one half times that of an adult. The trunk is considered approximately two-thirds that of an adult. The Lund-Browder classification is considered more accurate for all patients because it divides the body into more sections and makes adjustments for age-related changes in body size. To use the Lund-Browder classification, the nurse should note the red- and blue-colored areas, find the column that reflects the patient's age, and then add the percentages for each area of the body burned. A 2-year-old child with burns on the right upper arm, the right hand, and the anterior trunk would have burns on 26.5% of the body, whereas the percentage for an adult with burns in the same areas would be estimated at 22.5% TBSA.

Phases of Burn Care

The care of the burned patient is classified into three phases: the **emergent** period, the acute period, and the rehabilitative period. The emergent period begins with the burn injury and includes the first stage and initial care as determined by the severity of the injury. This period ends when the patient is stable and begins to diurese and no longer requires fluid therapy.

The acute period is directed toward continuous care of the wounds to prevent infection and promote healing. Rehabilitation involves all that is required to help that patient return to his or her previous or optimal level of functioning. Many aspects of rehabilitation, however, must be initiated from the time of admission and during the emergent care of the patient. The following sections on burn care deal with the total patient's needs throughout these periods.

Emergent phase

The first priority is to prevent further injury by extinguishing any flames still present or by removing the victim from the source of the burn, such as the electrical current in the event of an electricity burn. The patient must never be touched with metal or hands after an electrical burn. The current may still be active. Something nonmetallic such as a rope or broomstick handle should be used to move the victim away from the electrical current.

Flames should be smothered by wrapping the patient in a blanket, rug, or coat and rolling the victim on the ground. The rule of thumb is to *stop, drop, and roll* the patient until the flames are out.

In the case of a chemical burn, all contaminated clothing should be removed if it is not adhered to the skin. The skin is rinsed generously with cool water to remove the chemical. Any rings, watches, belts, ties, or other items that restrict circulation around any part of the body should also be removed because the patient will become edematous later from fluid shifts. The size of any burn can be decreased by the application of cool water, which reduces the temperature of the skin, lessens tissue destruction, and may prevent a full-thickness burn from occurring. The application of ice or ice water to the wound is now contraindicated because of the potential harm from hypothermia and frostbite. No attempt should be made to apply ointments (petroleum jelly, cold cream, butter, or lard) because ointments allow the heat from the burn to be contained and intensified. No medications should be given because the patient will probably go into *burn shock*. Burn shock is the combination of hypovolemic, cardiogenic, and neurogenic shock seen only in a patient who is burned. The victim should be wrapped in a clean sheet or blanket and taken immediately to the hospital or a burn center for emergency treatment. Eighty-five percent of all burns occur in the home—in the kitchen, bathroom, and bedroom. Fifteen percent occur in the work setting.

On the way to the burn center, a brief history on the victim should be taken. The following information should be obtained from the patient or a family member and given to the burn team:

1. The patient's previous state of health
2. Any allergies to drugs
3. Last tetanus toxoid immunization
4. Current height and weight
5. Detailed account of the accident identifying whether the victim was in an open or confined space at the time of contact with the flame, the duration of exposure to the burning agent, and the first aid treatment performed
6. The patient's age
7. Any other injuries that occurred

Once the cause of the burn has been identified and initially treated, the next priority is to maintain or provide a patent airway. Any bleeding that is present should be stopped. Burn shock may also be present and should be treated. The burn victim is usually conscious and in pain. The rescuer should reassure the victim and provide information about what is happening.

Assessment and intervention. During the emergent period, burn shock is a major problem for the victim. The shock can be treated with fluid therapy, which will be discussed later in this chapter. Suctioning may be necessary to remove aspirated secretions in maintaining a patent airway. Humidified oxygen at 100% should be administered.

Smoke inhalation by the victim may also result in damage to the respiratory tract and produce laryngeal edema. This type of damage is more likely when the victim inhales toxic chemical by-products from the combustion of synthetic materials. Early postburn pulmonary damage can be assessed by the following observations:

1. Look for burns around the neck and mouth.
2. Look for singed nasal hairs.
3. Inspect the mouth for burns of the oral and pharyngeal mucous membranes (they will look white in color).
4. Observe for continual coughing, **carbonaceous** (sooty) **sputum,** or voice changes such as hoarseness.

The patient with inhalation injuries is at great risk for developing bronchial pneumonia because the alveoli can be charred and destroyed.

Damage to the capillary system occurs in the burn area at the same time as damage to the body cells. Both injuries cause water and electrolytes to shift from the plasma to the interstitial fluid. This fluid accumulation causes edema, and in partial-thickness burns it is evidenced by blisters. In full-thickness burns the same process occurs, but the destroyed layers of the skin, or **eschar,** may trap the edema fluids beneath them. If the wounds are **circumferential,** covering all sides of an extremity, a tourniquet effect is created. Circumferential wounds on the torso can affect respiration by restricting diaphragmatic movements. Those involved in the neck may obstruct the airway. Pulses distal to the wound, respirations, and airway patency must be checked hourly. If edema causes complications in any of these areas, an **escharotomy**—cutting through the burned skin layers—is performed to relieve the constriction.

It can be expected that an adult with 15% of the body burned or a child with 10% burned will be suffering from some degree of shock. The accumulation of edema fluids in the burned area and the loss of fluids from injured tissues result in a decrease in the amount of circulating blood plasma. When the volume of the bloodstream falls, blood pressure drops, circulation decreases to the vital organs, and less oxygen is available to all body tissues. This process leads to shock. If treatment is not instituted, acute renal failure and damage to the kidneys and other organs will occur. Metabolic acidosis may result. This shift of fluids, electrolytes, and albumin from the capillaries to the burned tissues occurs in the first 24 to 48 hours following the injury.

The nurse caring for a newly burned patient must be constantly alert for symptoms of burn shock. Restlessness is a common sign of hypoxia and may indicate onset of shock. The pulse increases before the blood pressure falls, and respirations also increase. Urine flow is scant or absent. To prevent burn shock, administration of intravenous fluids is usually the first emergency treatment given to the severely burned patient. Many combinations of fluids may be used, depending on the physician's preference. Ringer's solution plus albumin may be given to combat protein loss. Fluids may be administered rapidly until urine flow is established, then regulated to maintain a urine output of 30 to 50 ml per hour. An indwelling catheter is inserted, and it is the nurse's responsibility to measure the output, urinary pH, and specific gravity each hour. The specific gravity and hematocrit value may be elevated because of the shift of fluid from the circulating blood in the vascular spaces to the burn tissue. Almost every burn patient is extremely thirsty but must not be allowed to drink water because this tends to dilute body electrolytes. The patient is given nothing by mouth; intravenous fluids are administered instead. Fluid resuscitation criteria are reviewed to determine whether the patient is adequately hydrated (Box 31-16). If hydrated, the patient should not complain of thirst.

BOX 31-16

CRITERIA FOR FLUID RESUSCITATION

Patient mentally alert and clear
Urine volume 30-50 ml/hr for an adult;
1 ml/kg body wt/hr for a child
Rectal body temperature = 99.6° F to 100° F
Central venous pressure normal (5-15 cm)
Slightly high pulse: < 120 bpm for an adult;
<160 bpm for a child
Slightly high but normal blood pressure
Absence of nausea, paralytic ileus, and thirst

Created by D. Starsiak, Loyola University, Chicago, 1994.

In patients with major burns, a nasogastric tube is inserted to prevent gastric dilation because peristalsis slows or stops altogether as a normal body response to stress.

With time, the capillary walls return to normal and the fluids accumulated in the tissues reenter the bloodstream. The electrolytes return with the fluid. This process is detected by a marked increase in urinary output or diuresis. If the kidneys are damaged or diseased, the patient is at great risk for kidney failure. This shift of fluid and electrolytes back into the vascular system also puts an extra volume load on the heart and lungs. Patients with a prior history of heart or lung problems should be monitored very closely for signs of congestive heart failure or pulmonary edema. Because electrolytes are also returning to the bloodstream, it would be dangerous to administer additional electrolytes to the patient in the intravenous fluids. The fluids, however, are still needed, so dextrose and water are administered. The onset of diuresis signals the end of the emergent period of care. The nurse, continuously observing the patient, notes this change in status and reports to the physician so the treatment plan can be modified. Formulas such as Parkland's and Brooke's have been developed to help determine the volume of fluid replacement. The use of these formulas depends on precise monitoring by the nurse. Determining the fluid needs of the burn patient requires accurate checking of intake, output, and vital signs every hour and frequent monitoring of weight and hematocrit levels.

Initial treatment of the wound involves cleansing with a dilute solution of povidone-iodine (Betadine), pHisoHex (one part povidone-iodine or pHisoHex to three or four parts water), or chlorhexidine gluconate (Hibiclens) solution. The wound should then be rinsed thoroughly and covered with moist saline dressings until the physician can thoroughly estimate the percentage of TBSA that is burned. If the wounds cover a great deal of the body, the saline should be warm and the patient should be kept covered with a sheet to prevent excessive heat loss. After all the wounds are cleansed, the saline dressings may be covered with dry dressings or may be replaced with dry sterile dressings. If the wound is a result of a chemical injury, it is washed with copious amounts of warm water before it is cleansed and covered with a dry dressing (Calistro, 1993).

Strict asepsis is essential to avoid wound contamination and subsequent infection. Morphine sulfate may be given to reduce pain and apprehension. Medications are not given intramuscularly because tissue absorption is poor in the burn patient as a result of the reduced blood supply to the tissues. Reduced dosages given intravenously have been found effective. Antibiotics and tetanus prophylaxis are usually given.

The initial treatment of the patient takes place in the hospital emergency room. If a burn treatment center is available, the patient with major burns is transferred there as soon as the initial needs are met. The patient's clothing should be placed in a bag and sent with the patient to the burn center, where the staff may need to examine its composition. If admitted to the general hospital, the patient is placed in an intensive care unit or a regular medical or surgical unit. The patient should be placed in reverse isolation in a private room in a clean area of the hospital (Box 31-17).

Expected outcomes. The following should be observed in the burn patient after proper interventions during this period:

- The burning process has stopped.
- A patent airway is maintained.
- Initial fluid resuscitation has been started using Ringer's Lactate solution.
- Arterial blood gases are within normal limits.
- Peripheral pulses are palpable.
- Urinary output is greater than 30 ml/hour.
- Blood pressure is above 100/70 mm Hg.
- Apical pulse is slightly tachycardic.
- Bowel sounds are present, with passing of flatus.
- Lungs sounds are clear, and respirations are within normal limits.
- Temperature is afebrile at 99° F to 100° F.
- The patient expresses feelings of safety and comfort.

The acute phase

During the acute, or initial hospitalization phase, the major burn victim is usually cared for in a special burn unit. The burn care team consists of the physician, nurse, social worker, physical therapist, occupational therapist, dietician, and other personnel who must coordinate activities to plan for the successful treatment of the patient.

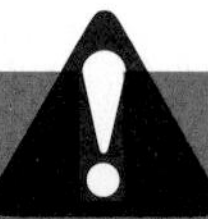

NURSE ALERT

Any patient under age 2 or over age 72 has less chance of surviving a burn injury than does a younger or middle-aged person.

Objectives of treatment. Each patient must be considered individually. The cause, depth, and extent of the burn; the patient's age; preexisting diseases or conditions; and the patient's emotional reaction to the injury determine the methods of treatment selected by the burn team. Although different methods are employed, the basic objectives are always the same:

1. Prevent and treat burn shock.
2. Relieve pain.
3. Prevent infection.
4. Heal open wounds.
5. Restore normal functioning and appearance.
6. Preserve emotional equilibrium.
7. Return to the social and work environment.

Methods of wound treatment—medical management. Initially the burn wounds are cleansed and debrided in the burn ICU or the tub room. Hair is clipped or shaved to reduce the risk of infection. If a burn wound is to heal without surgical intervention, various treatment plans are needed to keep the area free of dead tissue and bacteria. Wound healing is slow, taking anywhere from 2 weeks to 18 months, with the dangers of infection, scarring, and contracture formation ever present. This form of burn treatment generally includes the use of hydrotherapy, topical antimicrobials, and open or closed dressings.

Hydrotherapy. **Hydrotherapy,** or tubbing the burn victim, usually is used in combination with some other method. Once a day, for no more than 30 minutes, the patient is immersed in a solution of normal saline, plain water, or a balanced electrolyte solution. Nonirritating cleansing agents also may be used. Dressings are removed before the patient is placed in a tub unless they adhere to the wound. Immersion in the solution facilitates removal of dressings that have adhered and

BOX 31-17

Nursing Process

BURN INJURIES

ASSESSMENT

Burn area for drainage, evidence of healing, evidence of infection
Vital signs
Fluid volume status
Weight
Urine specific gravity
Respiratory status, including lung sounds
Overall skin color
Pain level on a scale of 0 to 10 (often)
Gastrointestinal function, bowel sounds, appetite
Level of orientation, anxiety, restlessness
Coping abilities and support systems
Laboratory studies: electrolytes, complete blood count, albumin, artrial blood gases

NURSING DIAGNOSES

Impaired skin integrity related to thermal injury
Risk for infection related to burn wound and inadequate nutrition for healing
Fluid volume deficit/excess related to fluid shifts, loss of skin integrity
Risk for impaired gas exchange related to inhalation injury, immobility
Pain related to tissue injury, wound care
Altered nutrition: less than body requirements related to increased metabolic needs, impaired gastrointestinal function, loss of body fluid
Fear related to pain, hospitalization, and unknown outcome of burn injury
Body image disturbance related to burn injury, potential long-term dependency, and therapy

NURSING INTERVENTIONS

Provide appropriate wound care (hydrotherapy, topical medications, dressings) as ordered.
Maintain aseptic technique with wound care.
Prevent trauma to the burn area.
Elevate extremities, if affected.
Obtain and monitor wound cultures if ordered.
Administer antibiotics if ordered.
Administer IV fluids as prescribed.
Encourage patient to drink prescribed fluid amounts.
Position patient for optimal breathing.
Administer oxygen as ordered.
Reduce oxygen need by using pain- and anxiety-reduction techniques.
Pace activities according to patient's tolerance.
Encourage use of incentive spirometer.
Administer analgesics as ordered.
Premedicate before dressing change.
Use a variety of comfort measures such as positioning and massage.
Teach relaxation, distraction, and guided imagery techniques.
Consult with the physician, occupational therapist, and others to assist in pain management.
Encourage high-protein, high-calorie diet, if permitted.
Arrange consultation with dietician.
Encourage family to bring in preferred foods, if allowed.
Modify environment to provide pleasant mealtime experience.
Encourage patient and family to verbalize feelings, fears, and grief.
Identify patient supports and coping strategies and use in planning care.
Explain hospital resources such as counseling, social service, and pastoral care and initiate referrals as requested.
Provide care that maintains privacy and personal dignity.

EVALUATION OF EXPECTED OUTCOMES

No evidence of fluid deficit:
- Vital signs within normal limits for individual
- Balanced input and output
- Serum electrolytes, hematocrit within normal limits
- Mucous membranes moist, denies thirst, supple tissue turgor

No evidence of fluid excess:
- No evidence of edema
- Weight constant
- Lung sounds clear
- Vital signs within normal limits for individual

Afebrile
WBC within normal limits
Burn area healing with no evidence of infection
Verbalizes signs and symptoms of infection and risk factors
Daily intake of 3000 to 5000 calories
Serum albumin, nitrogen levels within normal limits

continued

BOX 31-17 **Nursing Process**

BURN INJURIES—cont'd

Describes prescribed diet and indicates willingness to follow it
Lungs clear, no congestion or hoarseness
Skin pink, no cyanosis
Demonstrates ability to deep breathe and use supportive oxygen equipment if indicated
Able to rest, sleep 6 to 8 hours at night, and participate in care and decision making
States pain 0 to 3 on scale of 10 and reports relief after analgesic
Demonstrates ability to use noninvasive techniques for pain relief
Identifies strategies to reduce fear
Able to verbalize fears and concerns
Acknowledges actual change in appearance and function
Maintains relationship with significant others
States willingness to use identified resources after discharge

loosens slough, eschar, exudate, and topical medications. The tub also provides an excellent place for the patient to be bathed and exercise the extremities. A whirlpool provides the ideal form of hydrotherapy.

The tub must be cleaned thoroughly with bleach between uses, and the use of plastic liners for the tub can save time and prevent cross-contamination. The patient is placed on a narrow frame called a plinth, for which plastic covers are available. Long plastic gloves are worn by the person working with the patient in the tank, and plastic aprons, masks, and caps must be worn if the patient's wounds are exposed. The patient must be observed for chilling. Patients with newly grafted areas are not usually given full-body baths until the graft is healed, which takes 3 to 7 days. If there is a fine-mesh inner gauze over a fairly fresh grafted area, it should be left in place while the patient is in the tub. The gauze over a donor area also is not disturbed unless it loosens.

Topical antimicrobials.

Mafenide acetate (Sulfamylon Acetate). Organisms most often involved in infection of burn patients include *Staphylococcus aureus,* hemolytic streptococci, and *Pseudomonas aeruginosa.* Mafenide has been found to be a safe, effective adjunct in preventing infection, and some believe that it is more effective than silver nitrate.

Silver nitrate. The use of silver nitrate for treating burns is based on its bacteriostatic and infection-preventing properties. After thorough cleansing of the wounds, the burns are wrapped with dressings saturated with a solution of distilled water containing 0.5% silver nitrate. The dressings must be thoroughly soaked and thick enough to hold large amounts of solution. The entire dressing is then covered with two layers of prebleached stockinette. The dressings must be rewet every 2 to 4 hours so that the solution is in direct contact with the skin at all times. The silver nitrate solution hardens the eschar, which then serves as a pseudo-skin covering to protect the underlying tissues.

Povidone-iodine ointment. Povidone-iodine 10% ointment and solution (Betadine) are now being used in the care of burn wounds because of their broad spectrum of microbicidal action. The ointment can be used alone or in conjunction with the solution and may be used with or without dressings. This solution is used if a patient is allergic to sulfa drugs.

Silver sulfadiazine 1%. Silver sulfadiazine 1% (Silvadene) was approved for general use in the United States in 1974. It is a water-soluble cream that can be applied directly to the burn area by a sterile gloved hand. It can also be used to impregnate Kerlix rolls or thick back pads so it can be applied directly to the burned area without touching the patient with a gloved hand. Patients have reported that this method is preferred because less pressure is placed on the burn wound. The wounds may be left exposed, and the cream may be reapplied, as necessary, when it is rubbed off. A layer of cream 2 to 4 mm thick should be applied so that the wound is not visible through the cream. A single-layer gauze dressing can be impregnated with the cream and applied to the wound and secured with stretch gauze or tube dressings. If the wounds are draining heavily or are infected, the dressings may be changed as often as three times a day. Silver sulfadiazine cream can be bactericidal for up to 48 hours. It does annihilate *Pseudomonas* and *Candida.* The area covered by the cream must be cleansed thoroughly to prevent buildup (Table 29-2).

Surgical management. Surgical care of burn wounds may involve only periodic **debridement** (removal of dead tissue) of an area that is being treated by the medical methods above. If the burn wound is severe and no dermis remains to allow tissue regeneration, skin grafting is necessary. This involves removal of dead tissue and possibly the underlying fatty tissue and the application of a skin graft or an artificial covering. Closing a burn wound quickly decreases the potential for infection and scarring. It also results in decreased pain and fluid loss. The only permanent graft is an **autograft,** which is skin that is removed

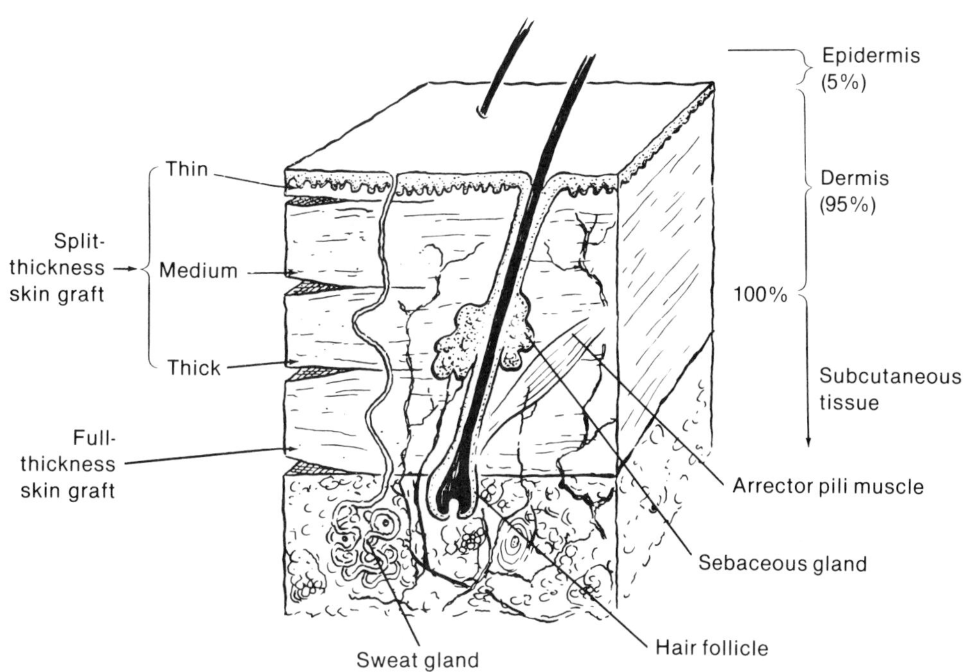

Figure 31-16 Layers of skin involved in various types of skin grafts. Thickness of epidermis and dermis shown here is typical of that found on lateral thigh of adult.

from a donor site on the burn victim. Any other form of wound cover is temporary and eventually will be rejected by the burn victim's immune system. Because the burn victim is initially medically unstable and unable to withstand autografting procedures, temporary grafts play a major role in early therapy. There are three major types:

- **Homograft** (allograft) is skin from another person. This skin may be from a living relative or, more commonly, from a cadaver or skin grown in a culture. These grafts may remain in place 3 to 5 weeks before rejection occurs.
- Xenograft **(heterograft)** is skin from another animal species. Pig skin is the most common, and the major disadvantage is early breakdown and potential for infection.
- Synthetic skin substitutes are substances such as collagen dressings (Biobrane). They have a long storage life and can provide wound cover for 2 months or longer until autograft is possible.

In addition to classification by material, grafts are also categorized by depth (Figure 31-16). A **full-thickness skin graft** includes the epidermis and all of the dermis and is the type used for reconstruction. When a full-thickness graft is taken, the donor site will also need grafting. **A split-thickness skin graft** leaves some dermis at the donor site, which allows that site to heal. The split-thickness graft may be applied without being altered to the burn wound as a sheet graft for the best cosmetic result. It may also be altered after removal from the donor site by a mechanical device that creates a mesh pattern of small slits. This mesh graft can be expanded to cover a larger surface area and allows drainage from the wound site.

The patient receives a general anesthetic for the grafting procedure, and on return from the operating room he or she will have two surgical sites that require care: the donor site and the grafted area. There are various types of dressings used for the grafted area, including fine-mesh petroleum gauze held in place by cotton pads and bandages. Some physicians prefer that the area be left open to the air. Most physicians apply a light pressure dressing to ensure that the graft remains in close contact with the burn site. Care must be taken by the nursing staff during the first 48 hours not to move the patient in any manner that would disrupt this surface contact. If dressings are used, the nurse never removes them unless told to do so by the physician. In other cases dressings are applied, and a daily inspection may be done for evidence of infection. Because many methods are used, the nurse will need to become familiar with the particular procedure desired by the surgeon.

The care of the donor site also varies. It may be covered with gauze and pressure bandages, or it may have a layer of fine-mesh gauze and be left open to the air. Analgesics may be needed for pain, and the ambulatory patient often finds that there is more discomfort from the donor site than from the grafted area. When the donor site is the thigh, walking may be difficult. Not all grafted skin may grow, and repeat grafts may be required.

The use of a Jobst pressure stocking or garment is necessary after the final grafting has taken place. This is measured specifically for the patient's body or body parts by the company. It is an elastic material that increases circulation of the blood to the grafted site, provides compression for the graft site itself, and prevents contractures. The patient must be instructed before discharge on the care of this garment. Each person receives two garments; one is to wear 23 hours a day while the other one is washed. The garment can be removed only once a day for the patient to inspect his or her skin and change into the other garment. These garments are worn by the patient for 1 to 2 years.

Nursing management.

Monitoring weight and intake and output. Careful measurement in recording fluid intake and urinary output is important for determining proper fluid replacement and preventing complications. The nurse should obtain and record a preburn weight for the patient because it will assist the burn team in determining the patient's fluid needs.

Positioning. Proper positioning of the patient is important in preventing contractures, decubitus ulcers, foot drop, and pulmonary complications. Care of the patient may be facilitated by using a specialty bed that alternates pressure on body surfaces. Flotation therapy also has been used successfully for severely burned patients. Flotation prevents pressure areas and allows blood flow to all areas of the body. This enhances nourishment of the cells, promotes healing, and helps to prevent pressure ulcers. The sensation of floating is soothing and relaxing and lessens pain and tension, and the patient is able to move about more freely. The physical therapist may assist with both passive and active range-of-motion exercises, and the patient should be encouraged to assist with his or her own exercises. The patient should not be placed in Fowler's position, and the knee gatch of the bed should not be elevated because both will contribute to contractures. When the patient is in the supine position, hyperextension of the head will help to prevent contractures when the neck is burned. Pillows should *not* be used under the patient's head because neck contracture could result. Splinting and exercise programs may be instituted to prevent deformities. A major objective of care is to encourage patients to participate actively in their own care when their individual condition has stabilized. If the patient's condition allows it, early ambulation is encouraged.

Prevention of infection. Some hospitals maintain rooms in which dressings are changed under aseptic conditions, or sometimes patients are taken to the operating room for dressing changes, and light anesthetics are administered. Medical centers and large hospitals are developing self-contained surgical suites in the burn units. Regardless of the method of treatment used, all personnel caring for the patient should observe the practice of thorough handwashing before providing any care. A gown, mask, and sterile gloves must be worn for all dressing changes and for all care if the burns are exposed (as in the exposure method). The patient also should wear a mask for protection against organisms present in his or her own respiratory tract. If visitors are allowed in the room, they should be required to follow the same gown-mask-gloves procedure. Antibiotics are usually administered to the patient to aid in preventing infection. Treatment depends partly on the conditions surrounding the injury. Persons with respiratory tract infections should not be allowed near the patient. When there are burns about the perineal area, care must be taken to prevent infection from fecal contamination. This may be especially important, and difficult, in children.

Relief of pain. When burns are severe, the patient will need medication for pain. When severe edema is present, medication to relieve pain should be given intravenously. Morphine or meperidine hydrochloride (Demerol) may be given intravenously as a continuous infusion. Medication should be given 15 to 30 minutes before any treatment or procedure that will be painful to the patient.

Diet. Nothing is given by mouth for the first 24 to 48 hours. Many burn patients have nausea and vomiting, and a nasogastric tube is usually inserted to prevent abdominal distention and paralytic ileus. After 24 hours, if there is no vomiting, oral fluids may be started. When the physician has ordered a clear-liquid diet, the nurse should offer 30 to 60 ml an hour and increase the amount as tolerated. If the patient can tolerate it, a high-calorie, high-protein diet is started in 7 to 10 days. Caloric requirements may exceed 5000 daily. Until the patient is able to consume a diet that can provide the required calories, parenteral hyperalimentation may be necessary. If the gastrointestinal tract is capable of absorbing nutrients, enteral hyperalimentation may be used. The oral fluids taken by the patient in the early days of treatment do not provide the required nutrients and calories, so enteral nutritional supplements are used to improve the patient's nutritional status and therefore the prognosis. Even the patient consuming a full, general diet may lack the appetite to eat the amount and variety of foods needed to deliver the total calorie requirement. Small, frequent feedings should be given. The use of between-meal, high-protein drinks is helpful in meeting caloric requirements.

Supportive care. After admission of the patient, the bed linens may be changed by using a sufficient number of persons to assist. Medication for pain should be administered 30 to 45 minutes before beginning the procedure. The patient needs special mouth care, and water and glycerin may be used. If the lips are not burned, cold cream or a water-soluble jelly should be applied. A retention catheter is usually inserted to measure hourly output, and care should be taken to prevent urinary tract infection by maintaining a sterile closed system of drainage.

If the feet have not been burned, ambulation is generally ordered as soon as possible for the patient. Ambulation helps to improve appetite and elimination. Soaks or tub baths may be ordered to remove dressings and to prevent damage to the tissues or to remove eschar before skin grafting. The tub should be thoroughly scrubbed with soap and water and disinfected with bleach, and the temperature of the water should be 100° F (37.8° C).

Emotional care. The burn patient has many emotional problems, especially fear of death and disfigurement. If the burn is the result of carelessness, there are bound to be feelings of guilt. Most patients realize that long weeks of recovery lie ahead, and the worry over loss of income and expenses may cause endless anxiety. The patient's family may have emotional problems and guilt feelings. Both the patient and the family need opportunities to talk about their problems, and these opportunities may be provided by the nurse, the hospital social worker, or a spiritual counselor. Plans to assist a family financially may relieve worry. Diversional activities should be provided for the patient to help fill unused time, and they may be helpful in preventing contractures by promoting muscle movement.

Expected outcomes. The following results should be seen in the burn patient during the acute period of hospitalization after proper intervention:

- Infection-free granulation tissue forms on burn sites.
- Graft sites and donor sites are free of infection.
- No pressure sores are formed.
- Patient consumes full diet without nausea or distention.
- Temperature, pulse, and respirations are normal.
- Patient has full range of motion in the burn area.
- Self-esteem is intact.
- Patient expresses concerns regarding changes in body image.

The Rehabilitation Period

The patient with major burns usually leaves the hospital with the prospect of a long period of rehabilitation. In addition to further pain, grafting, and reconstruction in the years ahead, the burn victim must deal with the social and emotional trauma of a profoundly altered body image and the changes in social relationships that may result. Many burn victims are young children and are particularly affected by the social stigma of being "different" from their peers. Long-term physical, social, and psychologic therapy, as well as the financial burdens that these services impose, require careful coordination and planning by the burn unit staff before discharge.

At the time of discharge a number of factors must be considered to smooth the transition. These are not solely nursing responsibilities, but the nurse may need to coordinate home care activities. Discharge planning should include consideration of the following areas (Boxes 31-18 and 31-19):

- *Emotional adjustment.* The patient and family may experience problems during the rehabilitative period. If the hospital social worker does not intervene, the nurse should arrange for psychologic follow-up.
- *Dressing procedures.* Instructions and supplies should be provided if the family is to continue changing dressings at home. What seems simple in the hospital setting may be problematic in the patient's kitchen or bathroom, so home care follow-up and supervision should be provided.
- *Exercise, splinting, and activities of daily living.* The nurse should observe the patient doing these activities before discharge. The physical therapist and/or occupational therapist may make follow-up visits to help with these programs.
- *Medications.* All medications, dosage, effects, and possible contraindications should be fully explained to the patient and family, and their level of understanding should be evaluated.
- *Return visits and phone numbers for problems.* The patient should be given written instructions for scheduling follow-up care. Arrangements for transportation should be made before discharge. Phone numbers of burn unit personnel should be given to the patient for use in case of questions or problems.
- *Home care or community agency followup.* If the hospital does not have a follow-up procedure, arrangements should be made with a community home care agency to provide these services.

ETHICAL DILEMMA

A 45-year-old woman has been admitted to the burn unit after suffering second- and third-degree burns on 85% of her total body surface area (TBSA) in a motor vehicle accident. She has no family or friends in this area. She has been fluid resuscitated and unconscious for the past 3 days. On the fourth day, she awakens and is obviously distressed when she becomes aware of all the technologic equipment and many doctors and nurses surrounding her bed. She frantically shakes her head to her primary nurse signifying, *"Stop! No more!"*

How would you analyze and resolve this dilemma?

BOX 31-18

DISCHARGE INSTRUCTIONS FOR BURN PATIENT

We on the burn team are happy to see that you are able to go home. To ensure you the speediest possible recovery, it is important that you are able to care for yourself and recognize problems that may interfere with your complete recovery.

If any of the following occur, please call the hospital and ask for the Burn Clinic. The nurse will be able to assist you.

1. Healed area breaking open. Cover with clean dressing.
2. Formation of blisters.
3. Signs of infection:
   a. Fever, temperature over 37.2° C (99° F).
   b. Redness, pain, swelling, hardness, or warmth in or around wound or any other part of body.
   c. Increased or foul-smelling drainage from wound.
4. Problems with your Ace bandages or Jobst garment such as improper fit, formation of blisters, or opening of healed area underneath.

Your first clinic appointment will be on ___. If a family member can come with you, they can register for you, and you may go to the Burn Clinic waiting room.

BATHING

Bathing or showering daily in your usual manner cleans the wounds, especially the ones that are still open.

1. Check the water and be sure to adjust the temperature to a warm and comfortable level. Your skin is more sensitive to extra heat or cold and can be easily injured.
2. Wash gently with a clean soft washcloth, using a mild detergent soap such as Dreft or Ivory Snow, approximately 2 tsp. Be careful not to rub too hard so as not to disturb the grafted areas. Avoid harsh or deodorant soaps.
3. Rinse skin thoroughly after washing.
4. Dry thoroughly.
5. Apply specific dressing as instructed.

CARE FOR BURN WOUND

These are your guidelines for the care of your burn wound. During this time, look at the involved areas and note if there are any changes that need to be reported.

1. Wash hands.
2. Remove dressing and dispose in paper bag or wrap in newspaper.
3. Wash hands.
4. Wash open area with gauze using solution of Dreft (or Ivory Snow) and water. Add 1 tbsp Dreft to a basin of water; 2 tbsp Dreft, if you use the bathtub. Use a clean towel and washcloth with each dressing change.
5. Rinse skin well.
6. Wash hands.
7. Apply dressings as described below.
8. Wear gloves. Wash basin or bathtub with a disinfectant such as Lysol.
9. Wash hands.

CARE OF CLOTHING

When you are discharged, you may find that healed burn areas are sensitive to harsh detergents, fabric softeners, and clothing dyes. If you are sensitive, we suggest the following:

1. Launder new clothing before use by machine or hand with Dreft or Ivory Snow.
2. Rinse clothes twice.
3. Do not use fabric softeners.
4. If you have open burns or a healed area that opens, wash all clothes separately from other family members.
5. Scarlet red ointment will permanently stain clothing.
6. If dyes used in clothing cause irritation, wear white articles.

ACE BANDAGES

You have been taught to put on your own Ace bandages while in the hospital, but if you have a problem with this, please notify the Burn Clinic. It is also important that you know how to care for them and understand problems that occur.

1. If they are too loose, they will be ineffective and must be rewrapped.
2. If they are too tight, they will cause discomfort, numbness, tingling, and puffiness and must be rewrapped.
3. They must be worn for a long period of time, probably 6-12 months to be effective, so please do not stop wearing them until your doctor tells you.
4. To care for your Ace bandages:
   a. Hand wash with Dreft or Ivory Snow in cold water.
   b. Towel dry.
   c. Lay flat or place over rod or clothesline.
   d. Do not use clothespins.

JOBST GARMENT

You have been taught to put on your Jobst garment while in the hospital, but if you have a problem with this, please notify the Burn Clinic. It is also important that you know how to care for it and understand problems that can occur.

1. If it is too loose, it will be ineffective and you will require a new garment.
2. If it is too tight, it will cause discomfort, numbness, and tingling. Do not wear it if this occurs, but notify the Burn Clinic as soon as possible.
3. To care for your Jobst garment:
   a. Hand wash with Dreft or Ivory Snow in cold water.
   b. Towel dry.
   c. Lay flat or place over rod or clothesline.
   d. Do not use clothespins.

Courtesy Burn Service, MetroHealth Medical Center, Cleveland. From Phipps WJ and others: *Medical-surgical nursing: concepts and clinical practice,* ed 5, St Louis, 1995, Mosby.

BOX 31-19

HOME CARE GUIDE

Burn Care

Before discharge, the patient and family or other caregiver must be taught proper care of the patient and his or her wounds to ensure proper healing and to help the patient begin readjustment into society.

GENERAL CARE

Patient or family should notify the clinic or physician if any of the following occur:

1. Change in wound status (open, draining, enlarging, blisters, edema, redness)
2. Signs of infection (temperature above 99° F, foul-smelling or copious wound drainage)
3. Difficulty with dressings or pressure garments

SKIN CARE

Daily care of the skin includes:

1. Daily gentle bathing with mild soap
2. Application of moisturizer to healed burn areas
3. Dressing changes on open areas
   - a. Wash hands
   - b. Wear gloves
   - c. Dispose of old dressing
   - d. Cleanse areas with mild soap and water and clean washcloth
   - e. Apply dressing as specified (may be open or closed method)
   - f. Disinfect basin or tub

DAILY LIVING

Activities are resumed in conjunction with the patient's ability and the physician's orders, but in general the patient is reminded to:

1. Take protective measures in sunlight because skin is much more sensitive
   - a. Use a sunscreen with a sun protection factor (SPF) higher than 15
   - b. Wear long-sleeved shirts, pants, and a hat
   - c. Avoid direct, intense sunlight
2. Avoid shearing of the skin
   - a. Wear soft clothing, and wash new clothing before wearing
   - b. Be aware of instances when the skin may be damaged and use caution (cleaning, cooking, ironing)
3. Eat a well-balanced diet
4. Avoid excess weight gain or loss because pressure garments will be affected
5. Take in ample fluids (64 ounces or more per day)
6. Exercise injured limbs and joints at least four times a day
7. Increase endurance with aerobic activity
8. Take medications as prescribed (side effects, indications, and dosages are reviewed before discharge)
9. Clean pressure garments daily in mild soap
10. Return to clinic or physician when scheduled

From Beare PG, Myers JL: *Adult health nursing,* ed 2, St Louis, 1994, Mosby.

KEY CONCEPTS

- The skin is a protective organ consisting of the epidermis, dermis, and subcutaneous tissue layers.
- The unbroken skin is the first line of defense against pathogenic organisms. It protects deeper tissue from injury and loss of body fluids and regulates body temperature.
- Skin lesions must be assessed by size, shape, color, distribution, and sequence or arrangement.
- Diagnosis of skin disorders requires a careful history that should include allergies, sleep habits, occupation, medications, recent travel or contact with others, level of anxiety, time or appearance of lesions, and direction of their spread.
- A therapeutic oatmeal bath can be prepared by placing 2 cups of oatmeal and 1 quart of boiling water in a double boiler to cook for 45 minutes, then placing the mixture in a gauze bag and swishing it in a tub of water at 100° F.
- Open wet dressings initiate vasoconstriction to cool the skin and relieve pruritus (itching).
- Closed wet dressings hydrate the epidermis and increase absorption of topical medications.
- Warm moist dressings can be wrapped in plastic to stay warm, but plastic should not be used if a heating pad is applied to keep temperature constant.
- Individuals with skin disorders may experience real or imagined feelings of being shunned, which may prompt withdrawal and lead to isolation.
- Sustained pressure over bony prominences cuts off blood supply to the tissue, which causes local areas of necrosis called pressure ulcers.
- Moisture, friction, and shear contribute to pressure ulcers and can be prevented.
- Specialty beds can be used to prevent and reduce pressure and should be selected with specific patient needs in mind.

KEY CONCEPTS—cont'd

- Wounds of pressure ulcers are treated by cleansing, debridement, and use of topical medications, exudate absorbers, and dressings. Patients who are at risk for formation of pressure ulcers can be identified by use of one of the three risk-assessment scales: Norton, Gosnell, or Braden. Specific measures can be instituted to reduce the risk of pressure ulcer formation.
- Decisions for wound care can also be made after classifying the wound as red, yellow, or black.
- Disorders of pigmentation include lentigo (freckles) and chloasma (patches of pigmentation).
- Disorders of the glands include seborrhea (oily skin), sebaceous cyst (wen), hyperhidrosis (excessive sweating), and anhidrosis (absence of sweating).
- Pruritus (itching) accompanies many skin disorders. Treatment involves removing the cause and reducing irritating factors.
- Skin tumors include keloids (overgrowth of fibrous tissue at scar sites), nevi (moles), and angiomas (benign tumors of dilated blood vessels). Keratoses are precancerous lesions.
- Basal cell carcinoma is seen most often in fair-skinned people who have had overexposure to the sun.
- Squamous cell carcinoma usually develops on areas exposed to radiation.
- Malignant melanoma is recognized by the ABCDs of melanoma: **A**symmetry, **B**order irregularity, **C**olor, **D**iameter greater than 6 mm.
- Pediculi (lice) are found on the head, on the body, and in the pubic area. Treatment is Nix, RID, or lindane lotion/shampoo.
- Scabies is an infectious skin disease caused by the itch mite, a parasite that burrows under the skin. It is recognized by intense itching and multiform lesions, papules, and vesicles, and a characteristic S-shaped burrow is sometimes present. Location of the lesion varies with age. It is treated with Elimite, Eurax, or 1% lindane.
- Skin infections require topical or systemic antibiotics, and the patient must receive instruction on use and side effects. Universal precautions should be employed when dealing with skin infections.
- Tinea capitis (ringworm of the scalp), tinea corporis (ringworm on the body, face, neck, and extremities), tinea barbae (barber's itch), tinea cruris (jock itch), and tinea pedis (athlete's foot) are caused by fungi.
- Viral infections can be confined to the skin, or they may be systemic and produce skin lesions, as in rubella and rubeola. The human papillomavirus causes warts. Those found in the genital area are transmitted through sexual contact.
- Herpes simplex 1 causes cold sores, and herpes simplex 2 causes genital herpes.
- Herpes zoster and varicella (chickenpox) are caused by the herpesvirus varicella. The characteristic lesion is described as a "dew drop on a rose petal" because it is a single vesicle on an erythematous base.
- The lesions of herpes zoster (shingles) are located in one or more of the spinal ganglia, and the skin area supplied by the affected nerve fibers becomes involved. Herpes zoster can occur when a dormant virus becomes activated or when there is contact with lesions of persons with herpes zoster. The lesions follow the dermatomes (nerve pathways).
- Dermatitis is an inflammatory condition of the skin; eczema is a reactive process. The terms are often used interchangeably.
- Psoriasis is a chronic, genetically determined disease of epidermal proliferation. It improves with exposure to ultraviolet rays of the sun and is exacerbated by emotional stress, infection, and alcohol. It appears as well demarcated erythematous patches or plaques with silver scale, generalized exfoliative dermatitis, or pustules.
- Acne is an inflammatory disorder of the pilosebaceous unit of the skin. It appears as eruptions of papules or pustules that are formed when oil delivered to the skin's surface meets with resistance. The nurse must assess the patient's reaction to the disorder and his or her understanding of the treatment prescribed. Severe cases are treated with a retinoid of vitamin A.
- Rosacea affects the blood vessels in the central part of the face. Rhinophyma (pronounced enlargement of the nose) may be seen in men in later stages of rosacea.
- Lupus erythematosus is a chronic inflammatory disease involving the connective tissues of the body. Discoid lupus erythematosus (DLE) is confined to the skin. Systemic lupus erythematosus (SLE) is generalized and affects many organs.
- Hypersensitivity reactions appear as urticaria identified by hives or wheals, or as erythema multiforme, characterized by iris or bull's-eye lesions. The underlying cause must be eliminated.

KEY CONCEPTS—cont'd

- Burns are classified by type or source as thermal, electrical, radiation, or chemical.
- Burns are classified by severity as minor, moderate, or major, depending on thickness (depth of the burn injury) and extent (amount of body surface involved).
- Extent of burn injury is estimated by either the Rule of Nines or the Lund and Browder Chart, which is more accurate because it accounts for differences in age.
- The care of the burned patient is divided into three phases: the emergent period, the acute period, and the rehabilitative period.
- The priorities in the emergent phase of burn care are to prevent further injury and maintain or provide a patent airway, stop bleeding, and treat burn shock.
- The goals of treatment during the acute phase of burn care are to relieve pain, prevent infection, heal open wounds, restore normal functioning and appearance, preserve emotional equilibrium, and return to the social and work environment.
- A severe burn wound that has no dermis remaining to allow tissue regeneration will require skin grafting. An autograft from the patient's own skin is the only graft that will not be rejected. Other grafts are used on a temporary basis until the patient's condition allows autografting.
- A full-thickness graft removes epidermis and dermis and is used for reconstruction. The donor site will require grafting eventually. A split-thickness graft leaves some dermis and allows that site to heal. A specially made elastic stocking or garment may be worn for 2 years to compress the graft site, increase circulation, and prevent contractures.
- The rehabilitation period can be lengthy and may include further pain, grafting, and reconstruction. The burn victim must deal with the social and emotional trauma of a profoundly altered body image and with the changes in social relationships that may result. Long-term physical, social, and psychologic therapy are required and must be coordinated before the patient is discharged.

CRITICAL THINKING EXERCISES

1 Explain the fact that patients with skin disorders are more likely to experience emotional problems that those with other types of disorders.
2 Develop a list of instructions to give a patient with pigmented moles.
3 Develop a list of instructions for the patient with impetigo. Include methods of treatment and methods of preventing spread of the disease to others.

REFERENCES AND ADDITIONAL READINGS

Agency for Health Care Policy and Research: *Urinary incontinence in adults,* Rockville, Md, March 1992. Public Health Service, US Department of Health and Human Services, AHCPR Publication No 92-0038.

Agency for Health Care Policy and Research: *Pressure ulcers in adults: prediction and prevention,* Rockville, Md, May 1992. Public Health Service, US Department of Health and Human Services, AHCPR Publication No 92-0047.

Beare PG, Myers JL: *Adult health nursing,* ed 2, St Louis, 1994, Mosby.

Bryant RA: *Acute and chronic wounds: nursing management,* St Louis, 1992, Mosby.

Calistro AM: Burn care basics and beyond, *RN* 56(3):26-32, 1993.

Carroll P: Bed selection: help patients rest easy, *RN* 58(5): 44-51, 1995.

Cuzzell J: Wound care forum: the new RYB color code, *Am J Nurs* 88(10):1342-1346, 1988.

Dyer C: Burn wound management: an update, *Plastic Surg Nurs* 8(1):6-12, 1988.

Eaglstein WH, Baxter C, Mertz PM, Oot-Giromini B, Rodeheaver G, Rudolph R, Shannon ML and Silane M: *New directions in wound healing,* Princeton, 1990, E.R. Squibb and Sons.

Erwin-Toth P, Hocevar BJ: Wound care: selecting the right dressing, *Am J Nurs* 95(2):46-51, 1995.

Hill MJ: The skin: anatomy and physiology, *Dermatol Nurs* 2(1):13-17, 1990.

Hill MJ: *Skin disorders: Mosby's clinical nursing series,* St Louis, 1994, Mosby.

Kinzie V, Lace C: What to do for the severely burned, *RN* 43:47-51, 1989.

Krasner D, editor: *Chronic wound care: a clinical source book for healthcare professionals,* King of Prussia, Pa, 1990, Health Management Publications.

Krasner D: Wound care: how to use the red-yellow-black system, *Am J Nurs* 95(5):44-47, 1995.

Krasner D: Managing pain from pressure ulcers, *Am J Nurs* 95(6):22-24, 1995.

Laudano JB, Leach EE, Armstrong RB: Acne: therapeutic perspectives with an emphasis on the role of isotretinon, *Dermatol Nurs* 2(6):328-336, 1990.

Makelbust J, Siegreen M, *Pressure ulcers: guidelines for prevention and management,* West Dundee, Ill, 1991, S-N Publications.

Marvin JA: Burn nursing history: the history of burn care, *J Burn Care Rehab,* 14(2pt2):252-256, 1993.

O'Hanlon-Nichols T: Commonly asked questions about wound healing, *Am J Nurs* 95(4):22-24, 1995.

Phipps WJ and others: *Medical-surgical nursing: concepts and clinical practice,* ed 5, St Louis, 1995, Mosby.

Trofino RB: *Nursing care of the burn-injured patient,* Philadelphia, 1991, FA Davis.

University of California at Berkeley: *Wellness Letter* 11(8):6, 1995, The School of Public Health, The University.

Whittington K: Debunking wound care myths, *RN* 58(8): 32-33, 1995.

Willey T: High-tech beds and mattress overlays: a decision guide, *Am J Nurs* 89(9):1105-1252, 1989.

Yotter M: Contact dermatitis: nursing intervention, *Dermatol Nurs* 2(5):267-269, 1990.

CHAPTER 32

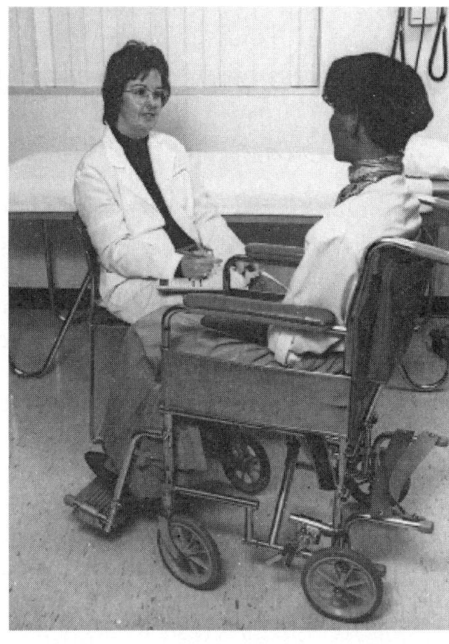

Mobility

CHAPTER OBJECTIVES

1. Describe the structure and function of the musculoskeletal system.
2. Discuss the physiology of fracture healing, including the role of hematomas, granulation tissue, and callus formation.
3. Compare the pathophysiology, findings, and nursing interventions for patients with rheumatoid arthritis and osteoarthritis.
4. Discuss the pathophysiology of gout, as well as the medical treatment, nursing process, and education for the patient with gout.
5. Define and describe the assessment of bursitis.
6. Differentiate between osteomyelitis and tuberculosis of bone.
7. Compare and contrast the interventions for sprains, dislocations, and fractures.
8. Discuss the nursing assessment, care, and education needs of the patient in a Thomas splint with a Pearson attachment.
9. Identify the various types of fractures, as well as their medical interventions.
10. Discuss the assessment of and interventions needed for patients with newly applied casts.
11. Discuss the psychosocial and teaching needs of patients with casts.
12. Discuss the nursing measures for preparing a patient who has had an amputation and is being fitted with a prosthesis.
13. Describe the psychosocial and teaching needs of a patient who has had an amputation.
14. Differentiate between the assessment of muscular dystrophy and of cerebral palsy.
15. Identify nursing measures, including psychosocial and teaching needs, that help prevent the complications associated with immobility.

KEY WORDS

abduction
adduction
arthrodesis
arthroplasty
arthrotomy
callus
compartment syndrome
contracture
countertraction
ecchymosis
external rotation
internal rotation
isometric
osteotomy
periosteum
prosthesis
remodeling
synovectomy
tophi
traction

STRUCTURE AND FUNCTION OF THE MUSCULOSKELETAL SYSTEM

Structure

The musculoskeletal system consists of bones, joints, and muscles. Within this system, muscles are attached to bones by fibrous cords called *tendons*. Bones are held together at the joints by bands of tough tissue called *ligaments*. *Cartilage* is a somewhat flexible tissue that connects bones and acts as a shock absorber. For example, cartilage is found between the vertebrae of the spinal column.

Bones are composed of living cells that are surrounded by an intercellular matrix. This intercellular substance is infiltrated with calcium salts, which makes bones hard and provides strength and rigidity. This *calcified intercellular substance* is permeated by a system of tiny canals that are filled with tissue fluid and through which bone cells are nourished and waste is removed.

Bones have various shapes. *Long bones* are found in the extremities, and *short bones* are found in the hands and feet. Flat bones protect vital structures such as the brain and thoracic organs. Irregular bones include the vertebrae and other small bones throughout the body.

Each long bone consists of six major parts. The *diaphysis* is the long shaft of the bone, and the two *epiphyses* are the ends. The *medullary cavity* is the space that is filled with bone marrow. In the adult, this cavity is filled with fatty, yellow marrow, and the ends of the long bones contain bloodforming red marrow. The medullary cavity is lined with the *endosteum*, which consists of cells that form new bone as needed. The **periosteum** is the fibrous membrane that covers the outside of the bone, except at the joints, and it contains blood vessels, lymphatic vessels, and nerves. The inner layer of the periosteum also contains bone-forming cells. Each end of a long bone is covered with *articular cartilage*, which cushions blows to the joint. *Bursae* (*bursa*, singular) are flattened sacs that are filled with synovial fluid. These sacs are located wherever it is necessary to reduce or eliminate the friction of a muscle or tendon against another muscle, tendon, or bone. The bursae also cushion certain muscles, as well as muscles that must move over bony prominences (Figure 32-1).

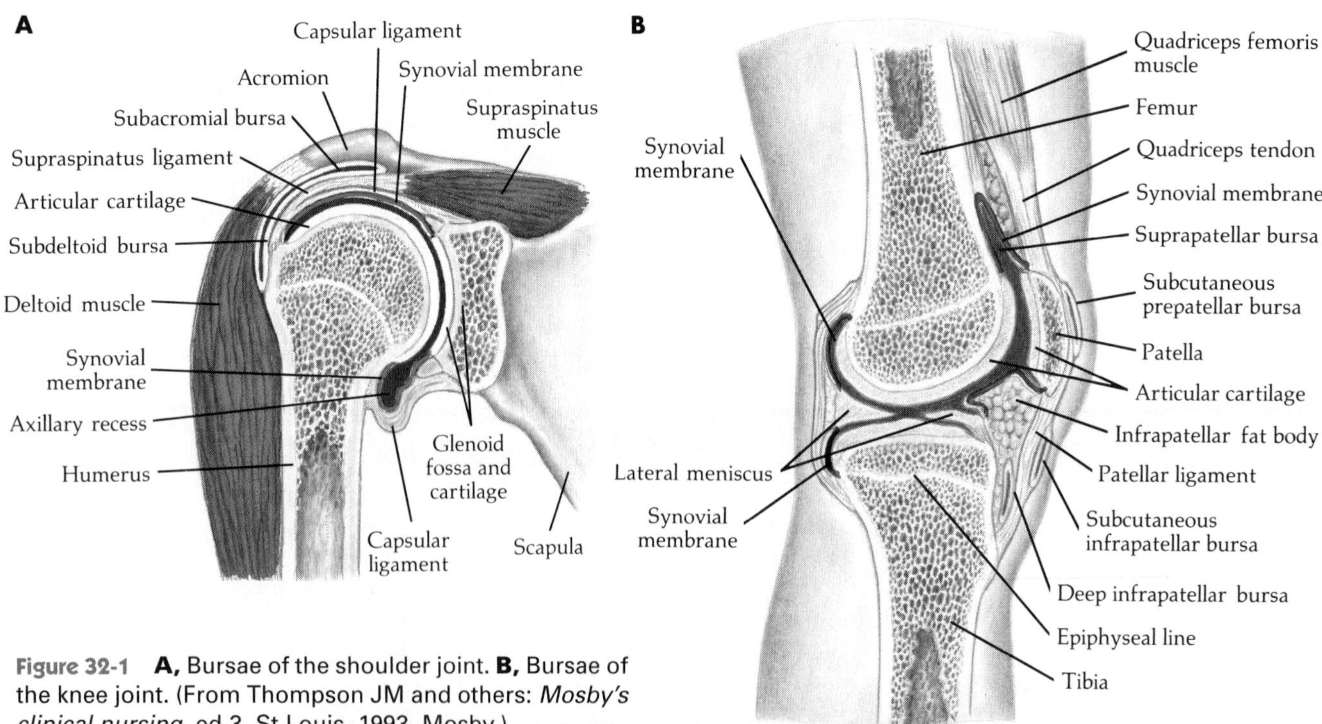

Figure 32-1 **A,** Bursae of the shoulder joint. **B,** Bursae of the knee joint. (From Thompson JM and others: *Mosby's clinical nursing*, ed 3, St Louis, 1993, Mosby.)

Bones in children are more flexible than those in adults. More calcium is deposited as bones grow, and they become rigid and inflexible. With advanced age, calcium may be lost from bones, which makes them porous and brittle.

To effectively put the patient's joints through a full range of motion, the nurse should have an understanding of joints. The range of motion for a joint is described as the degree or amount of motion that is possible for that joint (Figure 32-2). Some joints are

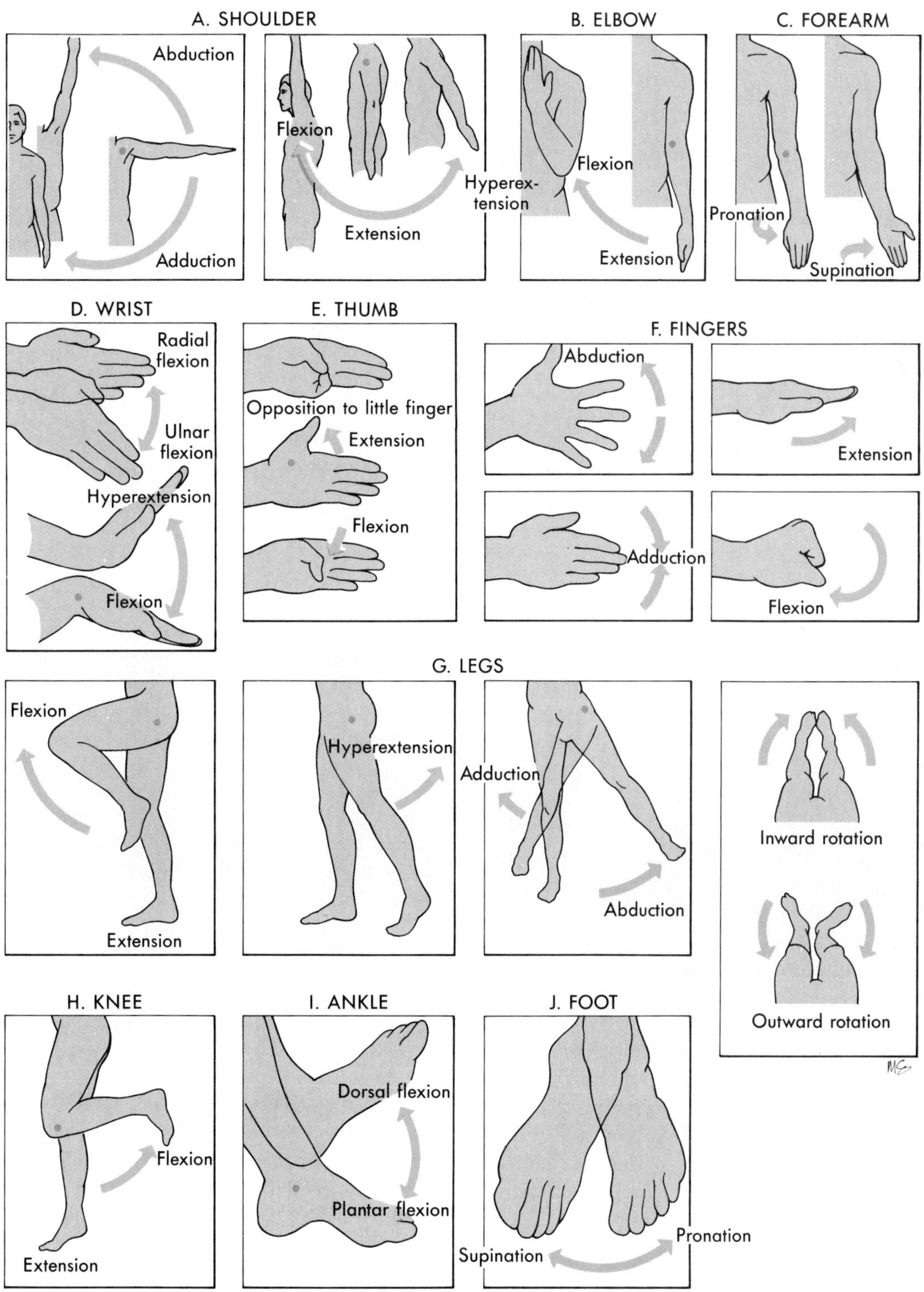

Figure 32-2 Range of motion for joints in the body. (From Beare PG, Myers JL: *Principles and practice of adult health nursing,* ed 2, St Louis, 1994, Mosby.)

K. WAIST

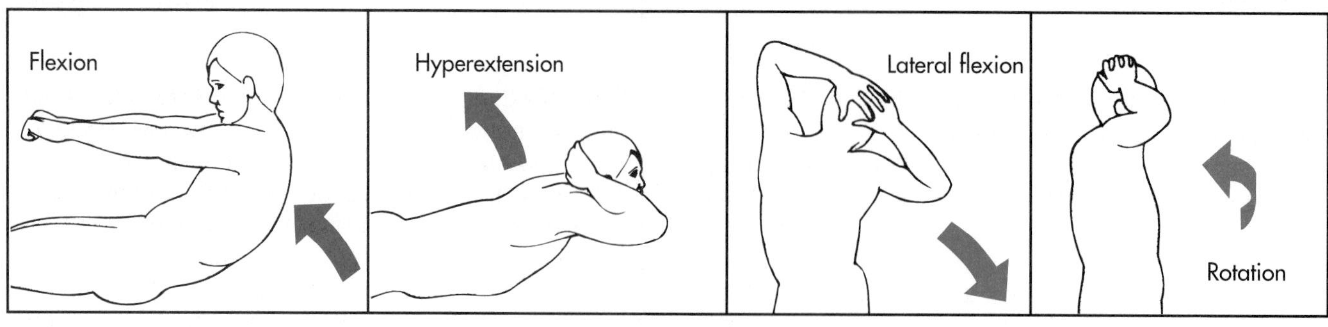

L. NECK

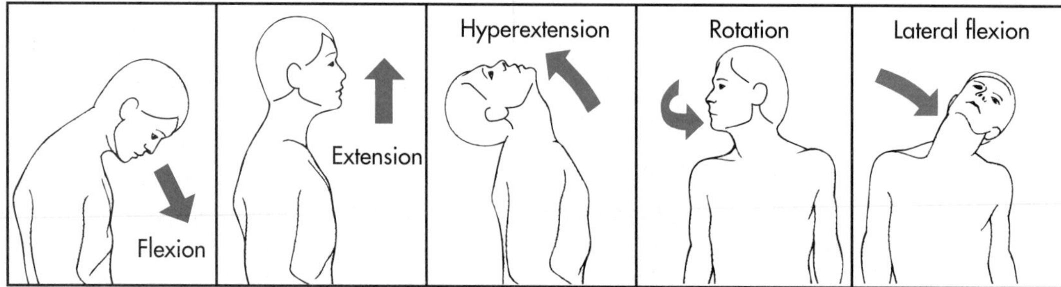

Figure 32-2, cont'd For legend see previous page.

freely movable, such as the hinge joints in the elbows and knees. The movements of these joints include flexion (bending at the joint) and extension (straightening the joint). Joint movement is also described by the terms **abduction,** which involves moving the extremity away from the midline of the body, and **adduction,** which involves moving the extremity toward the midline of the body. Shoulder and hip joints are ball-and-socket joints and have a rotating motion. The description of the rotating movement of a joint often includes information to indicate which way the joint is rotating, such as **external rotation** (away from the body midline) and **internal rotation** (toward the body midline). Other joints are slightly movable. For example, the joints between the vertebral bodies provide limited motion of the spine. Some joints are immovable and are found in places such as the cranium. Only those joints that are freely movable can be put through a full range of motion. Although movement of the body depends largely on muscle contraction, mobility is actually a cooperative function of bones, muscles, and joints.

Function

The musculoskeletal system has other functions in addition to locomotion. The bony framework supports the body in an upright position and protects vital organs. Blood cells are formed in the marrow of bones, and bones deposit calcium, which may be used to supply a deficiency in the body fluids. Injury and disease may affect any part of the system and may result in deformity or impairment of functions. Some disorders involve both nerves and muscles and are called *neuromuscular disorders.*

OLDER ADULT CONSIDERATIONS

Anatomic changes in the bones and joints

Age-related changes in the bones of the older adult include bones becoming porous and brittle as a result of lost calcium. Such changes make the bones easier to break or to fracture. There is also decreased range of motion in the joints as a result of degeneration of the cartilage in the joints, which makes them painful to move.

POSITION, EXERCISE, AND BODY MECHANICS

Proper positioning of a patient who is confined to a regimen of bedrest is essential. Properly positioning a patient is a nursing intervention, and medical orders are not necessary except in those surgical procedures in which physician's preferences vary. Orthopedic patients may be required to remain in plaster casts, traction, or other stabilization devices for prolonged periods. Nursing care must emphasize positioning to prevent **contractures,** deformities, or other complications of immobility. A contracture is a permanent shortening of muscles, tendons, and ligaments, and it reduces the range of motion in affected joints.

Active and passive exercise of the muscles of both the affected and unaffected extremities is essential for maintaining muscle tone, preventing complications, and preparing for ambulation. Active exercise is performed by the patient. Passive exercise does not involve muscle contraction, and the nurse or therapist often assists the patient with this type of exercise. An exercise program that is tailored to the individual is often initiated soon after immobilization. Active and passive movement of joints through their full ranges of motion should be incorporated into the daily activities of physical care and ambulation. Active range-of-motion exercises are performed by the patient, who moves the affected joint through its range of motion by using the muscles that surround that joint. Passive range-of-motion exercises require that the joint be moved through its range of motion by either the patient or someone else, but the muscles of the joint are not used. An example of passive range-of-motion would be a patient using his or her left arm to move the right elbow through its range of motion. Patients may fear that doing the prescribed exercises or moving an extremity that is in a cast will cause further injury. Many patients are afraid to wiggle their fingers and toes. The nurse should explain to these patients that the exercises stimulate bone growth and prevent muscle atrophy.

Specific exercises that prevent thrombophlebitis and help maintain muscle tone include *antithromboembolic* exercises of the calf muscle, as well as *quad-setting* and *gluteal-setting* **isometric** exercises. Isometric exercises require the patient to consciously tighten the muscles, but no movement is involved. Antithromboembolic and isometric exercises are to be performed in the supine position. To encourage circulation and to prevent thrombus and embolus development in the calf muscle, patients fully extend their legs and push the back of their knees down on the bed while dorsiflexing their feet. For quad-setting, patients tighten their quadriceps muscles, and for gluteal-setting, they tighten and pinch their buttocks together. With each of these exercises, patients may be advised to hold the position for a count of 10. They also may be advised to repeat these exercises 10 times every hour while awake.

Exercises that are designed to strengthen muscles in preparation for ambulation include prescribed weight-lifting and *bridging* exercises. To perform the bridging exercise, patients flex their unaffected leg at the knee. They push down on the bed with the sole of their foot while using the trapeze to lift their back and buttocks off the bed. They hold themselves in the lifted position with their backs straight for as long as possible. Patients also may be advised to do this 10 times an hour while awake.

Emphasis also has been placed on the importance of turning patients to prevent pulmonary complications. Too often a comfortable patient objects to being disturbed, and moving an obese or comatose patient or a patient who is in a body cast or in traction presents a special challenge for the nurse. However, research has confirmed that turning a patient as little as 12 degrees is sufficient to prevent pulmonary complications, stimulate circulation, and prevent decubitus ulcers. Therefore all immobilized patients should be turned at least every 2 hours.

The tilt table is a device that helps the patient adjust to an upright position before ambulation. Patients who have been confined to bedrest for long periods may develop hypotension when they sit or stand. Gradual elevation with a tilt table helps prevent this problem. The tilt table is used to prepare the patient for crutch walking and ambulation, as well as to reduce osteoporosis that develops from immobilization. The tilt table may also prevent urinary tract infections by decreasing the pooling of urine in the bladder, which results when the patient remains in a supine position.

After an injury to the musculoskeletal system, many patients need to be taught the proper methods of standing, sitting, walking, stooping, and lifting. Nurses who use their bodies skillfully are in a much better position to help teach their patients about body mechanics. The consideration of body mechanics conserves energy, prevents injuries to muscles, prevents fatigue, and promotes work efficiency.

NURSE ALERT

Nurses need to be very conscious about using good body mechanics because of the risk of injury to themselves while caring for their patients.

NEUROVASCULAR INTEGRITY

Neurovascular impairment is a threat to patients with orthopedic conditions and must be relieved promptly. Impairment of circulation or nerve function can result in tissue necrosis or the loss of the use of an extremity. Damage to nerves and blood vessels may result from trauma; surgery; or tight bandages, splints, and casts. Assessment and intervention for arterial vascular compromise is discussed later in this chapter in relation to the serious complications of compartment syndrome. Temporary impairment of the venous circulation in the extremities is more common and should be suspected when edema, coolness, pallor, cyanosis, pain, numbness, and tingling are observed in the fingers or toes. Edema is swelling that is caused by excess interstitial fluid. Pallor describes a whitish-grayish color of the skin. Cyanosis describes a bluish skin color. Cyanosis can be easily seen in the skin, nailbeds, and mucous membranes. These symptoms may be accompanied by slow capillary refill in the nailbeds, as well as by the absence of radial, pedal, or tibial pulses.

Assessment

To perform an accurate neurovascular assessment, the nurse should always compare the findings in the affected extremity with those in the unaffected extremity. Extremities should be positioned correctly, with the affected arm or leg elevated. An accurate description of sensations should be elicited from the patient. Using the same hand (rather than two hands) to access both extremities may provide a more accurate assessment. To determine true coolness in the affected extremity, the nurse must feel both feet because many people have cool feet under normal circumstances. The foot of the affected extremity may be warmer than the other extremity as a result of the normal inflammation that is associated with trauma and surgery.

Edema that is accompanied by warmth and a light, rosy flesh color usually does not indicate harmful circulatory impairment, particularly if other signs are absent or if the edema occurs within 48 to 72 hours after trauma or surgery. This type of warmth and edema gradually subsides. However, edema that is accompanied by pallor, cyanosis, and coldness is a sign of circulatory impairment. If swelling is difficult to determine, a comparison of the wrinkles on the toes or fingers of both feet or hands may show stretching of the tissue on the digits in question, which indicates slight edema (Box 32-1).

The *blanching sign* is a test of the rate of capillary refill, which signals the adequacy of circulation. When the nail of each toe or finger is compressed and immediately released, the nailbed should rapidly change from white to pink. Slow or sluggish capillary refill indicates decreased circulation.

Each digit should be checked for sensation and motion because not all digits are innervated by the same nerve. Localized numbness and the inability to flex and extend the digits indicate nerve compression. Increased pain may accompany circulatory impairment. A clear description of the pain with regard to its precise location (e.g., along a nerve, over a bony prominence), intensity, and response to movement should be obtained from the patient before pain medication is given. Palpating the pedal, tibial, or radial pulse may be difficult or impossible when a cast or bandage renders these areas inaccessible. Sometimes the nurse may be able to reach under a bandage to locate the pulse. However, caution must be used if an incision or open wound is underneath the bandage, and sterile gloves are required to protect the nurse from accidental contamination. The presence and strength of the pulse in the affected extremity should be identified and compared to that in the unaffected extremity.

Beginning immediately after surgery or the application of a cast, a neurovascular assessment should be performed every 30 minutes. Patients often describe a transient tingling and numbness in an extremity, which results from general immobility. Flexing the fingers and toes relieves this, and the patient should be encouraged to flex whenever these symptoms occur. Neurovascular assessments should be completely and accurately recorded. The previous assessment of the patient's circulation should be reviewed before each subsequent neurovascular assessment. This review provides a baseline for evaluating progress or deterioration of circulatory integrity.

The physician should be notified immediately when circulatory impairment is suspected. Repositioning, elevating, and applying ice packs to the extremity may alleviate the symptoms. The physician may loosen or remove a cast or bandage. Modification of a cast is discussed later in this chapter.

Pain

Specific types of musculoskeletal injuries or disorders produce specific types of pain. To effectively assess and alleviate the pain, the nurse must know the nature of the pain. The nurse must differentiate between pain as an expected outcome and pain as a diagnostic sign (see Chapter 9).

Patients with fractures often describe acute, deep, severe pain at the time of injury, which persists until the fracture is reduced and medication is given. When

BOX 32-1

Nursing Process

NEUROVASCULAR INTEGRITY

ASSESSMENT

Alignment of body
Peripheral tissue perfusion
Wound/fracture site
Pain/comfort level
Peripheral nerve sensation

NURSING DIAGNOSES

Altered peripheral tissue perfusion related to injury/treatment
Risk for injury related to neurovascular impairment

NURSING INTERVENTIONS

Position extremities in alignment; elevate affected extremity.
Compare affected extremity with unaffected extremity; use the same hand for palpation.
Test capillary refill.
Check *each* digit for sensation and motion.
Document the location and characteristics of pain.
Palpate pedal, tibial, or radial pulses and compare them to those of the unaffected extremity.
Look for edema with pallor, cyanosis, and coldness.
Elicit a description of sensations from the patient.

EVALUATION OF EXPECTED OUTCOMES

No impairment of neurovascular integrity.

the fracture is reduced, the bone ends and/or fragments are realigned and stabilized in the proper position. Reduction and stabilization prevents further soft tissue, nerve, and blood vessel damage by the ragged bone pieces, which is an expected outcome of traumatic fractures. The pain that accompanies a fractured hip can be severe because of muscle spasms and trauma to surrounding nerves. Once a fracture is reduced, the pain becomes more localized and gradually subsides as healing takes place.

A recurrence of severe pain after a fracture is reduced and stabilized is an indication that something is wrong. A constant, aching pain may be the first sign that neurovascular integrity is being compromised. This pain may be increased with passive movement of the extremity and is accompanied by other signs of neurovascular impairment such as numbness, paralysis, coolness, and paleness. These findings are diagnostic of a circulatory problem that must be corrected promptly.

Pain associated with spinal column disorders often accompanies a long-standing back problem. The pain ranges from being sudden and sharp to a constant or intermittent aching. The pain may extend down one or both extremities and often is influenced by voluntary movement or positioning of the patient. Ongoing precise assessment of the frequency, location, and influencing activity of the pain is necessary for determining progress in both the conservative and surgical treatment of spinal disorders.

Because pain associated with musculoskeletal disorders may be severe and persistent, the nurse can anticipate the patient's need for pain medications on a regular basis until the pain subsides. Pain medication should be given as soon as the pain has been assessed thoroughly. Additional measures to alleviate the pain by repositioning the affected body region should also be initiated.

THE PATIENT WITH A CAST

Casts are applied to fractured extremities or to other parts of the body to maintain correct alignment of bones during healing. Casts are most commonly applied to fractures that are reduced by closed manipulation. Closed manipulation involves realignment of the bone ends by manipulation and/or manual traction. Casts may also be applied following other surgical repairs, including realignments that involve surgical open reduction with internal fixation (ORIF) of the fracture (see the interventions for fractures later in this chapter). Usually the cast extends beyond the joints above and below the fracture site (Figure 32-3).

The application of a cast may be anticipated by the patient, but more often it accompanies an unexpected fracture. Once the cast is applied, the patient is faced with a frustrating limitation of movement and an interruption in fulfilling roles and responsibilities. The emotional adjustment may be difficult. The nurse should recognize the patient's and family's need to ask

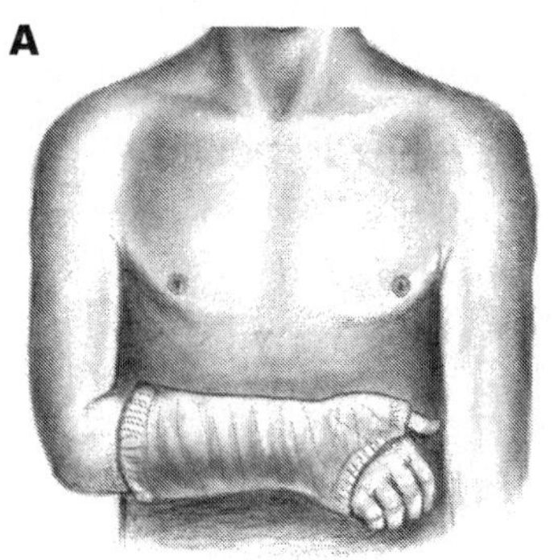

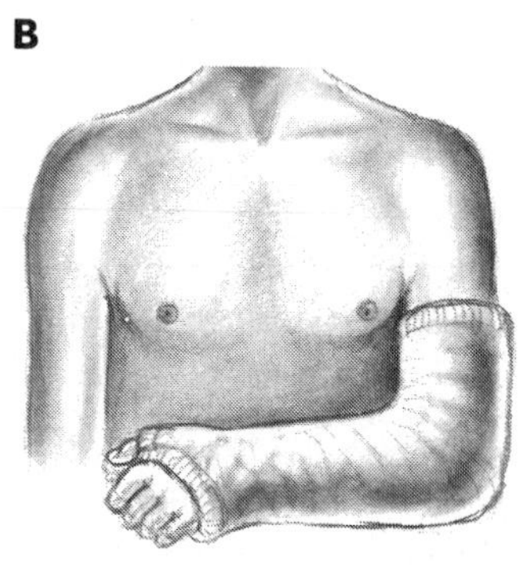

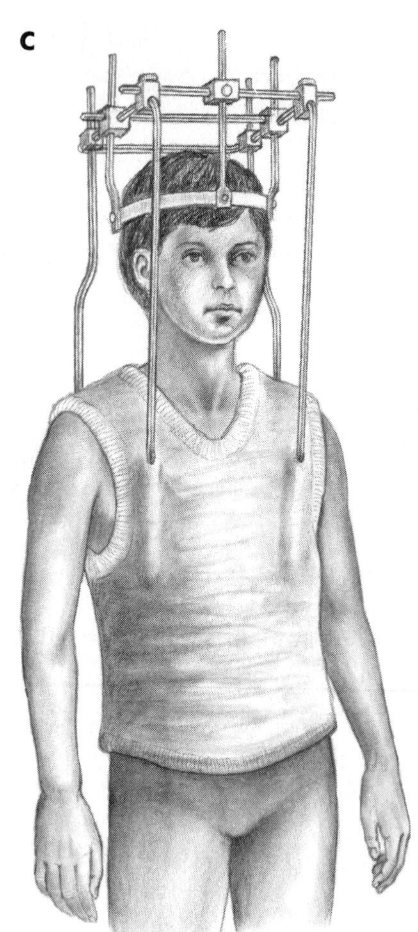

Figure 32-3 Examples of casts for upper extremity injuries. **A,** Short arm cast. **B,** Long arm cast. **C,** Body jacket with halo apparatus attached; it may be used with a brace, not a cast. (From Mourad LA: *Orthopedic disorders,* St Louis, 1991, Mosby.)

questions and to be supported in their adjustment to a changed level of function.

Care of the cast

A newly applied plaster cast sets quickly but takes as long as 48 hours to dry completely. During this drying time, the cast must be handled with the palms of the hands rather than with the fingers to prevent indentations that could create pressure. Casts are positioned and elevated on pillows to reduce swelling and to prevent pressure from the firm mattress (Figures 32-4, 32-5, and 32-6). The drying of the cast is accompanied by a considerable feeling of heat, which should be explained to the patient. To combat this heat and to help reduce swelling of the extremity, ice bags are placed beside the cast for 48 hours.

Once the cast has dried, it should be examined for rough edges that may need to be trimmed slightly or covered with adhesive *petals.* Petals are rectangular or oval pieces of adhesive with rounded corners and are approximately 1 inch × 3 inches. They are slipped under the edge of the cast, brought over the edge, and adhered to the top of the cast. Cotton wadding or a stockinette is applied under the cast during the application to provide smooth edges.

A plaster cast must be kept clean and dry. Moisture may soften the plaster and cause the cast to crack. A cast around the genital area can be protected from urine and stool by tucking plastic inside the cast and taping it to the outside. If this procedure is done, the skin beneath the plastic must be checked regularly for evidence of irritation or maceration. Using powder under the cast should be avoided because moisture from the patient's body may cause the powder to clump, which results in pressure against the skin. Cleaning a plaster cast is difficult, but small stains on the outside of the cast can be removed by gently rubbing it with

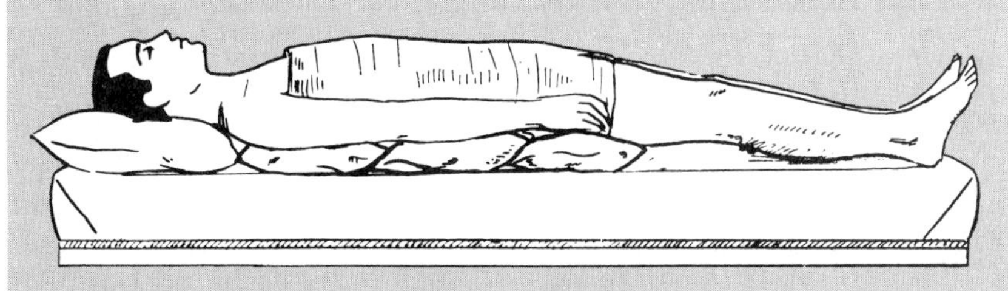

Figure 32-4 Placement of pillows to receive patient in wet body cast.

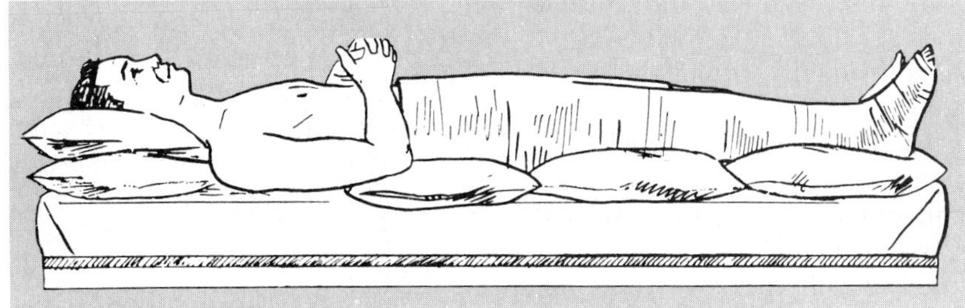

Figure 32-5 Placement of pillows to receive patient in wet hip spica cast.

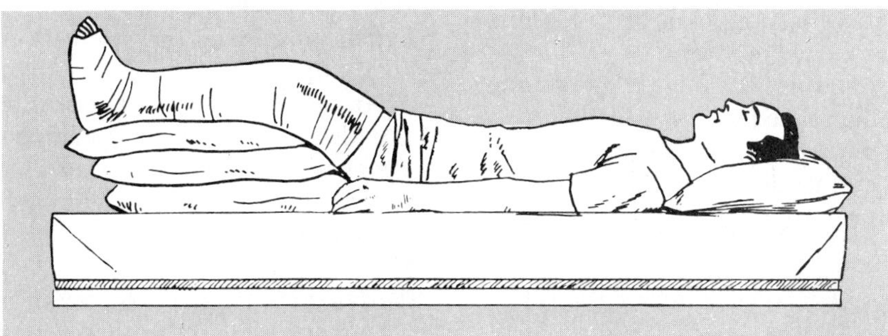

Figure 32-6 Placement of pillows to support extremity in long leg cast.

scouring powder that is on a slightly dampened cloth. Rubbing baby powder on a cast whitens it and gives it a pleasant smell. Spraying a cast with a plastic coating or painting it with white shoe polish is generally not recommended because such steps prevent the cast from "breathing." Bathing with a cast is possible if the cast is not submerged and if it is covered with a leakproof plastic bag such as a trash bag.

Fiberglass is the newest type of casting material that is used instead of plaster. A fiberglass cast is lighter and stronger than a traditional plaster cast and is also water-resistant and more durable. The fiberglass reaches full strength only minutes after it is applied. Fiberglass is also more expensive and is used for casts that do not require frequent changing.

Performing regular neurovascular assessments on all patients who have casts is a critical nursing function (Box 32-2). During the neurovascular assessment, the nurse should feel the entire cast for excessive local warmth and should sniff it for any foul odor. These signs, along with the patient's description of a localized burning sensation, signal the presence of tissue necrosis as a result of localized cast pressure. When a cast is applied, bony prominences and areas with nerves close to the skin are usually well padded. However, these sites are particularly susceptible to cast pressure, local necrosis, or neurovascular impairment. In the arm, susceptible sites are located at the condyles

BOX 32-2

Nursing Process

THE PATIENT WITH A CAST

ASSESSMENT

Neurovascular assessment of affected extremity
Skin assessment
Pain/comfort
Elimination patterns
Mobility
Self-concept/role disturbance
Home maintenance

NURSING DIAGNOSES

Pain related to bone displacement and muscle spasm
Constipation related to inactivity and altered position for elimination
Diversional activity deficit related to restrictions imposed by cast
Impaired home maintenance management related to restrictions on activity
Risk for injury related to falls, neurovascular impairment
Knowledge deficit related to diet to promote bone healing and correct use of ambulatory assistive devices
Impaired physical mobility related to cast
Altered nutrition: risk for more than body requirements related to reduced activity
Self-care deficit in feeding, bathing/hygiene, and dressing/grooming related to cast
Actual or risk for impairment of skin integrity related to trauma, cast irritation, or immobility
Altered tissue perfusion related to edema and cast constriction
Altered respiratory function related to imposed immobility or restricted respiratory movement secondary to body cast
Personal identity disturbance related to fracture

NURSING INTERVENTIONS

While plaster cast dries
Place patient on firm mattress.
Handle cast with palms of hands.
Explain to patient that he or she will feel heat as the cast dries.
Do not cover cast until it is completely dry.
Do not speed drying with heat or lamps; the cast may dry on the outside but remain weak on the inside and crack.
Elevate extremity on plastic-covered pillows, or support curves of body cast with small pillows.
Avoid weight bearing on walking leg cast for 48 hours.
When cast is dry
Attend to all complaints of pain, which may signal impending complications; do not medicate for pain until cause of pain is clearly identified.
Observe for signs of pressure such as pain, burning, and odor.
Check circulation; observe for pain, numbness, tingling, edema, color, blanching and capillary refill, skin temperature, inability to move fingers or toes, and presence and rate of pulse; compare these signs to the other extremity.
Use plastic sheeting to protect a cast in the perineal area from soiling.
Cleanse cast with an almost-dry cloth and abrasive soap or cleanser; whiten and freshen it by rubbing in baby powder.
Pull stockinette up and over edge of cast.
Cover edge of cast with adhesive tape petals.
Inspect skin under and at edge of cast for irritation.
Instruct patient not to insert wire hangers, knitting needles, or other sharp instruments under cast to scratch skin.
Assist patient with isometric exercises of affected extremities.
In addition to isometric exercises, actively exercise unaffected joints.
Allow patient to verbalize feelings about fracture, cast, and alterations in role performance and activity.
When cast is removed
Explain to patient that the cast cutter vibrates and cannot cut or injure skin.
After cast is removed, support affected body part with pillows in same position as when the part was in the cast.
Explain how affected extremity will appear when cast is removed.
Move extremity gently.
Wash skin with soap and water, followed by a gentle massage with lanolin or baby oil.
Assist patient in performing prescribed muscle-strengthening exercises.
If lower extremity is involved, instruct patient to elevate foot when sitting to prevent edema; apply an elastic bandage or elastic stocking as ordered to provide support; reinforce physician's instructions about weight bearing, which is usually limited after removal of leg cast.

EVALUATION OF EXPECTED OUTCOMES

Knows rationale for cast application
Cast integrity maintained
Neurocirculatory status normal
Cares for cast and observes condition of skin and extremities
Verbalizes feelings about altered self-concept and role performance
Identifies appropriate accommodations for self-care and home maintenance

and olecranon processes of the elbow and at the radial and ulnar styloids. In the leg, these sites are located at the popliteal space, the head of the fibula, the lateral aspect of the knee, the lateral and medial malleoli, and the heel. Specific measures to relieve circulatory impairment and localized pressure include splitting the cast lengthwise or cutting a window over the area of pressure. To accomplish these procedures, an oscillating saw (cast cutter) is used by the physician. The patient should be assured that the saw vibrates to cut the cast and is not a sharp blade that can cut into the skin.

A cast should also be observed for external bloody drainage, which may be expected with certain types of open reduction procedures. The area of drainage should be circled, dated, and timed on the cast with a permanent marker (not red ink); and its progression should be monitored, recorded, and reported. Because drainage may occur in the direction of gravity, careful examination of the underside of the cast is essential, even when the site of the incision is on the anterior surface of the extremity. The nurse should monitor the extremity carefully for other indicators of blood loss and tissue damage, because evidence of bleeding on the cast and development of odor from necrotic tissue may not occur until after considerable blood or tissue has been lost.

Skin care of the entire body and of areas that are close to the cast is important because casts can be heavy and patients may have difficulty moving in bed. Regular inspection of areas that usually rest on the bed is vital. Patients need assistance in regular turning and should be positioned in good body alignment with firm, supportive pillows. Itching under the cast as the wound heals is usually inevitable and is probably the patient's greatest annoyance. Little can be done to alleviate the itching unless a piece of gauze that runs the length of the cast and that the patient can pull back and forth was inserted at the time of application. Patients should be cautioned against using knitting needles, wire hangers, or foreign objects to scratch under the cast.

Hip spica and body casts

Hip spica and body casts are large, cumbersome casts (Figure 32-7). They are worn for long periods (5 months or longer) and require special techniques for turning and caring for the patient. These casts surround the entire trunk and may make the patient claustrophobic. The hip spica cast begins below the axilla and extends the entire length of one or both legs. It is applied to immobilize hip fusions, congenital hip dislocations, or fractures of the hip and femur. The body cast extends from the neck or upper chest to the groin or thigh. It is applied to immobilize spinal fractures, to protect the patient after spinal surgery, and to treat scoliosis. Confinement in these casts can be very frightening, and the patient must adjust to being confined within the cast. The patient may need to eat smaller or more frequent portions of food to be comfortable. A cast that is too tight can cause respiratory complications if the lungs cannot expand fully. The patient should be taught breathing exercises to prevent complications such as atelectasis while in the cast. The most serious complication of a tight cast is the development of "cast syndrome," which occurs when the superior mesenteric artery presses on or obstructs part of the duodenum. Symptoms of nausea, vomiting, abdominal pain, or intestinal obstruction require removal of the cast to alleviate the condition. Body casts generally have a window placed over the

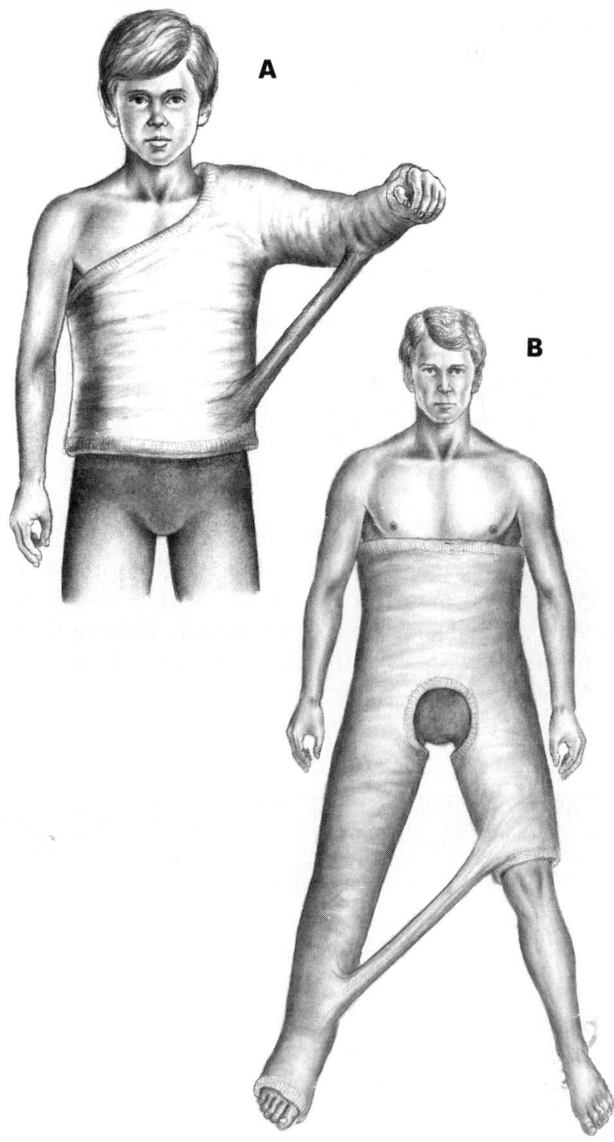

Figure 32-7 Spica casts. **A,** Shoulder spica. **B,** One and one-half leg-hip spica. (From Mourad LA: *Orthopedic disorders*, St Louis, 1991, Mosby.)

diaphragm to allow for expansion of the lungs and to prevent the development of cast syndrome.

Cast removal

When a cast is removed, the extremity should be moved carefully and supported at the joints. If the patient has been in a cast for a long time, some decalcification has occurred, and a spontaneous fracture is always a possibility. (A spontaneous fracture occurs when a bone breaks without any trauma, such as a blow or fall.) The patient may experience some discomfort once the external support has been removed. The patient should be told that the appearance of the casted limb will be different from the unaffected limb. The skin should be cleansed gently to remove the dead skin. Exercises to restore strength and mobility are begun. Weight bearing may be restricted until total bone healing has taken place.

THE PATIENT WITH AN ORTHOPEDIC DEVICE

Traction

Traction means "pulling." When traction is applied to a lower extremity because of a broken bone, the two ends of the bone are pulled into place (correct alignment). To relax or "stretch" the muscles of the affected extremity and allow the bone fragments to be brought into correct alignment, the force of the traction must be stronger than the force of the muscle contraction of the affected extremity. The physician decides on the type of traction, its placement, and the weight applied to achieve the desired results. When applied correctly, traction will be equal to countertraction. **Countertraction** is applied either by the patient's own body weight or by other weights or devices.

NURSE ALERT

Check that the weights are hanging free and not resting on the bed or the floor. Make sure that the knots are secure. Be sure that the patient is positioned properly and not pulled to the end of the bed where the traction is attached.

Traction may be applied to any of the extremities, the cervical area, or the pelvic region. *Cervical traction* may be needed when there has been severe injury to the cervical vertebrae or spinal cord (Figure 32-8). *Pelvic traction* may be used to relieve pain from injury of the lower back, often in the lumbar region (Figure 32-9). The purpose of traction may be to relieve muscle spasm, which often occurs as a result of disease or injury. For patients with certain types of fractures, traction may be necessary to keep bones in place while healing of the bones and soft tissue occurs. Traction may also be used to reduce dislocations or to correct or relieve contractures.

Traction may be applied as *skin traction,* in which some material with an adhesive surface is applied directly onto clean, dry skin; or as skeletal traction, in which various devices such as pins or wires are surgically placed through a bone. For cervical traction, tongs or pins, such as in the halo ring, are placed against the outer table of the skull.

NURSE ALERT

Monitor the skeletal pin sites for signs of infection. Perform pin care at least once daily. Occasionally patients are placed in balanced suspension with a splint. This type of traction is generally used to maintain an extremity in a specific position after surgery and may not involve skin or skeletal traction. In all types of traction, ropes, pulleys, weights, and countertraction are used.

Among the commonly used types of traction is *Buck's extension,* which is a form of running skin traction that is applied to the lower extremities (Figure 32-10). Adhesive material is attached to the skin at a point one inch above the malleolus and runs the length of the limb. The adhesive material is attached to a footplate, which is attached to a rope. The rope is placed over a pulley at the foot of the bed, and the desired weight is attached at the end. This is a simple type of traction and can be adapted for home use. Buck's extension cannot be used if there is an open wound in the area to be covered by the adhesive or if the patient is allergic to the adhesive material.

An innovation in the application of Buck's extension has been developed by the DePuy Company. The usual adhesive straps wrapped with Ace bandages are replaced with a foam rubber boot that is secured with a Velcro strap. This boot is commonly called a Buck's boot. The boot has a footplate at the bottom and comes in sizes to fit children and adults. The foam boot is ap-

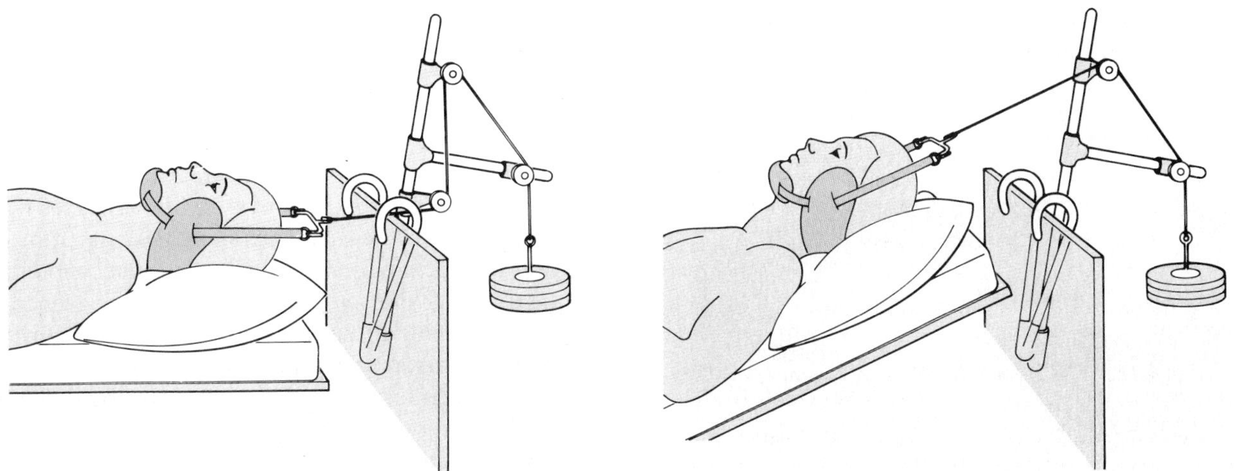

Figure 32-8 Cervical halter (skin traction). (From Beare PG, Myers JL: *Principles and practice of adult health nursing,* ed 2, St Louis, 1994, Mosby.)

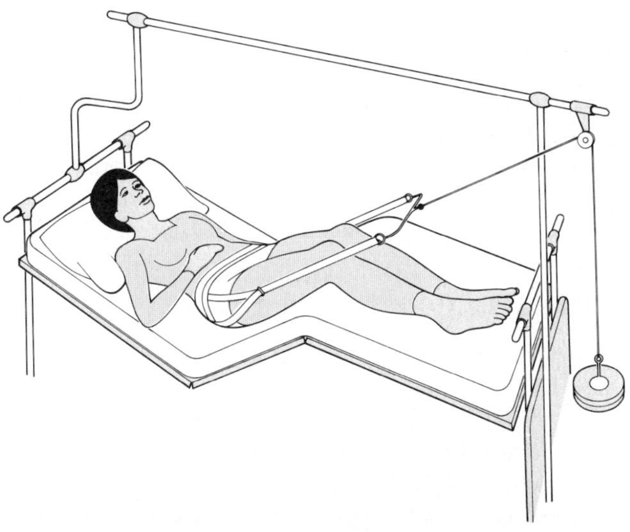

Figure 32-9 Pelvic belt traction (skin). (From Beare PG, Myers JL: *Principles and practice of adult health nursing,* ed 2, St Louis, 1994, Mosby.)

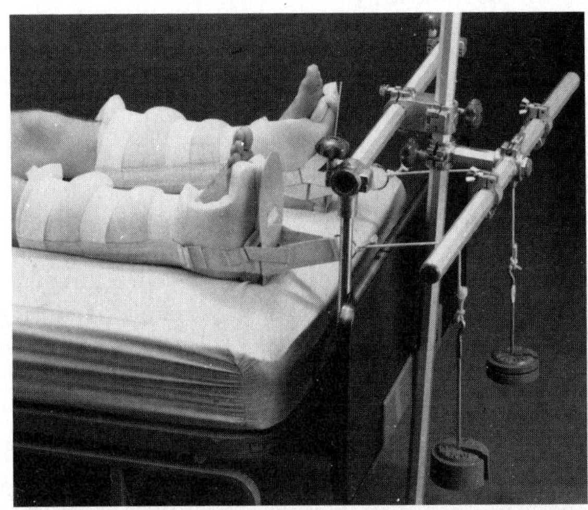

Figure 32-10 Buck's extension. Heel is supported off of bed to prevent pressure on heel. Weight hangs free of bed and floor. Foot is well away from footboard of bed. The limb should lie parallel to the bed unless prevented as in this case by a slight knee flexion contracture. (From Thompson JM and others: *Mosby's clinical nursing,* ed 3, St Louis, 1993, Mosby.)

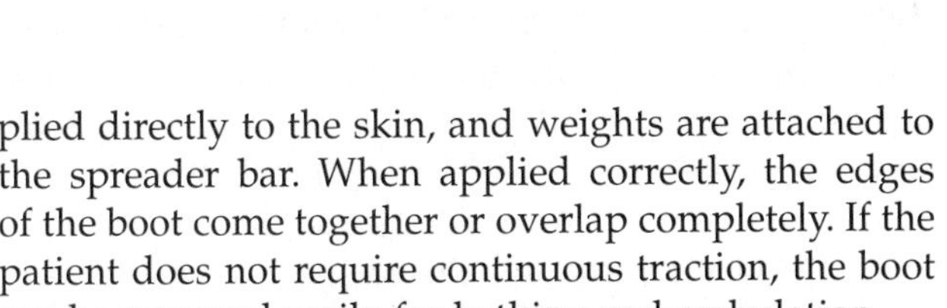

plied directly to the skin, and weights are attached to the spreader bar. When applied correctly, the edges of the boot come together or overlap completely. If the patient does not require continuous traction, the boot can be removed easily for bathing and ambulation.

Regardless of the materials and method used to apply Buck's extension, the nursing care of the patient's extremity is the same. Impaired circulation resulting from compression of the dorsalis pedis artery must be prevented. Decreased circulation to this area can result in ischemia (insufficient blood supply), which causes paralysis. The bony prominence of the foot and ankle must be observed for evidence of strap pressure, and cotton or felt should be used to protect the Achilles tendon, which is at the back of the ankle, from irritation.

The upper part of the calf should also be examined closely. The peroneal nerve lies close to the surface in this area, and compression against the bone can result in paralysis, plantar flexion (foot drop), and inversion of the foot. The area should be well padded before the tape is applied, and the foot should be observed daily

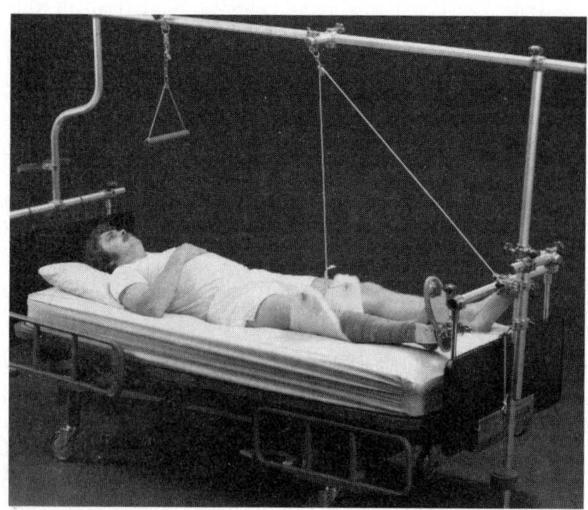

Figure 32-11 Balanced traction (Russell traction). Hip is slightly flexed. Pillows may be used under lower leg to provide support and keep the heel free of bed. (From Thompson JM and others: *Mosby's clinical nursing*, ed 3, St Louis, 1993, Mosby.)

for the tendency to turn inward toward the midline of the body. Any complaints of burning or pain under the tape should be reported immediately.

Balanced traction (Russell traction) consists of skin traction, often Buck's extension, as well as a sling under the knee that is attached to ropes and pulleys to provide suspension (Figure 32-11). The rope is brought overhead to a pulley and then down to a pulley at the foot of the bed. The same rope is brought back to a pulley on the footplate of Buck's extension and then back over the foot of the bed to a fourth pulley before dropping to the attached weight. This system of pulleys creates running traction plus a balanced traction or countertraction and may be used in fractures of the femur or hip. Countertraction is provided by elevating the foot of the bed.

Firm pillows should support the entire thigh and calf to maintain a 20-degree angle between the bed and the hip and to leave the heel free of the bed. The popliteal space under the sling should be examined often for irritation. A piece of felt placed in the sling may prevent wrinkling and reduce pressure areas. Because the affected limb is suspended above rather than resting on the bed, movement does not alter the position of the traction. The suspension apparatus takes up any slack in the traction caused by movement, and the line of the traction remains unchanged. This suspension provides greater freedom of movement for the patient and greater ease for the nurse who is providing care.

A *Thomas splint*, either half ring or full ring, is often used in another type of suspension traction (Figure 32-12). This type of traction is used preoperatively to stabilize the fracture until surgery. When the half-ring splint is used, the half ring is positioned over the anterior aspect of the thigh. Proper weights and adequate countertraction prevent the half ring from causing pressure in the groin and on the anterior aspect of the thigh. The full ring of a Thomas splint is covered with smooth, moisture-resistant leather. Pressure from the ring on the adductor and ischial area must be avoided at all times. A *Pearson attachment* can be fastened to a Thomas splint to support the leg down from the knee. The Pearson attachment usually is horizontal to and just high enough to swing clear of the bed. The patient's knee should correspond with the point where the Pearson attachment is fastened to the splint. The limb is usually held in a neutral position or in slight internal rotation and abduction. The patient must be positioned straight in bed because traction is lost if the patient lies diagonally. The patient in suspension traction may turn toward the limb in traction.

Skeletal traction

Traction can be applied directly to the bone by surgically inserting a pin or wire into the bone. The *Steinmann pin* and *Kirschner wire* are most commonly used. Weights are attached to the pin or wire while the patient is placed in suspension traction (Figure 32-13A).

Cervical traction

Cervical traction is a form of skeletal traction that is used to immobilize the cervical and upper thoracic spine. Tongs or a halo ring containing metal pins are placed against the patient's skull, and traction is applied. When tongs are used, the points of the tongs either rest against the skull or pierce it slightly (Figure 32-13B). With the halo ring, the pins are placed approximately .05 mm into the skull. Insertion of pins is generally performed with a local anesthetic.

The advantage of halo traction is that it can be attached to a rigid vest, which allows the patient to sit upright and to ambulate (see Figure 32-3C). However, caution must be used when the patient is upright because peripheral vision is restricted and the patient's balance is affected by the weight of the halo vest, which is approximately 7 pounds (Maher and others, 1994; Mikulaninec, 1992; Smeltzer, Bare, 1992).

Whenever skeletal traction is used, care of the pin or wire insertion site is required. Aseptic technique must be used to prevent infection, which can be severe if bacteria enters the wound and infects the underlying bone. Pin care consists of cleaning the surrounding area with sterile solution (usually normal saline) and drying it thoroughly. Evidence of redness, inflamma-

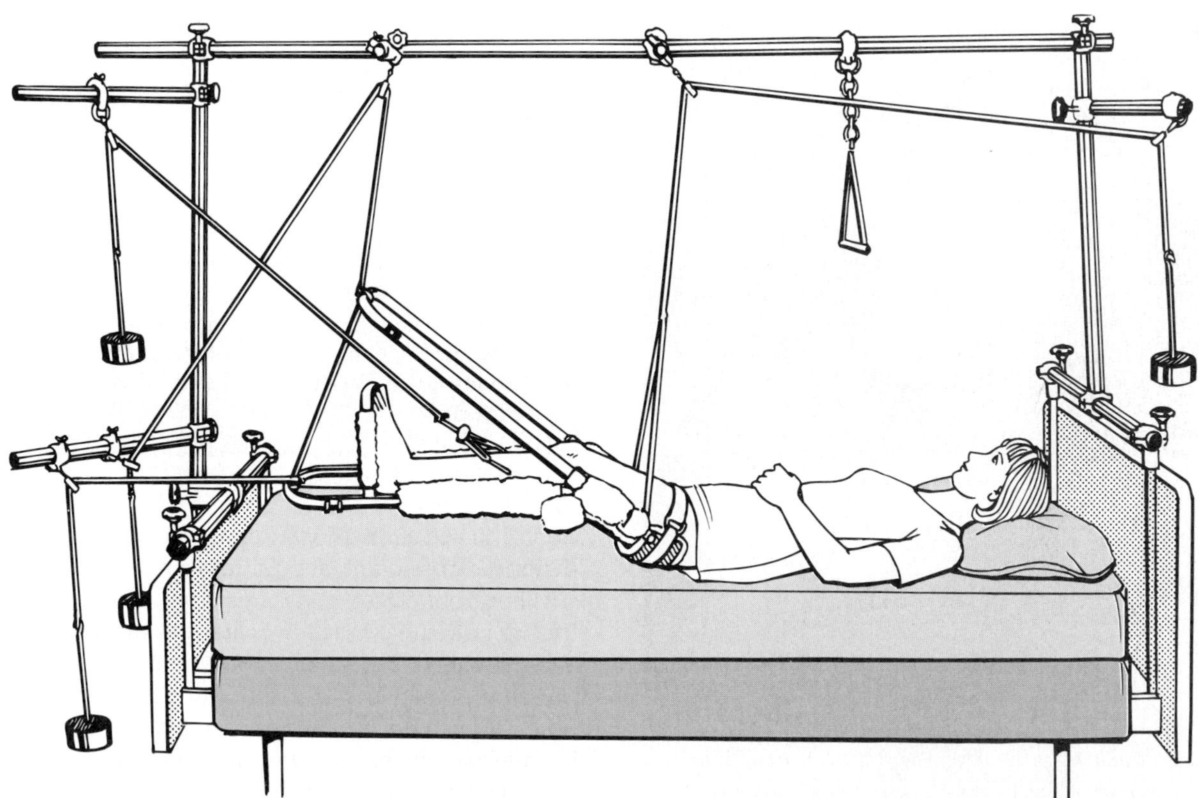

Figure 32-12 Balanced suspension with Thomas' splint and Pearson attachment. This apparatus can be used alone, or, as in this case, with skeletal traction. (From Phipps WJ and others: *Medical-surgical nursing: concepts and clinical practice,* ed 5, St Louis, 1995, Mosby.)

tion, or drainage from the pin site should be reported to the physician.

Pelvic traction

Pelvic traction is applied by using a canvas girdle that fits snugly over the crests of the ilia and the pelvis (see Figure 32-9). On either side are webbing straps that are joined to form one strap on each side at approximately midthigh. These straps are attached to ropes and weights. Light weights are applied at first and gradually increased. The iliac crests must be examined often for pressure, and padding may be necessary for thin patients.

Nursing intervention

The nurse is responsible for making sure that the traction is set up properly. Many hospitals have personnel who are trained and responsible for setting up the type of traction ordered by the physician. If such persons are not available, the nurse assumes responsibility for constructing the traction. The hospital procedure manual can be used as a reference for traction construction. The nurse is responsible for monitoring the traction equipment for effectiveness (e.g., the weights are not resting on the floor) and safety (e.g., the knots are tight and taped).

In many instances the patient is required to lie flat in bed and may not be permitted to sit up or to turn fully on either side. The nurse caring for patients in traction must be familiar with the amount of movement that the physician allows.

The skin around the edge of the adhesive tape must be observed for irritation or abrasion. If the tape seems to be pulling or loosening, it must be reinforced or replaced. Neurovascular assessment of the extremities should be performed several times a day. The skin over the ankles and the heel must be watched for pressure areas and irritation.

The patient's position and body alignment in bed, as well as the avoidance of internal or external rotation of the extremities, are extremely important. The patient should be positioned in good alignment at all times. The traction, height of backrest, knee elevator, and elevating blocks should not be changed unless

A

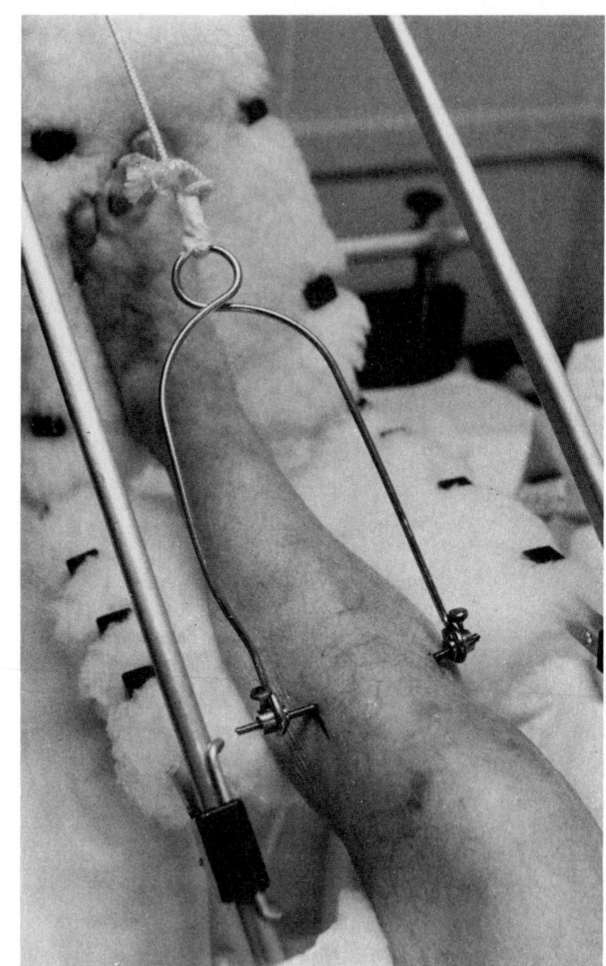

B

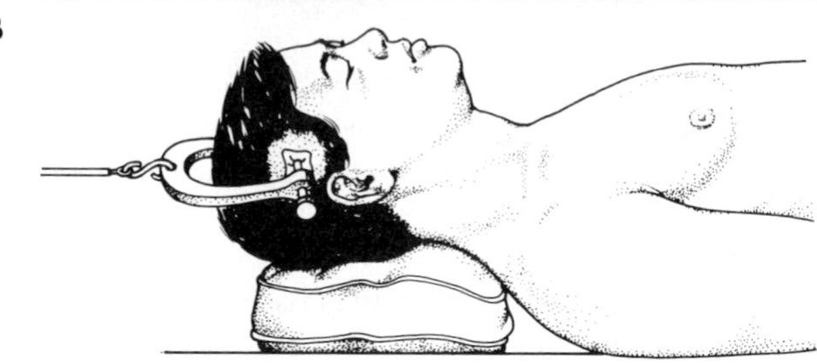

Figure 32-13 **A,** Tibial pin traction with Steinmann pin used in treatment of a distal femoral fracture. The bow attached to the pin provides a place of attachment for the rope that holds the traction weights. The pull exerted by the weight keeps the fracture fragments aligned. Pin sites must be inspected at least daily to detect signs of pin reaction or infection. **B,** Gardner-Wells tongs. (From Beare PG, Myers JL: *Principles and practice of adult health nursing,* ed 2, St Louis, 1994, Mosby.)

ordered by the physician. Although the patient usually is turned toward the affected side, specific turning instructions should be obtained from the physician before a regular turning schedule is begun. The skin beneath and around the traction splint or sling should be observed often for signs of pressure and irritation.

OLDER ADULT CONSIDERATIONS

Older adults with fractures have special needs that must be considered. The older adult's skin is more susceptible to skin irritation from traction or casts. The older adult has an increased need for position changes and skin care as a result of poor skin turgor, decreased mobility, and alterations in activity and in nutrition. The older adult must be monitored carefully to prevent any damage. Older adults may have chronic musculoskeletal disorders such as gout or osteoarthritis.

In addition, the traction weights should hang free of the frame or bed and should never rest on the floor.

When giving care, several persons may be needed to lift the patient so that his or her back can be washed and massaged. The sacral area should be inspected for pressure points. The area should be massaged several times a day, which may be accomplished without lifting the patient by running a hand under his or her back. The bottom of the bed is changed from the unaffected side, or top to bottom, and small blankets, sheets, or split linen may be used to cover the patient when large ones interfere with the placement of ropes or mechanical devices.

An orthopedic bedpan and female urinal may be desirable for bowel and bladder elimination. When a large pan is needed, as in the case of an enema, a plastic-covered pillow should be placed lengthwise along the patient's back when he or she is lifted onto the pan. An overhead trapeze should be provided, which allows patients to assist in lifting by lifting their hips.

Good oral care and a diet that is high in calcium, protein, iron, and vitamins are important. Foods high in roughage may help prevent constipation. Active and isometric exercises help prevent osteoporosis in the immobilized patient. Osteoporosis occurs when calcium leaves the bone of the immobilized patient. As it leaves the bone, it enters the serum and causes elevated levels of serum calcium. These high serum levels produce an alkaline urine, which can lead to the formation of urinary calculi. Fluids should be forced to help prevent this complication. The patient also should be encouraged to cough, deep breathe, and actively exercise the unaffected extremities. The affected extremity should not be exercised unless specifically ordered by the physician (Box 32-3).

Several new beds have been designed for the management of immobilized patients. The mattresses are filled with water, air, or air that is forced through sili-

BOX 32-3 **Nursing Process**

THE PATIENT IN TRACTION

ASSESSMENT

Neurovascular status
Body alignment
Traction apparatus
Skin assessment
Pain assessment
Need for diversional activities
Self concept/role alteration
Home maintenance
Elimination needs
Signs and symptoms of infection

NURSING DIAGNOSES

Pain related to bone displacement, muscle spasm, and tissue trauma
Constipation related to inactivity and altered position for elimination
Diversional activity deficit related to restrictions imposed by traction
Impaired home maintenance management related to hospitalization
Risk for injury related to accidental disturbance of line of pull and weight of traction
Knowledge deficit related to diet to promote healing and prevent urolithiasis and to exercises to promote circulation and bone healing
Impaired physical mobility related to traction
Altered nutrition: risk for more than body requirements related to decreased activity
Self-care deficit: feeding, bathing/hygiene, dressing/grooming, and toileting related to traction
Actual or risk for impaired skin integrity related to trauma, skin or skeletal traction, or immobility
Altered tissue perfusion related to edema

NURSING INTERVENTIONS

Keep patient in proper alignment.
Never change heights of backrest, knee elevators, or elevating blocks unless ordered by physician.
Never remove traction unless ordered by physician.
Place patient on firm mattress (use bedboards if needed).
Ensure that ropes and pulleys are in straight alignment with fracture site.
Check equipment often to ensure that ropes are not frayed, that the ropes are unobstructed and move freely in pulley grooves, that the knots are tied securely, and that the weights hang freely.
Weight applied in skin traction should not exceed tolerance of skin; the condition of the skin must be inspected at least every 2 hours.
Check pin or wire insertion site often when skeletal traction is used; be alert for odors, signs of local inflammation, or other evidence of osteomyelitis.
Check skin at least every 2 hours for evidence of pressure or friction over bony prominences.
Encourage active motion and exercise of unaffected joints.
Check for circulatory impairment (e.g., numbness, cyanosis, edema, color, and pain).
Encourage self-help and independence within limitations of traction.
Obtain specific orders on how patient can move; turning is not allowed with running traction; slight turning, usually to the affected side, is allowed with balanced suspension.

EVALUATION OF EXPECTED OUTCOMES

Knows rationale for traction and observes condition of skin and extremities
Traction alignment maintained
Neurocirculatory status normal
Elimination needs met
Performs exercises properly as ordered
No respiratory complications occur
Verbalizes that comfort needs are met
Verbalizes feelings about immobility, self-concept, and altered role performance
Assists with as much self-care as possible

cone beads. These beds help the patient move, yet they minimize the potential for constant pressure against skin and bony prominences. *Kinetic beds* also are available and provide constant side-to-side movement of the patient while also maintaining proper alignment of fractures in the thorax, pelvis, spine, or extremities. Each type of bed has distinct advantages and certain limitations. Because each type is expensive, the potential benefit to the patient should be evaluated carefully. A social worker should be contacted to help determine whether the patient's medical insurance will cover the cost of the bed. Whenever possible, the patient and family should participate in the final decision about the use of the bed.

PATIENT/FAMILY TEACHING

The patient in traction

The patient and family should be taught proper positioning and alignment of the affected body part. Diet and elimination needs for immobility and healing should be discussed. Effective pain relief measures such as ice packs, medications, diversional activities, and positioning of patient and weights should be identified for the patient and family.

Splints

Splints are used to support or immobilize an area of the body in a specific position. They are made of a variety of materials, such as plywood, lightweight aluminum, plastic, or casting materials. Plywood splints generally are used for first aid only. A tongue blade can be used to treat a fractured finger or an injury in which immobilization of the finger is desired. Aluminum splints are made for right or left extremities and support the foot or thumb. Many premolded splints are available for upper and lower extremities and are held in place by Velcro straps. Premolded splints are used for nondisplaced or incomplete fractures (such as a greenstick) and sprains. Other splints may be held in place by elastic bandages or gauze and have the advantage of allowing for the application of wet dressings to care for ulcers or other superficial injuries. These adjustable splints are also used when there is soft tissue swelling at the fracture site. Plaster or fiberglass casts are occasionally bivalved (cut in two along both sides) and made into removable shells. This allows access to the affected area while also maintaining mobilization. When splints of any type are used, the nurse must observe the skin for pressure areas and must use care when handling the extremity involved. The patient and family must be taught how to care for the cast and how to prevent and monitor for complications from the fracture and the cast.

Other Orthopedic Devices

External fixation devices are used to reduce complex fractures that have bone fragments that need stabilization. These devices can be used on extremities and pelvic fractures (Figure 32-14). Preoperative and postoperative care is the same as for internal fixation of fractures, with frequent and accurate neurovascular assessments of the affected extremity. Before discharge, the patient and family need to be taught pin care, as well as the signs and symptoms of infection at the sites.

Plastic or rubber heels may be incorporated into a cast to allow the patient to walk on the extremity. Sometimes a *walking iron,* which extends into the cast, is used. Walking casts can be used with only certain types of fractures, and the orthopedic surgeon decides if such a cast can be used safely. The patient must always be cautioned against outward rotation of the foot when walking.

Various types of *collars* or *neck supports* are designed to immobilize the head and to take the weight of the head off the spine. Collars and neck supports generally are used temporarily while healing occurs and may not be required at night. *Corsets* and *back braces* are used to immobilize the spine and to prevent the patient from engaging in activities that would cause further harm to the spine. Braces may have steel supports in the back, and corsets usually lace in front. Patients are measured for the supports, which are made specifically for their needs. A cotton t-shirt is worn under the brace to prevent skin irritation and to absorb perspiration. The brace or corset should be put on patients while they are in a recumbent position before they arise in the morning.

Interventions

The treatment of patients with orthopedic conditions is considered a surgical specialty because many require minor or major surgical procedures. Most patients are cared for in an orthopedic or surgical service. Certain basic aspects of nursing care apply to most orthopedic patients, and many of these procedures have been referred to in this and other chapters.

All patients with fractures should have a firm mattress (or bedboards) and an overhead trapeze. Cast care is the same for all patients regardless of the location of the cast. Extreme care must be taken to protect devices such as traction equipment, splints, or tongs so that the corrective procedure is not jeopardized. Skin care is a must for orthopedic patients, and because many patients are hospitalized for several weeks, the nurse should remember that good personal hygiene includes care of the nails and hair. Because the immobilized patient may have problems with elimination, a diet high in roughage, as well as the use of mild laxatives or enemas, may be necessary. Adequate fluid intake must be ensured to promote bowel function and to prevent a urinary tract infection and the formation

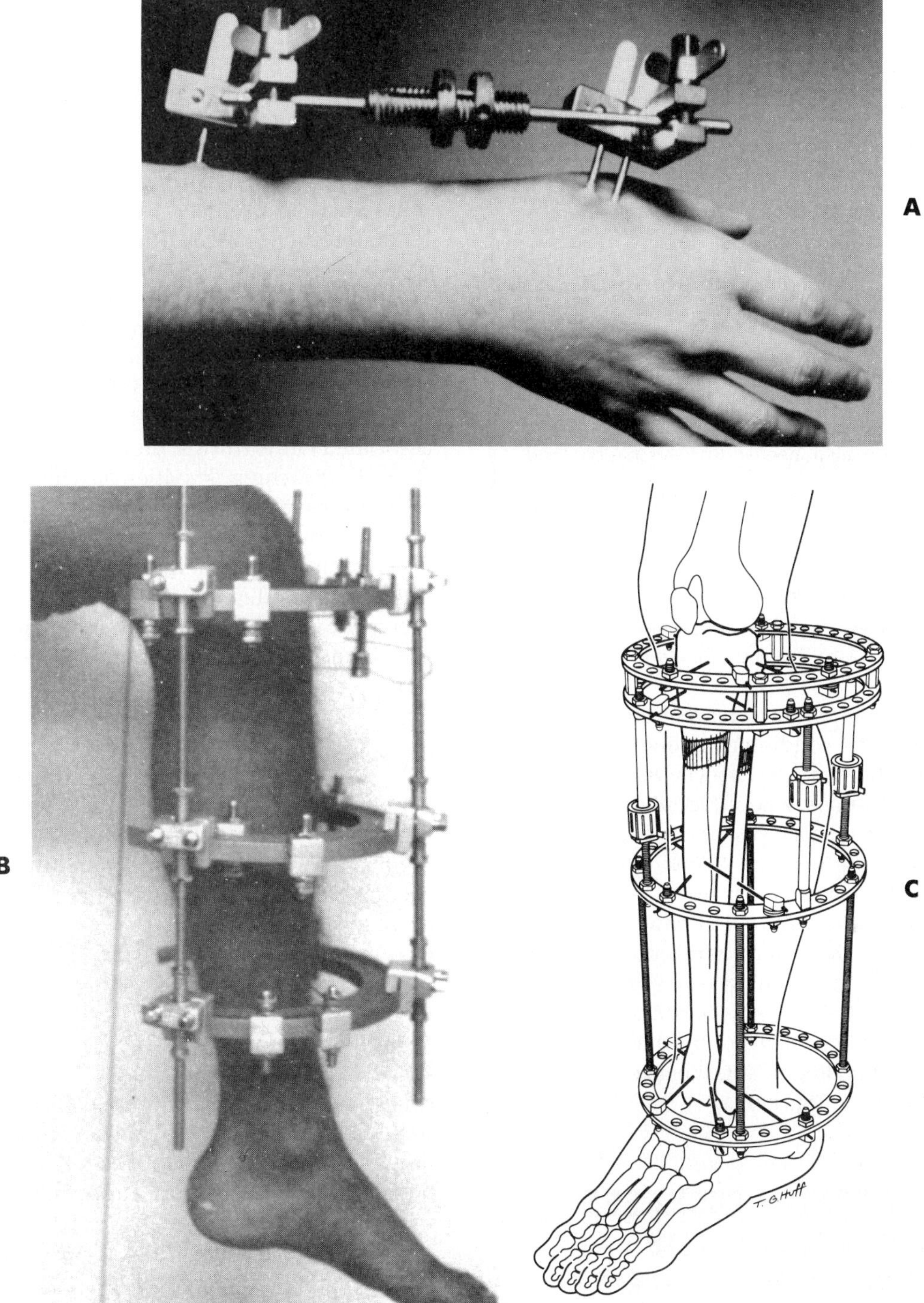

Figure 32-14 External fixation devices. **A,** Hoffman. **B,** Monticelli-Spinelli Circular Fixator. **C,** Ilizarov apparatus with corticotomies for lengthening lower leg. (From Thompson JM and others: *Mosby's clinical nursing,* ed 3, St Louis, 1993, Mosby.)

of urinary calculi (see Chapter 24). Isometric exercises slow the osteoporosis that accompanies immobility. Prescribed exercises should be carried out with the assistance of a physical therapist and members of the nursing staff. Maintaining muscle tone and function, as well as flexibility of unaffected joints, is important for preventing contractures and for fostering rehabilitation. Open surgery may be performed on bones, tendons, or muscles, and the immediate postoperative care is essentially the same as that for any surgical patient. All wounds must be protected from contamination.

PATIENT/FAMILY TEACHING

Patients with problems affecting mobility

Teaching needs vary according to the age of the patient and the particular problem that has occurred.
If there is a wound from trauma or surgery, signs and symptoms of infection need to be taught.
Knowledge of the medication regimen and pain relief techniques are also needed by the patient and family.
Ambulation techniques need to be discussed and demonstrated.
Ways to modify the patient's activities of daily living also need to be discussed.

One of the most important interventions for patients with musculoskeletal conditions involves the recognition and support of their psychosocial needs (Smeltzer, Bare, 1992). Individuals who suddenly are hospitalized as a result of injuries sustained during an accident, as well as those who are receiving medical care for chronic musculoskeletal disorders, are certain to have questions and concerns about how the injuries or illnesses will affect them and their families. In addition, patients who are elderly or who are hospitalized for long periods may show signs of confusion and disorientation. Consistent attention by the nurse to the patient's socialization and adaptation needs helps prevent or alleviate these concerns.

THE PATIENT WITH DISEASES AND DISORDERS OF THE MUSCULOSKELETAL SYSTEM

Arthritis

Arthritis belongs to a group of diseases commonly called *rheumatic disorders,* which involve inflammation of a joint. Although it is unknown exactly how many persons have some form of arthritis, it is the most crippling disease in the United States. Between one and three out of every 100 people are affected, and most of these people are between the ages of 20 and 40 (Black, Matassarin-Jacobs, 1993). Not all persons with arthritis are completely incapacitated. Many perform their daily activities, both at home and at work, with only varying degrees of discomfort. Many types of arthritis exist, but the most common are rheumatoid arthritis, rheumatoid spondylitis, and osteoarthritis (degenerative joint disease). Forms of arthritis often accompany other diseases such as psoriasis (see Chapter 31), rheumatic fever, infectious diseases (e.g., gonorrhea), and gout, which is a metabolic disease. In providing care and services for a patient who has arthritis, goals should be established, including medical and nursing care during the acute stages and long-range plans to maintain the patient in the best possible condition. Emphasis should be placed on preventing infectious diseases that may be associated with arthritis, preventing and correcting deformities, teaching activities of daily living, and providing a psychosocial environment in which the patient and family can comfortably accept and live with the chronic disability. To accomplish these goals, the physician, psychiatrist, psychologist, nurse, physical therapist, occupational therapist, religious counselor, social worker, vocational counselor, and public health nurse may need to be involved.

Rheumatoid arthritis

Rheumatoid arthritis is the most serious form of arthritis and leads to severe crippling. The disease may occur at any age but most commonly affects persons between ages 20 and 45. Rheumatoid arthritis in infants and children is a chronic systemic disease that affects many organs and tissues, including the joints. Children between 2 and 4 years of age are most commonly affected.

Pathophysiology. Research has failed to find a specific cause of rheumatoid arthritis, but it is now considered to be an autoimmune disease. Most people with rheumatoid arthritis have an unusual antibody in their bloodstream, and it appears that they make antibodies against their own antibodies. An individual with this disease is believed to damage his or her own antibodies while defending against infection. These damaged antibodies are then interpreted by the body's defense system as foreign and are attacked, which causes the inflammatory response (Mudge-Grout, 1992). This theory would explain why patients with rheumatoid arthritis often have a history of some type of recent infection. The disease may develop insidiously, or it may have an acute onset. Remissions occur and symptoms subside, but subsequent attacks follow, and a chronic state slowly develops. The disease affects the joints and initially causes an inflammation of the joint membrane. As the disease progresses, granulation tissue fills the joint, and the normal joint cartilage is destroyed. The joint cavities fill with scar tissue and adhesions, which causes stiffness, pain, and complete immobility. Swan-neck deformities of the hands and fingers also occur.

Assessment. The early symptoms of rheumatoid arthritis are loss of weight; loss of appetite; muscle aches; malaise; fever; and swollen, painful joints. Complaints of joint stiffness, especially on rising in the morning, are common. During the early course of the disease, considerable muscle spasm occurs, and any effort to move the affected joints is painful. The diagnosis is established by a variety of findings. The rheumatoid factor (RF) titer is elevated, which indicates the presence of an abnormal serum protein concentration. The erythrocyte sedimentation rate is elevated, and x-ray films show progressive damage to the joints.

Intervention. The care of the patient with rheumatoid arthritis is directed toward maintaining function, relieving pain, and preventing deformities. One of the most distressing factors in the treatment of rheumatoid arthritis is that some patients obtain unprofessional advice in hopes of relieving their symptoms. As a result, they may wear copper bracelets, drink potions of vinegar and honey, wear beans or potatoes around their necks, or sit in uranium mines. Patients hear about these "cures" through well-meaning friends and relatives who may be acquainted with someone whose symptoms seemingly disappeared with similar therapy. Because the disease is characterized by alternating periods of exacerbation and remission, a patient who adopts quackery as treatment may experience a normal remission and attribute the improvement to the "cure." As a result, the supposed cure is believed to be valuable despite medical advice to the contrary. Patients should seek medical attention early so that pain and joint deformity can be minimized.

Rest is important during acute attacks, and the nurse should give special attention to good body alignment. The mattress should be firm to provide adequate support. The extremities should be straight without pillows under the knees, and the knee gatch on the bed should not be raised. A bed cradle should be used to keep bedclothing off painful joints. Sandbags or trochanter rolls should be used to prevent outward rotation of the extremities. The patient should be positioned so that the back is straight, and a small pillow should be placed under the head. Hip and knee flexion must be avoided. Some of the most severe joint deformities are caused by patients assuming a comfortably flexed position.

Ibuprofen is generally considered to be the drug of choice to decrease both pain and inflammation. It may be given in fairly large doses and should be taken with food to avoid gastric upset. Other antiinflammatory drugs may be tried if the ibuprofen is ineffective. Gold compounds are selected for some patients, usually those who are not responding to other forms of treatment. These medications are slow acting, and the patient must be watched carefully for side effects while receiving the drug. Adrenocorticoids (cortisone, prednisone, hydrocortisone) are given if more conservative treatment fails. These drugs may produce dramatic relief of symptoms but do not cure the disease. However, somewhat severe side effects can result, and once the medication is discontinued, the patient may have a full return of original symptoms. Usually the patient is maintained on the lowest dose of corticosteroids that will produce an improvement in the condition. Hydrocortisone acetate injected into the joints results in immediate relief of pain and a temporary halt to the destructive process, which usually lasts for several weeks (Table 32-1).

The use of heat is helpful in relieving pain and may include hot, moist packs; hot tub baths; electric blankets; heat cradles; paraffin baths; and whirlpool baths.

Once the acute stage is passed, a program of physical therapy must be established. A planned program of rest and activity is important. Active exercise should be a part of the therapeutic plan so that normal functioning of the joints is maintained. Exercises should be simple and may be taught by the nurse or physical therapist. No special diet is required for the patient with arthritis, but a well-balanced diet and adequate fluid intake should be encouraged. After recovery from acute attacks, the patient may return to work and should be encouraged to remain active. Many patients with rheumatoid arthritis remain independent and self-sufficient for 20 or 30 years.

PATIENT/FAMILY TEACHING

The patient with rheumatoid arthritis

The disease process and treatments need to be discussed with the patient and family.
Medication dosages, schedules, and side effects need to be discussed.
Comfort measures during exacerbation periods should be identified.
Ways to maintain function and independence should be demonstrated.
Emotional support for the patient and family will be necessary as they recognize that this form of arthritis is chronic and progressively debilitating.

TABLE 32-1

Pharmacology of Drugs Used in Mobility

Drug (Generic and Trade Name); Route and Dosage	Action/Indication	Common Side Effects and Nursing Considerations
ALLOPURINOL (Zyloprim) **ROUTE:** PO **DOSAGE:** 200-800 mg/day (doses > 300 mg should be divided in bid doses)	Used in the prevention and treatment of gouty arthritis; inhibits the production of uric acid	Rash; use cautiously in renal disease and dehydration
CALCIUM SALTS **ROUTE:** PO **DOSAGE:** 1-2 g/day	Used as an adjunct in the prevention of postmenopausal osteoporosis; used in the treatment and prevention of hypocalcemia associated with vitamin D deficiency	Constipation; contraindicated in hypercalcemia, renal calculi, and ventricular fibrillation; use with caution in renal, cardiac, and respiratory disease
COLCHICINE **ROUTE:** PO **DOSAGE:** In acute gouty arthritis 0.5-1.3 mg, then 0.5-0.65 mg q 1-2 hr until relief; prophylaxis of recurrent gouty arthritis 0.5-0.6 mg/day, 3-4 times/week, up to 1.8 mg/day	Antigout agent used in the treatment of acute attacks of gouty arthritis (large doses) and the prevention of recurrence (small doses)	Nausea, vomiting, and diarrhea; contraindicated in severe renal or GI disease; use with caution in elderly or debilitated patients
ERGOCALCIFEROL (Vitamin D_2) **ROUTE:** PO **DOSAGE:** Osteomalacia from anticonvulsants, 1000-4000 units/day; vitamin D deficiency 1000-2000 units/day initially, then 400 units/day maintenance; rickets 12,000-60,000 units/day (vitamin D resistant), 10,000-60,000 (vitamin D dependent)	Prophylaxis and treatment of vitamin D deficiency; also used in treatment of osteodystrophy, rickets, and osteolmalacia secondary to chronic anticonvulsant therapy	Contraindicated in hypercalcemia and vitamin D toxicity
HYDROCORTISONE (Solu-Cortef) **ROUTE:** PO, IV, IM **DOSAGE:** PO, 10-320 mg/day in 1-4 divided doses; IV, IM, 100-500 mg q 2-6 hr	Short-term management of a variety of inflammatory conditions	Depression, nausea, petechiae, decreased wound healing, decreased growth in children, adrenal suppression, hypokalemia, and sodium retention; do not discontinue abruptly; use lowest dose possible; use of this drug may mask signs of infection
IBUPROFEN (Motrin) **ROUTE:** PO **DOSAGE:** 1200-3200 mg/day in three or four divided doses	Used for rheumatoid arthritis, osteoarthritis, osteoporosis, osteitis deformans, osteomalacia, and epicondylitis	Gastrointestinal irritation, hypersensitivity rash, rash, and dermatitis; therapeutic response may occur in a few days to 2 weeks
INDOMETHACIN (Indocin) **ROUTE:** PO **DOSAGE:** Rheumatoid arthritis and osteoarthritis, 25-50 mg tid, not to exceed 200 mg/day; 75-150 mg/day in divided doses for bursitis; 50 mg tid for gout	Used for rheumatoid arthritis, osteoarthritis, osteoporosis, bursitis, gout, osteitis deformans, osteomalacia, and epicondylitis	Headache, drowsiness, psychic disturbances, dizziness, nausea, dyspepsia, vomiting, and constipation; contraindicated in active GI bleeding and ulcer disease

TABLE 32-1

Pharmacology of Drugs Used in Mobility—cont'd

Drug (Generic and Trade Name); Route and Dosage	Action/Indication	Common Side Effects and Nursing Considerations
NAPROXEN (Naprosyn, Anaprox) **ROUTE:** PO **DOSAGE:** Analgesic, 500 mg initially followed by 250 q 6-8 hr; antiinflammatory, 250-500 mg bid	Management of mild-to-moderate pain; management of inflammatory disorders, including rheumatoid arthritis and osteoarthritis	Headache, drowsiness, dizziness, nausea, dyspepsia, and constipation; contraindicated in active GI bleeding and ulcers
PROBENECID (Benemid) **ROUTE:** PO **DOSAGE:** 250 mg bid for 1 week, increase to 500 mg bid, then may increase by 500 mg/day q 4 weeks (not to exceed 3 g/day)	Used in prevention of gouty arthritis	Headache, nausea, vomiting, and diarrhea; contraindicated in high-dose salicylate therapy; use with caution in renal impairment
SALICYLATE (aspirin) **ROUTE:** PO, rectal **DOSAGE:** Analgesia, PO, rectal, 325-1000 mg every 4-6 hours; antiinflammatory, PO 1.3 g/daily in 2-4 divided doses	Used as mild analgesic and in the management of many inflammatory disorders	Dyspepsia, heartburn, epigastric distress, and GI bleeding; contraindicated if bleeding disorders present; use with caution in history of ulcers or GI bleeding; use with caution in severe renal or hepatic disease

Rheumatoid (ankylosing) spondylitis

Rheumatoid (ankylosing) spondylitis is an inflammation of the vertebrae and sacroiliac joints and may affect part or all of the spine and lead to complete rigidity. The rheumatoid process may cause the thoracic spine to bow outward (kyphosis). Treatment of the condition is similar to that for rheumatoid arthritis, except that the program of exercise is designed to prevent kyphosis. Exercises are planned to keep the spine straight and to maintain range of motion in the cervical spine. The patient should be positioned on a firm mattress and should not use a pillow.

Osteoarthritis (degenerative joint disease)

Osteoarthritis is the result of the normal wear and tear that is placed on joints over the years (Figure 32-15). The process may be hastened by obesity or joint trauma. It is the most common form of arthritis and begins to appear in persons who are past middle age. Most people have some degree of osteoarthritis by the time they reach 60 years of age. The disease damages the cartilage in the joints, but although pain and stiffness result, it usually does not cause crippling. Several factors contribute to development of osteoarthritis. Engaging in occupations in which prolonged strain is placed on joints, as well as obesity, poor posture, and injury to a joint can lead to early development of osteoarthritis. The joints most often affected are the spine, knees, fingers, and hips.

Treatment for osteoarthritis should include a reduction in weight (if obesity is present) and a regular program of exercise to maintain range of motion. Analgesics may be given three or four times daily to relieve pain. In patients with severe joint pain, hydrocortisone acetate may be injected into the synovial cavity and usually provides pain relief for several weeks. The patient should have a program of rest, and the joints should be protected from continuing wear and strain. The application of moist heat with baths, soaks, packs, or paraffin baths may provide temporary relief.

Surgical intervention for arthritis

A variety of surgical procedures are available to prevent progressive deformities, to relieve pain, to improve function, and to correct deformities that result from rheumatoid arthritis or osteoarthritis. Tendon transplants can be done to prevent the progressive deformity caused by muscle spasm. The excision of the synovial membrane of a joint **(synovectomy)** is helpful to maintain joint function in rheumatoid

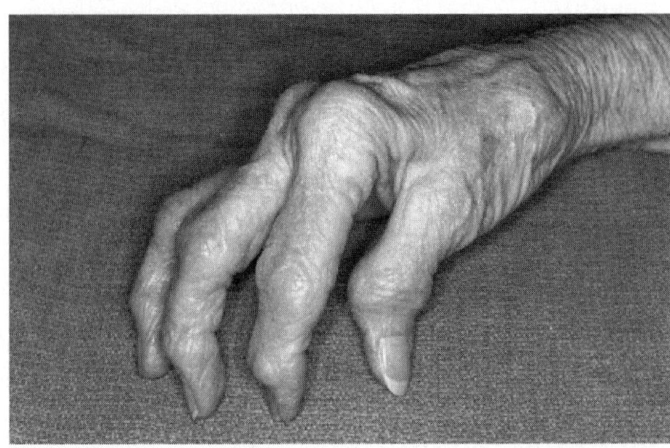

Figure 32-15 Osteoarthritis of hand. (Courtesy Michael Clement, MD, Mesa, Ariz.)

arthritis. An **osteotomy,** which is a cutting of bone to correct bone or joint deformities, may be performed to improve function or to relieve pain. Severe joint destruction may be treated with **arthrodesis,** which is a surgical fusion of the joint in a functional position. **Arthroplasty** involves plastic surgery on a diseased joint, such as the elbow, hip, knee, or shoulder, to increase mobility. Sometimes an arthroplasty involves removing a portion of the joint and replacing it with a metal or synthetic **prosthesis. Arthrotomy** is a broad term that refers to the surgical opening of a joint. *Arthroscopy* involves the introduction of an instrument or scope into a joint to examine it. Some surgical procedures can be performed through the arthroscope.

Total hip replacement

A hip arthroplasty is a common procedure that is performed when arthritis involves the head of the femur and the acetabulum. In this type of surgery a Vitallium cup is cemented into the arthritic acetabulum to receive the head of the femur. Many patients are candidates for total hip replacement, which involves removing and replacing the acetabulum and the femoral head. A white plastic cup is cemented in place to replace the damaged acetabulum. A stainless steel or Vitallium ball on a stem replaces the head of the femur. The stem is cemented into the femoral canal, and the new head fits precisely into the plastic acetabulum to provide friction-free movement in the joint. The cement is a soft, surgical bone cement that hardens quickly and stabilizes the prosthesis to prevent future erosion of the surrounding bone. If the patient experiences an adverse reaction to the cement, which is a remote possibility, the prosthesis must be surgically removed. Total hip replacement is performed for damage that results from trauma or congenital deformities, as well as for arthritis. The joint replacement may need to be repeated in 10 or 12 years if the prosthesis becomes too worn to be effective. Figure 32-16 shows examples of joint prostheses used in arthroplasty. Before surgery, the patient is taught to use the overhead trapeze to elevate the buttocks. The affected hip and groin are scrubbed twice daily with a surgical scrub to minimize the risk of postoperative infection. In addition to coughing and deep breathing, the patient is taught to perform isometric exercises of the quadriceps and gluteal muscles, to keep the toes pointed up, to flex the ankles often, and to flex and extend the knee of the unaffected extremity. These exercises are continued after surgery to improve circulation, prevent emboli, and reduce joint stiffness and muscle weakness. Thigh-high antiembolism stockings are applied before or during surgery. A hemovac is usually placed in the wound during surgery to provide closed wound suction. The patient is moved directly from the operating table to a bed to reduce the chance of dislocation during transfer at a later time. If traction is used, it is applied at this time.

After surgery, the affected leg must be maintained in abduction. Some surgeons apply traction, whereas others order the use of an abduction pillow between the legs. An *abduction pillow* is a large, hard, triangular pillow with Velcro straps on each side to attach to each leg. The straps must be fastened firmly while turning the patient to maintain the extremity in abduction. The patient may not be turned unless ordered by the physician. If turning is allowed, the patient is turned to the unaffected side, and additional pillows support the affected extremity in abduction.

After surgery, the affected extremity must be maintained in a position that will not dislocate the operative hip. The safest position depends on the position maintained during surgery. Two surgical positions are commonly used. One position is the anterior approach, in which the patient is supine and the operative hip is externally rotated and extended with the knee flexed. The other position is the posterolateral position, in which the patient lies in the lateral position with the operative hip internally rotated, adducted, and flexed. The operative hip is dislocated during surgery, and if the same position is repeated postoperatively, there is great danger of dislocating the hip prosthesis. Thus the safest position when the anterolateral position has been used is to maintain the hip in a flexed position with limited external rotation. The safest position for the patient who had a posterolateral approach is to maintain the hip in external rotation, abduction, and extension (Altizer, 1995).

If the hip is to be maintained in a flexed position with limited external rotation, pillows must be used to maintain position. If the affected leg must be maintained in abduction, the surgeon may apply traction. Other surgeons may order the use of an abduction pillow between the legs.

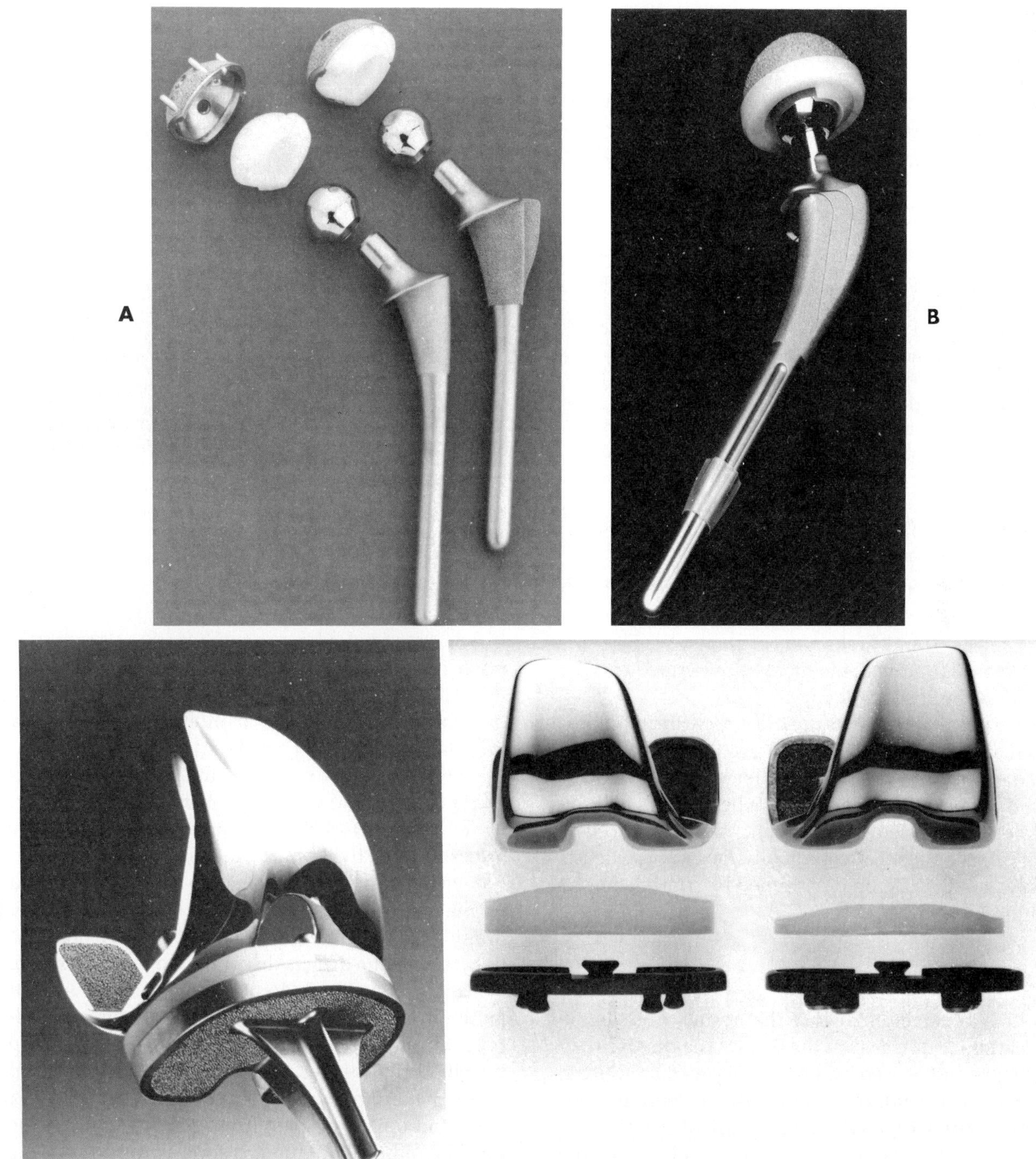

Figure 32-16 **A** and **B,** Total hip replacement prostheses. **C,** Total knee replacement prostheses. (**A,** Courtesy Zimmer, Warsaw, Ind. **B,** Courtesy Biomet, Warsaw, Ind. **C,** Courtesy Zimmer, Warsaw, Ind. From Mourad LA: *Orthopedic disorders,* St Louis, 1991, Mosby.)

The patient must be observed for phlebitis, urinary retention, infection, and circulation and sensation in the affected leg, as well as any adverse reaction to the cement. Some elevation in temperature is expected, but a fever that persists longer than 5 to 8 days indicates an infection. A plan of weight bearing and physical therapy is ordered by the physician, and some patients get out of bed very soon after surgery. Patients experience an immediate relief of joint pain after surgery and have relatively normal range of motion in the hip.

The patient must not sleep on the affected side for 2 months and should maintain the limb in extension and abduction when getting out of bed. Sitting on a high chair is allowed by the second or third day of the postoperative period. Extreme flexion of the hip, such as sitting in a low chair or stooping, must be avoided for several weeks to reduce the chance of dislocation. Exercises are performed while the patient is supine or standing (Maher and others, 1994). Because prosthetic devices for hip replacement are continually being de-

PATIENT/FAMILY TEACHING

The patient with a hip replacement

Signs and symptoms of postoperative complications should be reviewed with the patient and family.
Nutritional and elimination needs should be individualized for the patient.
Level of activity and exercises should be properly demonstrated by the patient.
Environmental modifications such as entrance ramps, removal of scatter rugs, and elevated commode seats at home should be discussed and adjusted before discharge if possible.
Wound care, activity levels, and medication schedules should be written and verbally reinforced.

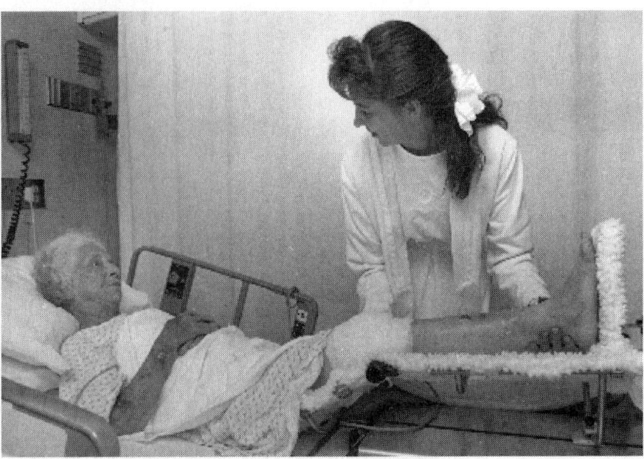

Figure 32-17 CPM machine (continuous passive motion therapy device). (From Elkin and others: *Nursing interventions and clinical studies,* St Louis, 1996, Mosby.)

veloped and improved, the therapy prescribed and the restrictions imposed will vary.

Total knee replacements are done for arthritic conditions that involve the knee, and procedures have also been developed to replace shoulder, elbow, and finger joints (Gregory, 1994; Maher and others, 1994). Following knee replacement, the extremity may be placed in a motorized splint that continually flexes and extends the knee to an angle predetermined by controls on the machine (Figure 32-17).

Gout (gouty arthritis)

Gout is a metabolic disease that results from an accumulation of uric acid in the blood. The disease may be primary and caused by a hereditary metabolic error, or it may be secondary to some other disease process and to certain drugs. The disease usually appears in middle life. It does not occur before puberty in the male or before menopause in the female. The disease almost exclusively attacks men (Wyngaarden and others, 1992). When the disease is primary, it takes approximately 20 years for sufficient urates to accumulate in the body before causing symptoms. However, when gout is the result of a negative response to drugs, its symptoms may develop rapidly over several days. Gouty arthritis can affect any joint in the body, but 20% of all first attacks occur in a joint of the great toe. First attacks may occur in other joints, but the great toe is involved in 80% of all persons with the disease (Figure 32-18). Typically the onset occurs at night, with excruciating pain, swelling, and inflammation in the affected joint. The pain may be of short duration and return at intervals, or it may be severe and continuous for 5 to 10 days. The patient may never have more than one attack throughout his or her entire life, or attacks may continue at intervals of months and gradually occur closer together.

The diagnosis is made on the basis of finding the blood level of uric acid above normal (normal range is 2.5 to 8 mg/dl) (Smeltzer, Bare, 1992). Several drugs are used in the treatment of the disease (see Table 32-1). For acute attacks, colchicine is administered orally or may be given intravenously. When administered orally, .5 mg may be given hourly until 12 doses have been given. The drug is discontinued if gastrointestinal symptoms develop. Indomethacin (Indocin) is a potent antiinflammatory drug that is useful for controlling gout in patients who suffer frequent attacks despite prophylactic dosages of colchicine. Because the high doses that are required tend to cause headache, dizziness, and epigastric pain, dosages should be reduced quickly and discontinued as soon as possible. In some cases, daily doses prevent acute attacks (Wyngaarden and others, 1992).

One factor in the treatment of gout is the prevention of tophi and gouty arthritis. **Tophi** are deposits of uric acid that may form in various parts of the body, including the kidneys. Uric acid stones may develop here and destroy kidney tissue. Drugs may be given to prevent these disorders from occurring or to relieve them when they are present. Drugs in use include allopurinol (Zyloprim), probenecid (Benemid), and sulfinpyrazone (Anturane) (Wyngaarden and others, 1992). Allopurinol decreases the production of uric acid in the body and must be taken regularly to prevent acute attacks and tophi formation. Probenecid increases the excretion of uric acid by the kidney, thus reducing

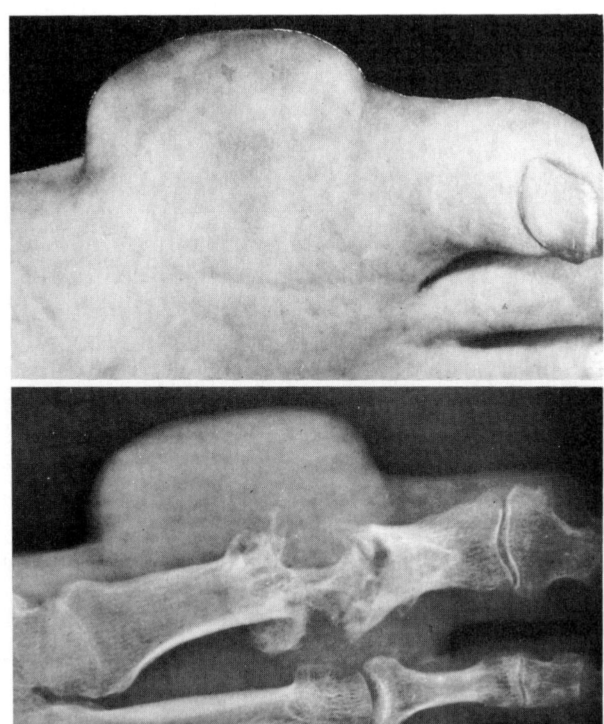

Figure 32-18 Gout of long duration. Tophaceous mass at base of great toe, as well as destructive bone and joint changes shown in x-ray film, are associated with extensive urate deposits. (From Phipps WJ and others: *Medical-surgical nursing: concepts and clinical practice,* ed 5, St Louis, 1995, Mosby.)

the amount in the body. It must be taken daily to be effective. Each patient is treated on an individual basis, and the period during which these drugs are to be administered depends on the stage of the disease and the practices of the individual physician. The patient may need to continue receiving drugs over several years. Although no special diet has been found to be effective, foods high in purine, such as liver, kidneys, anchovies, sardines, and sweetbreads, should be avoided. The diet should be well balanced, and water intake should be high. During an acute attack, the patient should be prescribed a regimen of bedrest, and painful joints should be protected from bedcovers by a bed cradle.

Bursitis

The bursae are small sacs that are located in the shoulder, elbow, knee, hip, and foot. They contain a small amount of fluid that lubricates areas in which movement may cause friction. The bursae may become inflamed and cause acute bursitis, or inflammation may extend over a long period and result in chronic bursitis and the formation of calcium salt deposits. Bursitis generally is the result of injury, strain, or prolonged use of the bursae, such as in active exercise. It also may occur secondary to infection elsewhere in the body. The subdeltoid region is the most common location of inflammation (see Figure 32-1). Subdeltoid bursitis is characterized by severe pain that may radiate down the arm and into the fingers. Treatment consists of supporting the arm in a sling and administering an analgesic for pain. Hydrocortisone may be injected into the bursae. Several other methods of treatment may be used, including administering a local anesthetic before inserting needles and washing out the calcium deposits. Range-of-motion exercises should be started as soon as possible. In chronic bursitis, pain occurs during use of the affected part, and treatment includes analgesics and physical therapy. Surgical removal of hardened calcium deposits may be necessary.

Infectious Diseases and Disorders—Osteomyelitis

Osteo- is the prefix that means *bone.* Therefore osteomyelitis is inflammation of the bone. The most common cause of the disease is the introduction of pathogenic bacteria into the bone as a result of penetrating injuries, such as gunshot wounds, or as a result of compound fractures with protruding bones. Acute osteomyelitis may also result from infections elsewhere in the body when the pathogenic bacteria are carried to the bone by the bloodstream. Because many infections are now treated with chemotherapeutic drugs, fewer cases of osteomyelitis result from bloodstream infection.

Chronic osteomyelitis may recur throughout life. No uniform method of treating patients with osteomyelitis exists. For some patients, surgery may be performed to remove necrotic bone. Antibiotics generally are given, and immobilization may be helpful. Treatment depends on the age and condition of the patient (Maher and others, 1994).

Because the wounds caused by osteomyelitis are painful, the nurse should be gentle when moving the affected part. Wounds often are irrigated with an antiseptic or antibiotic solution, and strict asepsis must be maintained. Contractures may occur unless care is taken to see that the patient is positioned properly. Because new foci of infection may develop, the patient should be observed for any sudden elevation of temperature, which should be reported at once. The diet should be high in calories, protein, and vitamins. Because osteomyelitis patients often are children, diversional activities should be planned.

Traumatic Injuries

Among all age groups, traumatic injuries to the musculoskeletal system are responsible for a large number of hospital admissions. Many less severe injuries, including contusions, sprains, and strains, are cared for in outpatient clinics or in a physician's office.

Contusions

Contusions are the most common and the simplest type of injury to the musculoskeletal system. *Contusion* is synonymous with *bruise* and is the result of an external injury to the soft tissues. A sharp blow to the eye, arm, or thigh are examples of injuries that can cause a simple contusion. The injury causes a rupture of small blood vessels and subsequent bleeding into tissues, which results in an **ecchymosis,** or the familiar discoloration that is often called a bruise or "black-and-blue spot." When the contusion is severe, a large amount of blood may collect in the tissue, resulting in a hematoma.

Treatment for contusions generally includes elevation of the part and the application of cold, which may be in the form of cold compresses or an ice cap. If there is no further bleeding after 24 hours, heat may be applied to relieve muscle soreness.

Sprains

A sprain involves ligaments, tendons, and muscles and occurs as the result of twisting or wrenching a joint beyond its normal range of motion. When this occurs, ligaments are torn, and tendons may be pulled from the bone. Blood vessels are ruptured, which causes contusions with ecchymosis. Pressure on nerve endings results in pain. As the result of a disturbance of circulation and lymph drainage, muscle spasm occurs, and there is a tendency for edema to occur. Sprains of the ankle or wrist joint are common examples.

Immediately after the injury, weight bearing or other pressure on the joint should be avoided. Walking on a sprained ankle causes further bleeding into soft tissues. The involved extremity should be elevated to promote drainage away from the injury. Ice bags should be applied for the first 24 hours to constrict blood vessels and to ensure control of further bleeding. After 24 hours, mild heat may be applied to encourage circulation and healing and to relieve soreness in the area. Treatment should include an x-ray examination to rule out the possibility of a fracture. The joint is then immobilized by a splint and Ace bandage, or a cast if the sprain is severe. Taping the foot occasionally provides enough immobilization for healing to occur. The support is removed in 2 to 3 weeks. If the ankle joint is involved, minimum weight bearing is permitted at first and is increased gradually as the discomfort subsides. If the ankle has been casted, active exercises should be performed after cast removal and before full weight bearing begins.

Dislocations

A dislocation may be congenital, as in the case of a congenitally dislocated hip; it may be caused by a disease process in the joint; or it may be caused by trauma. A dislocation results in the temporary displacement of a bone from its normal position within a joint. It is accompanied by a stretching and tearing of ligaments and tendons, and a fracture may sometimes occur at the same time. A dislocation results in severe pain, deformity, and loss of function. The treatment of dislocations is usually done with the patient under sedation or general anesthesia. The displaced parts are manipulated manually into normal position. Sometimes the fluoroscope may be used to assist the surgeon. The affected joint is immobilized in splints, bandages, or a cast until the injured tissues have healed. When a fracture accompanies a dislocation, achieving an effective outcome may be more difficult than with dislocation alone.

Nursing care of the patient includes observing for signs of impaired circulation, such as pain, tingling, numbness, or loss of sensation. Cast care is reviewed earlier in this chapter.

Fractures

A fracture is the same as a break and results from some force (blow, crushing, twisting) that places more stress on the bone than it can absorb. Decalcification and brittleness of bones (osteoporosis) occur in the aging process and make the bones increasingly unable to withstand external stresses. In elderly persons, this process may lead to fractures that occur with very little stress to bones and joints. Metastatic cancer and bone tumors also weaken bones and may result in fractures with little or no stress. These types of fractures are called *pathologic fractures.* Fractures may occur directly at the point at which stress is applied, or they may be some distance away from this point. Various types of fractures exist, and the method of treatment varies with the location and type. Some injury to the soft tissues and some bleeding occurs whenever a fracture occurs because the bones have their own blood supply.

Fractures are classified in four general categories. First, they are described as either *open* or *closed,* which means that the fracture either does or does not protrude through a break in the skin (Figure 32-19). Open fractures generally are more serious because they are

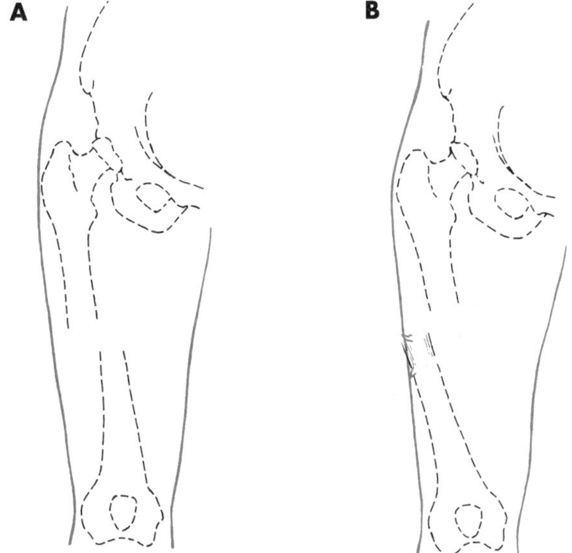

Figure 32-19 **A,** Closed fracture. **B,** Open fracture with bone protruding through skin.

accompanied by considerable soft tissue damage, require surgical treatment to repair, and involve a break in the body's first line of defense against infection—the skin. An open fracture is compounded by injury to the skin and by the possibility of infection. Because closed fractures do not involve a break in the skin, bones may be realigned by external manipulation only.

Fractures are also described according to their appearance. Greenstick, complete, comminuted, impacted, transverse, oblique, and spiral fractures are examples of various types of fractures (Box 32-4; Figure 32-20). Third, fractures are described according to their location on the bone, namely, proximal, midshaft, or distal (Figure 32-21). Fourth, fractures are described according to their displacement. Figure 32-22 shows that fragments may be displaced sideways, may override the opposite fractured surface, may angulate or create a bend in the bone, and may rotate away from the fracture site. Any displacement of bone fragments results in soft tissue damage, and the patient is likely to experience severe pain, swelling, and muscle spasm in the early stages of healing.

Assessment. Signs and symptoms of a fracture vary with the type and location and may include pain and swelling (particularly at the time of injury), tenderness, muscle spasm, deformity, and loss of function. Sometimes symptoms may not be present at the time of injury. Often injury to other body parts occurs simultaneously, and the patient may be admitted unconscious and in severe shock. The treatment of any general systemic condition takes precedence over treatment of the fracture. Immobilization of the fracture as soon as possible prevents further injury.

BOX 32-4

TYPES OF FRACTURES

greenstick fracture Incomplete fracture that is common in children because their bones are softer and more flexible than adult bones; bone is broken and bent but still secured on one side

complete fracture Bone is completely broken through and severed on all sides

comminuted fracture Bone is splintered into three or more fragments at the site of the break

colles' fracture A classic fracture of the wrist in which the distal end of the radius is broken off and displaced backward so that the wrist drops down; usually caused by breaking a fall with the outstretched hand

impacted fracture One broken end of a bone is driven or wedged into the opposite end of the fractured bone by external force; creates a shortening of the extremity in long bones

transverse fracture Break runs directly across the bone

oblique fracture Break runs along a slant the length of the bone

spiral fracture Break coils around the bone

An accurate diagnosis of the fracture is made by x-ray examination or by fluoroscopic examination. The physician will want to know exactly how the accident happened, because this information has a bearing on the type of fracture and the method of treatment.

Intervention. To treat a fracture, the bone segments must be realigned. The realignment of a fracture is termed *reduction.* Fractures are reduced by closed or open methods. In *closed reduction,* the bones are externally manipulated into position and immobilized with external devices such as casts, splints, or traction. In *open reduction,* the bones are exposed and aligned through a surgical incision and may be fixed in position with wires, nails, plates, screws, bolts, or any combination of these. The use of these devices is called *internal fixation.* As with closed reduction, external devices may be used for immobilization of the extremity.

NURSE ALERT

After open reduction, check for drainage *under* the cast. Because of gravity, drainage from the wound flows around the extremity and soaks through the underside of the cast or dressing before appearing on the anterior surface of the extremity.

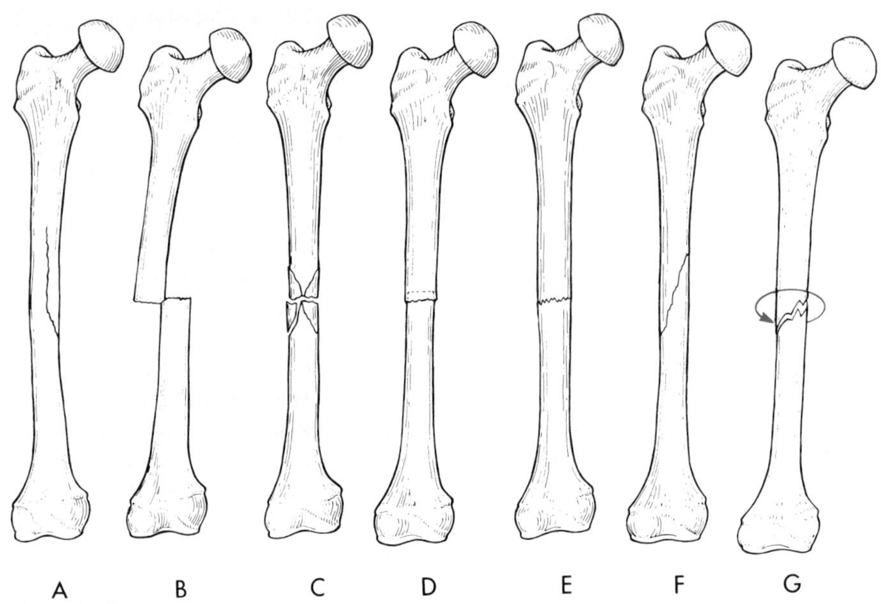

Figure 32-20 Description of fracture by appearance. **A,** Greenstick. **B,** Complete. **C,** Comminuted. **D,** Impacted. **E,** Transverse, **F,** Oblique. **G,** Spiral.

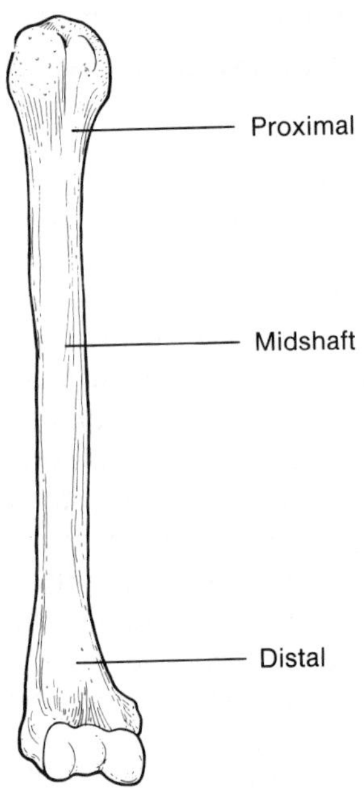

Figure 32-21 Location of fractures.

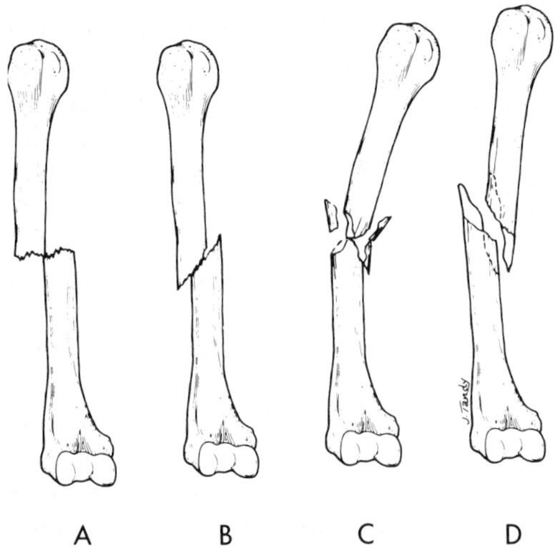

Figure 32-22 Displacement of fragments. **A,** Sideways. **B,** Override. **C,** Angulate. **D,** Rotate.

Fracture healing. Whereas other parts of the body heal by the formation of scar tissue, bones heal by the formation of new bone. When a fracture occurs, the bone is broken, soft tissues are damaged, and the periosteum is torn. The bleeding that occurs results in the formation of a hematoma, which surrounds the area within 24 hours. The coagulation of this blood forms a loose fibrin mesh, which acts as a framework for the early stages of new bone growth. An inflammatory reaction follows, which causes the fibrin mesh to be replaced by granulation tissue. Within 6 to 10 days the granulation tissue contains calcium, cartilage, and osteoblasts and is termed **callus.** Callus unites the bone so the cast can be removed, but the bone cannot withstand unprotected stress. The bone is immature and is gradually replaced by mature bone in the process of ossification. **Remodeling** of the bone is the process in which bone tissue consolidates and compacts the bone in relation to its function. This final step in fracture healing requires the stresses of muscle action and weight bearing. After remodeling, the bone is considered to be in union and may be used unprotected.

PATIENT/FAMILY TEACHING

The patient with a fracture

The patient and family should be taught the signs and symptoms of infection.
Nutritional needs of bone healing and decreased mobility should be discussed.
Cast care, pin care, and/or wound care should be properly demonstrated by the patient and or family before discharge.
Isometric exercises and the activity level of the patient should be reviewed and the home environment assessed to identify any obstacles that need to be modified to accommodate walkers, crutches, or other assistive devices.

The time required for the healing of fractures varies and is influenced by the type of fracture, the bone involved, and the age and condition of the patient and his or her bones. For example, displaced fractures take longer to heal than those with no displacement of fragments. Bones of the arms heal in 3 months, but long bones of the leg take 6 months to heal. A solid callus may be present in the fracture of a child within 3 weeks but may take 6 to 8 weeks in a young adult, and that same fracture may not develop good callus formation for 3 to 4 months in an elderly person.

The complete union of fractured bones may be prevented or delayed by infection, poor circulation, inadequate nutrition, necrosis, and improper immobilization or fixation. When a fracture does not form a bony union within the usual amount of time, *delayed union* occurs, which requires extended immobilization. *Nonunion* results when healing fails to occur, which requires revision or bone grafting to stimulate callus formation. Faulty reduction or improper immobilization may cause *malunion* of a fracture and result in deformity and disability and require surgery for repair. *Aseptic* or *avascular necrosis* is literally a clean death of the bone that results from loss of blood supply to the fracture site.

Fractures of the hip. Because more people are living longer now, the incidence of hip fractures among older persons is increasing. Because of the brittleness of their bones, older people need only a slight fall to sustain a fracture of the hip or arm. Hip fractures occur spontaneously in older people, which means that the patient falls as a result of the fracture rather than suffering the fracture as a result of the fall. A spontaneous fracture usually occurs in the neck of the femur. Regardless of the cause, the patient with a fractured hip experiences pain in the fracture site, the affected extremity shortens, and the foot turns outward (external rotation). Healing of a bone as large as the hip takes a long time in the elderly, which predisposes them to numerous complications. They are at risk for atelectasis and pneumonia, deep vein thrombosis, decubitus ulcers, urinary retention, constipation, and mental confusion or depression (Box 32-5).

Newer methods of treatment allow for earlier and greater mobility than was previously possible after hip fracture. Because different types of fractures occur, methods of treatment vary. The surgeon determines the method to be used on the basis of an x-ray examination. The care of patients in casts and traction is reviewed earlier in this chapter.

Nailing. *Nailing* means that a nail or rod made of stainless steel and Vitallium is inserted through the marrow cavity of one bone fragment and driven across the site of the fracture into the marrow cavity of another bone, thus holding the fractured bones in correct anatomic position. Not all fractures can be nailed, but when this procedure is possible, it allows many patients to be out of the hospital and walking on crutches in a few weeks. In some types of fractures a prosthetic device may be used. They are usually inserted when the neck of the femur has been fractured and the blood supply that is necessary for healing has been disrupted. The head and neck of the femur are surgically removed and replaced with a ball and stem (Austin Moore or Batemann prosthesis), which fits into the shaft of the femur. This procedure enables the patient to bear weight directly on the leg in a short time. Nailing and prosthetic devices offer the advantage of early ambulation and help to prevent complications commonly associated with immobility.

Intervention. The patient with internal fixation is given a general anesthetic for the procedure, after which vital signs are checked often until the patient is stabilized. After internal fixation, turning and moving the patient can begin. The patient's position should be changed from side to side every 2 hours. When the patient is turned on the unaffected side, the fractured extremity should be supported with pillows and should remain in the same line as the rest of the body. When the patient is in the supine position, the knee may be slightly flexed, and the extremity should be supported from the hip to the ankle with sandbags or a trochanter roll to prevent outward rotation. Pillows may be used to support the legs and keep the heels off the bed. Because physicians vary in what activity they permit, the nurse should understand exactly what the physician wishes to be done.

An orthopedic or pediatric bedpan may be more comfortable for the patient. The elderly patient should be observed for fecal impaction, and mild laxatives or small enemas may be ordered. Intake and output records should be maintained. With the physician's

BOX 32-5 **Nursing Process**

HIP FRACTURE
TOTAL HIP REPLACEMENT
TOTAL KNEE REPLACEMENT

ASSESSMENT

Vital signs (often)
Fluid volume status
Dressing for evidence of bleeding
Wound for healing and evidence of infection
Drain output
Tissue perfusion to affected extremity (often)
Respiratory status
Level of comfort
Elimination patterns and bowel sounds
Level of consciousness, orientation
Leg position in bed and in chair and during ambulation
Laboratory studies (CBC, coagulation profile)
Self-care ability
Evidence of skin breakdown
Signs and symptoms of thrombophlebitis
Restlessness, confusion, sudden chest pain, dyspnea, tachycardia
Signs of dislocation of hip
Evidence of bleeding if on anticoagulants

NURSING DIAGNOSES

Pain related to bone and soft tissue trauma and physical therapy
Ineffective breathing pattern related to sedation, anesthesia, and immobility
Impaired physical mobility related to pain and surgical procedure
Risk for altered tissue perfusion to affected lower extremity related to surgical procedure, edema, immobility
Risk for infection related to implanted prosthesis
Risk for impaired skin integrity related to immobility, age, pain
Self-care deficit related to pain and immobility
Constipation related to analgesics and immobility
Risk for injury: dislocation, DVT, pulmonary embolism related to improper positioning, surgical procedure, immobility
Knowledge deficit related to new condition, mobility restrictions, memory impairment

NURSING INTERVENTIONS

Prevent skin breakdown.
Turn patient and encourage him or her to cough and deep breathe every 2 hours.
Maintain affected extremity in alignment.
Mobilize patient and weight bearing per physician's order and patient tolerance.
Use orthopedic bedpan.
Perform range-of-motion exercises on all joints except affected leg.
Provide trapeze.
Request physical therapy consult for transfer techniques and use of mobility aids.
Administer IV fluids as ordered.
Administer prophylactic anticoagualtion as ordered.
Apply antiembolism hose as ordered.
Encourage dorsiflexion and plantar flexion exercises.
Provide high protein, high roughage diet.
Provide diet and fluids as tolerated.
Discuss use of patient-controlled analgesia for pain control with physician if not ordered and if appropriate.
Administer analgesics as prescribed.
Provide comfort measures (massage, relaxation, diversion).
Administer medications before physical therapy.
Encourage isometric exercises (quadriceps, gluteal sets per physical therapist's order).
Maintain aseptic technique with dressing changes.
Encourage participation in self-care activities.
Encourage balance between rest and activities.
Refer to social services for home physical therapy and nursing if indicated.

Mobility for total hip replacement
Enforce mobility restrictions to prevent dislocation.
Use abduction pillow at all times.
Avoid extreme flexion of affected hip (>90 degrees), as well as adduction and external rotation.
Teach patient to not bend at waist, to not cross legs, and to not sleep on operative side for 2 months.
Use raised toilet seat and high, firm chair.
Reinforce hip positions/precautions often.

Mobility for hip fracture
When on unaffected side, support fractured extremity with pillows in alignment.
Maintain pillow between legs.
Prevent external rotation.
Avoid adduction (especially with prosthesis).

Mobility for total knee replacement
If prescribed, apply continuous passive motion machine.

BOX 32-5 **Nursing Process**

HIP FRACTURE
TOTAL HIP REPLACEMENT
TOTAL KNEE REPLACEMENT—cont'd

NURSING INTERVENTIONS—CONT'D

Maintain correct position and knee alignment at all times.
Elevate leg on pillow when not in continuous passive motion machine; place pillow under calf to promote leg extension.
Initiate weight bearing as prescribed.
Instruct patient to sit with legs dependent to promote knee flexion.

EVALUATION OF EXPECTED OUTCOMES

Meets discharge criteria for postsurgical patient (p. 487)
Affected extremity in alignment
No evidence of dislocation
No evidence of infection
Pain controlled with oral analgesics
Tolerating activity within limitations
Demonstrates understanding of mobility limitations
Demonstrates increased strength and function of affected extremity
No evidence of thrombophlebitis
Adequate tissue perfusion to affected extremity
Verbalizes understanding of rehabilitation program

permission, the patient may be taught muscle-setting exercises such as quadriceps-setting, gluteal and abdominal muscle tightening, plantar flexion, and dorsiflexion of the feet. All joints except the affected leg should be exercised, and the patient may be encouraged to use the trapeze to move and exercise the arms. Exercise of the affected leg must be ordered by the surgeon. In most instances the patient is out of bed and in a chair on the day after surgery. Elderly patients may tire easily and should not be left sitting for long periods. Usually 1 hour two or three times a day is sufficient. Because the appetite may be poor, allowing the patient to be up at mealtimes may improve intake. Non–weight-bearing ambulation is allowed as soon as possible, and weight bearing is allowed when healing is complete.

When a prosthesis such as the Austin Moore or Batemann is inserted into the femur, the limb is kept in a neutral position, with slight abduction to prevent dislocation. The patient may be placed in traction to maintain this position and is not turned unless ordered by the physician. In such a case the patient is lifted off the bed for back care. If turning is permitted, the patient is placed on his or her unaffected side, and abduction is maintained by placing pillows between his or her legs. Muscle exercises are encouraged. Partial weight bearing may be allowed in 10 to 14 days and full weight bearing in approximately 4 weeks. Specific exercises, activities, and weight-bearing restrictions must be ordered by the physician.

Complications. Serious complications of fractures include pulmonary embolism, fat embolism (mostly occur with long bone fractures), gas gangrene, tetanus, and compartment syndrome.

Because of prolonged immobility, patients with fractures of the lower extremities are particularly susceptible to pulmonary embolism, which may be secondary to thrombophlebitis or may occur spontaneously. Measures to prevent pulmonary embolism include prophylactic anticoagulation, early ambulation, exercises, and the use of elastic stockings. Sudden respiratory distress with acute substernal pain and signs of shock should alert the nurse to suspect pulmonary embolism. Treatment includes oxygen administration to support respiration, anticoagulant therapy, and general emergency measures.

Fat embolism develops most commonly in young adults who sustain multiple, crushing-type fractures, such as those occurring from motorcycle accidents or industrial injuries. Although rare, fat embolism is life threatening because the released fat droplets can effectively occlude capillaries of the pulmonary circulation and cause brain hypoxia and tissue death. Measures to prevent fat embolism include cautious and minimum manipulation of bone fragments with immediate immobilization. Mental disturbances, respiratory distress, and signs of shock that occur within 72 hours after injury are signs of fat embolism. The classic appearance of petechiae on the upper chest and axillae, as well as the appearance of blood-tinged sputum, may accompany these early signs. Treatment includes the administration of high concentrations of oxygen, the control of shock, and all symptomatic measures to sustain life (Black, Matassarin-Jacobs, 1993; Smeltzer, Bare, 1992).

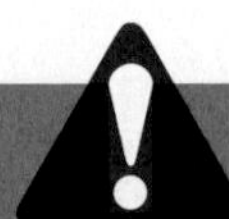

NURSE ALERT

The larger the bone involved, the higher the probability of fat embolism occurring. Watch for signs of respiratory distress when the femur is fractured.

Gas gangrene and *tetanus* occur rarely but must always be considered as possible complications when a compound fracture has been sustained through a small or puncture-type wound. Both gas gangrene and tetanus are caused by anaerobic bacteria, which produce rapid and life-threatening results. Gas gangrene is a rapid destruction of tissue and is signaled by an acute, fulminating infection with fever, wound pain, gas bubbles, and edema. If left untreated, the condition progresses to systemic toxemia and death. In tetanus, the bacteria affect the nerves, which causes muscle twitching, severe spasms, and inability to open the mouth (lockjaw). It progresses to severe seizures that can be stimulated by the slightest movement or noise. Treatment for both conditions includes wound debridement, hyperbaric oxygen, and antibiotic therapy. Anticonvulsive drugs are given for seizures. Amputation of the affected limb may be necessary.

Compartment syndrome is the progressive development of arterial vessel compression and circulatory compromise, which can rapidly result in a permanent contracture deformity of the hand or foot, called *Volkmann's contracture* (Figure 32-23). Fractures of the forearm or tibia usually can cause the onset of muscle swelling within the inelastic fascia, which forms compartments for the muscles of the forearm and lower leg. Entry and exit openings to each compartment are only large enough to allow passage of major arteries, nerves, and tendons. When the muscle within a compartment swells as a result of severe trauma or compression of a cast, blood vessels within the muscle are compressed, and muscle ischemia results. A vicious cycle is set in motion in which histamine is released, capillaries dilate, additional swelling occurs, blood flow is decreased further, and more ischemia results.

Within 6 hours the condition can progress to irreversible muscle ischemia, with compression of the arteries, nerves, and tendons that enter the compartment. Paralysis and loss of sensation follow, and contracture and permanent disability of the extremity may be complete within 24 to 48 hours. The nurse's careful assessment of the neurovascular integrity of fractured extremities can interrupt the development of compartment syndrome. Sharp pain that is unrelieved by analgesics increases with passive movement of the hand or foot and is the first symptom. This symptom is accompanied by an inability to flex the fingers or toes, numbness, coldness, and lack of pulse.

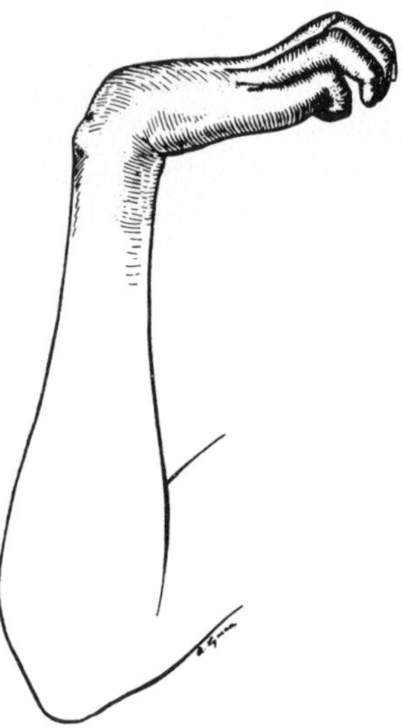

Figure 32-23 Well-established Volkmann's contracture with clawhand and flexion of wrist and fingers. (From Larson CB, Gould M: *Orthopedic nursing,* ed 9, St Louis, 1978, Mosby.)

Frequent assessment of the affected extremity is essential and should include observation of skin color and tension. Palpation detects changes in temperature, pulse rate, and capillary refilling time. Muscle strength of the extremity should be tested, and increased pain that is associated with muscle stretching should be reported. Tissue pressure measurements can be taken by a physician to determine the extent of tissue compression within the fascial compartment. Normally pressure is recorded at 0 mm Hg. Tissue ischemia begins when pressure rises to between 10 and 30 mm Hg less than the patient's diastolic blood pressure (Gregory, 1994; Maher and others, 1994; Mourad, 1991).

Continued elevated pressures in the presence of decreased sensory and motor function necessitate surgical intervention. A *fasciotomy* (surgical incision into the fascia) is performed to relieve pressure within the compartment and to allow return of normal blood flow to the area (Figure 32-24). After surgery, the patient is observed for signs and symptoms of infection in the open wound. The extremity is elevated above the level of the heart, and range-of-motion exercise is begun.

General nursing interventions. The patient with a fracture needs a well-balanced diet, and opinions differ on the value of vitamin and mineral supplements in hastening bone repair. Fluids should be provided. Exercise of the unaffected joints, muscle-setting exercises, skin care, and elimination are important considerations in patient care. Although internal fixation has

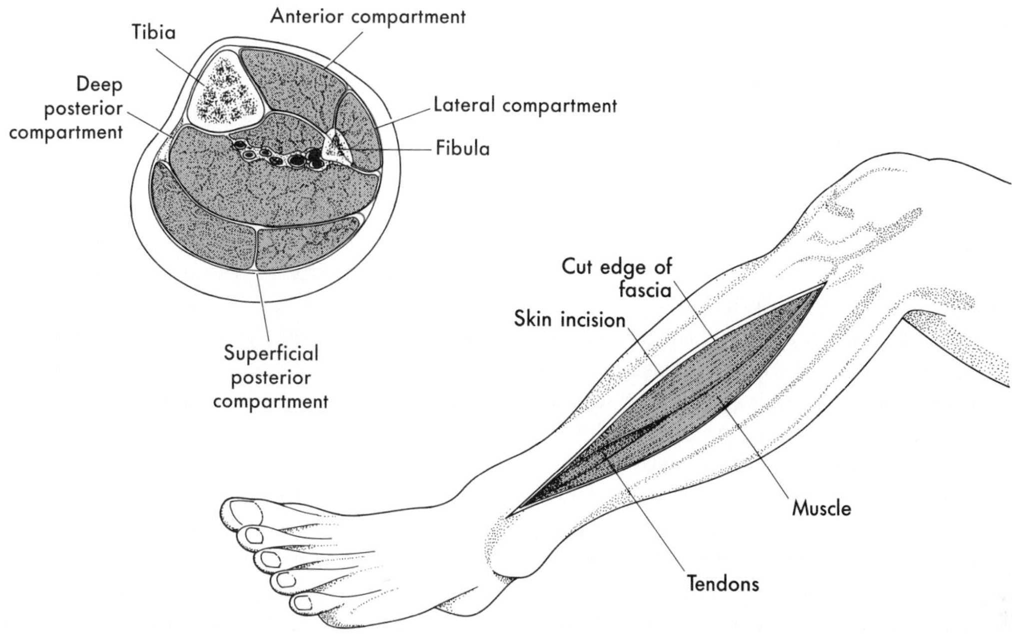

Figure 32-24 Compartment syndrome and fasciotomy to relieve pressure. Often more than one compartment is involved. (From Beare PG, Myers JL: *Principles and practice of adult health nursing,* ed 2, St Louis, 1994, Mosby.)

simplified nursing care for many patients with fractures and has shortened the period of hospitalization, many patients require several weeks of hospitalization. Some form of occupational therapy should be available for these patients. If activity is restricted, the complications that result from immobility must be anticipated and prevented.

Whiplash injuries

A whiplash injury to the musculoskeletal system is the result of a combination of severe flexion and extension of the neck. The injury may cause a compression fracture of the cervical vertebrae or result in tearing of muscles and ligaments. Although the injury can be severe enough to cause paralysis and loss of consciousness, most whiplash injuries do not produce immediate symptoms. Symptoms often do not appear until 4 or 5 days after the injury, at which time headache, spasm of neck muscles with loss of motion, and a drawing sensation in the back of the neck may be noticed. Pain may be referred from one side of the head to the base of the skull, and vision may be disturbed. If the injury has been severe enough to injure a nerve root, neurologic symptoms may occur.

Treatment should be obtained immediately after injury because without treatment, the condition may become chronic. Methods of treatment vary, but the patient may be admitted to the hospital for several days, and a regimen of bedrest may be prescribed. Cervical traction with a head halter, as well as the application of heat and massage, may be used. The patient may be fitted with a neck support that is to be worn when out of bed. After approximately 4 weeks, physical therapy and exercise are begun to strengthen neck muscles.

Bone Tumors

Tumors of the bone may be primary or secondary and may be benign or malignant. Several types of benign tumors exist, and their cause is not always known. Benign tumors do not metastasize to other parts of the body and usually produce few symptoms, with the most common symptom being pain from pressure exerted on surrounding anatomic structures. Benign tumors are diagnosed by x-ray examination and biopsy, and most are removed surgically.

Several different types of malignant bone tumors exist. One type of primary malignant tumor, *osteogenic sarcoma,* occurs in younger persons and metastasizes to the lungs, from which the malignant cells are carried throughout the body by the bloodstream. The long bones are usually affected, and amputation generally is required (Wyngaarden and others, 1992). Other types of malignant tumors affect the flat bones and often involve other types of tissues. Carcinoma of the prostate, lung, breast, thyroid, and kidney may metastasize to the bones, where destruction of the bone and spontaneous fractures result. In most cases of both benign and malignant bone tumors, pain and declining health are the primary symptoms. Anemia, temperature elevation, swelling, and platelet disturbance occur with some types of bone tumors. Treatment depends on the type of tumor, the extent of involvement, the location, and the presence of malignant lesions in other parts of the body.

Amputation

Amputation of an extremity or a portion of it may be necessary as a result of a malignant bone tumor, injury, diabetic gangrene, or any condition that threatens the patient's life unless the procedure is performed. Occasionally amputation is an emergency procedure that is performed when a severe accident has nearly severed the extremity, but generally it is an elective procedure, and the final decision rests with the patient. Deciding whether to exchange a leg for a life, particularly when life expectancy may not be too long, is not easy. Patients need as much emotional support and understanding as possible. Patients should know preoperatively about prostheses, and often a visit from a person who uses a prosthesis is helpful.

Advances in microsurgery techniques have made the reattachment of severed limbs possible. The equipment and skills for accomplishing this procedure are not available in many communities, and patients may need to be transferred to another hospital where these services are available.

Preoperative intervention

Before surgery, the patient's general physical condition is assessed carefully. If the patient has diabetes, an evaluation of his or her diabetic status is determined. Other examinations such as electrocardiograms and chest x-ray examinations may be ordered by the physician. Intravenous fluids may be given to combat dehydration, and a blood transfusion may be ordered if anemia is present. The skin is prepared according to the hospital procedure.

Postoperative intervention

The months of stump wrapping and conditioning before being fitted with a prosthesis have now been eliminated. Patients are fitted with a rigid temporary prosthesis either immediately after surgery or when the stump is healed and the sutures have been removed. Every patient who has had an amputation should receive a temporary prosthesis as soon as possible after surgery. The patient benefits psychologically from a temporary prosthesis, and complications are prevented. After returning from surgery, the patient should be watched for signs of shock, and the vital signs should be checked at frequent intervals until he or she is stabilized. The dressings should be observed for evidence of bright-red blood. In cases of severe bleeding, the nurse should apply manual pressure to the site and should contact the physician immediately. If oozing from the stump occurs, the nurse may reinforce the dressing but should never attempt to change it without a physician's order.

Because many amputations are performed on persons between 60 and 70 years of age, the patient must be observed carefully for shock, pulmonary complications, or cardiovascular collapse. Suction equipment and oxygen should be at the bedside, and intravenous fluids and emergency drugs should be available for immediate use. Patients may be cared for in an intensive care unit, where drugs and equipment are readily available. Because elderly patients may have problems with urinary incontinence, the dressing may need to be protected to prevent contamination of the wound.

The postoperative care of the patient with an amputation is directed toward preparing the stump for a prosthesis, preventing contractures of the hip or nearest joint, maximizing wound healing, and facilitating adaptation to an altered lifestyle. Providing support to the patient is an important component of nursing care. The loss of a limb results in grieving and fear about how to function and interact with others. When the psychologic response to the loss is severe, it can result in ineffective rehabilitation (Novotony, 1991).

If a temporary prosthesis has not been applied, the stump is wrapped with elastic compression bandages to shrink and shape the stump (Figure 32-25). Before healing occurs, every effort must be made to prevent infection of the wound. The stump may be elevated by raising the foot of the bed for the first 24 hours. When the patient is in the supine position, the stump should rest flat on the bed. The patient should be encouraged to spend some time each day in the prone position, with a pillow tucked under the lower trunk and the stump for support (Figure 32-26). The stump should not be flexed over the unaffected leg. When in the prone position, the patient may begin pushup exercises to strengthen arm and shoulder muscles. When in the supine position, the patient may begin leg exercises unless such exercises strain the suture line.

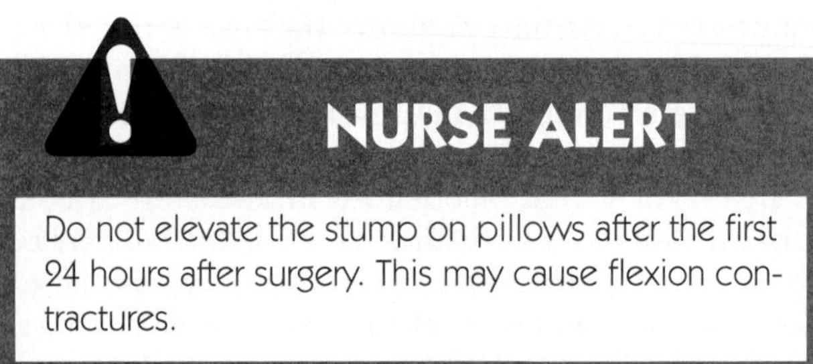

Do not elevate the stump on pillows after the first 24 hours after surgery. This may cause flexion contractures.

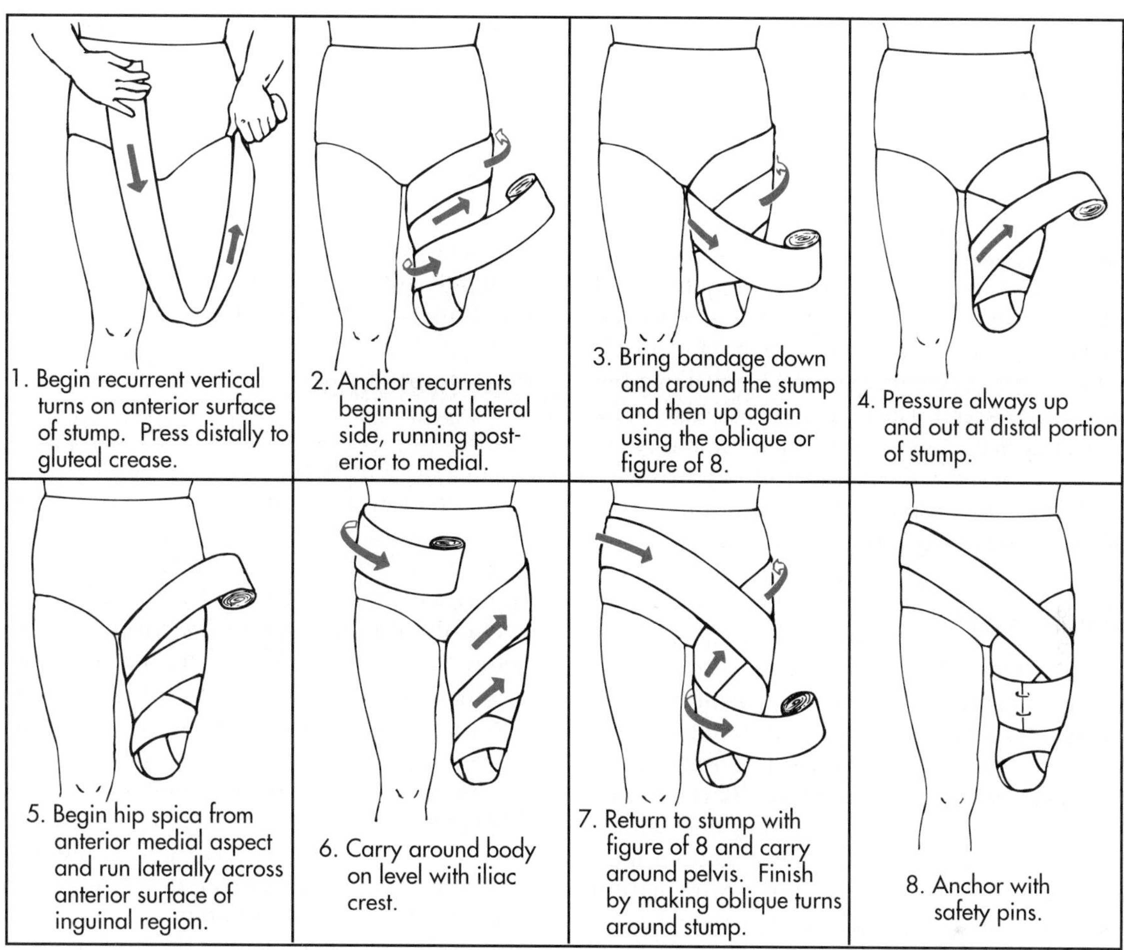

1. Begin recurrent vertical turns on anterior surface of stump. Press distally to gluteal crease.
2. Anchor recurrents beginning at lateral side, running posterior to medial.
3. Bring bandage down and around the stump and then up again using the oblique or figure of 8.
4. Pressure always up and out at distal portion of stump.
5. Begin hip spica from anterior medial aspect and run laterally across anterior surface of inguinal region.
6. Carry around body on level with iliac crest.
7. Return to stump with figure of 8 and carry around pelvis. Finish by making oblique turns around stump.
8. Anchor with safety pins.

Figure 32-25 Method of wrapping to help shape stump after above-the-knee amputation. (From Mourad LA: *Orthopedic disorders,* St Louis, 1991, Mosby.)

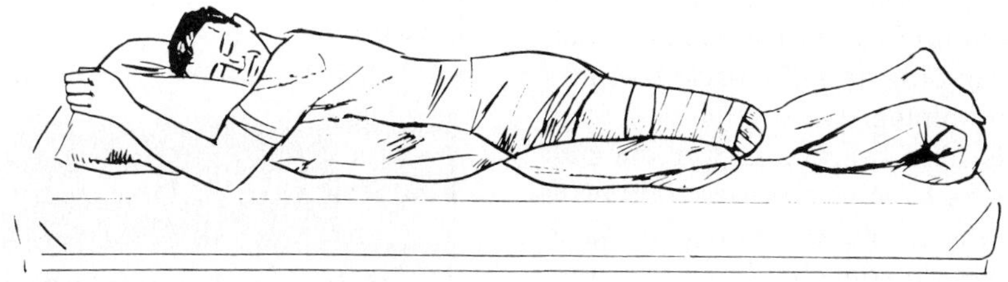

Figure 32-26 Patient in prone position following amputation. Note position of pillows.

If there is to be immediate postsurgical fitting of a prosthesis, a sterile stump sock is pulled over the stump when surgery is complete. Pressure areas are protected with felt pads. The stump is wrapped with elastic bandages to form a firm, snug dressing that prevents swelling and protects the stump from injury. The nurse must be alert for edema that may prevent weight bearing, and if the dressing comes off or is damaged, the physician must be notified immediately, and compression bandages should be applied until the physician arrives (Bending, 1993) Brief ambulation with limited weight bearing is possible within 24 hours. Gradually ambulation is increased, but weight bearing is limited until healing is complete (Black, Matassarin-Jacobs, 1993). Immediate postsurgical fitting of a prosthesis minimizes stump edema, reduces the risk of embolism, and prevents contractures that preclude subsequent use of a prosthesis. Pressure points must be inspected often for irritation that may progress to necrosis. The patient and/or family must be taught the signs and symptoms of infection at the incision site, as well as how to monitor the stump for pressure sores from the prosthesis.

If no complications occur and the wound has healed, the sutures are removed, and a temporary prosthesis that is made of plastic or plaster of Paris is provided 2 to 3 weeks after surgery. With the temporary prosthesis, the patient is allowed partial weight bearing. Unless complications develop, the patient may bear full weight on the prosthesis within 6 weeks, and a permanent prosthesis is supplied within 3 months. Patients may need to be taught balance and crutch walking before leaving the hospital. They often are referred to the physical therapy department. The patient should be instructed to wash and dry the stump thoroughly once a day when healing is complete. If any abrasion occurs, the physician should be consulted immediately.

Phantom limb pain

Patients may have little pain from the surgical procedure or may complain of pain in the amputated limb. This type of pain is referred to as phantom limb pain and often occurs during the first few weeks after surgery and is most intense during the initial 6 months after the amputation (Bowser, 1991; Davis, 1993; Rounseville, 1992). The exact mechanism of phantom limb pain is not completely understood, but a combination of physiologic and psychologic factors may be involved.

Until recently, the measures used to treat phantom limb pain have been ineffective. Consequently a number of individuals have been unable to completely rehabilitate because of the extreme discomfort associated with the application of the prosthesis and their inability to participate in programs of muscle strengthening and ambulation training.

Encouraging results have been seen over the past few years with the use of *transcutaneous electrical nerve stimulation* (TENS) for the relief of phantom pain (Katz, Melzack, 1991). Patients experiencing limb pain after amputation are now being instructed to attach a TENS unit to the nonamputated limb at a site that is comparable to where the pain is felt in the amputated limb. Relief from pain is believed to be the result of the inability of the cerebral cortex to distinguish the origin of the impulse. The impulses generated by the TENS unit "override" the pain impulses, which breaks the cycle of pain and relieves the discomfort (Katz, Melzack, 1991).

NEUROMUSCULAR CONDITIONS

A number of neurologic conditions affect the musculoskeletal system. Lower back pain may be caused by a ruptured intervertebral disk or may be caused by muscle strain that results from poor alignment of the vertebral column or excessive activity. *Carpal tunnel syndrome* and *thoracic outlet syndrome* both involve tingling and numbness of the upper extremities and impair function (see Chapter 28).

Cerebral Palsy

Cerebral palsy is a broad term that is applied to a variety of conditions that are characterized by impaired functional muscle control as a result of an abnormality in the cerebral areas that affect these functions. The cause may be any condition that produces cerebral anoxia and hemorrhage or trauma. The causal event may occur during the prenatal period, during or after delivery, or later in life. If the injury produces irreversible damage to any cerebral areas that affect neuromuscular function, cerebral palsy results. Many types of cerebral palsy exist, and the disease is classified on the basis of symptoms and the extent of involvement. The disease results in motor disability and is characterized by spasticity and involuntary movements related to walking, talking, or any activity that requires muscular coordination.

In addition to problems with motor function, the person with cerebral palsy may have multiple disabilities. Many have impairments of vision, hearing, and speech; convulsive disorders; and mental retardation. In addition, psychologic, emotional, and social problems occur.

ETHICAL DILEMMA

Mr. Thomas is admitted to your unit with gangrene of three toes. The surgical service is recommending amputation of the lower limb because of extremely poor circulation. However, Mr. Thomas is adamantly opposed to amputation. He appears to have a clear understanding of the risks and benefits of having surgery and of refusing surgery.

How would you analyze this case?

Nursing Care Plan

PATIENT WITH BELOW-THE-KNEE AMPUTATION

Mrs. Carter is an 88-year-old female with a history of noninsulin dependant diabetes mellitus (NIDDM type II). She enters the hospital for a below-the-knee amputation of the left leg as a result of gangrene and poor circulation. She states that she has enjoyed good health until this "circulation" problem. Additional medical data reveals that she has a history of hypertension. She has never smoked or used alcohol. She had her left below-the-knee amputation 2 days ago.

Past Medical History

- Appendectomy at age 17
- Total hysterectomy at age 46 because of fibroid tumors
- Fractured left femur at age 55 after fall from bicycle; healed without sequelae
- Denies any respiratory or cardiac disease
- Diabetes discovered during routine physical at age 62; takes Diabinese 250 mg daily in AM; follows ADA exchange diet with good control
- No known food or drug allergies; has received antibiotics and blood transfusions in the past without problems

Psychosocial Data

- Currently resides in an extended care facility because of increasing difficulty in performing activities of daily living and because of lack of available family resources
- Been a widow for 9 years; no children
- Retired elementary school teacher; engaged in physical sports until age 70

Assessment Data

- Patient alert and oriented × 3
- Blood pressure stable at 130/70
- Afebrile
- *Respiratory:* Lungs clear, able to demonstrate effective cough, rate 18-20, regular depth and rhythm
- *Abdominal:* Soft, nontender, nondistended, bowel sounds heard in all four quadrants
- *Skin:* Clear with the exception of a reddened area 2 cm × 3 cm on coccyx, with a 1 cm open area on left buttock
- *Cardiovascular:* Apical pulse 68-72, rate regular without thrills or murmurs, pulses on right leg palpable (femoral, popliteal, and pedal); pulses on left leg thready and weak (femoral and popliteal)
- *Wound assessment:* Stump dressing dry and intact and in good alignment; patient moving with only minor discomfort

Laboratory data

- Hgb 13.1, Hct 40
- Electrolytes within normal limits (WNL)
- Serum glucose 238
- Urinalysis and other laboratory data within normal limits
- Chest x-ray examination and ECG within normal limits

NURSING DIAGNOSIS

Body image disturbance related to left below-the-knee amputation as evidenced by statements of depression and periods of crying

NURSING INTERVENTIONS

- Inform patient that feelings of depression are expected after a loss of a body part.
- Provide time to listen.
- Discuss fears.
- Encourage expression of feelings.
- Explore resources among friends.
- Arrange for patient to interact with others who have similar problems.

EVALUATION OF EXPECTED OUTCOMES

- Acknowledges a change in body image
- Takes an active role in planning aspects of daily care
- Expresses her emotions associated with the change in body image
- Expresses at least one positive feeling about herself daily
- Participates in discussion with person who has had a similar change in body image

continued

NURSING DIAGNOSIS

Pain related to phantom sensations caused by nerve stimulation secondary to amputation as evidenced by complaint of soreness in left leg when moving and sensation of "feeling" blanket on missing foot

NURSING INTERVENTIONS	EVALUATION OF EXPECTED OUTCOMES
Explain the sensation of "phantom limb" pain. Assess patient's physical pain. Have patient describe the pain on a scale of 1 to 10. Provide comfort measures as indicated, including positioning, massage, ice packs, medications, diversional activities, relaxation techniques.	Expresses relief from pain Verbalizes understanding of phantom sensations

NURSING DIAGNOSIS

Impaired physical mobility related to left below-the-knee amputation as evidenced by need of assistance when moving and inability to assist with own ADLs

NURSING INTERVENTIONS	EVALUATION OF EXPECTED OUTCOMES
Maintain patient in proper body alignment, turn and position patient every 2 hours. Increase mobility by having patient move into chair, commode, and geriatric chair; teach patient how to assist with these transfers. Teach patient to move self in bed; encourage use of unaffected leg. Monitor deep breathing and coughing exercises. Perform range-of-motion exercises every 2 to 4 hours; teach these exercises to patient. Encourage and praise independent behaviors. Encourage active movement using trapeze and other assistive devices. Assess patient's physiologic response to increased activity (monitor vital signs).	Properly demonstrates isometric and range-of-motion exercises Explains rationale for maintaining activity level and states at least five risk factors for activity intolerance Performs self-care activities with as little assistance as possible Does not exhibit evidence of cardiovascular or respiratory complication during or after activities

NURSING DIAGNOSIS

Impaired skin integrity related to decreased mobility and bedrest as evidenced by reddened and open skin

NURSING INTERVENTIONS:	EVALUATION OF EXPECTED OUTCOMES
Change patient's position at least every 2 hours. Keep skin clean and dry. Avoid use of irritating soap; rinse skin well. Use preventive skin care devices as needed, such as sheepskin pads and heel protectors. Protect bony prominences and massage them gently every 2 hours to increase circulation. Keep linen clean, dry, and free of wrinkles or crumbs. Monitor nutritional intake; encourage adequate hydration. Leave reddened area exposed to air; turn patient from that area. Teach patient and friends the importance of preventing pressure sores.	No further breakdown in skin Reddened areas show signs of improved circulation Mucous membranes remain intact Eats at least 80% of each meal Drinks at least 100 ml of extra fluids every 2 hours while awake Remains clean and dry at all times Position is changed at least every 2 hours Weight remains within her established limits Lists preventive skin care measures

KEY CONCEPTS

- Proper patient positioning and active and passive exercises are essential for preventing permanent complications of prolonged immobility.
- Frequent assessment of neurovascular integrity of the injured limb will identify impairment of the neurovascular system and allow for early intervention to prevent damage.
- Edema with pallor, cyanosis, and coldness are signs of circulatory impairment.
- The blanching sign is a test of the rate of capillary refill, which is an indicator of adequacy of circulation in the extremity.
- A recurrence of severe pain after a fracture has been reduced and stabilized is an indication that something is wrong.
- When traction is applied to an extremity because of a broken bone, the two bone ends are pulled into place.
- Skin traction uses the skin to maintain the pull of traction. Skeletal traction uses pins or wires, which are placed in the bone to hold the traction on the affected extremity.
- Aseptic technique is used when caring for the pin or wire sites of skeletal traction.
- Patients in traction should have skin care performed on pressure points at frequent intervals to prevent skin irritations and pressure sores.
- External fixation devices are used to reduce complex fractures that have bone fragments that need stabilization.
- Patients with fractures should eat a diet high in calcium, minerals, and fiber to promote healing of the fracture and normal elimination habits.
- Arthritis involves inflammation of joints, which causes pain and restricts movement of the affected joint.
- Rheumatoid arthritis is considered an autoimmune disorder that affects the joints.
- Rheumatoid spondylitis is an inflammation of the vertebrae and sacroiliac joints and may affect part of all of the spine.
- Osteoarthritis is the result of wear and tear that has been placed on the joints over the years.
- A sprain involves ligaments, tendons, and muscles that have been torn or pulled from the bone as the result of twisting or wrenching a joint beyond its normal range of motion.
- A dislocation may be congenital or may be a result of disease or trauma. It is the temporary displacement of a bone from its normal position within a joint.
- Fractures are described as being open or closed. They are also described according to their appearance, location, and displacement.
- The time for healing of fractures varies and is influenced by the type of fracture, the bone involved, and the age and condition of the patient.
- Serious complications of fractures include pulmonary embolism, fat embolism, gas gangrene, tetanus, and compartment syndrome.
- Whiplash injury to the musculoskeletal system is the result of a combination of severe flexion and extension of the neck.
- Bone tumors may be primary or secondary and may be benign or malignant.
- An amputation of part or all of an extremity may be necessary because of a malignant bone tumor, injury, diabetic gangrene, or any condition that threatens the patient's life unless the procedure is performed.
- Cerebral palsy is a neuromuscular disorder that results in motor disability and is characterized by spasticity and involuntary movements related to walking, talking, or activities that require muscular coordination.

CRITICAL THINKING EXERCISES

1. Prepare a list of instructions for a patient who is going home with a cast on his or her arm.
2. Your 35-year-old patient has a fractured femur and will be placed in skeletal traction. He asks you why that is necessary. Explain to him what traction does and why it is necessary to keep the weights hanging free.
3. Describe three physiologic changes in the older adult that makes bone healing more difficult.

REFERENCES AND ADDITIONAL READINGS

Adams RD, Victor M: *Principles of neurology,* ed 5, New York, 1993, McGraw-Hill.

Agne RAC: Rehabilitating a loved one: a personal story, *Rehabil Nurs* 18(1): 23-25, 1993.

Altizer L: Total hip arthroplasty, *Orthop Nurs* 14(4):7-18, 1995.

Bending J: TENS relief of discomfort, *Physiother* 79(11):773-774, 1993.

Black JM, Matassarin-Jacobs E: *Luckman and Sorensen's medical-surgical nursing,* ed 4, Philadelphia, 1993, WB Saunders.

Bowser MS: Giving up the ghost: a review of phantom limb phenomena, *J Rehabil* 57(3):55-62, 1991.

Brewer S: The back injury battle, *Nurs Stand* 7(40):20-21, 1993.

Burke MM and others: *Gerontologic nursing: care of the frail elderly,* St Louis, 1992, Mosby.

Carpenito LJ: *Handbook of nursing diagnoses,* ed 5, Philadelphia, 1993, JB Lippincott.

Cole G: *Basic nursing skills and concepts,* St Louis, 1991, Mosby.

Davis RW: Phantom sensation, phantom pain, and stump pain, *Arch Phys Med Rehabil* 74(1):79-91, 1993.

Driscoll AH: When your patient wears an Ilizarov device, *Am J Nurs* 93(6):63-65, 1993.

Finley C: TENS: an adjunct to analgesia, *Can Nurse* 88(8): 24-26, 1992.

Gregory B: *Orthopaedic surgery,* St Louis, 1994, Mosby.

Harms M, Engstrom B: Continuous passive motion as an adjunct to treatment in the physiotherapy management of the total knee arthroplasty patient, *Physiother* 77(4):301-307, 1991.

Hazard RG and others: Helping your back pain patients make the most of spinal motion, *J Musculoskel Med* 11(1):24-6, 33-5 1994.

Jones-Walton P: Clinical standards in skeletal traction pin site care, *Orthop Nurs* 10(2):12-6, 1991.

Katz J, Melzack R: Auricular transcutaneous electrical nerve stimulation (TENS) reduces phantom limb pain, *J Pain Symptom Manage* 6(2):73-83, 1991.

Maher AB and others: *Orthopaedic nursing,* Philadelphia, 1994, WB Saunders.

McCarthy MR and others: The clinical use of continuous passive motion in physical therapy, *J Orthop Sports Phys Ther* 15(3):132-40, 1992.

Mikulaninec CE: An amputee critical path, *J Vasc Nurs* 10(2): 2-6, 1992.

Mourad LA: *Orthopedic disorders,* St Louis, 1991, Mosby.

Mudge-Grout CL: *Immunologic disorders,* St Louis, 1992, Mosby.

Nichol D: Preventing infection . . . patients with skeletal pins, *Nurs Time* 89(13):78-80, 1993.

Nissen SJ, Newman WP: Factors influencing reintegration to normal living after amputation, *Arch Phys Med Rehabil* 73(6):548-551, 1992.

Novotony MP: Psychosocial issues affecting rehabilitation, *Phys Med Rehabil Clin North Am* 2(2):373-393, 1991.

Rounseville C: Phantom limb pain: the ghost that haunts the amputee, *Orthop Nurs* 11(2):67-71, 1992.

Rudolphi D: Limb loss in the elderly peripheral vascular disease patient, *J Vasc Nurs* 10(3):8-13, 1992.

Smeltzer SC, Bare BG: *Brunner and Suddarth's textbook of medical-surgical nursing,* ed 7, Philadelphia, 1992, JB Lippincott.

Smith M: Two legs to stand on . . . left above the knee amputation, *Am J Nurs* 93(12):42-44, 1993.

Tucker SM and others: *Patient care standards,* St Louis, 1992, Mosby.

Williamson VC: Amputation of the lower extremity: an overview, *Orthop Nurs* 11(2):55-65, 1992.

Wyngaarden JB and others: *Cecil's textbook of medicine,* ed 19, Philadelphia, 1992, WB Saunders.

Appendix A

ABBREVIATIONS AND SYMBOLS FOR UNITS OF MEASUREMENT

<	Less than	mm^3	Cubic millimeter
≤	Less than or equal to	mM	Millimole
>	Greater than	mmHg	Millimeter of mercury
≥	Greater than or equal to	mm H_2O	Millimeter of water
C	Celsius	mol	Mole
cc	Cubic centimeter	mmol	Millimole
cg	Centigram	mOsm	Milliosmole
cm	Centimeter	mμ	Millimicron
cm H_2O	Centimeter of water	mU	Milliunit
cu	Cubic	mV	Millivolt
dl	Deciliter (100 ml)	ng	Nanogram
g	Gram	nmol	Nanomole
IU	International unit	Pa	Pascal
ImU	International milliunit	pg	Picogram (or micromicrogram)
IμU	International microunit	pl	Picoliter
K	Kilo	pm	Picomole
kg	Kilogram	S	Second (SI)
L	Liter	sec	Second
m	Meter	SI units	International System of Units
m^2	Square meter	μ	Micron
m^3	Cubic meter	μ^3	Cubic micron
mEq	Milliequivalent	μg	Microgram
mEq/L	Milliequivalent per liter	μIU	Microinternational unit
mg	Milligram	μmol	Micromole
min	Minute	μU	Microunit
ml	Milliliter	U	Unit
mm	Millimeter	yr	Year

From Pagana KD, Pagana TJ: *Diagnostic testing and nursing implications,* ed 4, St Louis, 1993, Mosby.

Appendix B

1994 NANDA-APPROVED NURSING DIAGNOSES

Activity intolerance
Activity intolerance, risk for
Adaptive capacity, decreased: intracranial
Adjustment, impaired
Airway clearance, ineffective
Anxiety
Aspiration, risk for
Body image disturbance
Body temperature, altered, risk for
Bowel incontinence
Breastfeeding, effective
Breastfeeding, ineffective
Breathing pattern, ineffective
Cardiac output, decreased
Caregiver role strain
Caregiver role strain, risk for
Communication, impaired verbal
Community coping, potential for enhanced
Community coping, ineffective
Confusion, acute
Confusion, chronic
Constipation
Constipation, colonic
Constipation, perceived
Coping, defensive
Coping, family: potential for growth
Coping, ineffective family: compromised
Coping, ineffective family: disabling
Coping, ineffective individual
Decisional conflict (specify)
Denial, ineffective
Diarrhea
Disuse syndrome, risk for
Diversional activity deficit
Dysreflexia
Energy field disturbance
Environmental interpretation syndrome: impaired
Family processes, altered
Family processes, altered: alcoholism
Fatigue
Fear
Fluid volume deficit
Fluid volume deficit, risk for
Fluid volume excess
Gas exchange, impaired
Grieving, anticipatory
Grieving, dysfunctional
Growth and development, altered
Health maintenance, altered
Health-seeking behaviors (specify)
Home maintenance management, impaired
Hopelessness
Hyperthermia
Hypothermia
Incontinence, functional
Incontinence, reflex
Incontinence, stress
Incontinence, total
Incontinence, urge
Infant behavior, disorganized
Infant behavior, disorganized, risk for
Infant behavior, organized: potential for enhanced
Infant feeding pattern, ineffective
Infection, risk for
Injury, perioperative positioning: risk for
Injury, risk for
Knowledge deficit (specify)
Loneliness, risk for
Management of therapeutic regimen, community: ineffective
Management of therapeutic regimen, families: ineffective
Management of therapeutic regimen, individuals: effective
Management of therapeutic regimen, individuals: ineffective
Memory, impaired
Mobility, impaired physical
Noncompliance (specify)
Nutrition, altered: less than body requirements
Nutrition, altered: more than body requirements
Nutrition, altered: risk for more than body requirements
Oral mucous membranes, altered
Pain
Pain, chronic
Parent/infant/child attachment, altered, risk for
Parental role conflict
Parenting, altered
Parenting, altered, risk for
Peripheral neurovascular dysfunction, risk for
Personal identity disturbance
Poisoning, risk for
Posttrauma response
Powerlessness
Protection, altered
Rape-trauma syndrome
Rape-trauma syndrome: compound reaction

Rape-trauma syndrome: silent reaction
Relocation stress syndrome
Role performance, altered
Self-care deficit, bathing/hygiene
Self-care deficit, dressing/grooming
Self-care deficit, feeding
Self-care deficit, toileting
Self-esteem, chronic low
Self-esteem, disturbance
Self-esteem, situational low
Self-mutilation, risk for
Sensory/perceptual alterations (specify) (visual, auditory, kinesthetic, gustatory, tactile, olfactory)
Sexual dysfunction
Sexuality patterns, altered
Skin integrity, impaired
Skin integrity, impaired, risk for
Sleep pattern disturbance
Social interaction, impaired
Social isolation
Spiritual distress (distress of the human spirit)
Spiritual well-being, potential for enhanced
Suffocation, risk for
Swallowing, impaired
Thermoregulation, ineffective
Thought processes, altered
Tissue integrity, impaired
Tissue perfusion, altered (specify type) (renal, cerebral, cardiopulmonary, gastrointestinal, peripheral)
Trauma, risk for
Unilateral neglect
Urinary elimination, altered
Urinary retention
Ventilation, inability to sustain spontaneous
Ventilatory weaning process, dysfunctional
Violence, risk for: self-directed or directed at others

Appendix C
NORMAL REFERENCE LABORATORY VALUES

Blood, plasma, or serum values

Determination	Reference Range: Conventional	SI
Acetoacetate plus acetone	0.3-2.0 mg/100 ml	3-20 mg/l
Aldolase	1.3-8.2 mU/ml	12-75 nmol · s $^{-1}$/l
Alpha-aminonitrogen	3.0-5.5 mg/100 ml	2.1-3.9 mmol/l
Ammonia	80-110 μg/100 ml	47-65 μmol/l
Ascorbic acid	0.4-1.5 mg/100 ml	23-85 μmol/l
Barbiturate	0	0 μmol/l
	Coma level: phenobarbital, approximately 10 mg/100 ml; most other drugs, 1-3 mg/100 ml	
Bicarbonate	24-32 mEq/L	
Bilirubin (van den Bergh test)	One minute: 0.4 mg/100 ml	Up to 7 μmol/l
	Direct: 0.4 mg/100 ml	
	Total: 1.0 mg/100 ml	
	Indirect is total minus direct	Up to 17 μmol/l
Blood volume	8.5%-9.0% of body weight in kg	80-85 ml/kg
Bromide	0	0 mmol/l
	Toxic level: 17 mEq/l	
Bromsulphalein (BSP)	Less than 5% retention 45 min after 5 mg/kg IV	<0.051
Calcium	8.5-10.5 mg/100 ml (slightly higher in children)	2.1-2.6 mmol/l
Carbon dioxide content	24-30 mEq/l	24-30 mmol/l
	20-26 mEq/l in infants (as HCO_3^-)	
Carbon monoxide	Symptoms with over 20% saturation	0(1)
Carotenoids	0.8-4.0 μg/ml	1.5-7.4 μmol/l
Ceruloplasmin	27-37 mg/100 ml	1.8-2.5 μmol/l
Chloride	100-106 mEq/l	100-106 mmol/l
Cholinesterase (pseudocholinesterase)	0.5 pH U or more/h	0.5 or more arb unit
	0.7 pH U or more/h for packed cells	
Copper	Total: 100-200 μg/100 ml	16-31 μmol/l
Creatine phosphokinase (CPK)	Female 5-35 mU/ml	0.08-0.58 μmol · s $^{-1}$/l
	Male 5-55 mU/ml	
Creatinine	0.6-1.5 mg/100 ml	60-130 μmol/l
Ethanol	0.3%-0.4%, marked intoxication; 0.4%-0.5%, alcoholic stupor; 0.5% or over, alcoholic coma	65-87 mmol/l 87-109 mmol/l >109 mmol/l
Glucose	Fasting: 70-110 mg/100 ml	3.9-5.6 mmol/l
Iron	50-150 μg/100 ml (higher in males)	9.0-26.9 μmol/l
Iron-binding capacity	250-410 μg/100 ml	44.8-73.4 μmol/l
Lactic acid	0.6-118 mEq/l	0.6-1.8 mmol/l
Lactic dehydrogenase	60-120 U/ml	1.00-2.00 μmol · s $^{-1}$/l
Lead	50 μg/100 ml or less	Up to 2.4 μmol/l
Lipase	2 U/ml or less	Up to 2 arb, unit

From Potter PA, Perry AG: *Basic nursing: theory and practice,* ed 3, St Louis, 1994, Mosby.
Modified from Kaye DA and Rose LF: *Fundamentals of internal medicine,* St Louis, 1983, Mosby. Adapted by permission from the New England Journal of Medicine, Vol 302, pages 37-48, 1980.
Abbrevations used: *SI,* Système international d/Unités (The SI for the Health Professions. World Health Organization, Office of Publications, Geneva, Switzerland, 1977); *d,* 24 hours, *P,* plasma; *S,* serum; *B,* blood; *U,* urine; *l,* liter; *h,* hour; and *s,* second.

continued

Blood, plasma, or serum values—cont'd

Determination	Reference Range: Conventional	SI
Lipids		
Cholesterol	120-220 mg/100 ml	3.10-5.69 mmol/l
Cholesterol esters	60%-75% of cholesterol	
Phospholipids	9-16 mg/100 ml as lipid phosphorus	2.9-5.2 mmol/l
Total fatty acids	190-420 mg/100 ml	1.9-4.2 g/l
Total lipids	450-1000 mg/100 ml	4.5-10.0 g/l
Triglycerides	40-150 mg/100 ml	0.4-1.5 g/l
Lithium	Toxic level 2 mEq/l	2 mmol/l
Magnesium	1.5-2.0 mEq/l	0.8-1.3 mmol/l
5′ Nucleotidase	0.3-3.2 Bodansky U	30-290 nmol · s^{-1}/l
Osmolality	285-295 mOsm/kg water	285-295 mmol kg
Oxygen saturation (arterial)	96%-100%	0.96-1.00 l
Pco_2	35-43 mm Hg	4.7-6.0 kPa
pH	7.35-7.45	Same
Po_2	75-100 mm Hg (dependent on age) while breathing room air	
	Above 500 mm Hg while on 100% O_2	10.0-13.3 kPa
Phenylalanine	0-2 mg/100 ml	0.120 μmol/l
Phenytoin (Dilantin)	Therapeutic level, 5-20 μg/ml	19.8-79.5 μmol/l
Phosphorus (inorganic)	3.0-4.5 mg/100 ml (infants in 1st yr up to 6.0 mg/100 ml)	1.0-1.5 mmol/l
Potassium	3.5-5.0 mEq/l	3.5-5.0 mmol/l
Primidone (Mysoline)	Therapeutic level 4-12 μg/ml	18-55 μmol/l
Protein: Total	6.0-8.4 g/100 ml	60-84 g/l
Albumin	3.5-5.0 g/100 ml	35-50 g/l
Globulin	2.3-3.5 g/100 ml	23.35 g/l
Electrophoresis	*% of total protein*	*Of total protein*
Albumin	52-68	0.52-0.68
Globulin:		
$Alpha_1$	4.2-7.2	0.042-0.072
$Alpha_2$	6.8-12	0.068-0.12
Beta	9.3-15	0.093-0.15
Gamma	13-23	0.13-0.23
Pyruvic acid	0-0.11 mEq/l	0.0.11 mmol/l
Quinidine	Therapeutic: 1.5-3 μg/ml	4.6-9.2 μmol/l
Salicylate:		
Therapeutic	20-25 mg/100 ml; 25-30 mg/100 ml to age 10 yr, 3 h post dose	1.4-1.8 mmol/l 1.8-2.2 mmol/l
Toxic	Over 30 mg/100 ml	Over 2.2 mmol/l
	Over 20 mg/100 ml after age 60	Over 1.4 mmol/l
Sodium	135-145 mEq/l	135-145 mmol/l
Sulfate	0.5-1.5 mg/100 ml	0.05-1.2 mmol/l
Sulfonamide	0 mg/100 ml	0 mmol/l
	Therapeutic: 5-15 mg/100 ml	
Transaminase (SGOT) (aspartate aminotransferase)	10-40 U/ml	0.08-0.32 μmol · s^{-1}/l
Urea nitrogen (BUN)	8.25 mg/100 ml	2.9-8.9 mmol/l
Uric acid	3.0-7.0 mg/100 ml	0.18-0.42 mmol/l
Vitamin A	0.15-0.6 μg/ml	0.5-2.1 μmol/l
Vitamin A tolerance test	Rise to twice fasting level in 3 to 5 h	

Urine values

Determination	Reference Range: Conventional	Reference Range: SI
Acetone plus acetoacetate (quantitative)	0	0 mg/l
Alpha amino nitrogen	64-199 mg/d not over 1.5% of total nitrogen	4.6-14.2 mmol/d
Amylase	24-76 U/ml	24-76 arb, unit
Calcium	150 mg/d or less	3.8 or less mmol/d
Catecholamines	Epinephrine: under 20 µg/d	<55 nmol/d
	Norepinephrine: under 100 µg/d	<590 nmol/d
Copper	0-100 µg/d	0-1.6 µmol/d
Coproporphyrin	50-250 µg/d	80-380 nmol/d
	Children under 80 lb 0-75 µg/d	0-115 nmol/d
Creatine	Under 100 mg/d or less than 6% of creatinine; in pregnancy: up to 12%; in children under 1 yr: may equal creatinine; in older children: up to 30% of creatinine	<0.75 mmol/d
Crystine or cysteine	0	0
Follicle-stimulating hormone:		
Follicular phase	5-20 IU/d	Same
Midcycle	15-60 IU/d	
Luteal phase	5-15 IU/d	
Menopausal	50-100 IU/d	
Men	5-25 IU/d	
Hemoglobin and myoglobin	0	
5-Hydroxyindole acetic acid	2-9 mg/d (women lower than men)	10-45 µmol/d
Lead	0.08 µg/ml or 120 µg or less/d	0.39 µmol/l or less
Phenolsulfonphthalein (PSP)	At least 25% excreted by 15 min; 40% by 30 min; 60% by 120 min	0.25 l
Phosphorus (inorganic)	Varies with intake; average 1 g/d	32 mmol/d
Porphobilinogen	0	0
Protein:		
Quantitative	<150 mg/d	<0.15 g/d
Steroids		
17-Ketosteroids (per day)	*Age* *Male* *Female*	*Male* *Female*
	(64) (mg) (mg)	(µmol/d) (µmol/d)
	10 1-4 1-4	3-14 3-14
	20 6-21 4-16	21-73 14-56
	30 8-26 4-14	28-90 14-49
	50 5-18 3-9	17-62 10-31
	70 2-10 1-7	7-35 3-24
17-Hydroxysteroids	3-8 mg/d (women lower than men)	8-22 µmol/d as hydrocortisone
Sugar:		
Quantitative glucose	0	0 mmol/l
Identification of reducing substances:		
Fructose	0	0 mmol/l
Pentose	0	0 mmol/l
Titratable acidity	24-40 mEq/d	20-40 mmol/d
Urobilinogen	Up to 1.0 Ehrlich U	To 1.0 arb. unit
Uroporphyrin	0	0 nmol/d
Vanillylmandelic acid (VMA)	Up to 9 mg/d	Up to 45 µmol/d

continued

Special endocrine tests

Determination	Reference Range: Conventional	Reference Range: SI
STEROID HORMONES		
Aldosterone	Excretion: 5-19 μg/d	14-53 nmol/d
Fasting, at rest, 210 mEq sodium diet	Supine: 48 ± 29 pg/ml	180 ± 64 pmol/l
	Upright: (2 h) 65 ± 23 ¶/ml	
Fasting, at rest, 110 mEq sodium diet	Supine: 107 ± 45 pg/ml	279 ± 125 pmol/l
	Upright: (2 h) 239 ± 123 pg/ml	663 ± 341 pmol/l
Fasting, at rest, 10 mEq sodium diet	Supine: 175 ± 75 pg/ml	485 ± 108 pmol/l
	Upright: (2 h) 523 ± 228 pg/ml	1476 ± 632 pmol/l
Cortisol		
Fasting	8 AM: 5-25 ≅g/100 ml	0.14-0.69 μmol/l
At rest	8 PM: Below 10 μg/100 ml	0-0.28 μmol/l
20 U ACTH	4 h ACTH test: 30-45 μg/100 ml	0.83-1.24 μmol/l
Dexamethasone at midnight	Overnight suppression test: Below 5 μg/100 ml	<0.14 nmol/l
	Excretion: 20-70 μg/d	≥0.22 ≅ mol/l
11-Deoxycortisol	Responsive; over 7.5 μg/100 ml (after metyrapone)	10.4-38.1 nmol/l >3.5 nmol/l
Testosterone	Adult male: 300-1100 ng/100 ml	0.87-3.12 nmol/l
	Adolescent male: over 100 ng/100 ml	106-832 pmol/l
	Female: 25-90 ng/100 ml	3.1-44.4 pmol/l
Unbound testosterone	Adult male: 3.06-24.0 ng/100 ml	
	Adult female: 0.09-1.28 ng/100 ml	
POLYPEPTIDE HORMONES		
Adrenocorticotropin (ACTH)	15-70 pg/ml	3.3-15.4 prmol/l
Calcitonin	Undetectable in normals	0
	>100 pg/ml in medullary carcinoma	>29.3 pmol/l
Growth hormone		
Fasting, at rest	Below 5 ng/ml	<233 pmol/l
After exercise	Child: over 10 ng/ml	>465 pmol/l
	Male: Below 5 ng/ml	<233 pmol/l
	Female: Up to 309 ng/ml	0-1395 pmol/l
After glucose	Male: Below 5 ng/ml	<233 pmol/l
	Female: Below 10 ng/ml	0-465 pmol/l
Insulin		
Fasting	6-26 μU/ml	43-187 pmol/l
During hypoglycemia	Below 20 μU/ml	<144 pmol/l
After glucose	Up to 150 μU/ml	0-1078 pmol/l
Leuteinizing hormone	Male: 6-18 mU/ml	6-18 μ/l
Preovulatory or postovulatory	Female: 5-22 mU/ml	5-22 μ/l
Midcycle peak	30-250 mU/ml	30-250 μ/l
Parathyroid hormone	<10 μl equiv/ml	<10 ml equiv/l
Prolactin	2-15 ng/ml	0.08-6.0 nmol/l
Renin activity		
Normal diet	Supine: 1.1 ± 0.8 ng/ml/h	0.9 ± 0.6 (nmol/Dh)
	Upright: 1.9 ± 17 ng/ml/h	1.5 ± 1.3 (nmol/Dh)
Low-sodium diet	Supine: 2.7 ± 118 ng/ml/h	2.1 ± 1.4 (nmol/Dh)
	Upright: 6.6 ± 2.5 ng/ml/h	5.1 ± 1.9 (nmol/Dh)
Low-sodium diet	Diuretics: 10.0 ± 3.7 ng/ml/h	7.7 ± 2.9 (nmol/Dh)
THYROID HORMONES		
Thyroid-stimulating hormone (TSH)	0.5-3.5 μU/ml	0.5-3.5 mU/l
Thyroxine-binding globulin capacity	15-25 μg T_4/100 ml	193-322 nmol/l
Total triiodothyronine by radioimmunoassay (T_3)		
Total thyroxine by RIA (T_4)	4-12 μg/100 ml	52-154 nmol/l
T_3 resin uptake	25%-35%	0.25-0.35
Free thyroxine index (FT_4I)	1-4 ng/100 ml	12.8-51.2 pmol/l

Cerebrospinal fluid values

	Reference Range	
Determination	**Conventional**	**SI**
Bilirubin	0	0 μmol/l
Chloride	120-130 mEq/l (20 mEq/l higher than serum)	
Albumin	Mean: 29.5 mg/100 ml ±2 SD: 11-48 mg/100 ml	0.295 g/l ±2 SD: 0.11-48
IgG	Mean: 4.3 mg/100 ml ±2 SD: 0-8.6 mg/100 ml	0.043 g/l ±2 SD: 0-0.086

	Reference Range	
Determination	**Conventional**	**SI**
Glucose	50-75 mg/100 ml (30%-50% less than blood)	2.8-4.2 mmol/l
Pressure (initial)	70-180 mm of water	70-80 arb. units
Protein:		
Lumbar	15-45 mg/100 ml	0.15-0.45 g/l
Cisternal	15-25 mg/100 ml	0.15-0.25 g/l
Ventricular	5-15 mg/100 ml	0.05-0.15 g/l

Hematologic values

	Reference Range	
Determination	**Conventional**	**SI**
Coagulation factors:		
Factor I (fibrinogen)	0.15-0.35 g/100 ml	4.0-10.0 μmol/l
Factor II (prothrombin)	60%-140%	0.60-1.40
Factor V (accelerator globulin)	60%-140%	0.60-1.40
Factor VII-X (proconvertin-Stuart)	70%-130%	0.70-1.30
Factor X (Stuart factor)	70%-130%	0.70-1.30
Factor VIII (antihemophilic globulin)	50%-200%	0.50-2.0
Factor IX (plasma thromboplastic cofactor)	60%-140%	0.60-1.40
Factor XI (plasma thromboplastic antecedent)	60%-140%	0.60-1.40
Factor XII (Hageman factor)	60%-140%	0.60-1.40
Coagulation screening tests:		
Bleeding time (Simplate)	3-9 min	18-540 s
Prothrombin time	Less than 2-s deviation from control	Less than 2-s deviation from control
Partial thromboplastin time (activated)	25-37 s	25-37 s
Whole-blood clot lysis	No clot lysis in 24 h	0/d
Fibrinolytic studies:		
Euglobin lysis	No lysis in 2 h	0 (in 2 h)
Fibrinogen split products	Negative reaction at greater than 1:4 dilution	0 (at >1:4 dilution)
Thrombin time	Control ± 5 s	Control ± 5 s
Complete blood count:		
Hematocrit	Male: 45%-52% Female: 37%-48%	Male: 0.42-0.52 Female: 0.37-0.48
Hemoglobin	Male: 13-18 g/100 ml Female: 12-16 g/100 ml	Male: 8.1-11.2 mmol/l Female: 7.4-9.9 mmol/l

continued

Hematologic values

Determination	Reference Range: Conventional	Reference Range: SI
Leukocyte count	4300-10,800/mm^3	4.3-10.8 × 10^9/1
Erythrocyte count	4.2-5.9 million/mm^3	4.2-5.9 × 10^{12}/1
Mean corpuscular volume (MCV)	80-94 μm^3	80-94 fl
Mean corpuscular hemoglobin (MCH)	27-32 pg	1.7-2.0 fmol
Mean corpuscular hemoglobin	32%-36%	19-22.8 mmol/l
Mean corpuscular hemoglobin concentration (MCHC)		
Erythrocyte sedimentation rate (Westergren method)	Male: 1-13 mm/h Female: 1-20 mm/h	Male: 1-13 mm/h Female: 1-20 mm/h
Erythrocyte enzymes:		
Glucose-6-phosphate dehydrogenase	5-15 U/gHb	5-15 U/g
Pyruvate kinase	13-17 U/gHb	13-17 U/g
Ferritin (serum)		
Iron deficiency	0.20 ng/ml	0-20 μg/l
Iron excess	Greater than 400 ng/l	>400 μg/l
Folic acid		
Normal	Greater than 1.9 ng/ml	>4.3 mmol/l
Borderline	1.0-1.9 ng/ml	2.3-4.3 mmol/l
Haptoglobin	100-300 mg/100 ml	1.0-3.0 g/l
Hemoglobin studies:		
Electrophoresis for A_2 hemoglobin	1.5%-3.5%	0.015-0.035
Hemoglobin F (fetal hemoglobin)	Less than 2%	<0.02
Hemoglobin, met- and sulf-	0	0
Serum hemoglobin	2-3 mg/100 ml	1.2-1.9 μmol/l
Thermolabile hemoglobin	0	0
LE (lupus erythematosus) preparation:		
Heparin as anticoagulant	0	0
Defibrinated blood	0	0
Leukocyte alkaline phosphatase:		
Quantitative method	1-40 mg of phosphorus liberated/h/ 10^{10} cells	15-40 mg/h
Qualitative method	Males: 33-188 U Females (off contraceptive pill): 30-160 U	33-188 U 30-160 U
Muramidase	Serum, 3-7 μg/ml Urine, 0-2 ≅ g/ml	3-7 mg/l 0-2 mg/l
Osmotic fragility of erythrocytes	Increased if hemolysis occurs in over 0.5% NaCl; decreased if hemolysis is incomplete in 0.3% of NaCl	
Peroxide hemolysis	Less than 10%	<0.10
Platelet count	150,000-350,000/mm^3	150-350 × 10^9/l
Platelet function tests:		
Clot retraction	50%-100%/2 h	0.50-1.00/2 h
Platelet aggregation	Full response to ADP, epinephrine, and collagen	1.0
Platelet factor 3	33-57 s	33-57 s
Prothrombin time	Less than 2 sec deviation from control	
Reticulocyte count	0.5%-1.5% red cells	0.005-0.015
Vitamin B_{12}	90-280 pg/ml (borderline: 70-90)	66-207 pmol/1 (borderline: 52-66)

Miscellaneous values

Determination	Reference Range: Conventional	SI
Autoantibodies in serum		
Thyroid collaid and microsomal antigens	Absent	
Stomach parietal cells	Absent	
Smooth muscle	Absent	
Kidney mitochondria	Absent	
Rabbit renal collecting ducts	Absent	
Cytoplasm of ova, theca cells, testicular interstitial cells	Absent	
Skeletal muscle	Absent	
Adrenal gland	Absent	
Carcinoembryonic antigen (CEA) in blood	0-2.5 ng/ml, 97% healthy nonsmokers	0-2.5 μg/l, 97% healthy nonsmokers
Cryoprecipitable proteins in blood	0	0 arb unit
Digitoxin in serum	17 ± 6 ng/ml	22 ± 7.8 nmol/l
Digoxin in serum		
0.25 mg/d	1.2 ± 0.4 ng/ml	1.54 ± 0.5 nmol/l
0.5 mg/d	1.5 ± 0.4 ng/ml	1.92 ± 0.5 nmol/l
Duodenal drainage:		
pH	5.5-7.5	5.5-7.5
Amylase	Over 1200 U/total sample	>1.2 arb. unit
Trypsin	Values from 35% to 160% "normal"	0.35-1.60
Viscosity	3 min or less	180 s or less
Gastric analysis	Basal:	
	Females: 2.0 ± 1.8 mEq/h	0.6 ± 0.5
	Males: 3.0 ± 2.0 mEq/h	0.8 ± 0.6 μmol/s
	Maximal: (after histalog or gastrin)	
	Females: 16 ± 5 mEq/h	
	Males: 23 ± 5 mEq/h	6.4 ± 1.4 μmol/s
Gastrin-I in blood	0-200 pg/ml	0-95 pmol/l
Alpha-fetoglobulin	Abnormal if present	
Alpha 1-antitrypsin	200-400 mg/100 ml	2.0-4.0 g/l
Antinuclear antibodies	Positive if detected with serum diluted 1:10	
Anti-DNA antibodies	Less than 15 units/ml	
Complement, total hemolytic	150-250 U/ml	
C3	Range 55-120 mg/100 ml	0.55-1.2 g/l
C4	Range 20-50 mg/100 ml	0.2-0.5 g/l
Immunoglobulins in blood:		
IgG	1140 mg/100 ml	11.4 g/l
	Range 540-1663	5.5-16.6 g/l
IgA	214 mg/100 ml	2.14 g/l
	Range 66-344	0.66-3.44 g/l
IgM	168 mg/100 ml	1.68 g/l
	Range 39-290	0.39-2.9 g/l
Viscosity	1.4-1.8 expressed as relative viscosity of serum compared with water	
Iontophoresis	Children: 0-40 mEq sodium/l	0-40 mmol/l
	Adults: 0-60 mEq sodium/l	0-60 mmol/l

continued

Miscellaneous values—cont'd

Determination	Reference Range: Conventional	Reference Range: SI
Propranolol (includes bioactive 4-OH metabolite) in serum 4h after last dose		
Stool fat	Less than 5 g in 24 hr or less than 4% of measured fat intake in 3-d period	<5 g/d
Stool nitrogen	Less than 2 g/d or 10% of urinary nitrogen	<2 g/d
Synovial fluid:		
Glucose	Not less than 20 mg/100 ml lower than simultaneously drawn blood sugar	See blood glucose mmol/l
Mucin	Type 1 or 2 Grades as: Type 1-tight clump Type 2-soft clump Type 3-soft clump that breaks up Type 4-cloudy, no clump	1-2 arb. unit
	5-8 g/5 h in urine	
D-Xylose absorption	40 mg/100 ml in blood 2 h after ingestion of 25 g of D-xylose	33-53 mmol 2.7 mmol/l

GLOSSARY

abduction Movement of the extremity away from the midline of the body.
abortion The termination of pregnancy before the fetus is viable.
abscess A localized infection with an accumulation of pus.
abuse To use wrongly or excessively.
acceptance Approval or the willingness to accept.
acetone A by-product of fat metabolism.
acidosis Increase in hydrogen ion concentration as a result of accumulation of acid products or depletion of bicarbonate reserves.
acquired immunodeficiency syndrome See AIDS.
acromegaly A chronic disease caused by an oversecretion of the growth hormone of the pituitary gland. In the adult it may be caused by a tumor.
active immunity Immunity acquired during a person's lifetime as a result of exposure to infectious organisms.
acute care Those services that treat the acute phase of illness or disability, the purpose of which is the restoration of normal life processes and functions.
acute pain Discomfort of relatively short duration; useful in that it provides information relating to injury or pathology.
acute renal failure Temporary loss of renal function; usually has a sudden onset.
adaptation Modification to meet a new or changed situation.
addiction Psychologic dependence on a drug; a behavioral pattern of compulsive drug use characterized by overwhelming involvement with getting and using the drug. Withdrawal symptoms specific to the drug occur after cessation of intake.
addictive disorders Physiologic dependence on a chemical or organic substance that results in withdrawal symptoms after cessation of intake.
adduction Movement of the extremity toward the midline of the body.
adhesion Joining of two parts by an abnormal fibrous band.
adjustment disorders An inability of the individual to adapt to new situations or changes in life, or an inability to modify behavior, which overwhelms the person's coping skills and defense mechanisms.
ADL Activities of daily living.
aerobic Describes a pathogen that requires free oxygen to live.
affective disorders One of a group of disorders that has a primary disturbance of emotions or mood as a major feature. It can be chronic or episodic.
agent A factor, such as a microorganism, where presence or relative absence is essential for the occurrence of a disease.
aging A nonpathologic process that gradually results in loss of cells and physiologic reserves.
agitation A state of anxiety accompanied by motor restlessness.
AIDS (acquired immunodeficiency syndrome) A manifestation of infection with the human immunodeficiency virus (HIV); characterized by the presence of one or more diseases as defined by the Centers for Disease Control and Prevention (CDC). These diseases occur following a depression of an individual's immune system function. The affected person becomes susceptible to unusual infections and malignancies.
AIDS-related complex See ARC.
airway A metal, plastic, or rubber device used to keep the tongue from obstructing the trachea.
aldosterone A steroid hormone produced by the adrenal cortex to regulate sodium and potassium in the blood.
alkalosis A condition in which the alkalinity of the body is increased.
alkylating agent A drug used in the treatment of cancer; examples include nitrogen mustard and cyclophosphamide (cytoxan).
allergen Any substance to which some individuals react abnormally.
allergist A physician trained in the diagnosis and treatment of allergic diseases and disorders.
Alzheimer's disease A chronic brain disorder that involves a progressive destruction of brain tissue. This disease can begin when a patient is in his or her forties and results in slurred speech, growing memory lapses, involuntary muscle movements, and gradual intellectual deterioration.
amblyopia Decrease in visual acuity without underlying cause; not correctable with lenses.
ambulation Not confined to bed; walking.
ambulatory care All health services provided on an outpatient basis to those who visit a hospital or other healthcare facility and depart after treatment on the same day.
amenorrhea Absence of menses; normal before puberty and during pregnancy.
Americans with Disabilities Act (Public Law 101-336) Passed in July 1990, this legislation establishes equal opportunity for persons with disabilities regarding employment, public accommodation, transportation, state and local government services, and telecommunications.
amputee A person who has lost one or more of his or her extremities.
anabolism A constructive process by which food is converted into living cells.
anaerobic Describes a pathogen that cannot live in the presence of oxygen.
analgesic A drug that relieves pain.
analysis Second step in the nursing process, sometimes combined with or implied as part of the first step (assessment). Involves the evaluation of data for the purpose of determining the patient's needs and problems and developing a nursing diagnosis.
anaphylaxis An immediate reaction that results from sensitivity to a foreign protein.
anastomosis Surgical connection between two normally distinct structures or segments of a structure (arteriovenous anastomosis); connection of an artery to a vein (intestinal anastomosis); connection of two previously distant parts of the intestine. Can also occur pathologically.
anemia A blood disorder caused by a reduction of erythrocytes and hemoglobin.
anesthesia Administration of a substance that causes loss of bodily sensations.
aneurysm Dilation of blood vessels into a saclike bulge.
anger An expression of anxiety resulting from real or perceived threats.
angina pectoris Paroxysms of pain caused by decreased blood supply to the myocardium.
angioplasty Percutaneous transfusional coronary angioplasty dilates the coronary vessel wall through mechanical compression.
anhidrosis Lack of sweating.
anion A negatively charged ion.
ankylosis Stiffening of a joint caused by infection or irritation and the development of fibrous tissue in the joint.
anorexia Loss of appetite.
antibody An immune substance produced within the body in response to a specific antigen.
anticipatory grief Expectation of loss of someone or something highly valued.
anticoagulant A drug that lengthens the prothrombin time and helps to prevent thrombosis and embolism.
antigen A substance that stimulates the immune process.

antihistamine A drug used in the treatment of allergic disorders and motion sickness.

antimetabolite An agent that is used primarily in treating leukemia in children.

antiseptic An agent that is used on the skin to inhibit or destroy microorganisms.

antispasmodic A drug used to relieve spasms of smooth muscles.

antitoxin A serum that is used to combat the toxin produced by a microorganism.

anuria Failure of the kidneys to secrete urine.

anxiety Feeling of uneasiness or apprehension in which the source is often unknown.

anxiety disorders Disorders that have anxiety as the most outstanding symptom. These disorders include posttraumatic stress disorder, phobic disorder, panic disorder, and obsessive-compulsive disorder.

aphasia Loss of the ability to speak.

apnea A temporary absence of breathing.

apoplexy Cerebrovascular accident.

appendicitis Acute inflammation of the appendix.

ARC (AIDS-related complex) The syndrome of general systemic infections (e.g., fever, diarrhea) that occur in an individual before the development of the opportunistic infections or malignancies of AIDS.

ARDS Adult respiratory distress syndrome.

arrhythmia Any deviation from the normal heartbeat rhythm.

arteriosclerosis Hardening of the arteries caused by the formation of fibrous plaques and loss of elasticity.

arthrodesis Surgical fusion of a joint in a functional position.

arthroplasty Plastic surgery on a diseased joint to increase mobility.

arthrotomy Incision of a joint.

articulation Point at which two bones are joined together, such as in a joint.

ascites Accumulation of fluid in the peritoneal cavity.

asepsis A condition of relative freedom from pathogenic organisms.

asphyxia Suffocation caused by a decrease of oxygen and an increase of carbon dioxide.

assessment The first step in the nursing process. It demands the collection and recording of data related to the patient and the family for the purpose of identifying patient problems. It includes the physical and emotional signs and symptoms presented by the patient, as well as information obtained from other sources (e.g., the patient's chart, laboratory report, and family visitors).

asthma A chronic bronchial disease that is caused by spasm of the bronchial tubes and is accompanied by edema.

astigmatism A defect in the curvature of the cornea or the lens of the eye.

ataxia A lack of coordination of motor movements.

atelectasis Collapse of the lung; may be total or partial.

atherosclerosis A degenerative process of the blood vessels that is characterized by fatlike deposits along the walls of the vessels.

atopic Pertaining to a state of hypersensitivity that is influenced by heredity.

atrial fibrillation An arrhythmia of the atria consisting of rapid, irregular, and ineffective contractions.

atrophic Wasting away of an organ or part of the body.

atrophy To waste away or decrease in size.

atropine An alkaloid of belladonna; may be administered with a narcotic as preoperative medication.

audiologist A person trained in the detection of hearing problems and the administration of hearing tests; a person who is trained in the use of hearing aids.

audiometry Hearing test using an audiometer, which is an instrument that produces tones of varying pitch and intensity; the tones are heard through earphones that are attached to the audiometer.

auditory canal Passage from the auricle or pinna of the external ear to the tympanic membrane.

aura A visual sensation experienced by a person with epilepsy before having a seizure.

auricle The visible portion of the external ear; also called the pinna.

auricular fibrillation An arrhythmia of the atria that is characterized by a rapid, irregular rate of contraction.

autoclave An apparatus that uses steam and pressure to sterilize.

autogenous Made from within the body. A vaccine made from organisms that are taken from a person is an autogenous vaccine.

autograft Tissue taken from the same donor as the recipient.

autoimmunity A condition in which antibodies are produced by one's own body, which causes immunization against the body's own proteins.

autologous blood transfusion Transfusion of blood that has either been donated by the patient in advance of surgery or collected from the surgical site during the procedure. Use of the patient's own blood rather than blood from a donor prevents possible exposure to the AIDS virus.

autonomy The ability or tendency to function independently.

BAC See Blood Alcohol Concentration.

bacteremia Presence of bacteria in the bloodstream.

bacterial endocarditis Infection that affects the valves and the lining of the heart.

bactericidal Describes an agent that kills bacteria.

bacteriophage A virus that attacks bacteria.

bacteriostatic Describes an agent that prevents multiplication of bacteria.

bargaining A mutual agreement.

barium A silver-white chemical agent used as a contrast medium in x-ray examination of the gastrointestinal tract.

bends Abdominal cramps caused by a rapid change from increased atmospheric pressure to normal atmospheric pressure.

benign Describes a nonmalignant growth or tumor.

benign prostatic hypertrophy Enlargement of the prostate gland.

bereavement Deprivation, such as in loss by death.

bilateral On both sides.

biliary Relating to the gallbladder, liver, and their ducts.

biliary colic Acute pain caused by obstruction of the cystic duct, usually as a result of a stone.

bioethics The application of normative ethics to issues in biology and medicine; sometimes referred to as healthcare ethics.

biologic response modifiers Natural products produced in large quantities by genetic engineering techniques. Proteins that stimulate and improve the cancer patient's biologic response against tumor cells.

biopsychosocial The interrelationship of physical, emotional, and social factors.

biotherapy Treatment of cancer using biologic response modifiers.

bleb An irregular elevation of the epidermis that is filled with serous fluid.

Blood Alcohol Concentration (BAC) The test is expressed in a blood alcohol concentration percentage. All states consider a level of 0.10 as legally intoxicated. Some mental and physical impairment is noticed.

blood dyscrasias Diseases of the blood and the blood-forming organs.

blood urea nitrogen (BUN) An end product of protein metabolism found in the blood.

body image The way in which a person views own body; may mean acceptance in the care of a deformity.

boil Cutaneous superficial infection of short duration.

bone marrow transplantation Replacement of bone marrow after chemotherapy and/or radiotherapy.

braces Mechanical device used for support, usually of an extremity.

bradycardia A cardiac arrhythmia that is marked by an unusually slow heartbeat.

brain stem Subdivision of the brain; located above the spinal cord and contains the midbrain, pons, and medulla.

bronchiectasis A chronic disease of the lungs in which there is a dilation of the bronchi; may affect both lungs or only a portion of one lung.

bronchitis An inflammatory condition of the bronchial tubes.

bronchography X-ray examination of the bronchi using a radiopaque substance.

bronchoscopy Examination of the bronchi and a portion of the lungs with a lighted instrument.

bulla A vesicle greater than 1 cm in diameter.

burnout A manifestation of physical and/or psychologic symptoms (e.g., hopelessness, helplessness, fatigue) that may occur in nurses who care for persons with AIDS or a terminal illness. It is an ongoing process in which nurses may have negative feelings toward life, careers, and other people. Stresslike symptoms are common.

bursitis Acute or chronic inflammation of a bursa caused by injury, disease, or an unknown factor.

calculus Many stones.

calibrated Marked or graduated to provide for accurate measurement.

callus (1) Thickening of skin from continuous irritation; (2) fibrous tissue formed at the site of a fracture.

candidiasis An infection with a fungus of the *Candida* family, generally *C. albicans,* that most commonly involves the skin (dermatocandidiasis), oral mucosa (thrush), respiratory tract (bronchocandidiasis), and vagina (vaginitis). Candidiasis of the esophagus, trachea, bronchi, or lungs is an indicator of AIDS.

cannulation Procedure of placing a cannula into the body, as into a vein.

capsule Mucilaginous envelope that surrounds some forms of bacteria.

carbuncle A boil with an infiltration into adjacent tissues that finally opens in several places on the skin.

carcinogenic Anything capable of producing cancer.

carcinoma A malignant tumor arising from epithelial cells. Tends to infiltrate or metastasize to other tissues.

cardiac output The volume of blood expelled by the ventricles of the heart.

cardiogenic shock Interference with pumping action of the heart, which causes insufficient vascular circulation.

cardiogram A tracing of the electric activity of the heart.

cardiopulmonary Pertaining to the heart and lungs.

cardiospasm A spasm of the cardiac valve between the esophagus and the stomach; generally a functional disorder.

Care Map A prewritten and adopted statement of specific activities to be achieved at each phase of the illness. It is broader in scope than nursing care plans; care maps include all activities, not just nursing activities.

carrier One who harbors germs of a disease and transmits the disease to others while having no symptoms of the disease.

case management Coordination and supervision of all aspects of healthcare for an individual patient, including delivery of care and evaluation of effectiveness.

catabolism Destructive process by which complex substances are broken down into simpler ones; opposite of anabolism.

cataract An opacity of the lens of the eye.

catecholamines Hormones that tend to increase and prolong the effects of the sympathetic nervous system.

cation A positively charged ion.

CD4 Cell Count (T4 count) The most characterized of all the surrogate markers of immunodeficiency; the number of CD4 (T4 helper) cells. As an HIV-infected individual's CD4 cells decline, the risk of developing opportunistic infections increases. The trend of several consecutive CD4 counts is more important than any one measurement.

cell-mediated immunity Acquired immunity characterized by the dominant role of small T-cell lymphocytes.

cellular immunity Acquired immunity that results in sensitization of whole lymphocytes to the invading agent.

central venous pressure A measurement to determine the ability of the right side of the heart to receive and pump blood.

cerebellum Part of the hindbrain; functions to coordinate movements.

cerebral edema Increased fluid accumulation in the interstitial areas of the cerebrum.

cerebral palsy A chronic neuromuscular disorder that affects motor coordination.

cerebrospinal fluid Fluid surrounding the brain and spinal cord.

cerebrum Main portion of the brain in the upper half of the cranium; forms the largest part of the central nervous system.

cerumen Earwax; a yellowish or brownish waxy secretion in the external ear canal.

chain of custody Tracing who handled evidence from the time it was obtained.

chancre Lesion of primary syphilis occurring at the point of inoculation.

chemotherapy Treatment of disease with drugs or medications. Most commonly refers to the treatment of cancer with antineoplastic drugs.

Cheyne-Stokes respiration Respiration in which the rhythm and depth vary with periods of apnea.

child abuse/maltreatment Any threat to a child's health or welfare.

cholangiography X-ray examination of the biliary tree after injection of a radiopaque dye.

cholecystectomy Surgical removal of the gallbladder.

cholecystitis Inflammation of the gallbladder.

cholecystography X-ray examination of the gallbladder by use of a radiopaque dye to determine the shape and position of the organ.

cholelithiasis A condition in which calculi are present in the gallbladder or one of its ducts.

cholesterol A substance present in all body tissues and fluids. It may be increased or is thought to be a factor in the development of atherosclerosis.

cholinergic Nerve fibers that liberate acetylcholine when an impulse passes through the nerve; a drug that resembles the action of acetylcholine.

chordotomy Surgical division of the anterolateral tracts of the spinal cord to relieve pain.

choreiform Resembling chorea.

chronic acute pain Acute pain lasting longer than 3 months; may be continuous or intermittent; examples include cancer or burn pain.

chronic benign pain Pain that persists for 3 months or longer and in which the pathologic cause is not progressive or life threatening. The pain serves no useful purpose and should be treated as a disease; examples include migraine headache, back pain, and arthritis.

chronic disease A disease involving structure or function or both; may be expected to continue over an extended period.

chronic malignant pain Pain associated with cancer or other progressive disorders.

chronic renal failure Loss of renal function; usually has a prolonged onset.

cilia Hairlike projections in nasal cavities, trachea, and bronchi.

CircOlectric bed A type of electrically operated bed that permits easy turning and moving of the patient.

circumcision A surgical procedure in which the prepuce of the penis is excised.

circumvent To go around or to prevent.

cirrhosis Disease characterized by death of liver cells and their replacement by scar tissue.

climacteric Synonymous with menopause.

clinical ethics The application of bioethics in the identification, analysis, and resolution of moral problems that arise in the care of a particular patient.

CMV (cytomegalovirus) A member of the herpes virus family that can cause fever, fatigue, enlarged lymph glands, aching, and a mild sore throat. In persons with AIDS, CMV infections can produce hepatitis, pneumonia, retinitis, and colitis. CMV infection may lead to blindness, chronic diarrhea, or death.

coalesce To run together, such as in measles.

coccidioidomycosis A disease of the lungs caused by inhaling spores of fungi from the soil.

cochlea Part of the inner ear. A snail-shaped tube containing the organ of Corti (the receptor end organ of hearing).

colectomy Surgical removal of part or all of the colon.

collagenase (ABC) ointment Ointment found to be effective in the treatment of decubitus ulcers.

colonization Presence of an infective agent in the body. Similar to infection.

colostomy A surgical procedure that provides an artificial passageway for fecal material from the colon to the outside.

colposcopy Examination of the cervix and vagina by means of a lighted instrument with a magnifying lens, which is called a colposcope and is inserted into the vagina.

coma A deep sleep from which a person cannot be aroused.

comedones Blackheads.

compartment syndrome The progressive development of arterial blood vessel compression and circulatory compromise (reduced blood supply). Can rapidly result in permanent contracture deformity of the hand or foot, which is called Volkmann's contracture; can occur with injury to forearm and lower leg, with or without fracture.

compromised host A person with deficient defense mechanisms and who is therefore at an increased risk for infection.

computerized tomography A computer-aided x-ray examination that visualizes soft tissues better than conventional x-ray examinations.

concurrent disinfection Daily handling and disposal of contaminated material or equipment.

concussion A violent jarring of the brain against the skull.

condom A sheath used to cover the penis during sexual intercourse to prevent conception and sexually transmitted diseases. Correct use of a rubber (latex) condom during every act of intercourse greatly reduces, but does not eliminate, the risk of infection with HIV. Lambskin or "natural" condoms do not offer protection because they are too porous.

confusion Altered orientation to time, person, or place.

congenital Existing at birth.

conization A surgical procedure in which a cone-shaped piece of tissue is removed from the cervix.

conjunctivitis Inflammation of the conjunctiva of the eye.

conscious The part of the mind that is one's awareness.

Consolidated Omnibus Reconciliation Act (COBRA) Legislation passed by Congress in 1986. Considered the "anti-dumping" law. Requires all hospitals that receive Medicare dollars to perform a medical examination on all patients to determine if a medical emergency exists. This law sets standards for transferring patients.

contamination Soiling with any infectious material.

continuity Uninterrupted connection, succession, or union.

contracture A shortening or tension of a muscle, which affects extension.

control Restricting the spread of infectious processes.

contusion Bruise; black-and-blue spot that is caused by rupture of small blood vessels.

convulsion Involuntary contraction of voluntary muscles.

corpuscle Blood cell; any small mass in the body.

coryza An acute upper respiratory infection; a common cold.

cotton-wool spots/patches Fluffy-looking white deposits on the retina that represent small areas that have lost their blood supply as a result of blockage of local vessels.

countertraction An opposing force or pulling in the opposite direction.

Cowper's gland Either of two round, pea-sized glands embedded in the male urethral sphincter. Also called the bulbourethral gland.

craniotomy A surgical opening of the cranium for exploration or removal of a tumor or blood clot.

creatinine Nonprotein substance in the blood; synthesized from three amino acids. Normally excreted by the kidney.

cretinism A condition resulting from complete absence of the thyroid gland or its secretions at birth.

cricothyroidotomy Incision made into the cricothyroid membrane to establish an emergency airway.

critical thinking A process used to make sound, accurate, and reasonable decisions on the basis of thorough data collection and analysis.

cross-infection Transmission of an infection from one patient to another who is already ill with another disease.

crust A dry exudate; commonly called a scab.

cryoprecipitate A fraction of fresh blood plasma; used to control bleeding in a person with hemophilia.

cryosurgery Surgical techniques that use an instrument to apply extreme cold either to destroy tissue or to cause tissues to adhere to one another. Used in retinal surgery.

cryptorchidism A condition of an undescended testicle.

culdoscopy A diagnostic procedure; involves making an incision through the posterior cul-de-sac and inserting a culdoscope to visualize the pelvic organs.

curettage A surgical procedure in which a cavity is scraped with an instrument called a curet.

cutdown Incision through the skin for the purpose of placing a needle or catheter into a vein.

cyanosis A bluish color of the skin; caused by inadequate oxygenation of the blood.

cyst Saclike, nonmalignant tumor; may contain fluid or cheeselike material.

cystectomy Removal of the urinary bladder.

cystitis Inflammation of the urinary bladder.

cystocele Protrusion of the bladder into the vagina.

cystography X-ray examination of the urinary bladder after injection of a radiopaque substance.

cystoscope Lighted instrument for examination of the inside of the urinary bladder.

cystostomy A surgical opening of the urinary bladder through an abdominal incision and drainage by a catheter through the abdominal wound.

cytomegalovirus See CMV.

deafness Hearing at 85-90 decibels below normal.

debridement Removal of infected or necrotic tissue from a wound.

decibel A ratio that compares the relationship between two sound intensities; used to measure hearing.

decomposition Dissolution into simpler chemical forms.

decompression Reduction of pressure.

decubitus ulcer Necrotic ulcer caused by pressure over bones, where there is little fat and subcutaneous tissue.

defense mechanisms Unconscious processes used to alleviate anxiety; physical structures or processes that protect against stresses from the environment.

defibrillation Application of a current countershock to the chest wall to stop ventricular fibrillation.

degeneration Gradual deterioration of the normal cells and body functions.

dehiscence Separation of a surgical incision.

delirium A global cognitive impairment of memory and organization of thought.

delirium tremens A form of alcoholic psychosis.

delusion False belief that contradicts the individual's knowledge or experience.

dementia A global cognitive dysfunction characterized by impairment in short-term and long-term memory, orientation, abstract thinking, and judgment, as well as by personality changes. Also referred to as organic brain syndrome.

demineralization A decrease of mineral or inorganic salts; occurs in some diseases.

denial Refusal to accept a situation.

depolarization The reduction of a membrane potential to a less negative value.

depression Feeling of inadequacy or sadness.

dermatologist A physician trained in the diagnosis and treatment of skin diseases and disorders.

dermatomycosis Superficial mycotic infections of the skin, hair, and nails.

dermis True skin just below the epidermis.

desensitization Injection of extracts of antigenic substances; causes immunization against specific antigens.

desquamation A scaling or flaking of the skin following certain infectious diseases, in psoriasis, or in reaction to radiation therapy.

diabetic A person with diabetes, which is caused by a deficiency of insulin secretin from the islets of Langerhans.

diagnosis-related group See DRG.

dialyzer A machine used to separate or remove certain substances from the blood when the kidneys fail to perform their normal function.

diffusion Movement of molecules from an area of higher concentration to an area of lower concentration.

digitalization Administration of digitalis in doses sufficient to achieve the maximum physiologic effect without toxic symptoms.

dignity Feeling of worth.

dilation Increasing the diameter of an opening either by normal physiologic processes, drugs, or mechanical means.

diplopia A condition of the eye in which a person sees double.

direct contact Touching of two individuals or organisms; done in association with a carrier in an infective state.

disease Any condition in which either the physiologic or psychologic functions of the body deviate from what is considered to be normal.

disinfectant A chemical that destroys microorganisms when applied to inanimate objects.

disinfection The elimination of many pathogenic organisms, with the exception of bacterial spores.

dislocation Separation of a bone in a joint from its normal position.

disseminated intravascular coagulation (DIC) An acute bleeding disorder that results in a hypercoagulable state.

dissociative disorders Disorders that involve the mental defense of splitting off some part of consciousness, identity, or particular behavior on a temporary basis.

distraction techniques Procedures that prevent or lessen the perception of pain sensations by focusing attention on sensations unrelated to pain.

distributive care The pattern of healthcare that concerns itself with environment, heredity, living conditions, lifestyle, and early detection; usually directed toward continuous care of persons who are not confined to healthcare institutions.

diuresis Increase in urinary output.

diuretic A drug used to increase urinary output.

diverticula Outpouching of weakened intestinal musculature.

diverticulitis Inflammation and perforation of a diverticular sac.

documentation The act of recording patient assessments and nursing interventions in the patient's chart. The chart is a permanent record, is considered a legal document, and is also audited to evaluate charges and quality of care.

domestic violence An abuse of power within an intimate relationship. Occurs when efforts are made to gain or maintain control over another person through intimidation.

donor A person who gives or furnishes blood, skin, or body organs for use by another person.

dorsiflexion A bending backward from a neutral position.

DRG (diagnosis-related group) A designation in a system that classifies patients by age, sex, diagnosis, treatment procedure, and discharge status to predict the use of hospital resources and length of stay. Currently used as the basis for a system of prospective payment under Medicare.

drug dependency Addiction to a drug.

dwarfism Abnormal smallness of body; caused by undersecretion of the growth hormone from the anterior pituitary gland.

dyscrasias Diseases of the blood.

dysmenorrhea Painful menstruation.

dysphagia Difficulty in swallowing.

dyspnea Shortness of breath; difficult, labored breathing.

dysrhythmia Any disturbance or abnormality in a normal rhythmic pattern; specifically irregularity in the brain waves or cadence of speech.

ecchymosis Large amount of bleeding into the tissues.

eclampsia A condition that can occur during pregnancy and is characterized by convulsions, hypertension, and edema.

ego In Freudian theory, the part of the personality structure that contains the instinctive drives and urges.

electrocardiogram Graphic recording of the electric potential resulting from the electric activity of the heart.

electroencephalograph Graphic recording of brain waves within the deep structures of the skull.

electrolytes Ions that play an important role in regulating body processes. Ions are substances that break apart into electrically charged particles when placed in a solution.

ELISA (Enzyme-linked immunosorbent assay) The most common assay for HIV antibodies. Used for screening donated blood, it is usually the first clinical screening test used to detect HIV infection. A positive ELISA or EIA test result should be confirmed with a Western Blot or an immunofluorescent assay test to conclusively diagnose HIV infection.

embolectomy Surgical removal of a blood clot from a vein.

embolism Foreign substance in the bloodstream; may be a fragment from a blood clot or an air bubble.

embryonic Pertaining to the embryo.

emmetropia Absence of refractive error; "normal" vision.

emphysema Overinflation and other destructive changes in alveolar walls; results in loss of lung elasticity and decreased gas exchange.

empyema Presence of pus in the pleural cavity.

endemic Describes the contiuous presence of a few cases of a disease in a community.

endogenous From within.

endogenous depression A depression that has no recognizable loss, stressor, or other identifiable cause; is seen as arising from intrapsychic sources.
endolymph Fluid in the inner ear (within the utricle, saccule, and a portion of the cochlea). Protects the cochlea and the semicircular canals.
endometriosis A disease caused by groups of cells growing in the pelvic cavity. The cells are similar to those of the uterine mucous membrane.
endorphins Substances produced by the brain that mimic the effects of opiates such as morphine.
endotoxin A toxin that is released when a cell disintegrates.
enteric fistula An abnormal communication between portions or loops of the bowel.
enteritis Inflammation of the intestines.
enucleation Surgical removal of the eyeball.
enuresis Involuntary voiding of urine; bedwetting.
environment All factors that influence the life and survival of a person.
enzyme-linked immunosorbent assay See ELISA.
eosinophils Granular leukocytes. Number is increased during an allergic reaction.
epidemic Occurrence of a large number of cases of a disease in a specific area at a given time.
epidemiology Study of factors related to epidemics of disease, their control, and their methods of spread.
epidermis The superficial layers of the skin; made up of an outer, dead portion and a deeper living, cellular portion.
epididymis One of a pair of long tightly coiled ducts that carry sperm from the seminiferous tubules of the testes to the vas deferens.
epididymitis Inflammation of the epididymis.
epidural analgesia The process of achieving regional anesthesia of the pelvic, abdominal, genital, or other area by the injection of a local anesthetic into the epidural space of the spinal column.
epinephrine A hormone secreted by the adrenal medulla; prepared commercially as Adrenalin.
epiphora Abnormal tearing; often associated with lacrimal system disorders, congenital glaucoma, or lid misalignment.
episodic care Care provided by the nurse to the medical or surgical patient who is hospitalized in an acute care or extended-care facility with a goal of cure or improvement in a specific illness or crisis.
epistaxis Nosebleed.
equilibrium A state of balance.
erythema A redness of the skin.
erythroblastosis A congenital blood disease of the newborn in which there is a reaction of the Rh-negative antibodies of the mother with the Rh-positive antibodies of the infant.
erythrocytes Red blood cells.
erythropoiesis Production of erythrocytes.
erythropoietin A glycoprotein hormone synthesized mainly in the kidneys and released into the bloodstream in response to anoxia. It stimulates red blood cell formation.
eschar Slough of tissue resulting from a burn.
Escherichia coli A species of organism found in the intestinal tract of humans and animals.
esophageal varices Fragile, collateral vessels that develop in the esophagus as a result of portal hypertension.
esophagogastroduodenoscopy Visualization of the upper gastrointestinal tract (esophagus, stomach, duodenum) by the use of an endoscope.
esophagoscopy Examination of the esophagus by the use of the endoscope.
estrogen A hormone excreted by the ovaries.
ethical dilemma A situation in which a choice must be made among two or more undesirable alternatives and in which the reasons for the alternatives are valid and important; no choice is obviously right or wrong. It occurs in a context in which the facts, as known, do not make it clear which is the right choice.
ethics A branch of philosophy that studies two facets of human existence: how people should act and what type of character they should have. Normative ethics involves principles and rules.
ethylene oxide A gas used in sterilization of surgical supplies and equipment.
etiologic Describes the cause of diseases or disorders.
eustachian tube Tube connecting the middle ear with the pharynx.
euthanasia The intentional death of a person who has been suffering from an incurable disease; mercy death.
evaluation The final stage of the nursing process. Patient progress is compared to previously identified expected outcomes of each nursing action prescribed for a problem. Evaluation requires the continued assessment of the patient.
evisceration Opening of a surgical incision, which permits the viscera to protrude to the outside.
excoriation An abrasion or a denuded area of the skin.
exfoliative cytology Microscopic study of the cell; used for diagnostic purposes.
exogenous From outside the body.
exotoxin A toxin or poison secreted by an organism.
expertise Skill and knowledge of a person by reason of special training.
extended-care facility Institution devoted to providing medical, nursing, or custodial care for an individual over a prolonged period of time. Includes intermediate- and skilled-care facilities.
external rotation Turning away of a limb from the midline of the body.
extracorporeal Outside the body; used to describe a method of bypassing a patient's heart and lungs by using the heart-lung machine; used in open heart surgery.
extrasystole A form of cardiac arrhythmia in which heartbeats occur sooner than expected.
exudate Pus containing dead cells, phagocytes, bacteria, and tissue fluids.
faces rating scale A series of faces ranging from very happy ones with smiles to very sad ones with tears; person points to the face that best describes how he or she feels at this time.
factitious disorders Symptoms or disorders voluntarily produced by a patient for unconscious reasons.
family Two or more persons who are related by blood, marriage, or adoption and who live together over a period of time.
fibrillation Tremor or rapid contraction of the heart.
fidelity Being faithful to one's duty, commitments, and promises.
filter A device for separating one substance from another.
filtration Movement of fluid and electrolytes by the pressure or force that is exerted as a result of the weight of the solution.
fimbriated Demonstrating fingerlike projections at the end of the fallopian tubes.
fissure A crack or slit in the skin.
flaccid Limp; cannot be controlled.
flagella Hairlike projections extending from some bacterial cells, which makes the cells capable of movement.
flotation therapy Semiweightlessness produced by various types of equipment; used in prevention and treatment of decubitus ulcers.
fomite Any object or material that may hold or transmit pathogenic organisms.
frostbite Freezing caused by exposure to extreme cold; seen as white patches on skin that do not redden on pressure or as deeper lesions that involve subcutaneous tissue.
functional assessment Admission examination of patient's functional abilities.

functional nursing An approach to nursing service that uses auxiliary health workers who are trained in a variety of skills. Each person is assigned specific duties or functions that are carried out for all patients on a given unit. Assignments are made in relationship to the skill levels of the worker. This type of nursing follows the "assembly line" approach.

functional psychosis Major emotional disorder characterized by derangement of the personality and loss of the ability to function in reality; not directly related to physical processes.

fungi Microbes from the plant kingdom, of which there are many different types. Some are harmless and some cause disease.

gangrene Necrosis of tissue caused by cutting off the blood supply.

gastrectomy Partial or complete surgical removal of the stomach.

gastritis Inflammation of the stomach; generally caused by ingestion of contaminated food.

gastroscopy A direct visualization of the stomach with a gastroscope.

gate control theory Proposes that pain impulses that are transmitted from nerve receptors, through the spinal cord, and to the brain can be altered or blocked in the spinal cord or brain.

genetic Pertaining to origin; inherited.

genitalia The reproductive organs.

geriatrics A medical specialty that deals with problems of aging and the aged.

germicide An agent that destroys bacteria.

gerontology The scientific study of the process of aging and of the problems of the aged. The science of gerontology is interdisciplinary and includes the social, biologic, and psychologic aspects of aging.

glans penis The conical tip of the penis; the urethral opening is usually located at the center of the distal tip of the glans penis.

glaucoma An eye disease characterized by increased intraocular pressure; leads to visual field loss, optic atrophy, and eventually blindness if untreated.

glomerular capillaries Cluster of blood vessels surrounded by Bowman's capsule.

glomerulonephritis A type of nephritis that involves the glomerulus of the kidney.

glucagon A hormone that is produced by the alpha cells in the islets of Langerhans and that stimulates the conversion of glycogen to glucose in the liver.

glycohemoglobin A type of hemoglobin that has a sugar attached (glycosylated) and that is increased in poorly controlled diabetes. It is an indicator of glucose levels over several weeks.

glycosuria Presence of sugar in the urine.

goiter Any abnormal enlargement of the thyroid gland.

gonads Sex glands; testes in the male and ovaries in the female.

gram-negative Term used in identifying bacteria after staining with a dye. Color can be removed with a solvent.

granulocytes Leukocytes identified by the shape of the nuclei and the coloring of their cytoplasm.

grief A severe emotional reaction to loss.

gumma A tumorlike lesion that is similar in appearance to an abscess.

gynecology A medical specialty concerned with diseases and disorders of the female reproductive system.

habitat The natural environment in which a plant or animal (including humans), resides.

hallucination A mental aberration that is based on seeing or hearing things that do not exist in reality.

hallucinogenic Describes an agent that causes hallucinations or changes in personality.

hashish A resinous mixture contained in the flowering tops of the *Cannabis sativa* plant.

health Defined by the World Health Organization as "a state of complete physical, mental, and social well-being and not merely the absence of disease."

health maintenance organization (HMO) Created by the Social Security Amendments of 1972 to provide comprehensive services to enrollees on the basis of a predetermined fixed cost or rate and without regard to the extent or frequency of services. These services may be given directly by the HMO or through arrangements with others and include the services of primary care, specialty physicians, and institutional services.

heat stroke Disturbance in the body heat–regulating mechanism; results in elevated body temperature and hot, dry skin; may be damaging to brain cells.

hematemesis Vomiting of blood.

hematocrit A measure of the volume of red blood cells and the plasma.

hematogenic shock A shock state caused by an internal or external loss of blood or plasma.

hematuria Blood in the urine.

hemianopia Defective vision or blindness in half the visual field.

hemiplegia Paralysis affecting one side of the body.

hemodialysis Artificial method of removing urea and nitrogenous wastes from the blood when the kidneys fail to function normally.

hemoglobin electrophoresis A test used to identify various abnormal hemoglobins in the blood; may indicate genetic disorders such as sickle cell anemia.

hemophilia A group of hereditary bleeding disorders.

hemoptysis Hemorrhage that may be from the lungs, trachea, or larynx.

hemorrhage Escape of blood from a broken vessel.

hemorrhoids Varicosities of the anal canal; may be internal or external.

hepatic coma Comatose condition caused by liver failure; believed to result from the accumulation of nitrogenous substances in the blood, especially ammonia.

hepatitis Inflammation of the cells of the liver; two types–hepatitis A and hepatitis B.

hernia A projection of a loop of an organ, tissue, or structure through a congenital or acquired defect.

herniorrhaphy Surgical repair of a hernia.

herpes simplex Cold sore or fever blister.

herpes zoster Shingles; caused by a virus that affects the nerve roots of the posterior ganglia; same virus that causes chickenpox.

heterograft Tissue taken from an animal or a species other than a human donor.

hiatus hernia Protrusion of a structure through the diaphragm around the esophageal opening.

High Efficiency Particulate Air Respirator (HEPA) Special mask that filters out dust that is one micron in size; is to be worn when caring for patients with tuberculosis. Presently the mask has not been tested for the TB bacillus.

high risk Applied to groups of persons considered to be more susceptible to infections or diseases than other individuals.

hirsutism Condition characterized by the excessive growth of hair or the presence of hair in unusual places.

histoplasmosis A benign disease of the lungs; caused by a fungus.

HIV (human immunodeficiency virus) The organism isolated and recognized as the etiologic agent of AIDS. HIV is classified as a lentivirus in a subgroup of the retroviruses. It infects and destroys a class of lymphocytes, CD4 cells, thereby causing progressive damage to the immune system. This family of retroviruses has RNA as its genetic material and makes an enzyme, reverse transcriptase, that converts viral RNA into viral DNA. The viral DNA is then incorporated into the host cell's DNA and is replicated along with it. There are two known types of HIV: HIV-1 is the most common in the United States; HIV-2 causes a milder immune suppression and is found primarily in West Africa.

HIV antibody (HIV-Ab) The antibody to HIV; usually appears within 6 weeks after infection. Antibody testing early in the infection process may not produce accurate results because recently infected people may have not yet begun producing antibodies and therefore test negative even though they are infected. Therefore a single negative antibody test result is not a guarantee that a person is free from infection. The change from HIV-negative to HIV-positive status is called seroconversion.

HIV infections A clinical spectrum of symptoms of an underlying immunodeficiency that predisposes an individual infected with the HIV virus.

Hodgkin's disease A malignant disease affecting the lymph nodes; was once considered highly fatal but can now be cured.

holistic care Care of the total or whole person, including physiologic, psychologic, and sociologic needs.

home healthcare Health services provided in the client's place of residence for the purpose of promoting, maintaining, or restoring health or minimizing the effects of illness and disability.

homemaker service A service to provide assistance in the home for elderly or sick persons; federal program under the Older Americans Act.

homeostasis A relative constancy in the internal environment of the body; naturally maintained by adaptive responses that promote health survival.

homograft A graft taken from a person other than the recipient.

hormone A chemical substance secreted by an endocrine gland; some are prepared commercially.

hospice An approach to providing support for the terminally ill patient and significant others; addresses physical, emotional, and spiritual needs.

host An organism, which may be a human, from which another obtains its nourishment.

human immunodeficiency virus See HIV.

human needs Those needs basic to every individual; identified by Maslow as physiologic, safety and comfort, love and belonging, esteem, and self-actualization.

humoral immunity Acquired immunity that results in lymphocytes forming antibodies that are specific to the invading agent.

Huntington's chorea A rare abnormal hereditary condition that is characterized by chronic, progressive chorea and mental deterioration that terminates in dementia.

hydrocele A collection of fluid in the testicle.

hydrolysis Splitting of a compound into parts by adding water. In digestion, enzymes reduce large molecules into small particles so that they may be absorbed.

hydronephrosis Distention of the kidney pelvis with urine; caused by an obstruction along the urinary route.

hypaxial Beneath the axis of the vertebral column.

hyperalimentation A method of providing complete nutritional requirements by the intravenous route.

hypercalcemia Excess of calcium in the extracellular fluid.

hypercapnia Excess of carbon dioxide in the blood.

hyperchloremia Excess of chloride in the blood.

hyperglycemia Excess of glucose in the blood.

hyperglycemic, hyperosmolar nonketotic coma A diabetic coma in which the level of ketone bodies is normal; caused by hyperosmolarity of extracellular fluid.

hyperkalemia Excess of potassium in the extracellular fluid.

hypernatremia Excess of sodium in the extracellular fluid.

hyperopia Farsightedness.

hyperplasia Increased number of cells, which causes a part to be enlarged.

hyperreflexia Exaggeration of reflexes.

hypersensitivity An abnormal sensitivity to certain substances.

hypertension A consistent elevation of blood pressure above normal.

hyperthermia Abnormally high body temperature.

hypertonic A solution having an osmotic pressure higher than the one with which it is being compared.

hypertrophy Enlargement of an organ that may or may not be caused by disease; increase in the size of the cells that comprise an organ.

hypervolemia Increase in the amount of extracellular fluid.

hypocalcemia Deficit of calcium in the extracellular fluid.

hypochloremia A decrease in the chloride level in the blood serum.

hypochromia Below normal color, as in a low index of the color of hemoglobin.

hypoglycemia A condition in which the glucose in the blood is abnormally low.

hyponatremia Deficit of sodium in the extracellular fluid.

hypospadias Congenital malformation of the male urethra.

hypostatic pneumonia Pneumonia caused by a patient remaining in the same position for long periods.

hypothermia A low body temperature as produced by exposure to cold weather or as an adjunct to anesthesia.

hypotonic A solution having an osmotic pressure lower than the one with which it is being compared.

hypovolemia Decrease in the amount of extracellular fluid.

hypovolemic shock A state of physical collapse and prostration; caused by massive blood loss and inadequate tissue perfusion.

hypoxia Deficiency of oxygen in the tissues.

hysterectomy Surgical removal of the uterus; may be abdominal or vaginal, total or partial.

iatrogenic A disorder produced inadvertently by a physician as a result of treatment for another disorder.

icterus index A test to measure the amount of yellowness in the blood serum.

id In Freudian theory, the part of the personality structure that contains the instinctive drives and urges.

IFA (immunofluorescence antibody) A serologic assay using an antibody tagged by a fluorescent molecule. There is an HIV-specific IFA assay available to confirm the results of a positive HIV ELISA test.

ileal conduit Method of urinary diversion. Ureters are implanted into a section of dissected ileum, which is then sewed to an opening in the abdomen.

ileostomy A surgical procedure in which an artificial passage from the ileum to the outside of the abdomen is constructed.

ileus Failure of peristalsis, which leads to intestinal obstruction.

immunity Resistance to a specific disease.

immunization Process of becoming immune to certain diseases; usually refers to injections that are given to develop active acquired immunity.

immunofluorescence antibody See IFA.

immunoglobulins (Ig) Serum proteins that include several groups of globulins; formerly called gamma globulins.

immunologist A person trained in the science of immunity.

immunotherapy A special treatment of allergic responses; administers increasingly large doses of the offending allergens to gradually develop immunity.

impetigo Contagious skin disease.

implementation Category of nursing behavior. One of five steps in the nursing process in which the actions necessary for accomplishing the healthcare plan are initiated and completed. Includes performance of or assistance in the performance of activities of daily living, counseling and teaching, caregiving, supervising and evaluating staff members, and recording and exchanging information relevant to the client's continued healthcare.

incontinence Inability to retain urine in the bladder.

incubation period The interval between initial infection and the appearance of the first symptom or sign of disease.
incus One of three small bones in the middle ear; shaped like an anvil and lies between the malleus and the stapes.
independence Capable of performing activities of daily living without assistance.
indirect contact Touching an object contaminated with an infective organism.
infection Entry and multiplication of an infective agent in the body of man or animal. May or may not cause infectious disease.
infectious disease A disease that may be transmitted from person to person, either by direct or indirect contact.
infiltration Passing of fluid through, as when intravenous fluid passes into the tissues; usually caused by a needle being displaced from the vein.
inner child Refers to the child ego state as described by the Redecision Theory, which states that it is found in any person, regardless of chronologic age.
insulin reaction Syndrome caused by too much circulating insulin.
intermediate-care facility A facility that provides care for chronically ill or disabled individuals; room and board are provided, but skilled nursing care is not.
internal rotation Turning of the limb toward the midline of the body.
intervention One step in the nursing process. The actual implementation of the most suitable actions chosen for a given situation, which may include direct patient care, health teaching, or other activities for the benefit of the patient or the supervision of such activities.
intracranial pressure Pressure within the cranium.
intrathecal analgesia Injection into the subarachnoid space of the spinal cord; a lumbar puncture must be performed.
intravenous therapy Administration of fluids, drugs, or both into the general circulation through a venipuncture.
intussusception Telescoping of the intestine; may involve any part of the small or large intestine.
iodophor An antiseptic or disinfectant agent that combines iodine with another agent (usually a detergent).
ion An atom or group of atoms that carry an electric charge.
ionizing radiation Rays of energy that break atoms into smaller, electrically charged particles called ions.
iridectomy Surgical procedure in which a small hole is made in the iris to provide drainage of aqueous humour when acute, narrow-angle glaucoma has caused the angle to narrow and obstruct drainage.
ischemia A temporary interruption of the blood supply to any area.
ischemic heart disease Pathology of the heart resulting from lack of oxygen.
isoenzyme An enzyme that may appear in multiple forms with slightly different chemical or other characteristics; can be produced in different organs, although each enzyme performs essentially the same function.
isolation Use of barriers to interrupt the transmission of infectious organisms.
isometric exercise Exercise done by a patient in which he or she contracts and relaxes a muscle.
isotonic Solution that is compatible with the normal tissue by having the same osmotic pressure.
isotope A chemical element that has been made radioactive.
jaundice A condition in which a yellow color affects the skin and the sclera of the eyes; caused by an accumulation of bile pigments in the blood.
Kaposi's sarcoma A painless tumor of the wall of blood vessels or of the lymphatic system; usually appears on the skin as pink-to-purple spots. It may also occur internally, independent of skin lesions.
keloid A benign overgrowth of fibrous tissue.
keratitis Inflammation of the cornea of the eye with formation of ulcers.
keratoplasty Corneal transplant. Can be full thickness or partial thickness graft.
ketoacidosis Acidosis resulting from the body's inability to neutralize keto acids from abnormal fat metabolism.
ketonuria Presence in the urine of excessive amounts of ketone bodies.
ketosis The abnormal accumulation of ketones in the body as a result of a deficiency or inadequate use of carbohydrates.
Klebsiella A genus of bacteria that lives in the intestinal tract and may cause serious infections.
Koplik's spots White spots on a reddened base; found in the throat in measles.
labyrinthitis Inflammation of the labyrinth of the inner ear.
lacrimal fluid Tears secreted by the lacrimal glands.
lacrimation Increased secretion from the lacrimal glands.
laminectomy Surgical procedure for a ruptured intervertebral disk or for fusion.
laparoscopy Examination of the interior of the abdomen with a laparoscope.
laparotomy Any surgical procedure in which the abdomen is opened.
laryngectomy Surgical procedure for the removal of the larynx.
laser surgery Procedures that use an instrument to create a narrow, highly focused beam of light that can cut, coagulate, or vaporize tissue.
leukapheresis Selective removal of leukocytes from blood that has been withdrawn from and reinfused into the patient.
leukemia Neoplastic disorder resulting in widespread proliferation of white blood cells and their precursors throughout the body.
leukocyte White blood cell.
leukocytopenia A reduction in the number of leukocytes.
leukocytosis Great increase in leukocytes; occurs in many types of infections.
leukopenia An abnormal decrease in the number of white blood cells to fewer than 5000 cells per cubic millimeter.
leukoplakia White spots formed on the mucous membrane of the mouth; may become malignant.
leukorrhea White or yellow vaginal discharge.
life-island A plastic bubble enclosing a bed; used to provide a germ-free environment.
life span The longest period of time for which a typical individual can be expected to live.
ligature Suture used in surgery to tie or ligate a blood vessel.
lipodystrophy Atrophy of subcutaneous fat at the site of injection of insulin.
lithiasis Formation of stones of calculi.
living will A written agreement between a patient and his or her physician to withhold heroic measures if the patient's condition is irreversible.
lobectomy Surgical removal of a lobe of a lung.
long-term care Those services designed to provide symptomatic treatment, maintenance, and rehabilitative services for patients of all age groups in a variety of healthcare settings.
lumen Passageway within a tube, such as the lumen of blood vessels.
lymph nodes Small structures of lymphatic tissue containing lymphocytes, the function of which is filtration and phagocytosis.
lymphangitis Inflammation of one or more lymph vessels.
lymphocytes A lymph cell or white blood cell; develops in the bone marrow.
lymphoma A malignant tumor involving abnormal lymphocyte production.

lysergic acid diethylamide (LSD) A hallucinogenic agent that causes changes in mood and personality.
lysis A gradual decrease of symptoms of a disease; also a laboratory procedure to indicate decomposing of an agent by another agent.
MAC (mycobacterium avium-intracellular complex) An acid-fast microorganism that causes lung and other organ system infections in individuals whose immune systems are severely damaged. Evidence of MAC has been found in approximately 50 percent of adult AIDS patients at autopsy.
macrophage Large phagocyte cell that wanders.
macule A discolored spot on the skin that may be of various colors and shapes. It is neither raised nor depressed.
magnetic resonance imaging An imaging method that provides superior visualization of soft tissue. Uses harmless low-energy radio waves to create a magnetic field. When introduced into the hydrogen nuclei of soft tissues, a complex series of events occurs and is assembled as a tomogram.
malaria A disease caused by a protozoan and transmitted by the *Anopheles* mosquito.
malignant Describes a disease that is a threat to life; usually applied to cancer.
malleus Hammer-shaped bone in the middle ear; attached to the tympanic membrane and the incus; transmits sound vibrations.
mammary gland Synonymous with the female breast.
mammography X-ray examination of the breast.
marijuana *(Cannabis sativa)* Same plant as hashish but contains less resin and is less psychoactive.
mastectomy Surgical removal of the breast. A simple mastectomy removes only breast tissue. A modified radical mastectomy removes the breast and axillary lymph nodes.
mastitis Inflammation of the breast.
mastoiditis Inflammation of the cells of the mastoid process.
Meals on Wheels Program designed to prepare food and take hot meals to elderly or physically handicapped persons.
mediastinum Space between the lungs that contains the heart.
Medicaid Federal- and state-supported program to provide hospital and medical care for certain eligible persons.
medical-surgical nursing The nursing care of patients whose conditions or disorders are treated pharmacologically or surgically.
Medicare Federal program to provide hospital and medical care for persons 65 years of age or older.
menarche First menstruation; occurs at puberty.
Meniere's syndrome A condition involving an increase in pressure following an increase in the endolymph in the inner ear; produces the symptoms of vertigo, nausea and vomiting, and ringing in the ears.
meninges Membrane enclosing the brain and spinal cord.
meningitis Infection and inflammation of the meninges.
menopause Climacteric or the cessation of menses; represents the end of the reproductive period.
menorrhagia Excessive menstrual flow either in quantity or duration.
mental health A state of being in which a person has a reasonably satisfactory balance of personality structure.
mental illness Any psychiatric illness that has been identified by various recognized authorities. A condition in which the person experiences enough psychic pain to cause interference with successful life functioning.
mental retardation A condition in which there is an absence of normal mental growth and development.
mental status The degree of competence shown by a person in intellectual, emotional, psychologic, and personality functioning (as measured by psychologic testing) with reference to a statistic norm.
mescaline Derivation of peyote cactus; classified as a hallucinogenic agent.
metabolism Sum of all processes within the body, including the breaking-down and wearing-out processes and the regeneration and building-up processes.
metastasis Spreading of cancer cells by the bloodstream or lymph from one part of the body to another.
methadone Synthetic narcotic analgesic agent used to replace heroin; considered addictive.
metrorrhagia Bleeding between regular menstrual periods.
miotic A drug that causes constriction of the pupil of the eye.
molecule Smallest particle of an element or compound.
monocyte A large mononuclear leukocyte.
mononucleosis An infectious disease characterized by swelling of the lymph nodes, especially the cervical nodes.
morals The set of values or principles to which a person is committed, often used interchangeably with ethics.
motivation Providing an incentive to cause a person to move or to act in a particular way.
MTB (mycobacterium tuberculosis) The microorganism that causes tuberculosis.
multisystem A corporation that manages a group of hospitals. Hospitals may or may not be owned by the managing system.
muscle spasm A severe muscular contraction.
myasthenic crisis Acute episode of muscular weakness.
mycobacterium avium-intracellular complex See MAC.
mycobacterium tuberculosis See MTB.
mycotic Pertaining to a disease caused by a fungus.
mydriatic A drug that dilates the pupils of the eyes.
myelin Fatlike substance forming a sheath around certain nerve fibers.
myelography X-ray examination of the spinal column after injection of a radiopaque substance.
myelosuppression Inhibition of the function of the bone marrow.
myocardial infarction Disorder caused by obstruction or thrombus of a coronary artery or its branches; deprives the myocardium of its blood supply and causes death of the affected tissue.
myopia Nearsightedness.
myringotomy A surgical incision of a portion of the tympanic membrane.
myxedema Condition resulting from hypofunction of the thyroid gland; characterized by large tongue, slow speech, puffiness of hands and face, coarse and thickened skin, mental apathy, and sensitivity to cold.
narcotic A drug that may be an opium derivative or synthetic, narcoticlike agent used to relieve pain and produce sleep. All narcotic drugs are habit forming and under government control.
natural immunity Immunity acquired by an infant as a result of maternal antibodies crossing the placental barrier and entering fetal circulation.
nebulization A method of spraying a drug into the respiratory passages; may be used with or without oxygen to carry the drug to the lungs.
necrosis Death of tissue.
necrotic tissue Dead tissue or small groups of cells.
neobladder Urinary diversion resulting from transplantation of the ureters into a constructed segment of the sigmoid colon.
neoplasm Abnormal tumor growth; may be benign or malignant.
nephrectomy Surgical removal of a kidney.
nephritis Inflammation of the kidney; may be acute or chronic.
nephron Nephron and its component parts comprise the structural and functional unit of the kidney.
nephrosclerosis Sclerosis of the blood vessels of the kidney, usually associated with hypertension.
nephrosis (nephrotic syndrome) Degeneration of renal tissue with inflammation; may occur with glomerulonephritis.

nephrostomy Surgical wound on the flank and placement of a catheter into the kidney pelvis for the purpose of drainage.
nephrotoxin A substance that is destructive to the kidney.
neurectomy Surgical division of the sensory portion of a peripheral or spinal nerve to relieve pain.
neurogenic shock Shock resulting from peripheral vascular dilation as a result of neurologic injury.
neurotransmitters The chemicals responsible for message transmission across the synapse. Examples include dopamine, substance P, endorphins, and enkephalins.
nodule Small, solid node that can be detected by touch.
normal flora Microscopic cells normally present on skin and mucosal surfaces that may include *Staphylococcus* organisms, *Streptococcus* organisms, and other bacteria.
normovolemic shock Shock resulting from a disproportion between the normal volume of blood and the size of the vascular bed.
nosocomial Hospital-acquired infection.
nursing care plan The proposed plan of care for each patient, preferably written; intended to communicate, prevent complications, ensure continuity of care, identify and ensure patient teaching, and provide for discharge planning. It must include statements that identify the patient's problems and proposed nursing interventions, as well as measurable expected outcomes.
nursing diagnosis A concise statement describing a combination of signs and symptoms that indicate an acute or potential health problem that nurses are licensed to treat and are capable of treating.
nursing history The documented findings of a thorough patient assessment, including the physical and emotional signs and symptoms presented by the patient, as well as information obtained from other sources.
nursing home A long-term or extended-care facility that provides nursing, medical, and rehabilative care, as well as furnishes residential and personal services.
nursing process A dynamic interpersonal problem-solving process that facilitates a person's potential for health. The steps in the process include assessment, planning, intervention, and evaluation.
nystagmus A continuous movement of the eyeball; may be associated with labyrinthitis.
occlusion Blockage of a passageway.
occult blood A minute or hidden quantity of blood that can be detected only by means of a chemical test or by microscopic or spectroscopic examination. Often present in stools of patients with gastrointestinal lesions.
oncogenes Certain genes in the cell that can somehow be activated and cause cells to become malignant.
oncology Branch of medicine dealing with tumors.
oophorectomy Surgical removal of an ovary.
opacity Omitting light, or opaque to light rays.
ophthalmia neonatorum Infection of the eyes of the newborn with the gonococcus organism.
ophthalmologist A medical doctor who has completed 4 years of residency and, in some instances, 1 to 3 years additional training in a subspecialty. Ophthalmologists diagnose and treat patients with eye diseases and vision problems. They perform surgery and prescribe medications, glasses, and contact lenses.
opiate Drug derived from opium.
opisthotonos Arching of the body caused by rigidity of the spine.
opportunistic infections Illnesses caused by organisms that do not usually cause disease in a person with a healthy immune system. When an individual's immune system is compromised, such organisms may cause serious, even life-threatening illness.
opportunistic pathogen A microbe that produces illness only in the compromised host.
optometrist Has a degree in optometry after attending optometry school for 4 years postbaccalaureate degree. Optometrists examine eyes, prescribe glasses and contact lenses, check intraoccular-pressure, and prescribe exercises for various eye muscle problems. They provide low-vision examinations, visual devices, and adaptive training for patients with limited vision.
orchitis Inflammatory condition of the testes caused by infection, injury, or malignancy.
organic psychosis Major emotional disorder characterized by derangement of the personality and loss of the ability to function in reality; caused by an underlying physical process, resulting in damage to the brain.
orthopedic Describes disorders of the musculoskeletal system.
orthopnea Ability to breathe only in the upright position.
oscilloscope An instrument that records a visual wave on a screen.
osmolarity The osmotic pressure of a solution expressed in osmols or milliosmols per kilogram of solution.
osmosis Diffusion of water through a semipermeable membrane.
osmotic pressure Pressure of a fluid that determines its ability to pass through a semipermeable membrane.
osseous Pertaining to bone.
osteoarthritis A degenerative type of arthritis affecting the joints; characteristic of the aging process.
osteomyelitis Infection and inflammation of a bone.
osteotomy Cutting of bone to correct joint or bone deformities.
otitis media Infection of the middle ear.
otologist A physician trained in the diagnosis and treatment of diseases and disorders of the ear.
otosclerosis A disease of the middle ear in which new growth of bone forms in the stapes and prevents transmission of sound to the inner ear.
otoscopy Direct visualization of the external auditory canal and the tympanic membrane using an otoscope.
outcomes The desired specific behaviors or results.
ovulation Discharge of a mature ovum from the ovarian follicle.
oxygenation The process of combining or treating with oxygen.
pacemaker A mechanical device used to provide electric stimulation in heart block; may be temporary or permanent.
pain Whatever the patient experiencing it says it is, existing whenever he or she says it exists.
pain threshold The point at which a sensation is perceived as pain.
pain tolerance The point at which a pain sensation is no longer voluntarily endured.
palliative Therapy designed to relieve or reduce discomfort of symptoms but not produce a cure.
pancreatitis Inflammation of the pancreas.
pandemic A disease that is widespread in a geographic area or throughout the world.
panhysterectomy Surgical removal of the uterus and the cervix.
Papanicolaou's smear test A cytologic test for the detection of cancer cells. Best known as the cervical Pap smear.
papule A small, solid elevation on the skin that varies in size from a pinhead to a pea.
paralytic ileus A decrease or absence of intestinal peristalsis.
paraplegia Paralysis of the lower part of the body below a point of injury to the spinal cord.
paresthesia Numbness, tingling, "pins and needles."
paroxysm Spasmodic attacks that recur at intervals.
paroxysmal atrial tachycardia Very rapid heartbeat that begins suddenly and ends abruptly.
passive immunity Immunity acquired by injecting into the body a serum that produces an immediate but temporary immune response.
pathogen An organism capable of causing disease.

pathophysiology Changes in the physiologic function as a result of pathologic disease.
patient The individual who initiates, plans, and actively participates in his or her healthcare.
patient-controlled analgesia Self-administration of pain medications by means of a mechanical device.
PCP (*Pneumocystis carinii* pneumonia) Form of pneumonia seen in persons with an impaired immune system, such as those who are HIV infected. PCP is the leading cause of death in patients with AIDS. It is caused by the opportunistic pathogen *P. carinii* (unclear whether fungal or protozoan), which can infect the eyes, skin, spleen, liver, and heart, as well as the lungs.
pelvic exenteration Removal of all reproductive organs and adjacent tissues.
penicillinase An enzymelike substance that is produced by some bacteria and that affects the antimicrobial properties of penicillin.
peptic ulcer An ulcer occurring in the wall of the stomach or the duodenum.
perfusion Procedure of introducing a chemical drug to an isolated part of the body by way of the bloodstream.
perilymph Inner ear fluid contained within the space between the bony and membranous labyrinths, as well as in a portion of the cochlea.
periosteum Specialized connective tissue covering all bones.
peristalsis Involuntary wavelike contraction of muscles of the gastrointestinal tract.
peritoneal dialysis A method of removal of waste products from the blood by way of the peritoneal membrane.
personality The unique combination of behavior patterns, attitudes, and traits of an individual.
personality disorders A group of mental disorders in which there are maladaptive patterns of behavior, often identifiable by adolescence or earlier.
pertussis Whooping cough.
pessary A device used to support the uterus in a normal position.
petechiae Small, pinpoint hemorrhagic spots on the skin.
Peyer's patches Areas of lymphoid tissue on the mucous membrane of the small intestine that become elevated and inflamed in typhoid fever; may become ulcerated and rupture, causing hemorrhage.
phacoemulsification Technique of extracapsular cataract extraction in which the lens nucleus is broken into pieces ultrasonically and then aspirated through a small incision.
phagocyte Cell that engulfs and ingests bacteria or other material.
phagocytosis Ingestion and digestion of bacteria at the scene of an infection.
phantom pain Painful sensations in an amputated body part, such as a leg or breast.
phenylketonuria Hereditary disease in which there is a faulty utilization of the amino acid phenylalanine.
phimosis A narrowing of the prepuce opening so that the foreskin of the penis cannot be retracted.
phlebotomy Incision of a vein for the purpose of removing blood.
phobia Abnormal fear.
photophobia Abnormal sensitivity to light; often found in congenital glaucoma, corneal abrasions, and conjunctivitis.
physical dependence The altered state produced by the repeated administration of a drug. When the drug is stopped, withdrawal symptoms occur.
pica A craving to eat substances that are not foods, such as dirt, clay, chalk, glue, or hair.
pinna Auricle of the ear, or the cartilaginous external ear.
pinworm Small parasitic worm that matures in the large intestine and crawls to the outside of the rectum to deposit its eggs.
placebo Any substance or procedure that is used as a supposedly effective treatment and that produces an effect in the patient because of its intent and not because of its specific physical or chemical properties. It is used to satisfy a patient's need for therapy or as a means of control in research studies.
planning That stage of the nursing process that involves the development of an orderly mental or written design of action on the basis of needs and the real or potential problems that have been identified in the patient. It is this stage in which nursing actions or interventions are proposed and goals or expected outcomes are identified.
plaques Atherosclerotic fatty deposits found in the intima of blood vessels; often the coronary arteries are affected.
plasmapheresis Process of separating the plasma and the red blood cells.
Platyhelminthes Flatworms.
pleurisy Inflammation of the pleura.
***Pneumocystis carinii* pneumonia** See PCP.
pneumonectomy Surgical removal of a lung.
pneumonia An acute inflammation of the lungs; often caused by inhaled pneumococci.
pneumothorax A collection of air or gas in the pleural space, which causes the lung to collapse.
poikilothermy Variations in body temperature in relation to the environment as a result of a loss of sympathetic nerve activity.
pollinosis An allergic condition; same as hay fever.
polycythemia An abnormal increase in the number of erythrocytes in the blood.
polyp A small, tumorlike growth that projects from a mucous membrane.
polyuria Increased urinary output.
populations Aggregation of individuals, often with specific characteristics in common.
porcine graft Temporary biologic heterograft taken from the skin of a pig.
Post Anesthesia Care Unit (PACU) Specifically equipped unit where a patient recovers from anesthesia; airway reflexes return and breathing is satisfactory.
posttraumatic stress disorder An anxiety disorder that originates with a traumatic event and is characterized by nightmares, flashbacks, physiologic symptoms, and acute anxiety attacks. This disorder can occur soon after the traumatic event or can occur years later.
preferred provider organization (PPO) An organization of physicians, hospitals, and pharmacists whose members discount their healthcare services to subscriber patients.
prepuce A fold of skin that forms a retractable cover as the foreskin of the penis.
presbycusis Impairment of hearing as a result of degenerative changes; a common cause of sensorineural loss associated with aging.
primary care The first contact in a given episode of illness that leads to a decision of what must be done to help resolve the problem. It is provided by the individual who is responsible for the continuum of care and includes maintenance of health, evaluation and management of symptoms, and appropriate referral. Primary care is usually provided by a physician; however, some primary care functions are now handled by nurses with advanced education and experience.
primary nursing An approach to nursing service that closely resembles the original case method. The primary nurse assumes complete responsibility for the total care of the patient from admission to discharge. When off duty, the primary nurse is assisted by other nurses, who follow the directives of the plan of care established. Each primary nurse is assigned a group of patients, preferably no more than five.
primary prevention Involves activities that promote general well-being, as well as specific protection for selected diseases, such as immunizations for diphtheria, measles, and tetanus.

priority Order of importance.

problem-oriented medical record (POMR) A system of record-keeping that involves the identification and numbering of patient problems. All progress notes and orders aredirectly related to patient problems, and each entry must consist of four parts designated by the acronym SOAP—subjective data, objective data, assessment, and plan.

problem-oriented record (POR) See problem-oriented medical record.

proctoscopy Examination of the rectum with an endoscope that is passed through the anus (proctoscope).

proctosigmoidoscopy Visualization of the sigmoid colon and rectum.

prognosis Expected outcome of a disease.

proprietary Operated for profit.

proprioception The brain's ability to know the spatial relation of the body's parts.

prospective payment Third party reimbursement on the basis of predetermined cost rather than actual costs incurred.

prostate gland A chestnut-sized gland in men that surrounds the neck of the bladder and the urethra. The ejaculatory ducts pass through the prostate to the urethra.

prostatitis Inflammation of the prostate gland.

prosthesis Any artificial device used to replace a missing part of the body.

prosthetist A person skilled in making and fitting prostheses.

Proteus morganii A species of bacteria that may cause infectious diarrhea in infants.

Proteus vulgaris A species of bacteria found in feces, water, and soil; a frequent cause of urinary tract infection.

Protozoa A phylum of unicellular organisms.

pruritus Itching of the skin.

Pseudomonas Microorganism found on the skin or in the intestinal tract of humans; may be the cause of hospital-acquired infections. It is resistant to most antibiotics.

pseudophakia The condition of the eye after the lens is removed and an artificial lens has been implanted. (IOL—intraocular lens implant)

psilocybin Active agent of the *Psilocybe mexicana* mushroom; classified as a hallucinogenic agent.

psoriasis A chronic skin disease characterized by scaly patches and desquamation.

psychoneurosis An emotional maladaptation in which the chief characteristic is anxiety.

psychophysiologic reactions Physical disorders resulting from an inward bodily channeling of anxiety and stress.

psychoses A major organic or emotional disorder resulting in an inability to function effectively in life; there may be loss of contact with reality.

psychosomatic Refers to disorders for which no pathologic condition can be found.

ptosis A dropping from the normal position, such as ptosis of the eyelid in facial paralysis.

puberty Period at which the ability to reproduce begins.

pulmonary edema A condition in which left ventricular heart failure occurs, which causes a slowing of the systemic circulation and backup of returning blood; a serious condition.

pulmonary embolism A condition that is usually caused by a blood clot that breaks away from its place of origin and travels by the bloodstream to the lungs, where it lodges in a small vessel.

pulmonary emphysema A chronic obstructive disease of the lungs in which there is an overdistention of the alveoli.

pulse deficit Difference between the radial pulse rate and apical pulse rate.

Purkinje's fibers Continuation of the bundle of His that extends into the muscle walls of the ventricles.

purpura Bleeding into the skin.

purulent Describes a discharge that contains pus.

pustule An elevated skin lesion that contains pus.

pyelitis Inflammatory condition of the kidney pelvis.

pyelography X-ray examination of the kidney pelvis; may include the ureters after injection of a radiopaque medium.

pyelonephritis An inflammatory condition that involves the kidney pelvis and extends into kidney tissue.

pyloric spasm Severe and painful spasm of the pyloric valve.

pyuria Pus in the urine.

quadriplegia Paralysis of all four extremities.

quality of life Expression used in speaking of issues relating to normalizing the life of a chronically ill individual. In defining quality of life, healthcare providers must consider not only the physical responses to medical therapy but also the psychologic implications of illness for both the patient and family. The overriding goal of care should be to relieve suffering and increase patient well-being. This concept varies among individuals but may include autonomy, security, and freedom in interpersonal relationships.

quarantine Isolation for a given time that prohibits person-to-person contact; used in infectious diseases.

Queckenstedt's test A test used in diagnosing an obstruction of the spinal cord.

radiation therapy Treatment of neoplastic disease by use of gamma rays or x-rays.

radioactive substance Any substance that is capable of giving off rays as a result of disintegration, such as radium.

radioisotope A chemical element that has been made radioactive and that emits rays of energy.

radiopaque A substance that cannot be penetrated by any form of radiation; used in x-ray examination of internal structures.

reaginic antibody IgE immunoglobulin that is elevated in hypersensitive individuals.

reality orientation A small group activity in which the group leader emphasizes such concepts as time, day, month, and weather.

referred pain Pain felt at a site other than its origin.

reflex An involuntary act.

refraction Bending of light rays entering the eye; also used to describe the technique of selecting lenses to correct optical defects of the eye (e.g., myopia, hyperopia).

regression Going backward.

regurgitation Usually applied to the return of food or fluids from the stomach.

rehabilitation Process of assisting an individual after a disabling event has occurred.

reimbursement Repayment for an expense or loan.

relaxation techniques Procedures that help the patient achieve freedom from mental and physical tension or stress.

reminiscing Recalling past events or experiences.

remission Relief from or temporary improvement of symptoms; opposite of exacerbation.

remodeling Reorganization or renovation of a preexisting structure, such as a bone or joint.

remotivation The use of special techniques that stimulate patients to become motivated to learn and interact.

renal threshold The maximum amount of a substance that can be reabsorbed by the renal tubules, at which point the excess is excreted into the urine.

residual Refers to the part remaining, such as urine remaining in the bladder after catheterization.

respite Period of relief from responsibilities for the care of a patient.

resuscitation The restoration of life or consciousness of one apparently dead.

reticuloendothelial system Main bodily defense to protect humans from harmful agents; responsible for phagocytosis and elimination of cellular debris in inflammatory conditions.
retinopathy Noninflammatory condition resulting in small vessel changes in the eyes.
retirement Period in one's life when one leaves a job and enters another phase of life.
retrospective payment Reimbursement payment to agencies after service has been provided.
rhinitis Inflammation of the nasal mucosa.
rhizotomy A neurosurgical procedure in which the anterior or posterior root of a spinal nerve is resected either by surgery or radiofrequency electrodes to relieve pain.
rickettsiae Small bodies that occupy an intermediate position between bacteria and viruses.
rigidity Inflexibility.
ringworm A skin disorder caused by a fungus.
risk factors A factor that causes a person or a group of people to be particularly vulnerable to an unwanted, unpleasant, or unhealthy event.
roentgen Unit for measuring radiation, such as in x-rays.
rose spots Small rose-colored spots on the abdomen; occur in typhoid fever.
Ryan White Act (Comprehensive AIDS Resources Emergency) Act Passed in 1990 to provide services for persons with HIV infection, this act seeks "to improve the quality and availability of care for individuals and families with HIV disease." It directs financial assistance for emergency services to metropolitan areas that have the largest numbers of reported cases of AIDS and to all states for improved care, support, and early intervention services.
saccule One of two small sacs that separate the semicircular canals from the cochlea. Serve as vestibular receptors.
sarcoma A type of malignant tumor that arises from connective tissue such as bone, muscle, and cartilage.
scale A small, thin flake of dry epidermis.
scar A mark left on the skin after repair of tissue.
Schick's test A subcutaneous skin test to determine immunity to diphtheria.
schizophrenia Psychotic behavior in which there are a variety of subgroups; consists of alterations in association, affect, ambivalence, autism, and attention.
scintillator A device used to measure the amount of radioactive material in a part of the body.
scolex Segment of the tapeworm that forms the head with hooks or suckers.
scrotum The pouch of skin containing the testes and spermatic cords.
sebaceous glands Oil glands that secrete sebum.
seborrhea An increased secretion of sebum from the sebaceous glands.
sebum Secretion from the sebaceous glands.
secondary prevention The level of prevention of illness that focuses on making early diagnoses and implementing measures to stop the progression of disease processes or handicapping disabilities.
sedimentation rate Rate at which red blood cells settle when blood is placed in a test tube.
seizure A sudden loss of consciousness, such as in epilepsy.
self-actualization The fundamental tendency toward the maximum realization and fulfillment of one's human potential. Highest need in Maslow's hierarchy of human needs.
semen Thick, whitish secretion of male reproductive organs; discharged from the urethra during ejaculation.
semicircular canals Part of the inner ear. Contain fluid and hair cells; help to maintain a sense of balance.
senescence Process of becoming old, or old age.
sensitized Describes tissues that have been made susceptible to antigenic substances.
septicemia A bloodstream infection resulting from invasion of the blood by bacteria or their toxins.
sexual assault Any sexual act done without permission.
sexuality A person's need for comfort, touch, companionship, and love that may or may not be expressed through sexual activity.
shearing force Causing two contacting parts to slide on one another.
shearlings Sheepskins used on the bed to help prevent decubitus ulcers.
sickle-cell disease Congenital disease marked by sickle-shaped red blood cells; occurs most commonly in blacks.
sigmoidoscopy Examination of the sigmoid colon with a sigmoidoscope.
sinoatrial node Cells located in the right atrial wall that contract to set the rate of the heartbeat; initiated electric conduction system of the heart; called the pacemaker.
sinus bradycardia A slowing of the heart action to 60 or fewer beats per minute.
sinus tachycardia Rapid beating of the heart in excess of 100 beats per minute.
situational depression A depression that occurs as a result of a specific, identifiable event or events in which feelings of sadness and loss do not resolve within a normal period of time.
skilled-nursing facility (SNF) A nursing home that provides 24-hour nursing services, regular medical supervision, and rehabilitation therapy.
SOAP The acronym that designates the four parts of each entry in a problem-oriented record—subjective data, objective data, assessment, and plan.
socioeconomic Interaction of social and economic factors.
sordes A foul accumulation of secretions and crusts around the teeth and gums; caused by lack of oral care.
spastic Describes involuntary muscular contractions that result in rigidity.
specificity theory Proposes that there is a fixed, straight-through pain transmission system from a pain receptor to a pain center in the brain.
spermatogenesis The process of development of spermatozoa.
sphincter Muscles that are circular in shape and that constrict an anatomic opening, such as the anal sphincter.
spinal shock Syndrome directly following acute spinal cord injury.
spirometer Mechanical device to measure vital capacity.
splenectomy Surgical removal of the spleen.
splenomegaly Enlargement of the spleen.
spores Bacilli that are capable of changing into resistant forms and that can exist at high temperatures and in the presence of ordinary disinfectants.
stabilization The creation of a stable state.
standardized care plan A prewritten plan of care that includes outcomes, interventions, and evaluation that can be adapted or tailored to fit a particular patient situation.
standards An evaluation that serves as a basis for comparison when evaluating similar phenomena or substances; also serves as a standard for the practice of a profession.
stapedectomy Surgical procedure to correct otosclerosis, a disorder that prevents sound from reaching the inner ear.
stapes One of three small bones in the middle ear—attached to the incus bone on one side and to the oval window on the other to transmit sound vibrations.
staphylococcus Species of bacteria that are often responsible for hospital-acquired infections.
stasis Slowing or stopping the normal flow.
stenosis Narrowing or constriction of a passageway, such as in the valves of the heart—mitral stenosis.

sterilization Process of destroying all pathogenic microorganisms.

stigma A mark of disgrace.

stimulus Any action or agent that causes changes or action in an organ or part.

stoma An opening onto the skin that is created by an artificial passageway; may also apply to the normal opening of a pore.

stomatitis Inflammation of the mucous membranes of the mouth.

strabismus Condition in which the muscles of the eyes are not aligned properly for three-dimensional vision. Eyes can turn inward, outward, upward, or downward.

strawberry tongue Strawberrylike appearance of the tongue in scarlet fever.

streptococcus Species of bacteria that probably causes the most illness in man.

stump Distal portion of an extremity after amputation.

stuporous Describes deep sleep with a diminished sense of feeling and responsiveness.

subconscious Partial responsiveness of the mind to impressions made by the senses.

subculture An ethnic, regional, economic, or social group with characteristic patterns of behavior that distinguish it from the larger culture or society.

substance P A chemical secreted by pain nerves; a neurotransmitter.

suicide Self-destruction.

sunstroke Disorder caused by overexposure to the sun.

superego In Freudian theory, that part of the personality structure that contains society's mores. It may often be self-critical.

surgical asepsis The complete absence of organisms (germs).

surveillance Supervising or watching a person or a condition.

synovectomy Excision of the synovial membrane of a joint.

tachycardia A cardiac arrhythmia that results in a very rapid heartbeat.

team A decentralized system in which the care of a patient is distributed among the members of a team of various professionals and/or family and friends.

team nursing A nursing service approach that uses the skills of a variety of nursing personnel in providing comprehensive care for the patient. The leader, a registered nurse, is assisted in the care of a group of patients by other nurses, LVN/LPNs, nursing assistants, and orderlies. The leader assigns and directs patient care on the basis of input from team members.

tenacious Describes secretions that are sticky and stringy and tend to hold together.

terminal disinfection Cleaning of equipment and airing of room after the release of a person who has had an infectious disease.

tertiary prevention The level of prevention of illness that deals with rehabilitation of a disabled patient to return the person to a level of maximum usefulness.

tetany A condition characterized by cramps, convulsions, muscle twitching, and sharp flexion of the wrist and ankle joints (carpopedal spasm).

thanatology Study of death and dying.

therapist A person skilled in various therapeutic techniques.

thermography Technique of determining surface temperature of the body through photography.

third spacing The accumulation of fluid in areas that normally have no fluid or a minimal amount of fluid, as seen in ascites or in the edema associated with burns.

thoracotomy A surgical opening into the thoracic cavity.

thrombocytopenia Decreased number of platelets in the circulating blood.

thrombophlebitis Inflammation of a vein; caused by a thrombus.

thrombosis Presence of a blood clot.

thrush An infection of the mouth and throat; caused by a fungus and usually occurs in infants.

tinea Ringworm; disease is further differentiated by the area of body affected. Tinea capitis—scalp; tinea barbae—beard and mustache; tinea corporis—body; tinea cruris—groin (jock itch); tinea manus—hand; tinea pedis—foot (athlete's foot).

tinnitus Ringing in the ears.

tissue macrophage Any phagocytic cell of the reticuloendothelial system, including cells in the liver, spleen, and connective tissue.

tolerance State in which increasingly larger doses of a drug are needed to provide the same effect as was produced by the original dose.

tonic Refers to tension of contraction.

tonometry Measurement of intraocular pressure.

tonsillectomy Surgical removal of tonsils.

tophus A deposit of urates in tissues around joints; seen in gout.

total parenteral nutrition An intravenous technique to provide for nutritional needs.

toxemia Presence of toxins or poisons in the blood.

toxicity State of being poisonous.

trabeculae Portion of the eye in front of Schlemm's canal and within the angle created by the iris and the cornea.

trabeculectomy Surgical removal of a section of corneoscleral tissue, usually including Schlemm's canal and the trabecular meshwork. Increases outflow of aqueous humor in patients with chronic side-angle glaucoma.

trabeculoplasty Use of the laser to apply burns in the trabecular meshwork to improve aqueous humour outflow in chronic, open-angle glaucoma.

tracheostomy Permanent opening into the trachea after a tracheotomy.

tracheotomy An incision is made into the trachea through the neck and below the larynx to gain access to the airway below the blockage that has been caused by a foreign body, tumor, or edema of the glottis.

traction Exerting a force that pulls or draws on a muscle or organ.

transcutaneous electrical neural stimulation (TENS) Alteration of pain sensations by stimulating peripheral nerves with electric current that is applied to the skin.

transected Cut across or severed.

transplantation Surgical transfer of an organ from a donor to a recipient.

tremor Involuntary trembling of the body or the extremities.

triage System of assigning priorities in treating patients in a disaster or emergency situation.

trichinosis Infection with trichina, a worm found in pork.

trichomoniasis Infection with the *Trichomonas* parasite.

tuning fork A metal, two-pronged fork that vibrates to test hearing.

tympanic membrane (eardrum) A thin, semitransparent membrane in the middle ear that transmits sound vibrations to the inner ear by means of the auditory vessicles.

tympanoplasty A group of surgical procedures to restore hearing; involves the eardrum or the bones of the middle ear.

type I diabetes Insulin-dependent diabetes mellitus.

type II diabetes Noninsulin-dependent diabetes mellitus.

ulcer An open lesion on the skin with loss of deep tissue.

ultrasonogram An instrument that measures and records the reflection of pulsed or continuous high-frequency sound waves to detect abnormalities.

unconscious The part of the mind that is only rarely in one's awareness. It contains experiences or data that may be too painful to recall.

unfinished business Concerns of the dying patient that require resolution before death can be accepted; range from financial factors to interpersonal relationships.

universal precautions CDC-recommended "universal blood and body fluid precautions." Includes preventing injury from needles and sharp objects; wearing protective devices during resuscitation; avoiding patient and equipment contact if a draining lesion exists in healthcare worker.

urea Chief end-product of protein metabolism; excreted by the kidney.

uremia Accumulation of urinary constituents in the blood; causes a general toxic condition.

ureterotomy Incision into a ureter.

urinalysis Analysis of components of urine.

urine osmolality Measurement of the concentration of urine.

urticaria Hives; an allergic reaction characterized by the appearance of wheals on the skin.

uveitis Inflammation of one or more parts of the uveal tract, which includes the ciliary body, iris, and cornea.

vaccine A pathogen whose virulence has been reduced and which is used as prophylaxis against a disease.

vaginitis Inflammation of the vagina.

values Used subjectively to identify what a person considers worthwhile; used objectively to identify the intrinsic quality (good) of a thing.

varicocele A varicosity or dilation of veins in the spermatic cord.

varicosities Dilated veins.

vasogenic shock Shock resulting from peripheral vascular dilation; caused by factors (toxins) that directly affect blood vessels.

vector An insect, rodent, or arthropod that carries disease and transmits it to humans.

vegetative bacteria Bacteria that do not form spores.

vehicle Mode of transmission of an infective agent from its source to a susceptible host.

venous access device An intravenous pump that patients use to give themselves limited doses of fast-acting analgesics at the onset of pain.

ventilation The movement of air into and out of the lungs.

ventricles Small cavities, such as in the heart or brain.

ventricular fibrillation Disorganization of the heartbeat; may cause cardiac arrest without prompt treatment.

ventricular tachycardia Rapid contraction of the ventricle with reduced cardiac output.

ventriculogram A diagnostic procedure in which air is injected into the cerebral ventricles and x-ray films are taken.

veracity Telling the truth habitually.

vertigo A sensation characterized by the movement of objects or of self-movement; an extreme form of dizziness.

vesicant A drug that induces blistering. Vesicant chemotherapeutic agents cause tissue damage if they leak out of the vein during administration.

vesicle A blisterlike elevation on the skin that contains serous fluid.

vesiculation Formation of vesicles.

vestibule A cavity in the inner ear that contains two small sacs, the utricle and saccule.

virology Study of viruses.

virulence Strength of an organism to produce disease.

viruses Infective agents that cause several diseases.

viscosity Thickness of a fluid that causes it to resist flow.

visual analog scale A rating scale that uses a line to represent a continuum; the ends are marked for the two extremes of pain.

vital capacity Amount of air that can be retained in the lungs after a full inspiration.

vitrectomy Removal of blood, opacities, or disease from the posterior segment of the eye; vitreous gel is replaced with an isotonic solution.

vulvovaginitis Inflammation of the vagina, the vulva, and usually the vulvovaginal glands.

Wangensteen suction A suction-siphonage method to remove secretions from the stomach.

wen A cyst that often occurs on the back of the scalp.

Western Blot A test for the presence of antibodies to multiple antigens of HIV; used to confirm HIV infection following a positive ELISA test. The Western Blot displays antibodies to specific HIV viral proteins in a separate, well-defined band. A positive result shows stripes at the locations for two or more viral proteins. A negative result is blank at these locations.

wheal An elevated type of rash on the skin, such as in urticaria.

withdrawal syndrome A syndrome of serious symptoms that occurs when the use of a drug is discontinued.

wound healing Repair of a break in the skin.

wound infection Invasion of a wound by pathogenic microorganisms that reproduce and multiply, causing injury.

INDEX

A

A2 Hong Kong influenza, 563
AA; see Alcoholics Anonymous
Abdomen, quadrants of, 692*f*
Abdominal distention, postoperative care and, 484-485
Abdominal hysterectomy, 848-849
Abdominal thrust, 496-497
Abdominal x-ray examination, 693
Abducens nerve, 924*t*
Abduction pillow, 1114
Abortion, 857-860, 860*t*, 861
  ectopic, 861
  types of, 857-858
Abortion counseling, 859
Above-the-knee amputation, 1127
Abrasions, 507
  corneal, 1003
Absence seizures, 949
Absorption, digestion and, 690-691
Absorption dressings, pressure ulcers and, 1048
Absorption poisoning, 517
Acceptance, dying process and, 85
Accommodation of eyes, 976
Accreditation, nursing practice and, 11
Accutane; *see* Isotretinoin
Ace bandages, burns and, 1085
Acetaminophen (Liquiprin; St. Joseph's tablets; Tempra; Tylenol), 212*t*
    and codeine (Tylenol #3), 212*t*
Acetazolamide (AK-Zol; Diamox), 983*t*
Acetone, diabetes mellitus and, 901
Acetylcysteine (Mucocil), 571*t*
Acetylsalicylic acid, 212*t*
Achromatopsia, 978
Achromycin; *see* Tetracycline
Acid-base imbalance, 185-190
Acid-base regulation, 185-186
Acid-fast bacilli (AFB) isolation, 313, 315, 333
Acidosis, 173, 186
  diabetic, 910-911
  metabolic, 186, 187, 189
  respiratory, 187-189

f indicates figures; *t* indicates tables.

Acids, 185
ACLS; *see* Advanced cardiac life support
Acne, 1069-1070
Acne rosacea, 1070-1071
Acne vulgaris, 1069-1070
Acoustic nerve, 924*t*
Acquired active immunity, 269-271
Acquired immunity, 139
Acquired immunodeficiency syndrome (AIDS), 135, 278, 290, 325-344, 579, 584, 953-954, 1000
  legal issues and, 338-339
  nursing interventions for, 340-343
  pharmacology and, 330*t*-332*t*
Acquired passive immunity, 271-272
Acromegaly, 898
ACS; *see* American Cancer Society
Actinomycin-D; *see* Dactinomycin
Activated charcoal, drug overdose and, 516
Active immunity, 269
Active transport, fluid and electrolyte exchange and, 164, 165*f*
Activities of daily living (ADLs), 347, 365, 382, 429
Acupuncture, 475
Acute bronchitis, 577-578
Acute confusional state, 441
Acute coryza, 562-563, 564
Acute follicular tonsillitis, 563
Acute laryngitis, 563
Acute leukemia, 677-678
Acute lymphoblastic leukemia, 677
Acute lymphocytic leukemia (ALL), 677
Acute mastitis, 850
Acute myelocytic leukemia (AML), 677, 678
Acute nonlymphocytic leukemia, 678
Acute pharyngitis, 563
Acute phase reactants, 613
Acute poststreptococcal glomerulonephritis (APSGN), 779-780, 781
Acute pulmonary edema, 639-641
Acute renal failure, 787-788, 789
Acyclovir (Zovirax), 330*t*, 1041*t*
ADA; *see* Americans with Disabilities Act
Adalat; *see* Nifedipine
Adaptation, 381
Adaptive equipment, rehabilitation and, 409-414
Addiction, 97, 216-217
Addisonian crisis, 897
Addison's disease, 897
Adenoids, enlarged, 565-566
Adenoma, bronchial, 588
Adenosine triphosphate (ATP), 164
ADH; *see* Antidiuretic hormone
Adjuvant therapy, 238
ADLs; *see* Activities of daily living
Admission, patient, surgery and, 457
Adolescents, female, psychosocial development in, 817-818
Adrenal cortex, 896
Adrenal glands, 886, 896-898
Adrenal medulla, 897
Adrenal steroids, 158
Adrenalectomy, 898
Adrenaline; *see* Epinephrine
Adriamycin; *see* Doxorubicin
Adult Children of Alcoholics, 114
Adult respiratory distress syndrome (ARDS), 591-592
Adult-onset diabetes, 899
Adults, older; *see* Older adults
Advanced cardiac life support (ACLS), 647
Advanced medical directives, 36, 82, 366
Advanced practice nurse, 12
Adventitious sounds, 536
Advocate, patient, nurse as, 9
Aerobic bacteria, 125-126
Aerosol spray, topical medications and, 1040*t*
Aerosol therapy, bronchial infections and, 547-548
Aerosporin; *see* Polymyxin B sulfate
AFB isolation; *see* Acid-fast bacilli isolation
Affective disorders, 52

Agency for Health Care Policy and Research (AHCPR), 402, 403, 992, 993
Agent, infections and, 267-268, 268*f*
Age-related macular degeneration (ARMD), 998
Aging; *see* Older adults
Agitation, 515
Agnosia, 441
Agranulocytes, 658
AHCPR; *see* Agency for Health Care Policy and Research
AICD; *see* Automatic implantable cardioverter-defibrillator
AIDS; *see* Acquired immunodeficiency syndrome
AIDS-related complex (ARC), 329
Air embolism, 194, 667
Air mattress, pressure ulcers and, 1046*f*
Air swallowing, 740
Airborne transmission, infections and, 268, 269, 302
Air-fluidized therapy, pressure ulcers and, 1046
Airway
  artificial, 477*f*
  assessment of, 494-496, 500-501, 503-504, 646, 648-649, 932
  postoperative care and, 476-477, 477*f*
  upper, obstruction and trauma to, 564-566
Airway management, 552-554
Airway obstruction, 648*f*, 648-649
AK-Dilate; *see* Phenylephrine
AK-Pentolate; *see* Cyclopentolate hydrochloride
AK-Pred; *see* Prednisolone
Ak-tracin; *see* Bacitracin ointment
AK-Zol; *see* Acetazolamide
Alanine aminotransferase (ALT), 698-699
Al-Anon, 114
Alateen, 114
Alatot, 114
Albumin, 659*t*, 699
  abnormal levels of, 179*t*
  serum, 661
Alcohol, 100-104
Alcohol substance abuse, 98, 100-104
  fetal development and, 132
  nursing interventions for, 114-119
  physiologic effects of, 102
  psychosocial signs and symptoms of, 114
Alcohol withdrawal, 101-102, 103
Alcoholic cirrhosis, 743
Alcoholics Anonymous (AA), 113-114
Alcoholism, Jellinek's stages of, 101
Aldactone; *see* Spironolactone
Aldosterone, 167, 896
Alimentary tract, 689
Alkaline phosphatase, 698
Alkalosis, 173, 186
  metabolic, 186-187, 188, 189
  respiratory, 187, 188, 189
Alkeran; *see* Melphalan
Alkylating agents, 245
ALL; *see* Acute lymphocytic leukemia
Allergen, 141
Allergic conjunctivitis, 980, 986*t*
Allergic contact dermatitis, 146
Allergic reaction, 505
Allergy, 141-149
  atopic, 147-149
  nursing interventions and, 149-156
Allergy shots, 156
Allergy survey sheet, 147*f*-148*f*
Allogenic bone marrow transplantation, 256
Allograft, 1083
Allopurinol (Zyloprim), 1112*t*
Alopecia, 254, 1055, 1071
Alopecia areata, 1055
Alpha cells, 887
Alpha-adrenergic receptors, 600
Alpha-hemolytic streptococci, 126-127
Alprazolam (Xanax), 60*t*, 105*t*
ALS; *see* Amyotrophic lateral sclerosis
ALT; *see* Alanine aminotransferase
Altered states of cerebral functioning, 927-928
Aluminum acetate (Burow's Solution; Domeboro), 1020, 1022*t*, 1038, 1041*t*, 1067
Aluminum hydroxide (Amphojel), 713*t*
  and magnesium hydroxide (Maalox), 713*t*
  magnesium hydroxide, and simethicone (Mylanta), 713*t*
Alveoli, 530
Alzheimer's Association, 426
Alzheimer's disease, 53, 359-360, 362, 434, 956
Amantadine (Symmetrel), 950*t*
Amblyopia, 977
Ambulation, 480
  cardiac surgery and, 633
  in older adults, 372-373
  postoperative care and, 481-482
Ambulatory care, 6, 8-9
Ambulatory electrocardiography, 616
Amebiasis, 287-288
Amenorrhea, 814
American Academy of Ophthalmology, 1005
American Association of Diabetes Educators, 912
American Burn Association, 1074-1075
American Cancer Society (ACS), 227, 231, 232, 233, 568, 840, 841, 851, 853, 854
American College
  of Emergency Physicians, 493
  of Surgeons, 305
American Diabetes Association, 891, 899, 902, 903, 911, 996
American Dietetic Association, 903
American Foundation for the Blind, 999
American Heart Association, 496, 499, 645, 648
American Hospital Association, 17, 308
American Medical Association, 1017-1018
American Nurses Association (ANA), 10, 37, 117, 382
American Operating Room Nurses (AORN), 11
American Printing House for the Blind, 999
American Psychiatric Association, 99
American Red Cross, 492, 496, 499, 645, 648, 662
American Rheumatic Association, 1071
American Society of Anesthesiology (ASA), 305
Americans with Disabilities Act (ADA), 338, 382, 388
Aminoglycosides, 158
Aminophylline; *see* Theophylline ethylenediamine
Amitriptyline (Elavil), 60*t*, 105*t*
AML; *see* Acute myelocytic leukemia
Ammonia, serum levels of, 699
Amoxicillin (Augmentin), 150*t*, 713*t*, 1022*t*
Amphetamines, 109
Amphojel; *see* Aluminum hydroxide
Amphotericin B (Fungizone), 330*t*, 982*t*
Ampicillin (Omnipen; Polycillin; Principen; Totacillin), 150*t*
Amputation, 410-414, 507, 1126-1128
  above-the-knee, 1127
  below-the-knee, 1129-1130
  phantom limb pain and, 1128
Amsler's grid test in vision assessment, 974, 974*f*
Amyotrophic lateral sclerosis (ALS), 954-955
ANA; *see* American Nurses Association; Antinuclear antibody
Anaerobic bacteria, 125-126
Anal sphincter spasm, 740
Analgesics, 211-221
Analysis in nursing process, 22-31
Anaphylactic shock, 137, 144-145, 145*t*, 146, 197, 503-504
Anaprox; *see* Naproxen
Anasarca, 780
Ancef; *see* Cefazolin sodium
Andro 100; *see* Testosterone
Androgens, 878, 896

Anectine; *see* Succinylcholine
Anemia, 668-669, 675
aplastic, 673-675, 682-685
hemorrhagic, 669
iron-deficiency, 670-671
pernicious, 664, 671-672, 717
sickle cell, 672-673, 674, 680
vitamin B_{12} deficiency, 671-672
Anesthesia
alternative forms of, 475-476
surgery and, 465, 471-476
types of, 471-475
Anesthesiologist, 476
Anesthetist, 476
Aneurysm, 641-642, 947-948
Anger, dying process and, 85
Angina pectoris, 622, 623*f*
Anginal syndrome, 622
Angioedema, 1074
Angiography, 616
cerebral, 925
fluorescein, 974
pulmonary, 542
Angioma, 1053
spider, 743, 1053
Angioplasty, percutaneous transluminal coronary, 633, 635*f*
Angiotensin, 195
Angiotensin II, 619
Angiotensinogen, 763
Angle-closure glaucoma, 991, 1003
Anhidrosis, 1052
Anion gap, 186
Anions, 162-163
Ankylosing spondylitis, 1113
Anorexia, 711
Anorexia nervosa, 130, 715
Antabuse; *see* Disulfiram
Antibiotics, 150*t*, 157-158, 246, 254, 982*t*
Antibodies, 140, 269
Antidepressants, 59, 214, 351
Antidiuretic hormone (ADH), 167, 763, 770, 898, 932
Antidotes, drug overdose and, 516
Antiembolic stockings, 644
Antifungals, vision and, 982*t*-983*t*
Antigen, 139-140, 141, 269
Antigen-antibody reaction, 140, 144
Antihemophilic factor, 658, 661
Antihistamines, 153*t*, 155
Antimetabolites, 245-246
Antimicrobial agents
cephalosporin, 157-158
topical, for burns, 1082
Antinuclear antibody (ANA), 1072
Antipsychotic drugs, 59-62
Antisepsis, nosocomial infections and, 312
Antiseptic agents, 306, 310
Antisocial personality, 53
Antitoxins, 271
Antitubercular agents, 572*t*
Antivert; *see* Meclizine
Antivirals, vision and, 983*t*
Anuria, 779-780
Anxiety, 45-49, 50
Anxiety disorders, 49, 49*t*
AORN; *see* American Operating Room Nurses
Aortic vessel injury, 503
A-P transfer, 397
Aphakic eye, 994
Aphasia, 441, 944, 945
Apheresis, 256
Aphthous ulcers, 1063
APIC; *see* Association for Professionals in Infection Control and Epidemiology
Aplastic anemia, 673-675, 682-685
Appendages, disorders of, 1055-1056
Appendectomy, 721, 722
Appendicitis, 720-722
Applanation tonometer, 972
APSGN; *see* Acute poststreptococcal glomerulonephritis
AquaMEPHYTON; *see* Phytonadione
Aquathermia pack, wound healing and, 138
Ara-C; *see* Cytarabine
ARC; *see* AIDS-related complex
ARDS; *see* Adult respiratory distress syndrome
Argon laser iridectomy, 991
Aristocort, 154*t*
Arm exercises after mastectomy, 857
ARMD; *see* Age-related macular degeneration
Arrhythmia, 605, 606-607
Artane; *see* Trihexyphenidyl
Arterial blood gas studies, respiratory system and, 539, 541*t*
Arterial occlusive disease, 642-643
Arterial pulses, 603-604
Arteries, diseases and disorders of, 641-646
Arteriography, 889
Arteriosclerosis, 354-355, 617-618
Arteriovenous fistula, 792
Arteriovenous malformation (AVM), 944
Arteritis, temporal, 1003
Arthritis, 1110-1117
gouty, 1116-1117
rheumatoid, 1110-1111
surgical interventions for, 1113-1116
Arthritis Foundation, 1073
Arthrodesis, 1114
Arthroplasty, 1114
Arthropod-borne encephalitis, 953
Arthroscopy, 1114
Arthrotomy, 1114
Artificial airways, 477*f*
Artificial eye, 411-414, 1001, 1004, 1004*f*
ASA; *see* American Society of Anesthesiology
A-scan, cataracts and, 993
Ascaris, 289
Ascites, 184, 636, 744
Asepsis, surgical, 469-470
Aseptic necrosis, 1121
Asepto syringe, 1038
Asherman's syndrome, 860
Asiatic cholera, 127
Asparaginase (Elspar), 247*t*
Aspartate aminotransferase (AST), 698
Aspiration, silent, 408
Aspirin, 158, 212*t*, 212-214, 215, 1113*t*
Assistive devices, rehabilitation and, 410-414
Associate degree in nursing, 12
Associated primary nurse, 492
Association
for Professionals in Infection Control and Epidemiology (APIC), 308
of Rehabilitation Nurses, 382
AST; *see* Aspartate aminotransferase
Asthma, 575-577
Astigmatism, 973, 976
Ataxia, 949
Atelectasis, 485, 584-585
Atenolol (Tenormin), 624*t*
Atherosclerosis, 354-355, 614, 617-618, 618*f*, 631
Athlete's foot, 128, 1061
Ativan; *see* Lorazepam
Atopic allergies, 147-149
Atopic dermatitis, 1066-1067
ATP; *see* Adenosine triphosphate
Atrial fibrillation, 608*f*, 608-609
Atrial flutter, 607-608, 608*f*
Atrial rate, 606
Atrial rhythm, 606
Atrium, 607-609
Atrophic urethritis, 402
Atrophy
of adrenal gland, 897
skin lesions and, 1036
Atropine (Atropisol; Isopto Atropine), 984*t*
Atropisol; *see* Atropine
Atrovent; *see* Ipratropium
Attorney, power of, for healthcare, 36, 82, 83*f*, 84*f*, 366
Audiologist, 1016
Audiometry in assessment of hearing loss, 1015-1016
Auditory canal, 1013, 1021
Auditory tests in assessment of hearing loss, 1015-1019
Augmentin; *see* Amoxicillin

Aura, seizures and, 949
Auricle, 1013
Auro Ear Drops; *see* Carbamide peroxide
Auscultation
  in assessment of cardiovascular system, 602, 602*f*
  in assessment of respiratory system, 536-537, 538*f*
Austin Moore prosthesis, 1121, 1123
Autoclaving, sterilization and, 470
Autograft, 1082-1083
Autoimmune disease, 156
Autoimmune thrombocytopenic purpura, 681
Autologous blood, 662
Autologous bone marrow transplantation, 256
Automatic implantable cardioverter-defibrillator (AICD), 611
Automatic speech, 945
Automatism, 949
Autonomic hyperreflexia, 938-939
Autonomic nervous system, 922
Autonomy, 33, 427
Avascular necrosis, 1121
Aveeno, 1037
Avlosulfon; *see* Dapsone
AVM; *see* Arteriovenous malformation
Axid; *see* Nizatidine
Azetazolamide (Diamox), 771*t*
Azmacort; *see* Triamcinolone
Azo Gantanol; *see* Sulfamethoxazole
Azo Gantrisin; *see* Sulfisoxazole
AZT; *see* Zidovudine

B

B & O Supprettes; *see* Belladonna and extract of opium
Babinski reflex, 924
BAC; *see* Blood alcohol concentration
Bachelor of science in nursing (BSN), 12
Bacillary dysentery, 282
Bacille Calmette-Guérin (BCG), 277, 786
Bacilli, 126, 127, 127*f*
Bacitracin, 1022*t*
Bacitracin ointment (Ak-tracin), 982*t*
Back braces, 1108
Background diabetic retinopathy (BDR), 996
Back-lying position, patient in, 395-396
Bacteremia, 302, 306-307
Bacteria, 125-128
Bacterial conjunctivitis, 980, 986*t*
Bacterial endocarditis, 613, 621-622
Bacterial infections, 273-283, 1058-1059
Bactericidal chemotherapeutic drugs, 156-157
Bacteriostatic chemotherapeutic drugs, 156-157
Bacteriostatic tetracyclines, 158
Bactrim, 332*t*
Bactroban; *see* Mupirocin
BAL; *see* Blood alcohol level
Balance
  hearing and, 1014
  in long-term care, 430
Balanced traction, 1104, 1104*f*, 1105
Baldness, 1056
Balneotherapy, 1038*t*
Bandage contact lenses, 977, 986
Barber's itch, 128, 1061
Barbiturates, 107-108, 473*t*
Bargaining, dying process and, 85
Barium enema, 236-237, 695-696
Baroreceptors, 600
Barrier methods of contraception, 829-831
Barthel Index, 391
Bartholinitis, 842
Basal body temperature (BBT), 833
Basal cell carcinoma, 1053
Basal skull fracture, 930
Bases, 185
Basic cardiac life support (BCLS), 499-501, 646-647, 647*f*
Basic first aid for poisoning, 517
Basophils, 133, 658
Batemann prosthesis, 1121, 1123
Baths
  burns and, 1085
  older adults and, 369
  therapeutic, 1037-1038
Battered patients, 513
BBT; *see* Basal body temperature
BCG; *see* Bacille Calmette-Guérin
BCLS; *see* Basic cardiac life support
BCNU; *see* Carmustine
BDR; *see* Background diabetic retinopathy
Beauchamp, Tom, 33
Bed
  kinetic, 1046, 1106-1107
  specialty, 1046
Beef tapeworm, 288
Behavioral techniques, urinary incontinence and, 406
Behavioral-cognitive theory, substance abuse and, 98-99
Beijerinck, Martinus W., 128
Beliefs, cultural, 68-69
Belladonna and extract of opium (B & O Supprettes), 771*t*
Below-the-knee amputation, 1129-1130
Benadryl; *see* Diphenhydramine
Bends, 130
Beneficence, 33
Benemid; *see* Probenecid
Benign prostatic hypertrophy (BPH), 872
Benign tumors, 228
Benzocaine (Solarcaine), 474*t*
Benzodiazepines, 104, 107
Benztropine (Cogentin), 950*t*
Bereavement, 85-86
Berkow's formula, burns and, 1076-1078
Beta cells, 887
Beta-adrenergic receptors, 600
Beta-blockers, 431
Betagan; *see* Levobunolol
Beta-hemolytic streptococci, 126-127
Beta$_2$-adrenergic receptors, 600
Betaxolol (Betoptic), 983*t*
Bethanechol (Urecholine), 771*t*
Bethesda System, Pap smears and, 838
Betoptic; *see* Betaxolol
Biaxin; *see* Clarithromycin
Bicillin; *see* Penicillin G benzathine
Bifocal glasses, 976
Bilateral amputee transfer, 398
Bilateral oophorectomy, 847
Bilateral salpingectomy, 847
Biliary cirrhosis, 743
Biliary function, assessment of, 698-699
Biliary system, diseases and disorders of, 748-752
Bilirubin tests, 698
Binging, 716
Bioethics, 32
Biologic environment, infections and, 268
Biologic response modifiers (BRMs), 255, 256-257
Biologic theory, substance abuse and, 98
Biology of aging, older adults and, 350
Biopsy
  in assessment of cancer, 234
  cervical, 838
  needle localization, 840
  renal, 769-770
  stereotactic, 840
Biopsychosocial factors, older adults and, 350-352
Biot's breathing, 535*t*
Bipolar disorder, 52
Birth control, female reproductive system and, 819-831
Birthmark, 1053
Bisacodyl (Dulcolax; Fleet laxative), 714*t*
Bites, 507, 517
Black wounds, pressure ulcers and, 1049, 1051
Blackheads, 1069
Blackouts, alcoholism and, 101
Bladder, 761, 761*f*
  and bowel reconditioning, 436-437
    bladder training and, 405
    spinal cord injuries and, 939

Bladder—cont'd
  exstrophy of, 868
  tumors of, 786
Bladder catheterization, 765
Bladder incontinence, stroke and, 947
Bladder irrigation, continuous, 874
Bladder studies, 768-769
Blanching sign, 1096
Blasts, 677
Bleb, 1036
Bleeding time, 664
Blenoxane; *see* Bleomycin sulfate
Bleomycin sulfate (Blenoxane), 247*t*
Blepharitis, marginal, 1001
Blindness
  color, 977-978
  cultural, 70
  river, 977
Blood, 598, 655-687, 660*t*
  autologous, 662
  blood dyscrasias and, 668-681
  collection of, 662
  diagnostic tests and, 662-666
  function of, 656
  occult, 696
  pharmacology and, 659*t*-660*t*
  respiratory system and, 539
  structure of, 656-658
  therapeutic blood fractions and, 658-662
  therapeutic procedures and, 666-668
Blood alcohol concentration (BAC), 504-505
Blood alcohol level (BAL), 101-102
Blood chemistry, 614, 666, 888
Blood clotting factors, 699
Blood cultures, 613
Blood dyscrasias, 668
Blood gas analysis, 189, 190, 614, 664
Blood glucose testing, 901, 902
Blood loss; *see* Hemorrhage
Blood plasma, 656, 658
Blood pressure, 602-603, 618, 619
  older adults and, 372
  shock and, 195, 196
Blood transfusion therapy, 666-668
Blood typing, 666, 666*t*
Blood urea nitrogen (BUN), 767
Blood vessels, 598
Blood/body fluid precautions, 313-314, 317
Blood-brain barrier, passage of drugs across, 370
Body casts, 1100-1102
Body fluids; *see* Fluids and electrolytes
Body image, 388
Body image changes, potential, surgery and, 455
Body mechanics, mobility and, 1095
Body substance isolation (BSI), 318-319
Boiling, sterilization and, 470
Boils, 1020-1021, 1058-1059
Bone marrow aspiration, 664, 665*f*
Bone marrow transplantation, 256, 674, 678
Bone tumors, 1125-1126
Bones, anatomic changes in, in older adults, 1094
Boots, paste, 1039
Boric acid, 1038-1039
Bowel function
  altered, 407
  postoperative care and, 480
Bowel incontinence, stroke and, 947
Bowman's capsule, 762, 762*f*, 763
BPH; *see* Benign prostatic hypertrophy
Braces, 414, 1108
Brachytherapy, 239
Braden Risk Assessment Scale, 400*f*, 1049
Brain, structure and function of, 922, 922*f*
Brain tumors, 941-942
Brainstem, 922
Breast cancer, 227, 850-857
  inoperable, 856-857
  screening for, 841*t*
  treatment options for, 855*t*
Breast conservation surgery, 851
Breast prosthesis, 854-856
Breast reconstruction after mastectomy, 852, 853*f*, 854*f*, 855*t*
Breast self-examination (BSE), 236, 236*f*, 839, 840*f*
Breasts
  female, 811
    conditions affecting, 850-857
    development of, 816*f*
    tumors of, 850
  male, 866
Breath sounds, 536-537, 539*t*, 540*t*
Breathing
  assessment of, 495, 496-499, 500-501, 501*f*, 503-504, 646, 923
  Biot's, 535*t*
  control of, 530
  deep; *see* Deep breathing
  postoperative care and, 477
Brevital; *see* Methohexital
Brewster, Mary, 445
Bris, 869
Brittle diabetes, 915
BRMs; *see* Biologic response modifiers
Broad openings, communication and, 57*t*
Broca's area, 944
Bronchial adenoma, 588
Bronchial breath sounds, 536, 539*t*
Bronchiectasis, 573-575, 576
Bronchitis
  acute, 577-578
  chronic, 570-573, 575
Bronchodilating drugs, 554
Bronchogenic carcinoma, 588, 590
Bronchoscopy, 235, 542-543
Bronchovesicular breath sounds, 536, 539*t*
Brooke Army Medical Center, 1074
Bruises, 507, 1118
B-scan ultrasonography, vitrectomy and, 995
BSE; *see* Breast self-examination
BSI; *see* Body substance isolation
BSN; *see* Bachelor of science in nursing
Buccal cavity, 689
Buck's extension, 1102-1104
Buerger's disease, 643
Buffer systems, hydrogen ion concentration and, 185
Bulimia, 715-716
Buliminia, 130
Bulla, 1036
Bullous impetigo, 1058
Bumetanide (Bumex), 771*t*
Bumex; *see* Bumetanide
BUN; *see* Blood urea nitrogen
Bundle-branch block, 611
Bupivacaine (Marcaine), 474*t*
Burn centers, 1074-1075
Burn shock, 1078
Burnout, nursing care of human immunodeficiency virus patients and, 339
Burns, 508-509, 1074-1087
  acute phase of care of, 1080-1087
  depth of, 1075-1076
  determination of extent of, 1076-1078
  emergent phase of care of, 1078-1080
  emotional care and, 1086
  home care guide for, 1086
  nursing interventions for, 1081-1082
  phases of care of, 1078-1087
  rehabilitation and, 1087
  severity of, 1075
  types of, 1075
Burow's Solution; *see* Aluminum acetate
Bursae, 1092, 1092*f*, 1117
Bursitis, 1117
Busulfan (Myleran), 247*t*

C

CABG; *see* Coronary artery bypass graft
Caffeine, 131, 132
Calcitonin, 178
Calcium, 177-181
Calcium deficit, 178-180
Calcium excess, 178, 181
Calcium salts, 1112*t*
Calculi, 784-786, 785*f*
Cancer, 226-265
  breast; *see* Breast cancer
  causes of, 230-231

Cancer—cont'd
cervical, 846
checkups for, 232
classification of, 234
colon, 719
colorectal, 227, 729-730
diagnostic tests and procedures for, 233-238
emotional care of patient with, 258-259
esophageal, 727-728
of larynx, 566
lung, 227, 261-263, 588-590
modes of dissemination of, 229*f*
oral, 726-727
ovarian, 846
pathophysiology of, 228-230
pharmacology and, 247*t*-253*t*
prevention and control of, 231-233
of prostate gland, 227, 871-872, 876
rehabilitation and, 259-260
risk factors for, 231, 233
self-help groups for, 260
seven warning signals of, 233
skin, 230
of small intestine, 729
stomach, 728-729
testicular, 869
thyroid, 895
treatment of, 238-257
tumors and; *see* Tumors
unproven methods of treatment of, 257
uterine, 846
vaginal, 845
vulvar, 843-845
Candida albicans, 129, 716, 841
Candidiasis, 329, 716
Candlelighters Childhood Cancer Foundation, 260
Canker sores, 1063
Cannabis, 109
CAPD; *see* Continuous ambulatory peritoneal dialysis
Capillary fluid movement, 165-166
Capoten; *see* Captopril
Capsules, bacteria and, 126, 126*f*
Captopril (Capoten), 624*t*
Caput medusae, 743
Carafate; *see* Sucralfate
Carbachol intraocular (Miostat), 984*t*
Carbamazepine (Tegretol), 950*t*
Carbamide peroxide (Auro Ear Drops; Debrox Drops; Murine Ear Drops), 1022*t*
Carbidopa (Sinemet), 950*t*
Carbon dioxide, partial pressure of, 539
Carbon monoxide poisoning, 131
Carbonaceous sputum, 1078
Carboplatin (Paraplatin), 247*t*
Carbuncle, 1058-1059
Carcinoembryonic antigen (CEA), 238, 697-698
Carcinogens, 230
Carcinoma, 230
bronchogenic, 588, 590
Cardiac anatomy, 597, 597*f*
Cardiac arrhythmia, 606
Cardiac catheterization, 616-617
Cardiac conduction, electrical, 599-600
Cardiac cycle, 599-600
Cardiac isoenzymes, 613
Cardiac output, 636
Cardiac rehabilitation, 635
Cardiac surgery, 631-633, 634
Cardiac tamponade, 503
Cardinal fields of gaze in vision assessment, 975, 975*f*
Cardiogenic shock, 196, 627, 636
Cardiopulmonary bypass, 631
Cardiopulmonary resuscitation (CPR), 428, 492, 496, 499-501, 500*f*, 646*f*, 646-647, 647*f*
Cardiopulmonary unit, 612-617
Cardiospasm, 739-740
Cardiovascular syphilis, 292
Cardiovascular system, 596-654
advanced cardiac life support and, 647
airway obstruction and, 648-649
arteries and, 641-646
basic life support and, 646-647
cardiac rehabilitation and, 635
coronary care unit and, 612-617
diseases and disorders of, 617-629
angina pectoris, 622
anginal syndrome, 622
arteriosclerosis, 617-618
atherosclerosis, 617-618
bacterial endocarditis, 621-622
congestive heart failure and, 650-653
coronary artery disease, 622-623
heart disease, 622-623
hypertension, 618-620
hypertensive heart disease, 618-620
myocardial infarction, 623-629, 636-641
oliguria and, 650-653
rheumatic heart disease, 620-621
subacute bacterial endocarditis, 621
disorders of rate and rhythm of heart and, 606-612
electrocardiography and, 604-606
lymphatics and, 641-646
nursing assessment of, 600-604
in older adults, 353-355
operative conditions of, 629-635
pharmacology and, 624-627
Cardiovascular system—cont'd
pregnancy and, 641
spinal cord injuries and, 937
structure and function of, 597-600
veins and, 641-646
Cardioversion, 608
Carditis, 621
Care maps, 23, 26*f*-30*f*
Care plans, nursing, 23, 24*f*-25*f*
Carmustine (BCNU), 248*t*
Carpal spasm, 179
Carpal tunnel syndrome, 1128
Carpopedal spasm, 179, 180*f*
Carrier, infections and, 268
Case management model of nursing, 13-14
Cast(s)
body, 1098*f*, 1099, 1100-1102
care of, 508, 1098-1100
hip spica, 1100-1102
mobility and, 1097-1102
nursing interventions for patient with, 1101
nursing process and, 1101
removal of, 1100
Cast syndrome, 1102
Catapres; *see* Clonidine
Cataract extraction, 988
Cataracts, 992-995, 993*f*, 994*f*
senile, 993
Catatonic schizophrenia, 51-52
Catecholamines, 897
Category-specific isolation precautions, 312-313
Cathartics, drug overdose and, 516
Catheter
care of, 773-774
cystostomy, 774-775, 776*t*-777*t*
inserting, 773
irrigation of, 775, 776*f*
nephrostomy, 774-775, 776*t*-777*t*
over-the-needle, 193*f*
peripherally inserted central, 194
pyelostomy, 774-775, 776*t*-777*t*
removal of, 775-777
ureteral, 774-775, 776*t*-777*t*
Catheterization, cardiac, 616-617
Cations, 162-163
Cat's eye reflex, 1000
CBC; *see* Complete blood count
CCNU; *see* Lomustine
CCRCs; *see* Continuing care retirement communities
CCU; *see* Coronary care unit
CD4 cell counts, acquired immunodeficiency syndrome and, 326, 327
CDC; *see* Centers for Disease Control and Prevention
CDC Guidelines for Isolation Prevention in Hospitals, 312

CEA; *see* Carcinoembryonic antigen
Cefazolin sodium (Ancef; Kefzol), 150*t*
Cefoxitin (Mefoxin), 150*t*
Cell, structures of, 131*f*
Cell membrane, 132
Cell organelles, 132
Cell-mediated hypersensitivity, 145-146
Cellular abnormalities, 132
Cellular immunity, 140, 140*f*
Cellulitis, 1058-1059
Centers for Disease Control and Prevention (CDC), 271, 300, 308, 492, 583, 814
Central cyanosis, 533
Central nervous system, 922, 954-958
Central nervous system depressants, 100-109
Central nervous system infection, 952-954
Central nervous system stimulants, 109-110
Central venous lines, 194, 194*f*
Central venous pressure (CVP), 614-615
Cephalexin (Keflex), 150*t*
Cephalosporin antimicrobial agents, 157-158
Cerebellum, 922
Cerebral angiography, 925
Cerebral artery aneurysm, 947-948
Cerebral contusion, 931
Cerebral edema, 932
Cerebral functioning, altered states of, 927-928
Cerebral hematoma, 509*f*, 509-510
Cerebral palsy, 1128
Cerebral vasospasm, 947
Cerebrospinal fluid (CSF), 923
Cerebrovascular accident (CVA), 355, 944, 944*f*, 946
Cerebrovascular disease, 942-947
  assessment of, 944, 945
  intervention in, 944-945
  pathophysiology of, 942-944
Cerebrum, 922
Cerespan; *see* Papaverine
Certification, nursing practice and, 11
Certified home health aide, 447
Cerubidine; *see* Daunorubicin
Cerumen, 1013, 1021
Ceruminous glands, 1013
Cervical biopsy, 838
Cervical cancer, 846
Cervical cap, contraception and, 830-831, 831*f*
Cervical spine, assessment of, 494-496
Cervical spine preparations in trauma victim, 498
Cervical traction, 1102, 1103*f*, 1104-1105
Cervicitis, 292, 845
Cervix, conditions affecting, 845-846, 847-850
Chafing, 1073
Chain of custody in sexual assault, 514
Chair, positioning patient in, 396-397
Chalazion, 1001
Chaplain, hospital, 456
Charcoal, activated, drug overdose and, 516
Chemical agents, disease and, 130-131
Chemical burns, 1002, 1075, 1078
Chemical face peeling, 1070
Chemical restraints, 433, 515
Chemically impaired nurses, 118-119
Chemistry, blood, 614, 666, 888
Chemoreceptors, 600
Chemotherapeutic agents, 156-158, 245-256
Chest
  conditions of, 568-577
  flail, 498-499, 499*f*, 590-591
Chest drainage, 556*f*, 556-559, 557*f*, 558*f*
Chest pain of pulmonary origin, 531
Chest wounds, 497, 590-591
Chickenpox, 285, 1064
Child abuse; *see* Child maltreatment
Child maltreatment, 511-512
Childress, James, 33
Chlorambucil (Leukeran), 248*t*
Chlorazepate (Tranxene), 105*t*
Chlordiazepoxide (Librium), 60*t*, 105*t*
Chloride, 183-184
Chloride deficit, 183
Chloride excess, 183-184
Chlorpheniramine (Chlor-Trimeton; Tildrin), 153*t*
Chlorpromazine (Thorazine), 60*t*, 105*t*
Chlorpropamide (Diabinese), 890*t*
Chlor-Trimeton; *see* Chlorpheniramine
Choasma, 1050
Choking, universal distress signal for, 497, 648*f*
Cholangiography, 697
Cholecystectomy, 749, 750-752, 753
Cholecystitis, 748, 749
Cholecystography, oral, 696-697
Cholecystostomy, 752, 753
Choledochostomy, 750, 752, 753
Cholelithiasis, 748, 749-750
Cholera, Asiatic, 127
Cholesterol, 614, 618
Cholestyramine (Questran), 624*t*
Cholinergic crisis, 958
Chordotomy, 220
Chorionic gonadotropin (HCG), 841
Choroid, 967
Choroidal melanoma, 1000
Christmas disease, 679
Chronic airflow limitation, 568-577
Chronic bronchitis, 570-573, 575
Chronic leukemia, 678
Chronic lymphocytic leukemia (CLL), 678
Chronic myelocytic leukemia, 678
Chronic myelogenous leukemia (CML), 678
Chronic obstructive pulmonary disease (COPD), 531, 568-577
Chronic renal failure, 788-790, 801-804
Chvostek's sign, 179, 180*f*
Chyme, 690
Cigarette smoking, 131, 227, 233
Cilia, 133, 530
Cilliary body, 968
Ciloxan; *see* Ciprofloxacin
Cimetidine (Tagamet), 713*t*
Ciprofloxacin (Ciloxan), 982*t*
Circulating nurse, 472
Circulation, 596-654
  assessment of, 495, 499-504, 646, 923
  pharmacology and, 624*t*-627*t*
  postoperative care and, 477
Circulation overload, blood tranfusion and, 667
Circulatory system, 655-687
Circumcision, 869
Circumferential wound, 1079
Cirrhosis, 742-748, 755-757
Cisapride (Propulsid), 713*t*
Cisplatin (Platinol), 248*t*
Clarification, communication and, 57*t*
Clarithromycin (Biaxin), 330*t*
Climacteric
  female, 834-835
  male, 867
Clinical ethics, 32
Clinical nurse specialist (CNS), 492
Clinton, Bill, 3
Clitoris, 808
CLL; *see* Chronic lymphocytic leukemia
Clomid; *see* Clomiphene
Clomiphene (Clomid), 820*t*
Clonidine (Catapres), 820*t*
Clorazepate (Tranxene), 60*t*
Closed fracture, 1118-1119, 1119*f*
Closed head injury, 930
Closed reduction of fracture, 1119
Closed tracheal suctioning catheter system (CTSS), 546
Clostridium difficile, 280
Clostridium infections, 279-280
Clostridium tetani, 280
Clotrimazole (Lotrimin), 822*t*, 1022*t*
CML; *see* Chronic myelogenous leukemia
CMV retinitis; *see* Cytomegalovirus retinitis
CNS; *see* Clinical nurse specialist
Coagulation tests, 614, 663-664
Cobalt-60, radiation therapy and, 239
Cocaine, 109-110
Cocci, 126
Cochlea, 1014

Cochlear implant, 1018, 1020*f*
Code of ethics of American Nurses Association, 37
Codeine, 212*t*, 571*t*
Codependency, substance abuse and, 100
Cogentin; *see* Benztropine
Cognitive impairment disorder, 959
Cognitively impaired nursing home resident, 434
Cogwheel movements, Parkinson's disease and, 955
Colace; *see* Docusate sodium
Colchicine, 1112*t*
Cold
  common, 562-563
  wound healing and, 138-139
Cold emergencies, 518-519
Cold sores, 293, 1063
Colles' fracture, 1119
Colloidal osmotic pressure, 165
Colloids, 165
Colon, 690
  cancer of, 719
Colonoscopy, 235, 693-694
Color blindness, 977-978
Colorectal cancer, 227, 729-730
Colostomy, 705-710, 706*f*
Colporrhaphy, 843, 844
Colposcopy, 838
Coma, 927, 928
  hepatic, 748
  hyperglycemic hyperosmolar nonketotic, 900, 911
Comedones, 1069
Comfort, postoperative care and, 479
Comminuted fracture, 1119, 1120*f*
Comminuted skull fracture, 930
Common cold, 562-563
Communication
  nonverbal, 58-59, 59*f*
  therapeutic relationship and, 56-59, 57*t*-58*t*
  verbal, 56-59
Community services
  disaster preparedness and, 519-520
  home healthcare and, 447
Community-acquired infections, 266-298, 300
  bacterial, 273-283
  control of, 269-273
  emerging, 294-295
  helminthic infestations and, 288-289
  infectious process and, 267-269
  protozoal, 287-288
  sexually transmitted diseases and, 289-294
  viral, 283-287
Compartment syndrome, 1124, 1125
Compazine; *see* Prochlorperazine
Compensation, 48*t*, 190
Complement, 140
Complete abortion, 858
Complete blood count (CBC), 613, 662, 663*t*
Complete fracture, 1119, 1120*f*
Compliance, noncompliance and, 76
Compromised host, 301
Computerized tomography (CT) scan, 541-542, 889, 926
  in assessment of cancer, 237
  in assessment of gastrointestinal system, 695
  in assessment of renal function, 769
Comtrex; *see* Dextromethorphan
Concern for Dying, 82
Concussion, 930-931
Condom
  female, 830, 831, 832*f*
  male, 337, 830, 831
Conductive hearing loss, 1018, 1018*f*, 1026
Condyloma latum, 292
Confidentiality, respect for, 36-37
Configuration, electrocardiography and, 606
Confused patient, 440, 515, 927-928, 960-964
Congenital malformations, male reproductive system and, 868
Congenital syphilis, 292
Congestion, rebound, 155-156
Congestive heart failure, 636-639, 650-653
Conization, cervicitis and, 845
Conjunctiva, 967
Conjunctivitis, 980-981
  allergic, 980
  bacterial, 980, 986*t*
  viral, 980, 986*t*
Conscious sedation, 508
Consciousness, 45, 371-372, 927
Consent, informed
  in emergency department, 492-493
  surgery and, 457-458
Constipation, 215, 739, 947
  in long-term care, 437-438
  in older adults, 360
Contact dermatitis, 1067
  allergic, 146
Contact isolation, 312-313, 315
Contact lenses, 977, 978, 978*f*, 986, 1004
Contact transmission, infections and, 268-269, 302
Continent pouch ileostomy, 710*f*, 710-711
Continent urostomy, 796
Continuing care retirement communities (CCRCs), 8
Continuity of care, rehabilitation and, 418
Continuous ambulatory peritoneal dialysis (CAPD), 793-794
Continuous bladder irrigation, 874
Contraception
  barrier methods of, 829-831
  emergency, 825-826, 826*t*
  female reproductive system and, 818-831
  surgical, 829
Contracture, 392-393, 1095
  Volkmann's, 1124
Contrast sensitivity testing in vision assessment, 973-974
Contusions, 507, 1118
  cerebral, 931
Conversion, 48*t*
Conversion disorder, 49*t*
Convoluted foam mattress, pressure ulcers and, 1046*f*
COPD; *see* Chronic obstructive pulmonary disease
Cor pulmonale, 570
Cornea, 967, 981, 987
Cornea safety, 989
Corneal abrasions, 506, 981, 987*f*, 1003
Corneal diseases, degenerative, 986-987
Corneal disorders, 981-986
Corneal donor criteria, 989
Corneal dystrophies, 987
Corneal transplantation, 987-989, 989*f*
Coronary artery bypass, 631
Coronary artery bypass graft (CABG), 633
Coronary artery disease, 622-623
Coronary care unit (CCU), 612-617
Corpus luteum, 810, 811
Corsets, 1108
Cortef; *see* Hydrocortisone
Corticosteroids, 153*t*-154*t*, 156, 158, 1043*t*
Cortisol, 985*t*
Cortisone, 158, 896
Coryza, acute, 562-563, 564
Cough(ing), 531-532
  and deep breathing, 479, 545-546, 556
  postoperative care and, 479
  tuberculosis and, 582
Coumadin therapy, 589
Counseling
  abortion, 859
  vocational, 387
Countertraction, 1102
Cover/uncover test in vision assessment, 975
CPK; *see* Creatine phosphokinase
CPR; *see* Cardiopulmonary resuscitation
Crack cocaine, 110
Crackles, 536, 540*t*

Cranial nerves, 924*t*
Craniotomy, 942, 943
Cranium, 923
Creams, topical medications and, 1040*t*
Creatine phosphokinase (CPK), 613
Creatinine, 763, 767
Creatinine clearance, 767
Creatinine tests, 787
Cretinism, 893, 895
Cricothyroidotomy, 496
Critical incidence stress debriefing, 520
Critical instruments, 310-311
Critical thinking/decision making, 22
Crohn's disease, 717-719
Cross-matching, blood typing and, 666
Cross-tolerance, substance abuse and, 98
Crush injuries, 507
Crust, skin lesions and, 1035, 1036
Crutches, 414, 415*f*, 416*f*, 417*f*
Cryoprecipitate, 659*t*, 661, 679
Cryosurgery, 238, 871, 992
Cryosurgical ablation for prostate cancer, 876
Cryotherapy, cervicitis and, 845
Cryptococcosis, 329
Cryptorchidism, 869, 870
Crysticillin; *see* Penicillin G procaine
CSF; *see* Cerebrospinal fluid
CT scan; *see* Computerized tomography scan
CTSS; *see* Closed tracheal suctioning catheter system
Culdoscopy, 838-839
Cultural blindness, 70
Cultural conflict, 69
Cultural considerations, 66-78
  cultural variability and, 71-75
  nursing diagnoses and, 75-76
  older adults and, 348
  patient and family teaching and, 76-78
  phenomenon of culture and, 67-69
  surgery and, 458-459
  transcultural nursing and, 69-71
Cultural imposition, 70
Cultural relativity, 68
Cultural variability, 71-75
Culturally congruent care, 67
Culture
  customs, beliefs, and values and, 68-69
  definition of, 67-68
  phenomenon of, 67-69
Cupping of disc, 991
Curare, 469*t*
Cushing's syndrome, 897-898
Customs, cultural, 68-69
CuT 380A intrauterine copper contraceptive, 828
Cutaneous disorders, 1071-1073
Cutaneous ureterostomy, 795, 796, 796*f*
CVA; *see* Cerebrovascular accident
CVP; *see* Central venous pressure
Cyanosis, 533
Cyclocryopexy, glaucoma and, 992
Cyclogyl; *see* Cyclopentolate hydrochloride
Cyclopentolate hydrochloride (AK-Pentolate; Cyclogyl), 985*t*
Cyclophosphamide (Cytoxan), 248*t*
Cycloplegics, vision and, 984*t*-985*t*
Cyclosporine (Sandimmune), 771*t*
Cyclothymic disorder, 53
Cystectomy, 795
Cystitis, 781-782
Cystocele, 842-843
Cystography, 768-769
Cystoscopy, 768
Cystostomy, 775
Cystostomy catheter, 774-775, 776*t*-777*t*
Cystotomy, 797
Cytarabine (Ara-C; Cytosar), 249*t*
Cytology, exfoliative, 233-234
Cytomegalovirus (CMV), 293, 329, 579, 995
Cytoplasm, 132
Cytosar; *see* Cytarabine
Cytotoxic hypersensitivity, allergy and, 145
Cytoxan; *see* Cyclophosphamide

D

D & C; *see* Dilation and curettage
Dacarbazine (DTIC-Dome), 249*t*
Dacryocystitis, 1002
Dactinomycin (Actinomycin-D), 249*t*
Dakin's solution, 1038, 1046
Dalkon Shield, 828
Danazol (Danocrine), 820*t*
Dandruff, 1001
Danocrine; *see* Danazol
Dapsone (Avlosulfon), 330*t*
Daraprim; *see* Pyrimethamine
Dark-skinned persons, assessment of skin in, 1036
Darvocet-N; *see* Propoxyphene/acetaminophen
Darvocet-N-100; *see* Propoxyphene-N/acetaminophen
Darvon; *see* Propoxyphene
Darvon-N; *see* Propoxyphene
DAT; *see* Dementia of Alzheimer's type
Daunorubicin (Cerubidine), 249*t*
Day hospital, older adults and, 373-374
dB; *see* Decibels
DCA; *see* Directional coronary atherectomy
Deafness, 1018, 1019, 1026
Death, 80-85
  care of family following, 92
  causes of, 5
  and dying, 79-95
    fear of, 82, 83
    nursing care and, 86-94
    nursing interventions and, 86-94
  following traumatic injury, 87-88
  grief and bereavement and, 85-86
  natural, 366
  preparation for, 366
  religious practices at time of, 81
  sudden, 521
  time of, 80-81
Debridement, 1047, 1082
Debrox Drops; *see* Carbamide peroxide
Decadron; *see* Dexamethasone
Decibels (dB), hearing loss and, 1017-1018
Decision making
  ethical, nursing process and, 21-39
  patient involvement in, 36
Decongestants, topical, 155-156
Decubitus, 399
Decubitus ulcers; *see* Pressure ulcers
Deep breathing
  coughing and, 545-546
  postoperative care and, 479
Deep pain, 207
Deep vein thrombosis (DVT), 585, 589, 644
Defense mechanisms, 47, 48*t*
  physiologic, 132-140
Defibrillation, 605
Degeneration, macular, 998-999, 999*f*
Degenerative diseases
  of central nervous system, 954-958
  corneal, 986-987
  joint, 1110, 1113, 1114
Dehiscence, postoperative care and, 486, 486*f*
Dehydration, 72*f*, 168, 169
Delayed union of bone, 1121
Delirium, 359, 361*t*, 441
Delirium tremens (DTs), 102
Delta-Cortef; *see* Prednisolone
Deltasone; *see* Prednisone
Delusions, 52
Dementia, 53-54, 359, 361*t*, 371, 430
  Alzheimer's disease and, 956
  of Alzheimer's type (DAT), 441
  in long-term care, 441-442
  senile, 53
Demerol; *see* Meperidine
Demographics, older adults and, 346-347
Demulcents, 545
Denial, 48*t*
  dying process and, 85
  substance abuse and, 112
Dentures, 369-370

Deontology, 34
Department
 of Health and Human Services, 308, 347, 999
 of Veterans Affairs, 9
Dependent patient, 50-51
Dependent transfer of patient, 397-398
Depolarization, electrocardiography and, 604
Depo-Provera; *see* Medroxyprogesterone acetate
Depressed skull fracture, 930
Depression, 52, 54-56, 63-64, 351, 361*t*, 515
 dying process and, 85
 endogenous, 54
 in long-term care, 429-430, 441
 nursing assessment of, 55
 situational/reactive, 54
 success, 54
Depro-Provera (DMPA), 827-828, 830, 859-860
Dermabrasion, 1070
Dermatitis, 1066-1069
 allergic contact, 146
 drug, 1067
 irritant, 1066
 seborrheic, 1066
Dermatitis medicamentosa, 1067
Dermatitis venenata, 1067
Dermatomycosis, 128
Dermis, 1032
DES; *see* Diethylstilbestrol
DES syndrome, 845
Desensitization, 149, 156
Desquamation, radiation therapy and, 240
Detached retina, nursing interventions for, 1006-1008
Detoxification, substance abuse and, 113
Detrusor hyperreflexia, 403
Deviated septum, 565
Dexamethasone (Decadron; Hexadrol; Maxidex), 985*t*
Dextromethorphan (Comtrex; Dimetane-DX; Humidid-DM; Rondec-DM; Tylenol Cold Medication), 571*t*
Diabetes
 brittle, 915
 surgical patient with, 459
Diabetes Control and Complication Study, 911
Diabetes insipidus, 899
Diabetes mellitus, 899-915, 900*t*
Diabetic acidosis, 910-911
Diabetic diet, 903
Diabetic ketoacidosis (DKA), 889, 910-911
Diabetic retinopathy, 996
Diabetic triopathy, 911
Diabinese; *see* Chlorpropamide
Diagnosis-related group (DRG) system, 6, 373, 451
Diagnostic and Statistical Manual of Mental Disorders IV, 99
Diagnostic and Therapeutic Criteria Committee of the American Rheumatism Association, 1071
Dialysate, 792-793
Dialysis, 791-794
 continuous ambulatory peritoneal, 793-794
 peritoneal, 792-793
Dialyzer, 791
Diamox; *see* Acetazolamide
Diapering, urinary incontinence and, 406, 779
Diaphragm, contraception and, 830, 831, 831*f*
Diaphragmatic hernia, 737-738
Diarrhea, 712-715
Diastole, 599
Diastolic blood pressure, 602, 618
Diazepam (Valium), 60*t*, 105*t*, 466*t*
Diclofenac (Voltaren), 984*t*
Diet; *see* Nutrition
Diethylstilbestrol (DES), 230, 250*t*, 838, 845, 877*t*
Diffusion
 facilitated, 164
 fluid and electrolyte exchange and, 164
Diflucan; *see* Fluconazole
Digestive system, 360-363, 690-691
Digitalis, hypokalemia and, 176
Digitalis toxicity, 176, 610, 638
Digoxin (Lanoxicaps; Lanoxin), 624*t*
Dilantin; *see* Phenytoin
Dilation and curettage (D & C), 841, 859
Dilaudid; *see* Hydromorphone
Dilemma, ethics and, 32, 36
Dimenhydrinate (Dramamine), 1022*t*
Dimetane-DX; *see* Dextromethorphan
Diphenhydramine (Benadryl), 153*t*
Diphenoxylate and atropine (Lomotil), 713*t*
Diphtheria tetanus toxoid (dT), 506
Diplococci, 126-127, 127*f*
Diploma schools, hospital-based, 12
Dipyridamole (Persantine), 625*t*
Direct visualization in assessment of cancer, 234-235
Directional coronary atherectomy (DCA), 633
Disability
 definition of, 381-382
 emotional response to, 388-390
Disaster
 psychologic reactions to, 520
 role of triage during, 493
Disaster preparedness, 519-520
Disc, cupping of, 991
Discharge, emergency and trauma care and, 521
Discoid lupus erythematosus (DLE), 1071
Disease-specific isolation precautions, 313
Disinfection, 310-312
Diskectomy, 940
Dislocations, 507-508, 1118
Disorganized schizophrenia, 51
Displacement, 48*t*
Disseminated intravascular coagulation, 197-198
Distraction, pain and, 219
Disulfiram (Antabuse), 103
Diuresis, 770
Diuretics, 431, 770
 loop, 174, 176
 thiazide, 174, 176
Diverticula, 722-725, 723*f*
Diverticular disease, 722-725
Diverticulitis, 722-725
Diverticulosis, 722-725
Dizziness, 1027
DKA; *see* Diabetic ketoacidosis
DLE; *see* Discoid lupus erythematosus
DMPA; *see* Depro-Provera
DNR orders; *see* Do-not-resuscitate orders
DNS; *see* Dysplastic nevus syndrome
Documentation
 nursing process and, 31
 of sexual assault, 514
Docusate sodium (Colace), 713*t*
Dolophine; *see* Methadone
Domeboro; *see* Aluminum acetate
Dome-paste bandage, 1039
Domestic violence, 513
Do-not-resuscitate (DNR) orders, 36, 81, 428
Dopar; *see* Levodopa
Double-barreled stoma, 705
Douching, 817
Doxorubicin (Adriamycin), 250*t*
Doxycycline (Vibramycin), 150*t*
Drainage, 316, 477, 481*f*
Dramamine; *see* Dimenhydrinate
Dressings
 eye, 980
 foam, 1048
 postoperative care and, 480, 481*f*, 482*f*
 pressure ulcers and, 1048
 wet, 1038-1039
DRG; *see* Diagnosis-related group system

Drip-o-meter, 775
Droperidol (Inapsine; Innovar), 466*t*, 473*t*
Droplet contact, infections and, 269
Drug dermatitis, 1067
Drug interactions, 371
Drugs; *see* Medications
Dry desquamation, radiation therapy and, 240
Dry drunk, 112
Dry heat sterilization, 470
Dry pleurisy, 582
Dry-eye syndrome, 1002
dT; *see* Diphtheria tetanus toxoid
DTIC-Dome; *see* Dacarbazine
DTs; *see* Delirium tremens
Dulcolax; *see* Bisacodyl
Dullness, percussion and, 536
Dumping syndrome, 736
Duodenal ulcer, 731*t*
Duodenoscopy, 693
Duodenostomy, 702
Durable power of attorney, 36, 82, 83*f*, 84*f*, 366
Duragesic; *see* Fentanyl
DVT; *see* Deep vein thrombosis
Dwarf tapeworm, 288
Dwarfism, 898-899
Dying; *see* Death and dying
Dypsnea, 531
Dyscrasias, blood, 668
Dysentery, bacillary, 282
Dysfunctional family, substance abuse and, 99-100
Dysmenorrhea, 813*f*, 813-814, 814*t*
Dyspareunia, 866, 869
Dysphagia, 407-409, 410, 727, 944, 945
Dysplastic nevus syndrome (DNS), 1053-1054
Dyspnea, 623
Dystrophies, 986-987

E

E chart in vision assessment, 970, 970*f*
Ear
  external
    disorders of, 1020-1023
    structure and function of, 1013, 1013*f*
  hearing and; *see* Hearing
  inner
    disorders of, 1027-1028
    structure and function of, 1013*f*, 1014
  middle
    disorders of, 1023-1027
    structure and function of, 1013, 1013*f*
Eardrum, 1013, 1021-1023
Eastern equine encephalitis, 953
Eating disorders, 715-716
EB virus; *see* Epstein-Barr virus
Ecchymosis, 681, 1118
ECF; *see* Extracellular fluid
ECG; *see* Electrocardiography
Echocardiogram, 616
Echothiophate iodide (Phospholine Iodide), 984*t*
ECT; *see* Electroconvulsive therapy
Ectoparasites, 1056*t*, 1056-1058
Ectopic abortion, 861
Ectopic pacemaker, 600
Ectopic pregnancy, 860-861
Ectopic testes, 870
Ectropion, 1002
Eczema, 1021, 1066-1069
ED; *see* Emergency department
Edema, 166, 604
  cerebral, 932
  of cornea, 987
  pitting, 604
  pulmonary, 621, 639-641
Edrophonium test, 958, 975, 1002
EEG; *see* Electroencephalography
EGD; *see* Esophagogastroduodenoscopy
Ego, 45
Ejection click, 602
ELA; *see* Excimer laser angioplasty
Elase, 439
Elavil; *see* Amitriptyline
Elder maltreatment, 512-513
Elderly; *see* Older adults
Electrical burns, 1075
Electrical cardiac conduction, 599-600
Electrocardiography (ECG), 604-606
  ambulatory, 616
  interpretation of, 605-606
Electroconvulsive therapy (ECT), 62
Electroencephalography (EEG), 81, 926
Electrolytes
  fluids and; *see* Fluids and electrolytes
  heart rate and, 600
Electromyography (EMG), 926-927
Electronic cardiac pacemakers, 611-612
Electronystagmography, 1017
Electrophoresis, hemoglobin, 663
Electrophysiology study (EPS), 617
Elephantiasis, 645
Elimination
  postoperative care and, 478
  surgery and, 462
Elimination tests, allergy and, 149
ELISA; *see* Enzyme-linked immunoabsorbent assay
Elspar; *see* Asparaginase
Embolectomy, 633-635
Embolic stroke, 943
Embolism
  air, 194, 667
  fat, 1123, 1124
Embolism—cont'd
  postoperative care and, 485-486
  pulmonary, 194, 485-486, 585-588, 588*f*, 589, 644, 1123
Emergency and trauma care, 489-525
  burns and, 508-509
  consent and, 492-493
  disaster preparedness and, 519-520
  discharge and teaching and, 521
  emergency department in, 490, 491
  emergency nursing and, 491-492
  environmental emergencies and, 517-519
  fractures and dislocations and, 507-508
  head injuries and, 509-510
  overdose management and, 515-517
  patient arrival and, 492-493
  physical assessment and, 494-506
  poisonings and, 517
  psychiatric emergencies and, 514-515
  sudden death and, 521
  trends in, 521
  triage and, 493-494
  violence and, 510-514
  wound care and, 507
Emergency care team, 490, 491*f*
Emergency contraception, 825-826, 826*t*
Emergency department (ED), 490, 491
  violence in, 510-511
Emergency nurse manager, 492
Emergency nurse practitioner, 492
Emergency Nurses Association (ENA), 491
Emergency Nurses Cancel Alcohol-Related Emergencies (ENCARE), 521
Emergency nursing, 491-492
Emerging infections, 294-295
EMG; *see* Electromyography
Emmetropia, 975, 976*f*
Emotional child maltreatment, 511, 512
Emotional disorders, 49-51
Emotional response to disability, 388-390
Emotional stages in dying process, 85
Emotional support
  cancer and, 258-259
  dying process and, 91
  nosocomial infections and, 319
Empathy, communication and, 57
Emphysema, pulmonary, 568-570
Empyema, 584
ENA; *see* Emergency Nurses Association
Enabling, substance abuse and, 99-100
Enalapril (Vasotec), 625*t*
ENCARE; *see* Emergency Nurses Cancel Alcohol-Related Emergencies

Encephalitis, 953
End stoma, 705
Endemic goiter, 891-892
Endocarditis, 597-598, 613, 621-622
Endocrine glands, 885*f*, 885-887
Endocrine system, 884-920
  diagnostic tests and procedures and, 888-889
  diseases and disorders of, 891-915
    disorders of adrenal glands, 896-898
    disorders of pancreas, 899-915
    disorders of parathyroid glands, 895-896
    disorders of pituitary gland, 898-899
    disorders of thyroid gland, 891-895
    pharmacology of drugs used for, 890*t*-891*t*
  endocrine glands and, 885-887
  nursing assessment of, 887
  pharmacology and, 890*t*-891*t*
  therapeutic procedures and, 889-891
End-of-life decision-making, 428
Endogenous depression, 54
Endogenous glucagon, 910
Endogenous infections, 135, 301
Endogenous insulin, 900
Endolymph, 1014
Endometriosis, 845-846
Endophthalmitis, 995
Endorphins, 206
Endoscopy, 542-543, 693
Endotoxins, 135
Endotracheal intubation, 472-473, 552
Enema, 437, 462, 694, 704
  barium, 236-237, 695-696
  preoperative, 462
Enflurane (Ethrane), 473*t*
Engraftment, 256
Enlarged tonsils and adenoids, 565-566
Enteral feeding, 304-305, 702-703
Enteric fistula, 705
Enteric precautions, 313, 316
Enteritis, 717
Enterostomal therapy (ET) nurse, 707, 708-710
Entropion, 1001-1002
Enucleation, 998, 1001
Environment, infections and, 267, 268, 268*f*
Environmental emergencies, 517-519
Enzyme-linked immunoabsorbent assay (ELISA), 326
Enzymes
  liver, 698-699
  serum, 613
Eosinophils, 133, 141, 658
Epi pen, 504
Epidermal origins, diseases of, 1066-1071
Epidermis, 1032
Epididymitis, 868-869
Epidural anesthesia, 218, 221-223, 475
Epidural hematoma, 509, 931, 932*f*
Epilepsy, 948
Epilepsy Foundation of America, 952
Epinephrine (Adrenaline), 155, 504, 600, 897, 985*t*
Epiphora, 981
Epispadias, 868
Epistaxis, 564-565
Epoetin alfa (Epogen), 659*t*, 771*t*, 790
EPS; *see* Electrophysiology study
Epstein-Barr (EB) virus, 286, 293, 676
Equilibrium, vestibular system and, 1014
Erectile dysfunction, 878
Erectile function, male reproductive system and, 878-879
Ergocalciferol, 1112*t*
Erikson, Erik, 45, 46*t*-47*t*, 351
Erysipelas, 1021
Erythema intertrigo, 1073
Erythema multiforme, 1074
Erythroblastosis fetalis, 666
Erythrocytes, 656-657, 668-676
Erythroderma, 1067, 1069
Erythromycin (Ilotycin), 151*t*, 158, 982*t*
Erythropoiesis, 656
Erythropoietin, 656
Eschar, 1047, 1049, 1079
Escharotomy, 1079
Escherichia coli, 294
Esophageal cancer, 727-728
Esophageal speech, 568
Esophageal varices, 743
Esophagogastroduodenoscopy (EGD), 693
Esophagogastrostomy, 727
Esophagoscopy, 235, 693
Esotropia, 976
Esteem needs, 44
Estradiol, 820*t*
Estradiol cypionate, 820*t*
Estradiol valerate, 820*t*
Estrogen, 230, 825, 835, 896
ESWL; *see* Extracorporeal shockwave lithotripsy
ET nurse; *see* Enterostomal therapy nurse
Ethambutol (Myambutol), 572*t*
Ethanol, 101
Ethical decision making, 32-35, 33*f*
  ANA code of ethics and, 37
  ethics committee and, 37
  in long-term care, 427-428
  nursing process and, 21-39
  patient respect and, 35-37
Ethical theory, 32-34
Ethics, 32
  clinical, 32
  code of, of American Nurses Association, 37
  in daily practice, 34-35
Ethics committee, 37
Ethnic factors, older adults and, 348
Ethnocentric attitudes, culture and, 68, 70
Ethosuximide (Zarontin), 950*t*
Ethrane; *see* Enflurane
Ethylene oxide, sterilization and, 470
Etoposide (VePesid), 250*t*
ETT; *see* Exercise tolerance test
Eulexin; *see* Flutamide
Eustachian tube, 1013
Evaluation in nursing process, 31-32
Eversion of upper eyelid, 506, 506*f*, 979, 979*f*
Evil eye, 74
Evisceration
  pelvic, 849-850, 879
  postoperative care and, 486, 486*f*
Examination
  breast, 839, 840*f*
  pelvic, female reproductive system and, 836-837
  physical; *see* Physical examination
Excimer laser angioplasty (ELA), 633
Excisional biopsy, 234
Excoriation, 1036
Excretory urography, 767-768
Exenteration, pelvic, 849-850, 879-880
Exercise(s)
  arm, after mastectomy, 857
  diabetes mellitus and, 908
  Kegel, 405, 406, 436, 776, 843
  mobility and, 1095
  postoperative care and, 480-481
  range-of-motion, 392-393, 394*f*, 1093-1094, 1095
Exercise tolerance test (ETT), 615
Exfoliative cytology, 233-234
Exfoliative dermatitis, 1067
Exhalation, ventilation and, 530
Exogenous androgens, 878
Exogenous glucagon, 910
Exogenous infections, 135, 301
Exogenous insulin, 900
Exophthalmic goiter, 892
Exophthalmometry, 974-975
Exophthalmos, 892, 892*f*, 893, 975
Exotoxins, 135
Exotropia, 976
Expectorants, 545
Exploitation, 511
Exposure of patient in primary assessment, 504-505
Expressed consent, 492
Expressive aphasia, 945
Exstrophy of bladder, 868

Extended-care facilities, 5, 7-8
External fixation devices, 1108, 1109*f*
External otitis, 1021
External radiation therapy, 239-241, 242, 243
Extracapsular cataract extraction, 993-994
Extracellular fluid (ECF), 162
Extracellular fluid excess, 169, 170, 171
Extracellular fluid volume imbalances, 167-170
Extracorporeal shock-wave lithotripsy (ESWL), 750, 786
Extraocular muscles, 968, 968*f*
Extraocular surgery, 998
Extrinsic asthma, 575
Exudate absorbers, pressure ulcers and, 1048
Eye
  aphakic, 994
  artificial, 410-414, 1001, 1004, 1004*f*
  diseases and disorders of, 975-978
    nursing assessment of, 969-975
    nursing interventions for, 979-1002
  emergencies and trauma to, 1002-1003
  evil, 74
  foreign bodies in, 506, 1003
  irrigation of, 1002, 1002*f*
  lazy, 977
  normal aging and, 1005
  pink, 980
  pseudophakic, 994
  red, 981, 986*t*
  refractive errors of, 975-977
  structure and function of, 967*f*, 967-969
  trauma to, 1003
  vision and; *see* Vision
Eye contact, cultural variability and, 75
Eye dresssings, 980
Eye drops, instillation of, 980
Eye examination; *see* Visual examination
Eye injuries, 1003-1004
Eye irrigation/cleansing, 981
Eye muscles, surgery and, 998
Eye safety, 1003-1004
Eyelid lacerations, 1003
Eyelids
  disorders and defects of, 1001-1002
  eversion of, 506, 506*f*
  surgery and, 998

F

Face mask, 548*f*, 548-549, 549*f*, 550*f*
Faces rating pain scale, 209, 211*f*
Facial nerve, 924*t*
Facilitated diffusion, fluid and electrolyte exchange and, 164
Factor VIII, 659*t*
Falling test, 1017
Fallopian tubes, conditions affecting, 846-850
Falls
  in long-term care, 430, 431*f*, 432, 432*t*
  rehabilitation and, 384
Familial adenomatous polyposis (FAP), 710
Family
  rehabilitation and, 390
  support of, dying process and, 91
Family violence, 511
Famotidine (Pepcid), 714*t*
FAP; *see* Familial adenomatous polyposis
Farsightedness, 976, 976*f*
Fascia, superficial, 1032-1033
Fasciotomy, 1124
Fat, saturated, foods high in, 618
Fat embolism, 1123, 1124
Fear of death and dying, 82, 83
Federal Emergency Management Agency (FEMA), 519
Federal Housing Act, 348
Federal Rehabilitation Act, 338
Feeding, enteral, 304-305, 702-703
Felon, 1058-1059
FEMA; *see* Federal Emergency Management Agency
Female condom, 830, 831, 832*f*
Female genitalia; *see* Reproductive system, female
Female reproductive system; *see* Reproductive system, female
Female sterilization, 829, 829*f*
Femoral hernia, 737
Fentanyl (Duragesic; Sublimaze), 212*t*, 466*t*, 473*t*
Ferrous salts, 659*t*
Fever, 130, 254
  rheumatic, 621, 641
  Rocky Mountain spotted, 127-128, 283
  scarlet, 274
  typhus, 127
Fiberglass casts, 1099
Fibrillation, ventricular, 610, 610*f*
Fibrinogen, 661
Fibrocystic breast disease, 850
Fibroid, 846
Fibroplasia, retrolental, 999
Fidelity
  ethics and, 32, 34
  respect as application of, 35-36
Field registered nurse, 492
Fight or flight response, 47, 731, 897, 922
Filtration, fluid and electrolyte exchange and, 164
FIM; *see* Functional Independence Measure
Finasteride (Proscar), 877*t*
First aid, basic, for poisoning, 517
First responder, role of, 501
First spacing, 162
First-degree burn, 1076
First-trimester legal abortion, 859-860
Fish tapeworm, 288-289
Fissure, 1036
Fistula
  arteriovenous, 792
  enteric, 705
  mucous, 705
  rectovaginal, 842
  vesicovaginal, 842
Flagella, bacteria and, 126, 126*f*
Flagyl; *see* Metronidazole
Flail chest, 498-499, 499*f*, 590-591
Flap reconstruction, breast reconstruction after mastectomy and, 852, 853*f*, 854*f*
Flashbacks, hallucinogens and, 111-112
Flashing lights, vitreous and, 995
Flatworms, 288-289
Fleet laxative; *see* Bisacodyl
Fleet mineral oil, 714*t*
Fleming, Alexander, 157
Flight nurse (FN), 492
Floaters, vitreous and, 995, 1005
Florinef; *see* Fludrocortisone acetate
Flow-rate measurements, 540
Fluconazole (Diflucan), 330*t*
Fludrocortisone acetate (Florinef), 890*t*
Fluid resuscitation, 1079
Fluid shifts, fluid and electrolyte exchange and, 166
Fluids and electrolytes, 161-203, 163*t*
  acid-base imbalance and, 185-190
  compartments of, 162
  exchange of, 164-167
  imbalances in, 167-184
  intravenous therapy and, 190-194
  protein imbalances and, 184-185
  psychosocial support and, 198
  regulation of, 167
  shock and, 195-198
  spacing of, 162
Fluocinonide (Lidex; Topsyn), 1022*t*
Fluorescein angiography in vision assessment, 974
Fluoroscopy, 235, 616
5-Fluorouracil (5-FU), 250*t*
Fluothane; *see* Halothane
Fluoxetine (Prozac), 61*t*, 106*t*
Flurbiprofen (Ocufen), 984*t*
Flutamide (Eulexin), 251*t*
FN; *see* Flight nurse
Foam dressings, pressure ulcers and, 1048

Foam mattress, pressure ulcers and, 1046*f*
Focusing, communication and, 58*t*
Focussed assessment in emergency and trauma care, 506
Folate, 659*t*
Folic acid, 659*t*
Folinic acid, 331*t*
Folk practices, culture and, 68
Follicle-stimulating hormone (FSH), 811, 866-867
Follicular tonsillitis, acute, 563
Folliculitis, 1058
Folstein Mini-Mental Status Examination (MMSE), 352-353
Fomite, 269
Food guide pyramid, 904
Food poisoning, 279, 280-282, 281*t*
Forane; *see* Isoflurane
Foreign bodies
  in external ear, 1021
  in eye, 506, 1003
  in throat, 566
Foster home, older adults and, 374
Fourth-degree burn, 1076
Fractionation, radiation therapy and, 239
Fractures, 507-508, 1118-1125
  assessment of, 1119
  complications of, 1123-1124
  healing of, 1120-1121
  of hip, 1121-1123
  laryngeal, 495-496, 649
  in older adults, 1106
  rib, 508
  skull, 930
  types of, 1119
Franklin bifocals, 976
Freckles, 1050
Freebase cocaine, 110
Fremitus, 535, 537*t*
Freud, Sigmund, 45
Friction, pressure ulcers and, 1043-1044
Friction rubs, 540*t*
Frostbite, 519
Frozen-section biopsy, 234
FSH; *see* Follicle-stimulating hormone
5-FU; *see* 5-Fluorouracil
Full-thickness burns, 1075-1076
Functional assessment
  in long-term care, 429
  in older adults, 365
  rehabilitation and, 390
Functional disorders of gastrointestinal system, 739-740
Functional hypoglycemia, 915
Functional Independence Measure (FIM), 391, 391*f*
Functional nursing, 14
Functional psychoses, 51
Fundus of eye, 973, 973*f*
Fundus photography in vision assessment, 972
Fungal infections of skin, 1059-1061, 1062
Fungi, 128-129
Fungizone; *see* Amphotericin B
Furosemide (Lasix), 772*t*
Furuncle, 1058-1059
Fusiform aneurysm, 641, 642, 642*f*

G

Gag reflex, 235, 693, 945
Gait
  in assessment of cerebellar function, 924
  crutch walking and, 414, 417*f*
  in long-term care, 430
  propulsive, Parkinson's disease and, 955
Gallbladder, 690
Gamma benzene hexachloride, 1041*t*
Gamma-glutamyl transpeptidase (GGTP), 699
Gangrene, gas, 279-280, 1124
Gantanol; *see* Sulfamethoxazole
Gantrisin; *see* Sulfisoxazole
Garamycin; *see* Gentamicin
Gardner-Wells tongs, 1106*f*
Gas gangrene, 279-280, 1124
Gas pains, 484
Gastrectomy, 702, 734-736
Gastric analysis, 696
Gastric decompression, 699-700
Gastric emptying, drug overdose and, 516
Gastric lavage, 515, 699
Gastric resection, 734-736
Gastric ulcer, 731*t*
Gastritis, 716-717
Gastroenteritis, 717
Gastroesophageal sphincter, 689
Gastrointestinal decompression, 699-700
Gastrointestinal (GI) series, 237, 695-696
Gastrointestinal system, 688-759
  anorexia and, 711
  assessment of, 691
  colostomy and, 705-710
  continent pouch ileostomy and, 710-711
  diagnostic procedures and, 691-697
  diarrhea and, 712-715
  digestion and absorption and, 690-691
  diseases and disorders of, 711-715, 716-754
    biliary system, 748-752
    functional, 739-740
    hemorrhoids, 738-739
Gastrointestinal system—cont'd
  diseases and disorders of—cont'd
    hernia, 737
    hiatus hernia, 737-738
    inflammatory, 716-725
    intestinal obstruction of, 725-726
    liver and, 740-748
    pancreatitis, 752-754
    peptic ulcer, 730-737
    tumors of, 726-730, 754
  eating disorders and, 715-716
  ileoanal reservoir and, 710-711
  ileostomy and, 705-710
  laboratory studies in assessment of, 697-699, 698*t*
  nausea and vomiting and, 711-712
  pharmacology and, 713*t*-714*t*
  spinal cord injuries and, 937-938
  structure and function of, 689*f*, 689-690
  surgery of, 704-705
  therapeutic techniques and, 699-703
Gastroscopy, 235, 693
Gastrostomy, 702, 727-728, 728*f*
Gastrostomy tube, 702
Gate control theory of pain, 206, 207*f*
Gaze, cardinal fields of, 975, 975*f*
GCS; *see* Glasgow Coma Scale
Geiger counter, 888
Gels, topical medications and, 1040*t*
Gemfibrozil (Lopid), 625*t*
Gender development, female reproductive system and, 818
Gender identity, 867
General anesthesia, 471-474, 473*t*
Generalized seizures, 949
Genitalia
  female; *see* Reproductive system, female
  male; *see* Reproductive system, male
Genitourinary system, spinal cord injuries and, 938-939
Genoptic; *see* Gentamicin
Gentamicin (Garamycin; Genoptic), 151*t*, 982*t*
Geriatric abuse, 512-513
Geriatric Depression Scale, 441
Geriatrics; *see* Older adults
German measles, 132, 271, 284, 1061
Gerontology; *see* Older adults
Geropsychiatric units, 351
GGTP; *see* Gamma-glutamyl transpeptidase
GI series; *see* Gastrointestinal series
Giardiasis, 287-288
GIFT, infertility and, 834
Gigantism, 899
Glands, disorders of, 1050-1052
Glare testing in vision assessment, 973

Glasgow Coma Scale (GCS), 504, 505, 927
Glaucoma, 109, 972, 990*f*, 990-992, 991*f*, 1003
  acute, 986*t*
  medications for, 983*t*-984*t*
Glioma, 941
Glipizide (Glucotrol), 890*t*
Globe, lacerations of, 1003
γ-Globulin, 661
Glomerular filtration, urine formation and, 763
Glomerular filtration rate, 763
Glomerulonephritis, 779
Glossopharyngeal nerve, 924*t*
Glucagon, 887, 910
Glucocorticoids, 896
Glucosuria, 900
Glucotrol; *see* Glipizide
Glycerin (Osmoglyn), 983*t*
Glycerine suppository, 438
Glycohemoglobin, 903
Glycopyrrolate (Robinul), 466*t*
Glycosuria, 767
Glycosylated hemoglobin, 903
GnRH; *see* Gonadotropin-releasing hormone
Goggles, 318
Goiter
  endemic, 891-892
  nodular, 895
  simple, 891-892
  toxic, 892
Goldmann perimeter, 972-973
Gomco thermotic pump, 701*f*
Gonadotropin-releasing hormone (GnRH), 811
Gonococcus, 127
Gonorrhea, 292-293
Gosnell scale, pressure ulcers and, 1049
Gout, 1116-1117
Gouty arthritis, 1116-1117
Government health departments, 9
Graduate education in nursing, 12
Graft, skin, 1083, 1083*f*
Graft-versus-host disease, 256, 674
Gram negative stain, 126
Gram positive stain, 126
Granulation tissue, 134
Granulocytapheresis, 661
Granulocytes, 133, 658, 660*t*, 662
Granulocytopenia, 657
Graves' disease, 892-893
Great vessel injury, 503
Greenstick fracture, 1119, 1120*f*
Grief, 85-86
Griseofulvin, 1041*t*
Group work with older adults, 366
Guaifenesin (Robitussin), 571*t*
Guide Dogs for the Blind, 999
Guillain-Barre syndrome, 956-957
Gumma, 1036
Gummatous syphilis, 292
Gynecomastia, 866

H

Habitual abortion, 857
Habituation, substance abuse and, 97
Hair, 1033
  loss of, 1055
  pubic, development of, 817
Hair transplant, 1056
Haldol; *see* Haloperidol
Halfway house, substance abuse and, 114
Hall, Edward T., 71
Hallucinations, 53
Hallucinogens, 111-112
Halo brace, 935, 937*f*, 938
Halo vest, 1104
Haloperidol (Haldol), 61*t*, 106*t*
Halothane (Fluothane; Somnothane), 466*t*, 473*t*
Handicap, 381, 382
Handwashing, 268-269, 303, 307, 309-310, 310*f*, 310*t*
Hantavirus pulmonary syndrome (HPS), 295
Haptens, 140
Hartmann's pouch, 705
Hashish, 109
Havighurst, 45, 46*t*-47*t*
Hay fever, 141
HCFA; *see* Health Care Financing Agency
HCG; *see* Human chorionic gonadotropin
Head injuries, 495-496, 509-510, 930-932, 933
  child maltreatment and, 512
Health
  definition of, 3
  mental; *see* Mental health
Health Care Financing Agency (HCFA), 6
Health maintenance organizations (HMOs), 5, 8, 450
Health Security Act, 3
Healthcare
  cost of, 5-6
  delivery of, 6-9
  home; *see* Home healthcare
  nursing and, 2-20
  nursing practice and, 10-16
  patient rights and, 16-18
  primary, rehabilitation in, 382-383
  reform of, 3-6
  rehabilitation in each phase of, 382-385
  reimbursement and, 5-6
Healthcare—cont'd
  secondary, rehabilitation in, 383
  tertiary, rehabilitation in, 383-385
  trends affecting, 4-5
Healthcare team, 9-10, 10*f*
Healthy People 2000, 3, 272, 293-294, 451
Hearing, 1012-1030
  external ear and, 1013, 1020-1023
  inner ear and, 1014, 1027-1028
  maintenance of balance and, 1014
  middle ear and, 1013, 1023-1027
  in older adults, 356
  pharmacology and, 1022*t*-1023*t*
  process of, 1014
  structure and function of ear and, 1013-1014
Hearing aid, 1019, 1019*f*
Hearing loss, 1017-1020
  behavioral signs and symptoms of, 1018
  diagnostic testing of, 1015-1017
  management of, 1019-1020
  nursing assessment of, 1014, 1015
  types of, 1018-1019
Heart
  anatomy of, 597, 597*f*
  neurohumoral controls of, 600
Heart block, 610-611
Heart disease, 622-623, 641
Heart muscle, 597-598
Heart rate
  disorders of, 606-612
  electrocardiography and, 606
Heart rhythm
  disorders of, 606-612
  electrocardiography and, 606
Heart sounds, 599, 603*t*
Heart valves, 598
Heartburn, 738, 740
Heat
  prickly, 1073
  rheumatoid arthritis and, 1111
  sterilization and, 470
  wound healing and, 138
Heat cramps, 518
Heat emergencies, 517-518, 522-523
Heat exhaustion, 518
Heat syncope, 518
Heatstroke, 517-518
Heave, 601
Heimlich, Harry J., 494-495
Heimlich chest drainage system, 558
Heimlich maneuver, 494-495, 497, 498*f*, 566, 648, 648*f*
Helicobacter pylori, 716, 728
Helminthic infestations, 288-289
HELP, violence and, 510, 521
"Help Yourself to Recovery," 854
Helper cells, 140

Hemarthrosis, 679
Hematocrit, 598, 663
Hematogenic shock, 669
Hematoma, 932, 1118, 1120
  cerebral, 509*f*, 509-510
  epidural, 509, 931, 932*f*
  intracerebral, 510
  subdural, 509-510, 931, 932*f*
Hematuria, 766, 777
Hemianopia, 944, 947
Hemilaminectomy, 940
Hemiplegia, 935*f*
Hemiplegic transfer, 398
Hemodialysis, 791*f*, 791-793, 792*f*
Hemoglobin (Hgb), 185, 598, 657, 662-663, 903
Hemoglobin electrophoresis, 663
Hemophilia, 679-680
Hemoptysis, 275, 532, 669
Hemorrhage, 457, 657
  intracerebral, 943-944
  intracranial, 932
  postoperative care and, 485
  subarachnoid, 943-944
  traumatic intracranial, 931
  uncontrolled, 501-503
Hemorrhagic anemia, 669
Hemorrhagic disorders, 668, 679-681
Hemorrhagic stroke, 942-944
Hemorrhoidectomy, 739
Hemorrhoids, 644, 738-739, 743
Hemothorax, 499, 500
Henderson, Virginia, 9, 15*t*
HEPA respirator; *see* High-efficiency particulate air respirator
Heparin, 625*t*
Hepatic coma, 748
Hepatitis, 135, 287, 492, 740-742
Hepatitis A, 287, 740
Hepatitis B, 287, 740
Hepatitis C, 287, 740
Hepatitis D, 740
Hepatitis E, 740
Hep-Lock, 625*t*
Hernia, 737-738
Herniation, increased intracranial pressure and, 930
Hernioplasty, 737
Herniorrhaphy, 737
Hero, dysfunctional family and, 100
Heroin, 108
Herpes simplex, 293, 981, 1063*f*, 1063-1064
Herpes zoster, 285, 1064*f*, 1064-1066
Herpesvirus, 1063*f*, 1063-1066
Herpesvirus hominus, 1063
Herplex; *see* Idoxuridine
Heterograft, 1083
Heterophil antibody test, 676
Hexadrol; *see* Dexamethasone
HHNC; *see* Hyperglycemic hyperosmolar nonketotic coma
Hiatal hernia, 737-738
Hiatus hernia, 737-738
High anion gap acidosis, 186
High-efficiency particulate air (HEPA) respirator, 492-493
High-level disinfection (HLD), 311
High–air-loss beds, pressure ulcers and, 1046
Hip arthroplasty, 1114
Hip replacement, 115*f*, 1114, 1116, 1122-1123
Hip spica casts, 1100*f*, 1100-1102
Hirsutism, 897
Histamine test, 696
Histerone 100; *see* Testosterone
Histoplasmosis, 128-129
History, 333, 456
  hearing loss and, 1014
  nursing, 22
  respiratory system and, 533
  surgery and, 457
HIV infection; *see* Human immunodeficiency virus infection
Hives, 143
HLA; *see* Human lymphocyte antigen
HLD; *see* High-level disinfection
HMOs; *see* Health maintenance organizations
Hodgkin's disease, 676-677
Hoffman device, 1109*f*
Holistic patient care, 3
Holter, Norman J., 616
Home, foster, older adults and, 374
Home health agencies, 8-9
Home health aide, 446
Home healthcare, 444-453
  community services and, 447
  long-term, 452
  nursing in, 447-451
  of older adults, 373
  reform in, 451
  team in, 447
Homeostasis, 43, 656, 885
Homograft, 1083
Honvol, 250
Hookworms, 289
Hormone replacement therapy (HRT), 834-835
Hormones, 230, 246, 885
  heart rate and, 600
  regulation of fluids and electrolytes and, 167
  renal, 763-764
  sex, 896
Hospice, 9, 80, 88-89, 89*f*
Hospital, 7
  day, older adults and, 373-374
Hospital infections, 300-302
Hospital-based diploma schools, 12
Hospitalized elderly patients, 371-373
Host
  compromised, 301
  infections and, 267, 268, 268*f*
Hostile patient, 50
HPS; *see* Hantavirus pulmonary syndrome
HPV; *see* Human papillomavirus
HRT; *see* Hormone replacement therapy
Human chorionic gonadotropin (HCG), 811-813
Human immunodeficiency virus (HIV) infection, 115, 278, 311, 313-318, 325-344, 492, 514, 582, 953-954, 1065-1066
  burnout and, 339
  clinical manifestations of, 328-333
  legal issues and, 338-339
  nursing process and, 333-337
  ocular conditions and, 1000
  pharmacology and, 330*t*-332*t*
  physical signs of, 334*t*
  prevention of transmission of, 337
Human lymphocyte antigen (HLA), 661, 674
Human papillomavirus (HPV), 833, 837, 1061
Humidid-DM; *see* Dextromethorphan
Humidification, bronchial infections and, 547-548
Humidifiers, 304, 548, 548*f*
Humor, communication and, 57*t*
Humoral immunity, 140, 140*f*
Humulin, 904, 906
Huntington's chorea, 53
Hyde Amendment, 858
Hydraulic lifts, patient transfer and, 398
Hydrocele, 869
Hydrochlorothiazide (Hydro-chlor; Hypodiuril; Thiuretic Esidrex), 772*t*
Hydrocolloids, pressure ulcers and, 439, 1048, 1049
Hydrocortisone (Cortef; Hydrocortone; Hytone; Solu-Cortef), 104*t*, 153*t*, 158, 896, 985*t*, 1112*t*
Hydrogels, pressure ulcers and, 1048, 1049
Hydrogen ion concentration, 185
Hydrogen peroxide, 1022*t*
Hydromorphone (Dilaudid), 212*t*
Hydronephrosis, 783-784
Hydrostatic pressure, 165, 166, 166*f*, 763
Hydrotherapy for burns, 1080-1082
Hydroureter, 784
Hygiene
  diabetes mellitus and, 908
  menstruation and, 816-817
  personal, older adults and, 369-370

Hyperacidity, 740
Hyperalbuminemia, 179*t*
Hyperaldosteronism, 743
Hyperalimentation, 703
Hyperbaric oxygen, 551-552
Hypercalcemia, 178, 181
Hyperchloremia, 183-184
Hyperemia, 980
Hyperglycemia, 167, 767, 899, 900, 909*t*, 910
Hyperglycemic hyperosmolar nonketotic coma (HHNC), 900, 911
Hyperhidrosis, 1052
Hyperkalemia, 176-177, 178
Hypermagnesemia, 183, 184
Hypernatremia, 171, 173
Hyperopia, 976, 976*f*
Hyperosmolar fluid, 165, 191
Hyperparathyroidism, 895
Hyperphosphatemia, 184
Hyperproteinemia, 184
Hyperreflexia, autonomic, 938-939
Hyperresonance, 497
Hypersensitivity, 141, 1073-1074
  cell-mediated, 145-146
  cytotoxic, 145
  immediate, 142*t*, 142-143
  immune complex, 145
Hypersplenism, 674
Hypertension, 383, 618-620
  intracranial, 928-930
  in older adults, 353
  portal, 743
Hyperthermia, 130, 476, 517-518, 935
Hyperthyroidism, 892*f*, 892-893, 894, 916-918
Hypertonic extracellular fluid deficit, 168-169
Hypertonic fluid, 165, 191
Hypertrichosis, 1055-1056
Hypertropia, 976
Hypervolemia, 169, 170
Hypnosis, 475
Hypoadrenalism, secondary, 897
Hypoalbuminemia, 179*t*
Hypocalcemia, 178-180
Hypochloremia, 183
Hypochromia, 670
Hypodiuril; *see* Hydrochlorothiazide
Hypoglossal nerve, 924*t*
Hypoglycemia, 907-908, 909*t*, 915
Hypoglycemic drugs, oral, 907-908
Hypoglycemic reaction, 908-910
Hypokalemia, 173, 174-176, 199-201, 638, 770
Hypomagnesemia, 182-183
Hyponatremia, 171, 172
Hypoosmolar fluid, 165, 191
Hypoparathyroidism, 895-896
Hypophosphatemia, 184
Hypophysis, 898
Hypoproteinemia, 184
Hypopyon, 995
Hypospadias, 868
Hypotension, orthostatic, 669
Hypothalamus, 167
Hypothermia, 130, 476, 518-519, 935
Hypothyroidism, 893-895, 896
Hypotonic fluid, 165, 191
Hypotonicity, 170
Hypotrichosis, 1055-1056
Hypotropia, 976-977
Hypovolemia, 167-168
Hypovolemic shock, 195-196, 485, 501, 669
Hypoxemia, 548
Hysterectomy, 847-849
  abdominal, 848-849
  subtotal, 847
  vaginal, 849
Hysterosalpingography, 839
Hytone; *see* Hydrocortisone
Hytrin; *see* Terazosin

I

I Can Cope, 260
IADLs; *see* Instrumental activities of daily living
IAR; *see* Ileoanal reservoir
IBD; *see* Inflammatory bowel disease
Ibuprofen (Motrin; Nuprin), 112*t*, 213*t*
ICF; *see* Intermediate care facility
ICF; *see* Intracellular fluid
Icing the scalp, 254
ICP; *see* Intracranial pressure
ICU; *see* Intensive care unit
Id, 45
IDDM; *see* Insulin dependent diabetes mellitus
Identification, 48*t*
Idiopathic epilepsy, 948
Idiopathic thrombocytopenic purpura (ITP), 681
Idoxuridine (Herplex; Stoxil), 983*t*
IFEX; *see* Ifosfamide
Ifosfamide (IFEX), 251*t*
Ig; *see* Immunoglobulins
ILD; *see* Intermediate-level disinfection
Ileal conduit, 795-796, 796*f*, 797, 798*f*, 799
Ileoanal reservoir (IAR), 705, 710-711
Ileobladder, 797
Ileostomy, 705-710, 711
  continent pouch, 710*f*, 710-711
  pouch, 710
Illness
  causes of, 125-132
  impact of, on patient respect, 35
  manic-depressive, 52
  mental, 43
Ilotycin; *see* Erythromycin
Immobile patient, rehabilitation of, 392
Immune complex hypersensitivity, 145
Immune responses, excessive, 141-156
Immunity, 139-140, 269-271
  acquired active, 269-271
  acquired passive, 271-272
  cellular, 140, 140*f*
  humoral, 140, 140*f*
Immunization, 269, 270, 506
  contraindications for, 271
  schedules for, 270*t*
Immunoglobulin (Ig), 140, 141, 269, 271
Immunology, human immunodeficiency virus infection and, 327-328
Immunosuppressants, 156
Immunotherapy, 149, 156
Imodium-A-D; *see* Loperamide
Impacted fracture, 1119, 1120*f*
Impetigo, 1058-1059
Impetigo contagiosa, 1058*f*, 1058-1059
Implementation in nursing process, 31
Implied consent, 492
Inactivated poliovirus vaccine (IPV), 271
Inapsine; *see* Droperidol
Incarcerated hernia, 737
Incentive spirometry (IS), 545, 545*f*, 556
Incisional biopsy, 234
Incisional hernia, 737
Incomplete abortion, 857-858
Incontinence
  in long-term care, 432
  overflow, 403, 435-436, 437, 778
  stress, 403, 434, 436, 778
  stroke and, 947
  urge, 403, 434-435, 436, 778
  urinary; *see* Urinary incontinence
Incontinence record, 404*f*
Increased intracranial pressure, 928-930, 931
Incus, 1013
Inderal; *see* Propanolol
Indigestion, 739
Individuality in older adults, 367-368
Indomethacin (Indocin), 1112*t*
Induced abortion, 857
Indwelling catheter, 405-406, 479-480, 774, 776*t*
Inevitable abortion, 857
Infection control committee, nosocomial infections and, 308
Infection control practitioner, nosocomial infections and, 308-309
Infections, 125, 135-139, 266-298
  bacterial, 273-283
  burns and, 1084
  central nervous system, 952-954

Infections—cont'd
 classification of, 136
 clostridium, 279-280
 community-acquired; *see* Community-acquired infections
 emerging, 294-295
 endogenous, 135, 301
 exogenous, 135, 301
 of external ear, 1020-1021
 hospital, 300-302
 human immunodeficiency virus, 325-344
 manifestations of, 136
 of musculocutaneous system, 1117
 nosocomial; *see* Nosocomial infections
 pelvic, 846-847
 postoperative care and, 486
 respiratory, 577-584
 rickettsial, 283
 Salmonella, 280-282
 skin, 1058-1066
 staphylococcal, 273-274
 streptococcal, 274
 surgery and, 455
 surgical wound, 305-306
 upper airway, 559-564
 urinary tract, 302-303
 viral, 283-287, 1061-1066
Infectious disease precautions, 492-493
Infectious mononucleosis, 286, 676
Infertility, female reproductive system and, 831-834
Infestations, 267, 1056-1058
Infiltration anesthesia, 475
Inflamase; *see* Prednisolone
Inflammation, 133-134, 134*f*
Inflammatory bowel disease (IBD), 717-720
Inflammatory diseases of gastro-intestinal system, 716-725
Inflated air mattress, pressure ulcers and, 1046*f*
Influenza, 286-287, 563, 564
Informed consent; *see* Consent, informed
Informing, communication and, 58*t*
Infundibulum, 810
Ingestion poisoning, 517
Inguinal hernia, 737
INH; *see* Isoniazid
Inhalants, 111, 473*t*
Inhalation, ventilation and, 530
Inhalation anesthesia, 471-473
Inhalation poisoning, 517
Injury
 to external ear, 1021
 head, 495-496, 512, 930-932, 933
Injury—cont'd
 needlestick, 337
 prevention of, in older adults, 367
 spinal cord; *see* Spinal cord injuries
 traumatic, death following, 87-88
Innovar; *see* Droperidol
Insects
 allergic reactions to, 143-144, 517
 in auditory canal, 1021
Inspection
 in assessment of cardiovascular system, 601, 601*f*
 in assessment of respiratory system, 533-534
Instrumental activities of daily living (IADLs), 365, 429
Insufflation, tubal, 840-841
Insulin, 600, 885, 887, 900, 903-907, 905*t*, 906*f*, 907*f*, 908, 913, 913*f*
Insulin reaction, 889, 908-910, 909*t*
Insulin-dependent diabetes mellitus (IDDM), 899, 900*t*
Intake and output
 burns and, 1084
 in older adults, 372
Integumentary system in older adults, 357-358
Intelligence, older adults and, 352
Intensive care unit (ICU), 478, 613
Interdisciplinary team, rehabilitation and, 385*f*, 387, 387*f*
Interferon, 257
Interferon Alfa-2A (Roferon-A), 330*t*
Intermediate care facility (ICF), 7-8
Intermediate-level disinfection (ILD), 311
Intermittent pneumatic compression (IPC), 588
Internal fixation of fracture, 1119-1120
Internal radiation therapy, 239, 241-245
International Association
 of Laryngectomees, 260
 for the Study of Pain, 205
Interstitial fluid, 162
 shifts of, to plasma, 166-167
 shifts of plasma to, 166
Interstitial oncotic pressure, 166
Intervertebral disk trauma, 939-941, 940*f*
Interviewing techniques, 23
Intestinal decompression, 700-702, 701*f*
Intestinal obstruction, 725-726
Intimate space, 74
InTouch, 111
Intracapsular cataract extraction, 993-994
Intracellular fluid (ICF), 162
Intracerebral hematoma, 510
Intracerebral hemorrhage, 943-944
Intracranial hemorrhage, 931, 932
Intracranial pressure (ICP), increased, 928-930, 931
Intradermal test, 148-149
Intraocular lens implant (IOL), 994
Intraocular pressure (IOP), 971-972
Intraocular surgery, 988
Intraoperative care, 469-476
Intraoperative complications, 476
Intraspinal analgesia, 217-218
Intrathecal analgesia, 218
Intrauterine device (IUD), 819, 828, 828*f*, 830
Intravascular fluid, 162
Intravenous drugs, anesthesia and, 473*t*, 473-474
Intravenous pyelography, 767
Intravenous therapy, 190-194, 478
Intrinsic asthma, 575
Intubation, endotracheal, 552
Involuntary consent, 492
Involutional melancholia, 52
Iodine, radioactive, radiation therapy and, 245
Iodine solution, strong, 891*t*
IOL; *see* Intraocular lens implant
Ionizing radiation, 230
Ions, 162-163
IOP; *see* Intraocular pressure
IPC; *see* Intermittent pneumatic compression
Ipratropium (Atrovent), 571*t*
IPV; *see* Inactivated poliovirus vaccine
Iridectomy, argon laser, 991
Iris, 967
Iron preparations, oral, 669
Iron salts, 659*t*
Iron-deficiency anemia, 670-671
Irrigation, continuous bladder, 874
Irritant dermatitis, 1066
IS; *see* Incentive spirometry
Ischemic heart disease, 617
Ischemic stroke, 942-943
Ishihara test, 978
Islets of Langerhans, 690, 887
Isoflurane (Forane), 466*t*, 473*t*
Isolation
 body substance, 318-319
 category-specific, 312-313
 disease-specific, 313
 nosocomial infections and, 312, 314
 reverse, 254
Isomolar fluid, 165
Isoniazid (INH), 331*t*, 572*t*
Isoosmolar fluid, 190-191
Isopropyl alcohol, 1023*t*
Isopto Atropine; *see* Atropine
Isopto-Hyoscine; *see* Scopolamine
Isotonic extracellular fluid deficit, 167-168
Isotonic fluid, 165, 190-191

Isotretinoin (Accutane), 1041*t*
Itch mite, 1057-1058
Itching, 1052
ITP; *see* Idiopathic thrombocytopenic purpura
Itraconazole (Sporanox), 331*t*
IUD; *see* Intrauterine device
IVF, infertility and, 834
Ivy poisoning, 1067

J

Jackson-Pratt (JP) drains, mastectomy and, 854
Jaeger chart in vision assessment, 970, 971, 976
Japanese B encephalitis, 953
Jaundice, 741
Jaw-thrust maneuver, 495, 498
JCAHO; *see* Joint Commission on Accreditation of Healthcare Organizations
Jejunostomy, 702
Jellinek's stages of alcoholism, 101
Jobst garment, burns and, 1084, 1085
Jock itch, 1061
Johnson, Vernon, 112
Joint Commission on Accreditation of Healthcare Organizations (JCAHO), 13, 308
Joints
  anatomic changes in, in older adults, 1094
  range of motion of, 1093-1094
Joslin, Elliot, 908
Journal of Transcultural Nursing, 69
Justice, 33-34
Juvenile Diabetes Association, 891
Juvenile myxedema, 893, 894-895

K

Kangaroo care, 67-68
Kaposi's sarcoma, 329, 333*f*, 1000
KCl; *see* Potassium chloride
Keflex; *see* Cephalexin
Kefzol; *see* Cefazolin sodium
Kegel exercises, 405, 406, 436, 776, 843
Keloid, 1052
Kenacort, 154*t*
Kenalog, 154*t*
Keratin, 1032
Keratitis, 1000
Keratoconjunctivitis sicca, 1002
Keratoconus, 986
Keratometry
  cataracts and, 993
  in vision assessment, 973
Keratopathy, pseudophakic bullous, 987
Keratoplasty, 987
  lamellar, 987
  penetrating, 987, 988
Keratoscopy, 973
Keratoses, 1053
Keratotomy, radial, 976
Kerion, 1060
Kerr's sign, 503
Ketaject; *see* Ketamine
Ketalar; *see* Ketamine
Ketamine (Ketaject; Ketalar), 473*t*
Ketoconazole (Nizoral), 331*t*, 1041*t*
Ketonuria, 901, 902
Ketosis, 900
Kidneys, 761, 761*f*
  tumors of, 786
  ureters, and bladder (KUB) x-rays, 767
Killer cells, 140
Kinetic beds, 1046, 1107
Kirschner wire, 1104
Kissing disease, 286
Klebsiella pneumoniae, 578
Knee replacement, 115*f*, 1122-1123
Koch, Robert, 274
Koch's pouch, 710, 796
Koch-Weeks bacillus, 980
Koplik's spots, 284, 1061
Korotkoff's sounds, 602
KUB x-rays; *see* Kidneys, ureters, and bladder x-rays
Kübler-Ross, Elisabeth, 80, 82
Kussmaul's respirations, 186, 535*t*, 911
Kwashiorkor, 130
Kwell shampoo, 1056
Kyphosis, 1112

L

Labia majora, 808
Labia minora, 808
Laboratory tests
  cancer and, 238
  cardiovascular system and, 613-614
  drug overdose and, 516
  female reproductive system and, 837-838
  gastrointestinal system and, 697-699, 698*t*
  male reproductive system and, 868
  respiratory system and, 539-544
Labyrinth, 1014
Labyrinthitis, 1027
Lacerated liver, 503
Lacerations, 507
  of globe, 1003
  lid, 1003
Lacrimal system disorders, 1002
Lacrimal-duct probing, 998
Lacrimation, mucous membrane sensitivity tests and, 149
Lactic dehydrogenase (LDH), 613, 628, 699
Laennec's cirrhosis, 743
Lamaze method of childbirth, 219
Lamellar keratoplasty, 987
Laminaria, abortion and, 859
Laminectomy, 940, 941
Lanoxicaps; *see* Digoxin
Lanoxin; *see* Digoxin
Laparoscopy, 238, 839
Laparotomy, 704
Large intestine, 690
Larodopa; *see* Levodopa
Laryngeal fracture, 495-496, 649
Laryngectomy, 566-568, 567*t*, 569
Laryngitis, 563, 564
Larynx, cancer of, 566
Laser laparoscopic cholecystectomy, 750
Laser surgery, 469
Laser trabeculoplasty, 991
Lasix; *see* Furosemide
Late syphilis, 292
Latent syphilis, 292
Lateral position, patient in, 396
Latex condoms, 337, 831
Lavage, gastric, 699
Laxatives, 437
Lazy eye, 977
LDH; *see* Lactic dehydrogenase
Lead poisoning, 131
LEDs; *see* Light-emitting diodes
Legal abortion, 858, 859-860
Legal issues, AIDS/HIV, 338-339
Legionellosis, 279
Legionnaire's disease, 279, 304, 578
Legislation
  affecting prehospital and emergency care, 490*t*
  rehabilitation, 387-388
Leininger, Madeleine, 16*t*, 67, 69, 70
Lens of eye, 968
Lenses, contact, 977, 978, 978*f*, 986, 1004
Lentigo, 1050
Lesions, skin, 1034-1036
Lethargy, 928
Leucovorin calcium, 331*t*
Leukapheresis, 661
Leukemia, 230, 238, 256, 285, 677-679
  acute, 677-678
  acute lymphoblastic, 677
  acute lymphocytic, 677
  acute myelocytic, 677, 678
  acute nonlymphocytic, 678
  chronic, 678
  chronic lymphocytic, 678
  chronic myelocytic, 678
  chronic myelogenous, 678
Leukeran; *see* Chlorambucil
Leukocytes, 133, 656, 657-658, 661-662
Leukocytosis, 139, 657, 676
Leukopenia, 240, 254, 657, 674, 676
Leuprolide (Lupron), 820*t*
LeVeen shunt, 745, 745*f*

Levobunolol (Betagan), 983*t*
Levodopa (Dopar; Larodopa), 950*t*
Levo-Dromoran; *see* Levorphanol
Levonorgestrel implant, 821*t*
Levonorgestrel IUD, 828
Levorphanol (Levo-Dromoran), 213*t*
Levothroid; *see* Levothyroxine
Levothyroxine (Levothroid; Synthroid), 890*t*
Librium; *see* Chlordiazepoxide
Lice, 1056-1057
Licensed practical nurse (LPN), 11-12, 447, 492
Licensed vocational nurse (LVN), 11-12
Licensure, nursing practice and, 11
Lichenification, 1067
Lidex; *see* Fluocinonide
Lidocaine (Xylocaine), 219-221, 467*t*, 474*t*
Lids; *see* Eyelids
Life, prolonging, 81
Lifestyle, disruption of, surgery and, 456
Lift, 601
Light, refraction of, 969
Light-emitting diodes (LEDs), 544
Lighthouse sweep, eye contact and, 75
Lindane, 1041*t*, 1057-1058
Linear skull fracture, 930
Lipodystrophy, 907
Liquiprin; *see* Acetaminophen
Listening, communication and, 57, 57*t*
Lister, Joseph, 469
Lithiasis, 784
Lithium, 52, 61*t*, 106*t*
Lithotomy, 797-798, 800
Lithotomy position, 837
Liver, 690, 691
  diseases and disorders of, 740-748
  lacerated, 503
Liver enzymes, 698-699
Liver function, assessment of, 698-699
Liver transplantation, 748
Living will, 36, 82, 83*f*, 84*f*, 366
LLD; *see* Low-level disinfection
Lobectomy, 554, 555, 555*f*
Lockjaw, 280, 1124
Lomotil; *see* Diphenoxylate and atropine
Lomustine (CCNU), 251*t*
Long-term care, 373-374, 425-443, 452
  assessment guidelines for, 428-430
  ethical dilemmas in, 427-428
  risk and, 430-442
Loop diuretics, 174, 176
Loop stoma, 705
Loperamide (Imodium-A-D; Pepto Diarrhea Control), 714*t*
Lopid; *see* Gemfibrozil
Lopressor; *see* Metoprolol
Lorazepam (Ativan), 61*t*, 106*t*
Lost child, dysfunctional family and, 100
Lost Cord Club, 568
Lotion, topical medications and, 1040*t*
Lotrimin; *see* Clotrimazole
Love, need for, 44
Lower GI series, 695-696
Lower respiratory system, conditions of, 568-577
Low-level disinfection (LLD), 311
Low–air-loss beds, pressure ulcers and, 1046
LPN; *see* Licensed practical nurse
Lues, 291-292
Lugol's solution, 891*t*
Lumbar puncture, 924-925, 925*f*
Lumpectomy, 851
Lund and Browder classification of burns, 1076-1078
Lung cancer, 227, 261-263, 588-590
Lung scans, 542
Lungs, 529*f*
Lupron; *see* Leuprolide
Lupus erythematosus, 1071
Lupus Foundation of America, 1073
Luteinizing hormone, 811
LVN; *see* Licensed vocational nurse
Lyme disease, 127, 273, 278*f*, 278-279
Lymph nodes, 133, 604
Lymphangitis, 645-646
Lymphatic circulation, 598
Lymphatics, diseases and disorders of, 641-646
Lymphedema, 645
Lymphoblasts, 677
Lymphocytes, 133, 134, 140, 658
Lymphoma, 230
Lysozyme, 132-133

M

Maalox; *see* Aluminum hydroxide and magnesium hydroxide
Ménière's syndrome, 1028
Macrolides, 158
Macrominerals, 129, 129*t*
Macrophages, 134
Macular degeneration, 998-999, 999*f*
Macule, 1035, 1036
Mafenide acetate (Sulfamylon), 1042*t*, 1082
Magnesium, 182-183
Magnesium citrate, 714*t*
Magnesium deficit, 182-183
Magnesium excess, 183, 184
Magnetic resonance imaging (MRI), 235, 889, 926
  in assessment of cancer, 237-238
  in assessment of gastrointestinal system, 695
  in assessment of renal function, 769
Makeup, surgery and, 463
Malaria, 135, 287-288
Male climacteric, 867
Male condom, 830, 831
Male genitalia; *see* Reproductive system, male
Male reproductive system; *see* Reproductive system, male
Malignant hyperthermia, 476
Malignant lesions, 234, 843-845
Malignant melanoma, 1053
Malignant tumors, 228-229, 1053-1054
Malleus, 1013
Malunion of bone, 1121
Mammography, 235-236, 839-840
Manic-depressive illness, 52
Manipulative patient, 50
Mannitol (Osmitrol), 772*t*, 984*t*
Mantoux test, 276, 583
MAP; *see* Mean arterial pressure
Marasmus, 130
Marcaine; *see* Bupivacaine
Marginal blepharitis, 1001
Marijuana, 109
Mascot, dysfunctional family and, 100
Masks, 318
Maslow, A., 14-16, 43*f*, 43-45
MAST; *see* Military AntiShock Trousers
Mastectomy, 851-856, 855*t*, 857
  breast reconstruction after, 852, 853*f*, 854*f*
Masters and Johnson, 368
Master's degree in nursing, 12
Mastication, 690
Mastitis, acute, 850
Mastoidectomy, 1026
Mastoiditis, 1025
Mattress overlays, pressure ulcers and, 1045-1046
Maxidex; *see* Dexamethasone
McBurney's point, 721
MDR-TB; *see* Multiple–drug-resistant strains of tuberculosis
MDS; *see* Minimum Data Set
Meal plan, diabetes mellitus and, 903, 905*t*
Meals on Wheels, 369, 447, 448
Mean arterial pressure (MAP), 620
Measles, 270, 283-284
  German, 132, 284
Measles-rubella (MR) vaccine, 270, 286
Mechanical ventilation, 554
Mechlorethamine, 251*t*
Meclizine (Antivert), 1023*t*
Medicaid, 5-6, 7-8, 31, 450, 452, 672
Medical abortion, 860
Medical ethics in long-term care, 427-428
Medical social work, home healthcare and, 447

Medical-surgical nursing, 10-11
Medical-surgical problems, 527-1132
Medicare, 5-6, 7-8, 31, 347, 373, 388, 450, 452, 672
Medications
 falls and, 432
 in long-term care, 431-432
 older adults and, 370-371
 pharmacology and; *see* Pharmacology
 topical; *see* Topical medications
Medroxyprogesterone acetate (Depo-Provera), 821*t*
Mefoxin; *see* Cefoxitin
Megace; *see* Megestrol acetate
Megakaryocytes, 658
Megastron, radiation therapy and, 245
Megestrol acetate (Megace), 251*t*
Melancholia, involutional, 52
Melanin, 1032
Melanoma
 choroidal, 1000
 malignant, 1053
Melasma, 1050
Melphalan (Alkeran), 252*t*
Memory, older adults and, 352-353, 371-372
Men, reproductive health of; *see* Reproductive system, male
Menarche, 811-813, 816
Meninges, 923
Meningioma, 941
Meningitis, 279, 952-953
Meningococcal meningitis, 279, 952-953
Meningococcus, 127
Menopause, 834-835
Menorrhagia, 814
Menstrual cycle, 811-813, 812*f*
 disturbances of, 813-816
 hygiene and, 816-817
Mental health, 43, 45
 definition of, 45
 older adults and, 350-352
Mental illness, 43
Mental status
 assessment of, 923
 in long-term care, 429, 440-442
 in older adults, 371-372
Meperidine (Demerol), 213*t*, 467*t*, 473*t*
mEq/L; *see* Milliequivalents per liter
6-Mercaptopurine (6-MP), 252*t*
Mesh graft, 1083
Mesocaval shunt, 747
Metabolic acidosis, 186, 187, 189
Metabolic alkalosis, 186-187, 188, 189
Metamorphopsia, 974
Metamucil; *see* Psyllium
Metastasis, 229
Methadone (Dolophine), 106*t*, 108, 213*t*
Methamphetamine, 109
Methohexital (Brevital), 473*t*
Methotrexate (MTX), 252*t*
Metoprolol (Lopressor), 625*t*
Metronidazole (Flagyl), 713*t*, 822*t*
Metrorrhagia, 814
MI; *see* Myocardial infarction
MICN; *see* Mobile intensive care nurse
Miconazole, 822*t*
Miconazole nitrate, 822*t*
Microhematocrit test, 663
Microorganisms, 125-129
Microscopy, specular, in vision assessment, 973
Midazolam (Versed), 467*t*
Midriatics, vision and, 984*t*-985*t*
Mifepristone (RU-486), 821*t*
Miliaria, 1073
Military antishock trousers (MAST), 196, 502-503, 508
Milliequivalents per liter (mEq/L), 164
Milliosmoles (mOsm), 165
Mineral oil, 714*t*
Mineralocorticoids, 896
Mini pills, contraception and, 822-825
Minimum Data Set (MDS), 428
Minipress; *see* Prazosin
Minoxidil (Rogaine), 1042*t*
Miosis, senile, 356
Miostat; *see* Carbachol intraocular
Miotics, vision and, 984*t*
Missed abortion, 858
Mite, itch, 1057-1058
Mitomycin C (Mutamycin), 253*t*
Mitoxantrone (Novantrone), 253*t*
Mixed diarrhea, 712
MMSE; *see* Folstein Mini-Mental Status Examination
Mobile intensive care nurse (MICN), 492
Mobility, 1091-1132
 neuromuscular conditions and, 1128
 neurovascular integrity and, 1096-1097
 patient with cast and, 1097-1102
 patient with disorders of musculoskeletal system and, 1110-1128, 1129-1130
 patient with orthopedic device and, 1102-1110
 pharmacology and, 1112-1113
 position, exercise, and body mechanics and, 1095
 rehabilitation and, 392-393
 structure and function of musculoskeletal system and, 1092-1094
Mobitz type I heart block, 610-611
Mobitz type II heart block, 611
Mohs, Frederich, 1054
Mohs' surgery, 1054
Mole, 1052-1053
Monilial vaginitis, 716
Monistat, 822*t*
Monistat 3, 822*t*
Monochronic time, culture and, 71-72
Monocytes, 133, 134, 658
Mononuclear leukocytes, 133
Mononucleosis, infectious, 286, 676
Mono-vacc test, 276
Monro-Kellie hypothesis, 929
Montgomery straps, 481, 482*f*
Montgomery's glands, 811
Monticelli-Spinelli Circular Fixator, 1109*f*
Mood disorders, 52-53
Morals, ethics and, 32
Morphine, 213*t*, 216*t*, 467*t*, 473*t*
mOsm; *see* Milliosmoles
Motivation, rehabilitation and, 389-390
Motrin; *see* Ibuprofen
Mouth problems, 241
6-MP; *see* 6-Mercaptopurine
MR vaccine; *see* Measles-rubella vaccine
MRI; *see* Magnetic resonance imaging
MS; *see* Multiple sclerosis
MTX; *see* Methotrexate
Mucocil; *see* Acetylcysteine
Mucocutaneous candidiasis, 329
Mucous fistula, 705
Mucous membrane sensitivity tests, allergy and, 149
Mucus patches, syphilis and, 291-292
Müllerian-duct inhibiting factor, 867
Multiple myeloma, 230
Multiple sclerosis (MS), 954
Multiple–drug-resistant strains of tuberculosis (MDR-TB), 582
Mummy wrap, 1039
Mumps, 270-271, 285-286
Mupirocin (Bactroban), 1042*t*
Murine Ear Drops; *see* Carbamide peroxide
Muscle relaxants, 474
Muscle spasms, intervertebral disk trauma and, 939
Muscle strength in long-term care, 431
Musculoskeletal system
 amputation and, 1126-1128, 1129-1130
 bone tumors and, 1125-1126
 diseases and disorders of, 1110-1128
  ankylosing spondylitis, 1113
  arthritis, 1110-1117
  bursitis, 1117
  degenerative joint disease, 1113, 1114
  gout, 1116-1117
  gouty arthritis, 1116-1117
  infectious, 1117
  osteoarthritis, 1113, 1114
  osteomyelitis, 1117
  rheumatoid arthritis, 1110-1111
  rheumatoid spondylitis, 1113

Musculoskeletal system—cont'd
  mobility and, 1092-1094
  neuromuscular conditions and, 1128
  in older adults, 358-359
  spinal cord injuries and, 937
  traumatic injuries to, 1118-1125
    contusions, 1118
    dislocations, 1118
    fractures, 1118-1125
    sprains, 1118
    whiplash injuries, 1125
Mustargen; *see* Nitrogen mustard
Mutamycin; *see* Mitomycin C
Myambutol; *see* Ethambutol
Myasthenia gravis, 954, 957-958, 975
Myasthenia Gravis Foundation, Inc., 958
Myasthenic crisis, 958
Mycifradin; *see* Neomycin sulfate
Myciguent; *see* Neomycin sulfate
Mycobacterium tuberculosis, 274, 332-333, 582
Mycobutin; *see* Rifabutin
Mycostatin; *see* Nystatin
Mydfrin; *see* Phenylephrine
Mydriacyl; *see* Tropicamide
Myeloblasts, 677
Myelography, 925-926
Myeloma, multiple, 230
Myelosuppression, 254
Mylanta; *see* Aluminum hydroxide, magnesium hydroxide, and simethicone
Myleran; *see* Busulfan
Myocardial infarction (MI), 623-629, 630
  complications of, 636-641
Myonecrosis, 279-280
Myopia, 976, 976*f*
Myringoplasty, 1026
Myringotomy, 1025
Myxedema, 893-894

N

Nafcillin sodium (Unipen), 151*t*
Nagi, Saad, 381
Nail disorders, 1056
Nailing, fractures of hip and, 1121
Nails, 1033
Naloxone (Narcan), 467*t*
NANDA; *see* North American Nursing Diagnosis Association
Naproxen (Anaprox; Naprosyn), 213*t*, 1113*t*
Narcan; *see* Naloxone
Narcotics, 108, 473*t*
Narrow-angle glaucoma, 991
Nasal cannula, oxygen by, 549
Nasal polyps, 565
Natamycin (Natacyn), 983*t*
National Association for Home Care, 446
National Cancer Act, 227
National Cancer Advisory Board, 227
National Cancer Institute, 227, 228, 233, 257
National Coalition for Cancer Survivorship (NCCS), 260
National Conference Group on the Classification of Nursing Diagnosis, 23
National Diabetes Data Group of the National Institutes of Health, 901
National Disaster Medical System (NDMS), 519
National Foundation of Ileitis and Colitis, 54
National Heart, Lung, and Blood Institute, 588
National Hemophilia Foundation, 680
National Institute of Burn Medicine, 1074-1075
National Institutes of Health, 901
National Multiple Sclerosis Society, 954
National Nosocomial Infections Study (NNIS), 300, 301, 305
National Society for the Prevention of Blindness (NSPB), 999, 1003
Natural death, 366
Natural family planning, 831
Natural immunity, 139, 269
Nausea and vomiting, 484, 711-712
NCCS; *see* National Coalition for Cancer Survivorship
NCLEX; *see* State board licensing examination
NDMS; *see* National Disaster Medical System
Nearsightedness, 976, 976*f*
Nebulizers, 304, 548
Necrosis, aseptic, 1121
Necrotizing fasciitis, 294
Need satisfaction, 44
Needle localization biopsy, 840
Needlestick injury, 337
Neglect, child, 511, 512
Neisseria gonorrhoeae, 292
Nematoda, 289
Neomycin sulfate (Mycifradin; Myciguent), 151*t*, 1023*t*
Neoplasms, 228, 229*t*
Neostigmine (Prostigmin), 771*t*, 950*t*
Neo-Synephrine; *see* Phenylephrine
Nephrectomy, 798-800
Nephrolithiasis, 784
Nephrolithotomy, 797, 800
Nephron, 762
Nephrosis, 780
Nephrostomy, 774, 774*f*, 774-775, 776*t*-777*t*, 798-800
Nephrotic syndrome, 780
Nephrotoxicity, 768
Nerve block, peripheral, 475
Nerve deafness, 1018, 1019
Nervous system
  structure and function of, 922-923
  trauma to, 930-941
Neuralgia, postherpetic, 1065
Neurectomy, peripheral, 220
Neurogenic shock, 196-197
Neurohumoral controls of heart, 600
Neuroleptic malignant syndrome, 59-62
Neurologic disorders
  pharmacology and, 950-951
  rehabilitation for, 958-959
Neurologic dysfunction, 923-927
Neurologic examination, 923-924
Neurologic function, 921-965
  assessment of, 923-927
  brain tumors and, 941-942
  central nervous system infections and, 952-954
  cerebral artery aneurysm and, 947-948
  cerebrovascular disease and, 942-947
  degenerative diseases involving central nervous system and, 954-958
  nursing interventions and, 927-930
  in older adults, 359
  rehabilitation and, 958-959
  seizure disorders and, 948-952
  structure and function of nervous system and, 922-923
  trauma to nervous system and, 930-941
  tumors of spinal cord and, 941-942
Neuromuscular conditions, 1128
Neuroradiologic studies, 925-927
Neurosyphilis, 292
Neurotransmitters, pain and, 206-207
Neurovascular integrity
  mobility and, 1096-1097
  nursing interventions for, 1097
Neutrophils, 133, 134, 658
Nevus, 1052-1053
New Voice Club, 568
Nicotine, 110
NIDDM; *see* Noninsulin-dependent diabetes mellitus
Nifedipine (Adalat; Procardia; Procardia XL), 626*t*
Nightingale, Florence, 10, 11, 15*t*, 67
Nitro Ointment; *see* Nitroglycerin
NitroBid; *see* Nitroglycerin
Nitro-Dur Patches; *see* Nitroglycerin
Nitrogen mustard (Mustargen), 251*t*
Nitroglycerin (Nitro Ointment; NitroBid; Nitro-Dur Patches; Nitrolingual Spray; Nitrostat), 626*t*

Nitrolingual Spray; *see* Nitroglycerin
Nitroprusside, 198
Nitrostat; *see* Nitroglycerin
Nitrous oxide, 467*t*, 473*t*
Nizatidine (Axid), 714*t*
Nizoral; *see* Ketoconazole
NNIS; *see* National Nosocomial Infections Study
Nocturnal seminal emissions (NSEs), 866-867
Nodular goiter, 895
Nodularity, physiologic, 850
Nodule, 1035, 1036
Nolvadex; *see* Tamoxifen citrate
Nonadherence, noncompliance and, 76
Noncritical instruments, 311
Noninotropic drugs, 198
Noninsulin-dependent diabetes mellitus (NIDDM), 899, 900*t*
Nonmaleficence, 33
Nonsteroidal antiinflammatory agents, 158, 212-214
  dysmenorrhea and, 814*t*
  vision and, 984*t*
Nonunion of bone, 1121
Nonverbal communication, 58-59, 59*f*
Norcuron; *see* Vecuronium
Norepinephrine, 198, 897
Norethindrone, 821*t*
Norgestrel, 822*t*
Normal anion gap acidosis, 186
Normovolemic shock, 196-198
Norms, cultural, 68-69
Norplant System, contraception and, 821*t*, 826-827, 827*f*, 830
North American Nursing Diagnosis Association (NANDA), 23, 75-76
Norton scale, 401, 1049
Nosocomial bacteremia, 306-307
Nosocomial infections, 135, 299-324
  emotional support for patient with, 319
  high-risk patients and, 301-302
  hospital, 300-302
  incidence of, 300-301
  methods of transmission of, 302
  nursing interventions for, 320-322
  prevention and control of, 308-319
  types of, 302-307
Nosocomial pneumonia, 303-305
Novantrone; *see* Mitoxantrone
Novocain; *see* Procaine
Novolin, 904, 906
NP; *see* Nurse practitioner
NSEs; *see* Nocturnal seminal emissions
NSPB; *see* National Society for the Prevention of Blindness
Nuccal rigidity, 953
Nummular eczema, 1066
Nuprin; *see* Ibuprofen
Nurse
  advanced practice, 12
  chemically impaired, 118-119
  circulating, 472
  collaboration between doctors and, 9-10
  licensed practical, 11-12
  licensed vocational, 11-12
  registered, 11
  rehabilitation and, 386, 390-414
  scrub, 470-471, 471*f*
  transcultural, 69
Nurse practitioner (NP), emergency, 492
Nursing
  definition of, 10
  emergency, 491-492
  functional, 14
  within healthcare system, 2-20
  home healthcare and, 447-451
  as inherently moral enterprise, 34
  medical-surgical, 10-11
  personal values and, 34
  primary, 14
  professional values and, 34
  rehabilitation, 382, 390-414
  skilled, home healthcare and, 446
  total patient care and, 3
  transcultural, 69-71
Nursing Agenda for Health Care, 3-4
Nursing assessment
  of cardiovascular system, 600-604
  constipation and, 437
  depression and, 55
  in emergency and trauma care, 494-506
  of eye problems, 969-975
  of female reproductive system, 835-836
  in long-term care, 428-430
  in nursing process, 22
  of problems of male reproductive system, 866
  of suicide, 55-56
  surgery and, 458-459, 463
  of urinary system, 764-765
Nursing care decisions and actions, 70-71
Nursing care plans, 23, 24*f*-25*f*, 31
Nursing delivery systems, 13-14
Nursing diagnosis, 22-31, 75-76
Nursing education, 11-12
Nursing ethics, 34-35
Nursing history, 22
Nursing homes; *see* Long-term care
Nursing interventions
  abortion and, 861
  acquired immunodeficiency syndrome and, 335, 340-343
Nursing interventions—cont'd
  acute head injury and, 933
  acute poststreptococcal glomerulonephritis and, 781
  acute renal failure and, 789
  adult respiratory distress syndrome and, 592
  allergy and, 149-156
  Alzheimer's disease and, 362
  anaphylactic shock and, 137, 146, 504
  anemias and, 675
  aplastic anemia and, 682-685
  appendectomy and, 722
  appendicitis and, 722
  asthma and, 577
  bacterial skin infections and, 1059
  below-the-knee amputations and, 1129-1130
  biologic response modifiers and, 257
  bronchiectasis and, 576
  burns and, 1081-1082
  calcium deficit and, 180
  cardiac surgery and, 634
  cardiovascular system and, 355
  casts and, 1101
  cataract extraction and, 988
  cerebral artery and, 948
  cerebrovascular accident and, 946
  in cerebrovascular disease, 944-945
  chemotherapy and, 255
  cholecystectomy and, 753
  cholecystostomy and, 753
  choledochostomy and, 753
  chronic bronchitis and, 575
  chronic obstructive pulmonary disease and, 574
  chronic renal failure and, 801-804
  cirrhosis and, 744, 755-757
  colporrhaphy and, 844
  community-acquired infections and, 295-296
  conditions of pregnancy and, 858-859
  confused patient and, 960-964
  congestive heart failure and, 637, 650-653
  constipation and, 437-438
  craniotomy and, 942, 943
  death and dying and, 86-94
  decline in mental status and, 441-442
  dehydration and, 169
  depression and, 63-64
  detached retina and, 1006-1008
  diabetes mellitus and, 914
  digestive system and, 362-363
  discharge instructions and, 1085
  disease of epidermal origins and, 1069
  diverticulitis and, 724
  diverticulosis and, 724
  dysphagia and, 410

Nursing interventions—cont'd
ectopic pregnancy and, 861
enucleation and, 998
epidural analgesia and, 221-223
external radiation therapy and, 242
extraocular surgery and, 998
eye disorders and, 979-1002
eye muscle surgery and, 998
eyelid surgery and, 998
food poisoning and, 282
fractures and, 1122-1123, 1124-1125
fungal infections of skin and, 1062
gastrectomy and, 736
glaucoma and, 992
hearing loss and, 1014
heat-related emergency and, 522-523
hepatitis and, 742
hip fractures and, 1122-1123
hypermagnesemia and, 184
hyperthyroidism and, 894, 916-918
hypertonic fluid deficit and, 169
hypervolemia and, 170
hypocalcemia, 180
hypokalemia and, 174-176, 199-201
hypomagnesemia and, 182
hyponatremia and, 172
hypothyroidism and, 896
hypotonic fluid excess and, 171
hypovolemia and, 168
hysterectomy and, 848
immobile patient and, 392
for implantation of penile prosthesis, 880-882
increased intracranial pressure and, 931
infections and, 137-139
inflammatory bowel disease and, 718
influenza and, 563, 564
insect stings and, 144
integumentary system and, 357-358
for intervertebral disk trauma, 940
intraocular surgery and, 988
isotonic fluid deficit and, 168
isotonic fluid excess and, 170
lacrimal-duct probing and, 998
laminectomy and, 941
leukemia and, 679
lithotomy and, 800
lung cancer and, 261-263
magnesium deficit and, 182
magnesium excess and, 184
mastectomy and, 856
metabolic acidosis and, 187
metabolic alkalosis and, 188
musculoskeletal system and, 358-359
myocardial infarction and, 630
nephrolithotomy and, 800
neurologic disorders and, 927-930
neurovascular integrity and, 1097
normovolemic shock and, 197

Nursing interventions—cont'd
nosocomial infections and, 320-322
orbit surgery and, 998
orthopedic devices and, 1105-1107, 1108-1110
otitis media and, 1024-1025
overhydration and, 171
pain and, 90
pain relief and, 211-221
Parkinson's disease and, 957
patient in traction and, 1107
penetrating keratoplasty and, 988
peptic ulcer disease and, 732
permanent pacemaker placement and, 612
pneumonia and, 580-582
postoperative care and, 483
potassium deficit and, 174-176
pressure ulcers and, 402, 439-440, 1048-1049, 1050, 1051
primary water imbalance and, 171
prostatectomy and, 873
psychotic patient and, 51
pulmonary embolism and, 587
pyelolithotomy and, 800
radiation therapy and, 242, 245, 246
rehabilitation and, 392-414
renal calculi and, 785
reproductive system and, 364
respiratory acidosis and, 189
respiratory alkalosis and, 188
respiratory system and, 364
scleral buckling and, 998
sealed internal radiation therapy and, 244
seizure disorders and, 949-951, 952
sexually transmitted diseases and, 291
skin and, 1034, 1036-1043
sodium deficit and, 172
spinal cord injury and, 936-937
stroke and, 419-422
substance abuse and, 113, 114-119
thoracotomy and, 560-562
total hip replacement and, 1122-1123
total knee replacement and, 1122-1123
total parenteral nutrition and, 703
trabeculectomy and, 988
tuberculosis and, 277, 583
unconscious patient and, 928
unsealed internal radiation therapy and, 246
ureterolithotomy and, 800
urinary diversion and, 799
urinary incontinence and, 403, 436-437
urinary system and, 363
urinary tract infections and, 303
viral infections and, 1065
vitrectomy and, 988
water intoxication and, 171

Nursing practice, 10-16
collaboration between nursing education and, 12
regulation of, 11
standards of, 12-13
Nursing process and ethical decision making, 21-39, 22*f*
Nursing theory, 14-16, 15*t*-16*t*
Nutrition
assessment of, 457, 699
burns and, 1084
cancer and, 230
colostomy and, 708
congestive heart failure and, 639
diabetes mellitus and, 903
older adults and, 368-369, 372
peptic ulcer disease and, 733
postoperative care and, 480
surgery and, 462
total parenteral, 703
Nutritional imbalance, 129-130
Nystagmus, 1015, 1017
Nystatin (Mycostatin), 331*t*, 823*t*

O

Oatmeal bath, 1037
Obese patient, 459
Obesity, 129-130
Oblique fracture, 1119, 1120*f*
OBRA 87; *see* Omnibus Reconciliation Act
Obsessive-compulsive disorder, 49*t*
Obsessive-compulsive personality, 53
Obstruction
of airway, 494-496
in external ear, 1021
intestinal, 725-726
punctal, 1002
of urinary system, 783-786
Obtunded patient, 928
Occult blood, 696
Occupational Safety and Health Administration (OSHA), 318, 339, 492
Occupational therapist (OT), 386
OCPs; *see* Oral contraceptive pills
Ocufen; *see* Flurbiprofen
Ocular malignancies, 1000
Ocular ultrasonography, 974
Oculomotor nerve, 924*t*
OHAs; *see* Oral hypoglycemic agents
Oily skin, 1050
Ointments, 1040*t*
Older adults, 345-376
abuse of, 512-513
acquired immunodeficiency syndrome in, 333
adrenal insufficiency in, 897
alcoholism in, 104
anatomic changes in bones and joints in, 1094

Older adults—cont'd
- anemia in, 670
- bronchodilator therapy in, 573
- cancer in, 258
- cardiovascular disease in, 603
- demographics and, 346-347
- diuretics and, 174
- dysphagia in, 408
- enlarged prostate gland in, 871
- factors affecting aging and, 348-353
- fluid overload in, 193*f*
- fractures in, 1106
- grief and, 86
- hearing loss in, 1019
- heritage consistency and, 76
- hospitalized, 371-373
- human immunodeficiency virus infection in, 333
- infections in, 138
- kidneys and, 764
- neurologic dysfunction in, 924
- nosocomial infections in, 301
- nursing care of, 364-371
- nursing homes and; *see* Long-term care
- pain in, 216
- physiology of aging and, 353-364
- pneumonia in, 578-579
- presbycusis in, 1019
- progress and research and, 347-348
- respiratory assessment of, 536
- skin conditions in, 1055
- skin integrity in, 1037
- surgery and, 460
- swallowing problems in, 408
- tuberculosis in, 276, 584
- urinary incontinence in, 436
- vision in, 1005

Older Americans Act, 347, 451
Olfactory nerve, 924*t*
Oligomenorrhea, 814
Oliguria, 168, 650-653, 779
Omnibus Reconciliation Act (OBRA 87), 433
Omnipen; *see* Ampicillin
ONC; *see* Over-the-needle catheter
Onchocerciasis, 977
Oncogenes, 230
Oncology unit, 256
Oncotic pressure, 165, 166
Oncovin; *see* Vincristine
Oophorectomy, bilateral, 847
Open fracture, 1118-1119, 1119*f*
Open head injury, 930
Open pneumothorax, 497-498, 499*f*
Open reduction
- of fracture, 1119
- with internal fixation (ORIF), 1097

Open-angle glaucoma, 991
Operative team, 470-471
Ophthalmia neonatorum, 981
Ophthalmic medications, 979-980
Ophthalmologist, 969
Ophthalmoscope, 973
Ophthalmoscopy, 973
Opiate drugs, 214, 215, 217-218
Opioids, 214, 215, 217-218
Optic nerve, 924*t*
Optician, 969
Optometrist, 969
OPV; *see* Oral poliovirus vaccine
Oral cancer, 726-727
Oral cavity, 689
Oral contraceptive pills (OCPs), 819-831
Oral hypoglycemic agents (OHAs), 907-908
Oral iron preparations, 669
Oral poliovirus vaccine (OPV), 271
Orbit, surgery and, 998
Orchiectomy, 871
Orchitis, 869
Orem, Dorothy, 10, 16*t*
Organ donation, 88
Organ of Corti, 1014
Organelles, 132
Organic brain syndrome, 53-54, 441
ORIF; *see* Open reduction with internal fixation
Orinase; *see* Tolbutamide
Orthodiagraphy, 616
Orthopedic devices, 1102-1110
- cervical traction and, 1104-1105
- nursing interventions for patient with, 1105-1107, 1108-1110
- pelvic traction and, 1105
- skeletal traction and, 1104, 1106
- splints and, 1108
- traction and, 1102-1104, 1105-1107, 1108

Orthostatic hypotension, 669
Oscilloscope, 694
OSHA; *see* Occupational Safety and Health Act
Osler's nodes, 621
Osmitrol; *see* Mannitol
Osmoglyn; *see* Glycerin
Osmolality, 165, 191
Osmolarity, 165
Osmosis, 164, 164*f*
Osmotic diarrhea, 712
Osmotic movement of fluids, 165
Osmotic pressure, 165, 661
Osteoarthritis, 1110, 1113, 1114
Osteogenic sarcoma, 1125
Osteomyelitis, 1117
Osteoporosis, 1106, 1108, 1118
Osteotomy, 1114
Ostomy clubs, 880
Ostomy equipment, 709, 709*f*
Ostomy "takedown," 705
Ostomy Visitor Program, 707
OT; *see* Occupational therapist
Otitis media, 1014, 1021, 1024-1025
Otologist, 1016
Otosclerosis, 1018, 1026
Otoscope, 1014, 1015*f*
Otoscopy, 1014
Outcomes in nursing process, 31
Outpatient surgery, 456-457, 487
Ovarian cancer, 846
Ovaries, 810, 846-850, 887
Overdose emergency management, 515-517
Overflow incontinence, 403, 435-436, 437, 778
Overhydration, 171
Over-the-needle catheter (ONC), 193*f*
Ovulation, 811
Oxazepam (Serax), 61*t*, 106*t*
Oximeter, 544
Oxycodone (Percodan), 214*t*
Oxygen
- hyperbaric, 551-552
- by mask, 548*f*, 548-549, 549*f*, 550*f*, 551
- by nasal cannula, 549
- partial pressure of, 539
- precautions for use of, 552

Oxygen saturation, 539, 543
Oxygen therapy, 548*f*, 548-552, 549*f*, 550*f*, 551*t*
Oxytocin, 857-858, 860

P

P wave, electrocardiography and, 606
PAC; *see* Premature atrial contraction
Pacemaker
- ectopic, 600
- electronic cardiac, 611-612

Pachymetry, 973
Packed red blood cells, 660*t*, 661
Pain, 204-225
- acute, 207
- assessment of, 209, 210*f*, 211*f*, 494
- burns and, 1084
- chest, 531
- definition of, 205-206
- ethical issues and, 36-37
- function of, 206
- gas, 484
- interventions for relief of, 211-221
- nature of, 205-209
- neurosurgical interventions for, 219-221
- neurovascular integrity and, 1096-1097
- noninvasive interventions for, 219
- nursing interventions and, 90, 220
- phantom limb, 411, 1128
- pharmacology and, 212*t*-214*t*
- postoperative care and, 478, 482-484

Pain—cont'd
 referred, 207-209, 208*f*
 substance abuse and, 115
 thoracic-pulmonary chest, 532*t*
 types of, 207-209
Pain theories, 206-207
Pain threshold, 205
Pain tolerance, 205
Palpation
 in assessment of cardiovascular system, 601, 601*f*
 in assessment of respiratory system, 534-535, 537*f*
Palsy, cerebral, 1128
Pamate, 107*t*
Pancreas, 690, 887, 899-915
Pancreatectomy, total, 754
Pancreatitis, 752-754
Pancuronium (Pavulon), 468*t*
Pancytopenia, 674
Panhysterectomy, 847
Panhysterosalpingo-oophorectomy, 847
Panic disorder, 49*t*
Panretinal photocoagulation (PRP), 996
Papanicolaou cytologic test (Pap smear), 233, 540, 837-838, 838*t*
Papaverine (Cerespan; Pavabid), 877*t*
Papillomaviruses, human, 833, 837, 1061
Papule, 1035, 1036
PAR; *see* Postanesthesia Recovery
Paragard intrauterine contraceptive, 828
Parainfluenza, 563
Paralytic ileus, 484, 704
Paranoid disorders, 53
Paranoid personality, 53
Paranoid schizophrenia, 52
Paraplatin; *see* Carboplatin
Paraplegia, 934, 935*f*
Paraplegic amputee transfer, 398
Parasites, 288-289
Parasympathetic nervous system, 922
Parathormone, 167, 895
Parathyroid glands, 886, 895-896
Parathyroid hormone, 177-178
Parenteral solutions, 191
Parietal pleura, 530
Parkinson's disease, 53, 351, 955*f*, 955-956, 957
Parnate, 62*t*
Paronychia, 1056
Parotitis, 285
Paroxetine (Paxil), 61*t*, 107*t*
Paroxysmal nocturnal dyspnea (PND), 636
Pars plana vitrectomy, 995
Partial pressure of oxygen, 539
Partial seizures, 949
Partial thromboplastin time (PTT), 664, 699
Partially dependent transfer of patient, 398
Partial-thickness burns, 1075-1076
PASG; *see* Pneumatic AntiShock Garment
Passive immunity, 139, 271
Passive transport, fluid and electrolyte exchange and, 164
Passive-aggressive personality, 53
Paste, topical medications and, 1040*t*
Paste boots, 1039
Past-pointing test, 1017
Patch test, 149, 150
Pathogen, 267
Pathologic fracture, 1118
Patient advocate, nurse as, 9
Patient arrival in emergency department, 492-493
Patient care, total, 3
Patient history; *see* History
Patient respect, 35-37
Patient rights, 16-18
Patient Self-Determination Act, 82, 428
Patient-controlled anesthesia (PCA), 217, 218*f*, 484
Patient's Bill of Rights, 16, 17-18
Paul-Bunnell test, 676
Pavabid; *see* Papaverine
Pavulon; *see* Pancuronium
Paxil; *see* Paroxetine
PCA; *see* Patient-controlled anesthesia
PCP; *see* Phencyclidine; *Pneumocystis carinii* pneumonia
PCU; *see* Postanesthesia care unit
PDR; *see* Proliferative diabetic retinopathy
PE; *see* Pulmonary embolism
Pearson attachment, 1104, 1105
Pediculi, 1056-1057
PEG; *see* Percutaneous endoscopic gastrostomy
Pelvic evisceration, 849-850, 879
Pelvic examination, 836-837
Pelvic exenteration, 849-850, 879-880
Pelvic floor exercises, 405, 406, 436, 776, 843
Pelvic infection, 846-847
Pelvic inflammatory disease (PID), 846-847
Pelvic musculature, relaxation of, 842-843
Pelvic sweep, 849-850, 879
Pelvic traction, 1102, 1103*f*, 1105
Pelvic ultrasonography, 839
Penetrating keratoplasty (PKP), 987, 988
Penicillin, 157
Penicillin G benzathine (Bicillin), 152*t*
Penicillin G potassium (Pentids), 152*t*
Penicillin G procaine (Crysticillin; Wycillin), 152*t*
Penile implant, 878*f*, 878-879, 879*f*
Penile prosthesis, implantation of, 880-882
Penile tumors, 869
Penile ulceration, 870
Penrose drain, 480, 481*f*
Pentamidine, aerosolized, 331*t*
Pentazocine (Talwin), 214*t*
Pentids; *see* Penicillin G potassium
Pentothal; *see* Thiopental sodium
Pepcid; *see* Famotidine
Peptic ulcer, 730-737
Pepto Diarrhea Control; *see* Loperamide
Pepto-Bismol, 713*t*
Perceptions, sharing, communication and, 58*t*
Perceptual problems, stroke and, 947
Percodan; *see* Oxycodone
Percussion
 in assessment of cardiovascular system, 601
 in assessment of respiratory system, 535-536, 538*f*
 postural drainage and, 547, 547*f*
Percutaneous cholangiography, 697
Percutaneous endoscopic gastrostomy (PEG), 702
Percutaneous renal biopsy, 769
Percutaneous transluminal coronary angioplasty (PTCA), 633, 635*f*
Perforation of eardrum, 1021-1023
Pericardiocentesis, 503
Pericarditis, 598
Perilymph, 1014
Perimetry, 972-973
Perineal prostatectomy, 875-876
Periosteum, 1092
Peripheral cyanosis, 533
Peripheral nerve block, 219-221, 475
Peripheral nervous system, 922
Peripheral neurectomy, 220
Peripheral veins, venous insufficiency and, 604
Peripheral vision, 356
Peripherally inserted central catheter, 194
Peristalsis, 480, 690
Peritoneal dialysis, 792-793
Peritoneovenous shunt, 745
Peritonitis, 725
Pernicious anemia, 664, 671-672, 717
PERRLA, 979
Persantine; *see* Dipyridamole
Personal hygiene, older adults and, 369-370
Personal space, 74
Personality, 45
Personality disorders, 53
Perspiration, 132
Pessary, 842-843

PET scan; *see* Positron emission tomography scan
Petals, casts and, 1098
Petechiae, 621, 681
PFT; *see* Pulmonary function test
pH, acid-base balance and, 539, 699-700
Phacoemulsification, cataracts and, 993-994
Phagocytes, 134
Phagocytosis, 134
Phantom limb pain, 411, 1128
Phantom pain, 209
Pharmacology
  acquired immunodeficiency syndrome and, 330*t*-332*t*
  blood and, 659*t*-660*t*
  cancer and, 247*t*-253*t*
  circulation and, 624*t*-627*t*
  congestive heart failure and, 638
  endocrine disorders and, 890*t*-891*t*
  female reproductive system and, 820*t*-823*t*
  gastrointestinal system and, 713*t*-714*t*
  hearing and, 1022*t*-1023*t*
  human immunodeficiency virus infection and, 330*t*-332*t*
  male reproductive system and, 877*t*
  medications and; *see* Medications
  mobility and, 1112*t*-1113*t*
  neurologic disorders and, 950*t*-951*t*
  ophthalmic, 979*t*-980*t*
  pain and, 212*t*-214*t*
  peptic ulcer disease and, 733-734
  physiologic responses and, 150*t*-155*t*, 155-156
  psychosocial effects and, 60*t*-62*t*
  respiratory system and, 571*t*-572*t*
  shock and, 198
  skin integrity and, 1041*t*-1042*t*
  substance abuse and, 105*t*-107*t*
  surgery and, 466-469
  tuberculosis and, 276
  urinary disorders and, 771*t*-772*t*
Pharyngitis, 563, 564
Phenazopyridine (Pyridium), 772*t*
Phencyclidine (PCP), 112, 113
Phenergan; *see* Promethazine
Phenobarbital, 951*t*
Phenylephrine (AK-Dilate; Mydfrin; Neo-Synephrine), 155-156, 985*t*
Phenytoin (Dilantin), 951*t*
Pheochromocytoma, 898
Pheresis, 661
Philadelphia chromosome, 678
Phimosis, 867, 869
Phlebotomy, 676
Phobic disorder, 49*t*
Phonocardiogram, 616
Phoria, 977
Phoropter in vision assessment, 971
Phosphates, 184
Phospholine Iodide; *see* Echothiophate iodide
Photocoagulation, panretinal, 996
Photography, fundus, in vision assessment, 972
Photophobia, 953, 981
Physical activities of daily living, 429
Physical agents, disease and, 130
Physical assessment in emergency and trauma care, 494-506
Physical child maltreatment, 511, 512
Physical dependence, addiction and, 216-217
Physical environment, infections and, 268
Physical examination
  in assessment of female reproductive system, 836-837
  in assessment of respiratory system, 533-537
  male reproductive system and, 867-868
  in vision assessment, 969
Physical restraints, 433
Physical therapist (PT), 386
Physician
  collaboration between nurses and, 9-10
  home healthcare and, 447
  rehabilitation and, 386
Physiologic aspects of patient care, 123-378
Physiologic defense mechanisms, 132-140
Physiologic nodularity, 850
Physiologic responses, 124-160
  aging and, 353-364
  causes of disease and, 125-132
  chemotherapeutic agents and, 156-158
  excessive immune responses and, 141-156
  pharmacology and, 150*t*-155*t*, 155-156
  physiologic defense mechanisms and, 132-140
Phytonadione (AquaMEPHYTON; Vitamin K_1), 659*t*
PID; *see* Pelvic inflammatory disease
Pigmentation, disorders of, 1050
Piles, 738-739
Pink eye, 980
Pinna, 1013
Pinworms, 288-289
Pitressin; *see* Vasopressin
Pitting edema, 604
Pituitary gland, 886, 887*f*, 898-899
Pivot transfer, 398
PKP; *see* Penetrating keratoplasty
Placebos, pain medications and, 217
Planning in nursing process, 31
Plant alkaloids, 245
Plant poisoning, 1067
Plantar response, 924
Plaque, 617, 1035
Plasma, 598, 656, 658, 660*t*
  shifts of, to interstitial fluid, 166
  shifts of interstitial fluid to, 166-167
Plasma bicarbonate concentration, 539
Plasma creatinine, 767
Plasma oncotic pressure, 166
Plasma pheresis, 661
Plasma protein fractions, 661
Plasma proteins, 656
Plasmapheresis, 958
Plasmodium falciparum, 288
Plaster casts, 1098-1099
Platelets, 660*t*, 661
Platinol; *see* Cisplatin
Platyhelminthes, 288-289
Pleural conditions, 584-588
Pleural friction rub, 537
Pleur-Evac system, 557, 558, 558*f*
Pleurisy, 582, 584
Plinth, 1082
PMI; *see* Point of maximum impulse
PMMA; *see* Polymethylmethacrylate
PMS; *see* Premenstrual syndrome
PND; *see* Paroxysmal nocturnal dyspnea
Pneumatic antishock garment (PASG), 196, 502-503
Pneumatic retinopexy, 997
Pneumococcus, 127
Pneumocystis carinii pneumonia (PCP), 329, 579, 584
Pneumonectomy, 554, 555, 555*f*
Pneumonia, 303-305, 578*f*, 578-579, 580-582
Pneumothorax, 544
  open, 497-498, 499*f*
  tension, 497, 498, 499*f*, 558, 649
Poikilothermy, 935
Point of maximum impulse (PMI), 601
Poison control centers, 131
Poisoning, 517
  absorption, 517
  carbon monoxide, 131
  food, 279, 280-282, 281*t*
  ingestion, 517
  inhalation, 517
  ivy, 142*f*, 1067
  lead, 131
  plant, 142*f*, 1067
  sumac, 1067
Poliomyelitis, 271, 382-383
Polychronic perceptions of time, 72-73
Polycillin; *see* Ampicillin
Polycythemia, 676

Polydipsia, 900, 911
Polymethylmethacrylate (PMMA), lens implants and, 994
Polymorphonuclear leukocytes, 133
Polymyxin B sulfate (Aerosporin), 982*t*
Polyphagia, 900, 911
Polyps, nasal, 565
Polyuria, 770, 900, 911
Pontocaine; *see* Tetracaine
Portacaval shunt, 747
Portal hypertension, 743
Portosystemic shunts, 747, 747*f*
Port-wine stain, 1053
Position
  of immobile patient, 393-399
  lithotomy, 837
  mobility and, 1095
Positron emission tomography (PET) scan, 926
Postanesthesia care, 476-478
Postanesthesia care unit (PCU), 476
Postanesthesia Recovery (PAR), 476
Postcoital pill, 825-826
Postherpetic neuralgia, 1065
Postnecrotic cirrhosis, 743
Postpartum depression, 52-53
Posttraumatic stress disorder, 49*t*
Postural drainage, 546-547, 547*f*
Postviral encephalitis, 953
Postvoiding residual (PVR) urine, 874
Potassium, 173-177
  effect of stress on serum levels of, 174
  foods rich in, 638
  sources of, 175
Potassium chloride (KCl), 175
Potassium deficit, 174-176, 175*f*
Potassium excess, 176-177, 178
Pouch ileostomy, 710
Pouchitis, 711
Povidine iodine, 1082
Povidone iodine, 439
Powder, topical medications and, 1040*t*
Power of attorney for healthcare, 36, 82, 83*f*, 84*f*, 366
PPD; *see* Purified protein derivative
PPOs; *see* Preferred provider organizations
PQRST pain assessment, 494
PR interval, electrocardiography and, 606
Prazosin (Minipress), 877*t*
Prealbumin, 699
PredMild; *see* Prednisolone
Prednisolone (AK-Pred; Delta-Cortef; Inflamase; PredMild), 154*t*, 985*t*
Prednisone (Deltasone), 154*t*, 890*t*
Preeclampsia, 1071
Preferred provider organizations (PPOs), 8
Pregnancy, 857-861
  ectopic, 860-861
  heart disease and, 641
  human immunodeficiency virus infection and, 317
  rubella and, 284
  tubal, 860-861
Pregnancy tests, 841
Preload, 614-615
Premature atrial contraction (PAC), 607
Premature ventricular contraction (PVC), 609
Prematurity, retinopathy of, 999-1000
Premenstrual syndrome (PMS), 815-816, 835
Premenstrual tension, 815
Prentif cervical cap, 830-831, 831*f*
Preoperative check list, 464*f*
Preoperative checklist, 463, 464*f*, 465
Preoperative preparation, surgery and, 458-462
Prepuce, 808
Presbyopia, 976
Pressure points, 501-502, 502*f*
Pressure sores; *see* Pressure ulcers
Pressure ulcers, 438, 1043-1049, 1051
  debridement and, 1047
  devices that augment nursing care of, 1045-1046
  dressing materials and, 1048
  exudate absorbers and, 1048
  in long-term care, 438*f*, 438-440
  mattress overlays and, 1045-1046
  nursing interventions for, 402, 1048-1049, 1050, 1051
  prevention of, 1045
  risk factors for, 1043-1045
  specialty beds and, 1046
  topical medications and, 1047-1048
  treatment of, 1046-1048
  wound cleansing and, 1047
Priapism, 878
Prickly heat, 1073
Primary assessment in emergency and trauma care, 494-505, 495*t*
Primary healthcare, rehabilitation in, 382-383
Primary nursing, 14, 492
Primary syphilis, 291
Primitive speech, 945
Principen; *see* Ampicillin
Principles, ethics and, 32
Privacy, respect for, 36-37
Probenecid (Benemid), 1113*t*
Problem-oriented record, 31
Procaine (Novocain), 468*t*, 474*t*
Procardia; *see* Nifedipine
Procardia XL; *see* Nifedipine
Prochlorperazine (Compazine), 1023*t*
Proctoscopy, 693, 694
Progestasert System, 828
Progesterone, 811
Progestin-only pills, contraception and, 822-825
Projectile vomiting, 711, 942
Projection, 48*t*
Proliferative diabetic retinopathy (PDR), 996
Prolonging life, 81
Promethazine (Phenergan), 468*t*, 1023*t*
Prone position, patient in, 396
Propanolol (Inderal), 626*t*
Propoxyphene (Darvon; Darvon-N), 214*t*
Propoxyphene/acetaminophen (Darvocet-N), 214*t*
Propoxyphene-N/acetaminophen (Darvocet-N-100), 214*t*
Propulsid; *see* Cisapride
Propulsive gait, Parkinson's disease and, 955
Proscar; *see* Finasteride
Prospective payment systems (PPSs), 6
Prostate gland
  cancer of, 227, 871-872, 876
  conditions affecting, 870-877
  enlargement of, 866
  transurethral resection of, 872-875
Prostatectomy, 872-876
  perineal, 875-876
  retropubic, 875
  suprapubic, 875
Prostate-specific antigen (PSA), 238, 871
Prostatitis, 870-871
Prostatosis, 871
Prostheses, 1114
  breast, 854-856
  penile, 880-882
  rehabilitation and, 410-414
  surgery and, 463
Prostigmin; *see* Neostigmine
Protective custody, child maltreatment and, 511
Protein imbalances, 184-185
Proteins, serum, 699
Proteinuria, 763
Prothrombin time (PT), 664, 699
Protoplasm, 132
Protozoal diseases, 129, 287-288
Proxemics, 73-74
Prozac; *see* Fluoxetine
PRP; *see* Panretinal photocoagulation
Pruritus, 1052
PSA; *see* Prostate-specific antigen
Pseudocysts, 754
Pseudomonas aeruginosa, 578, 1047
Pseudophakic bullous keratopathy, 987
Pseudophakic eye, 994
Psoralen and ultraviolet light A (PUVA), 1068

Psoriasis, 1067-1069, 1068*f*
Psychiatric emergencies, 514-515
Psychiatric examination, drug overdose and, 517
Psychic vomiting, 740
Psychoanalysis, 45
Psychologic preparation, surgery and, 461
Psychologic reactions to disaster, 520
Psychologic status, surgery and, 458
Psychologic theory, substance abuse and, 98
Psychologist, 387
Psychopharmacology, 59-62
Psychosis, 51-53
Psychosocial development in adolescence, 817-818
Psychosocial effects, 41-120
  anxiety and, 45-49
  dementia and, 53-54
  depression and, 54-56, 63-64
  electroconvulsive therapy and, 62
  emotional disorders and, 49-51
  mental health and, 45
  needs of individuals and, 43-45
  organic brain syndromes and, 53-54
  personality and, 45
  personality disorders and, 53
  pharmacology and, 60*t*-62*t*
  psychopharmacology and, 59-62
  psychoses and, 51-53
  somatic disorders and, 54
  therapeutic relationship in nursing and, 56-59
Psychosocial support, 198
Psychosomatic disorders, 54
Psychotropic drugs, 59
Psyllium (Metamucil), 714*t*
PT; *see* Physical therapist; Prothrombin time
PTCA; *see* Percutaneous transluminal coronary angioplasty
Ptosis, 975, 1002
PTT; *see* Partial thromboplastin time
Puberty
  female reproductive system and, 816-818
  male reproductive system and, 866-867
Pubic hair, development of, 817*f*
Public Health Service, 903
Public space, 74
Pulmonary angiography, 542
Pulmonary artery pressure, 615
Pulmonary artery wedge pressure, 615
Pulmonary edema, 621, 639-641
Pulmonary embolism (PE), 194, 485-486, 585-588, 588*f*, 589, 644, 1123
Pulmonary emphysema, 568-570
Pulmonary function test (PFT), 540-541, 542
Pulmonary infarction, 585-588
Pulmonary system, hydrogen ion concentration and, 185
Pulmonary tuberculosis, 274-278
Pulmonary ventilation, 554
Pulse oximetry, 473, 543-544, 544*f*
Pulses, arterial, 603-604
Puncta, 969
Punctal obstruction, 1002
Puncture wounds, 507
Pupil, 923, 967
Purging, 716
Purified protein derivative (PPD), 276, 583
Purkinje fibers, 599
Purpura, 157, 680-681
Purulent otitis media, 1025
Pustular psoriasis, 1069
Pustule, 1035, 1036
PUVA; *see* Psoralen and ultraviolet light A
PVC; *see* Premature ventricular contraction
PVR urine; *see* Postvoiding residual urine
Pyelitis, 782
Pyelography, 767-768
Pyelolithotomy, 797, 800
Pyelonephritis, 782-783
Pyelostomy, 774-775, 776*t*-777*t*
Pyloric sphincter, 689
Pylorospasm, 739-740
Pyridium; *see* Phenazopyridine
Pyridoxine, 331*t*
Pyrimethamine (Daraprim), 332*t*

Q

QA; *see* Quality assurance
QI; *see* Quality improvement
Quadrants of abdomen, 692*f*
Quadriplegia, 934, 935, 935*f*
Quality assurance (QA) in nursing, 13
Quality improvement (QI) in nursing, 13
Quality of life in older adults, 365-366
Quelicin; *see* Succinylcholine
Questran; *see* Cholestyramine

R

R factor, 186
Rabies, 128, 507
Radial keratotomy (RK), 976, 987-988, 989*f*
Radiation, ionizing, 230
Radiation burns, 1075
Radiation therapy, 239-245
Radical mastectomy, 851-852, 855*t*
Radioactive iodine, radiation therapy and, 245, 888, 889, 893
Radioallergosorbent technique (RAST) test, 141
Radiography in assessment of respiratory system, 541-542
Radioisotope studies, 235
  in assessment of cancer, 237
  of renal function, 769
Radiotherapy, 239-245
Ragweed pollen, allergic responses to, 143, 144*f*
Rales, 536
Range-of-motion exercises, 392-393, 394*f*, 1093-1094, 1095
Ranitidine (Zantac), 714*t*
RAP; *see* Right atrial pressure
Rape, 513-514
Rape trauma syndrome, 514
RAST test; *see* Radioallergosorbent technique test
Rationalization, 48*t*
Raynaud's disease, 643
RBCs; *see* Red blood cells
Reach to Recovery, 260, 853
Reaction formation, 48*t*
Reaginic IgE antibody, 142
Reality female condom, 831
Reality orientation, older adults and, 366
Rebound congestion, 155-156
Rebound hyperglycemia, 910
Rebound tenderness, 721, 721*f*
Receptive aphasia, 945
Recovery room, 476
Recreational therapist, 387
Rectocele, 842-843
Rectovaginal fistula, 842
Red blood cells (RBCs)
  disorders of, 668
  packed, 660*t*, 661
Red eye, 981, 986*t*
Red measles, 1061
Red reflex of eye, 973
Red wounds, pressure ulcers and, 1049, 1051
Redness, sudden loss of vision, or pain (RSVP), 987
Reduction of fracture, 1119
Reed-Sternberg cells, 677
Referred pain, 207-209, 208*f*
Reflection, communication and, 57*t*
Reflex(es)
  in assessment of cerebellar function, 924
  cat's eye, 1000
  gag, 235, 693, 945
  red, of eye, 973
Refraction of light, 969
Refractive errors of eye, 975-977
Refractometry in vision assessment, 971
Regional anesthetics, 474*t*, 474-475

Regional enteritis, 717
Registered nurse (RN), 11, 492
Regression, 48*t*, 51
Rehabilitation, 380-424
burns and, 1087
cancer and, 259-260
cardiac, 635
continuity of care and, 418
disability and, 381-382
in each phase of healthcare, 382-385
emotional response to disability and, 388-390
home healthcare and, 446-447
legislation and, 387-388
mastectomy and, 854, 857*f*
for neurologic disorders, 958-959
nursing approaches to, 390-414
in older adults, 372-373
patient teaching in, 415-418
rehabilitation team and, 385-387
spinal cord injuries and, 939
substance abuse and, 112-114
Rehabilitation Act, 388
Rehabilitation nursing, 382
Rehabilitation team, 385*f*, 385-387
Reimbursement, home healthcare and, 450-451
Relapse, substance abuse and, 103, 113
Relationship, therapeutic, 56-59, 57*t*-58*t*
Relaxation
pain and, 219
of pelvic musculature, 842-843
Religious practices at time of death, 81
Reminiscing groups, older adults and, 366
Remodeling of bone, 1120
Remotivation groups, older adults and, 366
Renal biopsy, 769-770
Renal calculi, 784-786, 785*f*
Renal failure, 787-790
acute, 787-788, 789
chronic, 788-790, 801-804
Renal hormones, 763-764
Renal impairment, 788
Renal insufficiency, 788
Renal system, hydrogen ion concentration and, 186
Renal threshold, diabetes mellitus and, 901, 902
Renal transplantation, 794-795
Renal trauma, 786-787, 787*f*
Renin-angiotensin system, hypertension and, 619
Renin-angiotensin-aldosterone system, 763-764
Renography, 769
Renoscan, 769
Repolarization, electrocardiography and, 604
Repression, 48*t*
Reproductive system
female, 807-863, 808*f*
diagnositic procedures and, 836-841
diseases and disorders of, 841-857
breast and, 850-857
cervix and, 845-846, 847-850
fallopian tubes and, 846-850
female external genitalia and, 841-845
ovaries and, 846-850
uterus and, 845-846, 847-850
vagina and, 841-845
nursing assessment of, 835-836
pharmacology and, 820*t*-823*t*
phases of, throughout life cycle, 816-835
pregnancy and, 857-861
structure and function of, 808-816
male, 864-883, 865*f*
conditions affecting, 868-880
congenital malformations, 868
prostate gland and, 870-877
testes and, 868-870
erectile function and, 878-879
nursing assessment of, 866
pelvic exenteration and, 879-880
pharmacology and, 877*t*
phases of, throughout life cycle, 866-867
physical examination in assessment of, 867-868
structure and function of, 865-866
in older adults, 364
Resonance, percussion and, 535
Respiration, Kussmaul's, 186, 535*t*, 911
Respirator, high-efficiency particulate air, 492-493
Respiratory acidosis, 187-189
Respiratory alkalosis, 187, 188, 189
Respiratory assistance, cardiac surgery and, 632
Respiratory infections, 577-584
Respiratory isolation, 313, 314
Respiratory patterns, 535*t*
Respiratory syncytial virus (RSV), 304
Respiratory system, 528-595
adult respiratory distress syndrome and, 591-592
airway management and, 552-554
chest wounds and, 590-591
diseases and disorders of, 559-577
infections, 577-584
pleural conditions, 584-588
postoperative care and, 485
tumors, 566-568, 588-590
laboratory tests in assessment of, 539-544
lower, diseases and disorders of, 568-577
Respiratory system—cont'd
nursing assessment of, 531-537
nursing strategies for problems of, 544-552
in older adults, 363-364
pharmacology and, 571*t*-572*t*
spinal cord injuries and, 937
structure and function of, 529-530
thoracic surgery and, 554-559
upper, diseases and disorders of, 559-566
Rest
congestive heart failure and, 637-638
peptic ulcer disease and, 733
Restating, communication and, 57*t*
Restraints, 433, 515
Resuscitation
cardiopulmonary, 428, 492, 496, 499-501, 500*f*, 646*f*, 646-647, 647*f*
emergency nursing and, 491
Retina, 967
Retin-A; *see* Retinoic acid
Retinal detachment, 997, 997*f*, 1006-1008
Retinal pathology, 996
Retinitis, cytomegalovirus, 995
Retinoblastoma, 1000
Retinoic acid (Retin-A), 1042
Retinopathy
background diabetic, 996
diabetic, 996
of prematurity (ROP), 999-1000
proliferative diabetic, 996
Retinopexy, pneumatic, 997
Retinoscope, 971
Retinoscopy, 971
Retirement, older adults and, 349-350
Retrograde urography, 768
Retrolental fibroplasia (RLF), 999
Retropubic prostatectomy, 875
Retrovir; *see* Zidovudine
Reverse isolation, 254
RF; *see* Rheumatoid factor
Rh factor, 666
Rhegmatogenous detachment, 997
Rheumatic disorders, 1110-1117
Rheumatic fever, 621, 641
Rheumatic heart disease, 620-621
Rheumatoid arthritis, 1110-1117
Rheumatoid factor (RF), 1111
Rheumatoid spondylitis, 1110, 1113
Rhinophyma, 1071
Rhizotomy, 220
Rho(D) immune globulin, 859-860
Rhonchi, 536-537
Rib fractures, 508, 590-591
Rickettsial infections, 127-128, 283
Rifabutin (Mycobutin), 332*t*, 572*t*
Rifampin (Rifadin; Rimactane), 332*t*, 572*t*

Right atrial pressure (RAP), 614-615
Rigidity of muscles, Parkinson's disease and, 955
Rimactane; *see* Rifampin
Ringworm of scalp, 128, 1060
Rinne test, 1016*f*, 1016-1017, 1017*f*
Risk in long-term care, 430-442
River blindness, 977
RK; *see* Radial keratotomy
RLF; *see* Retrolental fibroplasia
RN; *see* Registered nurse
Robinul; *see* Glycopyrrolate
Robitussin; *see* Guaifenesin
Rocky Mountain spotted fever, 127-128, 283
Roferon-A; *see* Interferon Alfa-2A
Rogaine; *see* Minoxidil
Rogers, Carl, 56
Rondec-DM; *see* Dextromethorphan
R-on-T phenomenon, 609, 610
ROP; *see* Retinopathy of prematurity
Rosacea, 1070-1071
Rotating tourniquets, 640
Roto Rest Kinetic Treatment Table, 935
Roundworms, 289
RSV; *see* Respiratory syncytial virus
RSVP; *see* Redness, sudden loss of vision, or pain
RU-486; *see* Mifepristone
Rubella, 284-285, 1018, 1061
Rubella virus vaccine, 271
Rubeola, 283-284, 1061
Rubin's test, 840-841
Rule of nines, burns and, 1076-1078
Rupture of globe, 1003
Ruptured spleen, 503
Rush, Benjamin, 99
Russell traction, 1104, 1104*f*, 1105
Ryan White Act, 338

S

SA node; *see* Sinoatrial node
Saccular aneurysm, 641-642, 642*f*
Saccule, 1014
Safety, postoperative care and, 479
Salicylate, 1113*t*
Salmonella infections, 280-282
Salpingectomy, bilateral, 847
Salt tablets, 518
Sandimmune; *see* Cyclosporine
SANE; *see* Sexual assault nurse examiner
Sarcoma, 230
  Kaposi's, 329, 333*f*, 1000
  osteogenic, 1125
Saturated fat, foods high in, 618
Saturated solutions of potassium iodide (SSKI), 892
Scabies, 1057-1058
Scale, skin lesions and, 1035, 1036
Scalp, ringworm of, 1060
Scapegoat, dysfunctional family and, 100
Scar, 1036
Scarlet fever, 274
Scaulded skin syndrome, 273
Schiller's test, 838
Schilling test, 664
Schirmer's test, 974, 1002
Schizoid personality, 53
Schizophrenia, 51-52, 52*t*
Scintilator, 888
Sclera, 967
Scleral buckling, 997, 997*f*, 998
Scolex, tapeworms and, 288
Scopolamine (Isopto-Hyoscine; Transderm-Scōp), 468*t*, 985*t*, 1023*t*
Scott Inflatable Prosthesis, 879*f*
Scratch test, 148
Scrotum, 867-868
Scrub nurse, 470-471, 471*f*
Sealed internal radiation therapy, 241-245
Seatworms, 289
Sebaceous cyst, 1052
Sebaceous glands, 1033
Seborrhea, 1050
Seborrheic blepharitis, 1001
Seborrheic dermatitis, 1066
Sebum, 1033, 1052
Second spacing, 162
Secondary assessment in emergency and trauma care, 496*t*, 505-506
Secondary healthcare, rehabilitation in, 383
Secondary hypoadrenalism, 897
Secondary syphilis, 291-292
Second-degree burn, 1076
Secondhand smoke, 131
Second-trimester abortion, 860
Secretory diarrhea, 712
Sedation
  conscious, 508
  surgery and, 462
Sedative hypnotics, 431
Sedimentation rate, 664
Seizure disorders, 948-952
Seldane; *see* Terfenadine
Self-actualization, need for, 44
Self-care, patient participation in, 398-399
Self-help cancer groups, 260
Self-worth, pelvic exenteration and, 850
Semicircular canals, 1014
Semicritical instruments, 311
Senescence, 346
Sengstaken-Blakemore tube, 746, 746*f*
SENIC; *see* Study of the Efficacy of Nosocomial Infection Control
Senile cataracts, 993
Senile dementia, 53
Senile miosis, 356
Senility, 53
Sensorineural hearing loss, 1018, 1019
Sensory system
  in long-term care, 431
  in older adults, 355-357
Septic abortion, 858
Septic shock, 197
Septum, deviated, 565
Serax; *see* Oxazepam
Sertraline (Zoloft), 62*t*, 107*t*
Serum albumin, 661
Serum enzymes, 613
Serum glutamic-oxaloacetic transaminase (SGOT), 627-628
Serum proteins, 699
Sex hormones, 896
Sexual abuse, 511, 512
Sexual assault, 513-514
Sexual assault nurse examiner (SANE), 511
Sexual assessment
  female reproductive system and, 835-836
  male reproductive system and, 866
Sexual counseling, spinal cord injuries and, 939
Sexual dysfunction, colostomy and, 708
Sexual role behavior, male reproductive system and, 867
Sexuality
  older adults and, 368
  rehabilitation and, 390
Sexually transmitted diseases (STDs), 289-294, 290*t*
SGOT; *see* Serum glutamic-oxaloacetic transaminase
Shaken baby syndrome, child maltreatment and, 512
Sharing perceptions, communication and, 58*t*
Shaving in preoperative preparation, 462
Shearing force, pressure ulcers and, 1044-1045
Shielding, radiation therapy and, 245
Shigellosis, 282-283
Shingles, 285, 293, 1064-1066
Shock, 195-198, 389
  assessment of, 195
  body response to, 195
  pharmacology and, 198
  postoperative care and, 485
  types of, 195-198
Shriner's Hospital for Children, 1074
Sick sinus syndrome, 607
Sickle cell anemia, 672-673, 674, 680
Sickle Cell Foundation, 673

Sickle cell trait, 672
Side-lying position, patient in, 396, 397*f*
Sigmoidoscopy, 235, 693, 694
Silence, communication and, 58*t*
Silent aspiration, 408
Silvadene; *see* Silver sulfadiazine
Silver nitrate, 1042*t*, 1082
Silver sulfadiazine (Silvadene), 1042*t*, 1082
Simple goiter, 891-892
Simple skull fracture, 930
Simulation, radiation therapy and, 239
Sinemet; *see* Carbidopa
Sinoatrial (SA) node, 599, 606
Sinus arrhythmia, 606-607
Sinus bradycardia, 607
Sinus node, 599
Sinus tachycardia, 607
Sinusitis, 563
Situational/reactive depression, 54
Skeletal traction, 1102, 1104, 1106
Skilled nursing, home healthcare and, 446
Skilled nursing facility (SNF), 7-8
Skin
  assessment of, in dark-skinned persons, 1036
  cutaneous disorders of, 1071-1073
  diseases and disorders of, 1050-1074
  diseases of epidermal origin, 1066-1071
  disorders of appendages and, 1055-1056
  disorders of glands of, 1050-1052
  disorders of pigmentation of, 1050
  hypersensitivity reactions of, 1073-1074
  infections of, 1058-1066
    bacterial, 1058-1059
    fungal, 1059-1061, 1062
    viral, 1061-1066
  infestations of, 1056-1058
  nursing assessment of, 1034
  oily, 1050
  in older adults, 1037
  pruritus and, 1052
  structure and function of, 1032-1034
  tumors of, 1052-1054, 1055
Skin breakdown, prevention of, 399-401
Skin cancer, 230, 1053
Skin expansion with implant, breast reconstruction after mastectomy and, 852, 853*f*
Skin grafts, 1083, 1083*f*
Skin integrity, 1031-1090
  burns and, 1074-1087
  diagnostic tests and procedures and, 1036-1037
  diseases and disorders of, 1050-1074
  emotional support and, 1039-1043
Skin integrity—cont'd
  nursing assessment of, 1034
  pharmacology and, 1041*t*-1042*t*
  pressure ulcers and, 1043-1049
  skin lesions and, 1034-1036
  structure and function of skin and, 1032-1034
  therapeutic procedures and, 1037-1043
Skin lesions, 1034-1036
Skin preparation, surgery and, 462
Skin protection factor (SPF), 1054
Skin sealants, pressure ulcers and, 1048
Skin tests, allergy and, 148-149
Skin traction, 1102
Skin turgor, 168, 169*f*
Skull, 923
Skull fractures, 930
SLE; *see* Systemic lupus erythematosus
Sliding board transfer, 398
Slit-lamp examination, 971
Small intestine, 690, 729
Smell in older adults, 356-357
Smoking, 131, 227, 233, 573
Snellen's eye chart, 970, 970*f*, 974, 976
SNF; *see* Skilled nursing facility
Snuff, 230
Snuffles, 292
Soaks, 1039
SOAP system, 31, 32
SOAPIE system, 31
Soapsuds enema, 694
Social and Rehabilitation Service, 388
Social Security Act, 5-6, 347-348
Social space, 74
Social work, medical, home healthcare and, 447
Social worker, 386
Society for the Prevention of Blindness, 991
Sociocultural theory, substance abuse and, 98
Socioeconomic environment, infections and, 268
Socioeconomic factors, older adults and, 348-349
Sodium, 171-173, 619, 620
Sodium deficit, 172
Sodium excess, 171, 173
Sodium-potassium pump, 164, 165*f*
Solarcaine; *see* Benzocaine
Solu-Cortef; *see* Hydrocortisone
Solutes, 162-163
Solutions, topical medications and, 1040*t*
Somatic disorders, 54
Somnothane; *see* Halothane
Sooty sputum, 1078
Space, cultural variability and, 73-74
Spasm, 179, 738, 740
Spasticity, 393
Special care settings, 379-525
Specialty beds, pressure ulcers and, 1046
Specialty care, home healthcare and, 447
Specific gravity, urine, 766
Specificity theory of pain, 206
Specular microscopy, 973
Speech, esophageal, 568
Speech center, 944
Speech therapist, 386-387
Spermatic cord, torsion of, 870
SPF; *see* Skin protection factor
Spica casts, 1100, 1100*f*
Spider angioma, 743, 1053
Spinal accessory nerve, 924*t*
Spinal anesthesia, 475
Spinal cord, 922-923, 923*f*
  tumors of, 941-942
Spinal cord injuries, 932-939
  daily care of, 935-939
  early intervention in, 934-935, 936-937
  emergency intervention in, 934
  rehabilitation and, 939
  spinal shock and, 935
Spinal cord micturition reflex, 764
Spinal shock, 935
Spinnbarkheit mucus, 811
Spiral fracture, 1119, 1120*f*
Spirilla, 126, 127, 127*f*
Spiritual distress
  death and, 80-81, 88
  surgery and, 456
Spiritual support, dying process and, 91
Spirochetes, 127
Spirometry, 540, 541, 545, 545*f*, 556
Spironolactone (Aldactone), 772*t*
Spleen, ruptured, 503
Splenectomy, 681
Splenomegaly, 681
Splenorenal shunt, 747
Splints, 1108
Spondylitis
  ankylosing, 1113
  rheumatoid, 1110, 1113
Spontaneous abortion, 857
Spontaneous fracture, 1100
Sporanox; *see* Itraconazole
Spore, bacteria and, 126, 126*f*, 310
Spots, vitreous, 1005
Spousal abuse, 513
Sprains, 1118
Sputum
  carbonaceous, 1078
  examination of, 539-540
  production of, 532
Squamocolumnar junction, 810
Squamous cell carcinoma, 1053
SSKI; *see* Saturated solutions of potassium iodide
St. Joseph's tablets; *see* Acetaminophen

St. Louis encephalitis, 953
Stabilization, emergency nursing and, 491
Staghorn calculi, 784-785
Standard nursing care plans, 23
Standard precautions, 319
Standards of Clinical Nursing Practice, 13
Stapedectomy, 1026-1027
Stapes, 1013, 1014
Staphylococcal enteric intoxication, 280
Staphylococcal infections, 273-274
Staphylococci, 126-127, 127*f*, 307
Staphylococcus aureus, 127, 273, 578
Staphylococcus epidermidis, 127, 300
State board licensing examination (NCLEX), 11
State Nurses Association, 117
Status asthmaticus, 577
Status epilepticus, 949
STDs; *see* Sexually transmitted diseases
Steam, sterilization and, 470
Steinmann pin, 1104, 1106*f*
Stem cell transplants, 256
Stenosis, 602
Stereotactic biopsy, 840
Stereotactic surgery, Parkinson's disease and, 956
Stereotyping, culture and, 68
Sterilization
  female, 829, 829*f*
  intraoperative care and, 470
  nosocomial infections and, 310-312
Steroidal antiinflammatory agents, 985*t*
Steroids, adrenal, 158
Stevens-Johnson syndrome, 157, 1074
Stilbestrol, 250*t*
Stilphostrol, 250*t*
Stoma, care of, 705-710
Stomach, 689
Stomach cancer, 728-729
Stomatitis, Vincent's, 716
Stool analysis, 696
STOP, violence and,521, 510
Stoxil; *see* Idoxuridine
Strabismus, 975, 976-977
Strangulated hernia, 737
Strawberry tongue, 274
Street names for commonly abused drugs, 99
Streptococcal diseases, 294
Streptococcal infections, 274
Streptococcal sore throat, 274
Streptococci, 126-127, 127*f*
Streptococcus pneumoniae, 127, 294, 578
Streptococcus pyogenes, 274
Streptomycin, 158, 572*t*
Stress
  effect of, on serum potassium levels, 174
  surgery and, 455
Stress incontinence, 403, 434, 436, 778
Stress response, 455
Stress ulcer, 727
Strict isolation, 312
Stroke, 355, 419-422, 943, 945-947
  hemorrhagic, 942-943
  ischemic, 942-943
Strontium-89, radiation therapy and, 245
Study of the Efficacy of Nosocomial Infection Control (SENIC), 300-301, 305, 306
Stupor, 928
Sty, 1001
Subacute bacterial endocarditis, 621
Subarachnoid hemorrhage, 943-944
Subconsciousness, 45
Subculture, 68, 352
Subdural hematoma, 509-510, 931, 932*f*
Sublimation, 48*t*
Sublimaze; *see* Fentanyl
Submucous resection, 565
Substance abuse, 96-120
  central nervous system depressants and, 100-109
  central nervous system stimulants and, 109-110
  chemically impaired nurses and, 117
  as disease, 99
  dysfunctional family and, 99-100
  etiology of, 98-99
  hallucinogens and, 111-112
  inhalants and, 111
  nursing management of, 114-118
  pharmacology and, 105*t*-107*t*
  psychosocial signs and symptoms of, 114
  terminology of, 97-98
  treatment and rehabilitation and, 112-114
Substance dependence, 97
Subtotal hysterectomy, 847
Success depression, 54
Succinylcholine (Anectine; Quelicin; Sucostrin), 468*t*
Sucking chest wound, 497
Sucostrin; *see* Succinylcholine
Sucralfate (Carafate), 714*t*
Suction curettage, abortion and, 859
Suctioning, 546
Sudden death, 521
Suggesting, communication and, 58*t*
Suicidal emergencies, 515
Suicide, nursing assessment of, 55-56
Sulfa drugs, 157
Sulfamethoxazole (Azo Gantanol; Gantanol), 155
Sulfamylon; *see* Mafenide acetate
Sulfamylon Acetate; *see* Mafenide acetate
Sulfisoxazole (Azo Gantrisin; Gantrisin), 155*t*
Sulfonamides, 155*t*, 157
Sulfonylureas, 907-908
Sumac poisoning, 1067
Superego, 45
Superficial fascia, 1032-1033
Supine position, patient in, 395-396
Suppressor cells, 140
Suprapubic aspiration, 765
Suprapubic prostatectomy, 875
Suprarenal glands, disorders of, 896-898
Surfactant, 530
Surgery
  aseptic, 469
  laser, 469
  negative effects of, 455-456
  outpatient, 456-457
  types of, 455
Surgical asepsis, intraoperative care and, 469-470
Surgical care, 454-488
  admission of patient and, 457
  on day of surgery, 463-469
  informed consent and, 457-458
  intraoperative, 469-476
  patient and family teaching and, 487
  pharmacology and, 466*t*-469*t*
  postoperative, 476-486
  preoperative preparation for, 458-462
  surgical experience and, 455-457
Surgical contraception, 829
Surgical wound infections, 305-306
Surital; *see* Thiamylal
Surveillance, infection control and, 308, 309
Survivor of violence, 513-514
Swallowing
  air, 740
  impaired, 407-409, 410
Swan-neck deformities, 1111
Sweat glands, 1033
Sweating
  absence of, 1052
  excessive, 1052
Swimmer's ear, 1021
Sycosis barbae, 1058
Symmetrel; *see* Amantadine
Sympathetic nervous system, 619, 922
Sympathetic ophthalmia, 990
Sync time, cultural variability and, 71-73
Syngeneic bone marrow transplantation, 256
Synovectomy, 1113-1114
Synthroid; *see* Levothyroxine
Syphilis, 291-292
  cardiovascular, 292
  gummatous, 292

Systemic lupus erythematosus (SLE), 1071-1073
Systole, 599
Systolic blood pressure, 602, 618

T

T_3 resin uptake test; *see* Triiodothyronine resin uptake test
Tachycardia, ventricular, 609-610, 610*f*
Tactile fremitus, 535
Tagamet; *see* Cimetidine
TAH BSO; *see* Total abdominal hysterectomy with bilateral salpingo-oophorectomy
Talwin; *see* Pentazocine
Tamoxifen citrate (Nolvadex), 253*t*, 822*t*
Tampons, guidelines for use of, 815
Tapeworms, 288
Taste in older adults, 356-357
Taxonomy, 23
TB; *see* Tuberculosis
TBSA; *see* Total body surface area
TCNs; *see* Transcultural nurses
Tegretol; *see* Carbamazepine
Telangiectasia, 1071
Telephone triage, 493
Teletherapy, 239
Temperature, heart rate and, 600
Temporal arteritis, 1003
Temporal lobe seizures, 949
Temporary incontinence, 402
Tempra; *see* Acetaminophen
Tenderness, rebound, 721, 721*f*
Tenormin; *see* Atenolol
TENS; *see* Transcutaneous electrical neural stimulation
Tensilon test, 958, 975, 1002
Tension, premenstrual, 815
Tension pneumothorax, 497, 498, 499*f*, 558, 649
Terazol 3; *see* Terconazole
Terazol 7; *see* Terconazole
Terazosin (Hytrin), 877*t*
Terconazole (Terazol 3; Terazol 7), 823*t*
Terfenadine (Seldane), 153*t*
Tertiary healthcare, rehabilitation in, 383-385
Tesamone; *see* Testosterone
Test(s)
  Amsler's grid, 974
  blood, 662
  coagulation, 663-664
  contrast sensitivity, 973-974
  cover/uncover, 975
  edrophonium, 958, 975, 1002
  elimination, allergy and, 149
  exercise tolerance, 615
  falling, 1017
  glare, 973
Test(s)—cont'd
  heterophil antibody, 676
  intradermal, 148-149
  Ishihara, 978
  Mantoux, 276, 583
  microhematocrit, 663
  Mono-vacc, 276
  mucous membrane sensitivity, 149
  past-pointing, 1017
  patch, 149, 150
  Paul-Bunnell, 676
  pregnancy, 841
  radioallergosorbent technique, 141
  Rinne, 1016*f*, 1016-1017, 1017*f*
  Rubin's, 840-841
  Schiller's, 838
  Schilling, 664
  Schirmer's, 974, 1002
  scratch, 148
  skin, allergy and, 148-149
  Tensilon, 958, 975, 1002
  tine, 276
  tuberculin skin, 146, 275-276, 277
  Weber, 1016, 1016*f*
Testes, 865, 867, 887
  conditions affecting, 868-870
  ectopic, 870
  undescended, 869, 870
Testicular carcinoma, 869
Testicular self-examination (TSE), 869, 870*f*
Testicular tumors, 869
Testosterone (Andro 100; Histerone 100; Tesamone), 253*t*, 865, 867, 877*t*
Tetanus, 280, 1124
Tetanus immunoglobulin (TIG), 506
Tetany, 179, 893
Tetracaine (Pontocaine), 474*t*
Tetracycline (Achromycin), 713*t*, 982*t*
Tetracyclines, 158
Thanatology, 80
Theme identification, communication and, 58*t*
Theophylline ethylenediamine (Aminophylline), 571*t*
Therapeutic abortion, 858
Therapeutic baths, 1037-1038
Therapeutic blood fractions, 658-662
Therapeutic relationship, 56-59, 57*t*-58*t*
Therapist
  occupational, 386
  recreational, 387
  speech, 386-387
Thermal burns, 1075
Thiamylal (Surital), 473*t*
Thiazide diuretics, 174, 176
Thiopental sodium (Pentothal), 469*t*, 473*t*
Third spacing, 162, 184
Third-degree burn, 1076
Thirst, hypothalamus and, 167
Thiuretic Esidrex; *see* Hydrochlorothiazide
Thomas splint, 1104
Thoracentesis, 543, 543*f*, 544
Thoracic cage, 530
Thoracic outlet syndrome, 1128
Thoracic surgery, 554-559
Thoracic-pulmonary chest pain, 532*t*
Thoracostomy, 497
Thoracotomy, 554, 560-562, 582, 704
Thorax, 529*f*, 533*f*, 534*f*
Thorazine; *see* Chlorpromazine
Threadworms, 289
Threatened abortion, 857
Three-day measles, 284, 1061
Throat irrigations, bronchial infections and, 547-548
Throat problems, 241
Thrombectomy, 644
Thromboangiitis obliterans, 643
Thrombocytes, 656, 658
Thrombocytopenia, 240, 254, 658, 674
Thrombocytopenic purpura, 681
Thrombocytosis, 658
Thrombophlebitis, 643-644
Thrombosis, 485-486
Thrombotic stroke, 943
Thrush, 716
Thymic tumors, 958
Thyroid, carcinoma of, 895
Thyroid crisis, 893
Thyroid gland, 886
  disorders of, 891-895
  tumors of, 895
Thyroid scan, 889
Thyroid storm, 893
Thyroid ultrasonogram, 888-889
Thyroidectomy, 179, 893
Thyroid-stimulating hormone (TSH), 891
Thyrotoxic crisis, 893
Thyrotoxicosis, 892
TIAs; *see* Transient ischemic attacks
Tick, Rocky Mountain spotted fever and, 127-128, 283
TIG; *see* Tetanus immunoglobulin
Tildrin; *see* Chlorpheniramine
Time, cultural variability and, 71-73
Timolol maleate (Timoptic), 984*t*
Tine test, 276
Tinea barbae, 1059, 1061
Tinea capitis, 1059, 1060*i*, 1060-1061, 1062*t*
Tinea corporis, 1059, 1060*i*, 1060-1061, 1062*t*
Tinea cruris, 1059, 1062*t*
Tinea manuum, 1061
Tinea pedis, 1059, 1061, 1062*t*

Tinea unguium, 1062*t*
Tinnitus, 1017
TIPS; *see* Transiugular intrahepatic portosystemic shunt
Tissue sampling, 233-234
TMP/SMX; *see* Trimethoprim and sulfamethoxazole
Tobacco, 131
Tobramycin (Tobrex), 982*t*
Tobrex; *see* Tobramycin
Tolazamide (Tolinase), 891*t*
Tolbutamide (Orinase), 891*t*
Tolerance, substance abuse and, 97-98
Tolinase; *see* Tolazamide
Tonic-clonic seizure, 949
Tonometer, 972, 991
Tonometry, 971-972
Tonsillectomy, 563
Tonsillitis, 563
Tonsils, enlarged, 565-566
Tophi, 1116
Topical anesthesia, 475
Topical medications, 1040*t*, 1042*t*, 1043*t*, 1047-1048
Topsyn; *see* Fluocinonide
Torsion of spermatic cord, 870
Totacillin; *see* Ampicillin
Total abdominal hysterectomy with bilateral salpingo-oophorectomy (TAH BSO), 847
Total body surface area (TBSA), burns and, 1075, 1076-1078
Total hip replacement, 1114, 1115*f*, 1116, 1122-1123
Total knee replacement, 1115*f*, 1115-1116, 1122-1123
Total lift, 397-398
Total pancreatectomy, 754
Total parenteral nutrition (TPN), 703
Total patient care, 3
Total quality management (TQM), 13
Touch
  cultural variability and, 74-75
  in older adults, 357
Tourniquet, 502, 640
Toxic goiter, 830, 892
Toxic shock syndrome (TSS), 273-274, 294, 814-815, 816-817
Toxoids, 230
Toxoplasmosis, 287-288, 329, 332
TPN; *see* Total parenteral nutrition
TQM; *see* Total quality management
Trabeculectomy, 988, 991
Trabeculoplasty, laser, 991
Tracer dose, radioactive iodine uptake and, 888
Tracheostomy, 304, 567*f*, 568, 568*f*
Tracheostomy tube, 552
Tracheotomy, 552-553, 553*f*
Trachoma, 981
Traction, 1102-1104, 1105-1107, 1108
  cervical, 1104-1105
  nursing interventions for patient in, 1107
  pelvic, 1105
  skeletal, 1104, 1106
Tranquilizers, 59, 104-107, 108
Transcultural nurses (TCNs), 69-71
Transcultural Nursing Society, 69
Transcultural triadic relationship, 70
Transcutaneous electrical neural stimulation (TENS), 218, 219*f*, 1128
Transderm-Scōp; *see* Scopolamine
Transdermal nicotine patches, 110
Transfer
  patient, 397-398
  postoperative, to patient's room, 478
Transfer belt, 397
Transferrin, 699
Transformation zone, 810
Transfusion, blood, 666-668
  reactions to, 667, 667*t*, 678
Transient incontinence, 402
Transient ischemic attacks (TIAs), 943
Transiugular intrahepatic portosystemic shunt (TIPS), 747-748
Transmission, infections and, 268-269
Transmission-driven precautions, 319
Transplant
  bone marrow, 256
  corneal, 987-989, 989*f*
  hair, 1056
  liver, 748
  renal, 794*f*, 794-795
  stem cell, 256
  ureteral, 795-797
Transport
  active, 164, 165*f*
  passive, 164
  surgery and, 465-469
Transurethral resection of prostate (TURP), 872-875
Transverse fracture, 1119, 1120*f*
Tranxene; *see* Chlorazepate
Tranylcypromine, 62*t*, 107*t*
Trauma
  emergency care and; *see* Emergency and trauma care
  to eye, 1002-1003
  intervertebral disk, 939-941
  to musculocutaneous system, 1118-1125
  to nervous system, 930-941
  renal, 786-787, 787*f*
Trauma center designations, 491
Traumatic
  death following, 87-88
Traumatic intracranial hemorrhage, 931
Treponema pallidum, 291
Tretinoin, 1042*t*
Triage, 493-494
Triage nurse, 492
Triamcinolone (Azmacort), 572*t*
Triamcinolone acetonide (Aristocort; Kenacort; Kenalog), 154*t*
Trichina, 289
Trichinella, 289
Trichinellosis, 289
Trichinosis, 289
Trichomonas vaginalis, 841
Trichomoniasis, 288
Tricyclic antidepressant drugs, 214
Trifluridine (Viroptic ophthalmic solution 1%), 983*t*
Trigeminal nerve, 924*t*
Trihexyphenidyl (Artane), 951*t*
Triiodothyronine (T_3) resin uptake test, 889
Trimethoprim and sulfamethoxazole (TMP/SMX), 332*t*
Trocar, 793
Trochlear nerve, 924*t*
Tropia, 977
Tropicacyl; *see* Tropicamide
Tropicamide (Mydriacyl; Tropicacyl), 985*t*
Trousseau's sign, 179, 180*f*
Truss, 737
TSE; *see* Testicular self-examination
TSS; *see* Toxic shock syndrome
T-tube cholangiography, 697
Tubal insufflation, 840-841
Tubal ligation, 829, 829*f*
Tubal pregnancy, 860-861
Tubercle bacillus, 582
Tuberculin skin test, 146, 275-276, 277
Tuberculosis (TB), 140, 274-278, 275*f*, 492, 579-584
  nursing interventions in, 277
  pharmacology and, 276
Tubocurarine chloride, 469*t*
Tubular processes, urine formation and, 763
Tumors
  benign, 228
  of bladder, 786
  bone, 1125-1126
  brain, 941-942
  of breast, 850
  cancer and; *see* Cancer
  of cervix, 846
  of gastrointestinal system, 726-730, 754
  of kidneys, 786
  of lung, 588-590
  male reproductive system and, 869, 870
  malignant, 228-229
  ovarian, 846

Tumors—cont'd
penile, 869
of respiratory system, 566-568
of skin, 1052-1054
of spinal cord, 941-942
testicular, 869
thymic, 958
of urinary tract, 786
of uterus, 846
Tuning forks in assessment of hearing loss, 1016*f*, 1016-1017
TURP; *see* Transurethral resection of prostate
Tylenol; *see* Acetaminophen
Tylenol #3; *see* Acetaminophen and codeine
Tylenol Cold Medication; *see* Dextromethorphan
Tympanic cavity, 1013
Tympanic membrane, 1013
Tympanic sound, percussion and, 536
Tympanoplasty, 1026
Typhus fever, 127

U

Ulcer
duodenal, 731*t*
gastric, 731*t*
peptic, 730-737
skin lesions and, 1036
stress, 727
Ulceration, penile, 870
Ulcerative colitis, 717, 719-720
Ulcer
pressure; *see* Pressure ulcers
Ultrasonography, 694, 889
in assessment of cancer, 238
in assessment of renal function, 769
B-scan, 995
ocular, 974
pelvic, 839
thyroid, 888-889
Umbilical hernia, 737
Unconsciousness, 45, 927, 928
Undescended testes, 869, 870
Undoing, 48*t*
Uniform Anatomical Gift Act, 501
Uniform Determination of Death Act, 81
Unipen; *see* Nafcillin sodium
United Ostomy Association, 260, 707
United States, population statistics in, 4
Universal precautions, 312-318, 337, 338, 668, 773, 979, 980, 1059
Unna's boot, 1039
Unsealed internal radiation therapy, 245, 246
Upper airway
obstruction and trauma to, 564-566
infections of, 559-564
Upper GI series, 695
Upper respiratory system, conditions of, 559-566
Urea, 766
Urecholine; *see* Bethanechol
Uremia, 788
Ureteral catheter, 768, 774-775, 776*t*-777*t*
Ureteral colic, 785
Ureteral transplants, 795-797
Ureterolithotomy, 797, 800
Ureterosigmoidostomy, 795
Ureterostomy, cutaneous, 795, 796, 796*f*
Ureterotomy, 797-798
Urethra, 761, 761*f*
Urethritis, 292, 402
Urge incontinence, 403, 434-435, 436, 778
Urinalysis, 765-767, 888
Urinary diversion, 795-797, 799
Urinary drainage, 770-777, 776*t*
Urinary incontinence, 370, 401-406, 778*t*, 778-779
in long-term care, 433-437, 435*t*
stroke and, 947
Urinary system, 760-806
diagnostic tests and, 765-770
dialysis and, 791-794
diseases and disorders of, 779-790
acute poststreptococcal glomerulonephritis, 779-780, 781
cystitis, 781-782
infectious, 780-783
nephrosis, 780
nephrotic syndrome, 780
noninfectious, 779-780
nursing assessment of, 764-765
obstructions of, 783-786
renal calculi, 784-786
in older adults, 363
operative conditions of, 795-800
pharmacology and, 771*t*-772*t*
pyelonephritis, 782-783
renal failure and, 787-790
renal transplantation and, 794-795
structure and function of, 761-764
therapeutic procedures and, 770-777
traumatic injuries to, 786-787
tumors of, 786
urinary incontinency and, 778-779
tumors of, 786
Urinary tract infection (UTI), 302-303, 304, 768, 782*f*
Urination, 764
Urine
collection of specimens of, 765
formation of, 763
retention of, postoperative care and, 484
Urine osmolality, 766
Urine smear, 766
Urine urea nitrogen (UUN), 669
Urine-collecting devices, urinary incontinence and, 406
Urodynamic studies of bladder function, 769
Urography
excretory, 767-768
retrograde, 768
Urologist, 867
Urostomy, continent, 796
Urticaria, 1073-1074
Uterine cancer, 846
Uterine prolapse, 842-843
Uterus, 809-810, 810, 810*f*, 845-846, 847-850
UTI; *see* Urinary tract infection
Utilitarianism, 34
Utricle, 1014
UUN; *see* Urine urea nitrogen
Uveal tract, 967
Uveitis, 989-990

V

Vaccines, 270-271, 286-287
Vacuum pump device, erectile dysfunction and, 878, 878*f*
Vagina, conditions affecting, 841-845
Vaginal cancer, 845
Vaginal contraceptive film (VCF), 829
Vaginal hysterectomy, 849
Vaginitis, 841-842
monilial, 716
pharmacology and, 822*t*-823*t*
Vagotomy, 734
Vagus nerve, 924*t*
Valium; *see* Diazepam
Valuables, surgery and, 463
Values
cultural, 68-69
ethics and, 32
Varicella, 285, 1064
Varicella-zoster (V-Z) virus, 285, 293
Varicocele, 644, 869
Varicose veins, 644-645, 645*f*
Vascular hemophilia, 679
Vascular purpuras, 680-681
Vascular system, 598
Vasectomy, 829
Vasoactive drugs, 198
Vasogenic shock, 196-197
Vasopressin (Pitressin), 680, 891*t*
Vasospasm, cerebral, 947
Vasotec; *see* Enalapril
VCF; *see* Vaginal contraceptive film
Vectorborne transmission, infections and, 268, 269, 302
Vectorcardiogram, 616
Vecuronium (Norcuron), 469*t*
Vehicle transmission, infections and, 268, 269, 302
Vein ligation and stripping, 644-645

Veins
diseases and disorders of, 641-646
peripheral, venous insufficiency and, 604
varicose, 644-645, 645*f*
Velban; *see* Vinblastine
Venipuncture, 193*f*
Venous hydrostatic pressure, 166
Venous measurement, 604
Ventilation, 530
mechanical, 554
Ventilation/perfusion lung scans, 542
Ventricle, 609-610
Ventricular fibrillation, 610, 610*f*
Ventricular rate, 606
Ventricular rhythm, 606
Ventricular tachycardia, 609-610, 610*f*
Venturi mask, 549, 550*f*, 551
VePesid; *see* Etoposide
Veracity, ethics and, 32, 34
Verbal communication, 56-59
Vernix caseosa, 1033
Versed; *see* Midazolam
Vertebral column, 923
Vertigo, 1014, 1017, 1027
Vesicle, 1035, 1036
Vesicovaginal fistula, 842
Vesicular breath sounds, 536, 539*t*
Vestibular tests, 1017
Vestibule, 808-809, 1014
Veterans Administration, 388
Vibramycin; *see* Doxycycline
Vibration, postural drainage and, 547
Victim of violence, 513-514
Vidarabine (Vira-A Ophthalmic), 983*t*
Videofluoroscopy, 409
Vinblastine (Velban), 253*t*
Vincent's stomatitis, 716
Vincristine (Oncovin), 253*t*, 332*t*
Violence, 510-514
Vira-A Ophthalmic; *see* Vidarabine
Viral conjunctivitis, 980, 986*t*
Viral encephalitis, 953
Viral hepatitis, 287, 740-742
Viral infections, 283-287, 1061-1066
Viridans streptococci, 126-127
Virology, 128
Viroptic ophthalmic solution 1%; *see* Trifluridine
Virulence, 136
Viruses, 128, 230
Visceral pleura, 530
Vision, 966-1011
normal, 975-976
nursing assessment of, 969-975
in older adults, 355-356
peripheral, 356
pharmacology and, 982-985
structure and function of eye in, 967-969
Vision loss, 977
Visiting nurse association, 8-9
Visitors, surgery and, 463
Visual acuity, 970, 971
Visual analog pain scale, 209, 211*f*
Visual examination, 969, 1014, 1015
Visual impairment, 999
Vital signs
cardiac surgery and, 632
in older adults, 371-372
Vitallium cup, hip arthroplasty and, 1114
Vitamin A acid, 1042*t*
Vitamin B, 659*t*
Vitamin B_6, 331*t*
Vitamin B_{12} deficiency anemia, 671-672
Vitamin D, 177
Vitamin D_2, 1112*t*
Vitamin K, 699
Vitamin K_1, 659*t*
Vitamins, cancer and, 230
Vitrectomy, 995*f*, 995-996, 997
nursing interventions for, 988
pars plana, 995
Vitreous floaters, 1005
Vitreous pathology, 995
Vocal fremitus, 535
Vocational counselor, 387
Vocational Rehabilitation Act, 387
Vocational Rehabilitation Department, 388
Voice tests in assessment of hearing loss, 1015
Voiding
prompted, 405
postoperative care and, 478, 479-480
record of, in long-term care, 436
surgery and, 462
Volkmann's contracture, 1124
Voltaren; *see* Diclofenac
Volvulus, 725
Vomiting
nausea and; *see* Nausea and vomiting
projectile, 711, 942
psychic, 740
von Willebrand's disease, 664, 679, 680
Vulva, 808, 843-845
Vulvectomy, 843-844
Vulvitis, 841
V-Z virus; *see* Varicella-zoster virus

W

Wald, Lilian, 445
Walking iron, 1108
Warts, 1061-1063
Water content of body, 162
Water excess with hypotonicity, 169-170
Water intoxication, 169-170
Weber test, 1016, 1016*f*
Weight, burns and, 1084
Wen, 1052
Wenckebach block, 610-611
Wernicke's area, 944
Western equine encephalitis, 953
Wet desquamation, radiation therapy and, 240
Wet dressings, 1038-1039
Wet pleurisy, 582
Wheal, 143, 1035, 1036
Wheezes, 532, 536-537, 540*t*
Whiplash injuries, 939-940, 1125
Whipple procedure, 702, 754, 754*f*
White blood cells, disorders of, 668, 676-678
White House Conference on Aging, 347
WHO; *see* World Health Organization
Will, living, 36, 82, 83*f*, 84*f*, 366
Withdrawal
alcohol, 101-102
substance abuse and, 97
Women, reproductive health of; *see* Reproductive system, female
Wood, Philip, 381
World Health Organization (WHO), 3, 271, 326, 382, 981
Wounds
care of, 507
chest, 590-591
circumferential, 1079
cleansing of, 1047
healing of, 134, 135*f*, 481
postoperative care and, 486
pressure ulcers and, 1049, 1051
puncture, 507
Wycillin; *see* Penicillin G procaine

X

Xanax; *see* Alprazolam
Xenograft, 1083
Xerophthalmia, 977, 986-987
X-ray examination
abdominal, 693
in cardiovascular assessment, 235, 616
Xylocaine; *see* Lidocaine

Y

Yellow wounds, pressure ulcers and, 1049, 1051

Z

Zantac; *see* Ranitidine
Zarontin; *see* Ethosuximide
Zidovudine (AZT; Retrovir), 332*t*, 334-336
Zollinger-Ellison syndrome, 730
Zoloft; *see* Sertraline
Zovirax; *see* Acyclovir
Zovirax Ointment; *see* Acyclovir
Zyloprim; *see* Allopurinol

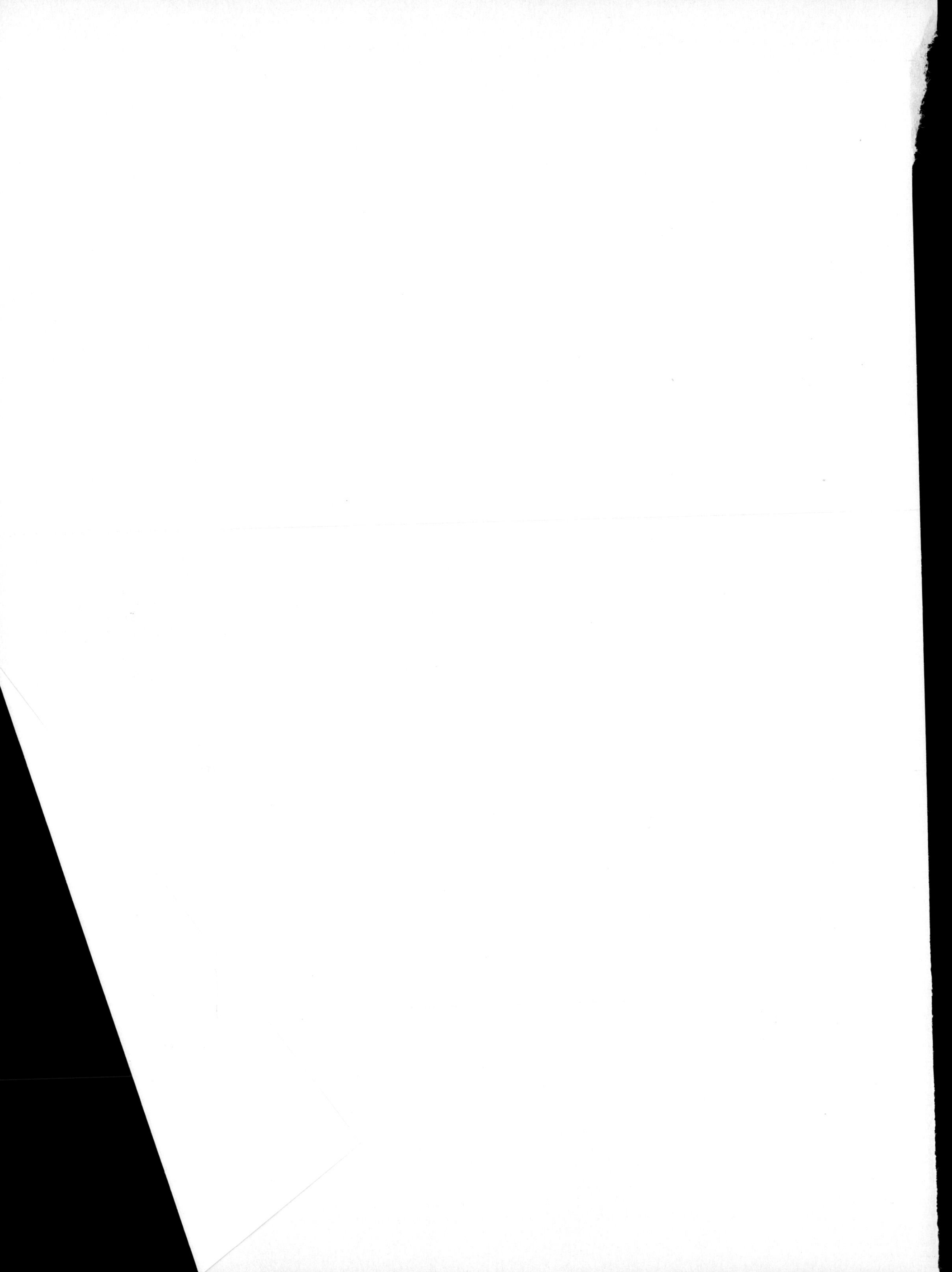

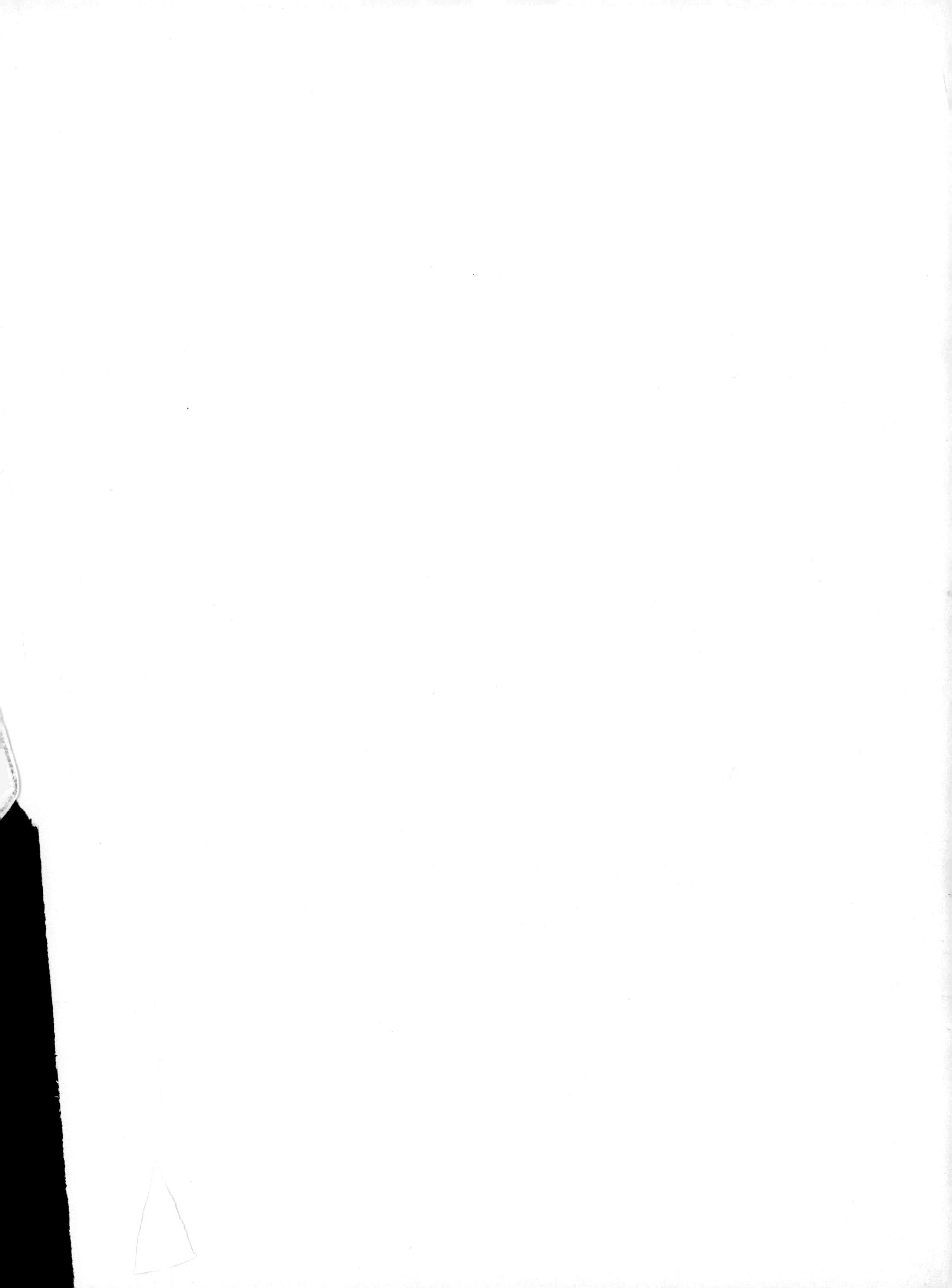

Commonly Used Abbreviations for Diagnostic and Laboratory Tests

ABEP	Auditory brainstem evoked potentials
ABG	Arterial blood gases
ACE	Angiotension converting enzyme
ACTH	Adrenocorticotropic hormone
ADH	Antidiuretic hormone
AFB	Acid-fast bacilli
AFP	Alpha fetoprotein
A/G ratio	Albumin/globulin ratio
AIDS	Acquired immunodeficiency syndrome
AIT	Agglutination inhibition test
ALA	δ-aminolevulinic acid
ALP	Alkaline phosphatase
ALT	Alanine aminotransferase
ANA	Antinuclear antibodies
APTT	Activated partial thromboplastin time
ARC	AIDS-related complex
ASO	Antistreptolysin O titer
AST	Aspartate aminotransferase
BE	Barium enema
BE	Base excess
BUN	Blood urea nitrogen
C & S	Culture and sensitivity
CATT	Computerized axial transverse tomography
CBC	Complete blood count
CDE	Common duct exploration
CEA	Carcinoembryonic antigen
CI	Cardiac index
CK	Creatinine kinase
Cl	Chloride
CMV	Cytomegalovirus
CO	Cardiac output
CO	Carbon monoxide
CO_2	Carbon dioxide
COHb	Carboxyhemoglobin test
CPK	Creatinine phosphokinase
CRF	Corticotropin-releasing factor
CRP	C-reactive protein
CSF	Cerebrospinal fluid
CST	Contraction stress test
CT	Computed tomography
Cu	Copper
CVB	Chorionic villi biopsy
CVS	Chorionic villi sampling
CXR	Chest x-ray examination
D & C	Dilation and curettage
DIC	Disseminated intravascular coagulation
DSA	Digital subtraction angiography
DST	Dexamethasone suppression test
EBV	Epstein-Barr virus
ECG	Electrocardiogram
ECHO	Echocardiography
EEG	Electroencephalogram
EF	Ejection fraction
EGD	Esophagogastroduodenoscopy
EKG	Electrocardiogram
ELISA	Enzyme-linked immunosorbent assay
EMG	Electromyography
ENG	Electroneurography
EP	Evoked potentials
ERCP	Endoscopic retrograde cholangiopancreatography
ERP	Estrogen receptor positive
ERV	Expiratory reserve volume
ESR	Erythrocyte sedimentation rate
ESV	End systolic volume
EUG	Excretory urography
FBS	Fasting blood sugar
FDP	Fibrin degradation products
Fe	Iron
FEV	Forced expiratory volume
FSH	Follicle-stimulating hormone
FTA-ABS	Flourescent treponemal antibody absorption test
FTI	Free thyroxine index
FUT	Fibrinogen uptake test
FVC	Forced vital capacity
G-6-PD	Glucose-6-phosphate dehydrogenase
GB series	Gallbladder series
GE reflux	Gastroesophageal reflux scan
GFR	Glomerular filtration rate
GGT	Gamma-glutamyl transferase
GGTP	Gamma-glutamyl transpeptidase
GH	Growth hormone
GHb, GHB	Glycosylated hemoglobin
GI series	Gastrointestinal series
GTT	Glucose tolerance test
HAA	Hepatitis-associated antigen
HAI	Hemagglutination inhibition test
HAT	Heterophile antibody titer
HAV	Hepatitis A virus
HbA	Glycohemoglobin
HBcAb	Hepatitis B core antibody
HBcAg	Hepatitis B core antigen
HBeAb	Hepatitis B e-antibody
HBeAg	Hepatitis B e-antigen
HBsAb	Hepatitis B surface antibody
HBsAg	Hepatitis B surface antigen
HBV	Hepatitis B virus
HCG	Human chorionic gonadotropin
HCO_3^-	Bicarbonate
HCS	Human chorionic somatomammotropin
Hct	Hematocrit
HDL	High-density lipoprotein